Pediatric Orthopedics

Volume 2

SECOND EDITION

Volume 2

Pediatric Orthopedics

SECOND EDITION

MIHRAN O. TACHDJIAN, M.S., M.D.

Professor of Orthopedic Surgery,
Northwestern University Medical School
Attending Orthopedic Surgeon and Former Head
Division of Orthopedics
Children's Memorial Hospital
Chicago, Illinois

1990

W.B. SAUNDERS COMPANY
Harcourt Brace Jovanovich, Inc.

Philadelphia ■ London ■ Toronto ■ Montreal ■ Sydney ■ Tokyo

W. B. SAUNDERS COMPANY
Harcourt Brace Jovanovich, Inc.

Independence Square West
Philadelphia, PA 19106

Library of Congress Cataloging-in-Publication Data

Tachdjian, Mihran O.

Pediatric orthopedics.

Includes bibliographies and index.

1. Pediatric orthopedia.   I. Title. [DNLM: 1. Orthopedics—in
infancy & childhood. WS 270 T117p]

RD732.3.C48T33 1990   617′.3   87-13006

ISBN 0–7216–8726–1 (set)

Listed here is the latest translated edition of this book together with the language of the translation and the publisher.

Spanish (*1st Edition*)–Nueva Editorial Interamericana S.A. de C.V., Mexico 4 D.F., Mexico

Editor: Edward H. Wickland, Jr.
Developmental Editor: Kathleen McCullough
Designer: Bill Donnelly
Production Manager: Bill Preston
Manuscript Editors: Ruth Barker, Constance Burton, Tina Rebane
Mechanical Artist: Karen Giacomucci
Illustration Coordinator: Peg Shaw
Indexer: Julie Schwager

Pediatric Orthopedics

Volume 1 ISBN 0–7216–8722–9
Volume 2 ISBN 0–7216–8723–7
Volume 3 ISBN 0–7216–8724–5
Volume 4 ISBN 0–7216–8727–X
Complete Set ISBN 0–7216–8726–1

© 1990 by W. B. Saunders Company. Copyright 1972 by W. B. Saunders Company. Copyright under the Uniform Copyright Convention. Simultaneously published in Canada. All rights reserved. This book is protected by copyright. No part of it may be reproduced, stored in a retrieval system, or transmitted in any form or by any means, electronic, mechanical, photocopying, recording, or otherwise, without written permission from the publisher. Made in the United States of America. Library of Congress catalog card number 87-13006.

Last digit is the print number: 9 8 7 6 5 4 3 2 1

Dedicated With Love to
My Wife
Vivian B. Tachdjian

Preface

During the past 18 years, great strides have been made in pediatric orthopedics. A new edition of this book is long overdue. The gestation period of such an *Arbeit* has been prolonged because of the tremendous amount of labor involved in writing a single-author book. The objectives and format of the textbook have not changed from the first edition. I have attempted to present a thorough and comprehensive treatise on the affections of the neuromusculoskeletal system in children.

I have expressed my preferred methods of treatment and surgical procedure based upon my personal experience and the privilege of association with the leaders in pediatric orthopedics throughout the world who have participated in the faculty of the Pediatric Orthopedic International Seminars, which I have directed annually since 1972. The names of the faculty appear in the acknowledgments in the following pages.

The illustrations and operative plates are all original; the majority represent the superb artistry of Mr. Ernest Beck, to whom I am greatly indebted. I also wish to acknowledge Miss Patricia Piescinski for her beautiful drawings.

I wish to thank the entire staff of the W.B. Saunders Company, particularly Miss Ruth Barker, Mr. Albert Meier, Mrs. Kathleen McCullough, and Mr. Edward H. Wickland, Jr.

I would also like to express my gratitude to Mrs. Mikie Boroughf, who assisted in the preparation of this book.

A question frequently posed to me over the years has been, "How do you write such an extensive book?" Every word has been handwritten in my illegible handwriting, readable only by Mrs. Lynn Ridings, without whose assistance and editorial support this work would not have been possible.

MIHRAN O. TACHDJIAN, M.D.

Acknowledgments

I would like to give special thanks to the following people for their help in writing certain sections of this book: Ellen Chadwick, M.D., and Stanford Shulman, M.D.—infectious diseases; Ramiro Hernandez, M.D.—CT scan of the hip; James Donaldson, M.D.—ultrasonography in congenital dislocation of the hip; Andrew Poznanski, M.D.—assistance in imaging findings in various skeletal disorders, especially bone dysplasias; Steven Hall, M.D.—orthopedic aspects of pediatric anesthesia; David McLone, M.D., and Thomas Naidich, M.D.—neurosurgical aspects of myelomeningocele and spinal dysraphism; Dror Paley, M.D.—Ilizarov limb lengthening; George Simons, M.D.—complications of talipes equinovarus; David H. Sutherland, M.D.—gait; and Mary Weck, R.P.T.—physical therapy for cerebral palsy.

I also wish to express my gratitude to the members of the faculty of the Pediatric Orthopedic International Seminars over the past 18 years.

Robert Abrams, M.D.
James Aronson, M.D.
Marc Asher, M.D.
R. Kirklin Ashley, M.D.
Henry H. Banks, M.D.
Riad Barmada, M.D.
Melvin H. Becker, M.D.
Henri Bensahel, M.D.
Anthony Bianco, M.D.
Eugene E. Bleck, M.D.
Prof. Alexander Bliskunov
Walter P. Blount, M.D.
J. Richard Bowen, M.D.
David W. Boyer, M.D.
Robert Bright, M.D.
Prof. Dieter Buck-Gramcko
Wilton H. Bunch, M.D.
Aloysio Campos da Paz, Jr., M.D.
S. Terry Canale, M.D.
Henri Carlioz, M.D.
Nils Carstam, M.D.
Prof. Robert Cattaneo

Mr. Anthony Catterall, F.R.C.S.
Prof. Paul L. Chigot
Eldon G. Chuinard, M.D.
Robert G. Chuinard, M.D.
Stanley M.K. Chung, M.D.
Sherman S. Coleman, M.D.
Mr. Christopher L. Colton, F.R.C.S.
Clinton L. Compere, M.D.
James J. Conway, M.D.
Henry R. Cowell, M.D.
Alvin H. Crawford, M.D.
Burr H. Curtis, M.D.
Prof. George Dall, F.R.C.S.
Prof. G. DeBastiani
Prof. Julio dePablos
Luciano Dias, M.D.
Harold M. Dick, M.D.
Alain Dimeglio, M.D.
James Donaldson, M.D.
John Dorst, M.D.
James Drennan, M.D.
Denis S. Drummond, M.D.

Prof. Jean Dubousset
Mr. Denis M. Dunn, F.R.C.S.
Peter M. Dunn, M.D.
Robert E. Eilert, M.D.
Richard E. Eppright, M.D.
John J. Fahey, M.D.
Albert B. Ferguson, Jr., M.D.
J. William Fielding, M.D.
Mr. John Fixsen, F.R.C.S.
Victor Frankel, M.D.
Nicholas Giannestras, M.D.
Prof. Alain Gilbert
J. Leonard Goldner, M.D.
Neil E. Green, M.D.
William T. Green, M.D.
Paul P. Griffin, M.D.
Donald Gunn, M.D.
John E. Hall, M.D.
Judith G. Hall, M.D.
John E. Handelsman, M.D.
Robert Hensinger, M.D.
Ramiro Hernandez, M.D.
Charles Herndon, M.D.
John A. Herring, M.D.
M. Mark Hoffer, M.D.
Walter A. Hoyt, Jr., M.D.
Mr. J. Rowland Hughes, F.R.C.S.
Prof. Sean P. F. Hughes
Prof. Gabriel Abramovich Ilizarov
Roshen Irani, M.D.
Francois Iselin, M.D.
Preston James, M.D.
Prof. Lutz F.H. Jani
Ali Kalamchi, M.D.
William J. Kane, M.D.
Buni'chiro Kawamura, M.D.
Theodore E. Keats, M.D.
Armen S. Kelikian, M.D.
Hampar Kelikian, M.D.
Mr. J.A. Kenwright, F.R.C.S.
Ara Y. Ketenjian, M.D.
Eugene Kilgore, M.D.
Richard E. King, M.D.
Prof. Predrag Klisiç
Steven Kopits, M.D.
Warren G. Kramer, M.D.
Mr. Douglas Lamb, F.R.C.S.
Prof. Anders F. Langenskiöld
Loren Larsen, M.D.
Franco Lavini, M.D.
Richard E. Lindseth, M.D.
Mr. George Lloyd-Roberts, F.R.C.S.
John E. Lonstein, M.D.
Wood Lovell, M.D.
G. Dean MacEwen, M.D.
John B. McGinty, M.D.
Douglas W. McKay, M.D.
Mr. Brian McKibbin, F.R.C.S.
David McLone, M.D.
John E. Madewell, M.D.
Roger A. Mann, M.D.
Prof. P.G. Marchetti
Prof. S. Matsuno

Peter L. Meehan, M.D.
Malcolm B. Menelaus, M.D.
Michael Michelson, M.D.
Lee W. Milford, M.D.
Edward A. Millar, M.D.
Mr. George P. Mitchell, F.R.C.S.
Prof. Giorgio Monticelli
Raymond T. Morrissy, M.D.
Colin F. Moseley, M.D.
Alf S. Nachemson, M.D.
Ann Nachemson, M.D.
John J. Niebauer, M.D.
John A. Ogden, M.D.
Michael B. Ozonoff, M.D.
Lauren M. Pachman, M.D.
Dror Paley, M.D.
Arsen Pankovich, M.D.
Arthur M. Pappas, M.D.
Klausdieter Parsch, M.D.
Sir Dennis Paterson
Hamlet A. Peterson, M.D.
Guillermo de Velasco Polo, M.D.
Ignacio V. Ponseti, M.D.
Melvin Post, M.D.
Jean-Gabriel Pous, M.D.
Andrew K. Poznanski, M.D.
Charles T. Price, M.D.
Mercer Rang, M.D.
Mr. A.H.C. Ratliff, F.R.C.S.
Inge Reimann, M.D.
L. Renzi-Brivio, M.D.
B. Lawrence Riggs, M.D.
Veijo A. Ritsila, M.D.
John M. Roberts, M.D.
Charles Rockwood, M.D.
Robert B. Salter, M.D.
Robert L. Samilson, M.D.
Shahan K. Sarrafian, M.D.
Michael F. Schafer, M.D.
William L. Schey, M.D.
Keith Schroeder, M.D.
Mr. W.J.W. Sharrard, F.R.C.S.
Stanford T. Shulman, M.D.
Robert S. Siffert, M.D.
Michael A. Simon, M.D.
George W. Simons, M.D.
Clement B. Sledge, M.D.
Wayne O. Southwick, M.D.
Donald P. Speer, M.D.
Prof. Renato Spinelli
Jurgen Spranger, M.D.
Lynn T. Staheli, M.D.
Stanko Stanisavljevic, M.D.
Herbert H. Stark, M.D.
Howard Steel, M.D.
David H. Stulberg, M.D.
Y. Sugioka, M.D.
David H. Sutherland, M.D.
Alfred B. Swanson, M.D.
Prof. W. Taillard
David J. Thompson, M.D.
Georges R. Thuilleux, M.D.
Dietrich Tonnis, M.D.

Levon K. Topouzian, M.D.
Miguel Ferrer Torrelles, M.D.
Prof. Naoichi Tsuyama
Prof. Raoul Tubiana
Vincent J. Turco, M.D.
Prof. M.V. Volkov
Prof. Heinz Wagner
Prof. Isidor Wasserstein
R.S. Watanabe, M.D
Hugh G. Watts, M.D.
Prof. B.G. Weber
Stuart L. Weinstein, M.D

Prof. S. L. Weissman
Dennis R. Wenger, M.D.
G. Wilbur Westin, M.D.
Harvey White, M.D.
Mr. Peter Williams, F.R.C.S.
John C. Wilson, M.D.
Robert Winter, M.D.
Miss Ruth Wynne-Davies, F.R.C.S.
Yasuo Yamauchi, M.D.
Prof. Eduardo Zancolli
Seymour Zimbler, M.D.

Preface to the First Edition

This work was undertaken upon the invitation of its publisher and begun with interest and great personal involvement that have never faltered. Now that its manuscript is complete, I must seize the occasion of this prefatory statement to answer the reader's natural question: Why was it done?

I began with the perhaps-simplistic idea of providing a detailed technical presentation of surgical treatment of disorders of the neuromuscular and skeletal systems in children. I intended to write primarily for the orthopedic surgeon but I hoped also to interest physicians and surgeons of other specialties involved in the care of children.

I had no sooner set out on what proved a long and tortuous path than I began to appreciate that one cannot describe the techniques of surgery without considering also the biological principles of surgery, the dynamics of trauma, and the rationale for surgical intervention. That rationale is itself dependent upon knowledge of neuromuscular physiology and of the biomechanics of motion. One cannot speak of the management of disorder or of the amelioration of congenital defect without understanding disease process and the genesis of musculoskeletal anomaly. The surgeon who operates well performs not only with skill but also with reason; and that reason rests upon a diagnostic acumen fortified by physical examination, pathology, radiology and accurate classification. Similarly, the evaluation of surgery cannot be set out without attention to its possible complications and its aftercare.

On reflection, I realize the project I have undertaken is more ambitious than I had originally envisioned. And so I have written a long and complex book. Its very length and complexity must mean occasional omission and even error. I have tried to guard against them by citing for each important statement significant findings from the vast literature of pediatric orthopedics; but the opinions I have expressed concerning preferred methods of treatment and surgical procedure arise from personal experience and from the privilege of having learned and worked at fine teaching centers.

In another and perhaps more important way I have departed from original intent. I decided to omit chapters on the hand and on orthotics and prosthetics in the conviction that these highly individual subjects should be treated intensively and thoroughly in separate monographs.

I wish to express gratitude to John Dusseau, Editor of the W. B. Saunders Company, for the confidence he invested in me. Without his support, advice, and encouragement, this work would have been impossible.

I wish to express thanks also to the Trust Under Will of Helen Fay Hunter–Crippled Children's Fund, and to Mr. Carl A. Pfau and the Harris Trust and Savings Bank Trustees for their generous support.

The kind indulgence of the Board of Directors of Children's Memorial Hospital in allowing me the necessary time to complete this work is greatly appreciated. I also wish to thank certain of my professional colleagues and members of the orthopedic staff for their sincere cooperation during preparation of this manuscript.

With the exception of a few that have been reproduced from other works, the illustrations and operative plates are all original. The majority represent the superb artistry of Mr. Ernest Beck, to whom I am greatly indebted. I also wish to thank medical artists Wesley Bloom, Jean McConnell, Diane Nelson, and Laurel Schaubert. The diligent work of Miss Helen Silver and Mr. John Kelley of the Photography Department, Children's Memorial Hospital, must be particularly acknowledged.

The entire staff of W. B. Saunders Company, particularly Miss Ruth Barker and Mr. Raymond Kersey, are to be commended for their meticulous work during the preparation and production of the printed book.

Finally, I wish to thank Miss Eleanor Lynn Schreiner, who, in her role as my personal editor, has prepared and finalized the entire manuscript as it has been written during the past four years. Without her assistance and meticulous attention to clarity, this task would have been difficult, if not impossible, to achieve. For her unselfish dedication I shall always be grateful.

I shall conclude in the hope that if the reader learns as much from reading as the writer has from writing this monograph, its attendant trouble and trial will have been amply repaid in the better care of children.

MIHRAN O. TACHDJIAN

Contents

VOLUME 1

1

Introduction 1
   Definition and Scope of Orthopedics 1
   Diagnosis in Neuromusculoskeletal Disorders 2
   THE ORTHOPEDIC HISTORY 2
      Prenatal History 3
      Birth History 3
   THE ORTHOPEDIC EXAMINATION 4
      Stance and Posture 4
      Gait 5
      GAIT CYCLE 6
      GRAVITY 8
      DETERMINANTS OF GAIT 9
      AXIAL ROTATIONS 12
      MUSCLE ACTION IN GAIT 13
      DEVELOPMENT OF MATURE GAIT 14
      PATHOLOGIC GAIT 18
      GAIT ANALYSIS 26
      Deformities 27
      INEQUALITY OF LIMB LENGTH 27
      ANGULATION OF BOWING 31
      Range of Motion of Joints 32
      Motor Power—Muscle Testing 40
      Neurologic Assessment 42
      Motor Evaluation 55
   RADIOGRAPHY AND OTHER DIAGNOSTIC TOOLS 59
      Electrodiagnosis 59
      TESTS OF NEUROMUSCULAR EXCITABILITY 64
   Anesthetic Considerations 67
   GENERAL CONSIDERATIONS 67
   SPECIFIC ENTITIES 68
      Muscular Dystrophy 68
      Myotonias 68
      Osteogenesis Imperfecta 68
      Arthrogryposis 69
      Rheumatoid Arthritis 69
      Myelomeningocele 69

    Cerebral Palsy 70
    Kyphoscoliosis 70
    Hemophilia 71
    Sickle Cell Disease 71
    Malignant Hyperthermia Syndrome 71
PREOPERATIVE CONSULTATION 74
OUTPATIENT SURGERY 74
RISK OF ANESTHESIA 75
Appendix to Chapter 1 77

2

Congenital Deformities 104

CLASSIFICATION 104
  Failure of Formation of Parts (Arrest of Development) 105
  TERMINAL TRANSVERSE DEFICIENCIES (CONGENITAL
    AMPUTATIONS) 105
  LONGITUDINAL DEFICIENCIES 105
  Failure of Differentiation (Separation) of Parts 105
  Duplication 110
  Overgrowth (Gigantism) 110
  Undergrowth (Hypoplasia) 111
  Congenital Constriction Band Syndrome 111
  Generalized Skeletal Developmental Defects 111
CONGENITAL MUSCULAR TORTICOLLIS 112
  Etiology 112
  Pathology 112
  Clinical Findings 113
  Diagnosis 115
  Treatment 115
KLIPPEL-FEIL SYNDROME 128
  Etiology 128
  Clinical Features and Associated Anomalies 128
  Radiographic Features 132
  Treatment 133
CONGENITAL HIGH SCAPULA 136
(*Sprengel's Deformity*)
  Etiology 136
  Pathology 137
  Clinical Features 138
  Radiographic Findings 138
  Treatment 138
PSEUDARTHROSIS OF THE CLAVICLE 168
  Etiology 168
  Clinical Findings 168
  Radiographic Findings 169
  Treatment 169
CONGENITAL DISLOCATION OF THE SHOULDER 174
  Treatment 175
**RARE CONGENITAL AND DEVELOPMENTAL ANOMALIES OF SHOULDER
  GIRDLE** 175
  Congenital Glenoid Hypoplasia 175
  Aplasia of Scapula 176
  Retrotorsion or Antetorsion of Glenoid Cavity 176
  Nonunion of Ossific Centers of Scapula 176
  Congenital Varus Deformity of Proximal Humerus 176
  Excessive Retroversion or Anteversion of Humeral Neck 179
CONGENITAL SYNOSTOSIS OF ELBOW 179
CONGENITAL RADIOULNAR SYNOSTOSIS 180
  Etiology 180
  Clinical Findings 180
  Treatment 183

CONGENITAL DISLOCATION OF THE RADIAL HEAD 184
    Diagnosis 186
    Treatment 187
CONGENITAL LONGITUDINAL DEFICIENCIES OF THE RADIUS 188
    Incidence 188
    Etiology 188
    Genetics 188
    Associated Anomalies 188
    Pathologic Anatomy 189
        MUSCLES 194
        NERVES 194
        VESSELS 194
    Clinical Findings 194
    Treatment 198
CONGENITAL LONGITUDINAL DEFICIENCY OF THE ULNA 206
    Classification 207
    Treatment 207
ULNAR DIMELIA 209
    Clinical Picture 209
    Treatment 209
MADELUNG'S DEFORMITY 210
    Etiology 211
    Pathologic Anatomy 211
    Clinical Features 211
    Diagnosis 213
    Differential Diagnosis 213
    Treatment 213
SYNDACTYLY 222
    Incidence 222
    Inheritance 222
    Classification 222
    Treatment 222
ACROCEPHALO-SYNDACTYLISM 236
(Apert's Syndrome)
    Clinical Features 236
    Treatment 236
POLYDACTYLY 240
    Incidence 240
    Postaxial Polydactyly 241
        TYPES 241
        INHERITANCE 241
        ASSOCIATED ANOMALIES AND SYNDROMES 241
    Preaxial Polydactyly 242
    (Duplication of the Thumb)
    Central Polydactyly 244
    Treatment 244
TRIPHALANGEAL THUMB 258
    Treatment 259
CONGENITAL LONGITUDINAL DEFICIENCY OF THE THUMB 260
    Hypoplastic Thumb 260
    Floating Thumb (Pouce Flottant) 268
CONGENITAL CLASPED THUMB 270
    Classification 270
    Incidence 270
    Anatomic and Clinical Findings 270
    Treatment 271
TRIGGER THUMB 272
    Treatment 272
SYMPHALANGISM 273
    Treatment 276
MACRODACTYLY 277
CLEFT HAND 279
    Clinical Picture 280
    Treatment 282

HYPOPLASTIC HAND AND DIGITS 283
   Treatment 283
FINGER DEFORMITIES 284
   ETIOLOGY 284
   DIAGNOSIS 284
   TREATMENT 285
   Clinodactyly 285
   TREATMENT 286
   Kirner Deformity 286
   Congenital Absence of Flexor Pollicis Longus and
     Median-Innervated Intrinsic Muscles 288
   (Abductor Pollicis Brevis, Opponens, and Short Flexors)
CONSTRICTION RING SYNDROME 291
   Etiology 291
   Treatment 294
CONGENITAL DYSPLASIA OF THE HIP 297
   Embryology 297
   Definition 298
   Classification 298
   Incidence 300
   Etiology 301
   PERIODS AT WHICH THE HIP MAY BE DISLOCATED 301
   LIGAMENTOUS LAXITY 302
   THE CONCEPT OF PRIMARY ACETABULAR DYSPLASIA 302
   MALPOSITION IN UTERO AND MECHANICAL FACTORS 302
   GENETIC FACTORS 304
   POSTNATAL ENVIRONMENTAL FACTORS 306
   SEASONAL INFLUENCE 306
   Pathology 306
TYPICAL PERINATAL CONGENITAL DISLOCATION OF THE HIP 312
   Diagnosis 312
   BIRTH TO TWO MONTHS OF AGE 312
   BETWEEN THREE AND TWELVE MONTHS OF AGE 326
   AFTER WALKING AGE 327
   Treatment 330
   BIRTH TO TWO MONTHS OF AGE 330
   THREE TO TWELVE MONTHS OF AGE 341
HIP DYSPLASIA IN THE ADOLESCENT 468
   Indications for Surgical Treatment 470
   Preoperative Assessment 473
   Classification 474
   Treatment 474
   SURGICAL PROCEDURES 474
CONGENITAL ABDUCTION CONTRACTURE OF THE HIP AND PELVIC
   OBLIQUITY 549
CONGENITAL LONGITUDINAL DEFICIENCY OF THE FEMUR 553
PROXIMAL FEMORAL FOCAL DEFICIENCY 554
   Classification 554
   Associated Anomalies 561
   Clinical Picture 564
   Treatment 565
   BILATERAL PROXIMAL FEMORAL FOCAL DEFICIENCY 565
   UNILATERAL INVOLVEMENT 566
HYPOPLASIA OF THE FEMUR 582
   Treatment 583
APLASIA OF THE FEMUR 583
DEVELOPMENTAL COXA VARA 583
   Incidence 584
   Heredity 584
   Pathogenesis 584
   Biomechanics 584
   Clinical Features 588
   Radiographic Findings 588
   Coxa Breva 588

Treatment	588
CONGENITAL DISLOCATION AND SUBLUXATION OF THE KNEE	609
Incidence	609
Etiology	609
Heredity	610
Associated Deformities	610
Pathologic Findings and Clinical Features	610
Diagnosis	611
Treatment	612
GENU RECURVATUM	617
CONGENITAL DISLOCATION OF THE PATELLA	618
Treatment	618
CONGENITAL ABSENCE OF THE PATELLA	620
CONGENITAL BIPARTITE OR TRIPARTITE PATELLA	620
CONGENITAL LONGITUDINAL DEFICIENCY OF THE FIBULA (PARAXIAL FIBULAR HEMIMELIA)	620
Classification	621
Diagnosis	623
Treatment	624
CONGENITAL LONGITUDINAL DEFICIENCY OF THE TIBIA	637
Classification	637
Treatment	637
CONGENITAL POSTEROMEDIAL ANGULATION OF THE TIBIA AND FIBULA	651
Treatment	653
CONGENITAL PSEUDARTHROSIS OF THE TIBIA	656
Incidence	656
Etiology	656
Classification	658
Treatment	658
THE PRE-PSEUDARTHROSIS OR INCIPIENT PHASE	662
ESTABLISHED PSEUDARTHROSIS	667
CONGENITAL PSEUDARTHROSIS OF THE FIBULA	685
DUPLICATION OF LONG BONES	687

VOLUME 2

3

Bone 688
   Responses of Bone 688
     Response to Function 688
     Response to Muscular Action 688
     Response to Use and Disuse 688
     Response to Circulatory Disturbances 689
     Response to Injury—Bone Repair 689
     Reaction to Radiation 690
   Dysplasias of Bone 690
     Nomenclature and Classification 690
     References 695
     Diagnostic Considerations 695
   MULTIPLE EPIPHYSEAL DYSPLASIA 701
     Inheritance 701
     Pathology 701
     Clinical Features 701
     Radiographic Findings and Differential Diagnosis 703
     Treatment 703
     Conradi-Hünermann Disease 715
   HEREDITARY PROGRESSIVE ARTHRO-OPHTHALMOPATHY (STICKLER'S SYNDROME) 716
   DYSPLASIA EPIPHYSEALIS HEMIMELICA 716

  Pathology 719
  Clinical Features 719
  Radiographic Findings 719
  Prognosis 719
  Treatment 719
 ACHONDROPLASIA 720
  Etiology 721
  Pathology 721
  Clinical Picture 721
  Radiographic Findings 726
  Diagnosis 726
  Prognosis and Treatment 727
 HYPOCHONDROPLASIA 729
  Clinical Features 729
  Radiographic Findings 729
 LETHAL FORMS OF SHORT-LIMBED DWARFISM 730
 CHONDROECTODERMAL DYSPLASIA (ELLIS-VAN CREVELD
  SYNDROME) 730
  Clinical Features 730
  Treatment 736
 ASPHYXIATING THORACIC DYSPLASIA (JEUNE'S DISEASE) 737
 METAPHYSEAL CHONDRODYSPLASIA 737
  Treatment 740
 HYPOPHOSPHATASIA 741
  Inheritance 740
  Pathology 742
  Clinical and Radiographic Findings 742
  Laboratory Findings 743
  Differential Diagnosis 743
  Treatment 743
  Mild Hypophosphatasia in the Adult 745
 SPONDYLOEPIPHYSEAL DYSPLASIA 746
  Spondyloepiphyseal Dysplasia Congenita 746
  Spondyloepiphyseal Dysplasia Tarda 749
 PSEUDOACHONDROPLASIA 749
  Pathology 750
  Clinical Features 750
  Radiographic Features 750
  Differential Diagnosis 750
 DIASTROPHIC DYSPLASIA (DIASTROPHIC DWARFISM) 752
  Pathogenesis and Pathology 752
  Clinical Picture 752
  Radiographic Features 756
  Differential Diagnosis 756
  Treatment 756
 MISCELLANEOUS TYPES OF DWARFISM 757
 OSTEOGENESIS IMPERFECTA 758
  Classification and Heredity 758
  Incidence 759
  Pathology 759
  Clinical Picture 761
  Radiographic Findings 769
  Hyperplastic Callus Formation 774
  Laboratory Findings 775
  Differential Diagnosis 775
  Treatment 776
   "ATTEMPTED" MEDICAL TREATMENT
    ORTHOPEDIC TREATMENT 777
  Prognosis 782
 IDIOPATHIC JUVENILE OSTEOPOROSIS 787
  Etiopathology 787
  Clinical Picture 787
  Radiographic Findings 787
  Diagnosis 788

Treatment	789
IDIOPATHIC OSTEOLYSIS	790
Classification	790
Pathology	791
Differential Diagnosis	791
Treatment	791
OSTEOPETROSIS	792
Classification	792
Etiology and Pathology	793
Radiographic Features	794
Laboratory Findings	796
Differential Diagnosis	797
Problems and Complications	797
Treatment	798
PYCNODYSOSTOSIS	800
PROGRESSIVE DIAPHYSEAL DYSPLASIA (CAMURATI-ENGELMANN DISEASE)	804
Etiology and Heredity	804
Pathology	804
Clinical Features	804
Radiographic Features	806
Scintigraphic Findings with Technetium-99m Diphosphonate	806
Laboratory Findings	806
Differential Diagnosis	806
Treatment	806
MELORHEOSTOSIS	808
Etiology	808
Pathology	808
Clinical Features	809
Radiographic Features	809
Differential Diagnosis	809
Treatment	809
OSTEOPATHIA STRIATA	812
OSTEOPOIKILOSIS (SPOTTED BONES)	815
IDIOPATHIC HYPERPHOSPHATASIA	816
INFANTILE CORTICAL HYPEROSTOSIS (CAFFEY'S DISEASE)	817
Etiology	817
Pathology	817
Clinical Features	819
Radiographic Features	819
Diagnosis	819
Treatment	824
Complications	824
MISCELLANEOUS DYSPLASIAS	825
Metaphyseal Dysplasia (Pyle's Disease)	825
Craniometaphyseal Dysplasia	826
Craniodiaphyseal Dysplasia	826
Osteodysplasty (Melnick-Needles Syndrome)	826
MARFAN'S SYNDROME	829
Heredity	829
Etiology	829
Clinical Features	829
Differential Diagnosis	833
Treatment	834
CONGENITAL CONTRACTURAL ARACHNODACTYLY	837
Clinical Features	837
Differential Diagnosis	839
Treatment	839
CLEIDOCRANIAL DYSPLASIA (CLEIDOCRANIAL DYSOSTOSIS)	840
Inheritance	840
Etiology	840
Clinical and Radiographic Features	840
Treatment	843

HEREDITARY ONYCHO-OSTEODYSPLASIA
(NAIL-PATELLA SYNDROME) 844
    Incidence 845
    Inheritance 845
    Clinical Features 845
    Treatment 847
TRICHO-RHINO-PHALANGEAL DYSPLASIA 848
CRANIOCARPOTARSAL DYSPLASIA (FREEMAN-SHELDON OR
"WHISTLING FACE" SYNDROME) 852
LARSEN'S SYNDROME 852
    Differential Diagnosis 854
    Treatment 854
CRANIOFACIAL DYSPLASIAS (WITH OR WITHOUT INVOLVEMENT
OF THE LIMBS) 855
ACROCEPHALOSYNDACTYLY AND RELATED DYSPLASIAS 855
    Apert's Syndrome 855
    Carpenter's Syndrome 856
    Crouzon's Syndrome 856
FIBRODYSPLASIA OSSIFICANS PROGRESSIVA (MYOSITIS OSSIFICANS
PROGRESSIVA) 857
    Pathology 857
    Clinical Features 857
    Radiographic Findings 858
    Prognosis and Treatment 860
CORNELIA DE LANGE SYNDROME 861
EHLERS-DANLOS SYNDROME 861
MISCELLAENOUS DYSPLASIAS 864
    Menkes Syndrome 864
    Orofaciodigital Syndrome 864
    Otopalatodigital Syndrome 865
    Rubinstein-Taybi Syndrome 865
THE MUCOPOLYSACCHARIDOSES 865
    Mucopolysaccharidosis I (Hurler Syndrome) 867
    Mucopolysaccharidosis II (Hunter Syndrome) 875
    Mucopolysaccharidosis III (Sanfilippo Syndrome) 875
    Mucopolysaccharidosis IV (Morquio Syndrome) 875
    Mucopolysaccharidosis V (Scheie Syndrome) 878
    Mucopolysaccharidosis VI (Maroteaux-Lamy Syndrome) 878
GAUCHER'S DISEASE 883
    Etiology 882
    Heredity 882
    Clinical Features 882
    Bony Manifestations 883
    Treatment 885
NIEMANN-PICK DISEASE 887
HOMOCYSTINURIA 888
    Biochemical Defect and Pathophysiology 888
    Clinical Features 888
    Diagnosis 889
DOWN'S SYNDROME (TRISOMY 21 OR MONGOLISM) 890
    Radiographic Features 891
    Treatment 891
OTHER CHROMOSOMAL ABERRATIONS 896
    Sex Chromosome Anomalies 897
Metabolic and Endocrine Bone Diseases 897
RICKETS 897
    General Pathophysiology 897
    Simple Vitamin D Deficiency Rickets 898
    RICKETS ASSOCIATED WITH MALABSORPTION SYNDROME 903
    *Rickets Due to Renal Tubular Insufficiency (Hypophosphatemic or
    Vitamin D–Refractory Rickets)* 905
    HYPOPHOSPHATEMIC VITAMIN D–REFRACTORY RICKETS
    OF THE SIMPLE TYPE 905

OTHER TYPES OF VITAMIN D–REFRACTORY RICKETS	908
Renal Osteodystrophy	910
SCURVY	918
Pathology	918
Clinical Features	918
Radiographic Findings	918
Diagnosis	919
Treatment	920
HYPERVITAMINOSIS A	920
Clinical and Radiographic Findings	921
Diagnosis and Treatment	922
HYPERVITAMINOSIS D	923
Pathology	923
Clinical Findings	923
Radiographic Findings	923
Laboratory Findings	925
Treatment	925
IDIOPATHIC HYPERCALCEMIA IN INFANCY	925
PITUITARY DWARFISM	926
Clinical Picture	926
Radiographic Findings	927
Diagnosis	927
Treatment	927
GIGANTISM	927
HYPOTHYROIDISM	927
IDIOPATHIC HYPOPARATHYROIDISM	929
PSEUDOHYPOPARATHYROIDISM	930
PRIMARY HYPERPARATHYROIDISM	931
Osteochondroses and Related Disorders	932
LEGG-CALVÉ-PERTHES DISEASE	933
Incidence	934
Hereditary Factors	934
Constitutional Factors	934
Associated Anomalies	935
Etiology	935
Pathology	936
Clinical Picture	943
Radiographic and Imaging Features	943
Differential Diagnosis	956
Natural History	958
Prognosis	960
Classification	965
Treatment	970
INITIAL PHASE	971
SECOND PHASE—CONTAINMENT AND MAINTENANCE OR RESTORATION OF FULL RANGE OF MOTION OF HIP	971
THIRD PHASE—RECONSTRUCTIVE SURGERY	982
KÖHLER'S DISEASE OF THE TARSAL NAVICULAR	1003
Etiology	1003
Clinical Features	1005
Radiographic Findings	1005
Treatment	1005
FREIBERG'S INFRACTION	1006
Etiology	1006
Clinical and Radiographic Findings	1008
Treatment	1008
OSGOOD-SCHLATTER DISEASE	1010
Etiology	1010
Clinical Picture	1010
Radiographic Findings	1011
Treatment	1011
Complications	1012
PANNER'S DISEASE (OSTEOCHONDRITIS OF THE HUMERAL CAPITELLUM)	1013

Pathology	1014
Clinical Features	1014
Radiographic Features	1014
Treatment	1014
MISCELLANEOUS SO-CALLED OSTEOCHONDROSES	1016
Ischiopubic "Osteochondritis"	1016
SLIPPED CAPITAL FEMORAL EPIPHYSIS	1016
Incidence and Epidemiology	1016
Classification	1017
Etiology	1017
Inheritance	1022
Pathology	1022
Clinical Picture	1026
Radiographic Findings	1028
Measurement of the Amount of Slipping	1028
Treatment	1031
Problems and Complications	1062
Infections of Bone	1081
PYOGENIC OSTEOMYELITIS	1081
Etiology	1081
Pathology	1082
Sites of Involvement	1084
Clinical Picture	1084
Radiographic Picture	1085
Bone Scan	1087
Laboratory Findings	1092
Diagnosis	1092
Treatment	1093
ACUTE HEMATOGENOUS OSTEOMYELITIS	1093
SUBACUTE OSTEOMYELITIS	1097
CHRONIC OSTEOMYELITIS	1099
Complications	1103
Unusual Sites of Involvement	1106
SALMONELLA OSTEOMYELITIS	1120
Salmonella Bone Infection in Hemoglobinopathies	1120
Treatment	1122
Brucellar Osteomyelitis	1123
Syphilis of Bone	1124
TUBERCULOSIS OF BONE	1127
FUNGUS INFECTIONS OF BONE	1129
Actinomycosis	1129
Blastomycosis of Bone	1129
Coccidioidomycosis	1129
Sporotrichosis	1120
VIRAL OSTEOMYELITIS	1131
Vaccinial Osteomyelitis	1131
Cat-Scratch Fever	1133
CHRONIC GRANULOMATOUS DISEASE OF CHILDHOOD	1133
Bone Manifestations of Hematologic Disorders	1135
ANEMIA	1135
Fanconi's Anemia	1135
Hemoglobinopathies	1136
Thalassemias (Cooley's Anemia or Mediterranean Anemia)	1136
SICKLE CELL DISEASE	1139
SKELETAL MANIFESTATIONS	1140
TREATMENT	1144
RETICULOENDOTHELIAL NEOPLASIA	1146
Leukemia	1146
Lymphoma, Lymphosarcoma, and Hodgkin's Disease	1147
Tumors and Tumorous Conditions of Bone	1150
BONE TUMORS	1150
Classification	1150
Clinical Picture	1150

    Radiographic Features 1151
    Isotope Scans 1153
    Computed Tomography 1155
    Magnetic Resonance Imaging 1155
    Angiography 1155
    Ancillary Studies 1155
    Laboratory Tests 1155
    Staging 1156
    Principles of Surgical Management 1158
    Treatment 1159
    Operative Procedural Considerations 1161
OSTEOCHONDROMA 1163
    Etiology 1164
    Incidence and Anatomic Site 1164
    Pathology 1164
    Clinical Picture 1165
    Radiographic Findings 1165
    Treatment 1165
    Problems and Complications 1167
MULTIPLE CARTILAGINOUS EXOSTOSIS 1172
    Genetics and Sex Incidence 1172
    Localization 1172
    Pathology 1172
    Clinical Features 1173
    Radiographic Findings 1180
    Treatment 1180
    Sarcomatous Transformation 1184
SOLITARY ENCHONDROMA AND MULTIPLE ENCHONDROMATOSIS 1190
    Solitary Enchondroma 1191
    Multiple Enchondromatosis or Ollier's Disease 1195
PERIOSTEAL CHONDROMA 1199
    Pathology 1199
    Clinical Features 1199
    Radiographic Imaging and Findings 1199
    Treatment 1199
BENIGN CHONDROBLASTOMA 1200
CHONDROMYXOID FIBROMA 1203
    Pathology 1203
    Clinical Picture 1203
    Radiographic and Imaging Findings 1203
    Treatment 1205
OSTEOID OSTEOMA 1206
    Age and Sex Predilection 1206
    Sites of Involvement 1206
    Pathology 1207
    Clinical Findings 1207
    Radiographic and Imaging Findings 1207
    Natural History 1215
    Treatment 1215
BENIGN OSTEOBLASTOMA 1220
    Age and Sex Predilection 1220
    Location 1220
    Pathology 1224
    Clinical Findings 1224
    Radiographic and Imaging Findings 1225
    Differential Diagnosis 1225
    Treatment 1225
    Complications 1225
FIBROUS DYSPLASIA 1228
    Etiology 1228
    Incidence 1228
    Localization 1228
    Clinical Findings 1228
    Nonskeletal Manifestations 1229

Pathology	1230
Radiographic and Imaging Findings	1231
Natural Course	1234
Treatment	1234
Malignant Transformation	1239
OSTEOFIBROUS DYSPLASIA OF THE TIBIA AND FIBULA (CAMPANACCI SYNDROME)	1242
Age and Sex Predilection	1242
Localization	1242
Clinical Features	1242
Radiographic Features	1242
Pathology	1242
Differential Diagnosis	1245
Treatment	1246
FIBROUS DEFECTS OF BONE	1246
Fibrous Metaphyseal Defect	1247
Desmoplastic Fibroma	1250
ANEURYSMAL BONE CYST	1251
Etiology	1251
Age and Sex Distribution	1252
Sites of Involvement	1252
Pathology	1252
Clinical Features	1252
Radiographic and Imaging Findings	1252
Diagnosis	1255
Treatment	1255
UNICAMERAL BONE CYST	1258
Sites of Involvement	1258
Etiology	1258
Pathology	1259
Clinical Findings	1259
Radiographic and Imaging Findings	1259
Differential Diagnosis	1261
Treatment	1264
Complications	1270
HISTIOCYTOSIS X	1274
Etiology	1275
Pathologic Features	1275
Letterer-Siwe Disease	1276
Hand-Schüller-Christian Disease	1278
Eosinophilic Granuloma of Bone	1278
NEUROFIBROMATOSIS (VON RECKLINGHAUSEN'S DISEASE)	1289
Etiology	1289
Heredity	1289
Pathology	1289
Clinical Features	1290
Treatment	1294
ADAMANTINOMA	1301
Localization	1301
Age and Sex Predilection	1301
Clinical Features	1301
Radiographic and Imaging Findings	1301
Differential Diagnosis	1301
Pathologic Findings	1301
Treatment	1303
OSTEOGENIC SARCOMA	1305
Classic Osteogenic Sarcoma	1305
Parosteal Osteogenic Sarcoma	1386
EWING'S SARCOMA	1387
Pathologic Findings	1388
Clinical Picture	1388
Radiographic Findings	1389
Staging	1390
Diagnosis	1390

Prognosis 1390
Treatment 1390
CHONDROSARCOMA 1399
Radiographic and Imaging Findings 1400
Pathology 1400
Treatment 1400
FIBROSARCOMA AND MALIGNANT FIBROUS HISTIOCYTOMA 1403
METASTATIC TUMORS OF BONE 1403
Neuroblastoma 1403
Wilms' Tumor (Nephroblastoma) 1405

4

Joints 1410
DIAGNOSTIC CONSIDERATIONS 1411
Joint Fluid Analysis 1411
ACUTE SUPPURATIVE ARTHRITIS (SEPTIC JOINT) 1415
Pathogenesis 1415
Pathology 1416
Clinical Picture 1419
Imaging Findings 1419
Diagnosis 1420
Differential Diagnosis 1421
Treatment 1422
ANTIBIOTIC THERAPY 1422
DRAINAGE OF JOINT 1424
LOCAL CARE OF JOINT 1427
Prognosis 1427
Septic Arthritis of the Hip in the Newborn and Infant 1428
Septic Arthritis Superimposed on Pre-Existing Joint Disease 1435
LYME ARTHRITIS 1440
Clinical Features 1440
Diagnosis 1440
Treatment 1441
GONOCOCCAL ARTHRITIS 1441
TUBERCULOUS ARTHRITIS 1443
Pathology 1443
Clinical Features 1443
Radiographic Features 1445
Laboratory Findings 1445
Treatment 1445
Tuberculosis of the Spine 1449
SYPHILITIC JOINT DISEASE 1458
ARTHRITIS ASSOCIATED WITH VIRAL DISEASE 1459
FUNGUS INFECTIONS OF JOINTS 1460
ACUTE TRANSIENT SYNOVITIS OF THE HIP 1461
Etiology 1461
Clinical Picture 1462
Imaging Findings 1462
Laboratory Findings 1462
Differential Diagnosis 1462
Treatment 1463
Sequelae 1464
RHEUMATOID ARTHRITIS 1466
Incidence 1466
Etiology 1466
Pathology 1467
Clinical Features 1469
Radiographic Findings 1473
Laboratory Findings 1474
Treatment 1477
ORTHOPEDIC MANAGEMENT 1480

GOUT	1494
HEMOPHILIA	1494
Incidence	1495
Classification and Inheritance	1495
Clinical Picture	1495
Hemophilic Arthropathy	1495
Soft-Tissue Bleeding	1498
Nerve Palsy	1500
Hemophilic Pseudotumor	1500
Fractures	1501
Dislocations	1501
Myositis Ossificans	1502
Treatment	1502
MEDICAL MANAGEMENT	1502
SURGICAL TREATMENT	1505
Fractures	1507
Pseudotumors	1507
NEUROPATHIC JOINT DISEASE (Charcot's Joint)	1512
Clinicopathologic Findings	1512
Radiographic Findings	1513
Treatment	1513
OSTEOCHONDRITIS DISSECANS	1515
Historical Background	1515
Etiology	1515
Pathology	1517
Sex and Age Predilection	1517
Site of Involvement	1517
Clinical Picture	1518
Imaging Findings	1518
Osteochondritis Dissecans of the Talus	1522
Treatment	1524
NONSURGICAL MANAGEMENT	1524
ARTHROSCOPY	1526
OPEN SURGICAL TREATMENT	1534
Osteochondritis Dissecans of the Hip	1534
DISCOID MENISCUS	1539
Pathogenesis	1539
Pathology	1540
Clinical Features	1540
Imaging Findings	1542
Treatment	1542
SNAPPING OF POPLITEUS TENDON	1551
RECURRENT MOMENTARY LATERAL SUBLUXATION OF THE TIBIOFEMORAL JOINT	1551
Treatment	1551
RECURRENT SUBLUXATION OF DISLOCATION OF THE PATELLA	1551
Etiology	1551
Classification	1552
Pathology	1554
Clinical Picture	1554
Radiographic Findings	1556
Treatment	1560
THERAPEUTIC PROCEDURES	1562
POPLITEAL CYST	1582
Pathologic Findings	1582
Clinical Picture	1585
Diagnosis	1586
Treatment	1589
SYNOVIAL CHONDROMATOSIS	1592
PIGMENTED VILLONODULAR SYNOVITIS	1593
Treatment	1594
HEMANGIOMA OF SYNOVIAL MEMBRANE	1596
INTRA-ARTICULAR LIPOMA	1596

SYNOVIAL SARCOMA	1598
(Synovioma)	
Diagnosis and Staging	1598
Treatment	1599

VOLUME 3

5

The Neuromuscular System	1601
GENERAL CONSIDERATIONS	1601
Levels of Affection	1601
Neuromuscular System as a Functional Unit	1604
Responses of Muscles	1604
Affections of the Brain and Spinal Cord	1605
CEREBRAL PALSY	1605
Definition	1605
Classification	1605
Etiology and Pathology	1608
BIRTH INJURY	1608
DEVELOPMENTAL MALFORMATIONS	1609
CAUSES OF ACQUIRED CEREBRAL PALSY	1610
Neurophysiologic Considerations	1610
SPASTICITY	1610
ABNORMAL MOVEMENTS OR HYPERKINESIA	1611
ATHETOSIS	1612
ATAXIA	1612
RIGIDITY	1613
Prevalence	1613
Clinical Features	1614
SPASTIC HEMIPLEGIA	1614
SPASTIC DIPLEGIA	1616
SPASTIC QUADRIPLEGIA WITH TOTAL BODY INVOLVEMENT	1617
EXTRAPYRAMIDAL CEREBRAL PALSY	1617
Management	1620
GENERAL PRINCIPLES	1620
SURGICAL MANAGEMENT	1620
TYPE OF CEREBRAL PALSY	1620
REFLEX MATURATION AND MOTOR LEVEL DEVELOPMENT	1621
ADEQUACY OF POSTOPERATIVE CARE	1621
TYPE AND TIMING OF SURGICAL PROCEDURES	1622
INTERDEPENDENCE OF THE FOOT, ANKLE, KNEE, HIP, AND TRUNK	1622
KINETIC ELECTROMYOGRAPHY AND GAIT ANALYSIS	1623
NONOPERATIVE METHODS OF MANAGEMENT	1623
The Hip	1627
SURGICAL MANAGEMENT	1627
ADDUCTION-FLEXION DEFORMITY	1628
MEDIAL ROTATION DEFORMITY OF THE HIPS	1630
HIP SUBLUXATION AND DISLOCATION	1633
TREATMENT	1637
PROBLEMS AND COMPLICATIONS	1660
The Foot and Ankle	1660
CONSERVATIVE MANAGEMENT	1663
SURGICAL TREATMENT	1665
The Knee	1705
FLEXION DEFORMITY	1706
EXTENSION CONTRACTURE OF THE KNEE	1714
GENU RECURVATUM	1716
ELONGATED PATELLAR TENDON AND QUADRICEPS FEMORIS INSUFFICIENCY	1717

The Upper Limb	1717
THUMB-IN-PALM DEFORMITY	1722
FINGER DEFORMITIES	1738
FLEXION DEFORMITY OF WRIST AND PRONATION CONTRACTURE OF FOREARM	1744
PRONATION CONTRACTURE OF THE FOREARM	1746
FLEXION DEFORMITY OF THE ELBOW	1746
SHOULDER DEFORMITY	1747
Scoliosis	1747
TREATMENT	1755
INTRACRANIAL TUMORS	1771
Pathologic Considerations	1771
Clinical Features	1771
Diagnostic Considerations	1771
Treatment	1772
MYELOMENINGOCELE	1773
Incidence	1774
Embryology	1774
Etiology	1774
Pathogenesis	1775
Heredity	1775
Antenatal Diagnosis	1776
AMNIOCENTESIS	1776
Pathology	1776
SKIN	1777
MENINGES	1777
SPINAL CORD	1778
PERIPHERAL ROOTS	1778
VERTEBRAE	1778
BRAIN	1778
Clinical Features	1778
Associated Congenital Anomalies	1780
General Considerations and Principles of Treatment	1781
Neurosurgical Treatment	1786
REPAIR OF MENINGOCELE	1786
HYDROCEPHALUS	1790
INTELLIGENCE	1790
URINARY INCONTINENCE	1791
HINDBRAIN DYSFUNCTION	1791
MORTALITY	1791
Orthopedic Management	1792
AMBULATION	1792
Foot and Ankle	1795
PES CALCANEUS	1798
VALGUS ANKLE	1804
TALIPES EQUINOVARUS	1805
PES EQUINUS	1811
PARALYTIC CONGENITAL CONVEX PES VALGUS	1811
PES CAVUS AND CLAW TOES	1816
FLAIL ANKLE	1817
Torsional Deformities of the Tibia-Fibula	1817
Knee	1818
FLEXION DEFORMITY	1818
EXTENSION OR HYPEREXTENSION CONTRACTURE OF THE KNEE	1820
GENU VALGUM	1821
VARUS DEFORMITY	1821
The Hip	1821
HIP SUBLUXATION-DISLOCATION	1821
FLEXION DEFORMITY	1836
ABDUCTION AND LATERAL ROTATION DEFORMITY OF THE HIP	1839
HIP ADDUCTION DEFORMITY	1840
The Spine	1841
LORDOSIS	1841

SCOLIOSIS	1843
KYPHOSIS	1848
Fractures	1852
ETIOLOGY	1852
CLINICAL FEATURES	1853
Orthotic Management of Habilitation	1854
SPINAL DYSRAPHISM	1871
Lipomyelomeningocele and Lipomas of the Filum Terminale	1871
EMBRYOLOGY AND PATHOLOGY	1871
CLINICAL FEATURES OF SPINAL DYSRAPHISM	1873
DIAGNOSIS	1874
NEUROSURGICAL MANAGEMENT	1875
ORTHOPEDIC MANAGEMENT	1878
Myelocystocele	1879
Tethered Cord	1879
CLINICAL FEATURES	1879
TREATMENT	1880
DIASTEMATOMYELIA	1881
Clinical Picture	1881
Radiographic Findings	1882
Treatment	1885
SPINA BIFIDA OCCULTA	1886
Clinical Features	1886
Treatment	1887
INTRASPINAL TUMORS	1887
Clinical Picture	1887
Radiographic Findings	1888
Cerebrospinal Fluid Findings	1892
Differential Diagnosis	1892
Treatment	1893
SPINAL MUSCULAR ATROPHY	1903
Pathology	1903
Clinical Features	1903
Laboratory Findings	1904
Differential Diagnosis	1905
Treatment	1905
POLIOMYELITIS	1910
Pathology	1910
Treatment	1911
ACUTE PHASE	1911
CONVALESCENT PHASE	1913
CHRONIC PHASE	1915
The Hip	1921
SOFT-TISSUE CONTRACTURE	1921
GLUTEUS MEDIUS PARALYSIS	1925
GLUTEUS MAXIMUS PARALYSIS	1925
PARALYTIC DISLOCATION OF THE HIP	1928
The Knee	1930
QUADRICEPS FEMORIS PARALYSIS	1930
FLEXION DEFORMITY OF THE KNEE	1934
GENU RECURVATUM	1934
FLAIL KNEE	1937
SPECIFIC DEFORMITIES OF THE FOOT AND ANKLE	1937
Arthrodesis of the Foot and Ankle	1946
TRIPLE ARTHRODESIS	1946
EXTRA-ARTICULAR SUBTALAR ARTHRODESIS	1955
ANKLE FUSION AND PANTALAR ARTHRODESIS	1955
ANTERIOR OR POSTERIOR BONE BLOCKS TO LIMIT MOTION AT ANKLE	1956
The Trunk	1957
The Shoulder	1957
ARTHRODESIS OF THE SHOULDER	1959
The Elbow	1959
STEINDLER FLEXORPLASTY	1959

DYSTROPHIA MYOTONICA (MYOTONIC DYSTROPHY) 2138
MYOTONIA CONGENITA AND PARAMYOTONIA CONGENITA 2141
   Diagnosis 2141
   Treatment 2141
   ORTHOTIC SURGERY 2150
   SURGICAL MEASURES 2150
   Screening and Genetic Counseling 2151
MYOTONIA CONGENITA (THOMSEN'S DISEASE) 2157
   Etiology and Pathology 2157
   Clinical Features 2157
   Laboratory Findings 2158
   Differential Diagnosis and Treatment 2158
MYOSITIS 2159
POLYMYOSITIS AND DERMATOMYOSITIS 2159
   Age-Sex 2160
   Classification 2160
   Etiology 2160
   Pathology 2160
   Clinical Features 2161
   Laboratory Findings 2161
   Diagnosis 2163
   Treatment 2163
SUPPURATIVE MYOSITIS 2167
   Etiology 2167
   Clinical Features 2167
   Diagnosis 2167
   Treatment 2167
VIRAL MYOSITIS 2167
PARASITIC MYOSITIS 2168
TRAUMATIC MYOSITIS, "MUSCLE CRAMPS" 2168
TRAUMATIC MYOSITIS OSSIFICANS (MYOSITIS OSSIFICANS
   CIRCUMSCRIPTA) 2169
   Pathology 2169
   Clinical Features 2169
   Imaging Findings 2169
   Differential Diagnosis 2169
   Treatment 2170
Metabolic Diseases of Muscle 2172
PERIODIC PARALYSIS 2172
   Familial or Hypokalemic Periodic Paralysis 2172
   TREATMENT 2172
   Hyperkalemic Periodic Paralysis 2172
   Normokalemic Periodic Paralysis 2173
McARDLE'S SYNDROME (MYOPHOSPHORYLASE DEFICIENCY) 2174
IDIOPATHIC PAROXYSMAL MYOGLOBINURIA 2175
STIFF-MAN SYNDROME 2176
MYASTHENIA GRAVIS 2177
   Clinical Features 2178
   NEONATAL TRANSIENT MYASTHENIA GRAVIS 2178
   NEONATAL PERSISTENT (CONGENITAL) MYASTHENIA GRAVIS 2178
   JUVENILE MYASTHENIA GRAVIS 2178
   Diagnosis 2178
   Treatment 2179
   Prognosis 2179
Affections of Bursae 2181
BURSITIS 2181
   Traumatic Bursitis 2181
   Infectious or Suppurative Bursitis 2182
   Appendix 2182A

6
The Spine 2183

CLASSIFICATION OF SPINAL DEFORMITIES	2183
TERMINOLOGY	2184
Posture and Postural Defects	2186
Development of Posture	2186
Normal Posture	2187
Gradation of Posture	2189
Treatment of Postural Defects	2189
NONSTRUCTURAL SCOLIOSIS	2191
Postural Scoliosis	2191
Functional Scoliosis Due to Lower Limb Length Disparity	2191
Nonstructural Soloiosis Due to Pelvic Obliquity	2196
Hysterical Scoliosis	2196
Congenital Anomalies of the Spine	2196
Classification	2197
Heredity	2198
Associated Anomalies	2199
CONGENITAL SCOLIOSIS	2200
Natural History	2200
Treatment	2204
CONGENITAL KYPHOSIS	2207
Classification	2207
Clinical Picture	2208
Natural History	2209
Differential Diagnosis	2209
Treatment	2209
CONGENITAL ABSENCE OF THE SACRUM AND LUMBOSACRAL VERTEBRAE (LUMBOSACRAL AGENESIS)	2212
Etiology	2212
Pathologic Findings	2212
Classification	2213
Clinical Picture	2213
Radiographic Findings	2217
Treatment	2218
CONGENITAL LUMBAR PEDICLE APLASIA	2229
Treatment	2230
Congenital Anomalies of the Occiput and Cervical Spine	2230
OSSICULUM TERMINALE AND OCCIPITAL VERTEBRA	2231
BASILAR INVAGINATION, BASILAR IMPRESSION, AND PLATYBASIA	2231
CONGENITAL FUSION OF FIRST CERVICAL VERTEBRA AND OCCIPUT	2232
Embryologic Data	2232
Clinical Picture	2232
Radiographic Findings	2233
Treatment	2233
CONGENITAL ANOMALIES OF THE ODONTOID PROCESS	2233
The Separate Odontoid Process	2233
DIFFERENTIAL DIAGNOSIS	2234
TREATMENT	2234
Absence of the Odontoid Process	2234
CONGENITAL ABSENCE OF PEDICLES AND FACETS IN THE CERVICAL SPINE	2236
Radiologic Examination	2236
Differential Diagnosis	2236
Prognosis and Treatment	2236
SPONDYLOLISTHESIS OF THE CERVICAL SPINE	2236
Radiographic Findings	2236
Treatment	2236
Spondylolisthesis	2238
History and Terminology	2238
Types of Spondylolisthesis	2238
DYSPLASTIC (CONGENITAL) SPONDYLOLISTHESIS	2239
ISTHMIC SPONDYLOLISTHESIS	2241
Age Incidence	2242

      Etiology 2242
      Genetic Factors 2243
      Pathology 2245
      Level of Involvement 2245
      Forward Slipping 2245
      Clinical Features 2248
      Radiographic Findings 2251
      Treatment 2252
      SPONDYLOLYSIS 2254
      SPONDYLOLISTHESIS 2254
      OPERATIVE TREATMENT 2255
Scoliosis 2265
      Definitions 2265
    IDIOPATHIC SCOLIOSIS 2265
      Prevalence 2266
      Sex Predilection 2266
      School Screening 2266
      Genetic Aspects 2267
      Etiology 2268
      Pathology 2270
      Natural History and Risk Factors Related to Curve Progression 2272
      Clinical Features 2273
      Radiographic Assessment 2282
      Curve Pattern 2291
      Treatment 2293
      NONOPERATIVE TREATMENT 2293
      ORTHOTIC TREATMENT 2294
      OPERATIVE TREATMENT 2302
    INFANTILE IDIOPATHIC SCOLIOSIS 2356
      Prevalence 2356
      Natural History—Prognosis 2357
      Diagnosis 2358
      Treatment 2358
    JUVENILE IDIOPATHIC SCOLIOSIS 2360
      Treatment 2362
    PARALYTIC SCOLIOSIS 2362
    SCOLIOSIS IN NEUROFIBROMATOSIS 2362
    POSTIRRADIATION SCOLIOSIS 2362
    SCOLIOSIS IN THE MANAGEMENT OF BONE DYSPLASIAS 2362
Scheuermann's Juvenile Kyphosis 2380
      Definition 2380
      Incidence 2380
      Etiology and Pathogenesis 2380
      Pathology 2381
      Clinical Features 2381
      Radiographic Findings 2383
      Differential Diagnosis 2383
      Natural History, Course, and Prognosis 2385
      Treatment 2386
      ORTHOTIC TREATMENT 2386
      CAST TREATMENT—THE LYON METHOD 2386
      SURGICAL CORRECTION 2387
Disorders of Intervertebral Discs in Children 2391
    INTERVERTEBRAL DISC CALCIFICATION 2391
      Etiology 2391
      Clinical Picture 2391
      Radiographic Findings 2391
      Treatment 2391
    DISCITIS 2394
      Pathogenesis 2394
      Clinical Findings 2394
      Imaging Findings 2395
      Laboratory Findings 2396

Diagnosis	2397
Treatment	2399
HERNIATED INTERVERTEBRAL DISC	2402
SLIPPED VERTEBRAL APOPHYSIS	2404

VOLUME 4

7

The Foot and Leg — 2405

General Considerations — 2405

INTRODUCTION	2405
DEVELOPMENT AND OSSIFICATION OF THE FOOT AND LEG	2406
GROWTH OF THE NORMAL FOOT	2411
NORMAL VARIATIONS OF THE BONES OF THE FOOT AND ANKLE	2412
Accessory Bones of the Foot	2412
ACCESSORY TARSAL NAVICULAR	2412
OS TRIGONUM	2415
MISCELLANEOUS ACCESSORY BONES	2416
Congenital Deformities of the Foot	2421
POSTURAL DEFORMITIES OF THE FOOT AND LEG	2421
Talipes Calcaneovalgus	2423
Talipes Varus	2425
Postural Talipes Valgus	2425
Postural Metatarsus Adductus	2426
Postural Clubfoot	2426
CONGENITAL TALIPES EQUINOVARUS	2428
Incidence	2428
Heredity	2428
ARREST OF FETAL DEVELOPMENT	2431
PRIMARY GERM PLASM DEFECT	2433
Pathology	2433
BONE DEFORMITIES	2434
ARTICULAR MALALIGNMENTS	2437
SOFT TISSUE CHANGES	2440
Diagnosis	2447
Radiographic Assessment	2455
TECHNIQUE OF RADIOGRAPHY	2458
Treatment	2462
CLOSED NONOPERATIVE METHOD OF MANAGEMENT	2463
REDUCTION OF TALOCALCANEONAVICULAR JOINT BY OPEN SURGICAL METHODS	2475
Complications of Surgical Treatment	2524
COMPLICATIONS INVOLVING THE ANKLE	2525
COMPLICATIONS INVOLVING THE SUBTALAR JOINT	2527
COMPLICATIONS INVOLVING THE PROXIMAL TARSAL JOINT (TALONAVICULAR AND CALCANEOCUBOID)	2528
COMPLICATIONS AT THE METATARSOTARSAL JOINTS	2531
COMPLICATIONS AT THE METATARSOPHALANGEAL JOINT LEVEL	2539
BONE COMPLICATIONS	2539
NEUROVASCULAR COMPLICATIONS	2540
LOSS OF REDUCTION AND RECURRENCE OF DEFORMITY	2541
CONGENITAL CONVEX PES VALGUS	2557
Pathologic Anatomy	2561
BONE AND JOINT CHANGES	2561
LIGAMENTOUS CHANGES	2562
MUSCLE AND TENDON ABNORMALITIES	2562
Clinical Features	2563
Radiographic Findings	2566
Differential Diagnosis	2567

Treatment	2567
ELONGATION OF CONTRACTED SOFT TISSUE BY MANIPULATIVE STRETCHING	2568
OPEN REDUCTION	2569
TARSAL COALITION	2578
Incidence and Classification	2579
Etiology	2581
Heredity	2581
Clinical Features	2585
Radiographic Findings	2586
Treatment	2596
MEDIAL TALOCALCANEAL COALITION	2600
CALCANEONAVICULAR COALITION	2601
CONGENITAL METATARSUS VARUS	2612
Clinical Features	2612
Diagnosis	2614
Treatment	2614
NONOPERATIVE MANAGEMENT	2615
SURGICAL TREATMENT	2615
CONGENITAL METATARSUS PRIMUS VARUS AND HALLUX VALGUS	2626
Metatarsus Primus Varus	2626
Hallux Valgus and Bunion	2626
Treatment	2626
CONGENITAL BALL-AND-SOCKET ANKLE JOINT	2631
BRACHYMETATARSIA (CONGENITAL SHORT METATARSAL)	2633
CONGENITAL SPLIT OR CLEFT FOOT (LOBSTER CLAW)	2637
POLYDACTYLISM	2642
MACRODACTYLISM	2651
MISCELLANEOUS DEFORMITIES OF TOES	2651
Microdactylism	2651
Syndactylism	2653
Divergent or Convergent Toes	2653
Congenital Digitus Minimus Varus	2653
TREATMENT	2653
Hallux Valgus Interphalangeus	2661
Congenital Curly (or Varus) Toe	2661
TREATMENT	2665
HAMMER TOE	2667
Treatment	2670
MALLET TOE	2670
Pes Cavus and Claw Toes	2671
PES CAVUS	2671
Etiology and Pathogenesis	2671
Clinical Features	2674
Radiographic Findings	2676
Treatment	2680
SOFT-TISSUE PROCEDURES	2686
PROCEDURES ON BONE	2687
CLAW TOES	2715
Treatment	2716
Flexible Pes Planovalgus (Flatfoot)	2717
Analysis of Deformity and Radiographic Features	2717
Clinical Features	2724
Treatment	2728
CONSERVATIVE MANAGEMENT	2729
SURGICAL MANAGEMENT	2731
Acquired Affections of the Toes	2758
HALLUX RIGIDUS	2758
Etiology	2758
Clinical Features	2759
Radiographic Features	2760
Treatment	2760

Tumors of the Foot 2766
SOFT-TISSUE TUMORS 2766
    Lipoma 2766
    Ganglion 2766
    Hemangioma 2768
    Lymphangiectasis 2768
    Recurrent Digital Fibroma in Childhood 2770
    Nerve Sheath Tumors 2773
    Miscellaneous Tumors 2773
Skin and Nail Lesions 2789
HARD CORN (CLAVUS DURUS) 2789
SOFT CORN (CLAVUS MOLLIS) 2789
PLANTAR WART (VERRUCA PLANTARIS) 2789
TUMORS OF BONE 2780
    Treatment 2790
INGROWING TOENAIL 2790
Torsional (or Rotational) Deformities of the Lower Limbs 2791
    Pathophysiologic Considerations 2791
    Rotation of the Limb Bud 2792
    Etiologic Considerations 2792
    PERSISTENT FETAL ALIGNMENT 2792
    HEREDITY 2793
    PERSISTENT MALPOSTURE IN POSTNATAL LIFE 2793
    Torsional (or Rotational) Profile 2794
FEMORAL TORSION 2800
    The Natural Course 2800
    Clinical Features 2801
    Methods of Measurement 2803
    CLINICAL METHOD 2803
    IMAGING METHODS 2803
    RADIOGRAPHIC METHODS 2805
    Treatment 2805
    CONSERATIVE MEASURES 2805
    OPERATIVE MEASURES 2806
TIBIAL TORSION 2810
    Measurement of Tibial Torsion 2811
    CLINICAL METHODS 2812
    CALCULATION OF TIBIAL TORSION BY COMPUTED
      TRANSVERSE TOMOGRAPHY 2815
    MEASUREMENT OF TIBIAL TORSION BY ULTRASOUND 2815
    MEDIAL TIBIAL TORSION 2815
    ABNORMAL LATERAL TIBIAL TORSION 2816
    Differential Diagnosis 2816
    Treatment 2817
Angular Deformities of the Long Bones of the Lower Limbs 2820
PHYSIOLOGIC EVOLUTION OF ALIGNMENT OF THE LOWER LIMBS ... 2820
PHYSIOLOGIC GENU VARUM 2822
    Radiographic Features 2824
    Differential Diagnosis 2824
    Treatment 2826
DEVELOPMENTAL GENU VALGUM 2827
    Treatment 2828
    MEDIAL PHYSEAL RETARDATION BY STAPLING AND
      GROWTH ARREST BY EPIPHYSIODESIS OF THE
      DISTAL FEMUR AND/OR PROXIMAL TIBIA 2829
    OSTEOTOMY 2832
TIBIA VARA 2835
    Classification 2835
    Etiology 2836
    Pathology 2837
    Clinical Picture 2837
    Radiographic Features 2839
    Differential Diagnosis 2841

Treatment	2841
INFANTILE TYPE	2842
Nonsurgical Treatment	2842
Operative Treatment	2843
ADOLESCENT TYPE	2846
ADULT TIBIA VARA	2847
Limb Length Discrepancy	2850
Longitudinal Growth of Long Bones	2852
Patterns of Skeletal Growth	2852
RATE OF GROWTH	2852
RELATIVE SIZE	2854
RELATIVE MATURITY	2854
Growth Prediction Chart	2864
Radiographic Methods of Measuring Length of Long Bones	2867
TELEOROENTGENOGRAPHY	2867
SLIT SCANOGRAPHY	2867
ORTHOROENTGENOGRAPHY	2867
CT SCAN	2870
Treatment	2871
ARREST OR RETARDATION OF GROWTH OF THE LONGER LIMB BY EPIPHYSIODESIS	2871
GROWTH RETARDATION BY PHYSEAL STAPLING	2887
SHORTENING OF THE LONG LIMB	2888
LENGTHENING OF THE SHORT LIMB	2892
Current Techniques of Limb Lengthening	2893
BIOLOGIC PRINCIPLES	2893
INDICATIONS	2894
REQUISITES	2894
CONTRAINDICATIONS	2894
LIMB LENGTHENING BY CALLOTASIS (CALLUS DISTRACTION) (DEBASTIANI TECHNIQUE)	2896
ILIZAROV METHOD: LIMB LENGTHENING WITH DISTRACTION OSTEOGENESIS WITHOUT BONE GRAFTING	2896
Method of Limb Lengthening	2895
Problems and Complications	2991
INTRAOPERATIVE	2996
IMMEDIATE POSTOPERATIVE PERIOD	2996
DURING DISTRACTION PERIOD	2996
DELAYED CONSOLIDATION AND NONUNION	3001
STRESS FRACTURE AND PLASTIC BOWING OF THE ELONGATED BONE	3001
MENTAL DISTURBANCE	3001

8

Fractures and Dislocations	3013
ANATOMIC AND BIOMECHANICAL DIFFERENCES	3014
The Normal Physis and Its Response to Trauma	3014
Direct Trauma	3015
Loss of Circulation	3019
Compression	3021
Classification	3021
Incidence	3026
Principles of Management of Fractures Involving the Physis	3026
The Upper Limb	3030
Injuries to the Region of the Shoulder	3030
FRACTURES OF THE CLAVICLE	3030
Mechanism of Injury	3030
Pathologic Anatomy	3032
Diagnostic Features	3032
BIRTH FRACTURES	3032
INFANCY AND CHILDHOOD	3032

Treatment	3033
BIRTH FRACTURES	3033
YOUNG CHILDREN	3034
OLDER CHILDREN AND ADOLESCENTS	3034
RECUMBENT TREATMENT	3036
Complications	3036
PHYSEAL SEPARATION OF THE MEDIAL (STERNAL) END OF THE CLAVICLE	3038
ACROMIOCLAVICULAR DISLOCATION	3041
FRACTURES OF THE SCAPULA	3042
Fractures of the Body of the Scapula	3043
Fractures of the Scapular Neck	3043
Fractures of the Glenoid Cavity of the Scapula	3044
Fractures of the Acromion	3044
Fracture of the Coracoid Process	3044
Fracture-Separation of Epiphyses of Acromion and Coracoid Process	3044
FRACTURES INVOLVING THE PROXIMAL HUMERAL PHYSIS	3046
Fracture-Separation of Upper Epiphysis of Humerus	3046
Mechanism of Injury	3046
Pathologic Anatomy	3047
Diagnosis	3047
Treatment	3047
Injuries to the Arm	3052
FRACTURES OF THE SHAFT OF THE HUMERUS	3052
Mechanism of Injury	3052
Pathologic Anatomy	3054
Diagnosis	3054
SUPRACONDYLAR FRACTURE OF THE HUMERUS	3058
Mechanism of Injury and Classification	3058
Pathologic Anatomy	3062
EXTENSION TYPE	3062
FLEXION TYPE	3062
Diagnosis	3064
Treatment	3067
EMERGENCY SPLINTING	3067
UNDISPLACED OR MINIMALLY DISPLACED FRACTURES	3068
MODERATELY DISPLACED FRACTURES WITH INTACT POSTERIOR CORTEX	3068
SEVERELY DISPLACED FRACTURES	3070
MAINTENANCE OF REDUCTION BY LATERAL SKELETAL TRACTION	3075
OPEN REDUCTION	3075
Complications	3079
MALUNION AND CHANGES IN CARRYING ANGLE	3079
NEURAL COMPLICATIONS	3081
VASCULAR INJURY	3083
VOLKMANN'S ISCHEMIC CONTRACTURE (COMPARTMENT SYNDROME)	3099
FRACTURE-SEPARATION OF THE ENTIRE DISTAL HUMERAL PHYSIS	3105
FRACTURES OF THE LATERAL CONDYLE OF THE HUMERUS	3108
Mechanism of Injury and Pathology	3109
Diagnosis	3109
Treatment	3110
Problems and Complications	3116
FRACTURES OF THE MEDIAL EPICONDYLE OF THE HUMERUS	3121
Diagnosis	3121
Treatment	3121
DISLOCATION OF THE ELBOW	3124
Mechanism of Injury and Pathologic Anatomy	3125
Diagnosis	3125
Treatment	3128
Complications	3131
VASCULAR INJURIES	3131

NEURAL INJURIES	3131
HETEROTOPIC BONE FORMATION AND MYOSITIS OSSIFICANS	3133
RECURRENT DISLOCATION OF THE ELBOW	3133
FRACTURES INVOLVING THE PROXIMAL RADIAL PHYSIS AND RADIAL NECK	3137
Incidence	3137
Mechanism of Injury	3137
Classification	3139
Diagnosis	3139
Treatment	3140
Complications	3143
FRACTURES OF THE OLECRANON	3145
PULLED ELBOW (SUBLUXATION OF THE RADIAL HEAD)	3148
Mechanism of Injury and Pathologic Anatomy	3148
Diagnosis	3149
Treatment	3150
MONTEGGIA FRACTURE-DISLOCATION	3151
Classification	3158
Mechanism of Injury	3158
Diagnosis	3161
Treatment	3163
OPERATIVE TREATMENT	3163
Complications	3168
NERVE PALSY	3168
RECURRENCE OF RADIAL HEAD DISLOCATION	3168
MALUNION OF THE FRACTURE OF THE ULNAR SHAFT	3178
RADIOULNAR SYNOSTOSIS	3178
RADIOHUMERAL FIBROUS ANKYLOSIS	3178
PARA-ARTICULAR ECTOPIC OSSIFICATION	3178
VOLKMANN'S ISCHEMIC CONTRACTURE	3178
PROBLEMS AND COMPLICATIONS OF TREATMENT	3178
Monteggia Equivalent Lesions of the Forearm	3178
Injuries to the Forearm and Hand	3181
FRACTURES OF THE SHAFT OF THE RADIUS AND ULNA	3181
Mechanism of Injury and Pathologic Anatomy	3181
Diagnosis	3182
Treatment	3182
GREENSTICK FRACTURES OF MIDDLE THIRD OF RADIUS AND ULNA	3184
DISPLACED FRACTURES OF MIDDLE THIRD OF BOTH BONES OF FOREARM	3185
FRACTURES OF THE DISTAL THIRD OF THE RADIUS AND ULNA	3188
FRACTURES OF THE PROXIMAL THIRD OF THE SHAFT OF THE RADIUS AND ULNA	3194
PLASTIC DEFORMATION (OR TRAUMATIC BOWING) OF BOTH BONES OF THE FOREARM	3194
REMODELING OF MALUNION OF FRACTURES OF BOTH BONES OF THE FOREARM	3195
FRACTURE-SEPARATION OF THE DISTAL RADIAL PHYSIS	3202
Salter-Harris Type I Injuries	3202
Salter-Harris Type II Injuries	3202
FRACTURES OF THE PHALANGES AND METACARPALS IN THE HAND	3205
WRINGER INJURY TO THE UPPER LIMB	3210
Treatment	3211
The Lower Limb	3212
TRAUMATIC DISLOCATION OF THE HIP	3212
Types	3212
Mechanism of Injury	3214
Pathologic Anatomy	3216
Diagnostic Features	3216
Treatment	3219
CLOSED REDUCTION OF POSTERIOR DISLOCATION	3220

CLOSED REDUCTION OF ANTERIOR DISLOCATION 3224
Postoperative Care 3224
Treatment of Fracture-Dislocations of the Hip 3224
Central Dislocations of the Hip 3224
Complications and Problems 3226
ASEPTIC NECROSIS 3226
SCIATIC NERVE PALSY 3226
VASCULAR INJURY 3226
INCOMPLETE NONCONCENTRIC REDUCTION 3226
DEGENERATIVE ARTHRITIS 3226
RECURRENT POST-TRAUMATIC DISLOCATION OF THE HIP 3226
FRACTURES OF THE NECK OF THE FEMUR 3231
Classification 3231
Mechanism of Injury 3231
Diagnosis 3233
Treatment 3233
TRANSEPIPHYSEAL FRACTURES 3236
UNDISPLACED TRANSCERVICAL OR CERVICOTROCHANTERIC
  FRACTURES 3237
DISPLACED TRANSCERVICAL AND CERVICOTROCHANTERIC
  FRACTURES 3237
Complications 3237
ASEPTIC NECROSIS 3237
COXA VARA 3244
PREMATURE FUSION OF CAPITAL FEMORAL PHYSIS 3244
DELAYED UNION AND NONUNION 3244
**AVULSION FRACTURES OF THE GREATER AND LESSER
  TROCHANTERS** 3247
FRACTURES OF THE FEMORAL SHAFT 3248
Pathologic Anatomy 3248
Diagnosis 3255
Treatment 3255
INFANTS AND CHILDREN UP TO TWO YEARS OF AGE 3255
CHILDREN BETWEEN THREE AND TEN YEARS OF AGE 3262
PREADOLESCENT AND ADOLESCENT AGE GROUP 3266
Complications 3266
DISCREPANCY IN LIMB LENGTH 3266
ANGULAR DEFORMITIES OF FEMORAL SHAFT 3268
FRACTURES INVOLVING THE DISTAL FEMORAL EPIPHYSIS 3274
Mechanisms of Injury and Pathologic Anatomy 3274
Diagnosis 3275
Treatment 3275
ABDUCTION TYPE FRACTURES 3275
HYPEREXTENSION TYPE FRACTURES 3279
HYPERFLEXION TYPE FRACTURES 3279
**TRAUMATIC DISLOCATION OF THE PATELLA AND OSTEOCHONDRAL
  FRACTURES OF THE KNEE** 3282
Diagnosis 3282
Treatment 3283
FRACTURES OF THE PATELLA 3284
FRACTURES OF THE INTERCONDYLAR EMINENCE OF THE TIBIA 3286
Mechanism of Injury 3286
Classification 3286
Clinical Picture 3287
Radiographic Findings 3288
Treatment 3288
**FRACTURES INVOLVING THE PROXIMAL TIBIAL PHYSIS AND THE
  APOPHYSIS OF THE TIBIAL TUBERCLE AND AVULSION FRACTURES
  OF THE APOPHYSIS OF THE TIBIAL TUBERCLE** 3290
Fractures Involving the Proximal Tibial Physis 3290
TREATMENT 3291
Avulsion Fractures of Apophysis of the Tibial Tubercle 3291
MECHANISM OF INJURY 3291
CLASSIFICATION 3291

TREATMENT	3294
FRACTURES OF THE SHAFT OF THE TIBIA AND FIBULA	3295
Spiral Fracture of Tibia with Intact Fibula in Infancy and Early Childhood	3296
Greenstick Fracture of Proximal Metaphysis or Upper Shaft of Tibia	3297
FRACTURES OF THE ANKLE	3302
Classification and Mechanism of Injury	3303
ANATOMIC CLASSIFICATION	3303
MECHANISTIC CLASSIFICATIONS	3303
MISCELLANEOUS FRACTURES	3316
Treatment	3323
Complications	3331
FRACTURES OF THE FOOT	3339
Injuries to the Spine and Pelvis	3345
INJURIES TO THE SPINE	3345
Rotatory Subluxation of Atlantoaxial Joint	3345
Fracture of Odontoid Process with Anterior Dislocation of Atlas	3345
Compression Fractures of Vertebrae in Thoracic and Lumbar Spine	3345
FRACTURES OF THE PELVIS	3345
Unstable Fractures with Disruption of the Pelvic Ring	3347
Isolated Fractures with Stable Pelvic Ring	3347
Avulsion Fractures of the Pelvis	3347
Miscellaneous Fractures	3352
OBSTETRICAL OR BIRTH INJURIES	3352
Birth Fractures of Shafts of Long Bones	3353
Birth Fractures Involving Physes of Long Bones	3353
Traumatic Separation of Distal Femoral Epiphysis	3353
Traumatic Displacement of Distal Humeral Epiphysis	3354
Other Obstetrical Injuries	3354
STRESS FRACTURES	3359
Sites of Involvement	3360
Pathogenesis	3360
Clinical Findings	3360
Radiographic Findings	3360
Treatment	3363
PATHOLOGIC FRACTURES	3366
THE BATTERED CHILD	3366
Index	i

Volume 2

Pediatric Orthopedics

SECOND EDITION

Volume 2

3. Bone

Responses of Bone

The skeleton serves as the general framework of the body and provides the articulating mechanisms that permit mobility. Bone, though physically rigid, is a living and dynamic structure. It is biologically plastic, being constantly remodeled. In addition to its supportive function, it is involved in many metabolic processes and is thus subject to a multitude of local and generalized diseases and metabolic disorders, as well as to physiologic and mechanical forces.

The ultimate size and form of an adult bone is determined by intrinsic and extrinsic factors. A fetal bone in tissue culture develops a form predetermined by its inherent nature; in life, however, this form may be modified by a variety of external influences acting in utero or postnatally.

Response to Function

The fundamental biologic law that relates to the interdependence of structure and function, usually referred to as Wolff's law, describes the reaction of bone to forces acting upon it. It states, "Every change in the form and function of bones or their function alone is followed by certain definite changes in their internal structure and equally definite changes in their external configuration in accordance with mathematical laws."[3] Because of physiologic variables, Wolff was not able to reduce this observation to mathematical accuracy, which, nevertheless, does not alter the law's inherent fundamental truth. To illustrate Wolff's law, consider the healed fracture of the femur with overriding and bowing in a child (Fig. 3–1). Forces of weight-bearing and the action of muscles reshape and remodel the bone, gradually correcting the deformity. Hueter and Volkmann, in considering the effect of force on growth, proposed the thesis that compression inhibits growth whereas tension stimulates it.[1,2]

Response to Muscular Action

Muscular forces also influence bony configuration; in fact, normal skeletal development is dependent upon balanced muscle action. This is illustrated, for example, by the calcaneus deformity that results when the gastrocnemius and soleus muscles are paralyzed and thus no longer able to act on the back of the heel, but the anterior tibial and other dorsiflexors of the ankle are functioning. The ensuing abnormal development of the os calcis causes its posterior aspect to rotate plantarward. Following posterior transfer of the anterior tibial and peroneus brevis muscles, the calcaneal deformity may be reversed in the young growing foot.

Response to Use and Disuse

Normal use of bone is itself a stimulus for bone formation and growth. If bones are not used, however, they will demonstrate what is designated as disuse atrophy, consisting of de-

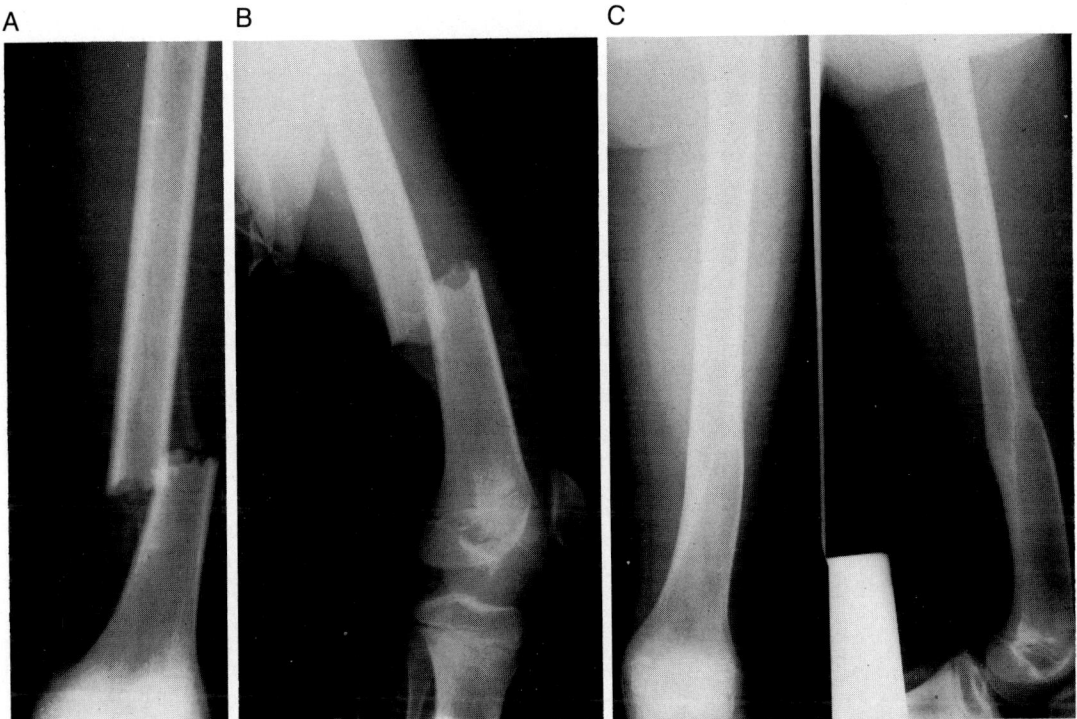

FIGURE 3–1. *Wolff's law as illustrated in remodeling of a malunited fracture of the femur.*

A and **B.** Note the overriding and bowing of the fracture fragments. **C.** One year later, remodeling and correction of the deformity.

calcification and a decrease in mass. This may become evident after a period of immobilization of a limb in a cast or following extensive flaccid paralysis and prolonged confinement to bed. The process may be quite rapid, causing complications such as pathologic fracture or more generalized metabolic disorders such as hypercalcemia, hypercalciuria, and nephrolithiasis, these being due to the extensive loss of calcium. In the case of a growing individual, disuse over long periods may cause the bone to be very much decreased in diameter and shortened because growth is inhibited.

Response to Circulatory Disturbances

Necrosis of bone results from an interruption of its blood supply, which may be due either to physical injury or to nontraumatic occlusion of its blood vessels. The femoral head is the most common site of aseptic necrosis following fracture of the neck of the femur or hip dislocation. Caisson disease is a well-known example of a nontraumatic lesion that produces necrosis by occlusion of the vessels of the epiphysis and diaphysis.

In aseptic necrosis in which there is some residual or returning blood supply the involved bone is invaded by a vascular fibrous stroma, by which the necrotic bone is gradually resorbed and replaced by new bone. After sufficient time has elapsed, the bone that has retained its blood supply undergoes atrophy with decalcification, whereas completely avascular bone, having no blood supply for removal of radiopaque mineral salts, shows increased density in the radiograms. This increased density may represent zones of hypertrophic living bone, necrotic bone with reactive bone about it, or simply necrotic bone. The sequestrum seen in osteomyelitis is another example of the effect of loss of blood supply on bone.

Bone responds to increased circulation by hypertrophy and an increase in length. This is well illustrated by the increased length of a lower limb in which there is an arteriovenous aneurysm or a prolonged inflammation near an epiphysis.

Response to Injury—Bone Repair

The basic reactive response of bone to injury is the formation of new bone, as is seen in a healing fracture, which is discussed in Chapter

8. Injury may produce other effects and responses as well, such as necrosis of bone resulting either from an interruption of its blood supply or from the local effect of trauma. Atrophy may be induced through the pain and subsequent disuse caused by the injury. Bone erosion or reactive sclerosis may occur at the site of chronic trauma.

Reaction to Radiation

Excessive radiation is injurious to bone, causing direct cellular damage or other indirect effects due to vascular injury. In the growing skeleton, the cartilage cells at the epiphyseal plate are particularly vulnerable to damage by heavy radiation, and skeletal growth is consequently disturbed. Pathologic fractures may occur following extensive radiation. Sarcomatous change has been observed in bones subsequent to heavy irradiation.

References

1. Hueter, C.: Anatomische Studien an den Extremitatengelenken Neugeborener und Erwachsener. Virchow. Arch. Pathol. Anat., 25:575, 1862.
2. Volkmann, R. von: Chirurgische Erfahrungen über Knochenverbiegungen und Knochen wachsthum. Arch. Pathol. Anat., 24:512, 1862.
3. Wolff, J.: Über die innere Architecture der Knochen und ihre Bedeutung fur die Frage von Knochenwachstum. Virchow. Arch. Pathol. Anat., 50:389, 1870.

Dysplasias of Bone

Generalized developmental disorders of the skeleton are rare, but have intrigued and been known to mankind for centuries, as depicted in primitive figurines and sculptures.

In the early medical literature there was semantic confusion because authors reported cases and syndromes by various names and eponyms. Many attempts were made to solve the problem, to derive a classification, and to produce a nomenclature acceptable to all the disciplines involved—radiology, genetics, pediatrics, and orthopedic surgery.

Nomenclature and Classification

Sir Thomas Fairbank was the pioneer—his *Atlas of General Affections of the Skeleton* set the groundwork.[8] It was followed by monumental contributions of other investigators—namely, Lamy and Maroteaux of France, Wiedemann and Spranger of Germany, and McKusick of the United States.[12-15, 18, 20] Rubin grouped the skeletal dysplasias according to the anatomic distribution of bone changes in his textbook *Dynamic Classification of Bone Dysplasias* (Table 3–1 and Figs. 3–2 and 3–3).[16]

The March of Dimes sponsored a series of meetings on birth defects in the United States, which set the stage for a classification to end the state of confusion about inherited bone dysplasias.[4]

The European Society of Paediatric Radiologists arrived at an International Nomenclature of Constitutional Disorders of Bone, an updated version of which is given in Table 3–2.

The term *dysplasia* was substituted for "dwarfism" and is used when the developmental changes in the skeleton are generalized; when the changes affect a single bone or segment of

Table 3–1. Dynamic Classification of Bone Dysplasias*

I. Epiphyseal Dysplasias
   A. Epiphyseal hypoplasias
      1. Failure of articular cartilage: spondylo-epiphyseal dysplasia, congenita and tarda
      2. Failure of ossification of center: multiple epiphyseal dysplasia, congenita and tarda
   B. Epiphyseal hyperplasia
      1. Excess of articular cartilage; dysplasia epiphysealis hemimelica
II. Physeal Dysplasias
   A. Cartilage hypoplasias
      1. Failure of proliferating cartilage: achondroplasia, congenita and tarda
      2. Failure of hypertrophic cartilage: metaphyseal dysostosis, congenita and tarda
   B. Cartilage hyperplasias
      1. Excess of proliferating cartilage: hyperchondroplasia
      2. Excess of hypertrophic cartilage: enchondromatosis
III. Metaphyseal Dysplasias
   A. Metaphyseal hypoplasias
      1. Failure to form primary spongiosa: hypophosphatasia, congenita and tarda
      2. Failure to absorb primary spongiosa: osteopetrosis, congenita and tarda
      3. Failure to absorb secondary spongiosa: craniometaphyseal dysplasia, congenita and tarda
   B. Metaphyseal hyperplasias
      1. Excessive spongiosa: multiple exostoses
IV. Diaphyseal Dysplasias
   A. Diaphyseal hypoplasias
      1. Failure of periosteal bone formation: osteogenesis imperfecta, congenita and tarda
      2. Failure of endosteal bone formation: idiopathic osteoporosis, congenita and tarda
   B. Diaphyseal hyperplasias
      1. Excessive periosteal bone formation: progressive diaphyseal dysplasia
      2. Excessive endosteal bone formation: hyperphosphatasemia

*From Rubin, P.: Dynamic Classification of Bone Dysplasias. Chicago, Year Book Medical Publishers, Inc., 1964, p. 82. Reprinted by permission.

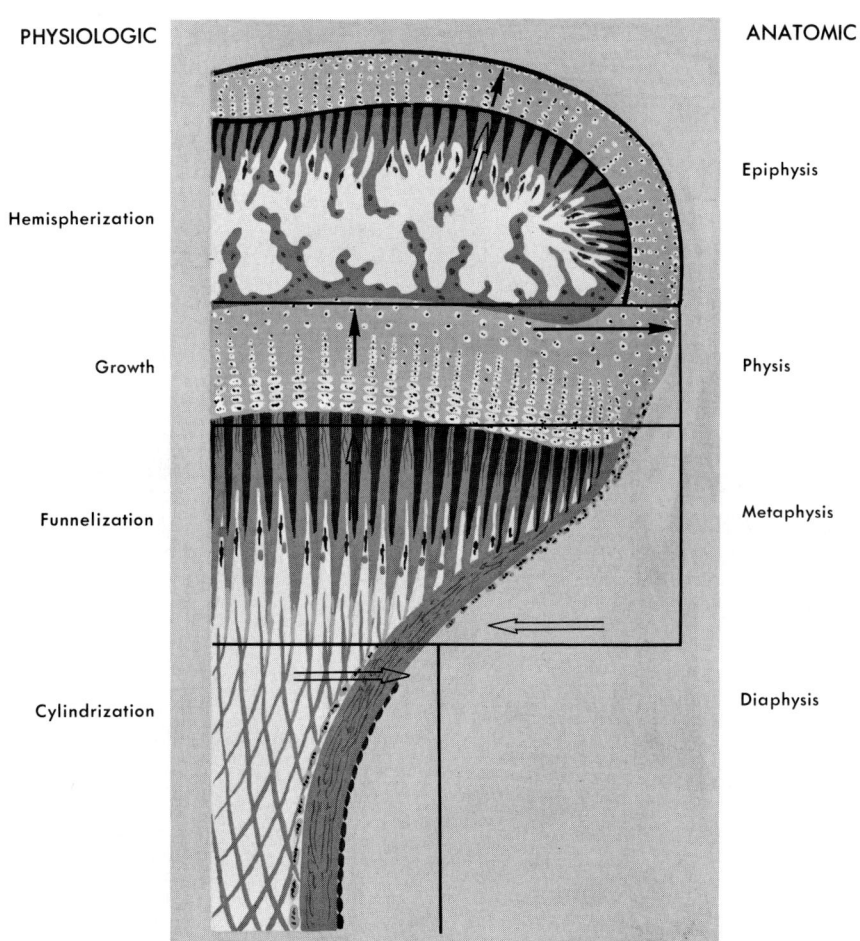

FIGURE 3–2. *Proposed terminology for normal bone modeling (anatomic-physiologic correlation).*

(Adapted from Rubin, P.: Dynamic Classification of Bone Dysplasias. Chicago, Year Book Medical Publishers, Inc., 1964.)

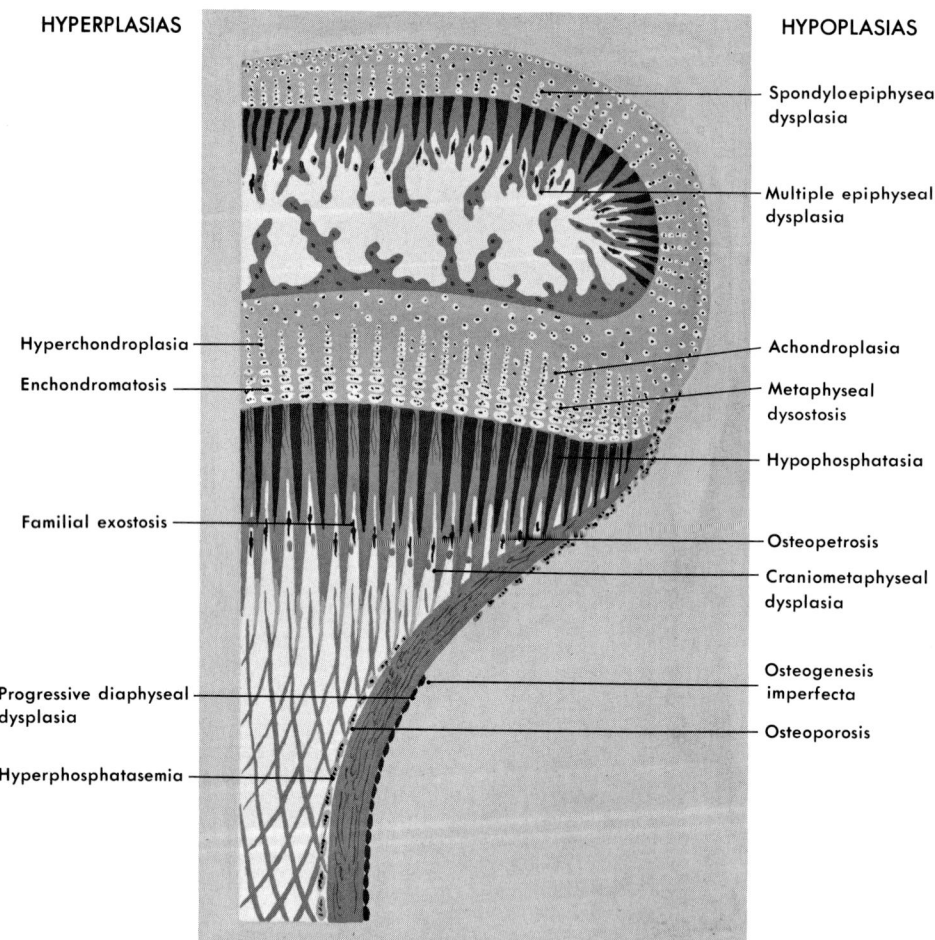

FIGURE 3–3. *Dynamic classification of bone dysplasias.*

(Adapted from Rubin, P.: Dynamic Classification of Bone Dysplasias. Chicago, Year Book Medical Publishers, Inc., 1964.)

Table 3-2. International Nomenclature of Constitutional Disease of Bone

Osteochondrodysplasias
Abnormalities of cartilage and/or bone growth and development.

Defects of Growth of Tubular Bones and/or Spine
A. Identifiable at birth
 1. Achondrogenesis type I, Parenti-Fraccaro
 2. Achondrogenesis type II, Langer-Saldino
 3. Thanatophoric dysplasia
 4. Thanatophoric dysplasia with clover-leaf skull
 5. Short rib-polydactyly syndrome type I, Saldino-Noonan (perhaps several forms)
 6. Short rib-polydactyly syndrome type II, Majewski
 7. Chondrodysplasia punctata
    a. Rhizomelic form
    b. Dominant form
    c. Other forms, excluding symptomatic stippling in other disorders (e.g., Zellweger syndrome, Warfarin embryopathy)
 8. Campomelic dysplasia
 9. Other dysplasias with congenital bowing of long bones (several forms)
 10. Achondroplasia
 11. Diastrophic dysplasia
 12. Metatropic dysplasia (several forms)
 13. Chondroectodermal dysplasia, Ellis Van Creveld
 14. Asphyxiating thoracic dysplasia, Jeune
 15. Spondyloepiphyseal dysplasia congenita
    a. Type Spranger-Wiedemann
    b. Other forms (see B, 11-12)
 16. Kniest dysplasia
 17. Mesomelic dysplasia
    a. Type Nievergelt
    b. Type Langer (probable homozygous dyschondrosteosis)
    c. Type Robinow
    d. Type Rheinhardt
    e. Other forms
 18. Acromesomelic dysplasia
 19. Cleidocranial dysplasia
 20. Larsen syndrome
 21. Otopalatodigital syndrome
B. Identifiable in later life
 1. Hypochondroplasia
 2. Dyschondrosteosis
 3. Metaphyseal chondrodysplasia type Jansen
 4. Metaphyseal chondrodysplasia type Schmid
 5. Metaphyseal chondrodysplasia type McKusick
 6. Metaphyseal chondrodysplasia with exocrine pancreatic insufficiency and cyclic neutropenia
 7. Spondylometaphyseal dysplasia
    a. Type Kozlowski
    b. Other forms
 8. Multiple epiphyseal dysplasia
    a. Type Fairbank
    b. Other forms
 9. Arthro-ophthalmopathy, Stickler
 10. Pseudoachondroplasia
    a. Dominant
    b. Recessive
 11. Spondyloepiphyseal dysplasia tarda
 12. Spondyloepiphyseal dysplasia, other forms (see A, 15-16)
 13. Dyggve-Melchior-Clausen dysplasia
 14. Spondyloepimetaphyseal dysplasia (several forms)
 15. Myotonic chondrodysplasia, Catel-Schwartz-Jampel
 16. Parastremmatic dysplasia
 17. Trichorhinophalangeal dysplasia
 18. Acrodysplasia with retinitis pigmentosa and nephropathy Saldino-Mainzer

Disorganized Development of Cartilage and Fibrous Components of Skeleton
 1. Dysplasia epiphysealis hemimelica
 2. Multiple cartilaginous exostoses
 3. Acrodysplasia with exostoses, Giedion-Langer
 4. Enchondromatosis, Ollier
 5. Enchondromatosis with hemangioma, Maffucci
 6. Metachondromatosis
 7. Fibrous dysplasia, Jaffe-Lichtenstein
 8. Fibrous dysplasia with skin pigmentation and precocious puberty, McCune-Albright
 9. Cherubism (familial fibrous dysplasia of the jaws)
 10. Neurofibromatosis

Abnormalities of Density of Cortical Diaphyseal Structure and/or Metaphyseal Modelling
 1. Osteogenesis imperfecta congenita (several forms)
 2. Osteogenesis imperfecta tarda (several forms)
 3. Juvenile idiopathic osteoporosis
 4. Osteoporosis with pseudoglioma
 5. Osteopetrosis with precocious manifestations
 6. Osteopetrosis with delayed manifestations (several forms)
 7. Pycnodysostosis
 8. Osteopoikilosis
 9. Osteopathia striata
 10. Melorheostosis
 11. Diaphyseal dysplasia, Camurati-Engelmann
 12. Craniodiaphyseal dysplasia
 13. Endosteal hyperostosis
    a. Autosomal dominant, Worth
    b. Autosomal recessive, Van Buchem
 14. Tubular stenosis, Kenny-Caffey
 15. Pachydermoperiostosis
 16. Osteodysplasty, Melnick-Needles
 17. Frontometaphyseal dysplasia
 18. Craniometaphyseal dysplasia (several forms)
 19. Metaphyseal dysplasia, Pyle
 20. Sclerosteosis
 21. Dysosteosclerosis
 22. Osteoectasia with hyperphosphatasia

Dysostoses
Malformation of individual bones singly or in combination.

Dysostoses with Cranial and Facial Involvement
 1. Craniosynostosis (several forms)
 2. Craniofacial dysostosis, Crouzon
 3. Acrocephalosyndactyly, Apert (and others)
 4. Acrocephalopolysyndactyly, Carpenter (and others)
 5. Mandibulofacial dysostosis
    a. Type Treacher Collins, Franceschetti
    b. Other forms
 6. Oculomandibulofacial syndrome, Hallermann-Streiff-Francois
 7. Nevoid basal cell carcinoma syndrome

Dysostoses with Predominant Axial Involvement
 1. Vertebral segmentation defects, including Klippel-Feil
 2. Cervico-oculoacoustic syndrome, Wildervanck
 3. Sprengel anomaly
 4. Spondylocostal dysostosis
    a. Dominant form
    b. Recessive forms
 5. Oculovertebral syndrome, Weyers
 6. Osteo-onychodysostosis
 7. Cerebrocostomandibular syndrome

Table 3–2. International Nomenclature of Constitutional Disease of Bone Continued

Dysostoses with Predominant Involvement of Extremities
1. Acheiria
2. Apodia
3. Ectodactyly syndrome
4. Aglossia-adactyly syndrome
5. Congenital bowing of long bones (several forms) (see also osteochondrodysplasias)
6. Familial radioulnar synostosis
7. Brachydactyly (several forms)
8. Symphalangism
9. Polydactyly (several forms)
10. Syndactyly (several forms)
11. Polysyndactyly (several forms)
12. Camptodactyly
13. Poland syndrome
14. Rubenstein-Taybi syndrome
15. Pancytopenia-dysmelia syndrome, Fanconi
16. Thrombocytopenia-radialaplasia syndrome
17. Orodigitofacial syndrome
    a. Type Papillon-Leage
    b. Type Mohr
18. Cardiomelic syndrome, Holt-Oram (and others)
19. Femoral facial syndrome
20. Multiple-synostoses (includes some forms of symphalangism)
21. Scapuloiliac dysostosis, Kosenow-Sinios
22. Hand-foot-genital syndrome
23. Focal dermal hypoplasia, Goltz

Idiopathic Osteolyses
1. Phalangeal (several forms)
2. Tarsocarpal
    a. Including Francois form (and others)
    b. With nephropathy
3. Multicentric
    a. Hajdu-Cheney form
    b. Winchester form
    c. Other forms

Chromosomal Aberrations
Specific entities not listed

Primary Metabolic Abnormalities
Calcium and/or Phosphorus
1. Hypophosphatemic rickets
2. Pseudodeficiency rickets, Prader, Royer
3. Late rickets, McCance
4. Idiopathic hypercalcuria
5. Hypophosphatasia (several forms)
6. Pseudohypoparathyroidism (normo- and hypocalcaemic forms, include acrodysostosis)

Complex Carbohydrates
1. Mucopolysaccharidosis, type I (alpha-L-iduronidase deficiency)
    a. Hurler form
    b. Scheie form
    c. Other forms
2. Mucopolysaccharidosis, type II, Hunter (sulfoiduronate sulfatase deficiency)
3. Mucopolysaccharidosis, type III San Filippo
    a. Type A (heparin sulfamidase deficiency)
    b. Type B (N-acetyl-alpha-glucosaminidase deficiency)
4. Mucopolysaccharidosis, type IV, Morquio (N-acetylgalactosamine-6-sulfate-sulfatase deficiency)
5. Mucopolysaccharidosis, type VI, Maroteaux-Lamy (aryl sulfatase B deficiency)
6. Mucopolysaccharidosis, type VII (beta-glucuronidase deficiency)
7. Aspartylglucosaminuria (aspartylglucosaminidase deficiency)
8. Mannosidosis (alpha-mannosidase deficiency)
9. Fucosidosis (alpha-fucosidase deficiency)
10. GMI-gangliosidosis (beta-galactosidase deficiency)
11. Multiple sulfatase deficiency, Austin, Thieffry
12. Neuraminidase deficiency (formerly mucolipidosis I)
13. Mucoplipidosis II
14. Mucolipidosis III

Lipids
1. Niemann-Pick disease
2. Gaucher disease

Nucleic Acids
1. Adenosine-deaminase deficiency and others

Amino Acids
1. Homocystinuria and others

Metals
1. Menkes kinky hair syndrome and others

From Horan, F., and Beighton, P.: Orthopaedic Problems in Inherited Skeletal Disorders. New York. Springer-Verlag, 1982. Reprinted by permission.)

the skeleton, the term *dysostosis* is used. A *malformation* denotes a primary abnormality of development, whereas a *deformity* means a change in structure of a previously normal bone.

The term *short stature* means height that is at the lower end of the normal range for a person's normal peers. *Dwarf*, a somewhat derogatory term commonly used by both the layman and members of the medical profession, denotes a pathologic diminution in stature (below the tenth percentile). Dwarfism may be subdivided into two general categories—disproportionate and proportionate (the proportionate dwarf is referred to as a midget by the layman).

The disproportionate type of dwarfism may be of either of two types—short-limb or short-trunk. The short-limb variety may be further subdivided according to the site of maximal shortening: rhizomelic (in the proximal portion), mesomelic (in the middle), and acromelic (in the distal portion).

Diagnosis and management of skeletal dysplasia in a child is best provided by a multidisciplinary clinic for skeletal dysplasia. The expertise of radiologist, geneticist, orthopedic surgeon, and pediatrician is essential for optimal care. The captain of the team is often the pediatrician with a background in genetics. The services of plastic surgeon, neurosurgeon, ophthalmologist, bronchologist, and other pediatric specialists should be available. Preventive psychologic counseling is crucial. Organizations like the "Little People of America" have provided contact and support with the goal of "problems shared are problems halved." Similar groups have been formed to deal with other disorders, such as the Brittle Bone Society for osteogenesis imperfecta. Such organizations have supported research and provided communication between physicians and patients.

A thorough discussion of bone dysplasia is beyond the scope of this book—this may be found in the excellent treatises cited. Only the more common bone dysplasias with special orthopedic problems are discussed here.

References

1. Bailey, J. A.: Disproportionate Short Stature. Philadelphia, Saunders, 1973.
2. Beighton, P.: Inherited Disorders of the Skeleton. New York, Churchill-Livingstone, 1978.
3. Beighton, P., and Cremin, B. J.: Sclerosing Bone Dysplasias. New York, Springer, 1980.
4. Bergsma, D. (ed.): Birth Defects Original Article Series, The National Foundation, March of Dimes. Limb malformations, Vol. 10, No. 5, 1974. Malformation syndromes, Vol. 10, No. 7, 1974. Skeletal dysplasias, Vol. 10, No. 9, 1974. Skeletal dysplasias, Vol. 10, No. 12, 1974. Disorders of connective tissue, Vol. 11, No. 6, 1975. Morphogenesis and malformation of the limb, Vol. 13, No. 1, 1977. The genetics of hand malformations, Vol. 14, No. 3, 1978.
5. Brailsford, J. F.: Radiology of Bones and Joints. 5th Ed. Baltimore, Williams & Wilkins, 1953.
6. Carter, C. O., and Fairbank, T. J.: The Genetics of Locomotor Disorders. London, Oxford University Press, 1974.
7. Cremin, B. J., and Beighton, P.: Bone Dysplasias of Infancy. New York, Springer, 1978.
8. Fairbank, H. A. T.: An Atlas of General Affections of the Skeleton. Edinburgh. Livingstone, 1951.
9. Hobaek, A.: Problems of Hereditary Chondrodysplasias. Oslo, Oslo University Press, 1961.
10. Haran, F., and Beighton, P.: Orthopaedic Problems in Inherited Skeletal Disorders. New York. Springer Verlag, 1982.
11. Kaufman, H. J. (ed.): Intrinsic diseases of bones. *In* Progress in Pediatric Radiology. Vol. 4. New York, Karger, 1973.
12. Lamy, M., and Maroteaux, P.: Les Chondrodystrophies Genotypiques. Paris, L'Expansion Scientifique Française, 1961.
13. McKusick, V. A.: Mendelian Inheritance in Man. Baltimore, Johns Hopkins Press, 1978.
14. McKusick, V. A.: Heritable Disorders of Connective Tissue. St. Louis, Mosby, 1972.
15. Maroteaux, P.: Bone Diseases of Children. Philadelphia, Lippincott, 1979.
16. Rubin, P.: Dynamic Classification of Bone Dysplasias. Chicago, Year Book, 1964.
17. Smith, D. W.: Recognizable Patterns of Human Malformations. Philadelphia, Saunders, 1976.
18. Spranger, J. W., Langer, L. O., and Wiedemann, H. R.: Bone Dysplasia. Philadelphia, Saunders, 1974.
19. Warkany, J.: Congenital Malformations. Chicago, Year Book, 1971.
20. Wiedemann, H. R.: Die grossen Konstitutions-Krankheiten des Skeletts. Stuttgart, G. Fischer, 1960.
21. Wynne-Davies, R., and Fairbank, T. J.: Fairbank's Atlas of General Affections of the Skeleton. Edinburgh, Churchill-Livingstone, 1976.
22. Wynne-Davies, R., Hall, C. M., and Apley, A. G.: Atlas of Skeletal Dysplasias. Edinburgh, Churchill-Livingstone, 1976.

Diagnostic Considerations

History and Physical Examination. Carefully and thoroughly done, these will often assist in making the diagnosis of bone dysplasia and metabolic bone disease, and will guide the physician to make the proper radiograms and perform the indicated biochemical investigations.

The common presenting complaints in bone dysplasia and endocrine and metabolic bone disease are shortness of stature (proportionate or disproportionate), deformities of the skull or flat or long bones, pain, and fractures.

Deformities include facial or ear abnormalities, deformation of the head such as dolichocephaly or bossing of the skull; enlargement of the epiphysis; angular deformities of the limbs such as genu varum, valgum, or recurvatum; lower limb length inequality; hand and foot abnormalities such as short fourth metacarpal or metatarsal, polydactyly, contracture of digits, or long and slender feet or fingers such as in Marfan's syndrome.

Pain is usually not a feature of bone dysplasia, but in metabolic bone disease such as rickets, deep bone pain may be present. It may be diffuse or localized—the latter when due to fractures in osteoporosis. The pain may be severe enough to keep the child awake at night and require analgesics. On palpation, the painful bones are tender, particularly if they are subcutaneous ones such as ribs or tibia.

Fractures may be the first sign of an osteoporotic bone. In rickets, *motor weakness* of proximal muscle groups may occur—it will manifest itself in a waddling gait and difficulty in getting up off the floor or raising the arms above the shoulders. It is crucial that the anamnesis include a detailed family history, as most of the bone dysplasias and metabolic bone disorders are heritable.

As dysplasias and metabolic and endocrine disorders of bone often affect normal growth, the skeleton is often involved in these processes. The patient may be of short stature (proportionate or disproportionate) or, occasionally, very tall. The first step, therefore, is to measure the child's standing and sitting heights and compare them with established normal ranges (see Tables 1–1 and 1–2 and Fig. 3–4).

Text continued on page 700

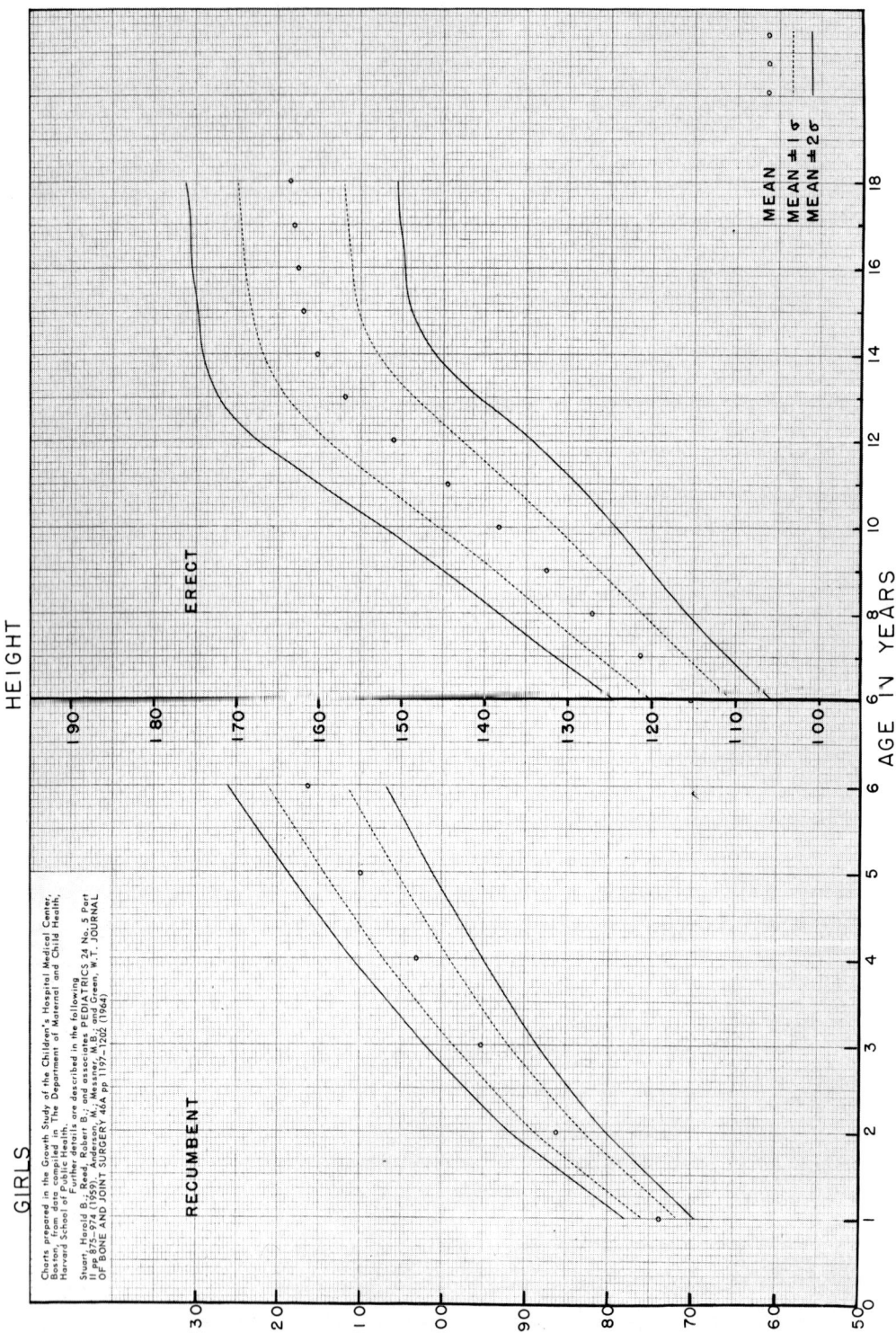

FIGURE 3–4. *Total and sitting heights between the ages of 1 and 18 years.*

A. Total height in girls. (Chart prepared in the Growth Study of the Children's Hospital Medical Center, Boston, from data compiled in The Department of Maternal and Child Health, Harvard School of Public Health, Boston, Massachusetts. Courtesy of R. B. Reed, M. Anderson, et al.)

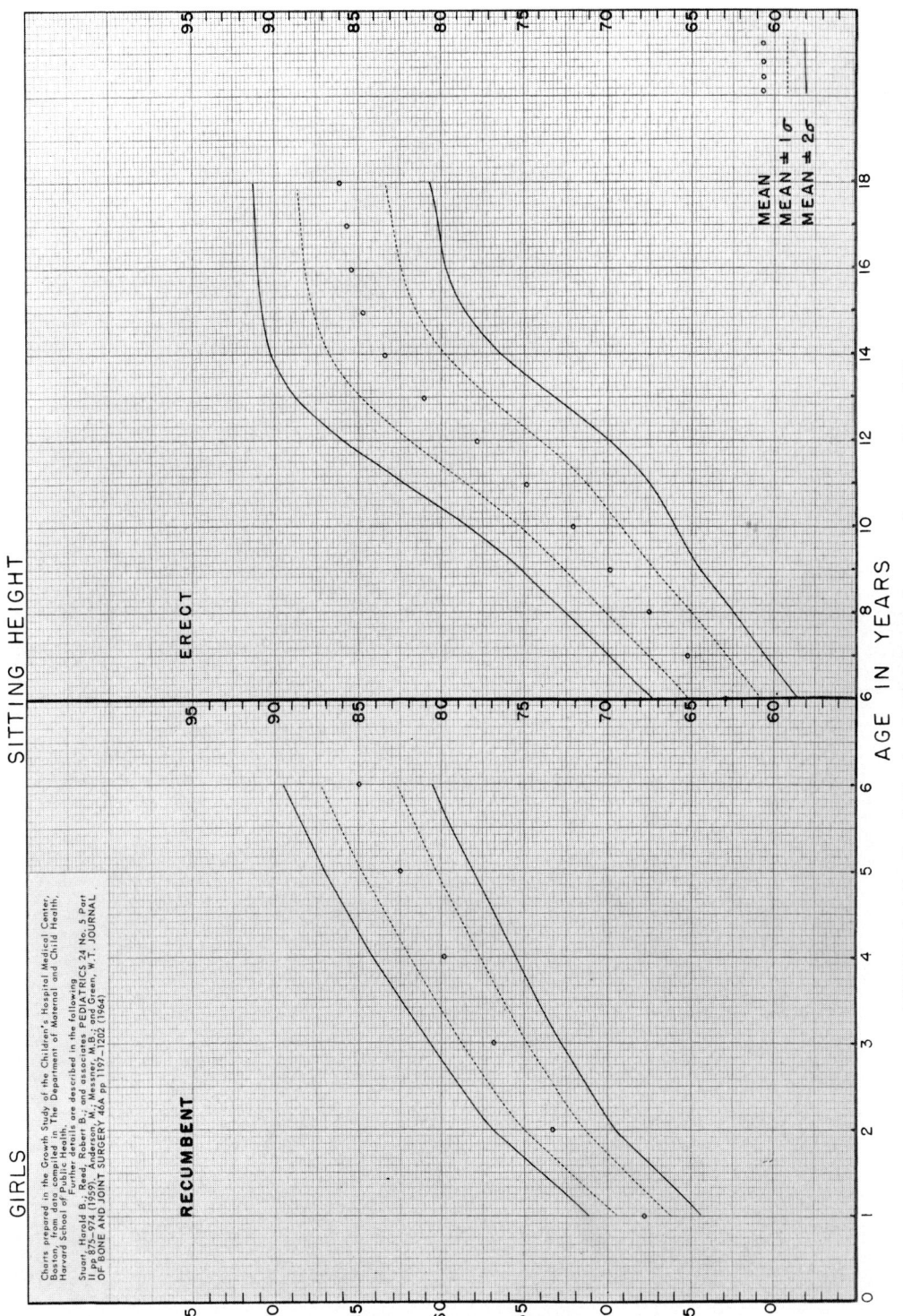

FIGURE 3–4 Continued. Total and sitting height between the ages of 1 and 18 years.

B. Sitting height in girls. (Chart prepared in the Growth Study of the Children's Hospital Medical Center, Boston, from data compiled in The Department of Maternal and Child Health, Harvard School of Public Health, Boston, Massachusetts. Courtesy of R. B. Reed, M. Anderson, et al.)

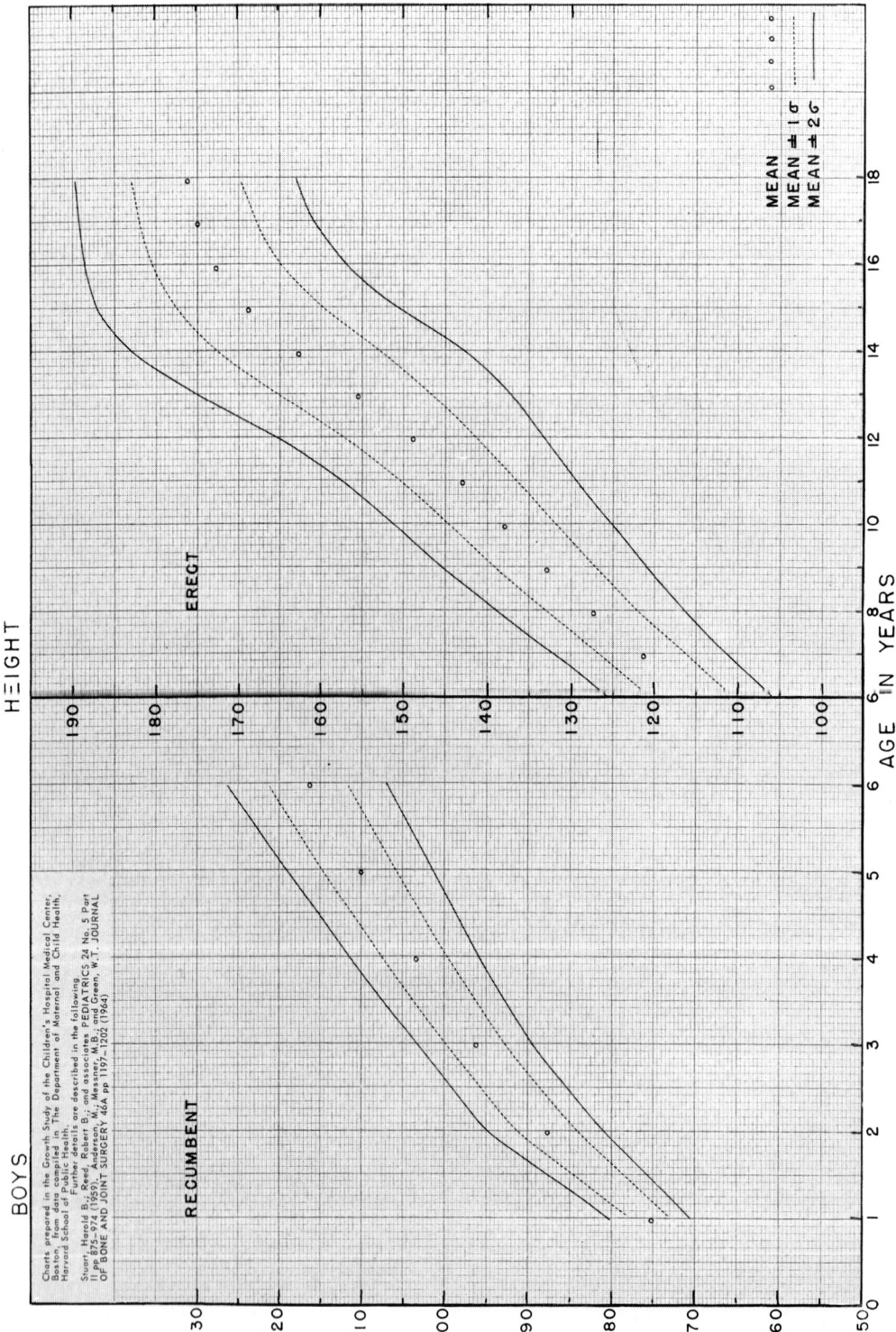

FIGURE 3–4 Continued. Total and sitting height between the ages of 1 and 18 years.

C. Total height in boys. (Chart prepared in the Growth Study of the Children's Hospital Medical Center, Boston, from data compiled in The Department of Maternal and Child Health, Harvard School of Public Health, Boston, Massachusetts. Courtesy of R. B. Reed, M. Anderson, et al.)

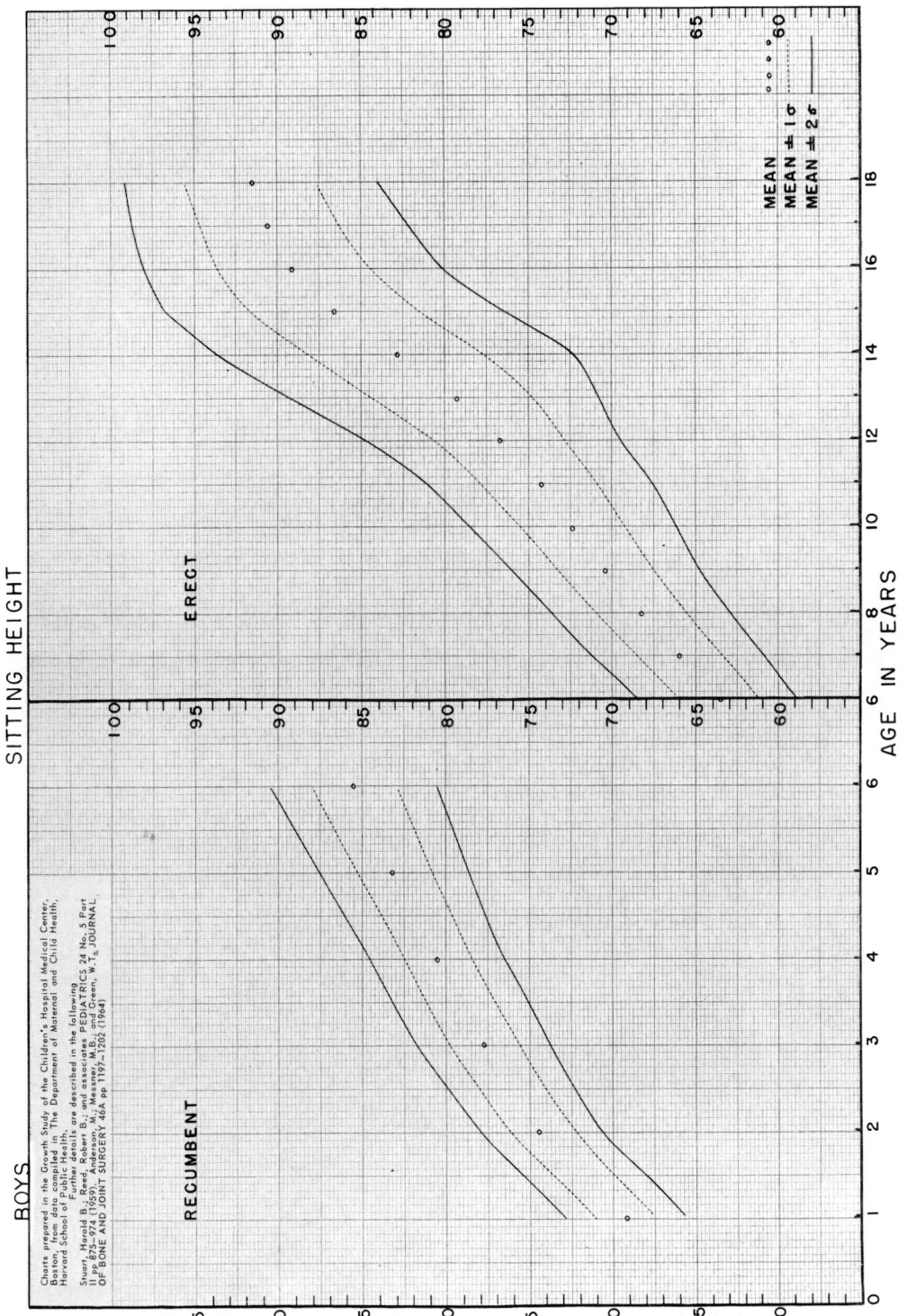

FIGURE 3–4 Continued. Total and sitting height between the ages of 1 and 18 years.

D. Sitting height in boys. (Chart prepared in the Growth Study of the Children's Hospital Medical Center, Boston, from data compiled in The Department of Maternal and Child Health, Harvard School of Public Health, Boston, Massachusetts. Courtesy of R. B. Reed, M. Anderson, et al.)

The measurements are recorded and expressed as standard deviations from the mean or in percentiles. Next, any disproportion between the length of the trunk and the length of the lower limbs is noted. The division between the upper and lower segments is at the top of the symphysis pubis. This ratio is approximately 1.7:1 at birth and gradually diminishes toward unity in late childhood. It should be noted, however, that in blacks, the lower segment is normally longer than the upper, whereas in most Chinese, this proportion is reversed. The span of the upper limbs is measured between the tips of the long fingers with the shoulders at 90 degrees of abduction and the elbows, wrists, hands, and fingers in neutral extension. Normally, the span of the upper limbs is approximately equal to the stature of the patient. In the proportionate type of short stature, such as pituitary dwarfism, the head, trunk, and limb proportions are normal, whereas in disproportionate short stature such as achondroplasia and vitamin D hypophosphatasic rickets, the limbs are disproportionately short. In Marfan's syndrome and homocystinuria, the limbs are relatively long.

The face and skull are inspected. In achondroplasia, the nasal bridge is low, the forehead bulges, and the maxillary area is small. In the trichorhinophalangeal syndrome, the hair is fine and sparse, and a large misshapen nose resembling a pear and a long philtrum are present. In Hurler's syndrome, there is a gargoyle appearance with a protruding tongue. In the hypogonadic male the skin is smooth and the hairline low, whereas in hypopituitarism, the face is rounded and wrinkled. In osteogenesis imperfecta and idiopathic hypercalcemia the face is elfin. These are a few examples illustrating the diagnostic value of inspection of the face and skull in bone dysplasias.

The eyes should be closely inspected for calcification of the cornea, the color of the sclerae, and corneal clouding. In osteogenesis imperfecta there may be a complete senile arcus, and in Marfan's syndrome the lens may be dislocated. In Down's syndrome the eyes are slanting with prominent epicanthal folds.

The teeth should be examined for abnormalities. Orthopedic surgeons should remember that dentin and bone matrix are chemically similar. The teeth are abnormal in osteogenesis imperfecta, whereas in juvenile osteoporosis and rickets, they are normal. Are the teeth late in developing?

Are the ears normal or abnormal? The cauliflower ear of diastrophic dwarfism and the crumpled ear of congenital contractural arachnodactyly are typical. In craniocarpotarsal dysplasia, or Freeman-Sheldon syndrome, the facies is distinctive—a whistling face with long philtrum and small nose. Is the neck webbed, as in Turner's syndrome?

The clavicles are inspected next. Are they defective, as in cleidocranial dysostosis? The spine is examined. Is there exaggerated lumbar lordosis, as seen in achondroplasia, or is there a thoracolumbar gibbus, suggesting mucopolysaccharidosis? Is there scoliosis? Are there café-au-lait spots to indicate neurofibromatosis? Are there multiple hemangiomata such as seen in Maffucci's syndrome? Are there any abnormal scars with poor healing to suggest collagen disorders? Is the skin hypermobile and hyperextensible, indicating Ehlers-Danlos syndrome?

The limbs are examined for contractural deformities, instability, and angular malalignment. Is there any limb length inequality? The hands and feet are examined. Are the digits abnormally long and thin—suggesting Marfan's syndrome? Are they short and wide like a starfish, suggesting achondroplasia? Is there a simian palmar crease to suggest Down's syndrome? Are the metacarpals short, especially the third and fourth, as seen in pseudohypoparathyroidism? Are there accessory digits, as in Ellis–van Creveld syndrome? Are the thumb and hallux short, as in fibrodysplasia ossificans progressiva? Is there a hitchhiker's thumb, which is present in diastrophic dwarfism owing to marked shortening of the first metacarpal? Are the nails dysplastic, as in hereditary osteoonychodysplasia? Is the hair coarse, as in cretinism and hyperthyroidism, or thin, as in the trichorhinophalangeal syndrome? Are there subcutaneous calcifications, as in hypoparathyroidism?

Radiographic Examination. The radiographic examination in skeletal dysplasias should ordinarily consist of eight views: (1) lateral of the skull; (2) anteroposterior and (3) lateral of the entire spine; (4) anteroposterior of the thoracic cage, which should show the shoulders and clavicles; (5) anteroposterior of the pelvis, which should include both hips and the symphysis pubis; (6) anteroposterior of one knee; (7) anteroposterior of one forearm to include the elbow and wrist; and (8) posteroanterior of one hand (preferably the left) to include all metacarpals and digits. Other radiologic studies such as scanning with technetium-99m or computed tomography are indicated in specific entities.

Biochemical Studies. Tests of the plasma include determination of values of calcium, inorganic phosphate, and alkaline phosphatase, and occasionally magnesium and other metals such as lead. It is important to remember that in the child normal values of *plasma phosphates* are higher than in the adult. In milligrams per 100 ml., in the age group birth to 12 months, the range is 3.7 to 8.5; in childhood it is 3.6 to 5.9; and in the adult 2.4 to 4.5. It is crucial to know this variation of the normal range of plasma phosphates with age because diagnosis of hypophosphatemic rickets depends upon it. The values of *alkaline phosphatase* increase during growth spurts, and reach a peak value of 30 K.A. units per 100 ml. in the adolescent. In the adult male, the normal value is 4 to 12 K.A. units per 100 ml. The *calcium values* remain virtually constant during childhood, with a range of 9.0 to 10.2 mg. per 100 ml.

Urine examination is crucial and should not be ignored as a diagnostic investigative tool in bone affections. This is usually not carried out, however, because of the difficulty of obtaining 24-hour urine collections. In the urine, the excretion rates of calcium, creatinine, and hydroxyproline are determined. Detailed descriptions of biochemical investigations in bone disease are given by Paterson and by Nordin.[3, 4]

Bone Biopsy. The bone sample is usually obtained with a trephine from the iliac crest under general anesthesia. In the older cooperative child, however, one may use intravenous diazepam (Valium). The specimen core should include both inner and outer tables of the ilium and trabecular cancellous bone. When assessment of the quantity of osteoid tissue is desired, it is essential to have a second specimen that is uncalcified. This author recommends that choice of the site of biopsy be guided by the pathologic changes seen radiographically. In some patients, biopsy must be obtained from bones other than the ilium.

References

1. Fourman, P., and Royer, P.: Calcium Metabolism and the Bone. 2nd Ed. Oxford, Blackwell, 1968.
2. Jowsey, J.: Metabolic Diseases of Bone. Vol. I. London, Saunders, 1977.
3. Nordin, B. E. C.: Calcium Phosphate and Magnesium Metabolism. London, Churchill-Livingstone, 1976.
4. Paterson, C. R.: Metabolic Disorders of Bone. Oxford, Blackwell, 1974.
5. Smith, R.: Biochemical Disorders of the Skeleton. London, Butterworth, 1979.

MULTIPLE EPIPHYSEAL DYSPLASIA

This common bone dysplasia is characterized by irregularity in development of the epiphysis that manifests itself as late appearance and mottling of the ossification centers, knobby joints, stubby digits, and minimal shortness of stature. There is little or no vertebral involvement.

Fairbank first delineated this entity, giving it the name *dysplasia epiphysealis multiplex*.[11-14] There is, however, more than one type; that described by Fairbank is the severe form. Ribbing, in 1937, reported a milder form with flattened epiphyses and only minimal involvement of the wrists and hands.[42] There are many gradations between these two extremes. The condition is very rare, though it is being detected with increasing frequency.[1-55] There is no sex predilection. According to Wynne-Davies and associates, there is a possible prevalence of 11 per million index patients; and 16 per million including affected relatives.[55]

Inheritance

Inheritance is almost always as an autosomal dominant trait.[2, 9, 20, 27] In some cases, however, it is autosomal recessive.[25, 42] Clinically these two genetic types are indistinguishable.

Pathology

The basic defect is a disturbance in the development of the epiphyseal ossification centers.[44] Enchondral ossification is disorganized, and epiphyseal cartilage cells are irregular with disordered columns and areas of degeneration.[22] Funnelization, diaphyseal cylindrization, and modeling are not affected. The articular cartilage is initially normal, but becomes secondarily misshapen later in life because underlying osseous support is lacking. The articular deformities are permanent, with degenerative changes and osteoarthritis developing early in adult life, especially in the weight-bearing joints (Fig. 3–5).

The number of epiphyses affected varies; the femoral and humeral heads are common sites. The short tubular bones of the hands and feet may also be involved. The vertebrae are normal in childhood, but development of secondary ossification centers in the spine may be irregular. The skull, facial bones, and pelvis are normal.

Histologic and biochemical analyses of the physes have failed to show any abnormality.[22]

Clinical Features

The condition is not suspected in infancy. Attention is first drawn to the disease when the

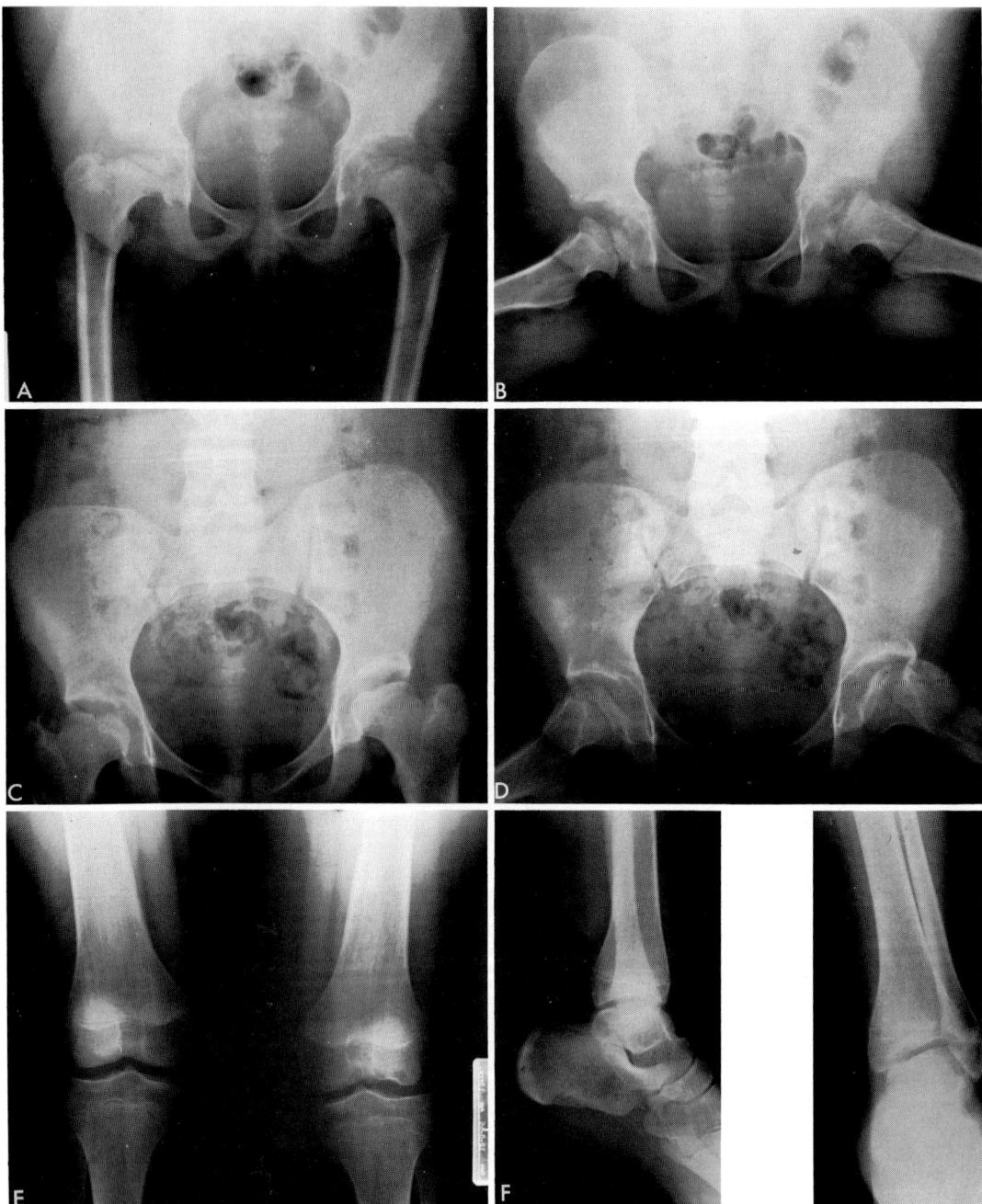

FIGURE 3–5. Multiple epiphyseal dysplasia in two sisters and their 40-year-old father.

Inheritance is almost always autosomal dominant. **A** and **B.** Anteroposterior and frog-leg lateral radiographs of both hips of a 12-year-old girl. Note the irregularity and flattening of the capital femoral epiphyses. Involvement is bilateral. **C** and **D.** Anteroposterior and lateral views of both hips of the 14-year-old sister, showing similar changes. **E** and **F.** Anteroposterior view of both knees and anteroposterior and lateral radiographs of the ankle of the 14-year-old girl. Note the irregularity and flattening of the epiphyses.

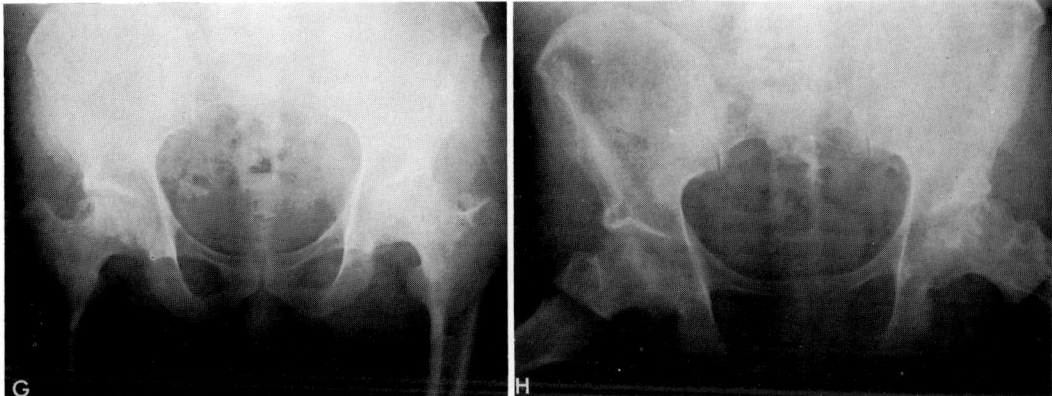

FIGURE 3–5 Continued. Multiple epiphyseal dysplasia in two sisters and their 40-year-old father.

G and H. Anteroposterior and lateral radiograms of the father's hips. Note the irregularity of the femoral heads and marked degenerative arthritis of both hips.

child is delayed in walking. Sometimes diagnosis is not made until early adolescence. The presenting complaints begin with joint stiffness, pain, a limp, or waddling gait. With growth, the progressively subnormal length of the limbs becomes more obvious. There is no true dwarfism. The deficiency in stature is of the short-limb type; the height of the trunk is normal.

The digits are short and stubby. Some limitation of motion of the affected joints, particularly flexion contracture of the knees and elbows, is usual. Genu valgum or varum is not uncommon. In general there is no marked deformity. In adolescence or early adult life, with onset of degenerative arthritis, pain in the hip, knee, or ankle may be a symptom. Motor musculature is of normal strength. The intelligence of these patients is normal.

Radiographic Findings and Differential Diagnosis

In the radiograms, the principal finding is the delay and irregularity of ossification of the epiphyses, which are markedly fragmented and mottled. They appear flattened (Fig. 3–6).

The capital femoral epiphyses are frequently affected. As involvement is usually bilateral, differentiation from bilateral Legg-Perthes disease is a common problem (Fig. 3–7).[38, 49] In multiple epiphyseal dysplasia, bone imaging with technetium-99m does not show a lack of uptake as it does in Legg-Perthes disease. Serial radiograms disclose that, in multiple epiphyseal dysplasia, there is no true avascular necrosis and that the progressive stages of necrosis, fragmentation, and regeneration seen in Legg-Perthes disease are not present. In bilateral Legg-Perthes disease, the degree and stage of involvement varies from one side to the other; the acetabula are normal or show minimal changes in response to the deformed femoral head. In multiple epiphyseal dysplasia the acetabula have loss of definition with a scalloped subchondral bony plate.

Multiple epiphyseal dysplasia is distinguished from *spondyloepiphyseal dysplasia* by the absence of severe vertebral changes; in the spondyloepiphyseal dysplasia the limbs, particularly the hands, are much less involved. *Cretinism* is differentiated from multiple epiphyseal dysplasia by its characteristic clinical and biochemical features.

Coxa vara may occur (Fig. 3–8). The femoral necks may be short. Mediolateral obliquity of the distal tibia with secondary adaptive changes in the talus is found in about 50 per cent of cases.[11–14, 39]

The metacarpals and phalanges are usually short with irregular epiphyses (Fig. 3–9). The feet are less often involved than the hands.

The secondary centers of ossification in the vertebrae may be irregular, but this should not be mistaken for the true platyspondyly of spondyloepiphyseal dysplasia. Laboratory studies in multiple epiphyseal dysplasia, especially in regard to abnormal mucopolysaccharide urinary excretion, are negative.

Treatment

In management of this disorder, excessive body weight should be avoided. A frequent pitfall is to misdiagnose the disease as Legg-Perthes disease and treat the hips unnecessarily with various orthotic containment devices.

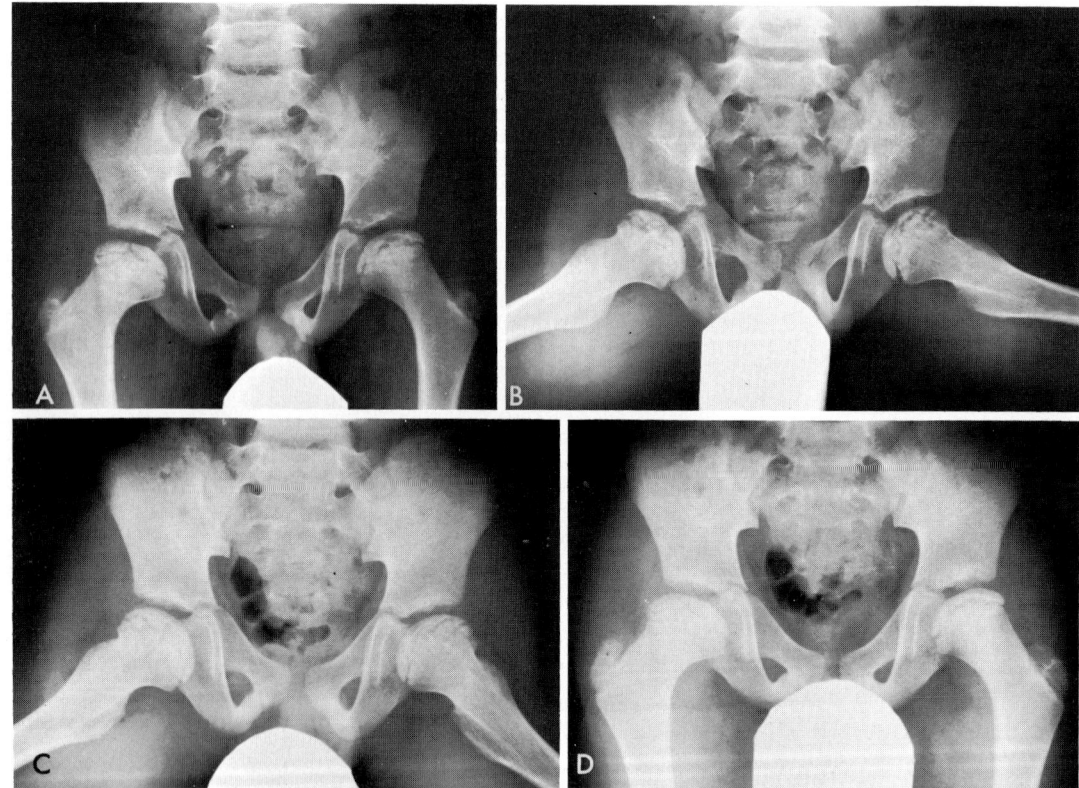

FIGURE 3–6. *Epiphyseal dysplasia of both femoral heads in a four-year-old boy.*

Original diagnosis was bilateral Legg-Perthes disease. **A** and **B**. Radiograms of hips showing irregular ossification and development of both femoral heads. **C** and **D**. Radiograms of hips of same patient a year later. There is no evidence of aseptic necrosis.

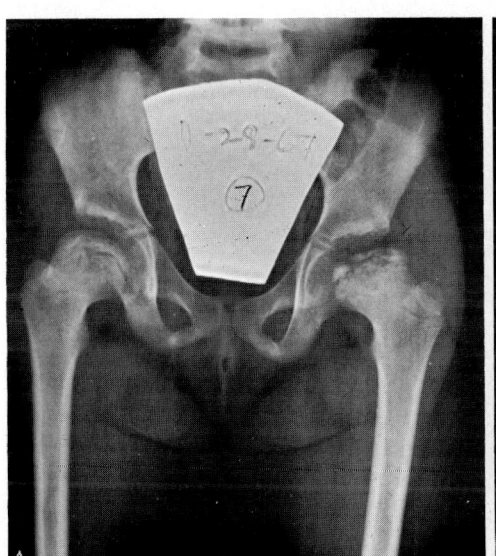
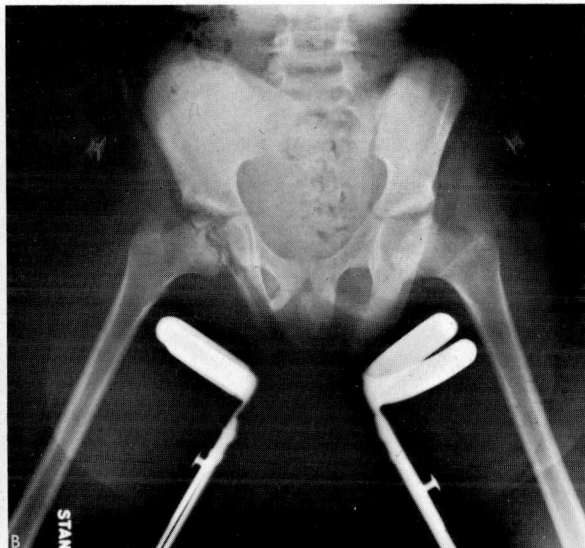
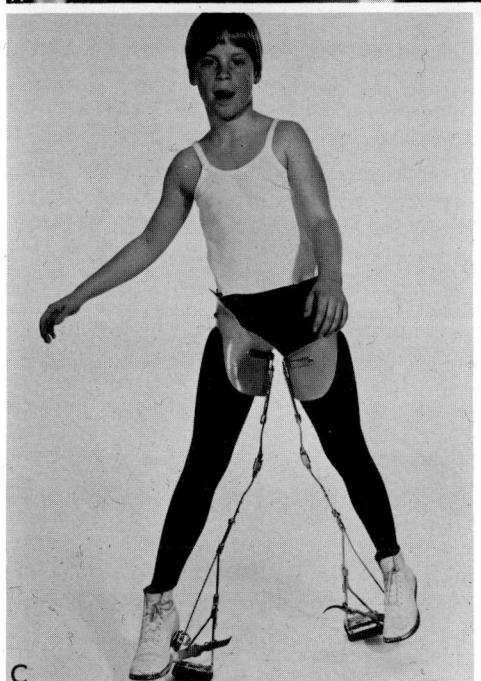

***FIGURE 3–7.** Multiple epiphyseal dysplasia of both femoral heads in a nine-year-old girl.*

This patient's problem was misdiagnosed as Legg-Perthes disease by this author and treated by bilateral trilateral socket hip orthoses. **A.** Anteroposterior view of both hips as the patient stands without the appliances. Note the flattening and lateral subluxation of both hips. **B.** Standing with the orthoses. The femoral heads are contained in the acetabula. **C.** The patient walking without assistance.

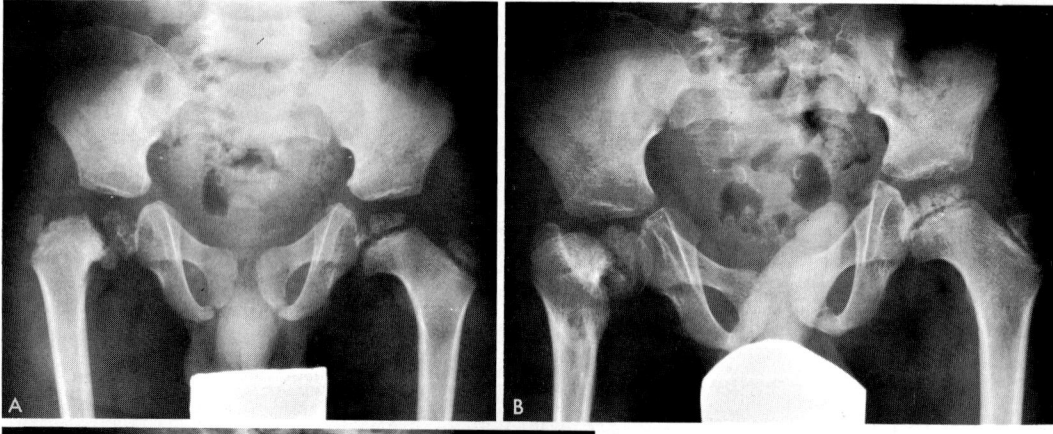
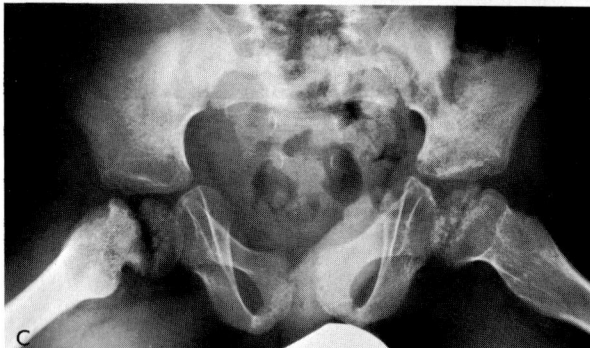

FIGURE 3–8. *Epiphyseal dysplasia of both hips in a five-year-old boy with a coxa vara deformity on the right.*

A and **B.** Preoperative radiographs. Irregularity of ossification and mottling of the femoral heads is evident. **C.** Radiogram one year following abduction subtrochanteric osteotomy of the right hip. Coxa vara deformity has recurred.

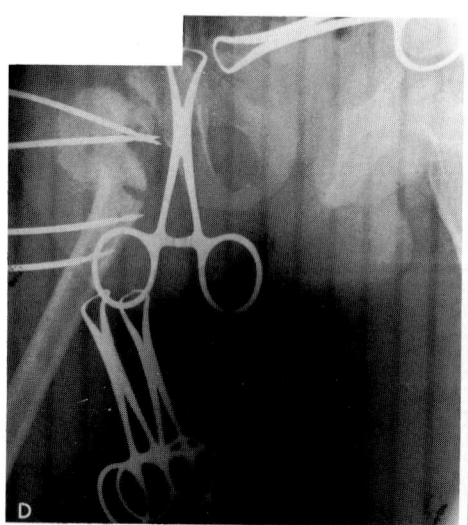
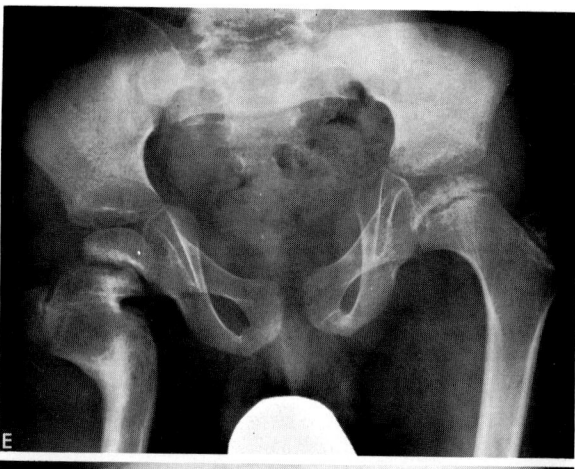
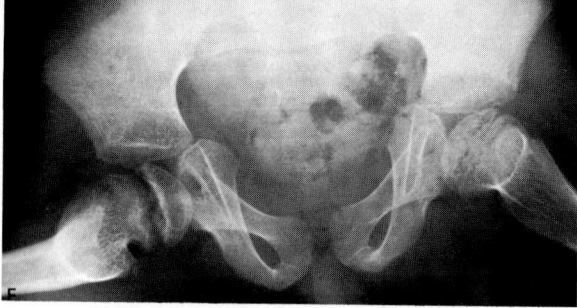

D. Radiogram of right hip taken in the operating room. The abduction osteotomy was repeated. **E** and **F.** Postoperative radiographs one year later. Note the normal ossification of the right femoral head.

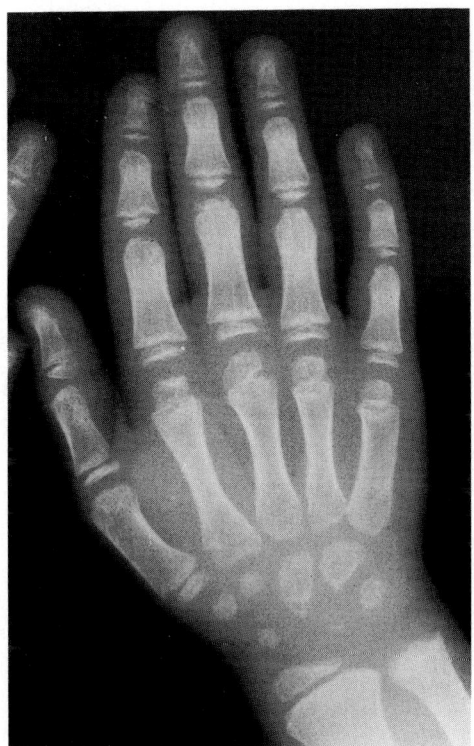

FIGURE 3-9. Anteroposterior view of the hand in multiple epiphyseal dysplasia.

Note the short metacarpals and phalanges with irregular epiphyses.

There is no evidence that such orthotic containment will alter the outcome. Continuous passive motion of major joints, particularly the hip and knee, may assist in remodeling. Pelvic osteotomy may be indicated when joint incongruity and pain and disability are severe. Degenerative arthritis is treated symptomatically, and later by total joint arthroplasty.

Lower limb inequality, if present, should be followed; if significant, an epiphysiodesis of the contralateral long limb is performed at the appropriate level and age to equalize limb lengths. Angulation osteotomy may be indicated to correct coxa vara and genu varum or valgum.

References

1. Anderson, C. E., Crane, J. T., Harper, H. A., and Hunter, J. W.: Morquio's disease and dysplasia epiphysealis multiplex. A study of epiphyseal cartilage in seven cases. J. Bone Joint Surg., 44-A:295, 1962.
2. Barrie, H., Carter, C., and Sutcliffe, J.: Multiple epiphyseal dysplasia. Br. Med. J., 2:133, 1958.
3. Beighton, P., Goldberg, L., and Op't Hof, J.: Dominant inheritance of multiple epiphyseal dysplasia, myopia and deafness. Clin. Genet., 14:173, 1978.
4. Berg, P. K.: Dysplasia epiphysealis multiplex. A case report and review of the literature. A.J.R., 97:31, 1966.
5. Christiansen, W. R., Lin, R. K., and Berghout, J.: Dysplasia epiphysealis multiplex. A.J.R., 74:1059, 1955.
6. Cowan, D.: Multiple epiphyseal dysplasia. Br. Med. J., 5373:1629, 1963.
7. Crossan, J. F., Wynne-Davis, R., and Fulford, G. E.: Bilateral failure of the capital femoral epiphysis. J. Pediatr. Orthop., 3:297, 1983.
8. Daentl, D. L., Siegel, R. C., Nevo, Z., Scheck, M., Parker, J. M., Smith, G., Sakovich, L., Ashley, R. K., and Larsen, L. J.: Auriculoepiphyseal dysplasia (multiple epiphyseal dysplasia and anomalous auricles): Clinical, structural and biochemical studies. Birth Defects, 11:217, 1975.
9. Dahners, L. E., Francisco, W. D., and Halleran, W. J.: Findings at arthrotomy in a case of double layered patellae associated with multiple epiphyseal dysplasia. J. Pediatr. Orthop., 2:67, 1982.
10. Elsbach, L.: Bilateral hereditary micro-epiphysial dysplasia of the hips. J. Bone Joint Surg., 41-B:514, 1959.
11. Fairbank, H. A. T.: Generalized diseases of the skeleton. Proc. R. Soc. Med., 28:1, 611, 1935.
12. Fairbank, H. A. T.: Dysplasia epiphysealis multiplex. Proc. R. Soc. Med., 39:315, 1946.
13. Fairbank, H. A. T.: Dysplasia epiphysialis multiplex. Br. J. Surg., 34:225, 1947.
14. Fairbank, H. A. T.: An Atlas of General Affections of the Skeleton. Baltimore, Williams & Wilkins, 1951.
15. Felman, A. H.: Multiple epiphyseal dysplasia. Three cases with unusual vertebral abnormalities. Radiology, 93:119, 1969.
16. Freiberger, R. H.: Multiple epiphyseal dysplasia: A report of three cases. Radiology, 70:379, 1958.
17. Herring, J. A.: Rapidly progressive scoliosis in multiple epiphyseal dysplasia. J. Bone Joint Surg., 58-A:703, 1976.
18. Hobaek, A.: Problems of Hereditary Chondrodysplasia. Oslo, Oslo University Press, 1961.
19. Hodkinson, H. M.: Double patellae in multiple epiphyseal dysplasia. J. Bone Joint Surg., 44-B:569, 1962.
20. Hoefnagel, D., Sycamore, L. K., Russell, S. W., and Bucknall, W. E.: Hereditary multiple epiphyseal dysplasia. Ann. Hum. Genet., 30:201, 1967.
21. Hulvey, J. T., and Keats, T.: Multiple epiphyseal dysplasia. A contribution to the problem of spinal involvement. A.J.R., 106:170, 1969.
22. Hunt, D. D., Ponseti, I. V., Pedrini-Mille, A., and Pedrini, V.: Multiple epiphyseal dysplasia in two siblings. Histological and biochemical analysis of epiphyseal cartilage plate in one. J. Bone Joint Surg., 49-A:1611, 1967.
23. Jackson, W. P. G., Hanelin, J., and Albright, F.: Multiple epiphyseal dysplasia, its relation to other disorders of epiphyseal development. Arch. Intern. Med., 94:886, 1954.
24. Jacobs, P. A.: Dysplasia epiphysialis multiplex. Clin. Orthop., 58:117, 1968.
25. Juberg, R. C., and Holt, J. F.: Inheritance of multiple epiphyseal dysplasia tarda. Am. J. Hum. Genet., 20:549, 1968.
26. Kaufman, E. E., and Coventry, M. B.: Multiple epiphysial dysplasia in a mother and son. Staff Meet. Mayo Clin., 38:115, 1963.
27. Kozlowski, K., and Lipska, E.: Hereditary dysplasia epiphysealis multiplex. Clin. Radiol., 18:330, 1967.
28. Lachman, R. S., Rimoin, D. L., and Hollister, D. W.: Hip arthrography in the epiphyseal dysplasias. Birth Defects, 10:186, 1974.
29. Lamy, M., and Maroteaux, P.: Les Chondrodystrophies Genotypiques. Paris, L'Expansion Scientific Française, 1961.
30. Leeds, N. E.: Epiphyseal dysplasia multiplex. A.J.R., 84:506, 1960.
31. Lehman, W. L., and Murray, D. M.: Multiple epiphy-

seal dysplasia: A longitudinal family study. Orthopedics, 4:38, 1981.
32. Lowery, R. B., and Wood, B. J.: Syndrome of epiphyseal dysplasia, short stature, microcephaly and nystagmus. Clin. Genet., 8:269, 1975.
33. Mansoor, I. A.: Dysplasia epiphysealis multiplex. Clin. Orthop., 72:287, 1970.
34. Maroteaux, R., Stanescu, R., and Cohen Solal, D.: Dysplasie polyépiphysaire probablement recessive autosomique. A propos de l'étude ultra-structurale dans l'isolement de cette forme autonome. Nouv. Presse Méd., 4:2169, 1975.
35. Marquardt, W.: Zur Klinik und Röntgenologie der atypischen chondrodystrophischen Wachstumsostorungen. Arch. Orthop. Unfallchir., 38:711, 1938.
36. Mau, H., and Schmitt, H. W.: Der konstitutionelldyostoitische Perthes und die Skelettreifungshemmungen beim eigentlichen Perthes. Z. Orthop., 93:515, 1960.
37. Maudsley, R. H.: Dysplasia epiphysialis multiplex. A report of fourteen cases in three families. J. Bone Joint Surg., 37-B:228, 1955.
38. Monty, C. P.: Familial Perthes disease resembling multiple epiphyseal dysplasia. J. Bone Joint Surg., 44-B:565, 1962.
39. Murphy, M. C., Shine, I. B., and Stevens, D. B.: Multiple epiphyseal dysplasia. Report of a pedigree. J. Bone Joint Surg., 55-A:814, 1973.
40. Patrone, N. A., and Kredich, D. W.: Arthritis in children with multiple epiphyseal dysplasia. J. Rheumatol., 12:1, 1985.
41. Pfeiffer, R. A., Junemann, G., Polster, J., and Bauer, H.: Epiphyseal dysplasia of the femoral head, severe myopia and perceptive hearing loss in three brothers. Clin. Genet., 4:141, 1973.
42. Ribbing, S.: Studien über hereditare multiple Epiphysenstorungen. Acta Radiol. (Stockholm), Suppl. 34, 1937.
43. Ribbing, S.: Hereditare multiple Epiphysenstorungen und osteochondrosis dissecans. Vortrag. Kongr. Nordisch. Med. Radiol., 6:397, 1951.
44. Rubin, P.: Dynamic Classification of Bone Dysplasias. Chicago, Year Book, 1964.
45. Shepard, E.: Multiple epiphyseal dysplasia. J. Bone Joint Surg., 38-B:458, 1956.
46. Spranger, J.: The epiphyseal dysplasias. Clin. Orthop., 114:46, 1975.
47. Vereanu, D., and Fruchter, Z.: Dysplasie polyépiphysaire multiple héréditaire. Maladie de Fairbank. Rev. Chir. Orthop., 54:33, 1968.
48. Walker, B.: Juvenile cataracts and multiple epiphyseal dysplasia in three sisters. Birth Defects, 5:315, 1969.
49. Wamoscher, Z., and Farhi, A.: Hereditary Legg-Calvé-Perthes disease. Am. J. Dis. Child., 106:131, 1963.
50. Watt, J. K.: Multiple epiphyseal dysplasia. Br. J. Surg., 39:533, 1952.
51. Waugh, W.: Dysplasia epiphysealis multiplex in three sisters. J. Bone Joint Surg., 34-B:82, 1952.
52. Weinberg, H., Frankel, M., Makin, M., and Vas, E.: Familial epiphysial dysplasia of the lower limbs. J. Bone Joint Surg., 42-B:313, 1960.
53. Wenger, D. R., and Ezaki, M.: Bilateral femoral head collapse in an adolescent with brachydactyly (multiple epiphyseal dysplasia tarda type 1c). J. Pediatr. Orthop., 1:267, 1981.
54. Wolfgang, G. L., and Heath, R. D.: Dysplasia epiphysealis hemimelica. A case report. Clin. Orthop., 116:23, 1976.
55. Wynne-Davies, R., Hall, C. M., and Apley, A. G.: Fairbank's Atlas of Skeletal Dysplasias. Edinburgh, Churchill-Livingstone, 1985, p. 19.

CHONDRODYSPLASIA CALCIFICANS PUNCTATA (CONRADI'S DISEASE)

This rare congenital bone dysplasia comprises a heterogeneous group of conditions characterized by stippling of the epiphyses, disordered longitudinal bone growth, mental retardation, and in some cases, cataracts. Since the original description of these entities by Conradi in 1914, a number of reports have appeared in the literature.[1-31] The condition is also referred to as chondrodystrophia fetalis ossificans and chondrodystrophia punctata. There are at least two clear types; in the first, a severe rhizomelic form, involvement is symmetrical with extremely short limbs, bilateral cataracts, psychomotor retardation, and death in early infancy. In the second type, often referred to as Conradi-Hünermann disease, shortening of the limbs is not marked but is asymmetrical, and mental retardation and cataracts are less frequent. There are gradations of involvement between these two extremes.

Severe Rhizomelic Form

Inheritance is as an autosomal recessive trait, and there are reported cases of parental consanguinity. There is no sex predilection. The disorder is usually recognizable in the immediate postnatal period. The limbs are very short, particularly the humeri and femora. The face is flat with a depressed ridge of the nose. In about 75 per cent of cases, there are bilateral cataracts. The skin is abnormal, often being dry and scaly. Mental retardation is common. Calcification of the cartilage in the trachea and larynx will produce stenosis and obstruction of the respiratory tract, necessitating tracheotomy. Other systemic abnormalities may include congenital heart disease, tracheoesophageal fistula, contracture of the joints, and congenital dislocation of the hips.[1, 12, 26]

Pathologic Findings. These include marked irregularity of vascularization of the epiphyses, disturbance of chondroblastic maturation, and mucoid degeneration of cartilage with irregular areas of amorphous calcification in chondroid tissue.[2, 8, 26, 31]

Laboratory findings are within normal limits, and no metabolic defect has thus far been demonstrated.

Radiographic Findings. These disclose multiple punctate opacities in the unossified cartilage (Figs. 3–10 and 3–11). There may be extra cartilaginous calcification about the vertebral column and pelvis. This punctate stippling of the epiphyses may disappear by the age of four to six years if the child survives; the epiphyses will, however, often be irregular. Cranial stenosis is a common feature. Congenital vertebral anomalies and scoliosis or kyphosis are often present. In the lateral projection, vertebral bodies may show separate centers of ossification anteriorly and posteriorly separated by a wide translucent band, the so-called butterfly vertebrae. There is no platyspondyly in the vertebrae of these patients, a finding that may serve to

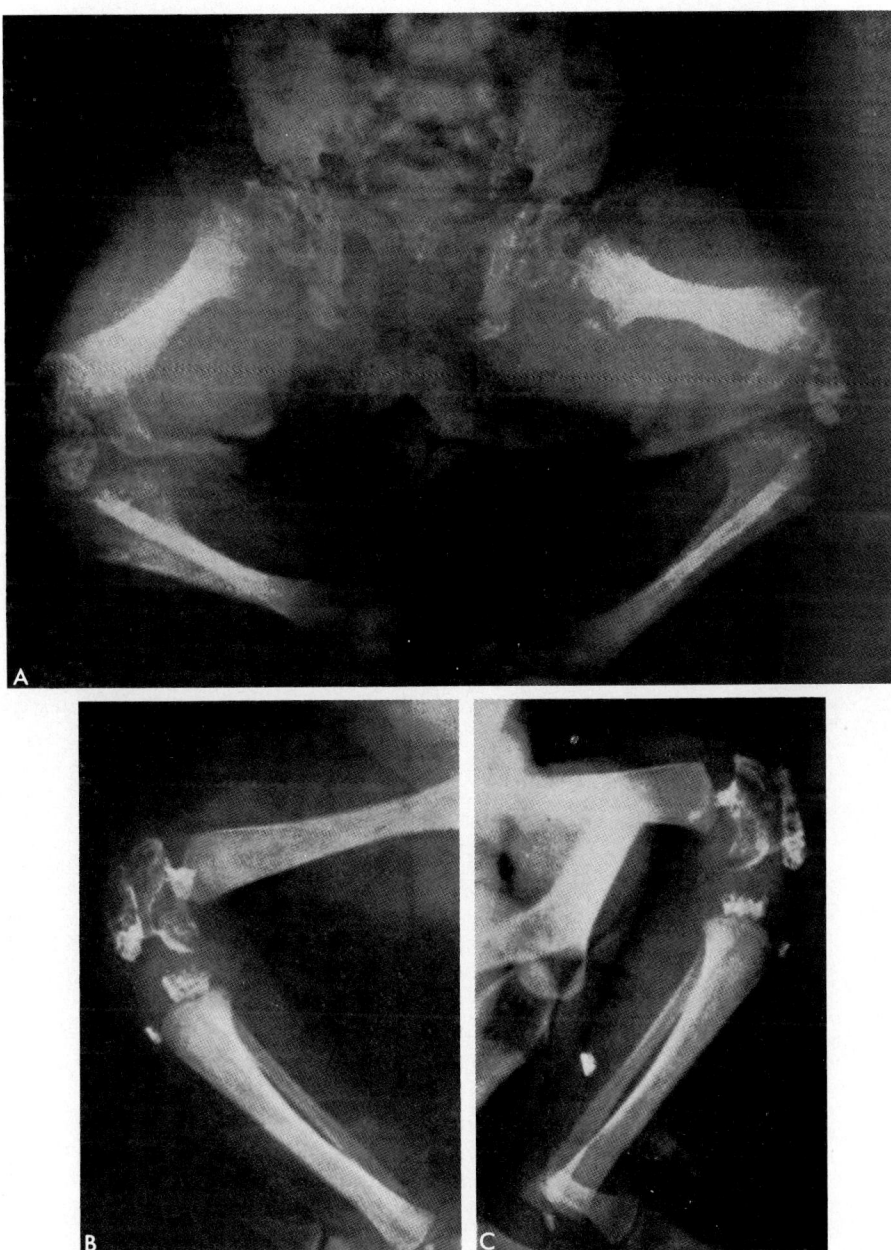

FIGURE 3–10. *Chondrodystrophia calcificans congenita (stippled epiphyses).*

Anteroposterior and lateral radiograms of both lower limbs in an infant. Irregularly shaped, densely stippled masses in the region of the epiphyses suggest calcified deposits. (From Coughlin, E. J., Guare, H. T., and Moskovitz, A. J.: J. Bone Joint Surg., 32-A:940, 1950. Reprinted by permission.)

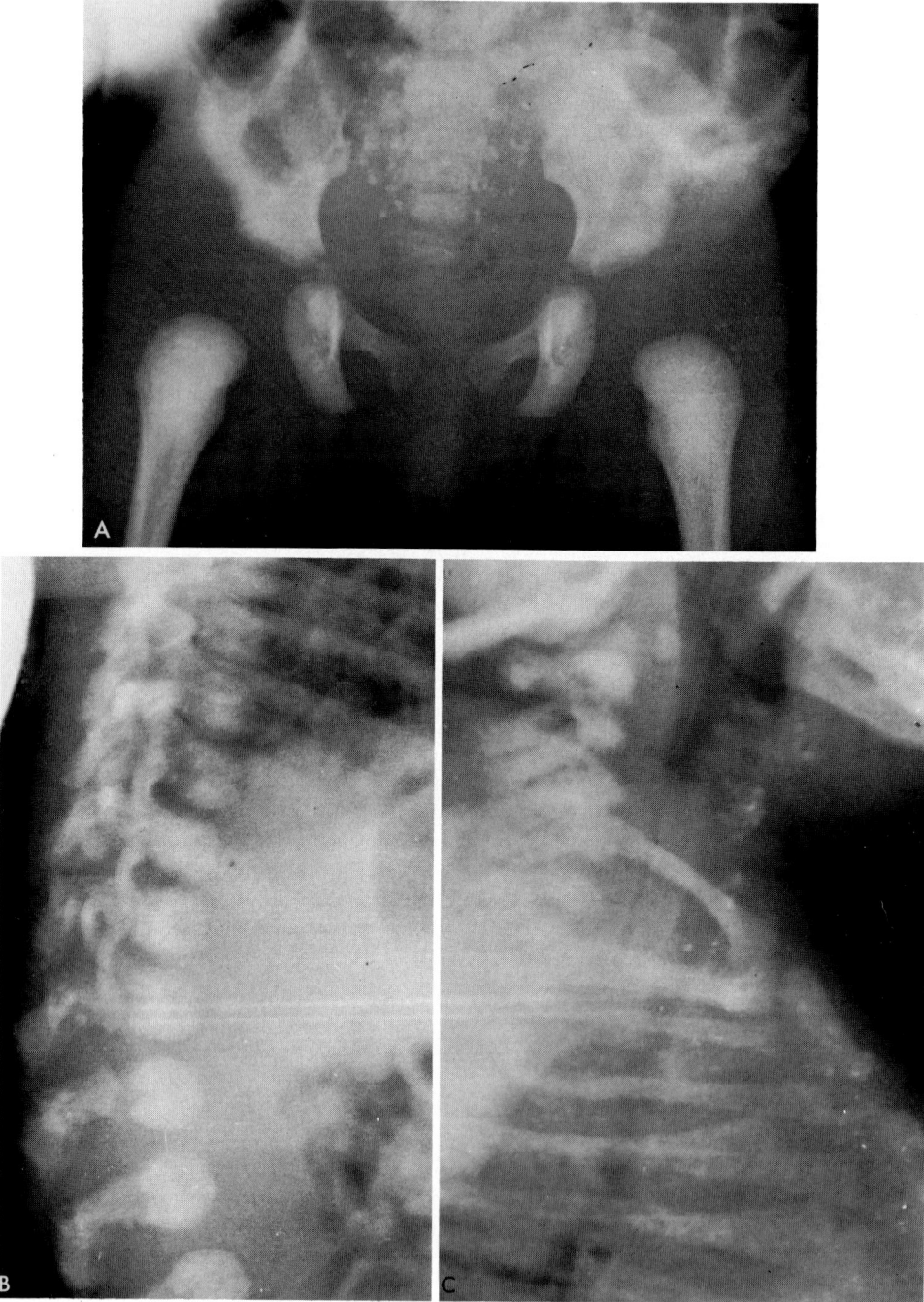

FIGURE 3–11. Stippled epiphyses.

A to **C.** Stippled epiphyses in a newborn infant. Anteroposterior view of pelvis and lateral views of spine and neck. Note the multiple areas of calcification in the trachea, sternum, spine, pelvis, and proximal femur. Because of difficulty of respiration, a tracheostomy was performed.

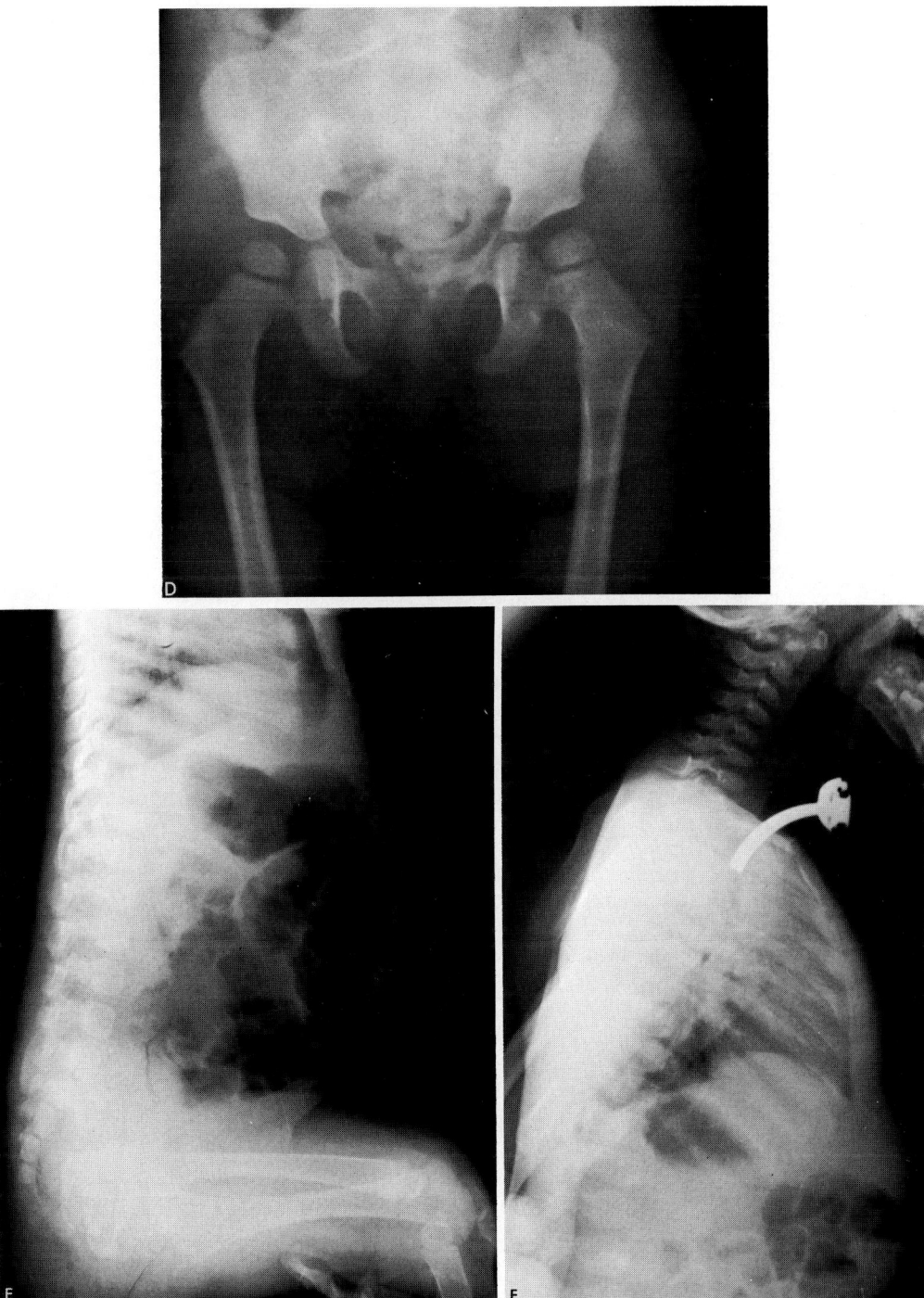

FIGURE 3–11 Continued. Stippled epiphyses.

D to **F.** Anteroposterior view of pelvis and lateral views of spine and neck showing disappearance of the calcified areas at one and one-half years of age.

differentiate it from spondyloepiphyseal dysplasia.

Prognosis and Complications. Most patients die within the first year of life as a result of secondary pulmonary infection or other associated anomalies. With modern respiratory and intensive care, the prognosis for these children has improved, and some of them will survive. They are, however, bedridden and markedly disabled. Severe scoliosis and kyphosis develop in the survivors.

Conradi-Hünermann Disease

Conradi-Hünermann disease is the mild form of this dysplasia in which the infant does survive. The mode of inheritance is variable: in some cases definitely autosomal dominant and in others autosomal recessive. Most cases are sporadic. It is more common in the female, with a female-to-male ratio of 3:1. As in the severe rhizomelic form, the face is flat with a depressed nasal bridge. The skin is dry and scaly, and congenital cataracts occur in about 20 per cent of cases. Involvement is often asymmetrical, one limb being short. The milder cases may go undetected in the perinatal period and early infancy.[14]

Pathologic Findings. Reports of examination of tissues are scanty because few cases have been recorded at autopsy. The epiphyseal cartilage shows irregular areas of calcification and cyst formation.

Radiographic Findings. Radiographs disclose punctate calcification at the ends of the long bones, primarily within the epiphyses, and also in the vertebrae and iliac bones. Cranial stenosis is common. Congenital deformities of the vertebrae are found, as in the severe rhizomelic form. Scoliosis and kyphosis may be severe.

Prognosis. The outlook is good in this milder form, with the epiphyseal stippling usually disappearing by the age of four years. Alcoholic fetopathy may be associated with punctate epiphyses.

Treatment. Orthopedic treatment consists of limb length equalization by epiphysiodesis at the appropriate skeletal age. The scoliotic spine is supported by orthosis and, if severe and progressive, by spinal fusion.

References

1. Allensmith, M., and Senz, E.: Chondrodystrophia congenita punctata (Conradi's disease). Am. J. Dis. Child., 100:109, 1960.
2. Bateman, D.: Two cases, and specimens from a third case of punctate epiphyseal dysplasia. Proc. R. Soc. Med., 29:745, 1936.
3. Bergstrom, K., Gustavson, K.-H., and Jorulf, H.: Chondrodystrophia calcificans congenita (Conradi's disease) in a mother and her child. Clin. Genet., 3:158, 1972.
4. Betoulieres, P., Ferran, J. L., Bassini, P., Del Socorro, P., and Jean, R.: Calcificans ponctuées épiphysaires localisées et dysmorphie nasale. J. Radiol. Electrol., 55:877, 1974.
5. Cohen-Solal, J., Faure, C., Sarrut, S., Loubry, P., Moreno, J. L., Lejeune, C., and Mande, R.: Un cas de forme majeure de maladie des épiphyses ponctuées avec étude histologique. Sem. Hôp. Paris, 44:2733, 1968.
6. Comings, D. E., Papazian, C., and Schoene, H. R.: Conradi's disease. J. Pediatr., 72:63, 1968.
7. Conradi, E.: Vorzeitiges Auftreten von Knochen- und eigenartigen Verkalkungskernen bei Chondrodystrophia fötalis hypoplastica. Histologische und Röntgenuntersuchungen. Jahrb. Kinderheilkd., 80:86, 1914.
8. Coughlin, E. J., Jr., Guare, H. T., and Moskovitz, A. J.: Chondrodystrophia calcificans congenita. J. Bone Joint Surg., 32-A:938, 1950.
9. Fairbank, H. A. T.: Some general diseases of the skeleton. Br. J. Surg., 15:120, 1927.
10. Fairbank, H. A. T.: Dysplasia epiphysialis punctata; synonyms—stippled epiphyses, chondrodystrophia calcificans congenita (Hünermann). J. Bone Joint Surg., 31-B:114, 1949.
11. Frank, W. W., and Denny, M. B.: Dysplasia epiphysialis punctata. J. Bone Joint Surg., 36-B:118, 1954.
12. Gilbert, E. F., Opitz, J. M., Spranger, J. W., Langer, L. D., Wolfson, J. J., and Visekul, C.: Chondrodysplasia punctata. Rhizomelic form. Eur. J. Pediatr., 123:89, 1976.
13. Hünermann, C.: Chondrodystrophia calcificans congenita als abortive Form der Chondrodystrophie. Z. Kinderheilkd., 51:1, 1931.
14. Josephson, B. M.: Chondrodystrophia calcificans congenita. Report of a case and review of the literature. Pediatrics, 28:425, 1961.
15. Mason, R. C., and Kozlowski, K.: Chondrodysplasia punctata: A report of 10 cases. Radiology, 109:145, 1973.
16. Melnick, J. C.: Chondrodystrophia calcificans congenita. Am. J. Dis. Child., 10:218, 1965.
17. Montlouis, H.: Contribution à l'étude de la maladie congénitale des épiphyses pointillées. Thèse Méd., Toulouse, 1961, No. 32.
18. Paul, L. W.: Punctate epiphyseal dysplasia (chondrodystrophia calcificans congenita). Report of a case with nine year period of observation. A.J.R., 71:941, 1954.
19. Raap, G.: Chondrodystrophia calcificans congenita. A.J.R., 49:77, 1943.
20. Silengs, M. C., Luzatti, L., and Silverman, F. N.: Clinical and genetic aspects of Conradi-Hünermann disease. J. Pediatr., 97:911, 1980.
21. Selakovich, W. G., and White, J. W.: Chondrodystrophia calcificans congenita; report of a case. J. Bone Joint Surg., 37-A:1271, 1955.
22. Sheach, J. M., and Middlemiss, J. H.: Dysplasia epiphysealis punctata. Br. J. Radiol., 29:11, 1956.
23. Silverman, F. N.: Discussion on the relation between stippled epiphyses and the multiplex form of epiphyseal dysplasia. Birth Defects Orig. Art. Series, 5:68, 1969.
24. Spranger, J., Opitz, J. M., and Bidder, U.: Heterogeneity of chondrodysplasia punctata. Humangenetik, 11:190, 1971.
25. Spranger, J., Bidder, U., Hansen, H. G., and Volz, C.: Die rhizomele Form der Chondrodysplasia punctata. Fortschr. Roentgenstr., 114:327, 1971.

26. Tasker, W. G., Mastri, A. R., and Gold, A. P.: Chondrodystrophia calcificans congenita (dysplasia epiphysealis punctata). Recognition of the clinical picture. Am. J. Dis. Child., 119:122, 1970.
27. Theander, G., and Pettersson, H.: Calcification in chondrodysplasia punctata. Relation to ossification and skeletal growth. Acta Radiol. [Diagn.] (Stockh.), 19:205, 1978.
28. Tisdall, F. F., and Erb, I. H.: Report of two cases with unusual calcareous deposits. Am. J. Dis. Child., 27:28, 1924.
29. Vinke, T. H., and Duffy, F. P.: Chondrodystrophia calcificans congenita. J. Bone Joint Surg., 29:509, 1947.
30. Viseskul, C., Opitz, J. M., Spranger, J. W., Hertman, H. A., and Gilbert, E. F.: Pathology of chondrodysplasia calcificans punctata. Rhizomelic type. Birth Defects Orig. Art. Series, 10:328, 1974.
31. Weber, A.: Zur Frage der Chondrodysplasia calcificans congenita. Helv. Paediatr. Acta, 13:228, 1958.

HEREDITARY PROGRESSIVE ARTHRO-OPHTHALMOPATHY (STICKLER'S SYNDROME)

This dysplasia was first described by Stickler and associates in 1965.[13] It is characterized by epiphyseal changes similar to those of multiple epiphyseal dysplasia with enlargement of the affected joints. The distinguishing feature of this syndrome is severe progressive myopia that leads to complete retinal detachment and blindness. There may be associated conductive hearing loss and cleft palate. Platyspondyly in the spine is usually minimal, but sometimes anterior wedging of the vertebrae causes thoracic kyphosis similar to that seen in Scheuermann's disease. It is of autosomal dominant inheritance.

Treatment consists of management of the eye complications by an ophthalmologist. Orthopedic treatment of the spinal deformity by orthosis and sometimes by fusion may be indicated.

References

1. Baraitser, M.: Marshall/Stickler syndrome. J. Med. Genet., 19:129, 1982.
2. Cohen, M. M., Knobloch, W. H., and Gorlin, R. J.: A dominantly inherited syndrome of hyaloideoretinal degeneration, cleft palate and maxillary hypoplasia (Cervenka syndrome). Birth Defects Orig. Art. Series, 8:83, 1971.
3. Haller, J., Berdon, W. E., Robinow, M., Slovis, T. L., Baker, D. H., and Johnson, G. F.: The Weissenbacher-Zweymuller syndrome of micrognathia and rhizomelic chondrodysplasia at birth with subsequent normal growth. A.J.R., 125:936, 1975.
4. Herrmann, J., France, T. D., Spranger, J., Opitz, J. M., and Wiffler, C.: The Stickler syndrome (hereditary arthroophthalmopathy). Birth Defects Orig. Art. Series, 11:76, 1975.
5. Kelly, T. E., Wells, H. H., and Tuck, K. B.: The Weissenbacher-Zweymüller syndrome. Possible neonatal expression of the Stickler syndrome. Am. J. Med. Genet., 11:113, 1982.
6. Kozlowski, K., and Turner, G.: Stickler syndrome. Report of a second Australian family. Pediatr. Radiol., 3:230, 1975.
7. Liberfarb, R. M., Hirose, T., and Holmes, L. B.: The Wagner-Stickler syndrome—a genetic study. Birth Defects Orig. Art. Series, 15:145, 1979.
8. Liberfarb, R. M., Hirose, T., and Holmes, L. B.: The Wagner-Stickler syndrome: A study of 22 families. J. Pediatr., 99:394, 1981.
9. Opitz, J. M., France, T., Herrmann, J., and Spranger, J. W.: The Stickler syndrome. N. Engl. J. Med., 286:546, 1972.
10. Say, B., Berry, J., and Barber, N.: The Stickler syndrome (hereditary arthro-ophthalmopathy). Clin. Genet., 12:179, 1977.
11. Spranger, J.: Arthroophthalmopathia hereditaria. Ann. Radiol., 11:359, 1968.
12. Stickler, G. B., and Pugh, D. G.: Hereditary progressive arthro-ophthalmopathy. II. Additional observations on vertebral anmalies, a hearing defect, and a report of a similar case. Mayo Clin. Proc., 42:495, 1967.
13. Stickler, G. B., Belau, P. G., Farrell, F. J., Jones, J. D., Pugh, D. G., Steinberg, A. G., and Ward, L. M.: Hereditary progressive arthro-ophthalmopathy. Mayo Clin. Proc., 40:433, 1965.
14. Turner, G.: The Stickler syndrome in a family with the Pierre Robin syndrome and severe myopia. Aust. Paediatr. J., 10:103, 1974.
15. Winter, R. M., Baraitser, M., Laurence, K. M., Donnai, D., and Hall, C. M.: The Weissenbacher-Zweymüller, Stickler and Marshall syndromes. Further evidence for their identity. Am. J. Med. Genet., 16:189, 1983.

DYSPLASIA EPIPHYSEALIS HEMIMELICA

Dysplasia epiphysealis hemimelica is characterized by asymmetrical abnormal cartilage proliferation and associated enchondral ossification (osteocartilaginous growth) in an epiphysis or in a tarsal, carpal, or flat bone. It is limited to the medial or lateral half of a single limb.

Mouchet and Belot were the first to describe this condition, giving it the name tarsomégalie.[39] In the English literature it was first reported by Trevor, who called it tarsoepiphyseal aclasis.[49] It is also referred to as benign epiphyseal osteochondroma. The most commonly used term, *dysplasia epiphysealis hemimelica*, was given by Fairbank.[16, 17] Kettelcamp and associates, in 1966, published a comprehensive review.[29] Many case reports have appeared in the literature.[1-53]

The etiology is unknown, and dysplasia epiphysealis hemimelica is extremely rare. The exact population incidence has not been determined, but according to Wynne-Davies, the prevalence is one per million.[53] No hereditary or familial factor has been demonstrated.[9] It is more common in the male, in a male to female ratio of 3:1.

Text continued on page 719

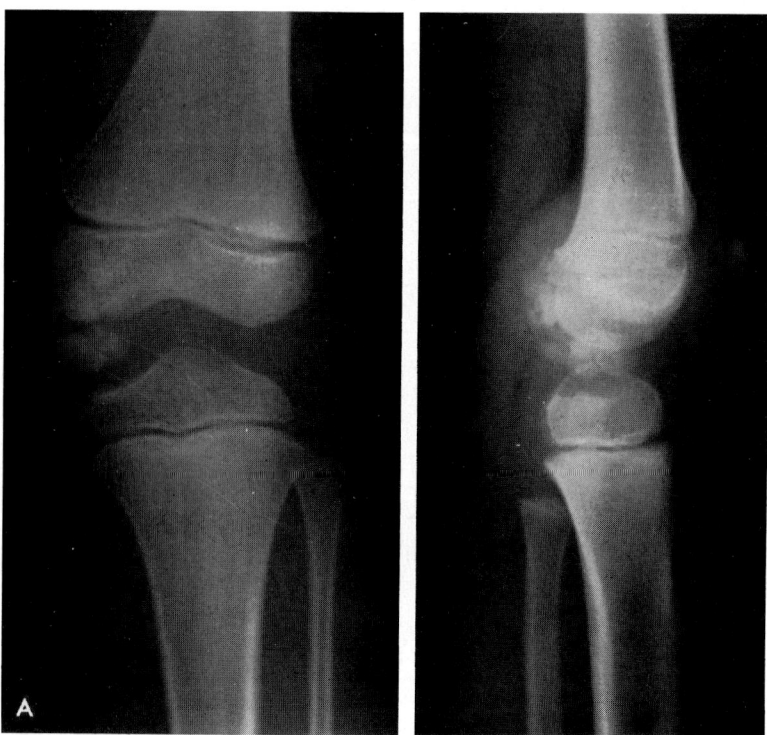

FIGURE 3–12. Dysplasia epiphysealis hemimelica.

A five-and-one-half-year-old boy presented with valgus deformities of the left knee and ankle. **A.** Initial radiograms of left knee. Note the multiple areas of accessory ossification in the medial part of the distal femoral epiphysis and a lesion of the medial part of the proximal femoral epiphysis. (From Kettelkamp, D. B., Campbell, C. J., and Bonfiglio, M.: J. Bone Joint Surg., 48-A:760–762, 1966. Reprinted by permission.)

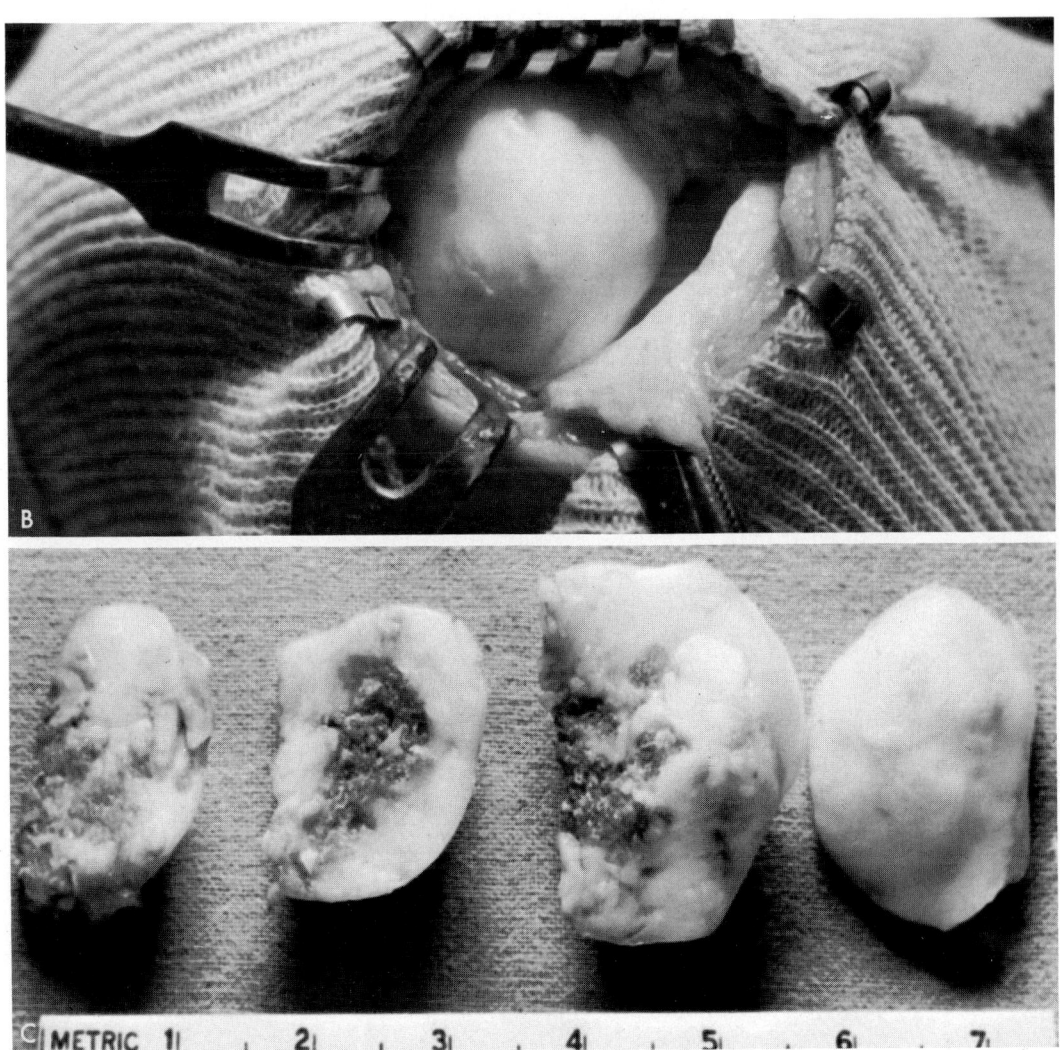

FIGURE 3–12 Continued. Dysplasia epiphysealis hemimelica.

B. Gross findings at operation. Note the enlarged and slightly irregular distal femoral epiphysis. **C.** The gross specimen. There was a cleavage area of cartilage between the ossification center in the lesion and the epiphysis. (From Kettelkamp, D. B., Campbell, C. J., and Bonfiglio, M.: J. Bone Joint Surg., 48-A:760–762, 1966. Reprinted by permission.)

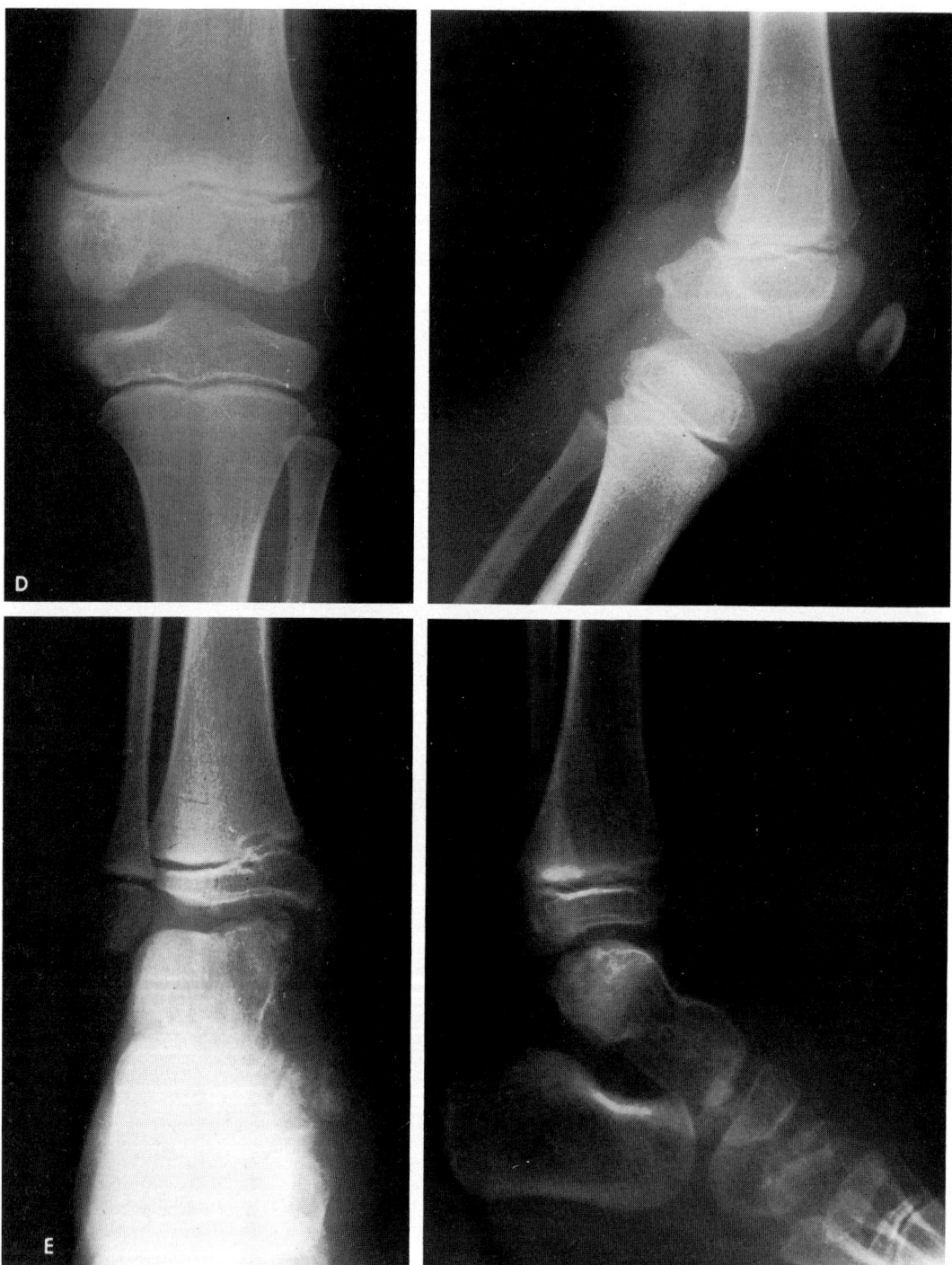

FIGURE 3–12 *Continued. Dysplasia epiphysealis hemimelica.*

D. Postoperative radiograms of the knee when the child was 11 years of age. **E.** Anteroposterior and lateral radiograms of the ankle and foot show involvement of the talus, the navicular, and the medial part of the cuneiform. (From Kettelkamp, D. B., Campbell, C. J., and Bonfiglio, M.: J. Bone Joint Surg., *48-A*:760–762, 1966. Reprinted by permission.)

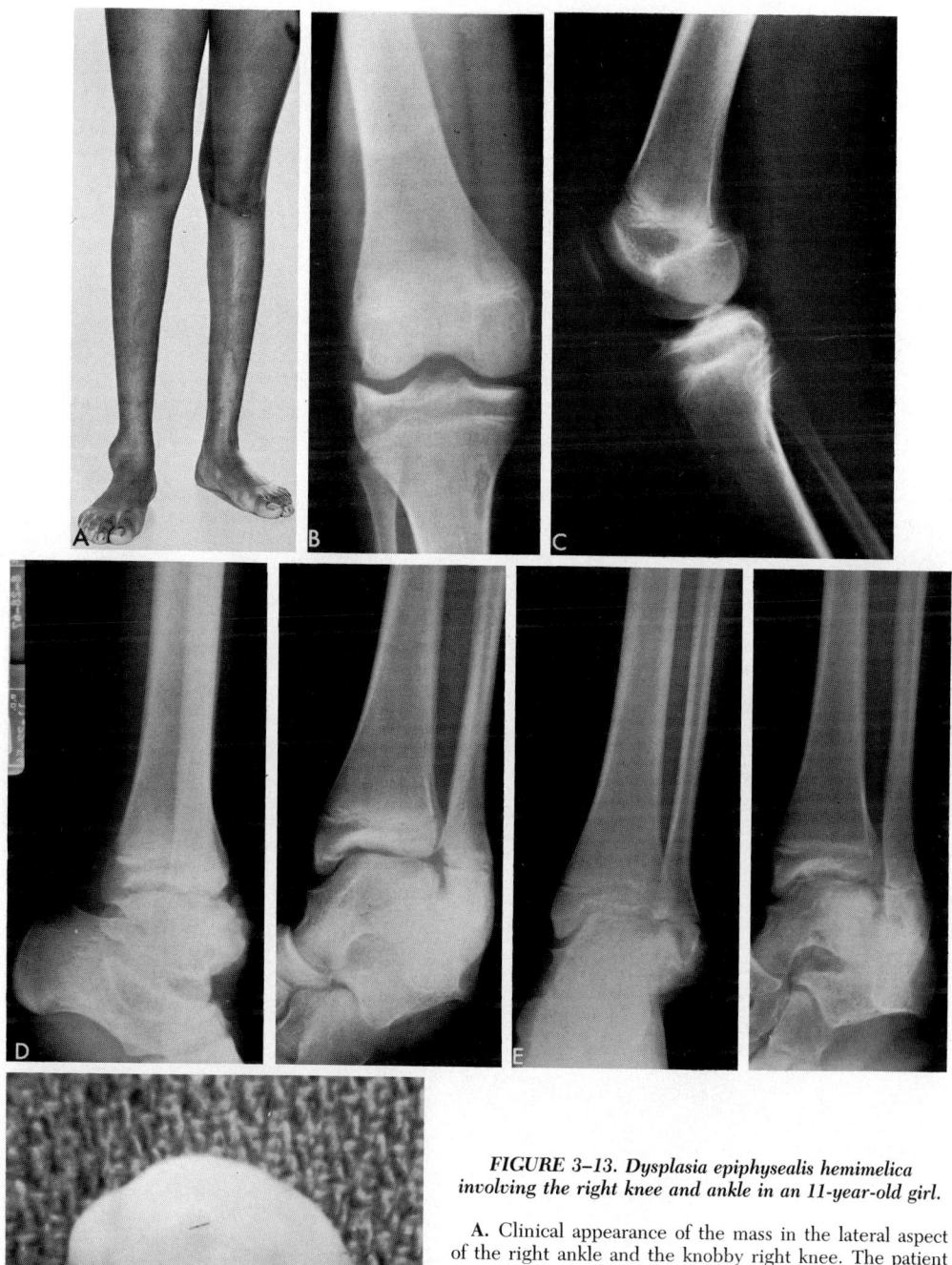

FIGURE 3–13. Dysplasia epiphysealis hemimelica involving the right knee and ankle in an 11-year-old girl.

A. Clinical appearance of the mass in the lateral aspect of the right ankle and the knobby right knee. The patient complained of pain in both joints. **B** and **C.** Anteroposterior and lateral radiograms of the right knee. Note the exostosis-like mass projecting from the lateral portion of the proximal tibial epiphysis. **D** and **E.** Views of right ankle showing the multicentric radiopacity on the lateral surface of the talus. **F.** Gross appearance of the lesion excised from the tibial plateau.

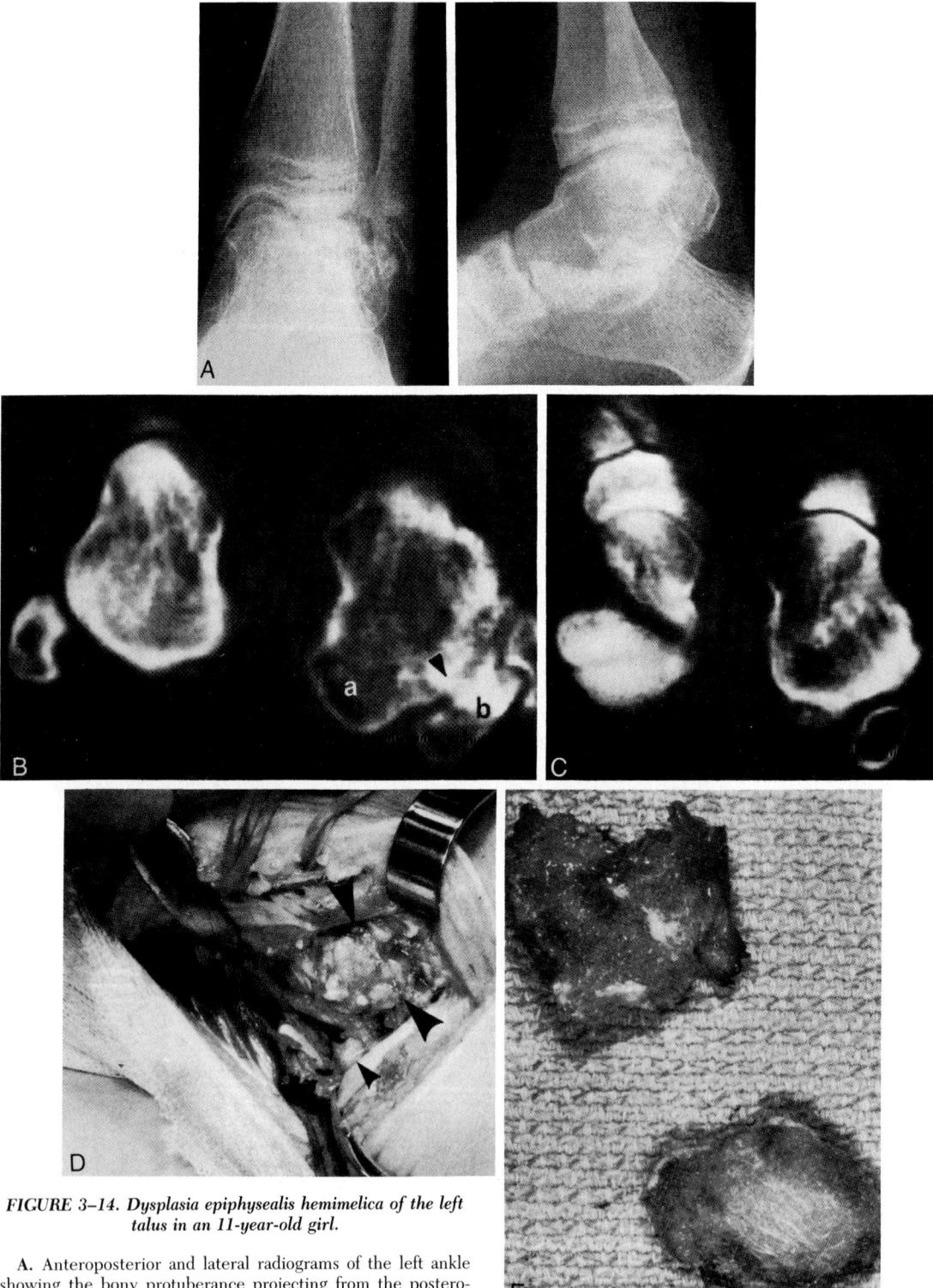

FIGURE 3–14. *Dysplasia epiphysealis hemimelica of the left talus in an 11-year-old girl.*

A. Anteroposterior and lateral radiograms of the left ankle showing the bony protuberance projecting from the posterolateral surface of the talus. Note the irregularity of the dome of the talus.

B and **C.** CT scans showing the bony protuberance projecting from the posterolateral surface of the talus and abutting the fibula. **D.** Operative photograph showing the cartilaginous surface of the two exostoses. **E.** Photograph of the gross specimens. (From Fisher, M. R., Hernandez, R. J., Poznanski, A. K., and Tachdjian, M. O.: Case report 262. Skeletal Radiol., *11*:147, 1984. Reprinted by permission.)

Pathology

The findings are similar to those of osteocartilaginous exostosis.[29] Grossly, the lesion appears as either a pedunculated mass with a cartilaginous cap or a somewhat irregular, enlarged articular surface. On section, the ossification center of the lesion is separated from that of the epiphysis by a cartilaginous area. Within the lesion there may be multiple centers of ossification. The histologic appearance of the lesions is indistinguishable from that of osteochondroma. Ossification of the tumor takes place by enchondral bone formation. Areas of necrosis may be encountered.

Clinical Features

The condition is not usually recognizable at birth, but becomes apparent in early childhood, usually after two years of age. Involvement is characteristically unilateral, affecting one limb. The most frequent sites of localization are the tarsus and the distal femoral and proximal tibial epiphyses. The exostoses protrude into the juxta-articular space, causing incongruity and distortion of the opposing joint surfaces. The lesions are multiple in about 70 per cent of cases. The exostoses may be lateral or medial, but sometimes the entire epiphysis may be involved. The medial side is involved twice as commonly as the lateral. It should be noted, however, that the lesions are not always hemimelic in distribution. The carpal bones, the patellae, and the scapulae are occasionally involved.[1, 16, 31]

The presenting complaint is commonly not pain, but rather deformity and limitation of motion of the affected joint. In the older patient pain is more frequent, usually in the ankle. Genu valgum or varum and pes valgus and equinus are common deformities that increase with growth. The affected portion of the epiphysis is enlarged, and a local mass may be palpable. Lower limb length inequality is not uncommon. The range of motion of the affected joints is limited, owing either to the presence of a mass or to the deformity. Increasing deformity or enlargement of the mass will cause progressive limitation of joint motion.

Radiographic Findings

The radiographic picture depends on the age of the patient. In infancy, radiograms may be normal or depict minimal metaphyseal widening. As the lesion matures, an irregular and often multicentric radiopacity develops adjacent to the affected epiphysis or tarsal bone. Appearance of the ossification centers of the affected bones is usually premature. In the adolescent and adult, the lesion appears as an irregular bony mass similar to an exostosis; the two may be differentiated, however, by the protrusion of the mass from the epiphysis rather than from the metaphysis or diaphysis (Figs. 3–12 and 3–13). CT scans will delineate the boundaries of exostoses (Fig. 3–14).

Prognosis

The lesion usually stops growing when the child reaches skeletal maturity, though occasionally it may increase in size during adult life. A protuberant exostosis may fracture and break loose into the joint. Incongruity of the joint will cause osteoarthritis later in life.

The condition is definitely benign. Malignant degeneration later in adult life has not been reported.

Treatment

Excision of the lesion is advised when it interferes with joint motion or produces severe deformity. Recurrence is common; repeated local excision is often required. Lower limb length discrepancy should be followed, and an epiphysiodesis should be performed at the appropriate skeletal age for limb length equalization. Arthrodesis of the ankle or knee joint may be required when disability is severe because of osteoarthritis.

References

1. Azouz, E. M., Slomic, A. M., and Archambault, H.: Upper extremity involvement in Trevor disease. J. Can. Assoc. Radiol., 35:209, 1984.
2. Balen, E.: Displasia epifisaria hemimelica. Rev. Esp. Cir. Ost., 6:91, 1971.
3. Barta, O., Schanzl, A., and Szepesi, J.: Dysplasia epiphysealis hemimelica. Acta Orthop. Scand., 44:702, 1973.
4. Bianchi, M., and Frassi, G.: Displasia epifisaria monomelica. Arch. Orthop., 76:15, 1963.
5. Bigliani, L. U., Neer, C. S., Parisien, M., and Johnston, A. D.: Dysplasia epiphysealis hemimelica of the scapula. J. Bone Joint Surg., 62-A:292, 1980.
6. Buckwalter, J. A., El-Khoury, G. Y., and Flatt, A. E.: Dysplasia epiphysealis hemimelica of the ulna. Clin. Orthop., 135:36, 1978.
7. Caffey, J.: Pediatric X-ray Diagnosis. 8th Ed. Chicago, Year Book, 1985.
8. Carlson, D. H., and Wilkinson, R. H.: Variability of unilateral epiphyseal dysplasia (dysplasia epiphysealis hemimelica). Pediatr. Radiol., 133:369, 1979.
9. Conor, J. M., Horan, F. T., and Beighton, P.: Dysplasia epiphysealis hemimelica: A clinical and genetic study. J. Bone Joint Surg., 65-B:350, 1983.

10. Cruz-Conde, R., Amaya, S., Valdivia, P., Hernandez, M., and Calvo, M.: Dysplasia epiphysealis hemimelica. J. Pediatr. Orthop., *4*:625, 1984.
11. D'Angio, G. J., Ritvo, M., and Ulin, R.: Clinical and roentgen manifestations of tarso-epiphyseal aclasis. A.J.R., *74*:1068, 1955.
12. Debrunner, H. U.: Dysplasia epiphysealis hemimelica. Helv. Paediatr. Acta, *17*:367, 1962.
13. DeSeze, S.: Dysplasie Epiphysaire Hémimélique. Maladie des Os et des Articulations. Paris, Flammarion, 1964.
14. Donaldson, J. S., Sankey, H. H., Girdany, B. R., and Donaldson, W. P.: Osteochondroma of the distal femoral epiphysis. J. Pediatr. *43*:212, 1953.
15. Enriquez, J., Quiles, M., and Torres, C.: A unique case of dysplasia epiphysealis hemimelica of the patella. Clin. Orthop., *160*:168, 1981.
16. Fairbank, T.: An Atlas of General Affections of the Skeleton. Baltimore, Williams & Wilkins, 1951.
17. Fairbank, T. J.: Dysplasia epiphysialis hemimelica (tarso-epiphysial aclasis). J. Bone Joint Surg., *38-B*:237, 1956.
18. Fasting, O. J., and Bjerkreim, I.: Dysplasia epiphysealis hemimelica. Acta Orthop. Scand., *47*:217, 1976.
19. Fèvre, M., and Rigault, P.: Fragmentation osseuse hypertrophiante. Rev. Chir. Orthop., *54*:525, 1968.
20. Finidori, G., Rigault, P., Padovani, J. P., and Naouri, A.: Dysplasie épiphysaire hémimélique. Rev. Chir. Orthop., *64*:367, 1978.
21. Fisher, M. R., Hernandez, R. J., Poznanski, A. K., and Tachdjian, M. O.: Case report 262. Skeletal Radiol., *11*:147, 1984.
22. Fontaine, G., Maroteaux, P., Farriaux, J.-P., and Saint-Aubert, P.: La dysplasie épiphysaire hémimélique. Etude d'une observation chez un nourrisson de 10 mois. Sem. Hôp. Paris, *14*:861, 1971.
23. Goldstein, W. B.: Dysplasia epiphysealis hemimelica with confirmation by knee arthrogram. Br. J. Radiol., *46*:470, 1973.
24. Gomar, F.: Displasias epifisarias hiperplasicas. In Patologia Quirurgica Osteoarticular. Valencia, Saber, 1973, p. 81.
25. Heiple, K. G.: Carpal osteochondroma. J. Bone Joint Surg., *43-A*:861, 1961.
26. Hensinger, R. N., Cowell, H. R., Ramsey, P. L., and Leopold, R. G.: Familial dysplasia epiphysealis hemimelica, associated with chondromas and osteochondromas. J. Bone Joint Surg., *56-A*:1513, 1974.
27. Ingelrans, P., and Lacheretz, M.: A propos d'un cas de chondrodystrophie épiphysaire. Rev. Chir. Orthop., *39*:242, 1953.
28. Keats, T. E.: Dysplasia epiphysealis hemimelica. Radiology, *68*:558, 1957.
29. Kettelkamp, D. B., Campbell, C. J., and Bonfiglio, M.: Dysplasia epiphysealis hemimelica. A report of fifteen cases and a review of the literature. J. Bone Joint Surg., *48-A*:746, 1966.
30. Lamesch, A.: Dysplasia epiphysealis hemimelica of the carpal bones. Report of a case and review of the literature. J. Bone Joint Surg., *65-A*:398, 1983.
31. Luck, V. J., and Smith, C. F.: Dysplasia epiphysealis osteochondromata: 22 cases correlated with 70 cases in medical literature. J. Bone Joint Surg., *54-A*:1351, 1972.
32. Mainzer, F., Minagi, H., and Steinbach, H. L.: The variable manifestations of multiple enchondromatosis. Radiology, *99*:377, 1971.
33. Maroteaux, P.: Dysplasies spondylo-épiphysaires. In Encyclopédie Medico-chirurgicale. Paris, Editions Techniques, 1969, p. 2.
34. Maroteaux, P.: Maladies osseuses de l'enfant. Paris, Flammarion, 1974, p. 107.
35. Martens, M., Tanghe, W., and Mulier, J. C.: Dysplasia epiphysealis hemimelica. Acta Orthop. Belg., *34*:625, 1968.
36. Mena-Bernal, R., Barbudo, R., Iturrate, C., and Fernandez, R.: Displasia epifisaria hemimelica. An. Med. Sevilla, *7*:393, 1968.
37. Milch, R. A.: Osteochondroma of the astragalus. Am. J. Surg., *87*:145, 1954.
38. Montminy, M., and Gagnon, P. A.: Dysplasie épiphysaire hémimélique. Union Méd. Can., *101*:1822, 1972.
39. Mouchet, A., and Belot, J.: La tarsomégalie. J. Radiol., *10*:289, 1926.
40. Mouraria, E., Jr., Koberle, G., Netto, J. R., and DeFaria, L. L.: Displasia epifisaria hemimelica. Relato de un caso. A.M.B., *24*:91, 1978.
41. Munthe, E.: Dysplasia epiphysealis hemimelica. Acta Rheum. Scand., *13*:222, 1967.
42. Rechnagel, K.: Dysplasia epiphysealis hemimelica. Acta Orthop. Scand., *29*:237, 1960.
43. Rook, F. R.: Intra-articular osteochondroma of the astragalus. Am. J. Surg., *85*:807, 1953.
44. Sauvegrain, J., and Sbihi, A.: Ostéochondrodysplasies. In Encyclopédie Médico-chirurgicale. RAD T. I squelette pathologique. 3133 A 10. Paris, Editions Techniques, 1967, p. 1.
45. Saxton, H. M., and Wilkinson, J. A.: Hemimelic skeletal dysplasia. J. Bone Joint Surg., *46-B*:608, 1964.
46. Spranger, J.: The epiphyseal dysplasia. Clin. Orthop., *114*:46, 1976.
47. Spranger, J. W., Langer, L. O., and Wiedemann, H. R.: Bone Dysplasia: An Atlas of Constitutional Disorders of Skeletal Development. Philadelphia, Saunders, 1974, pp. 191–194.
48. Theodorou S., and Lanitis, G.: Dysplasia epiphysealis hemimelica. Helv. Paediatr. Acta, *2*:195, 1968.
49. Trevor, D.: Tarso-epiphyseal aclasis: A congenital error of epiphysial development. J. Bone Joint Surg., *32-B*:204, 1950.
50. Wheble, V. H., and Connell, M. C.: Dysplasia epiphysealis hemimelica. Br. J. Radiol., *31*:637, 1958.
51. Wiedemann, H. R., Mann, M., Spreter, P., and Von Kreudenstein, P. S.: Dysplasia epiphysealis hemimelica—Trevor disease. Severe manifestations in a child. Eur. J. Pediatr, *136*:311, 1981.
52. Wolfgang, G. L., and Heath, R. D.: Dysplasia epiphysealis hemimelica. Clin. Orthop., *116*:32, 1976.
53. Wynne-Davies, R., Hall, G. M., and Apley, G. A.: Atlas of Skeletal Dysplasias. Edinburgh, Churchill-Livingstone, 1985.

ACHONDROPLASIA

Achondroplasia, the commonest type of dwarfism, is a developmental abnormality in which enchondral bone formation is defective; intramembranous bone formation, however, is normal. It is characterized by short limbs, a bulging cranium (especially the forehead), a low nasal bridge, a narrowed spinal canal in the lumbar region, and distinctive pelvic changes.

The term *achondroplasia* was proposed by Parrot in 1878, and its synonym, *chondrodystrophia foetalis*, was suggested by Kaufmann in 1892.[25, 49] During the past century, the term *achondroplasia* was used indiscriminately to describe any form of short-limb dwarfism. It is only during the past two decades that the distinctive features of achondroplasia have been delineated.

The depiction of the Egyptian goddess Ptah as an achondroplast and the discovery of an actual achondroplastic skeleton dating from the early Egyptian period indicate this type of dwarfism to be one known from the most ancient times. In the Middle Ages, court jesters were often typical achondroplastic dwarfs, as are the "midgets" in circuses and theaters today.

Achondroplasia also occurs in animals, the dachshund being a common example. A lethal form of the disease in rabbits was noted by Brown and Pearce.[10]

Etiology

Failure of enchondral ossification results from a primary germ plasm defect and is apparent toward the end of the second month of fetal life.

Achondroplasia is of autosomal dominant inheritance. Because most affected individuals do not reproduce, however, about 90 per cent of cases of achondroplasia appear sporadically in families with normal parents and siblings, the probable result of a new gene mutation.[41] An increased incidence of achondroplastic births has been correlated with increasing parental age.[8] It is rare that more than two generations of a family are involved. Sexes are equally affected. The incidence of achondroplasia is three per million.[19]

Pathology

The most striking findings are in the growth plate in the zone of cartilage proliferation.[1] Ponseti studied the growth plate of the fibula and found cartilage cell clusters separated by wide septa of fibrous matrix that appear to be very slowly resorbed.[53] There is a relative lack of cartilage production; the normal regular palisade arrangement of cartilage cells at the physis is absent, and provisional calcification is erratic. Mucoid degeneration of the cartilage cells takes place.[21] The trabeculae in the spongiosa are irregular. The abnormalities are in the metaphyseal area. Ossification remains undisturbed, the long bones increase in length, but the growth rate is very slow.

Because periosteal ossification remains unaffected, the diaphyses of long bones are of normal diameter. An apparent increase in width of the shaft is due to a reduction in length.

Occasionally, the connective tissue in the vascular channels from the periosteum to the physis may proliferate, forming a transverse fibrous band across the entire diameter of the bone. This seals the growth plate and prevents any further growth of the shaft.

Clinical Picture

The characteristic features of the achondroplast are obvious at birth. Dwarfism is the most conspicuous, the reduction in height being chiefly due to shortness of the lower limbs (Fig. 3–15 A to C). The trunk length (crown to pubis) is normal, but the lower limb length (pubis to heel) and the span length (fingertip to fingertip) are greatly diminished. The shortness of the limbs is greater in the proximal than in the distal segments. Adult standing height is usually slightly over 4 feet (males 131 cm., or 4′ 3½″, and females 124 cm., or 4′ 1″), but may be as little as 2 feet, 6 inches. The sitting height is around the tenth percentile value for normal individuals. The normal length of the trunk in contrast with the short limbs gives the impression of an adult body with four childlike limbs (Fig. 3–16 A to C). In erect posture, the fingertips may not reach below the greater trochanters, whereas in the normal individual, they extend to the lower part of the thigh. The midpoint of stature, normally at the umbilicus, is sometimes as high as the lower end of the sternum.

The head is disproportionately enlarged, suggesting hydrocephalus, which may be present to a mild degree in some cases. The skull is brachycephalic, its base shortened and its anteroposterior diameter decreased. The face is broad, with a prominent frontal region, protruding upper alveolar processes, and prognathous mandible. The bridge of the nose is depressed and flattened, giving a characteristic facies. Dentition is normal.

The chest, though normal in length, is flat, with flaring of the costal margins. There is markedly exaggerated lumbar lordosis that, along with the protrusion of the abdominal and gluteal regions, gives a characteristic posture. There may be increased thoracic kyphosis.

The hands are short and broad. The middle finger is shorter than that in the normal hand, resulting in all the digits being of equal length (sometimes referred to as "starfish hand"). The long and ring fingers are spread apart, forming a V-shaped space to which Marie applied the term "main en trident" (see Fig. 3–15 G).[38]

The lower limbs are often bowed, primarily in the tibia because the fibula is relatively longer. The ends of the long bones are enlarged, and the irregular shape of the epiphysis may limit the range of joint motion; there may be a waddling gait.

Muscular development is often above average. The skin and soft tissues are overabundant

Text continued on page 726

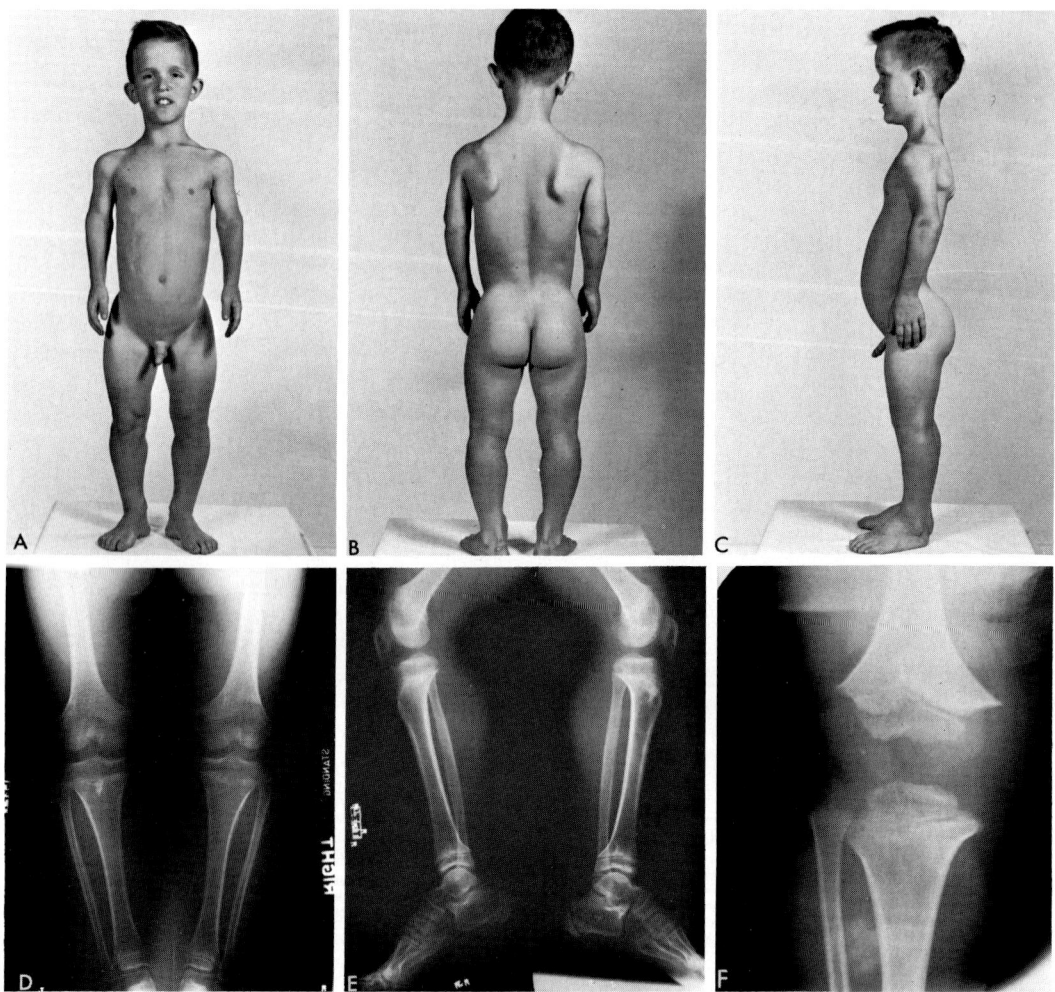

FIGURE 3-15. Achondroplasia in a ten-year-old boy.

A to C. Clinical appearance. D and E. Anteroposterior and lateral radiograms of lower limbs. F. Anteroposterior radiogram of the knee joint showing the centrally notched or U-shaped epiphyseal plates.

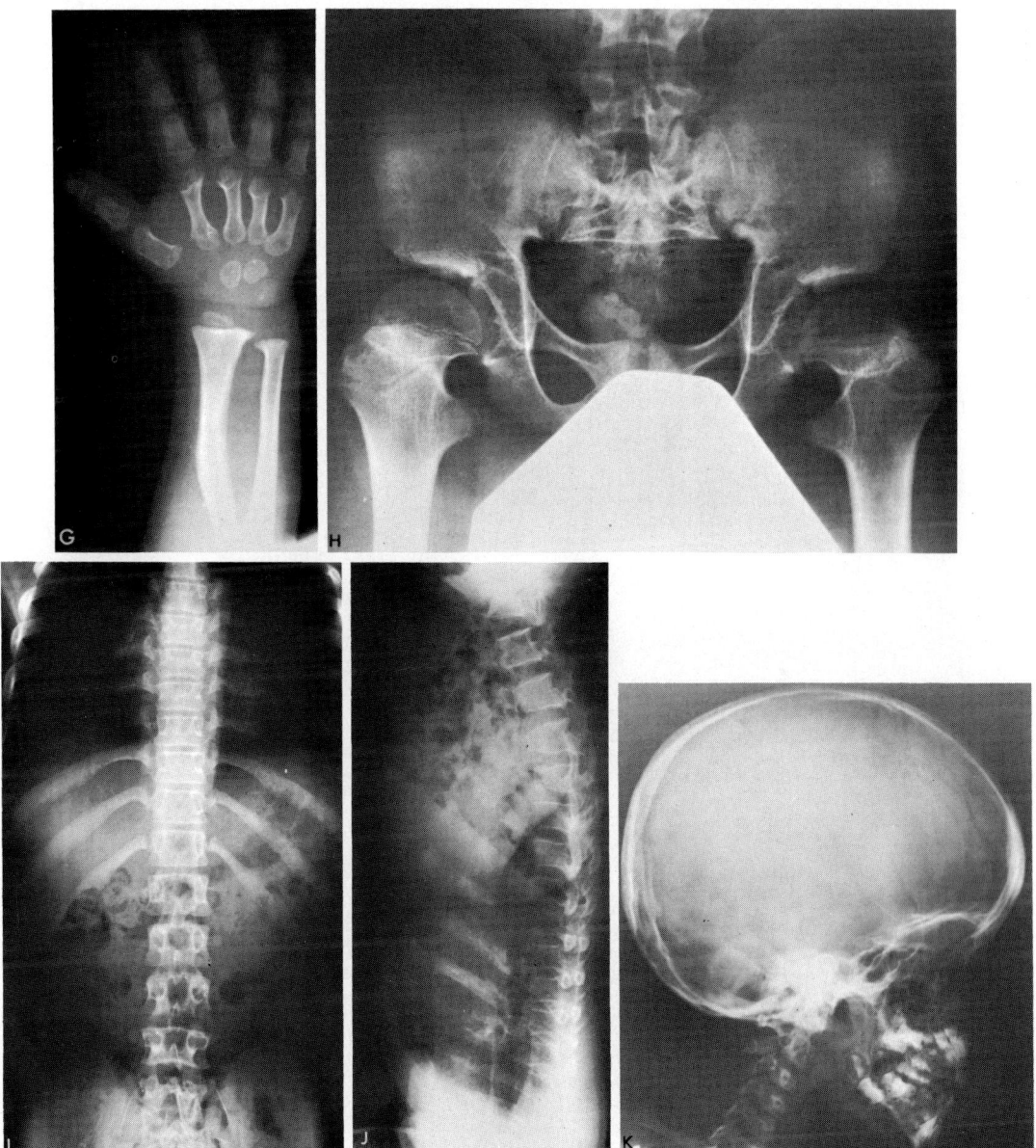

FIGURE 3–15 Continued. Achondroplasia in a ten-year-old boy.

G. Anteroposterior radiogram of the hand. Note the short thick metacarpals and phalanges. The long and ring fingers are spread apart, forming a V-shaped space ("main en trident"). **H.** Anteroposterior radiogram of the pelvis. Note the typical appearance of the inner pelvic contour and the squaring off of the iliac wings. **I** and **J**. Anteroposterior and lateral radiograms of the spine showing the progressive decrease in the size of the spinal canal in the lumbar vertebrae. Note the short thick pedicles. The vertebral bodies are smaller than normal and their posterior surface is concave. **K.** Lateral radiogram of the skull of the same patient.

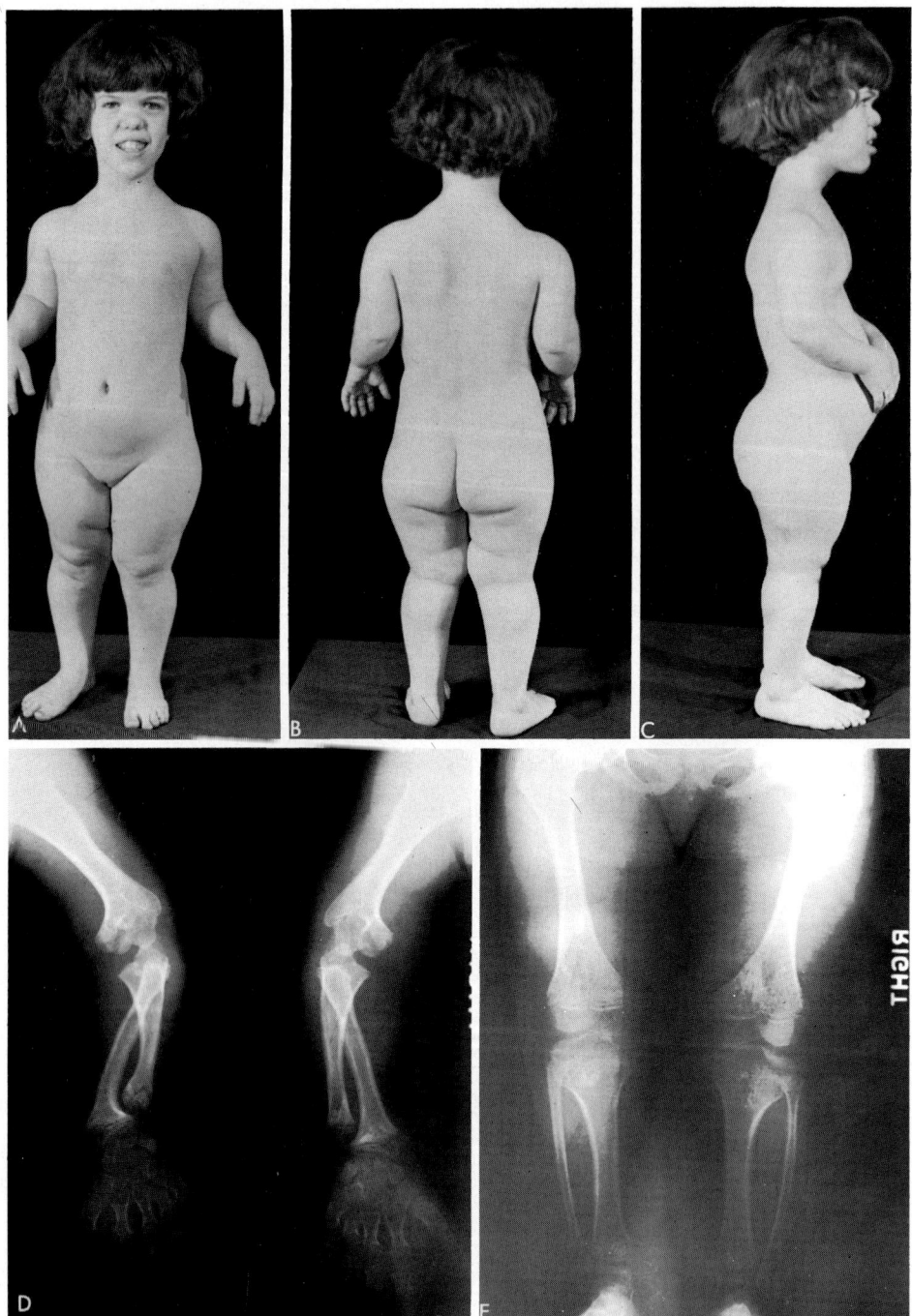

FIGURE 3–16. *Achondroplasia in an eight-year-old girl.*

A to **C.** Clinical appearance of a patient with typical deformities. **D** and **E.** Anteroposterior radiograms of upper and lower limbs.

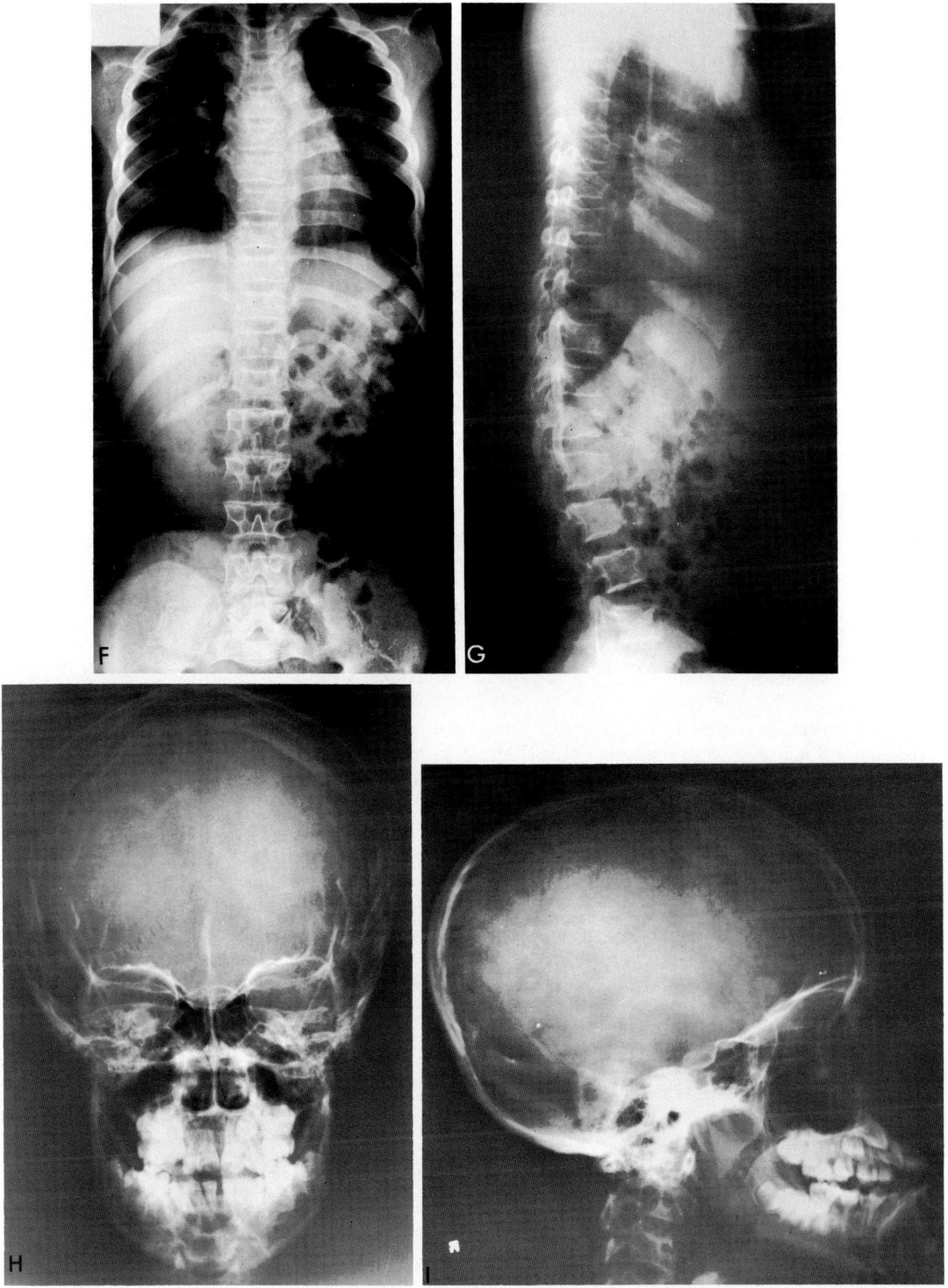

FIGURE 3-16 Continued. Achondroplasia in an eight-year-old girl.

F and **G**. Anteroposterior and lateral radiograms of the spine. **H** and **I**. Anteroposterior and lateral radiograms of the skull show marked shortness at its base.

for the length of the limb bones; transverse folds and furrows between rolls of fat form.

In general, endocrine function and sexual development remain undisturbed. Intelligence is usually normal or above average. Psychologically, however, because of their unusual appearance, achondroplasts often have strong feelings of inferiority.

Radiographic Findings

Shortness of the tubular bones with apparently increased diameter and density due to the reduction in length is the characteristic finding (Figs. 3–15 D and E, 3–16 D and E, and 3–17). All the long tubular bones are affected. The metaphyses are widened, but the epiphyses are normal. The proximal segments of the limbs, i.e., the humeri and femora, are more involved than the distal segments (rhizomelic micromelia). The clavicles and fibulae are less affected than other long bones. Thus, the fibula is longer than the tibia, its head at a higher level than normal and, at the ankle, the tip of its malleolus extending more distally than usual (Fig. 3–15 D and E).

The diaphyses of the long bones are of normal diameter. The cortex is thickened at the sites of muscle attachment. There is marked splaying and flaring of the metaphyses. The growth plates are centrally notched or U-shaped. This is best seen in the region of the knee joint (Fig. 3–15 F). The actual size of the epiphyses is within normal limits, but they appear enlarged. In young children, the ossific center of the epiphysis is located closer to the diaphysis, resulting in a considerable increase in depth of the articular cartilage space. The two limbs of the V of the metaphysis appear to embrace the epiphysis, giving them a ball-and-socket relationship. Long bones are frequently bowed. The metacarpal, metatarsal, and phalangeal bones are also short and thick.

The sacrum is narrow, and articulates low on the ilia, the sacral tilt being exaggerated and the sacral promontory protruding abnormally into the pelvic cavity. The greater sciatic notch is small. The iliac wings are squared off, and their height is less than normal because of poor growth at the base. The acetabular roofs are broad and flat. In infancy and early childhood there is sharp medial beaking of the acetabular roof at the superior border of the triradiate cartilage. In adolescence this medial beaking disappears. Because the width of the pelvic inlet exceeds its depth, the inner pelvic contour has a typical "champagne glass" appearance (Fig. 3–15 H). The upper femoral metaphyses are splayed, and the femoral necks are short.

The anteroposterior diameter of the thorax is decreased in the severe case because of the short ribs, which may be even less than half the normal length. The sternum is thick, broad, and short. Extreme deformity of the rib cage may cause marked respiratory distress. The scapulae have square angles.

The spine is of normal length, but the ossification centers of the vertebrae may be smaller than normal, as seen in the lateral projection. Often there is a long kyphosis. The achondroplastic spine is principally characterized by the progressive diminution of the interpedicular distances from the first lumbar vertebra through the fifth (Figs. 3–15 I and J and 3–16 F and G). In the normal spine the distance becomes greater through this area. The progressive decrease in the size of the spinal canal in the lumbar vertebrae is due to early synostosis between the vertebral body and its arch. The posterior surfaces of the vertebral bodies are concave (appearing scalloped), and the pedicles are thick and short. Computed tomography and contrast studies will demonstrate cephalocaudal tapering of the intraspinal canal. The carpal and tarsal bones are normal.

There is marked shortness of the base of the skull owing to retarded growth of the presphenoidal, postsphenoidal, and basioccipital cartilaginous centers of ossification. The foramen magnum is small and funnel-shaped; however, the remainder of the skull develops normally. Since the base of the skull provides little intracranial space, the vault and frontal regions are expanded to accommodate the enlarging brain. The face appears flattened and the root of the nose depressed because of the smallness of the base of the skull; otherwise, the facial bones are unaffected (Figs. 3–15 K and 3–16 H and I). There is no evidence of increased intracranial pressure except in the occasional case complicated by hydrocephalus. The circumferential growth of the head parallels that of normal, but is at a higher level.[12]

Diagnosis

There is usually little difficulty in diagnosis.[65] The cardinal features that characterize achondroplasia are typical appearance of the skull and facial bones; the vertebral column with its short pedicles, scalloping of the posterior borders of the vertebral bodies, and progressive narrowing of the interpedicular distance between the first lumbar and the fifth lumbar vertebrae; and the

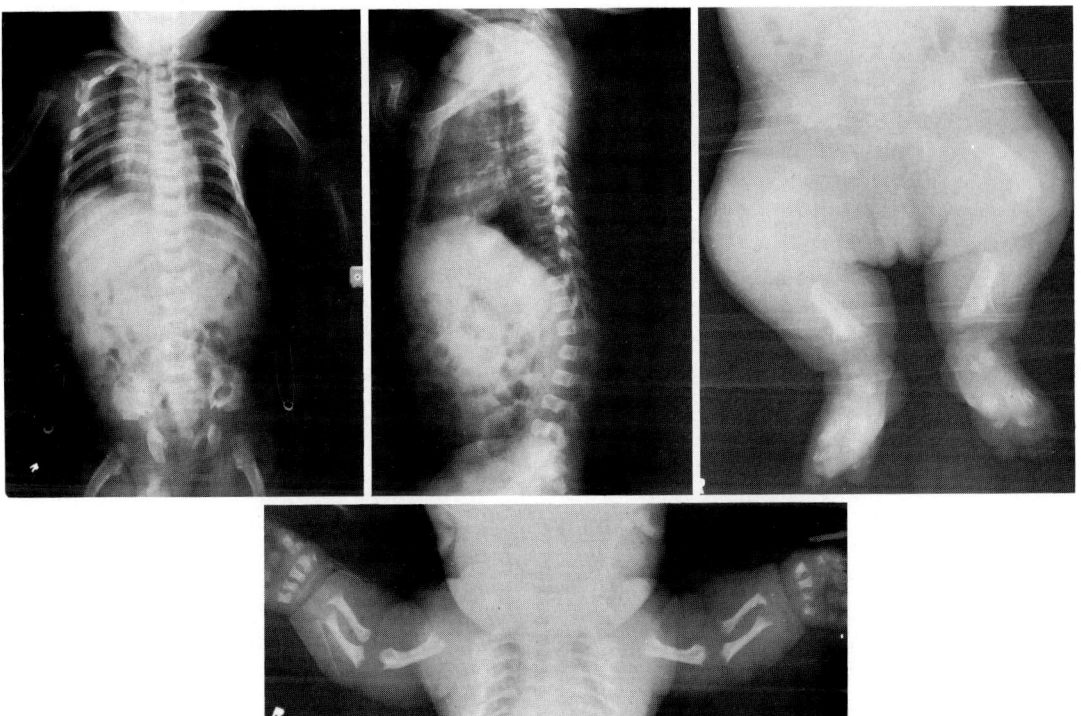

FIGURE 3–17. *Early radiographic findings in achondroplasia.*

Anteroposterior and lateral radiographs of the torso and upper and lower limbs of a six-month-old child.

typical pelvis. Achondroplasia does not affect the epiphysis. At birth, achondroplasia must be distinguished from lethal forms of short-limbed dwarfism such as thanatophoric dwarfism and achondrogenesis.

A severe prenatal case of osteogenesis imperfecta may simulate achondroplasia because the limbs are markedly short as compared with the trunk; however, the radiographic findings will differentiate the two. In infancy and early childhood, achondroplasia may be mistaken for rickets, cretinism, and various developmental affections of the skeletal system, such as the Morquio and Hurler syndromes. The radiographic features of these entities are characteristic, however. In older children, achondroplasia must be distinguished from hypochondroplasia, which is less severe and lacks the characteristic skull and pelvic changes of achondroplasia.

Prognosis and Treatment

The prognosis is excellent. Affected individuals usually have good general health and nearly normal longevity. Osteoarthritis in adult life is not a feature, because the epiphyses are normal.

In adulthood, the achondroplast may suffer from neurologic complications due to the small diameter of the intraspinal canal and multiple ruptures of the intervertebral discs. Pressure on the cord or spinal nerves or both may cause backache, sciatica, and even paraplegia (about 11 per cent), necessitating laminectomy and excision of ruptured discs. Hydrocephalus, if present, is not progressive, usually requiring no treatment.

There is no specific treatment for the disease. Correction of the varus deformity of the tibiae and femora may improve appearance, gait, and the biomechanics of the lower limbs. Limb lengthening procedures to increase height and upper limb length are performed in some medical centers; primarily in Europe and the Soviet Union. This author recommends limb lengthening in achondroplasts only when there is marked functional disability because of the short limbs or when there is marked deformity of a limb that is asymmetrically short.

References

1. Aegerter, E., and Kirkpatrick, J. A., Jr.: Orthopedic Diseases. 3rd Ed. Philadelphia, Saunders, 1965, p. 125.
2. Alexander, E., Jr.: Significance of the small lumbar spinal canal: Cauda equina compression syndromes due

to spondylosis. Part 5: Achondroplasia. J. Neurosurg., 31:513, 1969.
3. Bailey, J. A.: Orthopaedic aspects of achondroplasia. J. Bone Joint Surg., 52-A:1285, 1970.
4. Bailey, J. A.: Disproportionate Short Stature. Philadelphia, Saunders, 1973, p. 83.
5. Bargman, G. J., Mackler, B., and Shepard, T. H.: Studies of oxidative energy deficiency. I. Achondroplasia in the rabbit. Arch. Biochem., 150:137, 1972.
6. Bergstrom, K., Laurent, U., and Lundbert, P. O.: Neurological symptoms in achondroplasia. Acta Neurol. Scand., 47:59, 1971.
7. Bland, J. D., and Emery, J. L.: Unexpected death of children with achondroplasia after the perinatal period. Dev. Med. Child. Neurol., 24:489, 1982.
8. Bleyer, A.: Role of advancing maternal age in causing achondroplasia. Am. J. Dis. Child., 58:994, 1939.
9. Bouvet, J. P., Maroteaux, P., and Feingold, J.: Etude génétique de l'achondroplasie. Ann. Genet., 14:127, 1971.
10. Brown, W. H., and Pearce, L.: Hereditary achondroplasia in the rabbit. J. Exp. Med., 82:241, 1945.
11. Caffey, J.: Achondroplasia of the pelvis and lumbosacral spine. Some roentgenographic features. A.J.R., 80:449, 1958.
12. Cohen, M. E., Rosenthal, A. D., and Matson, D. D.: Neurological abnormalities in achondroplastic children. J. Pediatr., 71:367, 1967.
13. Duvoisin, R. C., and Yahr, M. D.: Compressive spinal cord and root syndromes in an achondroplastic dwarf. Neurology, 12:202, 1962.
14. Epstein, J. A., and Malis, L. I.: Compression of spinal cord and cauda equina in achondroplastic dwarfs. Neurology, 5:875, 1955.
15. Escamilla, R. F., Hutchings, J. J., Choh, H. L., and Forsham, P.: Achondroplastic dwarfism. Effects of treatment with human growth hormone. Calif. Med., 105:104, 1966.
16. Fairbank, H. A. T.: An Atlas of General Affections of the Skeleton. Edinburgh, Livingstone, 1951, p. 142.
17. Friedman, W. A., and Mickle, J. P.: Hydrocephalus in achondroplasia: A possible mechanism. Neurosurgery, 7:150, 1980.
18. Ganel, A., Horoszowski, H., Kahmine, M., and Farine, T.: Leg lengthening in achondroplastic children. Clin. Orthop., 144:194, 1979.
19. Gardner, R. J. M.: A new estimate of the achondroplasia mutation rate. Clin. Genet., 11:31, 1977.
20. Hall, J. G., Dorst, J. P., Taybi, H., Scott, C. I., Langer, L. O., and McKusick, V. A.: Two probable cases of homozygotes for the achondroplasia gene. Birth Defects Orig. Art. Series, 1969, pp. 29–34.
21. Harris, H. A.: Bone Growth in Health and Disease. London, Oxford University Press, 1833, p. 154.
22. Herring, J. A., and Winter, R. B.: Instructional Case. Kyphosis in an achondroplastic dwarf. J. Pediatr. Orthop., 3:250, 1983.
23. Horton, W. A., Rotter, D. L., Scott, C. I., and Hall, J. G.: Standard growth curves for achondroplasia. J. Pediatr., 93:435, 1978.
24. Ilett, S. J.: Achondroplasia (letter). Dev. Med. Child. Neurol., 25:100, 1983.
25. Kaufman, E.: Untersuchungen über die sogenannte foetale Rachitis (Chondro-dystrophie foetalis). Berlin, Reiner, 1892.
26. Kelly, T. E.: Probable case of achondroplasia-hypochondroplasia compound. Birth Defects, 10:360, 1974.
27. Kieny, M., and Abbott, U. K.: L'extrait d'embryon diplopode inhibe la croissance des ébauches cartilagineuses normales cultivées in vitro. C. R. Acad. Sci., 254:1520, 1962.
28. Konyukhov, B. V., and Paschin, Y. V.: Experimental study of the achondroplasia gene effects in the mouse. Acta Biol. Hung., 18:285, 1967.
29. Kopits, S. E.: Orthopedic implication of dwarfism. Clin. Orthop., 114:153, 1976.
30. Kopits, S. E.: Genetics clinics of The Johns Hopkins Hospital. Surgical intervention in achondroplasia. Correction of bowleg deformity in achondroplasia. Johns Hopkins Med. J., 146:206, 1980.
31. Langer, L. O., Jr., Baumann, P. A., and Gorlin, R. J.: Achondroplasia. A.J.R., 100:12, 1967.
32. Larson, S. E., Ray, R. D., and Kuettner, K. E.: Microchemical studies on acid glycosaminoglycans of the epiphyseal zones during enchondral calcification. Calcif. Tissue Res., 13:271, 1973.
33. Lefèbvre, J., Errara, A., and Chaurey, M.: Note préliminaire sur la mesure des distances interpédiculaires vertébrales chez l'enfant. J. Radiol. Electrol., 39:229, 1958.
34. Lutter, L. D., and Langer, L. O.: Neurological symptoms in achondroplastic dwarfs—surgical treatment. J. Bone Joint Surg., 59-A:87, 1977.
35. Lutter, L. D., Lonstein, J. E., Winter, R. B., and Langer, L. O.: Anatomy of the achondroplastic lumbar canal. Clin. Orthop., 126:139, 1977.
36. McKusick, V. A., Kelly, T. E., and Dorst, J. P.: Observations suggesting allelism of the achondroplasia and hypochondroplasia genes. J. Med. Genet., 10:11, 1973.
37. Mackler, B., Haynes, B., Inamdar, A. R., Pedegana, L. R., Hall, J. G., and Cohen, M. M., Jr.: Oxidative energy deficiency. II. Human achondroplasia. Arch. Biochem. Biophys., 159:885, 1973.
38. Marie, P.: L'achondroplasie dans l'adolescence et l'age adult. Presse Méd., 8:17, 1900.
39. Maroteaux, P., and Lamy, M.: Achondroplasia in man and animals. Clin. Orthop., 33:91, 1964.
40. Maynard, J. A., Ippolito, E. G., Ponseti, I. V., and Mickelson, M. R.: Histochemistry and ultrastructure of the growth plate in achondroplasia. J. Bone Joint Surg., 63-A:909, 1981.
41. Morch, E. T.: Chondrodystrophic Dwarfs in Denmark. Copenhagen, Munksgaard, 1941.
42. Morgan, D. F., and Young, R. F.: Spinal neurological complication of achondroplasia. Results of surgical treatment. Neurosurgery, 52:463, 1980.
43. Murdoch, J. L., Walker, B. A., Hall, J. G., Abbey, H., Smith, K. K., and McKusick, V. A.: Achondroplasia: A genetic and statistical survey. Ann. Hum. Genet., 33:227, 1970.
44. Nehme, A.-M. E., Riseborough, E. J., and Tredwell, S. J.: Skeletal growth and development of the achondroplastic dwarf. Clin. Orthop., 116:8, 1976.
45. Nelson, M. A.: Orthopaedic aspects of the chondrodystrophies. The dwarf and his orthopaedic problems. Ann. R. Coll. Surg., 47:185, 1970.
46. Nelson, M. A.: Spinal stenosis in achondroplasia. Proc. R. Soc. Med., 65:1028, 1972.
47. Oberklaid, F., Danks, D. M., Jensen, F., Stace, L., and Rosshandler, S.: Achondroplasia and hypochondroplasia: Comments on frequency, mutation rate, and radiological features in skull and spine. J. Med. Genet., 16:140, 1979.
48. Ozer, F. L.: Achondroplasia with spinal neurologic complications in mother and son: Case report. Birth Defects, 10:351, 1974.
49. Parrot, M. J.: Sur la malformation achondroplasique et le dieu Ptah. Bull. Soc. Anthropol. Paris, 1:296, 1878.
50. Pedrini-Mille, A., and Pedrini, V.: Studies of human iliac crest cartilage. III. Proteinpolysaccharides in human achondroplasia. Calcif. Tissue Res., 8:106, 1971.
51. Pedrini-Mille, A., and Pedrini, V.: Proteoglycans and glycosaminoglycans of human achondroplastic cartilage. J. Bone Joint Surg., 64-A:39, 1982.
52. Pfluger, W.: Leg lengthening in systemic skeletal disorders. Orthopaede, 6:16, 1977.

53. Ponseti, I. V.: Skeletal growth in achondroplasia. J. Bone Joint Surg., 52-A:701, 1970.
54. Porak, C., and Durante, G.: Les micromélies congénitales. Achondroplasie vraie et dystrophie periostale. Nouv. Iconogr. Salpet., 18:481, 1905.
55. Porter, R. W., Wicks, M., and Ottewell, D.: Measurement of the spinal canal by diagnostic ultrasound. J. Bone Joint Surg., 60-B:481, 1978.
56. Ravenna, F.: Achondroplasie et chondrohypoplasie. Contribution clinique. Nouv. Iconogr. Salpet., 26:157, 1913.
57. Rimoin, D. L.: Variable expressivity in the skeletal dysplasia. Birth Defects, 15:91, 1979.
58. Rimoin, D. L., Hughes, G. N., Kaufman, R. L., Rosenthal, R. E., McAlister, W. H., and Silverberg, R.: Endochondral ossification in achondroplastic dwarfism. N. Engl. J. Med., 283:728, 1970.
59. Rischbieth, H., and Barrington, A.: Dwarfism. Treas. Hum. Inher., VII–VIII:355, 1912.
60. Schergna, E., Saia, A., and Trevisan, C.: Achondroplasia is also a neurologic disease. Riv. Neurol., 50:212, 1980.
61. Schreiber, F., and Rosenthal, H.: Paraplegia from ruptured lumbar discs in achondroplastic dwarfs. J. Neurosurg., 9:648, 1952.
62. Shepard, T. H., and Bass, G. L.: Organ-culture studies of achondroplastic rabbit cartilage: Evidence for a metabolic defect in glucose utilization. J. Embryol. Exp. Morphol., 25:347, 1971.
63. Shepard, T. H., Fry, L. R., and Moffett, B. C., Jr.: Microscopic studies of achondroplastic rabbit cartilage. Teratology, 2:13, 1969.
64. Silberberg, R., Hasler, M., and Lesker, P.: Ultrastructure of articular cartilage of achondroplastic mice. Acta Anat., 96:162, 1976.
65. Silverman, F. N.: A differential diagnosis of achondroplasia. Radiol. Clin. North Am., 6:223, 1968.
66. Stanescu, V., Stanescu, R., and Maroteaux, P.: Etude morphologique et biochimique du cartilage de croissance dans les ostéochondrodysplasies. Arch. Fr. Pediatr., 34 (Suppl. 1):1–80, 1977.
67. Stanescu, V., Stanescu, R., and Szirmai, J. A.: Microbiochemical analysis of the human tibial growth cartilage in various forms of dwarfism. Acta Endocrinol., 69:659, 1972.
68. Stevenson, A. C.: Achondroplasia: An account of the condition in Northern Ireland. Am. J. Hum. Genet., 9:81, 1957.
69. Stokes, D. C., Phillips, J. A., Leonard, C. O., Dorst, J. P., Kopits, S. E., Trojak, J. E., and Brown, D. L.: Respiratory complications of achondroplasia. J. Pediatr., 102:534, 1983.
70. Todorov, A. B., Scott, C. I., Jr., Warren, A. E., and Leeper, J. D.: Developmental screening tests in achondroplastic children. Am. J. Med. Genet., 9:19, 1981.
71. Werner, A.: Compression de la queue de cheval dans l'achondroplasie. A propos de deux observations personnelles. Praxis, 53:374, 1964.
72. Winkielman, J., and Radelicka-Rajszys, H.: Achondroplasia. Pol. Przegl. Radiol., 45:267, 1981.
73. Wise, B. L.: Hydrocephalus in achondroplasia (letter). J. Neurosurg., 55:662, 1981.
74. Wynne-Davies, R., Walsh, W. K., and Gormley, J.: Achondroplasia and hypochondroplasia. Clinical variation and spinal stenosis. J. Bone Joint Surg., 63-B:508, 1981.

HYPOCHONDROPLASIA

Hypochondroplasia is a mild form of achondroplasia with much less severe changes, particularly in skull, pelvis, and vertebral column.[1–14]

It was first recognized as an entity in 1913 by Ravenna, who used the term *hypochondroplasia*.[11] Lamy and Maroteaux described the features of the disease in full detail in 1961.[6] Hypochondroplasia is inherited as an autosomal dominant trait; genetically, it is distinct and separate from achondroplasia. The true frequency is unknown, many cases being undiagnosed because of their mild clinical picture. It appears to be relatively common, its prevalence similar to that of achondroplasia—probably three or four per million.[13, 14] Both sexes are equally affected.

Clinical Features

The condition cannot be detected at birth or in infancy. The short stature becomes apparent when the child is five to six years of age. Shortness is the presenting complaint; the general appearance of the affected individuals in early childhood is rather normal. As the child matures, skeletal disproportion with mild rhizomelia becomes obvious. Soon flexion deformity of the elbows and knees develops, and ligamentous hyperlaxity and genu varum are common. Exaggeration of lumbar lordosis and prominence of the buttocks are mild. The facies and hands are normal. Intelligence is normal.

Radiographic Findings

In general, these are similar to achondroplasia, but of much less severity. The tubular bones are short and broad. In hypochondroplasia, the skull, pelvis, and hands are essentially normal. There may be slight enlargement of the frontal region of the calvarium and minimal decrease in size of the greater sciatic notch. The vertebral column is normal except for minimal decrease in interpedicular distance in the lumbar spine. Occasionally the vertebral pedicles are short. Posterior concavity of vertebral bodies is very rare.

Height at skeletal maturity is between 127 and 150 cm. (4 feet 2 inches to 5 feet). Life expectancy is normal, and usually there are no disabling symptoms. Orthopedic treatment is usually not required except for occasional correction of tibia vara. There are few complications, although occasionally neurologic symptoms due to spinal stenosis may develop.

References

1. Beals, R. K.: Hypochondroplasia. J. Bone Joint Surg., 51-A:728, 1969.
2. Glasgow, J. F. T., Nevin, N. C., and Thomas, P. S.: Hypochondroplasia. Arch. Dis. Child., 53:868, 1978.
3. Hall, J. G.: Hypochondroplasia. Birth Defects Orig. Art. Series, 5:267, 1969.
4. Heselson, N. G., Cremin, B. J., and Beighton, P.: The radiographic manifestations of hypochondroplasia. Clin. Radiol., 30:79, 1979.

5. Kozlowski, K., and Zychowicz, C.: Hypochondroplasie (ein weiterer Beitrag). Fortschr. Rontgenstr., *101*:531, 1964.
6. Lamy, M., and Maroteaux, P.: Les chondrodystrophies génotypiques. Paris, L'Expansion Scientifique Française, 1961.
7. Leri, A., and Linossier, Mlle.: Hypochondroplasie héréditaire. Bull Soc. Méd. Hôp. Paris, *48*:1780, 1924.
8. McKusick, V. A., Kelly, T. E., and Dorst, J. P.: Observations suggesting allelism of the achondroplasia and hypochondroplasia genes. J. Med. Genet., *10*:11, 1973.
9. Meerson, E. M., Iukina, G. P., and Nechvolodova, O. L.: The clinical, diagnostic and genetic aspects of study of hypochondroplasia. Ortop. Travmatol. Protez., 9:40, 1976.
10. Oberklaid, F., Danks, D. M., Jensen, F., Stace, L., and Rosshandler, S.: Achondroplasia and hypochondroplasia. Comments on frequency, mutation rate, and radiologic features in the skull and spine. J. Med. Genet., *16*:140, 1979.
11. Ravenna, F.: Achondroplasie et chondrohypoplasie. Nouv. Iconogr. Saltpetr., *26*:157, 1913.
12. Walker, B. A., Murdoch, J. L., McKusick, V. A., Langer, L. O., and Beals, R. K.: Hypochondroplasia. Am. J. Dis. Child., *122*:95, 1971.
13. Wynne-Davies, R., Gormley, J., and Walsh, K.: Clinical variation and spinal stenosis in achondroplasia and hypochondroplasia. J. Bone Joint Surg., *63-B*:508, 1981.
14. Wynne-Davies, R., Hall, C. M., and Apley, A. G.: Atlas of Skeletal Dysplasia. Edinburgh, Churchill-Livingstone, 1985, pp. 200–212.

LETHAL FORMS OF SHORT-LIMBED DWARFISM

These rare bone dysplasia with predominant metaphyseal involvement include *thanatophoric dwarfism*, which is characterized by a large head, very short limbs, and a narrow thorax with short horizontal ribs; *short-rib polydactyly syndromes*, such as Saldino-Noonan, Majewski, and Naumoff; and *achondrogenesis* with marked defective ossification (Fig. 3–18). These children die shortly after birth because of respiratory failure. There are no orthopedic implications. These chondrodysplasias are discussed in detail by Maroteaux and associates.[1]

Reference

1. Maroteaux, P., Stanescu, V., and Stanescu, R.: The lethal chondrodysplasias. Clin. Orthop., *114*:31, 1976.

CHONDROECTODERMAL DYSPLASIA (ELLIS–VAN CREVELD SYNDROME)

This syndrome was originally described in 1940 by Ellis and van Creveld, who reported on three cases, two of which were personal cases.[6] In 1962, Ellis and Andrew reviewed 40 previously reported cases and added two cases of their own.[5]

The mode of inheritance is autosomal recessive. There is a high incidence of consanguinity in the parents, and Ellis–van Creveld syndrome has been reported in identical twins.[11] This dysplasia is extremely rare, with a prevalence of under 0.1 per million.

Clinical Features

Salient components of the syndrome are chondrodysplasia; polydactyly; ectodermal dysplasia affecting the hair, teeth, and nails; and congenital heart disease (Fig. 3–19). Both mesodermal and ectodermal tissues are affected. The clinical features are present at birth, becoming more manifest with growth and maturation.

Chondrodysplasia. Manifest as progressive shortening of the long bones of the upper and lower limbs, chondrodysplasia typically affects the distal segment to a greater degree than it does the proximal one; i.e., the shortening is greater in the bones distal to the knees and elbows. The trunk is of normal height and shape for the patient's age. Lack of stature is primarily due to the shortness of the lower legs. The relative shortening of the tibia and fibula, as well as of the radius and ulna, is unequal. The head of the radius may be dislocated.

The proximal end of the tibia is widened and pointed.[3, 5, 6, 8] The ossification center of the proximal tibial epiphysis is hypoplastic and is displaced medially to lie opposite the shorter medial slope (Fig. 3–20 G and H). This results in severe genu valgum in most patients in adolescence. There may be an exostosis projecting from the medial aspect of the proximal tibial metaphysis.

The fibula is disproportionately short in relation to the tibia—in contrast to classic achondroplasia, in which the fibula is the bone least affected and is relatively long. Genu valgum is often present, as may be lateral subluxation or dislocation of the patella.

In both the upper and lower limbs, the long tubular bones are progressively shorter centrifugally from the spine toward the fingers and toes; the pattern of limb shortening is the converse of that seen in achondroplasia. The greatest shortening is found in the phalanges. Ossification centers of the distal phalanges may be absent. Often there is fusion of two or more of the carpal and tarsal bones. There may be an accessory carpal bone associated with the polydactyly.

The femora and humeri are often bowed, as well as shortened and thickened. The spine is normal. The ribs are short, and the thorax is long and narrow. The pelvis is distinctive; the iliac bones are small, with a decrease in their longitudinal measurement. In the region of the

Text continued on page 736

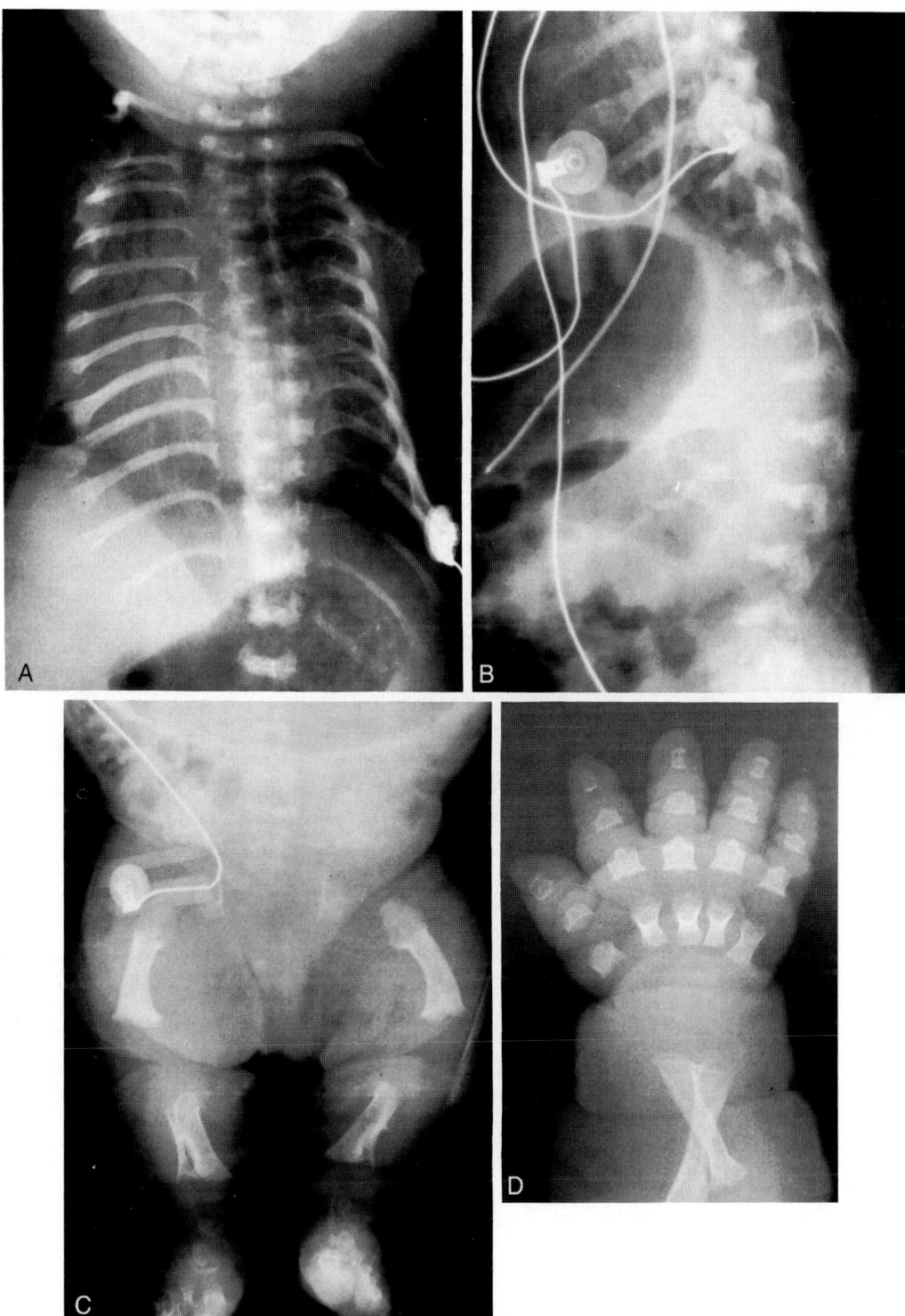

FIGURE 3–18. Thanatophoric dwarfism characterized by a large head, very short limbs, and a narrow thorax.

A and **B.** Anteroposterior and lateral views of the thorax. Note the short horizontal ribs and the platyspondyly with notched end-plates. **C.** Anteroposterior view of the femora and tibiae. The long bones are shortened and bowed. The femora are shaped like telephone receivers. **D.** Anteroposterior view of the right hand including the forearm. Note the short, broad phalanges, metacarpals, radius, and ulna.

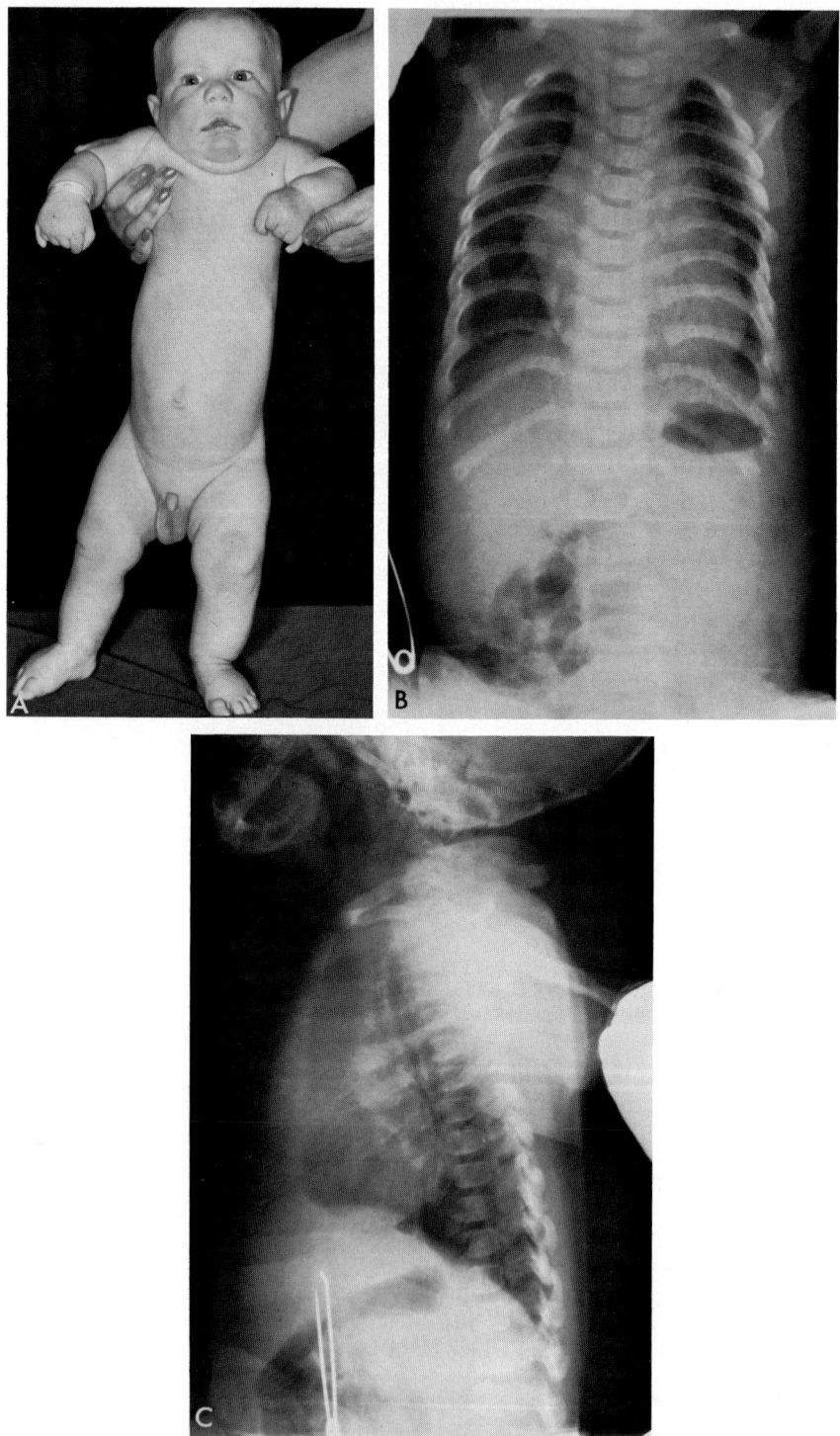

FIGURE 3–19. Ellis–van Creveld syndrome *(chondroectodermal dysplasia)* in a nine-month-old infant.

A. Clinical appearance. **B** and **C.** Radiograms of spine.

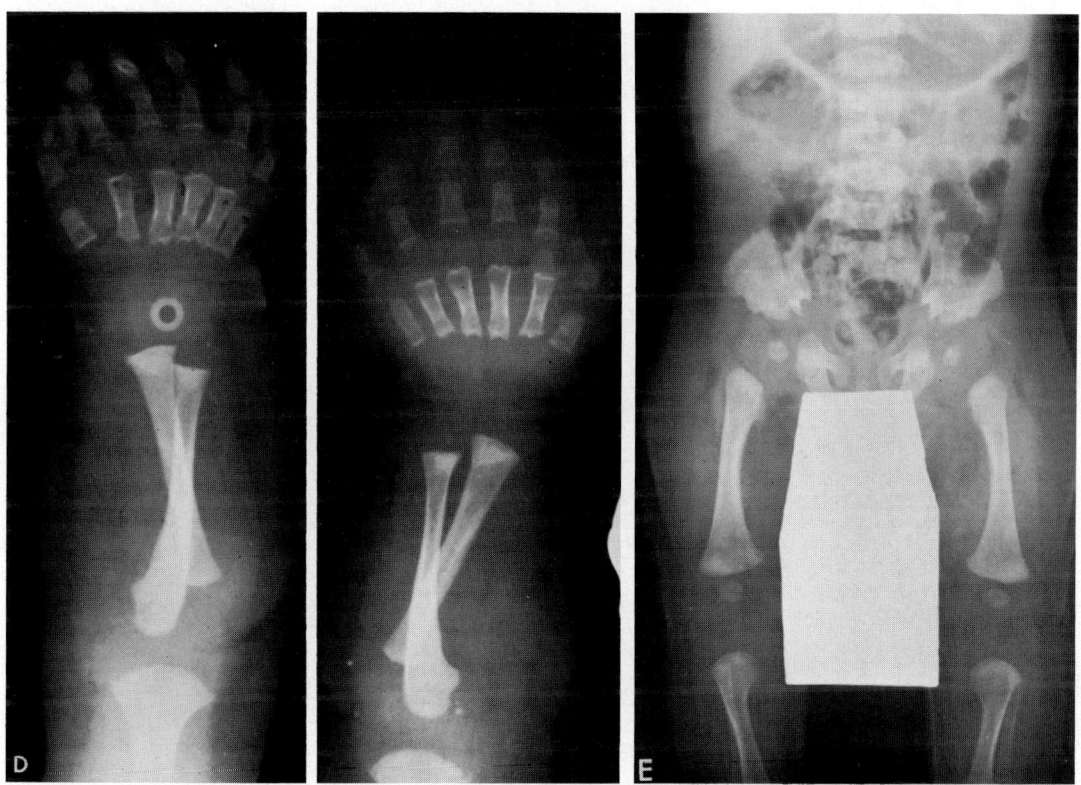

FIGURE 3–19 Continued. Ellis–van Creveld syndrome (chondroectodermal dysplasia) in a nine-month-old infant.
D. Anteroposterior radiograms of hands and forearm and **E,** of pelvis and lower limbs.

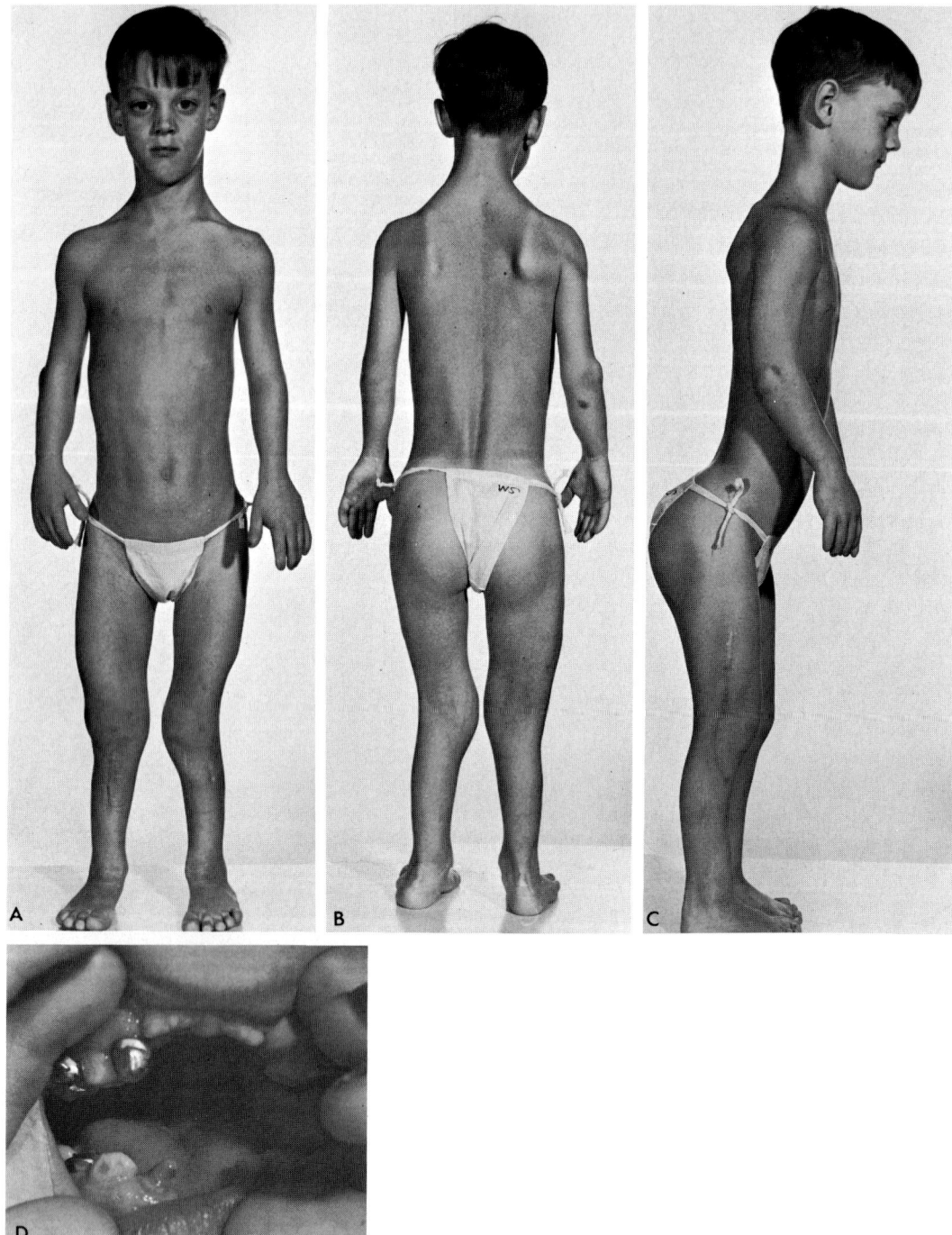

FIGURE 3–20. Ellis–van Creveld syndrome (chondroectodermal dysplasia) in a ten-year-old boy.

A to **C.** Characteristic clinical picture (see text for description). The extra toes and fingers were amputated at an early age. Bilateral osteotomies of the tibia and fibula were performed to correct genu valgum. **D.** The teeth are pointed, dystrophic, or absent.

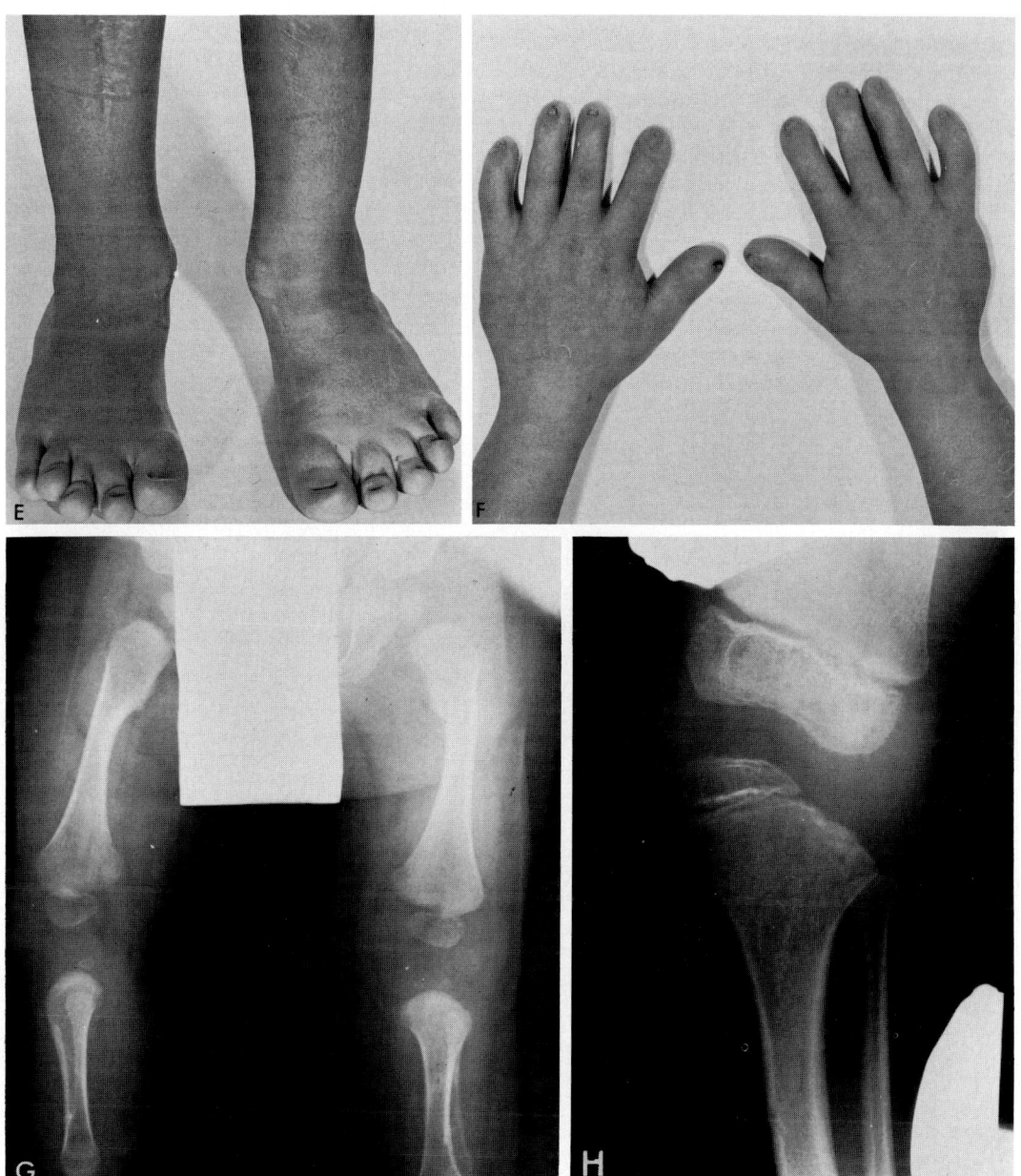

FIGURE 3–20 Continued. *Ellis–van Creveld syndrome (chondroectodermal dysplasia) in a ten-year-old boy.*

E and **F.** The nails are small, hypoplastic, and dystrophic and tend to be spoon-shaped. **G.** Anteroposterior radiograms of lower limbs, showing the shortened and thickened long bones. The fibula is disproportionately short in relation to the tibia. **H.** The proximal end of the tibia is widened and pointed. Note the genu valgum and slope of the tibial plateau. The hypoplastic proximal tibial epiphysis is displaced medially.

triradiate cartilage there is sometimes an inferiorly directed hook. The abnormal appearance of the pelvis gradually changes to normal with skeletal maturation. The skull and facies do not display any of the characteristics of classic achondroplasia.

Polydactyly. Polydactyly of the hands is invariably present (Fig. 3–19 A). The sixth and seventh digits are often on the ulnar side, although they may be on the radial side. Polydactyly of the feet occurs less frequently than that of the hands.

Ectodermal Dysplasia. The nails are small, hypoplastic, and dystrophic, and tend to be "spoon-shaped," the dorsal aspect being concave (Fig. 3–20 E and F). The teeth may be pointed, dystrophic, or absent (Fig. 3–20 D). Fusion of the maxillary gum pad may cause obliteration of the gingivolabial sulcus by the upper lip.

Congenital Heart Disease. A part of the complete syndrome, this is not a constant feature of the tetrad of symptoms (present in 22 of 38 patients). Often the lesion is an interatrial or interventricular septal defect, or may involve both. The heart may be trilocular or bilocular.[9, 10, 16, 37]

In the great majority of patients affected with the Ellis–van Creveld syndrome, intelligence is normal, although retardation has been reported in some cases. In individual cases, a variety of associated anomalies such as undescended testes and cleft palate have been described.

Treatment

The heart anomalies are treated by appropriate cardiac surgery. These require priority of treatment, as the cardiac complications may be lethal if untreated.

The accessory digits of the hands and feet are excised during the first two years of life. When genu valgum is severe, support of the limb with an above-knee knock-knee orthosis is indicated. If the valgus deformity is progressive, a varus osteotomy is performed. Parents should be warned that, because of asymmetrical growth, the deformity may recur and repeated operative measures may be required. At present this author recommends the Ilizarov technique for simultaneous correction of the valgus deformity at the knees and lengthening of the short femur and tibia. If there is dislocation of the patella, the quadriceps mechanism has to be realigned.

References

1. Aird, C., and McIntosh, R. A.: Shakespeare's Richard III and the Ellis–van Creveld syndrome. Practitioner, 220:656, 1978.
2. Blackburn, M. G., and Belliveau, R. E.: Ellis–van Creveld syndrome. A report of previously undescribed anomalies in two siblings. Am. J. Dis. Child., 122:267, 1971.
3. Caffey, J.: Chondroectodermal dysplasia (Ellis–van Creveld syndrome): Report of three cases. A.J.R., 68:875, 1952.
4. DaSilva, E. O., Janovitz, D., and DeAlbuquerque, S. C.: Ellis–van Creveld syndrome: Report of 15 cases in an inbred kindred. J. Med. Genet., 17:349, 1980.
5. Ellis, R. W. B., and Andrew, J. D.: Chondroectodermal dysplasia. J. Bone Joint Surg., 44-B:626, 1962.
6. Ellis, R. W. B., and van Creveld, S.: Syndrome characterized by ectodermal dysplasia, polydactyly, chondro-dysplasia and congenital morbus cordis: Report of three cases. Arch. Dis. Child., 15:65, 1940.
7. Engle, M. A., and Ehlers, K. H.: Ellis–van Creveld syndrome with asymmetric polydactyly and successful surgical correction of common atrium. Birth Defects, 5:65, 1969.
8. Ferrero, N. A., Pozo, O. O., and Morresi, E. S.: Chondroectodermal dysplasia (Ellis–van Creveld syndrome). Report of a case and review of the literature. J. Bone Joint Surg., 43-A:1230, 1961.
9. Franz, C., Mennicken, U., Butzler, H. O., and Henscher, L.: Angeborene Herzfehler beim Ellis–van Creveld syndrome. Literaturanalyse und Bericht über eine eigene Beobachtung. Z. Kinderheilkd., 117:127, 1974.
10. Giknis, F. L.: Single atrium and the Ellis–van Creveld syndrome. J. Pediatr., 62:558, 1963.
11. Goor, D., Rotem, Y., Friedman, A., and Neufeld, H. N.: Ellis–van Creveld syndrome in identical twins. Br. Heart J., 27:797, 1965.
12. Hill, R. D.: Two cases of Ellis–van Creveld syndrome in a small island population. J. Med. Genet., 14:33, 1977.
13. Kaufman, H. J.: The pelvis in the Ellis–van Creveld syndrome. Ann. Radiol., 8:146, 1965.
14. Kozlowski, K., Szmigiel, C., Barylak, A., and Stopyrowa, M.: Difficulties in differentiation between chondroectodermal dysplasia (Ellis–van Creveld syndrome) and asphyxiating thoracic dystrophy. Aust. Radiol., 16:401, 1972.
15. Kushnick, T., Paya, K., and Mamunes, P.: Chondroectodermal dysplasia. Ellis–van Creveld syndrome. Am. J. Dis. Child., 103:77, 1962.
16. Lynch, J. I., Perry, L. W., Takakuwa, T., and Scott, L. P.: Congenital heart disease and chondroectodermal dysplasia. Report of two cases, one in a Negro. Am. J. Dis. Child., 115:80, 1968.
17. McKusick, V. A., Egeland, J. A., Eldridge, R., and Krusen, D. E.: Dwarfism in the Amish. The Ellis–van Creveld syndrome. Bull. Johns Hopkins Hosp., 115:306, 1964.
18. Mahoney, M. J., and Hobbins, J. C.: Prenatal diagnosis of chondroectodermal dysplasia (Ellis–van Creveld syndrome) with fetoscopy and ultrasound. N. Engl. J. Med., 297:258, 1977.
19. Milgram, J. W., and Bailey, J. A., II: Orthopaedic aspects of the Ellis–van Creveld syndrome. Bull. Hosp. Joint Dis., 36:11, 1975.
20. Moore, T. C.: Chondroectodermal dysplasia (Ellis–van Creveld syndrome) with bronchial malformation and neonatal tension lobar emphysema. J. Thorac. Cardiovasc. Surg., 46:1, 1963.
21. Murdoch, J. L., and Walker, B. A.: Ellis–van Creveld syndrome. Birth Defects Orig. Art. Series, 5: Part 4:279, 1968.
22. Neiman, N., Pierson, M., Vidailhet, M., Worms, A. M., Plenat, F., and Fortier, G.: Le syndrome d'Ellis–van Creveld et ses rapports avec la dystrophie thoracique asphyxiante. A propos de 3 nouveaux cas chez le nourrisson. Pediatrie, 28:253, 1973.
23. Poznanski, A. K., Stern, A. M., and Gall, J. C., Jr.:

Skeletal anomalies in genetically determined congenital heart disease. Radiol. Clin. North Am., 9:435, 1971.
24. Renier, J. C., Larget-Piet, L., Boasson, M., Berthelot, J., and Fouillet, J. J.: Dysplasie chondro-ectodermique d'Ellis–van Creveld: Deux cas dans une même fratrie. Rev. Rhumat., 42:417, 1975.
25. Rosenberg, S., Carneiro, P. C., Zerbini, M. C. N., and Gonzalez, C. H.: Brief clinical report: Chondroectodermal dysplasia (Ellis–van Creveld) with anomalies of CNS and urinary tract. Am. J. Med. Genet., 15:291, 1983.
26. Smith, H. L., and Hand, A. M.: Chondroectodermal dysplasia (Ellis–van Creveld syndrome). Report of two cases. Pediatrics, 21:298, 1958.
27. Taylor, G. A., Jordan, C. E., Dorst, S. K., and Dorst, J. P.: Polycarpaly and other abnormalities of the wrist in chondroectodermal dysplasia: The Ellis–van Creveld syndrome. Radiology, 151:393, 1984.
28. Waldrigues, A., Grohmann, L. C., Takahashi, T., and Reis, H. M.: Ellis–van Creveld syndrome. An inbred kindred with five cases. Rev. Bras. Pesqui. Med. Biol., 10:193, 1977.

ASPHYXIATING THORACIC DYSPLASIA (JEUNE'S DISEASE)

In asphyxiating thoracic dystrophy, described by Jeune and associates in 1954, the thoracic cage is long, narrow, and cylindrical with both the anteroposterior and transverse diameters being markedly decreased. The limbs are short, and there may be associated postaxial polydactyly or cone epiphyses in the hands and feet with premature fusion (Fig. 3–21). Inheritance is as an autosomal recessive trait.

With intensive pulmonary care, these infants may survive the respiratory problems, but may, later on in adolescence or adult life, develop renal failure.

References

1. Jeune, M., Carron, R., Beraud, C., and Loaec, Y.: Polychondrodystrophie avec blocage thoracic d'évolution fatale. Pediatrie (Lyon), 9:390, 1954.
2. Oberklaid, F., Danks, D. M., Mayne, V., and Campbell, P.: Asphyxiating thoracic dysplasia. Arch. Dis. Child., 52:758, 1977.

METAPHYSEAL CHONDRODYSPLASIA

Metaphyseal chondrodysplasia is an extremely rare disease of the skeletal system in which dwarfism similar to that seen in achondroplasia is noted. This is caused chiefly by improper mineralization of the shafts of bones in the metaphyseal region, resulting in knobby segments of proliferating cartilage. Various clinical types have been differentiated, and an increasing number of varieties are being reported. It is beyond the scope of this book to attempt a comprehensive description of these disorders; only the well-known syndromes are presented. The disorder has been subclassified into four types, according to the degree of severity and the genetic mode of transmission.

Jansen Type. This is the most severe type and is extremely rare; its probable prevalence is less than 0.1 per million.[9, 14, 16, 18] Inheritance is most probably by an autosomal dominant trait; sporadic cases do occur. The disorder is usually apparent at birth because of the severe short stature (primarily due to shortness of the limbs and of their distal segments), the widely spaced exophthalmic eyes, and the prominence of the superciliary arches. The limb bones, especially the forearms and legs, are very short; they tend to develop angular deformity at the diaphyseal-metaphyseal junction, particularly in the weight-bearing lower limb bones. The striking finding in the radiogram is the bulbous expansion of the metaphyses of the long bones. The metaphyses are irregularly mottled and fragmented. The epiphyses are normal but delayed in appearance and markedly separated from the metaphyses because of the widened physes. The hands and feet are involved. The metacarpals and metatarsals show cupping with dense sclerotic bone on the side of the metaphysis.

Schmid Type. More common and much less severe, this type is often mistaken for achondroplasia.[9, 34, 43] It is characterized by predominant involvement of the proximal femora and moderate shortness of stature. Skeletal changes are not present at birth, but develop with weight-bearing at three to five years of age. Inheritance of this type is by the autosomal dominant mode. Again, the epiphyses are normal; the skull, spine, thorax, and pelvis remain unaffected. Growth of long bones is inhibited, and dwarfing is moderate. Progressive coxa vara with a tendency toward slipping of the capital femoral epiphyses, lateral bowing of the femora, and genu varum with a waddling gait are frequent. Severity of involvement varies and may be asymmetrical. Radiograms show splaying, irregularity, and cupping of the metaphyses similar to those in vitamin D–refractory rickets (Fig. 3–22). The condition cannot always be clearly differentiated; in metaphyseal chondrodysplasia, however, kidney function and serum chemistry are normal. The proximal femoral metaphysis is irregular, mottled, and splayed with medial beaking. The femoral neck-shaft angle is decreased, and in severe coxa vara there is an isolated triangular bone fragment on the inferior aspect of the femoral neck.

Spahr-Hartmann Type. This form of metaphyseal dysplasia is of autosomal recessive ori-

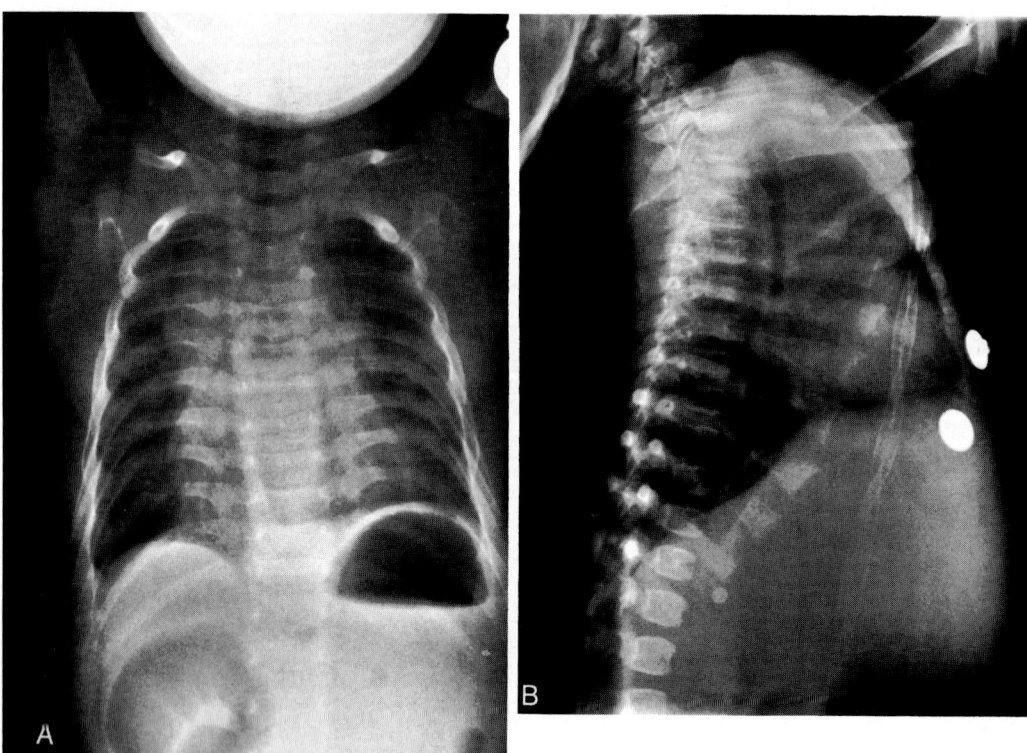
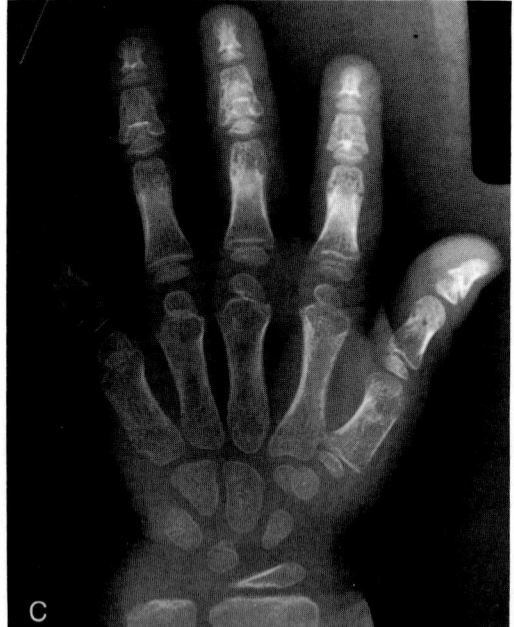

FIGURE 3-21. *Asphyxiating thoracic dysplasia.*

Jeune's disease. Radiographic findings in asphyxiating thoracic dysplasia. **A** and **B.** Anteroposterior and lateral radiograms of the chest. Note the long, narrow thoracic cage. **C.** Anteroposterior view of the hand showing the cone epiphyses of the phalanges with premature fusion of the physes.

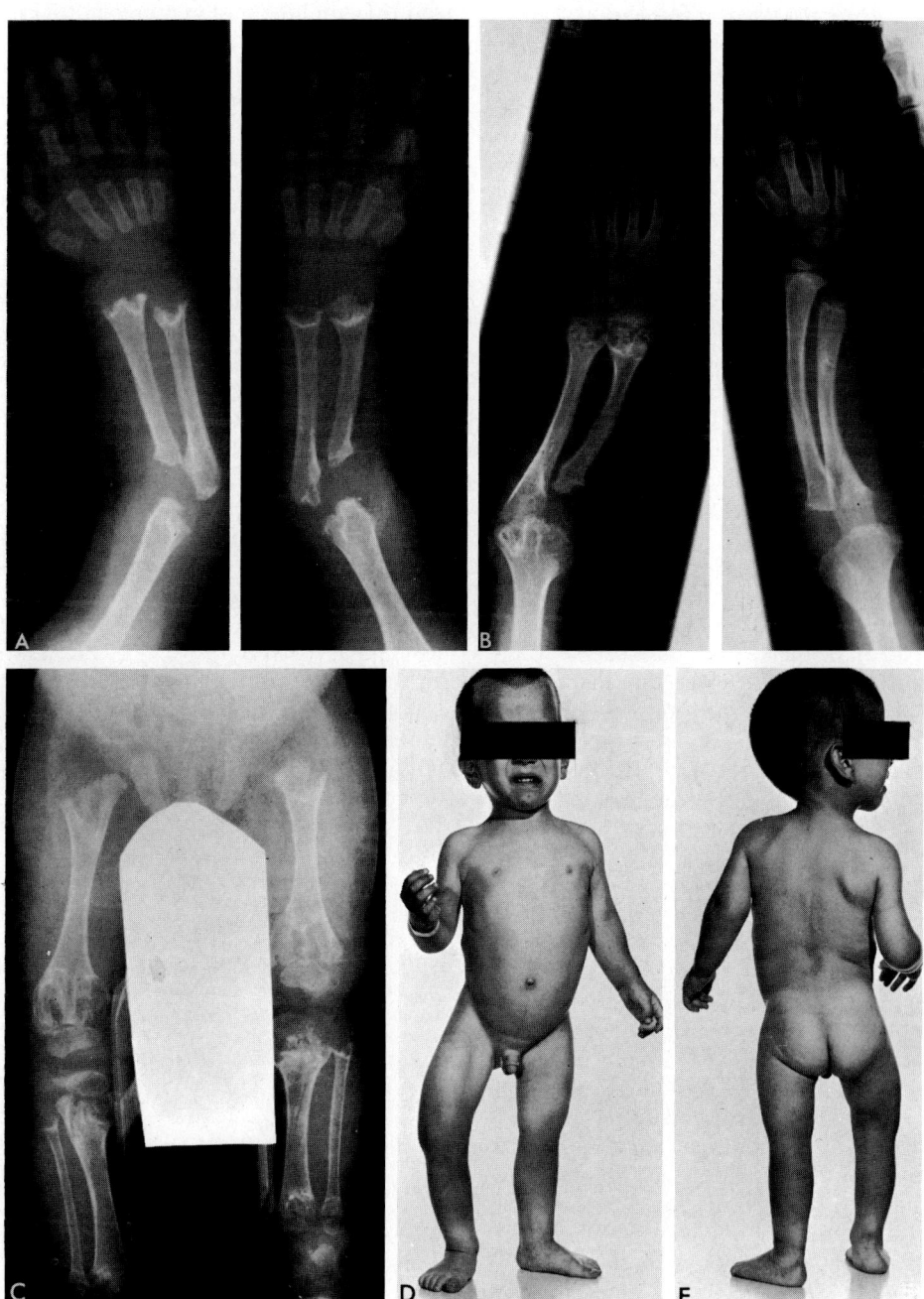

FIGURE 3-22. Metaphyseal chondrodysplasia (Schmid type).

A. Anteroposterior radiograms of both upper limbs at six months of age. The widening, cupping, and irregularity of the zone of provisional calcification at the metaphyseal ends is evident. This is often confused with rickets. **B.** Anteroposterior radiogram of both upper limbs at three years of age. **C.** Anteroposterior radiogram of the femora and tibiae at one year. The ossific nuclei of the distal femur and the proximal and distal tibia have calcified and are normal in appearance. The metaphyseal changes are characteristic. The left femur is short. An arthrogram of the left hip disclosed a cartilaginous anlage of the femoral head located in the acetabular socket. **D** and **E.** Clinical appearance of the patient. Shortening of the left lower limb is evident. The metaphyses of long bones are knobby.

gin, and severe bowlegs is the principal clinical finding.[37]

Cartilage-Hair Hypoplasia (McKusick Type). This chondrodysplasia is caused by a recessive gene.[25] The presence of fine, sparse, short, and brittle hair is a distinguishing feature. The eyelashes and eyebrows are also affected. An associated finding is excessive joint laxity. Radiographic findings somewhat resemble those of the Schmid type, but in the Schmid type the proximal femora are primarily involved and inheritance is by autosomal dominant transmission. Ankle deformity is caused by unusual length of the fibula. The hindfoot is in varus, but the midfoot and forefoot are in valgus. Shortened digits and hyperextensibility of the wrists and fingers may be noted. Extension of the elbow is limited. Dwarfing may be marked, an abnormally high upper segment to lower segment ratio giving an achondroplastic appearance. The range of stature is 105 to 157 cm. (3'5" to 5'2"). The epiphyses are normal. The skull has some tendency to brachycephaly with large fontanelles. Odontoid hypoplasia is sometimes present. In the lateral view of the spine the vertebral bodies are oval, the shape persisting into childhood. In the thorax the anterior ends of the ribs are widened with cupping. The sternum may be tilted forward. In the hands the metaphyses of the phalanges are cup-shaped, and the epiphyses may be delta-shaped.

Variations of the Disorder. Metaphyseal chondrodysplasia may be associated with pancreatic exocrine insufficiency, intestinal malabsorption, Hirschsprung's disease, and chronic neutropenia and lymphopenia. The immune deficiency can be serious; smallpox vaccination has been fatal, and reaction to varicella infection may be ominous.[33, 40] Kozlowski described a disorder with only a very mild form of metaphyseal chondrodysplasia and slight shortness of stature.[20] Maroteaux and associates reported a type similar to the Schmid type but in which not every metaphysis is involved.[27] Vaandrager described a form of metaphyseal chondrodysplasia in which the ossification defects were maximal in the metaphysis but extended for some distance into the diaphysis.[41] Pena reported a form in which all the metaphyses were affected with irregular ossification defects extending into the diaphysis and associated with dwarfism, scoliosis, and defective ossification or platyspondyly of the cervical spine.[30] Wiedemann and Spranger described a form of metaphyseal chondrodysplasia similar to the Schmid type with the exception that the hands and feet were normal; with growth, the dysplasia improved.[46]

In all these types, intelligence remains unimpaired. Radiographic findings are characterized by widening and cupping and an irregular zone of provisional calcification at the metaphyseal ends of the tubular bones. These changes in the growing ends of the bone resemble rickets. The diaphysis and epiphyseal centers of ossification, however, are normal.

Treatment

There is no specific therapy. Management is symptomatic. Supportive orthotic devices may relieve the stresses of body weight when deformity is very severe.

In the Schmid type, progressive coxa vara and tibia vara are deformities that require correction by valgus osteotomy—intertrochanteric or subtrochanteric in the proximal femur and in the diaphyseal-metaphyseal region in the upper tibia. In metaphyseal chondrodysplasia there is a primary growth abnormality, and the deformities tend to recur after surgery, requiring repeat osteotomy. The foot deformities, particularly varus hindfoot, may require surgical correction by lateral displacement osteotomy of the calcaneus. Excessive joint laxity is a problem; prior to foot surgery, stability of the ankle joint should be assessed.

References

1. Allemand, P.: A propos de deux cas d'une forme particulière de dysostose métaphysaire comportant des modifications des phanères et obéissant à un mode de transmission recessif autosomique. Thèse Méd., Paris, 1966.
2. Arroyo-Scotoliff, H.: Metaphyseal dysostosis, Jansen type. J. Bone Joint Surg., 55-A:623, 1973.
3. Beals, R. K.: Cartilage-hair hypoplasia. A case report. J. Bone Joint Surg., 50-A:1245, 1968.
4. Beluffi, G., Fiori, P., Notarangelo, C. D., Guarnaccia, S., Bozzola, M., Montanari, C., and Martini, A.: Metaphyseal dysplasia type Schmid. Early x-ray detection and evolution with time. Ann. Radiol. (Paris), 26:237, 1983.
5. Boothby, C. B., and Bower, B. T.: Cartilage-hair hypoplasia. Arch. Dis. Child., 48:918, 1973.
6. Cameron, J. A. P., Young, W. B., and Sissons, H. A.: Metaphyseal dysostosis. J. Bone Joint Surg., 36-B:622, 1954.
7. Cooper, R. R., and Ponseti, I. V.: Metaphyseal dysostosis: Description of an ultrastructural defect in the epiphyseal plate chondrocytes. Case report. J. Bone Joint Surg., 55-A:485, 1973.
8. Cooper, R. R., Pedrini-Mille, A., and Ponseti, I. V.: Metaphyseal dysostosis. A rough surfaced endoplasmic reticulum storage defect. Lab. Invest., 28:119, 1973.
9. Daeschner, C. W., Singleton, E. B., Hill, L. L., and Dodge, W. F.: Metaphyseal dysostosis. J. Pediatr., 57:844, 1960.
10. Dent, C. E., and Normand, I. C. S.: Metaphyseal dysostosis. Type Schmid. Arch. Dis. Child., 39:44, 1964.

11. Evans, R., and Caffey, J.: Metaphyseal dysostosis resembling vitamin D refractory rickets. Am. J. Dis. Child., 95:581, 1958.
12. Goor, M., Sauvage, D., Toursel, F., Farriaux, J. P., and Fontaine, G.: Contribution à l'étude de la dysostose métaphysaire (presentation d'une observation familiale). Rev. Pediatr., 6:531, 1970.
13. Gordan, S. L., Varano, L. A., Alandete, A., and Maisels, M. J.: Jansen's metaphyseal dysostosis. Pediatrics, 58:556, 1976.
14. Gram, P. B., Fleming, J. L., Frame, B., and Fine, G.: Metaphyseal chondrodysplasia of Jansen. J. Bone Joint Surg., 41-A:951, 1959.
15. deHaas, W. H. P., deBoer, W., and Griffioen, F.: Metaphysial dysostosis. J. Bone Joint Surg., 51-B:290, 1969.
16. Jansen, M.: Über atypische Chondrodystrophie (Achondroplasie) und über ein noch nicht beschriebene angeborene Wachsumstörung des Knochensystems: Metaphysäre Dysostosis. Z. Orthop. Chir., 61:253, 1934.
17. Kilburn, P.: A metaphyseal abnormality. Report of a case with features of metaphyseal dysostosis. J. Bone Joint Surg., 55-B:643, 1973.
18. Kiskuchi, S., Hasue, M., and Watanabe, M. F.: Metaphyseal dysostosis (Jansen's type). J. Bone Joint Surg., 58-B:102, 1976.
19. Kozlowski, K.: Metaphyseal dysostosis. Report of five familial and two sporadic cases of a mild type. A.J.R., 91:602, 1964.
20. Kozlowski, K.: Metaphyseal and spondylometaphyseal chondrodysplasias. Clin. Orthop., 114:83, 1976.
21. Kozlowski, K., and Sikorska, B.: Dysplasia metaphysaria, Typ Vaandrager-Pena. Z. Kinderheilkd., 108:165, 1970.
22. Kozlowski, K., and Zychowicz, C.: Metaphyseal dysostosis of mixed type in female child. A.J.R., 88:443, 1962.
23. Lenk, R.: Hereditary metaphyseal dysostosis. A.J.R., 76:569, 1956.
24. L'Hirondel, J., Caen, Daridon, and Tillet: Anémie de Blackfan-Diamond et dysostose métaphysaire recessif autosomique. Ouest Med., 20:1152, 1967.
25. McKusick, V. A.: Metaphyseal dysostosis and thin hair; a new recessively inherited syndrome. Lancet, 1:832, 1964.
26. McKusick, V. A., Eldridge, R., Hostetler, J. A., Ruangwin, U., and Egeland, J. A.: Dwarfism in the Amish. II. Cartilage-hair hypoplasia. Bull. Johns Hopkins Hosp., 116:697, 1965.
27. Maroteaux, P., Savart, P., Lefebvre, J., and Royer, P.: Les formes partielles de la dysostose métaphysaire. Presse Méd., 71:1523, 1963.
28. Maynard, J. A., Ippolito, E. G., Ponseti, I. V., and Mickelson, M. R.: Histochemistry and ultrastructure of the growth plate in metaphyseal dysostosis: Further observations on the structure of the cartilage matrix. J. Pediatr. Orthop., 1:161, 1981.
29. Nazara, Z., Hernandez, A., and Corona-Rivera, E.: Further clinical and radiographic features in metaphyseal chondrodysplasia, Jansen type. Radiology, 140:697, 1981.
30. Pena, J.: Disostosis metafisaria. Una revision. Con aportacion de una observacion familiar (una forma nueva de la enfermedad). Radiologia, 47:3, 1965.
31. Ray, H. C., and Dorst, J. P.: Cartilage-hair hypoplasia. In Kaufman, H. J. (ed.): Progress in Pediatric Radiology. Vol. 4. Basel, Karger, 1973, p. 270.
32. Rosenbloom, A. L., and Smith, D. W.: The natural history of metaphyseal dysostosis. J. Pediatr., 66:857, 1965.
33. Schmerling, D. H., Prader, A., Hitzig, W. H., Giedeon, A., Hadorn, B., and Kuhni, M.: The syndrome of exocrine pancreatic insufficiency, neutropenia, metaphyseal dysostosis and dwarfism. Helv. Pediatr. Acta, 24:547, 1969.
34. Schmid, F.: Beitrag zur Dysostosis enchondralis metaphysaria. Monatsschr. Kinderhilkd., 97:393, 1949.
35. Schmidt, B. J., Becak, W., Becak, M. L., Soibelman, I., Silva Queiroz, A. da, Lorga, A. P., Secaf, F., Antonio, C. F., and Andrade Carvalho, A. de: Metaphyseal dysostosis. J. Pediatr., 63:106, 1963.
36. Silva, E.: Disostosi metafisaria tip Jansen. Chir. Organi Mov., 54:400, 1966.
37. Spahr, A., and Spahr-Hartmann, I.: Dysostose métaphysaire familiale. Etude de 4 cas dans une fratrie. Helv. Paediatr. Acta, 16:836, 1961.
38. Stickler, G. B., Maher, F. T., Hunt, J. C., Burke, E. C., and Rosevear, J. W.: Familial bone disease resembling rickets (hereditary metaphyseal dysostosis). Pediatrics, 29:996, 1962.
39. Sutcliffe, J.: Metaphyseal dysostosis. Sem. Hôp. Paris, Ann. Radiol., 9:215, 1966.
40. Taybi, H., Mitchell, A. D., and Friedman, G. D.: Metaphyseal dysostosis and the associated syndrome of pancreatic insufficiency and blood disorders. Radiology, 93:563, 1969.
41. Vaandrager, G. J.: Metaphysial dysostosis. Ned. Tijdschr. Geneeskd., 104:547, 1960.
42. Virolaineu, M., Sarilahti, E., Kaitita, I., Perhentupa, J.: Cellular and humoral immunity in cartilage-hair hypoplasia. Pediatr. Res., 12:961, 1978.
43. Wasylenko, M. J., Wedge, J. H., and Houston, C. S.: Metaphyseal chondrodysplasia, Schmid type. J. Bone Joint Surg., 62-A:660, 1980.
44. Weil, S.: Die metaphysären Dysostosen. Z. Orthop., 89:1, 1957.
45. Wekselman, R.: Familial metaphyseal dysostosis. A case report. J. Bone Joint Surg., 59-A:690, 1977.
46. Wiedemann, H. R., and Spranger, J.: Chondrodysplasia metaphysaria (dysostosis metaphysaria)—ein neuer Type. Z. Kinderheilkd., 108:171, 1970.

HYPOPHOSPHATASIA

Hypophosphatasia, first described by Rathbun in 1948, is a genetically determined inborn error of metabolism characterized by low alkaline phosphatase activity in the plasma and tissues, abnormal mineralization of bone, and an increased urinary excretion of phosphoethanolamine.[34] There is a wide variation in the manifestation of this disorder, with its severity varying according to the age of onset.[13] Three forms are generally seen: first, the severe congenital form in which the baby is stillborn or dies shortly afterwards; second, an intermediate tarda form manifesting itself around six months of age; and third, the mild form presenting in the adult as osteomalacia.

The cause of the enzyme defect is unknown. It has not been determined whether it is primary or secondary to a cellular abnormality, e.g., in the osteoblast.

The exact frequency of the condition is unknown. Its incidence is extremely low.

Inheritance

Both the severe (lethal) congenital and the intermediate tarda varieties are of autosomal recessive inheritance; they have been reported in the same family and appear to be genetically similar. The very rare adult form is of autosomal dominant inheritance.[5, 44] Heterozygotes are traced in genetic studies by abnormally diminished alkaline phosphatase in the plasma and by the presence of phosphoethanolamine in the urine.[25]

Pathology

Deficiency of alkaline phosphatase results in disturbance of mineralization and defective ossification in cartilage. The histologic changes closely resemble those of rickets. In the skeleton there is a great amount of unmineralized osteoid tissue. The provisional zone of calcification is widened, with distortion and irregularity of the normal columnar arrangement of the cartilage cells. The degenerating cartilage fails to calcify. Nests of mature cartilage cells are present in the metaphyseal area. There is a large amount of osteoid tissue in all the bones. Hypercalcemia may cause renal calcinosis, evident in calcium deposits in the kidney tubules and interstitial tissues. The severity of pathologic findings varies according to the age at onset of the disorder, the congenital forms manifesting the more severe changes.

Clinical and Radiographic Findings

These vary according to the severity of the disease and the age of the patient at the time the disease becomes manifest.

Severe (Lethal) Congenital Form. The fetus may suffer from prenatal fractures and die in utero. If not stillborn, the newborn has bones that are very soft and deformed. The calvarium is soft and globular. The infant usually dies of respiratory failure in the neonatal period or in early infancy. Radiograms disclose diffuse severe demineralization of the entire skeleton with involvement of both cartilaginous and membranous bones. In the most severe form

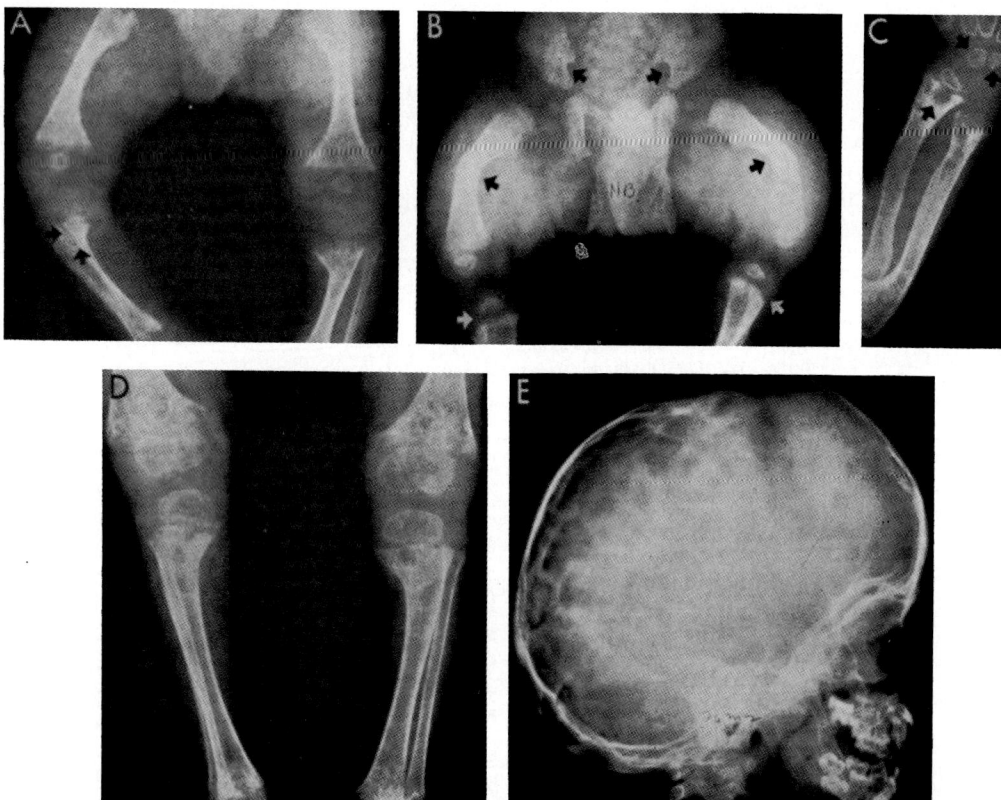

FIGURE 3–23. *Hypophosphatasia in an infant.*

A and **B.** Changes at two months of age. Note the flaring of the ends of the shafts and irregular calcification of the metaphyses. Both femora and tibiae are bowed. **C** and **D.** Two years later the deep segmented defects in the metaphyses indicate their disturbed and irregular calcification. **E.** Lateral view of the skull shows the increased digital markings caused by increased intracranial pressure due to premature synostosis of the sutures. (From Caffey, J.: Pediatric X-Ray Diagnosis. 5th Ed. Chicago, Year Book Medical Publishers, Inc., 1967, p. 982. Reprinted by permission.)

ossification will be absent in the greater portion of the skull bones; in the less severe forms there will be wide suture lines in the skull. The ribs are unossified at the ends and very slender in their middle parts (Figs. 3–23 and 3–24). The innominate bones are small and soft and poorly mineralized. In the spine the vertebral bodies are paper thin and the neural arches invisible because mineralization is lacking. The long bones show marked widening of the physis with large, jagged rarefied defects extending into the metaphysis. The congenital type may be diagnosed prenatally by ultrasound, which shows defective ossification of the skull. Amniocentesis is of no value because amniotic fluid alkaline phosphatase values may be normal in an affected pregnancy.[6, 28]

Intermediate Tarda Form. Onset of symptoms is later in infancy, usually after six months of age. The presenting complaint is failure to thrive with anorexia, vomiting, dehydration, fever, muscular hypotonia, and sometimes convulsions. Demineralization of the bones is less severe than in the congenital type but is still widespread; the radiographic appearance resembles that of rickets with bossing of the skull, bowing of the ribs, and flaring of the ends of long bones and costochondral junctions. In the long bones the physes are markedly widened, with jagged areas of rarefaction in the metaphysis extending into the diaphysis. The presence of fractures and angular deformity of long bones in association with the poor calcification may simulate severe osteogenesis imperfecta. In the infant the cranial sutures are wide, but as the child grows premature craniostenosis develops; the increased intracranial pressure may require craniotomy.[43] Premature loss of deciduous teeth is common. Hypercalcemia may cause renal calcinosis; calcium deposits may be found in the kidney tubules and interstitial tissues. Renal failure and hypertension may eventually ensue. Children who survive tend to improve with increasing maturation of the skeleton. Stature is normal in the infant, but shortness develops with defective enchondral bone formation and delay in skeletal maturation late in childhood.

Adult Form. The presenting picture of hypophosphatasia in the adult is that of osteomalacia.[1, 3, 5, 11, 18, 44] There may be a history of "rickets" in childhood. This disorder usually manifests itself in a fracture, most often of the weight-bearing long bones. In the radiogram there will be evidence of previous rachitic changes.

Laboratory Findings

The biochemical finding characteristic of the disease is the diminution or absence of alkaline phosphatase activity in the plasma, leukocytes, bones, kidneys, and spleen. The amount of alkaline phosphatase in the liver and intestines may be reduced or normal. Serum phosphorus levels are normal, but the serum calcium concentration is usually elevated. The urine of these patients contains phosphorylethanolamine; however, this finding is not particularly characteristic of hypophosphatasia, as the same compound may be found in patients with scurvy, hypothyroidism, and celiac disease.[13, 25] Other chemical changes in the urine are a decrease in the excretion of hydroxyproline and an increase in inorganic pyrophosphate.[40]

Differential Diagnosis

The severe (lethal) congenital form of hypophosphatasia may be mistaken for severe congenital osteogenesis imperfecta, thanatophoric dwarfism, or achondrogenesis. The characteristic low alkaline phosphatase level and absence of mineralization of the skull bones in hypophosphatasia will clarify the diagnosis.

The intermediate tarda form must be distinguished from various types of rickets. The low alkaline phosphatase level of hypophosphatasia is not a feature of rickets.

Treatment

There is no specific treatment. Vitamin D should not be administered because hypophosphatasia is mistaken for rickets. Vitamin D will increase the hypercalcemia, and metastatic calcification may result.[8, 43] If the patient survives into the juvenile period or early adolescence, osteotomy of long bones is performed to correct the severe angular deformities. One should, however, be cautioned that in hypophosphatasia, delayed union or nonunion may be a complication of fracture or osteotomy.[17] Enzyme replacement therapy for infantile hypophosphatasia has been attempted by intravenous infusions of alkaline phosphatase from patients with Paget's disease. The circulating alkaline phosphatase activity increased in each patient; in one patient the increase was maintained for two months. There was no radiographic evidence, however, for arrest of progression of osteopenia or improvement in the rachitic defect in any of the patients.[48, 49]

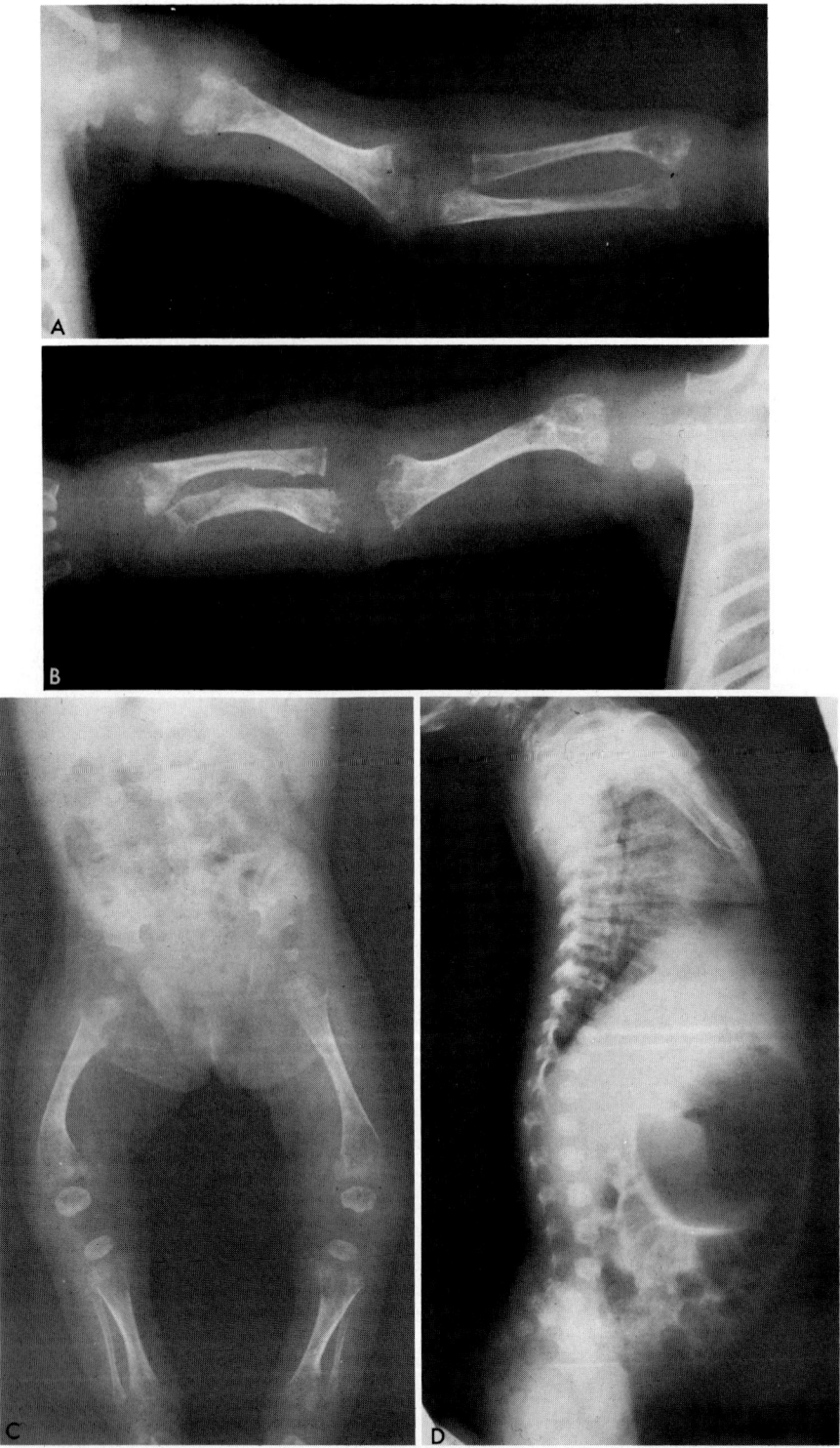

FIGURE 3–24. Typical radiographic changes of hypophosphatasia in a four-month-old infant.
A and **B.** Both upper limbs. **C.** Lower limbs. **D.** Spine. (See text for explanation.)

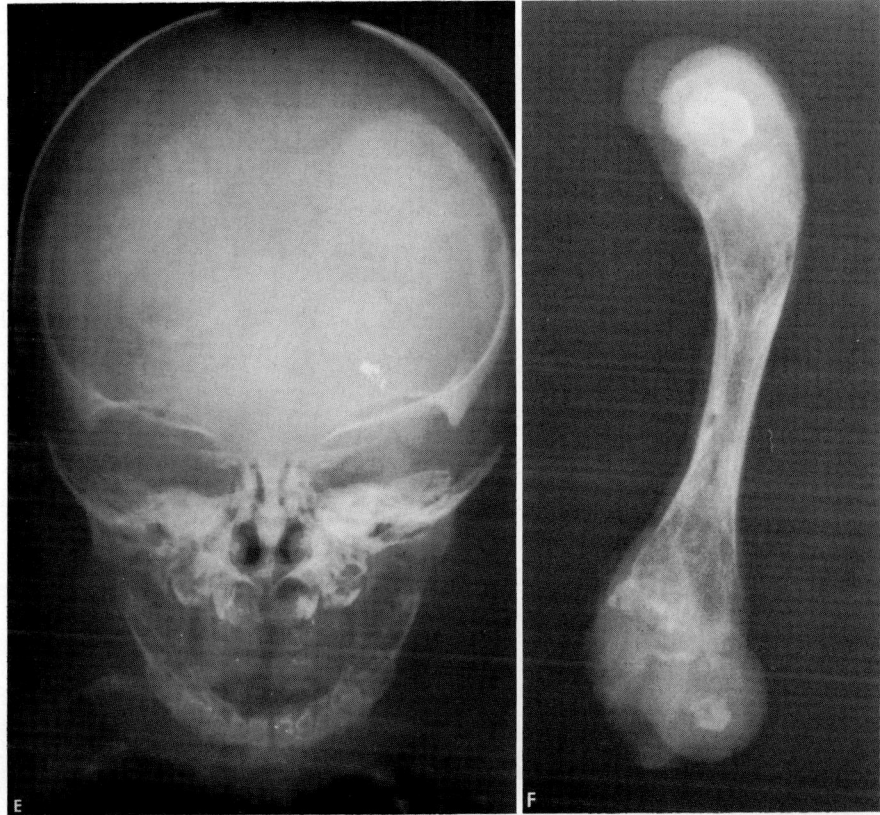

FIGURE 3–24 Continued. *Typical radiographic changes of hypophosphatasia in a four-month-old infant.*
E. Skull. F. Femur—obtained at autopsy. (See text for explanation.)

Mild Hypophosphatasia in the Adult

This presents with the signs and symptoms of osteomalacia. A pathologic fracture looking similar to Looser's zones may be the presenting complaint, but the partial fracture is on the lateral (convexity) rather than on the medial side of the long bone. These adult patients may give a history of so-called rickets in childhood.

References

1. Anderton, J. M.: Orthopedic problems in adult hypophosphatasia. A report of two cases. J. Bone Joint Surg., 61-B:82, 1979.
2. Bartter, F. C.: Hypophosphatasia. *In* Stanbury, J. B., Wyngaarden, J. B., and Frederickson, D. S. (eds.): The Metabolic Basis of Inherited Disease. 2nd Ed. New York, McGraw-Hill, 1966, p. 1015.
3. Beisel, W. R., Benjamin, N. R., and Austen, K. F.: Absence of leukocyte alkaline phosphatase activity in hypophosphatasia. Blood, 14:975, 1959.
4. Bessler, V. W., and Fanconi, A.: Die Röntgensymptome der Hypophosphatasie. Beobachtungen bei 2 Brudern mit maligner neonataler Verlaufsform. Fortschr. Röntgenstr., 117:58, 1972.
5. Bethune, L. D., and Dent, C. D.: Hypophosphatasia in the adult. Am. J. Med., 28:615, 1960.
6. Blau, K., Hoar, D. I., Rattenbury, J. M., and Rudd, N. L.: Prenatal diagnosis of hypophosphatasia. Lancet, 2:1139, 1977.
7. Bongiovanni, A. M., Album, M. M., Root, A. W., Hope, J. W., Marino, J., and Spencer, D. M.: Studies in hypophosphatasia and response to high phosphate intake. Am. J. Med. Sci., 255:163, 1968.
8. Currarino, G., Neuhauser, E. B., Keyersbach, G. C., and Sobel, E. H.: Hypophosphatasia. A.J.R., 78:392, 1957.
9. Currianio, G.: Hypophosphatasia. *In* Progress in Pediatric Radiology, Vol. 4, Intrinsic Diseases of Bones. Basel, S. Karger, 1973, p. 469.
10. Dickson, W., and Hurrocks, R. H.: Hypophosphatasia. J. Bone Joint Surg., 40-B:64, 1958.
11. Eisenberg, E., and Pimstone, B.: Hypophosphatasia in an adult. Clin. Orthop., 52:199, 1967.
12. Eyring, E., and Eisenberg, E.: Congenital hyperphosphatasia. J. Bone Joint Surg., 50-A:1099, 1967.
13. Fraser, D.: Hypophosphatasia. Am. J. Med., 22:730, 1957.
14. Fraser, D., and Laidlaw, J. C.: Treatment of hypophosphatasia with cortisone. Lancet, 2:553, 1956.
15. Fraser, D., Yendt, E. R., and Christie, F. H. E.: Metabolic abnormalities in hypophosphatasia. Lancet, 1:286, 1955.
16. Goyer, R. A.: Ethanolamine phosphate excretion in a family with hypophosphatasia. Arch. Dis. Child., 38:205, 1963.

17. Jacobson, D. P., and McLain, E. J.: Hypophosphatasia in monozygotic twins. J. Bone Joint Surg., 49-A:377, 1967.
18. Jardon, O. M., Burney, D. W., and Fink, R. L.: Hypophosphatasia in an adult. J. Bone Joint Surg., 52-A:1477, 1970.
19. Jelke, H.: Hypophosphatasia. Acta Paediatr., 49:297, 1960.
20. Kellsey, D. C.: Hypophosphatasia and congenital bowing of the long bones. J.A.M.A., 179:157, 1962.
21. Kovar, I., Mayne, P., and Barltrop, D.: Plasma alkaline phosphatase activity: A screening test for rickets in preterm neonates. Lancet, 1:308, 1982.
22. Kozlowski, K., Sutcliffe, J., Barylak, A., Harrington, G., Kemperdick, H., Nolte, K., Rheinwein, H., Thomas, P. S., and Uniecka, W.: Hypophosphatasia. Review of 24 cases. Pediatr. Radiol., 5:103, 1976.
23. Kretchner, N., Stone, M., and Bauer, C.: Hereditary enzymatic effects as illustrated by hypophosphatasia. Ann. N.Y. Acad. Sci., 75:279, 1958.
24. MacPherson, R. I., Kroeker, M., and Houston, C. S.: Hypophosphatasia. J. Can. Assoc. Radiol., 23:16, 1972.
25. McCance, R. A., Fairweather, D. V. I., Barrett, A. M., and Morrison, A. B.: Genetic, clinical, biochemical and pathological features of hypophosphatasia. Q. J. Med., 25:523, 1956.
26. McCance, R. A., Morrison, A. B., and Dent, C. D.: The excretion of phosphoethanolamine and hypophosphatasia. Lancet, 1:131, 1955.
27. Mehes, K., Klujber, L., Lassu, G., and Kajtar, D.: Hypophosphatasia: Screening and family investigations in an endogamous Hungarian village. Clin. Genet., 3:60, 1972.
28. Mulivor, R. A., Mennuti, M., Zackai, E. H., and Harris, H.: Prenatal diagnosis of hypophosphatasia: Genetic, biochemical, and clinical studies. Am. J. Hum. Genet., 30:271, 1978.
29. O'Duffy, J. D.: Hypophosphatasia associated with calcium pyrophosphate dihydrate deposits in cartilage Arthritis Rheum., 13:381, 1970.
30. Paterson, C. R. (ed.): Hypophosphatasia. In Metabolic Disorders of Bone. Oxford, Blackwell, 1974, p. 266.
31. Pimstone, B., Eisenberg, E., and Silverman, S.: Hypophosphatasia: Genetic and dental studies. Ann. Intern. Med., 65:722, 1966.
32. Rasmussen, K.: Phosphorylethanolamine and hypophosphatasia. Dan. Med. Bull., 15:1, 1968.
33. Rasmussen, H., and Bartter, F. C.: Hypophosphatasia. In Stanbury, J. B., Wyngaarden, J. B., and Fredrickson, D. S. (eds.): The Metabolic Basis of Inherited Diseases. 4th Ed. New York, McGraw-Hill, 1978, pp. 1340–1349.
34. Rathbun, J. C.: Hypophosphatasia. A new developmental anomaly. Am. J. Dis. Child., 75:822, 1948.
35. Rathbun, J. C.: Hypophosphatasia. Helv. Paediatr. Acta, 14:548, 1959.
36. Rathbun, J. C., MacDonald, J. W., Robinson, H. M. C., and Wanklin, J. M.: Hypophosphatasia: A genetic study. Arch. Dis. Child., 36:540, 1961.
37. Ritchie, G. MacL.: Hypophosphatasia: A metabolic disease with important dental manifestations. Arch. Dis. Child., 39:584, 1964.
38. Rosenthal, I. M., Bonting, S. L., Hogan, W., and Pirani, C. L.: Tissue alkaline phosphatase in hypophosphatasia. J. Dis. Child., 99:75, 1960.
39. Rudd, N. L., Miskin, M., Hoar, D. I., Benzie, R., and Doran, T. A.: Prenatal diagnosis of hypophosphatasia. N. Engl. J. Med., 295:146, 1976.
40. Russell, R. G. G.: Excretion of inorganic pyrophosphate in hypophosphatasia. Lancet, 2:461, 1965.
41. Russell, R. G. G., Bisaz, S., Donath, A., Morgan, D. B., and Fleisch, H.: Inorganic pyrophosphate in plasma in normal persons and in patients with hypophosphatasia, osteogenesis imperfecta and other disorders of bone. J. Clin. Invest., 50:961, 1971.
42. Scaglione, R. R., and Lucey, J. F.: Further observations on hypophosphatasia. Am. J. Dis. Child., 92:403, 1956.
43. Schlesinger, B., Luder, J., and Bodian, M.: Rickets with alkaline phosphatase deficiency: An osteoblastic dysplasia. Arch. Dis. Child., 30:265, 1955.
44. Silverman, J. L.: Apparent dominant inheritance of hypophosphatasia. Arch. Intern. Med., 110:191, 1962.
45. Smith, R.: Biochemical Disorders of the Skeleton. London, Butterworth, 1979, pp. 266–269.
46. Teree, T. M., and Klein, L.: Hypophosphatasia: Clinical and metabolic studies. J. Pediatr., 72:41, 1968.
47. Whyte, M. P., Teitbaum, S. I., and Murphy, W. A.: Adult hypophosphatasia. Clinical, laboratory and genetic investigations of a large kindred with review of literature. Medicine, 58:329, 1979.
48. Whyte, M. P., Valdes, R., Jr., Ryan, L. M., and McAlister, W. H.: Infantile hypophosphatasia: Enzyme replacement therapy by intravenous infusions of alkaline phosphatase–rich plasma from patients with Paget bone disease. J. Pediatr., 101:379, 1982.
49. Whyte, M. P., McAlister, W. H., Patton, L. S., Magill, H. L., Fallon, M. D., Lorentz, W. B., Jr., and Herrod, H. G.: Enzyme replacement therapy for infantile hypophosphatasia attempted by intravenous infusions of alkaline phosphatase–rich Paget plasma: Results in three additional patients. J. Pediatr., 105:926, 1984.

SPONDYLOEPIPHYSEAL DYSPLASIA

Spondyloepiphyseal dysplasia is characterized by disproportionate dwarfism with shortening predominantly of the trunk and primary progressive involvement of the spine and epiphyses of long bones, particularly of the upper femur.[17] In the past spondyloepiphyseal dysplasia has been confused with Morquio's disease. There are two types of spondyloepiphyseal dysplasia: the *congenita type*, which can be detected at birth, and the *tarda type*, which manifests itself later on in childhood. The congenita type is inherited as an autosomal dominant trait (however, most cases are sporadic); the tarda type is an X-linked recessive trait, occurring only in the male. The tarda type is more common, with a prevalence of three or four per million; the prevalence of the congenita type is one or two per million in the population.

Spondyloepiphyseal Dysplasia Congenita

Wynne-Davies has delineated two clinical variants of the congenita type: that with severe coxa vara, and that with mild coxa vara.[21] The two cannot be differentiated on clinical or radiologic grounds until the age of three or four years when the degree of coxa vara and the differences in shortness of stature become apparent.

In *spondyloepiphyseal dysplasia congenita with severe coxa vara* the stature is very short and the degree of varus deformity of femoral neck and shaft is marked (Figs. 3–25 and 3–26). Hip flexion deformity and hyperlordosis are marked. In the radiogram of the hips the femoral necks are seen to be defective and radiolucent, the greater trochanters being displaced proximally. The femoral heads are delayed in ossification and do not appear until five years of age. Often the radiographic appearance is mistaken for bilateral congenital hip dislocation; ultrasound or arthrography will, however, demonstrate the normal containment of the femoral heads in the acetabula.

In both clinical types of spondyloepiphyseal dysplasia congenita the vertebrae are flattened throughout and "pear-shaped" in early infancy; the odontoid process is dysplastic and delayed in ossification with risk of atlantoaxial instability (Fig. 3–25 C and D). Scoliosis and kyphosis develop in late childhood or early adolescence, and the thorax is deformed with pectus carinatum. Other epiphyses of the long bones show varying degrees of involvement.

Associated anomalies in spondyloepiphyseal congenita are cleft palate, myopia with retinal detachment, deafness, cataracts, talipes equinovarus, and occasionally herniae.

Treatment. The most serious problem is atlantoaxial instability. Flexion-extension lateral views of the cervical spine and CT scanning will demonstrate the instability. If cord compression is evident from the neurologic findings or is demonstrated by the CT scan or nuclear magnetic resonance imaging, occipital-cervical fusion must be performed.

Coxa vara is treated by abduction osteotomy

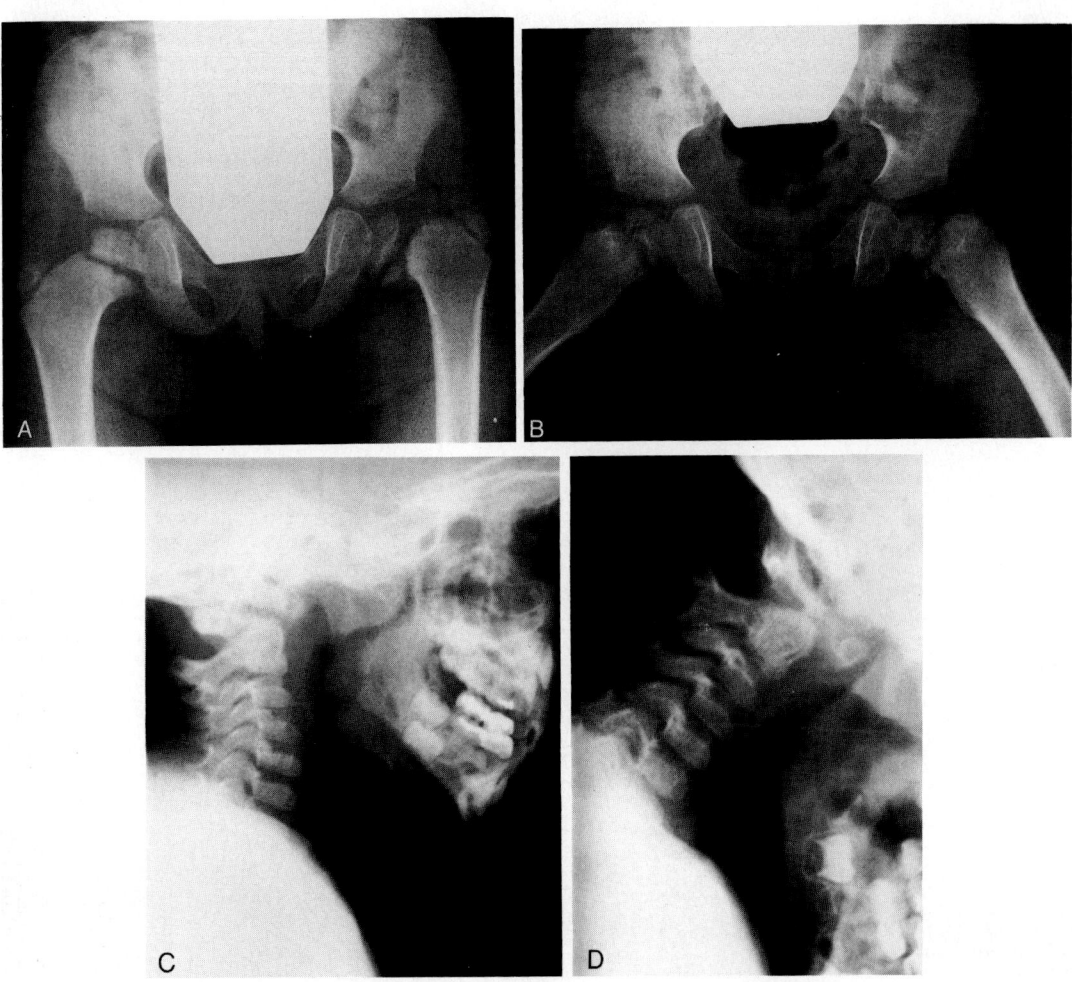

FIGURE 3–25. Spondyloepiphyseal dysplasia in a four-year-old girl.

A and **B.** Anteroposterior and lateral views of the pelvis showing the irregular ossification of the femoral heads. The left hip shows severe coxa vara deformity with elevation of the greater trochanter. **C** and **D.** Neutral and flexion lateral views of the cervical spine. Note the atlantoaxial instability.

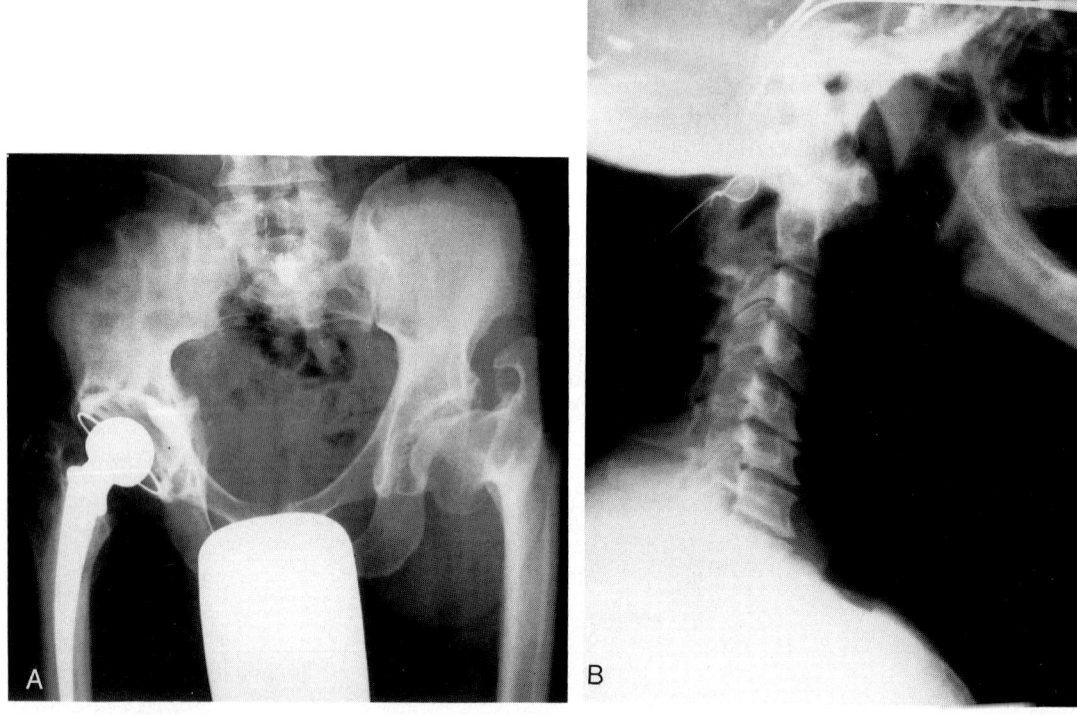

FIGURE 3-26. Spondyloepiphyseal dysplasia, severe type, in a 36-year-old man, the father of the girl shown in Figure 3-25.

A. Note the severe coxa vara of the left hip; he had a total joint replacement of the right hip because of severe degenerative arthritis. **B.** Lateral view of cervical spine. Note the upper cervical fusion for the hypoplasia of the odontoid process.

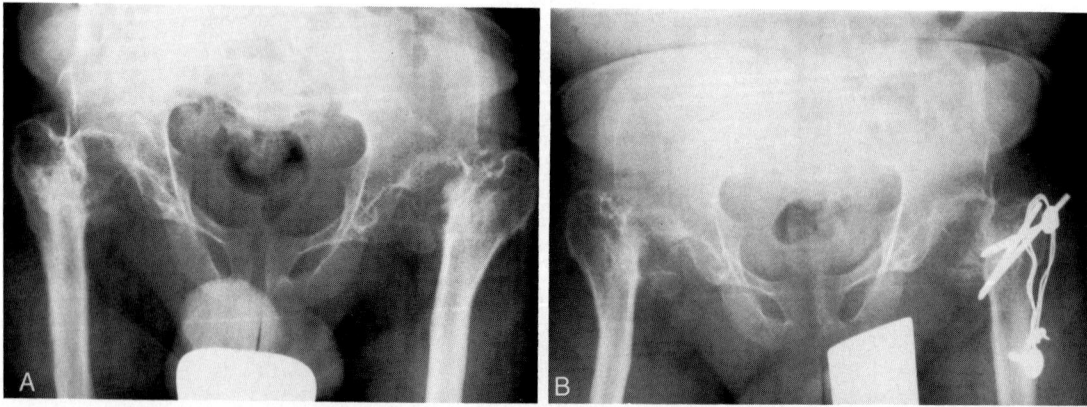

FIGURE 3-27. Severe bilateral coxa vara in spondyloepiphyseal dysplasia.

A. Preoperative radiogram. **B.** After treatment by abduction osteotomy and distal-lateral transfer of the greater trochanter of the left hip.

at the intertrochanteric level; the relatively overgrown greater trochanter is transferred distally and laterally (Fig. 3–27). Severe genu varum or valgum may require corrective angulation osteotomy or gradual correction by asymmetrical epiphysiodesis at the appropriate skeletal age.

Spondyloepiphyseal Dysplasia Tarda

This rare dysplasia, first described as an entity by Maroteaux, Lamy, and Bernard in 1957, is characterized by flattened vertebrae and narrowed disc interspaces.[13] In the lateral projection of the spine the posterior hump and the absence of ossification of the upper and lower anterior margins of the vertebral bodies are distinctive. The presenting complaint is back pain and stiffness, with onset in the five- to ten-year-old age group. The proximal epiphyses of the femora and humeri are minimally involved and show changes that resemble multiple epiphyseal dysplasia. The distal epiphyses of the long bones and hands and feet are not affected. Inheritance is by an X-linked recessive gene, being observed only in males. The dysplastic changes in the vertebral bodies and long-bone epiphyses are usually slowly progressive; increasing loss of joint motion due to degenerative arthritis may be noted in the third decade of life.

Treatment. Back pain is managed by conservative measures. Joint deformations usually are not severe enough to warrant surgery.

References

1. Al-Awadi, S. A., Farag, T. I., Naguib, K., El-Khalifa, M., Cuschieri, A., Hosny, G., Zahran, M., and Al-Ansari, A. G.: Spondyloepiphyseal dysplasia tarda with progressive arthropathy. J. Med. Genet., 21:193, 1984.
2. Bach, C., Maroteaux, P., Schaeffer, P., Bitan, A., and Crumiere, C.: Dysplasie spondylo-épiphysaire congénitale avec anomalies multiples. Arch. Fr. Pediatr., 24:23, 1967.
3. Battin, J., Serville, M. F., and Maroteaux, P.: Dysplasie spondylo-épiphysaire congenitale chez une fille de 14 ans. Ann. Pediatr., 22:175, 1975.
4. Borut, D., and Kogut, M.: Short stature in an adolescent due to spondyloepiphyseal dysplasia tarda. Am. J. Dis. Child., 129:1069, 1975.
5. Fisher, R. L.: Unusual spondyloepiphyseal and spondylometaphyseal dysplasias of childhood. Clin. Orthop., 100:78, 1974.
6. Fraser, G. R., Friedmann, A. I., Maroteaux, P., Glen-Bott, A. M., and Mittwochi, U.: Dysplasia spondyloepiphysaria congenita and related generalized skeletal dysplasias among children with severe visual handicaps. Arch. Dis. Child., 44:490, 1969.
7. Harper, P. S., Jenkins, P., and Laurence, K. M.: Spondyloepiphyseal dysplasia tarda: A report of four cases in two families. Br. J. Radiol., 46:676, 1973.
8. Kopits, S. E.: Orthopedic complications of dwarfism. Clin. Orthop., 114:153, 1976.
9. Kozlowski, K., Bittel-Dobrzynska, N., and Budsynska, A.: Spondylo-epiphyseal dysplasia congenita. Ann. Radiol., 11:367, 1968.
10. Kozlowski, K., Masel, J., and Nolte, K.: Dysplasia spondylo-epiphysealis congenita Spranger-Wiedemann. A critical analysis. Aust. Radiol., 21:260, 1977.
11. Kozlowski, K., Filipiak-Miastkowska, I., Narebska, E., Nowicki, S., and Chylinska, H.: Dysplasia spondylometaepiphysaria congenita und Dysplasia spondyloepiphysaria congenita mit Brachymetakarpie und-metarsie. Ein Beitrag zur Differentialdiagnose der Dysplasia spondyloepiphysaria congenita. Fortschr. Geb. Rontgenstr. Nuklearmed., 114:823, 1971.
12. Langer, L. O.: Spondyloepiphysial dysplasia tarda. Hereditary chondrodysplasia with characteristic vertebral configuration in the adult. Radiology, 82:833, 1964.
13. Maroteaux, P., Lamy, M., and Bernard, J.: La dysplasie spondylo-épiphysaire tardive. Description clinique et radiologique. Presse Méd., 65:1205, 1957.
14. Michaelis, E., Kemperdick, H., and Spranger, J. W.: Dysplasia spondyloepiphysaria congenita. Fortschr. Geb. Rontgenstr., 119:429, 1973.
15. Poker, N., Finby, N., and Archibald, R. M.: Spondyloepiphysial dysplasia tarda. Four cases in childhood and adolescence, and some considerations regarding platyspondyly. Radiology, 85:474, 1965.
16. Spranger, J.: Spondyloepiphyseal dysplasia. Birth Defects, 11:177, 1978.
17. Spranger, J., and Langer, L. O.: Spondyloepiphyseal dysplasia congenita. Radiology, 94:313, 1970.
18. Stanescu, R., Stanescu, V., and Maroteaux, P.: Dysplasie spondylo-épiphysaire avec accumulation de glycoproteines dans les chondrocytes. Arch. Fr. Pediatr., 41:185, 1984.
19. Sugiura, Y., Terashima, Y., Furukawa, T., and Yoneda, M.: Spondyloepiphyseal dysplasia congenita. Int. Orthop., 2:47, 1978.
20. Weinfeld, A., Ross, M. W., and Sarasohn, S. H.: Spondyloepiphyseal dysplasia tarda. A cause of premature osteoarthritis. A.J.R., 101:851, 1967.
21. Wynne-Davis, R., and Hall, C.: Two clinical variants of spondylo-epiphysial dysplasia congenita. J. Bone Joint Surg., 64-B:435, 1982.

PSEUDOACHONDROPLASIA

This dysplasia is characterized by short-limbed dwarfism in which both the epiphyses and metaphyses are involved. Craniofacial features are normal. The vertebrae are flat with a distinctive anterior central tonguelike protrusion and normal interpedicular distance in the lumbar region. Maroteaux and Lamy described it first in 1959; and Ford, Silverman, and Kozlowski, in 1961, clearly differentiated pseudoachondroplasia from classic achondroplasia and other forms of spondyloepiphyseal dysplasia.[3, 8]

Pseudoachondroplasia is a heterogeneous group genetically with both autosomal dominant and recessive forms of inheritance. Delineation of the two genetic types is not feasible radiographically, but it appears the more severely involved forms tend to be of autosomal recessive inheritance. Most cases are sporadic in occurrence. The prevalence of pseudoachondroplasia is possibly four per million population.

Pathology

Ultrastructural studies of the apophysis of the iliac crest and the physis of the fibula have shown a swelling of the endoplasmic reticulum cisternae due to accumulation of abnormal lipoprotein or glycoprotein.

Clinical Features

There is considerable variation in the severity of involvement. The dysplasia is not apparent at birth. The dwarfism and disproportionately short limbs become progressively apparent between two and four years of age, at which time the diagnosis is made.

The head and face are of normal appearance. Disproportionate shortness of stature with marked shortening of the limbs is the striking feature. Platyspondyly causes shortness of the trunk. Dwarfism may be quite severe, with adult height ranging between 82 and 130 cm. Excessive joint laxity causes hyperlordosis of the lumbar spine, hypermobility of the knee joint with genu recurvatum, ankle instability, and severe flexible pes planovalgus. Deformities of the knee and hip are common owing to growth irregularity of the epiphyses. Some children develop a "windswept" deformity of their lower limbs with valgus knee and adducted hip on one side and varus knee and abducted hip on the contralateral side. Progressive scoliosis and kyphosis may develop. Pseudoachondroplasts become disabled with severe degenerative arthritis of the weight-bearing joints in adult life. The hands are short and have a "trident" appearance in some patients. Intelligence and life expectancy are normal.

Radiographic Features

The cranium is normal. In the lateral projection of the spine the vertebrae appear flattened, with irrregular end-plates and a central tongue-like projection. The interpedicular distance in the lumbar spine is normal in width; it does not become narrow as in classic achondroplasia. Progressive scoliosis may develop in adolescence. Odontoid hypoplasia is common in pseudoachondroplasia. Lateral flexion-extension views of the cervical spine will show atlantoaxial instability if it is present.

The long bones are markedly short and broad, the metaphyses splayed and cupped, and the epiphyses delayed in ossification, irregular, and fragmented (Fig. 3-28). The distinguishing feature of pseudoachondroplasia is the involvement of both the epiphyses and metaphyses, whereas in achondroplasia the epiphyses are essentially normal. The hip and knee joints are most severely affected. The acetabula are shallow, with their roofs deficient superiorly, anteriorly, and posteriorly. The triradiate cartilages are wide and their ossification is delayed. The ischiopubic junction is wide and late to fuse. The sciatic notches are normal; this finding distinguishes pseudoachondroplasia from achondroplasia in which the greater sciatic notches are narrowed to a small aperture and the acetabular roofs are squared. The femoral necks are short with broad metaphyses. In the adult, degenerative arthritis results from incongruity of the hip joints with malformed and flattened femoral heads.

In the leg, the fibula is disproportionately long in relation to the tibia. Genu varum and varus ankle are common with irregularity of the epiphyses and eventual osteoarthritis. In the hands and feet, the small tubular bones are short, the metaphyses flaring and the epiphyses irregular and their ossification delayed.

Differential Diagnosis

Pseudoachondroplasia should not be mistaken for achondroplasia (Table 3-3). It is distinguished from multiple epiphyseal dysplasia, as in the latter the vertebrae and metaphyses are not affected or are minimally involved.

Diastrophic dwarfism is differentiated from pseudoachondroplasia by the presence of severe joint contracture in the former versus joint hyperlaxity in the latter. Severe scoliosis develops in infancy or early childhood in diastrophic dwarfism.

Treatment. There are a number of problems that require orthopedic management. Angular deformities at the knee (genu varum or valgum) are treated by appropriate corrective osteotomy, usually dome or closing-wedge. Timing of surgery is important; it is best to delay until adolescence because the deformity will recur with abnormal growth. Coxa vara or valga may also require surgical correction; the osteotomies of the proximal femur should be performed at the intertrochanteric level. Innominate osteotomy and/or shelf acetabular augmentation is performed to correct acetabular insufficiency and provide coverage of the femoral head.

Progressive scoliosis may be a problem and usually cannot be controlled by orthotic measures. Early spinal fusion should be performed; avoid procrastination.

Degenerative arthritis of the hips and knees

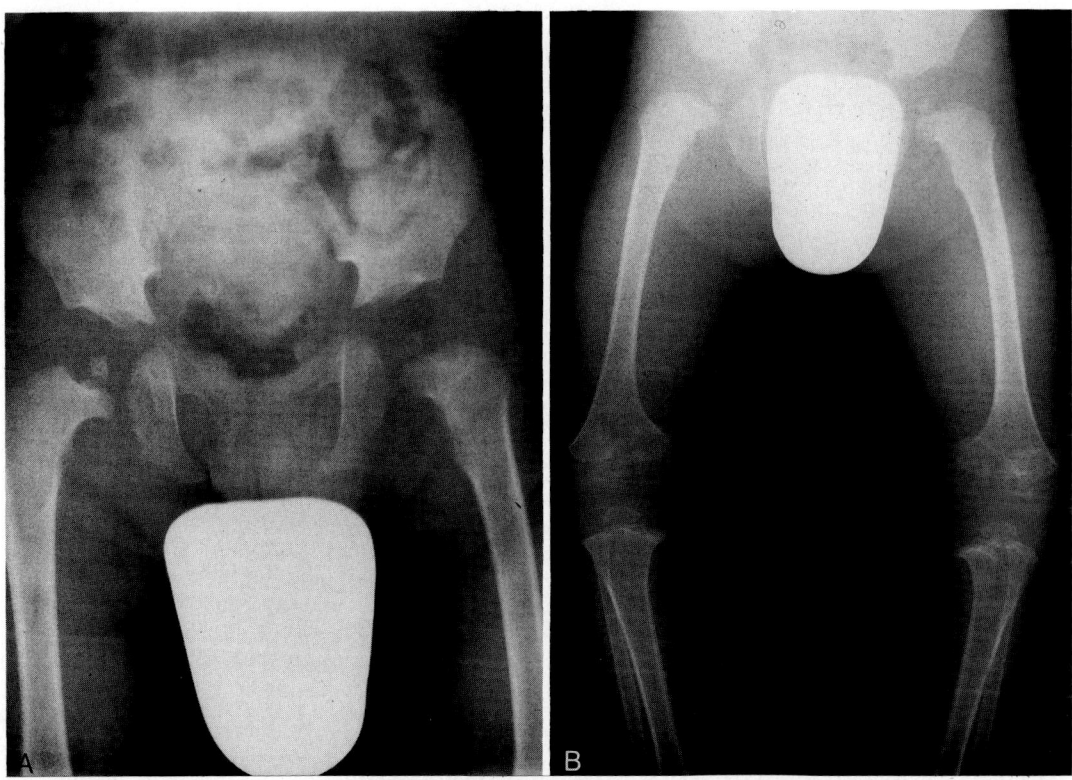

FIGURE 3–28. Pseudoachondroplasia.

A. Anteroposterior radiogram of the pelvis. Note the delayed ossification of the capital femoral epiphysis, the medial beaking of the femoral neck, and the marked widening of the triradiate cartilage. **B.** Anteroposterior radiogram of the femora and tibiae. Note the shortening of the long bones with the flared metaphyses. The epiphyses are abnormal and irregular in ossification. Both the epiphyses and the metaphyses are involved.

Table 3–3. Differential Diagnosis of Pseudoachondroplasia and Achondroplasia

Features	Pseudoachondroplasia	Achondroplasia
Inheritance	Heterogeneous; both autosomal dominant and recessive Most sporadic	Autosomal dominant Almost all new mutants
Skull and facies	Normal	Bulging forehead; low nasal bridge Sometimes hydrocephalic
Spine	Lumbar lordosis No progressive narrowing of interpedicular distance Platyspondyly with anterior central breaking	Severe lumbar lordosis Progressive narrowing of interpedicular distance at the lumbar spine, L_1, L_5 No platyspondyly; short pedicles
Long bones	Both epiphysis and metaphysis affected Epiphysis delayed in ossification, irregular, and fragmented Metaphysis flared	Epiphysis normal (only metaphysis affected) Metaphysis wide
Pelvis and sciatic notch	Shallow acetabulum Wide great sciatic notch Iliac wings flared	Horizontal acetabular roof Great sciatic notch narrowed to a slit Iliac wing squared
Problems and complications	Degenerative arthritis due to incongruous weight-bearing (hip and knee joints) Tibia vara—corrective osteotomy	Spinal stenosis due to narrow spinal canal Tibia vara—corrective osteotomy

may require total joint replacement in adult life.

References

1. Cooper, R. R., Ponseti, I. V., and Maynard, J. A.: Pseudoachondroplastic dwarfism: A rough surfaced endoplasmic reticulum storage disorder. J. Bone Joint Surg., 55-A:475, 1973.
2. Cranley, R. E., Williams, B. R., Kopits, S. E., and Dorst, J. P.: Pseudoachondroplastic dysplasia: Five cases representing clinical, roentgenographic and histologic heterogeneity. Birth Defects Orig. Art. Series, 11:205, 1975.
3. Ford, N., Silverman, F. N., and Kozlowski, K.: Spondyloepiphyseal dysplasia (pseudoachondroplastic type). A.J.R., 86:462, 1961.
4. Hall, J. G.: Pseudoachondroplasia. Birth Defects Orig. Art. Series, 11:187, 1975.
5. Hall, J. G., and Dorst, J. P.: Pseudoachondroplastic SED, recessive Maroteaux-Lamy type. Birth Defects Orig. Art. Series, 5:254, 1969.
6. Kopits, S. E.: Orthopedic complications of dwarfism. Clin. Orthop., 114:153, 1976.
7. Kozlowski, K.: Pseudoachondroplasia (Maroteaux-Lamy). Aust. Radiol., 20:255, 1976.
8. Maroteaux, P., and Lamy, M.: Les formes pseudoachondroplastiques des dysplasies spondylo-épiphysaires. Presse Méd., 10:383, 1959.

DIASTROPHIC DYSPLASIA (DIASTROPHIC DWARFISM)

Lamy and Maroteaux, in 1960, distinguished a very rare form of micromelic dwarfism from achondroplasia and named it *nanisme diastrophique*, deriving the word diastrophic from the Greek meaning "crooked or twisted," which denotes the associated talipes equinovarus, scoliosis, and "hitchhiker's" deformity of the hand—stigmata that so well identify the condition. Prior cases had been described in the literature.[19, 26] At the Second International Conference for Nomenclature for Congenital Diseases of Bone, in Paris in 1977, the term *diastrophic dwarfism* was changed to *diastrophic dysplasia*.

This disorder is inherited as an autosomal recessive trait.

Pathogenesis and Pathology

The cause of diastrophic dysplasia is unknown. It is a neuromesodermal defect resulting from failure of formation of normal collagen and chondroid tissue—skeletal changes are only a part of the total picture.

Pathologic studies have been reported in the literature by Salle, Kaplan, and Taber and their associates.[14, 24, 32] In the growth plate there is lack of normal columnization and calcification indicating a disorder of enchondral ossification.

Taber and his colleagues reported an autopsy study of the entire musculoskeletal system of a three-day-old infant with diastrophic dysplasia. They found diffuse abnormality of the chondrocytes in the entire skeleton. The cartilaginous matrix was abnormal, the chondrocytes were larger and clearer with more rounded nuclei than the hyperchromatic, almost pyknotic, nuclei of normal cartilage. The cartilage of the trachea was also defective.[32] These findings suggest an inborn error of chondrogenesis. To elucidate the pathogenesis of this diffuse neuromesodermal defect, further ultrastructural and histochemical investigations are necessary.

Laboratory studies of serum calcium, phosphorus, alkaline phosphatase, and electrophoretic protein patterns are normal. Abnormal amino acids have not been found in the urine.

Clinical Picture

The condition can be detected at birth. The afflicted newborn is severely dwarfed, with very short limbs and marked equinovarus deformity of both feet (Fig. 3–29). In the first ten days of life cystic swelling of the external ears develops, which subsequently calcifies and ossifies. The twisted and deformed ears have thickened and furrowed lobes as well as narrowed external auditory canals, giving a cauliflower appearance. Hearing is normal. The face appears "cherubic" owing to fullness of the cheeks around the mouth. The nasal bridge is narrow, the nostrils flared, and the mid-nose broad. Cleft palate is present in some patients.

The hands are short and broad. The thumb deformity is a distinctive feature of the dysplasia and is referred to as "hitchhiker's thumb" (Fig. 3–29A). It is caused by the excessive shortness of the first metacarpal, which is triangular in shape, and the radial subluxation of the metacarpophalangeal joint of the thumb, which is recessed proximally on the hand. The thumb is almost perpendicular to the other digits.

The equinovarus deformity of the foot is another distinctive and integral feature of the dysplasia. The first metatarsal is short and triangular in shape. The whole forefoot is medially deviated with the hallux in greater varus angulation than the lesser toes. The hindfoot and ankle are in extreme equinus posture; weight is borne on the toes. Often the deformity is referred to as a clubfoot, but the talocalcaneonavicular joint is not displaced medially and plantarly as in the true congenital talipes equinovarus. The Achilles tendon is a band of "fan-like" fibers and not a round cord, reflecting the

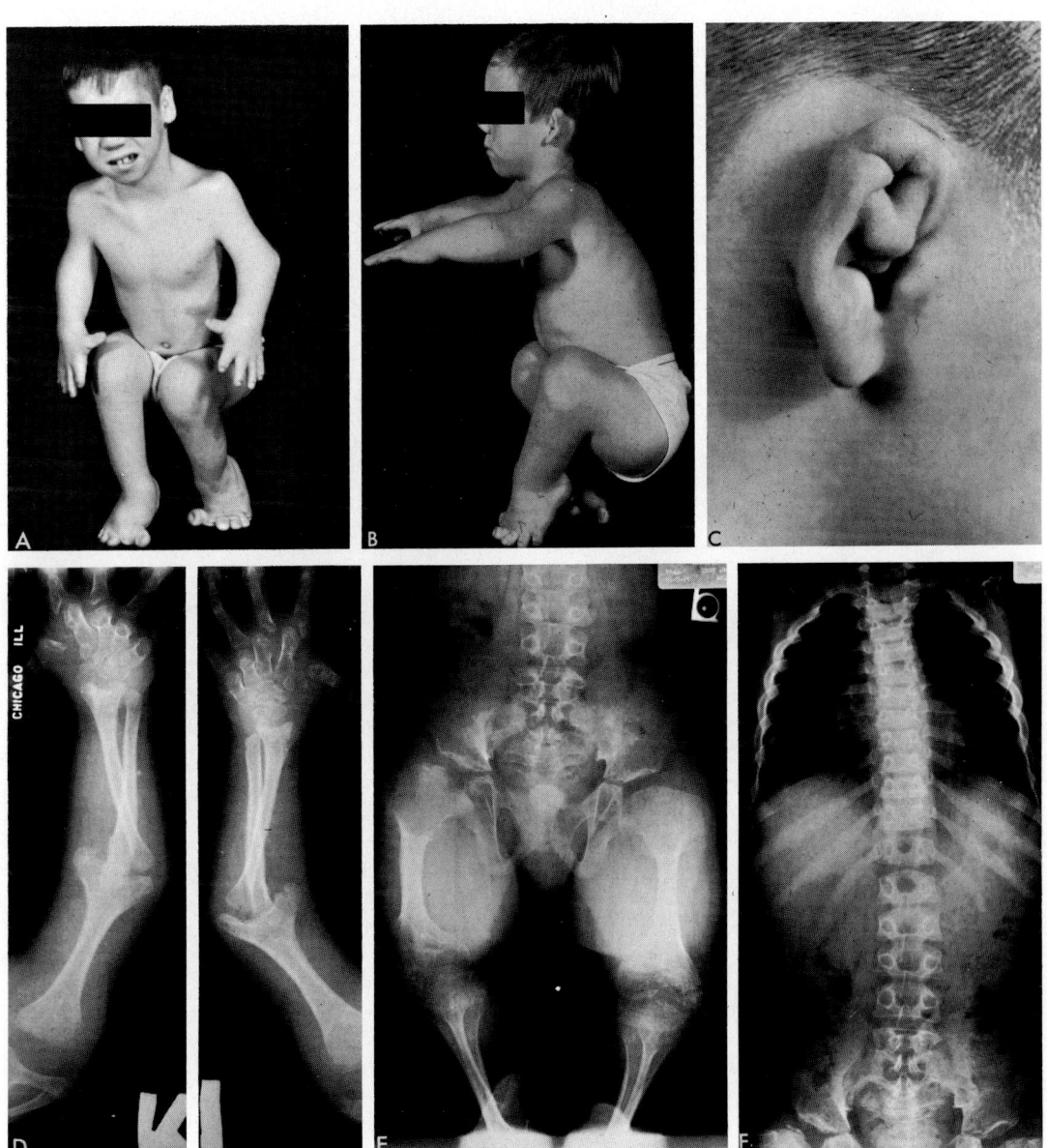

FIGURE 3–29. Diastrophic dysplasia.

A and **B.** Clinical appearance of a patient with the typical deformities. Note the severe flexion contractures of the hips and knees and the equinovarus deformities of the feet. "Hitch-hiker's thumb" is a principal feature. **C.** The deformed ears have thickened lobes, are furrowed, and have a narrow external auditory canal. **D.** Anteroposterior radiograms of both upper limbs. Note the excessive shortening of the first metacarpal and the radial subluxation of the metacarpophalangeal joint of the thumb. **E.** Anteroposterior radiogram of both lower limbs and pelvis. The metaphyses are broad and flared, and there is marked delay of ossification of the epiphyses. Coxa vara deformity is evident. **F.** Radiogram of the spine. The vertebrae are normal. There is no scoliosis.

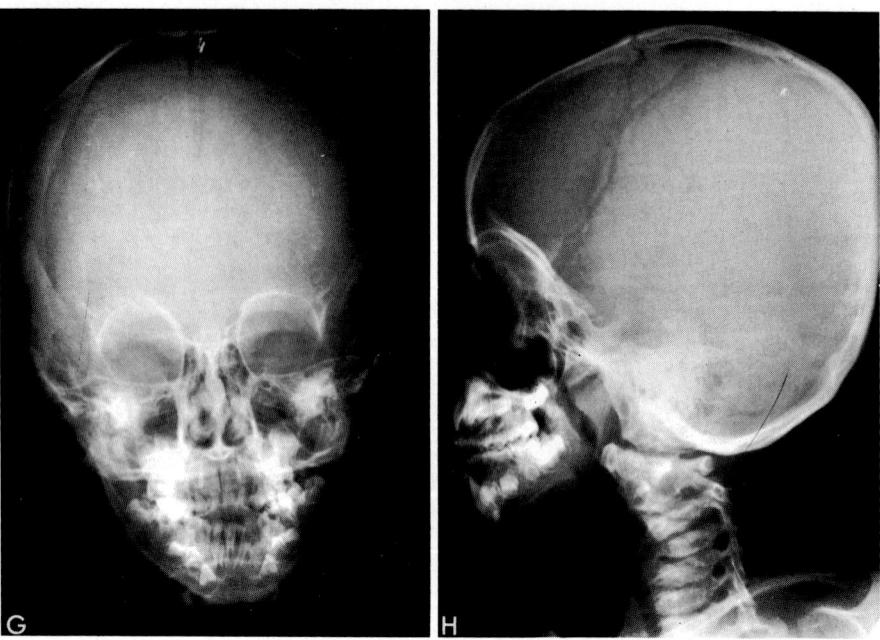

FIGURE 3–29 Continued. *Diastrophic dysplasia.*

G and **H.** Skull films are normal.

generalized mesodermal defect of diastrophic dysplasia. The foot deformity is progressive and becomes fixed and very resistant to correction.

The joints may be hyperextensible because of excessive ligamentous laxity or they may be limited in motion. The majority of cases are of the "stiff-joint" variety. In the "lax-joint" type the deformities of the limbs are not marked, and the prognosis for function is much better.

Flexion contractures of the hips, knees, and elbows are an integral part of the "stiff-joint" type of diastrophic dysplasia. They are present at birth and become progressively more severe and fixed to a degree that may impair standing and walking.

When the infant attempts to stand and walk progressive subluxation and dislocation of the hips and knees develops (Fig. 3–30). The contractural deformities are caused by structural osteocartilaginous deformities of the articulations and fixed fibrotic shortening of the soft tissues. Webbing of the joints may be present. Genu valgum commonly accompanies lateral subluxation of the patellofemoral joint.

In the elbows the radial heads may be dislocated. Contractural deformity of the shoulders is less frequent.

The trunk appears normal at birth, but when the child begins to walk, scoliosis and kyphosis gradually develop.[4, 10, 31, 37] Spinal deformity is progressive and present in all cases. This is explained by the fact that diastrophic dysplasia is caused by a neuromesodermal defect. The scoliosis becomes rapidly progressive in the preadolescent years; it has a large rotatory component and a strong tendency to become severe and fixed.

Cervical kyphosis is present in some cases and may become so severe that the odontoid process parallels the foramen magnum.[1, 4, 15] There is no abnormality of the odontoid process in diastrophic dysplasia, but the disorder has a high rate of association with hypoplasia of the cervical vertebral bodies. Defective neural arches at the cervico–upper thoracic level are present, but the development of cervical kyphosis cannot be correlated with spina bifida. Narrowing of the spinal canal will cause insidious myelopathy due to cord compression.[15]

Spinal stenosis is a variable feature of diastrophic dysplasia. The interpedicular distance may decrease caudally, remain constant, or increase slightly.[35] The lumbar pedicles are short, but there is no posterior bulging of the articular processes or thickening of the lamina.

Thoracolumbar kyphosis is present in almost all patients. The lumbar lordosis, which may be extreme, is secondary to the flexion contracture of the hips.

The stature of patients with diastrophic dysplasia is markedly reduced with an eventual adult height of 80 to 140 cm. (2'7" to 4'7"). The

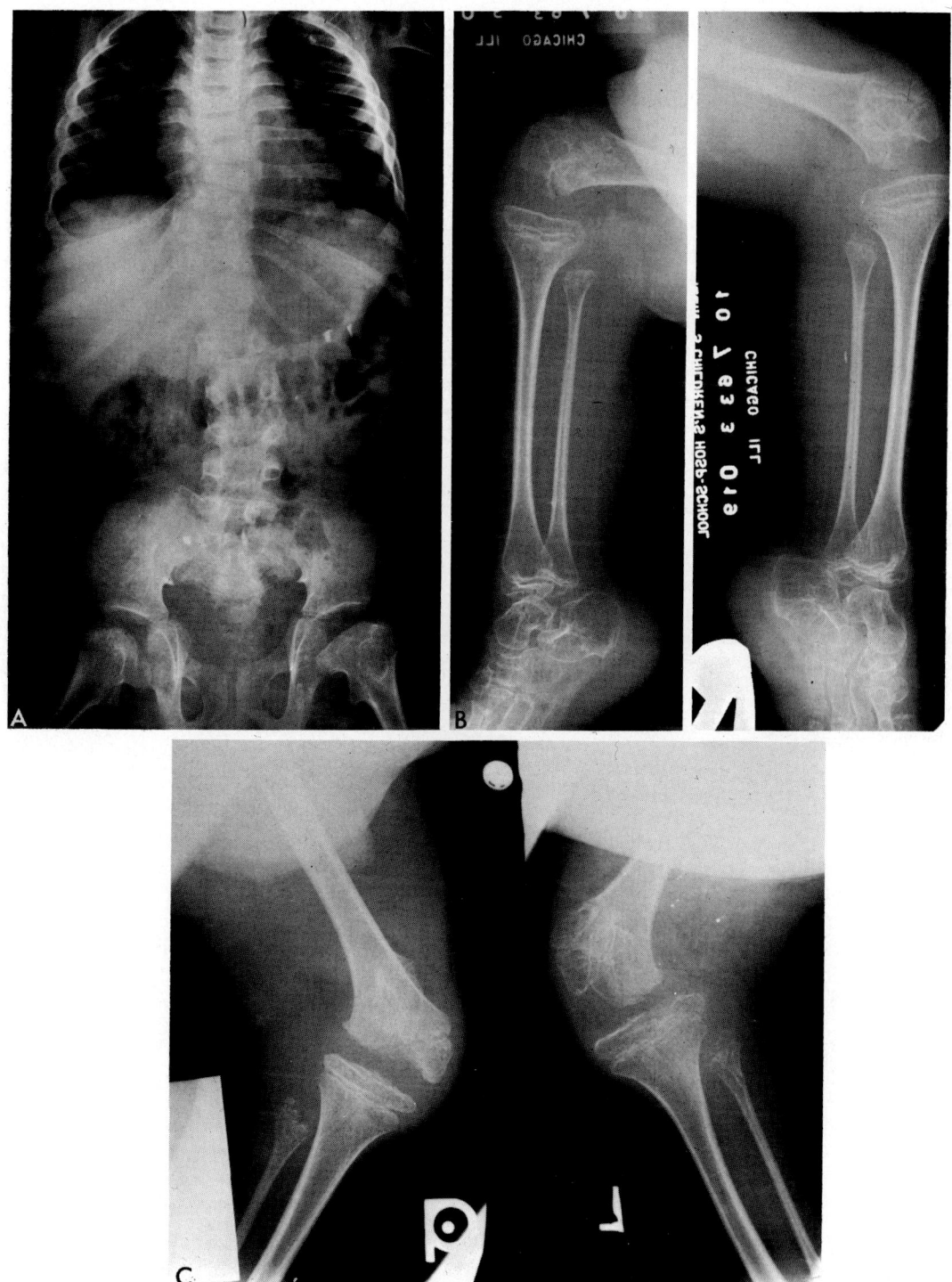

FIGURE 3–30. Diastrophic dysplasia in the brother of the patient in Figure 3–29.

A. Anteroposterior radiogram of spine, depicting scoliosis. **B** and **C.** Anteroposterior and lateral radiograms of both knees reveal lateral subluxation and severe flexion deformity. Note the delayed and irregular ossification of distal femoral epiphyses and flaring of the metaphyses.

dwarfism is disproportionate, the limbs being very short. The kyphoscoliosis and flexion contractures of the hips and knees accentuate the dwarfism.

Intelligence of these patients is normal; affected individuals have been employed in competitive professions.

Radiographic Features

These are not distinctive, are variable, and depend on the age of the patient and the severity of the dysplasia. The ossification centers of the epiphyses of long bones are delayed in appearance. Often the distal femoral epiphysis is not ossified at birth, and when it appears it is flattened, abnormally medial in its location, and triangular with its apex directed toward the metaphysis.[19] The metaphysis become broad and flared. Coxa vara occurs frequently, with broadening and irregularity of the femoral neck. Dislocation and other clinical deformities, especially of the hand and thumb, are apparent on the radiograms. The acetabula are shallow. In some cases there is coxa valga. The long bones are short and thick, resembling those of an achondroplast; the distinguishing feature of diastrophic dysplasia, however, is a marked delay in ossification of the epiphyses, which, when ossified, are misshapen and flattened.

In the spine the appearance of vertebrae varies; some are irregular, others flattened, some tall, and others showing scalloping of their posterior borders.

The flat bones and skull are essentially normal. In the hands and feet the first metacarpals and metatarsals are short, hypoplastic, and triangular in shape. The "hitchhiker's thumb" and foot deformities are evident.

Differential Diagnosis

In the infant one should rule out dysplasias with short-limbed dwarfism. These include such conditions as achondroplasia, chondrodystrophia calcificans congenita (Conradi's disease), spondyloepiphyseal dysplasia congenita, and others.

Arthrogryposis multiplex congenita may be mistaken for diastrophic dysplasia because of the multiple joint contractures and dislocations. Arthrogrypotic children do not have the features of short-limbed dwarfism—the hitchhiker's thumb and the cauliflower ears.

Treatment

Orthopedic problems in diastrophic dysplasia are formidable. The deformities are resistant, difficult to treat, and prone to recur. Often early surgical intervention may be necessary; diligent orthopedic care should be provided until the completion of growth.

Every attempt should be made to provide plantigrade feet. Soft-tissue release should be performed in early infancy, and use of a retentive orthotic device continued to prevent recurrence of the deformity.

Soft-tissue release at the knee should be combined with correction of flexion contracture of the hips. Ordinarily the flexion deformity of the knee recurs, and extension close-up wedge osteotomy of the distal femur is required.

The dislocated patella should be reduced early in life by release of the contracted iliotibial band and realignment of the quadriceps mechanism. With failure of early correction, the dislocation becomes irreducible.

The hip dislocations are very rigid, behaving like teratologic hip dislocation. Open reduction and femoral shortening are recommended. The poorly developed acetabula require subsequent innominate osteotomy with shelf augmentation. The hips are so resistant that sometimes it is good judgment to leave them dislocated.

Cervical kyphosis (if progressive and beginning to cause cord compression) is treated by anterior and posterior spinal fusion.[10]

Scoliosis and thoracolumbar kyphosis are treated by orthoses such as the Milwaukee brace. Often orthotic support is not effective in controlling the progressive scoliosis. In such cases this author strongly advises early surgery.

References

1. Amuso, S. L.: Diastrophic dwarfism. J. Bone Joint Surg., 50-A:113, 1968.
2. Bailey, J. A., II: Forms of dwarfism recognizable at birth. Clin. Orthop., 76:150, 1971.
3. Bailey, J. A., II: Disproportionate Short Stature. Diagnosis and Management. Philadelphia, W. B. Saunders, 1973.
4. Bethem, D., Winter, R. B., and Lutter, L.: Disorders of the spine in diastrophic dwarfism. A discussion of nine patients and review of the literature. J. Bone Joint Surg., 62-A:529, 1980.
5. Cremin, B. J., and Jarrett, J.: Diastrophic dwarfism. Aust. Radiol., 14:84, 1970.
6. Dallaire, L., and Fraser, F. C.: Diastrophic dwarfism. Birth Defects, 5:52, 1969.
7. Faucher, C., Regy, J. M., and Combe, P.: Nanisme diastrophique familial avec maladie de Hirschsprung. Ann. Pediatr. (Paris), 45:496, 1969.
8. Freedman, S. H., Taber, P., Hollister, D. W., and Rimion, D. L.: A lethal form of diastrophic dwarfism. Birth Defects, 10:43, 1974.
9. Herr, N., and Gulian, D.: Review of diastrophic dwarfism associated with cleft palate. Presentation of a case. Cleft Palate J., 11:299, 1974.
10. Herring, J. A.: The spinal disorders in diastrophic dwarfism. J. Bone Joint Surg., 60-A:177, 1978.

11. Horton, W. A., Hall, J. G., Scott, C. I., Pyeritz, R. E., and Rimion, D. L.: Growth curves for height for diastrophic dysplasia, spondyloepiphyseal dysplasia congenita, and pseudoachrondroplasia. Am. J. Dis. Child., 136:316, 1982.
12. Horton, W. A., Rimoin, D. L., Lachman, R. S., Skovby, F., Hollister, D. W., Spranger, J., Scott, C. I., and Hall, J. G.: The phenotypic variability of diastrophic dysplasia. J. Pediatr., 93:609, 1978.
13. Kaitila, I., Ammala, P., Karjalainen, O., Liukkonen, S., and Rapola, J.: Early prenatal detection of diastrophic dysplasia. Prenat. Diagn., 3:237, 1983.
14. Kaplan, M., Sauvegrain, J., Hayem, F., Drapeau, P., Maugey, F. and Boulle, J.: Etude d'un nouveau cas de nanisme diastrophique. Arch. Fr. Pediat., 18:981, 1961.
15. Kash, I. J., Sane, S. M., Samaha, F. J., and Briner, J.: Cervical cord compression in diastrophic dwarfism. J. Pediatr., 84:862, 1974.
16. Kopits, S. E.: Orthopedic complications of dwarfism. Clin. Orthop., 114:153, 1976.
17. Kozlowski, K., and Barylak, A.: Diastrophic dwarfism. Aust. Radiol., 18:398, 1974.
18. Lachman, R., Sillence, D., Rimoin, D., Horton, W., Hall, J., Scott, C., Spranger, J., and Langer, L.: Diastrophic dysplasia: The death of a variant. Radiology, 140:79, 1981.
19. Lamy, M., and Maroteaux, P.: Le nanisme diastrophique. Presse Méd., 52:1977, 1960.
20. Langer, L. O., Jr.: Diastrophic dwarfism in early infancy. A.J.R., 93:398, 1965.
21. Mantagos, S., Weiss, R. R., Mahoney, M., and Hobbins, J. C.: Prenatal diagnosis of diastrophic dwarfism. Am. J. Obstet. Gynecol., 139:111, 1981.
22. Mortensson, W.: Die Entwicklung der Skeletveränderungen beim diastrophischen Zwergwuchs. Radiology, 9:307, 1969.
23. Peytel, J.: Le nanisme diastrophique. Lyon, 1966.
24. Salle, B., Picot, C., Vauzelle, J.-L., Deffrenne, P., Monnet, P., François, R., and Robert, J.-M.: Le nanisme diastrophique. A propos de trois observations chez le nouveau-né. Pediatrie, 21:311, 1966.
25. Saule, H.: Diastropher Zwergwuchs. Bericht über ein Neugeborenes. Radiology, 15:50, 1975.
26. Schenk, A. K.: L'achondroplasia chez l'homme. Etude Clinique. Thèse de Saint Petersbourg, 1910.
27. Silverman, F. N.: Diastrophic dwarfism. Semin. Roentgenol., 8:152, 1973.
28. Spranger, J., and Gerken, H.: Diastrophischer Zwergwuchs. Z. Kinderheilkd., 98:227, 1967.
29. Stanescu, R., Stanescu, V., and Maroteaux, P.: Abnormal pattern of segment long spacing (SLS) cartilage collagen in diastrophic dysplasia. Coll. Relat. Res., 2:111, 1982.
30. Stanescu, V., Stanescu, R., and Maroteaux, P.: Etude histochimique et microchimique du cartilage de croissance tibial dans le nanisme diastrophique et la pycnodysostose. Ann. Histochim., 18:177, 1973.
31. Stover, C. N., Hayes, J. T., and Holt, J. F.: Diastrophic dwarfism. A.J.R., 89:914, 1963.
32. Taber, P., Freedman, S., and Lackey, D. A.: Diastrophic dwarfism. Progr. Pediatr. Radiol., 4:152, 1973.
33. Taybi, H.: Diastrophic dwarfism. Radiology, 80:1, 1963.
34. Vasquez, A. M., and Lee, F. A.: Diastrophic dwarfism. J. Pediatr., 72:234, 1968.
35. Walker, B. A., Scott, C. I., Hall, J. G., Murdoch, J. L., and McKusick, V. A.: Diastrophic dwarfism. Medicine, 51:41, 1972.
36. Walter, H.: Der diastrophische Zwergwuchs. Adv. Hum. Genet., 2:31, 1970.
37. Wilson, D. W., Chrispin, A. R., and Carter, C. O.: Diastrophic dwarfism. Arch. Dis. Child., 44:48, 1969.

MISCELLANEOUS TYPES OF DWARFISM

Metatropic dysplasia, first described by Maroteaux, Spranger, and Wiedemann in 1966, is characterized by severe short-limbed dwarfism with a distinctive "dumb-bell" appearance of the long bones due to diaphyseal constriction and widely flaring metaphyses.[12] In infancy the trunk is of normal length, but soon spinal deformity and trunk shortening develop. Scoliosis or kyphosis may be present at birth. On the radiograms the vertebrae appear flattened, almost paper thin, with apparent increase in disc interspace. The ribs are markedly shortened, and the thorax is narrow. In some patients there is a tail-like soft-tissue appendage over the sacrococcygeal region, extending to the anal cleft. The skull and facies are normal. Respiratory insufficiency may cause death in early infancy. If the child survives, cardiorespiratory embarrassment results from the severe kyphoscoliosis. Spinal cord compression due to atlantoaxial instability is another serious problem that may cause paralysis or death. Later on in adult life, degenerative arthritis of the hips and knees caused by the marked deformity of the joints is very disabling.[4, 6, 14]

In *pseudometatropic dysplasia*, also referred to as *Kniest disease*, the findings are similar to metatropic dysplasia, but its distinguishing features are the abnormal face with hypertelorism and depressed nasal bridge, deafness, and myopia with subsequent detached retina.[6–8, 11]

In *parastremmatic dysplasia*, first described by Langer, Petersen, and Spranger, the dwarfism is very severe and characterized by curving and twisting of the diaphyses of the long bones on their longitudinal axes, joints that are knobby and stiff, deformed epiphyses and metaphyses that have a distinctive flocculated appearance on the radiogram, and severe kyphoscoliosis.[9] This dysplasia is extremely rare. Inheritance appears to be as an autosomal dominant trait.[2, 5]

Dyggve-Melchior-Clausen disease is a short-trunk dwarfism, very similar to Morquio disease but characterized by the absence of mucopolysaccharides in the urine, mental retardation, disordered ossification of the iliac crest (which appears lacy), and marked platyspondyly of the vertebrae with a characteristic notched appearance on the lateral radiogram. Inheritance is as an autosomal recessive trait. The dysplasia is extremely rare. Most patients are of Lebanese origin.[1, 3, 15, 16] Severe genu valgum requires correction by varus osteotomy of the distal femur and/or the proximal tibia or by corticotomy and asymmetrical distraction by the Ilizarov apparatus.

References

1. Affifi, A. K., der Kaloustian, V. M., Bahuth, N. B., and Mire-Salman, J.: Concentrically laminated membranous inclusions in myofibres of Dyggve-Melchior-Clausen syndrome. J. Neurol. Sci., 21:335, 1974.
2. Apert, M. M., Liege, R., and Denet, J.: Dystrophie ostéo-articulaire grave chez une fille de 12 ans. Bull. Soc. Pediatr. Paris, 32:377, 1934.
3. Dyggve, H. V., Melchior, J. C., and Clausen, J.: Morquio-Ullrich's disease: An inborn error of metabolism? Arch. Dis. Child., 37:525, 1962.
4. Etesan, D. J., Adomian, G. E., Ornoy, A., Koide, T., Sugiura, Y., Calabro, A., Lungarotti, S., Mastrioacovo, P., Lachman, R. S., and Rimoin, D. L.: Fibrochondrogenesis. Radiologic and histologic studies. Am. J. Med. Genet., 19:277, 1984.
5. Horan, F., and Beighton, P.: Parastremmatic dwarfism. J. Bone Joint Surg., 58–B:343, 1976.
6. Jenkins, P., Smith, M. B., and McKinnell, J. S.: Metatropic dwarfism. Br. J. Radiol., 43:561, 1970.
7. Kniest, W.: Zur Abgrenzung der Dysostosis enchondralis von der Chondrodystrophie. Z. Kinderheilkd., 70:633, 1952.
8. Kozlowski, K., Barylak, A., Kobielowa, Z.: Kneist syndrome. Aust. Radiol., 21:60, 1977.
9. Langer, L. O., Petersen, D., and Spranger, J.: An unusual bone dysplasia: Parastremmatic dwarfism. A.J.R., 110:550, 1970.
10. Linker, A., Evans, L. R., and Langer, L. O.: Morquio's disease and mucopolysaccharide excretion. J. Pediatr., 77:1039, 1970.
11. Maroteaux, P., and Spranger, J.: La maladie de Kniest. Arch. Fr. Pediatr., 30:735, 1973.
12. Maroteaux, P., Spranger, J., and Wiedemann, H. R.: Der metatropische Zwergwuchs. Arch. Kinderheilkd., 173:211, 1966.
13. Rask, M. R.: Morquio-Brailsford osteochondrodystrophy and osteogenesis imperfecta: Report of a patient with both conditions. J. Bone Joint Surg., 45–A:561, 1963.
14. Rimoin, D. L., Siggers, D. C., Lachman, R. S., and Silberberg, R.: Metatropic dwarfism, the Kneist syndrome and pseudoachondroplastic dysplasias. Clin. Orthop., 114:70, 1976.
15. Schorr, S., and Legum, C.: The Dyggve-Melchior-Clausen syndrome. A.J.R., 128:107, 1977.
16. Toledo, S. P. A., Saldanha, P. H., Lamego, C., Mourao, P. A. S., Dietrich, C. P., and Mattar, E.: Dyggve-Melchior-Clausen disease: Genetic studies and report of affected sibs. Am. J. Med. Genet., 4:255, 1979.

OSTEOGENESIS IMPERFECTA

Osteogenesis imperfecta is a connective tissue disorder that is genetically heterogeneous and comprises a number of distinct syndromes, some inherited as autosomal dominant traits, others as recessive traits, some occurring as spontaneous mutations.[156–159] Manifestations of the syndrome have great variability; they consist of generalized osteoporosis—a nonspecific finding that may be clinically silent at one end of the spectrum or may be manifest as bowing and fragility of long bones with proclivity to fractures at the other end. Other stigmata are dentinogenesis imperfecta, blue sclerae, deafness, ligamentous hyperlaxity, herniae, easy bruising, and excessive sweating. In the literature, terms used to denote this disorder include *fragilis ossium*, *osteopsathyrosis idiopathica*, *brittle bone*, *Lobstein's disease*, and *Vrolik's disease*.[99, 180]

Classification and Heredity

Looser, in 1906, classified osteogenesis imperfecta into two types: osteogenesis imperfecta *congenita*, characterized by the presence of numerous fractures at birth, and osteogenesis imperfecta *tarda*, in which the fracture or fractures occurred after the perinatal period.[100] In the literature the former is referred to as Vrolik's disease, and the latter as Lobstein's disease, Ekman-Lobstein disease, or osteopsathyrosis idiopathica.[44, 99, 180] The prognosis in the osteogenesis imperfecta congenita type is poor with a high rate of mortality due to intracrural hemorrhage at birth or recurrent respiratory infection in infancy.

Seedorff, in 1949, subclassified osteogenesis imperfecta tarda into two types: *tarda gravis*, in which the first fracture occurs in the first year of life (these children subsequently develop severe deformities of the long bones and spine), and *tarda levis*, in which the first fracture occurs after the first year of life and deformity and disability are not so severe.[154]

In the tarda type age does not always correlate with the severity of the disease. Therefore, Falvo and associates subdivided this large and clinically variable tarda group according to the presence of bowing of the long bones; those cases with bowing were subclassified as tarda type I, and those without bowing as tarda type II.[51] Bowing of the long bones is a good measure of the severity of the disease because it correlates well with the number of fractures and the severity of the deformity. It is of therapeutic significance because it indicates the possible need to treat the tarda type I by surgery.

Sillence and Danks, in a comprehensive survey in Victoria, Australia, delineated at least four distinct *genetic types* of osteogenesis imperfecta, two inherited as autosomal dominant and two as autosomal recessive traits.[158] Variability of the dental abnormalities in dominantly inherited pedigrees suggests further heterogeneity in osteogenesis imperfecta. Because descriptive terms for the different osteogenesis imperfecta syndromes are cumbersome, Sillence proposed numerical classification (Table 3–4).

Osteogenesis Imperfecta Type I. It is characterized by generalized osteoporosis with abnormal bony fragility, distinct blue sclerae throughout life, and presenile conductive hearing loss. Genetic studies have shown an autosomal dominant inheritance.[154, 157-159] Dentinogenesis imperfecta is not present in all patients; in those without dentinogenesis imperfecta the disease is subclassified as OI Type IA, and in those with dentinogenesis imperfecta as OI Type IB. Otherwise these subtypes are indistinguishable clinically and radiographically.

Osteogenesis Imperfecta Type II. Type II is characterized by extreme bone fragility leading to death in the perinatal period or early infancy. The long bones are crumbled (accordion femora), and ossification of the skull is markedly delayed; on palpation the cranial vault feels like numerous small plates of bone. Inheritance is as an autosomal recessive trait.[154]

Osteogenesis Imperfecta Type III. This rare variety of osteogenesis imperfecta is of autosomal recessive inheritance. It is characterized by severe bone fragility, multiple fractures and progressive marked deformity of the long bones, and severe growth retardation. The sclerae are bluish at birth but become less blue with age. In the adolescent the sclerae are of normal hue.

Osteogenesis Imperfecta Type IV. This type is inherited through autosomal dominant transmission. At birth, the sclerae are of normal hue; if they are bluish they become progressively less so and are normal in the adolescent. The osteoporosis, bone fragility, and long bone deformities are of variable severity. Opalescent dentin is not present in all patients, indicating heterogeneity; those with normal dentition are classified as Type IVA and those with dentinogenesis imperfecta as Type IVB.

Some cases of osteogenesis imperfecta occur as spontaneous mutations.

Incidence

According to Wynne-Davies, possible prevalence in the population is 16 per million index patients (34 per million including affected relatives). Osteogenesis imperfecta can be identified at birth. It occurs in 1 in 20,000 live births.[187]

The incidence of the various types of osteogenesis imperfecta varies. The birth incidence and population frequency of Type I is 1:30,000; that of Type II in Victoria, Australia, is reported by Sillence and associates to be 1:62,487 live births.[157-159] Osteogenesis imperfecta Type III is extremely rare; at present the exact incidence of Type III and Type IV is unknown.

Pathology

The fundamental defect in osteogenesis imperfecta is failure of maturation of collagen beyond the reticulin fiber stage. The collagen fibers resemble reticulin fibers. The osteoblasts demonstrate normal or increased activity, but fail to produce and organize collagen.[53, 54, 127] Normally, following synthesis of collagen molecules, intermolecular cross links form between adjacent molecules; this progressive cross-linking is vital for maturation of collagen and provision of its chemical and physical properties. A defect in cross-linking will result in decreased stability of polymeric collagen. Instability of polymeric skin collagen in osteogenesis imperfecta has been reported by Francis and associates.[56-58] Cultured skin fibroblasts from patients with osteogenesis imperfecta fail to produce collagen polypeptide.[119] In Type II, Penttinen and associates found decreased proportions of Type I to Type III collagen from cultured fibroblasts.[123] Brown and colleagues reported abnormal distribution of glycosaminoglycans in dentin in Type I.[26]

Formation of both enchondral and intramembranous bone is disturbed. Histologic findings vary according to the type of osteogenesis imperfecta. The morphology of the cells and of the matrix is not consistent throughout the spectrum of the syndrome. The amount of woven bone is larger than in normal controls, and histometric analyses have shown that in the severe congenita form the proportion of primitive osseous tissue with a woven or irregular collagen matrix is significantly greater than in the less severe tarda form.[28, 50]

The bone trabeculae are thin and lack an organized trabecular pattern. Fractured spicules of trabeculae may be found. The spongiosa is scanty. The intracellular matrix is reduced, and as a result there is relative abundance of osteocytes (Fig. 3–31). The osteoclasts are morphologically normal, though they seem to be numerous and have an increased number of resorption surfaces.

Osteoid seams are wide and crowded by plump osteoblasts. The mineralized chondroid lattice is surrounded by wide seams of basophilic substance.[53, 54] This large number of osteoblasts and osteoclasts, the large size of the osteoblasts, and the plentiful osteoid tissue covering the thin bone trabeculae indicate in-

Table 3-4. Classification of Osteogenesis Imperfecta Syndromes (According to Sillence)

Type		Inheritance	Teeth	Bone Fragility	Deformity of Long Bones	Growth Retardation	Presenile Hearing Loss (per cent)
I	A	Autosomal dominant	Normal	Variable—less severe than other types	Moderate	Short stature, 2 to 3 per cent below mean	40
	B	Autosomal dominant	Dentinogenesis imperfecta	Variable—less severe than other types	Moderate	Short, 2 to 3 per cent below mean	40
II		Autosomal recessive	Unknown (because of perinatal death)	Very extreme	Crumbled bone (accordion femora) marked	Unknown (because of perinatal death)	
III		Autosomal recessive	Dentinogenesis imperfecta	Severe	Severe Progressive bowing of long bones and spine	Severe—smallest of all patients with osteogenesis imperfecta	
IV	A	Autosomal dominant	Normal	Moderate	Moderate	Short stature	Low frequency
	B	Autosomal dominant	Dentinogenesis imperfecta	Moderate	Moderate	Short stature	Low frequency

creased bone turnover. Tetracycline labeling studies have confirmed the increased bone turnover in osteogenesis imperfecta.[4, 128]

The lamellae in lamellar bone are thin and tenuous. On electromicroscopy the collagen fibrils do not aggregate in bundles of normal thickness; instead they are organized in thin, loosely compacted filaments.[175] The compact bone consists of a coarse fibrillary type of immature bone without haversian systems. Periosteum and perichondrium are normal. The physis is usually broad and irregular, the proliferative and hypertrophic zones are disorganized, and the typical columnar arrangement is lacking. The calcified zone of the growth plates is thinner, and metaphyseal blood vessels permeate the growth plate cartilage. Varying numbers of islands of cartilage are present in the juxtaphyseal metaphyseal region. The primary spongiosa in the metaphysis is sparse, with the osseous tissue almost always of the woven variety. The secondary centers of ossification in the epiphysis are delayed in maturation, and residual islands of cartilage remain in the epiphysis.

When a fracture is present the endosteal fracture callus is primarily cartilaginous and the periosteal reaction is abundant, consisting mainly of woven bone.

The bulk of cartilage in osteogenesis imperfecta consists of water and proteoglycans rather than collagen. The proteoglycans are normal. The cartilaginous ends of long bones are disproportionately large. At birth, the stature of children with osteogenesis imperfecta is within normal limits; with growth, however, it be-

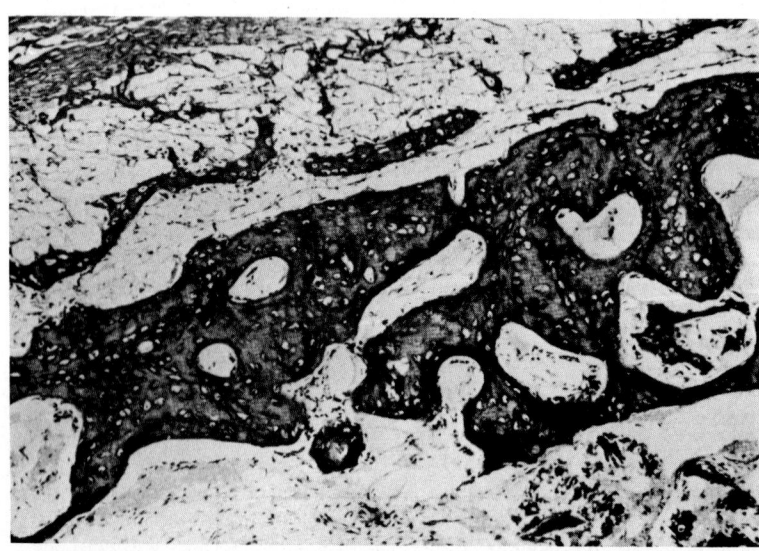

FIGURE 3-31. Histology of osteogenesis imperfecta.

There is relative abundance of osteocytes with decrease of intracellular matrix. Osteoclasts are normal, but number of resorption surfaces is increased. (From Bullough, P. G., Davidson, D. D., and Lorenzo, J. C.: The morbid anatomy of the skeleton in osteogenesis imperfecta. Clin. Orthop., 159:42, 1981. Reprinted by permission.)

Table 3-4. Classification of Osteogenesis Imperfecta Syndromes (According to Sillence) Continued

Prognosis	Sclerae	Spine	Skull	Other	Incidence
Fair	Distinctly blue throughout life	20 per cent scoliosis and kyphosis	Wormian bones in x-ray	Premature arcus senilis	1/30,000
Fair	Distinctly blue throughout life	20 per cent scoliosis and kyphosis	Wormian bones in x-ray	Premature arcus senilis	1/30,000
Perinatal death	Blue		Marked absence of ossification Wormian bones		1/62,000 live births
Nonambulatory, wheel-chair-bound May die in third decade	Bluish at birth, become less blue with age, white in adult	Kyphoscoliosis	Hypoplastic, more ossified than type II Wormian bones		Very rare
Fair	Normal	Kyphoscoliosis	Hypoplastic Wormian bones		Unknown
Fair	Normal	Kyphoscoliosis	Hypoplastic Wormian bones		Unknown

comes progressively short. It seems that when the cartilaginous skeleton is being replaced by bone, growth retardation develops and causes shortness. Dwarfing probably results from decreased matrix production by connective tissue cells. Another pathogenic factor is trauma, which will cause fragmentation and disruption of the physis, which is brittle because of the thin zone of calcification and is extremely susceptible to lateral compression.[27, 28]

Gross anatomic findings consist of porosis (osteopenia), diminution in size, and skeletal deformities secondary to fracture and asymmetrical physeal growth disturbance (Fig. 3–32). The long bones are slender and smaller than normal. The cortices are like eggshell, with paucity of medullary spongy bone (Fig. 3–33). There will be evidence of recent or healed fractures with varying degrees of angular or torsional deformities. The cartilaginous epiphyseal ends of the long bones in general retain a recognizable shape but are disproportionately large and have some irregularity of the articular surface (Fig. 3–34).

The spine may show varying degrees of deformity, usually scoliosis due to compression fractures and wedging of the vertebral bodies (Fig. 3–35). Kyphosis may be combined with scoliosis.

In the skull there are multiple centers of ossification, particularly in the occipital region, and wormian bones (Fig. 3–36).

In the skin, the collagen of the corium is immature, as indicated by the persistent metachromasia, argentophilia, and absence of adult collagen.

Clinical Picture

This varies according to the variety of the disease. In the severe congenital form, because of the multiple fractures, which may number

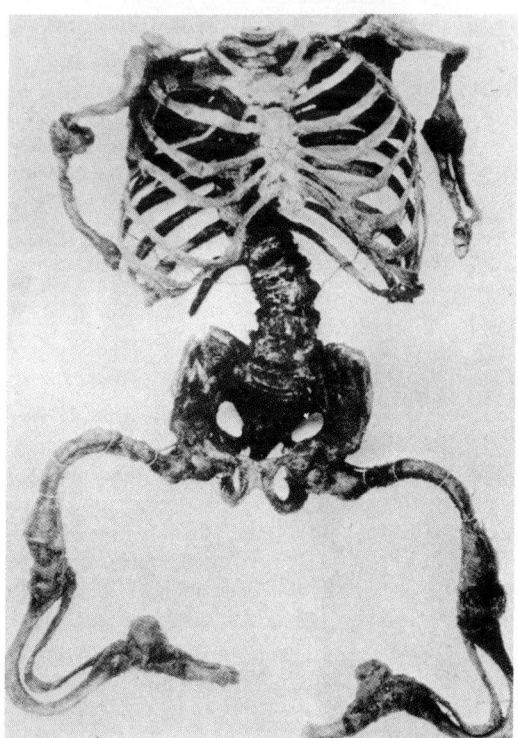

FIGURE 3–32. *Skeleton in osteogenesis imperfecta.*

(From Bullough, P. G., Davidson, D. D., and Lorenzo, J. C.: The morbid anatomy of the skeleton in osteogenesis imperfecta. Clin. Orthop., *159:*42, 1981. Reprinted by permission.)

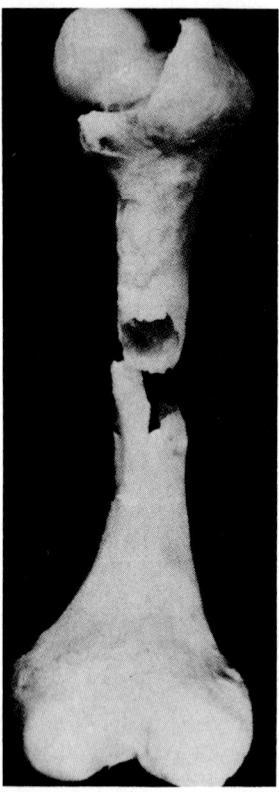

FIGURE 3–33. *Eggshell-thin cortex in osteogenesis imperfecta.*

(From Bullough, P. G., Davidson, D. D., and Lorenzo, J. C.: The morbid anatomy of the skeleton in osteogenesis imperfecta. Clin. Orthop., 159:42, 1981. Reprinted by permission.)

over 100, caused by minimal trauma during delivery or in utero, the limbs are deformed and short. Crepitation can be demonstrated by palpation at the fracture site. The skull is soft and membranous (Fig. 3–37). This type is often fatal owing to intracranial hemorrhage; the infant is stillborn or lives only a short time.

In the moderate and mild forms of the disease, fragility of the bones is the most outstanding feature, with fractures occurring on the slightest injury, such as a sudden muscle pull. The number of fractures varies according to the severity of the disease. In general, the earlier fractures occur, the more severe the disease. Lower limbs are more frequently affected, as they are more prone to trauma. The femur is more commonly fractured than the tibia. The fracture is usually located at the convexity of the bone and is usually transverse with minimal displacement. Fractures heal at a normal rate; the resultant callus may be very large and hyperplastic, resembling osteogenic sarcoma on the radiograms.[2, 11, 12, 90, 135, 178] Long bones may heal in various deformities, such as anterior, medial, lateral, or posterior bowing. Pseudarthrosis may occur if the fracture is not immobilized. Children usually complain of little pain on sustaining a fracture, as accompanying soft-tissue trauma is minimal and they are so accustomed to frequent fracture. A bone that has fractured once tends to do so repeatedly because of limb deformity with angulation of the fragments and disuse atrophy resulting from immobilization. Growth may be arrested by multiple microfractures at the epiphyseal ends. The frequency of fractures declines sharply after adolescence. Bowing results from multiple transverse fractures of long bones and the pull of strong muscles. In the distal half of the femur, the deformation is an anterolateral angulation; in the proximal end of the femur there is usually a decrease in the neck-shaft angle with a coxa vara deformity. Acetabular protrusion (Otto pelvis) may be present. The proximal part of the femur is angulated anterolaterally. The combined anterior angulation of the femur and the tibia gives an apparent flexion contracture of

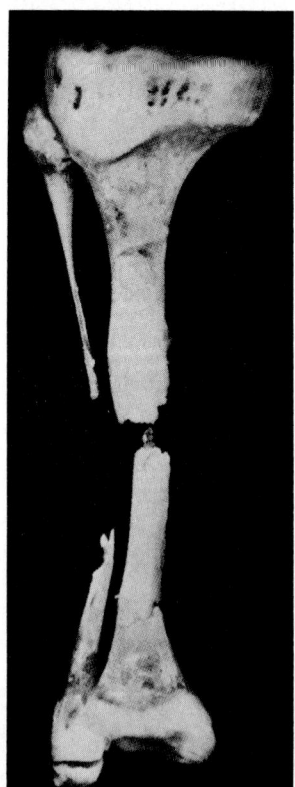

FIGURE 3–34. *Tibia in osteogenesis imperfecta.*

(From Bullough, P. G., Davidson, D. D., and Lorenzo, J. C.: The morbid anatomy of the skeleton in osteogenesis imperfecta. Clin. Orthop., 159:42, 1981. Reprinted by permission.)

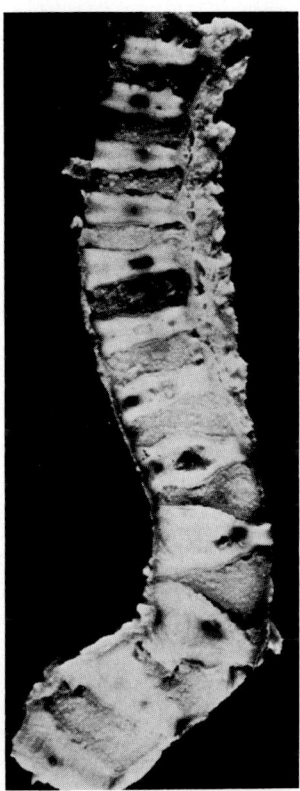

FIGURE 3–35. *Spine in osteogenesis imperfecta.*

(From Bullough, P. G., Davidson, D. D., and Lorenzo, J. C.: The morbid anatomy of the skeleton in osteogenesis imperfecta. Clin. Orthop., 159:42, 1981. Reprinted by permission.)

the knee that is in part compensated for by hyperextension deformity of the knee joint. The humerus is usually angulated laterally or anterolaterally. The forearm may be in minimal pronation; its rotation is often severely limited. Angulation is usually greater in the upper part of both bones of the forearm. The elbow joint has cubitus varus with flexion contracture. Hyperlaxity of ligaments is common with resultant hypermobility of joints. Atlantoaxial subluxation may be present. Deformity of the articular ends of the long bones may be another factor in contractural deformity of joints. Pes valgus is a frequent physical finding. Recurrent dislocation of the patellofemoral joint is not uncommon, predisposing the patient to falls and fractures (Fig. 3–38). The radial head and the hip joint may occasionally be dislocated.

The muscles are hypotonic, most probably because of the multiple fractures and deformities. The skin is thin. Subcutaneous hemorrhages may occur. The Rumpel-Leede test for capillary fragility may be positive. As a rule, scars of surgical incision are wide.

The forehead is broad, with prominent parietal and temporal bones and an overhanging occiput (Fig. 3–39 A to D). The bulging calvarium causes faciocranial disproportion, giving a triangular, elfin shape to the face. The ears are displaced downward and outward. The configuration of the skull in osteogenesis imperfecta has been likened to that of a soldier's helmet and called "helmet head."

Blue sclerae are one of the best-known manifestations of osteogenesis imperfecta but are not present in all types. In Type I, they are distinctly blue throughout life; in Type III, they are bluish at birth but become less blue with increasing age and white in the adult; and in Type IV, they are normal. Patients with Type II disease usually expire in the perinatal period, their sclerae are blue. The blueness of the sclera is caused by the thinness of its collagen layer, which has a low total collagen content but normal stability to depolymerization. Normal-colored sclerae in patients with osteogenesis imperfecta have a normal content of collagen in the connective tissue, but the collagen is very

Text continued on page 769

FIGURE 3–36. *Skull in osteogenesis imperfecta.*

(From Bullough, P. G., Davidson, D. D., and Lorenzo, J. C.: The morbid anatomy of the skeleton in osteogenesis imperfecta. Clin. Orthop., 159:42, 1981. Reprinted by permission.)

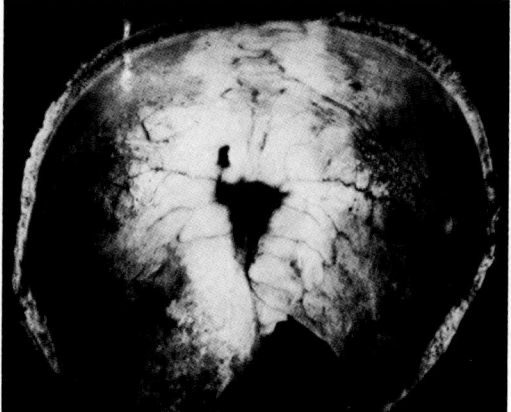

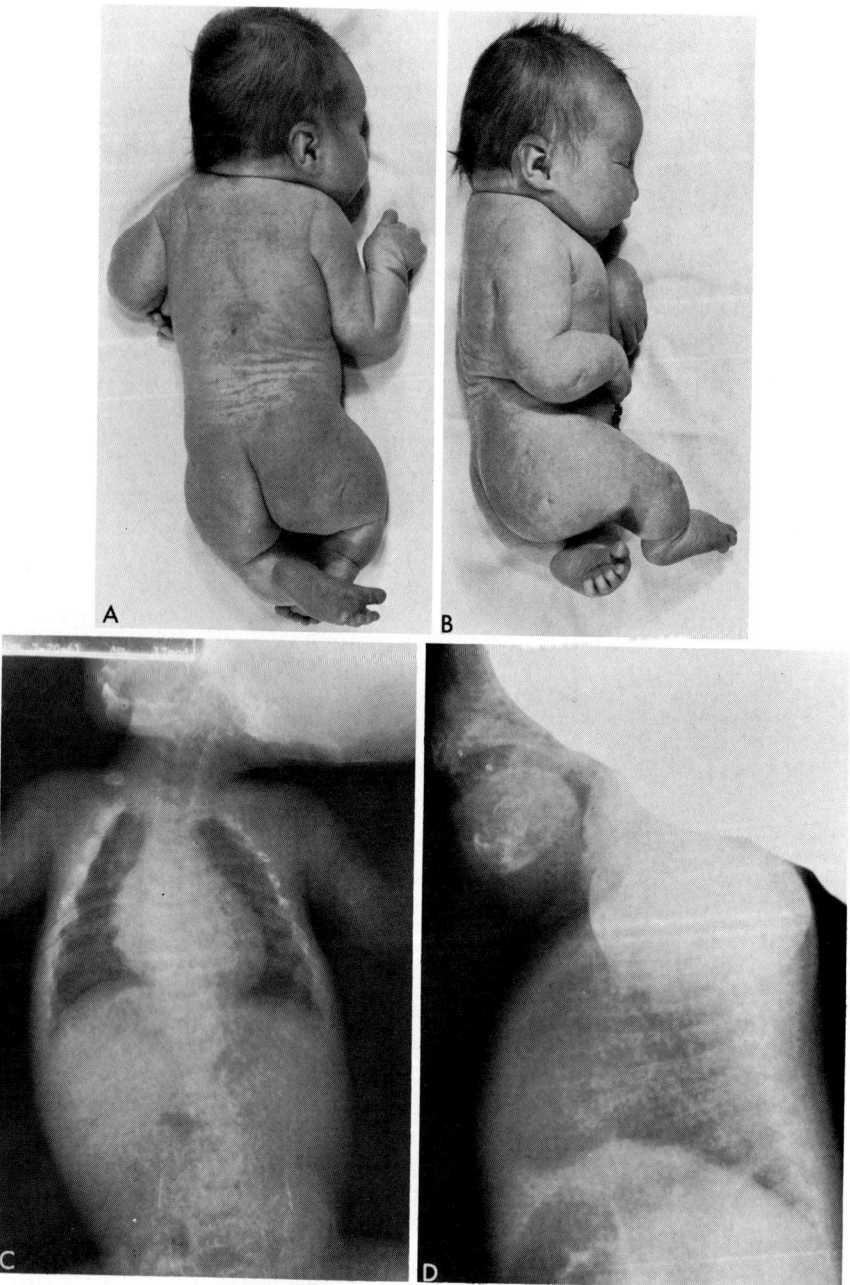

FIGURE 3–37. *Osteogenesis imperfecta congenita in a newborn.*

A and **B**. Clinical appearance. **C** and **D**. Anteroposterior and lateral radiograms of the trunk.

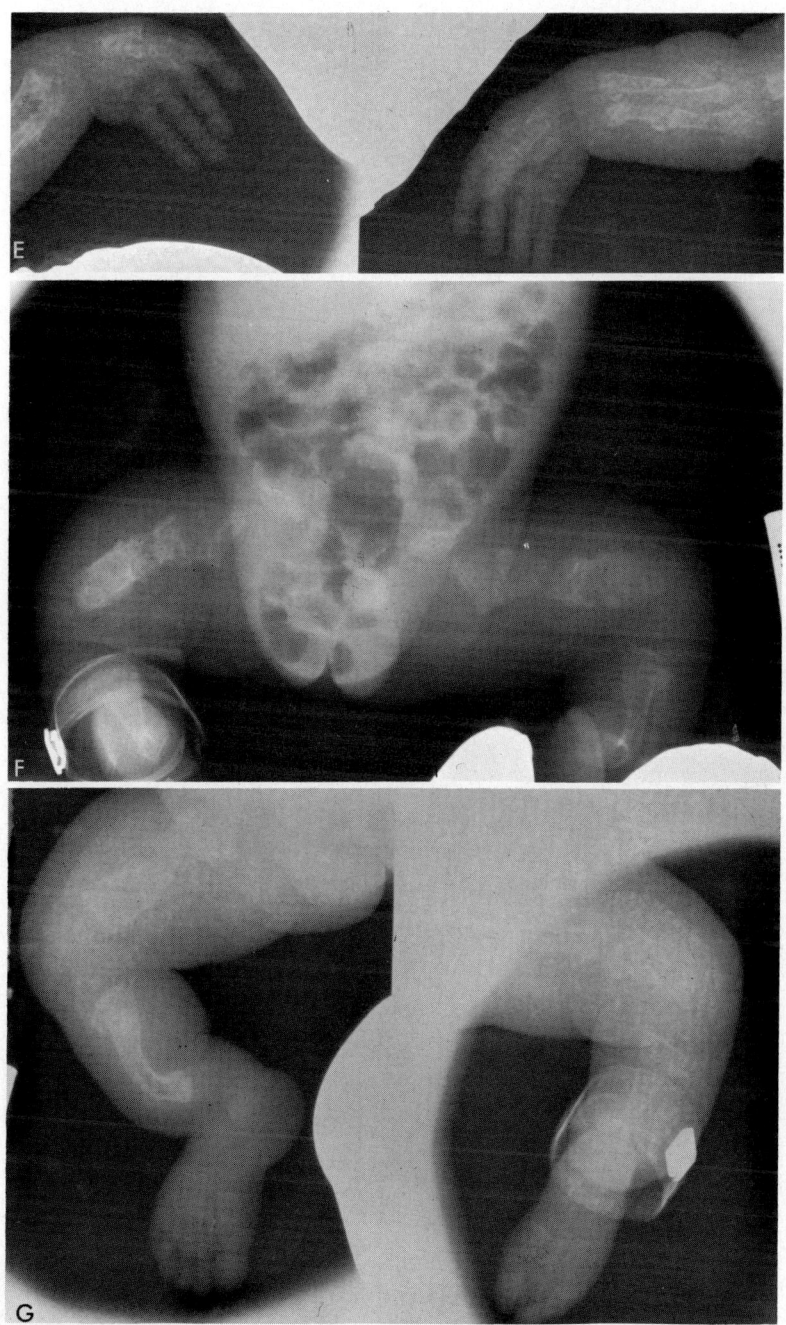

FIGURE 3–37 Continued. Osteogenesis imperfecta congenita in a newborn.

E. Radiograms of upper limbs and **F** and **G,** of lower limbs, showing multiple fractures.

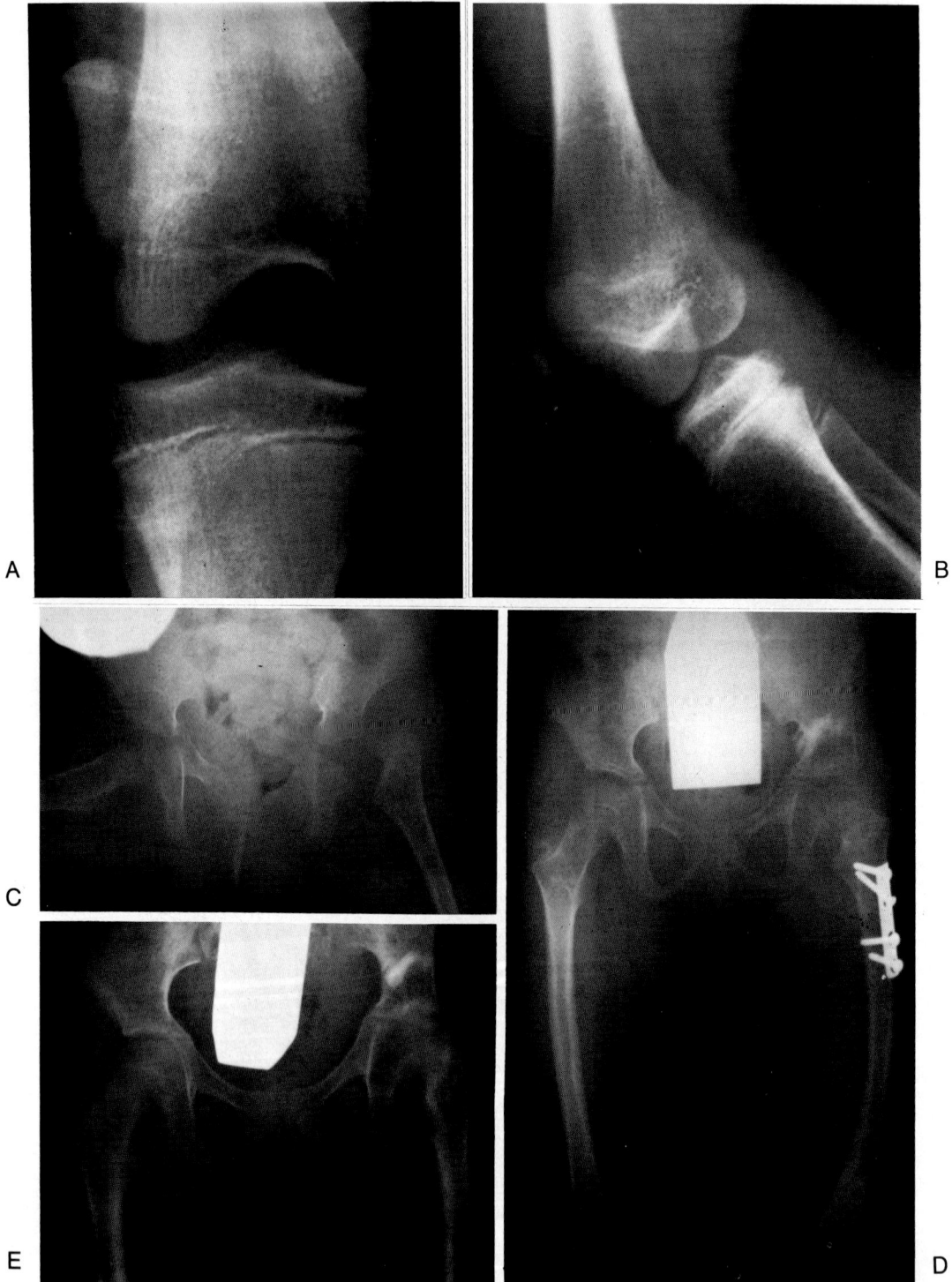

FIGURE 3-38. Osteogenesis imperfects.

A and **B.** Lateral dislocation of the patellofemoral joint in an adolescent with osteogenesis imperfecta. Anteroposterior (**A**) and lateral (**B**) views of the knees. **C** to **E.** Congenital dislocation of the left hip in an infant with osteogenesis imperfecta treated by open reduction, femoral shortening, innominate osteotomy, and capsular plication. The ilium was so soft that methylmethacrylate had to be used to glue the iliac fragments. **C.** Anteroposterior radiogram. Note the dislocation. **D.** Immediate postoperative anteroposterior view of the hip. **E.** Ten years later showing maintenance of reduction.

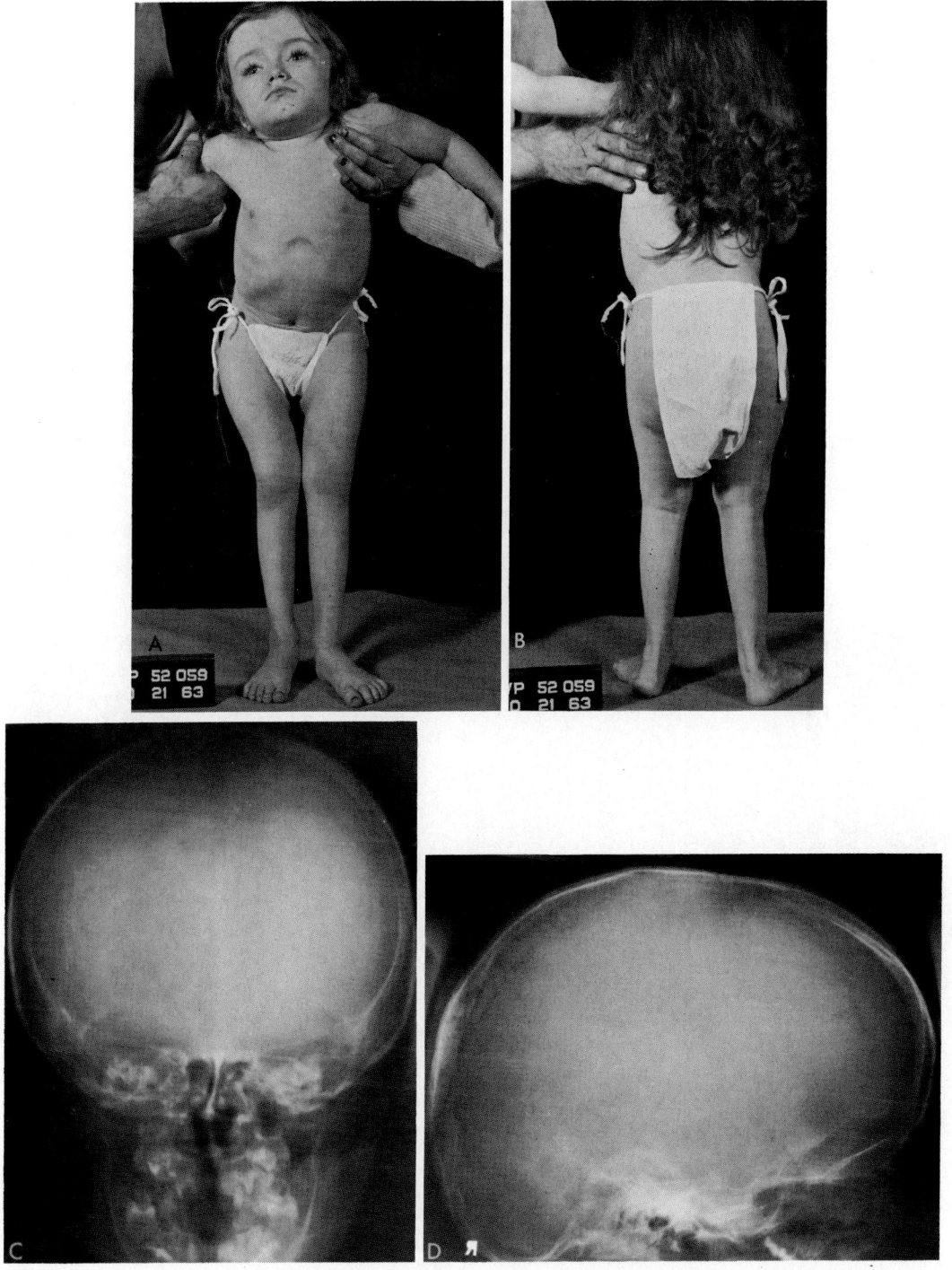

FIGURE 3–39. *Osteogenesis imperfecta in a five-year-old girl.*

A and **B.** Clinical appearance. Note the broad forehead and the prominent parietal and temporal bones. **C** and **D.** Anteroposterior and lateral radiograms of the skull.

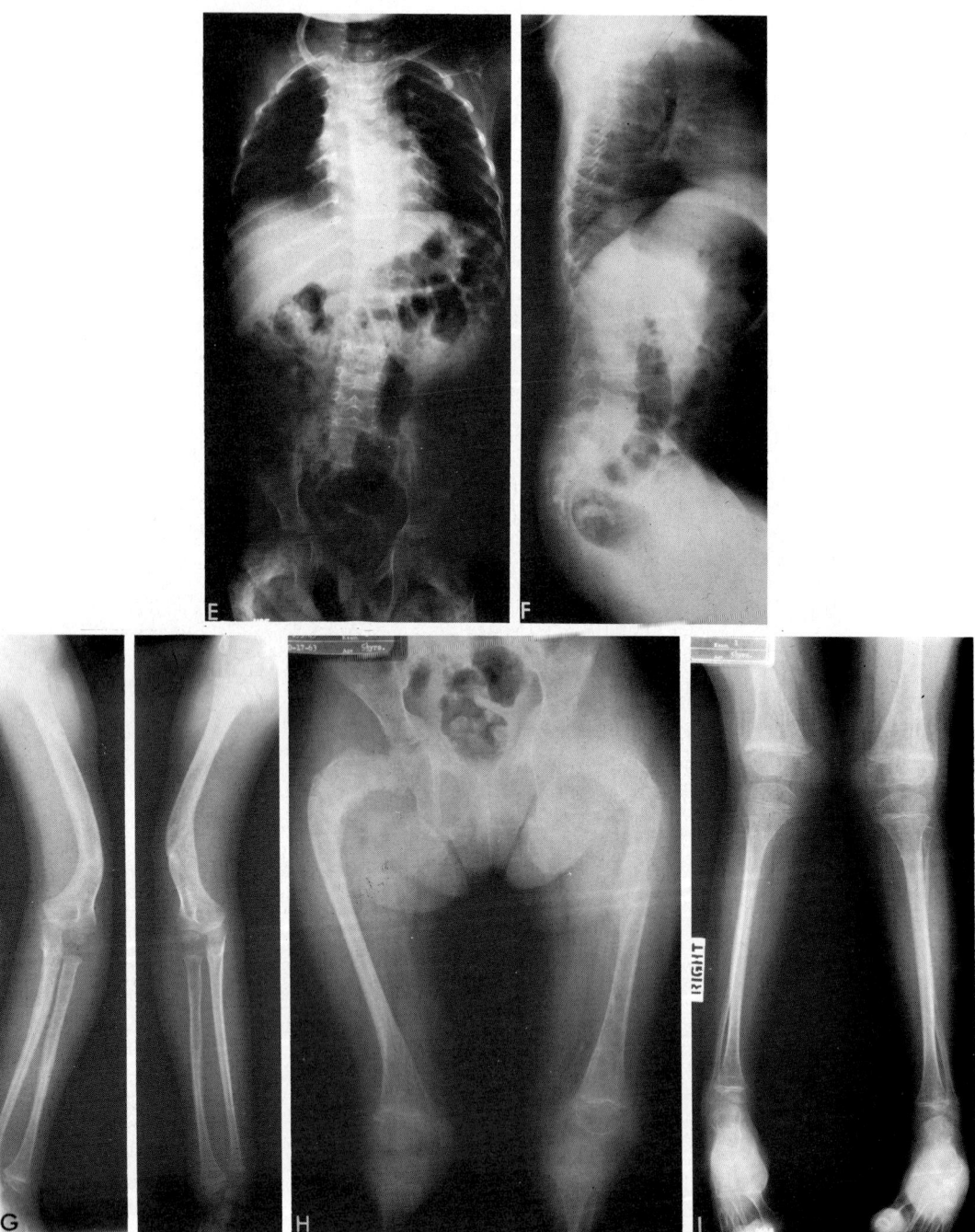

FIGURE 3–39 Continued. Osteogenesis imperfecta in a five-year-old girl.

E and **F.** Anteroposterior and lateral radiograms of the spine showing multiple compression fractures of the vertebral bodies and a left dorsolumbar scoliosis. **G** to **I.** Radiograms of upper and lower limbs. Note the multiple deformities, especially coxa vara and healed fractures.

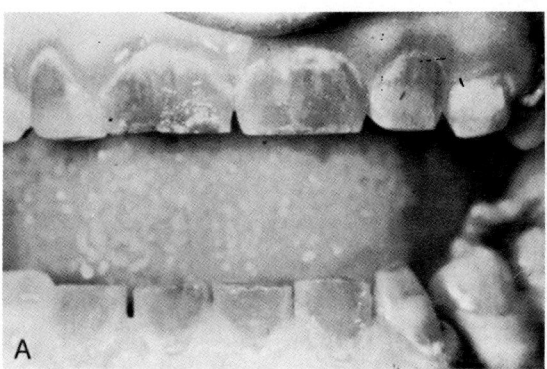 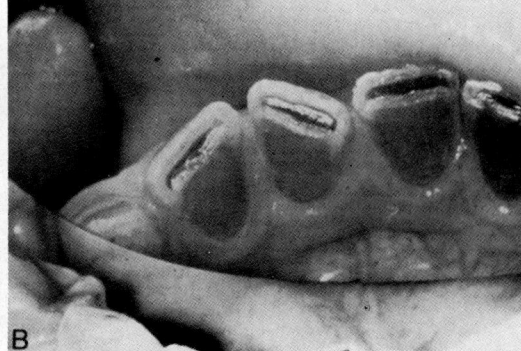

FIGURE 3–40. Teeth in osteogenesis imperfecta.

unstable to depolymerization. Abnormal thinness or translucency of the sclerae permits visibility of the intraocular pigment, which may vary from a "Wedgwood" or deep sky blue to a bluish-white tint. The so-called Saturn's ring, a frequent finding, is due to the white sclera immediately surrounding the cornea. Hyperopia is frequently present, but vision usually remains unaffected. An opacity in the periphery of the cornea, known as embryotoxon or arcus juvenilis, is common. Retinal detachment may occur.

The teeth are affected because of the deficiency of dentin. The enamel is essentially normal, as it is of ectodermal, not of mesenchymal, origin. Both deciduous and permanent teeth are involved. They break easily and are prone to caries, and fillings do not hold well. Yellowish brown or translucent bluish gray discoloration of the teeth is common (Fig. 3–40). The lower incisors, which erupt first, are the most severely affected. The terms *dentinogenesis imperfecta* and *hereditary opalescent dentin* or *hereditary hypoplasia of the dentin* have been used when the teeth alone are affected. Dentinogenesis imperfecta is not present in all types of osteogenesis imperfecta. It is present in Type IB and Type IVB, and may be present in Type III. In Type II it is unknown because of perinatal death. In Type IA and Type IVA the teeth are normal.

Deafness may occur in osteogenesis imperfecta, but it is not a major constant feature. It is present in 40 per cent of those with Type I and is lower in frequency in Type IV. Hearing loss may be either of the conduction type, due to otosclerosis, or of the nerve type, caused by pressure on the auditory nerve as it emerges from the skull. Otosclerosis results from abnormal proliferation of cartilage, which on calcification produces sclerosis of the petrous portion of the temporal bone. Onset of deafness is usually in adult life, occasionally in adolescence. The patient may also complain of tinnitus and vertigo.

A squeaky voice may be present in some patients.

Severe spinal deformity develops because of the combination of marked osteoporosis, compression fractures of the vertebrae, and ligamentous hyperlaxity. The resultant kyphoscoliosis may be very severe and disabling (Fig. 3–41). Kyphoscoliosis is present in 20 to 40 per cent of the patients. The most common type of curve is thoracic scoliosis. Some patients develop spondylolisthesis due to elongation of the pedicles without any actual break in the pars interarticularis.

Short stature is common. It is due to deformities of the limbs caused by angulation and overriding of fractures, growth disturbance at the physes, and the marked kyphoscoliosis.

A summary of the clinical characteristics of osteogenesis imperfecta as just described is illustrated in Figure 3–42.

Radiographic Findings

Severe Form. These radiographic findings in the severe congenital form of osteogenesis imperfecta are quite striking at birth. The long bones of the limbs are short and wide with thin cortices. The diaphyses are as wide as the metaphyses. There are numerous fractures, some recent and others in various stages of healing or healed (see Fig. 3–37 E, F, and G). Malunion of fractures results in angular deformation of the long bones; as the child begins to walk, the long bones may bend because of stress fractures. Multiple rib fractures and atrophy of the thoracic cage may simulate asphyxiating thoracic dysplasia.

Fairbank described three radiographic patterns: thick bone; slender, fragile bone; and

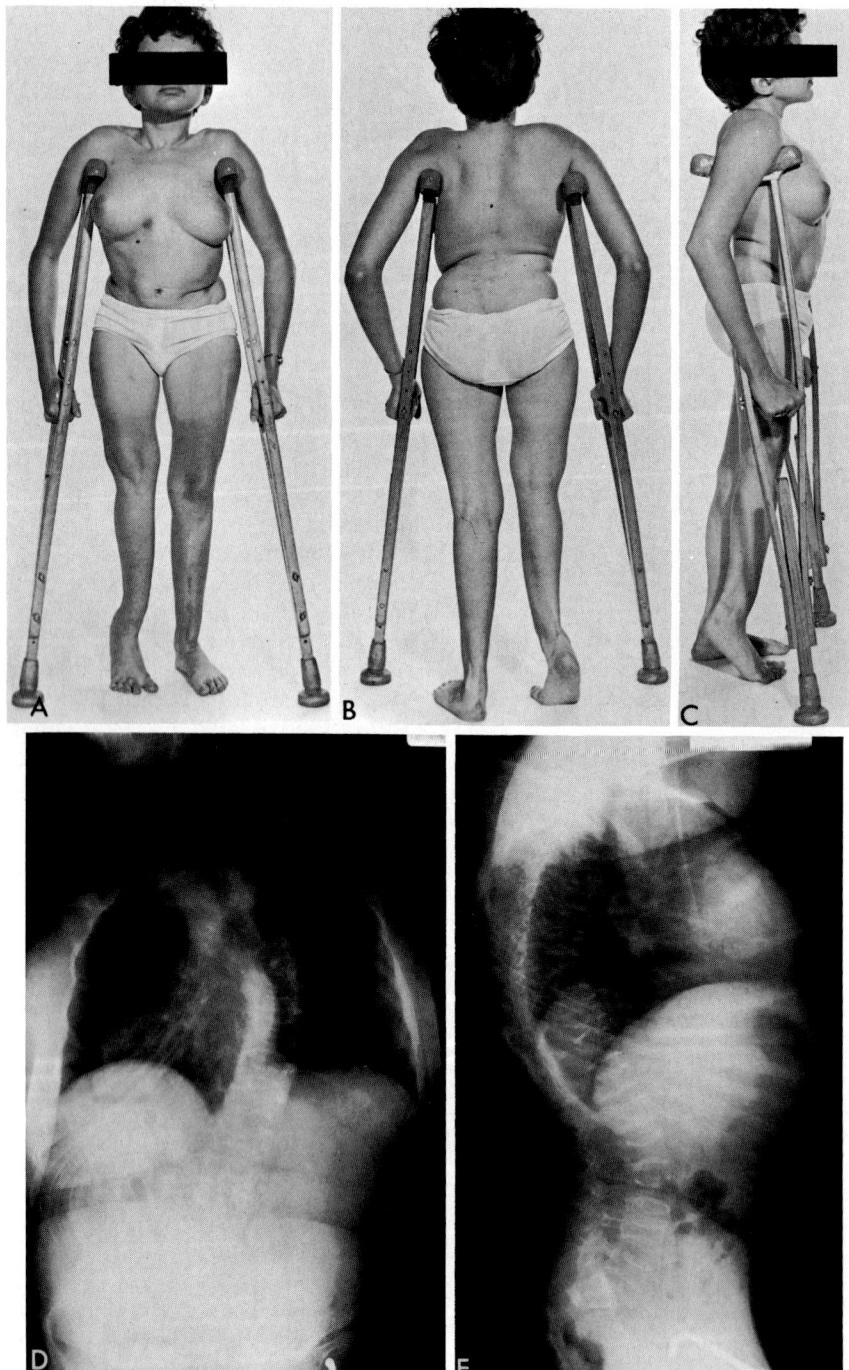

FIGURE 3–41. Osteogenesis imperfecta in a 15-year-old girl.

A to **C.** Clinical appearance of a patient with multiple deformities. **D** and **E.** Anteroposterior and lateral radiograms of the spine showing the kyphoscoliosis. Note the multiple compression fractures of the vertebral bodies. She was treated with a Milwaukee brace and had fragmentation, realignment, and intramedullary rod fixation of the malunited fractures of the long bones in the lower limbs.

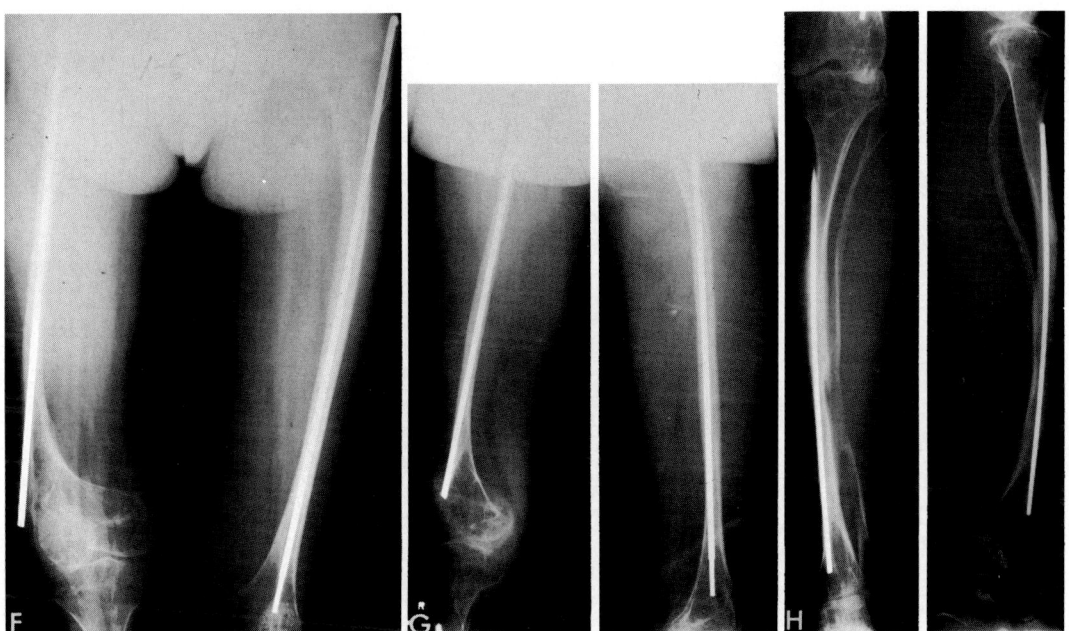

FIGURE 3–41 Continued. *Osteogenesis imperfecta in a 15-year-old girl.*

F to H. Anteroposterior and lateral radiograms of lower limbs.

cystic bone.[48] It has been shown that one radiographic pattern may progress to another. A *thick bone* appearance may be due to callus formation. Telescoping of fractures will give the bone a buttressed appearance. In the *thin bone* type, the shafts are very narrow with thin cortices, thin trabeculae in the medullary cavity, and marked osteopenia (see Fig. 3–39 G and I). The marrow cavity is very narrow and may be completely obliterated. In the fibula the diaphysis may be diminished to a thin sliver of bone. Its narrowness is due to failure of subperiosteal new bone formation. The metaphyses are trumpet-shaped, their relatively expanded appearance probably being due to a modeling defect. The normal width of the condyles indicates essentially normal lateral growth of the epiphysis. As the child grows but never walks, the lack of normal stress will give rise to a cystic honeycomb pattern in the long bones (Fig. 3–43). Goldman and associates described "popcorn" calcifications in the metaphyseal and epiphyseal areas of long bones close to the growth plate, appearing as clustered collections of rounded or scalloped radiolucencies, each with a sclerotic margin and some with central radiopacities (Fig. 3–44).[64] These have been referred to in the literature as "whorls of radiodensities." They probably represent traumatic fragmentation of the cartilaginous growth plate. The popcorn calcifications appear in childhood and usually resolve after completion of skeletal growth. They are more frequent in the lower than in the upper limbs and more common in the severe congenital type of disease. Their appearance parallels the development of growth plate irregularity. With a growth spurt, popcorn calcifications increase in number.

The skull has a mushroom appearance with a very thin calvarium. There is marked paucity and delay in ossification. Wormian bones (described by a Danish anatomist, Olaus Wormius, in 1643) are a salient radiographic feature of osteogenesis imperfecta.[38] They are detached portions of the primary ossification centers of the adjacent membrane bones. In order to be significant, wormian bones should be more than 10 in number, measure 6 mm. by 4 mm., and be arranged in a general mosaic pattern (Fig. 3–45). Cremin and associates studied the skull radiograms of 81 patients with osteogenesis imperfecta and 500 normal children for the presence of significant wormian bones, which they found in all cases of osteogenesis imperfecta but not in the normal skulls.[38] Significant wormian bones may be present in other bone dysplasias, such as cleidocranial dysplasia.

The spine shows marked osteoporosis; the vertebral bodies are compressed, becoming biconcave between bulging discs (Fig. 3–46). Scoliosis and kyphosis eventually develop in the majority of congenital severe forms of osteogenesis imperfecta.

Milder Forms. In the milder forms of osteogenesis imperfecta the radiographic picture is

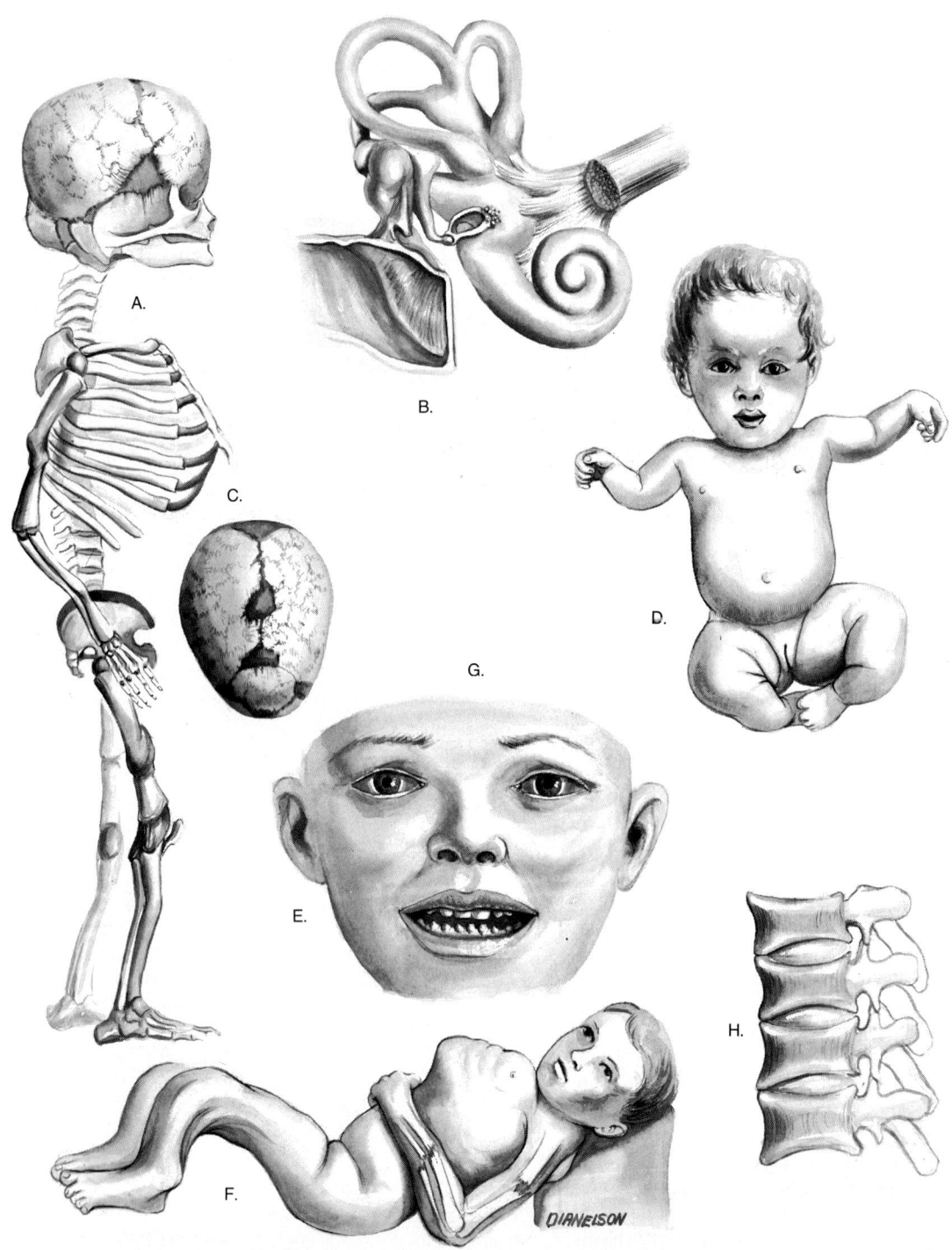

FIGURE 3–42. *Summary of clinical characteristics of osteogenesis imperfecta.*
A. Skeleton. **B.** Ear. **C.** Skull. **D.** Joints. **E.** Teeth. **F.** Bones. **G.** Eyes. **H.** Spine.

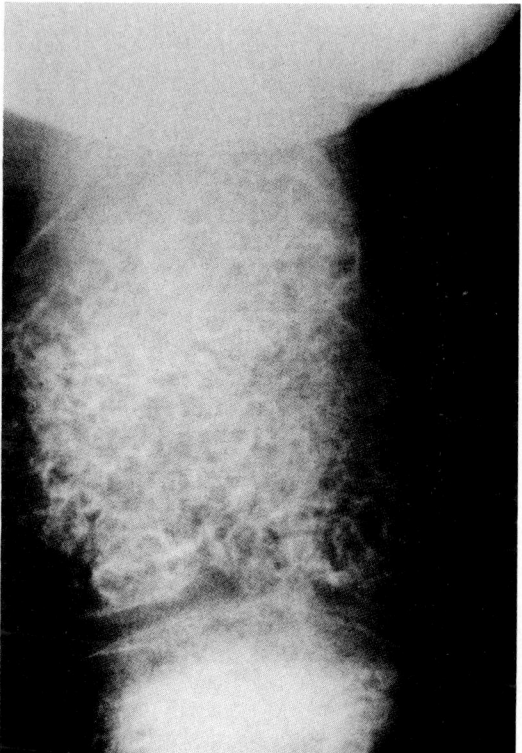

FIGURE 3-43. *Honeycomb appearance of end of long bones.*

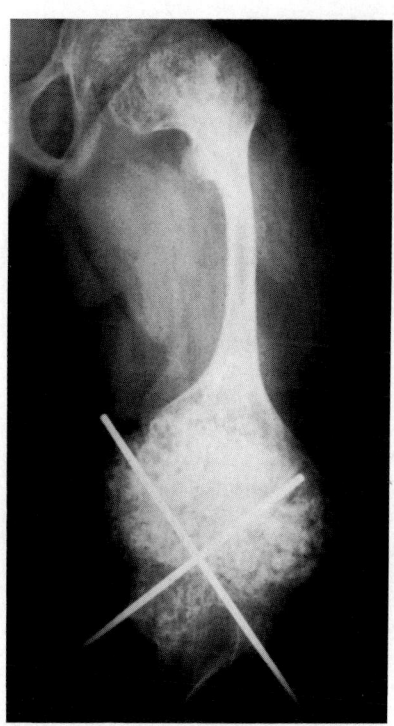

FIGURE 3-44. *Popcorn calcifications in osteogenesis imperfecta.*

that of osteoporosis—the cortices are thin, and in the medullary canal the bone trabeculae are thin with "feathering." There may be Harris lines, indicating transient periods of physeal growth arrest. Bone modeling impairment is evidenced in the metaphyseal region of long bones by the "Erlenmeyer flask" appearance in some and a trumpet shape in others. Fractures vary in frequency and age of occurrence. The radiogram may show fractures in various stages of healing. In contrast to the severe congenital form, in the milder form of osteogenesis imperfecta the fractures remodel quite adequately. Plastic bowing of long bones is common; this is due to microfractures and stress fractures or malunion of fractures. One lower limb may be in valgus deformation and the other in varus deviation. In the hip, coxa vara and acetabular protrusion may be found. The patellofemoral joint, the radial head, or the hip may dislocate. Platyspondyly and biconcave vertebrae are common. Varying degrees of scoliosis and kyphosis develop in about 40 per cent of cases.

In adolescence or adult life basilar impression—invagination of the foramen magnum into the posterior cranial fossa—may develop.[126] Ex-

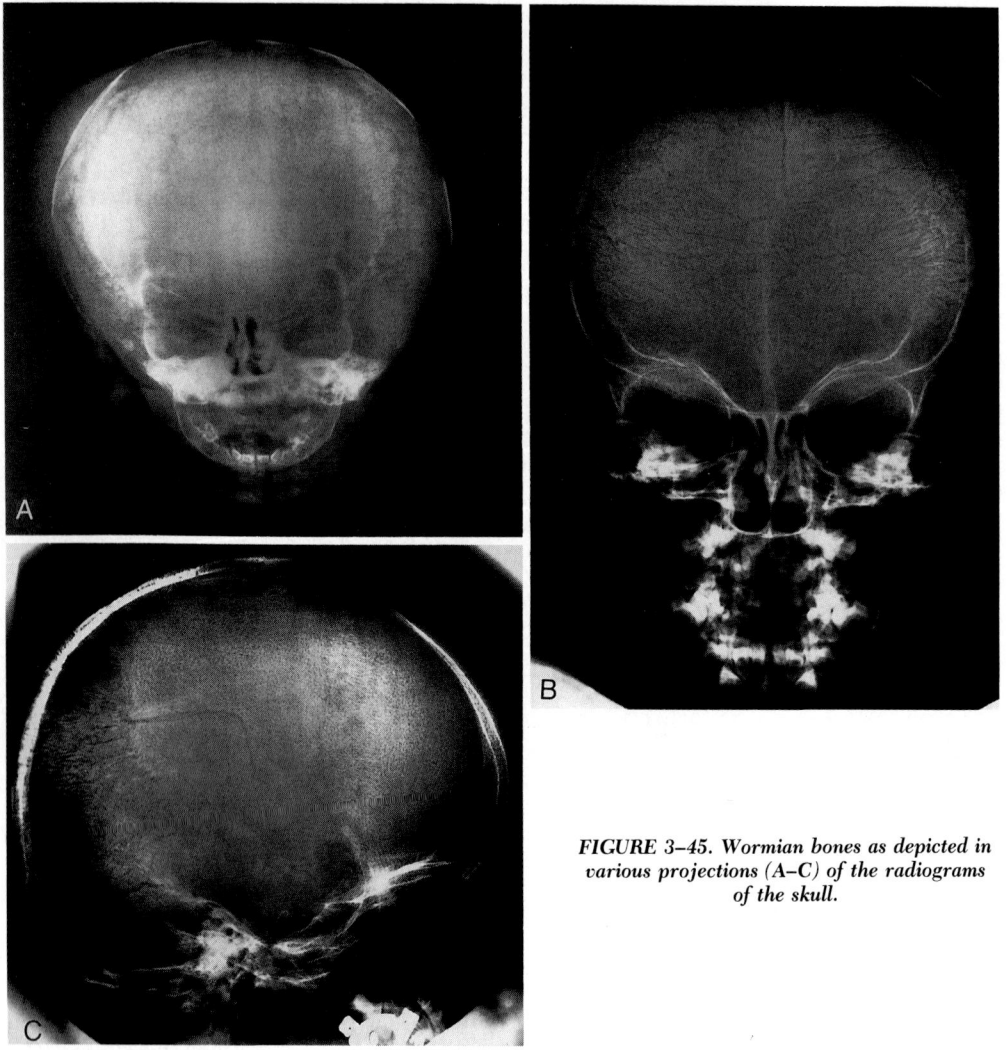

FIGURE 3–45. Wormian bones as depicted in various projections (A–C) of the radiograms of the skull.

cessive pneumatization of the frontal sinuses and mastoids may be present. The teeth show marked loss of enamel, hypoplastic pulp chambers, short roots, and bulbous crowns.

Hyperplastic Callus Formation*

This occurs very rarely in osteogenesis imperfecta but causes great concern because of diagnostic problems in distinguishing hyperplastic callus from osteogenic sarcoma. In the literature there are three cases reported in which amputation was performed but the subsequent findings and course showed the condition had been due to hyperplastic callus formation. Since the earliest description of its formation in osteogenesis imperfecta, numerous case reports have appeared in the literature, reviews of which have been presented by Strach in 1953 and later by Banta and associates in 1971.[12, 172]

It is more common in boys; the sclerae of affected patients are white, and family history is often negative for osteogenesis imperfecta. Hyperplastic callus formation may occur without fractures. These phenomena compound the difficulties of differential diagnosis. Furthermore, the development of osteosarcoma in patients with osteogenesis imperfecta has been reported.[84, 88]

The femur is the most common site; less frequently involved are the tibia and humerus. More than one bone may be affected at intervals of months or years. Often the patient gives a history of numerous fractures in the past without exuberant callus formation.

---

*See references 7, 11, 12, 49, 87, 90, 94, 101, 135, 152, 172.

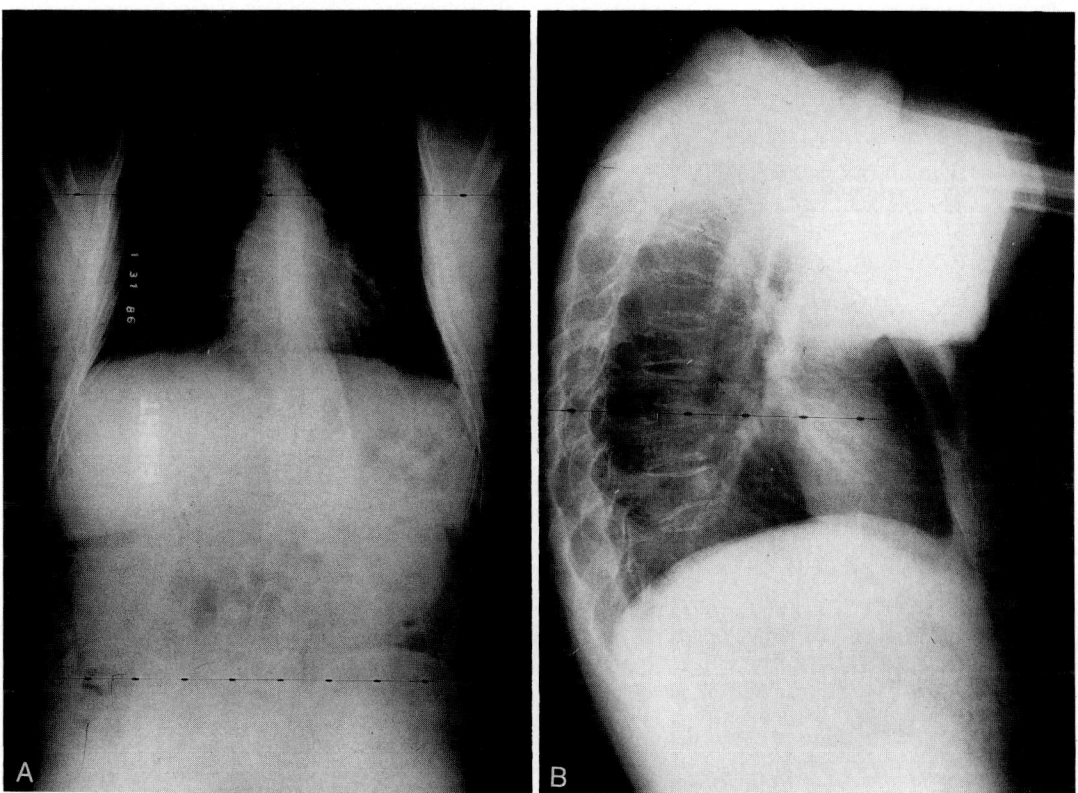

FIGURE 3–46. *Spine in an adolescent with osteogenesis imperfecta.*
Note the structural scoliosis and the collapsed vertebrae. **A.** Anteroposterior radiogram of the spine showing structural scoliosis. **B.** Lateral radiogram of dorsal spine showing osteoporosis and biconcave vertebrae.

The clinical features are those of acute localized inflammation. The involved limb progressively enlarges with alarming rapidity over the course of 10 to 20 days. The enlarging mass is painful, warm to touch, and tender to palpation. Overlying skin is tense, with loss of normal resiliency of the soft tissues. Prolonged low-grade fever is commonly present. Laboratory studies show an elevated erythrocyte sedimentation rate and alkaline phosphatase level. Radiograms reveal massive callus formation that is butterfly-shaped rather than fusiform (Fig. 3–47). A computed tomographic scan may be of value in distinguishing a hyperplastic callus formation from osteogenic sarcoma. In the former, fracture lines may be visible, and one can readily distinguish tumorous bone from callus. In doubtful cases, of course, biopsy is appropriate.

Histologic examination of the callus shows fibromucoid, cartilage-like tissue, or "chondroid," a transitional form between fibrous, mucoid, and cartilaginous tissue. In contrast a normal callus consists of a network of woven bone trabeculae lying in fairly dense connective tissue without mucoid or chondroid.[11, 49] The peripheral part of the mass shows undifferentiated tissue, while the central part is more differentiated, resembling normal callus.

Treatment is symptomatic. The part is splinted for comfort. Beneficial use of palliative radiation therapy has been reported in the literature.[11, 12, 94, 172] It is not, however, recommended by this author because of the danger of increasing the risk of future sarcomatous transformation.

Laboratory Findings

The serum calcium and phosphorus levels are normal. The alkaline phosphatase level may be elevated. There is no specific laboratory diagnostic abnormality in osteogenesis imperfecta. The diagnosis is made from clinical and radiographic features.

Differential Diagnosis

In the newborn and in early infancy, *congenital severe osteogenesis imperfecta* should be

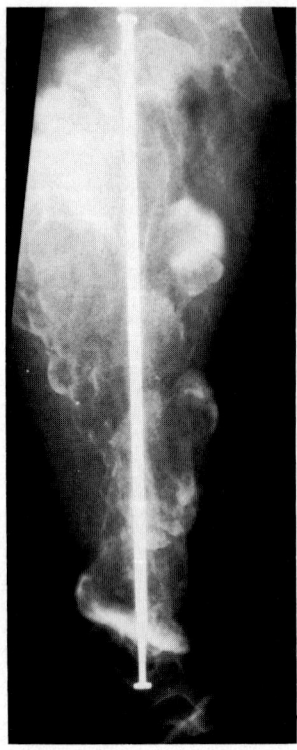

FIGURE 3–47. *Osteogenesis imperfecta with hyperplastic callus formation around fracture sites in the lower limb.*

Note the internal fixation with a Bailey rod

distinguished from *congenital hypophosphatasia*. In the latter, a lethal affection, the laboratory findings will show a low phosphatase level in the serum, a lack of alkaline phosphatase activity in the leukocytes, and excessive excretion of phosphorylethanolamine in the urine. In the infant, clinically, osteogenesis imperfecta and *achondroplasia* are frequently confused because the enlarged head and short limbs are common to both conditions. Radiographic findings will serve to distinguish between the two.

Camptomelic dwarfism may be mistaken for osteogenesis imperfecta because of the congenital bowing and angulation of the long bones. Fractures, however, are not a feature of this type of dwarfism.

The differential diagnosis of the *mild form of osteogenesis imperfecta* is more difficult. The presence of osteoporosis and a proclivity to fracture in *cystinosis* may suggest osteogenesis imperfecta.

Proneness to fracture is also characteristic of *pycnodysostosis*. This is distinguished from osteogenesis imperfecta by bone sclerosis, persistently wide cranial fontanelles, micrognathism with absence of the mandible, hypoplasia of the clavicles, and osteolysis of the terminal phalanges of the fingers.

A child presenting for the first time with a recent fracture or fractures and radiologic evidence of other fractures in various stages of healing may arouse suspicion of the *battered child*, or *Silverman, syndrome*. In the latter, dentinogenesis imperfecta, blue sclerae, and the typical shape of the skull of osteogenesis imperfecta are absent; however, osteogenesis imperfecta can occur without blue sclerae and tooth abnormalities. In the battered child, the fractures are more likely to occur at the metaphyses, and usually there is evidence of soft-tissue trauma. Bruising is a feature of osteogenesis imperfecta, but, in a battered baby, bruises will improve and disappear when the baby is in a protected environment.

The diffuse osteopenia in the early stages of *leukemia*, before the appearance of the typical blood picture, may be mistaken for osteogenesis imperfecta.

Idiopathic juvenile osteoporosis may be very difficult to distinguish from osteogenesis imperfecta; the former is characterized by being a self-limiting disorder and by its onset a year or so before puberty.

Osteoporosis and compression fractures of the vertebrae may also be caused by prolonged intake of steroids.

Treatment

There is no specific treatment to correct the basic defect in osteogenesis imperfecta. The cause of increased bone turnover is unknown at present; until the basic pathophysiology is determined, drugs are of dubious value.

"ATTEMPTED" MEDICAL TREATMENT

Sex hormones have been tried because of the clinical observation that the incidence of fracture diminishes at puberty and increases after menopause. They have, however, proved to be of no value. Anabolic steroids failed to increase deposition of calcium in bone and did not alleviate the disease. Their severe side effects—the masculinizing effect, premature closure of growth plates, and short stature—prohibit their empirical administration in osteogenesis imperfecta.

Fluoride therapy has been tried. Albright and Grunt administered 0.25 to 0.90 mg. per kilogram of body weight daily to 13 children with osteogenesis imperfecta; during this period of sodium fluoride therapy there were no significant changes in calcium and phosphorus balance studies. Although in some patients the incidence of fractures decreased, long-term results do not warrant the use of fluoride in the treatment of osteogenesis imperfecta.[3] It is true that bone density increased during fluoride therapy, but the new bone formed was poorly organized and mineralized. Fluoride depresses collagen formation and may be detrimental to bone growth.

The use of *magnesium oxide* was pioneered by the work of Solomons and associates, who found that the bone collagen of patients with osteogenesis imperfecta is an inhibitor of calcification in vitro; when osteogenesis imperfecta collagen was treated with pyrophosphatase in the presence of magnesium ions this inhibition was removed. It was also observed by Solomons's group that the serum and urinary levels of inorganic pyrophosphate were elevated in osteogenesis imperfecta. Oral administration of magnesium oxide reduced the serum and urinary levels of pyrophosphate. These investigators reported a decrease in fracture rate during the administration of magnesium oxide to patients with the disease, but later studies failed to support the beneficial effects of magnesium oxide in osteogenesis imperfecta.[163, 165, 166]

Calcitonin inhibits bone resorption and increases total bone mass. In osteoporosis in adults, administration of calcitonin has given favorable results. Castels and associates showed that calcitonin suppresses excessive bone turnover and suggested that long-term treatment with it might be helpful.[33] Definite clear-cut data as to the effectiveness of calcitonin in decreasing the incidence of fractures are not available at present. There are many variable factors, and it is difficult to assess its effectiveness. So far no medication has been proved to be of sufficient definite value to recommend its use in treatment of osteogenesis imperfecta. *Special diets* have not proved to be of value. Rather, the children should be on a well-balanced diet containing minimum daily vitamin requirements. The effectiveness of large doses of ascorbic acid is not established.

ORTHOPEDIC TREATMENT

The objective of treatment is to provide maximal possible function. The level of function attainable depends on the severity of the disease and the age of the patient. As the child matures the fracture rate progressively declines because of improvement in coordination, better emotional self-control, and increasing bone strength. As the patient matures, however, other problems (such as scoliosis) develop that require orthopedic attention. Since problems vary with the age of the child, treatment is discussed in relation to various age groups.

In the *newborn* infant multiple fractures, especially of the ribs and the skull, are the pressing problems; pulmonary insufficiency and infection are managed by the neonatologist, and the subdural hematoma by the neurosurgeon. Ordinarily the recent fractures do not require special treatment; splinting in a posterior plastic shell spica may be helpful. These fractures will heal within two weeks. The parents must be educated; they are instructed in techniques for handling the infant. Instinctively the mother develops rapid insight into how to handle the baby. Publications by the Osteogenesis Imperfecta Foundation are very informative. Parents are put in touch with parents of other patients. The baby is discharged to home as soon as the medical and neurologic status permits.

As the infant develops head and neck control and functional use of the upper limbs, a developmental therapist, who often is a physical therapist, shows the parents how to promote muscular development and normal developmental patterns. The occurrence of multiple fractures makes this a difficult task. Gentleness and patience are the cardinal principles. The family is given psychological support.

The orthopedic surgeon's task is to care for the fractures. As little immobilization as possible should be used in order to prevent exaggeration of osteopenia and further risk of fractures. At the same time, adequate bony alignment should be maintained. Osteoporosis is aggravated by inactivity due to fracture, and the danger of recurrent fracture is increased. A vicious circle may be created. The long bones may bend owing to the decreased strength of the osteoporotic bone. Once angulation develops, abnormal mechanical force tends to increase the deformity.

In severe osteogenesis imperfecta the multiplicity of fractures and the bowing of the long bones impair functional ability to stand and walk. Immobilization and lack of the stresses of loading cause progressive muscle atrophy and osteopenia. Abnormal mechanical stresses on the malaligned and porotic long bones increase their susceptibility to fractures. The fragile bones of severe osteogenesis imperfecta require support in order to maintain erect posture. Surgically, support may be provided by internal fixation with intramedullary rods; in such instances deformity of the long bones is corrected simultaneously by multiple osteotomies. An alternate means of providing support is by orthosis; conventional ones or pneumatic trouser splints.

Orthoses. These are manufactured of light plastic material and are utilized for external support and to promote stance and locomotion. An exercise program should be instituted; it is individually tailored to the patient. The goal is to develop maximal muscle strength.

Pneumatic Trouser Splints. Lightweight air-filled fluted trouser splints to support the osteoporotic fragile long bones of the lower limb in osteogenesis imperfecta were introduced by Morel and Houghton.[116] Definitely much lighter than conventional orthoses, in general the air splints are not cumbersome and are tolerated very well by children with osteogenesis imperfecta. They allow these severely affected children to stand upright, improving their mobility and general health and providing new psychological vistas. The pneumatic trouser splints do not eliminate gravitational weight-bearing stress and do stimulate osteogenesis in the affected bones; this is in contrast to the medullary rod fixation technique in which extreme osteoporosis invariably occurs around the rods.[115] There are no complications caused by the pneumatic splints. Morel recommends correction of long-bone deformities by closed osteotomy and traction; when the osteotomies are healed, the limbs are supported in the pneumatic external orthoses. Closed osteotomy obviates the problem of infection, it is relatively atraumatic, and blood transfusion is not required. The bones heal rapidly, and delayed union and nonunion are not problems. Other complications that occur with multiple osteotomies and intramedullary rodding—rod migration, fractures adjacent to rod ends, damage to the physis, and growth arrest—are obviated. Despite all these advantages, pneumatic trouser splints are not used in North America. Probably, commercial unavailability and lack of experience with them are factors in their unpopularity.

Fragmentation by Multiple Osteotomies, Realignment, and Intramedullary Rod Fixation

This technique was first described by Sofield and Millar.[162] Earlier, Springer had described multiple osteotomies and intramedullary rodding for the correction of long-bone deformity in rickets.[167] The indications for fragmentation and rodding are increasing deformity of long bones that is severe, interfering with the fitting of orthotic support and impairing function, and multiplicity of fractures. The parents of a severely involved child should understand that no surgical procedure will alter the basic disease process of bone fragility. The objectives of surgery, the problems, and the complications should be clearly appreciated. Most children affected with osteogenesis imperfecta have the potential for stance and assisted or independent walking if adequate support of their fragile long bones of the lower limbs is provided. The age of the patient and the size of the bone are determining factors in the timing of surgery. In general, fragmentation and intramedullary rod fixation should not be carried out until the child is at least two years of age; the surgical challenge of a short, fat thigh with soft bone and severe angulation may be insurmountable, even for the technically astute surgeon. It is best to postpone operation until after the fourth or fifth year of age.[113, 185] The propensity for fractures and deformity is less in the thick-bone type of disease; it is the thin bones that require the rods early, and these thin fragile bones present tremendous technical difficulties. Insertion of intramedullary rods in thin bones with very small medullary canals may be impossible. In such an instance closed osteoclasis is recommended to correct the deformity; alignment may be provided by percutaneous metaphysis-to-metaphysis rod fixation under image intensifier radiographic control or by skin traction for two to three weeks followed by support in plastic splints. Early weight-bearing should be initiated as soon as possible. Intramedullary rod fixation in long slender thin bones with expanded honeycombed ends is technically impossible. These children are best treated with Morel's pneumatic trouser splints.

Technical Considerations. The first decision to make is the choice between a solid and a telescoping rod. Factors to consider are the rate of the longitudinal growth of the long bone in which the rod is to be inserted and the diameter of the medullary canal. The drawback of the solid rod is that overgrowth of the long bone beyond the ends of the rod necessitates reoperation and replacement by a longer rod. Depending on the bone and the age of the patient, a new rod may be required every two to four years.[184] These children with severe osteogenesis imperfecta present a greater than normal anesthesia risk because of their diminished respiratory function due to the deformity of the thoracic cage and muscle atrophy. Bailey and Dubow introduced extensible intramedullary fixation devices to diminish the necessity for reoperation due to bone overgrowth. Their telescoping rod elongated commensurately with longitudinal bone growth without disturbing bone growth.[10] Rodriguez and Wickstrom reported their experience with fragmentation and use of the extensible intramedullary rod; in 13 of the 15 long bones operated on, the telescoping rod proved effective.[140] In the experience of Marafioti and Westin, the use of 47 Bailey-Dubow elongating rods increased the average length of time between replacement operations, yielded a lower removal rate, and showed no additional adverse effects.[107] Reoperation was required three and a half times less often with the telescoping rod than with the solid rod. In the experience of Millar, however, the extensible intramedullary rod may fail to extend by telescoping due to undetected bends, ridges, or corrugations. The extensible rods are more likely to bend, especially in a fall. After being straightened by closed manipulation, bent rods no longer keep extending with growth. Furthermore, they demand a larger medullary canal, precise central placement, and accurate sizing, and are much more difficult to tailor in the operating room than the solid rods, which are easier to fashion and insert. Extensible rods are more suitable for use in the femur and humerus than in the tibia or either bone of the forearm.[113] Another problem with the telescoping rods is disassembly of the epiphyseal fixation device, which damages the articular cartilage.[106] Lack of control of rotation is a definite drawback with the telescoping rods; therefore, postoperatively a hip spica cast must be applied for four to six weeks. Because the extensible rods are weak, external support with orthoses and a prolonged habilitation program are required. It is evident that the complication rate is definitely higher with the extensible rod than with the solid rod. The choice between a solid and an extensible rod should be individualized, depending on the preceding factors and the experience of the surgeon, who should appreciate the limitations of the extensible rod. At present this author favors the solid rod.

Prior to embarking upon surgery, the wise surgeon will measure the length and width of the bone in which the device is to be inserted and personally check the availability of a complete set of rods and instruments. It is best to have a wide selection of both extensible and solid rods, pending the surgical findings and difficulties, as last-minute decisions must often be made at the operating table. The rods should be of different diameters (preferably four) with a corresponding set of short and long drills. Other required instruments are an oscillating power saw, a heavy bolt cutter, and two parallel-acting heavy-duty pliers for bending the solid rods.

Children with osteogenesis imperfecta are prone to develop hyperthermia during surgery. The orthopedic surgeon should communicate with the anesthesiologist. Atropine as preoperative medication should be administered in minimal dosage if at all. The child should be on a thermally controlled mattress. Draping should be light, preferably sterile paper.

Blood should be available for replacement in all cases, as when the bones are subperiosteally exposed, bleeding always occurs, especially during the insertion of femoral and humeral rods where a tourniquet cannot be used. The surgeon should remember that easy bruising is a manifestation of osteogenesis imperfecta. Open surgery on both femora should not be performed at a single operation; death due to excess blood loss can occur. It is best to stage the procedures.

It is crucial to utilize radiographic control. A vital surgical prerequisite for any rod insertion is adequate exposure of the entire diaphysis—the bone should be visualized metaphysis to metaphysis. Any attempt to pass a rod blindly will end in disaster. Even radiograms may be deceiving; there are almost always imperceptible angular and rotatory deformations of the long bones in osteogenesis imperfecta.

Preservation of muscles is important. They surround and support the fragile bones and should be reflected and elevated at the intermuscular septum. The surgeon must resist the temptation to direct surgical approach and muscle splitting when bones are severely bowed. The femur is approached through a lateral approach, anterior to the intermuscular septum, and the tibia through an anterolateral approach. Meticulous hemostasis is crucial to minimize blood loss.

The periosteum is incised sharply with a scalpel and gently elevated with a moist sponge rather than a periosteal elevator. Elevate the periosteum first over intact bone and then proceed toward the fracture site. Bone retractors are placed subperiosteally, exposing the entire shaft of the bone. The cardinal rule is to be gentle—the soft bones of osteogenesis imperfecta can be easily crushed by bone holding forceps. Inspect and assess the deformity. How many cuts are required to achieve correction? The individual fragments should be as long and as few as possible, yet they should be straight enough to be strung on the rod. All cuts are made with an oscillating saw. In the femur and tibia the initial cut is distal, at the metaphyseal-diaphyseal junction. It is best to determine the exact level radiographically. Injury to growth plates should be avoided.

Intramedullary reaming is often required. Choose the narrowest bone fragment first and ream with a drill of appropriate diameter. There may be no medullary cavity. Meticulous technique is vital. Time is of the essence to minimize blood loss, the risk of anesthesia, and surgical complications; however, this is one stage of the operation in which the surgeon should not hurry. Technical ineptitude and surgical incompetence are not tolerated by the fragile deformed bones. Reaming can fracture and splinter them. The surgeon should understand the principles of carpentry; a vital prerequisite to rod insertion is the feasibility of placing all the fragments in a straight line.

Williams Modification of Sofield-Millar Technique. This is the technique for intramedullary rod insertion recommended by this author and is as follows (Fig. 3–48).[184-186] The first step is to determine the length of the rod to be used; this is achieved by adding three measurements. The first is the length of the gap between the two ends of the shaft with traction applied on the foot (for the tibia) or the knee (for the femur). Often this is less than the total length of the fragments, necessitating shortening or discarding of a bone fragment. The second and third measurements are the distances between the cuts at the proximal and distal diaphyseal-metaphyseal junction and the growth plate; these are obtained by pushing a rod into the open end of the shaft until the resistance of the physis is felt. A long smooth rod that traverses the physis and lies in the epiphysis ordinarily will not injure growth; as a general principle, however, violation of the growth plate should be avoided when possible. The rods should not penetrate the proximal or distal cortices of the metaphyses and should not enter the joints. A common pitfall is failure to discard sufficient bone. It is crucial that everything fall into a straight line without force. Inadequate bone shortening will tauten the soft tissues on the concave side, and when correction is attempted the excessive stress on the bone ends will displace the rods.

For the tibia, a rod with a "female" thread is cut to the measured length, and a rod of appropriate length with a "male" thread is screwed into it. The male end of the joined rods is driven into the open lower tibial metaphysis, across the ankle and tarsus, to exit from the sole of the foot. The osteotomized segments of the shaft are threaded snugly onto the rod with the female threads; then the rod is gently driven into the proximal tibial metaphysis until securely engaged. It is best to use image intensifier radiographic control and avoid injury to the upper tibial physis. In order to visualize the rod junction distally, the distal rod is unscrewed one or two turns. The ideal length of the rod is one that stops immediately short of the proximal tibial physis. The male rod is then unscrewed and withdrawn.

The technique of femoral rod insertion is similar to that of intramedullary nailing of a fractured femur with a Kuntschner or Schneider nail. A rod of the desired diameter and length is introduced from below. A hook should always be bent into the proximal end of the rod to prevent later migration. The male part of the rod is utilized to drive the rod into the distal femoral metaphysis. Radiograms are made to double-check the position of the rod; then the unwanted male part of the rod is unscrewed and removed from the gluteal region.

Placing the rod across the physis into the epiphysis adds length to the rod and postpones the problem of relative bone overgrowth and a rod that is too short. In order to minimize the problem of the rod cutting out, Tiley and Albright recommended that when coxa vara is present the position of the rod should be in the medial portion of the greater trochanter or in the base of the femoral neck. The most common deformity of the distal part of the femur is anterolateral angulation; it is crucial that during realignment osteotomy this deformity be com-

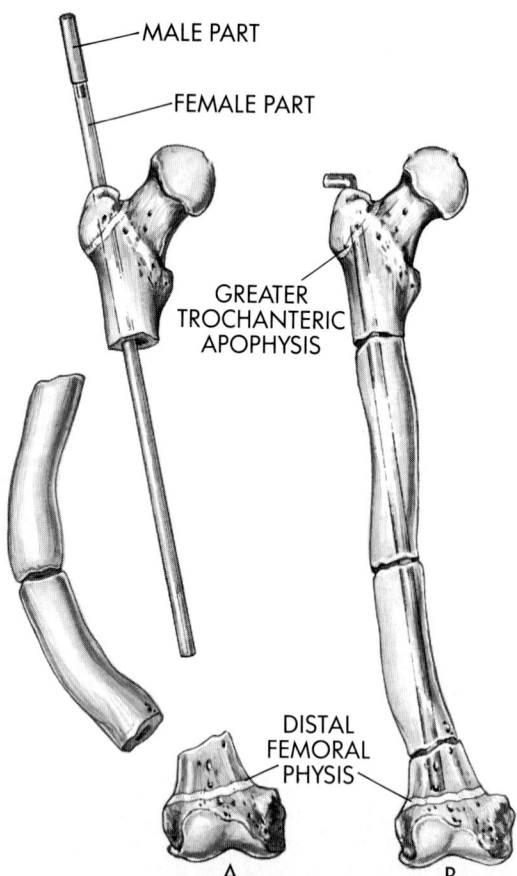

FIGURE 3–48. *Williams modification of Sofield-Millar intramedullary rod fixation.*

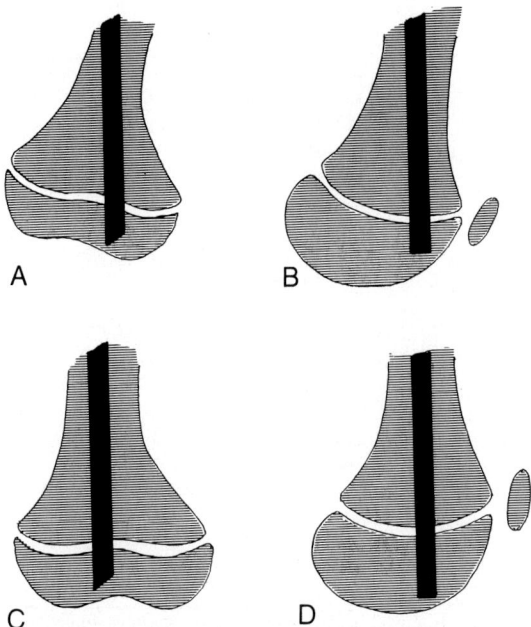

FIGURE 3-49. *Tiley-Albright technique of rod insertion.*

A and **B.** Incorrect position of the inferior end of the rod in the distal femoral epiphysis.

C and **D.** Correct position—note the distal end of the rod is centered and slightly anterolateral.

pletely corrected and the distal end of the rod be placed centrally or slightly anterolaterally (Fig. 3-49).[176] Other factors to consider in placing the rod in the distal femur are the deformity of the knee joint, the angular deformity of the upper end of the tibia, and future plans for surgery of the tibia. The deformity of the upper part of the tibia is usually anteromedial, and the most common site for rod protrusion is anterior; therefore Tiley and Albright recommended posterior placement of the rod on the upper tibia.

Tiley and Albright reported the results of 129 fragmentation and insertion operations in 13 patients with osteogenesis imperfecta. The follow-up was not long enough, but the operations were instrumental in preventing fractures to a degree. Eleven of the thirteen patients were ultimately able to walk, two without and nine with orthotic support.[176]

The periosteum, whenever possible, and the fascia are meticulously closed. External support by immobilization in a cast is always required until solid bony union is obtained. The hip spica or above-knee cast should be very light, preferably made of plastic. Leverage on adjacent long bones should be avoided. The hip, knee, ankle, and foot should be in functional stance position to allow early weight-bearing in the cast within a day or two postoperatively.

Use of the Extensible Intramedullary Rod. The telescoping intramedullary rod, described by Bailey and Dubow, is designed to allow elongation of the rod as the long bone grows. It consists of an outer tubular sleeve with a detachable T-shaped end that can be unscrewed and screwed in place with a drill bit, and an inner obturator rod with a solid T-shaped end. The inner rod is capable of telescoping totally into the sleeve. The T-shaped ends are anchored into the epiphyses away from the physes; with longitudinal bone growth the telescoping rod elongates.[8-10]

The surgical approach to the femur and tibia and the technique of fragmentation and stringing on the rod are similar to those of Sofield and Millar. The bowed bone is exposed subperiosteally from metaphysis to metaphysis. The deformed bone is removed, osteotomized into the appropriate number of fragments so that they can be lined up straight for insertion of the rod. The intercondylar notch of the femur and tibial plateau are exposed through a parapatellar incision. The ankle joint is exposed through a transverse incision. The rod is supposed to be long enough to extend from epiphysis to epiphysis with the inner rod completely within the outer sleeve. In order to allow for collapse of the bone fragments, however, it is wiser to have the total length of the rod 2 cm. shorter. This will ensure its proper anchorage in the upper and lower epiphyses of the long bone. The diameter of the outer sleeve is the widest that can be tolerated by the medullary canal. The bone fragments are reamed with progressively larger drill points. In the femur the outer tubular sleeve of the device (with the T-piece detached) is driven into the upper femoral segment in a retrograde fashion, through the medullary canal, exiting on the upper-lateral aspect of the femoral neck medial to the greater trochanteric notch. Through a separate small incision the upper end of the tubular sleeve is driven out through the skin; the T-piece is screwed in with a drill bit, and the sleeve is tapped into the upper femoral metaphysis until it is flush with and then countersunk into the cartilage of the superior aspect of the femoral neck. The separate bony fragments are threaded onto the outer sleeve portion of the rod. The inner obturator rod is driven upward through the intercondylar notch of the femur and articulated with the outer sleeve. The T-shaped end of the obturator rod is tapped into the cartilage of the lower femoral epiphysis. With needle-nose pliers, the T-end is rotated clockwise 90 degrees in the subchondral region; this will check the rod from sliding into the knee joint.

In the tibia the sleeve portion of the rod is placed distally; in the humerus it is placed in the upper humerus, exiting at the greater tuberosity, and the inner obturator rod is inserted through the lateral epicondyle.

Problems and Complications. Extreme osteoporosis may be associated with intramedullary rod fixation, with the bone almost disappearing because of lack of stress. Other problems and complications are bending and fracture of the rod, migration of the rod, growth arrest, nonunion, delayed union, and fractures adjacent to the rod ends. Blood loss is usually severe with significant morbidity and occasional death.

Scoliosis and Kyphosis

The incidence of scoliosis in the adolescent and adult with severe osteogenesis imperfecta is 80 to 90 per cent. The curves are usually severe and appear to continue to increase progressively in the adult. Orthotic devices are ineffective in controlling the scoliosis and kyphosis; the forces transmitted on the soft osteogenesis imperfecta bone cause progressive rib deformities resulting in a misshapen thoracic cage. Spinal fusion is performed in an attempt to control the scoliosis; it is questionable, however, whether a fused spine will maintain alignment over a period of time.[17] Instrumentation of the spine poses many problems.

Prognosis

In the congenital severe type, the fetus may not survive or the infant may die shortly after birth, although there have been instances of congenital cases in which the patients have lived through puberty but have been wheelchair-bound or bedridden. One patient with severe osteogenesis imperfecta is reported to have lived to the age of 95 years.[171]

Spranger and associates, in a clinical and radiographic study of 47 cases of newborns with osteogenesis imperfecta, devised a scoring system to code the degree of skeletal changes and to give an accurate prognosis (Table 3–5). A score of 2.7 or more carried a prospective mortality rate of 88 per cent, whereas scores of 2.6 or less had a survival rate of 90 per cent. Newborns with marked bowing of their lower limbs; less severe changes in the skull, ribs, vertebrae, and arms; and normal sclerae did survive and had fewer or no fractures as they grew older. In some of them, the bowed limbs straightened out spontaneously.[164]

In the moderate and mild type, the prognosis

Table 3–5. Scoring System for Osteogenesis Imperfecta Congenita

Skull	0 = normal
	1 = some wormian bones
	2 = multiple wormian bones
	3 = unossified calvaria
Ribs	0 = normal
	1 = 0–2 fractures, thin ribs
	2 = more than 2 fractures, thin ribs
	3 = innumerable fractures, thick ribs
Vertebrae	0 = normal
	1 = mild flattening of bodies
	2 = moderate flattening of bodies
	3 = severe flattening of bodies
Long Bones	0 = normal
	1 = osteopenia, normal or thin shaft, straight or slightly bowed, no fractures
	2 = same as 1, plus fractures
	3 = osteopenia, severe bowing of normally or excessively modeled (thin) shaft, with or without visible fractures
	4 = short, thick, "crumbled," or "telescoped" shaft

From Spranger, J. W., Cremin, B., and Beighton, P.: Osteogenesis imperfecta congenita. Pediatr. Radiol., *12*:21, 1982. Reprinted by permission.

varies. There is a gradual tendency toward improvement, with the incidence of fracture usually decreasing after puberty. This is due to the action of sex hormones, which play a role in bone matrix formation. With maturity, also, the patient learns how to prevent falls and fractures. In height, children with osteogenesis imperfecta are short—below the twenty-fifth percentile.

Schooling and Education. Children with osteogenesis imperfecta should be encouraged to receive optimal education and achieve the maximum in intellectual and academic development. The patient should be treated as a handicapped person and not one with a chronic disease.[22] Psychologic support and stimulation to master the environment are crucial. Most patients are capable of adapting to their problems and becoming useful, independent, productive members of society.

References

1. Aeschlimann, M. I., Grunt, J. A., and Crigler, J. F., Jr.: Effects of sodium fluoride on the clinical course and metabolic balance of an infant with osteogenesis imperfecta congenita. Metabolism, *15*:905, 1966.
2. Albright, J. A.: Management overview of osteogenesis imperfecta. Clin. Orthop., *159*:80, 1981.
3. Albright, J. A., and Grunt, J. A.: Studies of patients with osteogenesis imperfecta. J. Bone Joint Surg., 53-A:1415, 1971.
4. Albright, J. P., Albright, J. A., and Crelin, E. S.: Osteogenesis imperfecta tarda. The morphology of rib biopsies. Clin. Orthop., *108*:204, 1975.

5. Alston, J.: Children with brittle bones. Spec. Educ. Forward Trends, 9:29, 1982.
6. Apert, E.: Les hommes de verre. Presse Méd., 36:805, 1928.
7. Apley, A. G.: Hyperplastic callus in osteogenesis imperfecta. J. Bone Joint Surg., 33-B:591, 1951.
8. Bailey, R. W., and Dubow, H. I.: Studies of longitudinal bone growth resulting in an extensible nail. Surg. Forum, 14:455, 1963.
9. Bailey, R. W., and Dubow, H. I.: Experimental and clinical studies of longitudinal bone growth utilizing a new method of internal fixation crossing the epiphyseal plate. J. Bone Joint Surg., 47-A:1669, 1965.
10. Bailey, R. W., and Dubow, H. I.: Evolution of the concept of an extensible nail accommodating to normal longitudinal bone growth: Clinical considerations and implications. Clin. Orthop., 159:157, 1981.
11. Baker, S. L.: Hyperplastic callus simulating sarcoma in two cases of fragilitas ossium. J. Pathol. Bacteriol., 58:609, 1946.
12. Banta, J. V., Schreiber, R. R., and Kulik, W. J.: Hyperplastic callus formation in osteogenesis imperfecta simulating osteosarcoma. J. Bone Joint Surg., 53-A:115, 1971.
13. Baron, R., Gertner, J. M., Lang, R., and Vignery, A.: Increased bone turnover with decreased bone formation by osteoblasts in children with osteogenesis imperfecta tarda. Pediatr. Res., 17:204, 1983.
14. Barsh, G. S., David, K. E., and Byers, P. H.: Type I osteogenesis imperfecta: A non-functional allele for pro alpha-1(I) chains of type I procollagen. Proc. Natl. Acad. Sci. U.S.A., 79:3838, 1982.
15. Bauze, R. J., Smith, R., and Francis, M. J. P.: A new look at osteogenesis imperfecta. A clinical, radiological and biochemical study of forty-two patients. J. Bone Joint Surg., 57-B:2, 1975.
16. Beighton, P.: Familial dentinogenesis imperfecta, blue sclerae, and wormian bones without fractures: Another type of osteogenesis imperfecta? J. Med. Genet., 18:124, 1981.
17. Benson, D. R., and Newman, D. C.: The spine and surgical treatment in osteogenesis imperfecta. Clin. Orthop., 159:147, 1981.
18. Benson, D. R., Donaldson, D. H., and Millar, E. A.: The spine in osteogenesis imperfecta. J. Bone Joint Surg., 60-A:925, 1978.
19. Bergman, G., and Engfeldt, B.: Studies on mineralized dental tissues. IV. Biophysical studies in osteogenesis imperfecta. Acta Pathol. Microbiol. Scand., 35:537, 1954.
20. Bethge, J. F. J., Tolke, M., and Wiesinger, H.: Biochemische Untersuchungen bei Osteogenesis imperfecta. Bruns Beitr. Klin. Chir., 214:448, 1967.
21. Bilginturan, N., Ozsoylu, S., and Yordam, N.: Further experiences with sodium fluoride treatment in osteogenesis imperfecta. Turk. J. Pediatr., 24:151, 1982.
22. Bleck, E. E.: Nonoperative treatment of osteogenesis imperfecta: Orthotic and mobility management. Clin. Orthop., 159:111, 1981.
23. Bleckmann, H., Kresse, H., Wollensak, J., and Buddecke, E.: Glykosaminoglykan- und Kollagenanalysen bei Osteogenesis imperfecta. Z. Kinderheilkd., 110:74, 1971.
24. Blumcke, S., and Niedorf, H. R.: Histochemical and fine structural studies on the cornea with osteogenesis imperfecta congenita. Virchows Arch. B. (Cell Pathol.), 11:124, 1972.
25. Brailsford, J. F.: Osteogenesis imperfecta. Br. J. Radiol., 16:129, 1943.
26. Brown, D. M., Sauk, J. J., Corbin, K. W., Bradford, D. S., and Witkop, C. J.: Glycosminoglycans (GAG) of EDTA soluble and insoluble dentin in autosomal dominant osteogenesis imperfecta. Pediatr. Res., 9:312, 1975.
27. Bullough, P. G., and Davidson, D.: The morphology of the growth plate in osteogenesis imperfecta. Clin. Orthop., 116:259, 1976.
28. Bullough, P. G., Davidson, D. D., and Lorenzo, J. C.: The morbid anatomy of the skeleton in osteogenesis imperfecta. Clin. Orthop., 159:42, 1981.
29. Campbell, J. B.: Case report 217. Hyperostosis of the calvaria in osteogenesis imperfecta. Skeletal Radiol., 9:141, 1982.
30. Caniggia, A., Stuart, C., and Guideri, R.: Fragilitas ossium hereditaria tarda. Ekman-Lobstein disease. Acta Med. Scand., Suppl. 340, 1958.
31. Cassis, N., Gledhill, R. B., and Dubow, H.: Osteogenesis imperfecta: Its sociological and surgical implications, with a preliminary report on the use of a telescoping intramedullary nail. J. Bone Joint Surg., 57-B:533, 1975.
32. Castells, S.: New approaches to treatment of osteogenesis imperfecta. Clin. Orthop., 93:239, 1973.
33. Castells, S., Inamdar, S., Baker, R. K., and Wallach, S.: Effects of porcine calcitonin in osteogenesis imperfecta tarda. J. Pediatr., 80:757, 1972.
34. Cattell, H. S., and Clayton, B.: Failure of anabolic steroids in the therapy of osteogenesis imperfecta. Clinical, metabolic, and biochemical study. J. Bone Joint Surg., 50-A:123, 1968.
35. Chervenak, F. A., Romero, R., Berkowitz, R. L., Mahoney, M. J., Tortora, M., Mayden, K., and Hobbins, J. C.: Antenatal sonographic findings of osteogenesis imperfecta. Am. J. Obstet. Gynecol., 143:228, 1982.
36. Colbert, C., Mazess, R. B., and Schmidt, P. B.: Bone mineral determination in vitro by radiographic photodensitometry and direct photon absorptiometry. Invest. Radiol., 5:336, 1970.
37. Crawford, M. D., and Winter, R. M.: A new type of osteogenesis imperfecta (letter). J. Med. Genet., 19:158, 1982.
38. Cremin, B., Goodman, H., Spranger, J., and Beighton, P.: Wormian bones in osteogenesis imperfecta and other disorders. Skeletal Radiol., 8:35, 1982.
39. DalMonte, A., Manes, E., Capanna, R., and Andrisano, A.: Osteogenesis imperfecta: Results obtained with the Sofield method of surgical treatment. Ital. J. Orthop. Traumatol., 8:43, 1982.
40. Dorst, J. P.: Child abuse. Radiologe, 22:335, 1982.
41. Doty, S. B., and Matthews, R. S.: Electron microscopic and histochemical investigations of osteogenesis imperfecta tarda. Clin. Orthop., 80:191, 1971.
42. Eastoe, J. E., Martens, P., and Thomas, N. R.: The amino-acid composition of human hard tissue collagens in osteogenesis imperfecta and dentinogenesis imperfecta. Calcif. Tiss. Res., 12:91, 1973.
43. Eddowes, A.: Dark sclerotics and fragilis ossium. Br. Med. J., 2:222, 1900.
44. Ekman, O. J.: Descriptio et Casus Alliquot Osteomalaciae. Uppsala, J. F. Edman, 1788.
45. Engfeldt, B., Engstrom, A., and Zetterstrom, R.: Biophysical studies of the bone tissue in osteogenesis imperfecta. J. Bone Joint Surg., 36-B:654, 1954.
46. Engfeldt, B., Hjerpe, A., Mengarelli, S., Reinholt, F. P., and Wikstrom, B.: Morphological and biochemical analysis of biopsy specimens in disorders of skeletal development. Acta Paediatr. Scand., 71:353, 1982.
47. Fadli, M. E.: Neuropsychiatric complications of osteogenesis imperfecta: A case with cerebrovascular insufficiency. J. Egypt Med. Assoc., 51:528, 1968.
48. Fairbank, H. A. T.: Osteogenesis imperfecta and osteogenesis imperfecta cystica. J. Bone Joint Surg., 30-B:164, 1948.
49. Fairbank, H. A. T., and Baker, S. L.: Hyperplastic callus formation with or without evidence of a fracture in osteogenesis imperfecta. Br. J. Surg., 36:1, 1948.

50. Falvo, K. A., and Bullough, P. G.: Osteogenesis imperfecta: A histometric analysis. J. Bone Joint Surg., 55-A:275, 1973.
51. Falvo, K. A., Root, L., and Bullough, P. G.: Osteogenesis imperfecta: Clinical evaluation and management. J. Bone Joint Surg., 56-A:783, 1974.
52. Falvo, K. A., Klain, D. B., Krauss, A. N., Root, L., and Auld, P. A. M.: Pulmonary function studies in osteogenesis imperfecta. Am. Rev. Resp. Dis., 108:1258, 1973.
53. Follis, R. H., Jr.: Osteogenesis imperfecta congenita; a comnnective tissue diathesis. J. Pediatr., 41:713, 1952.
54. Follis, R. H., Jr.: Histochemical studies on cartilage and bone. III. Osteogenesis imperfecta. Bull. Johns Hopkins Hosp., 93:386, 1953.
55. Fontaine, G., Ingelrans, P., Dupont, A., Farriaux, J. P., Dubois, O., Richard, J., Walbaum, R., and Lejeune, J.: La fragilité osséuse constitutionnelle. Etude de 23 observations. Sem. Hôp. Paris, 44:380, 1968.
56. Francis, M. J. O., Smith, R., and Bauze, R. J.: Instability of polymeric skin collagen in osteogenesis imperfecta. Br. Med. J., 1:421, 1974.
57. Francis, M. J. O., Smith, R., and MacMillan, D. C.: Polymeric collagen of skin in normal subjects and in patients with inherited connective tissue disorders. Clin. Sci., 44:429, 1973.
58. Francis, M. J. O., Williams, K. J., Sykes, B. C., and Smith, R.: The relative amounts of the collagen chains alpha 1(I) alpha 2 and alpha 1(III) in the skin of 31 patients with osteogenesis imperfecta. Clin. Sci., 60:617, 1981.
59. Frank, E., Berger, T., and Tew, J. M., Jr.: Basilar impression and platybasia in osteogenesis imperfecta tarda. Surg. Neurol., 17:116, 1982.
60. Freda, V. J., Vosburgh, G. J., and Di Liberti, C.: Osteogenesis imperfecta congenita: A presentation of 16 cases and review of the literature. Obstet. Gynecol., 18:535, 1961.
61. Furey, J. G., and McNamee, D. C.: Air splints for long-term management of osteogenesis imperfecta. J. Bone Joint Surg., 55-A:645, 1973.
62. Gerber, B. E., and Jani, L.: Multiple pathologic fractures in osteogenesis imperfecta. Orthopade, 11:101, 1982.
63. Gitelis, S., Whiffen, J., and DeWald, R. L.: The treatment of severe scoliosis in osteogenesis imperfecta. Case report. Clin. Orthop., 175:56, 1983.
64. Goldman, A. B., Davidson, D., Pavlov, H., and Bullough, P. G.: "Popcorn" calcifications: A prognostic sign in osteogenesis imperfecta. Radiology, 136:351, 1980.
65. Gurlt, E.: Handbuch der Lehre von den Knochenbruchen. Berlin, 1862, Vol. I., p. 147.
66. Habekost, H. J., and Zichner, L.: Experiences with the operative therapy of osteogenesis imperfecta. Z. Orthop., 120:673, 1982.
67. Haebara, H., Yamasaki, Y., and Kyogoku, M.: An autopsy case of osteogenesis imperfecta congenita; histochemical and electron microscopical studies. Acta Pathol. Jpn., 19:377, 1969.
68. Hahnfeld, S.: Arteriopathia calcificans infantum associated with osteogenesis imperfecta. Zentralbl. Allg. Pathol., 125:31, 1981.
69. Hall, J. G., and Rohrt, T.: The stapes in osteogenesis imperfecta. Acta Otolaryngol., 65:345, 1968.
70. Hanck, A. B.: Vitamins in "malattie evolutive." Acta Vitaminol. Enzymol., 2:179, 1980.
71. Hathaway, W. E., Solomons, C. C., and Ott, J. E.: Abnormalities of platelet function in osteogenesis imperfecta. Clin. Res., 18:209, 1970.
72. Heise, A.: On osteogenesis imperfecta with special reference to the pathological and anatomical conditions. Acta Pathol. Microbiol. Scand., 2:972, 1944.
73. Herbage, D., Borsali, F., Buffevant, C., Flandin, F., and Aguercif, M.: Composition, cross-linking and thermal stability of bone and skin collagens in patients with osteogenesis imperfecta. Metab. Bone Dis. Relat. Res., 4:95, 1982.
74. Herndon, C. N.: Osteogenesis imperfecta: Some clinical and genetic considerations. Clin. Orthop., 8:132, 1956.
75. Herron, L. D., and Dawson, E. G.: Methylmethacrylate as an adjunct in spinal instrumentation. J. Bone Joint Surg., 59-A:866, 1977.
76. Hoek, K. J.: Scoliosis in osteogenesis imperfecta. J. Bone Joint Surg., 57-A:136, 1975.
77. Holmes, J. R., Baker, J. R., and Davies, E. T.: Osteogenesis imperfecta in lambs. Vet. Rec., 76:980, 1964.
78. Hreno, A., and Haust, D.: Osteogenesis imperfecta congenita. J. Pediatr., 62:908, 1963.
79. Humbert, J. R., and Solomons, C. C.: Increased leukocyte respiration in osteogenesis imperfecta. Soc. Pediatr. Res., April, 1970.
80. Humbert, J. R., Solomons, C. C., and Ott, J. E.: Increased oxidative metabolism by leukocytes of patients with osteogenesis imprefecta and of their relatives. J. Pediatr., 78:648, 1971.
81. Hurwitz, L. J., and McSwiney, R. R.: Basilar impression and osteogenesis imperfecta in a family. Brain, 83:138, 1960.
82. Jaffe, H. L.: Metabolic, Degenerative, and Inflammatory Diseases of Bones and Joints. Philadelphia, Lea & Febiger, 1972, pp. 162–177.
83. Jett, S., Ramser, J. R., Frost, H. M., and Villanueva, A. R.: Bone turnover and osteogenesis imperfecta. Arch. Pathol., 81:112, 1966.
84. Jewell, F. C., and Lofstrom, J. E.: Osteogenic sarcoma occurring in fragilitas ossium. Radiology, 31:741, 1940.
85. Keats, T. E.: Diffuse thickening of calvarium in osteogenesis imperfecta. Further observations. Radiology, 86:97, 1966.
86. Key, J. A.: Brittle bones and blue sclerae: Hereditary hypoplasia of the mesenchyme. Arch. Surg., 13:523, 1926.
87. King, J. D., and Bobechko, W. P.: Osteogenesis imperfecta. An orthopaedic description and surgical review. J. Bone Joint Surg., 53-B:72, 1971.
88. Klenerman, L., Ockenden, B. G., and Townsend, A. C.: Osteosarcoma occurring in osteogenesis imperfecta. J. Bone Joint Surg., 49-B:314, 1967.
89. Knaggs, L.: Osteogenesis imperfecta. Br. J. Surg., 11:737, 1924.
90. Koskinen, E. V. S.: Massive hyperplastic callus formation simulating osteogenic sarcoma in osteogenesis imperfecta. Report of a severe case. Ann. Chir. Gynaecol. Fenn., 47:271, 1958.
91. Langneso, U., and Behnke, H.: Collagen metabolites in plasma and urine in osteogenesis imperfecta. Metabolism, 20:456, 1971.
92. Laplane, R., Lasfargues, G., and Debray, P.: Essai de classification génétique des ostéogenèses imparfaites. Presse Méd., 67:893, 1959.
93. Laszio, A., and Sugar, E.: Sodium fluoride therapy of osteogenesis imperfecta in childhood. Kinderarztl. Prax., 50:416, 1982.
94. Laurent, L. E., and Salenius, P.: Hyperplastic callus formation in osteogenesis imperfecta. Report of a case simulating sarcoma. Acta Orthop. Scand., 38:280, 1967.
95. Lenzi, L., Brunelli, P. C., Vegetti, E., Cetta, G., and Tenni, R.: Osteogenesis imperfecta: Physiopathological, clinical and therapeutic aspects. Basic Appl. Histochem., 25:259, 1981.
96. Levin, L. S.: The dentition in the osteogenesis imperfecta syndromes. Clin. Orthop., 159:64, 1981.

97. Lièvra, J. A.: La fragilité osseuse constitutionnelle (étude de 25 familles comportant 53 malades). Rev. Rhum., 8:420, 1959.
98. Lindenfelser, R., Hasselkus, W., Haubert, P., and Kronert, W.: Zur Osteogenesis imperfecta congenita. Rasterelektronenmikroskopische Untersuchungen. Virchows Arch. B. (Cell Pathol.), 11:80, 1972.
99. Lobstein, J. F. G. C. M.: Lehrbuch der pathologischen Anatomie. Stuttgart, 1835, Vol. II, p. 179.
100. Looser, E.: Zur Kenntnis der Osteogenesis imperfecta congenita und tarda (sogenannte idiopathische Osteopsathyrosis). Mitt. Grenzgebieten Med. Chir., 15:161, 1906.
101. McCall, R. E., and Bax, J. A.: Hyperplastic callus formation in osteogenesis imperfecta following intermedullary rodding. Case report. J. Pediatr. Orthop., 4:361, 1984.
102. McKusick, V. A.: Osteogenesis imperfecta. In Heritable Disorders of Connective Tissue. 4th Ed. St. Louis, Mosby, 1972, pp. 390–454.
103. McKusick, V. A., and Scott, C. I.: A nomenclature for constitutional disorders of bone. J. Bone Joint Surg., 53-A:978, 1971.
104. Mackenzie, D. A., Labelle, P., and Burke, D.: Iatrogenic acute diaphyseal atrophy (disappearing bone disease). Paper read at the Annual Meeting of the Canadian Orthopedic Association, Ottawa, May 1975.
105. Manoria, P. C., Misra, M. P., and Bharagava, R. K.: Osteogenesis imperfecta with atrial septal defect. Indian Heart J., 34:173, 1982.
106. Marafioti, R. L., and Westin, G. W.: Twenty years experience with multiple osteotomies and intramedullary fixation in osteogenesis imperfecta (including the Bailey expandable rod) at the Shriners Hospital, Los Angeles, California. J. Bone Joint Surg., 57-A:136, 1975.
107. Marafioti, R. L., and Westin, G. W.: Elongating intramedullary rods in the treatment of osteogenesis imperfecta. J. Bone Joint Surg., 59-A:467, 1977.
108. Maroteaux, P., and Gilles, M.: Etude radiologique de l'ostéogenesis imperfecta. Ann. Radiol., 8:571, 1965.
109. Maroteaux, P., and Lamy, M.: L' "ostéogenesis imperfecta" et les difficultés de son diagnostic. Presse Méd., 73:1535, 1965.
110. Match, R. M., and Corrylos, E. V.: Bilateral avulsion fracture of the triceps tendon insertion from skiing with osteogenesis imperfecta tarda. A case report. Am. J. Sports Med., 11:99, 1983.
111. Messinger, A. L., and Teal, F.: Intramedullary nailing in correction of deformity in osteogenesis imperfecta. Clin. Orthop., 5:221, 1956.
112. Milgram, J. W., Flick, M. R., and Engh, C. A.: Osteogenesis imperfecta. A histopathological case report. J. Bone Joint Surg., 55-A:506, 1973.
113. Millar, E. A.: Observation on the surgical management of osteogenesis imperfecta. Clin. Orthop., 159:154, 1981.
114. Mirbaha, M.: Multiple osteotomies and intramedullary fixation of the radius and ulna to correct severe deformity and improve function in osteogenesis imperfecta. Report of a case. J. Bone Joint Surg., 48-A:523, 1966.
115. Moorefield, W. G., and Miller, G. R.: Aftermath of osteogenesis imperfecta. Disease in adulthood. J. Bone Joint Surg., 62-A:113, 1980.
116. Morel, G., and Houghton, G. R.: Pneumatic trouser splints in the treatment of severe osteogenesis imperfecta. Acta Orthop. Scand., 53:547, 1982.
117. Murray, D., and Young, B. H.: Osteogensis imperfecta treated by fixation with intramedullary rod. South. Med. J., 53:1142, 1960.
118. Neilson, H. E.: Familial occurrence of osseous fragility, blue sclerae, and deafness. Nord. Med., 15:2203, 1942.
119. Nichols, A. C., Pope, F. M., and Schlvon, H.: Biochemical heterogeneity in osteogenesis imperfecta. New variant. Lancet, 1:1193, 1979.
120. Niemann, K. M.: Surgical treatment of the tibia in osteogenesis imperfecta. Clin. Orthop., 159:134, 1981.
121. Nyhan, W. L., and Sakati, N. O.: Osteogenesis imperfecta. In Genetic Malformation Syndromes in Clinical Medicine. Disorders of Connective Tissue. Chicago, Year Book, 1976, pp. 181–185.
122. Passarge, E., and Kattner, E.: Lethal forms of hereditary collagen disorders: Ehlers-Danlos syndrome type IV and congenital osteogenesis imperfecta. Prog. Clin. Biol. Res., 104:237, 1982.
123. Penttinen, R. P., Lichtenstein, J. R., Martin, G. R., and McKusick, V. A.: Abnormal collagen metabolism in cultured cells in osteogenesis imperfecta. Proc. Natl. Acad. Sci. U.S.A., 72:586, 1975.
124. Penttinen, R., Sipola, E., Kouvalainen, K., Simila, S., and Remes, M.: An arthropathic form of osteogenesis imperfecta. Acta Paediatr. Scand., 69:263, 1980.
125. Pierog, S. H., Fontana, V. J., and Ferrara, A.: Osteogenesis imperfecta. Therapeutic challenge. N.Y. State J. Med., 69:310, 1969.
126. Pozo, J. L., Crockard, H. A., and Ransford, A. O.: Basilar impression in osteogenesis imperfecta. J. Bone Joint Surg., 66-B:233, 1984.
127. Ramser, J. R., and Frost, H. M.: The study of a rib biopsy from a patient with osteogenesis imperfecta. A method using in vivo tetracycline labeling. Acta Orthop. Scand., 37:229, 1966.
128. Ramser, J. R., Villanueva, A. R., and Pirok, D.: Tetracycline-based measurement of bone dynamics in 3 women with osteogenesis imperfecta. Clin. Orthop., 49:151, 1966.
129. Rebouillat, J., Revelin, P. L., and Brault, J. F.: Treatment of osteogenesis imperfecta with multiple diaphyseal osteotomies. Pediatrie, 24:411, 1969.
130. Reichelt, A.: Operative Behandlungsmoglichkeiten bei der Osteogenesis imperfecta. Langenbecks Arch. Chir., 330:238, 1972.
131. Remigio, P. A., and Grinvalsky, H. T.: Osteogenesis imperfecta congenita. Association with conspicuous extraskeletal connective tissue dysplasia. Am. J. Dis. Child., 119:524, 1970.
132. Riley, F. C., Jowsey, J., and Brown, D.: Connective-tissue ultrastructure and bone remodeling in osteogenesis imperfecta. J. Bone Joint Surg., 53-A:801, 1971.
133. Robert, J. M., Gremeau, J. L., Motter, A., and Guilhot, J.: La fragilité osseuse héréditaire. Lyon Med., 99:881, 1637, 1968.
134. Roberts, E., and Schour, I.: Hereditary opalescent dentine—dentinogenesis imperfecta. Am. J. Orthod., 25:267, 1939.
135. Roberts, J. B.: Bilateral hyperplastic callus formation in osteogenesis imperfecta. A case report. J. Bone Joint Surg., 58-A:1164, 1976.
136. Robichon, J., and Germain, J. P.: Pathogenesis of osteogenesis imperfecta. Can. Med. Assoc. J., 99:975, 1968.
137. Rodriguez, J. I., Perera, A., Regadera, J., Collado, F., and Contreras, F.: Lethal osteogenesis imperfecta. Anatomopathologic (optical and structural) study of 8 autopsy cases). An. Esp. Pediatr., 17:18, 1982.
138. Rodriguez, R. P.: Report of multiple osteotomies and intramedullary fixation by an extensible intramedullary device in children with osteogenesis imperfecta (abstract). Clin. Orthop., 116:261, 1976.
139. Rodriguez, R. P., and Bailey, R. W.: Internal fixation of the femur in patients with osteogenesis imperfecta. Clin. Orthop., 159:126, 1981.
140. Rodriguez, R. P., Jr., and Wickstrom, J. K.: Osteogenesis imperfecta: A preliminary report on resurfac-

ing of long bones with intramedullary fixation by an extensible intramedullary device. South. Med. J., 64:169, 1971.
141. Root, L.: Upper limb surgery in osteogenesis imperfecta. Clin. Orthop., 159:141, 1981.
142. Ropes, M. W., Rossmeisl, E. C., and Bauer, W.: The effect of estria medication in osteogenesis imperfecta. Conference on metabolic aspects of convalescence. Trans. 15th Meeting, Josiah Macy Jr. Foundation, New York, 1946, p. 87.
143. Ruedemann, A. D., Jr.: Osteogenesis imperfecta and blue sclerotics. A clinicopathologic study. Arch. Ophthalmol., 49:6, 1953.
144. Rush, A., and Burke, S. W.: Hangman's fracture in a patient with osteogenesis imperfecta. J. Bone Joint Surg., 66-A:778, 1984.
145. Russell, R. G. G., Bisaz, S., Donath, A., Morgan, D. B., and Fleisch, H.: Inorganic pyrophosphate in plasma in normal persons and in patients with hypophosphatasia, osteogenesis imperfecta and other disorders of bone. J. Clin. Invest., 50:961, 1971.
146. Ruth, E. B.: Osteogenesis imperfecta. Anatomic study of a case. Arch. Pathol., 3:111, 1943.
147. Rutkowski, R., Resnick, P., and McMaster, J. H.: Osteosarcoma occurring in osteogenesis imperfecta. A case report. J. Bone Joint Surg., 61-A:606, 1979.
148. Sauer, A. R., and Joyce, T. H., III: Management of a patient with osteogenesis imperfecta: A case study. A.A.N.A. J., 49:580, 1981.
149. Sbyrakis, S., Mengreli, C., Cote, G. B., and Morakis, A.: Vitamin D and related research in osteogenesis imperfecta. Prog. Clin. Biol. Res., 104:367, 1982.
150. Scherr, D. D.: A severely deformed patient with osteogenesis imperfecta at the age of fifty-four. J. Bone Joint Surg., 46-A:159, 1964.
151. Schroder, G.: Osteogenesis imperfecta. Z. Menschl. Vererb. Konstitutionslehre, 37:632, 1964.
152. Schwarz, E.: Hypercallosis in osteogenesis imperfecta A.J.R., 85:645, 1061.
153. Scott, P. P., McKusick, V. A., and McKusick, A. B.: The nature of osteogenesis imperfecta in cats. Evidence that the disorder is primarily nutritional, not genetic and therefore not analogous to the disease in man. J. Bone Joint Surg., 45-A:125, 1963.
154. Seedorff, K. S.: Osteogenesis imperfecta. A study of clinical features and heredity based on 55 Danish families comprising 180 affected persons. Copenhagen, Munksgaard, 1949.
155. Shapiro, F.: Consequences of an osteogenesis imperfecta diagnosis for survival and ambulation. J. Pediatr. Orthop., 5:456, 1985.
156. Sillence, D. O.: Bone Dysplasia. Genetic and ultrastructural aspects with special reference to osteogenesis imperfecta. M.D. Thesis. University of Melbourne, Australia, 1977.
157. Sillence, D. O.: Osteogenesis imperfecta: An expanding panorama of variants. Clin. Orthop., 159:11, 1981.
158. Sillence, D. O., and Danks, D. M.: The differentiation of genetically distinct varieties of osteogenesis imperfecta in the newborn period. Clin. Res., 26:178, 1978.
159. Sillence, D. O., Senna, A., and Danks, D. M.: Genetic heterogeneity in osteogenesis imperfecta. J. Med. Genet., 16:101, 1979.
160. Slavik, M., and Slacalkov, J.: Back pain as the main symptom in osteogenesis imperfecta tarda of a mild type. Acta Chir. Orthop. Traumatol. Cech., 48:288, 1981.
161. Smars, G.: Osteogenesis Imperfecta in Sweden. Clinical, Genetic, Epidemiological and Socio-medical Aspects. Stockholm, Svenska Boreforlaget, 1961.
162. Sofield, H. A., and Millar, E. A.: Fragmentation, realignment, and intramedullary rod fixation of deformities of the long bones of children. A ten-year appraisal. J. Bone Joint Surg., 41-A:1371, 1959.

163. Solomons, C. C.: Osteogenesis imperfecta. Biochemical defects (abstract). Clin. Orthop., 116:259, 1976.
164. Solomons, C. C., and Styner, J.: Osteogenesis imperfecta: Effect of magnesium administration on pyrophosphate metabolism. Calcif. Tiss. Res., 3:318, 1969.
165. Solomons, C. C., and Millar, E. A.: Osteogenesis imperfecta. New perspectives. Clin. Orthop., 96:299, 1973.
166. Solomons, C. C., Millar, E. A., Hathaway, W. E., and Ott, J. E.: Osteogenesis imperfecta. New perspectives in diagnosis and treatment. J. Bone Joint Surg., 53-A:1017, 1971.
167. Spranger, J., Cremin, B., and Beighton, P.: Osteogenesis imperfecta congenita. Pediatr. Radiol., 12:21, 1982.
168. Stein, R., Lazar, M., and Adam, A.: Brittle cornea; a familial trait associated with blue sclera. Am. J. Ophthalmol., 66:67, 1968.
169. Stevenson, C. J., Bottoms, E., and Shuster, S.: Skin collagen in osteogenesis imperfecta. Lancet, 1:860, 1970.
170. Stone, M. M.: Osteogenesis imperfecta. Orthopedics, 1:126, 1959.
171. Stool, N., Sullivan, C. R., and Bigelow, C. E.: Osteogenesis imperfecta in a 95-year-old woman. Proc. Mayo Clin., 34:523, 1959.
172. Strach, E. H.: Hyperplastic callus formation in osteogenesis imperfecta. J. Bone Joint Surg., 35-B:417, 1953.
173. Summer, G. K., and Patton, W. C.: Intravenous proline tolerance in osteogenesis imperfecta. Metabolism, 17:46, 1968.
174. Sykes, B., Francis, M. J. O., and Smith, R.: Altered relation of two collagen types in osteogenesis imperfecta. N. Engl. J. Med., 296:200, 1977.
175. Teitelbaum, S. L., Kraft, W. J., Land, R., and Avioli, L. V.: Bone collagen aggregation abnormalities in osteogenesis imperfecta. Calcif. Tiss. Res., 17:75, 1974.
176. Tiley, F., and Albright, J. A.: Osteogenesis imperfecta: Treatment by multiple osteotomy and intramedullary rod insertion. Report of thirteen patients. J. Bone Joint Surg., 55-A:701, 1973.
177. Trelstad, R. L., Rubin, D., and Gross, J.: Osteogenesis imperfecta congenita. Evidence of a generalized molecular disorder of collagen. Lab. Invest., 36:501, 1977.
178. Vandemark, W. E., and Page, M. A.: Massive hyperplasia of bone following fractures of osteogenesis imperfecta. J. Bone Joint Surg., 30-A:1015, 1948.
179. Villanueva, A. R., and Frost, H. M.: Bone formation in human osteogenesis imperfecta, measured by tetracycline bone labeling. Acta Orthop. Scand., 41:531, 1970.
180. Vrolik, W.: Tabulae ad illustrandam embryogenesin hominis et mammalium tam naturalem quam abnormem. Amstelodami, 1849.
181. Wallman, V. K.: Hyperplastische Kallusreaktion bei Osteogenesis imperfecta. Beitr. Orthop., 21:248, 1974.
182. Weber, M.: Osteogenesis imperfecta; A study of its histopathogenesis. Arch. Pathol., 9:984, 1930.
183. Werner, P., Metz, L., and Dubowski, F.: Nursing care of an osteogenesis imperfecta infant and child. Clin. Orthop., 159:108, 1981.
184. Williams, P. F.: Fragmentation and rodding in osteogenesis imperfecta. J. Bone Joint Surg., 47-B:23, 1965.
185. Williams, P. F.: Treatment of osteogenesis imperfecta. Personal communication, 1977.
186. Williams, P. F., Cole, W. H. J., Bailey, R. W., Dubow, H. I., Solomons, C. C., and Millar, E. A.: Current aspects of the surgical treatment of osteogenesis imperfecta. Clin. Orthop., 96:288, 1973.
187. Wynne-Davies, R., Hall, C. M., and Apley, A. G.:

Atlas of Skeletal Dysplasias. Edinburgh, Churchill-Livingstone, 1985, p. 411.
188. Yeoman, P. M.: Multiple osteotomies and intramedullary fixation of the long bones of osteogenesis imperfecta. Proc. R. Soc. Med., 53:946, 1960.
189. Yong-Hing, K., and MacEwen, G. D.: Scoliosis associated with osteogenesis imperfecta. J. Bone Joint Surg., 64-B:36, 1982.
190. Ziv, I., Rang, M., and Hoffman, H. J.: Paraplegia in osteogenesis imperfecta. A case report. J. Bone Joint Surg., 65-B:184, 1983.

IDIOPATHIC JUVENILE OSTEOPOROSIS

Idiopathic juvenile osteoporosis is a rare metabolic bone disease in childhood, characterized by profound reduction of bone mass of unknown etiology; the remaining bone is essentially of normal structure. The cardinal features of idiopathic juvenile osteoporosis are onset before puberty (usually between 8 and 15 years of age—earlier in girls than in boys); compression fractures of vertebrae and of the long bones, particularly in metaphyseal regions; and the formation of new but osteoporotic bone (this metaphyseal affection, termed "neo-osseous" osteoporosis, is unique to idiopathic juvenile osteoporosis).[1–37]

Etiopathology

Idiopathic juvenile osteoporosis is a nongenetic disorder whose exact cause is unknown. There is an imbalance between formation and resorption of osseous tissue. Is the decrease in bone mass due to excessive bone resorption or decreased bone formation? Jowsey and Johnson obtained bone from the ilium in seven patients with idiopathic juvenile osteoporosis for comparison with that of age-matched controls. In quantitative microradiographic studies, they found the linear surface involved in bone formation to be within the normal range, whereas the linear resorption surface was increased in all patients. The width of osteoid tissue was less in the osteoporotic specimens, but there were no qualitative abnormalities. They concluded the main abnormality in juvenile osteoporosis is excessive bone resorption.[23] This has, however, been questioned by Smith, who supported Kooh's proposal that primary osteoblastic failure may be the important change.[24, 33, 34]

Histologic examination of bone biopsy specimens from patients with idiopathic juvenile osteoporosis show the bone trabeculae to be thin and to have excessively scalloped edges with an increase in the number of Howship's lacunae.

Biochemical studies show no specific changes. The serum calcium and phosphorus values are within the normal range. The plasma alkaline phosphatase and urinary total hydroxyproline levels usually are normal, although in some patients they may be slightly elevated, which may reflect the normal temporary increase that coincides with the rapid prepubertal growth spurt.[23, 33, 34] The only metabolic abnormality found is a slightly positive to markedly negative calcium balance—the degree of which correlates with the clinical and radiologic severity of the osteoporosis. The abnormal balance may be due to intestinal malabsorption of calcium or hypercalciuria. The results of isotope studies have been conflicting: using calcium-47, Berglund and Lindquist found a normal accretion rate for age, whereas Lachman and associates reported the rate of intestinal absorption of calcium-47 to be high rather than low.[2, 25] With clinical recovery the calcium balance returns to normal positive.

Clinical Picture

This self-limiting transient form of osteoporosis may be manifest in varying degrees of severity and can occur in the young. Kooh and associates reported 11 children with the disorder, in 7 of whom the onset of symptoms was before the age of five years.[24] It seems the features of an attack are most clearly seen when the severe neo-osseous osteoporosis and the maximal growth rate coincide.

Symptoms consist of deep pain in the back, limbs, and feet, and difficulty and slowness in walking. Difficulty in rising from the ground without "climbing up oneself" is a sign of proximal muscle weakness. Compression fractures of vertebrae cause kyphosis and sometimes scoliosis.[1, 4, 5, 21] Recurrent multiple fractures of long bones are common and tend to occur in the metaphyseal regions of weight-bearing bones.

Radiographic Findings

Radiographs of the spine and limbs show diffuse, severe, generalized osteoporosis. The normal trabecular pattern is decreased or nonexistent, and the cortices are thin. In the lateral views of the spine the vertebral bodies show the typical "codfish" appearance. Thoracolumbar kyphosis is present to a varying degree in almost all cases. In some patients structural scoliosis is evident. Fractures of the long bones in various stages of healing are evident; typically they are metaphyseal in location and occur in the distal femur, proximal tibia, or femoral neck

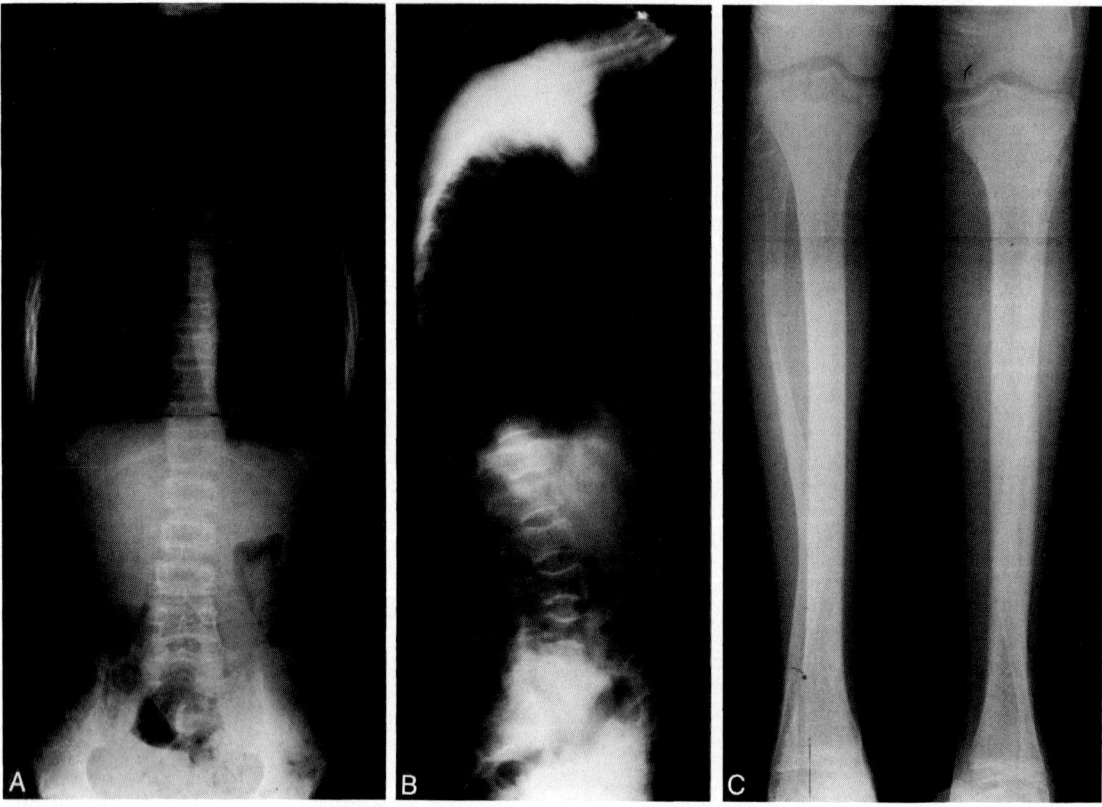

FIGURE 3–50. *Idiopathic juvenile osteoporosis.*

A and **B.** Anteroposterior and lateral radiogram of the spine showing the severe osteoporosis. Note the compression fractures of the vertebrae in the lumbar region. **C.** Anteroposterior radiogram of both tibiae. Note the plastic bowing of the fibulae and marked osteoporosis.

(Fig. 3–50). The skull is normal; there are no "significant" wormian bones. The lamina dura is normal.

Diagnosis

The diagnosis of idiopathic juvenile osteoporosis is made by ruling out secondary forms of osteoporosis in childhood, some of which are of known causes (Table 3–6).

The problem in differential diagnosis is to distinguish mild forms of osteogenesis imperfecta from idiopathic juvenile osteoporosis, which may be difficult and sometimes impossible. In *idiopathic juvenile osteoporosis* there is no positive family history of osteoporosis, the patients are normal at birth and usually until eight to ten years of age; the sclerae are not blue, and the teeth are normal (though these two features need not be present in osteogenesis imperfecta); the ligaments are not lax; and there is no easy bruising. In idiopathic juvenile osteoporosis, fractures of the long bones tend to be metaphyseal in location more often than they do in osteogenesis imperfecta. In *osteogenesis imperfecta tarda* the long bones are slender with thin cortices, whereas in idiopathic juvenile osteoporosis the osteoporosis is metaphyseal, and wherever new bone formation takes place it is osteoporotic. This "neo-osteoporosis" seems to be typical of idiopathic juvenile osteoporosis.

In the mild form of osteogenesis imperfecta there is defective formation of Type I alpha chain collagen, and there is an increased ratio of 1 (III) to 1 (I) collagen in the pepsin-digest of skin; however, unfortunately a normal ratio of Type III to Type I alpha chain collagen does not exclude osteogenesis imperfecta. In idiopathic juvenile osteoporosis the ratio is normal.

Quantitative histologic studies of biopsy specimens in idiopathic juvenile osteoporosis show an increase in resorption surface as compared with that in age-matched control subjects, whereas in osteogenesis imperfecta there is an abnormally excessive amount of primitive non-haversian bone.[23] These morphologic findings are helpful in distinguishing the two disorders.

Malignant disease of the bone marrow is the second most important cause of osteoporosis that should be ruled out. Any child with severe osteoporosis and multiple fractures of vertebrae

Table 3–6. Causes of Osteoporosis in Childhood

Endocrine disorders
    Hyperthyroidism
    Hyperparathyrodism
    Hypogonadism
    Glucocorticoid excess—Cushing's syndrome, steroid therapy
Metabolic disorders
    Homocystinuria
    Gastrointestinal malabsorption
    Idiopathic hypoproteinemia
    Vitamin C deficiency
    Rickets-osteomalacia
    Liver disease
Renal disease
    Chronic tubular acidosis
    Idiopathic hypercalciuria
    Lowe syndrome
    Uremia and regular hemodialysis
Bone affections
    Osteogenesis imperfecta
    Idiopathic juvenile osteoporosis
    Idiopathic osteolysis
    Turner syndrome (XO chromosome anomaly)
Malignant diseases
    Leukemia
    Lymphoma
Miscellaneous causes
    Disuse osteoporosis of paralyzed limbs as in myelomeningocele
    Generalized osteoporosis of Still's disease, especially after steroid therapy
    Heparin therapy
    Anticonvulsant drug therapy

and long bones should have a bone marrow examination by a competent hematologist to rule out *leukemia;* the marrow specimens should be obtained early in the course of the disease. Initial normal peripheral blood findings in leukemia may obscure the picture and delay early diagnosis. *Lymphoma* of bone is another possible cause of osteoporosis.

Treatment

There is neither specific nor effective treatment. There has been no improvement despite treatment with anabolic steroids, estrogens, androgens, and various forms of vitamin D.

Marder and associates reported an 11-year-old girl with diffuse osteoporosis and pathologic fractures. The diagnosis of idiopathic juvenile osteoporosis was supported by the onset of the disease prior to puberty and the characteristic metaphyseal location of fractures. The plasma calcitriol (1,25-dihydroxycholecalciferol) levels were low when the disease was active; calcitriol administration improved bone mineralization, the fractures diminished, and the calcitriol levels returned to normal after the disease remitted.[30] These investigators suggested a relationship between calcitriol deficiency and the pathogenesis of idiopathic juvenile osteoporosis. Calcitriol stimulates calcium absorption from the gut; a deficiency of calcitriol results in a negative calcium balance with high fecal calcium excretion. The only problem with the case report is that, in the natural history of idiopathic juvenile osteoporosis, there are periods when spontaneous resolution occurs. Further studies are needed to elucidate the relationship of calcitriol deficiency and its role in management of idiopathic juvenile osteoporosis.

Spinal deformity, especially kyphosis, should be treated with the Milwaukee brace. Early treatment until natural healing of the disease takes place is recommended by Jones and Hensinger.[21] The brace in itself may aggravate the osteoporosis because of immobilization. A gradually increasing physical therapy exercise program is important. Early weaning from the orthosis is recommended when there is evidence of reconstitution of the vertebral bodies. If a significant degree of kyphosis is allowed to develop the residual deformity will persist.

Fractures of long bones are managed in the conventional manner. Early weight-bearing is recommended. Prolonged immobilization should be avoided; otherwise disuse atrophy will trigger a vicious circle.

References

1. Bartal, E., and Gage, J. R.: Idiopathic juvenile osteoporosis and scoliosis. J. Pediatr. Orthop., *2*:295, 1982.
2. Berglund, G., and Lindquist, B.: Osteopenia in adolescence. Clin. Orthop., *17*:259, 1960.
3. Bordier, P., de Seze, S., Miravet, L., and Berbir, N.: Physiopathologie de l'ostéoporose de l'adulte jeune. Sem. Hôp. Paris, *50*:197, 1974.
4. Bradford, D. S., Brown, D. M., Moe, J. H., Winter, R. B., and Jowsey, J.: Scheuermann's kyphosis: A form of osteoporosis? Clin. Orthop., *118*:10, 1976.
5. Burner, W. L., Badger, V. M., and Sherman, F. C.: Osteoporosis and acquired back deformities. J. Pediatr. Orthop., *2*:383, 1982.
6. Catel, W.: Pubertätsfischwirbelkrankeit. Kinderaerztl. Prax., *22*:21, 1954.
7. Cloutier, M. D., Hayles, A. B., Riggs, B. L., Jowsey, J., and Bickel, W. H.: Juvenile osteoporosis: Report of a case including a description of some metabolic and microradiographic studies. Pediatrics, *40*:649, 1967.
8. Cumming, W. A.: Idiopathic juvenile osteoporosis. J. Can. Assoc. Radiol., *21*:21, 1970.
9. Dent, C. E.: Idiopathic juvenile osteoporosis. Birth Defects Orig. Art. Series, *5*:134, 1969.
10. Dent, C. E.: Osteoporosis in childhood. Postgrad. Med. J., *53*:450, 1977.
11. Dent, C. E., and Friedman, M.: Idiopathic juvenile osteoporosis. Q. J. Med., NS*34*:177, 1965.
12. Fanconi, A., Illig, R., Poley, J. R., Prader, A., Francillon, M., Labhart, A., and Uehlinger, E.: Idiopathische transitorische Osteoporose in Pubertätsalter. Helv. Paediatr. Acta, *21*:531, 1966.
13. Genssler, W., and Menzel, K.: Die juvenile Osteoporose (Fischwirbelkrankheit). Chir. Praxis, *21*:449, 1976.

14. Gooding, C. A., and Ball, J. H.: Idiopathic juvenile osteoporosis. Radiology, 93:1349, 1969.
15. Gorgenyi, A.: Idiopathic juvenile osteoporosis: Report of a case and review of the literature. Acta Paediatr. Acad. Sci. Hung., 10:315, 1969.
16. Grubbauer, H. M., Stogmann, W., and Wendler, H.: Differentialdiagnose und Verlauf der idiopathischen juvenilen Osteoporose. Klin. Paediatr., 188:353, 1976.
17. Guibaud, P., Larbre, F., Hermier, M., Frederich, A., and Meunier, P.: "Ostéoporose idiopathique" ou ostéogenèse imparfaite. Pediatrie, 5:553, 1970.
18. Hammel, H.: Über die Osteoporose der Wirbelsaule unklarer Ursache (Fischwirbelkrankheit). Arch. Orthop. Unfallchir., 44:412, 1951.
19. Houang, M. T. W., Brenton, D. P., Renton, P., and Shaw, D. G.: Idiopathic juvenile osteoporosis. Skeletal Radiol., 3:17, 1978.
20. Jackson, W. P. U.: Osteoporosis of unknown cause in younger people. J. Bone Joint Surg., 40-B:420, 1958.
21. Jones, E. T., and Hensinger, R. N.: Spinal deformity in idiopathic juvenile osteoporosis. Spine, 6:1, 1981.
22. Jowsey, J.: Metabolic Diseases of Bone. Philadelphia, Saunders, 1977, pp. 248–255.
23. Jowsey, J., and Johnson, K. A.: Juvenile osteoporosis: Bone findings in seven patients. J. Pediatr., 81:511, 1972.
24. Kooh, S. W., Cumming, W. A., Fraser, D., and Fornasier, V. L.: Transient childhood osteoporosis of unknown cause. In Frame B., Parfitt, A. M., and Duncan, H. (eds.): Clinical Aspects of Metabolic Bone Disease. Amsterdam, Excerpta Medica (International Congress Series No. 270), 1973, pp. 329–343.
25. Lachman, D., Willvonseder, R., Hofer, R., and Bugajer-Gleitmann, H. E.: A case report of idiopathic juvenile osteoporosis with particular reference to 47-calcium absorption. Eur. J. Pediatr., 125:265, 1977.
26. Lapatsanis, P., Kavadias, A., and Vretos, K.: Juvenile osteoporosis. Arch. Dis. Child., 46:66, 1971.
27. Lindemann, K.: Über die Osteoporose der Wirbelsaule unklarer Ursache (Fischwirbelkrankheit). Arch. Orthop. Unfallchir., 44:403, 1951.
28. Loirat, C., Houllemare, L., Lestradet, H., and Grenet, P.: L'ostéoporose idiopathique de l'enfant. Sem. Hôp. Paris, 43:2812, 1967.
29. McGrae, W. M., and Sweet, E. M.: Diagnosis of osteoporosis in childhood. Br. J. Radiol., 40:104, 1967.
30. Marder, H. K., Tsang, R. C., Hug, G., and Crawford, A. C.: Calcitriol deficiency in idiopathic juvenile osteoporosis. Am. J. Dis. Child., 136:914, 1982.
31. Schippers, J. C.: Over een geval van "spontane" algemeene osteoporose bij een klein meisje. Maandschr. Kindergeneeskd., 8:108, 1939.
32. Schwarz, G.: Orale calciumtherapie bei zwei Fallen von juveniler idiopatischer Osteoporose. Verh. Dtsch. Ges. Inn. Med., 71:884, 1965.
33. Smith, R.: Idiopathic juvenile osteoporosis. Am. J. Dis. Child., 133:889, 1979.
34. Smith, R.: Idiopathic osteoporosis in the young. J. Bone Joint Surg., 62-B:417, 1980.
35. Teotia, M., Teotia, S. P. S., and Singh, R. K.: Idiopathic juvenile osteoporosis. Am. J. Dis. Child., 133:894, 1979.
36. Towbin, R., and Dunbar, J. S.: Generalized osteoporosis with multiple fractures in an adolescent. Invest. Radiol., 3:171, 1981.

IDIOPATHIC OSTEOLYSIS

Idiopathic osteolysis, or "disappearing bones," is an extremely rare condition characterized by spontaneous onset, without previous causative factors, of rapid destruction and resorption of a single bone or often of several bones. This results in severe deformities with joint subluxation and instability.

The etiology is unknown.

Classification

The syndrome of idiopathic osteolysis consists of five types: idiopathic multicentric osteolysis with dominant inheritance, idiopathic multicentric osteolysis with recessive inheritance, idiopathic nonhereditary multicentric osteolysis with nephropathy, Gorham's massive osteolysis, and the Winchester syndrome.

Type I—Hereditary Multicentric Osteolysis With Dominant Transmission. *This type of osteolysis is characterized by the onset of spontaneous pain and swelling in the hands and feet in children between the ages of two and seven years. There may be a previous history of minor trauma. The disease gradually progresses over a period of a few years, resulting in partial or complete resorption of the carpal and tarsal bones. Initially, Beals and Bird referred to this as carpotarsal osteolysis, but the osteolytic process is more diffuse, involving the metacarpals distally and the distal epiphyses of the radius, ulna, and humerus proximally. The destruction of the carpal bones causes ulnar deviation of the wrist with gross instability (Fig. 3–51). The ankle joint may be in valgus or varus deviation, and there is pain and instability of the hindfoot. In cases in which the elbows are involved, the radial head will be subluxated, and restriction of joint motion will follow. The osteolytic process is self-limited, usually stopping in adolescence; there are, however, case reports of the reappearance of the osteolysis in adult life.

Type II—Hereditary Multicentric Osteolysis With Recessive Inheritance. This type was described by Torg and associates in 1969.[44] It is very similar to the dominant type with the exception that it is associated with generalized severe osteoporosis of the long bones of the appendicular skeleton.

Type III—Nonhereditary Multicentric Osteolysis With Nephropathy.† In this entity the tarsal bones are involved to a lesser degree than is the carpus. The pain and swelling of the carpal and tarsal bones begin between two and five years of age and eventually involve the metacarpals, which appear like the sucked end of a peppermint stick. The disorder is characterized by association with nephropathy, which

---

*See references 15, 24, 27, 37, 38, 41, 42, 45.
†See references 12, 25, 28–30, 32, 36, 44, 45.

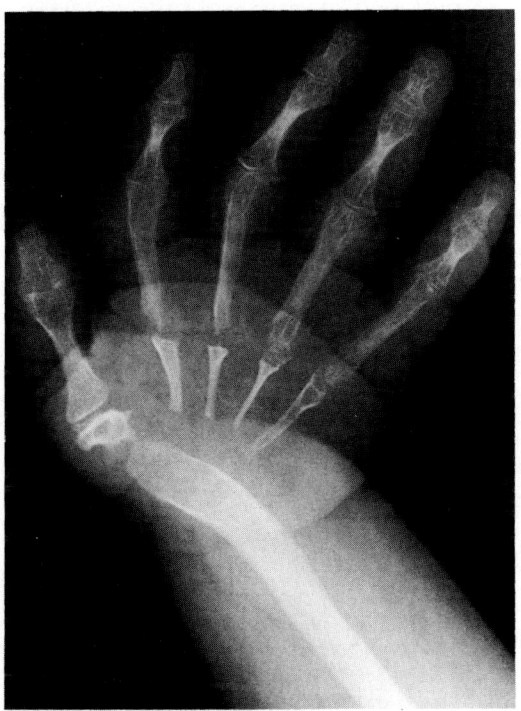

FIGURE 3–51. Osteolysis—carpotarsal form.

Note the marked erosion of the base of the metacarpals with absence of the carpal bones. The proximal phalanges appear bizarre and elongated. The hand is in marked ulnar deviation. (From Poznanski, A. K.: The Hand in Radiologic Diagnosis. Philadelphia, W. B. Saunders, 1984. Reprinted by permission.)

begins at the same time as the osteolysis, manifesting itself as proteinuria, severe chronic glomerulonephritis, and malignant hypertension. Death takes place, usually, in adolescence. Other occasional associated findings are atrophy of the shoulder girdle, thoracic scoliosis, and skull deformity.[21, 25, 44]

Type IV—Gorham's Massive Osteolysis. This monocentric massive osteolysis is associated with vascular abnormality, angiomatosis or hemangiomatosis. It is not a genetic condition and is not associated with nephropathy. It may appear in any part of the skeleton, and its course is benign, the osteolytic process stopping after a few years.[16]

Type V—The Winchester Syndrome. This extremely rare disorder has an inheritance pattern that is autosomal recessive. The symptoms begin in childhood. The carpotarsal osteolysis is associated with contractures of joints, shortness of stature, osteoporosis, corneal clouding, and skin lesions. The kidneys are normal.[47] Originally this was thought to be a type of mucopolysaccharidosis; the electron microscopic studies of Hollister and associates have, however, shown it to be a nonlysosomal collagenosis.[20]

Pathology

Osseous tissue is replaced by fibrous tissue with no regeneration of bone. In the *Gorham type* of osteolysis associated with vascular abnormality, there is marked proliferation of vascular spaces resembling hemangioendothelioma. Occasionally the vascular changes in bone resemble the proliferation of capillaries associated with an arteriovenous fistula.

Differential Diagnosis

One should consider inflammatory disorders of bone, malignant osteoclastic tumors, arterial vascular disease, post-traumatic osteolysis, and aseptic necrosis.

Treatment

Management is individualized according to the severity of involvement and the type of idiopathic osteolysis. Surgical measures employed depend upon the bone involved. Resection and prosthetic replacement have been successful in some patients.[46] Irradiation in small doses will stimulate new bone formation but does not arrest progression of the osteolysis.

References

1. Aston, J. N.: A case of "massive osteolysis" of the femur. J. Bone Joint Surg., *40-B*:514, 1958.
2. Beals, R. K., and Bird, C. B.: Carpal and tarsal osteolysis: A case report and review of the literature. J. Bone Joint Surg., *57-A*:681, 1975.
3. Berthoux, F., Robert, J. M., Zech, P., Fries, D., and Traeger, J.: Acro-ostéolyse essentielle à début carpien et tarsien avec néphropathie. Arch. Fr. Pediatr., *28*:615, 1971.
4. Blumdell, Jones, G., Midgley, R. L., and Smith, B. S.: Massive osteolysis—disappearing bones. J. Bone Joint Surg., *40-B*:494, 1958.
5. Branch, H. E.: Acute spontaneous absorption of bone. Report of a case involving a clavicle and a scapula. J. Bone Joint Surg., *27*:706, 1945.
6. Branco, F., and Horta, J.: Notes on a rare case of essential osteolysis. J. Bone Joint Surg., *40-B*:519, 1958.
7. Butler, R. W., McCance, R. A., and Barrett, A. M.: Unexplained destruction of the shaft of the femur in a child. J. Bone Joint Surg., *40-B*:487, 1958.
8. Campbell, J., Almond, H. G. A., and Johnson, R.: Massive osteolysis of the humerus with spontaneous recovery. J. Bone Joint Surg., *57-B*:238, 1975.
9. Cheney, W. P.: Acro-osteolysis. A.J.R., *94*:595, 1965.
10. Coste, F., and Gaucher, M.: Ostéolyses d'origine nerveuse. Rev. Rhum., *10*:51, 1943.
11. Crasselt, C.: Die Akroosteolyse. 2 Teil: Zur Differentialdiagnose der lokalisierten Akroosteolyse und die

Ätiologie des Akroosteolysesyndroms. Z. Orthop., 94:33, 1961.
12. Derot, M., Rathery, M., Rosselin, G., and Catellier, C.: Acro-ostéolyse due carpe, pied creux, scoliose et strabisme chez une jeune fille atteinte d'une insuffisance rénale. Bull. Soc. Med. Hôp. Paris, 77:223, 1961.
13. Erickson, C. M., Hirschberger, M., and Stickler, G. B.: Carpal-tarsal osteolysis. J. Pediatr., 93:779, 1978.
14. Fornasier, V. L.: Hemangiomatosis with massive osteolysis. J. Bone Joint Surg., 52-B:444, 1970.
15. Gluck, J., and Miller, J. J. III.: Familial osteolysis of the carpal and tarsal bones. J. Pediatr., 81:506, 1972.
16. Gorham, L. W., and Stout, A. P.: Massive osteolysis (acute spontaneous absorption of bone, phantom bone, disappearing bone): Its relation to haemangiomatosis. J. Bone Joint Surg., 37-A:985, 1955.
17. Gorham, L. W., Wright, A. W., Schultz, H. H., and Maxon, F. C.: Disappearing bones, a rare form of massive osteolysis. Am. J. Med., 17:674, 1954.
18. Hardeggar, F., Simpson, L. A., and Segmueller, G.: The syndrome of idiopathic osteolysis. J. Bone Joint Surg., 67-B:89, 1985.
19. Heyden, G., Kindblom, L. G., and Nielsen, J. M.: Disappearing bone disease. A clinical and histological study. J. Bone Joint Surg., 59-A:57, 1977.
20. Hollister, D. W., Rimoin, D. L., Lachman, R. S., et al.: The Winchester syndrome: a nonlysosomal connective tissue disease. J. Pediatr., 84:701, 1974.
21. Huke, B.: Ueberlegungen bei einer Langzeitstudie über eine progressive kranio-karpo-tarsale Osteolyse. Z. Orthop., 116:203, 1978.
22. Johnson, P. M., and McClure, J. G.: Observations on massive osteolysis. A review of the literature and report of a case. Radiology, 71:28, 1958.
23. Kery, L., and Wouters, H. W.: Massive osteolysis. J. Bone Joint Surg., 52-B:452, 1970.
24. Kohler, E., Babbitt, D., Huizenga, B., and Good, T. A.: Hereditary osteolysis: A clinical, radiological and chemical study. Radiology, 108:99, 1973.
25. Lagier, R., and Rutishauser, E.: Osteoarticular changes in a case of essential osteolysis. J. Bone Joint Surg., 47-B:339, 1965.
26. Lamy, M., and Maroteaux, P.: Idiopathic osteolysis (Lamy-Maroteaux). Arch. Fr. Pediatr., 18:693, 1961.
27. McManus, L. F., Ballard, A., Walton, S., and Omer, G. E.: Carpal and tarsal agenesis with features of essential and hereditary osteolysis: Follow-up notes on articles previously published in the Journal. J. Bone Joint Surg., 54-A:1099, 1972.
28. MacPherson, R. I., Walker, R. D., and Kowall, M. H.: Essential osteolysis with nephropathy. J. Can. Assoc. Radiol., 24:98, 1973.
29. Mahoudeau, D., Dubrisay, J., Elissalde, B., and Srear, C.: Ostéolyse essentielle et nephrite. Bull. Soc. Med. Hôp. Paris, 77:229, 1961.
30. Marie, J., Salet, J., and Leveque, B.: Polydystrophie squelettiques avec ostéolyse progressive. Arch. Fr. Pediatr., 8:752, 1951.
31. Marie, J., Salet, J., Leveque, B., and Sauvegrain, J.: Syndrome ostéodystrophique de nature congénitale probable: Réalisant l'association d'une ostéolyse essentielle progressive des extrémités des membres et d'anomalies malformatives vertébrales et costales. Presse Méd., 64:2173, 1956.
32. Marie, J., Leveque, B., Lyon, G., Bebe, M., and Watchie, J. M.: Acro-ostéolyse essentielle compliqué d'insuffisance rénale d'évolution fatale. Presse Méd., 71:249, 1963.
33. Milner, S. M., and Baker, S. L.: Disappearing bones. J. Bone Joint Surg., 40-B:500, 1958.
34. Mouchet, A.: Ostéolyses post-traumatiques. Rev. Rhum., 10:43, 1943.
35. Mouchet, A., and Rouvillois, H.: Ostéolyse du bassin d'origine indeterminée. Mem. Acad. Chir. (Paris), 63:277, 1937.
36. Neyroud, M., Baumgartner, J., and Lenoir, A.: Un cas d'ostéolyse essentielle. Helv. Paediatr. Acta, 11:155, 1956.
37. Normand, I. C. S., Dent, C. E., and Smellie, J. M.: Disappearing carpal bones. Proc. R. Soc. Med., 55:978, 1962.
38. Omer, G. E., and Nossman, D. L.: Bone agenesis. A case involving the carpus and tarsus. J. Bone Joint Surg., 40-A:917, 1958.
39. Poirier, H.: Massive osteolysis of the humerus treated by resection and prosthetic replacement. J. Bone Joint Surg., 50-B:158, 1968.
40. Sage, M. R., and Allen, P. W.: Massive osteolysis. Report of a case. J. Bone Joint Surg., 56-B:130, 1974.
41. Shurtleff, D. B., Sparkes, R. S., Clawson, D. K., Guntheroth, W. G., and Mottet, N. K.: Hereditary osteolysis with hypertension and nephropathy. J.A.M.A., 188:363, 1964.
42. Thieffry, S., and Sorell-Dejerine, J.: Forme spéciale d'ostéolyse essentielle héréditaire et familiale à stabilisation spontanée survenant dans l'enfance. Presse Méd., 66:1858, 1958.
43. Torg, J. S., and Steel, H. H.: Essential osteolysis and nephropathy. J. Bone Joint Surg., 50-A:1629, 1968.
44. Torg, J. S., DiGeorge, A. M., Kirkpatrick, J. A., Jr., and Trujillo, M. M.: Hereditary multicentric osteolysis with recessive transmission: A new syndrome. J. Pediatr., 785:243, 1969.
45. Tyler, T., and Rosenbaum, H. D.: Idiopathic multicentric osteolysis. A.J.R., 126:23, 1976.
46. Vitali, M.: The prosthetic management of a case of essential osteolysis. J. Bone Joint Surg., 44-B:652, 1962.
47. Winchester, P., Grossman, H., and Lim, W. N.: A new acid mucopolysaccharidosis with skeletal deformities simulating rheumatoid arthritis. A.J.R., 106:121, 1969.

OSTEOPETROSIS

Osteopetrosis is a bone dysplasia characterized by failure of bone resorption due to functional deficiency of the osteoclasts and persistence of calcified chondroid and primitive bone. Radiologically it is characterized by striking opacity of the bones, lack of cortical endothelial margins, and failure of bone modeling.

Albers-Schonberg first described it in 1904 in a 26-year-old patient.[2] It should be noted that the Albers-Schonberg disease was subsequently diagnosed in that patient's 80-year-old mother.[26] It was called *osteopetrosis* by Karshner in 1926.[36] Over 500 cases have been described in the literature.[5]

Classification

Osteopetrosis is a heterogeneous disorder that varies considerably in the severity of clinical manifestations and mode of inheritance. At least two distinct forms, the congenital and the tarda types, are recognized.

In the *congenital*, or *malignant*, *type* of osteopetrosis the clinical manifestations appear at birth or in early infancy. Obliteration of the marrow cavity by bone overgrowth results in marrow dysfunction and pancytopenia. The presenting symptoms are spontaneous bruising, abnormal bleeding, progressive and recalcitrant anemia, and failure to thrive. Compensatory hepatosplenomegaly develops. Dentition is delayed, and teeth are carious because of diminished resistance to infection. Palsies of the cranial nerves—optic, facial, or oculomotor—may occur because bony overgrowth, leading to narrowing of the cranial foramina, impinges on them.

Pathologic fractures of the fragile bones and osteomyelitis of the mandible are not uncommon. Death usually occurs in the first decade of life because of overwhelming infection or hemorrhage. Occasionally an affected patient may survive into adulthood. This severe congenital type is inherited as an autosomal recessive trait.

The second type, *benign* or *tarda*, is variable in its age of onset. Often the condition remains clinically silent and totally asymptomatic, being discovered incidentally when radiograms are made for some other reason. This tarda form is quite common and compatible with normal physical activity and life span. Mild anemia may be the only finding. Occasionally, there may be a pathologic fracture of the affected bone. Cranial nerve compression may cause facial palsy. Tooth extractions may be followed by osteomyelitis of the mandible or maxilla. The tarda form is autosomal dominant in inheritance.[34, 44]

In the literature, atypical cases have been reported that do not fall into either the congenital or tarda category; these have been grouped together as an *intermediate form* of osteopetrosis, that is of autosomal recessive inheritance.[6, 32, 35]

Etiology and Pathology

The exact cause of osteopetrosis is unknown. The basic defect appears to be cellular—the osteoclasts are abnormal and functionally unable to absorb cartilage and bone. Shapiro and associates performed histologic, ultrastructural, and biochemical studies of the tissue of a patient with osteopetrosis. The bone contained an increased number of osteoclasts, which, however, were not actively resorbing, as evidenced by the absence of ruffled borders and clear zones—the hallmarks of active resorption. In addition, the osteoclasts did not appear to respond to parathyroid hormone, as demonstrated by lack of tissue collagenase activity release. Also, in contrast with normal bone, tissue collagenase was not detected in the osteoporotic bone. The calcium secretion rate was low, and there was a marked reduction in the resorption rate. These findings further support the basic defect in osteopetrosis as being a functional deficiency of the osteoclast. There were no striking abnormalities of parathyroid hormone or calcitonin in the blood or parathyroid or thyroid glands.[64]

The pathologic changes in osteopetrosis are due to failure or diminution of resorption of enchondral cartilage and bone while their formation is proceeding at a normal rate. As a result large amounts of calcified cartilage and primitive bone persist and accumulate, first in the metaphysis and eventually in the diaphysis (Fig. 3–52). Bone remodeling is diminished. The metaphysis widens, and the cortex thickens. The structural stability of the bone, however, is diminished owing to the sparsity of collagen fibrils and failure of remodeling and normal regeneration of the bone matrix. As a result pathologic fractures do occur in osteopetrosis.

Pathologically the total lack of normal, organized bone structure is reflected by the characteristic histologic picture of irregular patches of immature chondro-osseous tissue embedded in matrices of coarse fiber bone with wide and prominent cement lines. In the central part of the disorganized cartilage bones there are areas of osseous metaplasia. Osteoblasts and osteoclasts are present but vary in quantity—they may be decreased, increased, or normal. The bone marrow spaces are almost obliterated by the dense bands of abnormal chondro-osseous tissue. There is marked paucity of bone marrow cells. This is compensated for by an intrinsic intramedullary hematopoiesis in the spleen, liver, and lymph nodes.

Failure of modeling of the long bones results in splaying of the metaphyseal regions and enlargement with bulbous clubbing of the ends of the diaphysis. These changes are more marked in areas of rapid growth, such as the distal femur. The short tubular bones, i.e., the metatarsals, metacarpals, and phalanges, exhibit changes similar to those found in long bones, but to a lesser degree.

Intramedullary bone formation is also abnormal, as noted in the partly nonlamellar nature of subperiosteal bone. The findings in the skull are more marked at its base, which is dense and sclerotic. The fossae are inadequately formed. The foramina for the cranial nerves are crowded with the unabsorbed bone, impinging on the nerves and causing nerve atrophy.

Rachitic changes may be associated with os-

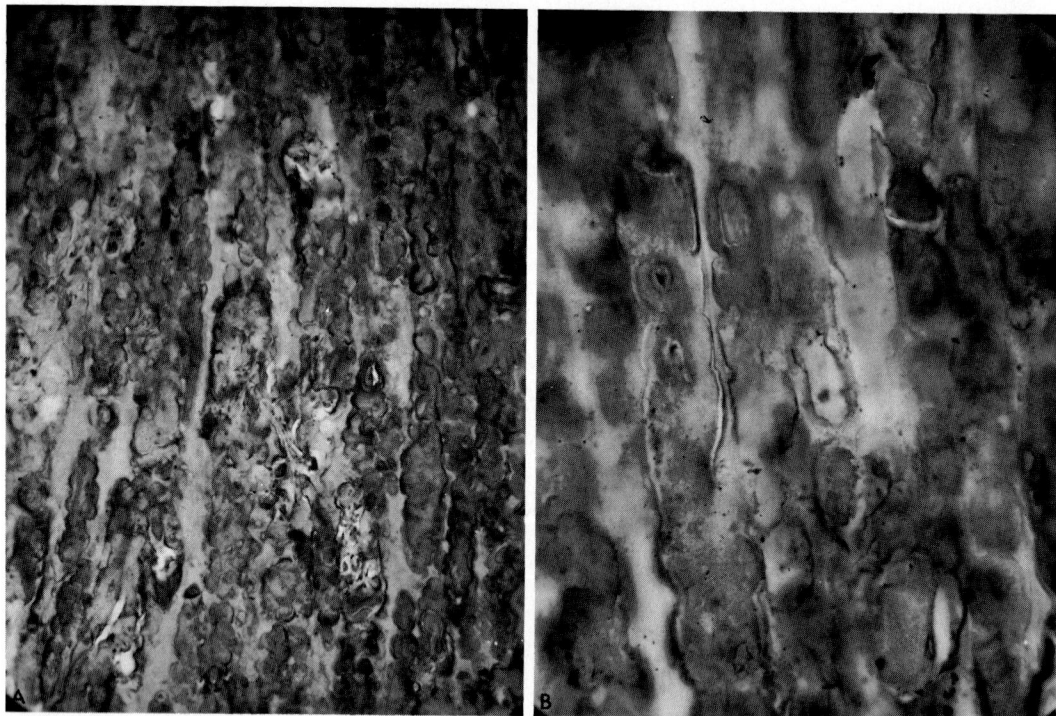

FIGURE 3–52. *Histologic findings in osteopetrosis.*

Note the irregular patches of immature chondro-osseous tissue embedded in matrix of coarse fiber bone with wide and prominent cement lines. **A.** × 100. **B.** × 400.

teopetrosis.[3, 9, 15, 43] This phenomenon is usually encountered in patients with the severe lethal form of the disease. Milgram and Jasty demonstrated that the previously formed hypertrophic cartilage (in the tissues obtained from patients with osteopetrosis and rickets) had calcified; there were no abnormally wide seams of osteoid on bone trabeculae surrounding the calcified cartilage cores. These findings indicate that the rickets in these patients developed secondarily and that the osteopetrosis was present prior to the onset of the rickets.[47]

Milhaud and associates described two forms of lethal osteopetrosis in the rat: "osteopetrosis" (op) and "toothless" (H) types. The thymus was precociously atrophic in both types, and both mutants died prematurely from the disease. The *op* mutant could be cured by normal bone marrow infusion, whereas the *H* mutant could not. The bone lesions in the two types were different. The *H* rat displayed several features of rickets in addition to the typical finding of osteopetrosis. The alpha-fetoprotein levels were high. Milhaud's findings in the rat suggest that a more generalized process is involved in the pathogenesis of this bone dysplasia.[49]

Radiographic Features

The hallmark of osteopetrosis is the increased radiopacity of the bones. The normal architecture is entirely obliterated so there is no distinction between cortical and cancellous bone (Fig. 3–53).

In underpenetrated films the bone appears uniformly dense; with better technique and adequately penetrated films, however, transverse (and sometimes longitudinal) striations and an *os-in-os* pattern will be visualized. The *transverse bands* are composed of alternating zones of sclerosis and lucency—caused by variations in the intensity of the resorption defect from time to time during growth in childhood (Fig. 3–54). The width of the bands in the different parts of the skeleton reflects the relative rates of growth at the different growth plates. Radiolucent zones are areas of more normal bone that was formed during times when the disease was less active. Longitudinal striations in the long bones represent shadows of vascular columns surrounded by connective tissue. The pattern of transverse and longitu-

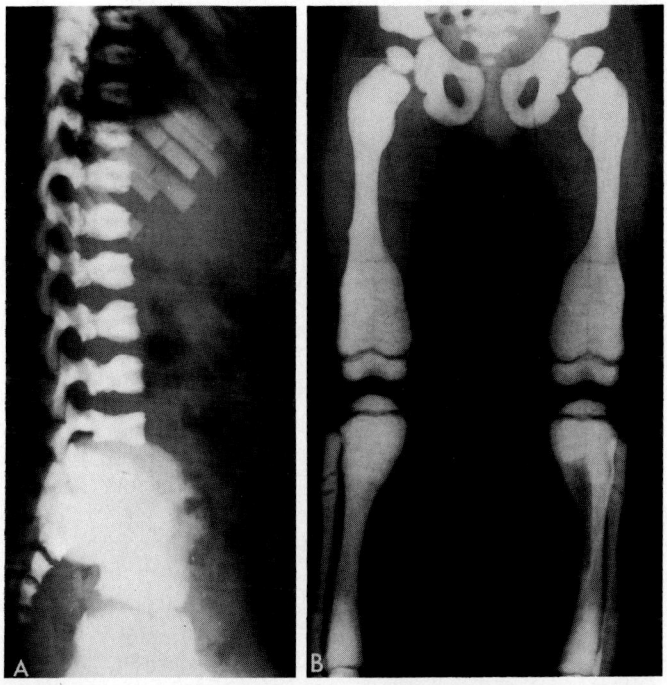
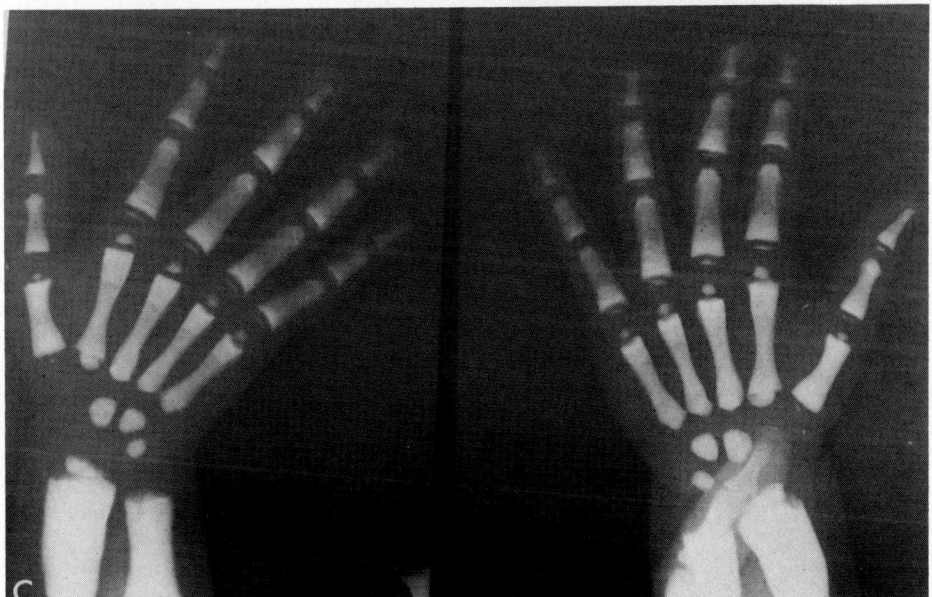

FIGURE 3–53. *Osteopetrosis.*

A. Lateral radiogram of the spine shows uniform opacity of vertebrae and obliteration of normal trabecular structure. There is no distinction between cortical and cancellous bone. **B.** Anteroposterior radiogram of both lower limbs and, **C**, anteroposterior radiograms of both hands show splaying of metaphyseal ends of diaphyses and transverse and longitudinal areas of rarefaction.

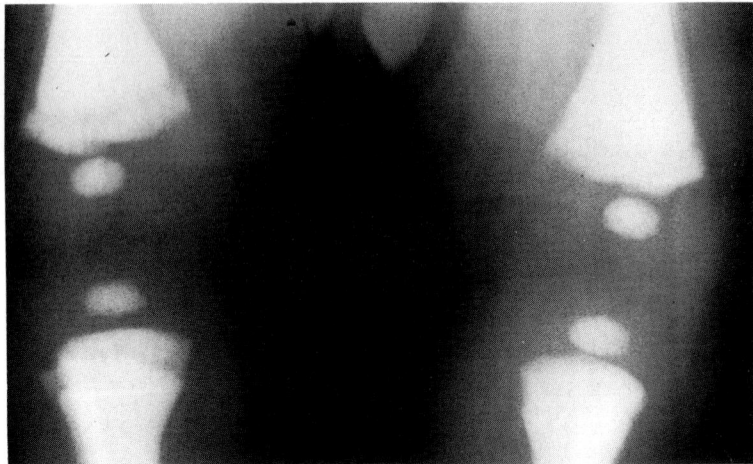

FIGURE 3–54. Transverse bands—alternating zones of sclerosis and lucency.

These are due to variations in intensity of resorption defect from time to time during skeletal growth.

dinal striations is disrupted by fracture or surgical intervention.

Endobone (also known as os-in-os, or bone-within-a-bone) is a core of primitive osseous tissue that resembles miniature fetal bone. This is separated from the cortex by an area of radiolucency (Fig. 3–55). The endobones are seen in childhood and gradually fade in adolescence. They are best visualized in the short tubular bones, tibia and fibula, radius and ulna, and the vertebrae and pelvic bones. In the long bones they are situated eccentrically away from the clubbed ends. The endobones are pathognomonic of osteopetrosis.

Splaying of the metaphysis and clubbing of the metaphyseal ends of the diaphysis are due to failure of normal bone modeling and tubulation. It is seen best at the rapid growth sites, such as the distal femur (see Fig. 3–53 B).

The *spine* shows uniform normal density in early childhood, but in the adolescent and adult the vertebrae have a *"sandwich"* appearance with bands of increased density superiorly and inferiorly adjacent to the vertebral end-plates (Fig. 3–56).

Skeletal imaging with technetium-99m in osteopetrosis demonstrates increased activity in the epiphyseal end of the splayed long bones and short tubular bones, and it is normal elsewhere. In sites of fracture and osteomyelitis, metabolic activity is increased. Reticuloendothelial imaging with sulfur colloid showed almost total lack of activity in the axial and appendicular skeleton. The role of bone imaging is to detect complications of osteopetrosis, namely, fracture and osteomyelitis.[54]

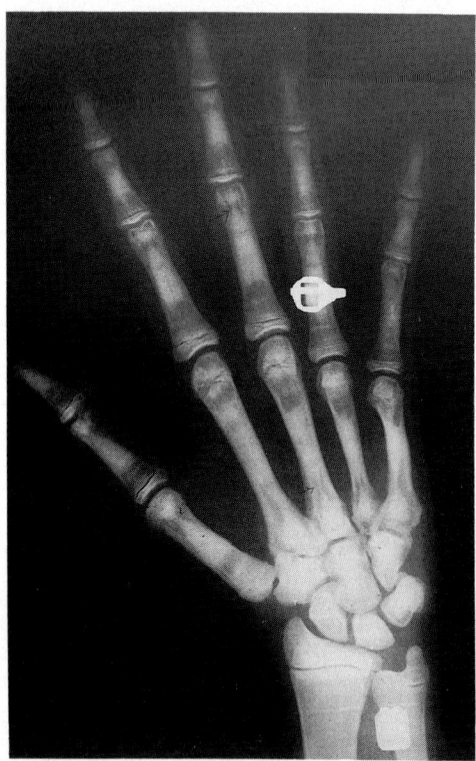

FIGURE 3–55. Endobone in osteopetrosis.

Anteroposterior radiogram of the hand showing increased bone density and the "bone within a bone" (os-in-os) appearance of the phalanges and metacarpals. (Courtesy of Dr. Michael Ozonoff.)

Laboratory Findings

Except for the hematologic changes of anemia and pancytopenia, these studies are essentially normal. The alkaline phosphatase level may be elevated with healing fractures. Serum calcium and phosphate values are normal. The acid phosphatase level may be elevated.[34]

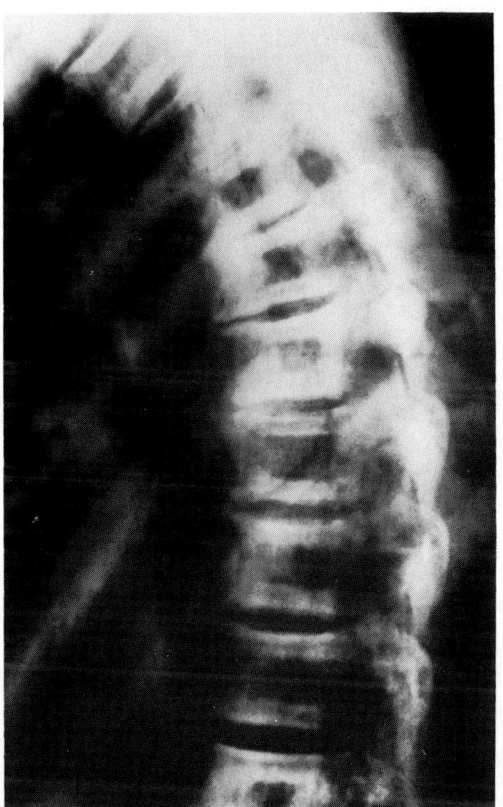

FIGURE 3–56. *Vertebrae in osteopetrosis.*

Increased density adjacent to the end-plates gives a "sandwich" appearance in the lateral projection of the vertebrae. (Courtesy of Dr. James W. Milgram.)

Differential Diagnosis

Osteopetrosis must be differentiated from a number of unrelated bone dysplasias that manifest increased bone density. In *pycnodysostosis* there are homogeneous osseous sclerosis and increased bone fragility. It is differentiated from osteopetrosis by the presence of hypoplasia of the *terminal phalanges* and *clavicles*; the obtuse angle of the *mandible* with the small maxilla; the appearance of the *skull* with open fontanelles, wide sutures, and wormian bones; and the absence of cranial nerve impingement, anemia, and hepatosplenomegaly.

In *progressive diaphyseal dysplasia* (Englemann's disease) the hyperostosis is almost entirely restricted to the diaphysis, the long-bone ends are not clubbed, and pathologic fractures and anemia are not features. The skull, however, may have a thickened vault and base with narrowed foramina, which sometimes causes cranial nerve impingement and palsies.

Craniometaphyseal dysplasia and *metaphyseal dysplasia* (Pyle's disease) show osteosclerosis and altered bone modeling, and cranial nerve palsies and pathologic fractures may occur. In these dysplasias hematopoiesis is normal, the vertebrae are not affected, and the pattern of tubular bone sclerosis is completely dissimilar to osteopetrosis. The *frontometaphyseal dysplasias* are readily differentiated by the massive thickening of the frontal bones.

Increased bone density may occur in metal poisoning, neoplasms, syphilis, and myelofibrosis; these conditions are distinguished by their clinical picture and appropriate laboratory studies.

Problems and Complications

Fractures, a common problem in osteopetrosis, occur because of excessive fragility of the "marble bones." The fracture line is usually transverse and sharply marginated (Fig. 3–57). The most common site is the femur, particularly in the hip region.[11, 28, 49] The callus formed by the healing fracture has the same characteristics as the original bone; it occurs through the same physiologic process, but the healing of osteo-

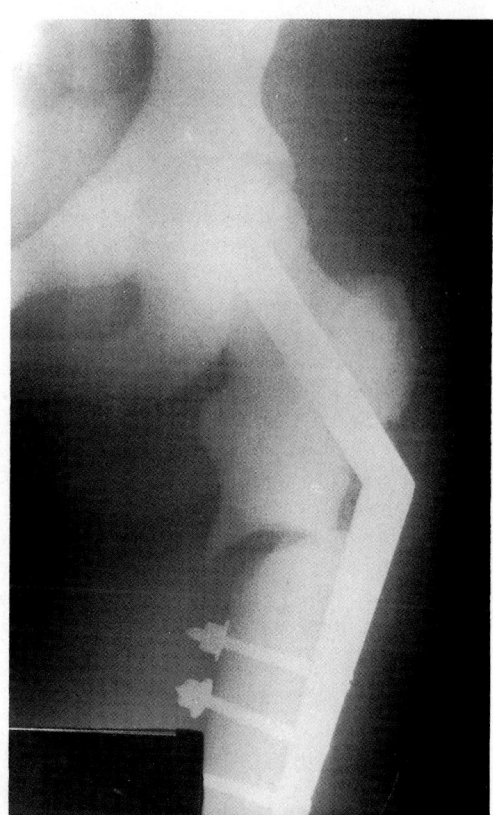

FIGURE 3–57. *Pathologic fracture of the femur is osteopetrosis.*

Note the transverse fracture line. (Courtesy of Dr. James W. Milgram.)

petrotic bone may be quite slow. Coxa vara may develop as a result of shearing stress on the abnormal bone in the femoral neck.[38]

Osteomyelitis is not uncommon, especially of the mandible and maxilla. A predisposing factor is the local decreased blood supply of the bone due to the crowding of the blood vessels by the bone-filled marrow spaces.

There is one reported case in the literature of sarcomatous degeneration in osteopetrotic bone.[37]

Treatment

In the congenital lethal form of osteopetrosis, treatment is directed toward controlling the life-threatening anemia. The only effective method of treatment is bone marrow transplantation. Coccia and associates reported the case of a five-month-old girl with autosomal recessive osteopetrosis who received a bone-marrow transplant from her five-year-old HLA-MLC-identical brother after preparation with cyclophosphamide and modified total-body irradiation. Anemia, thrombocytopenia, and leukoerythroblastosis were corrected within 12 weeks of transplantation. Serial radiographs demonstrated new nonsclerotic bone formation and bone remodeling.[14] The long-term effectiveness of this treatment, however, requires further assessment and experience.

In the past splenectomy has been attempted; its drawback is the removal of a large critical reservoir of extramedullary hematopoietic tissue.[50] Repeated blood transfusions are not the answer to the problem because of the potential for increasing immunization.

Cranial nerve palsies are managed by the neurosurgeon by relieving the bony impingement on the nerves at their foramina.

Fractures are treated by conventional methods. It should be remembered that hard bone is difficult to drill, causing problems with internal fixation. Fracture healing is usually slow. Osteomyelitis, which usually involves the mandible, may require hyperbaric oxygen therapy in addition to surgical incision and drainage.

References

1. Aarskog, D., Aksnes, L., and Markestad, R.: Effect of parathyroid hormone on vitamin D metabolism in osteopetrosis. Pediatrics, 68:109, 1981.
2. Albers-Schonberg, H.: Röntgenbilder einer seltenen Knochenerkrankung. Munchen. Med. Wochenschr., 51:365, 1904.
3. Alexander, W. G.: Report of a case of so-called "marble bones" with a review of the literature and a translation of an article. A.J.R., 10:280, 1923.
4. Ballet, J. J., Griscelli, C., Coutris, C., Milhaud, G., and Maroteaux, P.: Bone marrow transplantation in osteopetrosis. Lancet, 2:1137, 1977.
5. Beighton, P., and Cremin, B. J.: Sclerosing bone disease. Berlin, Springer, 1980.
6. Beighton, P., Hamersma, H., and Cremin, B. J.: Osteopetrosis in South Africa. The benign, lethal and intermediate forms. S. Afr. Med. J., 55:659, 1979.
7. Beighton, P., Horan, F., and Hamersma, H.: A review of osteopetrosis. Postgrad. Med. J., 53:507, 1977.
8. Besselman, D. M.: Splenectomy in the management of the anemia and thrombocytopenia of osteopetrosis. J. Pediatr., 69:455, 1966.
9. Bonucci, E., Sartori, E., and Spina, M.: Osteopetrosis fetalis. Report on a case with special reference to ultrastructure. Virchows Arch. Pathol. Anat., 368:109, 1975.
10. Brailsford, J. F.: Sclerosing conditions of bone. Br. J. Radiol., 23:83, 1950.
11. Breck, L. W., Cornell, R. C., and Emmett, J. E.: Intramedullary fixation of fractures of the femur in a case of osteopetrosis. J. Bone Joint Surg., 39-A:1389, 1957.
12. Callender, G. R., and Miyakawa, G.: Osteopetrosis in an adult. J. Bone Joint Surg., 35-A:204, 1953.
13. Cameron, H. U., and Dewar, F. P.: Degenerative osteoarthritis associated with osteopetrosis. Clin. Orthop., 127:148, 1977.
14. Coccia, P. F., Krivit, W., Cervenka, J., Clawson, C., Kersey, J. H., Kim, T. H., Nesbit, M. E., Ramsay, N. K., Warkentin, P. I., Teitelbaum, S. L., Kahn, A. J., and Brown, D. M.: Successful bone marrow transplantation for infantile malignant osteopetrosis. N. Engl. J. Med., 302:701, 1980.
15. Cohon, J.: Osteopetrosis. Case report, autopsy findings, and pathological interpretation: Failure of treatment with vitamin A. J. Bone Joint Surg., 33-A:923, 1951.
16. Dent, C. E., Smellie, J. M., and Watson, L.: Studies in osteopetrosis. Arch. Dis. Child., 40:7, 1965.
17. Enell, H., and Pehrson, M.: Studies on osteopetrosis. Clinical report of three cases with genetic considerations. Acta Paediatr., 47:279, 1958.
18. Engfeldt, B., Engstrom, A., and Zetterstrom, R.: Biophysical studies on bone tissue. III. Osteopetrosis (marble bone disease). Acta Paediatr., 43:152, 1954.
19. Engfeldt, B., Fajers, C. M., Lodin, H., and Pehrson, M.: Studies on osteopetrosis. III. Roentgenological and pathologic-anatomical investigations on some of the bone changes. Acta Paediatr., 49:391, 1960.
20. Enticknap, J. B.: Albers-Schonberg disease (marble bones). Report of a case with a study of the chemical and physical characteristics of the bone. J. Bone Joint Surg., 36-B:123, 1954.
21. Fairbank, H. A. T.: Osteopetrosis. J. Bone Joint Surg., 30-B:339, 1948.
22. Frost, H. M., Villanueva, A. R., Jett, S., and Eyring, E.: Tetracycline-based analysis of bone remodelling in osteopetrosis. Clin. Orthop., 65:203, 1969.
23. Glorieux, F. H., Pettifor, J. M., Marie, P. J., Delvin, E. E., Travers, R., and Shepard, N.: Induction of bone resorption by parathyroid hormone in congenital malignant osteopetrosis. Metab. Bone Dis. Rel. Res., 3:143, 1981.
24. Graham, C. B., Ridhe, U., and Eklof, O.: Osteopetrosis. In Intrinsic Diseases of Bones. Vol. 4. Basel, Karger, 1973.
25. Greene, W. B., and Torre, B. A.: Case report. Femoral neck fracture in a child with autosomal dominant osteopetrosis. J. Pediatr. Orthop., 5:483, 1985.

26. Hamersma, H.: Osteopetrosis (marble bone disease) of the temporal bone. Laryngoscope, 80:1518, 1970.
27. Hamersma, H.: Total decompression of the facial nerve in osteopetrosis. (Marble bone disease—morbus Albers-Schonberg.) J. Otolaryngol., 36:21, 1974.
28. Hasenhuttl, K.: Osteopetrosis. Review of the literature and comparative studies on a case with a twenty-four-year follow-up. J. Bone Joint Surg., 44-A:359, 1962.
29. Heine, J.: Beitrag zur Marmorknochenkrankheit. Fortschr. Geb. Rontgenstr., 64:121, 1941.
30. Hinkel, C. L., and Beiler, D. D.: Osteopetrosis in adults. A.J.R., 74:46, 1955.
31. Horan, F. T., and Beighton, P. H.: "Osteopetrosis" in the Fairbank Collection. J. Bone Joint Surg., 60-B:53, 1978.
32. Horton, W. A., Schimke, R. N., and Iyama, T.: Osteopetrosis: Further heterogeneity. J. Pediatr., 97:580, 1980.
33. Hoyt, C. S., and Billson, F. A.: Visual loss in osteopetrosis. Am. J. Dis. Child., 133:955, 1979.
34. Johnston, C. C., Lavy, N., Lord, T., Vellios, F., Merritt, A. D., and Deiss, W. P.: Osteopetrosis. A clinical, genetic, metabolic, and morphologic study of the dominant inherited, benign form. Medicine, 47:149, 1968.
35. Kaibara, N., Katsuki, I., Hotokebuchi, T., and Takagishi, K.: Intermediate form of osteopetrosis with recessive inheritance. Skeletal Radiol., 9:47, 1982.
36. Karshner, R.: Osteopetrosis. A.J.R., 16:405, 1926.
37. Kerr, H. J.: A case of osteopetrosis (marble bones) complicated by osteogenic sarcoma. A.J.R., 35:212, 1936.
38. King, R. E., and Lovejoy, J. F.: Familial osteopetrosis with coxa vara. A case report. J. Bone Joint Surg., 55-A:381, 1973.
39. Kleinberg, S.: Osteopetrosis. Am. J. Surg., 87:50, 1954.
40. Kneals, E., and Sante, L. R.: Osteopetrosis (marble bones). Am. J. Dis. Child., 81:693, 1951.
41. Loria-Cortes, R., Quesada-Calvo, E., and Cordero-Chaverri, C.: Osteopetrosis in children. A report of 26 cases. J. Pediatr., 91:43, 1977.
42. McCune, D. J., and Bradley, C.: Osteopetrosis (marble bones) in an infant. Am. J. Dis. Child., 48:949, 1934.
43. McPeak, C. N.: Osteopetrosis. Report of 8 cases occurring in three generations of one family. A.J.R., 36:816, 1936.
44. Mainous, E. G., Hart, G. B., Soffa, D. J., and Graham, G. A.: Hyperbaric oxygen treatment of mandibular osteomyelitis in osteopetrosis. J. Oral Surg., 33:288, 1975.
45. Majale, M., Hunt, S. C. M., and Huckstep., R. L.: Fracture in osteopetrosis. J. Bone Joint Surg., 49-B:595, 1967.
46. Mazur, J., and Wortsman, J.: Hypogonadotropic hypogonadism from osteopetrosis. Clin. Orthop., 162:202, 1982.
47. Milgram, J. W., and Jasty, M.: Osteopetrosis. A morphological study of twenty-one cases. J. Bone Joint Surg., 64-A:912, 1982.
48. Milhaud, G.: Thymus and osteopetrosis. Clin. Orthop., 135:260, 1978.
49. Milhaud, G., Labat, M. L., Litwin, I., Moricard, Y., Moutier, R., Rimbaut, C., Buffe, D., and Juster, M.: Osteopetro-rickets: a new congenital bone disorder. Metab. Bone Dis. Rel. Res., 3:91, 1981.
50. Moe, P. J., and Skjaeveland, A.: Therapeutic studies in osteopetrosis. Report of 4 cases. Acta Paediatr. Scand., 58:593, 1969.
51. Montgomery, R. D., and Standard, K. L.: Albers-Schonberg's disease. A changing concept. J. Bone Joint Surg., 42-B:303, 1960.
52. Morrow, G., Barness, L. A., Fost, A., and Rasmussen, H.: Calcium mobilization in osteopetrosis. Am. J. Dis. Child., 114:161, 1967.
53. Moss, A. A., and Mainzer, F.: Osteopetrosis: An unusual cause of terminal-tuft erosion. Radiology, 97:631, 1970.
54. Park, H.-M., and Lambertus, J.: Skeletal and reticuloendothelial imaging in osteopetrosis. J. Nucl. Med., 18:1091, 1977.
55. Pines, B., and Lederer, M.: Osteopetrosis: Albers-Schonberg disease (marble bones). Report of a case and morphologic study. Am. J. Pathol., 23:755, 1947.
56. Pirie, H.: The development of marble bones. A.J.R., 24:147, 1930.
57. Ragab, A. H., Ducos, R., Crist, W. M., and Duck, S. C.: Granulopoiesis in osteopetrosis. J. Pediatr., 87:422, 1975.
58. Reeves, J. D., August, C. S., Humbert, J. R., and Weston, W. L.: Host defense in infantile osteopetrosis. Pediatrics, 64:202, 1979.
59. Rousseau, J., Dupuy, J. P., Olivier, J. P., Pompon, J. P., Douvion, D., and Pascaud, J. L.: A propos d'un cas exceptionnel de maladie d'Albers-Schonberg. Ann. Radiol., 18:747, 1975.
60. Salzano, F. M.: Osteopetrosis: Review of dominant cases and frequency in a Brazilian state. Acta Genet. Med. Gemeliol., 10:340, 1961.
61. Schmidt, C. J., Marks, S. C., and Harves, L. E.: A radiographic and histologic study of fracture healing in rats. Radiology, 122:517, 1977.
62. Schneider, G. B., Cuenoud, M. L., and Marks, S. C., Jr.: The diagnosis and cure of neonatal osteopetrosis: Experimental evidence from congenitally osteopetrotic (ia) rats. Metab. Bone Dis. Rel. Res., 1:335, 1979.
63. Seifert, M. F.: The biology of macrophages in osteopetrosis. Structure and function. Clin. Orthop., 182:270, 1984.
64. Shapiro, F., Glimcher, M. J., Holtrop, M. E., Tashjian, A. H., Brickley-Parsons, D., and Kenzora, J. E.: Human osteopetrosis. A histological, ultrastructural, and biochemical study. J. Bone Joint Surg., 62-A:384, 1980.
65. Sief, C. A., Chessells, J. N., Levinski, R. J., Pritchard, J., Rodgers, D. W., Casey, A., Muller, K., and Hall, C. M.: Allogenic bone marrow transplantation in infantile malignant osteopetrosis. Lancet, 1:437, 1983.
66. Sjolin, S.: Studies in osteopetrosis. II. Investigations concerning the nature of the anemia. Acta Paediatr., 48:529, 1959.
67. Sly, W. S., Whyte, M. P., Sundaram, V., Tashian, R. E., Hewett-Emmett, D., Guibaud, P., Vainsel, M., Baluarte, H. J., Gruskin, A., Al-Mosawi, M., Sakati, N., and Ohlsson, A.: Carbonic anhydrase II deficiency in 12 families with the autosomal recessive syndrome of osteopetrosis with renal tubular acidosis and cerebral calcifications. N. Engl. J. Med., 313:139, 1985.
68. Solcia, E., Rondini, G., and Capella, C.: Clinical and pathological observations on a case of newborn osteopetrosis. Helv. Paediatr. Acta, 23:650, 1968.
69. Teitelbaum, S. L., Coccia, P. F., Brown, D. M., and Kahn, A. J.: Malignant osteopetrosis: A disease of abnormal osteoclast proliferation. Metab. Bone Dis. Rel. Res., 3:99, 1981.
70. Tips, R. L., and Lynch, H. T.: Malignant congenital osteopetrosis resulting from a consanguineous marriage. Acta Paediatr., 51:585, 1962.
71. Walker, D. G.: Osteopetrosis cured by temporary parabiosis. Science, 180:875, 1973.
72. Yu, J. S., Oates, R. K., Walsh, K. H., and Stuckey, S. J.: Osteopetrosis. Arch. Dis. Child., 46:257, 1971.
73. Zamboni, G., Cecchettini, M., Marradi, P., Foradori, M., and Zoppi, G.: Association of osteopetrosis and vitamin D–resistant rickets. Helv. Paediatr. Acta, 32:363, 1977.
74. Zawsch, C.: Marble bone disease. A study of osteogenesis. Arch. Pathol., 43:55, 1947.
75. Zetterstrom, R.: Osteopetrosis (marble bone disease). Clinical and pathological review. Mod. Probl. Paediatr., 3:488, 1957.

PYCNODYSOSTOSIS

Pycnodysostosis was first described as a distinct syndrome, in 1962, by Maroteaux and Lamy, who derived the term from the Greek *pycnos*, meaning "thick or dense," *dys*, "defective," and *osteon*, "bone".[17, 18]

This entity is characterized by short-limbed short stature; generalized osteosclerosis with proclivity to fracture of the long bones; hypoplasia or absence of the lateral portion of the clavicles; partial or total aplasia of the terminal phalanges of the digits; dysplasia of the cranium with widened suture lines, wormian bones, and persistent open fontanelles; and micrognathia with an obtuse mandibular angle, small maxilla, parrot nose, and delayed and disordered eruption of teeth (Fig. 3–58). In the spine there may be a failure of segmentation at the atlantoaxial level and lower lumbar vertebrae; spondylolisthesis may occur. The alternating bands of greater and lesser density associated with osteopetrosis do not appear on the spinal radiogram. It is said that the artist Henri de Toulouse-Lautrec was afflicted with pycnodysostosis.[19]

Pycnodysostosis is inherited as an autosomal recessive trait, and it is extremely rare, with a possible prevalence of less than one per million.

The medullary canal is consistently present, although it is small and imperfect. There is always evidence of hematopoiesis.[6] The formation and resorption of bone are simultaneously diminished.[12]

In the differential diagnosis, osteopetrosis and cleidocranial dysostosis should be considered (Table 3–7). Other rare conditions to rule out are progressive diaphyseal dysplasia and idiopathic nonfamilial acro-osteolysis.

Life expectancy of these patients is normal. The adult height varies from 130 to 150 cm. The orthopedic problem is the occurrence of pathologic fractures, which vary in frequency. Fracture healing is normal, and no special treatment is required.

References

1. Benz, G., and Schmid-Ruter, E.: Pycnodysostosis with heterozygous beta-thalassemia. Pediatr. Radiol., 5:164, 1977.
2. Bernard, R., Pinsard, N., Combes, J. C., Fieschi, J.

Table 3–7. Differential Diagnosis of Pycnodysostosis, Osteopetrosis, and Cleidocranial Dysplasia

Features	Pycnodysostosis	Osteopetrosis	Cleidocranial Dysplasia
Inheritance	Autosomal recessive	Congenital malignant type (autosomal recessive) Mild tarda type (autosomal dominant)	Autosomal dominant
Stature	Short stature—short-limbed type	Short in congenital type Normal in tarda type	Usually normal Sometimes minimal shortness
Prevalence	Under 1 per million	3 per million	Less than 1 per million
Facies	Micrognathia with obtuse mandible, small maxilla; delayed eruption of disorganized teeth	Normal	Low nasal bridge with bulging frontal and parietal regions teeth Disordered eruption of failure of fusion of mandibular symphisis
Paranasal sinus	Unaerated or closed	Unaerated	Normal
Skull	Dysplasia with widened sutures; wormian bones Persistent open fontanelles No cranial foramina impingement No cranial nerve palsy	Thickened vault, base Cranial foramina impingement with bone overgrowth Cranial nerve palsy	Wormian bones Open fontanelles in childhood No cranial nerve palsy
Clavicle	Hypoplastic, sometimes absent in lateral portion	Present and normal	Partially or completely absent
Hands, feet	Hypoplasia or absence of terminal phalanges of digits	Normal	Normal
Pelvis-hips	Flattened femoral heads, short and deformed femoral necks	Endobones and transverse bands of increased and decreased radiopacity Coxa vara may be present	Wide symphysis pubis Triradiate cartilages and sacroiliac joints wide
Bone texture	Osteosclerosis without obliteration of intermedullary canals	Osteosclerosis with obliteration of intramedullary canals	Normal
Hematologic picture	Normal	Aplastic anemia	Normal
Liver, spleen	Normal	Hepatosplenomegaly	Normal

FIGURE 3–58. *Pycnodysostosis.*

A. Typical appearance in a 15-year-old girl. **B.** A double row of teeth results from persistence of the deciduous teeth. (From Elmore, S. M.: Pycnodysostosis: A review. J. Bone Joint Surg., *49-A*:153, 1967. Reprinted by permission.)

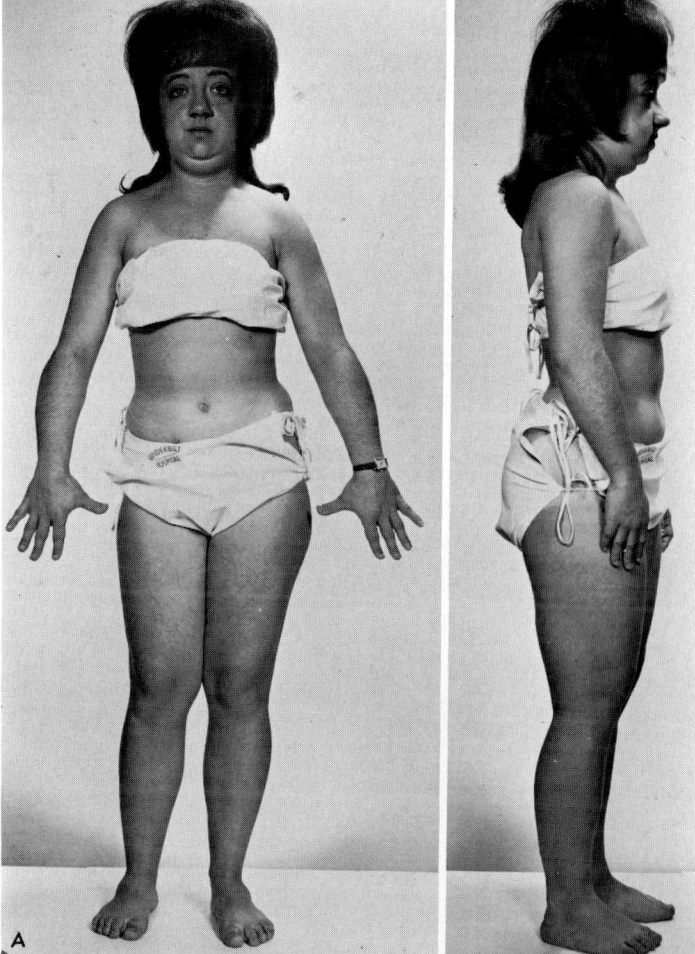
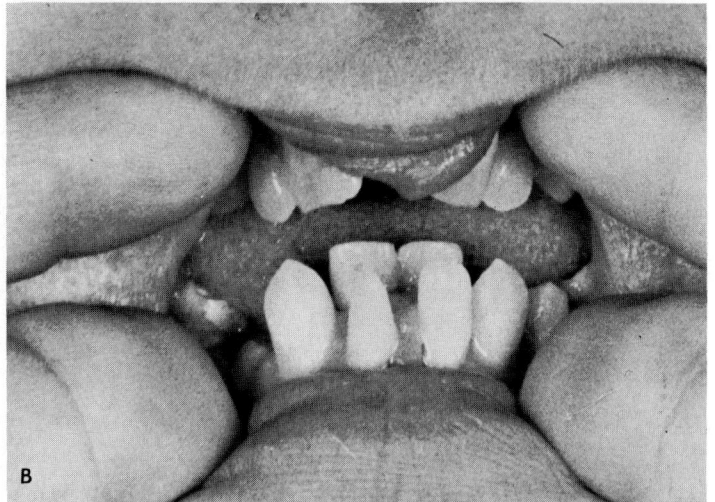

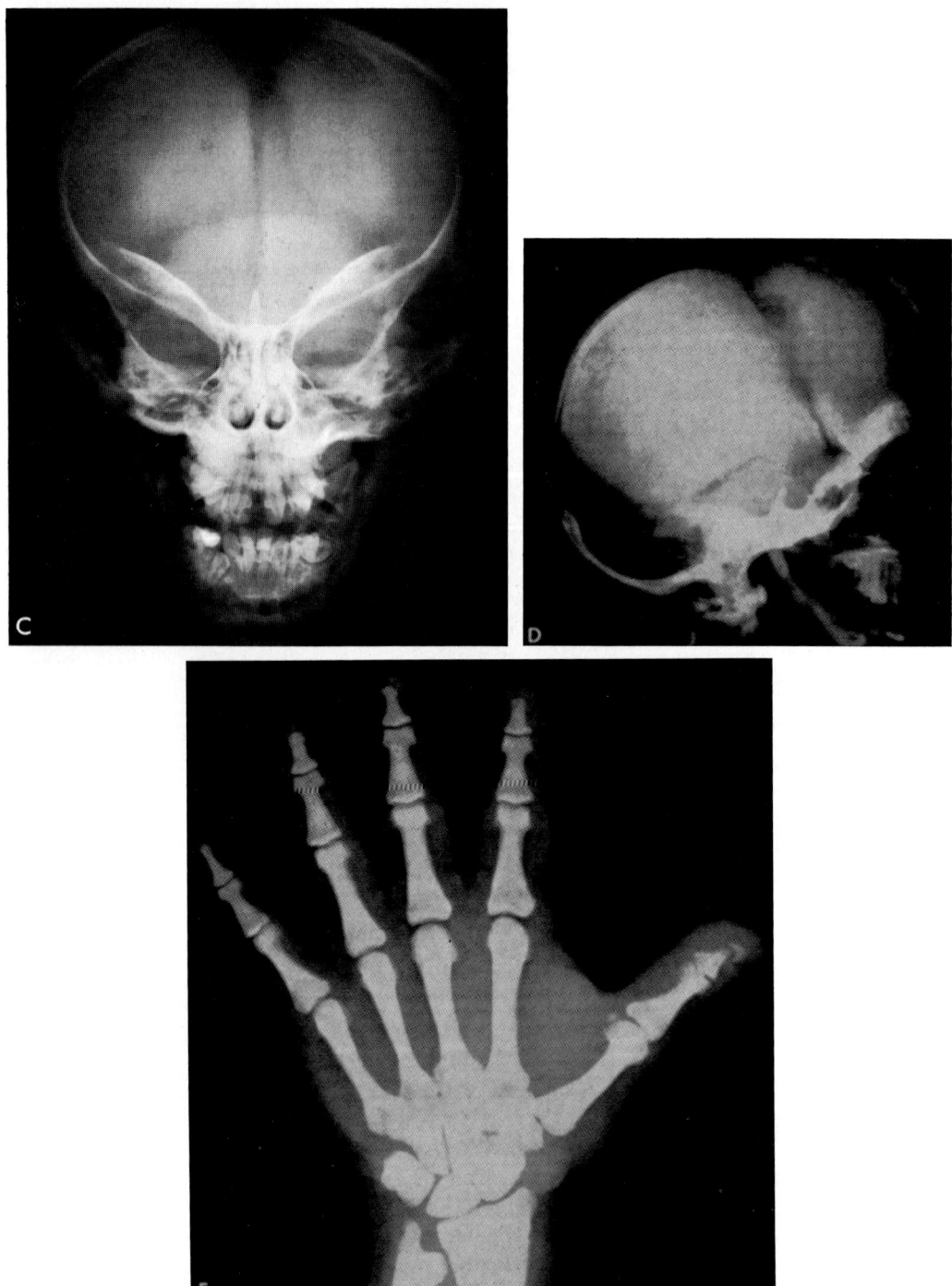

FIGURE 3–58 Continued. Pycnodysostosis.

C and D. Radiograms of the skull. Note the separation of the sagittal, coronal, and lambdoidal sutures. The anterior fontanelle is open, and the paranasal sinuses are hypoplastic and nonpneumatized. There is a wormian pattern in the parietal bone, and the facial bones are small with the mandible flattened to 180 degrees. The articulation between the skull and the atlas is abnormal. E. Anteroposterior radiogram of the hand showing the tapering of the distal phalanges and the absence of the ungual tufts. (From Elmore, S. M.: Pycnodysostosis: A review. J. Bone Joint Surg., 49-A:153, 1967. Reprinted by permission.)

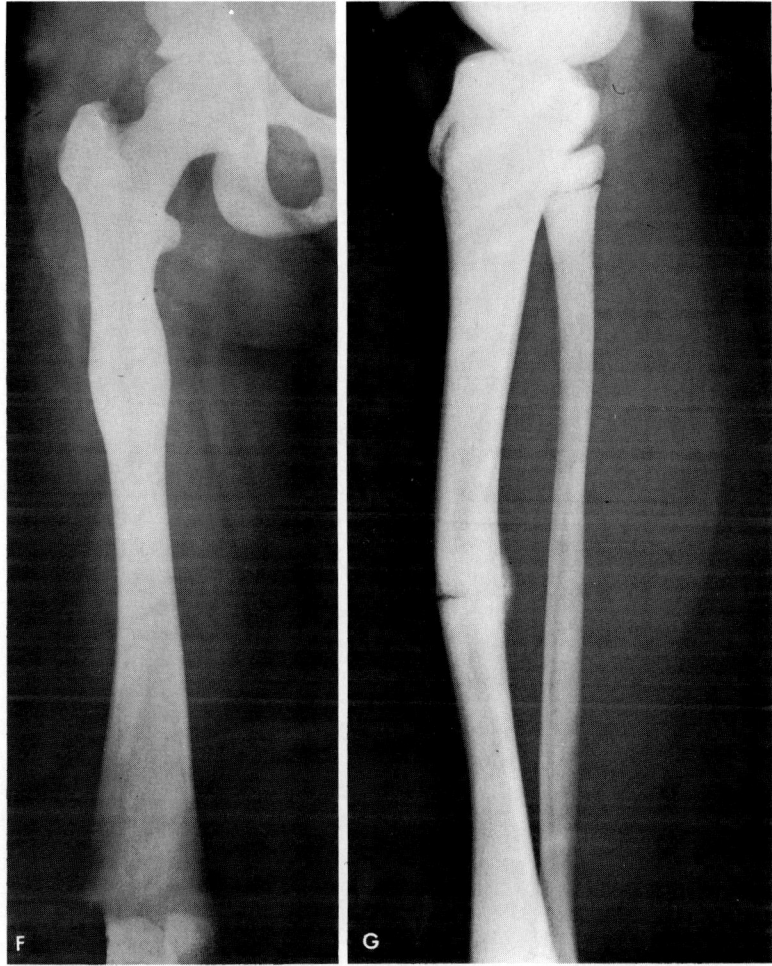

FIGURE 3–58 Continued. Pycnodysostosis.

F. Radiogram of right femur. There is a widened Erlenmeyer flask deformity of the distal third. Residuals of a healed fracture in the proximal third of the femoral shaft are evident. **G.** Lateral radiogram of the left tibia. Note the transverse fracture, which has persisted for three years, resembling an umbauzonen line. There is narrowing of the marrow spaces of the tibia and fibula. (From Elmore, S. M.: Pycnodysostosis: A review. J. Bone Joint Surg., 49-A:153, 1967. Reprinted by permission.)

B., and Youssef, M. E.: Pycnodysostose et craniostenose. Ann. Pediatr., 27:383, 1980.
3. Bressot, C., Meunier, P. J., Bard, J., and Vignon, G.: La pycnodysostose. Analyse histomorphometrique et dynamique de l'os dans une nouvelle observation. Rev. Rhumat., 47:425, 1980.
4. Clark, A. R. L.: Two cases of pycnodysostosis (the malady of Toulouse-Lautrec). Postgrad. Med. J., 45:684, 1969.
5. Dusenberry, J. F., Jr., and Kane, J. J.: Pycnodysostosis. Report of three new cases. A.J.R., 99:717, 1967.
6. Elmore, S. M.: Pycnodysostosis: A review. J. Bone Joint Surg., 49-A:153, 1967.
7. Elmore, S. M., Nance, W. E., McGee, B. J., Engel-de Montmollin, M., and Engel, E.: Pycnodysostosis with a familial chromosome anomaly. Am. J. Med., 40:273, 1966.
8. Emami-Ahari, Z., Zarabi, M., and Javid, B.: Pycnodysostosis. J. Bone Joint Surg., 51-B:307, 1969.
9. Fairbank, T. J., and Wynne-Davies, R.: Fairbank's Atlas of General Affections of the Skeleton. Edinburgh; Churchill-Livingstone, 1976, pp. 96–99.
10. Giaccai, L., Salaam, M., and Zellweger, H.: Cleidocranial dysostosis with osteopetrosis. Acta Radiol., 41:417, 1954.
11. Kozlowski, K., and Yu, J. S.: Pycnodysostosis. A variant form with visceral manifestations. Arch. Dis. Child., 47:804, 1972.
12. Lacey, S. H., Eyring, E. J., and Shaffer, T. E.: Pycnodysostosis: A case report of a child with associated trisomy X. J. Pediatr., 77:1033, 1970.
13. Lentle, B. C.: Pycnodysostosis: A case report. J. Can. Assoc. Radiol., 22:210, 1971.
14. Lievre, J. A., Chaput, A., and Camus, J. P.: Pycnodysostose de Maroteaux et Lamy. (Une observation.) Rev. Rhum., 31:282, 1964.
15. Lykkegaard, N. E.: Pycnodysostosis. Acta Paediatr. Scand., 63:437, 1974.
16. Maroteaux, P., Bone Diseases in Children. Philadelphia, J.B. Lippincott, 1979.

17. Maroteaux, P., and Lamy, M.: Deux observations d'une affection osseuse condensante la pycnodysostose. Arch. Fr. Pediatr., *19*:267, 1962.
18. Maroteaux, P., and Lamy, M.: La pycnodysostose. Presse Méd., *20*:99, 1962.
19. Maroteaux, P., and Lamy, M.: The malady of Toulouse-Lautrec. J.A.M.A., *191*:715, 1965.
20. Meredith, S. C., Simon, M. A., Laros, G. S., and Jackson, M. A.: Pycnodysostosis. J. Bone Joint Surg., *60-A*:1122, 1978.
21. Poznanski, A.: Pycnodysostosis. Birth Defects, *5*:312, 1969.
22. Roth, V. G.: Pycnodysostosis presenting with bilateral subtrochanteric fractures. A case report. Clin. Orthop., *117*:247, 1976.
23. Sedano, H. D., Gorlin, R. J., and Anderson, V. E.: Pycnodysostosis. Clinical and genetic considerations. Am. J. Dis. Child., *116*:70, 1968.
24. Shiraishi, S.: Pycnodysostosis. Acta Orthop. Scand., *42*:227, 1971.
25. Shuler, S. E.: Pycnodysostosis. Arch. Dis. Child., *38*:620, 1963.
26. Soto, R. J., Mautalen, C. A., Hojman, D., Codevilla, A., Pique, J., and Pangaro, J. A.: Pycnodysostosis: Metabolic and histologic studies. Birth Defects, *5*:109, 1969.
27. Sugiura, S., Yamada, Y., and Koh, J.: Pycnodysostosis in Japan: Report of six cases and a review of Japanese literature. Birth Defects, *10*:78, 1974.
28. Taylor, M. M., Moore, T. M., and Harvey, J. P., Jr.: Pycnodysostosis. A case report. J. Bone Joint Surg., *60-A*:1128, 1978.
29. Zachariades, N., and Koundouris, I.: Maxillofacial symptoms in two patients with pycnodysostosis. J. Oral Maxillofac. Surg., *42*:819, 1984.
30. Yousefzadeh, D. K., Agha, A. S., and Reinertson, J.: Radiographic studies of upper airway obstruction with cor pulmonale in a patient with pycnodysostosis. Pediatr. Radiol., *8*:45, 1979.

PROGRESSIVE DIAPHYSEAL DYSPLASIA (CAMURATI-ENGELMANN DISEASE)

This is a rare developmental syndrome of the skeleton characterized by widened fusiform diaphyses with excessive periosteal and endosteal new bone formation and sclerosis, but with no involvement of the epiphysis or physis. Over the involved part of the limb the muscles are atrophic and weak, with wasting of the subcutaneous fat. It was first described by Camurati in 1922, and by Engelmann in 1929.[9, 14] Perhaps the first patient reported was by Cockayne, who presented a case for diagnosis at the Royal Society for Medicine in 1920.[11] The eponym Engelmann's disease was given by Sear.[49] Extensive reviews of the literature with case presentations have been given by Neuhauser and associates, by Griffiths, and by Lennon and associates.[22, 34, 42]

Etiology and Heredity

Inheritance is often by autosomal dominant transmission. Sparkes and Graham reported eight individuals in three generations of one family, and Hundley and Wilson reported seven cases in three generations in a family.[25, 52] There is considerable variation in expression of this disorder. Sporadic cases do occur. There is no racial predilection. Prevalence is under one per million. It is more common in the male in the ratio of three to two.

Pathology

The changes are nonspecific. On gross inspection the bony cortex appears markedly thickened with some hypertrophy of the periosteum. Both endosteal and periosteal new bone are incorporated in it. Microscopic examination shows an increase in the fibrous component of the periosteum. There is marked osteoblastic as well as osteoclastic activity with evidence of progressive active bone resorption as well as deposition. The bone trabeculae are thickened, but otherwise normal (Fig. 3–59 D). The medullary cavity is eventually narrowed.

At a later stage in the course of the disease, as a result of combined resorption and deposition, the bone may change from compact to cancellous type. The marrow is normal in the beginning, but later consists of a loose mesenchymal type of fibrous tissue with occasional foci of hematopoiesis.[12, 40]

Clinical Features

Involvement of the long bones is usually bilateral and symmetrical. The bone most commonly affected is the tibia; next in order of frequency are the femur, fibula, humerus, radius, and ulna. With progression of the disease the base of the skull, other calvarial bones, the pelvis, and the vertebrae may be affected. The short tubular bones are rarely involved.

Clinically, pain in the limbs, usually in one or both legs, is the presenting complaint. Weakness of the musculature is common, manifested by a delay in walking, an inability to run, and easy fatigability. There is often a waddling gait. Exaggerated lumbar lordosis with a protuberant abdomen is commonly present. These children are tall and thin with reduced muscle mass and legs that are spindle-shaped (Fig. 3–59 A and B).

Other clinical findings include signs of delayed puberty, hypogonadism, diminution of secondary sex characteristics, dry hard skin, dental caries, and ocular proptosis. When skull bones are involved, the head becomes enlarged, and there may be frontal bossing. Neurologic deficit may result from impingement on cranial

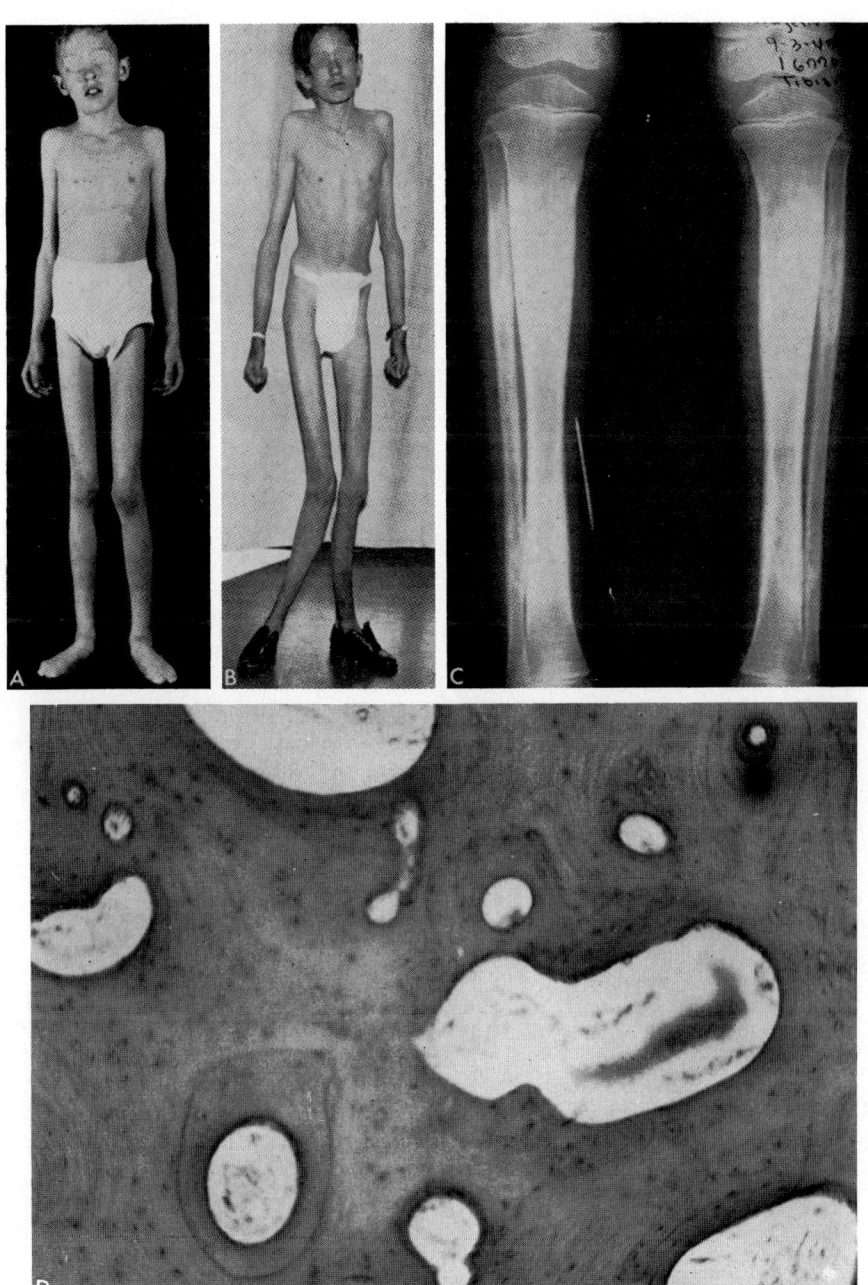

FIGURE 3–59. Engelmann's disease in a young boy.

A and B. Clinical appearance at 10 and at 18 years of age shows asthenic habitus, lack of physical development, marked genu valgum, and external tibial torsion. C. Anteroposterior radiograms of both tibiae at seven years of age show the diaphyseal sclerosis with both endosteal and periosteal thickening and the relatively normal epiphyses and metaphyses. D. Histologic section of specimen obtained at time of osteotomy reveals thickened trabeculae with normal haversian systems (×100). (From Clawson, D. K., and Loop, J. W.: Progressive diaphyseal dysplasia (Engelmann's disease). J. Bone Joint Surg., *46-A*:143, 1964. Reprinted by permission.)

nerves as they emerge from the neural foramina.

Radiographic Features

These depend on the stage of the disease, being more marked in patients who have a long history. Initial findings are increased density and widening of the cortex of the diaphyses of the long bones, commonly the tibia and femur, which are fusiform in shape (Fig. 3–59 C). The process begins in the middle third of the shaft and then extends proximally and distally toward the metaphyses. The physes and the epiphyses themselves are not affected. At first, the cortical surface is smooth, but later it becomes irregular. With progression of the disease, the diameter of the diaphysis enlarges, and the medullary cavity becomes increasingly narrowed and almost obliterated. Consequently, hematopoiesis may be disturbed, and secondary anemia may develop along with hepatosplenomegaly as a result of myeloid metaplasia.

Scintigraphic Findings with Technetium-99m Diphosphonate

These were reported in four patients and correlated with radiographic skeletal surveys by Kumar and associates.[31] Some affected bones were scintigraphically normal but radiographically abnormal, and vice versa. This discordance between radiographic and scintigraphic findings is explained by the activity in the disease process. A positive radiograph and a normal scintigram indicate a quiescent or "mature" lesion, whereas a normal radiograph with a positive scintigram is indicative of an early active lesion whose activity is insufficient to affect structural change in bone but that can be visualized by imaging with technetium-99m. The value of scintigraphy is in detection and evaluation of disease activity in progressive diaphyseal dysplasia.

Laboratory Findings

Biochemical studies by Smith and associates have shown that the blood alkaline phosphatase and urinary hydroxyproline excretion levels may be elevated. Occasionally there are hypocalcemia, hyperphosphatemia, and a positive calcium balance.[51] Electromyography of the atrophic muscles shows a normal pattern.

Differential Diagnosis

In the young patient progressive diaphyseal dysplasia should be distinguished from *infantile cortical hyperostosis;* the latter occurs at an earlier age (usually at eight weeks, but may be present at birth or in the fetus); the distribution of involvement differs (infantile cortical hyperostosis preferentially involves mandible, ribs, and clavicle, whereas Engelmann's dysplasia commonly affects the tibiae and femora); affection is asymmetrical (infantile cortical hyperostosis is asymmetrical, whereas Engelmann's dysplasia is symmetrical); and the course of the disease differs (infantile cortical hyperostosis is self-limited and regresses, but Engelmann's disease is progressive).

Other conditions to consider in the differential diagnosis are polyostotic fibrous dysplasia, multiple enchondromatosis, juvenile Paget's disease, heavy metal poisoning, and metaphyseal and craniometaphyseal dysplasia. When only one bone is affected, one should also consider osteomyelitis, osteoid osteoma, benign osteoblastoma, and Ewing's sarcoma. In the adult, Paget's disease and osteoblastic carcinomatosis must be excluded.

Treatment

There is no specific treatment. Management is symptomatic. Anti-inflammatory medications such as salicylates or naproxen (Naprosyn) can be given for pain. Physical therapy exercises are performed to increase the motor strength of wasting muscles in the affected limbs and the range of motion of the joints.

When there is increasing bone pain, muscle weakness and irritability, and failure to respond to the foregoing measures, steroids are administered. Royer and associates first reported the beneficial effects of steroids in Engelmann's disease in a five-and-one-half-year-old boy who was followed for five years. The patient was symptom free as long as he was kept on small doses of corticosteroids. Exacerbations of bone pain and fatigue recurred when the dosage of prednisone was inadequate or when its administration was stopped. The radiographic picture returned to normal.[46] Allen and associates reported beneficial effect of corticosteroids in three children with progressive diaphyseal dysplasia. There was complete remission of clinical symptoms. Histologic studies showed increased bone resorption and secondary remodeling with increased osteoclastic activity and decreased lamellar bone deposition. The corticosteroids produced a more normal histologic picture in bone. The mechanism of action of steroids in progressive diaphyseal dysplasia is unclear.[1]

Successful use of corticosteroids in Engelmann's disease with clinical relief of symptoms and radiologic improvement was reported by Lindstrom in a 16-year-old patient, and by Minford and associates in a 13-year-old girl.[35, 39] The initial dosage of prednisone, depending upon the age of the patient, is 15 to 60 mg., followed by a maintenance dose of 5 to 10 mg. daily, or 15 mg. on alternating days. The risk and complications of steroid therapy in children should be carefully weighed. Steroids should be given only in severe and recalcitrant cases.

Ribbing's disease also called hereditary multiple diaphyseal sclerosis, is a closely related disorder with a radiographic appearance similar to that of Engelmann's disease and may, it has been suggested, be its adult form.[45, 47] It is usually seen in the young adult and is distinguished by normal muscular development, high familial incidence, localization in the lower limbs, asymmetrical involvement, and nonprogressive clinical course.

References

1. Allen, D. I., Sanders, A. M., Northway, W. H., Williams, G. F., and Schafer, J. A.: Corticosteroids in the treatment of Engelmann's disease: Progressive diaphyseal dysplasia. Pediatrics, 46:523, 1970.
2. Altuna, E. A., Kunath, A., and Daneri, L. A. L.: Enfermedad de Camurati-Engelmann. A proposito de un caso observado. Rev. Argent. Radiol., 33:162, 1970.
3. Anderson, F. G.: Engelmann's disease. Br. J. Radiol., N. S., 26:603, 1953.
4. Battaglia, L., and Venturi, R.: La poliosteopatia addensante simmetrica ereditaria (malattia di Camurati-Engelmann). Studio clinico ed anatomo-patologico. Chir. Organi Mov., 49:179, 1960.
5. Benabderrahmane, M., Siegenthaler, P., Uhlmann, C., and Wettstein, P.: Le syndrome de Camurati-Engelmann. A propos d'un cas et revue de la littérature. Schweiz. Med. Wochenschr., 99:1204, 1969.
6. Bingold, A. G.: "Engelmann's disease," osteopathia hyperostotica (sclerotisans) multiplex infantilis: Progressive diaphysial dysplasia. Br. J. Surg., 37:266, 1950.
7. Braham, R. L.: Multiple congenital abnormalities with diaphyseal dysplasia (Camurati-Engelmann's syndrome). Oral Surg., 27:20, 1969.
8. Brodrick, J. D.: Luxation of the globe in Engelmann's disease. Am. J. Ophthalmol., 83:870, 1977.
9. Camurati, M.: Di un raro caso di osteite simmetrica ereditaria degli arti inferiori. Chir. Organi Mov., 6:662, 1922.
10. Clawson, D. K., and Loop, J. W.: Progressive diaphyseal dysplasia (Engelmann's disease). J. Bone Joint Surg., 46-A:143, 1964.
11. Cockayne, E. A.: Case for diagnosis. Proc. R. Soc. Med., 13:132, 1920.
12. Cohen, J., and States, J. D.: Progressive diaphyseal dysplasia: Report of a case with autopsy findings. Lab. Invest., 5:492, 1956.
13. Crisp, A. J., Brenton, D. P., and Shaw, D. G.: Case report 202. Skeletal Radiol., 8:239, 1982.
14. Engelmann, G.: Ein Fall von Osteopathia hyperostotica sclerotisans multiplex infantilis. Fortschr. Geb. Röntgenstr., 39:1101, 1929.
15. Fallon, M. D., White, M. D., and Murphy, W. A.: Progressive diaphysial dysplasia (Engelmann's disease). Report of a sporadic case of the mild form. J. Bone Joint Surg., 62-A:465, 1980.
16. Fairbank, H. A. T.: An Atlas of General Affections of the Skeleton. Edinburgh, Livingstone, 1951.
17. Farreras, V. P., Vilaseca, J. M., and de Caralt, M.: Osteosclerosis diafisaria multiple hereditaria tipo Camurati-Engelmann con sindrome de leontiasis osea. Rev. Esp. Reum., 5:354, 1954.
18. Fosmoe, R. J., Holm, R. S., and Hildreth, R. C.: Van Buchem's disease (hyperostosis corticalis generalisata familiaris). A case report. Radiology, 90:771, 1968.
19. Gillespie, J. B., and Mussey, R. D.: Progressive diaphyseal dysplasia (Engelmann's disease). J. Pediatr., 38:55, 1951.
20. Girdany, B. R.: Engelmann's disease (progressive diaphyseal dysplasia): A nonprogressive familial form of muscular dystrophy with characteristic bone changes. Clin. Orthop., 14:102, 1959.
21. Girdany, B. R., Sane, S., and Graham, C. B.: Engelmann's disease. In Progress in Paediatric Radiology. Vol. 4, Intrinsic Diseases of Bones. Basel, S. Karger, 1973, pp. 414–437.
22. Griffiths, D.: Engelmann's disease. J. Bone Joint Surg., 38-B:312, 1956.
23. Gulledge, H. W., and White, J. W.: Engelmann's disease (progressive diaphyseal hyperostosis). Report of a case. J. Bone Joint Surg., 33-A:793, 1951.
24. Gvozdanovic, V.: A new case of Engelmann's disease. Contribution to the knowledge of congenital osteodystrophy. Fortschr. Geb. Röntgenstr., 73:86, 1950.
25. Hundley, J. D., and Wilson, F. C.: Progressive diaphyseal dysplasia: Review of the literature and report of seven cases in one family. J. Bone Joint Surg., 55-A:461, 1973.
26. Jackson, W. P. U., Hanelin, J., and Albright, F.: Metaphyseal dysplasia, epiphyseal dysplasia, diaphyseal dysplasia, and related conditions: III. Progressive diaphyseal dysplasia. Arch. Intern. Med., 94:902, 1954.
27. Jammes, A., Seruz, R., Prouxet, J., and Duclos, G.: Maladie d'Engelmann: Ostéopathie hyperostosante et sclerosante infantile multiple: (A propos d'une nouvelle observation). Rev. Rhum., 20:406, 1953.
28. Johnston, C. E.: Progressive diaphyseal dysplasia. Pediatr. Orthop., 7:133, 1984.
29. Joseph, R., Lefebvre, J., Guy, E., and Job, J. C.: Dysplasie cranio-diaphysaire progressive. Ses relations avec la dysplasie diaphysaire progressive de Camurati-Engelmann. Ann. Radiol. (Sem. Hôp. Paris), 1:1, 1958.
30. Krohel, G. B., and Wirth, C. R.: Engelmann's disease. Am. J. Ophthalmol., 84:520, 1977.
31. Kumar, B., Murphy, W. A., and Whyte, M. P.: Progressive diaphyseal dysplasia (Engelmann's disease): Scintigraphic-radiographic-clinical correlations. Radiology, 140:87, 1981.
32. Lavine, L. S., and Koven, M. T.: Engelmann's disease (progressive diaphyseal dysplasia). J. Pediatr., 40:235, 1952.
33. LeBien, W. E., and Heilman, C.: Progressive diaphyseal dysplasia with report of a case. Lancet, 71:189, 1951.
34. Lennon, E. A., Schechter, M. M., and Hornabrook, R. W.: Engelmann's disease. Report of a case with a review of the literature. J. Bone Joint Surg., 43-B:273, 1961.

35. Lindstrom, J. A.: Diaphyseal dysplasia (Engelmann) treated with corticosteroids. Birth Defects, 10:504, 1974.
36. Lundy, M. M., Billingsley, J. L., Redwine, M. D., et al.: Scintigraphic findings in progressive diaphyseal dysplasia. J. Nucl. Med., 23:324, 1982.
37. Michaelis, L. S.: Engelmann's disease. Proc. R. Soc. Med., 42:271, 1949.
38. Mikity, V. G., and Jacobson, G.: Progressive diaphyseal dysplasia (Engelmann's disease). J. Bone Joint Surg., 40-A:206, 1958.
39. Minford, A. M. B., Hardy, G. J., Forsythe, W. I., Fitton, J. M., and Rowe, V. L.: Engelmann's disease and the effect of corticosteroids. A case report. J. Bone Joint Surg., 63-B:597, 1981.
40. Mottram, M. E., and Hill, H. A.: Diaphyseal dysplasia. Report of a case. A.J.R., 95:162, 1965.
41. Naveh, Y., Kaftori, J. K., Alon, U., Ben-David, J., and Berant, M.: Progressive diaphyseal dysplasia: Genetics and clinical and radiologic manifestations. Pediatrics, 74:399, 1984.
42. Neuhauser, E. B. D., Schwachman, H., Wittenborg, M., and Cohen, J.: Progressive diaphyseal dysplasia. Radiology, 51:11, 1948.
43. Ortolani, M., and Castagnari, G.: L'osteopatia di Camurati-Engelmann. Arch. Putti Chir. Organi Mov., 3:146, 1953. (Cited by Griffiths.)
44. Paul, L. W.: Hereditary multiple diaphyseal sclerosis (Ribbing). Radiology, 60:412, 1953.
45. Ribbing, S.: Hereditary multiple, diaphyseal sclerosis. Acta Radiol., 31:522, 1949.
46. Royer, P., Vermeil, G., Apostolides, P., and Engelmann, F.: Maladie d'Engelmann: Résultat du traitment par la prednisone. Arch. Fr. Pediatr., 24:693, 1967.
47. Rubin, P.: Dynamic Classification of Bone Dysplasia. Chicago, Year Book, 1964, p. 325.
48. Ruelle, M., and Dubois, J. L.: A propos de deux cas familiaux de sclerose diaphysaire multiple (syndrome de Camurati-Engelmann). Rev. Rhum., 7:345, 1964.
49. Sear, H. R.: Engelmann's disease. Osteopathia hyperostotica sclerotisans multiplex infantilis. Br. J. Radiol., 21:236, 1948.
50. Singleton, E. B., Thomas, J. R., Worthington, W. W., and Hild, J. R.: Progressive diaphyseal dysplasia (Engelmann's disease). Radiology, 67:233, 1956.
51. Smith, R., Walton, R. J., Corner, B. D., and Gordon, I. R. S.: Clinical and biochemical studies in Engelmann's disease (progressive diaphyseal dysplasia). Q. J. Med., 46:273, 1977.
52. Sparkes, R. S., and Graham, C. B.: Camurati-Engelmann disease. Genetics and clinical manifestations with a review of the literature. J. Med. Genet., 9:73, 1972.
53. Stegman, K. F., and Peterson, J. C.: Progressive hereditary diaphyseal dysplasia. Pediatrics, 20:966, 1957.
54. Stronge, R. F., and McDowell, H. B.: A case of Engelmann's disease. Progressive diaphysial dysplasia. J. Bone Joint Surg., 32-B:38, 1950.
55. Thelen, P. O.: Familiäres Auftreten einer Camurati-Engelmannschen Erkrankung. Fortschr. Geb. Röntgenstr., 94:713, 1961.
56. Thurmon, T. F., and Jackson, J.: Tumoral calcinosis and Engelmann disease. Birth Defects Orig. Art. Series, 12:321, 1976.
57. Trunk, G., Newman, A., and Davis, T. E.: Progressive and hereditary diaphyseal dysplasia. Arch. Intern. Med., 123:417, 1969.
58. Van Dalsem, V. F., Genant, H. K., and Newton, T. H.: Progressive diaphyseal dysplasia: Report of a case with thirty-four years of progressive disease. J. Bone Joint Surg., 61-A:596, 1979.
59. Wolf, B. H., and Ford, H. W.: An unusual radiographic manifestation of Engelmann's disease in a young Negro child. Radiology, 99:401, 1971.
60. Yen, J. K., Bourke, R. S., Popp, A. J., and Wirth, C. R.: Camurati-Engelmann disease (progressive hereditary craniodiaphyseal dysplasia): Case report. J. Neurosurg., 48:138, 1978.

MELORHEOSTOSIS

Melorheostosis is a rare condition in which involvement is usually unilateral and always asymmetrical; it is characterized by hyperostotic streaks extending longitudinally along the axes of long bones, associated with soft-tissue contracture, fibrosis, pain, and abnormalities of the skin, which tends to be tense, shiny, and erythematous. It was initially described in 1922 by Leri and Joanny, who derived the word melorheostosis from two Greek words, *melos*, meaning "member," and *rhein*, meaning "flow," because of the resemblance of its characteristic radiographic appearance to melting wax on the side of a candle.[20] The incidence in the population is very low, with a prevalence of one per million. Campbell and associates, in 1968, reviewed the literature and reported the clinical, radiographic, and pathologic findings in 14 cases.[5] Younge and colleagues reported the clinical features, natural history, and experience in the management of 14 children.[36]

Etiology

The disorder is congenital, affecting not only one bone but also many other tissues of mesodermal origin. The exact cause is unknown. The unique pattern and distribution of the lesions suggests an abnormality in embryogenesis, either prior to or during the actual formation of the limb buds between the fourth and seventh postovulatory weeks.[5, 37] It most probably is caused by a metameric disturbance in the proliferating mesodermal cells.

Distribution of the hyperostosis can be correlated to dermatomes, which are zones supplied by single sensory roots. An infectious etiology (similar to herpes zoster) was suggested by Murray and McCredie. The resultant scarring lesions spread along the distribution of nerve roots, and involvement of the dermatomes and myotomes causes the associated subcutaneous fibrosis and muscular contractures.[27] A hereditary pattern has not been established; the condition is nongenetic.

Pathology

The long bones are most commonly involved, but any bone in the body may be affected. The skull, spine, and ribs, however, are very rarely involved. The disease may be monostotic, polyostotic, or monomelic; on occasion, involvement is extensive, including several limbs and the trunk.

Pathologic examination of bone and soft tissues reveals no pathognomonic features: histologic findings consist of osteosclerosis and fibrosis.[10, 19]

Bone formation exceeds normal destruction. Pathologic changes consist of thickening of the cortex and bone trabeculae, with narrowing of the medullary cavity. The haversian canals are surrounded by condensed, thickened, and somewhat irregular laminae. There are varying degrees of membranous new bone formation and areas of enchondral ossification, the latter being more periarticular in location. The bone marrow may be fibrous or fatty. Periosseous fibrosis of soft tissues is common. The muscles are edematous and poor in texture. Fibrosis of the skin and subcutaneous tissues is frequently found. Other soft-tissue changes are calcifications, especially periarticular, and vascular tumors.[5, 19]

Clinical Features

Pain in the affected bones is the main symptom and is present in almost every patient. It is neither marked nor constant and may be aggravated by activity. Onset of pain usually follows several years after joint contracture is first noted. Limitation of joint motion is common. Rigid joint deformity is present in all patients and often is the presenting complaint. It is caused by contracture and soft-tissue fibrosis, by bony deformity of the articular surfaces, or by the presence of periarticular masses of ectopic bone. Deformities such as flexion contracture of the hips and knees, shown in Figure 3–60 A, pelvic obliquity due to contracture of the iliotibial band, genu valgum, pes equinus, pes varus or pes valgus, and flexion contractures of fingers or toes are not uncommon. The affected limb appears enlarged in circumference. Inequality of limb length is present in almost all patients; the affected limb is often shorter, but sometimes longer, than its opposite normal limb. If there is pressure on the nerves there may be sensory disturbance. Edema and induration of subcutaneous soft tissues are often present. The skin is tense, thickened, shiny, or erythematous; it has a woody firm texture with tethering by the underlying fascia. Contracture of palmar or plantar fascia results in flexion deformity of the digits (Fig. 3–60 B).

Radiographic Features

The classic radiographic finding in melorheostosis is radiopacity in longitudinal streaks along the axes of long bones with a distinct border between pathologic and normal bone. The sclerotic linear streaks appear like wax flowing down the side of a candle. In the adult, the pattern of sclerosis is subperiosteal or extracortical, the radiopaque streaks flowing on the outside of the diaphysis of the long bone (Fig. 3–61). In children, in contrast to the adult, the sclerosis in long bones is endosteal, and in flat bones, such as the pelvis, melorheostotic lesions manifest themselves as condensed foci in the medullary portion of the bone (Figs. 3–62 and 3–63). With skeletal maturation the sclerosis changes and progresses from endosteal to periosteal distributions.[36]

Differential Diagnosis

In the differential diagnosis, one should consider pyogenic osteomyelitis, osteopetrosis, osteopoikilosis, and osteopathia striata. In infancy, before bony changes have become manifest, the soft-tissue and joint contractures may be mistaken for arthrogryposis multiplex congenita; in arthrogryposis, however, the contractures are not painful, and the fixed joint deformities are present at birth. The thickened and erythematous skin with indurations of the subcutaneous tissue may be mistaken for scleroderma. Pain in the affected limb may mimic acute rheumatic fever, poliomyelitis, or myositis.

Treatment

Management of the deformed limb in melorheostosis is difficult and fraught with problems and complications. The biologic performance of the contractures of periarticular soft tissue is similar to that of arthrogryposis multiplex congenita. The same basic principles of treatment should be applied for both entities. In melorheostosis, however, failure is more common because the lesions progress in childhood, particularly during periods of rapid growth. The gloomy prognosis and hazards of surgery should be made clear to the family in the beginning. The dense fibrotic soft tissues do not stretch with growth; recurrence of deformity is common.

Treatment is directed toward relief of pain and prevention and correction of contractural deformity. Fixed contractures are corrected by radical release with wide capsulotomy and te-

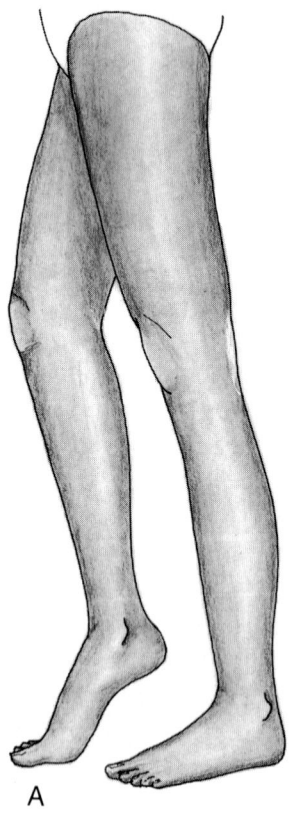
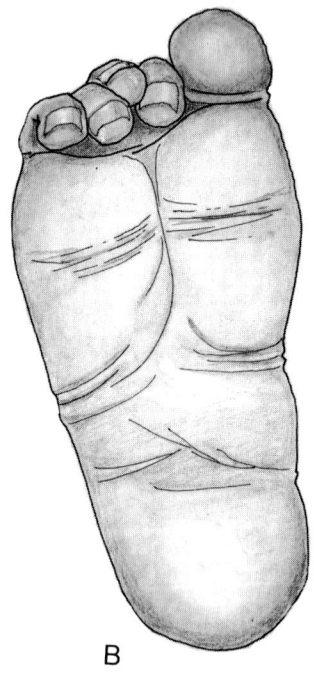

FIGURE 3–60. Clinical findings in melorheostosis.

A. Flexion deformity of the right knee, equinocavovarus deformity of the right foot, and lower limb length inequality of the affected leg. **B.** Plantar view of the foot showing woody, firm thickening of the plantar skin, contracture of the plantar fascia, and flexion contracture of the toes.

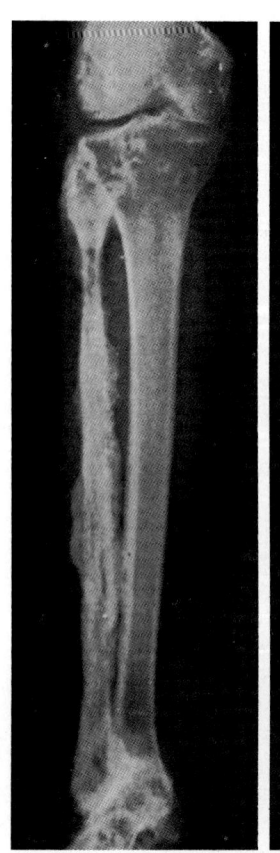
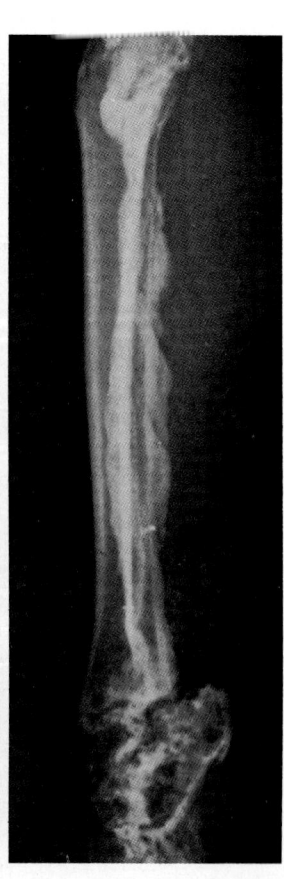

FIGURE 3–61. Melorheostosis of the fibula in a 39-year-old woman.

(From Campbell, C. J., Papademetriou, F., and Bonfiglion, M.: Melorheostosis. J. Bone Joint Surg., 50-A:1294, 1968. Reprinted by permission.)

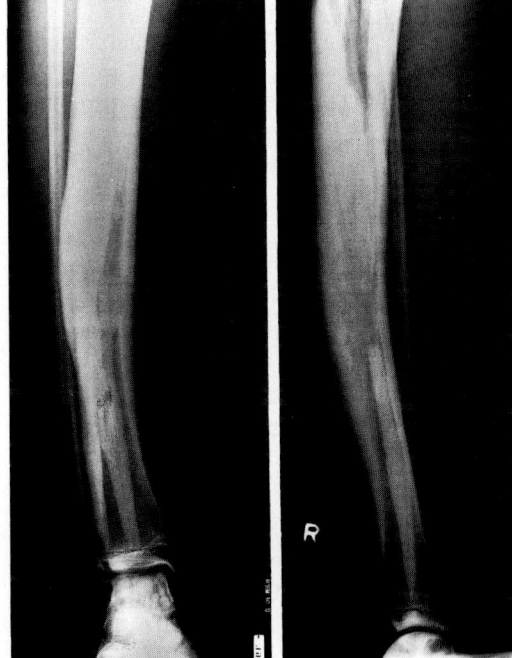

FIGURE 3-62. *Endosteal sclerosis of long bones in a child with melorheostosis.*

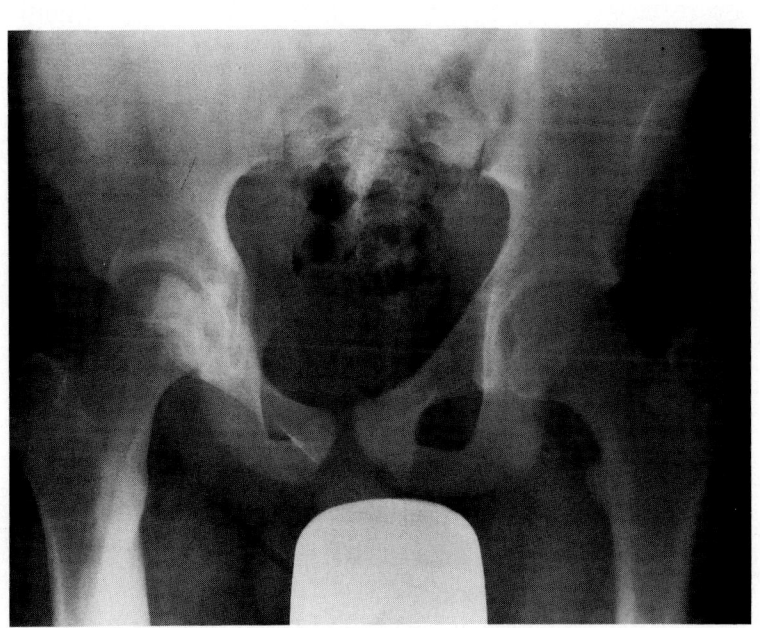

FIGURE 3-63. *Melorheostosis of the pelvis in a child.*

Note the condensed foci in the medullary portion.

notomy rather than tendon lengthening. Postoperatively the part should be splinted with an orthosis to prevent recurrence of deformity. Closing-wedge osteotomy is safer than open-up osteotomy. Shorten bone to gain soft-tissue length, in order to minimize distal ischemia. Younge and associates reported a case of distal ischemic gangrene requiring amputation.[36]

In the adult there may be slow progress of the lesions, but malignant changes have not been reported.

References

1. Abrahamson, M. N.: Disseminated asymptomatic osteosclerosis with features resembling melorheostosis, osteopoikilosis, and osteopathia striata. Case report. J. Bone Joint Surg., 50-A:991, 1968.
2. Aegerter, E. E., and Kirkpatrick, J. A.: Orthopedic Diseases. 4th Ed. Philadelphia, Saunders, 1975, pp. 162–165.
3. Beauvais, P., Faure, C., Montagne, J. P., Chigot, P. L., and Maroteaux, P.: Leri's melorheostosis: Three pediatric cases and a review of the literature. Pediatr. Radiol., 6:153, 1977.
4. Bostman, O. M., and Bakalim, G. E.: Carpal tunnel syndrome in a melorheostotic limb. J. Hand Surg., 10-B:101, 1985.
5. Campbell, C. J., Papademetriou, T., and Bonfiglio, M.: Melorheostosis. A report of the clinical, roentgenographic, and pathological findings in fourteen cases. J. Bone Joint Surg., 50-A:1281, 1968.
6. Dillehent, R. B., and Chuinard, E. G.: Melorheostosis Leri. J. Bone Joint Surg., 18:991, 1936.
7. Dissing, I., and Zafirovski, G.: Para-articular ossifications associated with melorheostosis Leri. Acta Orthop. Scand., 50:717, 1979.
8. Elkeles, A.: Melorheostosis in all limbs, pelvis and sacrum. X-ray. Trans. Med. Soc. London, 70:204, 1954.
9. Fryns, J. P., Pedersen, J. C., Vanfleteren, L., Vandeputte, F., and Van den Berghe, H.: Melorheostosis in a 3-year-old girl. Acta Paediatr. Belg., 33:185, 1980.
10. Garver, P., Resnick, D., Haghighi, P., and Guerra, J.: Melorheostosis of the axial skeleton with associated fibrolipomatous lesions. Skeletal Radiol., 9:41, 1982.
11. Gold, R. H., and Mirra, J. M.: Case report 35. Skeletal Radiol., 2:57, 1977.
12. Green, A. E., Ellswood, W. H., and Collins, J. R.: Melorheostosis and osteopoikilosis. A.J.R., 87:1096, 1962.
13. Hall, G. S.: A contribution to the study of melorheostosis: Unusual bone changes associated with tuberous sclerosis. Q. J. Med., 12:77, 1943.
14. Hoshino, T., and Mura Kami, Y.: Melorheostosis. Acta Orthop. Scand., 42:28, 1971.
15. Hove, E., and Sury, B.: Melorheostosis. Report on 5 cases with follow-up. Acta Orthop. Scand., 42:315, 1971.
16. Janousek, J., Preston, D. F., Martin, N., and Robinson, R. G.: Bone scan in melorheostosis. J. Nucl. Med., 17:1106, 1976.
17. Kawabata, H., Tsuyuguchi, Y., Kawai, H., and Yasui, N.: Melorheostosis of the upper limb: A report of two cases. J. Hand Surg., 9-A:871, 1984.
18. Kinzinger, H., Blaimont, P., and Wollast, R.: Un cas de melorheostose. Int. Orthop., 3:55, 1979.
19. Klumper, A., Wendt, H., Weller, S., and Plotner, E.: Entwicklung einer Melorheostose. Fortschr. Geb. Röntgenstr., 103:572, 1965.
20. Leri, A., and Joanny: Une affection non decrite des os. Hyperostose "en coulée" sur toute la longueur d'un membre ou "melorheostose." Bull. Soc. Méd. Hôp. Paris, 46:1141, 1922.
21. Leri, A., Loiseleur, and Lievre, J. A.: Une nouvelle observation de melorheostose. Etude clinique, anatomique et expérimentale. Bull. Soc. Hôp. Paris, 54:1210, 1930.
22. Maroteaux, P., and Lamy, M.: La melorheostose chez l'enfant. Sem. Hôp. Paris, 37:3470, 1961.
23. Maroteaux, P., and Lamy, M.: Melorheostose, ostéopoecilie et sclerodermie en bandes. Sem. Hôp. Paris, 37:3476, 1961.
24. Milleret, P., Comba, J., and Carbillet, J. P.: Une observation de melorheostose. Lyon Chir., 68:204, 1972.
25. Morris, J. M., Samilson, R. L., and Corley, C. L.: Melorheostosis. J. Bone Joint Surg., 45-A:1191, 1963.
26. Muller-Alberti, W.: Ein Beitrag zum Krankheitsbilde der Melorheostose. Z. Orthop., 72:194, 1941.
27. Murray, R. O., and McCredie, J.: Melorheostosis and the sclerotomes. Skeletal Radiol., 4:57, 1979.
28. Patrick, J. H.: Melorheostosis associated with arteriovenous aneurysm of the left arm and trunk: Report of a case with long follow-up. J. Bone Joint Surg., 51-B:126, 1969.
29. Putti, V.: L'osteosi eburneizzante monomelica (una nuova sindrome osteopatica). Chir. Organi Mov., 11:335, 1927.
30. Simon, L., Blotmaman, F., Calleus, J. P., Brousson, A., and Serre, H.: Melorheostose et pathologie articulaire de la hanche. Rev. Rhum., 43:737, 1976.
31. Soffa, D. J., Sire, D. J., and Dotson, J. H.: Melorheostosis with linear sclerodermatologic changes. Radiology, 114:577, 1975.
32. Thompson, N. M., Allen, C. E. I., Andres, G. S., and Gillwald, F. N.: Scleroderma and melorheostosis. J Bone Joint Surg., 33-B:430, 1951.
33. Todesco, S., Bedendo, A., Punzi, L., D'Angelo, A., and Romani, S.: Melorheostosis and rheumatoid arthritis. Clin. Exp. Rheumatol., 1:349, 1983.
34. Wagers, L. T., Young, A. W., and Ryan, S. F.: Linear melorheostotic scleroderma. Br. J. Dermatol. 86:297, 1972.
35. Wallenstein, S.: Melorheostosis Leri. Acta Chir. Scand., 102:463, 1952.
36. Younge, D., Drummond, D., Herring, J., and Cruess, R. L.: Melorheostosis in children. J. Bone Joint Surg., 61-B:415, 1979.
37. Zimmer, P.: Über einen Fall einer eigenartigen seltenen Knockenerkrankung. Osteopathia hyperostotica—Melorheostose. Beitr. Klin. Chir., 140:75, 1927.

OSTEOPATHIA STRIATA

Osteopathia striata, first described by Voorhoeve in 1924, is characterized by striations in the metaphyseal regions of cancellous bone with sclerosis and thickening of the base and vault of the skull.[21] The name *osteopathia striata* was proposed in 1935 by Fairbank, who had described a similar case in 1924.[6–8] The condition is very rare, with a prevalence of under 0.1 per million. Inheritance is autosomal dominant.[14]

There is usually bilateral symmetrical involvement of one bone or of the entire skeleton, depending on the stage of maturation. The

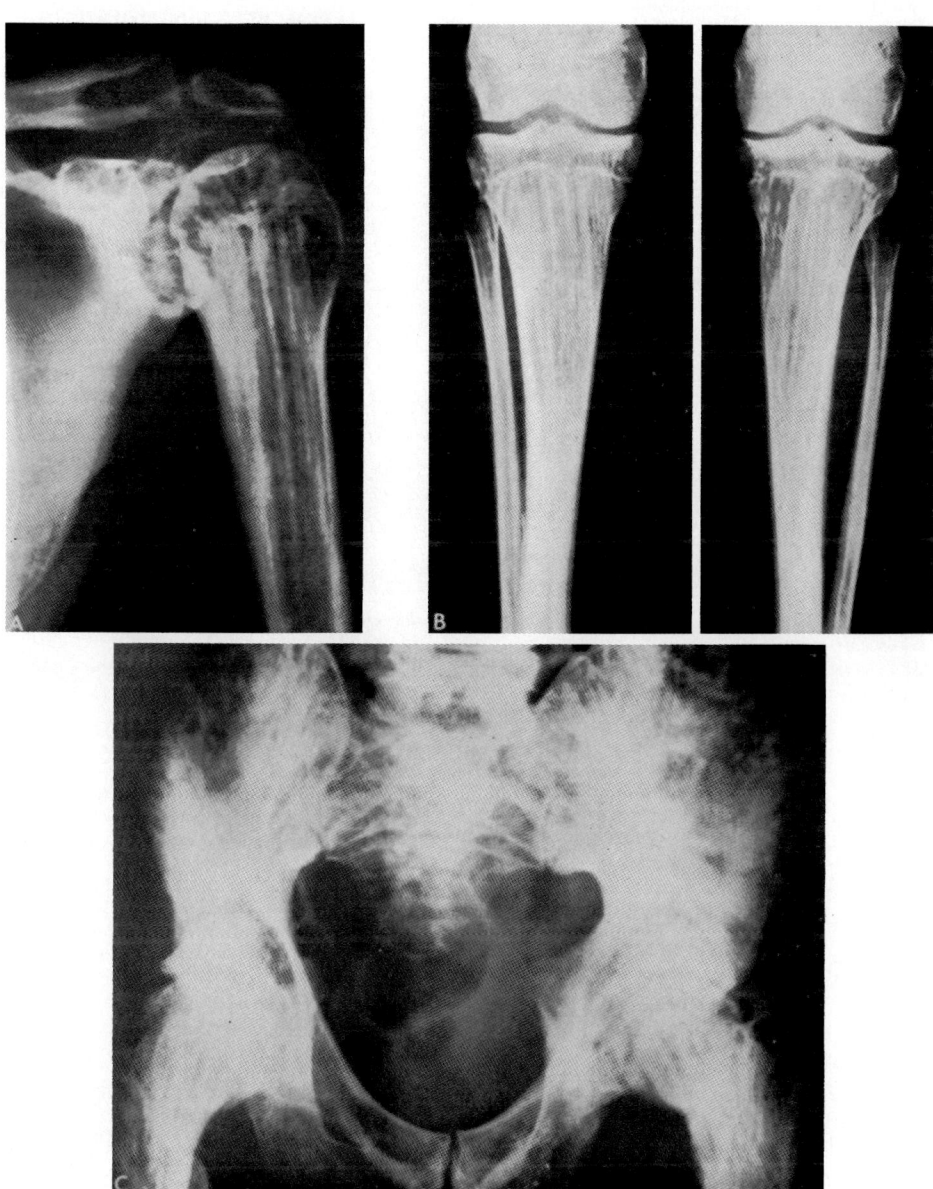

FIGURE 3–64. Osteopathia striata—radiographic appearance.

A and **B.** Radiograms of right proximal humerus and both tibiae and fibulae, showing the longitudinal striations. **C.** Radiogram of pelvis. Note the irregular fanlike striations in the ilium. (From Hurt, R. L.: Osteopathia striata—Voorhoeve's disease. J. Bone Joint Surg., 35-B:89, 1953. Reprinted by permission.)

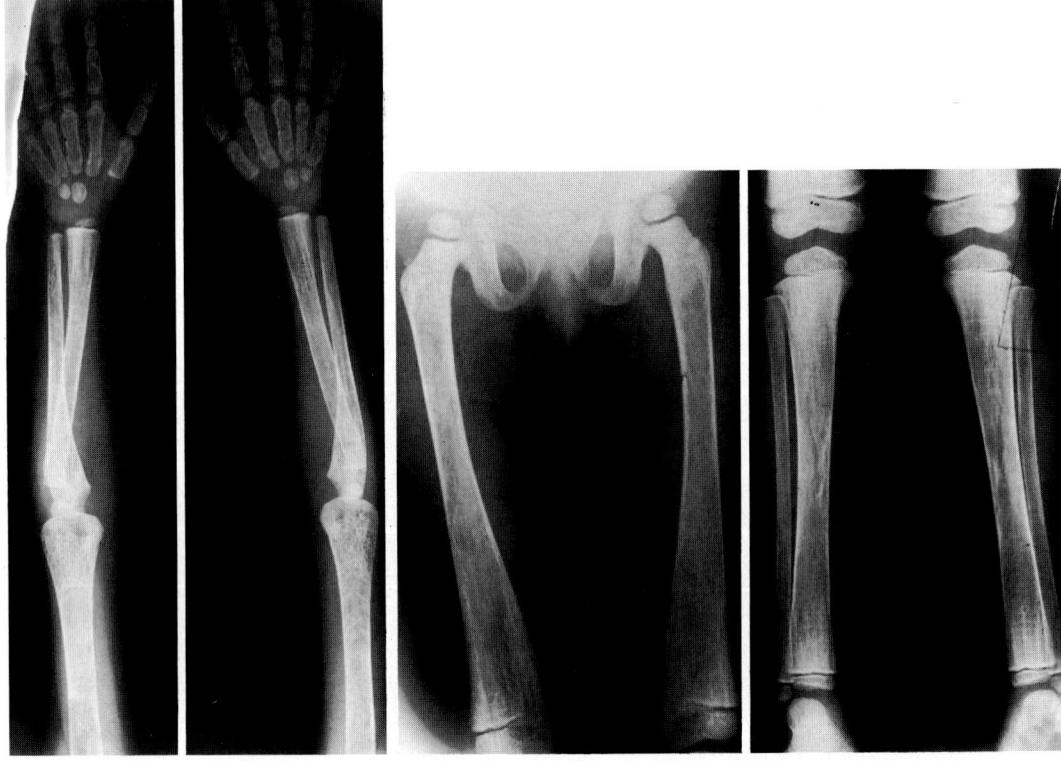

FIGURE 3-65. *Osteopathia striata.*

Anteroposterior radiograms of upper and lower limbs. Note the striations parallel to the longitudinal axis. They are especially marked in the metaphyseal areas.

striations are similar in density to the nodules seen in osteopoikilosis but are parallel to the long axis and may extend into the epiphysis (Figs. 3-64 and 3-65). When found in the ilia, the radiating lines have a fanlike "sunburst" arrangement.

In the differential diagnosis one should consider other bone dysplasias with striations of increased bone density. The pathognomonic feature of osteopathia striata is the association of cranial sclerosis with the striations. Focal dermal hypoplasia is distinguished by skin pigmentation, atrophy, and fat herniation associated with the sclerotic striations of bone.

The condition is clinically asymptomatic and of no pathologic significance. The bone striations do not change appreciably with age. There are no complications, and there is no specific treatment.

References

1. Albers-Schonberg, H. E.: Eine seltene, bisher nicht bekannte Strukturannomalie des Skelettes. Fortschr. Geb. Röntgenstr., 23:174, 1915.
2. Barthels, W., Boepple, D., and Petzel, H.: Die Osteopathia striata: Ein charakteristischer Röntgenbefund bei der fokalen dermalen Hypoplasie (Goltz-Gorlin Syndrom). Radiologe, 22:562, 1982.
3. Bloor, D. V.: A case of osteopathia striata. J. Bone Joint Surg., 36-B:261, 1954.
4. Culver, G. J., and Thumasathil, C.: Osseous changes of osteopathia striata and Pyle's disease occurring in a patient with an 11 year follow-up. A case report. A.J.R., 116:640, 1972.
5. De Keyser, J., Bruyland, M., De Greve, J., Leemans, J., Potvliege, R., Six, R., and Ebinger, G.: Osteopathia striata with cranial sclerosis. Report of a case and review of the literature. Clin. Neurol. Neurosurg., 85:41, 1983.
6. Fairbank, H. A. T.: A case of unilateral affection of the skeleton of unknown origin. Br. J. Surg., 12:594, 1925.
7. Fairbank, H. A. T.: Generalized disorders of the skeleton. Proc. R. Soc. Med., Clin. Sect., 28:1611, 1935.
8. Fairbank, H. A. T.: Osteopathia striata. J. Bone Joint Surg., 32-B:117, 1950.
9. Fermin, H. E. A.: Osteorhabdotose. Een voor het eerst door N. Voorhoeve beschreven bijzondere vorm van osteopathia condensans disseminata. Ned. Tydschr. Geneeskd., 106:1188, 1962.
10. Franklyn, P. P., and Wilkinson, D.: Two cases of osteopathia striata, deafness and cranial osteopetrosis. Ann. Radiol., 21:91, 1978.
11. Gehweiler, J. A., Bland, W. R., Carden, R. S., and Daffner, R. H.: Osteopathia striata—Voorhoeve's disease. Review of the roentgen manifestations. A.J.R., 18:450, 1973.

12. Goltz, R. W., Peterson, N. C., Gorlin, R. J., and Ravits, H. G.: Focal dermal hypoplasia. Arch. Dermatol. Syph. (Chicago), 86:708, 1962.
13. Hinkel, C. L.: Developmental affections of the skeleton characterized by osteosclerosis. Clin. Orthop., 9:91, 1957.
14. Horan, F. T., and Beighton, P. H.: Osteopathia striata with cranial sclerosis. An autosomal dominant entity. Clin. Genet., 13:201, 1978.
15. Hurt, R. L.: Osteopathia striata—Voorhoeve's disease. J. Bone Joint Surg., 35-B:89, 1953.
16. Larregue, M., Maroteaux, P., Michel, Y., and Faure, C.: L'ostéopathie striée, symptome radiologique de l'hypoplasie dermique en aires. Ann. Radiol., 15:287, 1972.
17. Ledoux-Lebard, R., Chabaneix, and Dessane: L'ostéopoecilie, forme nouvelle d'ostéite generalisée. J. Radiol. Electrol., 2:133, 1916.
18. Robinow, M., and Unger, F.: Syndrome of osteopathia striata, macrocephaly, and cranial sclerosis. Am. J. Dis. Child., 138:821, 1984.
19. Rucker, T. N., and Alfidi, R. J.: A rare familial systemic affection of the skeleton: Fairbank's disease. Radiology, 82:63, 1964.
20. Schnyder, P. A.: Osseous changes in osteopathia striata associated with cranial sclerosis. An autosomal dominant entity. Skeletal Radiol., 5:19, 1980.
21. Voorhoeve, N.: L'image radiologique non encore décrite d'une anomalie du squelette. Acta Radiol., 3:407, 1924.
22. Walker, B. A.: Osteopathia striata with cataracts and deafness. Birth Defects, 5:295, 1969.
23. Walker, G. F.: Mixed sclerosing bone dystrophies. Two case reports. J. Bone Joint Surg., 46-B:546, 1964.
24. Whyte, M. P., Murphy, W. A., and Siegel, B. A.: ^{99m}Tc-pyrophosphate bone imaging in osteopoikilosis, osteopathia striata, and melorrheostosis. Radiology, 127:439, 1978.

OSTEOPOIKILOSIS (SPOTTED BONES)

This bone dysplasia is characterized by dense ovoid or circular spots in cancellous bone, which may be noted at birth or which may appear during skeletal growth. Usually found in clusters in the metaphyseal and epiphyseal regions of long bones, they are rarely seen in the diaphyses. The most frequent locations are the carpals and tarsals, the ends of large tubular bones, or around the acetabula. The skull, face, ribs, sternum, and vertebrae are rarely involved.[1-24]

Osteopoikilosis is inherited as an autosomal dominant trait with a prevalance of under 0.1 per million.

Histologic examination discloses these condensed nodules to consist of laminated bone that merges with the surrounding spongiosa. The proportion of haversian spaces is the same as that seen in dense cortical bone.

Clinically, the condition is asymptomatic. Spontaneous fractures do not occur. Occasionally, it is associated with hereditary multiple exostosis. In about 10 per cent of cases there are skin lesions (dermatofibrosis lenticularis disseminata). These manifest themselves as small whitish-yellow fibrous dermal and subcutaneous nodules.[8]

In the radiograph these oval or lens-shaped densities measure 3 to 5 mm. in diameter and are characteristic in appearance (Fig. 3-66). The lesions do not affect the cortex or the contour of the bone.

The natural history of osteopoikilotic nodules follows the laws of normal bone growth. Over a period of years they may increase or diminish in size, and some of them may disappear. No treatment is indicated. A single case has been

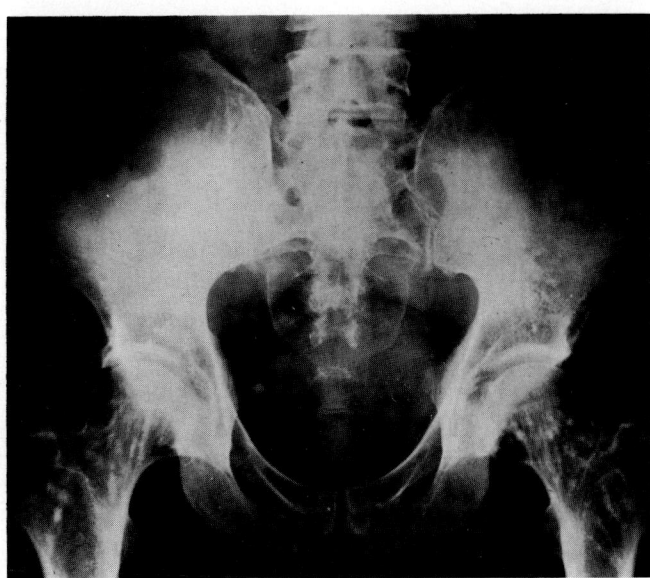

FIGURE 3-66. Osteopoikilosis of the proximal femora.

Note the numerous sclerotic fossae in the epiphyses and metaphyses.

reported of osteosarcoma developing in a 48-year-old man with osteopoikilosis.[16]

References

1. Agostinelli, J. R.: Osteopoikilosis. A case report. J. Am. Podiatry Assoc., 73:529, 1983.
2. Albers-Schonberg, H. E.: Einer seltene, bisher nicht bekannte Strukturanomalie des Skelettes. Fortschr. Geb. Röntgenstr., 23:174, 1915.
3. Archer, M. C., and Fox, K. W.: Osteopoikilosis. Radiology, 47:279, 1946.
4. Beighton, P., and Cremin, B. J.: Sclerosing bone dysplasias. Berlin, Springer, 1980.
5. Curth, H. O.: Dermatofibrosis lenticularis disseminata and osteopoikilosis. Arch. Dermatol. Syph., 30:552, 1934.
6. Dume, T., Schulte-Brinkmann, W., and Sturm, A., Jr.: Osteopoikilie mit Hyperostose. Dtsch. Med. Wochenschr., 96:422, 1971.
7. Fairbank, H. A. T.: Osteopoikilosis. Synonym—osteopathia condensans disseminata. J. Bone Joint Surg., 30-B:544, 1948.
8. Green, A. E., Ellswood, W. H., and Collins, J. R.: Melorheostosis and osteopoikilosis. A.J.R., 87:1096, 1962.
9. Harmston, G. J.: Osteopathia condensans disseminata. Radiology, 66:556, 1956.
10. Hinkel, C. L.: Developmental affections of the skeleton characterized by osteosclerosis. Clin. Orthop., 9:92, 1957.
11. Hinson, A.: Familial osteopoikilosis. Am. J. Surg., 45:566, 1939.
12. Holly, L. E.: Osteopoikilosis: A five-year study. A.J.R., 36:512, 1936.
13. Jancu, J.: Osteopoikilosis. A case report and a suggestion of its pathogenesis. Acta Orthop. Belg., 37:284, 1971.
14. Lagier, R., Mbakop, A., and Bigler, A.: Osteopoikilosis: A radiological and pathological study. Skeletal Radiol., 11:161, 1984.
15. Lippelt, C., and Petzel, H.: Dermatofibrosis lenticularis disseminata mit Osteopoikilie (Buschke-Ollendorff-Syndrom). Radiologe, 22:553, 1982.
16. Mindell, E. R., Northup, C. S., and Douglass, H. O., Jr.: Osteosarcoma associated with osteopoikilosis. J. Bone Joint Surg., 60-A:406, 1978.
17. Schimpf, A., Roth, W., and Kopper, J.: Dermatofibrosis lenticularis disseminata mit Osteopoikilie. Buschke-Ollendorf Syndrom. Dermatologica, 141:409, 1970.
18. Serre, H., Simon, L., Barjon, M. C., Sany, J., and Privat, J. M.: Ostéopoecilie familiale. A propos de 3 observations. Rhumatologie, 10:233, 1968.
19. Staniczek, J., and Szkandera, J.: Die Osteopoikilie bei einem Dizephalus-Thorakopagus. Roentgenologische und pathologish-anatomische Beobachtung. Fortschr. Geb. Röntgenstr., 120:116, 1974.
20. Stieda, A.: Uber umschriebene Knochenernichtungen in Bereich der Substantia. Spongiosa im Roentgenbilde. Beitr. Klin. Chir., 45:700, 1905.
21. Strigl, M., and Bohm, E.: Osteopoikilie klinische und pathologisch-anatomische Beobachtungen. Unfallchirurgie, 9:193, 1983.
22. Szabo, A. D.: Osteopoikilosis in a twin. Clin. Orthop., 79:156, 1971.
23. Weisz, G. M.: Lumbar spinal canal stenosis in osteopoikilosis. Clin. Orthop., 166:89, 1982.
24. Whyte, M. P., Murphy, W. A., and Siegel, B. A.: 99mTc-pyrophosphate bone imaging in osteopoikilosis, osteopathia striata, and melorheostosis. Radiology, 127:439, 1978.

IDIOPATHIC HYPERPHOSPHATASIA

This extremely rare bone dysplasia is characterized by bowing of the long bones with anterior concavity, extreme fragility due to osteoporosis, and failure to replace immature bone with compact haversian bone.[1-22] There is generalized diaphyseal expansion with subperiosteal deposits of disorganized new bone in which there is less differentiation between medulla and cortex. The patient's head is enlarged, the base and vault of the skull are thickened, and there is patchy sclerosis of the calvarium. The paranasal sinuses are obliterated. The spine and pelvis also show patchy areas of sclerosis. Biochemically, serum levels of alkaline phosphatase are high, and urinary excretion of hydroxyproline is minimal.

The etiology is unknown. Inheritance is by autosomal recessive transmission.

Pathologic studies of bone tissue show extensive fibrosis of the marrow with cellular hyperactivity. There may be a mosaic pattern of cement lines as seen in Paget's disease.

The presenting complaint is painful swelling of the limbs, which are bowed. The muscle mass is diminished, and the limbs may be warm. Fracture may be the first sign. Affected children have large heads and very short stature.

In the differential diagnosis one should consider Engelmann's disease, craniodiaphyseal dysplasia, and polyostotic fibrous dysplasia. In all these entities there are patchy areas of sclerosis, bowing, and fracture of long bones; however, in these conditions, serum alkaline phosphatase levels are not elevated. Osteogenesis imperfecta may pose a problem in diagnosis.

Treatment with human and porcine thyrocalcitonin has produced a favorable response in some patients.[1, 7]

A tarda form of idiopathic hyperphosphatasia with its onset in adolescence was described by Buchem and associates in 1955.[2] The main feature is involvement of the cranial nerves (the seventh most frequently) due to thickening of the base of the skull and obliteration of the foramina. The mandible is enlarged and sclerotic. The long tubular bones are sclerotic, involvement being in the diaphyses but not the epiphyses. Fractures of long bones do not occur. Pathologic findings are similar to those seen in the congenital type. Inheritance is as an autosomal recessive trait, but a dominant form has been reported by Maroteaux and associates.[14]

In the differential diagnosis one should rule out osteopetrosis. The serum alkaline phosphatase levels are elevated in Van Buchem's disease. Histologic examination of a bone biopsy will establish the diagnosis.

References

1. Blanco, O., Stivel, M., Mautalen, C., and Schajowicz, F.: Familial idiopathic hyperphosphatasia. A study of two young siblings treated with porcine calcitonin. J. Bone Joint Surg., 59-B:421, 1977.
2. Buchem, F. S. van, Hadders, H. N., and Ubbers, R.: An uncommon familial systemic disease of the skeleton: Hyperostosis corticalis generalisata familiaris. Acta Radiol., 4:109, 1955.
3. Buchem, F. S. van, Hadders, H. N., Hansen, J. F., and Woldring, M. G.: Hyperostosis corticalis generalisata. Report of seven cases. Am. J. Med., 33:387, 1962.
4. Caffey, J.: Familial hyperphosphatasemia with ateliosis and hypermetabolism of growing membranous bone; review of the clinical, radiographic and chemical features. Bull. Hosp. Jt. Dis., 33:81, 1972.
5. Choremis, C., Yannakos, D., Papadatos, C., and Baroutsou, E.: Osteitis deformans (Paget's disease) in an eleven year old boy. Helv. Paediatr. Acta, 13:185, 1958.
6. Desai, M. P., Joshi, N. C., and Shah, K. N.: Chronic idiopathic hyperphosphatasia in an Indian child. Am. J. Dis. Child., 126:625, 1973.
7. Doyle, F. H., Woodhouse, N. J. Y., Glen, A. C. A., Joplin, G. F., and MacIntyre, I.: Healing of the bones in juvenile Paget's disease treated by human calcitonin. Br. J. Radiol., 47:9, 1974.
8. Dunn, V., Condon, V. R., and Rallison, M. L.: Familial hyperphosphatasia: Diagnosis in early infancy and response to human thyrocalcitonin therapy. A.J.R., 132:541, 1979.
9. Eroglu, M., and Taneli, N. N.: Congenital hyperphosphatasia (juvenile Paget's disease). Eleven year follow-up of three sisters. Ann. Radiol., 20:145, 1977.
10. Eyring, E. J., and Eisenberg, E.: Congenital hyperphosphatasia. A clinical, pathological and biochemical study of two cases. J. Bone Joint Surg., 50-A:1099, 1968.
11. Iancu, T. C., Almagor, G., and Savir, H.: Ocular abnormalities in chronic familial hyperphosphatasemia. J. Pediatr. Ophthalmol. Strabismus, 17:220, 1980.
12. Iancu, T. C., Almagor, G., Friedman, E., Hardoff, R., and Front, D.: Chronic familial hyperphosphatasemia. Radiology, 129:669, 1978.
13. Jett, S., and Frost, H. M.: Tetracycline-based measurements of the bone dynamics in a rib of a girl with hyperphosphatasia. Henry Ford Hosp. Med. J., 16:325, 1968.
14. Maroteaux, P., Fontaine, G., Scharfman, W., and Farriaux, J. P.: L'hyperostose corticale généralisée: Transmission dominante. Arch. Fr. Pediatr., 28:685, 1971.
15. Melhem, R. E., Najjar, S. S., and Khachadurian, A. K.: Cortical hyperostosis with hyperphosphatemia: A new syndrome? J. Pediatr., 77:986, 1970.
16. Mikati, M. A., Melhem, R. E., and Najjar, S. S.: The syndrome of hyperostosis and hyperphosphatemia. J. Pediatr., 99:900, 1981.
17. Mitsudo, S. M.: Chronic idiopathic hyperphosphatasia associated with pseudoxanthoma elasticum. J. Bone Joint Surg., 53-A:303, 1971.
8. Romero, J. R., Diaz, L. G., Mateos, F. P., and Del Cuvillo, L. M.: Hiperfosfatasemia congenita. Rev. Clin. Esp., 157:211, 1980.
19. Swoboda, V. W.: Hyperostosis corticalis deformans juvenilis. Helv. Paediatr. Acta, 13:292, 1958.
20. Thompson, R. C., Jr., Gaull, G. E., Horwitz, S. J., and Schenk, R. K.: Hereditary hyperphosphatasia. Studies of three siblings. Am. J. Med., 47:209, 1969.
21. Whalen, J. P., Horwith, M., Krook, L., MacIntyre, I., Mema, E., Viteri, F., Torun, B., and Nunez, E. A.: Calcitonin treatment in hereditary bone dysplasia with hyperphosphatasemia: A radiographic and histologic study of bone. A.J.R., 129:29, 1977.
22. Woodhouse, N. J. Y., Fisher, M. T., Sigurdsson, G., Joplin, G. F., and MacIntyre, I.: Paget's disease in a 5-year-old: Acute response to human calcitonin. Br. Med. J., 4:267, 1972.

INFANTILE CORTICAL HYPEROSTOSIS (CAFFEY'S DISEASE)

Infantile cortical hyperostosis is a self-limiting disease of early infancy that is characterized by swelling of soft tissues, cortical thickening of the underlying bones, and hyperirritability. Caffey and Silverman, in 1945, thoroughly described this entity and gave it its name.[15] Similar cases had, however, been reported by Roske, in 1930, and by Ellis, in 1938.[22, 57]

The condition is rare. There is no sex or racial predilection.

Etiology

The cause of infantile cortical hyperostosis is unknown. Numerous reports of its familial occurrence suggest a possible hereditary factor.[7, 31, 63, 74, 75] The self-limiting nature of the condition makes it difficult to establish the exact mode of inheritance; most probably it is an autosomal dominant trait.[8, 23, 44, 45, 58] An inherited defect of the arterioles of the periosteum has been proposed.[62, 63] Because of the response of the disease to corticosteroids and the precipitation of symptoms with changes in diet, an allergic basis has also been postulated.[6] Infection has been considered by some because of the acute inflammatory findings. All attempts to isolate bacteria or viruses have failed, however, and serologic tests for infection have been negative.[24, 62, 63]

Pathology

The pathologic changes have been studies in biopsy specimens and, in three cases, at autopsy.[20, 24, 34, 40, 52, 62] In the early stages there is a marked inflammatory process involving the periosteum and the surrounding soft tissues. Gradually the inflammation subsides, leaving behind a thickened periosteum and subperiosteal immature lamellar bone (Fig. 3–67). A

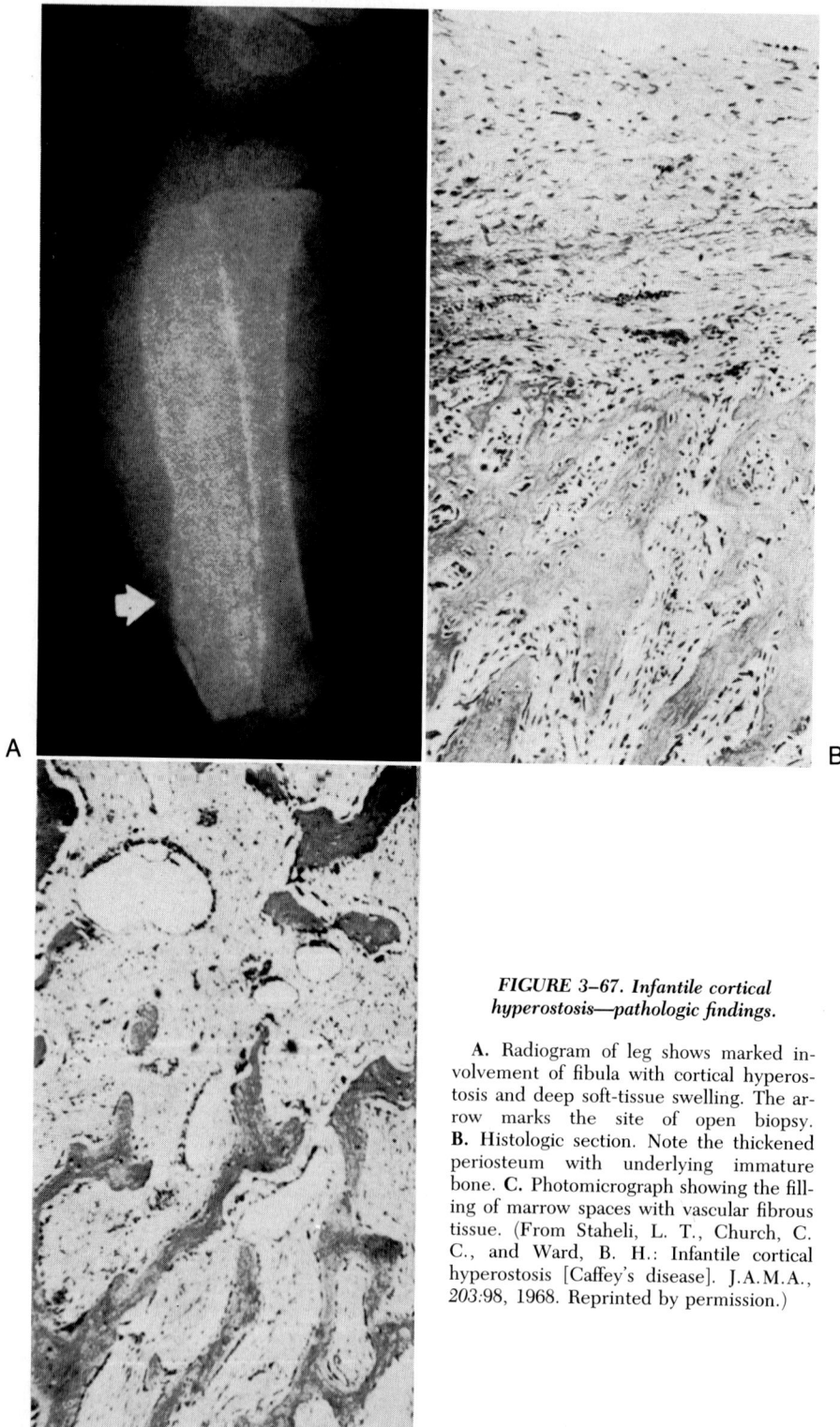

FIGURE 3-67. Infantile cortical hyperostosis—pathologic findings.

A. Radiogram of leg shows marked involvement of fibula with cortical hyperostosis and deep soft-tissue swelling. The arrow marks the site of open biopsy. **B.** Histologic section. Note the thickened periosteum with underlying immature bone. **C.** Photomicrograph showing the filling of marrow spaces with vascular fibrous tissue. (From Staheli, L. T., Church, C. C., and Ward, B. H.: Infantile cortical hyperostosis [Caffey's disease]. J.A.M.A., 203:98, 1968. Reprinted by permission.)

vascular fibrous tissue occupies the bone marrow spaces. Proliferation of the intima of the arterioles in the affected osseous and soft tissues was demonstrated by Sherman and Hellyer, a finding that suggested hypoxia as a causative agent of the reactive hyperostosis.[62]

In studying the ultrastructure of bone in infantile cortical hyperostosis, Beluffi and associates found that hydroxyapatite crystals were first deposited between the collagen fibers. The normal pattern of periosteal growth was then lost.[3]

Clinical Features

The mandible is the most common site of involvement. In the limbs, the ulna is most frequently affected. Next in frequency are the tibiae, clavicles, scapulae, and ribs. The humerus, femur, and fibula are less often involved. Occasionally, hyperostosis may occur in the frontal and parietal bones, the ilium, scapulae, and metatarsals.[33, 36] Involvement of neither the phalanges of the hand nor of the vertebrae has been reported. Affection of more than one bone is common, and if involvement is bilateral, it is often asymmetrical.

Onset of the disease usually occurs around the ninth week of postnatal life. It may, however, be present at birth, and has been demonstrated in utero as early as the twenty-fourth week of gestation. It rarely occurs after the fifth month of postnatal life.

The commonest clinical manifestations are hyperirritability and the presence of a local mass, often over the mandible. The swelling appears suddenly, is deep and firm, and may be tender initially; there is, however, no increased local heat or redness. Moderate fever is frequently present in the early stages. The sedimentation rate and serum alkaline phosphatase levels are elevated, and anemia is not uncommon.

Radiographic Features

The characteristic radiographic finding is formation of abundant new bone by the periosteum with enlargement of the diameter of the affected bones (Figs. 3–68, 3–69, and 3–70). In the long bones, the hyperostosis is primarily confined to the diaphysis, and the epiphysis and metaphyses are not involved. In the early stages, the external surface of the new bone is coarse and the underlying cortex is still visible. As the disease progresses, the new bone increases in density, becoming homogeneous with the cortex. At this time, overlying soft-tissue swelling will be visible. Several months, sometimes years, are required for complete resolution. Late recurrences of infantile cortical hyperostosis have been reviewed in the literature.[5, 56, 66]

Diagnosis

In the differential diagnosis, one should consider osteomyelitis, syphilis, scurvy, hypervitaminosis A, trauma, Ewing's sarcoma, and metastatic tumors such as neuroblastoma. Swelling in the mandibular region may be mistaken for parotitis; hyperostosis is not, however, produced by parotitis. The diagnostic features of infantile cortical hyperostosis are specific: (1) the narrow age group limitation between birth and five months; (2) the triad of irritability, swelling, and bone lesions; (3) and the mandibular involvement. Serologic, biochemical, and other laboratory tests will aid in ruling out other conditions. Biopsy of the lesion is usually not indicated; it is very rare that the question of malignancy must be ruled out by biopsy unless there is reason to doubt the clinical and radiographic features. The differential diagnosis of infantile hyperostosis from hypervitaminosis A is given in Table 3–8.

Text continued on page 824

Table 3–8. Differential Diagnosis of Infantile Cortical Hyerostosis and Hypervitaminosis A

Features	Infantile Cortical Hyerostosis	Hypervitaminosis A
Age at onset	Birth to six months	One year and older
Involvement of mandible	Present-almost always	Universally absent
Metatarsal involvement	Rare	Usual
Fever	Present	Absent
Cortical hyperostosis	Present	Present
Tender soft-tissue swelling	Present	Present
Vitamin A level	Normal	Elevated
Response to low vitamin diet	None	Amelioration of symptoms within one month
Response to corticosteroid therapy	Alleviation of acute system manifestation	No response
Inheritance	Possibly autosomal dominant	Nonhereditary

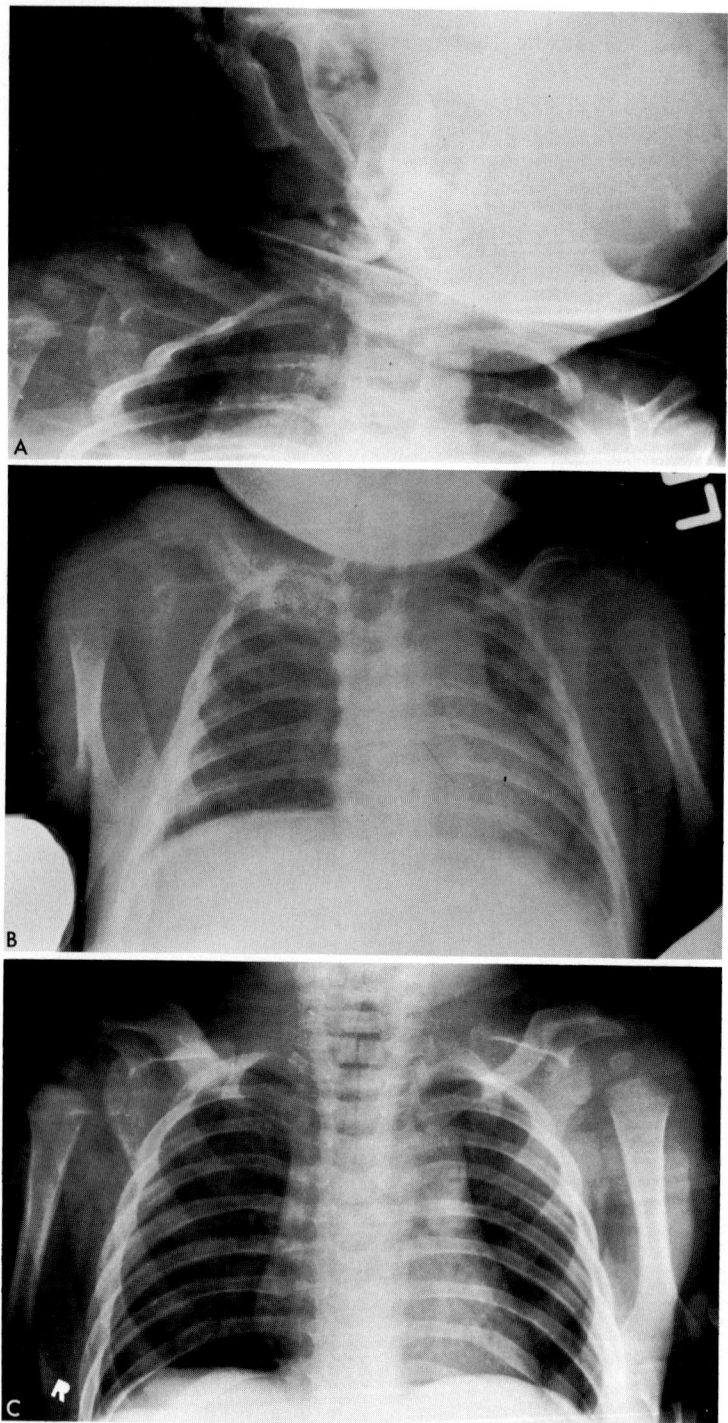

FIGURE 3–68. Infantile cortical hyperostosis in a two-month-old infant.

A. Radiogram of mandible. Note the thickened mandible with layers of newly formed bone over its inferior margins. **B.** Radiogram of shoulders. There is marked hyperostosis of the right clavicle. **C.** Four months later, radiogram shows healing of right clavicle.

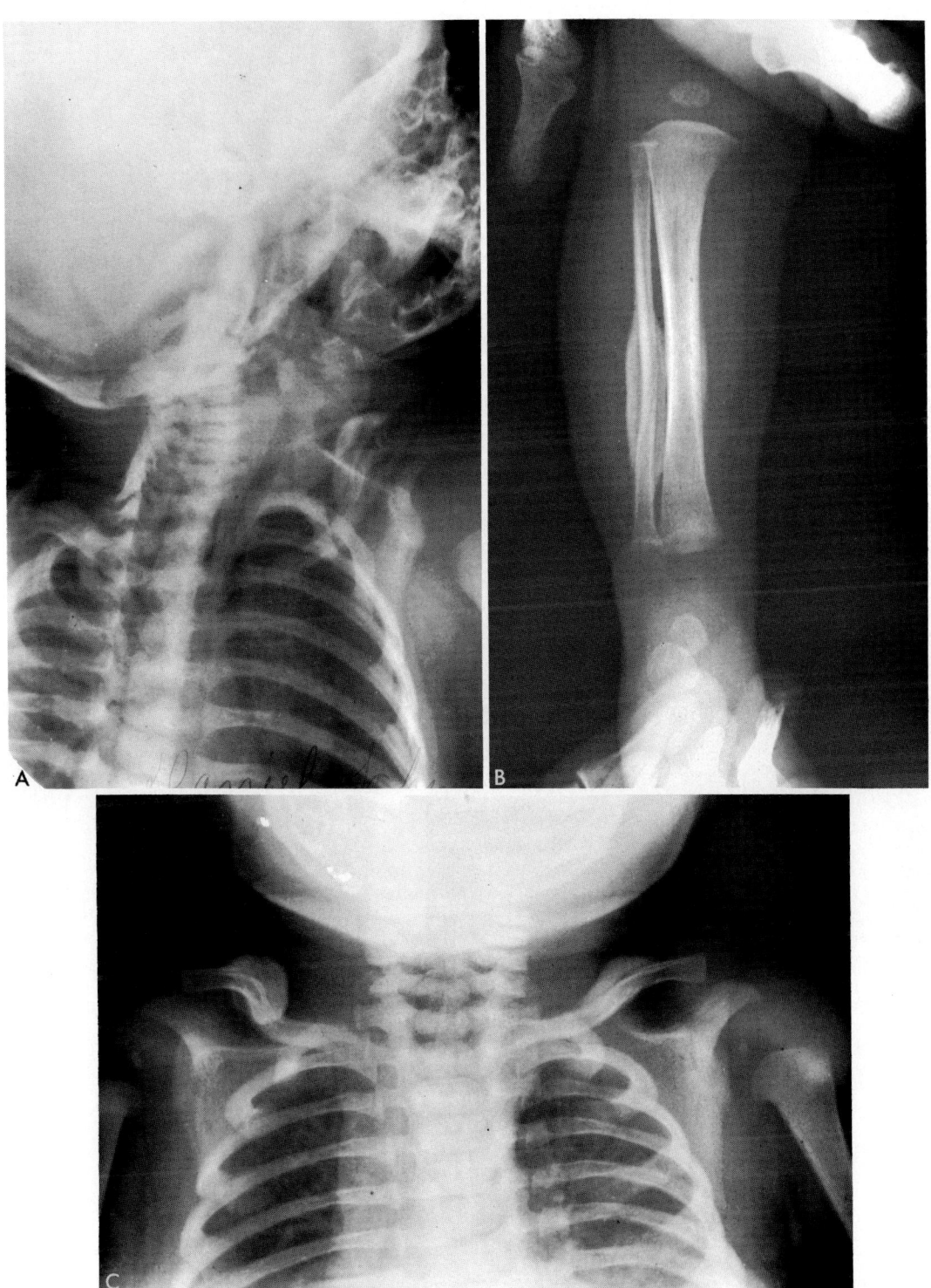

FIGURE 3–69. Infantile cortical hyperostosis in a one-month-old boy.

A. Radiogram of jaw shows involvement of mandible. **B.** The right fibula and tibia are also involved. **C.** The right scapula and both clavicles are affected.

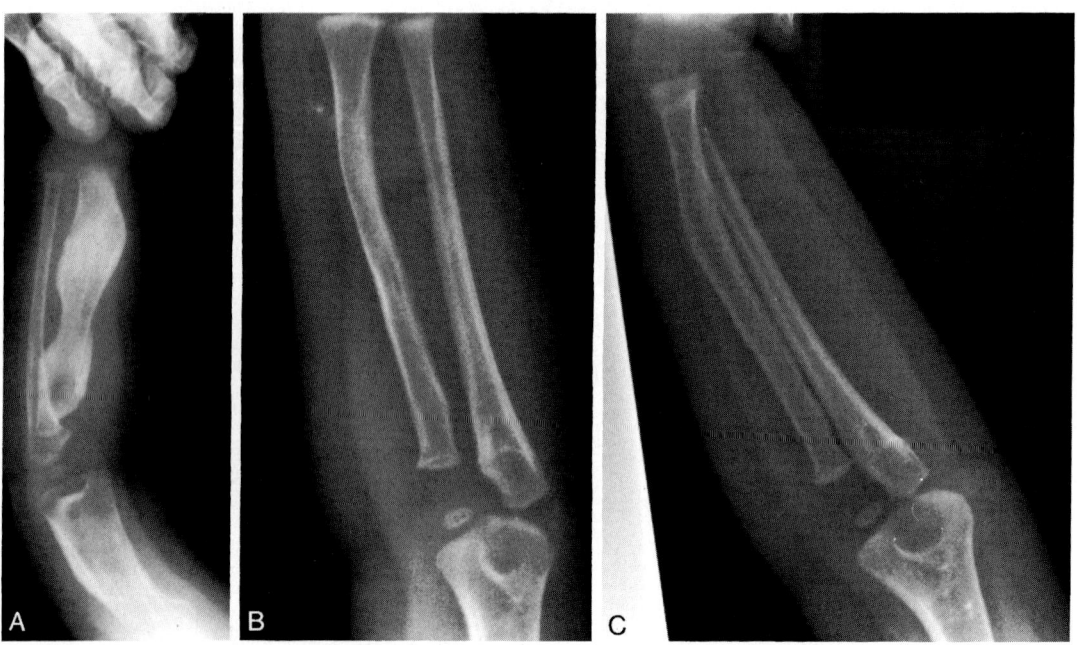

FIGURE 3–70. Four-month-old girl with infantile cortical hyperostosis (Caffey's disease).

A. Lateral view of the left forearm. **B** and **C.** Anteroposterior and lateral views of the left forearm 18 months later.

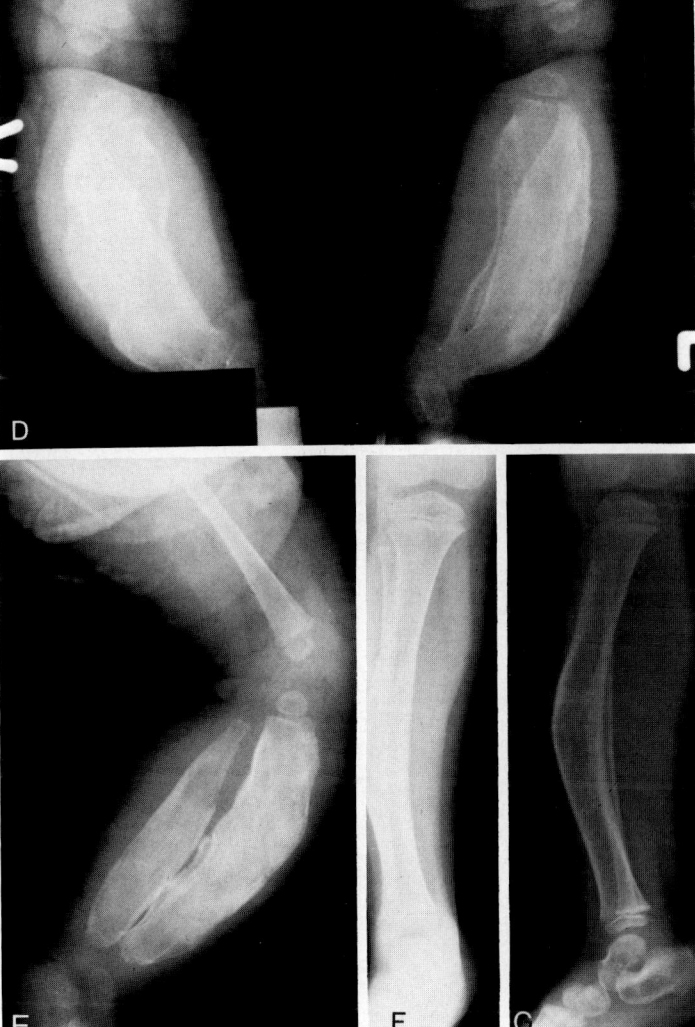

***FIGURE 3–70 Continued.** Four-month-old girl with infantile cortical hyperostosis (Caffey's disease).*

D and **E.** Anteroposterior and lateral views of the legs showing involvement of the tibiae and fibulae. **F** and **G.** Lateral views of both legs four years later, still involved. The clavicle and mandible were also involved.

Treatment

There is no specific treatment. The disease is self-limiting, and complete recovery within six to nine months is the rule. Spontaneous remissions and exacerbations may occur. Antibiotics and surgical measures are not indicated.

Corticosteroids are effective in alleviating the acute systemic manifestations but have no effect on the bone changes. Caffey recommends treatment with corticosteroids (100 mg. cortisone daily for 10 to 14 days, then gradual tapering of the dose).[14] It is more judicious, however, to reserve the use of corticosteroids for only those infants who have extensive and recurrent involvement.

Complications

Occasionally, when the disease is severe and active, with intermittent recurrences, a number of residual deformities of the affected limb may remain. Those reported in the literature include dilatation of the medullary cavity and thinning of the cortex; fusion of adjacent bones such as the ribs, tibia and fibula, and radius and ulna (with dislocation of the radial head); anterior bowing of the tibia or femur; lower limb length inequality; and persistent facial asymmetry. Pleural effusion, exophthalmos, and diaphragmatic paralysis are other rare complications.[10–15, 37, 61, 62, 69, 76]

References

1. Allen, D. H., Browne, F. S., and Pierce, A. W.: Infantile cortical hyperostosis: Report of two cases with review of points of differential diagnosis from hypervitaminosis A. A.J.R., 76:576, 1956.
2. Barba, W. P., II, and Freriks, D. J.: The familial occurrence of infantile cortical hyperostosis in utero. J. Pediatr., 42:141, 1953.
3. Beluffi, G., Chirico, G., Colombo, A., Ceciliani, L., Dell'Orbo, C., Fiori, P., Pazzaglia, U., and Quacci, D.: Report of a new case of neonatal cortical hyperostosis. Histological and ultrastructural study. Ann. Radiol., 27:2, 1984.
4. Bennett, H. S., and Nelson, T. R.: Prenatal cortical hyperostosis. Br. J. Radiol., 26:47, 1953.
5. Blank, E.: Recurrent Caffey's cortical hyperostosis and persistent deformity. Pediatrics, 55:856, 1975.
6. Bowman, J. R., Piston, R. E., and Meeks, E. A.: Further observations on the etiology of infantile cortical hyperostosis. Ann. Allergy, 19:1154, 1961.
7. Boyes, J. G., and Demy, N. G.: Infantile cortical hyperostosis: A familial disease? A.J.R., 65:924, 1951.
8. Bull, M. J., and Feingold, M.: Autosomal dominant inheritance of Caffey disease. Birth Defects Orig. Art. Series, 10:139, 1974.
9. Bush, L. G., and Merrell, O. E.: Infantile cortical hyperostosis. Report of a case responding to treatment with corticotropin. J. Pediatr., 40:330, 1952.
10. Bywaters, T. W., Jr., Bailey, R. W., Carrol, C. J., and O'Connor, G. A.: Infantile cortical hyperostosis presenting with exophthalmos: Case report. J. Mich. Med. Soc., 62:285, 1963.
11. Caffey, J.: Infantile cortical hyperostosis. J. Pediatr., 29:541, 1946.
12. Caffey, J.: On some late skeletal changes in chronic infantile cortical hyperostosis. Radiology, 59:651, 1952.
13. Caffey, J.: Infantile cortical hyperostosis. A review of the clinical and radiographic features. Proc. R. Soc. Med., 50:347, 1957.
14. Caffey, J.: Pediatric X-ray Diagnosis. 5th Ed. Chicago, Year Book, 1967.
15. Caffey, J., and Silverman, W. A.: Infantile cortical hyperostosis. Preliminary report in a new syndrome. A.J.R., 54:1, 1945.
16. Campbell, D. J., and Turner, E.: Aminoaciduria in a case of infantile cortical hyperostosis (Caffey's disease). Am. J. Clin. Pathol., 38:97, 1962.
17. Cayler, G. C., and Peterson, C. A.: Infantile cortical hyperostosis: Report of 17 cases. Am. J. Dis. Child., 91:119, 1956.
18. Claesson, I.: Infantile cortical hyperostosis. Report of a case with late manifestations. Acta Radiol. Diagn., 17:594, 1976.
19. Clement, A. R., and Williams, J. H.: The familial occurrence of infantile cortical hyperostosis. Radiology, 80:409, 1963.
20. Dickson, D. D., Luckey, C. A., and Logan, N. H.: Infantile cortical hyperostosis. J. Bone Joint Surg., 29:224, 1947.
21. Eik, S.: Infantile cortical hyperostosis. Development of a case in utero. Acta Paediatr., 44:Suppl. 103:135, 1955.
22. Ellis, R. W. B.: Vitamin C deficiency as periostitis of both ulnae: Scurvy. Proc. R. Soc. Med., 32:139, 1939.
23. Emmery, L., Timmerman, J., Christens, J., and Fryns, J. P.: Familial infantile cortical hyperostosis. Eur. J. Pediatr., 141:56, 1983.
24. Eversole, S. L., Jr., Holman, G. H., and Robinson, R. A.: Hitherto undescribed characteristics of the pathology of infantile cortical hyperostosis (Caffey's disease). Bull. Johns Hopkins Hosp., 101:80, 1957.
25. Faure, C., Beyssac, J. -M., and Montagne, J.-P.: Predominant or exclusive orbital and facial involvement in infantile cortical hyperostosis (de Toni-Caffey's disease). Pediatr. Radiol., 6:103, 1977.
26. Finsterbush, A., and Husseini, N.: Infantile cortical hyperostosis with unusual clinical manifestations. Clin. Orthop., 144:276, 1979.
27. Finsterbush, A., and Rang, M.: Infantile cortical hyperostosis. Follow-up of 29 cases. Acta Orthop. Scand., 46:727, 1975.
28. Frana, L., and Sekanina, M.: Infantile cortical hyperostosis. Arch. Dis. Child., 51:589, 1976.
29. Fried, K., Manor, A., Pajewski, M., Starinsky, R., and Vure, E.: Autosomal dominant inheritance with incomplete penetration of Caffey disease (infantile cortical hyperostosis). Clin. Genet., 19:271, 1981.
30. Gentry, R. R., Rust, R. S., Lohr, J. A., and Alford, B. A.: Infantile cortical hyperostosis of the ribs (Caffey's disease) without mandibular involvement. Pediatr. Radiol., 13:236, 1983.
31. Gerrard, J. W., Holman, G. H., Gorman, A. A., and Morrow, I. H.: Familial infantile cortical hyperostosis. J. Pediatr., 59:543, 1961.
32. Goluboff, N.: Infantile cortical hyperostosis (Caffey-Smyth syndrome). Can. Med. Assoc. J., 62:189, 1950.
33. Harris, V. J., and Ramilo, J.: Caffey's disease: A case originating in the first metatarsal and review of a 12 year experience. A.J.R., 130:335, 1978.
34. Holman, G. H.: Infantile cortical hyperostosis. Q. Rev. Pediatr., 59:543, 1961.
35. Holman, G. H.: Infantile cortical hyperostosis: A review. Q. Rev. Pediatr., 17:24, 1962.
36. Holtzman, D.: Infantile cortical hyperostosis of the

scapula presenting as an ipsilateral Erb's palsy. J. Pediatr., *81*:785, 1972.
37. Jackson, D. R., and Lyne, E. D.: Infantile cortical hyperostosis. Case report. J. Bone Joint Surg., *61-A*:770, 1979.
38. Jones, E. T., Hensinger, R. N., and Holt, J. F.: Idiopathic cortical hyperostosis. Clin. Orthop., *163*:210, 1982.
39. Kane, S. H., and Borzell, F. F.: Infantile cortical hyperostosis. Case report. A.J.R., *58*:629, 1947.
40. Katz, J. M., Kirkpatrick, J. A., Papanicolaou, N., and Desai, P.: Case report 139. Skeletal Radiol., *6*:77, 1981.
41. Kaufman, H. J., Mahboubi, S., and Mandell, G. A.: Case report 39. Skeletal Radiol., *2*:109, 1977.
42. Kitchin, I. D.: Atypical case of infantile cortical hyperostosis. J. Bone Joint Surg., *33-B*:248, 1951.
43. Kuhl, J., Harris, G. B. C., Maroteaux, P., and Hansen, H. G.: Ein Beitrag zum Krankheitsbild der infantilen kortikalen Hyperostose. Arch. Kinderheilkd, *179*:209, 1969.
44. Landthaler, G., Loizeau, A., Tron, P., Mallet, E., Le Dosseur, P., and De Menibus, C. H.: Maladie de Caffey chez une mère et ses deux enfants. Arch. Fr. Pediatr., *41*:275, 1984.
45. Langewisch, W. H.: Infantile cortical hyperostosis—familial occurrence in a mother and daughter. J. Pediatr., *87*:323, 1975.
46. MacGregor, M., and Davis, R.: Infantile cortical hyperostosis. Lancet, *2*:1176, 1949.
47. McSweeney, T.: Caffey's syndrome. J. Bone Joint Surg., *45-B*:623, 1963.
48. Marquis, J. R.: Infantile cortical hyperostosis. A report of an unusual case. Radiology, *80*:282, 1967.
49. Meadows, J. L., and Weens, H. S.: Infantile cortical hyperostosis. Acta Radiol., *42*:43, 1954.
50. Melhem, R. E., Najjar, S. S., and Khachadurian, A. K.: Cortical hyperostosis with hyperphosphatemia: A new syndrome. J. Pediatr., *77*:986, 1970.
51. Minton, L. R., and Elliott, J. H.: Ocular manifestations of infantile cortical hyperostosis. Am. J. Ophthalmol., *64*:902, 1967.
52. Mossberger, J. I.: Infantile cortical hyperostosis. Report of a case with observations at autopsy. Am. J. Dis. Child., *80*:610, 1950.
53. Neuhauser, E. B.: Infantile cortical hyperostosis and skull defects. Postgrad. Med., *48*:57, 1970.
54. Newberg, A. H., and Tampas, J. P.: Familial infantile cortical hyperostosis: An update. A.J.R., *137*:93, 1981.
55. Padfield, E., and Hicken, P.: Cortical hyperostosis in infants: A radiological study of 16 patients. Br. J. Radiol., *43*:231, 1970.
56. Pajewski, M., and Vure, E.: Late manifestations of infantile cortical hyperostosis (Caffey's disease). Br. J. Radiol., *40*:90, 1967.
57. Roske, G.: Eine eigenartige Knochenerkrankung im Sauglingsalter. Monatsschr. Kinderheilkd., *47*:385, 1930.
58. Saul, R. A., Lee, W. H., and Stevenson, R. E.: Caffey's disease revisited. Further evidence for autosomal dominant inheritance with incomplete penetration. Am. J. Dis. Child., *136*:56, 1982.
59. Sauterel, L., and Rabinowicz, T.: A new etiologic view of infantile cortical hyperostosis. Ann. Radiol., *4*:211, 1961.
60. Schmitt, M., Metaizeau, J. P., and Prevot, J.: Hyperostose corticale infantile. A propos de deux observations. Ann. Chir. Infant. (Paris), *18*:399, 1977.
61. Scott, E. P.: Infantile cortical hyperostosis: Report of an unusual complication. J. Pediatr., *62*:782, 1963.
62. Sherman, M. S., and Hellyer, D. T.: Infantile cortical hyperostosis. Review of the literature and report of five cases. A.J.R., *63*:212, 1950.
63. Sidbury, J. B., Jr., and Sidbury, J. B.: Infantile cortical hyperostosis. An inquiry into the etiology and pathogenesis. N. Engl. J. Med., *250*:309, 1954.
64. Staheli, L. T., Church, C. C., and Ward, B. H.: Infantile cortical hyperostosis (Caffey's disease). J.A.M.A., *203*:96, 1968.
65. Sutcliffe, J.: Vesico-ureteric reflux in Caffey's disease. (infantile cortical hyperostosis). Ann. Radiol., *10*:687, 1967.
66. Swerdloff, B. A., Ozonoff, M. B., and Gyepes, M. T.: Late recurrence of infantile cortical hyperostosis (Caffey's disease). A.J.R., *108*:461, 1970.
67. Swoboda, W.: Hyperostosis corticalis deformans juvenilis. Helv. Paediatr. Acta., *13*:292, 1958.
68. Taillefer, R., Danais, S., and Marton, D.: Scintigraphic aspect of infantile cortical hyperostosis (Caffey's disease). J. Can. Assoc. Radiol., *34*:12, 1983.
69. Tampas, J. P., Van Buskirk, P., Peterson, O., and Soule, A.: Infantile cortical hyperostosis. J.A.M.A., *175*:491, 1961.
70. Thoman, W. S., and Murphy, R. E.: Infantile cortical hyperostoses. A review of cases with a case report. Radiology, *54*:735, 1950.
71. Ueda, K., Saito, A., Nakano, H., Aosumna, M., Yokota, M., Muraoka, R., and Iwaya, T.: Cortical hyperostosis following long-term administration of prostaglandin E in infants with cyanotic congenital heart disease. J. Pediatr., *97*:834, 1980.
72. Van Biervliet, J. P., Hendrickx, G., and Kramer, P.: Infantile cortical hyperostosis. Caffey disease. Acta Pediatr. Belg., *29*:185, 1976.
73. Van Buchem, F. S., Hadders, H. N., Hansen, J. F., and Woldring, M. G.: Hyperostosis corticalis generalisata. Report of seven cases. Am. J. Med., *33*:387, 1962.
74. Van Buskirk, F. W., Tampas, J. P., and Peterson, O. S., Jr.: Infantile cortical hyperostosis: An inquiry into its familial aspects. A.J.R., *85*:613, 1961.
75. Van Zeben, W.: Infantile cortical hyperostosis. Acta Paediatr., *35*:10, 1948.
76. Veller, K., and Laur, A.: Etiology of infantile cortical hyperostosis (Caffey's syndrome). Fortschr. Geb. Röntgenstr., *79*:446, 1953.
77. Vialatte, J., and Nodot, A.: Hyperostose corticale infantile ou maladie de Caffey. Ann. Pediatr., *43*:699, 1967.
78. Walley, J.: A case of infantile cortical hyperostosis affecting only clavicle and scapula. J. Bone Joint Surg., *35-B*:426, 1953.
79. Wilson, A. K.: Infantile cortical hyperostosis: A review of the literature and report of a case without mandibular involvement. Clin. Orthop., *62*:209, 1969.
80. Yousefzadeh, D. K., Brosman, P., and Jackson, J. H.: Infantile cortical hyperostosis, Caffey's disease involving two cousins. Skeletal Radiol., *4*:141, 1979.

MISCELLANEOUS DYSPLASIAS

Metaphyseal Dysplasia (Pyle's Disease)

Metaphyseal dysplasia, one of the sclerosing bone dysplasias, is characterized by thickening of the medial ends of the clavicle, pubis, and ischium with poor modeling of all long bones with marked "Erlenmeyer-flask" flaring of the long bones, particularly in the distal portions of the femur and the proximal ends of the tibia and fibula. The bony cortices may be thin (Figs. 3–71 and 3–72). There is some sclerosis of the vault and base of the skull, which has caused semantic confusion between metaphyseal and craniometaphyseal dysplasia (in which there is

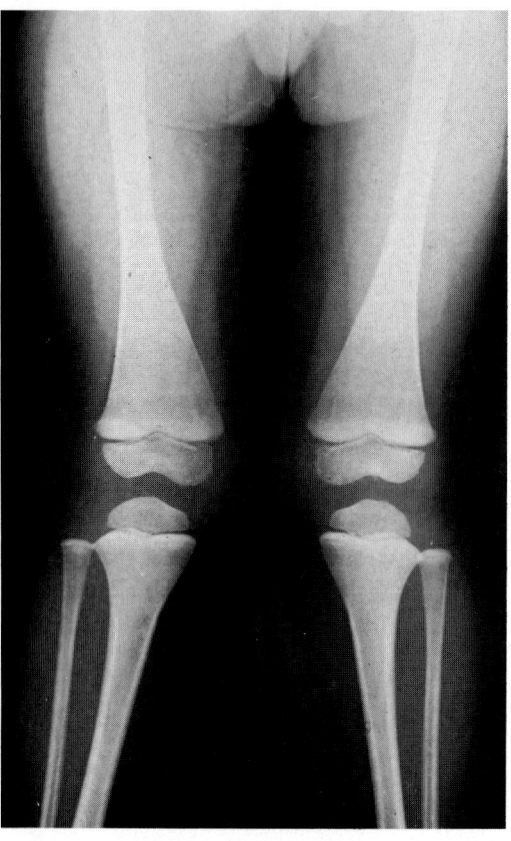

FIGURE 3–71. *Metaphyseal dysplasia of distal femora and proximal tibiae.*

Note the "Erlenmeyer flask" deformity due to a failure of normal cylindrical bone modeling.

massive thickening of the skull). Metaphyseal dysplasia is inherited as an autosomal recessive trait and has no clinical implications except the presence of genu valgum in some patients. Very occasionally there may be a minor degree of lower limb length inequality or minimal scoliosis. A stress fracture due to excessive bone fragility may occur. There is no special treatment. The genu valgum, if severe, may require orthopedic correction by asymmetrical growth arrest of the medial parts of the distal femur, the tibia, or both.[5, 16]

Craniometaphyseal Dysplasia

This dysplasia is characterized by metaphyseal "Erlenmeyer-flask"—type flaring of long bones (similar to Pyle's disease, but of a much lesser degree), and marked sclerosis and thickening of the skull and facial bones. The condition is heterogeneous. There are two forms: (1) an autosomal recessive type, which is very severe and rare; and (2) an autosomal dominant type, which is common and milder in its manifestations.

The severe form manifests itself in infancy with paranasal bossing and progressive distortion of the jaws and facies due to progressive sclerotic thickening of the skull and mandible. In addition to the objectionable cosmetic deformity, malocclusion of the teeth and cranial nerve palsies may be problems. Recurrent nasorespiratory infections develop owing to partial blocking of the paranasal sinuses. Intrasinal pressure may be elevated, requiring neurosurgical intervention.[8, 10, 17]

Craniodiaphyseal Dysplasia

In craniodiaphyseal dysplasia there is progressive thickening of all parts of the skull, leading to cranial nerve palsies, blocking of all sinuses, and mental retardation. The diaphyses of long bones are thickened and irregular. The clinical and therapeutic implications are primarily neurosurgical and maxillofacial.[20]

Osteodysplasty (Melnick-Needles Syndrome)

In osteodysplasty the base of the skull and frontal region are sclerotic, but the anterior fontanelle is large, closing late.

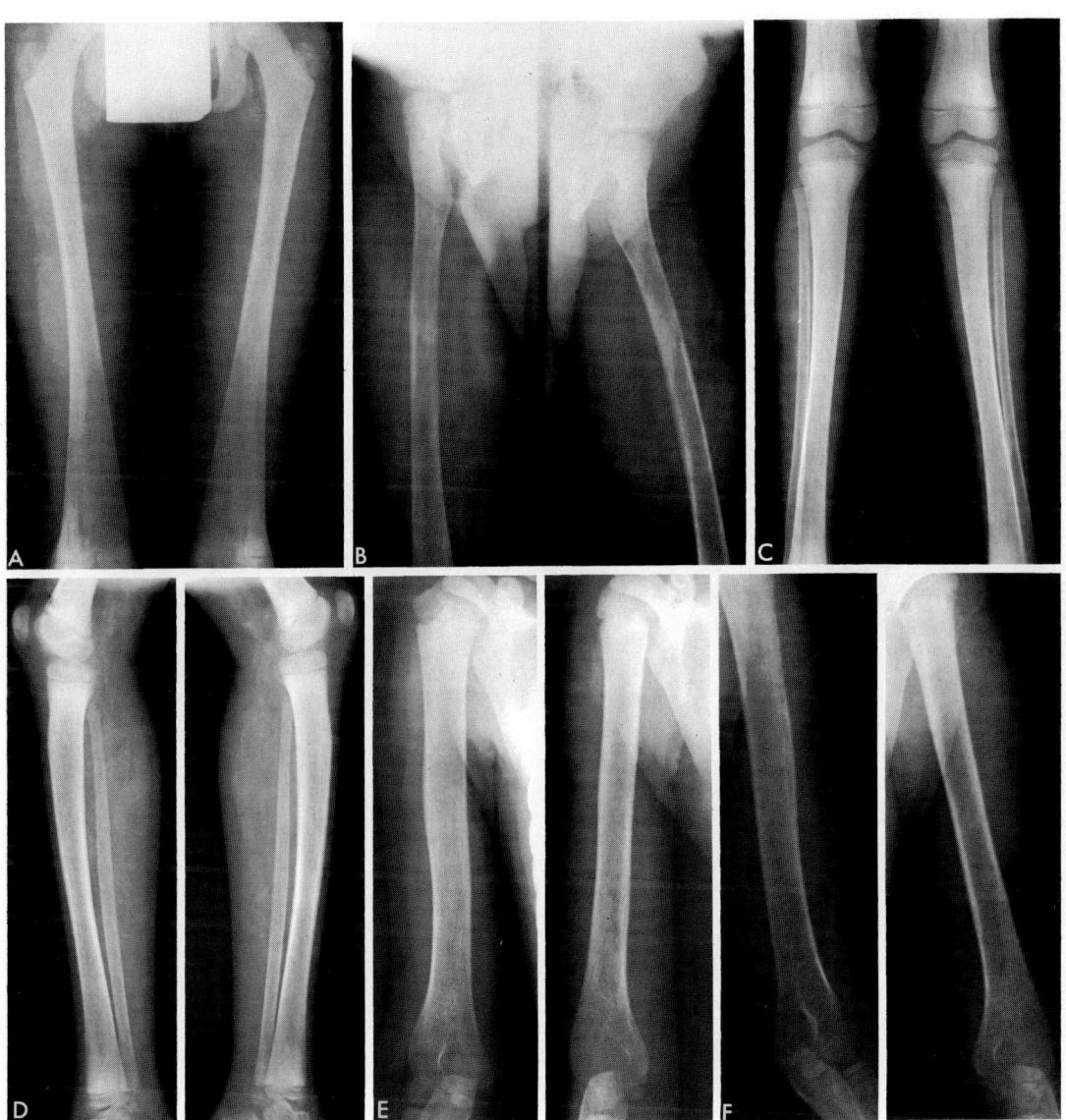

FIGURE 3–72. Metaphyseal dysplasia.

A to **D**. Anteroposterior and lateral views of both lower limbs. Note the flaring of the ends of the femur with "Erlenmeyer flask" deformity. The cortices are thin, and there is apparent narrowing of the mid-diaphysis. **E** and **F**. Anteroposterior and lateral radiograms of humeri.

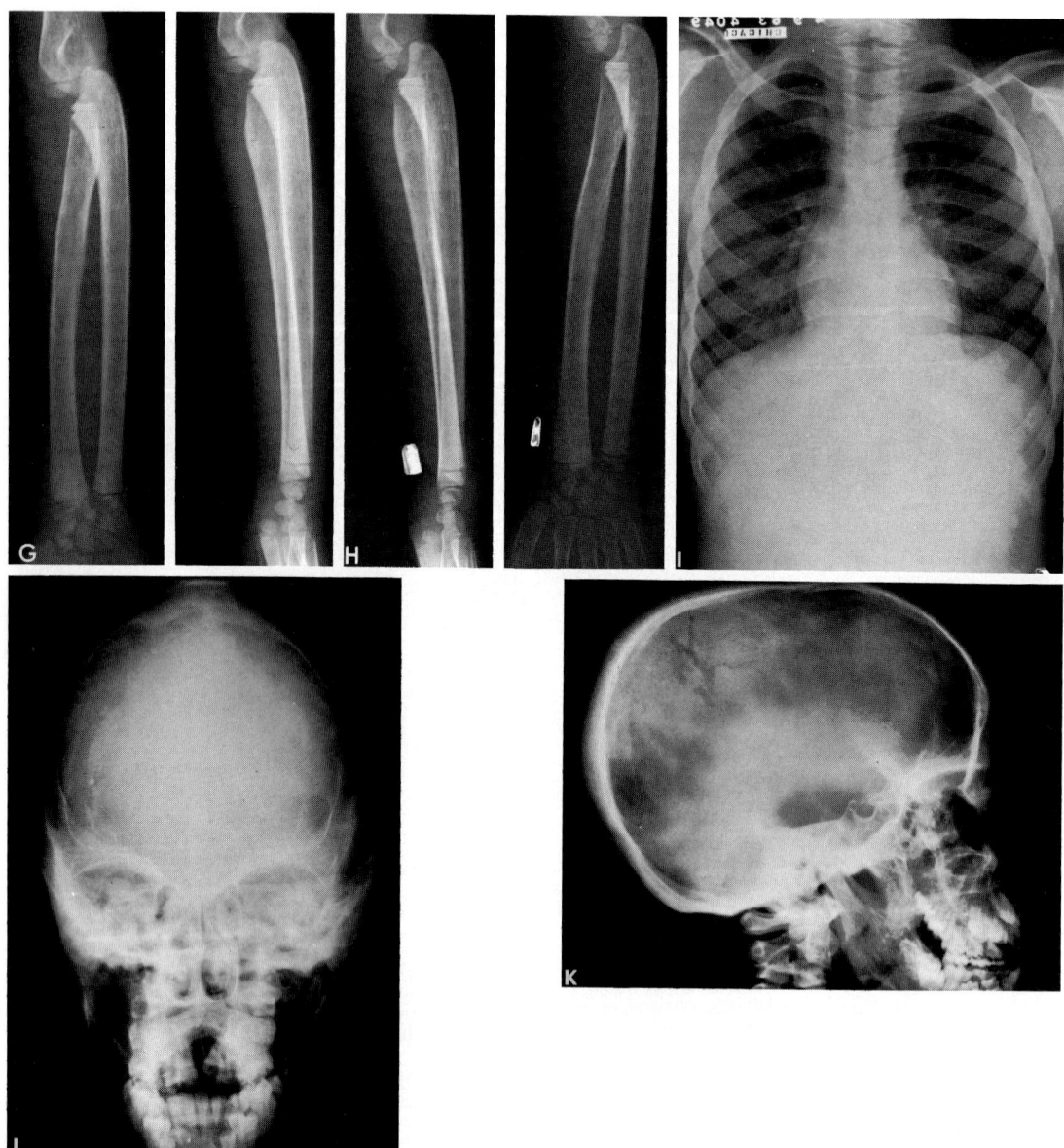

FIGURE 3-72 Continued. Metaphyseal dysplasia.

G and H. Anterior and lateral views of both forearms. I. Posteroanterior view of thoracic cage. Note the thickening of the medial ends of the clavicles. J and K. Skull views showing sclerosis of the base of the skull and of the facial bones.

Part of the syndrome is the metaphyseal flaring of long bones with irregular density, cortical thickening, and bowing (particularly of the humerus, femur, and tibia). Functional disability is minimal, and orthopedic intervention is not required.[13]

References

1. Bakwin, H., and Krida, A.: Familial metaphyseal dysplasia. Am. J. Dis. Child., 53:1521, 1937.
2. Beighton, P., and Cremin, B. J.: Sclerosing Bone Dysplasia. Berlin, Springer-Verlag, 1980.
3. Carlson, D. H., and Harris, G. B. C.: Craniometaphyseal dysplasia. Radiology, 103:147, 1972.
4. David, J. E. A., and Palmer, P. E. S.: Familial metaphyseal dysplasia. J. Bone Joint Surg., 40-B:86, 1958.
5. Gorlin, R. J., Koszalka, M. F., and Spranger, J.: Pyle's disease (familial metaphyseal dysplasia). J. Bone Joint Surg., 52-A:347, 1970.
6. Guibaud, P., Hermier, M., Ajacques, J. C., Boeuf, J. P., and Larbre, F.: La dysplasie cranio-métaphysaire. Pediatrie, 28:149, 1973.
7. Holt, J. F.: The evolution of cranio-metaphyseal dysplasia. Ann. Radiol., 9:209, 1966.
8. Jackson, W. P. U., Albright, F., Drewry, G., Hanelin, J., and Rubin, M. I.: Familial metaphyseal dysplasia and craniometaphyseal dysplasia; their relation to leontiasis ossea and osteopetrosis; disorders of "bone remodeling." Arch. Intern. Med., 94:871, 1954.
9. Komins, C.: Familial metaphyseal dysplasia (Pyle's disease). Br. J. Radiol., 27:670, 1954.
10. Lehman, E. C. H.: Familial osteodystrophy of the skull and face. J. Bone Joint Surg., 39-B:313, 1957.
11. Lievre, J. A., and Fischgold, H.: Leontiasis ossea chez l'enfant (ostéopétrose partielle probable). Presse Méd., 64:763, 1956.
12. Malpuech, G., Raynaud, E. J., Merle, J., and Espinasse, G.: La dysplasie cranio-métaphysaire. Etude clinique et génétique d'une observation. Arch. Fr. Pediatr., 31:71, 1974.
13. Melnick, J. C., and Needles, C. F.: An undiagnosed bone dysplasia. A two family study of four generations and three generations. A.J.R., 97:39, 1966.
14. Millard, D. R., Jr., Maisels, D. O., Batstone, J. H. F., and Yates, B. W.: Craniofacial surgery in craniometaphyseal dysplasia. Am. J. Surg., 113:615, 1967.
15. Pease, C. N., and Newton, G. G.: Metaphyseal dysplasia due to lead poisoning in children. Radiology, 79:233, 1962.
16. Pyle, E.: A case of unusual bone development. J. Bone Joint Surg., 13:874, 1931.
17. Rimoin, D. L., Woodruff, S. L., and Holman, B. L.: Craniometaphyseal dysplasia (Pyle's disease): Autosomal dominant inheritance in a large kindred. Birth Defects Orig. Art. Series, 5:96, 1969.
18. Schwarz, E.: Craniometaphyseal dysplasia. A.J.R., 84:461, 1960.
19. Spranger, J., Albrecht, C., Rohwedder, H. J., and Wiedemann, H. R.: Die Dysosteosklerose, eine Sonderform der generalisierten Osteosklerose. Fortschr. Geb. Röntgenstr., 109:504, 1968.
20. Tucker, A. S., Klein, L., and Antony, G. J.: Craniodiaphyseal dysplasia: Evolution over a 5 year period. Skeletal Radiol., 1:47, 1976.

MARFAN'S SYNDROME

Marfan, a French pediatrician, in 1896 described a developmental disorder of connective tissue that manifests itself in disproportionately long thin limbs, generalized joint laxity, dislocation of the lenses, dissecting aneurysm or prolapsed cardiac valves, and increased prevalence of hernias. He termed the condition *dolichostemelia*, meaning "long, thin limbs."[41] Achard named the syndrome "arachnodactyly" in 1902.[1] A thorough and detailed description of this entity is given by McKusick.[38]

Heredity

Marfan's syndrome is transmitted as an autosomal dominant trait. There is great variability in its clinical expression; many individuals are mildly affected. The term *forme fruste* has been used to designate manifestations of the disorder in a person who has a partial Marfan phenotype. This clinical heterogeneity of Marfan's syndrome has made it difficult to determine its frequency; probably 1.5 per million population is an approximate estimate of its prevalence.

Etiology

The reduced tensile strength of connective tissue in Marfan's syndrome is caused by defective collagen organization. Electromicrographic images have shown loosely organized collagen bundles, and in cell cultures there is a relatively large neutral salt-soluble collagen fraction. The primary abnormality seems to be due to a deficiency of chemically stable collagen cross links.[13]

Clinical Features

Clinical features are characteristic (Figs. 3–73 and 3–74). The physical findings of Marfan's syndrome, however, may be present in other syndromes and conditions (Table 3–9). Historically, photographs of Abraham Lincoln suggest that he was afflicted with Marfan's syndrome. The subjects of the painter El Greco resemble persons with Marfan's syndrome. Patients with the disorder are of tall stature with disproportionately long, thin limbs, usually attaining a height of over 6 feet in adult life. The distal bones of the limbs exhibit the excess length most strikingly (see Fig. 3–73). The ratio of the upper segment (US) of the body to the lower segment (LS) is most useful. The lower segment (measured from the top of the symphysis pubis to the sole) is greater than the upper segment (obtained by subtracting the LS from the total height). The arm span usually exceeds the patient's total height. The US:LS ratio of most patients with Marfan's syndrome falls in the abnormally low range.

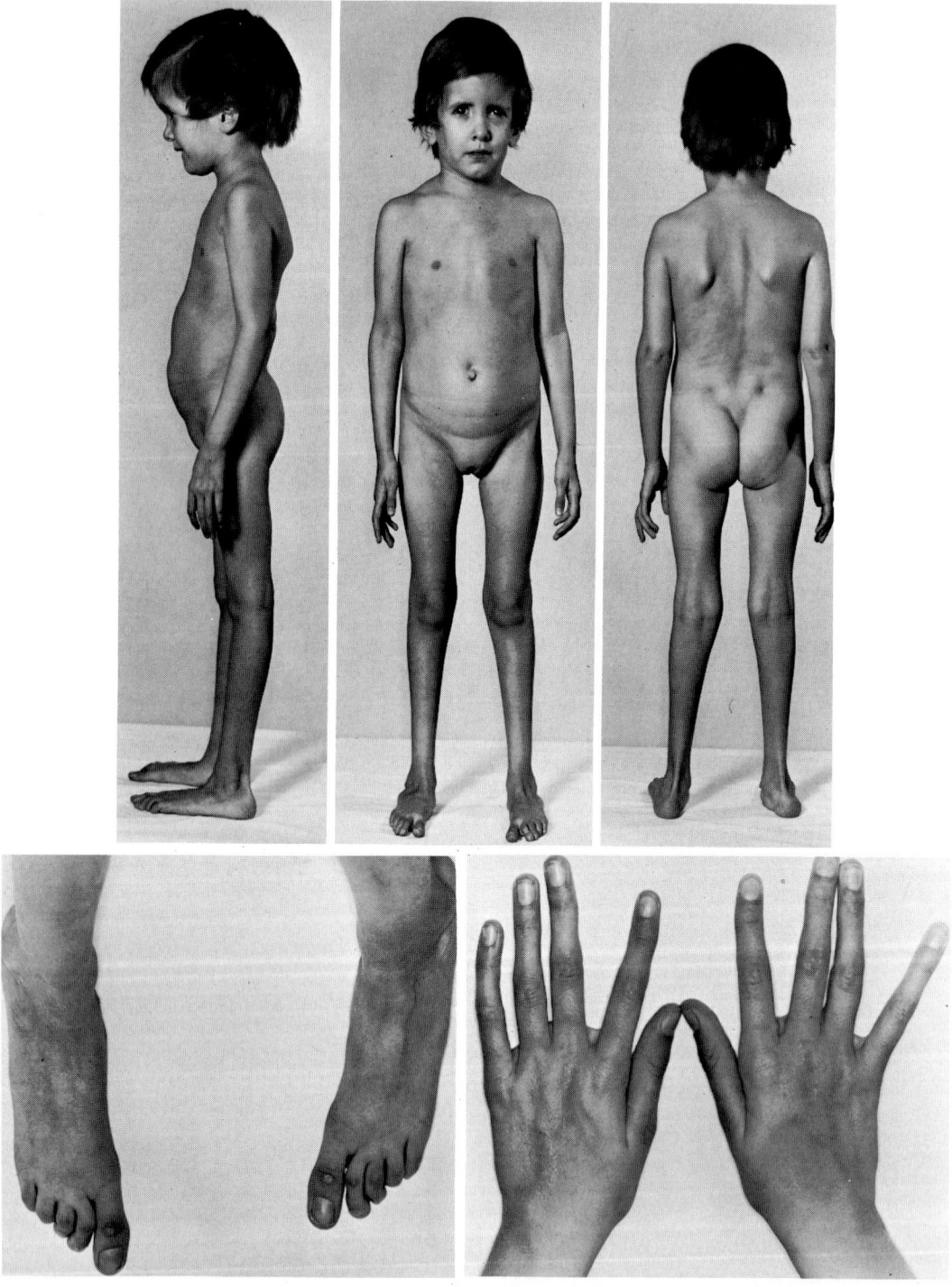

FIGURE 3–73. *Marfan's syndrome (arachnodactyly) in a five-year-old girl.*

Note the thin long limbs and sparse subcutaneous fat. She also has ectopia lentis, ventricular septal defect, and dilation of the ascending aorta.

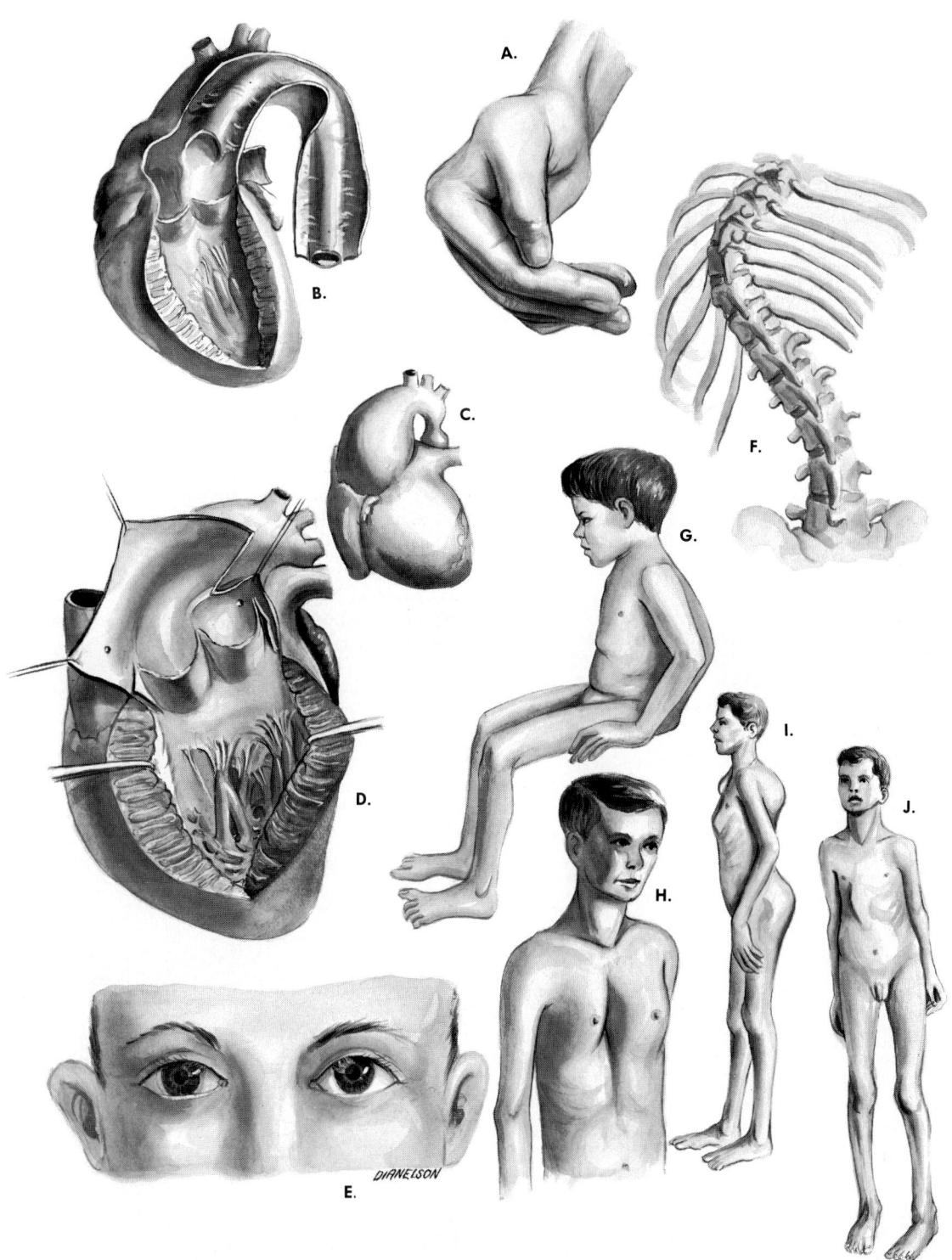

FIGURE 3–74. Marfan's syndrome.

A. Hands. **B** to **D.** Cardiovascular system. **E.** Eyes. **F** and **G.** Spine. **H.** Chest. **I** and **J.** Limbs. (See text for explanation.)

*Table 3–9. Clinical Features Common to Both the Marfan Syndrome and Other Syndromes**

Skeletal
  Homocystinuria
  Congenital contractural arachnodactyly
  Marfanoid hypermobility syndrome
  Eunuchism or delayed puberty
  Klinefelter syndrome (47,XXY)
  Sickle cell anemia
  Goodman camptodactyly syndrome B
  Stickler syndrome
  Syndrome of nerve deafness, eye anomalies, and marfanoid habitus
  Nemaline myopathy
  Syndrome of pigmentary retinal degeneration, cataract, microcephaly, and arachnodactyly
  Myotonic dystrophy
  Multiple endocrine adenomatosis, type III
  Megaduodenum-megacystis syndrome
  Fragilitis oculi
  Achard syndrome
Ocular
  Homocystinuria
  Familial ectopia lentis
  Weill-Marchesani syndrome
  Ehlers-Danlos syndrome, Type VI
  Congenital contractural arachnodactyly
  Marfanoid hypermobility syndrome
  Stickler syndrome
Cardiovascular
  Syphilitic aortitis
  Ehlers-Danlos syndrome, Type IV, and other Ehlers-Danlos variants
  Congenital contractural arachnodactyly
  Marfanoid hypermobility syndrome
  Familial bicuspid aortic valve
  Osteogenesis imperfecta
  Erdheim cystic medial necrosis
  Familial mitral valve prolapse
  Relapsing polychondritis
  Ankylosing spondylitis
  Reiter syndrome

*From Pyeritz, R. E., Murphy, E. A., and McKusick, V. A.: Clinical variability in the Marfan syndrome(s). Birth Defects Original Article Series, 15:155, 1979. Reprinted by permission.

Skull and Facies. Patients with Marfan's syndrome often have dolichocephaly, a high-arched palate, a long narrow face, and prognathism. The increased height of the skull is associated with enlargement of the frontal sinus.

Eyes. The hallmark of ocular involvement is ectopia lentis due to lax ligaments (Fig. 3–74 E). The dislocated lens is best visualized by a slit-lamp examination following dilatation of the pupil. There is usually extreme myopia. Other eye findings are strabismus, cataract, and detached retina.

Cardiovascular System. Dilatation of the ascending aorta, aortic or mitral valve insufficiency or both, septal defects, and aneurysms of the Valsalva sinus may be present (Fig. 3–74 B to D). Aneurysm formation, usually of the dissecting type, is the most common and serious complication, often causing death in early adult life.[3, 14]

Pectus excavatum is common, being caused by excessive longitudinal growth of the ribs (Fig. 3–75 H). The anteroposterior diameter of the thoracic cage is reduced.

Joint Laxity. Severe laxity of the ligaments and joint capsules causes marked pes valgus and genu recurvatum. The patellar tendon is elongated with patella alta. Recurrent dislocation of the patella and voluntary dislocation of the hips are not infrequent. Perilunate dislocations may occur because of excessive carpal ligamentous laxity.[51] The thumb protrudes beyond the ulnar border of the clenched fist as shown in Figure 3–75. This was first reported by Parker and Hare; the clenched fist test is, however, often referred to as the Steinberg sign (Steinberg recommended that it become a part of the routine physical examination as a screening test for Marfan's syndrome).[49, 71] The length of the metacarpal index is increased—this is measured as the average of the radiographic length of the second through fifth metacarpals and divided by the average width at the adjacent midjoint of the respective joints. Occasionally flexion contracture of the interphalangeal joints of the digits does occur in Marfan's syndrome. In the long fingers the greater elongation is in the proximal phalanges (Fig. 3–76). The feet are long and thin, with the greater elongation in the first metatarsal and hallux.

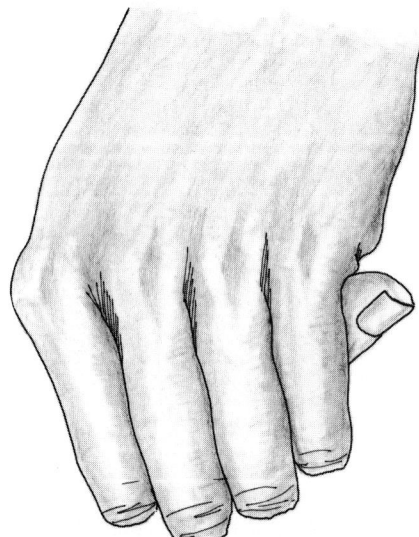

FIGURE 3–75. *Steinberg sign.*

Note the thumb protruding beyond the ulnar border of the hand.

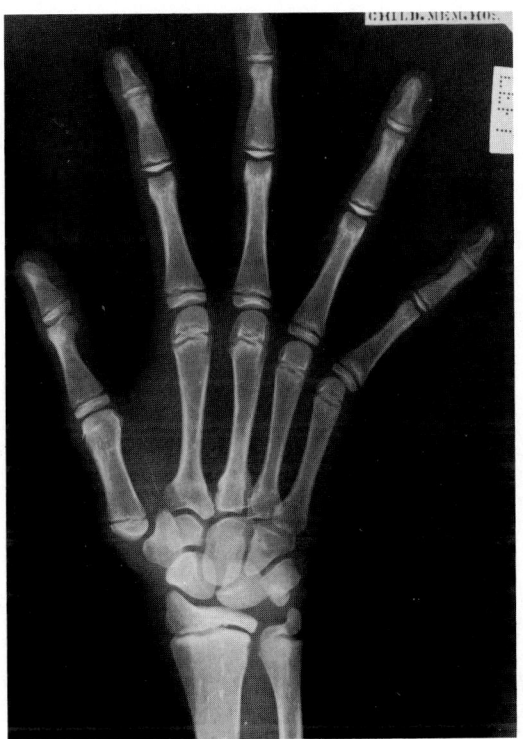

FIGURE 3-76. *Marfan's syndrome.*

Radiogram of the hand, showing the elongated phalanges and metacarpals in a child with Marfan's syndrome.

Muscular underdevelopment and hypotonia are common. Inguinal, femoral and diaphragmatic hernias may be present. Subcutaneous fat is usually sparse.

The vertebral column is elongated with tall vertebral bodies. The position of the sacrum is low in relation to the iliac crests. The spinal canal may appear widened in the lumbar region with concavity of the posterior borders of the vertebral bodies.[48]

Scoliosis. The reported incidence of scoliosis is high, an average 50 per cent (range from 30 to 70 per cent).[58, 75, 76] This is explained by the basic pathology of Marfan's syndrome, which is a connective tissue defect. The onset of Marfan scoliosis is at a younger age than that of idiopathic scoliosis, and often it increases markedly during the years of rapid vertebral growth (Figs. 3-74 F and 3-77). When first observed the degree of curvature varies; often it is not detected early, and the curves are rigid and severe. It behooves the surgeon to examine the spines of patients with Marfan's syndrome carefully for early diagnosis of scoliosis. The curve pattern in Marfan's syndrome is usually double structural (right thoracic and left lumbar) in contrast to the single pattern often seen in idiopathic scoliosis. The rigid severe curve in Marfan's syndrome is often painful. The poor musculature and the pectus excavatum deformity of the thoracic cage further aggravate the impaired cardiorespiratory function, which is frequently already compromised by mitral valve prolapse, aortic dilatation, or other heart anomalies. The importance of early detection and prevention of severe scoliosis in Marfan's syndrome cannot be overemphasized.

Spondylolisthesis, usually of L 5–S 1, is common in Marfan's syndrome; it should be ruled out by lateral and oblique views of the lower lumbar spine.

Associated anomalies, e.g., polysyndactyly, myopathy, and talipes equinovarus, are variable in occurrence.[27, 28]

Differential Diagnosis

There is great clinical heterogeneity and variability of expression in Marfan's syndrome. The diagnosis is made by the clinical findings. There is no biochemical test, as in homocystinuria. The partial Marfan phenotype is referred to sometimes as *forme fruste Marfan.*[55] Strict criteria must be used to make the diagnosis of Marfan's syndrome. These include: (1) tall stature with disproportionately long limbs with a lower upper to lower segment ratio and a higher

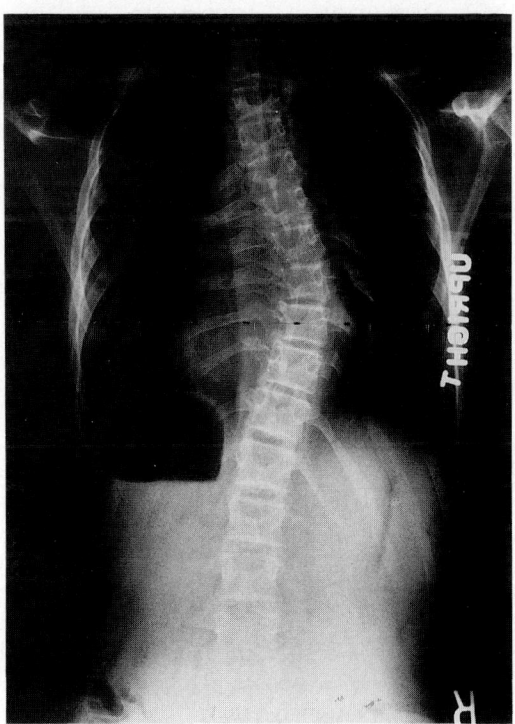

FIGURE 3-77. *Marfan's syndrome with right dorsolumbar scoliosis.*

Table 3–10. Differential Diagnosis of Congenital Contractural Arachnodactyly and Marfan's Syndrome

	Congenital Contractural Arachnodactyly	Marfan's Syndrome
Inheritance	Autosomal dominant	Autosomal dominant
Lens dislocation	Absent	Present
Cardiovascular disease	Absent	Aortic dilation
Joints	Contractural deformity present at birth, maximal at knees, spontaneous improvement with use	Lax patellofemoral joint dislocation, elongation of patellar tendon joint contracture may develop later in adolescence
Limbs	Dolichostenomelia (long, slender)	Dolichostenomelia (long, slender)
Arachnodactyly	Present, with flexion contracture of proximal interphalangeal joints in the hand	Present
Facies	Oval, retrognathia	Normal
Ears	Antihelix has crumpled appearance due to extra and prominant crura, partial obliteration and flattening of helix	Nondistinctive
Spine	Scoliosis	Scoliosis, may be progressive, very severe
Intelligence	Normal	Normal
Prognosis	Good	Variable, death may be due to aortic aneurysm rupture

arm span to height ratio; (2) slit lamp documentation of elongated suspensory ligaments or dislocation of the lens (ectopia lentis); (3) positive echographic and angiographic evidence of dilation of the aorta or of insufficiency of the aortic or mitral valve (or both); (4) arachnodactyly; (5) dolichocephaly, (6) pectus excavatum with decreased anteroposterior diameter of the chest, or scoliosis; (7) and a positive family history. There should be none of the cutaneous changes associated with Ehlers-Danlos syndrome, and homocystinuria should be ruled out by urine test. The differentiation of Marfan's syndrome from congenital contractural arachnodactyly is given in Table 3–10 and from homocystinuria in Table 3–12 (p. 889).

Treatment

There is no specific treatment. Multidisciplinary care is essential in the management of Marfan's syndrome. Orthopedic measures are directed toward control of the spinal deformity and joint laxity. The herniae are treated by the general surgeon. The serious problems due to the cardiovascular defects are managed by the cardiologist and the cardiac surgeon. The ophthalmologist treats the ectopia lentis and the eye defects. Genetic counseling should not be ignored.

Scoliosis. Curves of 15 degrees or less are observed closely for possible progression; if the degree of curvature is greater than 15 degrees and less than 40 degrees, orthotic treatment is indicated. The curves are usually flexible, and excellent alignment can be achieved. The incidence of recurrence of the scoliotic deformity is quite high after discontinuing the orthotic support, however; the curvature may relapse to the original degree or worse. It is best at the outset to make clear to the family the goals of orthotic treatment; i.e., it is an attempt to prevent progression of the scoliosis, if possible.

Spinal fusion with internal instrumentation is indicated when the degree of curvature is greater than 40 to 50 degrees. One can expect solid fusion and maintenance of correction as in idiopathic scoliosis; it is vital, however, to obtain a thorough cardiovascular study to exclude the presence of aortic aneurysm and valvular lesions with incipient cardiac failure.[58]

Spondylolisthesis, if progressive or symptomatic, is treated by lumbosacral fusion.

Joint Laxity. The severe flexible pes planovalgus is of the complex type with sagging at both the talocalcaneonavicular and naviculocuneiform joints (Fig. 3–78). Footwear is a problem, and as the child becomes older he complains of foot strain. Therefore, the feet should not be ignored in Marfan's syndrome. A foot orthosis (U.C.B.L.) is prescribed to support the feet. In the adolescent with painful feet, triple arthrodesis may be required; before it is performed, however, it is vital to make standing anteroposterior roentgenograms of the ankles and stress views to rule out ligamentous instability of the ankle joint. Occasionally the ankle instability and pain are so severe that an arthrodesis of the ankle is indicated.

The recurrent subluxation or dislocation of

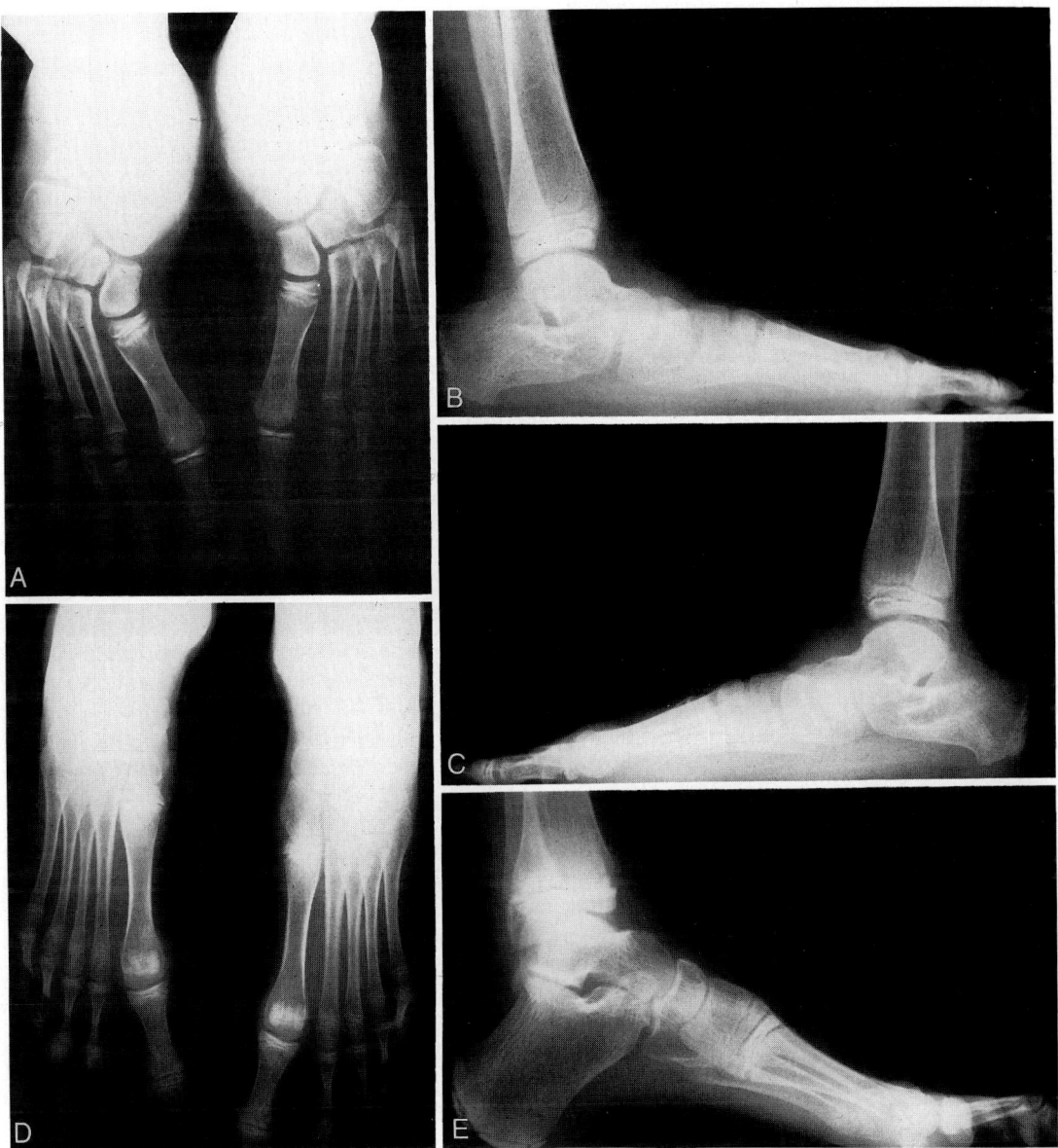

FIGURE 3–78. Deformities of the foot in Marfan's syndrome.

A to **C**. Anteroposterior and lateral radiograms of the feet showing serpentine foot with valgus hindfoot and varus forefoot. **D** and **E**. Severe calcaneocavus deformity. Note the long metatarsals and phalanges.

the patellofemoral joint is treated by the Gallezzi-Dewar operation. If the patella is riding high it should be lowered and anchored in its normal position by the semitendinosis tendon.

Management of recurrent dislocations of the hips, shoulder, acromioclavicular, and other joints is individualized. They pose horrendous problems.

References

1. Achard, C.: Arachnodactylie. Bull. Mem. Soc. Méd. Hôp. Paris, 19:834, 1902.
2. Ambani, L. M., Gelehrter, T. D., and Sheahan, D. G.: Variable expression of Marfan syndrome in monozygotic twins. Clin. Genet., 8:358, 1975.
3. Anderson, R. E., Grondin, C., and Amplatz, K.: The mitral valve in Marfan's syndrome. Radiology, 91:910, 1968.
4. Bailey, J. D., Park, E., and Cowell, C.: Estrogen treatment of girls and constitutional tall stature. Pediatr. Clin. North Am., 28:501, 1981.
5. Beals, R. K.: Hereditary arthro-ophthalmopathy (the Stickler syndrome). Report of a kindred with protrusio acetabuli. Clin. Orthop., 125:32, 1977.
6. Beals, R. K., and Hecht, F.: Congenital contractural arachnodactyly. A heritable disorder of connective tissue. J. Bone Joint Surg., 53-A:987, 1971.
7. Beals, R. K., and Mason, L.: The Marfan skull. Radiology, 140:723, 1981.
8. Becker, K. L.: Marfan's syndrome. Postgrad. Med., 53:216, 1973.
9. Beneux, J., Rigault, P., Pouliquen, J. C., Geffroy, J., Padovani, J. P., Merckx, J., and Guyonvarch, G.: Spine deformity in Marfan's syndrome in childhood. Rev. Chir. Orthop., 64:471, 1978.
10. Bijelic, A.: Cardiovascular changes in Marfan's syndrome. Reumatizam, 22:140, 1975.
11. Birkenstock, W. E., Louw, J. H., Maze, A., and Sladen, R. N.: Combined Ehlers-Danlos and Marfan's syndromes, with a case report. S. Afr. Med. J., 47:2097, 1973.
12. Bjerkreim, I., Skogland, L. B., and Trygstad, O.: Congenital contractural arachnodactyly. Acta Orthop. Scand., 47:250, 1976.
13. Boucek, R. J., Noble, N. L., Gunja-Smith, Z., and Butler, W. T.: The Marfan syndrome: A deficiency in chemically stable collagen cross-links. N. Engl. J. Med., 305:988, 1981.
14. Bowden, D. H., Favara, B. E., and Donahue, J. L.: Marfan's syndrome. Accelerated course in childhood associated with lesions of mitral valve and pulmonary artery. Am. Heart J., 69:96, 1965.
15. Bowers, D.: Marfan's syndrome: The S. family revisited. Can. Med. Assoc. J., 89:337, 1963.
16. Brenton, D. P., Dow, C. J., James, J. I. P., Hay, R. L., and Wynne-Davies, R.: Homocystinuria and Marfan's syndrome. A comparison. J. Bone Joint Surg., 54-B:277, 1972.
17. Carter, C. O., and Fairbank, T. J.: Marfan's syndrome. In The Genetics of Locomotor Disorders. London, Oxford University Press, 1974, p. 141.
18. Chemke, J., Nisani, R., Feigl, A., Garty, R., Cooper, M., Barash, Y., and Duksin, D.: Homozygosity for autosomal dominant Marfan syndrome. J. Med. Genet., 21:173, 1984.
19. Cooperman, E. M.: Letter: Marfan's syndrome and Sherlock Holmes. Can. Med. Assoc. J., 112:423, 1975.
20. Cooperman, E. M.: Letter: More on Sherlock Holmes. Can. Med. Assoc. J., 113:1024, 1975.
21. Edwards, R. H.: Congenital Marfan syndrome. Birth Defects, 11:329, 1975.
22. Fahey, J. J.: Muscular and skeletal changes in arachnodactyly. Arch. Surg., 39:741, 1939.
23. Fauchet, R., and Stagnara, P.: Scoliosis in arachnodactyly. Z. Orthop., 113:566, 1975.
24. Floret, D., Rosenberg, D., Robert, J. M., and Monnet, P.: Associated Duchenne's disease and Marfan disease. Pediatrie, 28:331, 1973.
25. Fournier, C.: Cardiovascular lesions in Marfan's syndrome. Coeur Med. Interne, 16:331, 1977.
26. Fried, K., and Krakowsky, D.: Probable autosomal recessive Marfan syndrome. J. Med. Genet., 14:359, 1977.
27. Fried, K., and Mundel, G.: Polysyndactyly and Marfan's syndrome. J. Med. Genet., 11:141, 1974.
28. Goebel, H. H., Muller, J., and DeMeyer, W.: Myopathy associated with Marfan's syndrome. Neurology, 23:1257, 1973.
29. Golden, R. L., and Lakin, H. M.: The forme fruste in Marfan's syndrome. N. Engl. J. Med., 260:797, 1959.
30. Gruber, M. A., Graham, T. P., Engel, E., and Smith, C.: Marfan syndrome with contractural arachnodactyly and severe mitral regurgitation in a premature infant. J. Pediatr., 93:80, 1978.
31. Halpern, B. L., Char, F., Murdoch, J. L., Horton, W. B., and McKusick, V. A.: A prospectus on the prevention of aortic rupture in the Marfan syndrome with data on survivorship without treatment. Johns Hopkins Med. J., 129:123, 1971.
32. Heldrich, F. J., and Wright, C. E.: Marfan's syndrome. Diagnosis in the neonate. Am. J. Dis. Child., 114:419, 1967.
33. Herrmann, J., France, T. D., Spranger, J. W., Opitz, J. M., and Wiffler, C.: The Stickler syndrome (hereditary arthroophthalmopathy). Birth Defects, 11:76, 1975.
34. Hohn, A. R., and Webb, H. M.: Cardiac studies of infant twins with Marfan's syndrome. Am. J. Dis. Child., 122:526, 1971.
35. Kontras, S. B.: Congenital contractural arachnodactyly. In: Bergsma, D. (ed.): Disorders of Connective Tissue. Birth Defects Orig. Art. Series, 11:63, 1975.
36. Lipson, E. H., Visekul, C., and Herrmann, J.: The clinical spectrum of congenital contractural arachnodactyly. Z. Kinderheilkd., 118:1, 1974.
37. McKusick, V. A.: Heritable disorders of connective tissue: Newer aspects. Birth Defects, 2:58, 1966.
38. McKusick, V. A.: The Marfan syndrome. In Heritable Disorders of Connective Tissue. 4th Ed. St. Louis, Mosby, 1972, p. 61.
39. McKusick, V. A.: The classification of heritable disorders of connective tissue. In: Bergsma, D. (ed.): Disorders of Connective Tissue. Birth Defects Orig. Art. Series, 11:1, 1975.
40. McKusick, V. A., Traisman, H. S., and Bianchine, J. W.: More speculation on Marfan syndrome. J. Pediatr., 80:530, 1972.
41. Marfan, A. B.: Un cas de déformation congénitale des quatre membres plus prononcée aux extrémités caractérisée par l'allongement des os avec un certain degré d'amincissement. Bull. Mem. Soc. Méd. Hôp. Paris, 13:220, 1896.
42. Mark, H., and Hershkowitz, M.: Letter: Endocarditis and the Marfan's syndrome. Ann. Intern. Med., 83:120, 1975.
43. Moe, J. P.: Marfan's disorder in scoliosis. In Zorab, P. A. (ed.): Scoliosis. 5th Symposium, September, 1976. London. Academic Press, 1977, p 257.
44. Murdoch, J. L.: Ectopia lentis as part of the Marfan's syndrome. Birth Defects, 7:167, 1971.
45. Murdoch, J. L., Walker, B. A., and Halpern, B. L.: Life expectancy and causes of death in the Marfan's syndrome. N. Engl. J. Med., 286:804, 1972.

46. Murdoch, J. L., Walker, B. A., and McKusick, V. A.: Parental age effects on the occurrence of new mutations for the Marfan syndrome. Ann. Hum. Genet., 35:331, 1972.
47. Neimann, N., Rauber, G., Marchal, C., Vidailhet, M., and Fall, M.: Maladie de Marfan chez un nouveau-né avec atteintes polyviscerales. Etude anatomo-clinique. Ann. Pediatr., 40:1, 1968.
48. Nelson, T. J.: Marfan syndrome with specific reference to congenital enlargement of the spinal canal. Br. J. Med., 31:561, 1958.
49. Parker, A. S., and Hare, H. F.: Arachnodactyly. Radiology, 45:220, 1945.
50. Penchaszadeh, V. B., Barreiro, C., and Grotso, J. A.: Marfan syndrome with congenital contractures. Birth Defects, 11:109, 1975.
51. Pennes, D. R., Braunstein, E. M., and Shirazi, K. K.: Carpal ligamentous laxity with bilateral perilunate dislocation in Marfan syndrome. Skeletal Radiol., 13:62, 1985.
52. Pernod, J., Gerbeaux, A., Gagnol, J. P., Richard, D., Gay, J., and Droniou, J.: Ultrasound echography in mitral insufficiency. Ann. Med. Interne (Paris), 128:939, 1977.
53. Phornphutkul, C., Rosenthal, A., and Nadas, A. S.: Cardiac manifestations of Marfan syndrome in infancy and childhood. Circulation, 47:587, 1973.
54. Polakowski, L., Pucher, A., and Wlodarczyk, R.: Scoliosis in Marfan's syndrome treated by Harrington instrumentation and spinal fusion. Chir. Narzadow Ruchu Ortop. Pol., 40:59, 1975.
55. Pyeritz, R. E., Murphy, E. A., and McKusick, V. A.: Clinical variability in the Marfan syndrome(s). Birth Defects, 15:155, 1979.
56. Redmond, D. A.: Letter: Marfan's syndrome and Sherlock Holmes. Can. Med. Assoc. J., 113:19, 1975.
57. Roberts, W. C., and Honig, H. S.: The spectrum of cardiovascular disease in the Marfan syndrome: A clinico-morphologic study of 18 necropsy patients and comparison to 151 previously reported necropsy patients. Am. Heart J., 104:115, 1982.
58. Robins, P. R., Moe, J. H., and Winter, R. B.: Scoliosis in Marfan's syndrome. Its characteristics and results of treatment in thirty-five patients. J. Bone Joint Surg., 57-A:358, 1975.
59. Rubisz-Brezezinska, J., Seferowicz, E., and Gruszczynski, J.: Marfan's syndrome with coexisting psoriasis. Przegl. Dermatol., 61:319, 1974.
60. Ruchti-Rous, M., and Hauser, H.: Syndrome de Marfan. Complications aortiques étudiées par scanographie. Arch. Mal. Coeur, 76:21, 1983.
61. Sanger, R. G., and Weiman, W. B.: The C.C.A. syndrome (congenital contractural arachnodactyly): A new differential syndrome for Marfan's syndrome and homocystinuria. Oral Surg., 40:354, 1975.
62. Savini, R., Cervellati, S., and Beroaldo, E.: Spinal deformities in Marfan's syndrome. Ital. J. Orthop. Traumatol., 6:19, 1980.
63. Schoenfeld, M. R.: Nicolo Paganini. Musical magician and Marfan mutant? J.A.M.A., 239:40, 1978.
64. Schwartz, H.: Abraham Lincoln and aortic insufficiency. The declining health of the president. Calif. Med., 116:82, 1972.
65. Sensenig, D. M., and LaMarche, P.: Marfan's syndrome and spontaneous pneumothorax. Am. J. Surg., 139:602, 1980.
66. Shahin, W., Eshkol, D., and Levy, M. J.: Valve replacement for mitral insufficiency in an infant with Marfan's syndrome. J. Pediatr. Surg., 4:350, 1969.
67. Sinclair, R. J. G., Kitchin, A. H., and Turner, R. W. D.: The Marfan syndrome. Q. J. Med., 54:19, 1960.
68. Skovby, F., and McKusick, V. A.: Estrogen treatment of tall stature in girls with the Marfan syndrome. Birth Defects, 13:155, 1977.
69. Smith, R.: Marfan's disorder and scoliosis. In Zorab, P. A. (ed.): Scoliosis 5th Symposium, London, September 1976. London, Academic Press, 1977, p. 301.
70. Steinberg, I.: Dilatation of the aortic sinuses in the Marfan syndrome: Roentgen findings in five new cases. A.J.R., 83:302, 1960.
71. Steinberg, I.: A simple screening test for the Marfan syndrome. A.J.R., 97:118, 1966.
72. Strand, R. D., and Eisenberg, H. M.: Anterior sacral meningocele in association with Marfan syndrome. Radiology, 99:653, 1971.
73. Walker, B., and Murdoch, J. L.: The wrist sign. A useful physical finding in the Marfan syndrome. Arch. Intern. Med., 126:276, 1970.
74. Wenger, D. R., Ditkoff, T. J., Herring, J. A., and Mauldin, D. M.: Protrusio acetabuli in Marfan's syndrome. Clin. Orthop., 147:134, 1980.
75. Wilner, H. I., and Finby, N.: Skeletal manifestations in the Marfan syndrome. J.A.M.A., 187:490, 1964.
76. Winter, R. B.: The surgical treatment of scoliosis in Marfan's syndrome. In Zorab, P. A. (ed.): Scoliosis 5th Symposium, London, September 1976. London, Academic Press, 1977, p. 283.
77. Winter, R. B.: Severe spondylolisthesis in Marfan's syndrome: Report of two cases. J. Pediatr. Orthop., 2:51, 1982.

CONGENITAL CONTRACTURAL ARACHNODACTYLY

This rare syndrome resembles and has been confused with Marfan's syndrome. In fact, the case Marfan described in 1896 was actually congenital contractural arachnodactyly.[17] Epstein and associates described a case in 1968.[5] In 1971, Beals and Hecht delineated this syndrome in a report of two kindred.[3] Congenital contractural arachnodactyly is differentiated from Marfan's syndrome by the absence of lens dislocation and heart disease, and the presence of joint contractures, maximal at the knee, which spontaneously improve with growth and walking (see Table 3–10). Inheritance of congenital contractural arachnodactyly is by autosomal dominant transmission.

Clinical Features

The head is oval. There is a tendency to retrognathia and a small mouth. The crumpled appearance of the antihelix is distinctive—it is caused by extra and prominent crura in the antihelix, partial obliteration of the concha, and flattening of the helix (Fig. 3–79 A). There may be mild restriction of range of motion of the temporomandibular joints. Intelligence is normal.

The joint contractures in congenital contractural arachnodactyly are present at birth (Fig. 3–79 B and C). The knee flexion contracture is the most severe; it may be as great as 90 degrees and delay walking. The hips are normal. The

Congenital contractural arachnodactyly. Acta Orthop. Scand., *47*:250, 1976.
5. Epstein, C. J., Graham, C. B., Hodgkins, W. E., Hecht, F., and Motulsky, A. G.: Hereditary dysplasia of bone with kyphoscoliosis, contractures, and abnormally shaped ears. J. Pediatr., *73*:379, 1968.
6. Grenier, B., Laugier, J., Soutoul, J., and Desbuquois, G.: Maladie de Marfan et arthrogrypose. A propos d'un cas chez un nouveau-né. Ann. Pediatr., *45*:1, 1969.
7. Hale, M. S., Rodman, H. D., and Lipshin, J.: Congenital contractural arachnodactyly. West. J. Med., *120*:74, 1974.
8. Hecht, F., and Beals, R. K.: "New" syndrome of congenital contractural arachnodactyly originally described by Marfan in 1896. Pediatrics, *49*:574, 1972.
9. Hernandez, R., Poznanski, A. K., and Hensinger, R.: Case Report 16. Skeletal Radiol., *1*:175, 1977.
10. Ho, N.-K., and Khoo, T.-K.: Congenital contractural arachnodactyly. Report of a neonate with advanced bone age. Am. J. Dis. Child., *133*:639, 1979.
11. Kontras, S. B.: Congenital contractural arachnodactyly. Birth Defects Orig. Art. Series, *11*:63, 1975.
12. Langenskiöld, A.: Congenital contractural arachnodactyly. Report of a case and of an operation for knee contracture. J. Bone Joint Surg., *67-B*:44, 1985.
13. Lipson, E. H., Viseskul, C., and Herrmann, J.: The clinical spectrum of congenital contractural arachnodactyly. A case with congenital heart disease. Z. Kinderheilkd., *118*:1, 1974.
14. Lowry, R. B., and Guichon, B. C.: Congenital contractural arachnodactyly: A syndrome simulating Marfan's syndrome. Can. Med. Assoc. J., *107*:531, 1972.
15. McKusick, V. A.: More speculation on Marfan syndrome. J. Pediatr., *80*:530, 1972.
16. MacLeod, P. M., and Fraser, F. C.: Congenital contractural arachnodactyly (a heritable disorder of connective tissue distinct from Marfan's syndrome). Am. J. Dis. Child., *126*:810, 1973.
17. Marfan, M.: Un cas de déformation congénitale des quatre membres, plus prononcée aux extrémités, caractérisée par l'allongement des os avec un certain degré d'amincissement. Bull. Soc. Méd. Hôp. Paris, *13*:220, 1896.
18. Meinecke, P., Schaefer, E., and Passarge, E.: Congenitale kontrakurelle Arachnodactylie (CCA Syndrom) eine autosomal dominant erbliche Bindegewebser Krankung. Klin. Paediatr., *195*:64, 1983.
19. Passarge, E.: A syndrome resembling congenital contractural arachnodactyly. Birth Defects Orig. Art. Series, *11*:53, 1975.
20. Penchaszadeh, V. B., Barreiro, C., and Groiso, J. A.: Marfan syndrome with congenital contractures. Birth Defects Orig. Art. Series, *11*:109, 1975.
21. Poznanski, A. K., and LaRowe, P. C.: Radiographic manifestations of the arthrogryposis syndrome. Radiology, *95*:353, 1970.
22. Steg, N. L.: Congenital contractural arachnodactyly in a Black family. Birth Defects Orig. Art. Series, *11*:57, 1975.

CLEIDOCRANIAL DYSPLASIA (CLEIDOCRANIAL DYSOSTOSIS)

This skeletal dysplasia is characterized by deficient or imperfect ossification of bones formed in membrane, principally the clavicles, cranium, and pelvis. The bones preformed in cartilage, however, are also affected, especially the short tubular bones in the hands and feet. The terminal phalanges are short and pointed, and there may be extra epiphyses at the proximal ends of the metacarpals and metatarsals. The name *hereditary cleidocranial dysostosis* was given by Marie and Sainton in 1898.[27] Rhinehart and Soule[33, 36] referred to the condition by a more general term, *mutational dysostosis.*

Inheritance

The dysplasia is inherited as an autosomal dominant trait.[10, 20] Approximately two thirds of the reported cases are familial, and one third, sporadic.[36] There is no sex predilection.

Etiology

This dysplasia results from failure of ossification at the midline junctions of bones, particularly those of membranous origin. The exact cause is unknown.

Clinical and Radiographic Features

The disease is usually evident in the first two years of life, though it may be discovered at any age. The typical appearance consists of a large head, a relatively small face, drooping shoulders, and a narrow chest (Fig. 3–81 A to D).

There is considerable variation in the distribution of the lesions.

Clavicles. One or both clavicles may be affected (Fig. 3–81 E). The most common defect is loss of the lateral (acromial) end of the clavicle; next in frequency is failure of development of the middle third of the clavicle, with the sternal and acromial portions present but unfused; on rare occasions, the sternal third or the entire clavicle may be absent.

Clinically, the defect may be palpable. When it is bilateral, the shoulders have abnormal mobility and can be approximated in front of the chest to the extent that they touch each other (Fig. 3–81 D). The scapulae are somewhat small and have a winged appearance. On occasion, subluxation of the humeral heads may be noted.

Skull. Ossification of the membranous portion of the cranium is imperfect, but the base is unaffected (Fig. 3–81 F and G). The membranous portion is poorly mineralized, and there are multiple wormian bones.

Closure of the sutures is delayed and may fail to take place. The anterior fontanelle is

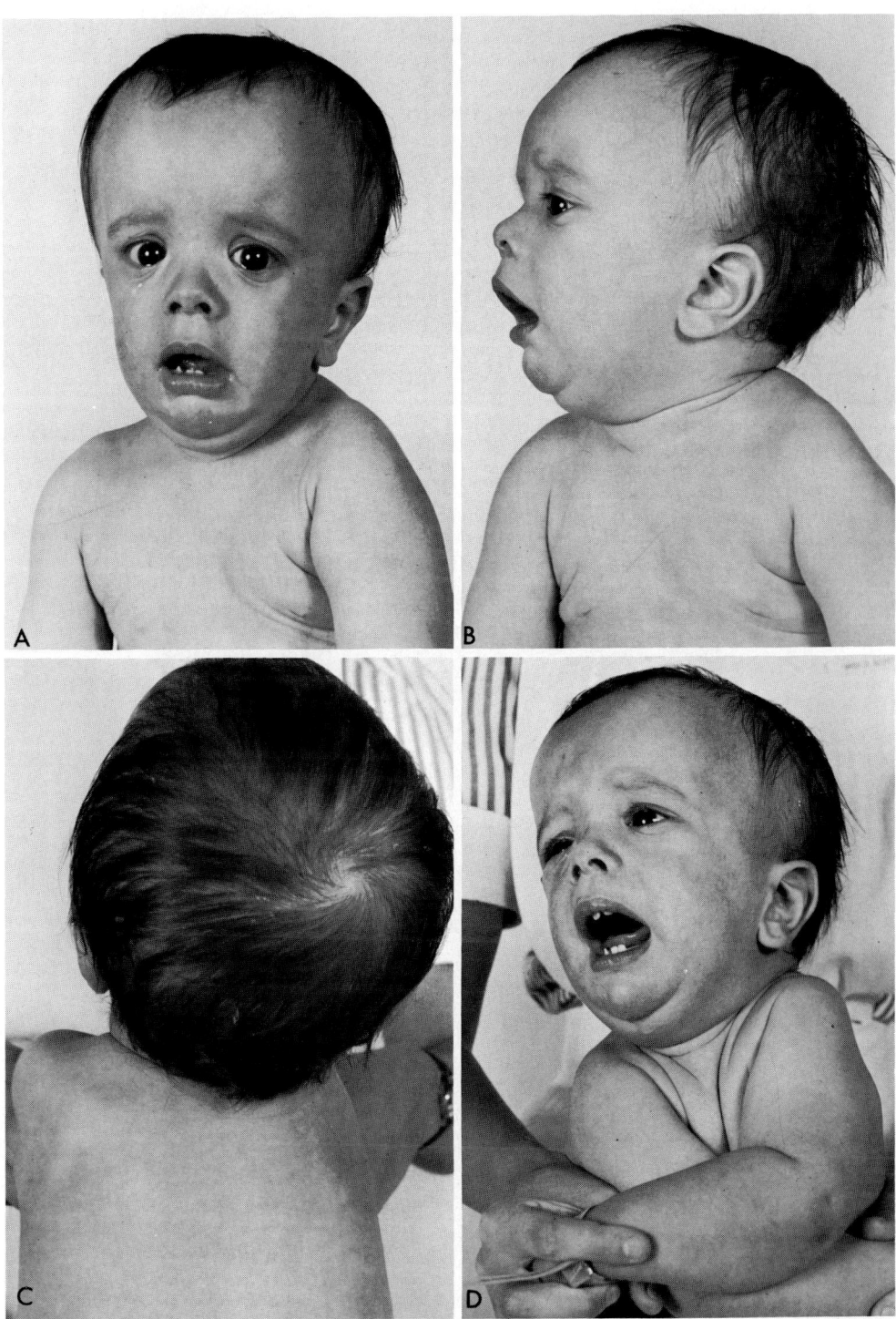

FIGURE 3–81. Cleidocranial dysostosis.

A to **D**. Clinical appearance of the patient. Note the enlarged head. The shoulders can be approximated because of the absence of the clavicles (**D**).

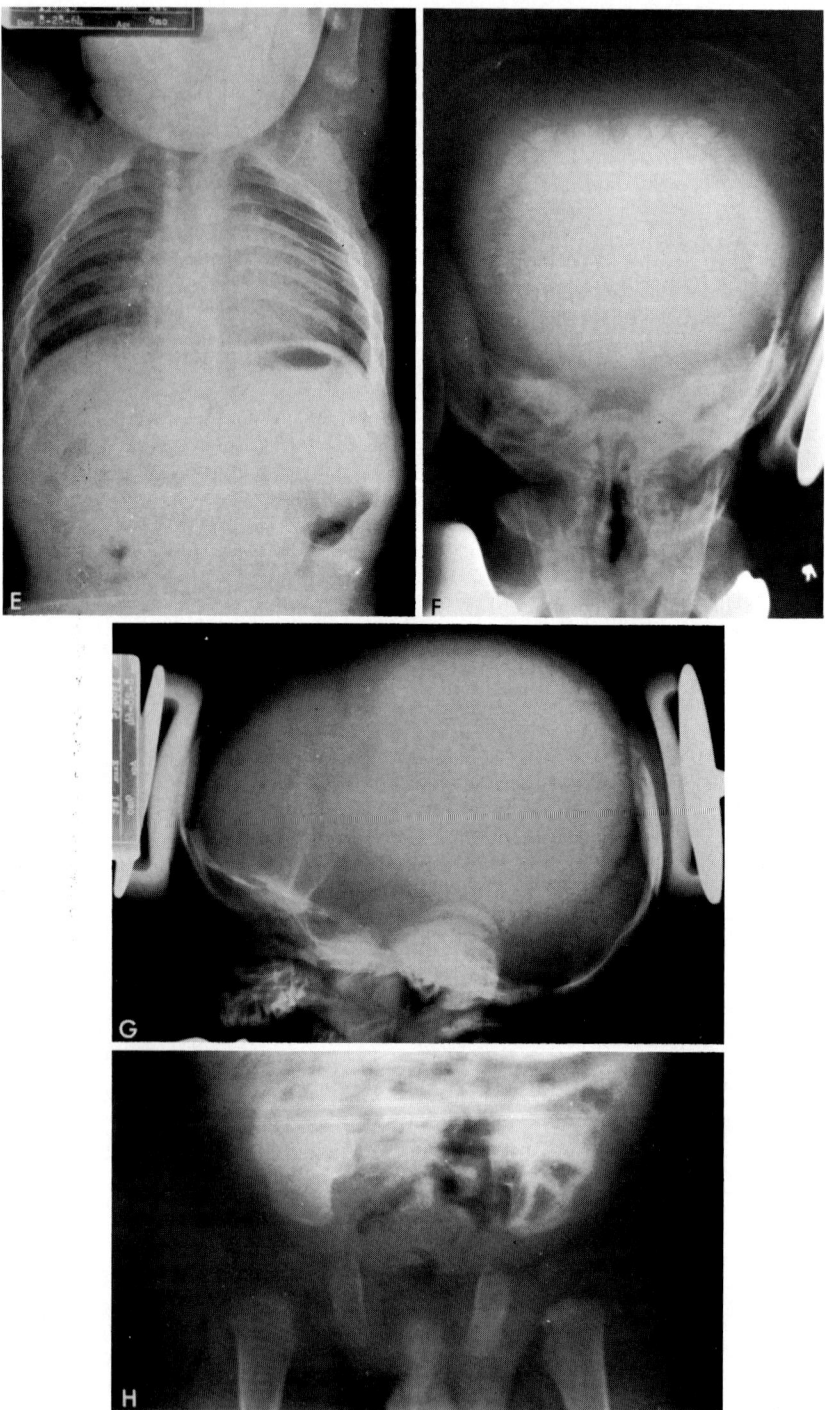

FIGURE 3–81 Continued. Cleidocranial dysostosis.

E. Radiogram of the thorax. Note the bilateral absence of the clavicles. **F** and **G.** Posteroanterior and lateral views of the skull. Note the enlarged anterior fontanelle as well as the sutures and bossing. **H.** Pelvis and hips. Note the absence of ossification of the bodies and descending rami of the pubis. There is also delayed ossification in the inferior rami of the ischium.

enlarged, sometimes in severe cases reaching to the level of the orbital ridges; in some cases, it may never close, persisting even to adult life. There may be a fontanelle in the sphenoid or mastoid region.

The frontal and paranasal sinuses are delayed in development—they are small or may be absent. The nasal, lachrymal, and malar bones may be hypoplastic or completely absent. The zygomatic bones are poorly developed. The maxilla is underdeveloped, and the mandible may fail to fuse at its symphysis.

Clinically, there is frontal, parietal, and occipital bossing. The head is brachycephalic, and its interparietal diameter is widened.

The face is small. The eyes are set wider apart than normal. The arch of the palate is high and narrow. The chin is prognathous. Deciduous teeth erupt normally, but they may be retained longer than usual. Commonly, the eruption of permanent teeth is delayed, and they are consequently maldeveloped.

Pelvis. Ossification of the pelvis may be faulty and incomplete in varying degrees (Fig. 3–81 H). Involvement is almost always bilateral. The symphysis pubis remains relatively wide. The conjoint rami are incompletely fused, with a decrease in their normal thickness. There may be widening of the sacroiliac joint.

Unilateral or bilateral coxa vara of the infantile type is not infrequently found associated with cleidocranial dysostosis. Occasionally the hips may be dislocated.

Spine. The neural arches in both the thoracic and lumbar spine may fail to unite (spina bifida occulta). Occasionally scoliosis is present.

Thoracic Cage. There may be an increase in the slant of the ribs and deficiency of the manubrium of the sternum.

Hands and Feet. Ossification of the carpal and tarsal bones is delayed. The terminal phalanges are short, pointed, hypoplastic, or even absent (Fig. 3–82). There are extra epiphyses at the proximal ends of the second through the fifth metatarsals and metacarpals, which thus have epiphyses at both proximal and distal ends. The second metacarpal is unusually long, with the additional epiphysis at its base enlarged.

Neuromuscular. The defective clavicle may be associated with muscular abnormalities, such as absence or hypoplasia of the clavicular portion of the sternocleidomastoid muscle and the anterior fibers of the deltoid. Irritation of the brachial plexus is rare, but can occur with resultant pain and numbness.

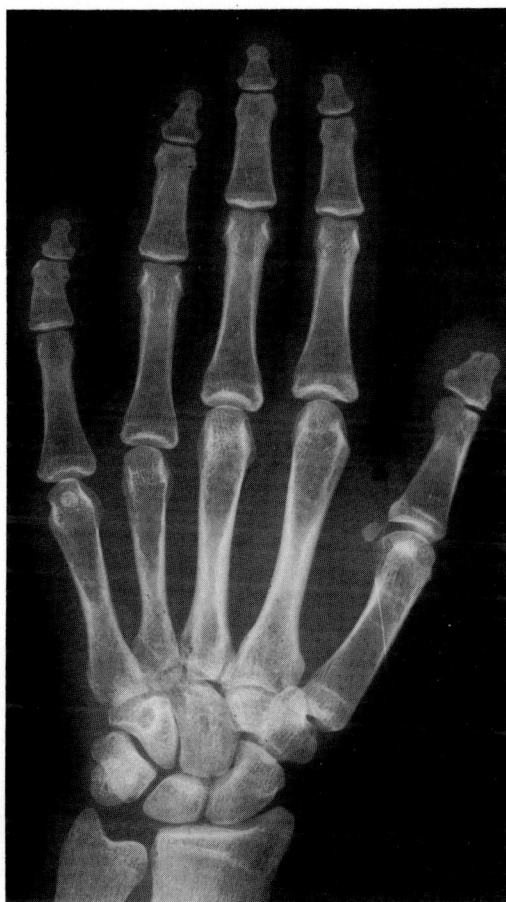

FIGURE 3–82. Radiograms of the hand in an adult with cleidocranial dysplasia.

Note the shortening of the distal phalanges and the minimal clinodactyly of the fifth finger. The second metacarpal is relatively long. (From Poznanski, A. K.: The Hand in Radiologic Diagnosis. Philadelphia, W. B. Saunders, 1984. Reprinted by permission.)

Treatment

Though the deformities are multiple and sometimes cosmetically not pleasing, the dysplasia causes little, if any, functional disability. If the clavicular fragments compress the brachial plexus, they may have to be excised to relieve the pressure. The associated coxa vara, if present, is treated by valgus osteotomy of the proximal femurs. The abnormal teeth require dental care.

References

1. Anspach, W. E., and Heupel, R. G.: Familial cleidocranial dysostosis (cleidal dysostosis). Am. J. Dis. Child., 58:786, 1939.
2. Broitman, H., Mancinelli, S., and Gallegos, X.: Cleidocranial dysostosis. Rev. Chil. Pediatr., 51:124, 1980.

3. Burdca, M., Wexler, T., and Negrescu, D.: Cleidocranial dysostosis. Rev. Pediatr. Obstet. Ginecol. (Pediatr.), 23:425, 1974.
4. Carter, C. O., and Fairbank, T. J.: Cleidocranial dysplasia. In The Genetics of Locomotor Disorders. London, Oxford Univ. Press, 1974, pp. 67–68.
5. Chung, S. M. K., and Nissenbaum, M. M.: Congenital and developmental defects of the shoulder. Orthop. Clin. North Am., 6:381, 1975.
6. Cole, W. R., Chir, B., and Levin, S.: Cleidocranial dysostosis. Br. J. Radiol., 24:549, 1951.
7. Delaire, J., and Le Diascorn, H.: Les dysostoses cleidocraniennes. Aspects cliniques. Actual. Odontostomatol. (Paris), 28:413, 1974.
8. Dionisio, A.: Nota su un caso di malattia di Marie e Sainton. Minerva Med., 53:141, 1962.
9. Eisen, D.: Cleidocranial dysostosis. Radiology, 61:21, 1953.
10. Eventon, I., Reider-Grosswasser, I., and Weiss, S.: Cleidocranial dysplasia. A family study. Clin. Radiol., 30:323, 1979.
11. Fairbanks, H. A. T.: Cranio-cleido dysostosis. J. Bone Joint Surg., 31-B:608, 1949.
12. Faur, E. C., Montagen, J. P., and Quemeneur, P.: Iconographic presentation. Arch. Fr. Pediatr., 37:465, 1980.
13. Faure, C., and Maroteaux, P.: Cleidocranial dysplasia. Prog. Pediatr. Radiol., 4:211, 1973.
14. Faure, C., Job, J.-C., and Nahum, M.: Anostéogenèse partielle (en particulier rachidienne). Entité nouvelle ou nouveau concept de la dysostose cleido-cranienne. Ann. Radiol., 8:154, 1965.
15. Fitzwilliams, D. C.: Hereditary cranio-cleido dysostosis. Lancet, 2:466, 1910.
16. Forland, M.: Cleidocranial dysostosis. Am. J. Med., 33:792, 1962.
17. Graillot, J., and Ramez, J.: Dysostose cleido-cranienne. J. Radiol., 44:855, 1963.
18. Jackson, W. P. U.: Osteo-dental dysplasia (cleidocranial dysostosis). The "Arnold head." Acta Med. Scand., 139:292, 1951.
19. Jarvinen, S.: Cephalometric findings in three cases of cleidocranial dysostosis. Am. J. Orthod., 79:184, 1981.
20. Jarvis, J. L., and Keats, T. E.: Cleidocranial dysostosis. A review of 40 new cases. A.J.R., 121:5, 1974.
21. Keats, T. E.: Cleidocranial dysostosis. Some atypical roentgen manifestations. A.J.R., 100:71, 1967.
22. Krawczynski, M., Stanska, M., Cichy, W., and Socha, J.: Marie-Sainton syndrome (cleidocranial dysostosis) associated with osseous changes in the hand. Endokrynol. Pol., 26:133, 1975.
23. Lasker, G. W.: The inheritance of cleidocranial dysostosis. Hum. Biol., 18:103, 1946.
24. Leopold, J. S., and Castrovinci, F.: Cleidocranial dysostosis. Am. J. Dis. Child., 46:113, 1933.
25. Leroy, D., Guerniou, H., Richier-Chevrel, M. E., and Richier, J. L.: Un cas de dysostose cleido-craniopelvienne. Bull. Acad. Natl. Méd. (Paris), 137:14, 1953.
26. Levin, E. J., and Sonnenschein, H.: Cleidocranial dysostosis. N.Y. State J. Med., 63:1562, 1963.
27. Marie, P., and Sainton, P.: Sur la dysostose cleidocranienne héréditaire. Rev. Neurol., 6:835, 1898.
28. Nazar, A. Z., Fragoso, R., Hernandez, A., and Cantu, J. M.: Letter: Cleidocranial dysplasia. Radiology, 132:238, 1979.
29. Oatis, G. W., Robertson, G. R., Sugg, W. E., and Firtell, D. N.: Cleidocranial dysostosis with mandibular cyst. Report of a case. Oral Surg., 40:62, 1975.
30. Palacios Mateos, J. M., Albarran, A. J., Moreno Esteban, B., and Lopez-Vidriero, E.: Case of Pierre Marie-Sainton cleidocranial dysostosis. Rev. Clin. Esp., 123:177, 1971.
31. Pancini, R., and Lurz, A.: A clinical and radiologic study of "cleido-cranial dysostosis" of Pierre Marie-Sainton, Crouzon. Ann. Radiol. Diagn., 37:275, 1964.
32. Piotrowski, R., and Winkielman, J.: Dysostosis cleidocranialis in siblings. Pol. Przegl. Radiol., 34:625, 1970.
33. Rhinehart, B. A.: Cleidocranial dysostosis (mutational dysostosis) with a case report. Radiology, 26:741, 1936.
34. Salmon, D. D.: Hereditary cleidocranial dysostosis. Radiology, 42:391, 1944.
35. Scott, R. B., and Banks, L. O.: Cleidocranial dysostosis syndrome. Am. J. Dis. Child., 81:394, 1951.
36. Soule, A. B.: Mutational dysostosis (cleidocranial dysostosis). J. Bone Joint Surg., 28:81, 1946.
37. Spranger, J. W., Langer, L. O., and Wiedemann, H. R.: Cleidocranial dysplasia. In Bone Dysplasia. Philadelphia, Saunders, 1974, p. 254.
38. Srivastava, K. K., Pai, R. A., Kolbhandari, M. P., and Kant, K.: Cleidocranial dysostosis. A clinical and cytological study. Clin. Genet., 2:104, 1971.
39. Tan, K. L., and Tan, L. K.: Cleidocranial dysostosis in infancy. Pediatr. Radiol., 11:114, 1981.
40. Thoms, J.: Cleidocranial dysostosis. Acta Radiol., 30:514, 1958.
41. Thomsen, G., and Guttadauro, M.: Cleidocranial dysostosis associated with osteosclerosis and bone fragility. Acta Radiol., 37:559, 1952.
42. Wildervanck, L. S., and Blickman, J. R.: Dysostosis cleido-cranialis in drie generaties. Ned. Tijdschr. Geneeskd., 115:5, 1971.
43. Witkop-Oostenrijk, G. A.: Contribution to the study of the inheritance of dysostosis cleidocranialis. Acta Genet., 7:223, 1957.
44. Wolstenholme, J., Booth, P. B., and Basset, D. J.: Cleido-dysostosis in a New Guinea family. J. Coll. Radiol. Aust., 8:272, 1964.
45. Yunis, E., and Varon, H.: Cleidocranial dysostosis, severe micrognathism, bilateral absence of thumbs and first metatarsal bone, and distal aphalangia: A new genetic syndrome. Am. J. Dis. Child., 1334:649, 1980.

HEREDITARY ONYCHO-OSTEODYSPLASIA (NAIL-PATELLA SYNDROME)

In 1820, Chatelain described a patient with congenital anomalies of the nails, elbows, and knees—the earliest report of nail dystrophy associated with skeletal dysplasia.[6] In 1897, Little quoted a description by Sedgwick of a family of which 18 members of four generations had no thumbnails and no patellae, thus suggesting the hereditary nature of this disorder.[22] Involvement of the elbows in this inherited defect was reported by Wrede in 1909.[48] A detailed study of this triad of anomalies was made by Osterreicher, in 1931.[31] Turner, in 1933, observed flaring of the iliac crests and prominence of the anterior superior iliac spines in some of the affected patients.[44] Fong, in 1946, during routine pyelography, noted conical bony projections on the dorsolateral aspects of the ilia, which he termed "iliac horns"; he did not, however, associate them with any syndrome.[13] A few years later, these iliac horns were observed in association with knee, elbow, and nail anomalies and reported by other authors.[29, 42] Thus iliac horns were established as an important constituent of this syndrome. The popular name of "nail-patella syndrome" has been applied to this triad of anomalies, but Love and Beiler, in 1957, coined the more correct term *hereditary osteo-onychodysplasia*.[23] Other terms applied to the condition are *hereditary onycho-osteodysplasia* and *hereditary onycho-osteoarthrodysplasia*.[28]

Incidence

The exact incidence of this syndrome is not known. Mino and associates, in 1948, collected over 100 cases from the literature.[29] Duncan and Souter, in 1963, found reports in the world literature of 44 families exhibiting the syndrome; the whole series comprised over 400 affected persons, details being available for only 252 of them.[9] In 1963, Duthie and Hecht reported one case among 800 boys examined at a boys' summer camp.[10] Wynne-Davies and associates report a birth incidence of one in 50,000 and probable prevalence of about one per million population.[50]

Inheritance

Onycho-osteodysplasia is transmitted as a simple autosomal dominant gene.[10]

There is a definite linkage between the locus of the nail-patella gene and that of the ABO blood groups.[37, 38] The syndrome in a given family will be transmitted in association with only one of the genes A, B, or O.

Clinical Features

Nail Dystrophy. In this commonest anomaly of the syndrome, the dystrophy is greatest in the thumbs and becomes less severe in the more ulnar digits (Fig. 3–83 E and F). The little finger is only very occasionally affected. Abnormalities of the toenails have been noted in some cases. The thumbnail may be absent, bifid, or hemiatrophic (the ulnar side of the nail is usually the part that is absent). In a very rare instance, the nail of the index finger may also be absent. The nails may be decreased in length and show numerous longitudinal cracks. Nail deformity is present in 98 per cent of cases. Bony abnormalities of the digits have not been demonstrated. Mesodermal tissues of the fingers appear to be involved to some extent. The terminal pulp may extend round from the volar aspect onto the dorsal surface. The dorsal skin creases over the distal interphalangeal joints may be absent or poorly developed. There may be laxity of the ligaments of the metacarpophalangeal and interphalangeal joints.

Knee Dysplasia. This abnormality is manifested as absence or hypoplasia of the patella (Fig. 3–83 G to K). The hypoplastic patella may be ovoid, triangular, or irregular in shape and may arise from several ossific centers. It may be located more distally than in the normal knee, superimposed on both the femoral and lateral tibial condyles.

The presenting complaint may be recurrent lateral dislocation of the patella, caused by hypoplasia of the lateral femoral condyle. Varying degrees of genu valgum are usually present. The medial femoral condyle is frequently large and prominent; the lateral condyle is underdeveloped. The medial tibial plateau may slip downward and medially, or even may be grooved. The medial margin of the proximal tibial metaphysis tends to sweep upward and medially in a characteristic arc.

Elbow Dysplasia. The carrying angle of the elbow joint is increased with varying degree of cubitis valgus. There is hypoplasia of the lateral side of the elbow joint, involving not only the capitellum and lateral condyle but also the radial head (Fig. 3–83 A to D). The radial head may articulate normally with the capitellum, or there may be subluxation or dislocation posteriorly. There may be a pointed exostosis of the lateral aspect of the coronoid process. Range of motion of the elbow joints is usually limited.

Pelvic Dysplasia. "Iliac horns" and flaring of the iliac crests with prominence of the anterior superior iliac spines are the two types of pelvic abnormalities encountered. Iliac horns, one of the most common characteristic features of onycho-osteodysplasia, are bilateral; they are present in 75 per cent of cases and may be visible, palpable, or impalpable, according to their size (Fig. 3–84). Secondary centers of ossification may occur at their tips. They are present quite early in life. When outflaring of the iliac crests with prominence of the anterior superior iliac spines is combined with iliac horns, the appearance of the pelvis has been likened to that of an elephant's ear.

Other purely coincidental anomalies may be found in association with the foregoing main lesions, such as clubfoot, congenital dislocation of the hips, spina bifida, congenital contracture of the little finger, abnormal pigmentation of the iris (which occurs in about 50 per cent of cases), and Plummer-Vinson syndrome (dysphagia, hypochromic anemia, and koilonychia).

Later in life, usually during the third or fourth decade, the patients develop nephropathy and proteinuria and subsequent renal failure.[8, 10, 17, 49]

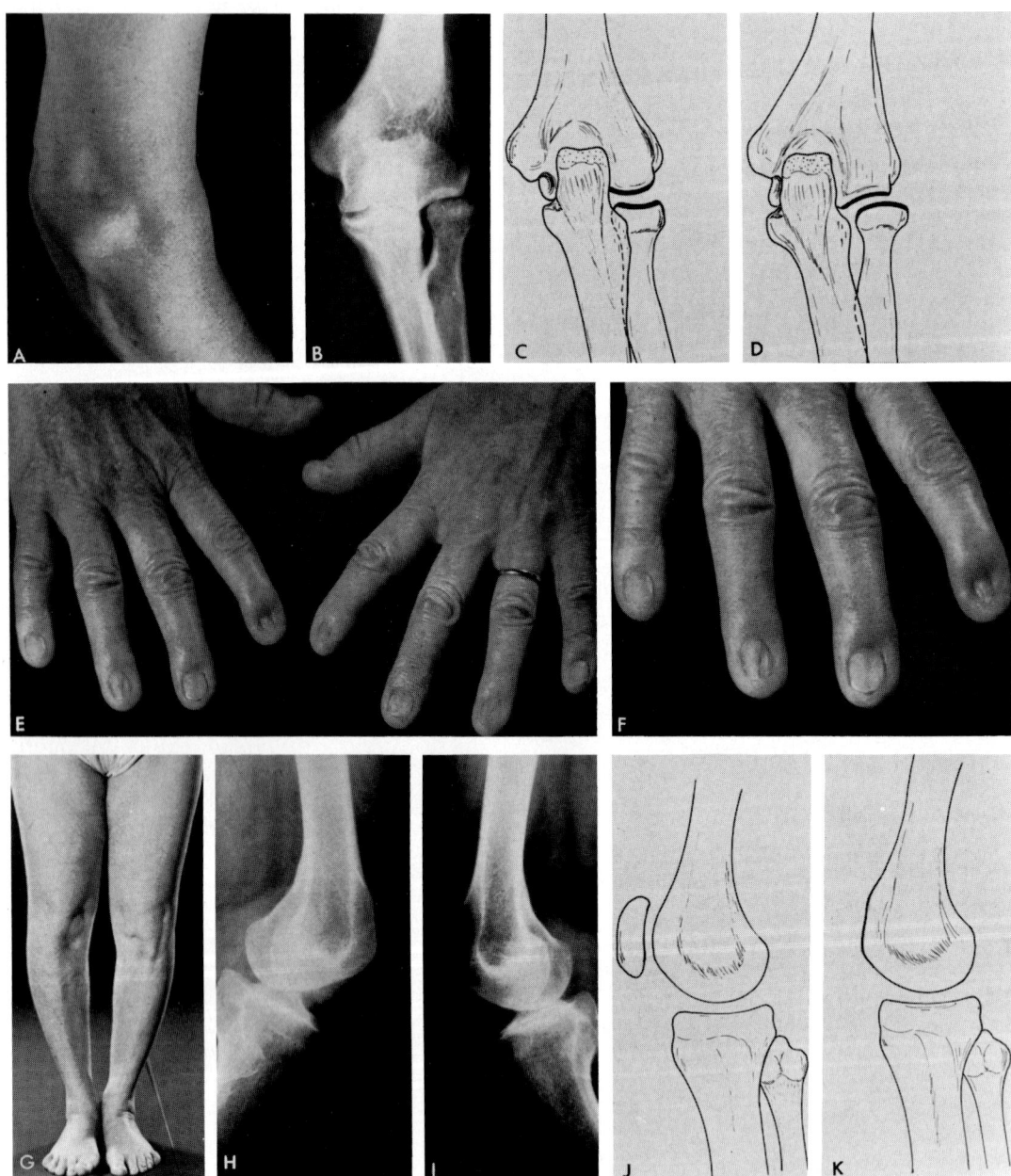

FIGURE 3–83. Hereditary onycho-osteodysplasia (nail-patella syndrome) in an adult.

A and **B**. Photograph and radiogram of right elbow showing hypoplasia of the capitellum, lateral condyle, and radial head. **C**. Drawing of a radiogram of a normal elbow and **D**, of that of the patient. **E** and **F**. the hand, showing dystrophy of the nails. Note that it gets less severe in the ulnar digits, and the little finger is not affected. **G** to **K**. The lower limbs and a lateral radiograph and line drawing of the knees. The patellae are absent and the femoral condyle is hypoplastic. **J** is a line drawing of a normal knee. (Courtesy of Dr. H. Kelikian.)

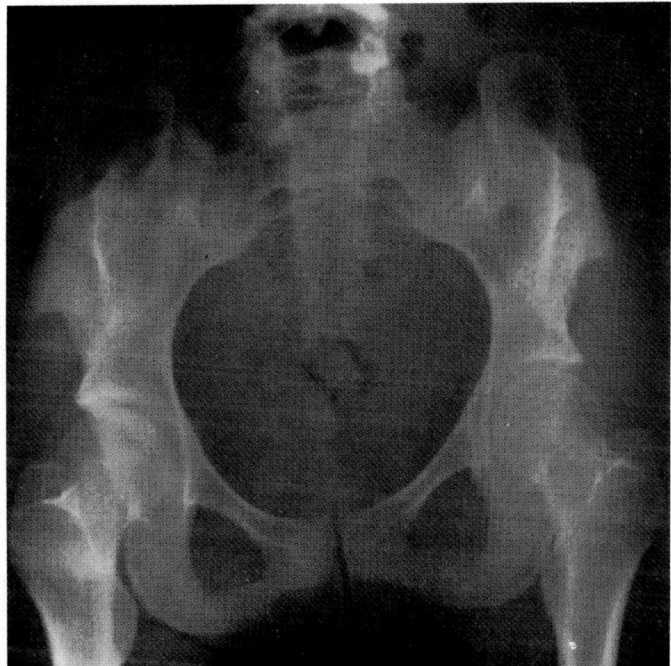

FIGURE 3–84. Hereditary onycho-osteodysplasia.

Radiogram of the pelvis and upper femora showing bilateral iliac horns. Note the severe valgus deformity of femoral necks. (From Duthie, R. B., and Hecht, F.: The inheritance and development of the nail-patella syndrome. J. Bone Joint Surg., 45-B:259, 1963. Reprinted by permission.)

Treatment

There is no specific treatment for the disorder. Recurrent dislocation of the patella may occur, which, if disabling, is treated by quadricepsplasty.

References

1. Aggarwal, D., and Mittal, R. L.: Nail-patella syndrome. J. Bone Joint Surg., 52-B:29, 1970.
2. Alain, J. L., and Rigault, P.: Hereditary onycho-arthro-dysplasia. Rev. Chir. Orthop., 58:623, 1972.
3. Bates, J. C.: Iliac horns. A manifestation of hereditary osteo-onychodysplasia. U.S. Armed Forces Med. J., 5:865, 1954.
4. Beals, R. K., and Eckhardt, A. L.: Hereditary osteo-onychodysplasia. J. Bone Joint Surg., 51-A:505, 1969.
5. Bernhang, A. M., and Levine, S. A.: Familial absence of the patella. J. Bone Joint Surg., 55:1088, 1973.
6. Chatelain (1820), quoted by Roeckerath, W.: Fortschr. Geb. Rontgenstr., 75:700, 1951.
7. Cowell, H. R.: Hereditary onycho-osteodysplasia. Report of a kindred with dysplasia of the fifth finger. Clin. Orthop., 76:43, 1971.
8. Darlington, D., and Hawkins, C. F.: Nail-patella syndrome with iliac horns and hereditary nephropathy. Necropsy report and anatomical dissection. J. Bone Joint Surg., 49-B:164, 1967.
9. Duncan, J. G., and Souter, W. A.: Hereditary onycho-osteodysplasia. The nail-patella syndrome. J. Bone Joint Surg., 45-B:242, 1963.
10. Duthie, R. B., and Hecht, F.: The inheritance and development of the nail-patella syndrome. J. Bone Joint Surg., 45-B:259, 1963.
11. Eisenberg, K. S., Potter, D. E., and Bovill, E. G.: Osteo-onychodystrophy with nephropathy and renal osteodystrophy. J. Bone Joint Surg., 54-A:1301, 1972.
12. Faure, C., and Petrel, P.: L'ostéo-onycho-dysplasie héréditaire. Ann. Radiol., 11:1, 1968.
13. Fong, E. E.: "Iliac horns" (symmetrical bilateral central posterior iliac processes). Radiology, 47:517, 1946.
14. Garces, M. A., Muraskas, J. K., and Abdel-Hameed, M.: Hereditary onycho-osteo-dysplasia (HOOD syndrome): Report of two cases. Skeletal Radiol., 8:55, 1982.
15. Goodman, R. M., Lockareff, S., and Gwinup, G.: Hereditary congenital deafness with onychodystrophy. Arch. Otolaryngol., 90:474, 1969.
16. Grunberg, J.: Onycho-arthro-dysplasie. Ann. Radiol., 13:877, 1970.
17. Hawkins, C. F., and Smith, O. E.: Renal dysplasia in a family with multiple hereditary abnormalities including iliac horns. Lancet, 1:803, 1950.
18. Hybbinette, C. H.: The nail-patella-elbow syndrome. A case report. Acta Orthop. Scand., 46:593, 1975.
19. Jansen, J., Hansen, E., Hobolth, N., Jacobsen, P., and Mikkelsen, M.: 48 XXXY Klinefelter syndrome and nail-patella syndrome in the same child. Clin. Genet., 9:163, 1976.
20. Leahy, M. S.: The hereditary nephropathy of osteo-onychodysplasia. Nail-patella syndrome. Am. J. Dis. Child., 112:237, 1966.
21. Leiba, S., Grunebaum, M., Savir, H., and Ber, A.: Oculootonasal malformations associated with osteoonychodysplasia. Birth Defects Orig. Art. Ser., 11:67, 1975.
22. Little, E. M.: Congenital absence or delayed development of the patella. Lancet, 2:781, 1897.
23. Love, W. H., and Beiler, D. D.: Osteo-onychodysplasia. J. Bone Joint Surg., 39-A:645, 1957.
24. Lucas, G. L.: Hereditary onycho-osteodysplasia (nail-patella syndrome) masquerading as arthrogryposis. South. Med. J., 60:751, 1967.
25. Lucas, G. L., and Opitz, J. M.: The nail-patella syndrome. Clinical and genetic aspects of 5 kindreds with 38 affected family members. J. Pediatr., 68:273, 1966.
26. McCluskey, K. A.: The nail-patella syndrome. (Hered-

itary onycho-mesodysplasia.) Can. J. Surg., 4:192, 1961.
27. Mace, J. W., and Gotlin, R. W.: Short stature and onychodysplasia. Report of a case resembling Senior syndrome. Am. J. Dis. Child., 125:114, 1973.
28. Maini, P. S., and Mittal, R. L.: Hereditary onycho-osteo-arthrodysplasia. J. Bone Joint Surg., 48-A:924, 1966.
29. Mino, R. A., Mino, V. H., and Livingstone, R. G.: Osseous dysplasia and dystrophy of the nails. Review of the literature and report of a case. A.J.R., 60:633, 1948.
30. Neuhold, A., Seidl, G., Stummvoll, H., Syre, G., and Brandstatter, G.: Nail-Patella-Syndrom. Radiologe, 22:568, 1982.
31. Osterreicher, W.: Family with anonychia, patella abnormalities and dislocation of the radius. Dominant characteristic over five generations. Z. Menschl. Vererb. Konstitutionsl., 15:465, 1931.
32. Pearce, R. L.: The nail-patella syndrome. Aust. Med. J., p. 994, 1970.
33. Pelizza, A., and Gobbi, U.: Arthro-onyco-osteodysplasia: Radiological diagnosis in a nursling. Gaslini, 6:155, 1974.
34. Pieron, R., Mafart, Y., Couderc, L. J., and Roussin, S.: Osteo-onychodysplasia (nail-patella syndrome): A case report. Sem. Hôp. Paris, 58:1039, 1982.
35. Pussell, B. A., Charlesworth, J. A., MacDonald, G. J., and Baker, W.: The nail-patella syndrome. A report of a family. Aust. J. Med., 7:20, 1977.
36. Renwick, J. H., and Izatt, M. M.: Some genetical parameters of the nail-patella locus. Ann. Hum. Genet., 28:369, 1965.
37. Renwick, J. H., and Lawler, S. D.: Genetic linkage between the ABO and nail-patella loci. Ann. Hum. Genet., 19:312, 1954.
38. Renwick, J. H., and Schulze, J.: Male and female recombination fractions for the nail-patella ABO linkage in man. Ann. Hum. Genet., 28:379, 1965.
39. Saha, M. M., and Bhardwaj, O. P.: Hereditary onycho-osteodysplasia (Fong's lesion). Indian J. Radiol., 23:199, 1969.
40. Sanchez, O., Mazas, J. J., Ortiz, I., and de DeMatos, F.: The deafness, onycho-osteo-dystrophy, mental retardation syndrome. Hum Genet., 58:228, 1981.
41. Simila, S., Vesa, L., and Wasz-Hockert, O.: Hereditary onycho-osteoplasia (the nail-patella syndrome) with nephrosis-like renal disease in a newborn boy. Pediatrics, 46:61, 1970.
42. Thompson, E. A., Walker, E. T., and Weens, H. S.: Iliac horns. An osseous manifestation of hereditary arthrodysplasia associated with dystrophy of the fingernails. Radiology, 53:88, 1949.
43. Tsuchiya, K., and Kameshita, K.: Hereditary osteo-onychodysplasia. Report of a family. Yokohama Med. Bull., 18:183, 1967.
44. Turner, J. W.: A hereditary arthrodysplasia associated with hereditary dystrophy of thumb nails. J.A.M.A., 100:882, 1933.
45. Valdueza, A. F.: The nail-patella syndrome. A report of three families. J. Bone Joint Surg., 55-B:145, 1973.
46. Vernier, R. L., Hoyer, J. R., and Michael, A. F.: The nail-patella syndrome—pathogenesis of the kidney lesion. Birth Defects Orig. Art. Series, 10:57, 1974.
47. Williams, H. J., and Hoyer, J. R.: Radiographic diagnosis of osteo-onychodysostosis in infancy. Radiology, 109:151, 1973.
48. Wrede: Kongenitale erbliche Luxation der Patells nach aussen. Berl. Klin. Wochenschr., 46:373, 1909.
49. Wright, L. A., and Fred, H. L.: Fatal renal disease associated with hereditary osteo-onychodysplasia. South. Med. J., 62:833, 1969.
50. Wynne-Davies, R., Hall, C., and Apley, A. G.: Atlas of Skeletal Dysplasias. Edinburgh, Churchill-Livingstone, 1985, p. 614.
51. Zimmerman, C.: Iliac horns: A pathognomonic roentgen sign of familial onycho-osteodysplasia. J. Roentgenol., 86:4789, 1961.

TRICHO-RHINO-PHALANGEAL DYSPLASIA

This dysplasia, first described by Giedion in 1966, consists of slow-growing very sparse hair with early balding, a characteristic face (with pear-shaped beaked nose, long philtrum, and wide mouth), and cone-shaped phalangeal epiphysis (principally at the base of the middle phalanx) with brachyphalangia (Fig. 3–85).[12] The fourth and fifth metacarpals are commonly shortened. In about two thirds of the patients the femoral heads are flattened and fragmented, with Perthes'-like changes (Fig. 3–86). Involvement of the hips is usually bilateral.[7]

In some patients associated anomalies are noted: cartilaginous exostosis of long bones, short distal phalanges of the thumb and hallux, scoliosis and lordosis, and delay in skeletal maturation with bone age several years behind chronological age. Inheritance is by autosomal dominant transmission.

References

1. Beals, R. K.: Tricho-rhino-phalangeal dysplasia. Report of a kindred. J. Bone Joint Surg., 55-A:821, 1973.
2. Camacho, F., Armijo, M., Naranjo, R., and Dulanto, F.: Le syndrome tricho-rhino-phalangien (Giedion). Ann. Dermatol. Venereol. (Paris), 105:17, 1978.
3. Colavita, N., Aluffi, A., Bock, E., De Palma, L., and Colagrande, C.: Individualisation d'une forme fruste du syndrome tricho-rhino-phalangien et follow-up à long terme dans une famille étudiée par "Profile Pattern Analysis." Pediatr. Radiol., Proc. 15th Intern. Cong. Radiol., Brussels, 1983, p. 180.
4. Cottin, S., Le Gall, G., and Lorgeas, J. M.: Le syndrome tricho-rhino-phalangien. A propos de quatre observations familiales. Rev. Rhumat., 47:169, 1980.
5. Cruz, M., and Frances, J.-M.: Le syndrome tricho-rhino-phalagien: Une forme nouvelle de dysostose périphérique. Arch. Fr. Pediatr., 27:649, 1970.
6. Cruz-Hernandez, M., Palomeque, A., Querol, X., and Conills-Santias, M.: Nueva aportacion clinica sobre el sindrome trico-rino-falangico. Arch. Pediatr. Barcelona, 127:393, 1971.
7. Felman, A. H., and Frias, J. L.: The trichorhinophalangeal syndrome: Study of 16 patients in one family. A.J.R., 129:631, 1977.
8. Ferrandez, J., Ramirez, J., Saenz, P., and Calvo, M.: The trichorhinophalangeal syndrome. Report of 4 familial cases belonging to 4 generations. Helv. Paediatr. Acta, 35:559, 1980.
9. Fontaine, G., Maroteaux, P., Farriaux, J.-P., Richard, J., and Roelens, B.: Le syndrome tricho-rhino-phalangien. Arch. Fr. Pediatr., 27:635, 1970.
10. Frias, J. L., Felman, A. H., Garnica, A. D., and Wallace, S. E.: Variable expressivity in the trichorhinophalangeal syndrome type I. Birth Defects Orig. Art. Series, 15:361, 1979.
11. Gaarsted, C., Madsen, E. H., and Friedrich, U.: A Danish kindred with tricho-rhino-phalangeal syndrome type I. Eur. J. Pediatr., 139:84, 1982.

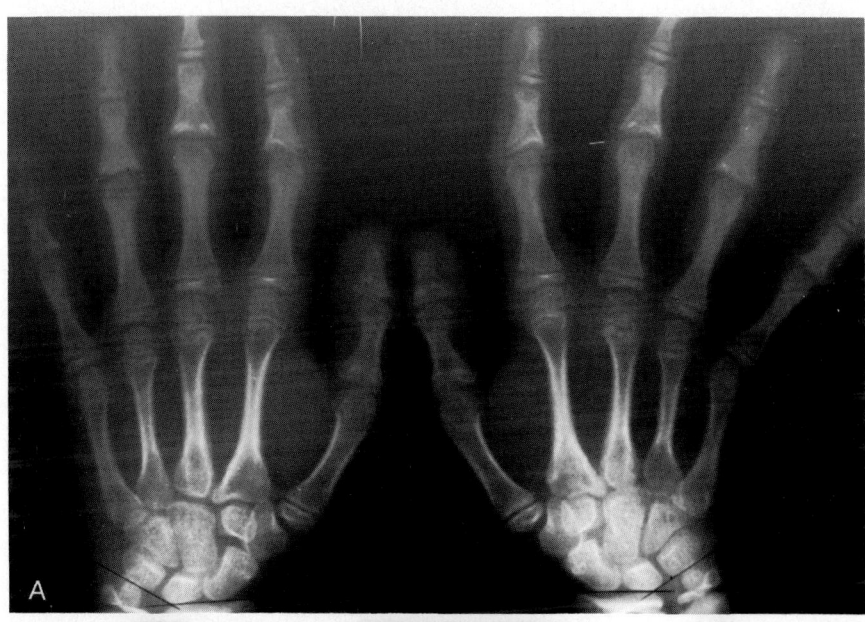

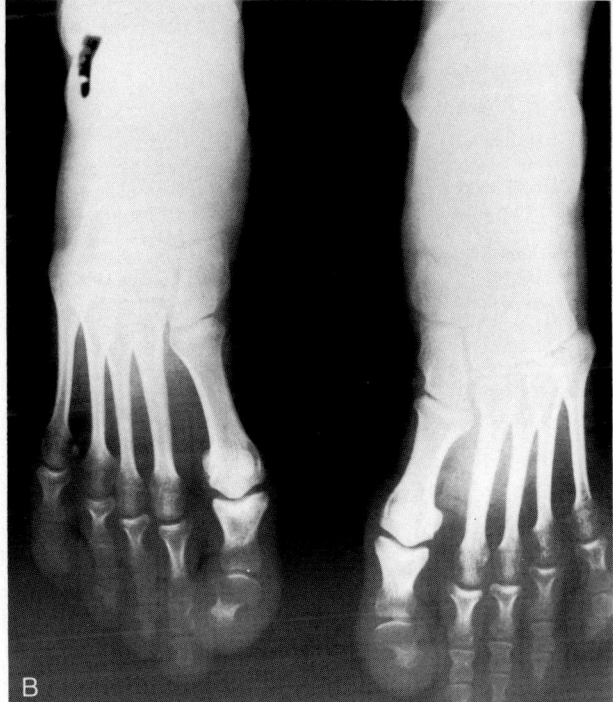

FIGURE 3–85. Tricho-rhino-phalangeal syndrome.

A. Anteroposterior radiograms of the hands (**A**) and the feet (**B**). Note the cone-shaped epiphyses of the phalanges and the shortening of the fourth and fifth metatarsals and metacarpals.

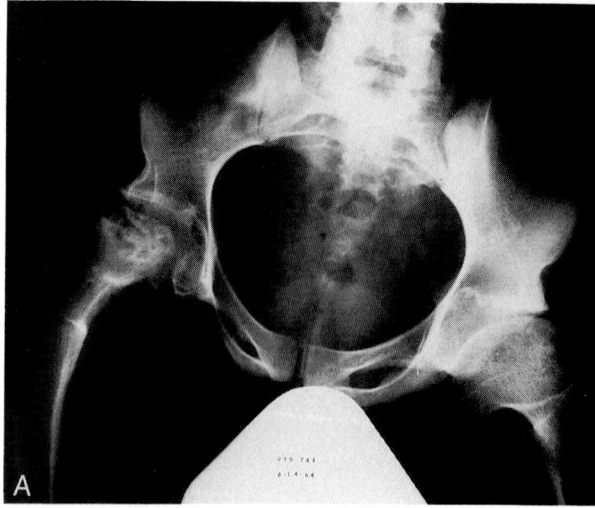
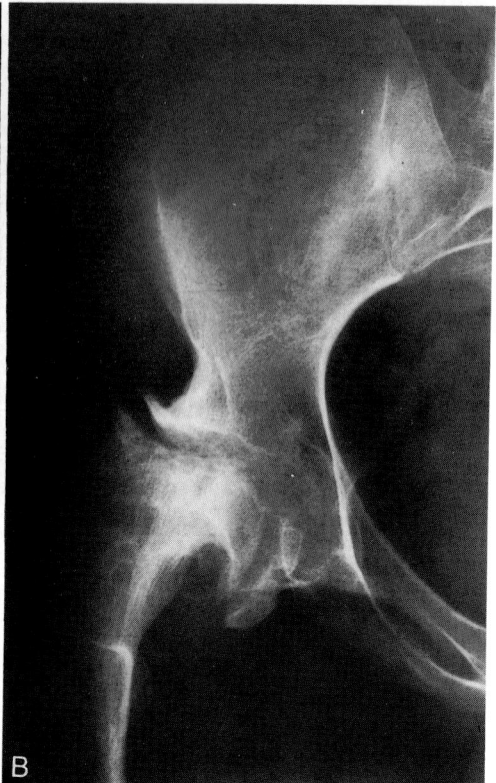

FIGURE 3–86. The hips in tricho-rhino-phalangeal syndrome.

A. Anteroposterior radiogram of both hips. Note the irregularity of the femoral head on the right resembling Legg-Calvé-Perthes disease. **B.** Severe degenerative arthritis of the hip due to deformity of the capital femoral epiphysis.

12. Giedion, A.: Das Tricho-Rhino-Phalangeale Syndrom. Helv. Paediatr. Acta, 21:475, 1966.
13. Giedion, A.: Cone-shaped epiphyses of the hands and their diagnostic value. The tricho-rhino-phalangeal syndrome. Ann. Radiol., 10:322, 1967.
14. Giedion, A., Burdea, M., Fruchter, Z., Meloni, T., and Trosc, V.: Autosomal-dominant transmission of the tricho-rhino-phalangeal syndrome. Report of 4 unrelated families, review of 60 cases. Helv. Paediatr. Acta, 28:249, 1973.
15. Gorlin, R. J., Cohen, M. M., Jr., and Wolfson, J.: Tricho-rhino-phalangeal syndrome. Am. J. Dis. Child., 118:595, 1969.
16. Gorlin, R. J., and Sedano, H.: Trichorhinophalangeal syndrome. Mod. Med., May, 1972, p. 98.
17. Jorgenson, R. J., Sallnas, C. F., Sujansky, E., and Belerie, L. E.: Heterogeneity in the trichorhinophalangeal syndromes. Birth Defects Orig. Art. Series, 19:167, 1983.
18. King, G. J., and Frias, J. L.: A cephalometric study of the craniofacial skeleton in trichorhinophalangeal syndrome. Am. J. Orthod., 75:70, 1979.
19. Kozlowski, K., and Mowbray, G.: Tricho-rhino-phalangeal syndrome with Perthes disease–like changes and coxa vara (report of a case). Aust. Radiol., 23:170, 1979.
20. Kozlowski, K., Blaim, A., and Malolepszy, E.: Tricho-rhino-phalangeal syndrome. Aust. Radiol., 16:411, 1972.
21. Kuna, G. B., Collipp, P. J., and Balsam, D.: Trichorhinophalangeal dysplasia (Giedion syndrome). Clin. Pediatr., 17:96, 1978.
22. Poznanski, A. K., Schmickel, R. D., Harper, H. A. S.: The hand in trichorhinophalangeal syndrome. Birth Defects Orig. Art. Series, 10:209, 1974.
23. Prens, E. P., Peereboom-Wynia, J. D. R., De Bruyn, W. C., Van Joost, T., and Stolz, E.: Clinical and scanning electron microscopic findings in a solitary case of trichorhinophalangeal syndrome type I. Acta Derm Venereol. (Stockh.), 64:249, 1979.
24. Ranke, M. B., and Heitkamp, H. C.: Tricho-rhino-phalangeales Syndrom. Bericht über 4 Falle in drei Generationen. Montatsschr. Kinderheilkd., 128:208, 1980.
25. Say, B., Barber, N., and Poznanski, A. K.: Pattern profile analysis of the hand in trichorhinophalangeal syndrome. Pediatrics, 59:123, 1977.
26. Scheffer, P., Verdier, M., and Finidori, G.: Syndrome tricho-rhino-phalangien. Analyse architecturale craniofaciale de six cas. Rev. Stomatol. Chir. Maxillofac., 4:230, 1981.
27. Stoll, C., Levy, J.-M., and Paira, M.: Le syndrome tricho-rhino-phalangien. Une nouvelle observation familiale. Pediatrie, 31:519, 1976.
28. Sugiura, Y.: Tricho-rhino-phalangeal syndrome associated with Perthes-disease-like bone change and spondylolisthesis. Jpn. J. Hum. Genet., 23:23, 1978.
29. Sugiura, Y., Shionoya, M., Inoue, T., and Tsuruta, T.: Tricho-rhino-phalangeal syndrome: Report on three unrelated families. Jpn. J. Hum. Genet., 21:13, 1976.
30. Tuzovic, S., Fiebach, B. J. O., Magnus, L., and Sauerbrei, H. U.: Das trichorhinophalangeale Syndrom. Bericht über eine Familie mit 14 Merkmalstragern in 5 Generationen. Röntgenblatter, 35:391, 1982.
31. Van Neste, D., and Dumortier, M.: Tricho-rhinophalangeal syndrome. Disturbed geometric relationships between hair matrix and dermal papilla in scalp hair bulbs. Dermatologica, 165:16, 1982.
32. Weaver, D. D., Cohen, M. M., and Smith, D. W.: The tricho-rhino-phalangeal syndrome. J. Med. Genet., 11:312, 1974.

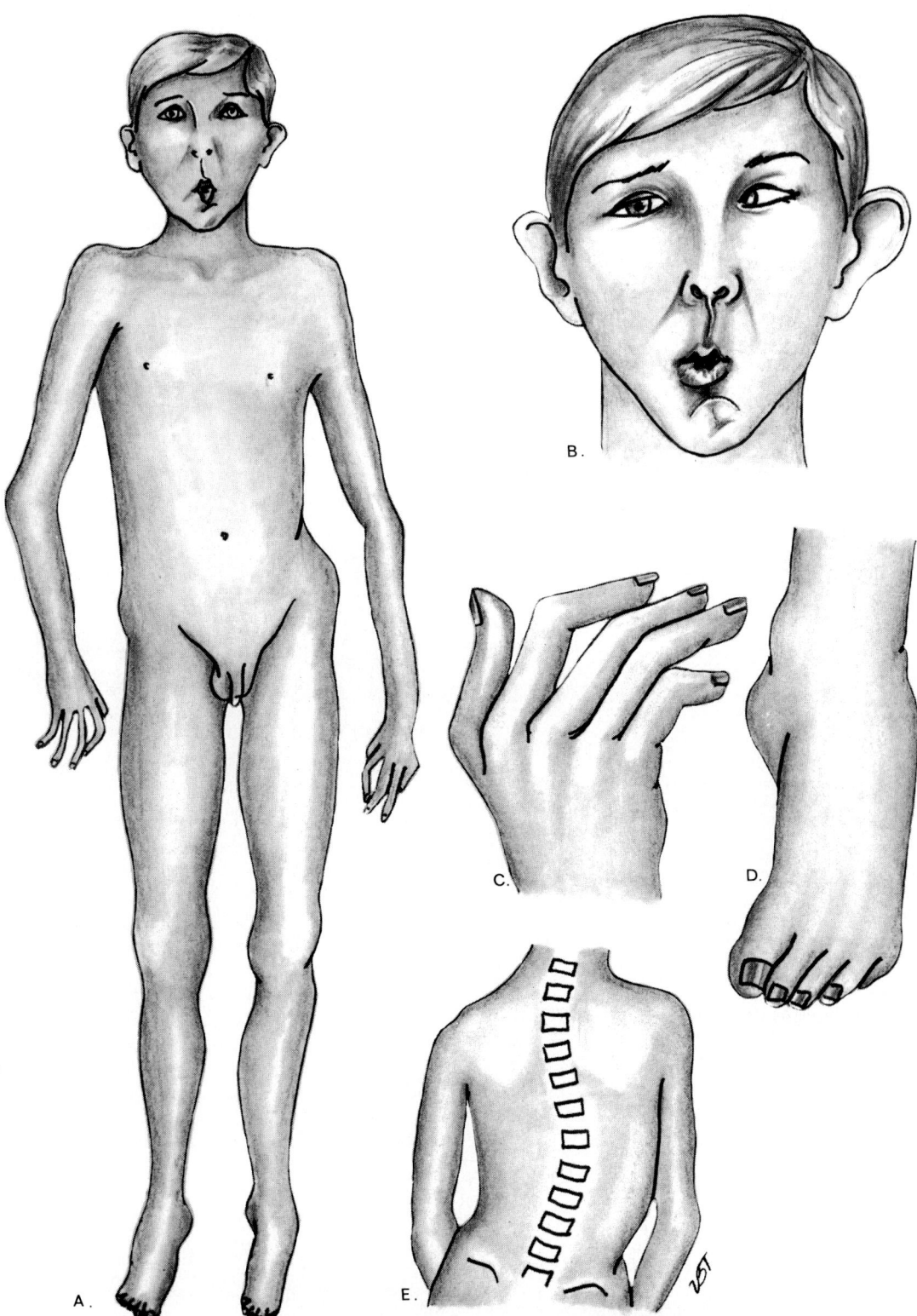

FIGURE 3–87. Craniocarpotarsal dysplasia.

A and **B**. Characteristic findings include full forehead, deeply set eyes, flattened midface, and small mouth with protuberant lips that give a "whistling" appearance. **C**. The fingers are deviated ulnarward, and there are equinovarus deformity and flexion contracture of the toes, **D**, and scoliosis, **E**.

CRANIOCARPOTARSAL DYSPLASIA (FREEMAN-SHELDON OR "WHISTLING FACE" SYNDROME)

This dysplasia was first described in 1938 by Freeman (an orthopedic surgeon) and Sheldon (a pediatrician).[10] It is characterized by a typical "whistling" *facies* (a small "pursed" mouth, long philtrum, small nose, deeply sunken eyes, and an H- or U-shaped scarlike contracture that extends from the middle of the lower lip to the chin); ulnar deviation and flexion contractures of the fingers without bony deformity; rigid talipes equinovarus, usually bilateral; and short stature, generally below the third percentile (Fig. 3–87).

Other associated anomalies are kyphosis, congenital dislocation of the hip, occasional spina bifida occulta, asymmetrical pinnae, mild pterygium colli, and pectus excavatum.

Inheritance is by both dominant and recessive autosomal transmission.

The foot and hand deformities often require surgical correction.

References

1. Aldinger, G., and Eulert, J.: Das Freeman-Sheldon Syndrom. Z. Orthop., *121*:630, 1983.
2. Alves, A. F. P., and Azevedo, E. S.: Recessive form of Freeman-Sheldon's syndrome or "whistling face." J. Med. Genet., *14*:139, 1977.
3. Antley, R. M., Uga, N., Burzynski, N. J., Baum, R. S., and Bixler, D.: Diagnostic criteria for the whistling face syndrome. Birth Defects Orig. Art. Series, *11*:161, 1975.
4. Barta, O., Bellyei, A., and Kranicz, J.: Über das Freeman-Sheldonsche Syndrom. Arch. Orthop. Unfallchir., *75*:69, 1973.
5. Burzynski, N. J., Podruch, P. E., Howell, J., and Shawder, K.: Craniocarpotarsal dysplasia syndrome (whistling face syndrome). Oral Surg., *39*:893, 1975.
6. Call, W. H., and Strickland, J. W.: Functional hand reconstruction in the whistling-face syndrome. J. Hand Surg., *6*:148, 1981.
7. Cervenka, J., Gorlin, R. J., Figalova, P., and Farkarova, J.: Craniocarpotarsal dysplasia or whistling face syndrome. Arch. Otolaryngol., *91*:183, 1970.
8. Estrada, R., Rosenfeld, W., Salazar, J. D., and Jhaveri, R.: Freeman-Sheldon syndrome with unusual hand and foot anomalies. J. Natl. Med. Assoc., *73*:664, 1981.
9. Fraser, F. C., Pashayan, H., and Kadish, M. E.: Cranio-carpo-tarsal dysplasia. Report of a case in father and son. J.A.M.A., *211*:1374, 1970.
10. Freeman, E. A., and Sheldon, J. H.: Cranio-carpo-tarsal dystrophy: An undescribed congenital malformation. Arch. Dis. Child., *13*:277, 1938.
11. Freilinger, G., Rett, A., and Killian, W.: Eine seltene Handfehlbildung. Freeman-Sheldon Syndrom. Handchirurgie, *12*:225, 1980.
12. Gorlin, R. J., and Sedano, H.: Craniocarpotarsal dysplasia. Whistling face syndrome. Mod. Med., April 1970, p. 130.
13. Gross-Kieselstein, E., Abrahamov, A., and Ben-Hur, N.: Familial occurrence of the Freeman-Sheldon syndrome: Cranio-carpotarsal dysplasia. Pediatrics, *47*:1064, 1971.
14. Kousseff, B. G., McConnachie, P., and Hadro, T. A.: Autosomal recessive type of whistling face syndrome in twins. Pediatrics, *69*:328, 1982.
15. MacLeod, P., and Patriquin, H.: The whistling face syndrome—cranio-carpo-tarsal dysplasia: Report of a case and a survey of the literature. Clin. Pediatr., *13*:184, 1974.
16. Martini, A. K., and Banniza u Bazan, U.: Die Handdeformitäten beim Freeman-Sheldon-Syndrom und ihre operative Behandlung. Z. Orthop., *121*:623, 1983.
17. O'Connell, D. J., and Hall, C. M.: Cranio-carpo-tarsal dysplasia. A report of seven cases. Radiology, *123*:719, 1977.
18. Rinsky, L. A., and Bleck, E. E.: Freeman-Sheldon ("whistling face") syndrome. J. Bone Joint Surg., *58-A*:148, 1976.
19. Rintala, A. E.: Freeman-Sheldon's syndrome, craniocarpo-tarsal dystrophy. Acta Paediatr. Scand., *57*:553, 1968.
20. Rosti, D.: Sindrome di Freeman-Sheldon distrophia: Cranio-carpo-tarsal. Minerva Pediatr., *23*:1091, 1971.
21. Walbaum, R., Lejeune, M., Poupard, B., Lacheretz, M., and Fontaine, G.: Le syndrome de Freeman-Sheldon (syndrome du siffleur). Ann. Pediatr., *20*:357, 1973.
22. Walker, B. A.: Craniocarpotarsal Dystrophy, First Conference on the Clinical Delineation of Birth Defects. Baltimore, The Johns Hopkins Hospital, May, 1968, pp. 26–37.
23. Weinstein, S., and Gorlin, R. J.: Cranio-carpo-tarsal dysplasia or the whistling face syndrome. I. Clinical considerations. Am. J. Dis. Child., *117*:427, 1969.

LARSEN'S SYNDROME

This rare syndrome was first described by Larsen and associates in 1950.[16] It is characterized by its flat facies with depressed nasal bridge, bulging forehead, and widely spaced eyes (hypertelorism); by multiple and bilateral congenital dislocations, usually of the hips, knees, and radial heads, as shown in Figure 3–88; and by a juxta-calcaneal accessory bone or bifid calcaneus, which, if present, is diagnostic (Fig. 3–89).[17] There are distinctive deformities of the hand consisting of spatulate distal phalanx of the thumb, long and cylindrical fingers that do not taper normally from the base to the tip and have extra creases, and relatively shortened metacarpals. The carpal bones often have multiple centers of ossification.

Inheritance of Larsen's syndrome is by both dominant and recessive autosomal transmission. The basis of the extensive abnormalities is probably a generalized mesenchymal defect involving connective tissue.

There may be other associated anomalies. *Abnormal segmentation of the cervical spine*, occurring in about 20 per cent of the reported cases, results in midcervical kyphosis, cervicothoracic lordosis, and progressive spinal instability. The cervical vertebrae are flattened and hypoplastic, more so posteriorly.[20]

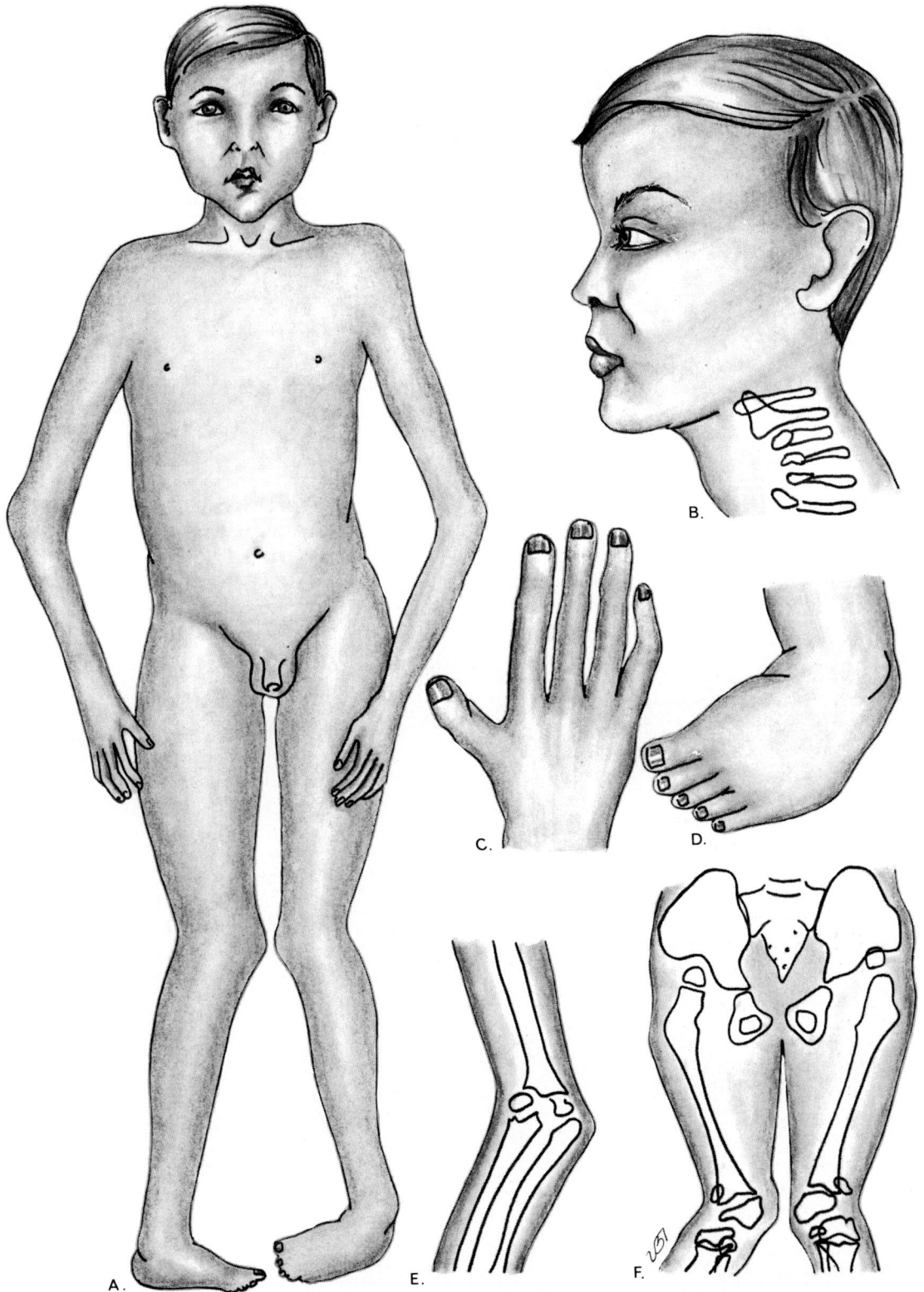

FIGURE 3-88. *Larsen's syndrome.*

Note the flat facies with depressed nasal bridge and prominent forehead, multiple joint dislocations (knees, hips, and elbows), and vertebral malformations (scoliosis).

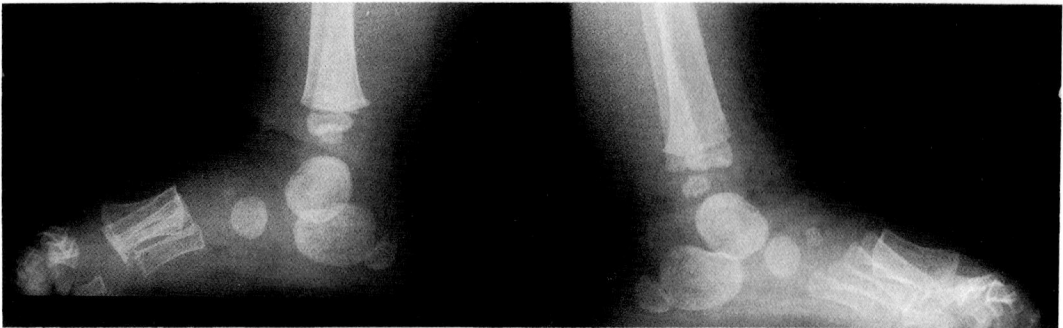

FIGURE 3–89. *Accessory ossification center next to calcaneus in Larsen's syndrome.*

It should be noted that one of the six patients of Larsen and associates died suddenly because of cardiopulmonary failure on the evening following surgery for a dislocated knee.[16] One of Micheli and associates' patients died as a result of the mechanically unstable cervical spine.[22] Muzumdar reported a case of quadriplegia in a patient with Larsen's syndrome who fell and sustained indirect injury to the neck.[23] Therefore, it is vital to evaluate the cervical spine carefully by flexion-extension lateral radiograms and if necessary by computed tomography or nuclear magnetic resonance imaging.

Segmental abnormalities and multiple vertebrae may cause progressive scoliosis.[35] In the *feet* talipes equinovarus or equinovalgus is quite common. Occasionally the first metatarsal is short and the cuboid bone is bifid. The presence of a juxtacalcaneal accessory bone or a bifid calcaneus is a characteristic radiologic finding of the syndrome. Cleft palate, often incomplete, may occur and is sometimes associated with cleft uvula but never with cleft lip.

Cardiovascular lesions are not uncommon. These consist of congenital anomalies, e.g., ventricular or atrial septal defect, patent ductus arteriosus, or auricular lesions, aortic dilation and insufficiency, mitral valve prolapse and insufficiency, and ductus arteriosus aneurysm.

Maldeveloped cartilage of the larynx and the tracheal rings ("flabby cartilage") may cause respiratory difficulty.

Affected children usually have normal intelligence and have minimal disability after correction of the orthopedic deformities. A few patients are mentally retarded.

Differential Diagnosis

Larsen's syndrome may masquerade as *arthrogryposis multiplex congenita*; the latter, however, is characterized by extreme stiffness and contracture of the joints and decreased muscle mass. Multiple bilateral joint dislocations may also be encountered in conditions associated with excessive ligamentous laxity of the joints such as *Ehlers-Danlos syndrome*, which is characterized by lax skin and other cutaneous changes. The facies of *otopalatodigital syndrome* may resemble that of Larsen's syndrome, but the digital and carpal anomalies (up to 12 carpal bones), the deafness, and the cleft palate are characteristic of the otopalatodigital syndrome.

Treatment

The infant with Larsen's syndrome is presented to the orthopedic surgeon because of multiple congenital dislocations and occasionally club feet. Prior to surgical intervention the whole infant should be carefully assessed. It is crucial to rule out cardiovascular anomalies, malacia of the trachea, and mechanical instability of the cervical spine prior to operation.

If the knees are dislocated the tibia is displaced anterolaterally on the femur. Open reduction is often required. This should be carried out prior to treating hip dislocations. Dislocated hips are antenatal, taking place in utero; they are best treated by open reduction with femoral shortening. Talipes equinovarus and congenital convex pes valgus are treated initially by manipulation and cast retention, but almost invariably open surgical reduction of the talocalcaneonavicular joints is necessary.

Instability of the cervical spine is treated by prophylactic bracing and early surgical stabilization.[22] Thoracolumbar fusion is indicated if significant scoliosis cannot be controlled by appropriate orthotic support.

References

1. Anderson, C. E., Bocian, M. E., Walker, A. P., Lachman, R., and Rimon, D. L.: A syndrome of short

stature, joint laxity and developmental delay. Clin. Genet., 22:40, 1982.
2. Avramova, S., and Denev, D.: Larsen's syndrome. Pediatr. (Sofia), 18:295, 1979.
3. Azimi, F., Edeiken, J., and MacEwen, G. D.: Larsen's syndrome. Congenital dislocation of multiple large joints of the extremities associated with an unusual flat facies. Aust. Radiol., 18:333, 1974.
4. Beluffi, G., and Segre, A.: Sindrome di Larsen in due fratelli. Minerva Pediatr., 30:293, 1978.
5. Buffatti, G., and Pannone, G.: Sindrome di Larsen: Lussazioni multiple congenite con anomalie facciali. Minerva Pediatr., 27:1171, 1975.
6. Colombo, M. L., Tosi, M. T., Magnetti, L., and Artesani, L.: La sindrome di Larsen. Descrizione di un caso con eccezionale dismaturita scheletrica. Minerva Pediatr., 31:1765, 1979.
7. Faure, C., Lascaux, J. P., and Montagne, J. P.: Le syndrome de Larsen. A propos de trois observations nouvelles. Ann. Radiol., 19:629, 1976.
8. Galanski, V. M., and Statz, A.: Radiologische Befunde beim Larsen Syndrom. Fortschr. Geb. Rontgenstr., 128:534, 1978.
9. Haberman, E. T., Sterling, A., and Dennis, R. I.: Larsen's syndrome: A heritable disorder. J. Bone Joint Surg., 58-A:558, 1976.
10. Harris, R., and Cullen, C. H.: Autosomal dominant inheritance in Larsen's syndrome. Clin. Genet., 2:87, 1971.
11. Herrmann, H. C., Kelly, B. A., Fried, M. P., and Strome, M.: The association of a hearing deficit with Larsen's syndrome. J. Otolaryngol., 10:1, 1981.
12. Houston, C. S., Reed, M. H., and Desautels, J. E. L.: Separating Larsen's syndrome from the "arthrogryposis basket." J. Can. Assoc. Radiol., 32:206, 1981.
13. Kaijser, R.: Ueber Kongenitale Kniegelenksluxationen. Acta Orthop. Scand., 6:1, 1935.
14. Kiel, E. A., Frias, J. L., and Victorica, B. E.: Cardiovascular manifestations in the Larsen syndrome. Pediatrics, 71:942, 1983.
15. Kozlowski, K., Robertson, F., and Middleton, R.: Radiographic findings in Larsen's syndrome. Aust. Radiol., 18:336, 1974.
16. Larsen, L. J., Schottstaedt, E. R., and Bost, F. C.: Multiple congenital dislocations associated with characteristic facial abnormality. J. Pediatr., 37:574, 1950.
17. Latta, R. J., Graham, C. B., Aase, J., Scham, S. M., and Smith, D. W.: Larsen's syndrome: A skeletal dysplasia with multiple joint dislocations and unusual facies. J. Pediatr., 78:291, 1971.
18. Lee, P. A.: Multiple joint dislocations and peculiar facies. Am. J. Dis. Child., 126:828, 1973.
19. Lopez-Sastre, J., Toral, J. F., Orense, M., Valdes-Hevia, J., and Crespo, M.: Sindrome de Larsen. Rev. Esp. Pediatr., 31:350, 1975.
20. Maroteaux, P.: L'Hétérogénéité du syndrome de Larsen. Arch. Fr. Pediatr., 32:597, 1975.
21. Masson, A., Buck, P., Pressager, A., Korn, R., and Schneegans, E.: Le syndrome de Larsen. A propos de deux observations. Pediatrie, 33:775, 1978.
22. Micheli, L. J., Hall, J. E., and Watts, H. G.: Spinal instability in Larsen's syndrome. J. Bone Joint Surg., 58-A:562, 1976.
23. Muzumdar, A. S.: Quadriplegia in Larsen syndrome. Birth Defects, 13:202, 1977.
24. Oki, T., Terashima, Y., Murachi, S., and Nogami, H.: Clinical features and treatment of joint dislocations in Larsen's syndrome. Clin. Orthop., 119:206, 1976.
25. Payet, G.: Nanisme et hyperlaxité dysmorphie faciale et luxations multiples. Syndrome de Larsen? Arch. Fr. Pediatr., 32:601, 1975.
26. Perez Trigrueros, A., Vilanova Vasquez, J. L., Diaz, D. E., and Miguel, G. F.: Larsen's syndrome. Report of 3 cases in one family, mother and two offsprings. Acta Orthop. Scand., 49:582, 1978.
27. Renault, F., Arthuis, M., Rethore, M. O., and Lafourcade, J.: Le syndrome de Larsen. Aspects cliniques et génétiques. Arch. Fr. Pediatr., 39:35, 1982.
28. Robertson, F. W., Kozlowski, K., and Middleton, R. W.: Larsen's syndrome. Three cases with multiple congenital joint dislocations and distinctive facies. Clin. Pediatr., 14:53, 1975.
29. Ronningen, H., and Bjerkreim, I.: Larsen's syndrome. Acta Orthop. Scand., 49:138, 1978.
30. Salmon, M. A., and Lindenbaum, R.: Hare-lip in Larsen's syndrome. Lancet, 1:318, 1973.
31. Samuel, A. W., and Davies, D. R. A.: The Larsen syndrome with multiple congenital dislocations and a normal facies. Int. Orthop. (SICOT), 5:229, 1981.
32. Silverman, F. N.: Larsen's syndrome: Congenital dislocations of the knees and other joints, distinctive facies, and, frequently, cleft palate. Ann. Radiol., 15:297, 1972.
33. Spranger, J. W., Langer, L. O., and Wiedemann, H. R.: Larsen syndrome. In Bone Dysplasias. An Atlas of Constitutional Disorders of Skeletal Development. Stuttgart, Fisher, 1974, p. 239.
34. Stanley, D., and Seymour, N.: The Larsen syndrome occurring in four generations of one family. Int. Orthop. (SICOT), 8:267, 1985.
35. Steel, H. H., and Kohl, J.: Multiple congenital dislocations associated with other skeletal anomalies (Larsen's syndrome) in three siblings. J. Bone Joint Surg., 54-A:75, 1972.
36. Sugarman, G. I.: The Larsen syndrome, autosomal dominant form. Birth Defects, 11:121, 1975.
37. Ventruto, V., Festa, B., Sebastio, L., and Sebastio, G.: Larsen syndrome in two generations of an Italian family. Case Report. J. Med. Genet., 13:538, 1976.

CRANIOFACIAL DYSPLASIAS (WITH OR WITHOUT INVOLVEMENT OF THE LIMBS)

Craniofacial syndromes are uncommon; they are caused by premature closure of the cranial sutures. The various types are distinguished by the mode of inheritance and whether the limbs are involved or not.

ACROCEPHALOSYNDACTYLY AND RELATED DYSPLASIAS

Apert's Syndrome

Apert's syndrome is characterized by premature closure of the cranial sutures and complex syndactyly of the hands and feet. Inheritance is autosomal dominant.

The clinical appearance of the patient is characteristic. The head is peaked and vertically elongated in its anteroposterior diameter, with the planes of the face and the back of the skull being parallel. The enlarging brain causes increased intracranial pressure. The protuberant eyes are wide spaced and bulging, with divergence of the transverse axis. Strabismus and progressive impairment of vision are common. Often the posterior palate is high arched, and there are fusion defects of the maxilla and mandible. Convolutional atrophy of the brain and mental retardation are not uncommon.

Syndactyly of digits, metacarpals, and metatarsals may be complete or partial. There may be synostosis of the phalanges of the same digit, owing to the failure of joint formation.

Treatment. Treatment is neurosurgical in the early months of life. An osteotomy of the cranial bones is performed to prevent an increase in intracranial pressure. Surgical separation of syndactyly, as described in the section on congenital deformities of the hand, is performed later if the infant survives the neurosurgical procedures.

Carpenter's Syndrome

Carpenter's syndrome is associated with syndactyly of the third and fourth digits, and polydactyly—usually postaxial in the hand and preaxial in the foot. It may be associated with cardiac malformations. Inheritance is as an autosomal recessive trait.

Crouzon's Syndrome

Crouzon's syndrome is characterized by dysplasia of the midface, wide-spaced eyes, proptosis, and nasal beaking, giving a froglike appearance. Deafness and malocclusion of the teeth are common. Inheritance is as an autosomal dominant trait. Treatment is by maxillofacial surgery. Orthopedic care is not required.

References

APERT'S SYNDROME

1. Anderson, C. E., Fernhoff, P. M., and Quan, L.: Dominant polysyndactyly: A report of two families. J. Pediatr., 90:961, 1977.
2. Beligere, N., Harris, V., and Pruzansky, S.: Progressive bony dysplasia in Apert syndrome. Radiology, 139:593, 1981.
3. Bergstrom, L., and Neblett, L. M.: Otologic manifestations of acrocephalosyndactyly. Arch. Otolaryngol., 96:117, 1972.
4. Blank, C. E.: Apert's syndrome (a type of acrocephalosyndactyly)—observations on a British series of thirty-nine cases. Ann. Hum. Genet., 24:151, 1960.
5. Blauth, W., vonTorne, O.: Der Apert-Fuss. Z. Orthop., 116:1, 1978.
6. Cohen, M. M.: Cardiovascular anomalies in Apert type acrocephalosyndactyly. Birth Defects Orig. Art. Series, 8:132, 1972.
7. Cohen, M. M.: An etiologic and nosologic overview of craniosynostosis syndromes. Birth Defects Orig. Art. Series, 12:137, 1975.
8. Dell, P. C., and Sheppard, J. E.: Deformities of the great toe in Apert's syndrome. Clin. Orthop., 157:113, 1981.
9. Green, S. M.: Pathological anatomy of the hands in Apert's syndrome. J. Hand Surg., 7:450, 1982.
10. Hogan, G. R., and Bauman, M. L.: Hydrocephalus in Apert's syndrome. J. Pediatr.: 79:782, 1971.
11. Hoover, G. H., Flatt, A. E., and Weiss, M. W.: Hand and Apert's syndrome. J. Bone Joint Surg., 52-A:878, 1970.
12. Kelikian, H.: Craniosynostosis. In Congenital Deformities of the Hand and Forearm. Philadelphia, Saunders, 1974, pp. 345–351.
13. Martsolf, J. T., Cracco, J. B., Carpenter, G. G., and O'Hara, A. E.: Pfeiffer syndrome: Unusual type of acrocephalosyndactyly with broad thumbs and great toes. Am. J. Dis. Child., 121:257, 1971.
14. Mohr, G., Hoffman, M. D., Munro, I. R., Hendrick, E. B., and Humphreys, R. P.: Surgical management of unilateral and bilateral coronal craniostenosis: 21 years of experience. Neurosurgery, 2:83, 1978.
15. Pilanzer, K.: Apert's syndrome. Radiol. Clin. North Am., 47:233, 1978.
16. Rubin, M. B., Pirozzi, D. J., and Heaton, C. L.: Acrocephalo-syndactyly. Report of a case with review of the literature. Am. J. Med., 53:127, 1972.
17. Schafer, M. E.: Upper airway obstruction and sleep disorders in children with craniofacial anomalies. Clin. Plast. Surg., 9:555, 1982.
18. Schauerte, E. W., and St. Aubin, P. M.: Progressive synostosis in Apert's syndrome (acrocephalosyndactyly) with a description of roentgenographic changes in the feet. A.J.R., 97:67, 1966.
19. Sherk, H. H., Whitaker, L. A., and Pasquariello, P. S.: Facial malformations and spinal anomalies. A predictable relationship. Spine, 7:526, 1982.
20. Shillito, J., Jr., and Matson, D. D.: Craniosynostosis. A review of 519 surgical patients. Paediatrics, 41:829, 1968.
21. Shons, A. R., Press, B. H., Waite, D. E., and Chou, S. N.: The use of methyl methacrylate in a two-stage correction of Crouzon's/Apert's deformity. Ann. Plast. Surg., 10:147, 1983.
22. Spranger, J. W., Langer, L. O., Jr., and Weidemann, H. R.: Acrocephalosyndactyly, Type I. In Bone Dysplasias. Philadelphia, Saunders, 1974, pp. 261–263.
23. Stewart, R. E., Dixon, J., and Cohen, A.: The pathogenesis of premature craniosynostosis in acrocephalosyndactyly. A reconsideration. Plast. Reconstr. Surg., 59:699, 1977.
24. Vanek, J., and Losan, F.: Pfeiffer's type of acrocephalosyndactyly in two families. J. Med. Genet., 19:289, 1982.
25. Walsh, R. J.: Acrosyndactyly: Study of twenty-seven patients. Clin. Orthop., 71:99, 1970.

ACROCEPHALOPOLYSYNDACTYLY (CARPENTER'S SYNDROME)

1. Balsamo, V., Corso, D., and Giuffre, L.: Un caso di sindrome di Carpenter (acrocefalopolisindattilia). Pediatria (Napoli), 76:407, 1968.
2. Bartowiak, K., Pionetek, E., and Pawlaczyk, B.: Zespol Carpentera U II—letniej dziewcznki. Pediatr. Pol., 47:349, 1972.
3. Carpenter, G.: Two sisters showing malformations of the skull and other congenital abnormalities. Rep. Soc. Dis. Child., 1:110, 1901.
4. Der Kaloustian, V. M., Sinno, A. A., and Nassar, S. J.: Acrocephalopolysyndactyly, type II (Carpenter syndrome). Am. J. Dis. Child., 124:716, 1972.
5. Eaton, A. P., Sommer, A., Kontras, S. B., and Sayer, M. P.: Carpenter syndrome—acrocephalopolysyndac-

tyly, type II. Birth Defects Orig. Art. Series, 10:249, 1974.
6. Kaler, S. G., Bixler, D., and Yu, P.-I.: Metacarpophalangeal pattern profile in ACPS type II (Carpenter syndrome). J. Craniofac. Genet., 1:373, 1981.
7. Pfeiffer, R. A., Seeman, K. B., Tunte, W., Gussone, J., and Klemm, E.: Akrozephalopolysyndaktylie (Akrozephalosyndaktylie, typ II McKusick (Carpenter-Syndrom) Bericht über 4 Falle und eine Beobachtung des Typs von Marshall-Smith. Klin. Pädiatr., 189:120, 1977.
8. Piussan, C., Van Poperinghe, M., Grumbach, Y., Audebert, M., Helsmans, C., and Risbourg, B.: Le syndrome de Carpenter. Arch. Fr. Pediatr., 34:891, 1977.
9. Temtamy, S. A.: Carpenter's syndrome: Acrocephalopolysyndactyly. An autosomal recessive syndrome. J. Pediatr., 69:111, 1966.

CROUZON'S SYNDROME

1. McCarthy, J., Coccaro, P., Epstein, F., and Converse, J.: Early skeletal release in the infant with craniofacial dysostosis. Plast. Reconstr. Surg., 62:335, 1978.
2. Tessier, P.: Osteotomes de la face. Syndrome de Crouzon. Syndrome d'Apert. Oxycephalies: Scaphocephalies; turricephalies. Ann. Chir. Plast., 12:273, 1967.
3. Tessier, P.: Relationship of craniostenosis to craniofacial dysostoses and to faciostenoses. Plast. Reconstr. Surg., 48:224, 1971.

FIBRODYSPLASIA OSSIFICANS PROGRESSIVA (MYOSITIS OSSIFICANS PROGRESSIVA)

This rare congenital affection, first described by Guy Patin in 1692, is characterized by progressive calcification and then ossification of the fasciae, aponeuroses, ligaments, tendons, and connective tissue in interstitial tissues of skeletal muscles; a short big toe (hallux); and less often a short thumb owing to absence of one or fusion of two phalanges. The skeletal muscles are fundamentally normal; the basic defect resides in the connective tissue.[30] Thus, the term *myositis ossificans progressiva* is a misnomer; the name *fibrodysplasia ossificans progressiva* is more appropriate to describe the condition. Rosenstirn, in 1918, collected 119 cases from the literature and added one of his own.[35] Other comprehensive reviews include those of Lutwak, McKusick, and Nutt.[22, 23, 29] Helferich was first to observe the constant association of microdactyly with fibrodysplasia ossificans progressiva.[18]

Inheritance. The condition is inherited as an autosomal dominant trait, but most cases are sporadic.[23] It has been reported in homozygotic twins.[11, 38] There is a preponderance in the male sex, the male to female ratio being 4:1 according to Ryan, and 3:2 according to Fairbank.[11, 38] Rosenstirn found 62 per cent of cases occurred in the male.[35]

Etiology. The exact cause of the disease is unknown.[1] The basic pathogenetic factor appears to be a hereditary defect of some element of connective tissue, leading to secondary calcification and ossification. High levels of alkaline phosphatase activity are found in areas of heterotopic ossification.[48] A congenital deficiency of an inhibitor substance or a relative excess of an inhibitor-destroying mechanism was postulated by Lutwak.[22]

Pathology

The early lesions are characterized by marked interstitial edema and connective tissue proliferation. The muscle fibers undergo secondary atrophic and degenerative changes. Later, calcification and ossification of the involved mesodermal tissues take place. On occasion, it may be difficult to distinguish fibrodysplasia ossificans progressiva from osteogenic sarcoma.

Clinical Features

Manifestations of the disease usually develop before the age of ten years; on occasion, however, the abnormalities in the fasciae and tendons may be present at birth, indicating onset of the pathologic process in fetal life. The short hallux and thumb definitely have a prenatal origin.

In a typical case, swellings first appear in the neck, on the dorsal aspect of the trunk, in the shoulder girdle, and eventually in the proximal parts of the limbs. The site of involvement may also be determined by local injury. These swellings are usually small, although at times, they may be as large as an egg or an apple. In the early acute phase they are painful, locally tender, slightly warm, and associated with a low-grade fever. Swellings may be cystlike and fluctuant, or they may be firm from onset. Often they are attached to the deep fascia, and the overlying skin is normal and loose; but on occasion, they may be ill-defined and not adherent to the deep fascia.

Torticollis is a common presenting complaint; the head is tilted to one side, and there are painful swellings in the region of the sternocleidomastoid muscle. Flexion of the neck is limited when the ligamentum nuchae is involved. Motion of the temporomandibular joint is diminished, with affection of the masseters (about 20 per cent of cases). Restriction of motion of the shoulder, elbow, hip, and knee eventually develops. The soft swellings subside within a few days or weeks, but the indurated swellings usually persist.

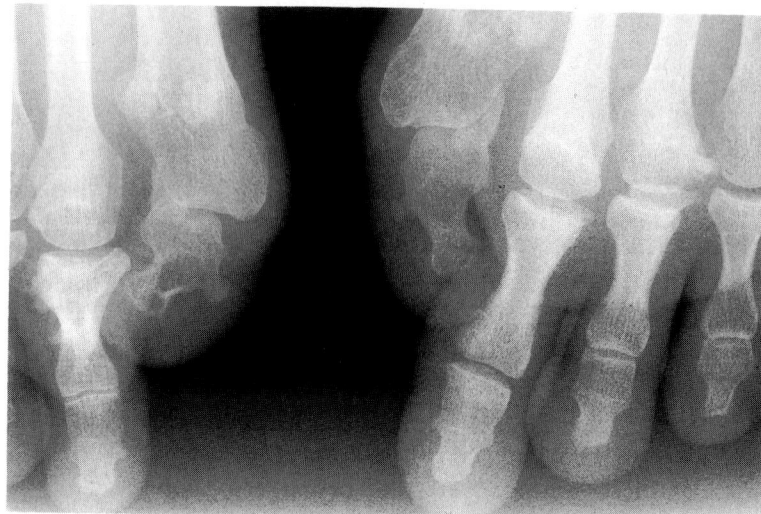

FIGURE 3–90. *Fibrodysplasia ossificans progressiva.*

Note characteristic short hallux in the anteroposterior radiogram of the forefoot.

Involvement of the limbs distal to the knees and elbows is rare. The tongue, heart, larynx, diaphragm, and sphincters are exempt from involvement.

In this early stage the finding of microdactyly of the big toe or the thumb will be of great help in diagnosis. Stunting of growth of the great toe (due to the reduced length of its phalanges) is present in almost all cases of true fibrodysplasia ossificans progressiva (Fig. 3–90). The proximal phalanx may be diminished to a mere wedge-shaped fragment. Rarely is the first metatarsal bone shortened. Hallux valgus is common. The thumbs are shortened less frequently (about 50 per cent of cases). On occasion other digits may be reduced in length. Other rare deformities include absence of a phalanx, fusion of a metacarpal or metatarsal to the proximal phalanx, and volar-radial deviation of the distal phalanx of the little finger.

Advanced ossification of the epiphyses and widening of the femoral necks may be present. Dystrophic calcification and ossification develop gradually in the involved areas. If a swelling is firm and persistent, ossification will usually take place within two to eight months. The ossific areas may be arranged in columns, lying along the course of muscles, tendons, or ligaments; or may take the form of irregular masses in the fasciae or aponeuroses. The skin may ulcerate over a protruding mass of bone. The spine and the joints in the vicinity of ossified areas become progressively stiff and then completely rigid. Eventually, the patient may be unable to sit.

Radiographic Findings

The columns and irregular masses of extraskeletal bone have varying densities on the radiogram. They may be connected to skeletal bone, or they may be entirely free (Figs. 3–91 and 3–92). The skeleton as a whole shows disuse atrophy. The microdactyly and digital anomalies are self-evident.

In the *differential diagnosis* several entities should be considered. In infancy and early childhood, the condition may be mistaken for *congenital muscular torticollis*; the short big toe or thumb, however, and the progressive nature of the disease should determine the diagnosis of fibrodysplasia ossificans progressiva. Prior to the stage of advanced ossification, the swellings may suggest *Weber-Christian syndrome* or *relapsing nodular nonsuppurative panniculitis*. The latter condition is very rare and is characterized by the appearance of crops of painful subcutaneous nodules of degenerating and inflamed adipose tissue on the trunk, thighs, and arms. It is commonly associated with fever, leukopenia, and an elevated sedimentation rate. Within one or two weeks, the nodules regress, leaving behind a pigmented depression. The etiology of this disease is unknown and there is no specific therapy.

Fibrodysplasia ossificans progressiva should also be distinguished from calcinosis universalis and dermatomyositis. In *calcinosis universalis* the calcification will cast a granular and fragmentary shadow on the radiogram. The lesions are more common in the limbs, beginning in the subcutaneous tissues and later extending to involve the ligaments, tendons, and connective tissue of the muscles. *Dermatomyositis* also initially affects the limbs and later involves the trunk. The skin and underlying muscle are inflamed, with local tenderness, induration, swelling, and weakness. The necrotic foci in the

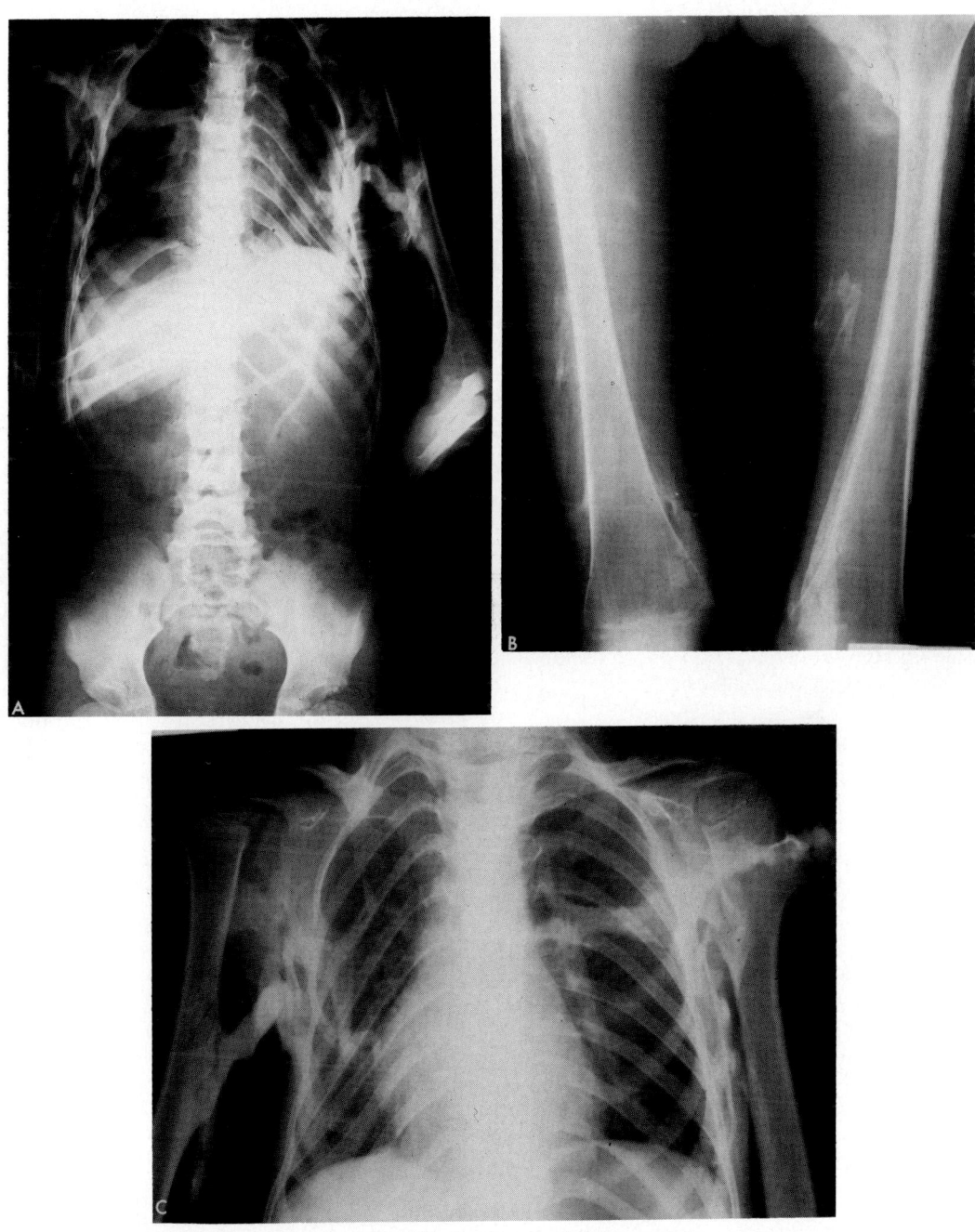

FIGURE 3-91. Fibrodysplasia ossificans progressiva.

A. Initial radiogram. **B** and **C.** Radiograms taken one year later, showing progression of the disease. Note the columns and plaques of ectopic bone.

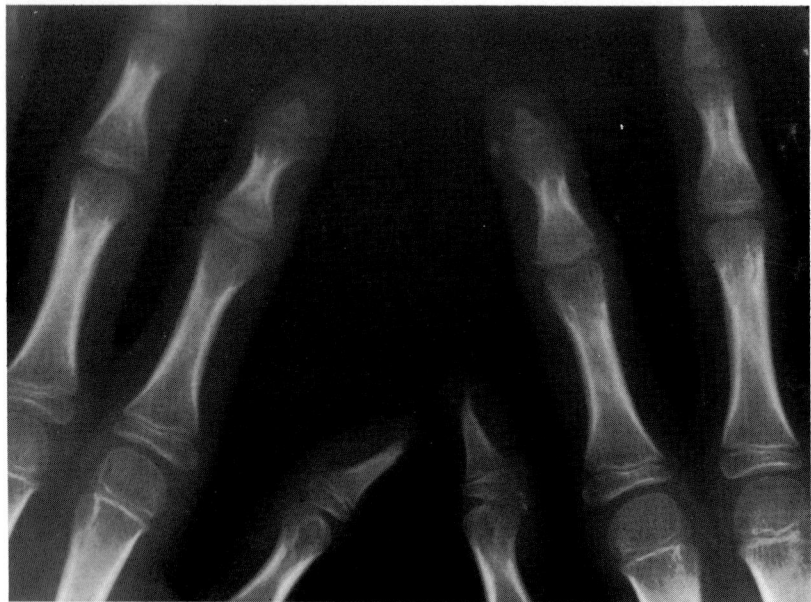

FIGURE 3-92. *Fibrodysplasia ossificans progressiva.*

Radiograms of the hands, showing microdactyly of the thumbs and index fingers. Note the tapered ends of the distal phalanx of the thumb.

muscle and subcutaneous fat may calcify and be visible on the radiogram. Skin and muscle biopsy will establish the diagnosis.

Prognosis and Treatment

The course of the disease is one of steady progression with periods of remission and acute exacerbations. Eventually the patient becomes totally disabled.

There is no specific therapy.[41] A trial of treatment with adrenocortical hormones has given dubious results.[10, 21] Beryllium has been tried and found to be of doubtful benefit.[43] Radiation therapy will aggravate the condition. The progress of the disease is not arrested by treatment with diphosponate.[2, 37, 47] Operative excision of the bony columns to relieve ankylosis has been disappointing, as the surgical trauma has aggravated the condition, and more extensive bone has reformed.

References

1. Ackerman, L. V.: Extra-osseous non-neoplastic bone and cartilage formation (so-called myositis ossificans). J. Bone Joint Surg., *40-A*:279, 1958.
2. Bassett, A. L., Donath, A., Macagno, F., Preisig, R., Fleisch, H., and Francis, M. D.: Diphosphonates in the treatment of myositis ossificans. Lancet, 2:845, 1965.
3. Burton-Fanning, F. W., and Vaughan, A. L.: A case of myositis ossificans. Lancet, 2:849, 1901.
4. Byers, W, M · Almost complete ossification of the human body. New Orleans J. Med., 23:122, 1870.
5. Cox, H. L.: Progressive myositis ossificans: Review of the literature and report of a case. North Carolina Med. J., *18*:459, 1957.
6. Cremin, B., Connor, J. B., and Beighton, P.: The radiological spectrum of fibrodysplasia ossificans progressiva. Clin. Radiol., 33:499, 1980.
7. Dixon, T. F., Mulligan, L., Nassim, R., and Stevenson, F. H.: Myositis ossificans progressiva. J. Bone Joint Surg., *36-B*:445, 1954.
8. Dobrzanieck, W.: The problem of myositis ossificans progressiva. Ann. Surg., *104*:987, 1936.
9. Eaton, W. L., Conkling, W. S., and Daeschner, C. W.: Early myositis ossificans progressiva occurring in homozygotic twins. J. Pediatr., 50:591, 1957.
10. Ellingsworth, R. S.: Myositis ossificans progressiva (Munchmeyer's disease). Brief review with report of two cases treated with corticosteroids and observed for 16 years. Arch. Dis. Child., 46:264, 1971.
11. Fairbank, H. A. T.: Myositis ossificans progressiva. J. Bone Joint Surg., *32-B*:108, 1950.
12. Frejka, B.: Heteropic ossification and myositis ossificans progressiva. J. Bone Joint Surg., *11*:157, 1929.
13. Gaster, D.: A case of myositis ossificans. W. Lond. Med. J., *10*:37, 1905.
14. Goto, S.: Pathologisch-anatomische und klinische Studien über die sogen. Myositis ossificans progressiva multiplex. (Hyperplasia fascialis ossificans progresiva.) Arch. Klin. Chir., 6:730, 1912–1913.
15. Grewal, K. S., and Das, N.: Myositis ossificans progressiva. J. Bone Joint Surg., *35-B*:244, 1953.
16. Griffith, G.: Progressive myositis ossificans. Arch. Dis. Child., *24*:71, 1949.
17. Hall, C. M., and Sutcliffe, J.: Fibrodysplasia ossificans progressiva. Ann. Radiol., *22*:119, 1979.
18. Helferich, H.: Ein Fall von sogenannter Myositis ossificans progressiva. Zerztliches Intelligenz-Blatt, 26:485, 1879.

19. Hutchinson, J.: Reports of hospital practice. Medical Times and Gazette, 1:March 31, 1960.
20. Koontz, A. R.: Myositis ossificans progressiva. Am. J. Med. Sci., 174:406, 1927.
21. Lockhart, J. D., and Burke, F. G.: Myositis ossificans progressiva—report of a case treated with corticotropin (ACTH). Am. J. Dis. Child., 87:626, 1954.
22. Lutwak, L.: Myositis ossificans progressiva: Mineral, metabolic, and radioactive calcium studies of the effects of hormones. Am. J. Med., 37:269, 1964.
23. McKusick, V. A.: Fibrodysplasia ossificans progressiva. In Heritable Disorders of Connective Tissue. 3rd Ed. St Louis, Mosby, 1966, p. 400.
24. Maini, P. S., and Singh, M.: Localized myositis ossificans progressiva. J. Bone Joint Surg., 49-A:955, 1967.
25. Mair, W. F.: Myositis ossificans progressiva. Edinburgh Med. J., 39:13,69, 1932.
26. Mandsley, R. H.: A case of myositis ossificans progressiva. Br. Med. J., 1:954, 1952.
27. Mather, J. H.: Progressive myositis ossificans. Br. J. Radiol., 4:207, 1931.
28. Michelsohn, J.: Ein Fall von Myositis ossificans progressiva. Z. Orthop. Chir., 12:424, 1904.
29. Nutt, J. J.: Report of a case of myositis ossificans progressiva with bibliography. J. Bone Joint Surg., 5:344, 1923.
30. Patin, G.: Lettres choisies de feu Mr. Guy Patin. Cologne, 1:28, 1692.
31. Peck, G. T., and Braund, R. R.: The development of sarcoma in myositis ossificans. J.A.M.A., 119:776, 1942.
32. Riley, H. D., and Christie, A.: Myositis ossificans progressiva. Pediatrics, 8:753, 1951.
33. Rolleston, H. D.: Progressive myositis ossificans with reference to other developmental disease of the mesoblast. Clin. J., 17:209, 1901.
34. Rosborough, D.: Ectopic bone formation associated with multiple congenital anomalies. J. Bone Joint Surg., 48-B:499, 1966.
35. Rosenstirn, J.: A contribution to the study of myositis ossificans progressiva. Ann. Surg., 68:485,591, 1918.
36. Royers, J. G., and Geho, W. B.: Fibrodysplasia ossificans progressiva: Survey of 42 cases. J. Bone Joint Surg., 61-A:909, 1979.
37. Russell, G. G., and Smith, R.: Diphosphonates: Experimental and clinical aspects. J. Bone Joint Surg., 55-B:66, 1973.
38. Ryan, K. J.: Myositis ossificans progressiva: Review of the literature with report of a case. J. Pediatr., 27:348, 1945.
39. Singleton, E. B., and Holt, J. F.: Myositis ossificans progressiva. Radiology, 62:47, 1954.
40. Smith, D. M., Zeman, W., Johnston, C. C., Jr., and Deiss, W. P., Jr.: Myositis ossificans progressiva. Metabolism, 15:521, 1966.
41. Smith, R., Russell, G. G., and Woods, C. G.: Myositis ossificans progressiva: Clinical features of eight patients and their response to treatment. J. Bone Joint Surg., 58-B:48, 1976.
42. Tunte, W., Becker, P. E., and Von Knorre, G.: Zur Genetik der Myositis ossificans progressiva. Humangenetik., 4:320, 1967.
43. Tutunjian, K. H., and Kegerreis, R.: Myositis ossificans progressiva. J. Bone Joint Surg., 19:503, 1937.
44. Uehlinger, E.: Myositis ossificans progressiva. Ergeb. Med. Strahlenforsch., 7:175, 1936.
45. Van Creveld, S., and Soeters, J. M.: Myositis ossificans progressiva. Am. J. Dis. Child., 62:1000, 1941.
46. Vastine, J. H., Vastine, M. F., and Arango, O.: Myositis ossificans progressiva in homozygotic twins. A.J.R., 59:204, 1948.
47. Weiss, I. W., Fischer, L., and Phang, J. M.: Diphosphonate therapy in a patient with myositis ossificans progressiva. Ann. Intern. Med., 74:933, 1971.
48. Wilkins, W. E., Regen, E. M., and Carpenter, G. K.: Phosphatase studies on biopsy tissue in progressive myositis ossificans. Am. J. Dis. Child., 49:1219, 1935.

CORNELIA DE LANGE SYNDROME

This very rare syndrome is characterized by short stature, microcephaly, distinctive facies (low hair line, bushy eyebrows meeting in the midline, small nose with anteverted nostrils, and in-turned upper lip), mental retardation, and congenital longitudinal deficiency of long bones, primarily on the ulnar side. Prognosis is poor because of failure to thrive.

References

1. DeLange, C.: Sur un type nouveau de dégénération (Typus Amstelodamensis). Arch. Med. Enfant., 36:713, 1933.
2. Jervis, G. A., and Stimson, C. W.: DeLange syndrome. The "Amsterdam type" of mental defect with congenital malformation. J. Pediatr., 63:634, 1963.
3. MacArthur, R. G., and Edwards, J. H.: DeLange syndrome. Report of 20 cases. Can. Med. Assoc. J., 96:1185, 1967.
4. Pashayan, H., Whelan, D., Guttman, S., and Fraser, F. C.: Variability of the DeLange syndrome: Report of three cases and genetic analysis of 54 families. J. Pediatr., 75:853, 1969.

EHLERS-DANLOS SYNDROME

This syndrome is a group of related disorders caused by defective collagen metabolism and characterized by skin changes consisting of hyperextensibility, fragility, and easy bruising with resultant "cigarette paper" scarring; extreme ligamentous laxity of the joints; bone fragility with varying degrees of osteopenia; and generalized friability of the tissues (Fig. 3–93). Of the various names given to this common heritable disorder of connective tissue, *Ehlers-Danlos syndrome* seems preferable. In 1682, Job van Meeckeren described the first definitive case, pointing out the "extraordinary dilatability of the skin."[22] Ehlers, in 1901, pointed out the associated loose-jointedness and subcutaneous hemorrhages, and Danlos, in 1908, added the subcutaneous tumors that may develop at pressure points.[7,8]

A rare disease, it is inherited as an autosomal dominant trait and is caused by faulty organization of collagen bundles into an intermeshing network, as shown in Figure 3–93 A.

Clinically, the skin is hyperextensible, fragile, and brittle, and bruises easily. Pseudotumors form at pressure points, such as the knees, heels, and elbows (Figs. 3–93 C and 3–94). It is hyperpigmented and has been described as

The condition is caused by diminished productions of type III collagen. Inheritance may be by autosomal dominant or recessive transmission.

Type V is characterized by marked fragility and hyperextensibility of the skin but limited joint hypermobility. Hereditary transmission is X-linked and recessive.

Type VI is characterized by deficiency of lysine hydroxylase and low concentrations of hydroxylysine in the collagen. The collagen fibers are loose and have minimal solubility. Joint and skin involvement are moderate. Eyes are affected with ectopia lentis. Inheritance is as an autosomal recessive trait.[16, 17]

Type VII is also known as *arthrochalasis multiplex congenita* because of the extreme hyperlaxity of the joints. The stature is short. The condition is caused by a deficiency of procollagen peptidase and an abnormal alpha-2-chain. It is inherited as an autosomal dominant trait.[12, 19]

Type VIII is characterized by progressive periodontal disease in addition to joint hyperlaxity and skin hyperextensibility. Inheritance is by autosomal dominant transmission.[15]

Treatment. There is no specific treatment for the disease. Management is symptomatic.

References

1. Baumer, J. H., and Hankey, S.: Transient pulmonary cysts in an infant with the Ehlers-Danlos syndrome. Br. J. Radiol., 53:598, 1980.
2. Beighton, P.: The Ehlers-Danlos Syndrome. London, Heinemann, 1970.
3. Beighton, P., and Horan, F.: Orthopedic aspects of the Ehlers-Danlos syndrome. J. Bone Joint Surg., 51-B:444, 1969.
4. Blickman, J. G., and Griscom, N. T.: Aortic rupture in a previously undiagnosed case of the Ehlers-Danlos syndrome. Pediatr. Radiol., 12:86, 1982.
5. Bowers, W. H., Spencer, J. B., and McDevitt, N. B.: Brachial-artery rupture in Ehlers-Danlos syndrome: An unusual cause of high median-nerve palsy. A case report. J. Bone Joint Surg., 58-A:1025, 1976.
6. Byers, P. H., Barsh, G. S., and Holbrook, K. A.: Disorders of connective tissue metabolism as related to the skin. Birth Defects, 17:147, 1981.
7. Danlos, M.: Un cas de cutis laxa avec tumeurs par contusion chroniques des coudes et des genoux (xanthome juvénile pseudodiabétique de MM. Hallopeau et Mace de Lepinary). Bull. Soc. Fr. Dermatol. Syph., 19:70, 1908.
8. Ehlers, E.: Cutis laxa, Neigung zu Haemorrhagien in der Haut, Lockerung mehrerer Artikulationen. Dermatol. Z., 8:173, 1901.
9. Hernandez, A., Aguirre-Negrete, M. G., Liparoli, J. C., and Cantu, J. M.: Third case of a distinct variant of the Ehlers-Danlos syndrome. Clin. Genet., 20:222, 1981.
10. Igarashi, M., Katsumata, M., Masu, S., Seiji, M., and Watanabe, N.: Clinical features and an ultrastructural study of Ehlers-Danlos syndrome Type II. J. Dermatol. (Tokyo), 9:309, 1982.
11. Krieg, T., Ihme, A., Weber, L., Kirsch, E., and Mueller, P. K.: Molecular defects of collagen metabolism in the Ehlers-Danlos syndrome. Int. J. Dermatol., 20:415, 1981.
12. Lichtenstein, J. R., Martin, G. K., Kohn, L. D., Byers, P. H., and McKusick, V. A.: Defect in conversion of procollagen to collagen in a form of Ehlers-Danlos syndrome. Science, 182:298, 1973.
13. McKusick, V. A.: Heritable Disorders of Connective Tissue. 3rd Ed. St. Louis, Mosby, 1966, pp. 17–22.
14. Nagashima, C., Tsuji, R., Kubota, S., and Tajima, K.: Atlanto-axial, atlanto-occipital dislocations. Developmental cervical canal stenosis in the Ehlers-Danlos syndrome. No Shinkei Geka, 9:601, 1981.
15. Piette, E., and Douniau, R.: Juvenile parodontolysis symptomatic of Ehlers-Danlos syndrome, a sporadic case? Acta Stomatol. Belg., 77:217, 1980.
16. Pinnell, S. R.: Molecular defects in the Ehlers-Danlos syndrome. J. Invest. Dermatol., 79:905, 1982.
17. Pinnell, S. R., Krane, S. M., Kenzora, J. E., and Glimcher, M. J.: A heritable disorder of connective tissue, hydroxylysine-deficient collagen disease. N. Engl. J. Med., 286:1013, 1972.
18. Salem, O. S., and Tomecki, K. J.: Ehlers-Danlos syndrome, Type II (mitis). Clev. Clin. Q., 49:265, 1982.
19. Steinmann, B., Tuderman, L., Peltonen, L., Martin, G. R., McKusick, V. A., and Prockop, D. J.: Evidence for a structural mutation of procollagen Type I in a patient with the Ehlers-Danlos syndrome Type VII. J. Biol. Chem., 255:8887, 1980.
20. Stevanovic, D. V., Duknic, V., Lalevic-Vasic, B., and Dimitrijevic, N.: Ehlers-Danlos syndrome—type unknown. Dermatol. Monatsschr., 168:87, 1982.
21. Sussman, M., Lichtenstein, J., Nigra, T., Martin, G. R., and McKusick, V.: Hydroxylsine-deficient skin collagen in a patient with a form of the Ehlers-Danlos syndrome. J. Bone Joint Surg., 56-A:1228, 1974.
22. van Meekeren, J. A.: De dilatabilitate extraordinaria cutis, Chap. 32, Observations medico-chirugicae. Amsterdam, 1682.
23. Wesley, J. R., Mahour, H., and Wooley, M. M.: Multiple surgical problems in two patients with Ehlers-Danlos syndrome. Surgery, 87:319, 1980.

MISCELLANEOUS DYSPLASIAS

Menkes Syndrome

Menkes syndrome is characterized by severe mental retardation due to cerebral and cerebellar degeneration. Inheritance is sex-linked and recessive.

Patients have peculiar hair that is kinky, stubbly, and whitish. Extensive skeletal changes consist of metaphyseal spurring and periosteal new bone formation in the long bones. These patients also have microcephaly with multiple wormian bones.

The disorder is caused by a defect in the intestinal absorption of copper, which can be detected by biochemical testing. Prognosis is poor.

Orofaciodigital Syndrome

This extremely rare syndrome is transmitted through an X-linked dominant inheritance that is lethal in the male. There is an autosomal recessive type (Mohr syndrome). Half the patients are mentally retarded. The facies are characteristic, marked by a central cleft of the upper lip and palate and a lobulated tongue.

Orofaciodigital syndrome is also associated with deformities of the hand: postaxial polydactyly and brachydactyly. In the Mohr syndrome, there is preaxial polydactyly.

Otopalatodigital Syndrome

This syndrome is characterized by deafness and cleft palate. There are anomalies of the hands and feet that result from defective modeling and fusion of the carpal or tarsal bones.

Inheritance is probably X-linked and dominant.

Rubenstein-Taybi Syndrome

This nonhereditary condition, in most cases, occurs sporadically. It is characterized by broadening of the thumb and hallux and severe mental retardation. The nose is large, and the philtrum extends below the alae. The palpebral fissures slope downward.

The orthopedic surgeon's primary concern is cervical spondylolisthesis, which may result in quadriplegia if not stabilized by fusion; the foot and hand deformities may require surgical correction.

References

MENKES SYNDROME

1. Danks, D. M., Campbell, P. E., Stevens, B. J., Mayne, V., and Cartwright, E.: Menkes' kinky hair syndrome. An inherited defect in copper absorption with widespread effects. Pediatrics, 50:188, 1972.
2. Menkes, J. H., Alter, M., Steigleder, G. K., Weakley, D. R., and Sung, J. H.: A sex-linked disorder with retardation of growth, peculiar hair and focal cerebral and cerebellar degeneration. Pediatrics, 29:764, 1962.
3. Williams, D. M., Atkin, C. L., Frens, D. B., and Bray, P. F.: Menkes kinky hair syndrome—studies of copper metabolism and long term copper therapy. Pediatr. Res., 11:823, 1977.

OROFACIODIGITAL SYNDROME

1. Burn, J., Dezateux, C., Hall, C., and Baraitser, M.: Orofaciodigital syndrome with mesomelic limb shortening. J. Med. Genet., 21:189, 1984.
2. Rimion, D. L., and Edgerton, M. T.: Genetic and clinical heterogeneity in the oral-facial-digital syndrome. J. Pediatr., 71:94, 1967.

OTOPALATODIGITAL SYNDROME

1. Gall, J. C., Stern, A. M., Poznanski, A. K., Garn, S. M., Weinstein, E. D., and Hayward, J. R.: Oto-palatal-digital syndrome. Comparison of clinical and radiographic manifestations in males and females. Am. J. Hum. Genet., 24:24, 1972.

RUBENSTEIN–TAYBI SYNDROME

1. Johnson, C. F.: Broad thumbs and broad great toes with facial abnormalities and mental retardation. J. Pediatr., 68:942, 1966.
2. Simpson, N. E., and Brissendon, J. E.: The Rubenstein-Taybi syndrome: Familial and dermatoglyphic data. Am. J. Med. Genet., 25:225, 1973.

THE MUCOPOLYSACCHARIDOSES

The mucopolysaccharidoses constitute the largest group of lysosomal storage diseases. The intracellular degradation of micromolecular compounds into smaller component units is carried out by lysosomes. Defective activity of any of the lysosomal enzymes will cause a block in the breakdown processes, with a consequent intracellular accumulation of semi-degraded compounds. The mucopolysaccharidoses are subclassified according to the type of substance that accumulates.

Clinical and Radiographic Features. Heparan sulfate, dermatan sulfate, and keratan sulfate are the mucopolysaccharides that accumulate in abnormal quantities and are excreted in the urine. The clinical type of the various mucopolysaccharides can be diagnosed by biochemical analysis of the urine. Recent and more accurate diagnostic tools are metabolic studies of cultured skin fibroblasts and identification of the specific enzyme defect. Most of the mucopolysaccharides have an effect on skeletal growth and development. Spranger and associates proposed the term *dysostosis multiplex* to embrace the main radiographic features of the mucopolysaccharidoses.[128] These include enlargement of the skull, a thick calvarium, and a sella turcica that is J-shaped (Fig. 3–95 A). The clavicles are broad, particularly at the medial end, and the ribs are oar-shaped, narrow, attenuated posteriorly, and broad anteriorly (Fig. 3–95 B). Scoliosis is frequently present. The vertebral bodies are ovoid when immature, underdevelopment of their anterosuperior portion giving the appearance of a broad hook (Fig. 3–95 D). (In Morquio's disease, the vertebrae are flat with a central tongue, as shown in Figure 3–95 E.) The iliac wings are flared and the acetabuli dysplastic with frequent increase of the femoral neck-shaft angle (Fig. 3–95 F). (In Morquio's disease the capital femoral epiphyses are irregular.) The long tubular bones are short, lack diaphyseal modeling, and have thick-

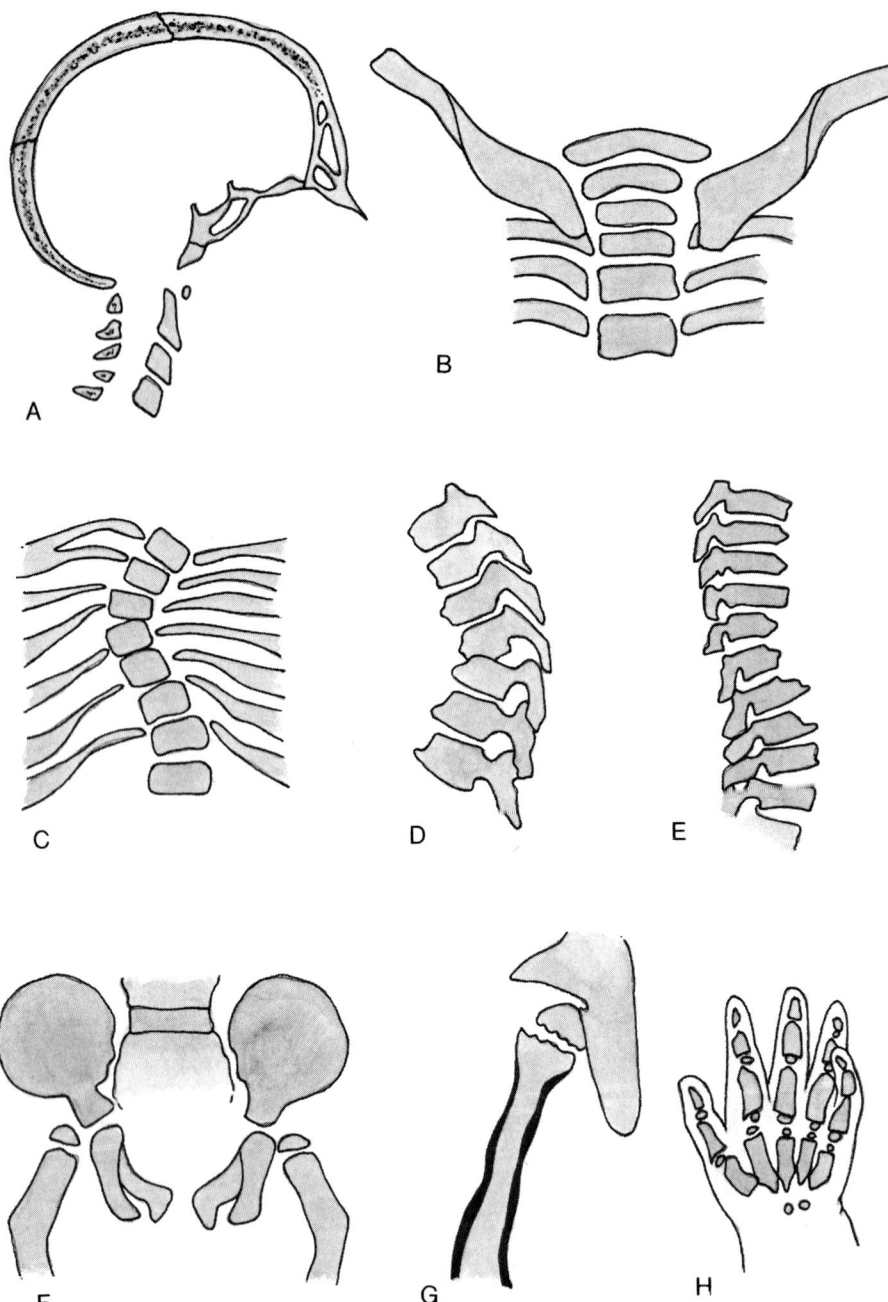

FIGURE 3–95. *Skeletal changes in the mucopolysaccharidoses.*

A. Thickening of the skull and enlarged sella turcica. **B.** Broad medial ends of the clavicles. **C.** Narrowing and attenuation of the ribs posteriorly, and widening anteriorly. Often there is associated scoliosis. **D.** Lateral projection of the vertebrae, showing underdevelopment of vertebral bodies anterosuperiorly, giving a broad hooked appearance. **E.** Lateral view of the spine in Morquio's disease. Note the platyspondyly with a central tongue. **F.** Anteroposterior view of the pelvis, showing the oblique acetabular roofs, the flaring of the iliac wings, and the coxa valga. **G.** The upper end of the humerus, demonstrating the lack of diaphyseal modeling of the long bones. The shaft is thicker than the metaphysis, and the scapula is short and stocky. **H.** Anteroposterior view of the hand. Note the second and fifth metacarpals, which are pointed proximally; the delayed ossification of the carpal bones; and the bullet shape of the phalanges. (Redrawn from Wynne-Davies, R., and Fairbank, T. J.: Fairbank's Atlas of General Affections of the Skeleton. 2nd Ed. New York, Churchill-Livingstone, 1976, p. 173.)

ened cortices. The scapulae are short and stubby (Fig. 3–95 G). The second to the fifth metacarpals are pointed at their proximal ends, the phalanges are bullet-shaped, and there is delay of ossification of the carpal bones (Fig. 3–95 H). (In Morquio's disease the metacarpals and phalanges have a central constriction.)

Differentiation between the various types of mucopolysaccharidoses is not feasible by the radiographic findings alone. Diagnosis is made by thorough assessment of the clinical and radiographic features, genetic studies, laboratory findings, and determination of the precise enzyme deficiency by urine studies and skin fibroblast cultures. Differentiation between various mucopolysaccharidoses is presented in Table 3–11.

Mucopolysaccharidosis I (Hurler Syndrome)*

This form of mucopolysaccharidosis was first described by Gertrude Hurler, in 1919, in infants with gibbus, corneal clouding, and mental retardation.[57] Because of the peculiar, repugnant appearance of these children, the term *gargoylism* was applied by Ellis, Sheldon, and Capon in 1936. They also suggested the possibility that a metabolic error might be responsible for the disease.[33] Brante, in 1952, considered Hurler's syndrome to be a mucopolysaccharidosis.[16] Dorfman and Lorincz, and Meyer and associates reported the presence of excessive amounts of dermatan sulfate and heparan sulfate in the urine and tissues in Hurler's syndrome, thus firmly establishing the nature of the disease as a mucopolysaccharidosis.[31, 97] Bach and associates, in 1972, showed the basic enzyme deficiency is of α-L-iduronidase.[4]

The disease is inherited as an autosomal recessive trait. Both parents of affected siblings may be normal, but consanguinity of parents is not uncommon. Danes and Bearn reported finding metachromatic granules in cultured fibroblasts stained with toluidine blue, in both homozygous patients and heterozygous parents.[24]

Hurler's syndrome, the most common of the mucopolysaccharidoses, has been reported in a wide variety of ethnic groups.[78]

Pathologic and Laboratory Findings. Cells of parenchymal and mesenchymal tissues are infiltrated with deposits of abnormal mucopolysaccharide. The deposits are found in the nerve cells of the central nervous system and peripheral ganglia, the nuclear layer of the retina, the Kupffer and parenchymal cells of the liver, the reticulum cells of the spleen and lymph nodes, and the epithelial cells of several endocrine organs such as the pituitary gland and the testes.[81] In the heart, nodular thickening and heavy deposits of yellow-orange material are found in the valves, and the coronary arteries show extensive intimal deposits. Enlargement and vacuolization of the chondrocytes and osteocytes have been noted. In the peripheral blood, on Wright's stain, the neutrophils, lymphocytes, and eosinophilic leukocytes show coarse, deeply staining violet granules (Reilly granules).[145]

There is increased urinary secretion of dermatan sulfate (+ +) and heparan sulfate (+). Toluidine blue stain of cultured fibroblasts shows metachromasia. The specific enzyme that is deficient is α-L-iduronidase.

Clinical Features. In the first few months of life, the infant appears to be normal, but soon there is increasing evidence of the disease. The facies is heavy and grotesque (Fig. 3–96 A and B). The head is enlarged, and hydrocephalus resulting from meningeal deposits is not uncommon. The skull is scaphocephalic (boat-shaped), and the forehead is low. The eyes are wide apart, suggesting hypertelorism. Clouding of the cornea, best shown by slit-lamp examination, is a universal feature of the disease and masks the associated progressive degeneration of the retina. Initially, eyesight is normal, but vision is impaired as corneal clouding and retinal degeneration increase. The nostrils are wide, and the nose has a broad tip as well as a saddle-shaped, depressed bridge. "Chronic rhinitis" with noisy mouth breathing is present in all cases; it is caused by narrowing of the nasopharyngeal airway by enlarged adenoids and deposits in the mucosa. The appearance of a cretin is given by the everted, patulous lips, the open mouth, and the enlarged thick tongue. The teeth are poorly formed, small, and widely spaced. The ears are set low on the head. Because of premature closure of the sagittal and metopic sutures and local hyperostosis, one may be able to palpate a prominent longitudinal ridge that may cross the forehead.

The neck is markedly shortened, and the rib cage is deformed, with flaring in its lower portion. The abdomen is protuberant, owing to enlargement of the liver and spleen (Fig. 3–96 C and D). Umbilical and inguinal hernias are frequent. There is a localized kyphosis in the

---

*See references 1, 4, 6, 9, 13, 16, 23, 29, 30, 33, 38–40, 49, 53, 57, 60, 70, 78, 84, 87, 91, 92, 97, 99, 106, 107, 112, 117, 119, 126, 145.

Table 3–11. Differential Diagnosis of Mucopolysaccharidosis

Type	Enzyme Defect	Increased Urinary Excretion of Acid Muccopolysaccharide	Inheritance	Age at Which Features Present	Facies	Corneal Clouding
Hurler syndrome MPS I	Deficient α-L-iduronidase	Dermatan sulfate ++ Heparan sulfate +	Ausotomal recessive	First few months May appear normal at birth	Grotesque Gargoyle	Present
Hunter syndrome MPS II	Low sulfoiduronate sulfatase	Heparan sulfate ++ Dermatan sulfate +	Sex-linked recessive All patients male	6–12 months	Similar to Hurler; less severe	Absent
San Filippo syndrome MPS III	Low N-heparan sulfatase or α-acetyl-glucosaminidase	Heparan sulfate ++	Autosomal recessive	Early childhood	Not coarse	Absent
Morquio syndrome MPS IV	N-Ac-Gal-6 sulfate sulfatase	Keratin sulfate ++ (diminishes with age)	Autosomal recessive	2–4 years	Not coarse Wide mouth Prominent maxilla	Present, slowly progressive
Scheie syndrome MPS I-S	α-L-Iduronidase	Heparan sulfate + Dermatan sulfate ++	Autosomal recessive	Late childhood	Somewhat coarse	Present
Maroteaux-Lamy syndrome MPS VI	N-Ac-Gal-4-sulfatase	Dermatan sulfate ++	Autosomal recessive	Early to late childhood	Coarse	Present, poor vision

dorsolumbar area (Fig. 3–96 G). Peripheral lymphadenopathy may be present.

Flexion contracture of joints is common. The little finger is curved, usually radially. The hands are broad, with short, stubby digits (Fig. 3–96 E and F). Genu valgum and pes planovalgus may be present.

Stature may be normal; dwarfism is not an essential feature of the disease.

Mental retardation is a striking and almost constant feature of the Hurler syndrome. This trait, if looked for, may be detected early. The highest intellectual level that can be achieved is idiocy.

Most patients with the Hurler syndrome die in childhood, before the age of ten years, from heart disease or respiratory infection, although some may live well into adult life.

Radiographic Features. The skeletal changes in the Hurler syndrome show a general similarity to those of the Morquio syndrome, but there are definite distinctions between the two conditions. The skull is normal in infancy, but in the second year of life it becomes deformed. It is enlarged in its anteroposterior diameter and is scaphocephalic because of premature closure of the sagittal and metopic sutures (Fig. 3–96 H). The sella turcica is elongated and shallow with anterior "pocketing," which gives it a J-shaped appearance (Fig. 3–97 A). There is no evidence of bony erosion, indicating that the shape of the sella turcica is caused by a malformation of the sphenoid bone rather than by an enlargement of the pituitary. The paranasal sinuses are maldeveloped and poorly aerated. The mandible is short and wide, with the articular surface of its condyle flattened or concave.[53]

In the first few months of life dysplastic changes in the vertebral bodies become evident. In the lateral projection the infantile biconvex shape persists, especially in the twelfth thoracic and first lumbar vertebrae; on careful inspection, a mild kyphosis can be discerned. Between one and two years of age, the

Table 3–11 *Differential Diagnosis of Mucopolysaccharidosis* Continued

Deafness	Hepatosplen-omegaly	Cardio-vascular Abnormality	Stature	Skeletal Changes	Mental Retardation	Prognosis
Present	Present	Present	Normal at birth, later may be moderately short	Moderate dorsolumbar kyphosis Anterior-inferior beaking of body of L2 or L1	Severe	Progressive disease; usually death by 10 years of age due to heart disease or respiratory infection
Frequent	Present	Present Pulmonary hypertension	Normal at birth; later may be moderately short	Moderate, absence of lumbar kyphosis	Late in onset, less severe than in Hurler	Survival usually into the third decade of life Eventual death from cardiopulmonary disease
Present	Minimal or moderate	Absent	Normal	Minimal widening of clavicles at medial ends, no kyphosis	Severe	Survival to third or fourth decade
Present	Usually absent	Minimal, if present aortic regurgitation	Markedly short (under 4 ft.)	Severe and diffuse platyspondyly with central tongue Capital femoral epiphyses irregular, eventually disappear	Absent	Normal longevity Respiratory failure due to rib cage rigidity
Present	Absent	Present; aortic valve disease	Normal	Small epiphysis on hands	Absent	Normal longevity
Present	Hepatomegaly rather than splenomegaly	Absent	Normal at birth, later markedly short	Severe (same as Hurler's)	Absent	Guarded, death from cardiovascular complications

marked localized kyphosis at the dorsolumbar junction is evident (Fig. 3–97 B and C). At the site of the gibbus, one vertebral body is hypoplastic and is displaced posteriorly, its anterior surface deficient in the superior part and its inferior portion projecting forward in a "beak" (Fig. 3–97 C). The second lumbar vertebra is the one that is most often beak-shaped and displaced, the first lumbar vertebra being next most frequently involved. The anterior inferior "beak" of the Hurler syndrome is quite distinct from the central "tongue" of the Morquio syndrome.

The distinctive shape of the pelvis with its flared iliac wings and shallow acetabular roofs is evident by six months of age. Coxa valga is marked (see Fig. 3–96 K). Ossification of the capital femoral epiphysis is delayed. Subluxation or dislocation of the hips is common in Hurler's syndrome. The ischium and pubis are thick and undermodeled. The radiographic findings in the thoracic cage are distinctive. The ribs are narrow posteriorly and broad anteriorly, giving an oar- or paddle-shaped appearance. The lateral ends of the clavicles are hypoplastic or even aplastic, but their medial ends are short and thick. The scapulae are high and decreased in their superoinferior dimension. The cardiac shadow is often enlarged because of associated cardiovascular problems.

The long bones are abnormal, with marked diaphyseal widening. The osseous changes are more marked in the upper limbs than in the lower. There is shortening and thickening of the humerus with widening of its medullary canal. The radius and ulna, though wide in their diaphyseal portions, taper distally, with their physes tilted toward each other (Fig. 3–97 D). Flattening of the ossific nuclei of the epiphyses may be present. The metacarpals are broad distally at their epiphyseal ends and are tapered proximally. The phalanges are short and broad, showing narrowing of their shafts away from the epiphyseal ends. The terminal phalanges are

Text continued on page 875

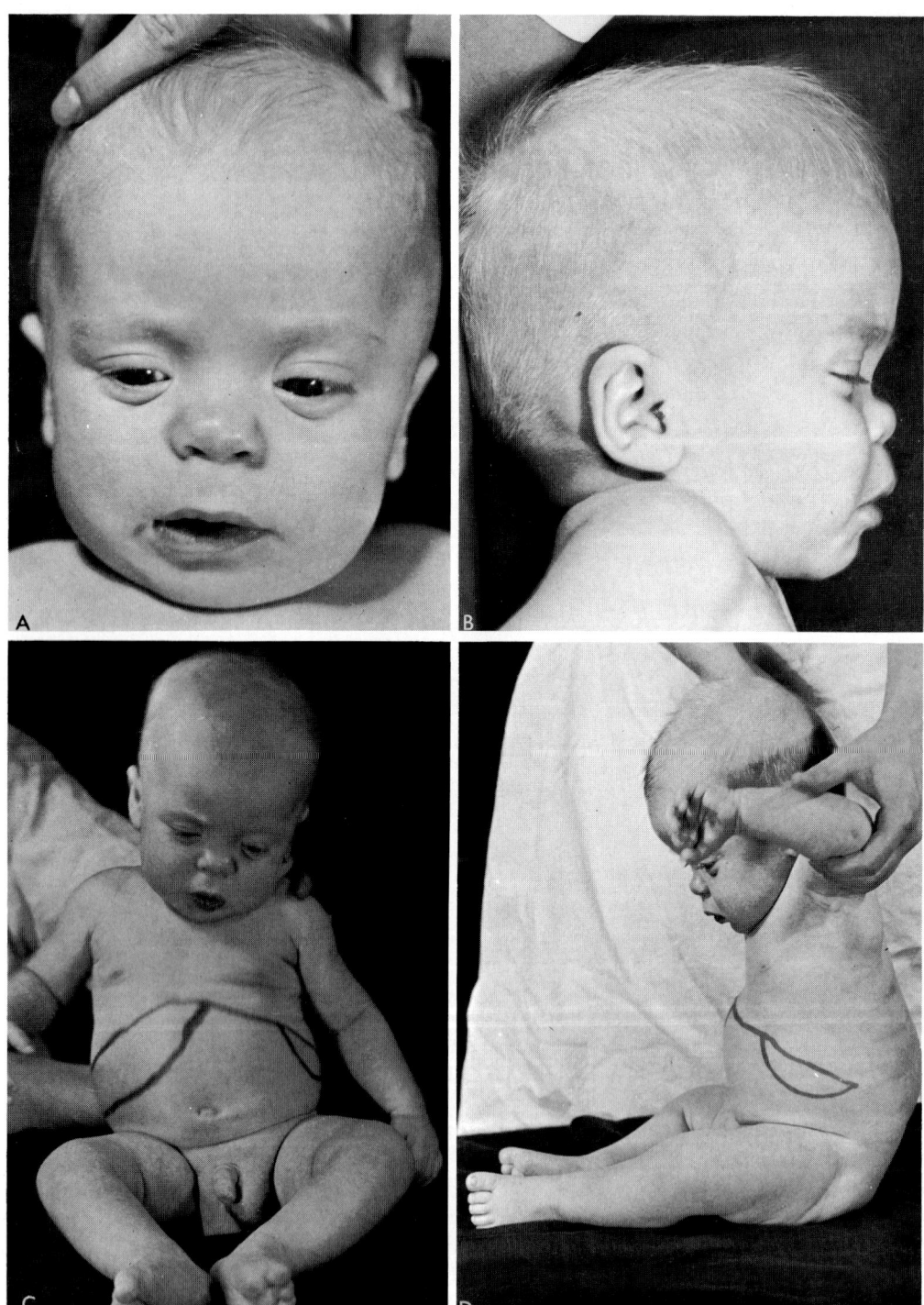

FIGURE 3–96. Hurler's syndrome (mucopolysaccharidosis I) in an infant.

A and **B.** Typical deformity of the head. **C** and **D.** Clinical appearance of the patient. The enlarged liver and spleen are outlined on the protuberant abdomen.

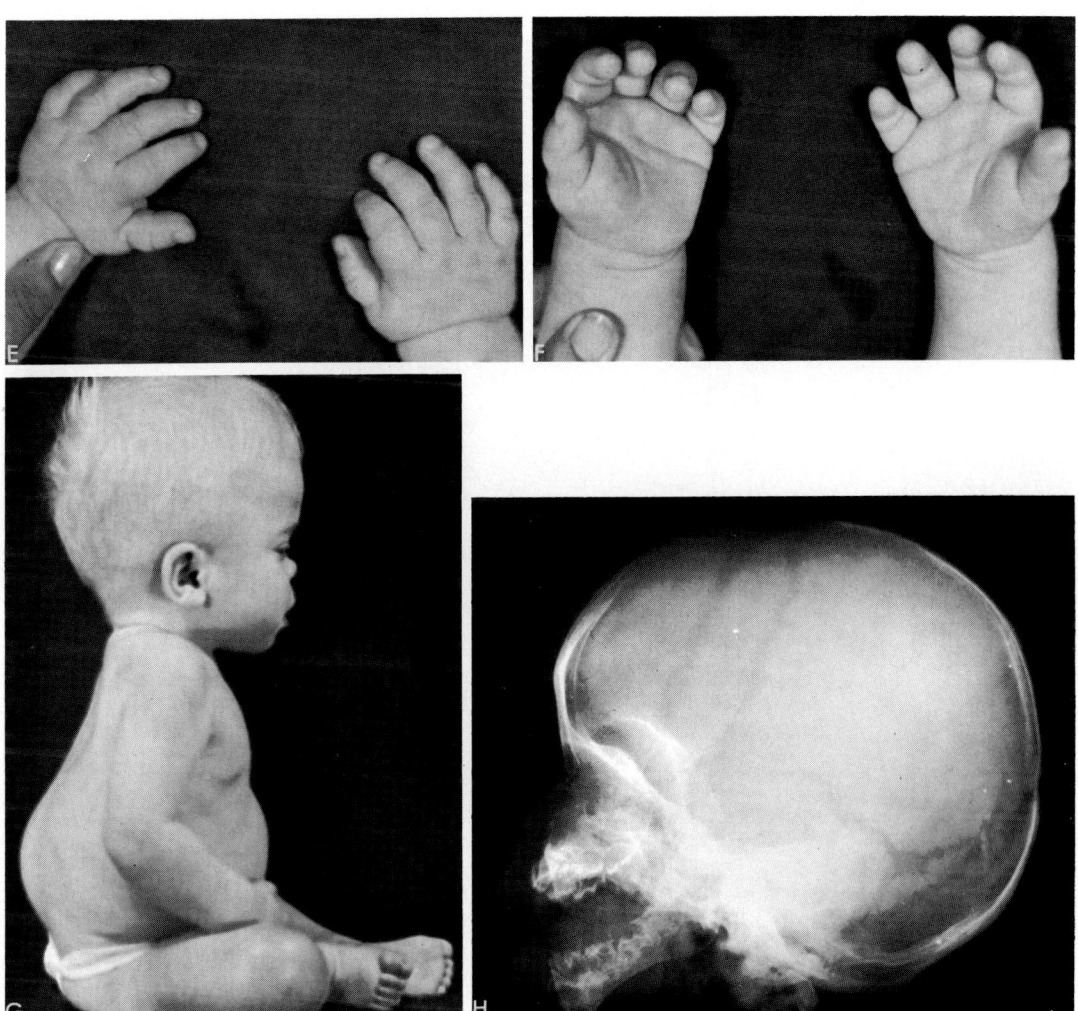

FIGURE 3–96 Continued. Hurler's syndrome (mucopolysaccharidosis I) in an infant.

E and F. The hands are broad and short, with stubby digits. G. Lateral view of the patient shows localized kyphosis at the dorsolumbar junction. H. Lateral radiogram of the skull, which is enlarged in its anteroposterior diameter.

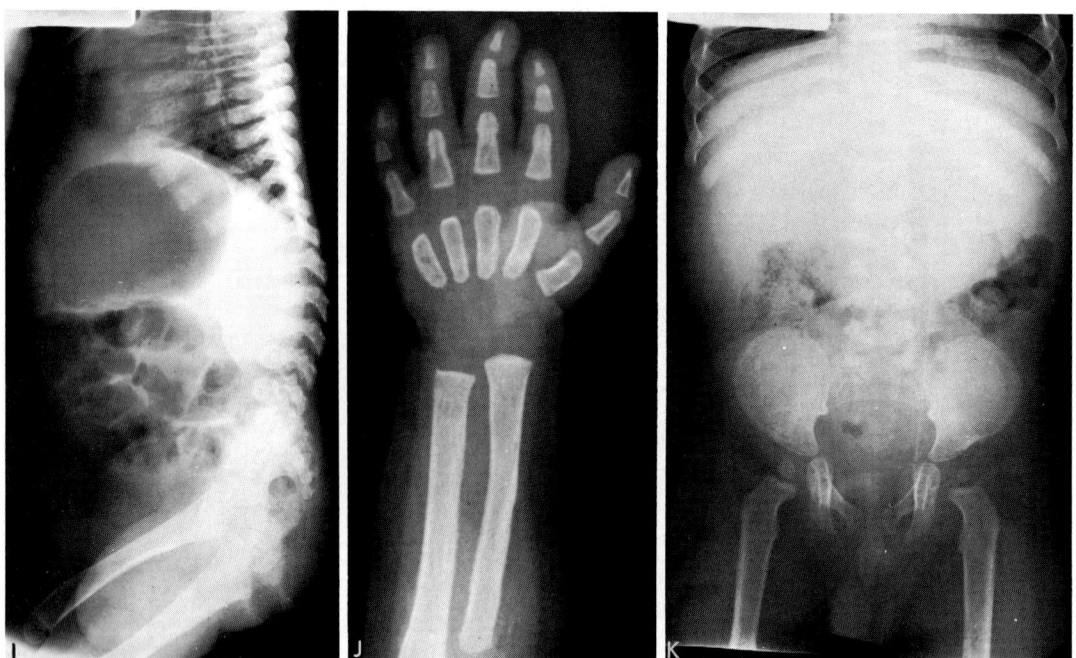

FIGURE 3-96 Continued. Hurler's syndrome (mucopolysaccharidosis I) in an infant.

I. Lateral radiogram of the spine. **J.** Anteroposterior radiogram of the hand. **K.** Radiogram of the pelvis and hips. Note the coxa valga.

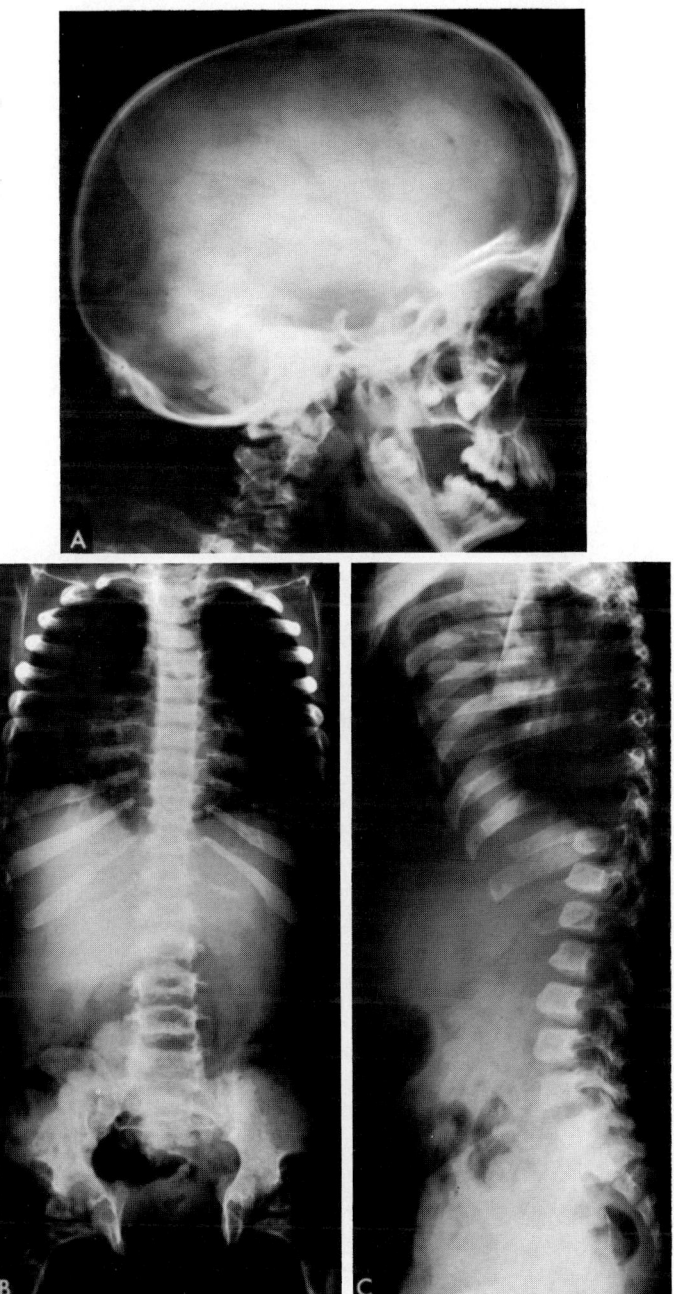

FIGURE 3–97. *Hurler's syndrome.*

Radiograms of a three-year-old child show the typical changes. **A.** Lateral view of the skull. Note the elongated and shallow sella turcica with anterior pocketing; it has a "shoe-shaped" appearance. **B** and **C.** Anteroposterior and lateral radiograms of the spine. Note in the upper lumbar area the hypoplastic vertebra that is beaked in its anteroinferior portion.

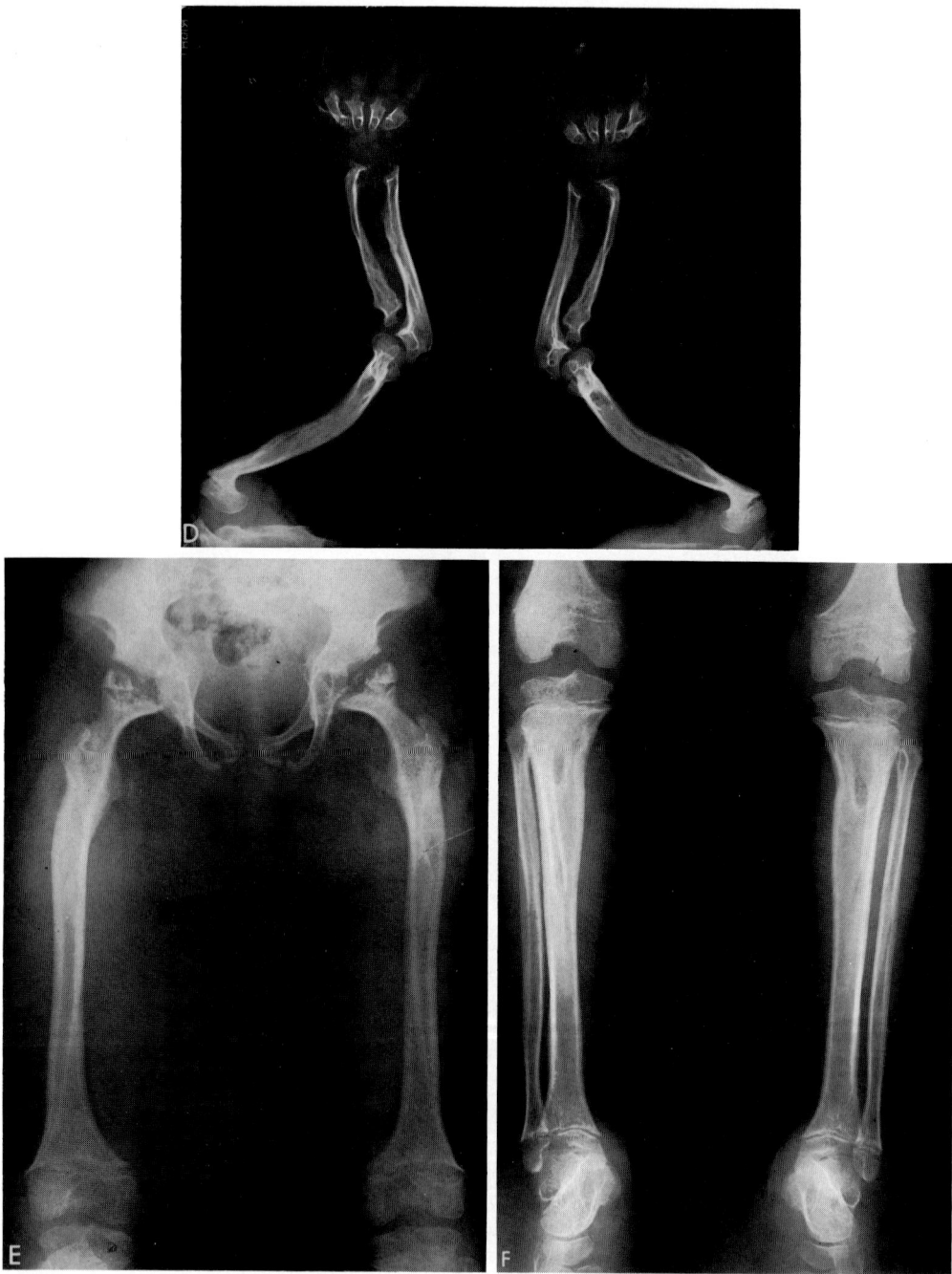

FIGURE 3–97 Continued. Hurler's syndrome.

D. Anteroposterior radiograms of upper limbs. The radius and ulna taper distally with their physes facing each other. The humeri are short and thick, with widening of their medullary canals. **E** and **F.** Radiograms of lower limbs. Note the severe coxa valga with narrowing of the femoral necks. The ossific nuclei of the epiphyses of the femoral heads are flattened and irregular.

not affected. The distinguishing features are summarized in Figure 3–98.

Treatment. There is no specific treatment for the disease. Management is symptomatic. Despite the poor prognosis, dislocated hips should be treated by conventional methods. Atlantoaxial instability due to odontoid hypoplasia may require support with a collar and occasionally by cervical fusion.

Mucopolysaccharidosis II (Hunter Syndrome)*

This disease was described by Hunter in 1917, before the description of Hurler's syndrome.[56] Inheritance is sex-linked and recessive; therefore, all patients are male.[107] Patients with mucopolysaccharidosis excrete large amounts of heparan sulfate (++) and dermatan sulfate (+). The enzyme defect is low sulfoiduronate sulfatase. Incidence of the disorder is said to be one fifth that of the Hurler syndrome. The distinguishing features are absence of clouding of the cornea and absence of lumbar kyphosis. Mental retardation is late in onset, less in severity, and slower in progress. Deafness is frequent, occurring in about 50 per cent of cases. Skin changes in the form of grooving or nodular lesions and hypertrichosis are common. Radiographic findings are similar to those of Hurler's syndrome but less severe. The clinical course is milder than that of the Hurler syndrome, most patients surviving to the third decade of life; some may have a normal life span and die of natural causes. Pulmonary hypertension is frequent; patients usually succumb to heart disease.

Mucopolysaccharidosis III (Sanfilippo Syndrome)†

First described by Harris in 1961, this type of mucopolysaccharidosis was reported in affected sibling pairs by Sanfilippo and associates in 1963.[49, 120]

The basic biochemical disturbance in this disorder is demonstrated in excessive urinary excretion of heparan sulfate, which is the only mucopolysaccharide excreted in large amounts. This particular mucopolysaccharidosis is caused by two enzyme deficiencies that are chemically indistinguishable: the first a deficiency of N-heparan sulfatase and the second a deficiency of α-acetylglucosaminidase. The condition is inherited as an autosomal recessive trait and is characterized by severe mental retardation. Corneal clouding and cardiac abnormalities are absent. Other somatic changes such as hepatosplenomegaly, stiffness of joints, skeletal deformities, and shortness of stature are less severe than in the Hurler syndrome, being minimal or, at the utmost, moderate. During the first few years of life these children appear normal, but soon mental retardation develops that becomes very severe. The minimal skeletal changes tend to revert to normal in adolescence. There are no specific musculoskeletal problems.

Mucopolysaccharidosis IV (Morquio Syndrome)*

The Morquio type of mucopolysaccharidosis is distinct from the other types. It is characterized by normal intelligence, severe dwarfing, platyspondyly with a central tongue, marked kyphosis, pectus carinatus, generalized joint laxity, deformation of the epiphyses (particularly of the femoral heads), and central constriction of the metacarpals and phalanges. It was independently described in 1929 by Morquio of Montevideo and Brailsford of Birmingham (England). Morquio called it "a form of familial osseous dystrophy" in his report of four members of a family of five.[100] Brailsford used the name *chondrodystrophy* in his single case report.[14] The eponym *Morquio's disease* is the most widely used and is retained here.

Inheritance is autosomal recessive.[39] Consanguinity may play a role, as the syndrome was reported in the parents as well as in the paternal grandparents of the family described by Morquio.[100] Additionally, Whiteside and Cholmeley reported that Morquio's disease appeared five times in 41 families of consanguineous marriage.[143] Sporadic cases do occur.

There is excess excretion of keratan sulfate in the urine, but this diminishes with age. The deficient enzyme is N-Ac-Gal-6-sulfate sulfatase.

Clinical Features. The developmental error is usually not apparent at birth, and affected infants are thought to be normal. Features of the disease often become recognizable between the ages of 12 and 18 months, when the child begins to walk. With growth and development the characteristic findings become increasingly

---

*See references 3, 14, 20, 21, 25, 26, 29, 39, 40, 56, 74, 78, 84, 106, 121.

†See references 2, 18, 27, 34–37, 41, 42, 47, 51, 64, 67, 71, 109, 116, 120, 126, 138.

*See references 8, 11, 15, 17, 19, 26, 31, 32, 44, 45, 55, 58, 59, 72, 75, 76, 87, 88, 90, 95, 100, 101, 104, 113–115, 118, 123, 124, 136, 137, 142, 144–146.

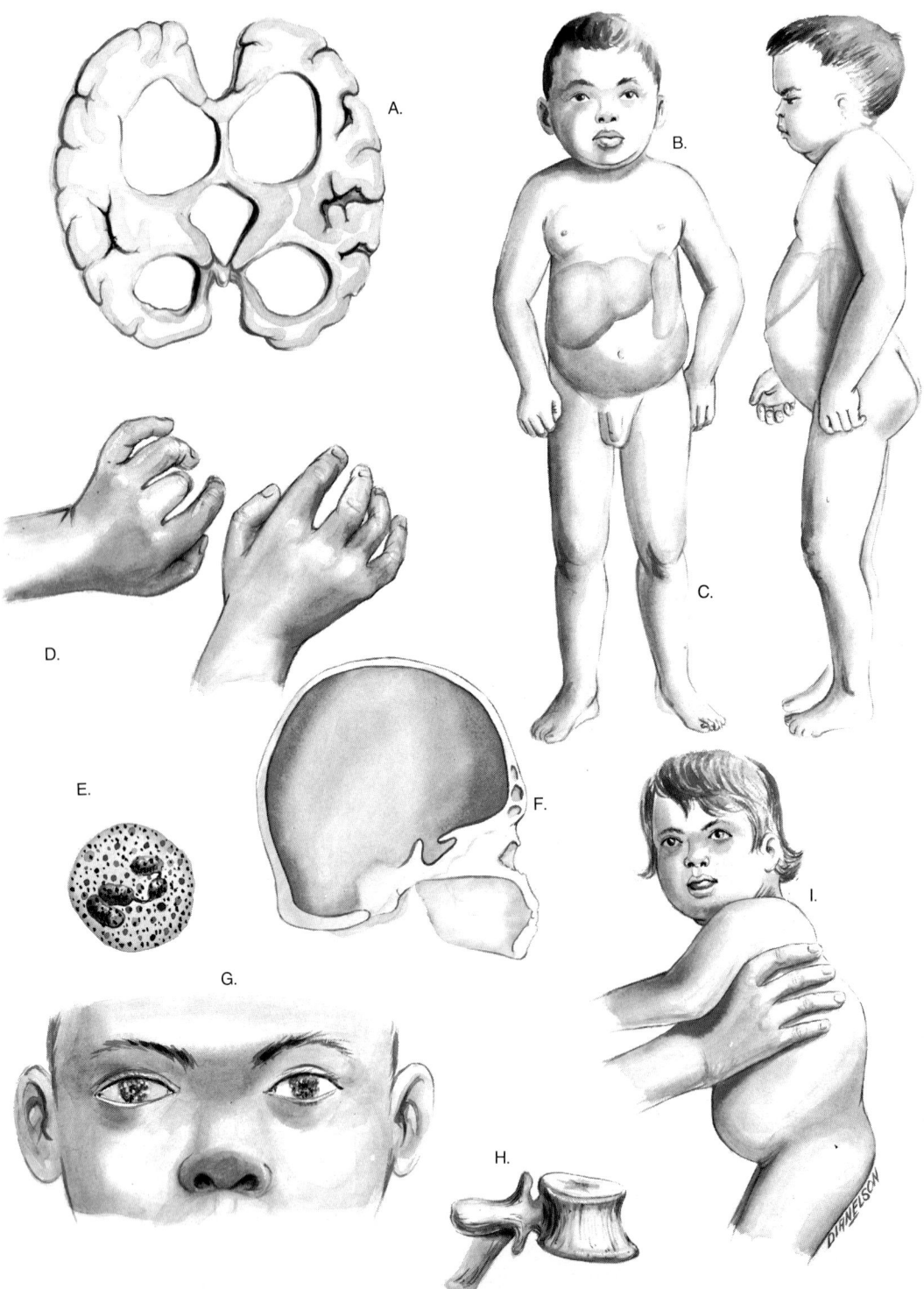

FIGURE 3–98. Summary of characteristic features of Hurler's syndrome.

A. Brain. **B.** Liver and spleen. **C.** Skeleton. **D.** Hands. **E.** Blood. **F.** Sella turcica. **G.** Eyes. **H.** Vertebrae. **I.** Spine.

evident, and by the age of four years the typical clinical features are established.

A dorsolumbar kyphosis is usually the deformity to first attract the parents' attention. Soon a number of generalized and symmetrical deformities of the skeleton appear. The child is round-backed and knock-kneed, and has pes valgus. Dwarfing is chiefly due to shortness of the trunk; the limbs are relatively long. The neck is short, and the patient stands with the knees and hips flexed in a crouched position with the head thrust forward and sunk between the high shoulders. The size and shape of the head are usually normal, though it may appear large because of the diminished growth of the trunk and limbs. The facies appear normal, though the eyes are widely spaced, the bridge of the nose is depressed, and the maxilla is prominent. The corneal opacities are mild and develop late. Unlike Hurler's syndrome, the disorder is associated with a level of intelligence within normal limits.

The anteroposterior diameter of the thorax is increased, with the sternum projecting forward (pectus carinatum) with a manubrial-sternal angle of about 90 degrees. Sternal segments fuse prematurely with consequent severe restriction of chest excursion and reduced vital capacity. In severe cases the thorax is practically immobile. There is marked kyphosis of the spine, usually accentuated at the dorsolumbar region with a short lordotic curve below. There may be associated scoliosis. The range of motion of the spine, particularly extension, is limited. The abdomen may protrude, but the spleen and liver are not enlarged.

The epiphyses, especially of the knees, elbows, shoulders, wrists, and ankles, are often enlarged, owing to hypertrophy of the bone ends, not to soft-tissue swelling of the joints. Generalized joint laxity is a feature of Morquio's syndrome—this is dissimilar to the other mucopolysaccharidoses in which the joints are stiff. Knock-knees are almost universal in Morquio's disease. Ligamentous hyperlaxity causes instability of the wrists, elbows, knees, and ankles and pes planovalgus. Muscle weakness may be present. The hands and feet are short, with broad digits. There is valgus deformity of the ankles, which causes difficulty in wearing shoes. The gait is waddling.

Radiographic Findings. The radiographic features of Morquio's disease are distinctive. The vertebral bodies in the thoracic and lumbar regions are ovoid in infancy and early childhood, but with aging they become flattened (platyspondyly) and have irregular and defective upper and lower surfaces that tend to approximate each other anteriorly, forming a central projection or tongue. This anterior beaking is more obvious in the lower dorsal and upper lumbar vertebrae. The intervertebral discs are narrower than normal, although in early cases, they may appear widened. Kyphosis is common and is aggravated by hypoplasia and posterior displacement of the twelfth dorsal and first lumbar vertebrae. Hypoplasia or absence of the odontoid process is a characteristic feature of Morquio's syndrome and causes atlantoaxial instability and spinal cord compression.

The epiphyses of the long tubular bones ossify irregularly; as a result, they are broad and flattened.

Ossification of the femoral heads is delayed, and the femoral necks are widened and flared. Coxa vara or valga deformity is common. The acetabula are poorly developed. In the weight-bearing joints, the epiphyses seem to be unable to withstand the strain and pressure of body forces, and compression and fragmentation of epiphyses are frequent. Delay in ossification of the lateral side of the proximal tibial epiphysis and metaphysis is commonly found.

The metaphyses are widened to accommodate the enlarged epiphyses. The diaphyses of the major long bones are usually normal, although at times they may be short and thick. In the hands and feet ossification of the carpal and tarsal bones is delayed and irregular. The short tubular bones, especially the metacarpals and metatarsals, are thicker and shorter than normal. The ends away from the epiphyses, i.e., the bases of the second, third, fourth, and fifth metacarpals, as well as the distal ends of their phalanges, tend to be pointed. The diaphyses of the metacarpals, phalanges, and metatarsals show central constriction.

The pelvis, which is normal at birth, becomes narrow with growth, resulting in equal depth and width of the inner pelvic contour. Rubin likens it to the shape of a wineglass.[119] The iliac wings are flared laterally and are more rounded than normal. The openings of the sacroiliac notches become prominent. The thoracic cage appears barrel-shaped, and the ribs tend to be broad and expanded at both their anterior and posterior extremities. Pectus carinatum is evident in the lateral projection.

Changes in the skull, if any, are usually minimal. The facial bones, likewise, develop normally.

Prognosis. This is variable; in general patients with Morquio's disease live for many years. Aortic regurgitation may cause cardiovascular complications.[80, 81] Marked rigidity of the rib cage and decrease of vital capacity will cause respiratory failure.

The disease is rarely fatal. Progression of the

deformities is usually arrested as growth is completed; with age, however, degenerative changes and arthritis in the joints develop.

Treatment. There is no specific treatment. The serious problems are atlantoaxial instability and upper cervical spinal cord compression and myelopathy. Gradual and progressive muscle weakness in the upper and lower limbs should alert the surgeon. Computed tomography and nuclear magnetic resonance imaging will demonstrate the cord compression. Occipito–upper cervical fusion is performed to stabilize the atlantoaxial joint.[65, 66]

Surgical correction of deformity should be undertaken only after careful evaluation and analysis. Pain and difficulty in walking should be the only indications for operative intervention. The cervical spinal cord is at risk in a patient with Morquio's syndrome. Intubation for general anesthesia should be performed very cautiously; flexion-extension of the neck should be minimized.

Triple arthrodesis for the correction of severe pes valgus and abduction osteotomy of the proximal femur for severe coxa vara are occasionally performed. Genu valgum is corrected by realignment osteotomy. Instability and subluxation of the wrist are treated by appropriate splinting and occasionally by wrist fusion.

Mucopolysaccharidosis V (Scheie Syndrome)*

This rare condition was first described by Scheie and colleagues as a forme fruste of Hurler's syndrome.[122] It is inherited as an autosomal recessive trait and characterized by the physical findings of clouding of the cornea, retinitis pigmentosa, limitation of motion of joints, claw hands, excessive body hair, and aortic valve disease (commonly aortic regurgitation). Intellectual deterioration does not occur, and stature is nearly normal. There is excessive urinary excretion of dermatan sulfate (+ +) and heparan sulfate (+). The enzyme deficiency is of α-L-iduronidase, as in Hurler's syndrome. Musculoskeletal problems do not develop, and orthopedic care is usually not required.

Mucopolysaccharidosis VI (Maroteaux-Lamy Syndrome)†

This very rare type of mucopolysaccharidosis was first delineated by Maroteaux and Lamy and their associates in 1963.[89] Spranger and associates reviewed 19 cases in 1970.[130] It is inherited as an autosomal recessive trait and characterized by excessive excretion of dermatan sulfate (and some heparan sulfate). The deficient enzyme is N-Ac-Gal-4-sulfatase. Clinically, the condition is suggested at an age of two or three years by shortness of the trunk and limbs, knock-knees, lumbar kyphosis, and anterior protrusion of the sternum. The ultimate stature of these patients is between three and four feet. Corneal opacities and hepatosplenomegaly are present. The skeletal abnormalities are quite marked and are the same as those of Hurler's syndrome. Polymorphonuclear and lymphocytic inclusions are found in the blood. Intellectual development is normal in this syndrome in distinction from Hurler's syndrome.

References

1. Aleu, F. P., Terry, R. D., and Zellweger, H.: Electronmicroscopy of two cerebral biopsies in gargoylism. J. Neuropathol. Exp. Neurol., 24:304, 1965.
2. Arvidsson, J., Chester, M. A., and Hecht, H.: The first case of the Sanfilippo type C syndrome in Scandinavia. Acta Paediatr. Scand., 72:313, 1983.
3. Bach, G., Eisenberg, F., Jr., Cantz, M., and Neufeld, E. F.: The defect in the Hunter syndrome. Deficiency of sulfoiduronate sulfatase. Proc. Natl. Acad. Sci. (U.S.A.), 70:2134, 1973.
4. Bach, G., Freidman, R., Weissman, B., and Neufeld, E. F.: The defect in the Hurler and Scheie syndromes: Deficiency of α-L-iduronidase. Proc. Natl. Acad. Sci. (U.S.A.), 69:2048, 1972.
5. Bao, S. C.: The ocular manifestations and differential diagnosis of the mucopolysaccharidoses (a report of 34 cases). Chung Hua Yen Ko Tsa Chih, 18:165, 1982.
6. Barton, R. W., and Neufeld, E. F.: The Hurler corrective factor, purification and some properties. J. Biol. Chem., 246:7773, 1971.
7. Barton, R. W., and Neufeld, E. F.: A distinct biochemical deficit in the Maroteaux-Lamy syndrome (mucopolysaccharidosis VI). J. Pediatr., 80:114, 1972.
8. Beighton, P., and Craig, J.: Atlanto-axial subluxation in the Morquio syndrome. J. Bone Joint Surg., 55-B:478, 1973.
9. Bhandari, B., and Ranka, S. L.: Hurler-Scheie compound—a variant of MPS-i (MPS-i H/S). A case report. Indian Pediatr., 17:971, 1980.
10. Bioulac, P., Coquet, M., Fontan, D., Micheau, M., Beylot, C., and Vital, C.: Interest of ultrastructural study of skin and muscle biopsies in inborn storage diseases. A report of 18 cases. Ann. Dermatol. Venereol., 107:137, 1980.
11. Blaw, M. E., and Langer, L. O.: Spinal cord compression in Morquio-Brailsford's disease. J. Pediatr., 74:593, 1969.
12. Booth, C. W., and Nadler, H. L.: Plasma infusions in an infant with Hurler's syndrome. J. Pediatr., 82:273, 1973.
13. Booth, C. W., and Nadler, H. L.: Demonstration of the heterozygous state in Hunter's syndrome. J. Pediatr., 53:396, 1974.
14. Brailsford, J. F.: Chondro-osteodystrophy. Roentgenographic and clinical features of a child with dislocation of vertebrae. Am. J. Surg., 7:404, 1929.

---

*See references 4, 5, 9, 60, 111, 122.
†See references 5, 7, 73, 85, 89, 110, 130, 134, 139.

15. Brailsford, J. F.: The Radiology of Bones and Joints. 5th Ed. Baltimore, Williams & Wilkins, 1953.
16. Brante, G.: Gargoylism: A mucopolysaccharidosis. Scand. J. Clin. Lab. Invest., 4:43, 1952.
17. Brovelli, A., Laterza, L., Lenzi, L., and Castellani, A. A.: Characterization of urinary peptoglycans in Morquio's disease. Calcif. Tiss. Res., 1:324, 1968.
18. Burrows, R., and Muzzo, S.: Sanfilippo's syndrome: Typing of mucopolysaccharides in urine and enzymatic determination in plasma. Rev. Chir. Pediatr., 51:129, 1980.
19. Campailla, E., and Martinelli, B.: Morquio's disease: Modification of mucopolysacchariduria with advancing age: Report of three cases. Birth Defects, 4:172, 1969.
20. Cantz, M., Chrambach, A., Bach, G., and Neufeld, E. F.: The Hunter corrective factor. Purification and preliminary characterization. J. Biol. Chem., 247:5456, 1972.
21. Coppa, G. V., Singh, J., Nichols, B. L., and Di Ferrante, N.: Urinary excretion of disulfated disaccharides in Hunter syndrome: Correction by infusion of a serum fraction. Anal. Let., 6:225, 1973.
22. Crow, J., Gibbs, D. A., Crozens, W., Spellacy, E., and Watts, R. W.: Biochemical and histopathological studies on patients with mucopolysaccharidoses, two of whom had been treated by fibroblast transplantation. J. Clin. Pathol., 36:415, 1983.
23. Danes, B. S., and Bearn, A. G.: Hurler's syndrome: Demonstration of an inherited disorder of connective tissue in cell culture. Science, 149:987, 1965.
24. Danes, B. S., and Bearn, A. G.: Cellular metachromasia, a genetic marker for studying mucopolysaccharidoses. Lancet, 1:241, 1967.
25. Dean, M. F., Muir, H., and Benson, P. F.: Mobilization of glycosaminoglycans by plasma infusion in mucopolysaccharidosis type III. Two types of response. Nature, 243:143, 1973.
26. Dean, M. F., Muir, H., and Ewins, R. J. F.: Hurler's, Hunter's and Morquio's syndromes. A biochemical study in the light of current views of the underlying defects. Biochem. J., 123:883, 1971.
27. Dean, M. F., Muir, H., Benson, P. F., and Button, L. R.: Enzyme replacement therapy by transplantation of HLA-compatible fibroblasts in Sanfilippo A syndrome. Pediatr. Res., 15:959, 1981.
28. Dekaban, A. S., and Constantopoulos, G.: Mucopolysaccharidoses. Relation of elevated cerebral spinal fluid to mental retardation. Arch. Neurol., 28:385, 1973.
29. Di Ferrante, N., Nichols, B. L., Donnelly, P. V., Neri, G., Hergovcic, R., and Berglund, R. K.: Induced degradation of glycosaminoglycans in Hurler's and Hunter's syndromes by plasma infusion. Proc. Natl. Acad. Sci. (U.S.A.), 68:303, 1971.
30. Dorfman, A., and Lorincz, A. E.: Occurrence of urinary acid mucopolysaccharides in the Hurler syndrome. Proc. Natl. Acad. Sci., 43:443, 1957.
31. Edwards, M. K., Harwood-Nash, D. C., Fitz, C. R., and Chuang, S. H.: CT metrizamide myelography of the cervical spine in Morquio syndrome. A.J.N.R., 3:666, 1982.
32. Einhorn, N. H., Moore, J. R., and Rowntree, L. G.: Osteochondrodystrophia deformans (Morquio's disease). Observation and autopsy in one case. Am. J. Dis. Child., 72:536, 1946.
33. Ellis, R. W. B., Sheldon, W., and Capon, N. B.: Gargoylism (chondro-osteo-dystrophy, corneal opacities, hepatosplenomegaly and mental deficiency). Q. J. Med., 5:119, 1936.
34. Escourolle, R., Berger, B., and Poirier, J.: Biopsie cérébrale d'un cas de mucopolysaccharidose H.S. (oligophrénie polydystrophique ou maladie de Sanfilippo). Etude histochimique et ultrastructurale. Presse Méd., 74:2869, 1966.
35. Federico, A., Robert, J., Zanetta, J. P., and Guazzi, G. C.: Sanfilippo A syndrome (mucopolysaccharidosis III A): A neurochemical study. Ital. J. Neurol. Sci., 2:119, 1981.
36. Federico, A., Capece, G., Cecio, A., D'Auria, N., Di Iorio, G., Ronsisvalle, L., and Di Natale, P.: Sanfilippo B syndrome (MPS III B): Case report with analysis of CSF mucopolysaccharides and conjunctival biopsy. J. Neurol., 225:77, 1981.
37. Figura, K. von, and Kresse, H.: The Sanfilippo B corrective factor: A N-acetyl-α-D-glucosaminidase. Biochem. Biophys. Res. Commun., 48:262, 1972.
38. Fratantoni, J. C., Hall, C. W., and Neufeld, E. F.: The defect in Hurler's syndromes: Faulty degradation of mucopolysaccharide. Proc. Natl. Acad. Sci. (U.S.A.), 60:699, 1968.
39. Fratantoni, J. C., Hall, C. W., and Neufeld, E. F.: Hurler and Hunter syndromes: Mutual correction of the defect in cultured fibroblasts. Science, 162:570, 1968.
40. Fratantoni, J. C., Hall, C. W., and Neufeld, E. F.: The defect in Hurler and Hunter syndromes. II. Deficiency of specific factors involved in mucopolysaccharide degradation. Proc. Natl. Acad. Sci. (U.S.A.), 64:360, 1969.
41. Fuster Siebert, M., Caamano Mata, J. M., Fraga Bermudez, J. M., and Couselo Sanchez, J. M.: Sanfilippo syndrome and shortened PR. Med. Clin. (Barc.), 79:387, 1982.
42. Gatti, R., Borrone, C., Durand, P., De Virgilis, S., Sanna, G., Cao, A., Von Figura, K., Kresse, H., and Paschke, E.: Sanfilippo type D disease: Clinical findings in two patients with a new variant of mucopolysaccharidosis III. Eur. J. Pediatr., 138:168, 1982.
43. Gehler, J., Cantz, M., Tolksdorf, M., Spranger, J., Gilbert, E., and Drube, H.: Mucopolysaccharidosis VII: β-Glucuronidase deficiency. Hum. Genet., 23:149, 1974.
44. Glossl, J., Lembeck, K., Gamse, G., and Kresse, H.: Morquio's disease type A: Absence of material cross reacting with antibodies against N-acetylgalactosamine-6-sulfate sulfatase. Hum. Genet., 54:87, 1980.
45. Goidanich, I. F., and Lenzi, L.: Morquio-Ullrich disease, a new mucopolysaccharidosis. J. Bone Joint Surg., 46-A:743, 1964.
46. Grossman, H., and Dorst, J.: The mucopolysaccharidoses and mucolipidoses. In Progress in Pediatric Radiology, Vol. 4, Intrinsic Diseases of Bones. Basel, Karger, 1973, p. 495.
47. Hadfield, M. G., Ghatak, N. R., Nakeneczna, I., Lippman, H. R., Myer, E. C., Constantopoulos, G., and Bradley, R. M.: Pathologic findings in mucopolysaccharidosis type IIIB (Sanfilippo's syndrome B). Arch. Neurol., 37:645, 1980.
48. Hall, C. W., Cantz, M., and Neufeld, E. F.: A β-glucuronidase deficiency mucopolysaccharidosis: Studies in cultural fibroblasts. Arch. Biochem. Biophys., 155:32, 1973.
49. Harris, R. C.: Mucopolysaccharide disorders. A possible new genotype of Hurler's syndrome (abstract). Am. J. Dis. Child., 102:741, 1961.
50. Hassler, A., Kirchner, M., Friedrich, H., and Machill, G.: Mucopolysaccharide storage diseases. II. Possibilities and problems in diagnostic typing as seen in patients in a pediatric hospital. Klinderaerztl. Prax., 48:455, 1980.
51. Haust, M. D., Gordon, B. A., Bryans, A. M., Wollin, D. G., and Binnington, V.: Heparitin sulfate mucopolysaccharidosis (Sanfilippo disease): A case study with ultrastructural, biochemical and radiological findings. Pediatr. Res., 5:137, 1971.
52. Hers, H. G., and Van Hoof, F.: Lysosomes and mucopolysaccharidoses. Biochem. J., 115:34, 1969.
53. Horrigan, W. D., and Baker, D. H.: Gargoylism: A

review of the roentgen skull changes with description of a new finding. A.J.R., 86:473, 1961.
54. Hors-Cayla, M. C., Maroteaux, P., and Grouchy, J. de: Fibroblastes en culture au cours des mucopolysaccharidoses: Influence du sérum sur la metachromasie. Ann. Genet., 11:265, 1968.
55. Humbel, R., Marchal, C., and Fall, M.: Diagnosis of Morquio's disease: A simple chromatographic method for the identification of keratosulfate in urine. J. Pediatr., 81:107, 1972.
56. Hunter, C.: A rare disease in two brothers. Proc. R. Soc. Med., 10:104, 1917.
57. Hurler, G.: Ueber einen Typ multipler Abartungen, vorwiegend an Skelettsystem. Z. Kinderheilkd., 24:220, 1919.
58. Ikeda, K., Burck, U., and Goebel, H. H.: Ultrastructure of lymphocytes and skin in mucopolysaccharidosis IV A (Morquio syndrome). Brain Dev., 3:329, 1981.
59. Jenkins, P., Davies, G. R., and Harper, P. S.: Morquio-Brailsford disease. A report of four affected sisters with absence of excessive keratan sulphate in the urine. Br. J. Radiol., 46:668, 1973.
60. Jensen, O. A., Pedersen, C., Vestermark, S., and Warburg, M.: The Hurler/Scheie phenotype in children from a consanguineous marriage: Case report with electronmicroscopy of the conjunctiva and ERG. Metab. Pediatr. Syst. Ophthalmol., 4:133, 1980.
61. Kint, J. A., Dacremont, G., Carton, D., Urye, E., and Hooft, C.: Mucopolysaccharidosis, secondarily induced abnormal distribution of lysosomal isoenzymes. Science, 181:352, 1973.
62. Kirchner, M., Hassler, A., and Machnick, G.: Mucopolysaccharide storage diseases. I. Clinical aspects and diagnosis. Kinderaerztl. Prax., 48:19, 1980.
63. Knudson, A. G., Di Ferrante, N., and Curtis, J. E.: Effect of leukocyte transfusion in a child with type II mucopolysaccharidosis. Proc. Natl. Acad. Sci. (U.S.A.), 68:1738, 1971.
64. Konyar, E., Tondeur, M., and Resibois, A.: Histochemical demonstrations of acid mucopolysaccharides in Sanfilippo's disease: An ultrastructural study of the liver. Virchows Arch. B, 11:224, 1972.
65. Kopits, S. E.: Orthopedic complications of dwarfism. Clin. Orthop., 114:153, 1976.
66. Kopits, S. E., Perovic, M. N., McKusick, V. A., Robinson, R. A., and Bailey, J. A.: Congenital atlantoaxial dislocations in various forms of dwarfism. J. Bone Joint Surg., 54-A:1349, 1972.
67. Kresse, H., Wiesman, U., Cantz, M., Hall, C. W., and Neufeld, E. F.: Biochemical heterogeneity of the Sanfilippo syndrome: Preliminary characterization of two deficient factors. Biochem. Biophys. Res. Commun., 42:892, 1971.
68. Lambotte, C., Winand, R., Chantraine, J. M., Biertho, G., and Leruth-Fafchamps, Y.: Le traitement des mucopolysaccharidoses par des perfusions de plasma humain. Modification des mucopolysaccharides de haut et de faible poids moléculaire. Acta Paediatr. Belg., 25:297, 1971.
69. Lamy, M., and Maroteaux, P.: Des chondrodystrophies génotypique. Paris, L'Expansion Scientifique Française, 1961.
70. Lamy, M., Maroteaux, P., and Bader, J. P.: Etude génétique du gargoylisme. J. Genet. Hum., 5:156, 1957.
71. Langer, L. O.: The radiographic manifestations of the HS-mucopolysaccharidosis of Sanfilippo. Ann. Radiol., 7:315, 1964.
72. Langer, L. O., and Carey, L. S.: The roentgenographic features of the KS-mucopolysaccharidosis of Morquio (Morquio-Brailsford's disease). A.J.R., 47:1, 1966.
73. Levy, L. A., Lewis, J. C., and Sumner, T. E.: Ultrastructures of Reilly bodies (metachromatic granules) in the Maroteaux-Lamy syndrome (mucopolysaccharidosis VI). A histochemical study. Am. J. Clin. Pathol., 73:416, 1980.
74. Lichtenstein, J. R., Bilbrey, G. L., and McKusick, V. A.: Clinical and probable genetic heterogeneity within mucopolysaccharidosis II, report of a family with a mild form. Johns Hopkins Med. J., 131:425, 1972.
75. Linker, A., Evans, L. R., and Langer, L. O.: Morquio's disease and mucopolysaccharide excretion. J. Pediatr., 77:1039, 1970.
76. Lipson, S. J.: Dysplasia of the odontoid process in Morquio's syndrome causing quadriparesis. J. Bone Joint Surg., 59-A:340, 1977.
77. Loeb, H., Jonniaux, G., Resibois, A., Cremer, N., Dodion, J., Tondeur, M., Gregoire, P. E., Richard, J., and Cieters, P.: Biochemical and ultrastructural studies in Hurler's syndrome. J. Pediatr., 73:860, 1968.
78. Lowrey, R. B., Renwick, S. H. G.: The relative frequency of the Hurler and Hunter syndromes. N. Engl. J. Med., 284:221, 1971.
79. McCallum, D. I., Macadam, R. F., and Johnston, A. W.: Angiokeratoma corporis diffusum with features of a mucopolysaccharidosis. J. Med. Genet., 17:21, 1980.
80. McKusick, V. A.: The nosology of the mucopolysaccharidoses. Am. J. Med., 47:730, 1969.
81. McKusick, V. A.: Heritable Disorders of Connective Tissue. 4th Ed. St. Louis, Mosby, 1972.
82. McKusick, V. A., Howell, R. R., Hussels, I. E., Neufeld, E. F., and Stevenson, R. E.: Allelism, non-allelism and genetic compounds among the mucopolysaccharidoses. Lancet, 1:993, 1972.
83. Markesbery, W. R., Robinson, R. O., Falace, P. V., and Frye, M. D.: Mucopolysaccharidoses: Ultrastructure of leukocyte inclusions. Ann. Neurol., 8:332, 1980.
84. Maroteaux, P.: Différenciation biochimique des maladies de Hurler et de Hunter par fractionnement de l'héparitine sulfate. Rev. Eur. Etud. Clin. Biol., 15:203, 1970.
85. Maroteaux, P.: Un nouveau type de mucopolysaccharidose avec athétose et élimination urinaire de keratan-sulfate. Nouv. Presse Méd., 2:975, 1973.
86. Maroteaux, P., and Hors-Cayla, M. C.: Le probléme biologique des mucopolysaccharidoses. Ann. Biol. Clin., 28:111, 1970.
87. Maroteaux, P., and Lamy, M.: Hurler's disease, Morquio's disease, and related mucopolysaccharidoses. J. Pediatr., 67:312, 1965.
88. Maroteaux, P., Lamy, M., and Fouchier, M.: La maladie de Morquio, étude clinique, radiologique et biologique. Presse Méd., 71:2091, 1963.
89. Maroteaux, P., Leveque, B., Marie, J., and Lamy, M.: Une nouvelle dysostose avec élimination urinaire de chondroitine-sulfate B. Presse Méd., 71:1849, 1963.
90. Maroteaux, P., Stanescu, V., Stanescu, R., Kresse, H., and Hors-Cayla, M. C.: Heterogeneity of formes frustes of Morquio's disease. Arch. Fr. Pediatr., 39:Suppl 2:761, 1982.
91. Matalon, R., and Dorfman, A.: The structure of acid mucopolysaccharides produced by Hurler fibroblasts in tissue culture. Proc. Natl. Acad. Sci. (U.S.A.), 60:179, 1968.
92. Matalon, R., and Dorfman, A.: Hurler's syndrome, an α-L-iduronidase deficiency. Biochem. Biophys. Res. Commun., 47:959, 1972.
93. Matalon, R., Wappner, R., Deanching, M., Brandt, I. K., and Horwitz, A.: Keratan and heparan sulfaturia: glucosamine-6-sulfate deficiency. Ann. Clin. Lab. Sci., 12:234, 1982.
94. Matteini, M., Cotrozzi, G., Relli, P., and Valenza, T.: Psuedo-Morquio type II syndrome. Arch. Putti Chir. Organi Mov., 31:225, 1981.

95. Maynard, J. A., Cooper, R. R., and Ponsetti, I. V.: Morquio's disease (mucopolysaccharidosis type IV). Ultrastructure of epiphyseal plates. Lab. Invest., 28:194, 1973.
96. Melet, J., Hooghwinkel, G. J., Giesberts, M. A., and Gelderen, H. H.: A semi-quantitative micromethod for the determination of free glycosaminoglycans in serum. Results from studies on serum of healthy children of various ages and patients affected by mucopolysaccharidosis. Clin. Chim. Acta, 108:179, 1980.
97. Meyer, K., Brumbach, M. M., Linker, A., and Hoffman, P.: Excretion of sulfated mucopolysaccharides in gargoylism (Hurler's syndrome). Proc. Soc. Exp. Biol. Med., 97:275, 1958.
98. Minami, R., Abo, K., Tsugawa, S., Oyanagi, K., and Nakao, T.: Acidic glycosaminoglycans in liver from five patients with mucopolysaccharidosis and mucolipidosis. Tohoku J. Exp. Med., 134:215, 1981.
99. Mittwoch, U.: Abnormal lymphocytes in gargoylism. Br. J. Haematol, 5:365, 1959.
100. Morquio, L.: Sur une forme de dystrophie osseuse familiale. Arch. Med. Enf. Paris, 32:129, 1929; Bull. Soc. Pediatr. Paris, 27:145, 1929.
101. Morquio, L.: Sur une forme de dystrophie osseuse familiale. Arch. Med. Enf., 38:5, 1935.
102. Muir, H.: The structure and metabolism of mucopolysaccharides (glycosaminoglycans) and the problem of the mucopolysaccharidoses. Am. J. Med., 47:673, 1969.
103. Munnich, A., Saudubray, J. M., Hors-Cayla, M. C., Poenaru, L., Ogier, H., Strecker, G., Aicardi, J., Frezal, J., and Maroteaux, P.: Enzyme replacement therapy by transplantation of HLA-compatible fibroblasts in Sanfilippo syndrome: Another trial. Pediatr. Res., 16:259, 1982.
104. Namiki, O., Masubushi, M., Toyoshima, H., Endo, M., and Yosizawa, Z.: Urinary keratan sulfate of Morquio's disease. Tohoku J. Exp. Med., 132:103, 1980.
105. Neufeld, E. F., and Fratantoni, J. C.: Inborn errors of mucopolysaccharide metabolism. Science, 169:141, 1970.
106. Neuhauser, E. B. D., Griscom, N. T., Gilles, F. H., and Crocker, A. C.: Arachnoid cysts in the Hurler-Hunter syndrome. Ann. Radiol. (Paris), 11:453, 1968.
107. Nja, A.: A sex-linked type of gargoylism. Acta Paediatr., 33:267, 1946.
108. O'Brien, J. S.: Sanfilippo's syndrome: Profound deficiency of α-acetyl-glucosaminidase activity in organs and skin fibroblasts from type B patients. Proc. Natl. Acad. Sci. (U.S.A.), 69:1720, 1972.
109. O'Brien, J. S., Miller, A. L., Loverde, A. W., and Veath, M. L.: Sanfilippo's disease type B: Enzyme replacement and metabolic correction in cultured fibroblasts. Science, 181:753, 1973.
110. Paterson, D. E., Harper, G., Weston, H. J., and Mattingley, J.: Maroteaux-Lamy syndrome, mild form—MPS VI B. Br. J. Radiol., 55:805, 1982.
111. Perks, W. H., Cooper, R. A., Bradbury, S., Horrocks, P., Baldock, N., Allen, A., Van't Hoff, W., Weidman, G., and Prowse, K.: Sleep apnoea in Scheie's syndrome. Thorax, 35:85, 1980.
112. Philippart, M., and Sugarman, G. I.: Chondroitin-4-sulphate mucopolysaccharidosis. A new variant of Hurler's syndrome. Lancet, 2:854, 1969.
113. Pouliquen, J. C., Pennecot, G. F., and Guyonvarch, G.: Cranio-spinal vertebra and Morquio disease. Rev. Chir. Orthop., 66:106, 1980.
114. Pouliquen, J. C., Pennecot, G. F., Beneux, J., Chadoutaud, F., Lacert, P., Duval-Beaupere, G., and Durand, J.: Cranio-vertebral junction and Morquio disease. Apropos of 6 cases. Chir. Pediatr., 23:247, 1982.
115. Pramuljo, H. S., Tamaela, L. A., and Karyomanggolo, W. T.: Morquio's disease. Paediatr. Indones., 20:130, 1980.
116. Rampini, S.: Das Sanfilippo-Syndrom (polydystrophe Oligophrenie, HS-Mucopolysaccharidose). Helv. Paediatr. Acta, 24:55, 1969.
117. Rampini, S., and Maroteaux, P.: Ein ungewohnlicher Phanotyp des Hurler-Syndroms. Helv. Paediatr. Acta, 21:376, 1966.
118. Randaccio, M., Patrucco, R., and Lanteri, C.: Cooley's anaemia in association with mucopolysaccharidosis (type IV) and enchondromatosis respectively. Pediatr. Radiol., 9:27, 1980.
119. Rubin, P.: Dynamic Classification of Bone Dysplasias. Chicago, Year Book, 1964.
120. Sanfilippo, S. J., Podosin, R., Langer, L. O., Jr., and Good, R. A.: Mental retardation associated with acid mucopolysacchariduria (heparitin sulfate type). J. Pediatr., 63:837, 1963.
121. Schaap, T., and Bach, G.: Incidence of mucopolysaccharidoses in Israel: Is Hunter disease a "Jewish disease"? Hum. Genet., 56:221, 1980.
122. Scheie, H. G., Hambrick, G. W., Jr., and Barness, L. A.: A newly recognized forme fruste of Hurler's disease (gargoylism). Am. J. Ophthalmol., 53:753, 1962.
123. Schenk, E. A., and Haggerty, J.: Morquio's disease. A radiologic and morphologic study. Pediatrics, 34:839, 1964.
124. Sengel, A., Stoebner, P., and Juif, J.: Les chondrocytes de la maladie de Morquio. Vacuoles ergastoplasmiques à inclusions spécifiques. Microscopie, 10:33, 1971.
125. Sewell, A. C., Gehler, J., Mittermaier, G., and Meyer, E.: Mucopolysaccharidosis type VII (beta-glucuronidase deficiency): A report of a new case and a survey of those in the literature. Clin. Genet., 21:366, 1982.
126. Silberberg, R., Rimoin, D. L., Rosenthal, R. E., and Hasler, M. B.: Ultrastructure of cartilage in the Hurler and Sanfilippo syndromes. Arch. Pathol., 94:500, 1972.
127. Sly, W. S., Quinton, B. A., McAlister, W. H., and Rimoin, D. L.: Beta glucuronidase deficiency: Report of clinical, radiologic and biochemical features of a new mucopolysaccharidosis. J. Pediatr., 82:249, 1973.
128. Spranger, J. W., Schuster, W., and Freitag, F.: Chondroitin-4-sulfate mucopolysaccharidoses. Helv. Paediatr. Acta, 26:387, 1971.
129. Spranger, J., Teller, W., Kosenow, W., Murken, J., and Eckert-Husemann, E.: Die HS-Mucopolysaccharidose von Sanfilippo (polydystrophe Oligophrenie). Z. Kinderheilkd., 101:71, 1967.
130. Spranger, J., Koch, F., McKusick, V. A., Natzschka, J., Wiedemann, H. R., and Zellweger, H.: Mucopolysaccharidosis VI (Maroteaux-Lamy's disease). Helv. Paediatr. Acta, 25:337, 1970.
131. Stanescu, V., Bona, C., and Ionescu, V.: The tibial growing cartilage biopsy in the study of growth disturbances. Acta Endocrinol., 64:577, 1970.
132. Strumpf, D. A., Austin, J. H., Crocker, A. C., and Lafrance, M.: Mucopolysaccharidosis type VI (Maroteaux-Lamy syndrome). Am. J. Dis. Child., 126:747, 1973.
133. Sugiura, Y., Terashima, Y., Furukawa, T., and Yoneda, M.: Spondyloepiphyseal dysplasia congenita. Int. Orthop., 2:47, 1978.
134. Tanase-Mogos, I., Turcanu, L., Petrescu, L., and Popescu, M.: Biochemical and clinical correlations in children suspected of having lysosomal diseases. Physiologie, 18:37, 1981.
135. Tondeur, M.: Etude ultrastructurale des mucopolysaccharidoses et d'affections apparentées. Thèse. Méd., Bruxelles, 1973.

136. Tondeur, M., and Loeb, H.: Etude ultrastructurale du foie dans la maladie de Morquio. Pediatr. Res., 3:19, 1969.
137. Trojak, J. E., Ho, C. K., Roesel, R. A., Levin, L. S., Kopits, S. E., Thomas, G. H., and Toma, S.: Morquio-like syndrome (MPS IV B) associated with deficiency of a beta-galactosidase. Johns Hopkins Med. J., 146:75, 1980.
138. van de Kamp, J. J., Niermeijer, M. F., von Figura, K., and Giesberts, M. A.: Genetic heterogeneity and clinical variability in the Sanfilippo syndrome (types A, B, and C). Clin. Genet., 20:152, 1981.
139. Van Dyke, D. L., Fluharty, A. L., Schafer, I. A., Shapiro, L. J., Kihara, H., and Weiss, L.: Prenatal diagnosis of Maroteaux-Lamy syndrome. Am. J. Med. Genet., 8:235, 1981.
140. Van Hoof, F., and Hers, H. G.: The abnormalities of lysosomal enzymes in mucopolysaccharidoses. Eur. J. Biochem., 7:34, 1968.
141. Watts, R. W., Spellacy, E., Kendall, B. E., du Boulay, G., and Gibbs, D. A.: Computed tomography studies on patients with mucopolysaccharidoses. Neuroradiology, 21:9, 1981.
142. Whiteside, J. D., and Cholmeley, J. G.: Morquio's disease: Review of literature with description of 4 cases. Arch. Dis. Child., 27:487, 1952.
143. Winchester, P., Grossman, H., Wan Ngo Lim, and Danes, B. S.: A new acid mucopolysaccharidosis with skeletal deformities simulating rheumatoid arthritis. A.J.R., 106:121, 1969.
144. Xia, R. G.: Clinical and roentgenographic diagnosis of mucopolysaccharidosis. II. Mucopolysaccharidosis type IV and VI—a report of 8 cases. Chung Hua Fang She Hsueh Tsa Chih, 15:146, 1981.
145. Zellweger, H., Giaccai, L., and Firzli, S.: Gargoylism and Morquio's disease. Am. J. Dis. Child., 84:421, 1952.
146. Zellweger, H., Ponseti, I. V., Pedrini, V., Stamler, F. S., and Von Noorder, G. K.: Morquio Ullrich's disease: Report of two cases. J. Pediatr., 59:549, 1961.

GAUCHER'S DISEASE

Gaucher's disease is an inborn disturbance of lipid metabolism characterized by a deficiency of the enzyme beta-glucocerebrosidase that results in the secondary accumulation of the glucocerebrosides in the reticuloendothelial system and sometimes in the central nervous system.

It was first described by Gaucher in 1882 as ". . . l'epithelioma primitif de la rate, hypertrophie idiopathique de la rate sans leucemie"—idiopathic hypertrophy of the spleen without leukemia.[21] The spleen was infiltrated with the pale-staining foam cells, now known as Gaucher cells, that are distinctive of the disease. They are roughly circular or polyhedral in outline and range in size from 20 to 40 μ. The nuclei appear small, there is often more than one, and they are seen in mitosis. Their cytoplasm is wrinkled and fibrillar, but not so much foamy or vacuolated (Fig. 3–99).

Etiology

The cause of Gaucher's disease was clarified by the extensive investigations of Brady and associates.[11] There is no abnormality in the formation of the glucocerebrosides—no overproduction. It is the deficient activity of the enzyme beta-glucocerebrosidase that causes the abnormal accumulation of the glucocerebroside. Similiar enzyme deficiency was demonstrated in Niemann-Pick disease, which is caused by lack or decreased activity of the sphingomyelin-clearing enzyme. They demonstrated that these enzyme defects are specific—i.e., deficiency of beta-glucocerebrosidase causes Gaucher's disease, and that of sphingomyelin-clearing enzyme, Niemann-Pick disease. Furthermore, Brady and associates showed intravenous infusions of purified human placental glucocerebrosidase diminished the quantity of accumulated glucocerebroside in the liver and erythrocytes of patients with Gaucher's disease; the glucocerebrosidase enzyme infusions had no effect on the quality of other lipids in these organs.[9–12]

Heredity

Gaucher's disease has a strikingly high incidence in Ashkenazi Jews of central and northern Europe; it is less preponderant among Jews whose ancestors lived in areas bordering the Mediterranean, the Sephardic Jews. There is a very high familial incidence.

The inheritance of Gaucher's disease is by autosomal recessive transmission. Gaucher cells have been found in the heterozygote parents and sibs of patients with Gaucher's disease.[65] There are, however, occasional instances of spontaneous mutation and affected cases in families in which there is evidence of some aberrant autosomal dominant trait.[35]

In utero diagnosis of Gaucher's disease can be made by examination of cultured amniotic fluid cells which show decreased activity of glucocerebrosidase enzyme.[32]

Clinical Features

Gaucher's disease manifests three distinct clinical forms.[10] The first is the *acute infantile neuropathic form*, which is rare and occurs in infants, in whom it primarily involves the central nervous system. It is fulminating and severe, resulting in death within 18 months in infancy and childhood. Significant bone lesions do not occur in the infantile form.[4] Brady and Barranger refer to this as Type II Gaucher's disease.[10] The extensive neuronal cell destruction appears to be caused by accumulation of the toxic glucosylsphingosine (psychosine) in the cerebrum and cerebellum.[49]

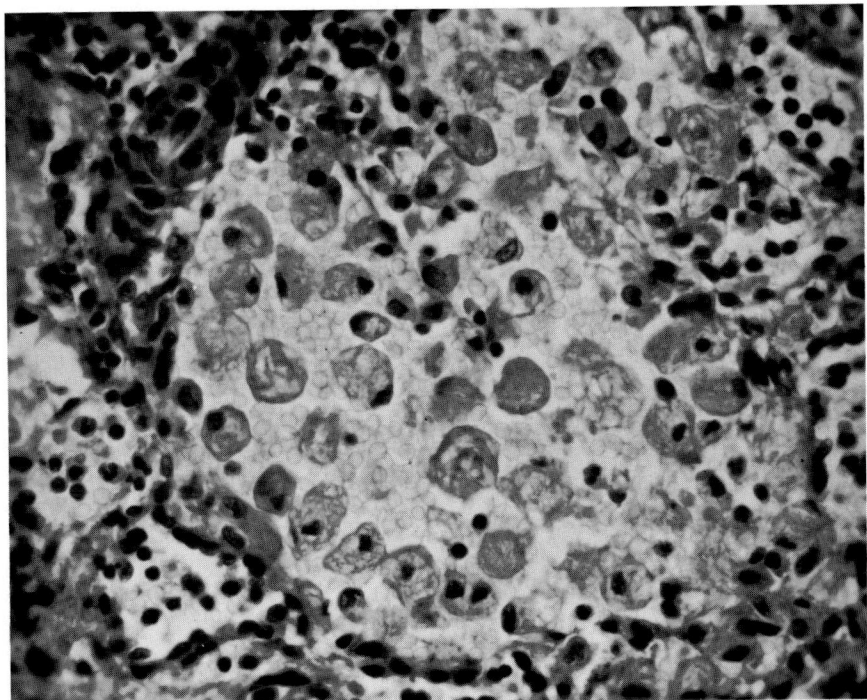

FIGURE 3–99. *Gaucher's cells, characteristic of Gaucher's disease.*

(Hematoxylin and eosin, ×400.)

The second is the *chronic, non-neuropathic form*: This is also referred to as the adult form, or Type I Gaucher's disease, by Brady and Barranger.[10] It is the most common clinical form and becomes manifest with an insidious onset during the first two decades of life. The severity and course of the disease are extremely variable, with a proclivity to be more severe in children. Splenomegaly, enlargement of lymph nodes, bone lesions, skin pigmentation, and pingueculae in the eyes are the physical findings. The central nervous system is not involved.

The third type is the *subacute neuropathic, or juvenile, form.* It has the features of the chronic form, but in addition, the central nervous system is involved. It manifests itself in childhood with slowly progressive neural dysfunction, hypertonicity of muscles with gait abnormality, strabismus, seizures, and mental retardation.

Clinical features vary with the type and age of onset of Gaucher's disease. Infiltration of the bone marrow causes anemia, leukopenia, and thrombocytopenia; these manifest clinically as fatigue, bleeding tendencies, and recurrent infections. Enlargement of the spleen causes asymmetrical abdominal protuberance and a feeling of heaviness. Enlarged liver and lymph nodes can be palpated. The neurologic findings in the infantile form are quite striking.

Bony Manifestations

The orthopedic surgeon is involved with the skeletal lesions and complications of the disease. On the basis of pathophysiology, these can be subgrouped into six categories: bone marrow infiltration, aseptic necrosis, bone crises, pathologic fractures, lytic bone lesions, and osteomyelitis.

First, the bone marrow is infiltrated by Gaucher cells, which multiply and replace the medullary cavity. Soon, the affected metaphysis and adjacent diaphysis expand, and the regional cortex becomes thinned and eroded from within. The distal femora are most frequently involved. Expansion of the distal diaphysis and metaphysis with failure of tubulation gives the bone the appearance of an Erlenmeyer flask on the radiogram (Fig. 3–100). Additional findings in the radiograph are decreased bone density with irregular wide trabeculae and cortical thinning. Expansion and erosion of the cortices is the cause of the chronic complaint of bone and joint pain. Bone changes, however, may be clinically asymptomatic, even though they are demonstrable in the radiogram.

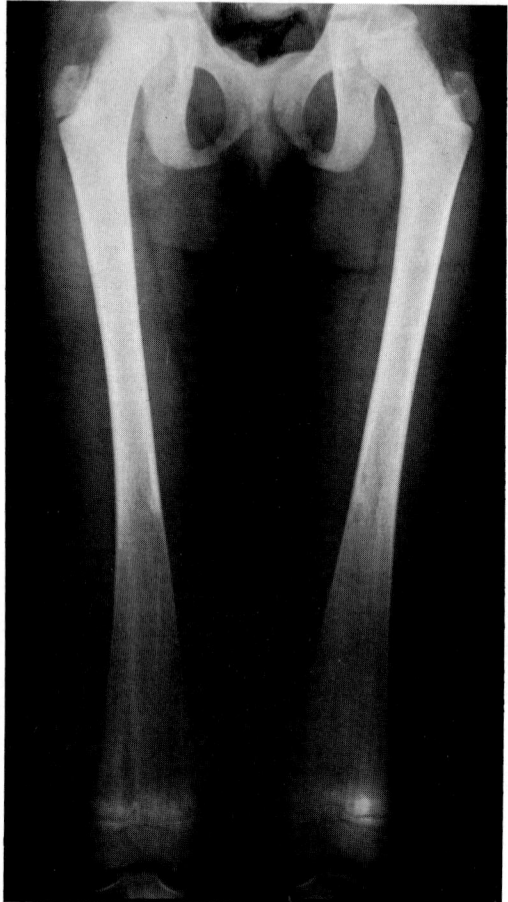

FIGURE 3–100. Bilateral "Erlenmeyer flask" deformity of the femora in Gaucher's disease.

The second group of skeletal manifestations is related to *aseptic necrosis,* caused by interruption of the blood supply mechanically from the expanding cell mass, vasospasm, thrombosis, and edema. Avascular necrosis of the femoral head is common; it occurred in 15 of the 20 patients of Amstutz and Carey.[2] Usually it is bilateral and may be either total or partial in type, with radiographic findings of fragmentation and collapse of the femoral head.

Histologic examination of these femoral heads has disclosed sheets of Gaucher cells and fibrous tissue filling the marrow spaces, causing cartilaginous and osseous necrosis. With the stress of weight-bearing, the articular cartilage space of the hip joint becomes narrowed, osteoarthritic changes develop, and the joint may disintegrate completely (Fig. 3–101). Recurrence of avascular necrosis later on in adult life may occur.[38]

Necrosis of the humeral head and pathologic fracture of the proximal shaft of the humerus may occur.[20] Any bone may be involved—the talus, radius, ulna, tibia, skull, or spine. Pathologic compression fractures of the vertebrae will cause backache and localized kyphosis.

Medullary infarction gives the radiographic picture of poorly defined diaphyseal lytic lesions, periosteal reaction, split cortices, and sometimes an "endobone" (os-in-os) appearance.

The third group are the *"bone crises"* in Gaucher's disease. They present as acute episodes of severe pain in a limb with localized tenderness, warmth, redness, inability to use the limb, fever, and leukocytosis. Radiograms show periosteal new bone formation and mottled rarefaction of the involved bone. These findings mimic osteomyelitis and present a difficult problem of differential diagnosis. In Gaucher's disease, the child is not acutely sick. There is radiographic evidence of multiple osseous involvement and hepatosplenomegaly. The serum acid phosphatase level may be elevated.

Bone imaging with technetium-99m may assist in differentiating between "bone crisis" and osteomyelitis. The Gaucher cell–packed bone marrow will show decreased uptake of the radionucleotide, whereas osteomyelitis will show increased uptake. In Gaucher's disease, however, microfracture of the thinned cortex with remodeling may show increased uptake on scintigraphy. Gallium-67 scintigraphy is useful in evaluating underlying osteomyelitis. Uptake will be decreased in the marrow packed with noninflammatory Gaucher cells, whereas in osteomyelitis it will be increased.[45]

The course of Gaucher's crises is self-limited, the episode gradually subsiding within days or weeks without specific treatment.[48, 68] Material obtained by repeated aspirations of the affected area is sterile on culture. The pathophysiology of "bone crises" in Gaucher's disease seems to be vascular compromise, very similar to sickle cell crises; in Gaucher's disease the infiltration of Gaucher's cells mechanically blocks the circulation, whereas in sickle cell disease the altered viscosity of the erythrocytes is the cause. The acuteness of symptoms probably is due to marked elevation of intramedullary pressure. Aspiration of a symptomatic long bone may be indicated to rule out infection; it is crucial that it be carried out under very strict aseptic conditions in the operating room and with antibiotic coverage provided empirically. The hazard of secondary contamination is very great.

The fourth group is *pathologic fractures,* usually of the proximal femur, either basal neck or subtrochanteric.[24] In children, these fractures heal with conservative treatment, but they tend to be displaced, with resultant coxa vara. In the spine, the vertebrae may collapse be-

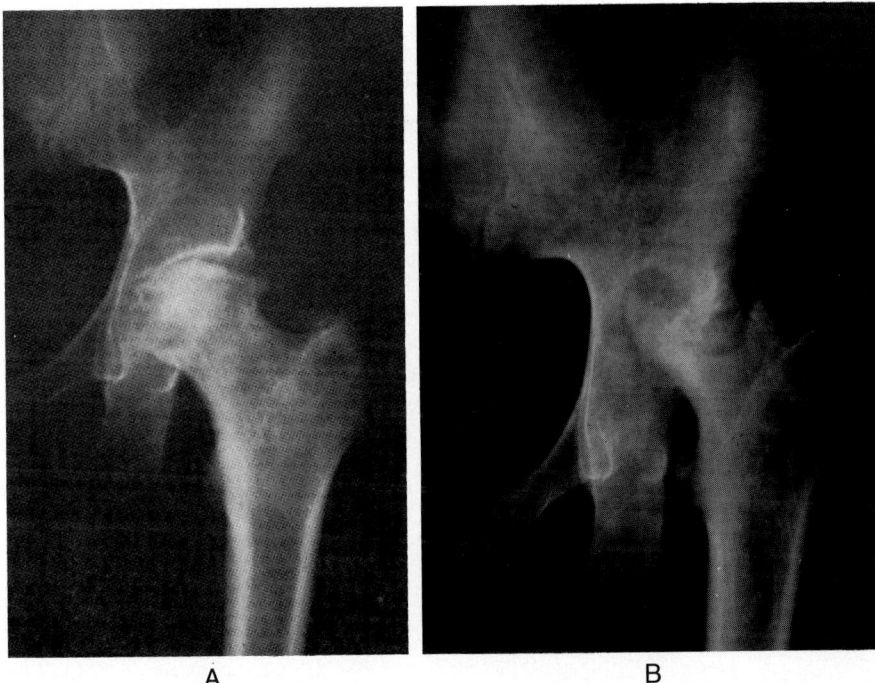

FIGURE 3–101. *Gaucher's disease in a 52-year-old woman.*

A. Necrosis of the left femoral head. The joint space is narrowed and the superior surface of the head is somewhat collapsed. **B.** The same hip 18 months later. Note the complete disintegration of the joint with severe collapse and superolateral migration of the femoral head. (From Amstutz, H. C., and Carey, E. J.: Skeletal manifestations and treatment of Gaucher's disease. J. Bone Joint Surg., 48-A:683, 1966. Reprinted by permission.)

cause of stress fractures, which results in vertebra plana with structural localized kyphosis. The discs may protrude into the vertebral bodies. The "H," or "step-off," vertebrae (so characteristic of sickle-cell hemoglobinopathy) may be seen in Gaucher's disease, but the pathogenesis of "H" deformation of the vertebral bodies is different.

The fifth group consists of large *bubbly expansile lytic lesions* in long bones, caused by marked aggregates of abnormal Gaucher cells. Tumor formation in Gaucher's disease is very rare. Watanabe and associates, however, reported a huge intraosseous tumor in the tibia with complete destruction of the overlying cortex.[64]

The sixth problem is pyogenic *osteomyelitis*. Gaucher bone is susceptible to infection because of the leukopenia, anemia, and hypoxia due to decreased blood supply in the bone. It is crucial that gallium-67 scintigraphy be performed to demonstrate the presence of inflammatory cells.[45] The temptation to emergency operation and drainage of bone must be resisted, as often the result is chronic osteomyelitis at the operative site.

Treatment

Treatment is individualized. Splenectomy is indicated if there is hypersplenism with thrombocytopenia and a hemorrhagic tendency. It will also relieve gastrointestinal symptoms and the abdominal distention and heaviness caused by the markedly enlarged spleen. The orthopedic complications, however, may be aggravated after splenectomy, because the destruction of blood cells taking place in the spleen will then occur in other organs, such as the bone marrow.[54, 55, 64]

The use of radiation therapy to control recalcitrant bone pain is controversial.[2, 35] It is not recommended by this author.

Management of pathologic fractures should be conservative in children. The fractures heal adequately in time. Open reduction and internal fixation have a high risk of secondary infection. It is better judgment to accept a certain degree of fracture displacement and deformity than risk chronic osteomyelitis.

Severe arthritis of the hip due to osteonecrosis of the femoral head is treated by hip arthroplasty or total hip replacement, depending on whether there are severe collapse and secondary involvement of the acetabulum.[40, 41]

Enzyme replacement therapy is advised by Brady and associates and by Bleutler and Dale.[6, 12] Preliminary reports are encouraging, but further experience, refinement of the enzyme, and delineation of various parameters are necessary.

References

1. Amstutz, H. C.: The hip in Gaucher's disease. Clin. Orthop., *90*:83, 1973.
2. Amstutz, H. C., and Carey, E. J.: Skeletal manifestations and treatment of Gaucher's disease. J. Bone Joint Surg., *48-A*:670, 1966.
3. Arkin, A. M., and Schein, A. J.: Aseptic necrosis in Gaucher's disease. J. Bone Joint Surg., *30-A*:631, 1948.
4. Banker, B. Q., Miller, J. Q., and Crocker, A. C.: The cerebral pathology of infantile Gaucher's disease. In Aronson, S. M., and Volk, B. W. (eds.): Cerebral Sphingolipidoses. New York, Academic Press, 1962, p. 73.
5. Berranger, P., Navel, M., Decobert, G., and Gillot, F.: La forme aigue infantile de la maladie de Gaucher. A propos d'une observation familiale. Ann. Pediatr., *22*:641, 1975.
6. Beutler, E., and Dale, G. L.: Gaucher's disease. A century of delineation and research; enzyme replacement therapy; model and clinical studies. Prog. Clin. Biol. Res., *95*:703, 1982.
7. Beutler, E., Dale, G. L., and Kuhl, W.: Replacement therapy in Gaucher's disease. Birth Defects, *16*:369, 1980.
8. Beutler, E., Kuhl, W., and Trinidad, F.: β-Glucosidase activity in fibroblasts from homozygotes and heterozygotes for Gaucher's disease. Am. J. Hum. Genet., *23*:62, 1971.
9. Brady, R. O.: Glucosyl ceramide lipidosis: Gaucher's disease. In Stanbury, J. B., Wyngaarden, J. B., and Fredrickson, D. S. (eds.): The Metabolic Basis of Inherited Disease. New York, McGraw-Hill, 1978, pp. 731–746.
10. Brady, R. O., and Barranger, J. A.: Glucosyl ceramide lipidosis: Gaucher disease. In Stanbury, J. B., Wyngaarden, J. B., Fredrickson, D. S., Goldstein, J. L., and Brown, M. S. (eds.): The Metabolic Basis of Inherited Disease. 5th Ed. New York, McGraw-Hill, 1983, pp. 842–856.
11. Brady, R. O., Kanfer, J. N., and Shapiro, D.: Metabolism of glucocerebrosides. II. Evidence of enzymatic deficiency in Gaucher's disease. Biochem. Biophy. Res. Commun., *18*:221, 1965.
12. Brady, R. O., Pentchev, P. G., Gal, A. E., Hibbert, S. R., and Dekaban, A. S.: Replacement therapy for inherited enzyme deficiency. Use of purified glucocerebrosidase in Gaucher's disease. N. Engl. J. Med., *291*:989, 1974.
13. Carbone, A. O., and Petrozzi, C. F.: Gaucher's disease. Case report with stress on eye findings. Henry Ford Hosp. Med. J., *16*:55, 1968.
14. Chen, T. H., and Holman, B. L.: Radionuclide assessment of Gaucher's disease. J. Nucl. Med., *19*:1333, 1978.
15. Crocker, A. C., and Landing, B. H.: Phosphatase studies in Gaucher's disease. Metabolism, *9*:341, 1960.
16. Crone, R. I., and Bergin, J. J.: Gaucher's disease in identical twins. Ann. Intern. Med., *49*:941, 1958.
17. Cushing, E. H., and Stout, A. P.: Gaucher's disease with report of a case showing bone disintegration and joint involvement. Arch. Surg., *12*:539, 1926.
18. Danes, B. S., and Bearn, A. G.: Gaucher's disease: A genetic disease detected in skin fibroblast cultures. Science, *161*:1347, 1968.
19. Davies, F. W. T.: Gaucher's disease in bone. J. Bone Joint Surg., *34-B*:454, 1952.
20. Epps, C. H., Jr.: Painful hematologic conditions affecting the shoulder. Clin. Orthop., *173*:38, 1983.
21. Gaucher, P. C. E.: De l'epithelioma primitif de la rate, hypertrophie idiopathique de la rate sans leucemie. Paris, 1882. (Thèse.)
22. Geddes, A. K., and Moore, S.: Acute (infantile) Gaucher's disease. Report of a case, the second in the family. J. Pediatr., *43*:61, 1953.
23. Goldblatt, J., Sacks, S., and Beighton, P.: The orthopedic aspects of Gaucher disease. Clin. Orthop., *137*:208, 1978.
24. Goldman, A. B., and Jacobs, B.: Femoral neck fractures complicating Gaucher disease in children. Skeletal Radiol., *12*:162, 1984.
25. Gordon, E. J.: Gaucher's disease in adults. South. Med. J., *69*:664, 1976.
26. Greenfield, G. B.: Miscellaneous diseases related to the hematologic system. Semin. Roentgenol., *9*:241, 1974.
27. Greenfield, G. B.: Bone changes in chronic adult Gaucher's disease. A.J.R., *110*:800, 1970.
28. Groen, J.: The hereditary mechanism of Gaucher's disease. Blood, *3*:1238, 1948.
29. Guibaud, P., Maire, I., Vanier, M.-T., Mathieu, M., Gilly, J., and Larbre, F.: La forme infantile de la maladie de Gaucher étude clinique et biologique d'une observation. Arch. Fr. Pediatr., *35*:949, 1978.
30. Harrison, W. E., Jr., and Louis, H. J.: Osseous Gaucher's disease in early childhood. Report of a case with extensive bone changes and pathological fractures without splenomegaly. J.A.M.A., *187*:997, 1964.
31. Herndon, C. N., and Bender, J. R.: Gaucher's disease: Cases in five related Negro sibships. Am. J. Hum. Genet., *2*:49, 1950.
32. Ho, M. W., Seck, J., and Schmidt, D.: Adult Gaucher's disease: Kindred studies and demonstration of a deficiency of acid β-glucosidase in cultured fibroblasts. Am. J. Hum. Genet., *24*:37, 1972.
33. Hodson, P., Goldblatt, J., and Beighton, P.: Non-neuropathic Gaucher disease presenting in infancy. Arch. Dis. Child., *54*:707, 1979.
34. Hsia, D. Y. Y., Naylor, J., and Bigler, J. A.: Gaucher's disease. Report of two cases in father and son and review of literature. N. Engl. J. Med., *261*:164, 1959.
35. Jaffe, H. L.: Metabolic Degenerative and Inflammatory Diseases of Bones and Joints. Philadelphia, Lea & Febiger, 1972, pp. 506–522.
36. James, N. E.: Gaucher's disease. Report of a case. J. Bone Joint Surg., *34-B*:464, 1952.
37. Kampine, J. P., Brady, R. O., Kanfer, J. N., Feld, M., and Shapiro, D.: Diagnosis of Gaucher's disease and Niemann-Pick disease with small samples of venous blood. Science, *155*:86, 1966.
38. Katz, J. F.: Recurrent avascular necrosis of the proximal femoral epiphysis in the same hip in Gaucher's disease. J. Bone Joint Surg., *49-A*:514, 1967.
39. Katz, M., Dorfmann, H., Hubault, A., Djian, A., Bard, M., and Seze, S. de.: Maladie de Gaucher. A propos d'une observation à manifestations ostéo-articulaires dominantes. J. Radiol. Electrol., *54*:61, 1973.
40. Lachiewicz, P. F., Lane, M. J., and Wilson, P. D.: Total hip replacement in Gaucher's disease. J. Bone Joint Surg., *63-A*:602, 1981.
41. Lau, M. M., Lichtman, D. M., Hamati, Y. I., and Bierbaum, B. E.: Hip arthroplasties in Gaucher's disease. J. Bone Joint Surg., *63-A*:591, 1981.
42. Levin, B.: Gaucher's disease. Clinical and roentgenologic manifestations. A.J.R., *85*:685, 1961.
43. Matoth, Y., and Fried, K.: Chronic Gaucher's disease.

44. Matoth, Y., Zaizov, R., Hoffman, J., and Klibansky, C.: Clinical and biochemical aspects of chronic Gaucher's disease. Isr. J. Med. Sci., 10:1523, 1974.
45. Miller, J. H., Ortega, J. A., and Heisel, M. A.: Juvenile Gaucher disease simulating osteomyelitis. A.J.R., 137:880, 1981.
46. Moseley, J. E.: Bone changes in hematologic disorders. In Roentgen Aspects. New York, Grune & Stratton, 1963, pp. 12–26, 179–198.
47. Nilsson, O., and Svennerholm, L.: Accumulation of glucosylceramide and glucosylsphingosine (psychosine) in cerebrum and cerebellum in infantile and juvenile Gaucher disease. J. Neurochem., 39:709, 1982.
48. Noyes, F. R., and Smith, W. S.: Bone crisis and chronic osteomyelitis in Gaucher's disease. Clin. Orthop., 79:132, 1971.
49. Peters, S. P., Lee, R. E., and Glew, R. H.: Gaucher's disease, A review. Medicine, 56:425, 1977.
50. Reiss, O., and Kato, K.: Gaucher's disease. A clinical study, with special reference to the roentgenography of bones. Am. J. Dis. Child., 43:365, 1942.
51. Rosenberg, A., and Charagaff, E.: A reinvestigation of the cerebroside deposited in Gaucher's disease. J. Biol. Chem., 233:1323, 1958.
52. Rourke, J. A., and Heslin, D. J.: Gaucher's disease. Roentgenologic bone changes over 20 year interval. A.J.R., 94:621, 1965.
53. Sacks, S.: Osteitis in Gaucher's disease. South Afr. J. Surg., 9:161, 1971.
54. Schein, A. J., and Arkin, A. M.: Hip-joint involvement in Gaucher's disease. J. Bone Joint Surg., 24:396, 1942.
55. Schein, A. J., and Arkin, A. M.: The classic hip joint involvement in Gaucher's disease. Clin. Orthop., 90:4, 1973.
56. Schneider, E. L., Ellis, W. G., Brady, R. O., McCulloch, J. R., and Epstein, C. J.: Infantile (Type II) Gaucher's disease: In utero diagnosis and fetal pathology. J. Pediatr., 81:1134, 1972.
57. Schwartz, A. M., Homer, M. J., and McCauley, R. G. K.: "Step-off" vertebral body: Gaucher's disease versus sickle cell hemoglobinopathy. A.J.R., 132:81, 1979.
58. Seinsheimer, F., and Mankin, H. J.: Acute bilateral symmetrical pathologic fractures of the lateral tibial plateaus in a patient with Gaucher's disease. Arthritis Rheum., 20:1550, 1977.
59. Silverstein, M. N., and Kelly, P. J.: Osteoarticular manifestations of Gaucher's disease. Am. J. Med. Sci., 253:569, 1967.
60. Todd, R. M., and Keidan, S. E.: Changes in the head of the femur in children suffering from Gaucher's disease. J. Bone Joint Surg., 34-B:447, 1952.
61. Tripp, J. H., Lake, B. D., Young, E., Ngu, J., and Brett, E. M.: Juvenile Gaucher's disease with horizontal gaze palsy in three siblings. J. Neurol. Neurosurg. Psychiatry, 40:470, 1977.
62. Tuchman, L. R., and Swick, M.: High acid phosphatase level indicating Gaucher's disease in patient with prostatism. J.A.M.A., 164:2034, 1957.
63. Tuchman, L. R., Suna, H., and Carr, J. J.: Elevation of serum acid phosphatase in Gaucher's disease. J. Mt. Sinai Hosp., 23:227, 1956.
64. Watanabe, M., Yanagisawa, M., Sonobe, S., Matsumoto, J., and Miura, H.: An adult form of Gaucher's disease with a huge tumour formation of the right tibia. Int. Orthop., 8:195, 1984.
65. Wiedeman, H. R., and Gerken, H.: Gaucher cells in healthy relatives of patients with Gaucher's disease. Lancet, 2:866, 1964.
66. Wolson, A. H.: Pulmonary findings in Gaucher's disease. A.J.R., 123:712, 1975.
67. Wood, H. L. C.: Gaucher's disease with pseudocoxalgia. Report of a case. J. Bone Joint Surg., 34-B:462, 1952.
68. Yossipouitch, Z. H., Herman, G., and Makin, M.: Aseptic osteomyelitis in Gaucher's disease. Isr. J. Med. Sci., 1:531, 1973.

NIEMANN-PICK DISEASE

The result of a deficiency of the enzyme sphingomyelinase, this rare inborn error of metabolism is characterized by accumulation of large foam cells containing phospholipids. In the central nervous system it is ganglioside that accumulates, whereas in the viscera the improperly metabolized phospholipid is sphingomyelin.[4] The disease was first described by Niemann in 1914, and its characteristic features were further delineated by Pick in 1926.[8,9]

The condition is hereditary with an autosomal recessive mode of inheritance. It occurs predominantly in inbred members of the Jewish race, affecting males and females equally.

Clinically, the disease manifests itself in infancy or early childhood with hepatosplenomegaly or jaundice. Mental retardation is universally present, resulting from extensive involvement of the central nervous system. It may be associated with amaurotic familial idiocy (Tay-Sachs disease), in which instance lecithin is demonstrated in nerve tissue, and a cherry-red macula is found in the retina.

Skeletal changes consist of osteoporosis and expansion of the lower diaphyses and metaphyseal regions of long bones, particularly the femur. Expansion of the metacarpals has been noted.[3,5] There may be coxa valga. Avascular necrosis is not a feature. Fractures and deformities of the bones usually do not occur.

There is no specific treatment. The prognosis is very poor, death occurring within a year following onset of the disease. Few subjects have survived into adult life.

References

1. Brady, R. O., Kanfer, J. N., Mock, M. D., et al.: The metabolism of sphingomyelin. II. Evidence of an enzymatic deficiency in Niemann-Pick disease. Proc. Natl. Acad. Sci., 55:366, 1966.
2. Crocker, A. C.: The cerebral defect in Tay-Sachs disease and Niemann-Pick disease. J. Neurochem., 7:69, 1961.
3. Crocker, A. C., and Farber, S.: Niemann-Pick disease: A review of eighteen patients. Medicine, 37:1, 1958.
4. Gilbert, E. F., Callahan, J., Viseskul, C., and Opitz, J. M.: Niemann-Pick disease type C. Pathological, histochemical, ultrastructural and biochemical studies. Eur. J. Pediatr., 136:263, 1981.
5. Greenfield, G. B.: Miscellaneous diseases related to the hematologic system. Semin. Roentgenol., 9:241, 1974.
6. Jaffe, H. L.: Metabolic Degenerative and Inflammatory Diseases of Bone and Joints. Philadelphia, Lea & Febiger, 1972, pp. 522–528.

7. Lachman, R., Crocker, A., Schulman, M., and Stroud, R.: Radiological findings in Niemann-Pick disease. Radiology, *108*:659, 1973.
8. Niemann, A. L.: Ein unbekanntes Krankenheitsbild. Jahrb. Kinderheilkd., 79:1, 1914.
9. Pick, L.: Der Morbus Gaucher und die ihm ahnlichen Erkrankungen. (Die lipoidzellige Splenohepatomegalie Typus Niemann und die diabetische Lipoidzellenhyperplasie der milz.) Ergeb. Inn. Med. Kinderheilkd., 29:519, 1926.
10. Schneider, P. B., and Kennedy, E. P.: Sphingomyelinase in normal human spleens and in spleens from subjects with Niemann-Pick disease. J. Lipid Res., 8:202, 1967.
11. Videbaek, A.: Niemann-Pick's disease. Acute and chronic type? Acta Paediatr. Scand., 37:95, 1949.

HOMOCYSTINURIA

Homocystinuria is an inborn error of methionine metabolism caused in its classic form by deficiency of the enzyme cystathionine-β-synthase. Clinically it is characterized by mental retardation, thrombotic tendency, lens dislocation, and various skeletal abnormalities that strongly resemble those of Marfan's syndrome. It is inherited as an autosomal recessive disorder. First described in 1962 by Field and associates, it was later reported independently in 1964 by Gerritsen and Waisman.[16, 17] Previously, cases of homocystinuria had been misdiagnosed as Marfan's syndrome.[28]

Biochemical Defect and Pathophysiology

The deficiency of the enzyme cystathionine synthase (or synthetase) blocks the conversion of homocysteine to cystathionine. The abnormally accumulated homocysteine is converted to homocystine, and as a result, the level of homocystine in the tissues and plasma is elevated, and homocystine is excreted in large quantities in the urine. The plasma concentration of methionine is also increased. Normally cystathionine is present in brain tissue; in the homocystinuric patient cystathionine cannot be found in the brain, and thereby, cystine becomes an essential amino acid.

There are other extremely rare causes of homocystinuria: vitamin B_{12} malabsorption syndrome (Imerslund-Gräsbeck syndrome); vitamin B_6 depletion; 5-methyltetrahydrofolate–homocysteine methyltransferase deficiency due to defective production of cofactor methylcobalamin; and 5,10,methylene tetrahydrofolate reductase deficiency. The latter two causes of homocystinuria are inheritable metabolic defects. In this text only the "classic" homocystinuria is discussed.

Clinical Features

These consist of a tendency to venous and arterial thrombosis; mental retardation; dislocation of the lens; and skeletal changes resembling those of Marfan's syndrome with the additional findings of osteoporosis and metaphyseal enlargement, particularly around the knee.

Vascular Changes. The lesions in the blood vessels consist of intimal fibrosis, abnormality of the elastic laminae, atherosclerosis, and thrombosis. Homocysteine, in itself, is a very toxic substance, causing endothelial lesions. Another factor in the pathogenesis of thrombosis is platelet stickiness. Venous and arterial thrombosis can become life-threatening. Death can occur because of myocardial infarction, pulmonary embolism, mesenteric thrombosis, or cerebral vascular accident. About 20 per cent of patients with homocystinuria develop serious thombosis. Following surgery the incidence of venous thrombosis is very high, and the operating surgeon should be wary, avoiding elective procedures.

Mental Retardation. This is common but not uniformly present. Some patients with homocystinuria have normal intelligence and are college graduates.[34] In those who are retarded, the I.Q. is usually about 50: it does deteriorate with age. Whether the mental retardation is due to the biochemical abnormalities or to intermittent cerebral thrombosis is not determined. In general, homocystinuric patients who respond to pyridoxine are less retarded. Adolescents with homocystinuria may exhibit schizophrenia-like states. Intracranial thrombosis may cause other central nervous system disorders such as "acute hemiplegia" and "cerebral palsy." Patients may develop seizures and have abnormal electroencephalograms.

Dislocation of the Lens. This is not observed in infancy, but develops later on in childhood. It appears to be caused by a defective suspensory ligament. Lens dislocation can produce glaucoma.

Skeletal Changes. The limbs are excessively long and thin (dolichostenomelia); the disproportionately long limbs make the arm span exceed the height of the patient, and the length from head to symphysis pubis is less than from the symphysis pubis to the heel. Arachnodactyly is present but is not as severe or frequent as in Marfan's syndrome. There may be fixed flexion deformity of the digits and flexion deformity of the elbow with limited supination. The feet and toes are long. Severe pes planovalgus is common. Most patients have scoliosis—usu-

Table 3-12. Differential Diagnosis of Homocystinuria and Marfan's Syndrome

	Homocystinuria	Marfan's Syndrome
Inheritance	Autosomal recessive	Autosomal dominant
Etiology	Deficiency of enzyme cystathionine synthase	No known biochemical defect
Clinical features	Mental retardation present in most but not all	Absent
Neurologic abnormality	Convulsions; schizophrenia-like state	Absent
Vascular changes	Tendency to thrombosis of veins and arteries	Dissecting aneurysm
		Rupture of aorta
	High incidence of thromboembolism	Prolapse of mitral valve
Lens dislocation	Present, usually downward	Present, usually upward
	Not present at birth	Present at birth
Skeletal changes	Osteoporosis with platyspondyly and biconcavity of vertebrae	Osteoporosis absent or very minimal
		Large vertebrae
	Dolichostenomyelia present	Dolichostenomyelia present
	Flaring of metaphysis with enlargement of epiphysis at knee	Epiphysis and metaphysis normal
	Joint laxity, dislocation rare (not a feature of the disease)	Joint laxity with patellofemoral dislocation
	Arachnodactyly, moderate	Severe arachnodactyly
	Pectus excavatum or carinatum present	Pectus excavatum or carinatum present

ally a left lumbar, right thoracic curve with the lumbar curve being the greater. Osteoporosis, especially in the spine, is often a striking feature.

Widening of the metaphyses and enlargement of the epiphyses of the long bones, particularly at the knee, are important features in homocystinuria.[6] These are usually not present in Marfan's syndrome.

Associated anomalies are pectus carinatum or excavatum, high-arched palate, a facial appearance characterized by malar flush, and light-colored hair.

Diagnosis

The urine is tested for homocysteine by the nitroprusside test. Sodium cyanide is added first, which reduces the homocystine to homocysteine. The latter reacts with sodium nitroprusside to form a dark red color. Cystine in the urine gives the same reaction as the homocysteine in the nitroprusside test. Electrophoresis will distinguish between homocysteine and cystine. As a screening method for homocystinuria the nitroprusside test has its pitfalls: it may be falsely negative in patients with homocystinuria and falsely positive in normal persons. It is, therefore, best to perform quantitative serum amino acid analyses and also to determine the cystathionine-β-synthase activity in a fibroblast culture obtained by skin biopsy for definitive diagnosis.

Differential diagnosis of homocystinuria from Marfan's syndrome is given in Table 3-12.

Treatment

An attempt should be made to reverse the biochemical abnormalities with pyridoxine (vitamin B_6), which may or may not overcome the enzyme block. Initially, the dosage is large, up to 250 mg. of pyridoxine daily with subsequent reduction to about 50 mg. daily. At present it is not clear whether this correction of the biochemical defect will improve the signs and symptoms or prevent their progression. McKusick's personal experience suggests that pyridoxine treatment can prevent thrombotic episodes or lens dislocation.[29] Folic acid should be given adjunctively. About 50 per cent of patients do not respond to pyridoxine therapy.

Progressive scoliosis is initially treated with a thoracolumbosacral or cervicothoracolumbar (CTLSO) orthosis such as the Milwaukee brace. Often, this fails to check progression, and spinal fusion and instrumentation is required.

References

1. Andlauer, A. C., David, M., Feit, J. P., Macabeo, V., Vibert, J., Collombel, C., Rolland, M. O., and Jeune, M.: Homocystinurie et insuffisance respiratoire chronique. A propos d'une observation. Pediatrie, 33:669, 1978.
2. Barber, G. W., and Spaeth, G. L.: The successful treatment of homocystinuria with pyridoxine. J. Pediatr., 75:463, 1969.
3. Beals, R. K.: Homocystinuria. A report of two cases and review of the literature. J. Bone Joint Surg., 51-A:1564, 1969.
4. Boers, G. H. J., Polder, T. W., Cruysberg, J. R. M., Schoonderwaldt, H. C., Peetoom, J. J., Van Ruyven, T. W. J., Smals, A. G. H., and Kloppenborg, P. W. C.: Homocystinuria versus Marfan's syndrome: The therapeutic relevance of the differential diagnosis. Neth. J. Med., 27:206, 1984.
5. Brenton, D. P.: Skeletal abnormalities in homocystinuria. Postgrad. Med. J., 53:488, 1977.
6. Brenton, D. P., Dow, C. J., James, J. I. P., Hay, R. L., and Wynne-Davies, R.: Homocystinuria and Marfan's syndrome. A comparison. J. Bone Joint Surg., 54-B:277, 1972.
7. Brill, P. W., Mitty, H. A., and Gaull, G. E.: Homocystinuria due to cystathionine synthase deficiency:

Clinical-roentgenologic correlations. A.J.R., *121*:45, 1974.
8. Carson, N. A., and Carre, I. J.: Treatment of homocystinuria with pyridoxine. Arch. Dis. Child., *44*:387, 1969.
9. Carson, N. A. J., and Neill, D. W.: Metabolic abnormalities detected in a survey of mentally backward individuals in Northern Ireland. Arch. Dis. Child., 37:505, 1962.
10. Cernea, P., and Zbranca, E.: L'homocystinurie et le syndrome de Marfan. Ann. Ocul., *205*:167, 1972.
11. Cusworth, D. C., and Dent, C. E.: Homocystinuria. Br. Med. Bull., *25*:42, 1969.
12. Cusworth, D. C., and Gattereau, A.: Inhibition of renal tubular reabsorption of homocystine by lysine and arginine. Lancet, 2:916, 1968.
13. Dehnel, J. M., and Frances, M. J. O.: Somatomedin (sulphation factor)-like activity of homocystine. Clin. Sci., *43*:903, 1972.
14. Drayer, J. I. M., Cleophas, A. J. M., Trijbels, J. M. F., Smals, A. G. H., and Kloppenborg, P. W. C.: Symptoms, diagnostic pitfalls and treatment of homocystinuria in seven adult patients. Neth. J. Med., *23*:89, 1980.
15. Dunn, H. G., Perry, T. L., and Dolman, C. L.: Homocystinuria. A recently discovered cause of mental defect and cerebrovascular thrombosis. Neurology, *16*:407, 1966.
16. Field, C. M. B., Carson, N. A. J., Cusworth, D. C., Dent, C. E., and Neill, D. W.: Homocystinuria, a new disorder of metabolism. Abstr. 10th International Congress of Pediatrics, Lisbon, 1962, p. 274.
17. Gerritsen, T., and Waisman, H. A.: Homocystinuria, an error in the metabolism of methionine. Pediatrics, 33:413, 1964.
18. Gibson, J. B., Carson, N. A., and Neill, D. W.: Pathologic findings in homocystinuria. J. Clin. Pathol., *17*:497, 1964.
19. Grieco, A. J.: Homocystinuria: Pathogenetic mechanisms. Am. J. Med. Sci., *273*:120, 1977.
20. Gaull, G., Sturman, J. A., and Schaffner, F.: Homocystinuria due to cystathionine synthase deficiency: Enzymatic and ultrastructural studies. J. Pediatr., *84*:381, 1974.
21. Hagberg, B., and Hambraeus, L.: Some aspects of the diagnosis and treatment of homocystinuria. Dev. Med. Child. Neurol., *10*:479, 1968.
22. Harker, L. A., Slichter, S. J., Scott, C. R., and Ross, R.: Homocystinuria, vascular injury and arterial thrombosis. N. Engl. J. Med., *291*:537, 1974.
23. Kang, A. H., and Trelstad, R. L.: A collagen defect in homocystinuria. J. Clin. Invest., *52*:257, 1973.
24. Kennedy, C., Shih, V. E., and Rowland, L. P.: Homocystinuria: A report in two siblings. Pediatrics, *36*:736, 1965.
25. Komrower, G. M., Lambert, A. M., Cusworth, D. C., and Westall, R. G.: Dietary treatment of homocystinuria. Arch. Dis. Child., *41*:666, 1966.
26. Kurczynski, T. W., Muir, W. A., Fleisher, L. D., Palomaki, J. F., Gaull, G. E., Rassin, D. K., and Abramowsky, C.: Maternal homocystinuria: Studies of an untreated mother and fetus. Arch. Dis. Child., *55*:721, 1980.
27. MacCarthy, J. M. T., and Carey, M. C.: Bone changes in homocystinuria. Clin. Radiol., *19*:128, 1968.
28. McKusick, V. A.: Homocystinuria. In McKusick, V. A. (ed.): Heritable Disorders of Connective Tissue. St. Louis, Mosby, 1972, pp. 224–281.
29. McKusick, V. A.: Heritable disorders of connective tissue. New clinical and biochemical aspects. In Peters, D. K. (ed.): 12th Symposium on Advanced Medicine. New York, McGraw-Hill, 1976, pp. 458–503.
30. Morreels, C. W., Fletcher, B. D., Weilbaecher, R. G., and Dorst, J. P.: The roentgenographic features of homocystinuria. Radiology, *90*:1150, 1968.
31. Mudd, S. H., and Levy, H. L.: Disorders of transsulphuration. In Stanbury, J. B., Wyngaarden, J. B., and Fredrickson, D. S. (eds.): The Metabolic Basis of Inherited Disease. New York, McGraw-Hill, 1982, pp. 522–559.
32. Sardharwalla, I. B., Fowler, B., Robins, A. J., and Komrower, G. M.: Detection of heterozygotes for homocystinuria. Arch. Dis. Child., *49*:553, 1974.
33. Schedewie, H., Willich, E., Grobe, H., Schmidt, H., and Muller, K. M.: Skeletal findings in homocystinuria: A collaborative study. Pediatr. Radiol., *1*:12, 1973.
34. Schimke, R. N., McKusick, V. A., Huang, T., and Pollack, A. D.: Homocystinuria. Studies of 20 families with 38 affected members. J.A.M.A., *193*:711, 1965.
35. Smith, R.: Biochemical Disorders of the Skeleton. London, Butterworth, 1979, pp. 210–217.
36. Smith, S. W.: Roentgen findings in homocystinuria. A.J.R., *100*:147, 1967.
37. Spaeth, G. L., and Barber, G. W.: Prevalence of homocystinuria among mentally retarded: Evaluation of a specific screening test. Pediatrics, *40*:586, 1967.
38. Thomas, P. S., and Carson, N. A. J.: Homocystinuria: The evolution of skeletal changes in relation to treatment. Ann. Radiol., *21*:95, 1978.
39. Uhlemann, E. R., Tenpas, J. H., Lucky, A. W., Schulman, J. D., Mudd, S. H., and Shulman, N. R.: Platelet survival and morphology in homocystinuria due to cystathionine synthase deficiency. N. Engl. J. Med., *295*:1283, 1976.
40. Wilcken, B., and Turner, B.: Homocystinuria: Reduced folate levels during pyridoxine treatment. Arch. Dis. Child., *48*:58, 1973.
41. Wong, P. W. K., Justice, P., Hruby, M., Weiss, E. B., and Diamond, E.: Folic acid nonresponsive homocystinuria due to methylenetetrahydrofolate reductase deficiency. Pediatrics, *59*:749, 1977.
42. Zavala, C., Cobo, A., Lisker, R., and Chavez, Y.: Frequency of homocystinuria amongst the blind. Clin. Genet., *4*:98, 1973.

DOWN'S SYNDROME (TRISOMY 21 OR MONGOLISM)

Down's syndrome is characterized by mental retardation, slanted eyes with prominent epicanthal folds (mongoloid appearance), general hypotonia, hands that are short and stubby with a single palmar crease, incurving of the little finger, a wide space between the hallux and second toe in the feet, and a distinctively abnormal pelvis with lateral flaring of the iliac wings, resembling an elephant's ear.[4, 6, 7, 13] It is frequently associated with congenital heart disease (particularly septal defect) and anomalies of the gastrointestinal tract (typically duodenal atresia and Hirschsprung's disease). Orthopedic problems are common and causally related to the ligamentous hyperlaxity. The most important deformities requiring care are atlantoaxial instability, dislocation of the patella, spontaneous habitual dislocation of the hip, genu valgum, and severe flexible pes planovalgus.

Table 3–13. Increasing Chances of Nondisjunction for Down's Syndrome with Increasing Maternal Age*

Maternal Age	Chance of Nondisjunction
20 years	1 in 1000
40 years	1 in 100
45 years	1 in 40

*From Uchida, I. A.: Epidemiology of mongolism: The Manitoba Study. Ann. N.Y. Acad. Sci. *171*:361, 1970. Reprinted by permission.

With effective and successful surgical correction of the congenital heart anomalies, the survival of children with Down's syndrome has increased; the orthopedic surgeon therefore faces formidable problems in the management of the musculoskeletal deformities.

Down's syndrome occurs in approximately one in every 700 births. It is more common in girls with a 3:1 female to male ratio. Most often, Down's syndrome is caused by trisomy 21 in the G group, the result of nondisjunction. There is uneven allocation of chromosomes during normal reduction and division. Consequently, the ovum may end up with an extra G chromosome—the zygote having 47 instead of 46 chromosomes. The probability of nondisjunction increases with increasing maternal age (Table 3–13). A less common form of Down's syndrome is due to translocation of the extra 21 chromosome to another location, such as D. Such a person has 46 chromosomes in his karyotype, but one of the chromosomes is larger.

It is important to differentiate between the causes of Down's syndrome, because of the implications in genetic counseling.

If a mother has a translocated chromosome with a modal number of 45 chromosomes, her chances of having a child with Down's syndrome are one in three. If a mother has a child with Down's syndrome because of nondisjunction, however, her chances of having another child with Down's syndrome are 1 in 50.

Radiographic Features

The appearance of the pelvis is characteristic. The acetabular angle (the acute angle of intersection between an oblique straight line drawn between upper lateral and lower medial ends of the acetabulum and Hilgenreiner's horizontal line drawn between the triradiate cartilages) is markedly decreased owing to flattening of the lower edge of the ilium (Fig. 3–102 A). The iliac wings are wide and flared, causing a decrease of the *iliac angle* (formed by the intersection of the horizontal line with an oblique straight line drawn through the most lateral point of the iliac wing above and the iliac body below (Fig. 3–102 B). The ischial rami bilaterally are small in caliber, tapering distally, and there is bilateral coxa valga (Fig. 3–103).[6, 7]

The hand shows brachymesophalangism, dysplastic phalanges, and incurving of the little finger (Fig. 3–104).

In the lateral projection, the lumbar spine shows the vertebral bodies increased in height and decreased in anteroposterior diameter. The anterior border of the vertebral body has an increased posterior concavity.[37] These radiographic changes are suggestive but not pathognomonic of Down's syndrome. The thoracic cage usually has 11 pairs of ribs, and the sternal manubrium has doubled ossification centers.[3, 10]

Treatment

Atlantoaxial Instability. Ten to twenty per cent of patients with Down's syndrome have atlantoaxial instability.[17, 24, 30, 46, 48, 49, 51] It is partly due to laxity of the transverse ligament as a part of generalized ligamentous hyperlaxity, but abnormal development of the odontoid process

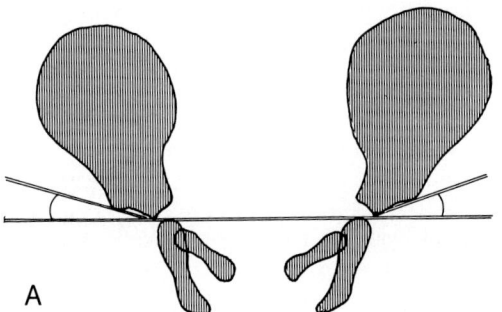
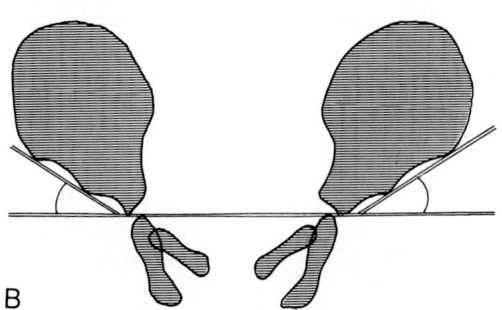

FIGURE 3–102. *Diagram illustrating the typical changes in the pelvis in Down's syndrome.*

A and **B.** Note the marked decrease in acetabular angle, wide and flared iliac wings, ischial rami that are tapered and small in caliber, and coxa valga.

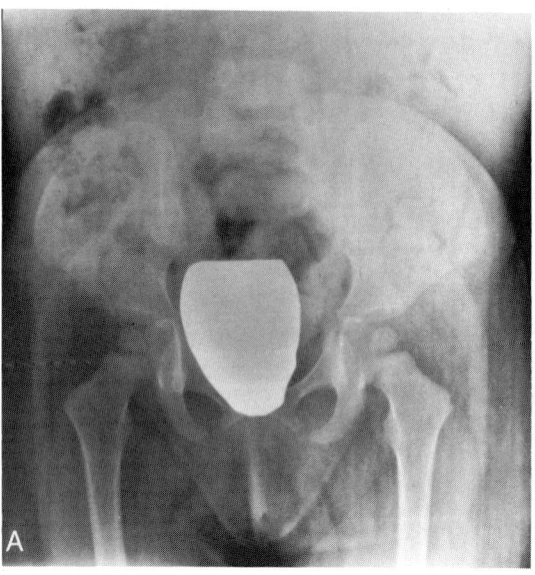 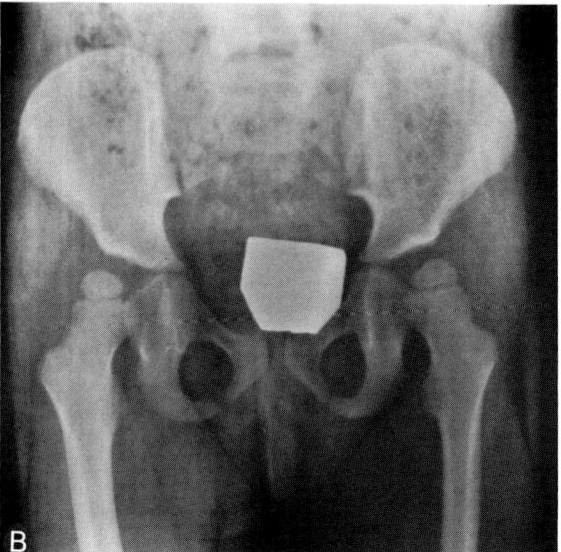

FIGURE 3–103. Anteroposterior radiograms of the pelvis and hips in Down's syndrome showing characteristic changes.

Note (1) the marked decrease of the acetabular angle, (2) the wide and flared iliac wings (decreased iliac angle), (3) narrow tapered ischii, and (4) severe coxa valga

(such as dysplasia or hypoplasia) may also be a predisposing factor. The presenting complaint may be neck pain, torticollis, motor weakness, gait abnormality, change in bowel or bladder function, spasticity, or quadriparesis. There is usually delay between onset of symptoms and diagnosis because children with Down's syndrome are retarded and do not vocalize their complaints. The foregoing symptoms should alert the physician to assess stability of the atlantoaxial joint by lateral views of the cervical spine in neutral position, flexion, and extension (Fig. 3–105). If the joint is unstable, neurosurgical consultation should be obtained, and after appropriate computed tomographic, myelographic, and nuclear magnetic resonance imaging studies, the upper cervical spine should be fused.

The Committee on Sports Medicine of the American Academy of Pediatrics has issued the following guidelines for patients with Down's syndrome who desire to participate in sports that could result in head and neck injury, such as gymnastics, diving, soccer, and high jumping.[1] (The same guidelines apply to persons with rheumatoid arthritis, some forms of bone dysplasia, and anomalies of the odontoid process in which atlantoaxial instability can also occur.)

The recommended guidelines are: (1) All children with Down's syndrome who wish to participate in sports that could involve head or neck trauma should have lateral view x-ray films taken of the cervical region in neutral, flexion, and extension positions before beginning training or competition. (2) A patient should not participate in sports that could result in neck or head trauma if the distance between the odontoid process of the axis and the anterior arch of the atlas is more than 4.5 mm. or if the odontoid process is abnormal. (3) It is not necessary to repeat x-ray films on patients who have had normal findings. Some physicians may want to screen children with Down's syndrome routinely at five and six years of age for atlantoaxial instability. (4) Children with atlantoaxial subluxation or dislocation and neurologic signs or symptoms should not participate in any strenuous activity. (5) Children with Down's syndrome who have no evidence of atlantoaxial instability can participate in all sports.

Spontaneous Habitual Dislocation of the Hip.[5, 21, 33, 38, 45] This occurs in 4.5 per cent of children with Down's syndrome. These children are usually delayed in walking; their hips are hypermobile but not dislocatable until at two to four years of age the affected hip spontaneously becomes dislocated and relocated. Presenting complaints are a click in the hip, an increasing limp or "giving way," and refusal to walk. With recurrent dislocation physical activity diminishes. The dislocations are not painful (Fig. 3–106). If untreated, eventually subluxation or dislocation may become fixed.

In treatment of habitual dislocation of the hip, nonoperative measures are usually not successful because of the underlying pathologic ligamentous laxity. A hip abduction orthosis, such as the Scottish-Rite brace, may be tried, but its deleterious effects on the knee joints, which are in valgus posture and susceptible to

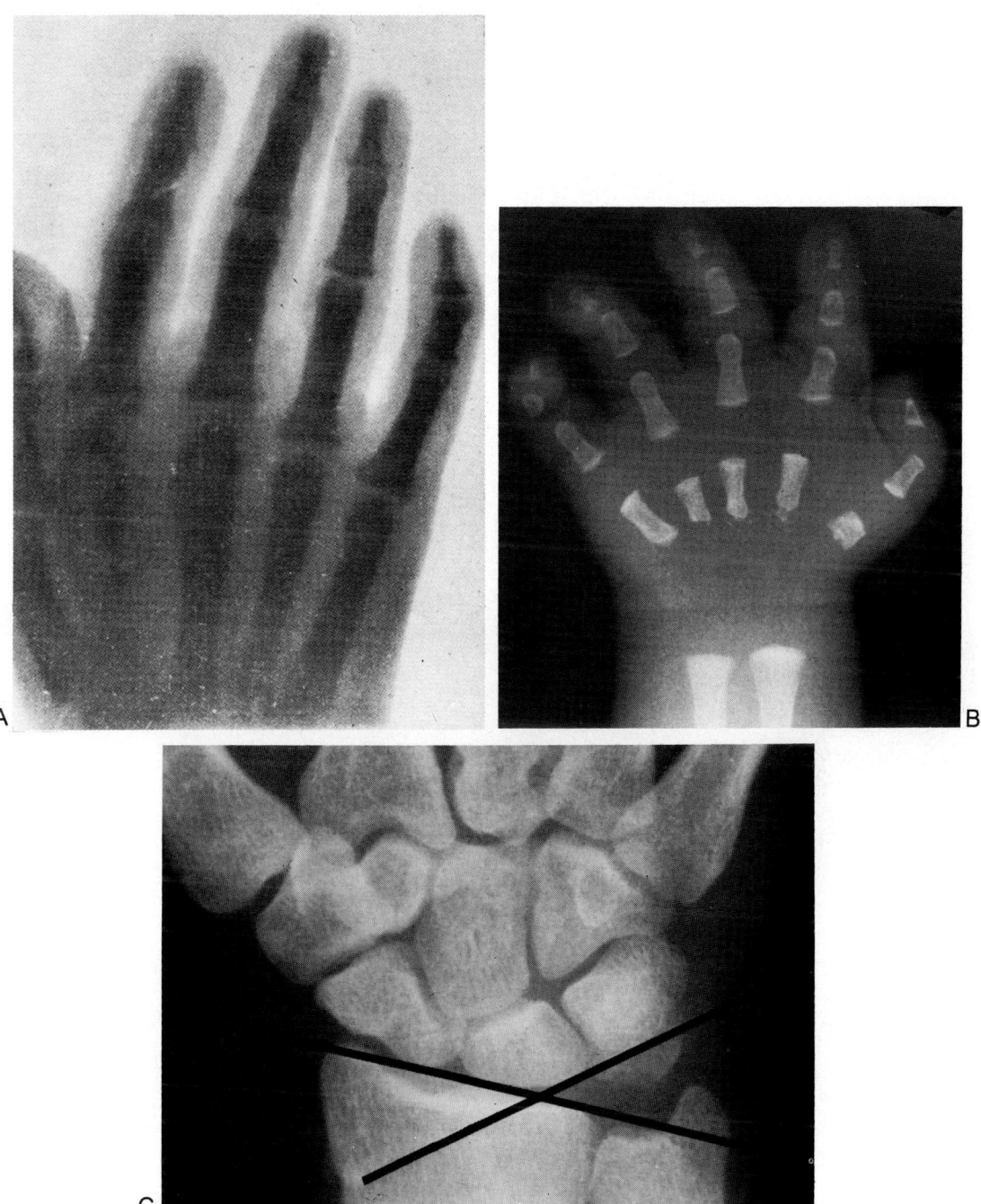

FIGURE 3–104. *Radiograms of the hand in Down's syndrome.*

A. Clinodactyly of the little finger. This was published in 1896, one year after the discovery of roentgen rays. **B.** Anteroposterior radiogram of the hand of an infant showing punctate epiphyses in Down's syndrome. Note the punctate calcification at the base of the markedly shortened metacarpals. (Punctate epiphyses are seen in other conditions besides Down's syndrome.) **C.** Radiogram of the wrist of an adult with Down's syndrome showing the increase in the carpal angle (143 degrees) and the hypoplastic carpal, navicular, and lunate bones. (From Poznanski, A. K.: The Hand in Radiologic Diagnosis. Philadelphia, W. B. Saunders, 1984. Reprinted by permission.)

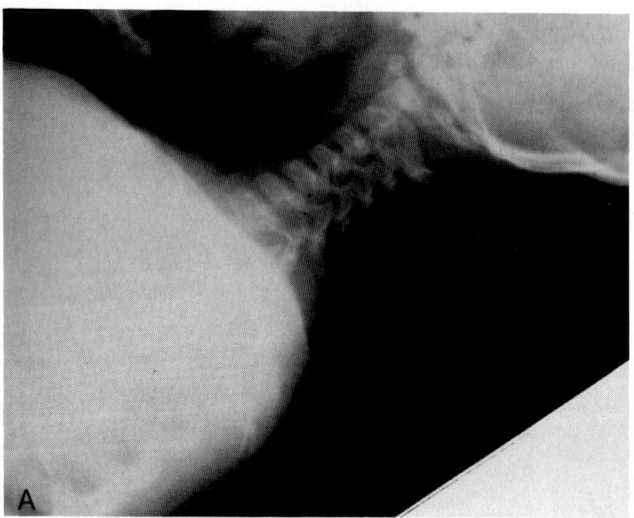 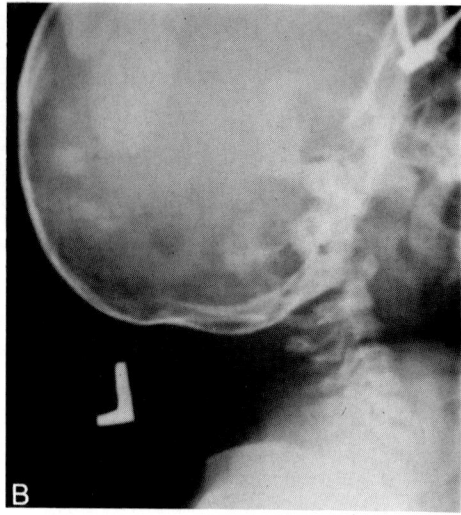

FIGURE 3–105. Atlantoaxial instability in Down's syndrome.

Lateral flexion and extension views of the cervical spine show that the distance between the odontoid process of the axis and the anterior arch of the atlas is greater than 4.5 mm.

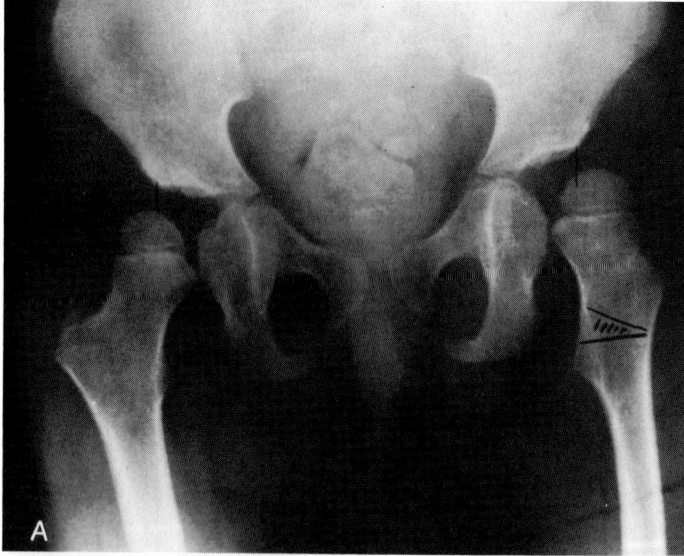

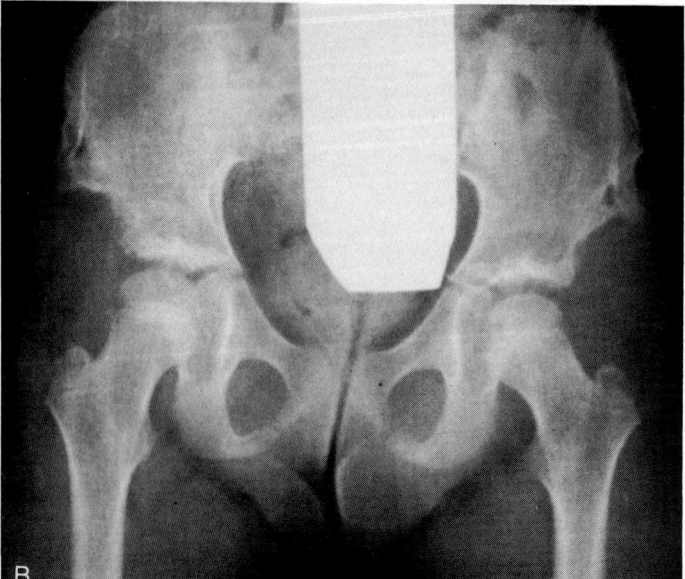

FIGURE 3–106. Spontaneous habitual dislocation of the hip in Down's syndrome in a four-year-old girl.

A. Preoperative radiogram showing dislocation of the left hip and subluxation of the right hip. **B.** Postoperative radiogram following open reduction and bilateral Pemberton's innominate osteotomy. The hips are very stable.

patellofemoral joint subluxation, should be considered. This author has had no success with orthotic or cast containment. The recurring dislocated hip is usually treated surgically. CT scans are performed to determine the degree of acetabular and femoral torsion, in order to delineate the pathologic changes. Open reduction, capsular plication, and innominate or femoral osteotomy are usually required to maintain reduction. Postoperative splinting is crucial; the recurrence rate is high because of the persisting ligamentous hyperlaxity.

Patellofemoral Joint Dislocation. This occurs in about 5 per cent of cases. The knee gives way, causing frequent falls. Quadriceps strengthening exercises are used, but often surgery is required. The Galleazzi-Dewar operation is the procedure of choice.

Severe Flexible Pes Planovalgus. This is treated with the University of California Biomechanics Laboratory (U.C.B.L.) foot orthosis.

References

1. American Academy of Pediatrics Committee on Sports Medicine: Guidelines for Down's syndrome patients active in sports. News and Comments, 35:8, 1984.
2. Armendares, S., Urrusti-Sanz, J., and Diaz-del-Castillo, E.: Iliac index in newborns. Comparative values at term, in prematurity and in Down's syndrome. Am. J. Dis. Child., 113:229, 1967.
3. Beber, B. A., Litt, R. E., and Altman, D. H.: A new radiographic finding in mongolism. Radiology, 86:332, 1966.
4. Benda, C. E.: Down's Syndrome. New York, Grune & Stratton, 1969.
5. Bennet, G. C., Rang, M., Roye, D. P., and Aprin, H.: Dislocation of the hip in trisomy 21. J. Bone Joint Surg., 64-B:289, 1982.
6. Caffey, J., and Ross, S.: Mongolism (mongoloid deficiency) during early infancy—some newly recognized diagnostic changes in the pelvic bones. Pediatrics, 17:642, 1956.
7. Caffey, J., and Ross, S.: Pelvic bones in infantile mongoloidism. Roentgenographic features. A.J.R., 80:458, 1958.
8. Chumlea, W. C., Malina, M., and Rarick, G. L.: Brachymesophalangia of the fifth finger, stature and weight in children with Down syndrome. J. Ment. Defic. Res., 25:7, 1981.
9. Chumlea, W. C., Malina, R. M., Rarick, G. L., and Seefeldt, V. D.: Communalities for rates of diaphyseal elongation of short bones of the hand of children with Down syndrome. Am. J. Physic. Anthropol., 53:129, 1980.
10. Currarino, G., and Swanson, G. E.: A developmental variant of ossification of the manubrium sterni in mongolism. Radiology, 82:916, 1964.
11. Curtis, B. H., Blank, S., and Fisher, R. L.: Atlantoaxial dislocation in Down's syndrome: Report of two patients requiring surgical correction. J.A.M.A., 205:212, 1968.
12. Dingan, S. J.: Polydactyly in Down's syndrome. Am. J. Ment. Defic., 77:486, 1973.
13. Down, J. L. H.: Observations on an ethnic classification of idiots. London Hosp. Clin. Lect. Rep., 3:259, 1866.
14. Engler, M.: Mongolism. Bristol, John Wright & Sons, 1949.
15. Evison, G., and Oliver, M.: Acetabulum excavatum in adult Down's syndrome. Br. J. Radiol., 54:340, 1981.
16. Fabia, J., and Drolette, M.: Malformations and leukemia in children with Down's syndrome. Pediatrics, 45:60, 1970.
17. Finerman, G. A. M., Sakai, D., and Weingarten, S.: Atlantoaxial dislocation with spinal cord compression in a Mongoloid child. J. Bone Joint Surg., 58-A:408, 1956.
18. Garn, S. M., Gall, J. C., Jr., and Nagy, J. M.: Preliminary radiogrammetric analysis of the bone recovery phase in adolescents with Down's syndrome. Invest. Radiol., 7:97, 1972.
19. Gerald, B. E., and Silverman, F. N.: Normal and abnormal interorbital distances, with special reference to mongolism. A.J.R., 95:154, 1965.
20. Gerard, Y., Segal, P., and Bedoucha, J.-S.: Instabilité de l'atlas sur l'axis dans le mongolisme. Presse Méd., 79:573, 1971.
21. Gore, D. R.: Recurrent dislocation of the hip in a child with Down's syndrome. J. Bone Joint Surg., 63-A:823, 1981.
22. Hall, B.: Mongolism in newborns. A clinical and cytogenic study. Acta Paediatr. [Suppl.], 154:41, 1964.
23. Hefke, H. W.: Roentgenologic study of anomalies of the hands in one hundred cases of mongolism. Am. J. Dis. Child., 60:1319, 1940.
24. Hreidarsson, S., Magram, G., and Singer, H.: Symptomatic atlantoaxial dislocation in Down syndrome. Pediatrics, 69:568, 1982.
25. Hungerford, G. D., Akkaraju, V., Rawe, S. E., and Young, G. F.: Atlanto-occipital and atlanto-axial dislocations with spinal cord compression in Down's syndrome: A case report and review of the literature. Br. J. Radiol., 54:758, 1981.
26. Kaufman, H. J., and Taillard, W. F.: Pelvic abnormalities in mongols. Br. Med. J., 1:948, 1961.
27. Kleinman, P. K.: Case report 224. Radiological studies. Skeletal Radiol., 10:192, 1983.
28. Levinson, A., Friedman, A., and Stamps, F.: Variability of mongolism. Pediatrics, 16:43, 1955.
29. Martel, W., and Tishler, J. M.: Observations on the spine in mongoloidism. A.J.R., 97:630, 1966.
30. Martel, W., Uyham, R., and Stimson, C. W.: Subluxation of the atlas causing spinal cord compression in a case of Down's syndrome with a "manifestation of an occipital vertebra." Radiology, 93:839, 1969.
31. Mortensson, W., and Hall, B.: Abnormal pelvis in newborn infants with Down's syndrome. Acta Radiol., 12:847, 1972.
32. Nicolis, F. B., and Sacchetti, G.: A nomogram for the x-ray evaluation of some morphological anomalies of the pelvis in the diagnosis of mongolism. Pediatrics, 32:1074, 1963.
33. Packer, J. W., Lefkowitz, L. A., and Ryder, C. T.: Habitual dislocation of the hip treated by innominate osteotomy: A report of three cases. Clin. Orthop., 83:184, 1972.
34. Peterson, C. D., and Luzzatti, L.: The role of chromosome translocations in the recurrence risk of Down's syndrome. Pediatrics, 85:463, 1965.
35. Poznanski, A. K., Garn, S. M., Nagy, J. M., and Gall, J. C., Jr.: Metacarpophalangeal pattern profiles in the evaluation of skeletal malformations. Radiology, 104:1, 1972.
36. Pozsonyi, J., Gibson, D., and Zarfas, D. E.: Skeletal maturation in mongolism (Down's syndrome). J. Pediatr., 64:75, 1964.
37. Rabinowitz, J. G., and Moseley, J. E.: The lateral lumbar spine in Down's syndrome: A new roentgen feature. Radiology, 83:74, 1964.
38. Rang, M.: Dislocation of the hip in Down's syndrome. J. Bone Joint Surg., 54-B:770, 1972.
39. Rarick, G. L., Rapaport, I. F., and Seefeldt, V.: Bone

development in Down's disease. Am. J. Dis. Child., *107*:45, 1964.
40. Rarick, G. L., Rapaport, I. F., and Seefeldt, V.: Long bone growth in Down's syndrome. Am. J. Dis. Child., *112*:566, 1966.
41. Roche, A. F.: Skeletal maturation rates in mongolism. A.J.R., *91*:979, 1964.
42. Roche, A. F.: The stature of Mongols. J. Ment. Defic. Res., 9:131, 1965.
43. Rochels, R., and Schmid, F.: Morphologische und metrische Abweichungen der Handknochen beim Down-syndrom—eine radiologische studie. Fortschr. Geb. Rontgenstr., *133*:30, 1980.
44. Rowe, R. D., and Uchida, I. A.: Cardiac malformation in mongolism. A prospective study of 184 mongoloid children. Am. J. Med., *31*:726, 1961.
45. Rundle, A. T., Donoghue, E., Abbas, K. A., and Krstic, A.: A catch-up phenomenon in skeletal development of children with Down's syndrome. J. Ment. Defic. Res., *16*:41, 1972.
46. Semine, A. A., Ertel, A. N., Goldberg, M. J., and Bull, M. J.: Cervical-spine instability in children with Down syndrome (trisomy 21). J. Bone Joint Surg., *60-A*:649, 1978.
47. Shapiro, B. L., Gorlin, R. J., Redman, R. S., and Bruhl, H. H.: The palate and Down's syndrome. N. Engl. J. Med., *276*:1460, 1967.
48. Sherk, H. H., and Nicholson, J. T.: Rotatory atlantoaxial dislocation associated with ossiculum terminale and mongolism. A case report. J. Bone Joint Surg., *51-A*:957, 1969.
49. Shield, L. K., Dicksens, D. R., and Jensen, F.: Atlantoaxial dislocation with spinal cord compression in Down syndrome. Aust. Paediatr. J., *17*:114, 1981.
50. Smith, T. T.: A peculiarity in the shape of the hand in idiots of the "mongol" type. Pediatrics, 2:315, 1896.
51. Tishler, J., and Martel, W.: Dislocation of the atlas in mongolism. Preliminary report. Radiology, *84*:904, 1965.
52. Uchida, I. A.: Epidemiology of mongolism: The Manitoba study. Ann. N.Y. Acad. Sci., *171*:361, 1970.
53. Whaley, W. J., and Gray, W. D.: Atlantoaxial dislocation and Down's syndrome. Can. Med. Assoc. J., *123*:35, 1980.
54. Zangeneh, F., and Steiner, M. M.: Oxandrolone therapy in growth retardation of children. Am. J. Dis. Child., *113*:234, 1967.

OTHER CHROMOSOMAL ABERRATIONS

Trisomy 18. There are multiple congenital malformations in trisomy 18. The orthopedic surgeon is consulted because of the severe talipes equinovarus and congenital convex pes valgus. The posturing of the fingers is characteristic—the index finger is elongated and overlaps the middle and ring fingers, and the little finger incurves with contracture of the proximal interphalangeal joint (Fig. 3–107). The pelvis is narrow, the lower jaw is recessed, and the chest is small. The neck is short and the maxilla hypoplastic. The ears resemble those of a faun, and the skull is elongated. Congenital abnormalities of the spine are commonly present. The prognosis is very poor in these patients; death usually occurs before one year of age.[1, 2]

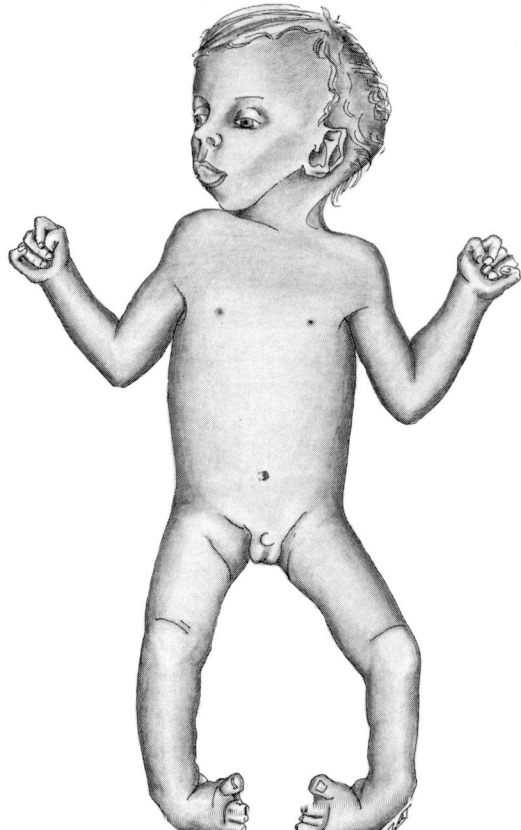

FIGURE 3–107. *Clinical features of trisomy 18.*

Trisomy 13–15. The hand and foot deformities in trisomy 13–15 will be the presenting complaint to the orthopedic surgeon. These include polydactyly, syndactyly, flexion contracture of the interphalangeal joints, or pes varus or valgus. The craniofacial deformities (microcephaly with cleft lip and palate) with small eyes are the most striking features. The outlook for life is very gloomy because of the associated heart and kidney anomalies. These infants die before one year of age. Their limb deformities should not be treated.[3, 7]

Trisomy 8. Talipes equinovarus with flexion deformity of the hallux and generalized contractural deformities of other joints are the concern of the orthopedic surgeon treating trisomy 8 patients. These infants have diffuse abnormalities of the skeletal system including 13 ribs, congenital deformities of the vertebrae (wedged with neural arch defects), coxa valga, camptodactyly, and clinodactyly. The head is large with a short neck and long trunk.[5]

Cri-du-Chat Syndrome. Chromosome 5 short arm deficiency is the cause of the syndrome. The skeletal deformities consist of dislocation of the radial head, clinodactyly, short metacarpals, and malformations of the spine. These children are severely retarded mentally and fail to thrive. Their kitten-like cry makes diagnosis very simple. Orthopedic measures should not be taken because of the poor prognosis.[6]

Sex Chromosome Anomalies

Turner's Syndrome. One X chromosome is missing in Turner's syndrome, and the ovaries are absent, with resultant infantilism and amenorrhea. The condition is manifest at birth by webbing of the neck and peripheral lymphedema. Cubitus valgus, short fourth metacarpals, and the short neck with a low hairline are the presenting complaints to the orthopedic surgeon. There may be multiple other defects—of the heart, kidney, or spine. The prognosis depends on the nature of the cardiac and renal anomalies. Most of these children survive. Orthopedic treatment is individualized according to the nature of the deformity.

Klinefelter's Syndrome. XXY syndrome occurs in the male, who presents at puberty with small testicles and lack of spermatogenesis. The patients are very tall with a long lower body segment. Radioulnar synostosis may occur in these children.[4]

References

1. Edwards, J. W., Harnden, D. G., Cameron, A. H., Crosse, U. M., and Wolff, O. H.: A new trisomic syndrome. Lancet, 1:787, 1960.
2. James, A. E., Jr., Belcourt, C. L., Atkins, L., and Janower, M. L.: Trisomy 18. Radiology, 92:36, 1969.
3. James, A. E., Jr., Belcourt, C. L., Atkins, L., and Janower, M. L.: Trisomy 13–15. Radiology, 92:44, 1969.
4. Klinefelter, H. F., Jr., Reifstein, E. C., and Albright, F.: Syndrome characterized by gynecomastia, aspermatogenesis, without a-Leydigism, and increased excretion of follicle-stimulating hormone. J. Clin. Endocrinol., 2:615, 1942.
5. LeJeune, J., and Rethore, M. O.: Trisomies of chromosome no. 8. Nobel 23, Chromosome Identification, 1973, pp. 214–216.
6. LeJeune, J., LaFourcade, J., DeGrouchy, J., Berger, R., Gautien, F., Salmon, C., and Turpin, R.: Deletion partielle du bras court du chromosome 5. Individualisation d'un novel état morbide. Sem. Hôp. Paris, 40:1069, 1964.
7. Patau, K., Smith, D. W., Thorman, E., Inhorn, S. L., and Wagner, H. P.: Multiple congenital anomalies caused by an extra autosome. Lancet, 1:790, 1960.
8. Turner, H. H.: A syndrome of infantilism, congenital webbed neck, and cubitus valgus. Endocrinology, 23:566, 1935.

Metabolic and Endocrine Bone Diseases

RICKETS

General Pathophysiology

Rickets is a disease process of the growing skeleton, caused by a disturbance in calcium and phosphorus metabolism and characterized by inadequate mineralization of bone matrix. Because, in children, the epiphyseal ends of the bones are the sites of the most active osteogenesis, the disease is more apparent in these areas. The term *osteomalacia* refers to the same disease process in the adult, in whom the entire skeleton is affected, and in whom pathologic changes require a much longer period to manifest themselves. The forms of osteomalacia that occur in adults are not discussed here.

Pathogenesis.* During the past two decades there have been great advances in our understanding of vitamin D metabolism. When vitamin D is given it increases intestinal absorption of calcium; there is, however, a lag of several hours before its action takes place. This is because the vitamin requires conversion to various biologically active metabolites before it can exert its specific effects on tissues. The sources of vitamin D are diet and the skin (provitamin 7-dehydrocholesterol). Dietary sources of vitamin D are fish, eggs, and fortified foods (such as milk and other dairy products). Its two important physiologic forms are vitamin D_2 (calciferol) and vitamin D_3 (cholecalciferol). Ultraviolet light converts 7-dehydrocholesterol into vitamin D_3. Both forms are fat soluble, and their absorption may be impaired in steatorrhea with resultant vitamin D malabsorption. The hydroxylated derivative of vitamin D_3, 25-hydroxycholecalciferol (25-HCC), is manufactured by the parenchymal cells of the liver. In the plasma, the active circulating forms of vitamin D are vitamin D_3 itself and 25-hydroxycholecalciferol. The kidney converts the 25-hydroxycholecalciferol into 1,25-dihydroxycholecalciferol (1,25-DHCC). In glomerular and tubular renal disease this conversion may not take place. This is the pathophysiologic basis of renal rickets—which is subdivided into renal glomerular and renal tubular rickets. The action of 1,25-dihydroxycholecalciferol on the small in-

---

*See references 2, 3, 7, 15, 17–19, 24, 25, 33, 45, 46, 50, 62.

testine is to enhance calcium absorption. In the state of vitamin D deficiency, intestinal absorption of calcium is very poor, with resultant hypocalcemia. The low serum calcium level stimulates parathyroid function (PTH), which partially raises the serum calcium level and markedly decreases the phosphate resorption in the kidney. The resultant low serum phosphorus and low to low-normal serum calcium concentrations cause poor mineralization of bone matrix and failure of calcification of cartilage and osteoid tissues.

Poor absorption of calcium from the gastrointestinal tract may be caused by deficiency states of vitamin D, primarily nutritional, occasionally by the presence of chelates in the diet, or by liver or gastrointestinal disease.[16, 67] In liver damage, there is decreased production of 25-hydroxycholecalciferol, and the excess fat in the stools (as in steatorrhea) interferes with absorption of fat-soluble vitamin D.

The second pathophysiologic cause of rickets is a decrease in the phosphate available for bone mineralization. This group of disorders is classically referred to as vitamin D–resistant or –refractory rickets, which can be further subdivided into four pathophysiologic types. The *first* is due to failure of reabsorption of phosphate filtered by the glomerulus. The result is marked hypophosphatemia and hyperphosphaturia. *Second* is failure of synthesis of adequate amounts of the biologically active 1,25-dihydroxycholecalciferol (1,25-DHCC). *Third* is the biologic insensitivity of the cells in the small intestine. There is ample 1,25-dihydroxycholecalciferol, but the intestinal cells do not synthesize the transport system, and intestinal absorption of calcium is impaired. The *fourth* is referred to as renal tubular acidosis, which is characterized biochemically by hypochloremic, hyponatremic, hypokalemic acidosis and an alkaline urine. The impairment of the handling of fixed base and bicarbonate in the kidney may be genetic or acquired.

In *renal osteodystrophy*, due to chronic renal insufficiency, there is hyperphosphatemia that induces hypocalcemia.

Simple Vitamin D Deficiency Rickets

This type rarely occurs before the sixth month or after the third year of life. It results from insufficient intake of vitamin D and inadequate exposure to sunlight. Since it was demonstrated by Mellanby and Park that it is possible to prevent rickets, its incidence has greatly diminished.[42, 43, 50] Milk and dairy products are rich in calcium and phosphorus, and are often supplemented with synthetic preparations of vitamin D. It is only in starvation areas and in groups with dietary eccentricities that simple vitamin D deficiency rickets presents a clinical problem.

Premature infants are more prone to rickets, as they are born without a normal store of calcium in the skeleton, which is normally mineralized in the last three months of intrauterine life.*

Pathology.[22, 23, 51, 54] In rickets, the primary disturbance in bone is a failure of calcification of cartilage and osteoid tissue. In vitro studies have demonstrated that rachitic cartilage can be calcified if immersed in a solution containing adequate concentrations of calcium and phosphate.

Normally, the cartilage cells at the provisional zone of calcification proliferate in columns, the oldest parts of which are calcified, invaded, reabsorbed, and replaced by new bone. In rickets, however, there are failure of deposition of calcium along the mature cartilage cell columns, disorderly invasion of cartilage by blood vessels, lack of reabsorption at the zone of provisional calcification, and increased thickness of the epiphyseal plate (Fig. 3 108). Cellular growth is not disturbed. The chondrocytes multiply normally, but the normal process of maturation of cartilage columns fails to take place, with lack of calcification of their matrix and their eventual resorption. The thickening of the physis is not caused by hypertrophy of cartilage cells.

Osteoblastic activity in both the endosteal and periosteal tissues is normal, forming abundant osteoid tissue. Phosphatase production is normal. With defective mineralization, however, osteoclastic resorption of the uncalcified osteoid does not take place. Hence, the overabundance of osteoid produced by the normal osteoblasts is laid down irregularly around anything that will serve as a scaffolding in the metaphysis. Some osteoid islets may even be encountered in the diaphysis, where normally only calcified osseous tissue is present. The sparsity of osteoclasts is striking; they are only found adjacent to calcified bone. There is no normal lattice formation.

In rickets, there is an abnormality in the arrangement of bundles of collagen fibers in

---

*See references 8–10, 12–14, 28, 29, 34, 35, 37, 39, 41, 48, 56.

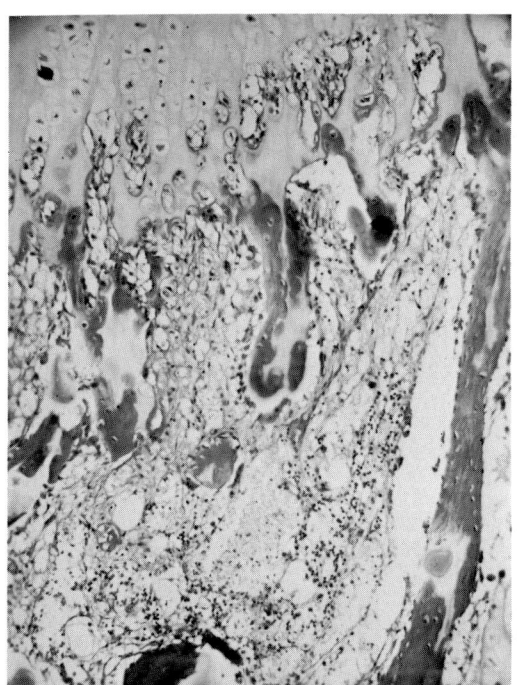

FIGURE 3–108. Histologic appearance of rickets.

Photomicrograph through the epiphyseal-metaphyseal junction. Note the uncalcified osteoid tissue, failure of deposition of calcium along the mature cartilage cell columns, and disorderly invasion of cartilage by blood vessels (×25).

compact bone; they run perpendicularly, rather than parallel to the haversian canal.[22]

Grossly, rachitic bone is soft in its active phase and becomes distorted in shape under the loading of body weight and other stresses. If the disease remains untreated and continues to persist, angular deformities of the long bones (particularly the tibia and femur), scoliosis, and deformities of the thoracic cage and pelvis develop.

The histopathology of healing of rickets has been studied in enchondral bone by Dodds and Cameron, and in membranous bone by Bailie and Irving.[5, 21] On administration of vitamin D, calcium absorption increases, and calcification of the cartilage columns in the provisional zone of calcification and in osteoid tissue takes place. Osteoclastic resorption of calcified cartilage and osteoid with remodeling of bone follows, and a normal pattern of ossification is established.

Clinical Features. Clinical findings depend on the severity and duration of the disease. Generalized muscular weakness and lethargy are early signs. The infant with rickets has a protuberant abdomen and is delayed in sitting, standing, and walking.

Early bony manifestations of active rickets are craniotabes, "rachitic rosary," and slight thickening of the ankles, knees, and wrists. The craniotabes is due to softening and thinning of the skull, and is easily detectable over the occipital and posterior parietal bones, which, on firm palpation, have a parchment-like consistency. Beading of the ribs is due to enlargement at the costochondral junctions.

With continuation of the activity of rickets, there is progressive enlargement of the bony prominences of the wrists, ankles, and knees (Fig. 3–109). The pull of the diaphragm on the rib cage produces a horizontal depression that is called "Harrison's groove." "Pigeon-breast deformity" is caused by forward projection of the sternum. Closure of the anterior fontanelle is delayed. The softened skull is usually larger than normal; it may flatten and become asymmetrical. Prominences or bosses develop as a result of thickening of parietal and frontal bones. Dentition is also affected, with defects in the enamel and a delay in normal eruption of teeth.

The softened long bones of the lower limbs tend to bend under the stress of body weight, giving rise to genu valgum. In severe rickets, coxa vara may occur, and the child will walk with a waddling gait. Greenstick fractures of the femoral or tibial shafts may be present. Later on, kyphoscoliosis may develop. The deformities of the lower limbs and spine will cause a reduction in total height.

Radiographic Findings.[55, 65, 68] The failure of calcification of osteoid tissue and cartilage is depicted in the radiograms. The physis is thickened, with haziness of the provisional zone of calcification (Fig. 3–109 F). The epiphyseal borders of the metaphyses are frayed and have a brushlike pattern due to islands or columns of uncalcified cartilage. The epiphyses are widened. The density of the cortices of the diaphysis is diminished. The bone trabeculae are coarse, widely separated, and not aligned along the lines of stress.

As the rachitic process progresses, deformities of the long bones, ribs, pelvis, and spine are evident.

With healing of the rickets, calcification in the provisional zone of calcification and osteoid tissue takes place. The epiphyseal plate thins, and the bone density is increased.[59–61]

Treatment. Rickets can be prevented by intake of 400 I.U. of vitamin D per day. Whole milk and evaporated milk are fortified as a public health measure by the addition of vitamin D concentrate, so that one quart of fresh

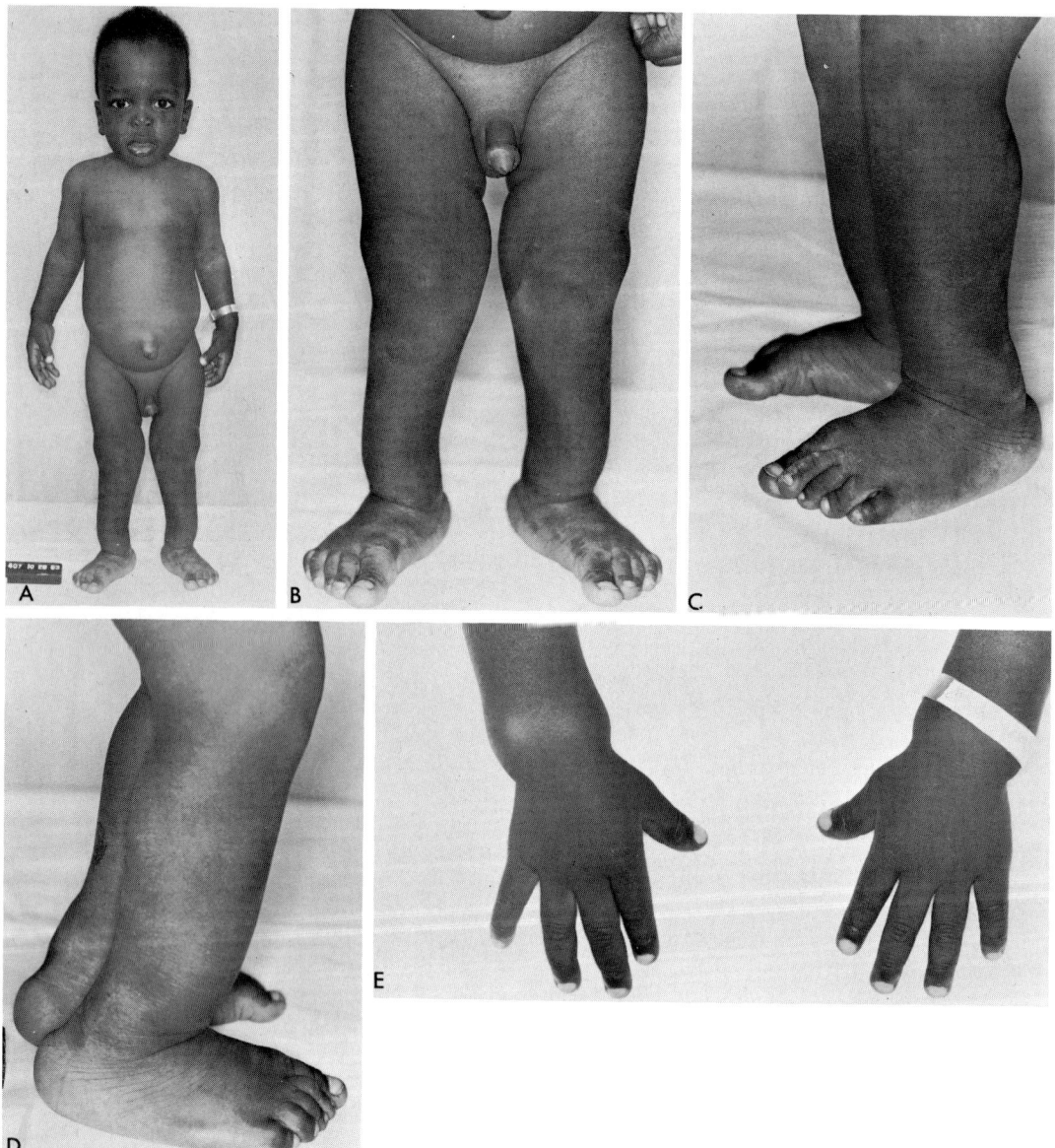

FIGURE 3–109. Simple vitamin D deficiency rickets.

A to **E.** Clinical appearance of patient. The bony prominences of the wrists, knees, and ankles are enlarged. The legs are bowed anterolaterally. Note the protuberant abdomen with the umbilical hernia.

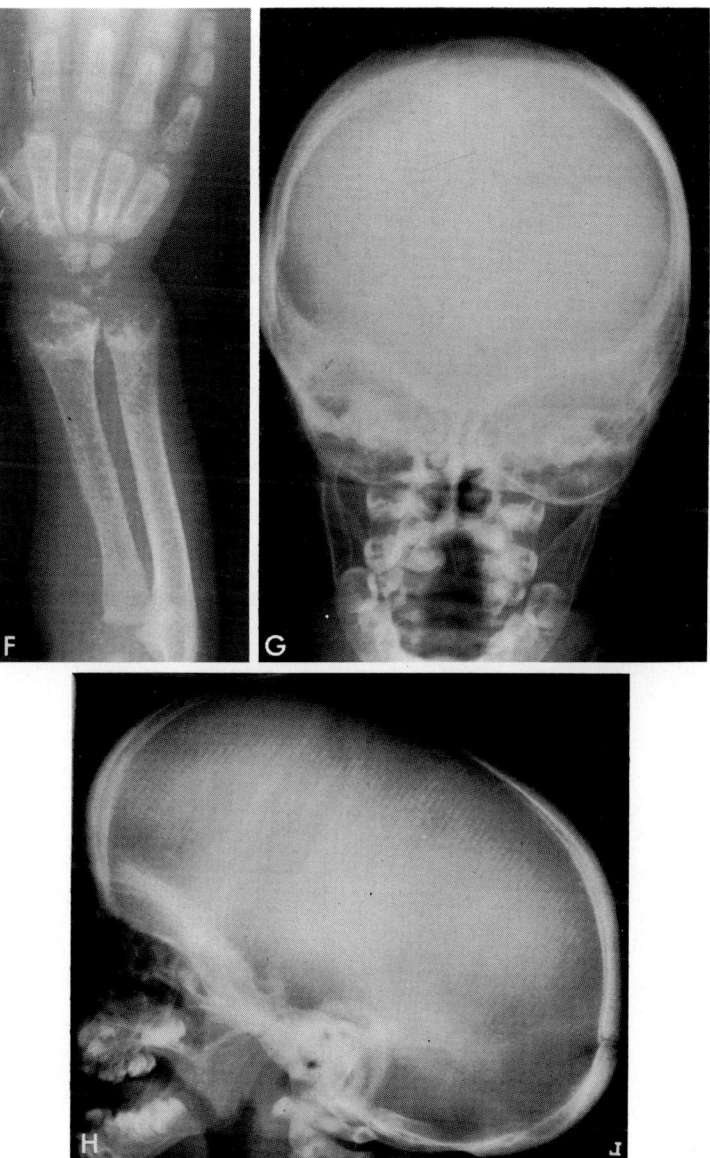

FIGURE 3–109 Continued. Simple vitamin D deficiency rickets.

F. Anteroposterior radiogram of wrist and forearm showing thickening of the physis and haziness of the provisional zone of calcification. Note the fraying and brushlike pattern of the epiphyseal border of the metaphyses. **G** and **H.** Radiograms of skull. There is external thickening of the frontal and parietal eminences. The coronal suture is relatively radiolucent as a result of lack of thickening of the edges of the bones.

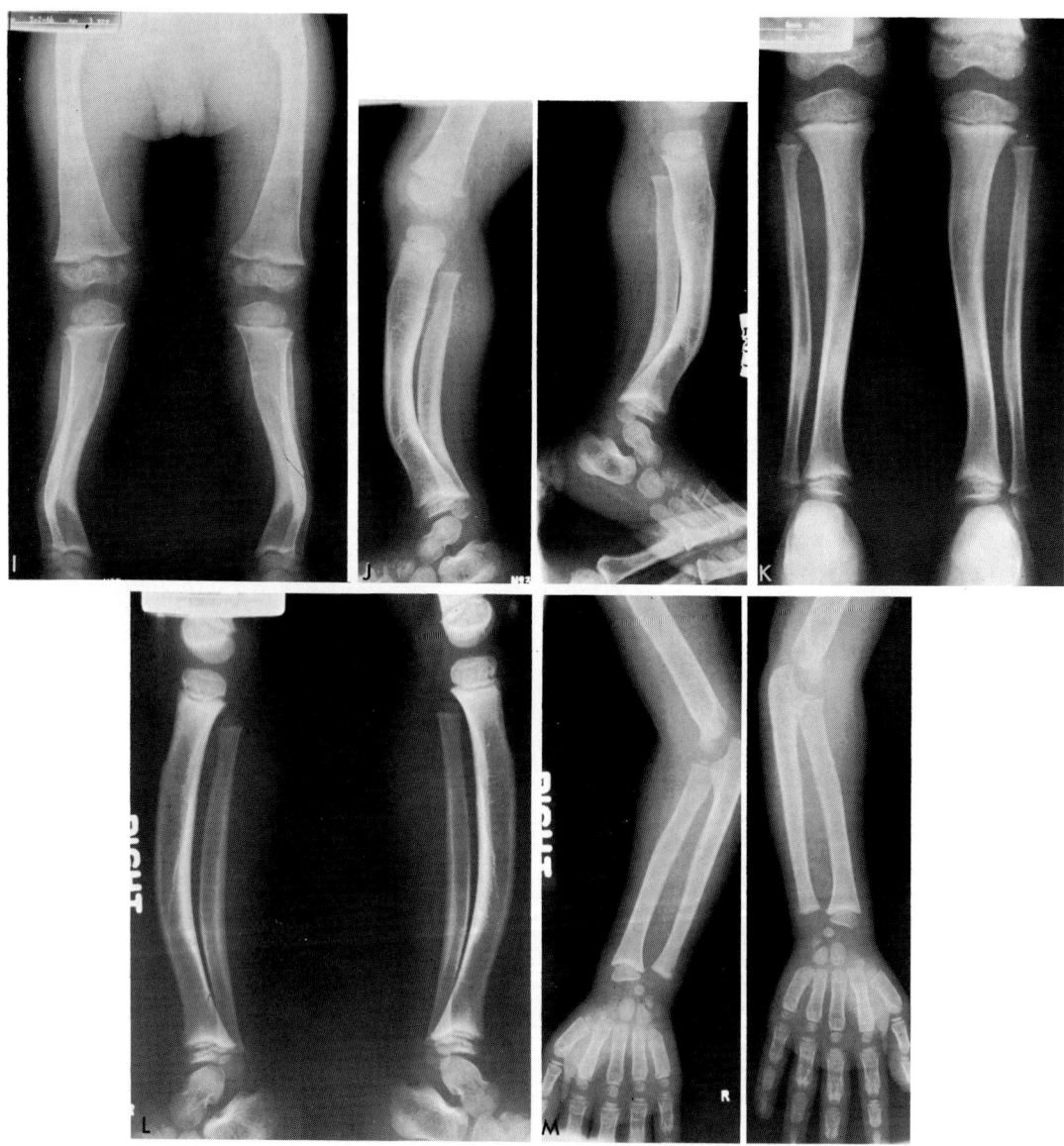

FIGURE 3–109 Continued. Simple vitamin D deficiency rickets.

I and **J**. Radiograms of legs ten months following treatment with vitamin D. Note the persistence of anterolateral angulation of the tibiae; the epiphyseal-metaphyseal areas are healed. **K** and **L**. Radiograms of the legs two years later show improvement of the angular deformities of the tibiae. **M**. Radiograms of upper limbs three years following initial treatment. There is no evidence of rickets.

whole milk or one can of evaporated milk contains 400 I.U. of vitamin D. There is no store of the vitamin at birth; therefore, it should be administered to breast-fed as well as bottle-fed infants, beginning at five or ten days of age. Premature infants require a larger dosage of about 2000 I.U. of vitamin D daily for the first three months.

Several difficulties, however, deter uniform prevention of rickets. These include poor standards of living in certain geographic areas, and lack of medical supervision, as well as genetic variations in individual requirements for vitamin D.

Treatment of simple vitamin D deficiency rickets consists of daily oral administration of 2000 to 5000 I.U. of vitamin D for six to ten weeks. Within two to four weeks, radiograms will demonstrate evidence of healing (Fig. 3–110). In depressed areas or when parents cannot be depended upon, a dose of 600,000 I.U. vitamin D may be given. If within three weeks there is no evidence of healing, the dose may be repeated once. If the child does not respond to this regimen of therapy, he probably has vitamin D–refractory rickets.

RICKETS ASSOCIATED WITH MALABSORPTION SYNDROME

In children, this is usually seen in gluten-sensitive enteropathy (celiac disease). Infants present with wasting and bulky, pale stools. Iron-deficiency anemia may be present. Radiograms show the same typical findings of rickets as in the vitamin D deficiency type plus the features of generalized osteoporosis. If fecal fat

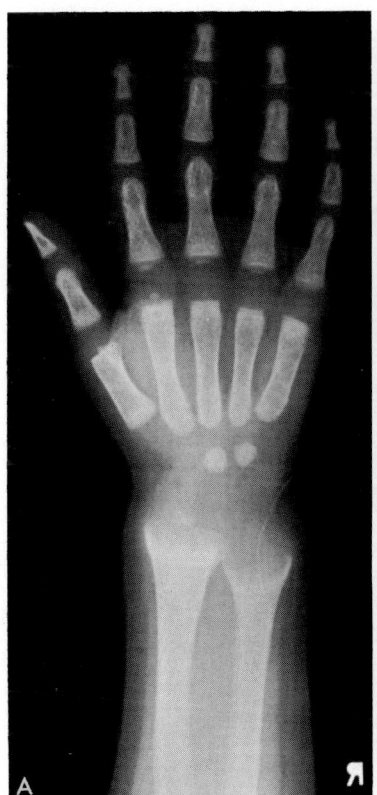
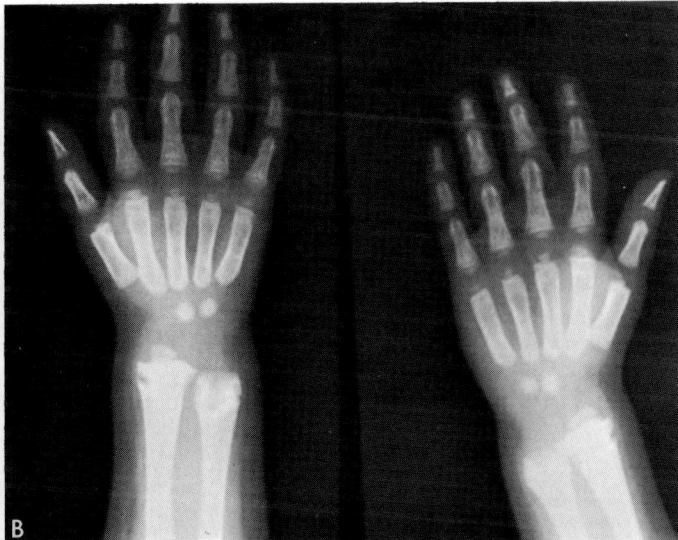
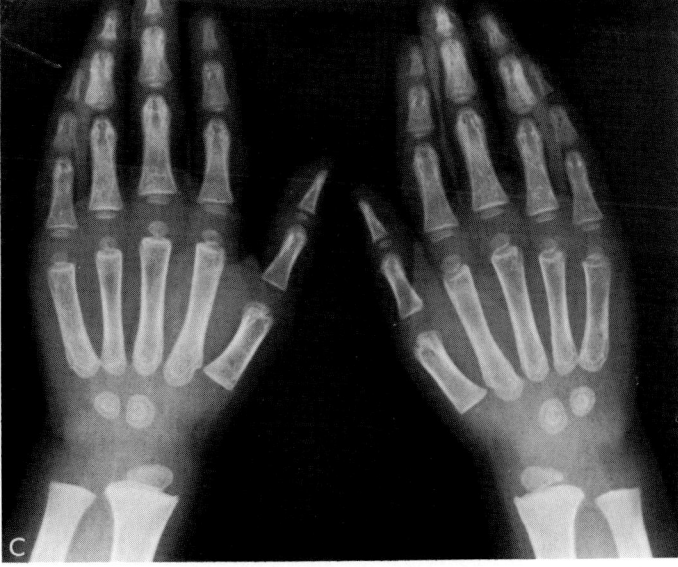

FIGURE 3–110. Simple vitamin D–deficiency rickets.

Radiographic evidence of healing is apparent following daily oral administration of 3000 I.U. vitamin D for a period of ten weeks. Failure of such response indicates probable vitamin D–refractory rickets. **A.** Initial radiogram showing florid rickets. **B.** Three weeks following therapy with vitamin D. **C.** Six months later. There is no evidence of active rickets.

is more than 5 gm. per day, it indicates steatorrhea. In addition to lack of absorption of vitamin D, rapid transit of intestinal contents is another factor in the decrease of extracellular compartment calcium. Congenital biliary atresia and fibrocystic disease are other rare causes of rickets in children.

References

1. Andrews, W. S., Pau, C. M., Chase, H. P., Foley, L. C., and Lilly, J. R.: Fat soluble vitamin deficiency in biliary atresia. J. Pediatr. Surg., 16:284, 1981.
2. Arnaud, C. D., Tsao, H. S., and Littledike, T.: Calcium homeostasis, parathyroid hormone and calcitonin: Preliminary report. Mayo Clin. Proc., 45:125, 1970.
3. Arnstein, A. R., Frame, B., and Frost, H. M.: Recent progress in osteomalacia and rickets. Ann. Intern. Med., 67:1296, 1967.
4. Avioli, L. V., and Haddad, J. G.: Progress in endocrinology and metabolism. Vitamin D: Current concepts. Metabolism, 22:507, 1973.
5. Bailie, J. M., and Irving, J. T.: Development and healing of rickets in intramembranous bone. Acta Med. Scand., 306:Suppl. 1, 1955.
6. Barnes, M. J., Constable, B. J., Morton, L. F., and Kodicek, E.: Bone collagen metabolism in vitamin D deficiency. Biochem. J., 132:113, 1973.
7. Beal, V. A.: Calcium and phosphorus in infancy. Am. Diet. Assoc., 53:450, 1968.
8. Bosley, A. R., Verrier-Jones, E. R., and Campbell, M. J.: Aetiological factors in rickets of prematurity. Arch. Dis. Child., 55:683, 1980.
9. Callenbach, J. C., Sheehan, M. B., Abramson, S. J., and Hall, R. T.: Etiologic factors in rickets of very low-birth-weight infants. J. Pediatr., 98:800, 1981.
10. Chesney, R. W., Hamstra, A. J., and DeLuca, H. F.: Rickets of prematurity. Supranormal levels of serum 1,25-dihydroxyvitamin D. Am. J. Dis. Child., 135:34, 1981.
11. Chesney, R. W., Zimmerman, J., Hamstra, A., DeLuca, H. F., and Mazees, R. B.: Vitamin D metabolite concentrations in vitamin D deficiency. Are calcitriol levels normal? Am. J. Dis. Child., 135:1025, 1981.
12. Chudley, A. E., Brown, D. R., Holzman, I. R., and Oh, K. S.: Nutritional rickets in 2 very low-birth-weight infants with chronic lung disease. Arch. Dis. Child., 55:687, 1980.
13. Cifuentes, R. F., Kooh, S. W., and Radde, I. C.: Vitamin D deficiency in a calcium-supplemented very low-birth-weight infant. J. Pediatr., 96:252, 1980.
14. Cleghorn, G. J., Tudehope, D. I., and Masel, J. P.: Rickets in extremely low-birth-weight infants. Aust. Paediatr. J., 17:285, 1981.
15. Cousins, R. J., and DeLuca, H. F.: Vitamin D and bone. In Bourne, G. F. F. (ed.): The Biochemistry and Physiology of Bone. Vol. 2. New York, Academic Press, 1971, p. 281.
16. Curtis, J. A., Kooh, S. W., Fraser, D., and Greenberg, M. L.: Nutritional rickets in vegetarian children. Can. Med. Assoc. J., 128:150, 1983.
17. DeLuca, H. F.: Current concepts: Vitamin D. N. Engl. J. Med., 281:1103, 1969.
18. DeLuca, H. F.: Vitamin D: New horizons. Clin. Orthop., 78:4, 1971.
19. DeLuca, H. F.: The vitamin D system: A view from basic science to the clinic. Clin. Biochem., 14:213, 1981.
20. Delvin, E. E., Glorieux, F. H., Marie, P. J., and Pettifor, J. M.: Vitamin D dependency: Replacement therapy with calcitrol? J. Pediatr., 99:26, 1981.
21. Dodds, G. S., and Cameron, H. C.: Studies on experimental rickets in rats. II. The healing process in the head of the tibia and other bones. Am. J. Pathol., 14:273, 1938.
22. Engfeldt, B., and Zetterstrom, R.: Biophysical studies of the bone tissue of dogs with experimental rickets (Biophysical studies of bone tissue No. II). Arch. Pathol., 59:321, 1955.
23. Engfeldt, B., Zetterstrom, R., and Winberg, J.: Primary vitamin-D-resistant rickets. III. Biophysical studies of skeletal tissue. J. Bone Joint Surg., 38-A:1323, 1956.
24. Fourman, P., and Royer, P.: Calcium Metabolism and the Bone. 2nd Ed. Philadelphia, F. A. Davis, 1968, pp. 104, 153, 444.
25. Fraser, D. R.: Biochemical and clinical aspects of vitamin D function. Br. Med. Bull., 37:37, 1981.
26. Fraser, D., and Salter, R. B.: The diagnosis and management of the various types of rickets. Pediatr. Clin. North Am., 5:417, 1958.
27. Galante, L., Colston, K. W., MacAuley, S. J., and MacIntyre, I.: Effects of calcitonin on vitamin D metabolism. Nature, 238:271, 1972.
28. Gefter, W. B., Epstein, D. M., Anday, E. K., and Dalinka, M. K.: Rickets presenting as multiple fractures in premature infants on hyperalimentation. Radiology, 142:371, 1982.
29. Glass, E. J., Hume, R., Hendry, G. M., Strange, R. C., and Forfar, J. O.: Plasma alkaline phosphatase activity in rickets of prematurity. Arch. Dis. Child., 57:373, 1982.
30. Goel, K.: Rickets. I. An old enemy returns. Nurs. Mirror, 152:16, 1981.
31. Goel, K. M.: Rickets in Asian children in Britain. Indian J. Pediatr., 48:763, 1981.
32. Goldsmith, R. S.: Laboratory aids in the diagnosis of metabolic bone diseases. Orthop. Clin. North Am., 3:545, 1972.
33. Harrison, H. E., and Harrison, H. C.: Vitamin D and permeability of intestinal mucosa to calcium. Am. J. Physiol., 208:370, 1965.
34. Kien, C. L., Browning, C., Jona, J., and Starshak, R. J.: Rickets in premature infants receiving parenteral nutrition: A case report and review of the literature. J.P.E.N., 6:152, 1982.
35. Kulkarni, P. B., Hall, R. T., Rhodes, P. G., Sheehan, M. B., Callenbach, J. C., Germann, D. R., and Abramson, S. J.: Rickets in very low-birth-weight infants. J. Pediatr., 96:249, 1980.
36. Lawson, D. E.: Dietary vitamin D: Is it necessary? J. Hum. Nutr., 35:61, 1981.
37. Lewin, P. K., Reid, M., Reilly, B. J., Sawyer, P. R., and Fraser, D.: Iatrogenic rickets in low-birth-weight infants. J. Pediatr., 78:207, 1971.
38. McIntosh, N., Brooke, O. G., and Livesey, A.: Prevention of rickets in preterm infants (letter). Lancet, 1:685, 1982.
39. McIntosh, N., Livesey, A., and Brooke, O. G.: Plasma 25-hydroxyvitamin D and rickets in infants of extremely low-birth-weight. Arch. Dis. Child., 57:848, 1982.
40. Marie, P. J., Pettifor, J. M., Ross, F. P., and Glorieux, F. H.: Histological osteomalacia due to dietary calcium deficiency in children. N. Engl. J. Med., 307:584, 1982.
41. Masel, J. P., Tudehope, D., Cartwright, D., and Cleghorn, G.: Osteopenia and rickets in the extremely low-birth-weight infant—a survey of the incidence and a radiological classification. Australas. Radiol., 26:83, 1982.
42. Mellanby, E.: Experimental rickets. The effect of cereals and their interaction with other factors of diet and environment in producing rickets. Spec. Rep. Ser. Med. Res. Coun. (London), 93:48, 1925.
43. Mellanby, E.: The part played by an accessory factor

in the production of experimental rickets. LII-LIV. A further demonstration of the part played by accessory food factors in the aetiology of rickets. J. Physiol. Soc. XI-XII, 52:106, 1918.
44. Morii, H., and DeLuca, H. F.: Relationship between vitamin D deficiency, thyrocalcitonin and parathyroid hormone. Am. J. Physiol., 213:358, 1967.
45. Nordin, B. E. C.: Effect of malabsorption syndrome on calcium metabolism. Proc. R. Soc. Med., 54:497, 1961.
46. Norman, A. W.: Recent studies on vitamin D and parathyroid hormone regulation of calcium and phosphorus metabolism. Clin. Orthop., 52:249, 1967.
47. Norman, M. E.: Vitamin D in bone disease. Pediatr. Clin. North Am., 29:947, 1982.
48. Ozsoylu, S.: Rickets in low-birth-weight infants (letter). J. Pediatr., 98:672, 1981.
49. Ozsoylu, S.: Rickets and deficiency of vitamin D metabolites (letter). Am. J. Dis. Child., 136:754, 1982.
50. Park, E. A.: The etiology of rickets. Physiol. Rev., 3:106, 1923.
51. Park, E. A.: Observations on the pathology of rickets with particular reference to the changes at the cartilage-shaft junction of the growing bones. Harvey Lect., 34:157, 1938–39.
52. Paterson, C. R.: Vitamin D deficiency rickets simulating child abuse. J. Pediatr. Orthop., 1:423, 1981.
53. Pettifor, J. M., and Ross, F. P.: Low dietary calcium intake and its role in the pathogenesis of rickets (letter). S. Afr. Med. J., 63:179, 1983.
54. Pick, L.: Pathologic, anatomic and clinical considerations concerning malacic diseases of the bones. Harvey Lect., 27:179, 1932.
55. Rudolf, M., Arulanantham, K., and Greenstein, R. M.: Unsuspected nutritional rickets. Pediatrics, 66:72, 1980.
56. Seino, Y., Ishii, T., Shimotsuji, T., Ishida, M., and Yabuuchi, H.: Plasma activity vitamin D concentration in low-birth-weight infants with rickets and its response to vitamin D treatment. Arch. Dis. Child., 56:628, 1981.
57. Sevastikoglou, J. A., Ray, R. D., Hjertquist, S. O., and Berquist, E.: Vitamin D and skeletal metabolism. Acta Orthop. Scand., Suppl. 136, 1970.
58. Sima, E., and Sauciuc, M.: Surveillance and follow-up of the child for the prevention and control of rickets due to vitamin D deficiency. Viata Med. (Medii Sanit), 29:175, 1981.
59. Simmons, D. J., and Kunin, A. S.: Development and healing of rickets in rats. I. Studies with tritiated thymidine and nutritional considerations. Clin. Orthop., 68:251, 1970.
60. Simmons, D. J., and Kunin, A. S.: Development and healing of rickets in rats. II. Studies with tritiated proline. Clin. Orthop., 68:261, 1970.
61. Simmons, D. J., and Kunin, A. S.: RNA and mucopolysaccharide metabolism in rachitic cartilage and bone. Isr. J. Med. Sci. 7:412, 1971.
62. Smith, R.: The pathophysiology and management of rickets. Orthop. Clin. North Am., 3:601, 1972.
63. Smith, R., and Dick, M.: Total urinary hydroxyproline excretion after administration of vitamin D to healthy volunteers and a patient with osteomalacia. Lancet, 1:279, 1968.
64. Smythe, P. M.: Respiratory distress in rickets (letter). S. Afr. Med. J., 57:1067, 1980.
65. Steinback, H. L., and Noetzli, M.: Roentgen appearance of the skeleton in osteomalacia and rickets. A.J.R., 91:955, 1964.
66. Toomey, F., Hoag, R., Batton, D., and Vain, N.: Rickets associated with cholestasis and parenteral nutrition in premature infants. Radiology, 142:85, 1982.
67. Warrier, R. P., Kini, K. R., and High, R. H.: Nutritional rickets due to food fadism. Indian J. Pediatr., 48:345, 1981.
68. Weiss, A.: The scapular sign in rickets. Radiology, 98:633, 1971.

Rickets Due to Renal Tubular Insufficiency (Hypophosphatemic or Vitamin D–Refractory Rickets)

Rachitic changes in bone may result from a derangement in function of the renal tubule without loss of glomerular function and, therefore, without signs of glomerular failure and retention of urea. The mechanisms by which rickets is produced by renal tubular dysfunction are, commonly, increased renal clearance of phosphate (hyperphosphaturia) and severe hypophosphatemia. As a result there is a decrease in the phosphate avaliable for mineralization of bone. In addition to failure of phosphate resorption, there may be other reabsorptive defects, such as for glucose, amino acids, water, or fixed base.

HYPOPHOSPHATEMIC VITAMIN D–REFRACTORY RICKETS OF THE SIMPLE TYPE

Vitamin D–refractory rickets is one of the most common metabolic bone diseases of children in North America. The only demonstrable kidney defect is the diminished resorption of phosphate from glomerular filtrate in the renal tubules.

The clinical and radiographic features are quite similar to those of simple vitamin D deficiency rickets. Vitamin D–refractory rickets, however, does not respond to the usual dosage of vitamin D and heals only following administration of phosphate in relatively large dosages.

Heredity. In about two thirds of cases, the inheritance is sex-linked and dominant with the abnormal gene carried on the long arm of the X chromosome.[40] In one third of cases, the syndrome is sporadic and possibly represents new mutations. An autosomal dominant transmission has been described.[5, 16, 65] Hypophosphatemia and reduced absorption of phosphate by the kidney may be found in the nonrachitic kindred of the proband. It is twice as common in girls as in boys.

Clinical Features. These usually become manifest around two years of age. In its severe form, the disease may be recognized as early as three months of age. The initial presenting complaints are delay in walking and deformities of the limbs. In contrast to vitamin D deficiency rickets, systemic manifestations such as apathy, irritability, and muscular hypertonia are minimal or absent.

The overt physical findings are the skeletal deformities, which are more or less like those seen in vitamin D deficiency rickets, but because of the chronicity of the disorder, they are more severe. The type of angular deformity of the lower limbs depends on the ambulatory status and muscle tone of the patient. If the child has normal muscle tone and is ambulatory, marked genu varum occurs; the varus deformity is mild or not present if the child does not walk. Children who have hypotonia and are ambulatory develop genu valgum. Legs are straight in patients who have hypotonia and are nonambulatory.[58] Other physical findings are "rachitic rosary" and enlargement of the epiphyses.

Radiographic Features. The same changes seen in vitamin D deficiency rickets are depicted in the radiograph. In hypophosphatemic rickets, however, the skeletal changes are predominant in the *lower limbs*, particularly around the knee. In the presence of genu varum, the physes of the distal femur and proximal tibia are markedly widened medially (Fig. 3–111 A and B). Similar changes, but to a lesser degree, are found in the proximal femur and distal tibia (Fig. 3–111 E and F). In the *upper limbs*, such physeal changes are minimal or absent; there the physeal abnormality consists of slight broadening or cupping of the ulna. The distal radial physis usually remains unaffected.

Swischak and Hayden, however, identified a group of patients with hypophosphatemic vitamin D–refractory rickets in whom the knee and wrist were equally affected. In this group of patients an additional finding was the short, squat long bones due to deficient tubulation.[65a] Identification of these two types has certain therapeutic complications. In those patients in whom upper limbs are not affected, the dosage of vitamin D required for bony healing is considerably less than in those in whom the upper limbs are affected.[58]

Biochemical Findings. Serum analysis will reveal hypophosphatemia, usually between 1 and 3 mg. per 100 ml. Alkaline phosphatase activity is increased. The serum calcium level is normal or slightly diminished. The plasma urea level, electrolytes, and pH are normal.

The constant finding of hypophosphatemia that can be rarely, if ever, reversed by administration of vitamin D indicates that the primary defect is in the tubular reabsorption of phosphate.

Treatment

Medical Treatment. Large doses of vitamin D (50,000 to 500,000 I.U. daily) are given, with the object of raising the plasma phosphate level without increasing the urinary excretion of calcium beyond 6 mg. per day and without raising the plasma level of calcium beyond 10.5 mg. per 100 ml. The nature of resistance to vitamin D is not yet determined. Large doses of vitamin D are, however, effective in diminishing the excessive phosphate clearance.

These patients present a multidisciplinary problem and are usually followed jointly by the pediatrician or endocrinologist and the orthopedic surgeon. Medical treatment should be provided by a pediatric endocrinologist. Close supervision is necessary to determine the optimal subtoxic dose of vitamin D. In the beginning, these children are seen at biweekly intervals; once the effective maintenance dose is established, they are examined every three months. The parents and patient should understand that this is a chronic metabolic bone disease that must be followed throughout life, especially during growth.

During physical examination, the parents are questioned concerning the symptoms of vitamin D intoxication, such as anorexia, thirst, and polyuria. The earliest evidence of vitamin D poisoning is an abnormal increase in urinary excretion of calcium, which is grossly determined by the Sulkowitch test. The Sulkowitch reagent consists of 2.5 gm. oxalic acid, 2.5 gm. ammonium oxalate, 5 ml. glacial acetic acid, and distilled water added to 150 ml. Equal volumes (about 5 ml.) of Sulkowitch reagent and urine are mixed and left to stand for two minutes. The density of the cloud of precipitated calcium oxalate is noted. A slight precipitate is normal. In untreated rickets or hypoparathyroidism there is no precipitate. A dense precipitate, graded + + to + + + +, indicates hypercalciuria. The results of the Sulkowitch test, however, are not reliable and are of no great value in determining the presence of intoxication. Twenty-four-hour urinary calcium excretion studies are useful but not practical in day-to-day general management of these children. The author relies more on clinical signs and utilizes the Sulkowitch test as a rough method to keep the parents aware of the possibility of vitamin D intoxication. The most valuable determination is the serum calcium concentration, which, when elevated over 10.5 mg. per 100 ml., is an indication for intensive evaluation. When mild poisoning is present,

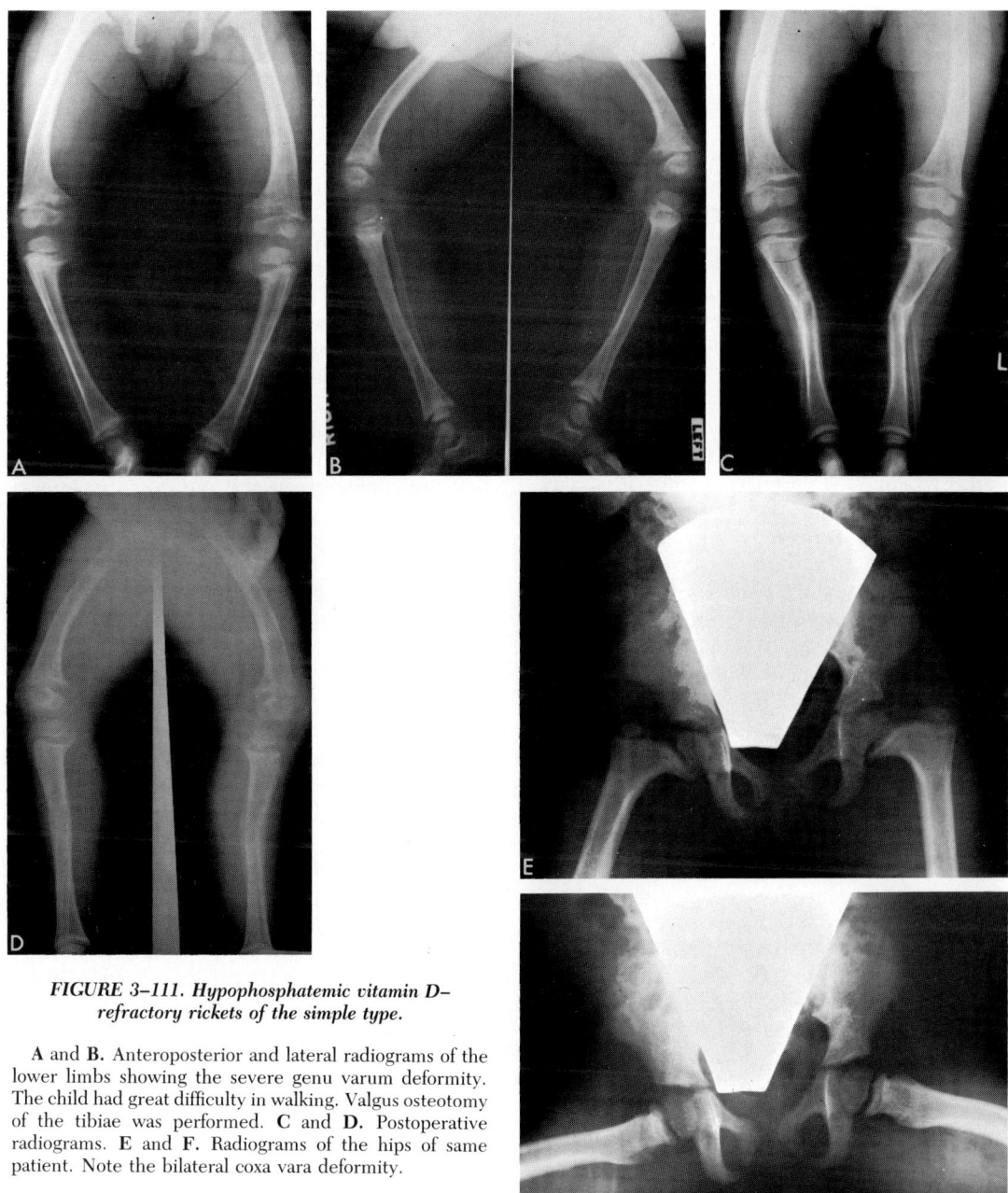

FIGURE 3–111. *Hypophosphatemic vitamin D–refractory rickets of the simple type.*

A and **B.** Anteroposterior and lateral radiograms of the lower limbs showing the severe genu varum deformity. The child had great difficulty in walking. Valgus osteotomy of the tibiae was performed. **C** and **D.** Postoperative radiograms. **E** and **F.** Radiograms of the hips of same patient. Note the bilateral coxa vara deformity.

administration of vitamin D is discontinued for two to three weeks. With subsidence of all signs of intoxication, the vitamin therapy is reinstituted at a daily dosage of 25,000 I.U. less than previously. Administration of vitamin D should be discontinued in the case of a febrile bedridden child.

It is imperative to realize that careless administration of vitamin D in large doses can be very dangerous, causing irreversible renal damage and possibly death.

Phosphates may be administered orally in large quantities, particularly to a child whose plasma phosphate level is less than 1.5 mg. per 100 ml. Savill and associates, as well as other authors, have shown that a dietary supplement of phosphate led to healing and reversed the metabolic defects toward normal, making it feasible to reduce the dose of vitamin D to 50,000 to 100,000 I.U.[60a] The dosage of phosphorus varies from 0.6 to 1.2 gm. daily.[46]

Vitamin D treatment must be continued until completion of growth. In adults, requirements for the vitamin vary, and each case should be individualized.

Orthopedic Treatment. The deformities requiring orthopedic attention are usually in the lower limbs and include genu varum or valgum, anterior angulation of the femur, anterolateral angulation of the tibia, coxa vara, and intrapelvic protrusion of the acetabulum; in the spine, kyphoscoliosis may be a problem. In the upper limbs, the bones are less deformed, as they are not subjected to the stresses of body weight.

In mild lower limb deformities, supportive shoes are all that is required. Under adequate medical management, the skeletal deformities will correct themselves spontaneously with growth.

For moderate or severe deformities, the use of supportive orthotic devices is indicated, the type and extent of which depend on the severity of the disease and the deformity. When there is excessive medial tibiofibular torsion with distal tibia vara, an 8 to 12 inch Fillauer bar that holds the feet in about 25 to 30 degrees of lateral rotation may be used. This is worn at night only for 8 to 10 hours. Such night splinting may improve the deformity. In severe or recalcitrant cases, a Blount tibia vara knee-ankle-foot orthosis is worn at night; during the day a knee-ankle-foot tibia vara orthosis is used.

Surgical Treatment. Surgical alignment of the limbs may be indicated prior to bracing when the deformity is severe. This is especially indicated when genu varum or valgum is so severe that pain and instability of the knee joint develop because of the abnormal stress on the collateral ligaments. On occasion, even pathologic fractures may occur at points of maximum stress (Looser's zones).

Four to six weeks prior to operation, the vitamin D is discontinued. This is imperative because the demineralization and hypercalciuria resulting from immobilization in a plaster cast and inactivity augmented by the action of vitamin D cause severe hypercalcemia and hypercalcinuria, consequent kidney damage, and central nervous system depression. Usually, it is a varus or valgus deformity that is to be corrected, and a curve or "dome" type of osteotomy through the metaphyseal region is the most satisfactory technique (Fig. 3–112). Internal fixation with two staples or preferably a four- or six-hole plate with screws is utilized.

Resistive active exercises of the limbs that have not been operated on are initiated immediately, and ambulation is begun as soon as possible. Vitamin D therapy is reinstituted following removal of the cast and resumption of normal activities. Use of a supportive orthosis may be indicated in the postoperative period until the osteotomy is healed solidly and vitamin D has substantially controlled the activity of rickets.

Slipped capital femoral epiphysis, a rare complication, may require pinning.

OTHER TYPES OF VITAMIN D–REFRACTORY RICKETS

Hypophosphatemic Vitamin D–Refractory Rickets with Aminoaciduria. This rare form of rickets has been referred to as the "Fanconi syndrome." It consists of two types that differ in their mode of genetic transmission, clinical findings, and prognosis. It has been suggested that use of the eponym "Fanconi syndrome" be discontinued.[18, 19, 23, 24]

The form of hypophosphatemic vitamin D–refractory rickets with aminoaciduria is differentiated from simple hypophosphatemic vitamin D–refractory rickets by an earlier onset, a greater severity of rachitic bone lesions, marked muscular weakness, and the presence of glucosuria and generalized aminoaciduria. The serum calcium level may be normal or lowered. The prognosis is good, provided the condition is diagnosed and treated in its early stages with large doses of vitamin D (100,000 I.U. daily), which results in rapid and almost complete restoration of radiographic and chemical blood changes to normal, as well as disappearance of the aminoaciduria.

Hypophosphatemic Vitamin D–Refractory Rickets with Aminoaciduria and Acidosis. In

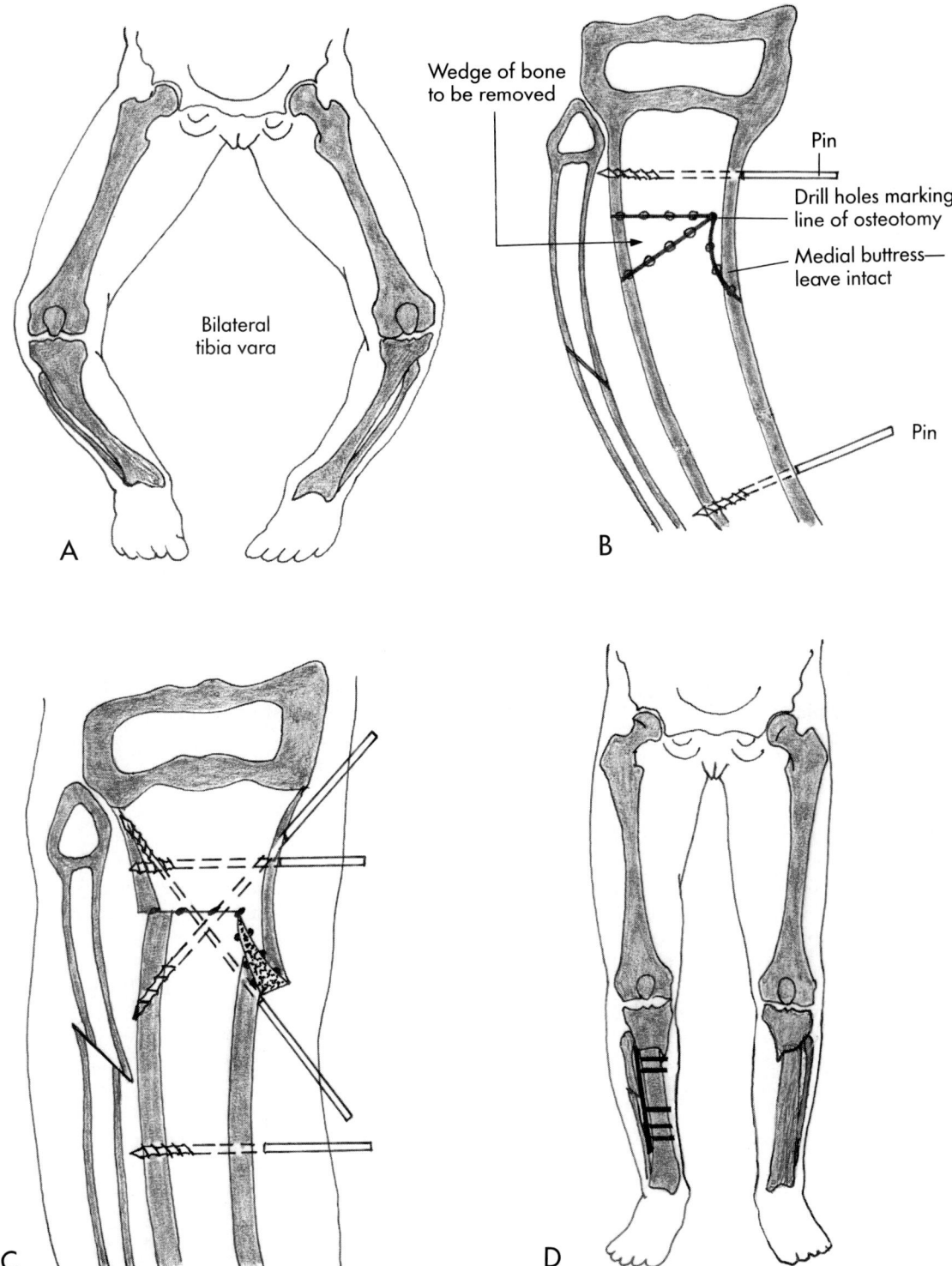

FIGURE 3–112. *Osteotomy through the metaphyseal-diaphyseal juncture to correct tibia vara.*

A. Bilateral tibia vara. **B.** Note the threaded Steinmann pins in the proximal and distal segments and the drill holes marking the line of osteotomy. The medial buttress should be left intact. **C.** Steinmann pins transfixing the proximal and distal tibial segments in the corrected position. Note that the excised wedge of bone is used as a graft to fill the medial defect. Note also the osteotomy of the fibula. **D.** Bilateral tibia vara corrected. Internal fixation is by plate and screws placed on the lateral side.

this type of rickets, acidosis is an additional finding due to a disturbance of the conservation of a fixed base. Favorable results are obtained by treatment with alkalis and large doses of vitamin D.

Cystine Storage Disease with Rickets. In this rare condition, also known as Fanconi syndrome, Debre–De Toni–Fanconi syndrome, Lignac's disease, Lignac-Fanconi syndrome, cystinosis, or cystinuria with rickets, there is, in addition to the renal tubular insufficiency, an inborn error of cystine metabolism with deposition of cystine in various tissues. The disease is transmitted by a recessive gene, with most affected patients being the offspring of consanguineous marriages.[4]

At birth, the infant appears to be normal; at about six months of age, the initial symptoms become manifest in the form of failure to thrive, lack of appetite, vomiting, and polyuria. Soon bouts of dehydration and high fever make the infant seriously ill. Photophobia is common.

In the second or third year of life, severe and crippling rachitic deformities develop. Radiograms disclose the usual findings of rickets. Diagnosis is established by demonstration of insoluble cystine crystals in various tissues, such as the cornea, sternal marrow, or lymph nodes.

Histologic changes in bone are those of rickets and renal osteodystrophy. Microdissection techniques have demonstrated certain lesions in proximal tubules of the kidneys in cystinosis.

There is no specific treatment for the disordered metabolism of cystine and the prognosis is poor. The glomeruli eventually become involved, uremia develops, and the child dies in the first decade of life. The rachitic bone lesions usually respond to large doses of vitamin D. Correction of acidosis by administration of oral alkalis (sodium citrate) and of hypokalemia by large doses of potassium does much to improve the general condition of the patient.

Hypophosphatemic Vitamin D–Refractory Rickets with Hyperglycinuria. Severe rachitic bone lesions, marked muscle weakness, a low concentration of phosphate in the serum, acidosis, and excessive urinary excretion of calcium and glycine are the manifestations of this rare syndrome, which has its onset in late adolescence. It responds to large doses of vitamin D.

Oculocerebral Syndrome with Hypophosphatemic Vitamin D–Refractory Rickets. In this very rare syndrome, described by Lowe and associates in 1952, the hypophosphatemic vitamin D–refractory rickets is associated with congenital glaucoma, cataracts, mental deficiency, hypotonia, diminished reflexes, acidosis, and aminoaciduria.[30, 38a] It is seen in the male as a sex-linked recessive trait.

Rickets Due to Renal Tubular Acidosis. This is very uncommon in children and is not discussed here. Depletion of calcium in bone develops as a result of protracted loss of a fixed base. The bone changes respond to control of acidosis.

Renal Osteodystrophy

This is a chronic disease of bone caused by generalized kidney failure involving both glomeruli and tubules. Lucas and Davies-Colley are credited with having first called attention to the association of kidney and bone disease.[14, 39] Since then, the skeletal complications of chronic renal failure have been well described. In the literature, this disease is known by a number of names—renal rickets, renal osteodystrophy, rickets due to glomerular insufficiency, glomerular rickets, secondary hyperparathyroidism, uremic osteodystrophy, and pan-nephritic osteodystrophy.

The condition is usually seen in children whose bones are still growing and metabolically very active, and in whom the natural course of renal failure is more chronic than in adults. The principal causes of kidney failure in children are chronic pyelonephritis complicating various congenital abnormalities of the urinary tract, such as polycystic kidney disease, congenital absence or hypoplasia of the kidney, chronic glomerulonephritis, and late stages of cystine storage disease with vitamin D–refractory rickets and rickets due to renal tubular acidosis.

Etiology. The pathogenesis of bone lesions in chronic renal failure is still not determined. Various factors must be considered. In chronic renal failure, secondary parathyroid hyperplasia develops, and there is a high concentration of parathormone in the serum. Parathyroid hyperplasia has been produced in rats experimentally by removal of two thirds of the kidneys.[32] Renal damage and failure caused by administration of platinum, copper, lead, or uranium has also resulted in secondary parathyroid hyperplasia and bone lesions. Removal of the parathyroid glands prevented the bone changes. The stimulus for the parathyroid hyperplasia of renal failure is most likely hypocalcemia; acidosis, however, may be another factor. Because administration of ammonium chloride to animals has resulted in bone changes similar to those found in osteitis fibrosa, some of the skeletal

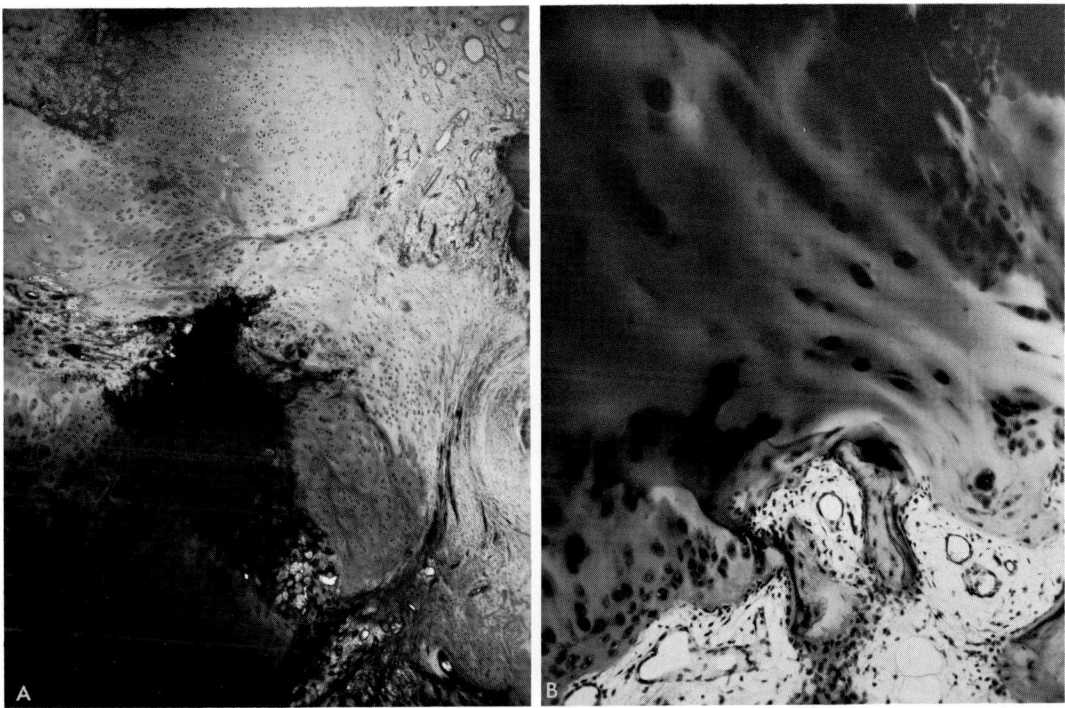

FIGURE 3–113. *Histologic findings of osteodystrophy due to chronic renal insufficiency.*

A. Photomicrography of a section through the widened physis showing extension of cartilage cells into the metaphysis (×25). **B.** Higher magnification (×100) of same area. Note the uncalcified osteoid tissue and the replacement of the normal fatty bone marrow by hyperplastic fibrous tissue.

lesions of renal failure have been thought to arise directly from the acidosis.[31] Studies of the composition of bone in uremia have shown increasing loss of bone bicarbonate, a homeostatic mechanism used to neutralize the "acid."[55]

In renal failure there is another possible factor that disturbs the intrinsic process of bone calcification; this is suggested by the experimental work of Yendt and associates, who found that sera from patients with kidney failure failed to calcify rachitic rat cartilage in vitro with levels of calcium and phosphate that normally produced calcification.[70]

Pathology. Features of both rickets and hyperparathyroidism are present in varying degrees in the skeleton.[27, 28, 65] The characteristic lesions are best seen in the epiphyseal-metaphyseal area of the growing long bones (Fig. 3–113). The rachitic changes consist of a failure of replacement of proliferating cartilage cells by new bone. Mature cartilage cells persist, forming islands in the metaphyseal area. The provisional zone of calcification is widened and irregular. There is an abundance of osteoid tissue laid down along the bone trabeculae and remaining nests of cartilage cells. The amount of osteoid tissue is somewhat less in renal osteodystrophy than in true rickets; histologically, however, on the basis of the preceding findings, the two conditions cannot be differentiated.

The characteristic histologic feature of hyperparathyroidism is osteoclastic resorption of bone with fibrous osteitis, the normal fatty bone marrow being replaced by hyperplastic fibrous tissue. There are also areas of patchy formation of new bone, particularly at the base of the skull and in the vertebrae, resulting in osteosclerosis.[29]

The parathyroid glands are enlarged and hyperplastic. The kidneys and urinary tract show the primary pathologic lesions. There may be metastatic calcification in cardiopulmonary, renal, arterial, and subcutaneous tissues.

Clinical Picture. Polyuria, albuminuria, inability to concentrate the urine, nitrogen retention, and metabolic acidosis are present and precede symptoms and signs of bone disease by at least two years. Children with renal osteodystrophy are stunted in growth, and dwarfism is common. The bones of the lower limbs are more severely involved than those of the upper limbs, as they are more subject to the mechanical stresses of weight-bearing. Aching of the bones is a frequent complaint. Skeletal deformities may consist of genu valgum, enlargement of the ends of the long bones, and slipping of the epiphyses, especially of the femoral head (Fig. 3–114). A "rachitic rosary" at the costochondral junction may be palpable. The mandible and maxilla may be overgrown, making the inferior part of the face appear widened and protuberant.

Radiographic Findings. Generalized osteoporosis with thinning of the cortices and bone trabeculae is the common finding, as shown in Figure 3–114. This imparts a "ground glass" appearance in the radiograms. The coarsely granular pattern of the skull bones looks "wooly" or like "salt and pepper" (Fig. 3–114 N). The physes are increased in thickness, and the metaphyses are frayed at the zone of provisional calcification (Fig. 3–114 L and M). The physeal lines are not cupped like those in vitamin D deficiency rickets but instead are rather oblique. Slipping of the epiphyses may be present (Fig. 3–114 D, E, J, and K). Skeletal maturation may be delayed, and the ossification centers of the epiphyses are late to appear.

Later in the course of the disease, bone changes similar to those of hyperparathyroidism develop. Subperiosteal cortical resorption takes place, beginning in the terminal phalanges and spreading proximally to involve the metacarpals and the distal ends of the radius and ulna (Fig. 3–114 O). Subperiosteal resorption of the lamina dura and mandible, identical to that of parathyroid adenoma, may be present. The irregular, coarse, and thin bone trabeculae and the eroded and poorly defined cortex impart a "ground glass" appearance in the radiogram.

Osteosclerosis can be recognized at the base of the skull and in the vertebrae. In the lateral radiogram of the spine, the sclerotic vertebral end-plates are seen as transverse bands of increased density. The horizontal striped appearance is called "rugger-jersey spine" (Fig. 3–114 Q).[13, 70]

Biochemical Findings. Serum analysis shows an elevated level of urea and an increase in the concentration of inorganic phosphate and alkaline phosphatase in the blood. The serum calcium level is usually diminished. Increased hydrogen ion concentration is common in uremic bone disease. Urinary excretion of calcium is very minimal.

Treatment

The life span of children with chronic renal

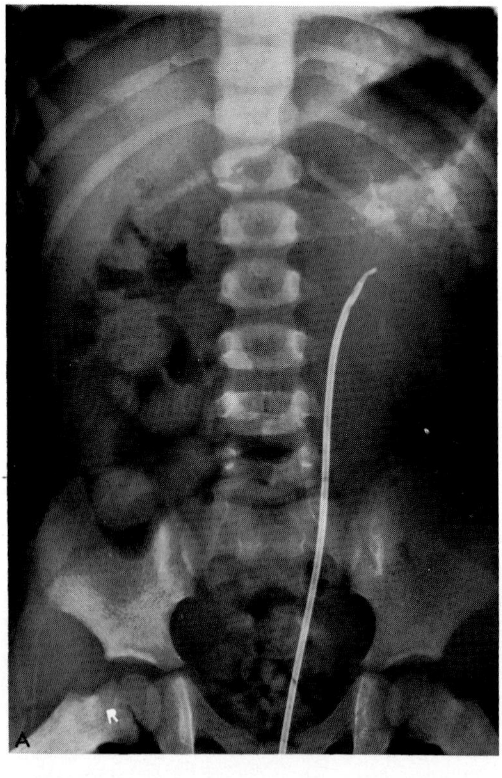

FIGURE 3–114. Osteodystrophy due to chronic renal insufficiency in a young girl with progressive slipped capital femoral epiphyses.

A. Anteroposterior radiogram of pelvis showing normal relationship of femoral heads to the necks.

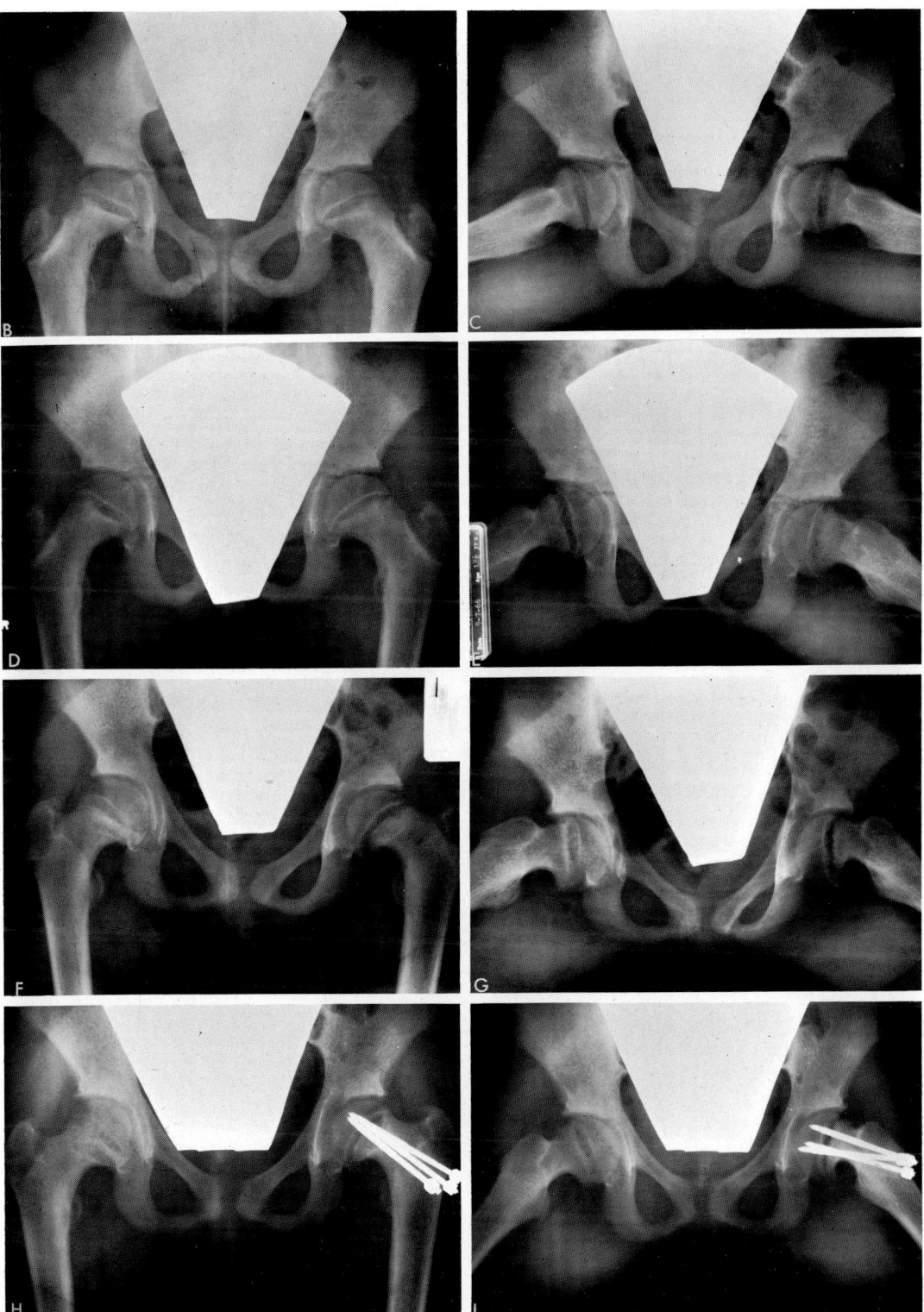

FIGURE 3–114 Continued. *Osteodystrophy due to chronic renal insufficiency in a young girl with progressive slipped capital femoral epiphyses.*

B and **C.** At age of 12 years, anteroposterior and lateral radiograms of the hips disclose increased thickening of the physes, but there is no slipping. **D** and **E.** Six months later. Note early slip on the left. **F** and **G.** Fifteen months later. Note the moderate slip on the left. Patient had pain and an antalgic limp on the left side. Left hip was pinned in situ when kidney function and general condition permitted following dialysis. **H** and **I.** Postoperative radiograms of the hips.

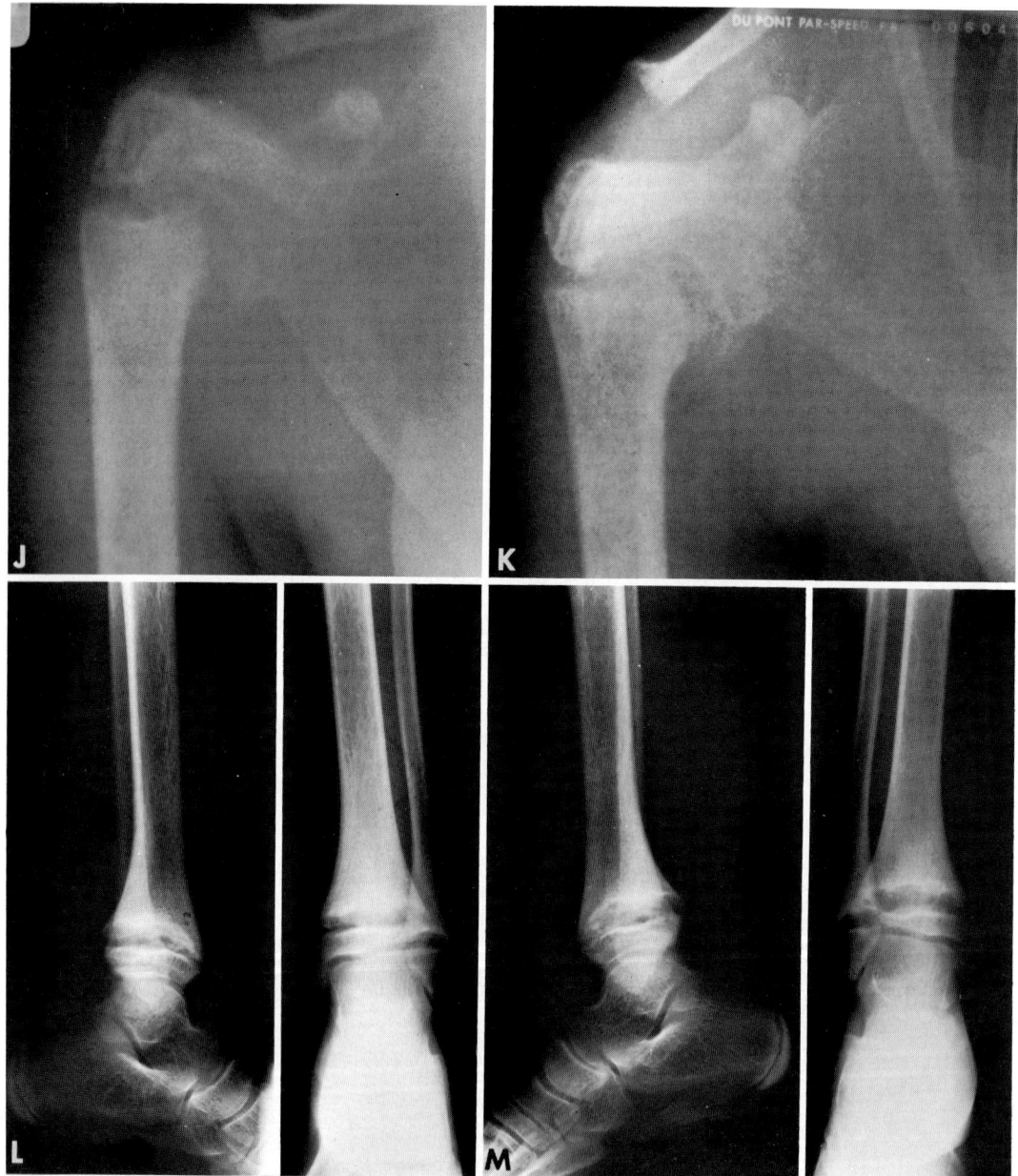

FIGURE 3–114 Continued. Osteodystrophy due to chronic renal insufficiency in a young girl with progressive slipped capital femoral epiphyses.

J and **K**. Anteroposterior radiograms of both shoulders show slipping of humeral head. **L** and **M**. Anteroposterior and lateral radiograms of both ankles at age of 12 years show increased thickness of the physes and irregularity of the metaphysis at the zone of provisional calcification.

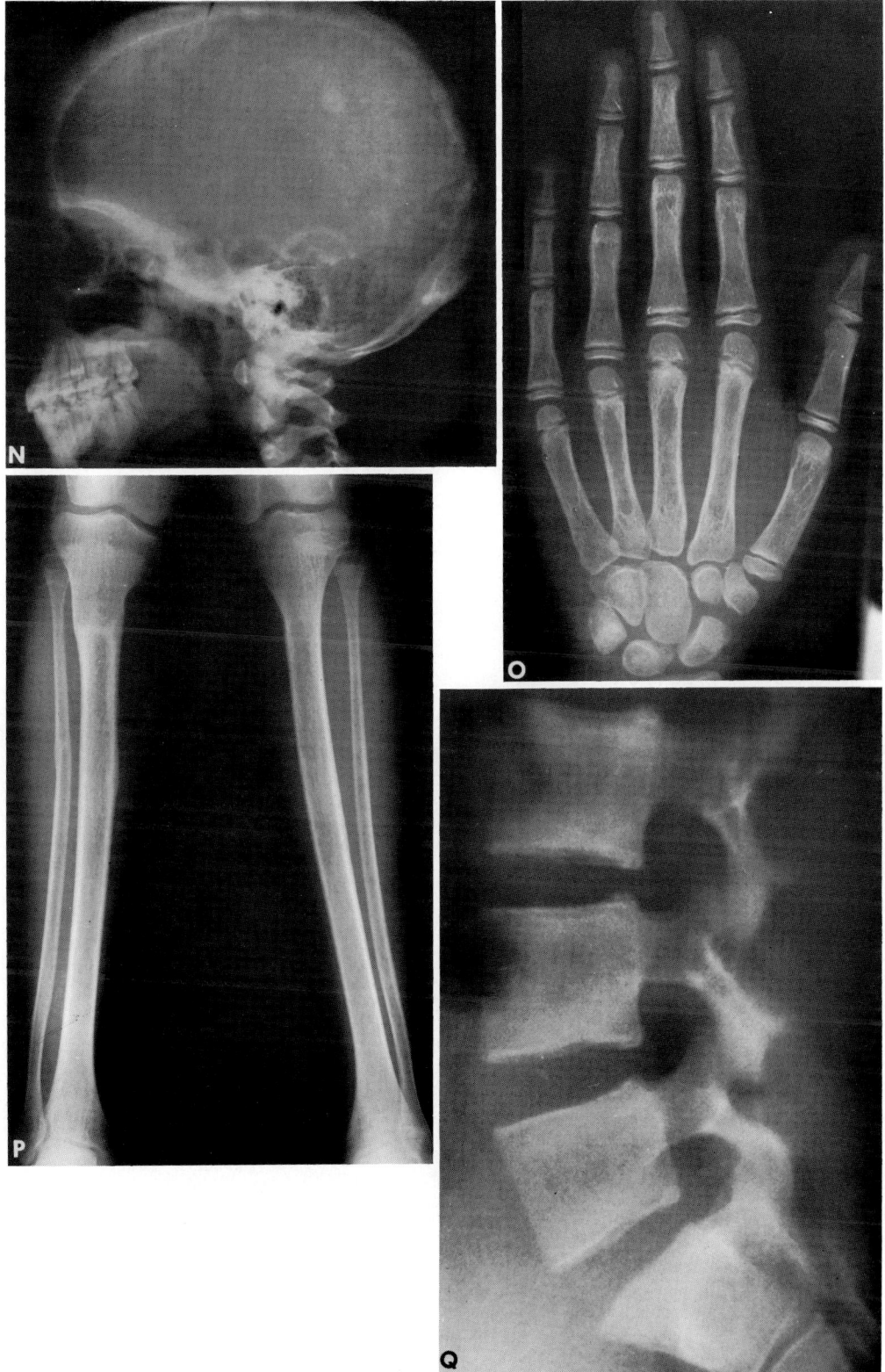

FIGURE 3–114 Continued. Osteodystrophy due to chronic renal insufficiency in a young girl with progressive slipped capital femoral epiphyses.

N. Lateral view of skull showing "ground-glass" appearance. Note the absence of the lamina dura of the teeth. **O.** Anteroposterior view of hand showing thinning of the cortices of the phalanges due to subperiosteal bone resorption. The trabeculae are coarse and irregular. **P.** Standing anteroposterior radiograms of both lower limbs show the bilateral genu valgum. On the right the healed line of osteotomy is evident. **Q.** Lateral radiogram of fourth and fifth lumbar vertebrae. Note the transverse bands of osteosclerosis.

failure has been considerably prolonged with dialysis and renal transplantation. With improvement of the prognosis, these children are participating in normal physical activities and applying stress on the lesions of the skeleton. Their management requires continued and meticulous orthopedic care.

Medical Treatment. This is provided by the pediatric endocrinologist and nephrologist. Administration of vitamin D daily in large doses (100,000 to 200,000 I.U.) has proved effective. A good index of positive response is a gradual decrease in the formerly elevated alkaline phosphatase activity. Increasing nitrogen retention may occur, and during the initial period of treatment it is best to observe the child daily in a metabolic unit as an inpatient. Serum calcium levels are determined regularly. Hypercalcemia as a result of vitamin D administration should be avoided. As soon as the bones begin to heal, the dosage of vitamin D should be decreased to 50,000 I.U. three times a week. Ectopic calcification and ossification may occur and cause further renal damage.

Sufficient sodium bicarbonate and citrate are administered to raise the plasma bicarbonate level to normal, as there is indication that the bone lesions will improve if the acidosis of renal insufficiency is corrected.

Orthopedic Treatment. Children with renal failure should be encouraged to be ambulatory as long as possible. In correction of orthopedic deformities, the hazards and complications of surgical intervention should be carefully weighed because of the possible presence of anemia, hypertension, bleeding tendencies, and electrolyte abnormalities. In general, surgical measures to correct bony deformities should be delayed until medical therapy has given the rachitic changes a chance to heal. For treating slipped capital femoral epiphysis in renal osteodystrophy, Shea and Mankin suggest conservative management with partial or total non-weight-bearing. In the three cases they reported, progression of epiphyseal displacement did not occur.[63] Each patient should be individually considered, however. With modern advances in renal dialysis and anesthesia, as well as excellent intensive care, surgery is tolerated by these patients. This author recommends pinning to prevent further progression of slipping of the capital femoral epiphysis.

References

1. Alfrey, A. C., Jenkins, D., Groth, C. G., Schorr, W. S., Geceiter, L., and Ogden, D. A.: Resolution of hyperparathyroidism renal osteodystrophy and metastatic calcification after renal homotransplantation. N. Engl. J. Med., 279:1349, 1968.
2. Ashcroft, G. V.: Renal rickets. J. Bone Joint Surg., 8:279, 1926.
3. Barber, H.: Renal dwarfism. Q. J. Med., 14:205, 1921.
4. Barber, H.: Renal dwarfism. A study of the course of the disease from seventeen cases. Guys Hosp. Rep., 76:307, 1926.
5. Brailsford, J. F.: Slipping of the epiphysis of the head of the femur. Its relation to renal rickets. Lancet, 1:16, 1933.
6. Brockman, E. P.: Some observations on the bone changes in renal rickets. Br. J. Surg., 14:634, 1927.
7. Cameron, H. C.: Case of osteomalacia and infantilism with renal deficiency. Proc. R. Soc. Med., 11:22, 1918.
8. Castleman, B., and Mallory, T. B.: Parathyroid hyperplasia in chronic renal insufficiency. Am. J. Pathol., 13:553, 1937.
9. Cattell, H. S., Levin, S., Kopits, D., and Lyne, E. D.: Reconstructive surgery in children with azotemic osteodystrophy. J. Bone Joint Surg., 53-A:216, 1971.
10. Chan, J. C.: Vitamin D disorders in children with chronic renal failure. Va. Med., 109:255, 1982.
11. Chan, J. C., and Hsu, A. C.: Vitamin D and renal diseases. Adv. Pediatr., 27:117, 1980.
12. Clay, R. D., Darmady, E. M., and Hawkins, M.: The nature of the renal lesions in the Fanconi syndrome. J. Pathol. Bacteriol., 65:551, 1953.
13. Crawford, T., Dent, C. E., Lucas, P., Martin, N. H., and Nassim, J. R.: Osteosclerosis associated with chronic renal failure. Lancet, 2:981, 1954.
14. Davies-Colley, N.: Bones and kidneys from a case of osteomalacia in a girl aged 13. Trans. Pathol. Soc. Lond., 35:285, 1884.
15. Dent, C. E.: Rickets and osteomalacia from renal tubule defects. J. Bone Joint Surg., 34-B:266, 1952.
16. Dent, C. F., and Harris, H.: Hereditary forms of rickets and osteomalacia. J. Bone Joint Surg., 38-B:204, 1956.
17. Dent, C. E., Harper, C. M., and Philpot, G. R.: The treatment of renal glomerular osteodystrophy. Q. J. Med. (N.S.), 30:1, 1961.
18. DeToni, G.: Remarks on the relations between renal rickets (renal dwarfism) and renal diabetes. Acta Paediatr. (Uppsala), 16:479, 1933.
19. DeToni, G.: Renal rickets with phospho-gluco-amino renal diabetes. De Toni-Debré-Fanconi syndrome. Ann. Paediatr. (Basel), 187:42, 1956.
20. Donckerewolcke, R. A.: Diagnosis and treatment of renal tubular disorders in children. Pediatr. Clin. North Am., 29:895, 1982.
21. Eil, C., Liberman, U. A., Rosen, J. F., and Marx, S. J.: A cellular defect in hereditary vitamin-D-dependent rickets type II: Defective nuclear uptake of 1,25-dihydroxyvitamin D in cultured skin fibroblasts. N. Engl. J. Med., 304:1588, 1981.
22. Engfeldt, B., Zetterstrom, R., and Winberg, J.: Primary vitamin-D-resistant rickets. III. Biophysical studies of skeletal tissue. J. Bone Joint Surg., 38-A:1323, 1956.
23. Fanconi, G.: Der fruhinfantile nephrotischglykosurische Zwergwuchs mit hypophosphatamischer Rachitis. Jb. Kinderheilkd., 147:299, 1936.
24. Fanconi, G., and Girardet, P.: Familiärer persistierender Phosphatdiabetes mit D Vitamin resistenter Rachitis. Helv. Paediatr. Acta, 7:14, 1952.
25. Fletcher, R. F., Jones, J. H., and Morgan, D. B.: Bone disease in chronic renal failure. Q. J. Med. (N.S.), 32:321, 1963.
26. Follis, R. H.: Renal rickets and osteitis fibrosa in children and adolescents. Bull. Johns Hopkins Hosp., 87:593, 1950.
27. Follis, R. H., and Jackson, D. A.: Renal osteomalacia and osteitis fibrosa in adults. Bull. Johns Hopkins Hosp., 72:232, 1943.

28. Gilmour, J. R.: The Parathyroid Glands and Skeleton in Renal Disease. Oxford, Oxford Medical Publications, 1947.
29. Hampers, C. L., Katz, A. I., Wilson, R. E., and Merrill, J. P.: Calcium metabolism and osteodystrophy after renal transplantation. Arch. Intern. Med., 124:282, 1969.
30. Haust, M. D., Landing, B. H., Holmstrand, D., Currarino, G., and Smith, B. X.: Osteosclerosis of renal disease in children. Comparative pathologic and radiographic studies. Am. J. Pathol., 44:141, 1964.
31. Jaffe, H. L., Bodansky, A., and Chandler, J. P.: Ammonium chloride decalcification, as modified by calcium intake. The relation between generalized osteoporosis and ostitis fibrosa. J. Exp. Med., 56:669, 1930.
32. Jarrett, W. A., Peters, H. L., and Pappenheimer, A. M.: Parathyroid enlargement in rats following experimental reduction of kidney substance. Proc. Soc. Exp. Biol. Med., 32:1211, 1935.
33. Kaye, M., Pritchard, J. E., Halpenny, G. W., and Light, W.: Bone disease in chronic renal failure with particular reference to osteosclerosis. Medicine, 39:157, 1960.
34. Kristiansen, J. H., and Pedersen, V. F.: Treatment of hypophosphataemic vitamin D-resistant rickets (letter). Arch. Dis. Child, 56:76, 1981.
35. Lalli, A. F., and Lapides, J.: Osteosclerosis occurring in renal disease. A.J.R., 93:924, 1965.
36. Lanfmead, F. S., and Orr, J. W.: Renal rickets associated with parathyroid hyperplasia. Arch. Dis. Child., 8:265, 1933.
37. Lightwood, R., and Butler, N. R.: Decline in primary infantile renal acidosis. Aetiological implications. Br. Med. J., 534:855, 1963.
38. Loeffler, R. D., Jr., and Sherman, F. C.: The effect of treatment on growth and deformity in hypophosphatemic vitamin D-resistant rickets. Clin. Orthop., 162:4, 1982.
38a. Lowe, C. V., Terry, M., and MacLachlan, E. A.: Organic aciduria, decreased from renal ammonia production, hydrophthalmus, and mental retardation. Am. J. Dis. Child., 83:164, 1952.
39. Lucas, R. C.: On a form of late rickets associated with albuminuria. Rickets of adolescents. Lancet, 1:933, 1883.
40. Lumb, G. A., Mawer, E. B., and Stanbury, S. W.: The apparent vitamin-D resistance of chronic renal failure. Am. J. Med., 50:421, 1971.
41. Lyles, K. W., Clark, A. G., and Drezner, M. K.: Serum 1,25-dihydroxyvitamin D levels in subjects with X-linked hypophosphatemic rickets and osteomalacia. Calcif. Tissue Int., 34:125, 1982.
42. Lyes, K. W., Harrelson, J. M., and Drezner, M. K.: The efficacy of vitamin D2 and oral phosphorus therapy in X-linked hypophosphatemic rickets and osteomalacia. J. Clin. Endocrinol. Metab., 54:307, 1982.
43. McNair, S. L., and Stickler, G. B.: Growth in familial hypophosphatemic vitamin-D resistant rickets. N. Engl. J. Med., 281:511, 1969.
44. Mankin, H. J.: Rickets, osteomalacia, and renal osteodystrophy. Part I. J. Bone Joint Surg., 56-A:101, 1974.
45. Mankin, H. J.: Rickets, osteomalacia and renal osteodystrophy. Part II. J. Bone Joint Surg., 56-A:352, 1974.
46. Marie, P. J., and Glorieux, F. H.: Stimulation of cortical bone mineralization and remodeling by phosphate and 1,25-dihydroxyvitamin D in vitamin-D resistant rickets. Metab. Bone Dis. Relat. Res., 3:159, 1981.
47. Mason, R. S., Rohl, P. G., Lissner, D., and Posen, S.: Vitamin D metabolism in hypophosphatemic rickets. Am. J. Dis. Child., 136:909, 1982.
48. Mehls, O., Ritz, E., Kreusser, W., and Krempien, B.: Renal osteodystrophy in uraemic children. Clin. Endocrinol. Metab., 9:151, 1980.
49. Mitchell, A. G.: Nephrosclerosis (chronic interstitial nephritis) in childhood, with special reference to renal rickets. Am. J. Dis. Child., 40:101, 1930.
50. Morgan, B.: Osteomalacia, Renal Osteodystrophy and Osteoporosis. Springfield, Thomas, 1973.
51. Ogura, Y., Imamura, N., and Tsukui, I.: Disorders of calcium and phosphorus metabolism in Fanconi syndrome and renal tubular acidosis. Nippon Rinsho, 40:2680, 1982.
52. Pappenheimer, A. M., and Wilens, S. L.: Enlargement of the parathyroid glands in renal disease. Am. J. Pathol., 11:73, 1935.
53. Parfitt, A. M.: Renal osteodystrophy. Orthop. Clin. North Am., 3:681, 1972.
54. Pederson, H. E., and McCarroll, H. R.: Vitamin-resistant rickets. J. Bone Joint Surg., 33-A:203, 1951.
55. Pellegrino, E. D., and Blitz, R. M.: The composition of bone in uremia. Observations on the reservoir function of bone and demonstration of a labile fraction of bone carbonate. Medicine, 44:397, 1965.
56. Pierce, D. S., Wallace, W. M., and Herndon, C. H.: Long-term treatment of vitamin D-resistant rickets. J. Bone Joint Surg., 46-A:978, 1964.
57. Pollak, V. E., Schneider, A. F., Freund, G., and Kark, R. M.: Chronic renal disease with secondary hyperparathyroidism. Arch. Intern. Med., 103:200, 1959.
58. Rasmussen, H., Pechet, M., Anast, C., Mazur, A., Gertner, J., and Broadus, A. E.: Long-term treatment of familial hypophosphatemic rickets with oral phosphate and 1 alpha-hydroxyvitamin D3. J. Pediatr., 99:16, 1981.
59. Ryan, W. G., Nibbe, A. F., Schwartz, R. B., and Ray, R. D.: Fibrous dysplasia of bone with vitamin D resistant rickets: A case study. Metabolism, 17:988, 1968.
60. Sagy, M., Birenbaum, E., Balin, A., Orda, S., Barzilay, Z., and Brish, M.: Phosphate-depletion syndrome in a premature infant fed human milk. J. Pediatr., 96:683, 1980.
60a. Saville, P. D., Nassim, J. R., and Stevenson, F. H.: Osteomalacia in von Recklinghausen's neurofibromatosis: Metabolic study of a case. Br. Med. J., 1:1311, 1955.
61. Schoen, E. J.: Growth in familial hypophosphatemic rickets. N. Engl. J. Med., 281:1195, 1969.
62. Schoen, E. J., and Reynolds, J. B.: Severe familial hypophosphatemic rickets. Normal growth following early treatment. Am. J. Dis. Child., 120:58, 1970.
63. Shea, D., and Mankin, H. J.: Slipped capital femoral epiphysis in renal rickets. Report of three cases. J. Bone Joint Surg., 48-A:349, 1966.
64. Short, E. M., Binder, H. J., and Rosenberg, L. E.: Familial hypophosphatemic rickets: Defective transport of inorganic phosphate by intestinal mucosa. Science, 179:700, 1973.
65. Stanbury, S. W., and Lumb, G. A.: Metabolic studies of renal osteodystrophy. I. Calcium, phosphorus and nitrogen metabolism in rickets, osteomalacia and hyperparathyroidism complicating chronic uremia and in the osteomalacia of the adult Fanconi syndrome. Medicine, 41:1, 1962.
65a. Swischuk, L. E., and Hayden, C. K.: Rickets: A roentgenographic scheme for diagnosis. Pediatr. Radiol., 8:203, 1979.
66. Weller, M., Edeikin, J., and Hodes, P. J.: Renal osteodystrophy. A.J.R., 104:354, 1968.
67. West, C. D., Blanton, J. C., Silverman, F. N., and Holland, N. H.: Use of phosphate salts as an adjunct to vitamin D in the treatment of hypophosphatemic vitamin D refractory rickets. J. Pediatr., 64:469, 1964.
68. Willis, M. R.: Biochemical Consequences of Chronic Renal Failure. Hallsbury, Harvey, Miller, Metcalf, 1971.

69. Wolf, H. L., and Denko, J. V.: Osteosclerosis in chronic renal disease. Am. J. Med. Sci., 235:3, 1958.
70. Yendt, E. R., Connor, T. B., and Howard, J. E.: In vitro calcification of rachitic rat cartilage in normal and pathological human sera with some observations on the pathogenesis of renal rickets. Bull. Johns Hopkins Hosp., 96:1, 1955.
71. Zimmerman, H. B.: Osteosclerosis in chronic renal disease. Report of 4 cases associated with secondary hyperparathyroidism. A.J.R., 88:1152, 1962.

SCURVY

The clinical manifestations of scurvy have been well depicted in the pages of history. One of the earliest accounts is that of Joinville's *Chronicle of the Crusade of St. Louis, in 1250*.[17] In 1757 James Lind published a "Treatise on the Scurvy," recommending the inclusion of lemon juice in naval diets.[24]

In children, scurvy was mistaken for rickets until 1883, when Sir Thomas Barlow distinguished between the two conditions.[3] Not infrequently, scurvy in children is referred to as "Barlow's disease." That the guinea pig could be rendered scorbutic was discovered by Holst and Frolich, who also demonstrated that boiling fresh vegetables could destroy their preventive power.[18] Vitamin C was chemically identified by Szent-Gyorgi.[36]

Pathology

Skeletal changes in scurvy have been studied in the bones of both animals and humans.[1, 12, 16, 18, 37] Ascorbic acid deficiency causes a dysfunction of the osteoblasts; this has been ascribed by Follis to a loss of ribose nucleic acid and the disappearance of phosphatase and cystochrome oxidase activity in the cytoplasm of osteoblasts.[12] The result is a failure to produce osteoid tissue and form new bone. The chondroblasts, however, continue to proliferate normally, align in columns, and form chondroid tissue. There is no disturbance in mineralization; the degenerating cartilage columns calcify normally, but are not converted into bone. A broad zone of calcified chondroid is produced by the persisting cartilage cells, which accumulate in great numbers and are pushed toward the metaphysis. In the radiogram this calcified cartilage appears as a densely opaque thick white shadow immediately to the diaphyseal side of the epiphyseal plate (Fraenkel's line).

Generalized osteoporosis results from lack of formation of osteoid tissue and new bone. Osteoclasts are normal, and resorption continues. The plump osteoblasts become flattened, resembling connective tissue fibroblasts. The bone trabeculae and the cortices of long bones are thin and fragile.

Hemorrhages and fractures from minimal injury are common; the attempt at repair is disorderly. The provisional zone of calcification is fragile, and complete separation of the epiphyses may occur. Collagen synthesis is interfered with in ascorbic acid deficiency. Instead of normal collagenized fibrous tissue, a primitive type of connective tissue is formed. In the teeth, lack of dentin formation from the odontoblasts corresponds to the failure of osteoid formation from the osteoblasts.

In protracted scurvy in guinea pigs, Banks demonstrated a suppression of the entire growth zone leading eventually to complete cessation of enchondral ossification.[1] The scorbutic bone lesions in young guinea pigs are similiar to those in the human child, except that calcified cartilage cells do not accumulate in the metaphysis as a "lattice" because chondrocyte growth is more markedly inhibited in the guinea pig than in man.

Clinical Features

Scurvy develops following 6 to 12 months of vitamin C deficiency in the diet. Early manifestations consist of a loss of appetite, irritability, and a slow gain in weight. With the progression of scurvy the typical scorbutic signs appear.[17] Hemorrhage of the gums, particularly about the upper incisors, is common. The gingival mucous membrane is swollen and bluish purple in color. Subperiosteal hemorrhage is another distinctive sign, the lower ends of the femur, tibia, and humerus being frequent sites. The affected limbs are tender on palpation. The infant screams with pain when being lifted from his crib or when his diaper is being changed. His facies is very apprehensive, and he prefers to lie supine in frog-leg position—a pseudoparalytic posture in response to pain. The legs are swollen and edematous. Spontaneous epiphyseal separation may take place.[29, 33, 34] "Beading" of the ribs at costochondral junctions may develop. The sternum may be depressed. Hemorrhages may occur in subcutaeous tissues, in or between the muscles, in the urinary or gastrointestinal tract, or in the subchondral space. The capillary resistance test is positive. Anemia and delayed wound healing are common.

Radiographic Findings

The radiographic changes are best visualized at the knees, wrists, proximal ends of the

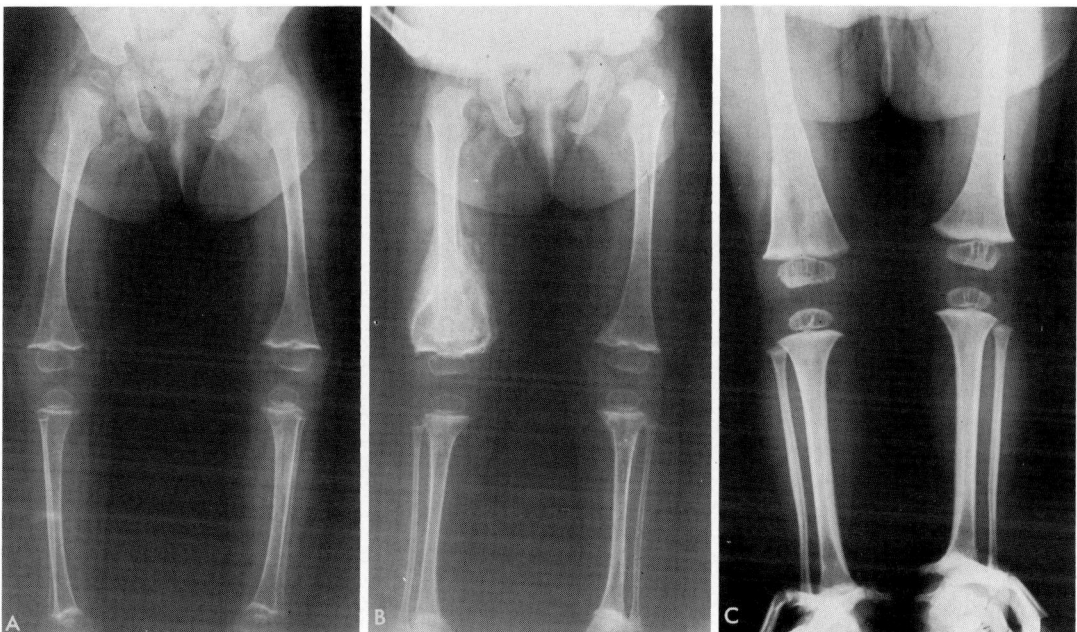

FIGURE 3-115. *Scurvy in a ten-month-old infant.*

A. Anteroposterior radiograms of both lower limbs demonstrate early changes in the scorbutic bones. Note the generalized osteoporosis with rarefaction of the spongiosa and atrophy of the cortex. There is relatively increased opacity of the provisional zones of calcification at the ends of the metaphyses and around the margins of the epiphyseal centers of ossification ("ringing of the epiphyses"). **B.** Two weeks after treatment with ascorbic acid, marked calcification of subperiosteal hematoma of the right femur has occurred. Such minimal calcification is also evident in the medial aspects of the distal left femoral shaft and proximal left tibia. Note the multiple metaphyseal spur formation. **C.** Three months later there are further radiographic signs of healing scurvy. The cortices have become thicker and the spongiosa are of almost normal density. Note the persistence of rarefaction in the epiphyseal centers.

humerus, and costochondral junctions—sites of rapid bone growth. The initial picture is that of generalized osteoporosis of the spongiosa and thinning of the cortex. Atrophy takes place in the metaphyses, epiphyseal centers of ossification, and diaphyses. With the normal formation and calcification and the failure of resorption of the calcified cartilaginous matrix, there is increased width and opacity of the zone of provisional calcification at the ends of the metaphyses (Fraenkel's line) and around the margins of the epiphyseal centers of ossification ("ringing of the epiphyses") (Fig. 3–115 A). Lateral spur formation at the ends of the metaphysis is produced by the outward projection of the zone of provisional calcification, beyond the limits of the shaft, and by new bone formation under the raised periosteum at that angle (Fig. 3–115 B). The "scurvy line," or the so-called "scorbutic zone," is seen as a transverse band of diminished density adjacent to the dense provisional zone. The "corner," or "angle," sign of scurvy is a peripheral metaphyseal cleft due to a defect in the spongiosa and cortex just adjacent to the provisional zone of calcification.

Subperiosteal hematomas may occur at any site, but most commonly occur over the femora, tibiae, and humeri. They are seen as local increases in the soft-tissue density.

Upon administration of ascorbic acid, the subperiosteal hemorrhage calcifies (see Fig. 3–115 B). Soon the cortex thickens, and the osteoporosis of the spongiosa diminishes. With growth the thickened zone of provisional calcification recedes from the epiphyseal plate. Central areas of rarefaction in the epiphyses may persist for years (Fig. 3–115 C).

Diagnosis

The pain, local tenderness, and pseudoparalysis of acute scurvy may suggest acute osteomyelitis, septic arthritis, or acute poliomyelitis. Hematologic disorders, such as Henoch-Schönlein purpura, thrombocytopenic purpura, and leukemia, are other conditions to consider in the differential diagnosis. Syphilis may be suspected, but it occurs at an earlier age, and other stigmata of lues will be present. Rheumatic fever is very rare under two years of age.

The typical radiographic findings and a history of poor intake of ascorbic acid combined with the characteristic clinical picture will establish the diagnosis of scurvy. Laboratory tests for levels of ascorbic acid are usually not useful. A fasting serum level of vitamin C of over 0.6 mg. per 100 ml. will rule out scurvy; a lowered level of vitamin C does not, however, indicate its deficiency. An absence of vitamin C in the white cell platelet layer of centrifuged oxalated blood is a more reliable index.

Treatment

Rapid recovery occurs following daily oral or parenteral administration of 100 to 200 mg. of vitamin C. Pain and tenderness will disappear, subperiosteal hemorrhages will gradually subside, and body growth will resume.

Scurvy is prevented by an adequate intake of vitamin C (50 mg. per day for infants and children, 75 to 100 mg. per day for adults). The human body tolerates vitamin C well, and massive doses have not resulted in intoxication or in any pathologic state.

References

1. Banks, S. W.: Bone changes in acute and chronic scurvy; experimental study. J. Bone Joint Surg., 25:553, 1943.
2. Barlow, T.: On cases described as "acute rickets" which are probably a combination of scurvy and rickets, the scurvy being an essential, and the rickets a variable, element. Med. Chir. Trans., 48:159, 1883.
3. Barlow, T.: Infantile scurvy and its relation to rickets. Lancet, 2:1075, 1894.
4. Bartley, W., Krebs, H. A., and O'Brien, J. R. P.: Vitamin C requirements of human adults. Spec. Rep. Ser. Med. Res. Counc., London, No. 280, 1953.
5. Beraud, C., Sobotska, F., and Cret, M.: Scorbut osseux chez un nourisson de 11 mois. Evolution radiologique. J. Radiol. Electrol., 56:527, 1975.
6. Bourne, G. H.: Vitamin C and bone. In Bourne, G. H. (ed.): The Biochemistry and Physiology of Bone. London, Academic Press, 1956, Chap. 18, p. 539.
7. Brailsford, J. W.: Some radiological manifestations of early scurvy. Arch. Dis. Child., 28:31, 1953.
8. Bromer, R. S.: A critical analysis of the roentgen signs of infantile scurvy. A.J.R., 49:575, 1943.
9. Burns, R. R.: The unusual occurrence of scurvy in an eight week old infant. A.J.R., 89:923, 1963.
10. Douglas, N. L., Liakakos, D., and Vlachos, P.: Scurvy in a 4 year old child. Am. J. Dis. Child., 126:712, 1973.
11. Evans, P. R.: Infantile scurvy: The centenary of Barlow's disease. Br. Med. J., 287:1862, 1983.
12. Follis, R. H.: Histochemical studies on cartilage and bone. II. Ascorbic acid deficiency. Bull. Johns Hopkins Hosp., 89:9, 1951.
13. Follis, R. H., Jr., Jackson, B., and Park, E. A.: Prevalence of scurvy at autopsy during the first two years of life. Bull. Johns Hopkins Hosp., 87:569, 1950.
14. Greuar, D.: Scurvy and its prevention by vitamin C fortified evaporated milk. Can. Med. Assoc. J., 80:977, 1959.
15. Gross, J.: Studies on the formation of collagen. IV. Effect of vitamin C deficiency on the neutral salt-extractable collagen of the skin. J. Exp. Med., 109:557, 1959.
16. Ham, A. W., and Elliott, H. C.: The bone and cartilage lesions of protracted moderate scurvy. Am. J. Pathol., 14:323, 1938.
17. Hess, A. F.: Scurvy, Past and Present. Philadelphia, Lippincott, 1920.
18. Holst, A., and Frolich, T.: Experimental studies relating to ship beri-beri and scurvy. II. On the etiology of scurvy. J. Hyg., 7:634, 1907.
19. Ingalls, T. H.: Ascorbic acid requirements in early infancy. N. Engl. J. Med., 218:872, 1938.
20. Kato, K.: Critique of the roentgen signs of a infantile scurvy. Radiology, 18:1096, 1932.
21. Lee, R. V.: Scurvy: A contemporary historical perspective. Conn. Med., 47:629, 1983.
22. Lee, R. V.: Scurvy: A contemporary historical perspective. Conn. Med., 47:703, 1983.
23. Lee, R. V.: Scurvy: A contemporary historical perspective. Conn. Med., 48:33, 1984.
24. Lind, J.: A Treatise on the Scurvy. 2nd Ed. London, Millar, 1757.
25. MacLean, A. D.: Spinal changes in a case of infantile scurvy. Br. J. Radiol., 41:385, 1968.
26. McKibbon, B., and Porter, R. W.: The incidence of vitamin-C deficiency in meningomyelocele. Dev. Med. Child. Neurol., 9:338, 1967.
27. McLean, S., and McIntosh, R.: Healing in infantile scurvy as shown by x-ray. Am. J. Dis. Child., 36:875, 1928.
28. Meiklejohn, A. P.: The physiology and biochemistry of ascorbic acid. Vitam. Horm., 11:61, 1953.
29. Nerubay, J., and Pilderwasser, D.: Spontaneous bilateral distal femoral physiolysis due to scurvy. Acta Orthop. Scand., 55:18, 1984.
30. Ossofsky, H. J.: Infantile scurvy. Am. J. Dis. Child., 109:173, 1965.
31. Park, E. A., Guild, H. G., Jackson, D., and Bond, M.: Recognition of scurvy, with especial reference to the early x-ray changes. Arch. Dis. Child., 10:265, 1935.
32. Ruffa, G., Cottafave, F., Bonioli, E., Mangiante, G., and Matterella, F.: Lo scorbuto conclamato in eta pediatrica. An cora due casi. Minerva Pediatr., 35:885, 1983.
33. Silverman, F. N.: An unusual osseous sequel to infantile scurvy. J. Bone Joint Surg., 35-A:215, 1953.
34. Silverman, F. N.: Recovery from epiphyseal invagination: Sequal to an unusual complication of scurvy. J. Bone Joint Surg., 52-A:384, 1970.
35. Sprague, P. L.: Epiphyseo-metaphyseal cupping following infantile scurvy. Pediatr. Radiol., 4:122, 1976.
36. Szent-Gyorgi, A.: Identification of vitamin C. Nature, 131:225, 1933.
37. Wollbach, S. B., and Bessey, O. A.: Tissue changes in vitamin deficiencies. Physiol. Rev., 22:233, 1942.

HYPERVITAMINOSIS A

Vitamin A is a fat-soluble vitamin whose primary biologic functions are concerned with skeletal growth, maintenance and regeneration of epithelial tissues, and preservation of visual purple in the retina. It is also necessary for membrane stability. The chemistry and metabolism of vitamin A are not discussed here; they are comprehensively set forth in the symposium by Karrer.[19] The normal level of vitamin A in human plasma is between 80 and 100 international units (I.U.) per 100 ml.

Experimental studies of the toxic effects of vitamin A have shown bone and cartilage to be predilected target tissues. Using radioactive sulfate, McElligott demonstrated that vitamin A disturbs the metabolism of chondrocytes and interferes with the synthesis of chondroitin sulfate.[22] Fell and associates' research into its effect on bone in organ cultures suggested that the chondrocytes most probably synthesize an enzyme that forms a soluble sulfated mucopolysaccharide instead of chondroitin sulfate.[13, 14]

Administration of excessive amounts of vitamin A causes rats to develop abnormal fragility of bone.[25] This proclivity to fracture is the result of increased osteoclasis stimulated by the large dosage of the vitamin.[2] In dogs, the excess causes premature closure of the epiphyseal plate.[41]

The orthopedist is mainly interested in the skeletal manifestations of excessive administration of vitamin A.

Clinical and Radiographic Findings

Hypervitaminosis A in human beings is rare, and the osseous lesions produced are quite dissimilar to those seen in animals. Skeletal changes in children develop when there is chronic overdosage of vitamin A (100,000 units or more daily) for six months or more. Consequently, bone lesions are not encountered in infants under 12 months of age. In hypervitaminosis A, there is periosteal hyperostosis and thickening of the cortex of certain long bones (Fig. 3–116). The ulna, radius, metacarpals, and metatarsals are particularly affected. The mandible and other facial bones, however, are not

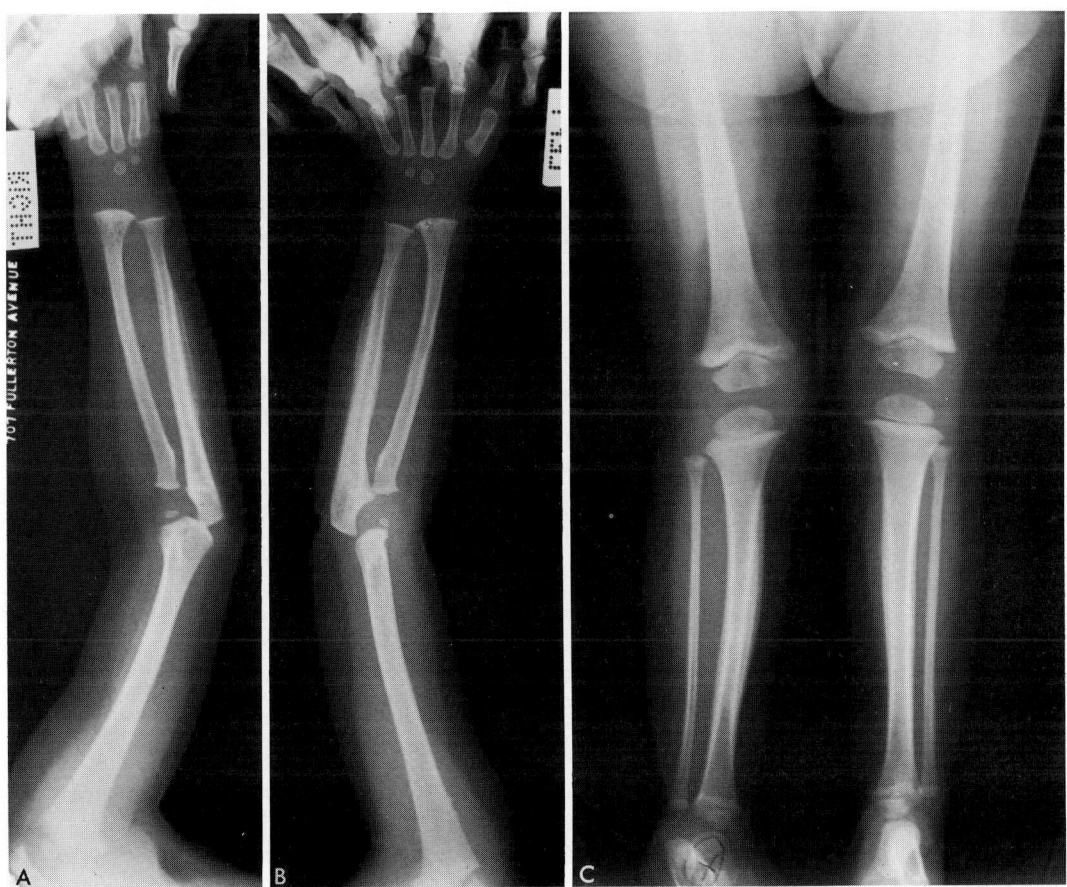

FIGURE 3–116. Hypervitaminosis A in a two-year-old child.

Note the subperiosteal new bone formation and cortical thickening of both tibiae and both ulnae. The mandible and other facial bones are not affected. **A** and **B**. Radiograms of right and left forearms. **C**. Radiogram of both lower limbs.

involved, a finding that distinguishes this condition from infantile cortical hyperostosis. Clinically, the soft tissues over the hyperostotic bones are swollen and tender. Proliferation of basal cells and hyperkeratinization cause dry and itchy skin. Anorexia, vomiting, and lethargy are caused by increased intracranial pressure.[11, 27] The child fails to thrive.

Hepatosplenomegaly with cirrhosis-like liver damage or splenomegaly may be present. Premature partial or complete closure of the physis causes growth retardation.[28, 34]

Radiograms will disclose increased density of the cortices of the affected bones and a varying degree of subperiosteal new bone formation as shown in Figure 3–116. Bone scanning with technetium-99m will show increased uptake over the involved bones.

Hypervitaminosis A must be distinguished from congenital syphilis, scurvy with calcified subperiosteal hematoma, and infantile cortical hyperostosis.

Diagnosis and Treatment

The diagnosis is established on determination of the plasma level of vitamin A, which will be elevated to 5 to 15 times the normal value. Hypercalcemia can be present.[15] Treatment consists of total cessation of administration of vitamin A, including all food elements that may contain it, such as butter, milk, animal liver, and fish oils, as well as certain green vegetables and fruits that are carotenoid precursors. Because of the great body reserves of vitamin A, the hyperostosis will disappear only after a long period of time, although other symptoms will subside rapidly. Growth of the long bones should be followed; early closure of the growth plates will not become manifest until years after the initial insult.

Measures should be taken to prevent vitamin A intoxication. The general public can buy over-the-counter multiple vitamin preparations containing more than the recommended daily dosage (3000 I.U. in children and 5000 I.U. in adults). Preparations containing more than 5000 I.U. per dose should be dispensed only by prescription.

Retinoids and synthesized retinoid congeners (13-cis-retinoic acid) are used in a variety of keratinizing dermatologic disorders (such as ichthyosis) and cystic acne. These drugs are chemically similiar to vitamin A and can cause skeletal hyperostosis and premature fusion of growth plates.[24, 29]

References

1. Arena, J. M., Sarazen, P., and Baylin, C. J.: Hypervitaminosis A. Pediatrics, 8:788, 1951.
2. Barnicot, N. A.: Local action of vitamin A on bone. J. Anat., 84:374, 1950.
3. Bernhardt, I. B., and Dorsey, D. J.: Hypervitaminosis A and congenital renal anomalies in a human infant. Obstet. Gynecol., 43:750, 1974.
4. Caffey, J.: Chronic poisoning due to excess of vitamin A. Description of clinical and roentgen manifestations in seven infants and young children. A.J.R., 65:12, 1951.
5. Clark, I.: Effects of hypervitaminosis A and D on skeletal metabolism. J. Biol. Chem., 239:1266, 1964.
6. Clark, L., and Seawright, A. A.: Long bone abnormalities in kittens following vitamin A administration. J. Comp. Pathol., 80:113, 1970.
7. DiBenedetto, R. J.: Chronic hypervitaminosis A in an adult. J.A.M.A., 201:700, 1967.
8. Dingle, J. T.: Studies on the mode of action of excess vitamin A. 3. Release of a bound protease by the action of vitamin A. Biochem. J., 79:509, 1961.
9. Dingle, J. T., Lucy, J. A., and Fell, H. B.: Studies on the mode of action of excess vitamin A. 1. Effect of excess of vitamin A on the metabolism and composition of embryonic chick-limb cartilage grown in organ culture. Biochem. J., 79:497, 1961.
10. Drablos, A., and Slordahl, J.: Chronic vitamin A poisoning. Acta Paediatr., 48:507, 1959.
11. Feldman, M. H., and Schlezinger, N. S.: Benign intracranial hypertension associated with hypervitaminosis A. Arch. Neurol., 27:1, 170.
12. Fell, H. B., and Mellamby, E.: Effects of hypervitaminosis A on foetal mouse bones cultivated in vitro. Br. Med. J., 2:535, 1950.
13. Fell, H. B., Dingle, J. T., and Webb, M.: Studies on the mode of action of vitamin A: IV. Specificity of effect of embryonic chick limb cartilage in culture and on isolated rat-liver lysosomes. Biochem. J., 83:63, 1962.
14. Fell, H. B., Mellamby, E., and Pele, R.: The influence of excess of vitamin A on the sulfate metabolism of bone rudiments grown in vitro. J. Physiol., 134:179, 1956.
15. Fisher, G., and Skillern, P. G.: Hypercalcemia due to hypervitaminosis A. J.A.M.A., 227:1413, 1974.
16. Frame, B., Jackson, C. E., Reynolds, W. A., and Umphrey, J. E.: Hypercalcemia and skeletal effects in chronic hypervitaminosis A. Ann. Intern. Med., 80:44, 1974.
17. Joseph, H. W.: Hypervitaminosis A and carotenemia. Am. J. Dis. Child., 67:33, 1944.
18. Jowsey, J., and Riggs, B. L.: Bone changes in a patient with hypervitaminosis A. J. Clin. Endocrinol., 28:1833, 1968.
19. Karrer, P.: Symposium on vitamin A and metabolism. Vitam. Horm., 18:291, 1960.
20. Knudson, A. G., and Rothman, P. E.: Hypervitaminosis A. Am. J. Dis. Child., 85:316, 1953.
21. Lippe, B., Hensen, L., Mendoza, G., Finerman, M., and Welch, M.: Chronic vitamin A intoxication. A multisystem disease that could reach epidemic proportion. Am. J. Dis. Child., 135:634, 1981.
22. McElligott, T. F.: Decreased fixation of sulfate (SO) chondrocytes in hypervitaminosis A. J. Pathol. Bacteriol., 83:347, 1962.
23. Mahoney, C. P., Margolis, M. T., Knauss, T. A., and Labbe, R. F.: Chronic vitamin A intoxication in infants fed chicken liver. Pediatrics, 65:893, 1980.
24. Milstone, L. M., McGuire, J., and Ablow, R. C.: Premature epiphyseal closure in a child receiving oral 13-cis-retinoic acid. J. Med. Acad. Dermatol., 7:663, 1982.

25. Moore, T., and Wang, Y. L.: Hypervitaminosis A. Biochem. J., *39*:222, 1945.
26. Oliver, T. K., Jr.: Chronic vitamin A intoxication. Report of a case in an older child and review of the literature. Am. J. Dis. Child., *95*:57, 1958.
27. Pasquariello, P. S., Schut, L., and Borns, P.: Benign increased intracranial hypertension due to chronic vitamin A overdose in a 26-month-old child. Clin. Pediatr., *16*:379, 1977.
28. Pease, C. N.: Focal retardation and arrestment of growth of bones due to vitamin A intoxication. J.A.M.A., *182*:980, 1962.
29. Pennes, D. R., Ellis, C. N., Madison, K. C., Voorhees, J. J., and Martel, W.: Early skeletal hyperostosis secondary to 13-cis-retinoic acid. A.J.R., *141*:979, 1984.
30. Persson, B., Tunell, R., and Ekengren, K.: Chronic vitamin A intoxication during first half year of life. Description of five cases. Acta Paediatr., *54*:49, 1965.
31. Pickup, J. D.: Hypervitaminosis A. Arch. Dis. Child., *31*:229, 1956.
32. Pittsley, R. A., and Yoder, F. W.: Retinoid hyperostosis. Skeletal toxicity associated with long-term administration of 13-cis-retinoic acid for refractory ichthyosis. N. Engl. J. Med., *308*:1012, 1983.
33. Rubin, E., Florman, A. L., Degnan, T., and Diaz, J.: Hepatic injury in chronic hypervitaminosis A. Am. J. Dis. Child., *119*:132, 1970.
34. Ruby, L. K., and Mital, M. A.: Skeletal deformities following chronic hypervitaminosis A. A case report. J. Bone Joint Surg., *56-A*:1283, 1974.
35. Searwright, A. A., English, P. B., and Gartner, R. J. W.: Hypervitaminosis A and hyperostosis of the cat. Nature, *206*:1171, 1965.
36. Seibert, J. J., Byrne, W. J., and Golladay, E. S.: Development of hypervitaminosis A in a patient on long-term parenteral hyperalimentation. Pediatr. Radiol., *10*:173, 1981.
37. Soler-Bechara, J., and Soscia, J. L.: Chronic hypervitaminosis A. Report of a case in an adult. Arch. Intern. Med., *112*:462, 1963.
38. Toomey, J. A., and Morissette, R. A.: Case report. Hypervitaminosis A. Am. J. Dis. Child., *73*:473, 1947.
39. Voorhees, J. J., and Orfanos, C. E.: Oral retinoids: Broad spectrum dermatologic therapy for the 1980's. Arch. Dermatol., *117*:478, 1981.
40. Wason, S., and Lovejoy, F. H., Jr.: Vitamin A toxicity. Am. J. Dis. Child., *136*:174, 1982.
41. Wolbach, S. B.: Vitamin A deficiency and excess in relation to skeletal growth. J. Bone Joint Surg., *29*:171, 1947.
42. Wolke, R. E., Eaton, H. D., Nielson, S. W., and Hemboldt, C. F.: Qualitative and quantitative osteoblastic activity in chronic porcine hypervitaminosis A. J. Pathol., *97*:677, 1969.
43. Woodard, W. K., Miller, L. J., and Legant, O.: Acute and chronic hypervitaminosis in a 4-month-old infant. J. Pediatr., *59*:260, 1961.

HYPERVITAMINOSIS D

The toxic effects of excessive vitamin D were shown first by Harris and Stewart in young rats, and later by Harris in humans.[19, 20] In the past, vitamin D intoxication was not uncommon, as it was customary to treat arthritis, psoriasis, skin tuberculosis, and chilblains with large doses. The incidence of hypervitaminosis D declined, however, when the vitamin's lack of effectiveness in the treatment of these diseases was demonstrated, and as the medical profession's awareness of its toxic effects increased.

At present, hypervitaminosis D occurs as a complication of treatment of vitamin D–refractory rickets with large doses of the vitamin.

Susceptibility of children to vitamin D varies. To determine definitely what would constitute a toxic dose, the daily dosage, the duration of treatment, and the intake of calcium must all be considered. A dosage of 2000 I.U. per day or 2,000,000 I.U. per month is dangerous. Hypervitaminosis D usually arises from excess intake of ergocalciferol (vitamin D_2) and cholecalciferol (vitamin D_3).

The effect of vitamin D is to enhance the absorption of calcium from the intestinal wall and elevate the serum calcium level. The resultant hypercalcemia is followed by hypercalciuria and excessive urinary phosphate secretion.

Pathology

Histologically, wide osteoid seams are found around the trabeculae, suggesting rickets.[18] The physis, however, is normal and well calcified. The osteoid seams are probably the result of normal functioning of the osteoblasts, which form abundant matrix at a period when the dynamics of calcium metabolism tend to mobilize calcium from bone rather than to deposit it.

Metastatic calcification may be found in the kidneys, arteries, thyroid, pancreas, lungs, stomach, and brain. Deposition of calcium salts in the kidneys and degenerative changes in the arteries are the more serious pathologic changes.

Clinical Findings

Anorexia, constipation, nausea and vomiting, polyuria, and thirst are the early clinical manifestations. The child feels very tired and has no energy. Soon mental depression and stupor develop, simulating encephalitis. Renal failure and arterial hypertension are common.

Radiographic Findings

The long bones disclose dense metaphyseal bands due to an increase in the proximal zone of calcification (Fig. 3–117). The diaphyses show increased rarefaction due to demineralization of the skeleton. Osteosclerosis is clearly visible at the base and vault of the skull. Craniostenosis may result from premature fusion of sutures. Vertebral end-plates become dense. Metastatic calcifications are seen in soft tissues (Fig. 3–117 A and C).

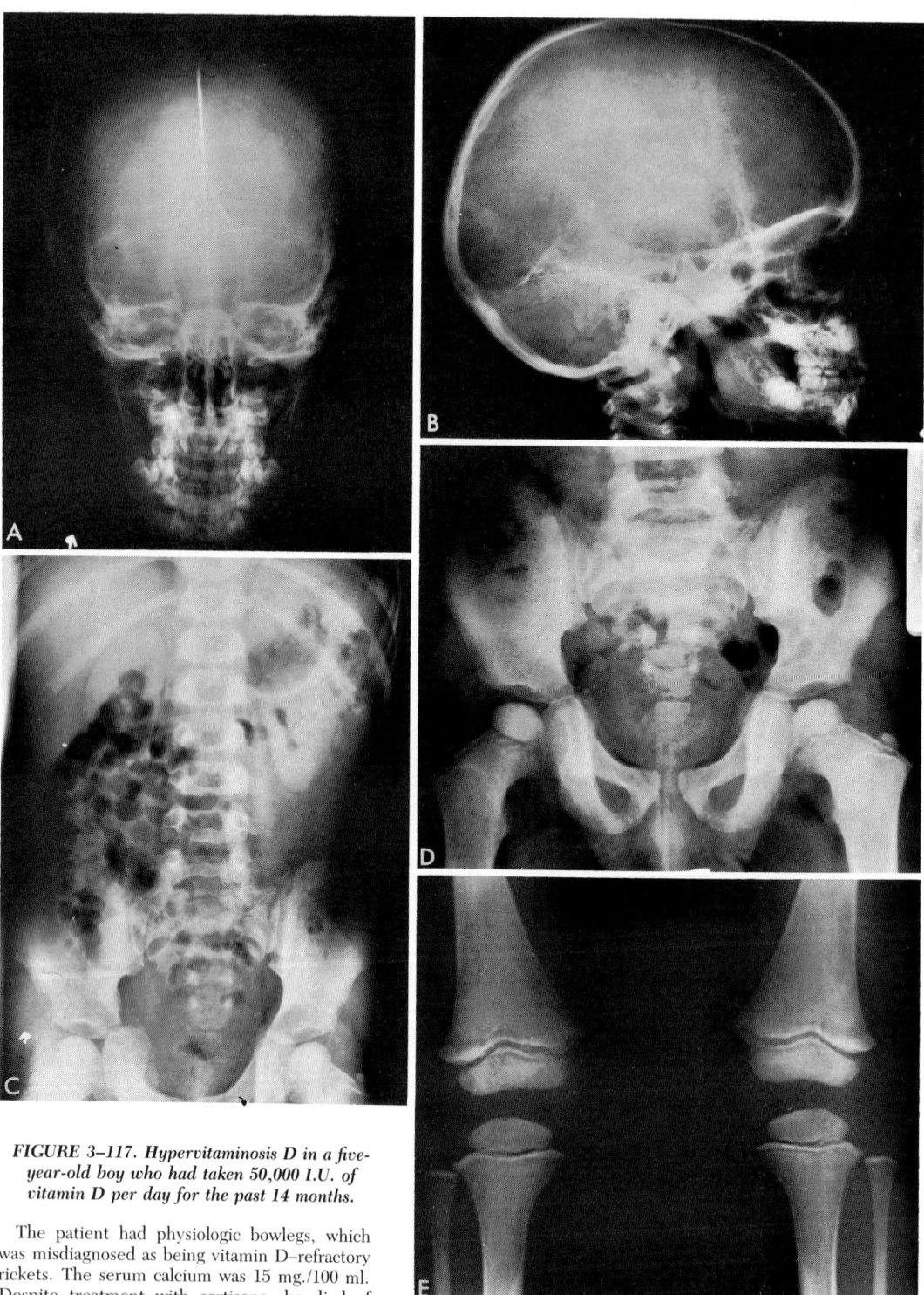

FIGURE 3–117. Hypervitaminosis D in a five-year-old boy who had taken 50,000 I.U. of vitamin D per day for the past 14 months.

The patient had physiologic bowlegs, which was misdiagnosed as being vitamin D–refractory rickets. The serum calcium was 15 mg./100 ml. Despite treatment with cortisone, he died of renal failure and arterial hypertension. **A** and **B.** Anteroposterior and lateral views of skull showing metastatic calcification of the cerebral and cerebellar falces. **C.** Anteroposterior view of spine showing metastatic calcification of the kidneys. **D** and **E.** Anteroposterior views of both hips and lower limbs. Note the increased radiopacity of metaphyses.

Laboratory Findings

The level of plasma calcium is elevated, reaching as high as 15 mg. per 100 ml. The serum phosphate level is usually normal, and the plasma phosphatase activity is usually diminished.

Treatment

Administration of vitamin D is discontinued promptly, and the ingestion of calcium is diminished to a minimum. Sodium sulfate may be given orally or parenterally to inhibit absorption of calcium from the intestinal tract. EDTA infusion is usually not indicated.

Cortisone is effective in treatment of the hypercalcemia of vitamin D poisoning; it is given until the serum calcium level is lowered to normal. Cortisone and vitamin D seem to compete in some metabolic process, but the exact mechanism of the action is yet unknown.

Dehydration and electrolyte imbalance should be corrected immediately, as they may be serious and cause death.

If the condition is diagnosed and treated early, the prognosis is good, although vitamin D action continues for some time, as it is stored in the body. Within seven to ten days, nausea and anorexia subside, and the metastatic calcium deposits gradually resorb. If the condition is recognized late, permanent damage in the form of renal insufficiency, arterial hypertension, and cerebral softening may result.

References

1. Adams, F. D.: Reversible uremia with hypercalcemia due to vitamin D intoxication. N. Engl. J. Med., *244*:590, 1951.
2. Anning, S. T., Dawson, J., Dolby, D. E., and Ingram, J. T.: Toxic effects of calciferol. Q. J. Med., N.S., *17*:203, 1948.
3. Bosman, C.: Hypervitaminosis D and pneumocystis pneumonia in an infant. Helv. Paediatr. Acta, *20*:300, 1965.
4. Caffey, J.: Chronic poisoning due to excess of vitamin D. Pediatrics, *5*:672, 1950.
5. Caffey, J.: Pediatric X-Ray Diagnosis. 7th ed. Chicago, Year Book, 1978.
6. Castello, F., Callis, L., Nieto, J. L., and Vilaplana, E.: Hipervitaminosis D. Revision de 15 casos. An. Esp. Pediatr., *12*:207, 1979.
7. Chaplin, H., Clark, L. D., and Ropes, M. W.: Vitamin D intoxication. Am. J. Med. Sci., *221*:369, 1951.
8. Chesney, R. W.: Current clinical applications of vitamin D metabolite research. Clin. Orthop., *161*:285, 1981.
9. Christensen, W. B., Liebman, C., and Sosman, M. C.: Skeletal and periarticular manifestations of hypervitaminosis D. A.J.R., *65*:27, 1951.
10. Clark, I., and Bassett, C. A. L.: The amelioration of hypervitaminosis D in rats with vitamin A. J. Exp. Med., *115*:147, 1962.
11. DeWind, L. T.: Hypervitaminosis D with osteosclerosis. Arch. Dis. Child., *36*:373, 1961.
12. Dupont, B., Dupont, A., Bliddal, J., Holst, E., Melchior, J. C., and Ottersen, O. E.: Idiopathic hypercalcemia of infancy: The elfin face syndrome. Dan. Med. Bull., *17*:33, 1965.
13. Fanconi, G., and Chastonay, E.: Die D Hypervitaminose in Sauglings Alter. Helv. Paediatr. Acta, 5:Suppl.:5, 1950.
14. Fanconi, G., Girardet, P., Schlesinger, P., Butler, N., and Black, J.: Chronische Hyperkalzamie, kombiniert mit Osteosklerose, Hyperazotamie, Minderwuchs und kongenitalen Missbildungen. Helv. Paediatr. Acta, *7*:314, 1952.
15. Follis, R. H.: Studies on hypervitaminosis D. Am. J. Pathol., *31*:568, 1955.
16. Fraser, D., Kidd, B. S. L., Kooh, S. W., and Paunier, L.: A new look at infantile hypercalcemia. Pediatr. Clin. North Am., *13*:503, 1966.
17. Freedman, P.: Renal colic and persistent hypercalciuria following self-administration of vitamin D. Lancet, *1*:668, 1957.
18. Ham, A. W., and Lewis, M. D.: Hypervitaminosis D rickets: The action of vitamin D. Br. J. Exp. Pathol., *15*:228, 1934.
19. Harris, L. J.: The mode of action of vitamin D. The "parathyroid" theory: Clinical hypervitaminosis. Lancet, *1*:1031, 1932.
20. Harris, L. J., and Stewart, C. P.: The effect of excess doses of irradiated ergosterol on the calcium and phosphorous content of the blood. Biochem. J., *23*:206, 1929.
21. Holman, C. B.: Roentgenologic manifestations of vitamin D intoxication. Radiology, *59*:805, 1952.
22. Kowarski, A., Shapiro, T. R., Biezunski, N., and Kowarski, C.: Hypervitaminosis D. Effect of treatment with sodium sulfate. Pediatrics, *27*:1004, 1961.
23. Lightwood, R.: Idiopathic hypercalcemia in infants with failure to thrive. Arch. Dis. Child., *7*:193, 1932.
24. Payne, W. R.: The blood chemistry in idiopathic hypercalcemia. Arch. Dis. Child., *27*:302, 1952.
25. Ross, S. G.: Vitamin D intoxication in infancy. A report of four cases. J. Pediatr., *41*:815, 1952.
26. Scharfman, W. P., and Propp, S.: Anemia associated with vitamin D intoxication. N. Engl. J. Med., *255*:1207, 1956.
27. Scherrer, H., Koehl, G., Passa, P., and Canivet, J.: Hypercalcémie sévère due à une intoxication volontaire et dissimulée par la vitamine D. Nouv. Presse Med., *30*:2379, 1976.
28. Winberg, J., and Zetterstrom, R.: Cortisone treatment in vitamin D intoxication. Acta Paediatr. (Uppsala), *45*:96, 1956.

IDIOPATHIC HYPERCALCEMIA IN INFANCY

Idiopathic hypercalcemia is caused by hypersensitivity to vitamin D, or an inborn error of cholesterol metabolism.

Clinical, radiographic features, and treatment are similar to those of hypervitaminosis D.[1-7]

References

1. Creery, R. D. C.: Idiopathic hypercalcemia of infants. Lancet, 2:17, 1953.
2. Feinberg, S., and Margolis, A. R.: Severe idiopathic hypercalcemia of infancy. A.J.R., *80*:468, 1958.
3. Fraser, D., Kidd, L., Kooh, S. W., and Pannier, L.: A

new look at infantile hypercalcemia. Pediatr. Clin. North Am., 13:503, 1961.
4. Lightwood, R.: Idiopathic hypercalcemia in infants and failure to thrive. Arch. Dis. Child., 7:193, 1932.
5. Lightwood, R.: Report of a case of hypercalcemia. Proc. R. Soc. Med., 45:401, 1952.
6. Lowe, K. G., Henderson, J. L., Park, W. W., and McGreal, D. A.: Idiopathic hypercalcemia syndrome of infancy. Lancet, 2:101, 1954.
7. Singleton, E. B.: The radiologic features of severe idiopathic hypercalcemia of infancy. Radiology, 68:721, 1957.

PITUITARY DWARFISM

Deficiency of the somatotrophic hormone is due to congenital hypoplasia or aplasia of the eosinophilic cells in about two thirds of the cases of hypopituitarism. The pituitary hormone deficiency is balanced in such cases. It is often a hereditary disorder and is transmitted by an autosomal recessive gene, although sporadic cases do occur. In the remaining cases cessation of growth may result from destructive lesions of the anterior pituitary, such as craniopharyngioma, tuberculosis, syphilis, sarcoidosis, reticuloendotheliosis, toxoplasmosis, or intracranial aneurysm.

Clinical Picture

In the congenital forms, the infant is of normal size and weight at birth; between the ages of two and four years, growth retardation becomes evident. The limbs are proportioned normally in relation to the head and trunk (Fig. 3–118). Pituitary dwarfs are of normal intelligence. The condition may be associated with hypogonadism and delay or absence of sexual maturation.

In the acquired form due to destructive lesions of the anterior pituitary, signs of neurologic deficit, such as impaired vision, ocular disturbances, and pathologic somnolence, are present.

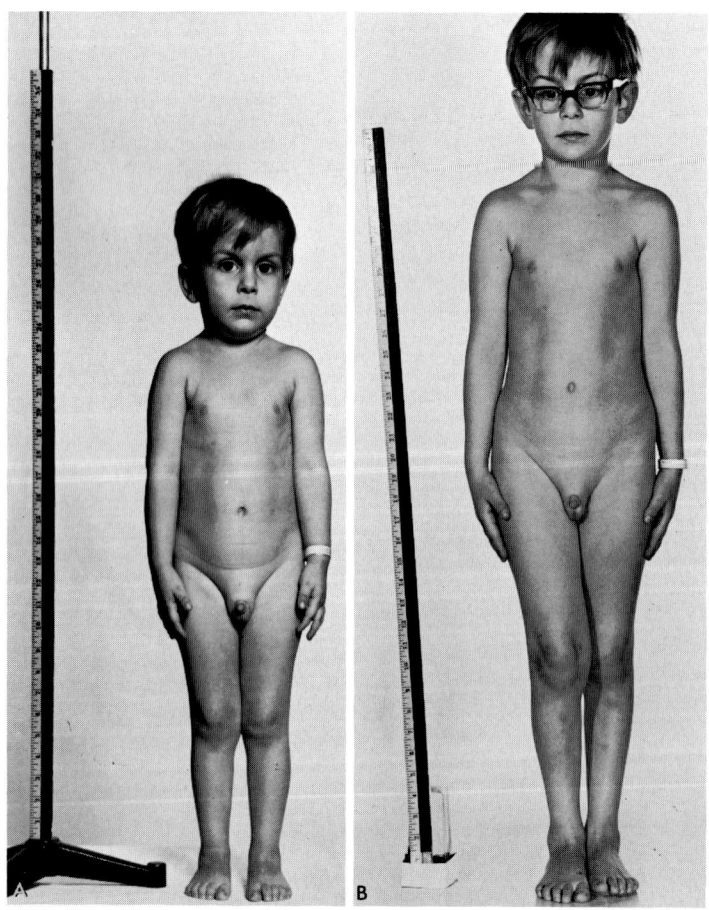

FIGURE 3–118. Pituitary dwarf.

A. The patient at five years of age and **B**, at eight years of age, two years following treatment with growth hormone.

Radiographic Findings

In the congenital, or idiopathic, hypopituitarism, skeletal maturation is delayed, the ossification centers of the epiphysis appearing and closing late. The long bones and skull are osteoporotic. There is also a delay in closure of the fontanelles.

In the presence of organic lesions of the pituitary, the skull radiograms disclose certain changes. Tumors enlarge the sella turcica, and the clinoid process may be deformed or destroyed. Intrasellar or suprasellar calcification suggests craniopharyngioma.

Diagnosis

Growth hormone in the serum will be at a low level or absent. Because the amount in normal children is very small, in order to evaluate it increased secretion of growth hormone may have to be stimulated by inducing hypoglycemia with insulin or by intravenous infusion of L-arginine. In response to this stimulus, the circulating growth hormone level will increase in normal children, but not in pituitary dwarfs.

Treatment

Growth hormone of human origin administered in doses of 1 to 2 mg. twice a week, has proved to be effective in inducing somatic growth. It is difficult to predict the ultimate stature that can be obtained with this treatment. It is the pediatric endocrinologist who administers the therapy; it should, however, be remembered that slipped capital femoral epiphysis can occur in these children.

References

1. Bartolotta E., Giacomozzi, E., Migliori, C., and Conti, S.: Pituitary dwarfism. Evaluation of our cases. Minerva Med., 73:1421, 1982.
2. Bohles, H.: Treatment of short stature with growth hormone from the human hypophysis. Pathologe, 2:48, 1980.
3. Endo, Y.: Marfan syndrome and pituitary dwarfism. Jinrui Idengaku Zasshi, 26:91, 1981.
4. Evain-Brion, D., Donnadieu, M., Roger, M., and Job, J. C.: Simultaneous study of somatotrophic and corticotrophic pituitary secretions during ornithine infusion test. Clin. Endocrinol. (Oxf.), 17:119, 1982.
5. Goodman, H. G., Grumbach, M. B., and Kaplan, S. L.: Growth and growth hormone. II. A comparison of isolated growth hormone, hormone deficiency, and multiple pituitary hormone deficiencies in 35 patients with idiopathic hypopituitary dwarfism. N. Engl. J. Med., 278:57, 1968.
6. Greenwood, I. C., Hunter, W. M., and Marrian, V. J.: Growth hormone levels in children and adolescents. Br. Med. J., 1:25, 1964.
7. Gruneiro de Papendieck, L., Iorcansky, S., Rivarola, M. A., Heinrich, J. J., and Bergada, C.: Patterns of TSH response to TRH in children with hypopituitarism. J. Pediatr., 100:387, 1982.
8. Henneman, P. H.: The effect of human growth hormone on growth of patients with hypopituitarism. A combined study. J.A.M.A., 205:828, 1968.
9. Hernandez, R. J., Poznanski, A. W., and Hopwood, N. J.: Size and skeletal maturation of the hand in children with hypothyroidism and hypopituitarism. A.J.R., 133:405, 1978.
10. Hernandez, R. J., Poznanski, A. W., and Hopwood, N. J., et al.: Incidence of growth lines in psychosocial dwarfs and idiopathic hypopituitarism. A.J.R., 131:477, 1978.
11. Kirkland, R. T., Harrist, R. B., and Clayton, G. W.: Results of four years of intermittent human growth hormone (hGH) and fluoxymesterone therapy in hypopituitary dwarfism. Pediatrics, 65:562, 1980.
12. Martin, M. M., and Wilkins, L.: Pituitary dwarfism: Diagnosis and treatment. J. Clin. Endocrinol., 18:679, 1958.
13. Martinez, A., Coianis, L., Heinrich, J. J., Rodriguez, A., and Bergada, C.: Evaluation of short stature in children. Helv. Paediatr. Acta, 37:563, 1982.
14. Raiti, S.: Short stature: Evaluation and treatment. Pediatr. Ann., 9:135, 1980.
15. Rosenfeld, R. G., Kemp, S. F., Gaspich, S., and Hintz, R. L.: In vivo modulation of somatomedin receptor sites: Effects of growth hormone treatment of hypopituitary children. J. Clin. Endocrinol. Metab., 52:759, 1981.
16. Sorgo, W., Zachmann, M., Tassinari, D., Fernandez, F., and Prader, A.: Longitudinal anthropometric measurements in patients with growth hormone deficiency. Effect of human growth hormone treatment. Eur. J. Pediatr., 138:38, 1982.

GIGANTISM

Gigantism is caused by two different conditions—hypogonadism (eunuchoid) and hyperpituitarism in childhood. In the hypogonadic giant, testicular function is destroyed by castration, or the testes do not mature because the testicles remain undescended. In the hypogonadic giant the lower span is much greater than the upper, the physes remain open for a very long time, and the external genitalia are underdeveloped.

Pituitary gigantism is caused by eosinophilic adenoma of the anterior pituitary; this is extremely rare in childhood and beyond the scope of this book.

HYPOTHYROIDISM

Deficient production of thyroid hormone may be of congenital or acquired origin. The degree of this insufficiency, its age of onset, and its duration are all factors that determine the severity of clinical and skeletal manifestations.

"Cretinism" is the severe form of hypothyroidism that is characterized by dwarfism and mental retardation, the result of congenital thy-

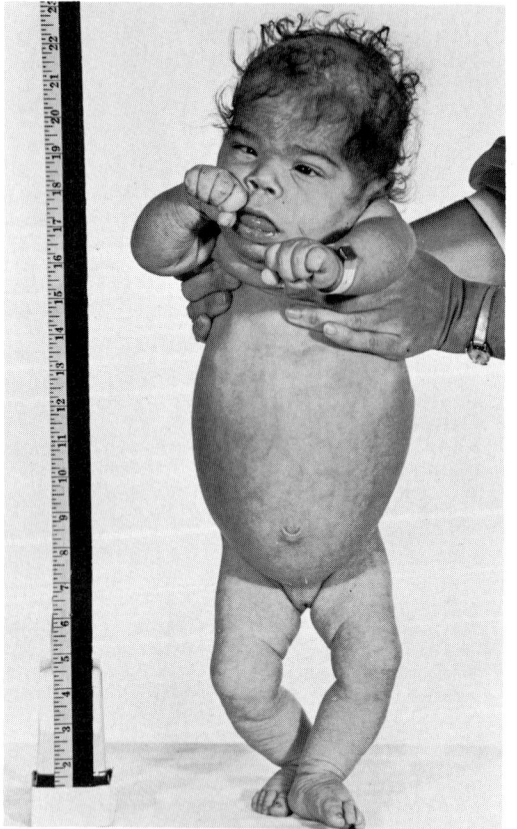

FIGURE 3–119. Typical clinical appearance of a cretin.

roid hormone insufficiency. It is three times as common in girls as in boys. The condition may be suspected in early infancy because of such signs as overweight, prolongation of physiologic icterus, somnolence, general sluggishness, poor appetite, feeding difficulties, and obstinate constipation. If these symptoms are mild, diagnosis is usually not made until the latter half of the first year of life. Other typical features of cretinism in addition to the considerable dwarfism and mental retardation include dry skin, scanty and coarse hair, an enlarged tongue, narrowed palpebral fissures, expressionless facies, an enlarged abdomen with umbilical hernia, and general lethargy (Fig. 3–119). Cretins are slow to sit and stand.

The skeletal manifestations are the primary concern of the orthopedic surgeon. Enchondral bone formation is greatly disturbed. The skeleton is immature for the chronological age. *Epiphyseal dysgenesis* was the term used by Reilly and Smyth to describe the ossific nuclei, which are fragmented by the persistence of cartilaginous islands.[13] Looser correlated the anatomic and radiographic findings.[10] Wilkins studied skeletal changes in seven-day-old kittens following surgical removal of their thyroid glands.[18] The exact pathogenesis of epiphyseal dysgenesis is yet unknown; Aegerter postulates a disturbance in water metabolism, as chondroid is very similar to collagen in chemical consistency.[1]

The ossification centers are late to appear in radiograms, and when they do, they are mottled, fragmented, and smaller than normal. These epiphyseal changes are particularly marked in the hip joint, which may suggest Legg-Perthes disease or multiple epiphyseal dysplasia. The physis may be irregular and widened, resembling that seen in rickets.

The ratio of bone age to height age (BA:HA) is greater than unity because the delay in epiphyseal maturation is less than the delay in longitudinal growth. As intramembranous bone formation remains undisturbed, the long bones become abnormally widened in relation to their length, making these children appear heavier than normal.

The head is comparatively large for the rest of the body. Retarded ossification and shortening of the base of the skull are common. The angle between the clivus and the sphenoid is abnormally increased (over 110 degrees). The sella turcica may be enlarged and is in the same plane as the base of the skull. Closure of the fontanelles and sutures is delayed. The sinuses and air spaces in the petrous bone are late to appear. A delay in normal dentition is common.

In the spine the second lumbar vertebra is wedge-shaped, with beaking of its anterior margin. The first and third lumbar vertebrae may also be affected. The bony end-plates of the vertebral bodies are convex. When the child begins to sit and stand, a lumbar kyphosis develops. Spondylolisthesis may also occur.[16]

Some patients with hypothyroidism have hypercalcemia and osteosclerotic bones. In the radiograms, radiopaque transverse bands appear in the metaphyseal areas, and the cortices are thickened. Metastatic calcifications in the kidneys, brain, and soft tissues have been observed.[2]

Calcium balance studies have shown abnormal retention of calcium in hypothyroidism. Absorption of calcium from the intestine is increased, and excretion of endogenous calcium is diminished.[7]

When the condition is diagnosed early and treated with thyroid hormone by a competent endocrinologist, the prognosis is good for normal mental development and skeletal maturation. If cretinism remains untreated, however, the mental retardation will increase with age, and these children will usually die as a result of infection or respiratory complications.

References

1. Aegerter, E., and Kirkpatrick, J. A., Jr.: Orthopedic Diseases. 3rd. Ed. Philadelphia, Saunders, 1968, p. 432.
2. Bateson, E. M., and Chander, S.: Nephrocalcinosis in cretinism. Br. J. Radiol., 38:581, 1965.
3. Birrell, J., Frost, G. J., and Parkin, J. M.: The development of children with congenital hypothyroidism. Dev. Med. Child Neurol., 25:512, 1983.
4. Braid, F.: Hypothyroidism in childhood. Br. Med. J., 1:1169, 1951.
5. Dieterle, T.: Die Athyreosis unter besonderer Berucksichtigung der dabei auftretenden Skelettveranderungen, sowie differential-diagnostisch vornehmlich in Betracht kommende Storungen des Knochenwachstums. Virchows Arch. Pathol. Anat., 174:56, 1906.
6. Hulse, J. A.: Outcome of congenital hypothyroidism. Arch. Dis. Child., 59:23, 1984.
7. Krane, S. M., Brownell, G. L., Stanbury, J. B., and Corrigan, H.: The effect of thyroid disease on calcium metabolism in man. J. Clin. Invest., 35:874, 1956.
8. Langhans, T.: Anatomische Beitrage zur Kenntnis der Kretinen. Virchow. Arch. Pathol. Anat., 149:155, 1897.
9. Lobovits, A.: Early recognition of congenital hypothyroidism. J. Pediatr., 103:662, 1983.
10. Looser, E.: Über Ossifikationsstorungen bei Kretinismus. Verh. Dtsch. Pathol. Ges., 24:352, 1929.
11. Lyon, I. C.: Screening of congenital hypothyroidism: A three year experience. N.Z. Med. J., 97:175, 1984.
12. Puliyel, J. M., and Thomas, P. G.: Hypothyroidism with multiple congenital anomalies. Indian Pediatr., 20:865, 1983.
13. Reilly, W. A., and Smyth, F. S.: Cretinoid epiphyseal dysgenesis. J. Pediatr., 11:786, 1937.
14. Royer, P., Lestradet, H., Frederich, A., and Dartois, A. M.: Les rachitismes vitamino-résistants hypophosphatémiques idiopathiques de l'enfant. (Essai de dissociation de deux maladies différentes par l'étude clinique, radiologique, biologique et génétique). Arch. Fr. Pediatr., 18:41, 1961.
15. Silverman, F. N., and Currarino, G.: Roentgen manifestations of hereditary metabolic diseases in childhood. Metabolism, 9:248, 1960.
16. Swoboda, W.: Angulare dorsolumbale Kyphose als unbekanntes Skelettzeichen beim kongenitalen Myxodem. Fortschr. Geb. Rontgenstr., 73:740, 1950.
17. Swoboda, W.: Typische Ossifikationsstorungen der Wirbelsaule beim angeborenen Myxodem. Helv. Paediatr. Acta, 10:462, 1955.
18. Wilkins, L.: Epiphyseal dysgenesis associated with hypothyroidism. Am. J. Dis. Child., 61:13, 1941.

IDIOPATHIC HYPOPARATHYROIDISM

This disorder is caused by deficient function of the parathyroid glands and failure to produce sufficient parathyroid hormone. Some cases are familial; X-linked recessive inheritance is reported by Whyte and Weidon.[5, 15]

Idiopathic hypoparathyroidism should be distinguished from pseudohypoparathyroidism in which production of parathormone is increased but the end organs do not respond to the hormone (hormone-resistant hypoparathyroidism).

The principal symptoms of hypoparathyroidism are tetany, laryngismus, lassitude, and mental depression. Changes in tissues of ectodermal origin include dryness and coarseness of the skin, scanty hair, brittleness of the nails, late eruption and premature loss of teeth, and cataract. Papilledema may occur, suggesting the presence of an intracranial neoplasm.

The serum calcium level is low, and urinary secretion of calcium may be greatly diminished, with elevation of serum phosphorus. Radiograms of the skeleton may be normal, or there may be increased radiopacity of the cortices of long bones. Soft-tissue calcification, particularly in the basal ganglia, may occur.

Hypoparathyroidism is treated by the pediatric endocrinologist by administration of vitamin D and parathormone. Infants who have hypoparathyroidism complicated with tetany may require calcium infusion.

References

1. Albright, F., and Ellsworth, R.: Studies on the physiology of the parathyroid glands. I. Calcium and phosphorus studies in a case of idiopathic hypoparathyroidism. J. Clin. Invest., 7:183, 1929.
2. Allen, E. H., Millard, F. J. C., and Nassim, J. R.: Hypo-hyperparathyroidism. Arch. Dis. Child., 43:295, 1968.
3. Auidi, L. V.: The therapeutic approach to hypoparathyroidism. Am. J. Med., 57:34, 1974.
4. Benderly, A., Etzioni, A., and Levy, J.: Idiopathic hypoparathyroidism and anticonvulsive treatment as possible cause for cardiac failure. Helv. Paediatr. Acta, 35:501, 1980.
5. Bronsky, D., Kiamo, R. T., and Waldstein, S.: Familial idiopathic hypoparathyroidism. J. Clin. Endocrinol., 18:61, 1968.
6. Bronsky, D., Kushner, D. S., Dubin, A., and Snapper, I.: Idiopathic hypoparathyroidism and pseudohypoparathyroidism: Case reports and review of literature. Medicine, 37:317, 1958.
7. Daneman, D., Kooh, S. W., and Fraser, D.: Hypoparathyroidism and pseudohypoparathyroidism in childhood. Clin. Endocrinol. Metab., 11:211, 1982.
8. Glatthaar, C., Smith, R., Espiner, E. A., Donald, R. A., and Hinton, D.: 1,25-dihydroxy-vitamin D3: A new treatment for hypoparathyroidism. N.Z. Med. J., 92:267, 1980.
9. Gupta, M. M., Kuppuswamy, G., and Suri, R. K.: Hypoparathyroidism. J. Indian Med. Assoc., 75:89, 1980.
10. Ishida, M., Seino, Y., Simotsuji, T., Ishii, T., Yamaoka, K., Harada, T., Yabuuchi, H., and Nishimura, K.: Differential diagnosis of hypoparathyroid disorders during childhood. Calcif. Tissue Int., 31:203, 1980.
11. Kruse, K., Scheunemann, W., Baier, W., and Schaub, J.: Hypocalcemia myopathy in idiopathic hypoparathyroidism. Eur. J. Pediatr., 138:280, 1982.
12. Lund, B., Sorensen, O. H., Lund, B., Bishop, J. E., and Norman, A. W.: Vitamin D metabolism in hypoparathyroidism. J. Clin. Endocrinol. Metab., 51:606, 1980.

13. Richards, G. E., Brewer, E. D., Conley, S. B., and Saldana, L. R.: Combined hypothyroidism and hypoparathyroidism in an infant after maternal ^{131}I administration. J. Pediatr., 99:141, 1981.
14. Steinberg, H. L., and Waldron, B. R.: Idiopathic hypoparathyroidism. An analysis of 52 cases including the report of a new case. Medicine, 31:133, 1952.
15. Whyte, M. P., and Weidon, V. V.: Idiopathic hypoparathyroidism presenting with seizures during infancy. X-linked recessive inheritance in a large Missouri kindred. J. Pediatr., 99:608, 1981.

PSEUDOHYPOPARA-THYROIDISM

Pseudohypoparathyroidism is a disease whose clinical and radiographic manifestations are similar to those of hypoparathyroidism; it is, however, distinguished from that entity by the fact that it does not respond to parathyroid hormone. It was first described by Albright, Burnett, Smith, and Parson in 1942.[1] The condition is genetically determined, as it is familial with more than one generation affected. Three patterns of inheritance have been reported in the literature: X-linked dominant inheritance with a 2 : 1 female to male ratio, autosomal dominant, and autosomal recessive.[5, 17, 19] The disease is more severe in the male.

Parathyroid glands are hyperplastic or normal on pathologic examination. The cause of failure of response of the end organs to the action of parathormone is unknown. Two possible mechanisms are primary excessive tubular reabsorption of phosphate and production of an excess of thyrocalcitonin.[18]

At birth, the infant appears to be normal. Skeletal changes gradually become manifest at the age of two to four years. The hands are deformed owing to shortening of the metacarpals, mainly the first, fourth, and fifth, most probably caused by premature closure of the epiphysis (Fig. 3–120). When the hands are clenched, dimples are present at the sites of the knuckles of the shortened digits. There may be multiple exostoses, and the radius may be abnormally curved. Dwarfism and a moon-shaped facies are common. Deposits of calcium are sometimes noted in the subcutaneous tissues, particularly around large joints.

If the disease has not been treated in its early stages, dentition may also be affected, the teeth being abnormally small in size with large pulp chambers and blunt roots.

Pseudohypoparathyroidism may be associated with hypothyroidism, Turner's syndrome, and diabetes. Short metacarpals may be seen in Turner's syndrome and in myositis ossificans progressiva.

Laboratory confirmation of the clinical diagnosis is made following injection of 200 units of parathyroid hormone daily for five to seven days. When pseudohypoparathyroidism is present, there will be no change in the serum level of calcium. The Ellsworth-Howard test was used in the past; it is, however, not reliable.

Pseudopseudohypoparathyroidism is the condition in which the stigmata of pseudohypoparathyroidism of short metacarpals and subcutaneous calcification are present but the

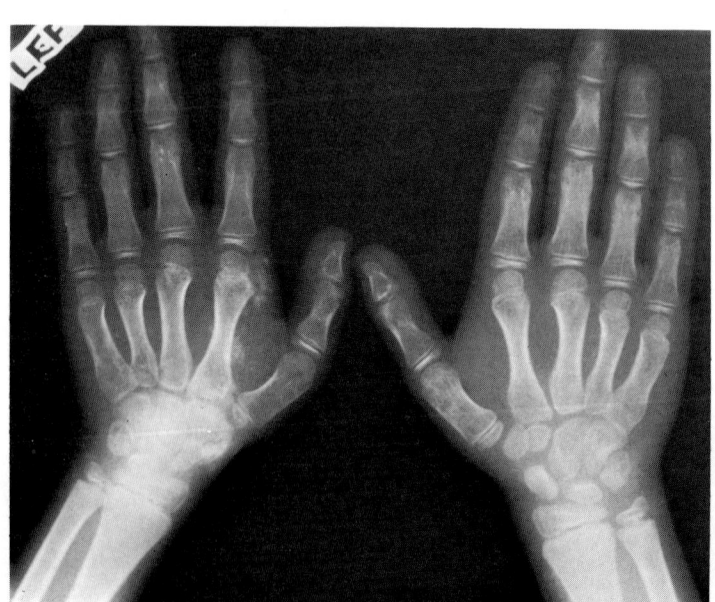

FIGURE 3–120.
Pseudohypoparathyroidism.

Anteroposterior radiogram of the hands shows shortening of the first, fourth, and fifth metacarpals.

abnormalities of low levels of serum calcium and high levels of serum phosphate are absent.

References

1. Albright, F., Burnett, C. H., Smith, P. H., and Parson, W.: Pseudo-hypoparathyroidism, an example of "Seabright-bantam" syndrome, report of three cases. Endocrinology, *30*:922, 1942.
2. Aurbach, G. D.: Pseudohypoparathyroidism and related disorders. Henry Ford Hosp. Med. J., *31*:233, 1983.
3. Bartter, F. C.: Pseudohypoparathyroidism and pseudopseudohypoparathyroidism. In Stanbury, J. B., Wyngaarden, J. B. and Fredrickson, D. S. (eds.): The Metabolic Basis of Inherited Disease. 2nd Ed. New York, McGraw-Hill, 1966.
4. Bell, N. H., Gerald, E. S., and Bartter, F. C.: Pseudohypoparathyroidism with osteitis fibrosa cystica and impaired absorption of calcium. J. Clin. Endocrinol., *23*:759, 1963.
5. Cederbaum, S. D., and Lippe, B. M.: Probable autosomal recessive inheritance in a family with Albright's hereditary osteodystrophy and an evaluation of the genetics of the disorder. Am. J. Hum. Genet., *25*:638, 1973.
6. Chase, L. R., Melson, G. L., and Aurbach, G. D.: Pseudohypoparathyroidism: Defective excretion of 3',5'-AMP in response to parathyroid hormone. J. Clin. Invest., *48*:1832, 1969.
7. Cohen, M. C., and Donnell, G. N.: Pseudohypoparathyroidism with hypothyroidism. Pediatrics, *56*:369, 1960.
8. Drezner, M., Neelon, F. A., and Lebovitz, H. E.: Pseudohypoparathyroidism Type II. A possible defect in the reception of the cyclic A.M.P. signal. N. Engl. J. Med., *289*:1056, 1973.
9. Elrick, H., Albright, F., Bartter, F. C., Forbes, A. P., and Reeves, J. D.: Further studies on pseudohypoparathyroidism: Report of four new cases. Acta Endocrinol. (Copenh.), *5*:199, 1950.
10. Farfel, Z., Brickman, A. S., Kaslow, H. R., Brothers, V. M., and Bourne, H. R.: Defect of receptor-cyclase coupling protein in pseudohypoparathyroidism. N. Engl. J. Med., *303*:237, 1980.
11. Frame, B., Hanson, C. A., Frost, H. M., Block, M., and Arnstein, A. R.: Renal resistance to parathyroid hormone with osteitis fibrosa. "Pseudohypoparathyroidism." Am. J. Med., *52*:311, 1972.
12. Gentili, A., and Bottone, E.: Pseudohypoparathyroidisme. Helv. Paediatr. Acta, *15*:115, 1960.
13. Kruse, K., Gutekunst, B., Kracht, U., and Schwerda, K.: Deficient prolactin response to parathyroid hormone in hypocalcemic and normocalcemic pseudohypoparathyroidism. J. Clin. Endocrinol. Metab., *52*:1099, 1981.
14. Macgregor, M. E., and Whitehead, T. P.: Pseudohypoparathyroidism. Description of 3 cases and critical appraisal of earlier accounts of disease. Arch. Dis. Child., *29*:398, 1954.
15. Nouailhat, F.: Albright's hereditary osteodystrophy: Its two clinical aspects, pseudohypoparathyroidism and pseudopseudohypoparathyroidism. Presse Méd., *71*:121, 1963.
16. Ritchie, G. MacL.: Dental manifestations of pseudohypoparathyroidism. Arch. Dis. Child., *40*:565, 1965.
17. Spranger, J. W.: Skeletal dysplasias and the eye; Albright's hereditary osteodystrophy. Birth Defects Orig. Art. Series, 5:122, 1969.
18. Tachdjian, A. H., Frantz, A. G., and Lee, J. B.: Pseudohypoparathyroidism: Assays of parathyroid hormone and thyrocalcitonin. Proc. Natl. Acad. Sci. U.S.A., *56*:1138, 1966.
19. Weinberg, A. G., and Stone, R. T.: Autosomal dominant inheritance in Albright's osteodystrophy. J. Pediatr., *79*:996, 1972.
20. Zampa, G. A., and Zucchelli, P. C.: Pseudohypoparathyroidism and bone demineralization: Case report and metabolic studies. J. Clin. Endocrinol., *25*:1616, 1965.

PRIMARY HYPERPARATHYROIDISM

This is caused by diffuse hyperplasia or neoplasm of the parathyroid gland. It is extremely rare in children.[1-6] The increased secretion of parathormone, through its action on bone and renal tubules, elevates the serum calcium level, lowers the serum phosphorus level and elevates the serum alkaline phosphatase level. Hypercalcemia and hypercalcinuria precipitate calcium and phosphorus in the urinary tract. The osteoclastic bone resorption causes bone pain, and inhibition of smooth muscle action in the gastrointestinal tract results in constipation and abdominal pain. Mental behavior may change with lethargy.

Radiograms show generalized osteoporosis, cortical thinning of long bone, and bone resorption in the phalanges.

Direct assay of levels of PTH will establish the diagnosis of hyperparathyroidism. Treatment is surgical—for the adenoma and hyperplasia.

References

1. Anast, C. S.: Parathyroid disorders in children. Pediatr. Ann., *9*:376, 1980.
2. Bergman, L., and Hagberg, S.: Primary hyperparathyroidism in a child investigated by determination of ultrafiltrable calcium. Am. J. Dis. Child., *123*:174, 1972.
3. Bjernulf, A., Hall, K., Sjogren, I., and Werner, I.: Primary hyperparathyroidism in children. Acta. Pediatr. Scand., *59*:249, 1970.
4. Cohen, R. D., and Vince, F. P.: Pseudohypoparathyroidism with raised plasma phosphatase. Arch. Dis. Child., *44*:96, 1969.
5. Cutler, R. E., Reisse, E., and Ackerman, L. U.: Familial hyperparathyroidism. N. Engl. J. Med., *270*:859, 1964.
6. Singleton, E. B., and Teng, C. T.: Pseudohypoparathyroidism with bone changes simulating hyperparathyroidism. Report of a case. Radiology, *78*:388, 1962.

Osteochondroses and Related Disorders

Osteochondroses are a group of idiopathic, self-limited conditions characterized by disturbance of enchondral ossification in which both chondrogensis and osteogenesis of a previously normal growth process are deranged. Siffert proposed a classification of osteochondroses based on the anatomic site of involvement of the growth mechanism (Table 3–14).[22] Disorders of enchondral ossification may occur at the *articular epiphysis*, the *apophysis* (i.e., nonarticular epiphysis), and the *physis* (i.e., the longitudinal growth plate).

The original mass of epiphyseal cartilage at the ends of the long bones subdivides into two separate growth areas—the "epiphyseal" and the "physeal" growth plates. The *"epiphyseal" growth plate* contributes to the enlargement of the epiphysis by multiplication of the cartilage cells that cover the dome-shaped hemispheric cartilaginous caps. These growth cartilage cells derive their nutrition from the synovial fluid. In addition, there are deeper proliferating cartilage cells within the epiphysis that are nourished via vessels within the ossific nucleus of the epiphysis. The *"physeal" growth plate* is the horizontal growth plate that contributes to the longitudinal growth of the long bones; it receives its nutrition from the epiphyseal blood vessels within the bony epiphysis that penetrate the bony end-plate. Growth of the short tubular bones in the hands and feet is similar to that of long tubular bones. The bony nucleus of the carpal and tarsal cuboid bones is completely surrounded by proliferating cartilage throughout growth; nutrition is through blood vessels that penetrate at sites of synovial sheaths of tendons, ligament, or tendon attachments. In the vertebrae the bony centrum enlarges as in an epiphysis of a long bone; the superior and inferior cartilage surfaces adjacent to each intervertebral disc remain in the vertebral growth plate; they derive their nutrition through vascular channels that traverse the layer of small cartilage cells adjacent to the disc. Osteochondroses occur only at the superior and inferior vertebral growth plates.[22]

Osteochondroses can occur in any bone that grows by enchondral ossification. Historically, each bone is designated by the name of the person who first described it, a practice that has resulted in a voluminous list of eponyms (Table 3–15). The situation is further confused because some of the osteochondroses are caused by aseptic necrosis of bone and stress fracture, and others by simple stress fracture or stress on normal bone, whereas some are simple physiologic variations of growth with minor irregularities of normal ossification. For the sake of convenience a few of these latter conditions are discussed in this section.

*Table 3–14. Classification of Osteochondroses (According to Siffert)**

I. Articular Osteochondroses
  A. Primary involvement of articular and epiphyseal cartilage and subjacent enchondral ossification (e.g., capitellum of humerus (Panner's disease) or metatarsal head (Freiberg's infraction)
  B. Secondary involvement of articular and epiphyseal cartilage as a consequence of avascular necrosis of subjacent bone (e.g., Legg-Calvé-Perthes' disease, Köhler's disease, osteochondritis dissecans)
II. Nonarticular osteochondroses
  A. At tendon attachments (e.g., Osgood-Schlatter disease)
  B. At ligament attachments (e.g., vertebral ring and epicondyles)
  C. At impact sites (e.g., Sever's disease)
III. Physeal Osteochondroses
  A. Long bones (e.g., tibia vara)
  B. Vertebrae (Scheuermann's disease)

*From Siffert, R. S.: Classification of osteochondroses. Clin. Orthop., 158:10, 1981. Reprinted by permission.

Table 3–15. Sites in Which "Osteochondrosis" Has Been Described

Lower limb
  Femoral head—Legg[13], Calvé[5], Perthes[19]
  Ischiopubic syndesmosis—Van Neck[27]
  Greater trochanter—Mandl[15], Hall[8]
  Primary ossification center of patella—Köhler[12]
  Secondary ossification center of the patella—Sinding-Larsen[24], Wolf[28]
  Superior tibial epiphysis—Boldero and Mitchell[2]
  Posteromedial part of upper tibial physis—Blount[1]
  Distal tibial epiphysis—Siffert and Arkins[23], Hassler, Heyman, and Bennett[9]
  Internal cuneiform of tarsus—Meilstrup[17]
  Tarsal navicular—Köhler[12]
  Metatarsal head (2, 3, or 4)—Freiberg[6]
  Epiphysis of fifth metatarsal—Iselin[10]

Upper limb
  Capitellum of humerus—Panner[18]
  Distal ulnar epiphysis—Burns[4]
  Distal radial epiphysis—Madelung[14]
  Carpal lunate—Kienbock[11]
  Heads of metacarpals—Mauclaire[16]
  Epiphysis of phalanges—Thiemann[26], Shaw[21], Staples[25]

Spine
  Vertebral end plates—Scheuermann[20]

References

1. Blount, W. P.: Tibia vara. Osteochondrosis deformans tibiae. J. Bone Joint Surg., *19*:1, 1937.
2. Boldero, J. L., and Mitchell, G. P.: Osteochondritis of the superior tibial epiphysis. J. Bone Joint Surg., *36-B*:114, 1954.
3. Breck, C. W.: An Atlas of the Osteochondroses. Springfield, Ill., Thomas, 1971.
4. Burns, B. H.: Osteochondritis juvenilis of the lower ulnar epiphysis. Proc. R. Soc. Med., *24*:912, 1931.
5. Calvé, J.: Sur une forme particulière de coxalgie greffée. Sur des déformations caracteristique de l'extrémité superieure du fémur. Rev. Chir. (Paris), *42*:54, 1910.
6. Freiberg, A. H.: Infraction of the second metatarsal bone; a typical injury. Surg. Gynecol. Obstet., *19*:191, 1914.
7. Goff, C. W.: Legg-Perthes Syndrome and Related Osteochondroses of Youth. Springfield, Ill., Thomas, 1954.
8. Hall, T. D.: Osteochondritis of the greater trochanteric epiphysis. J. Bone Joint Surg., *40-A*:644, 1958.
9. Hassler, W. L., Heyman, C. H., and Bennett, G. W.: Osteochondrosis of the distal tibial epiphysis. A report of two cases. J. Bone Joint Surg., *42-A*:1261, 1960.
10. Iselin, H.: Wachstumsbeschwerden zur Zeit der knochernen Entwicklung der Tuberositas metatarsi quinti. Dtsch. Z. Chir., *117*:529, 1912.
11. Kienbock, R.: Über Osteochondritis an der Tuberositas tibiae und die sogenannte Osgood-Schlatter'sche Erkrankung. Fortschr. Geb. Rontgenstr., *15*:135, 1910.
12. Kohler, A.: Über eine haufige, bisher anscheinend unbekannte Erkrankung einzelner kindlicher knochen. Münch. Med. Wochenschr., *55*:1923, 1908.
13. Legg, A. T.: An obscure affection of the hip joint. Boston Med. Surg. J., *162*:202, 1910.
14. Madelung, O. W.: Die spontane Subluxation der Hand nach vorne. Verh. Dtsch. Ges. Chir., *7*:259, 1878.
15. Mandl, F.: Die "Schlatter'sche Krankheit" als "Systemerkrankung." Beitr. Klin. Chir., *126*:707, 1922.
16. Mauclaire, P.: Epiphysitis der Metacarpuskopfchen mit Hohlbildung der Hand. Fortschr. Geb. Rontgenstr., *37*:425, 1928.
17. Meilstrup, D. B.: Osteochondritis of the internal cuneiforms. A.J.R., *58*:329, 1947.
18. Panner, H. J.: An affection of the capitelum humeri resembling Calvé-Perthes disease of the hip. Acta Radiol., *8*:617, 1927.
19. Perthes, G. C.: Über Arthritis deformans juvenilis. Dtsch. Z. Chir., *107*:111, 1910.
20. Scheuermann, H. W.: Deforming osteochondritis of the spine. Ugeskr. Laeger., *82*:385, 1920.
21. Shaw, E. W.: Avascular necrosis of the phalanges of the hands (Thiemann's disease). J.A.M.A., *156*:711, 1954.
22. Siffert, R.: Classification of osteochondroses. Clin. Orthop., *158*:10, 1981.
23. Siffert, R. S., and Arkin, A. M.: Post-traumatic aseptic necrosis of the distal tibial epiphysis. J. Bone Joint Surg., *32-A*:691, 1950.
24. Sinding-Larsen, C. M. F.: A hitherto unknown affection of the patella in children. Acta Radiol., *1*:171, 1921.
25. Staples, O. S.: Osteochondritis of the epiphyses of the terminal phalanx of the fingers. J. Bone Joint Surg., *25*:917, 1943.
26. Thiemann, H.: Juvenile Epiphysenstörungen. Fortschr. Geb. Röntgenstr., *14*:79, 1909.
27. van Neck, M.: Osteochondrite du pubis. Arch. Franco-Belges Chir., *27*:238, 1924.
28. Wolf, J.: Larsen-Johansson disease of the patella. Br. J. Radiol., *23*:335, 1950.

LEGG-CALVÉ-PERTHES DISEASE

Legg-Calvé-Perthes disease is a self-limited disease of the hip produced by ischemia and varying degrees of necrosis of the femoral head. Subchondral stress fracture of the necrotic bone initiates the clinical onset of the disease and the process of resorption of dead bone. Legg-Calvé-Perthes disease is not aseptic necrosis of bone per se, because in the absence of subchondral fracture, aseptic necrosis of the femoral head will resolve without bone resorption, subluxation, or deformation. It is the subchondral fracture and the subsequent bone resorption and repair with growth disturbance that characterize Legg-Calvé-Perthes disease.[578]

Coxa plana was described in 1910, independently, by Legg of the United States, Calvé of France, and Perthes of Germany, as a nontuberculous disease of the hip in children.[89, 420, 527] Waldenström, in 1909, reported a similar disorder of the hip in ten children, calling it "der obere tuberkulöse Collumherd."[672] The clinical and radiologic features of these cases were quite characteristic of coxa plana. Because all his patients had a positive tuberculin skin test, Waldenström regarded the disease as tuberculous in nature. In 1910, he described it in great detail, still drawing the same conclusions.[673]

Legg titled his first paper "An Obscure Affection of the Hip Joint," basing his report on five cases having clinical and radiographic signs that were not typical of any condition previously reported.[420] Calvé described ten cases of a disorder of the hip that he termed "pseudocoxalgie."[89] Perthes, in his initial report of six cases, called the disease "arthritis deformans juvenilis."[527]

Phemister, in 1921, described the disease histologically as "bone necrosis."[530] In 1922, Waldenström presented his well-known classification of its different stages, based on a study of 22 cases that he had followed from onset until completion of healing.[674] Catterall, in 1971, described the four degrees of involvement of the femoral head, stressing the "heads at risk" sign, and in 1982 published his definitive textbook on Legg-Calvé-Perthes disease.[103, 107] The pathogenetic importance of the subchondral fracture of the avascular bone in the resorption and subsequent repair of the dead bone, and its prognostic significance as to extent of involvement, were described by Salter in 1984.[578]

Table 3-16. Incidence of Legg-Calvé-Perthes Disease

Author	Geographic Location	Overall	Male	Female
Molloy and MacMahon[482]*	Massachusetts, U.S.A.	1:1200	1:740	1:3700
Helbo[312]*	Denmark	1:2300		
Gray et al.[274]*	British Columbia	1:1400	1:820	1:4500
Harper et al.[296]	South Wales, Wales	1:4750	1:3000	1:11,800
Catterall[107]	Scotland	1:5590	1:4060	1:14,830
Barker et al.[21]	England	1:12,500	1:8064	1:30,300

*In the studies of Molloy and MacMahon, Helbo, and Gray and associates the conclusions are derived from summed annual "attack rates" rather than a longitudinal study of a population at risk (as in the Harper and associates study).

Incidence

The exact incidence of Legg-Calvé-Perthes disease is difficult to determine because some cases are undiagnosed. It is definitely more predominant in the male, with a male to female ratio of four to one. The overall incidence reported by authors from different parts of the world varies: according to Molloy and McMahon, it is 1:1200 in Massachussetts; to Gray and associates, 1:1400 in British Columbia; to Helbo, 1:2300 in Denmark; to Harper and associates, 1:4750 in South Wales; to Catterall, 1:5590 in Scotland; and to Barker and associates, 1:12,500 in England (Table 3–16).[21, 107, 274, 296, 312, 482] There is regional variation, the rate being higher in urban than in rural areas.

The clinical onset of Legg-Calvé-Perthes disease occurs within a narrow age range, about 80 per cent of the patients being between 4 and 9 years, with an average of 6 years and a span of about 2 to 13 years. The age of onset is earlier in the female. In about 10 per cent of cases, involvement is bilateral.

Hereditary Factors

In the literature, there are several reports of familial occurrence of coxa plana. The disease was traced by Stephens and Kerby through four generations in one family in which 28 of the 63 members investigated were affected.[625] Wansborough and associates found that Legg-Calvé-Perthes disease occurred in 1 in 35 (3 per cent) of the siblings born after the index patient.[679] Goff reported a 20 per cent familial incidence of coxa plana.[259] Gray and associates noted occurrence of Legg-Calvé-Perthes disease in 0.8 per cent of parents, 3.8 per cent of siblings, and 0.3 per cent of second- and third-degree relatives, suggesting polygenic inheritance.[274]

Upon close scrutiny, however, many of the cases in which there is a strong family history are of bilateral involvement and are not true Legg-Calvé-Perthes disease; they are cases of skeletal dysplasia involving the hip joint (such as multiple epiphyseal dysplasia, spondyloepiphyseal dysplasia, or trichorhinophalangeal syndrome).[144, 705] On elimination of these misdiagnosed cases, the incidence of Legg-Calvé-Perthes disease among first-degree relatives (parents, siblings, and children of adult patients) is very low. Fisher studied first-degree relatives of 203 patients and found only one father, two brothers, and two sisters who were affected. He concluded that there is no definite genetic predisposition to coxa plana.[217] Wynne-Davies and Gormley studied the proportion of near relatives affected with Legg-Calvé-Perthes disease and found the incidence to be extremely low with no obvious pattern of inheritance.[705] There are a few reports of the occurrence of the disorder in identical twins.[169, 246, 340] These reports were selected, however, because of their concordance. In unselected reports in the literature, only one of each pair described is affected.[217, 705]

In summary, the evidence, as published, is that genetic factors do not play a role in the etiology of Legg-Calvé-Perthes disease. This conclusion is based on the findings that the frequency of the disease among near relatives is extremely low, that the proportion of affected second- and third-degree relatives is the same as that of the normal population, that it rarely involves identical twins, and that there is no genetic pattern of inheritance. There is no evidence of single-gene inheritance, and if Legg-Calvé-Perthes disease were of multifactorial inheritance, one would expect that the more rarely affected sex would have a higher proportion of affected relatives. The studies of Wynne-Davies and Gormley have demonstrated that this is not the case.[705]

Constitutional Factors

The growth of children with Legg-Calvé-Perthes disease is abnormal. They are generally shorter than average. Cameron and Izatt found that affected boys were about one inch shorter, and affected girls about three inches shorter, than unaffected children of corresponding age.[92] The short stature of these children also has been reported by Weiner and O'Dell in 1970, and by Fischer in 1972.[217, 687] Their weight, however, is about or above average. Burwell and associates, in 1978, noting that the shortening affects primarily the lower legs and forearms, suggested that the growth disturbance occurs during distal limb development.[82] Neither the parents nor the siblings of patients are shorter than normal, indicating that the short stature is not familial. Goff attributed it to delay of skeletal maturation existing for months or years prior to the onset of the disease.[259] The skeletal age of affected children in Ralston's series was delayed by an average of 21 months.[545] Fisher, Harrison and associates, and Girdany and Osman also noted the delay in skeletal age of children with Legg-Calvé-Perthes disease.[217, 253, 303]

The bone age returns to normal for chronologic age after healing of the disease. Some children remain shorter than average throughout life, but others do not differ significantly from normal. Wynne-Davies and Gormley reported that 14 per cent of children who developed Legg-Calvé-Perthes disease before three years of age were of short stature later, whereas 33 per cent of those who developed it after the age of seven remained conspicuously undersized. It seems that when a child is affected at an early age there is time for growth to catch up.[705]

Molloy and MacMahon found that the birth weight of children with Legg-Calvé-Perthes disease was significantly lower compared with that of unaffected children. The data they presented suggested that male infants with a birth weight under 5½ pounds are five times as susceptible to coxa plana as male infants weighing 8½ pounds or more at birth.[483]

Wynne-Davies and Gormley, however, could not show low birth weight as a particular feature of coxa plana and could not correlate low birth weight with subsequent short stature. They noted children who were third-born or later in the family and those who had older than average parents were more at risk for the disease; approximately 10 per cent of the affected patients had been born by breech presentation, had shown other malposition, or had undergone version late in pregnancy.[705] It seems environmental factors that make a child's hip more susceptible to injury increase the risk of developing Legg-Calvé-Perthes disease.

Associated Anomalies

There are high incidences of hernia, undescended testicles, and kidney abnormalities in children with Legg-Calvé-Perthes disease.[108, 217, 451, 697, 705] Renal abnormalities are more frequent in bilateral disease and in the female. Other concomitant anomalies reported are pyloric stenosis, congenital heart disease, and epilepsy.[288]

Etiology

Legg-Calvé-Perthes disease is produced by avascularity of the femoral head; biopsy specimens taken from the femoral head have shown bone necrosis in different stages of repair.[16, 232, 251, 307, 356, 530, 538, 554, 709] The reason for this impairment of blood supply to the femoral head, however, has not yet been determined.

Various experiments on animals have been performed in order to produce necrosis of the femoral head by blocking or dividing its blood supply. Division of the ligamentum teres in young dogs failed to result in necrosis (Iselin); when the periosteum around the femoral neck was divided and the ligamentum teres severed, however, necrosis of the femoral head did result (Nussbaum).[343, 509]

Other methods used to induce necrosis of the femoral head included injection of alcohol into the area surrounding the metaphysis in young rabbits and goats (Bentzon); excision of the periosteum of the femoral neck in rabbits (Bergmann); local trauma to the femoral head in rabbits (Nagura); division of the ligamentum teres, nutrient vessels to the epiphysis, and the anterior circumflex artery in rabbits (Lemoine); tight ligation of the femoral neck with steel wire and division of the ligamentum teres in rabbits (Rokkanen); and experimental dislocation of the hip in rabbits (Langenskiöld and associates).[35, 38, 409, 425, 498, 559] These experimental studies in which there was a single episode of interruption of blood supply did not reproduce the anatomic changes seen in Legg-Calvé-Perthes disease. Other animal studies by Freeman and England, Sanchis and associates, and Inoue and associates have demonstrated that multiple episodes of infarction are required to produce the characteristic pathologic picture of the disease.[225, 342, 582]

The epiphyseal vessels traverse the femoral neck between the bone and the inelastic capsule. This unique anatomic feature makes the retinacular vessels vulnerable to increased hydrostatic pressure in the hip joint. An attractive and plausible theory is that synovitis of the hip will increase intra-articular pressure, cause tamponade (occlusion) of the retinacular vessels, and thereby obstruct the vascular supply to the femoral head. Tachdjian and Grana produced avascular necrosis of the femoral head by increasing the pressure in the hip joints of puppies with intra-articular injection of silicone, which is inert, of high viscosity, nonirritating, nonabsorbable, and which maintains an elevated pressure. The normal arteriolar pressure in the retinacular vessels of the hip is about 40 mm. of mercury. These investigators demonstrated experimentally that 80 and 100 mm. of mercury of increased intra-articular pressure caused partial vascular occlusion; complete avascular necrosis of the femoral head was produced when the initial level of increased intra-articular pressure was 200 mm. of mercury or over and the increased pressure lasted for ten hours or more.[643]

A number of other investigators have produced avascular necrosis of the femoral head by tamponade compression of the retinacular vessels around the femoral neck.[314, 383, 607]

A causal relationship between transient synovitis of the hip and Legg-Calvé-Perthes disease has been proposed because 1.5 to 18 per cent of cases with a preceding episode or episodes of transient synovitis later develop coxa plana.[347, 620, 666] Gershuni and associates questioned the significance of hip joint tamponade in producing osteonecrosis in Legg-Calvé-Perthes disease. In experimental work on the hip in the immature pig, they demonstrated that the elevated intra-articular pressure declined within a maximum of 132 minutes to 35 mm. of mercury. This is much less than the ischemic time required to cause the death of the osteocytes. It seems that the decrease of intra-articular pressure resulted from capsular distention and diffusion of the infusate from the hip joint.[243] This author has performed technetium-99m bone scans of 40 hips with acute transient synovitis; all have been normal, and the patients at follow-up had not developed Legg-Calvé-Perthes disease. It is improbable that acute transient synovitis is the cause of the disease; this author believes it is the subchondral fracture of the avascular femoral head (heralding the onset of Legg-Calvé-Perthes disease) that is the cause of the acute synovitis of the hip.

Kleinman and Bleck determined blood viscosity and percentage of platelet aggregation in 22 patients with Legg-Calvé-Perthes disease and 21 control normal persons. The blood viscosity in the patients was definitely increased over that of the normals. There was no difference in the platelet aggregation studies. They proposed that the increased blood viscosity may lead to decreased blood flow to the femoral head and may be a contributory factor in the pathogenesis of the disease.[397]

Studies of the arterial and venous circulation of the femoral neck have shown that the venous drainage is disturbed in the active stage of Legg-Calvé-Perthes disease.[638] Green and Griffin studied the intraosseous venous pressure in 23 diseased hips and 23 normal hips. The intraosseous venous pressure, as measured in the femoral neck, was slightly higher in the hips with Legg-Calvé-Perthes disease, and after intraosseous injection of 5 ml. of saline solution, became significantly higher. In the diseased hips the intraosseous venogram was abnormal, but the etiology of the venous obstruction is unknown.[275]

Pathology

In Legg-Calvé-Perthes disease there are varying degrees of avascular necrosis of the femoral head in different stages of repair. This was first reported by Phemister in 1922, and later was confirmed by Zemansky.[531, 709]

Jonsäter performed core biopsies of the femoral head in various stages of the disease. He demonstrated in the *initial stage* (avascular necrotic) the histologic picture is dominated by marked necrosis of bone and bone marrow (Figs. 3–121 and 3–122). The trabeculae may be crushed. The nuclei in the osteocytes are absent or pyknotic. A necrotic mass consisting of dead marrow and pulverized particles of dead bone (Trümmermehl) accumulates in the marrow spaces. Occasional remnants of living bone may be encountered. There is no evidence of bone regeneration. The basal layer of articular cartilage may show degenerative changes in areas where the bone necrosis reaches as far as the cartilage-bone junction. The peripheral cartilaginous cap is thickened because it continues to proliferate, being nourished by synovial fluid. The physis may show some irregularity in the columnization of the cartilaginous growth cells. Grossly, the bone is softer than normal. Arthrographic studies by Jonsäter have shown that the cartilaginous head retains it spherical shape in this initial stage.[356]

In the second, or *resorption, stage* revitalization of the femoral head takes place by "creeping substitution" and apposition. This stage ordinarily lasts from one to three years. On histologic examination there will be vascular connective tissue invading the dead bone, which is resorbed actively by osteoclasts and

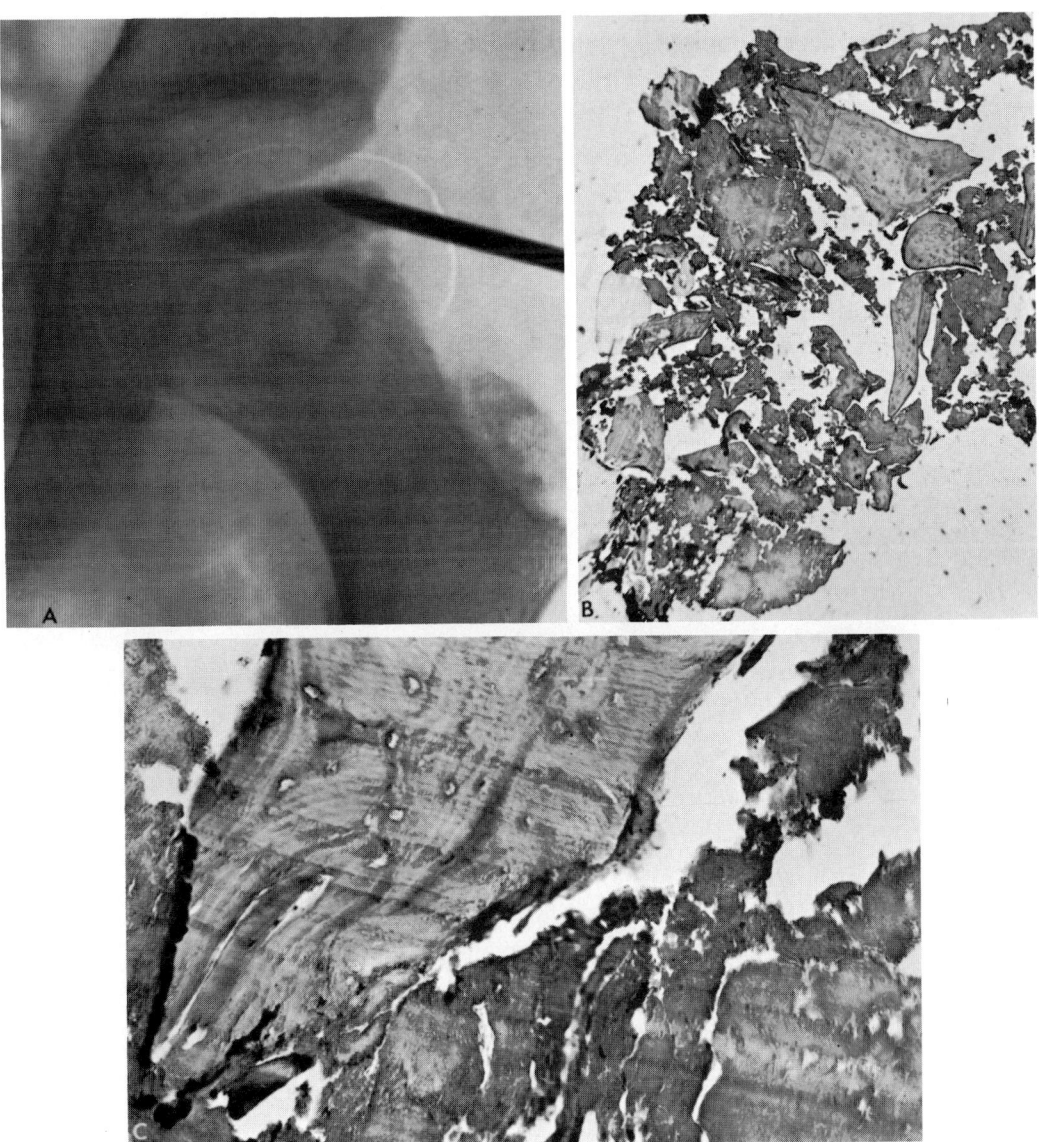

FIGURE 3–121. Histopathologic findings in the avascular or necrotic stage of coxa plana (the initial stage of Waldenström).

A. Radiogram of the hip shows increased density and minimal compression. The puncture needle marks the site of biopsy. **B.** Photomicrograph showing the dead bone trabeculae, which are partially retained (×35). The marrow spaces are filled with dead marrow and pulverized pieces of dead bone. There is no sign of regeneration. **C.** Photomicrograph (×200). Note the absence of pyknosis of the nuclei in the lacunar spaces of the osteocytes. (From Jonsäter, S.: Coxa plana. A histopathologic and arthrographic study. Acta Orthop. Scand., Suppl. 12, p. 29, 1953. Reprinted by permission.)

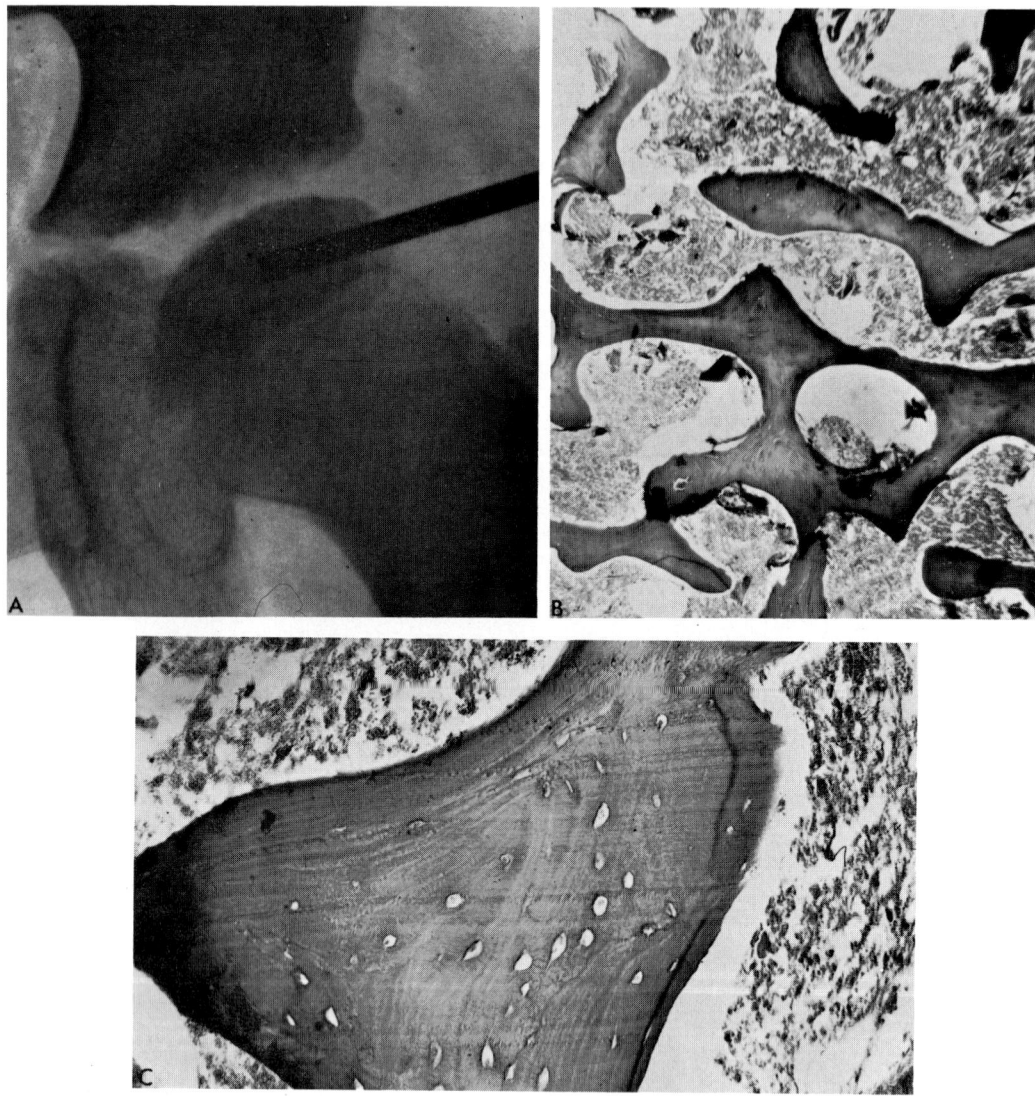

FIGURE 3–122. Histopathologic findings in the avascular or necrotic stage of coxa plana (the initial stage of Waldenström).

A. Radiogram of the hip showing the markedly dense and flattened head. **B.** Photomicrograph (×35). Note the crushed trabeculae, which are totally necrotic. Bone marrow is absent; there is no sign of reaction. **C.** Greater magnification (×200) shows the absence of nuclei in the dead trabeculae surrounded by amorphous necrotic masses. (From Jonsäter, S.: Coxa plana. A histo-pathologic and arthrographic study. Acta Orthop. Scand., Suppl. 12, p. 29, 1953. Reprinted by permission.)

replaced by newly formed immature bone (Figs. 3–123 and 3–124). The stage of repair may vary in different parts of the femoral head because of repeated periods of infarction.[110] The cartilage changes are similar to those seen in the necrotic stage.

The epiphysis loses height as a result of collapse of the bony trabeculae and, in part, of the progressive resorption of the fragmented necrotic bone from its deep surface.[110]

Enchondral ossification in the viable portions of the femoral head (usually the posteromedial segment) proceeds normally. When the necrotic and collapsed anterolateral part revascularizes, an area of ossification develops in the articular cartilage. In the radiograms this appears as "specks of calcification," one of Catterall's signs of "head-at-risk."[103, 106]

Metaphyseal changes are present in both the moderate and severely involved cases. In the early active stage of the disease the metaphyseal trabeculae are essentially normal; the central part of the metaphysis contains adipose tissue. Later on in the course of the disease, the radiolucent areas correspond histologically to areas of fibrocartilage that undergo disorganized ossification. The physis may extend inferiorly on the side of the metaphysis of the femoral neck.

In the *reparative stage* normal bone appears, replacing the diseased bone (Fig. 3–125).

Catterall and associates described the morphology of Legg-Calvé-Perthes disease in six whole femoral heads and five core biopsies. The spectrum of findings ranged from an ischemic arrest of ossification in the capital articular cartilage without infarction to multiple infarction of the ossific nucleus of the femoral head. It is the reparative process through resorption of bone that leads to the pathologic changes of the disease. Pathologic fracture causes collapse of the avascular bone trabeculae; "creeping substitution" and apposition of viable bone in dead trabeculae give sclerosis and chondrification by metaplasia of reactive fibrous tissue formed by resorption of loose necrotic bone, giving rise to radiolucencies.[110]

Ponseti and associates studied the histochemical and ultrastructural changes of the epiphyseal cartilage and physis that were obtained from the femoral head and neck in five patients with Legg-Calvé-Perthes disease. Beneath the articular cartilage cap there was a thick zone of hyaline (epiphyseal) cartilage in which were found sharply demarcated areas of hypercellular and fibrillated cartilage with prominent blood vessels. Electron microscopic examination of these areas showed numerous irregularly oriented collagen fibrils and many areas of proteoglycan granules. Histochemical examination showed the fibrillated cartilage to be strongly positive to alcian blue, weakly positive to periodic acid–Schiff, and positive to aniline blue. In the hypercellular areas the interterritorial matrix was weakly positive to both alcian blue and periodic acid–Schiff. These findings indicate that the fibrillar areas have a high proteoglycan content, a decrease in structural glycoproteins, and a different size of collagen fibrils from normal epiphyseal cartilage. The hypercellular areas had decreased proteoglycans, glycoproteins, and collagen. The lateral physeal margin was often irregular, showed a marked reduction of collagen and proteoglycan granules, and contained numerous large lipid inclusions.[540] These cartilage lesions are similar to those seen in the vertebral end-plates of Scheuermann's juvenile kyphosis. Whether the cartilage abnormalities are primary or secondary to ischemia is uncertain. In patients with unilateral Legg-Calvé-Perthes disease, the studies of the epiphyseal cartilage of the opposite normal hip have shown irregularities of ossification and thick epiphyseal cartilage with areas of calcification.[110] These observations suggest the probability that Legg-Calvé-Perthes disease could be a localized expression of a generalized, transient disorder of the epiphyseal cartilage. It is possible that the collapse and necrosis of the femoral head may be caused by the breakdown and disorganization of the matrix of the epiphyseal cartilage. The persistence of abnormally soft cartilage through which the vascular channels must traverse to penetrate into the femoral head may cause repeated episodes of ischemia.

The pathogenesis of Legg-Calvé-Perthes disease according to Salter and as shown in Figure 3–126 is as follows. First, avascular necrosis of the femoral head takes place. This causes temporary cessation of growth of the ossific nucleus of the femoral head; the articular cartilage cells on the periphery of the femoral head, however, continue to grow as they derive nutrition from the synovial fluid. At this stage there is no collapse of the femoral head, which is structurally intact. Revascularization and enchondral ossification take place peripherally and progress centrally. There are simultaneous resorption of avascular bone and laying down of immature new bone (primarily woven bone). The pathologic changes of Legg-Calvé-Perthes disease, until this stage, are silent. There are no symptoms. Legg-Calvé-Perthes disease is "potential" but not "true" according to Salter.

If the "potential" Legg-Calvé-Perthes disease is *not* complicated by trauma and subchondral

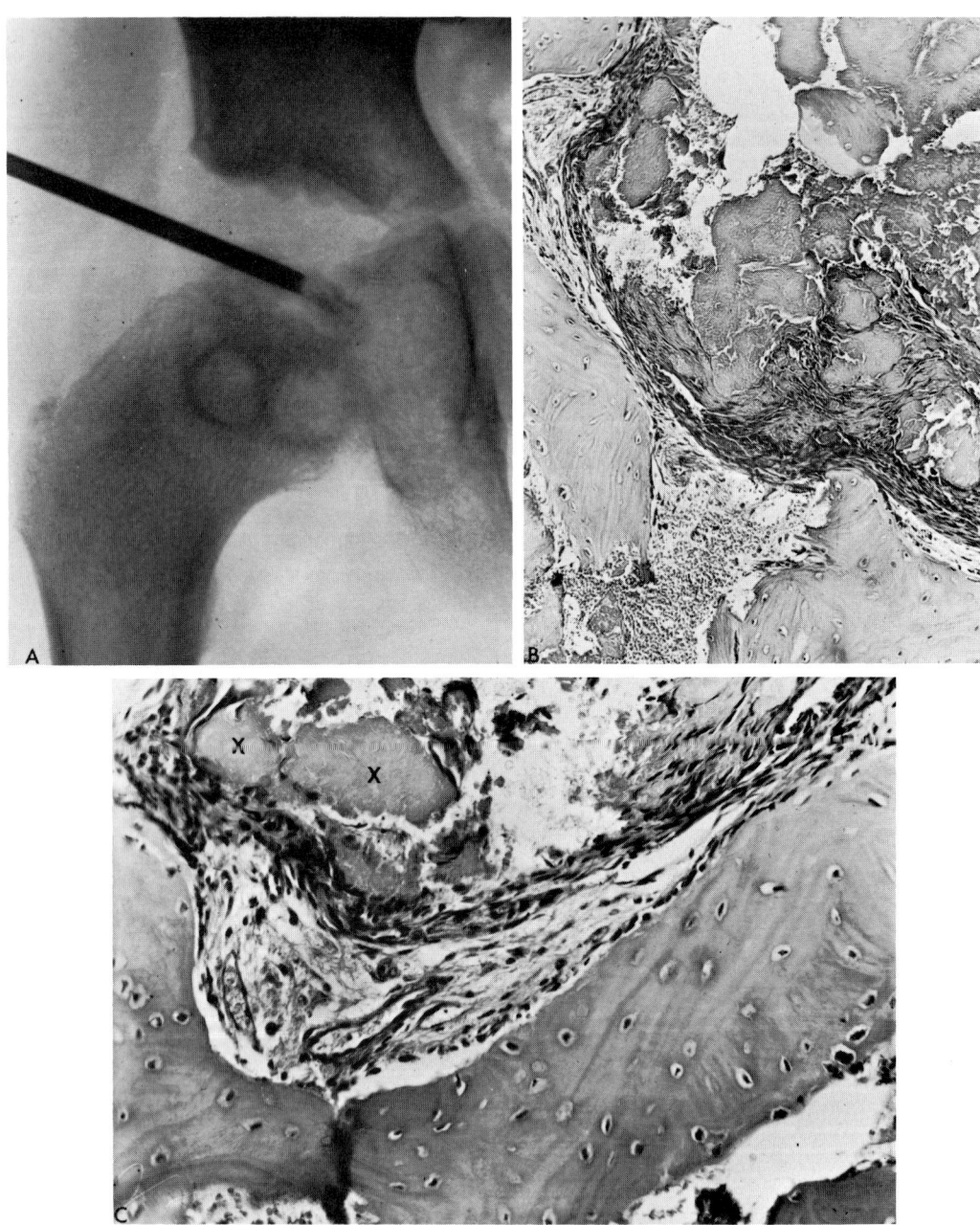

FIGURE 3-123. *Histopathologic findings in the regenerative stage of coxa plana (the fragmentation stage of Waldenström).*

A. Radiogram of the hip showing the fragmented and flattened femoral head. **B.** Photomicrograph (×100). Note, in the upper right portion, the vascular connective tissue growing into the dead bone. Newly formed bone is seen at lower left. **C.** Photomicrograph (×200). X's mark the remnants of necrotic bone, below which is the markedly vascular connective tissue. Immature bone with large, well-stained nuclei is seen in the lower part of the picture. (From Jonsäter, S.: Coxa plana. A histo-pathologic and arthrographic study. Acta Orthop. Scand., Suppl. 12, p. 39, 1953. Reprinted by permission.)

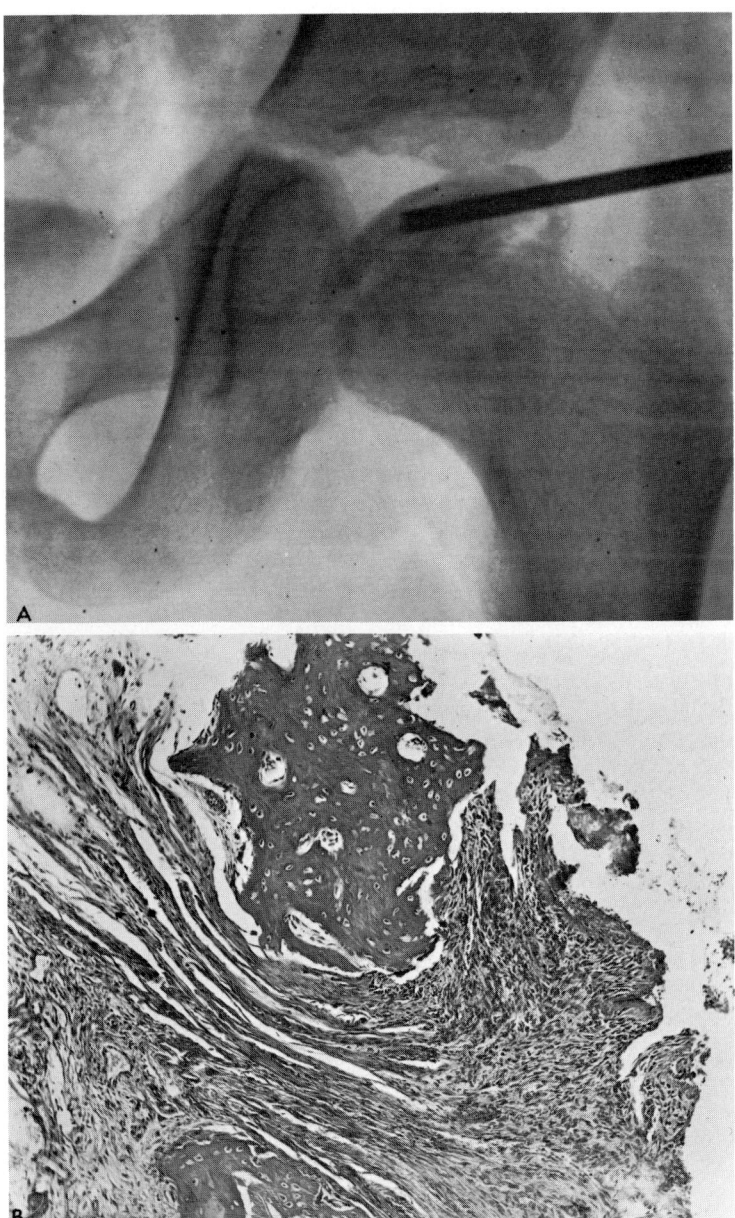

FIGURE 3–124. *Histologic changes in the regenerative stage of coxa plana (the fragmentation stage of Waldenström).*

A. Radiogram of the hip. Note the compressed and fragmented ossific nucleus of the femoral head. **B.** Photomicrograph (×100). The vascular connective tissue is forming immature bone. (From Jonsäter, S.: Coxa plana. A histo-pathologic and arthrographic study. Acta Orthop. Scand., Suppl. 12, p. 40, 1953. Reprinted by permission.)

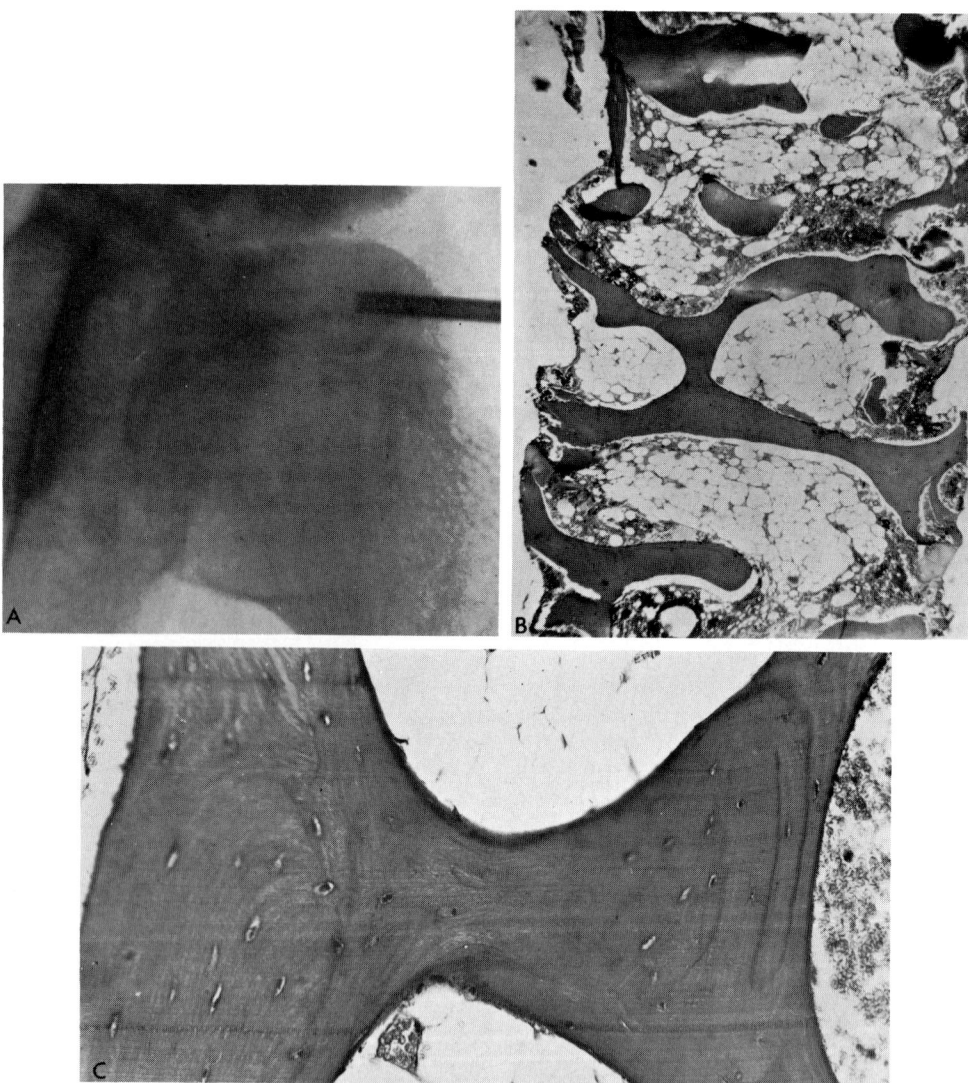

FIGURE 3–125. Histopathology of residual stage of coxa plana.

A. Radiogram of the hip. Note the normal bony structure. The epiphyses are somewhat flattened. **B.** Photomicrograph (×35) showing the normal bone trabeculae and marrow spaces. There is no necrosis or active regeneration. **C.** Photomicrograph (×200). Note the well-stained nuclei of the osteocytes in the trabeculae. (From Jonsäter, S.: Coxa plana. A histo-pathologic and arthrographic study. Acta Orthop. Scand., Suppl. 12, p. 51, 1953. Reprinted by permission.)

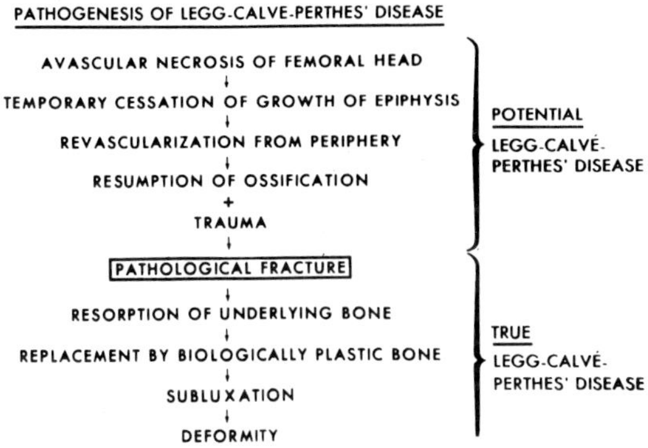

```
PATHOGENESIS OF LEGG-CALVE-PERTHES' DISEASE

  AVASCULAR NECROSIS OF FEMORAL HEAD
               ↓
TEMPORARY CESSATION OF GROWTH OF EPIPHYSIS   ⎫
               ↓                             ⎪   POTENTIAL
   REVASCULARIZATION FROM PERIPHERY          ⎬   LEGG-CALVÉ-
               ↓                             ⎪   PERTHES' DISEASE
      RESUMPTION OF OSSIFICATION             ⎭
               +
             TRAUMA
               ↓
       ┌─────────────────────┐
       │ PATHOLOGICAL FRACTURE│                  ⎫
       └─────────────────────┘                  ⎪
               ↓                                ⎪
    RESORPTION OF UNDERLYING BONE               ⎪   TRUE
               ↓                                ⎬   LEGG-CALVÉ-
 REPLACEMENT BY BIOLOGICALLY PLASTIC BONE       ⎪   PERTHES' DISEASE
               ↓                                ⎪
           SUBLUXATION                          ⎪
               ↓                                ⎭
            DEFORMITY
```

FIGURE 3–126. *Pathogenesis of Legg-Calvé-Perthes disease.*

(From Salter, R. B., and Thompson, G. H.: Legg-Calvé-Perthes disease. The prognostic significance of the subchondral fracture and a two-group classification of the femoral head involvement. J. Bone Joint Surg., 66-A:479, 1984. Reprinted by permission.)

fracture, the process is resolved by reconstitution of the femoral head with no subluxation and no deformity. The part of the ossific nucleus that was ossified at the time of interruption of blood supply is outlined by a growth arrest line. The subsequent ossification of the surrounding cartilage gives a "head-within-a-head" appearance in the radiogram.

Trauma to the femoral head will cause a subchondral stress fracture. This triggers the onset of *"true" Legg-Calvé-Perthes disease*. The stress fracture is usually due to vigorous normal activity and not to acute trauma. It manifests itself clinically by pain, muscle spasm with limitation of hip motion, and antalgic limp. The subchondral fracture begins anteriorly and extends posteriorly for a varying distance. It is best observed in the lateral radiogram of the hip.

The cancellous bone beneath the fracture collapses owing to loss of structural stability and sustains a second episode of vascular compromise because vascular channels are obliterated. Revascularization of the involved bone is slow because the capillaries are obstructed by trabecular and marrow debris. Resorption of fibroosseous tissue and subsequent reossification of the epiphysis with primary woven bone make the femoral head "biologically plastic"; i.e., it is not physically soft but can be molded into round or flat surfaces depending on the concentricity of its containment in the acetabulum and the biomechanical forces acting on it. Collapse and flattening of the femoral head may occur with its anterolateral subluxation (Fig. 3–127 C). Range of motion of the hip is restricted because of muscle spasm and soft-tissue contracture. Adduction-flexion deformity of the hip will develop; this will further displace the femoral head superiorly and laterally (Fig. 3–127 D). A dent will form in the anterolateral aspect of the femoral head by the rim of the acetabulum in the weight-bearing position of the femoral head (Fig. 3–127 E). On abduction of the hip the femoral head will hinge and displace laterally, increasing medial joint space (Fig. 3–127 F).[570-581]

Clinical Picture

The presenting complaints are a limp and pain of several weeks' to months' duration. The pain is usually mild and referred to the knee region, the anteromedial aspect of the thigh, and the groin, following the sensory distribution of the obturator nerve. It is usually aggravated by activity and relieved by rest. In some cases, pain may be absent or very minimal.

Symptoms are usually insidious in onset. A history of trauma can be obtained in about one fourth of cases, with acute onset from the date of injury.

The antalgic limp is associated with limitation of hip motion, especially hip abduction and medial rotation. There may be flexion-adduction contracture of the affected hip. In the acute synovitis stage, local tenderness may be elicited on the anterior aspect of the hip joint on deep palpation. Atrophy of the muscles of the thigh is common. There may be slight shortening of the affected lower limb. Adduction contracture of the hip will aggravate the apparent lower limb shortening.

Radiographic and Imaging Features

Radiography. The radiographic findings depend on the stage in the natural course of the disease and the extent of involvement. Waldenström divided the natural history of coxa plana into four stages according to the radiographic changes.

The *incipient stage* is characterized in the radiogram by a widened articular cartilage space (Fig. 3–128). According to Waldenström, this stage lasts one to three weeks.

In the *aseptic necrotic, or avascular, stage* there is homogeneous increased radiopacity of the femoral head without areas of rarefaction; subchondral rarefaction and varying degrees of flattening of the femoral head may be visualized (Fig. 3–129). According to Waldenström, this stage may last several months to a year.

Text continued on page 949

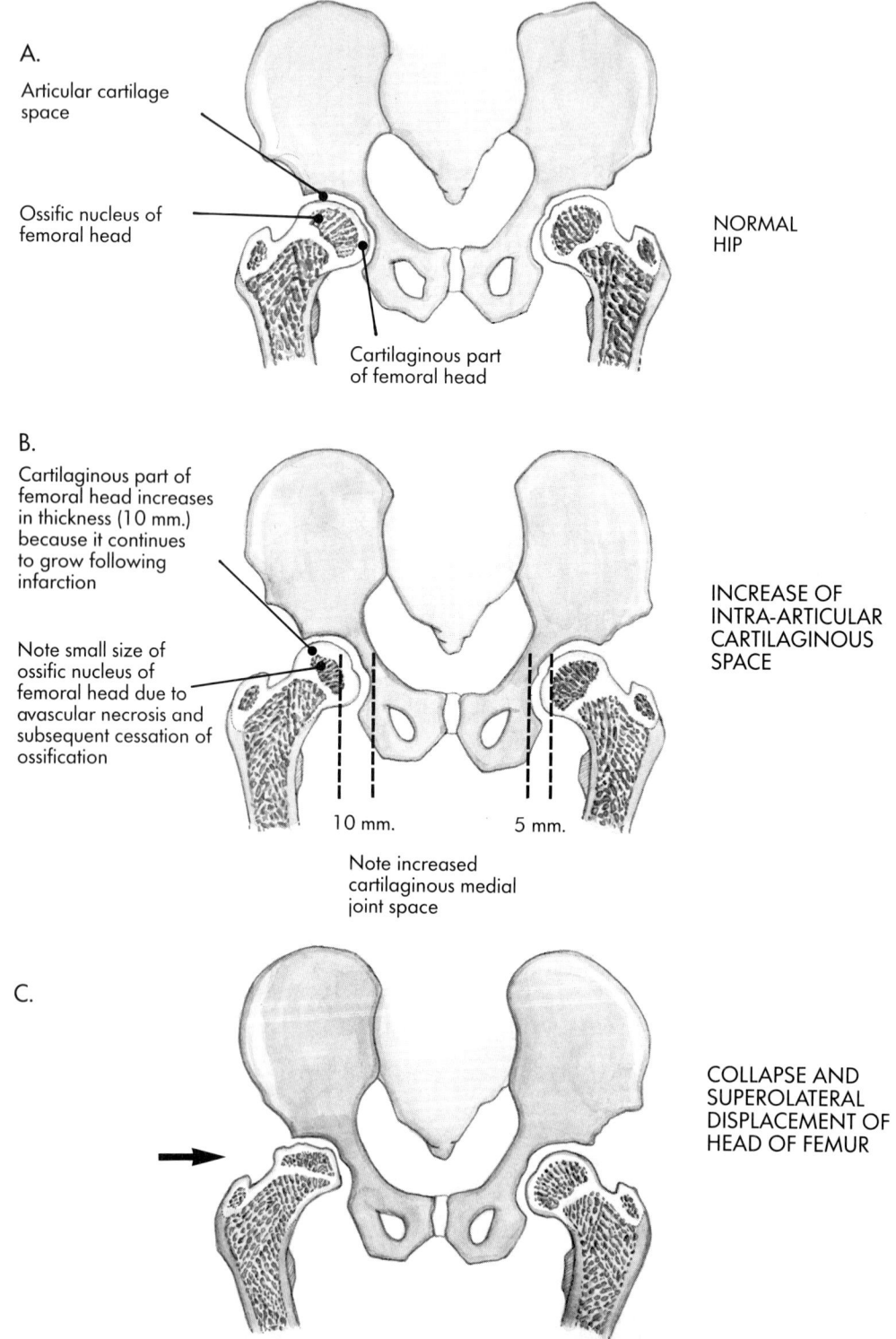

FIGURE 3–127. Pathogenesis of deformity of the femoral head in Legg-Calvé-Perthes disease.

A. Normal hips. **B.** Widening of the medial cartilaginous joint space due to hypertrophy of the cartilage covering of the femoral head. Note the smaller ossific nucleus due to cessation of bone growth as a result of avascular necrosis. **C.** Collapse of the femoral head with superolateral displacement.

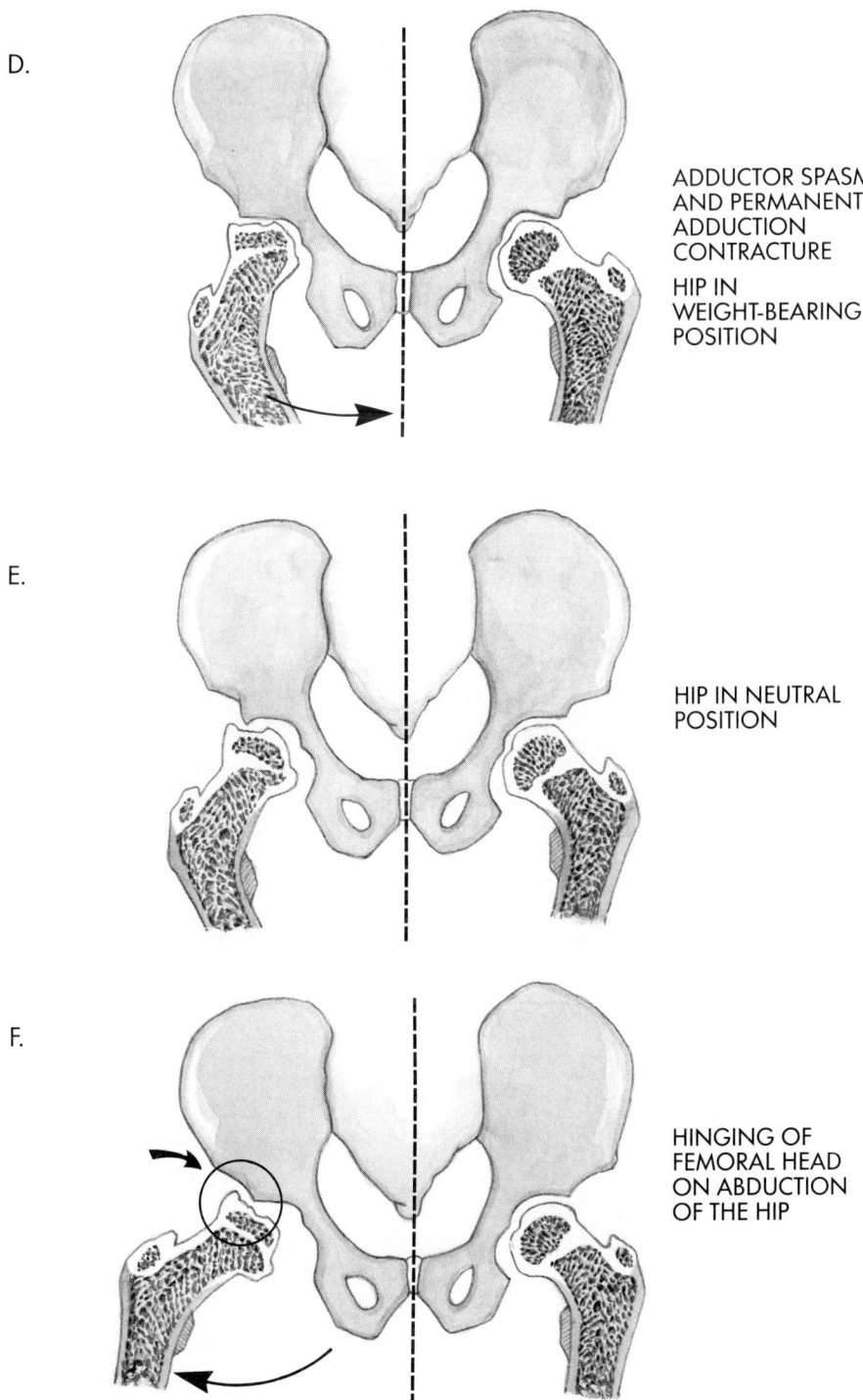

FIGURE 3–127 Continued. *Pathogenesis of deformity of the femoral head in Legg-Calvé-Perthes disease.*

D. The hip is adducted in weight-bearing position. Note in **E** the dent in the lateral part of the femoral head blocking concentric reduction of the hip. **E** and **F.** Hinged abduction. On abduction of the hip (**F**) the femoral head is displaced farther laterally with increase in the medial joint space.

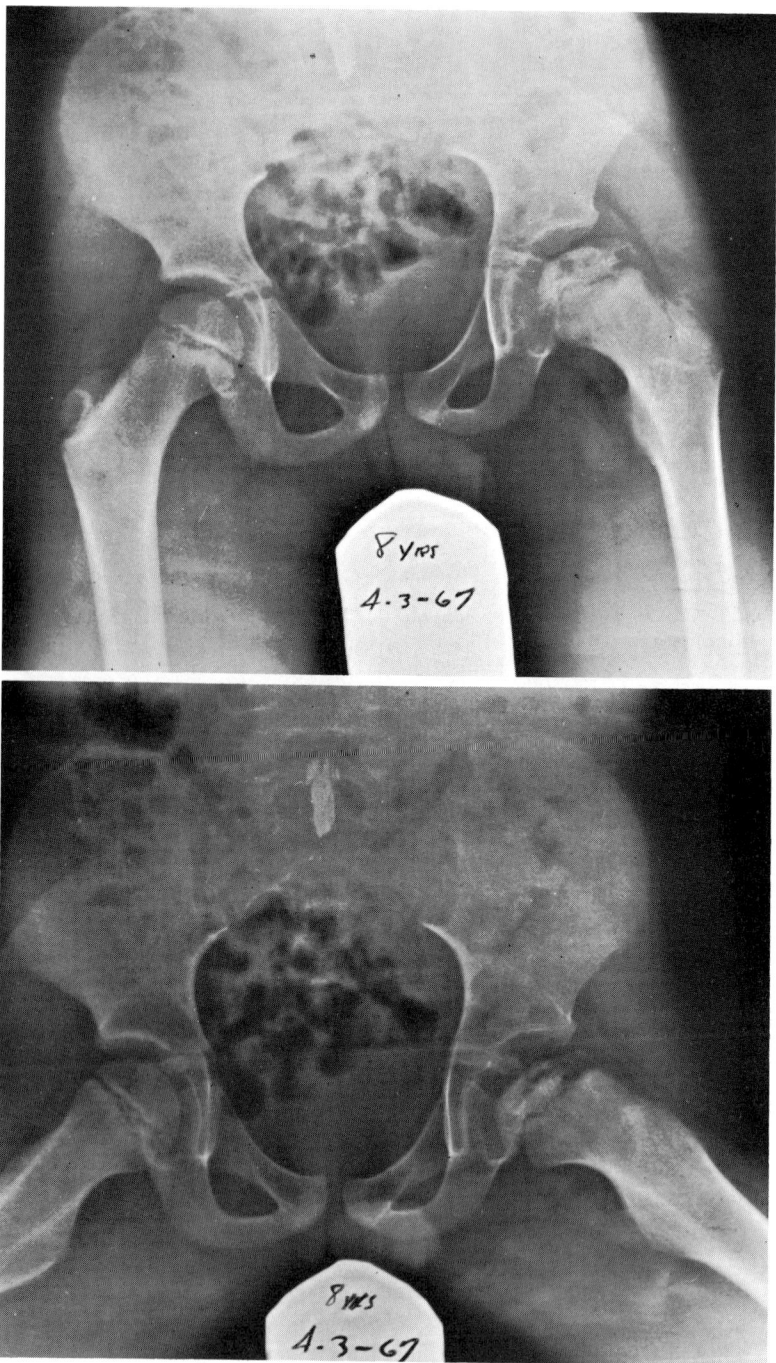

FIGURE 3–130. Regenerative stage of coxa plana.

Note the presence of radiolucent areas and fragmentation of the condensed epiphysis. Revitalization of the femoral head is taking place by "creeping substitution."

The *regenerative, or fragmentation, stage* is distinguished by areas of rarefaction and fragmentation, which correlate with sites of bone resorption by ingrowth of fibrous vascular tissue and laying down of immature bone that is not yet calcified (Fig. 3–130). The femoral neck may be widened with varying degrees of anterolateral extrusion of the femoral head.

The *residual stage* is demonstrated by the gradual disappearance of the rarefied areas and replacement with normal trabecular bone. The eventual shape of the femoral head may be spherical or flattened. In a certain percentage of cases, residual coxa magna of variable degree will be the outcome (Fig. 3–131). Aspherical congruity (a flat femoral head in a normal acetabulum) and anatomic incongruity of the femoral head and acetabulum, if present, will result in degenerative arthritis of the hip later on in adult life (Fig. 3–132).[672–677]

In the past two decades there have been great advances in our understanding of the pathogenesis and pathology of Legg-Calvé-Perthes disease. It has become evident that Waldenström's classification of the radiographic stages of the disease, though pragmatic, is not scientifically valid. Legg-Calvé-Perthes disease results from more than one ischemic episode, and there are varying stages of repair in the different parts of the femoral head. This is well documented by the pathologic findings of biopsy specimens from 57 hips with the disease.[342]

The complex, varying nature of Legg-Calvé-Perthes disease is becoming increasingly elucidated by bone scan and magnetic resonance imaging findings. In the light of current knowledge and the state of the art of bone imaging, it is best to present the radiographic features as follows:

The *first radiographic sign* is the smaller size of the ossific nucleus of the femoral head combined with the widened articular cartilage space of the affected hip as compared with the opposite normal hip (Fig. 3–133). This is due to temporary cessation of enchondral ossification of the ossific nucleus of the femoral head (due to ischemia) while the deeper layer of the articular cartilage (the growth plate of the epiphysis) continues to grow because it derives its nutrition from the synovial fluid.

The *second sign* is the subchondral fracture line in the femoral head. This subchondral lucency was first observed by Waldenström, but he thought it was caused by bone resorption rather than by pathologic fracture.[672, 677] In the adult avascular femoral head, the radiolucent crescent line was attributed to pathologic fracture by Norman and Bullough.[508] Caffey is credited with being the first to describe the nature of the crescentic subchondral line in children with Legg-Calvé-Perthes disease as due to fracture and to recognize it as one of the early radiographic signs of coxa plana.[84] It is therefore referred to as "Caffey's sign." Salter and Thompson later described the prognostic significance of Caffey's crescent line.[578] The subchondral fracture line heralds the clinical onset of the disease, and it is a relatively transient finding seen early in the course of the disease, with an average duration of two to nine months. Later on, with bone resorption and enchondral ossification, the fracture cannot be detected. The older the patient and the more severe the avascular necrosis, the longer the subchondral fracture will be present. The fracture line is best seen in the Lowenstein lateral view. It begins in the anterior margin of the femoral head and traverses posteriorly in the subchondral zone to a varying extent (Fig. 3–134). It can almost always be detected when appropriate radiograms are made within four months of the onset of symptoms. When it can no longer be visualized on the radiograms because of progressive resorption, the extent of involvement can be assessed by Catterall's parameters, and the extent of the fracture line is no longer necessary as a prognostic sign.

In the natural course of the disease, the *third radiographic finding* is increased radiopacity of the femoral head (see Fig. 3–129). This is present to a varying degree. The sclerotic radiographic image is produced primarily by appositional new bone being laid down on avascular trabeculae, in part by calcification of the necrotic marrow, and in the early stages, by collapse and crushed crowding of the avascular trabeculae in the dome of the epiphysis.[53, 166]

In the process of repair, the avascular trabeculae are resorbed by ingrowth of fibrous vascular tissue from the periphery. In this "creeping substitution," immature bone is apposed to the avascular bone trabeculae. The reparative stage is depicted in the radiograms as fragmentation of the condensed epiphysis by radiolucent areas (see Fig. 3–130). With the progressive formation of normal bone trabeculae, the rarefied areas gradually disappear.

The various radiographic parameters that influence the shape of the femoral head and neck and the final outcome are discussed later.

Bone Scan With Technetium-99m. The findings obtained by bone scan with technetium-99m in Legg-Calvé-Perthes disease are distinctive; they show a marked decrease in or lack of uptake of the nuclide at the site of avascular necrosis of the femoral head (Fig. 3–135). The

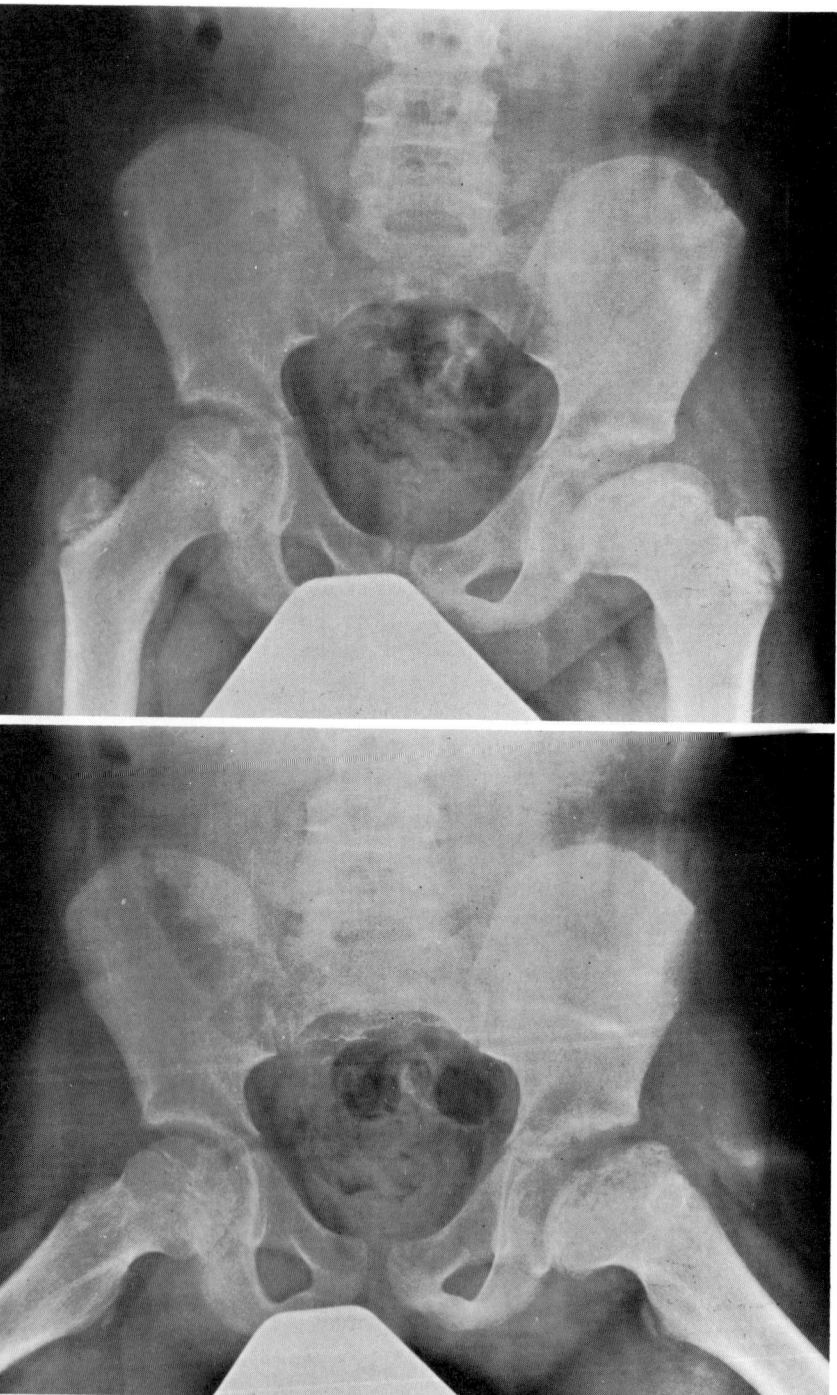

FIGURE 3–131. Residual stage of coxa plana.

Note the flattening and mushrooming of the epiphysis and the broadening of the femoral neck.

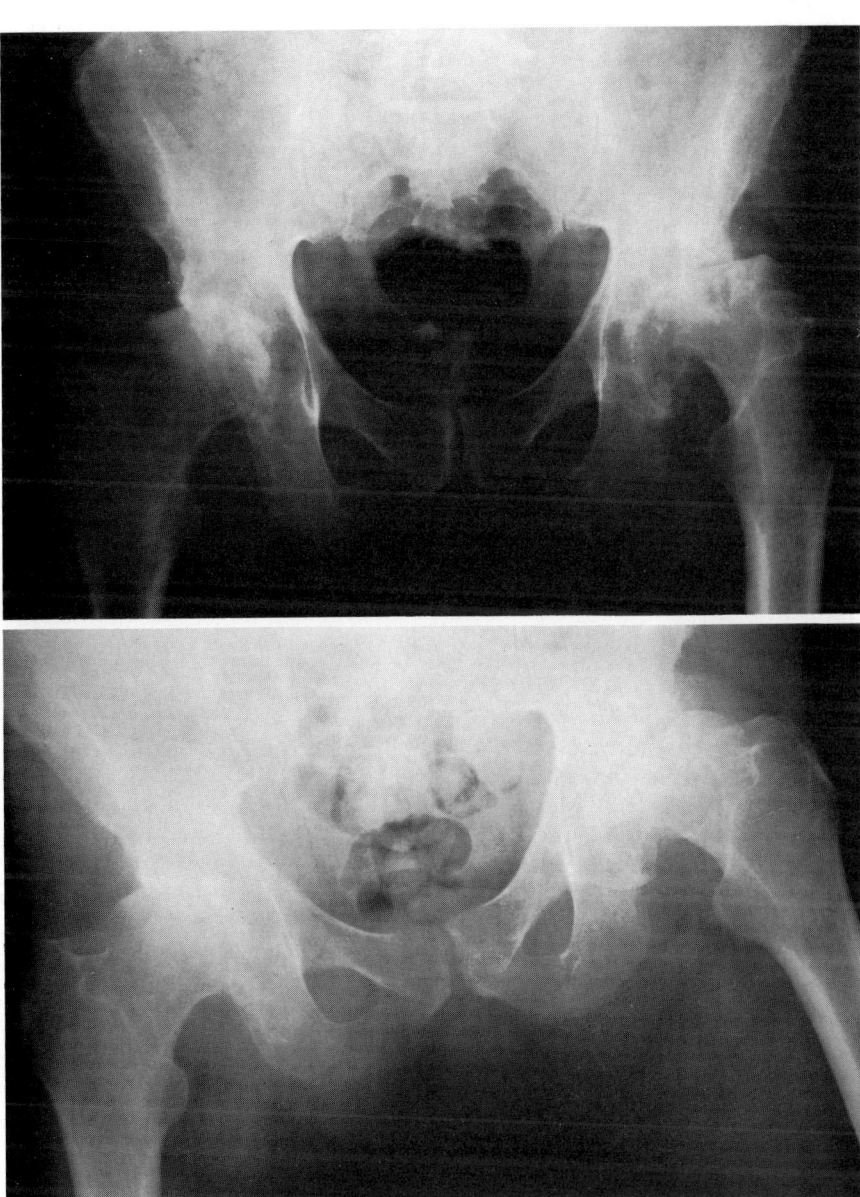

FIGURE 3–132. Legg-Perthes disease in an adult.

Anteroposterior and lateral radiograms of both hips. Note the coxa magna senilis with severe degenerative changes.

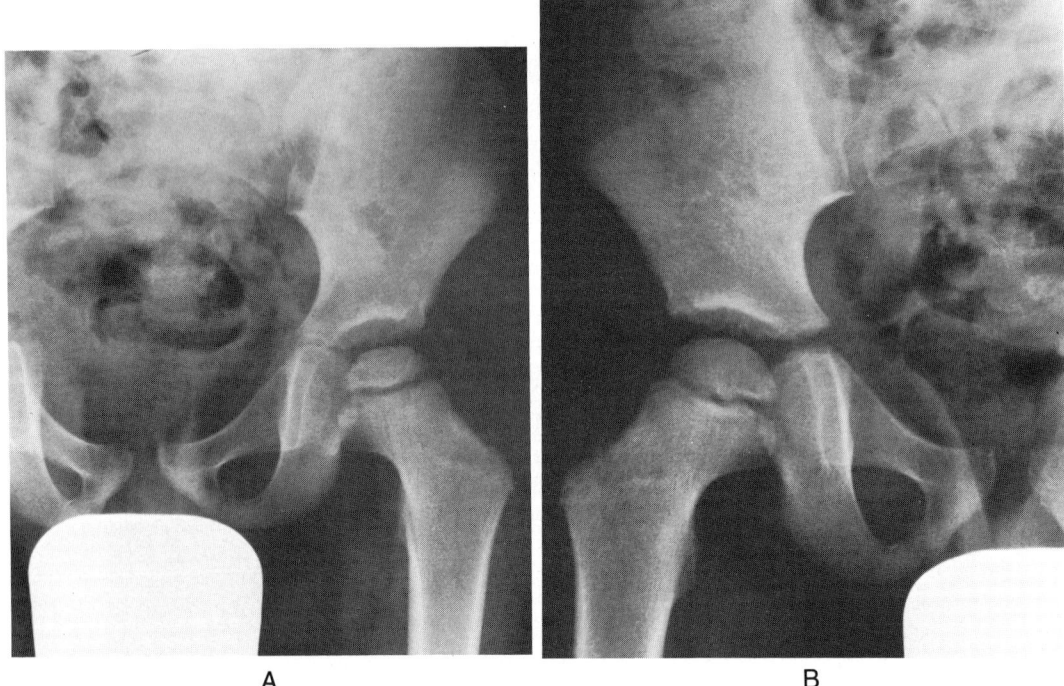

FIGURE 3–133. Early radiographic signs of Legg-Calvé-Perthes disease.

A and **B.** Anteroposterior radiograms. Left femoral ossific nucleus is slightly smaller than the right; otherwise the hips appear to be normal.

concentration of the radionuclide in bone depends on regional blood flow and bone metabolism. The capital femoral physis and the acetabular rim are biologically and metabolically active. Sites of necrosis show defective uptake. With revascularization of necrotic bone there is increased radioisotope marginal activity, progressive decrease in size of localized defects, and full vascularization of the femoral head. The scan will reliably diagnose Legg-Calvé-Perthes disease with a sensitivity of 0.98 and a specificity of 0.95. Furthermore, diagnosis is possible some months before radiographic signs develop.[639] Revascularization can be detected in the bone scan before there is radiographic evidence.[32, 33, 201, 219]

Scintigraphy should be performed with pinhole imaging. Both anteroposterior and lateral projections should be made.[152, 153] This is crucial to determine the degree of epiphyseal involvement. Conway and associates have classified the following scintigraphic stages in the course of Legg-Calvé-Perthes disease (Table 3–17).[137]

In the *first stage* the epiphysis appears totally avascular (Fig. 3–136). At this stage radiograms of the hips are normal; however, the ossific nucleus of the femoral head may be smaller than normal size, and the medial joint space may be increased. In the *second stage*, revascularization appears as a lateral column (Figs.

3–137 and 3–138). This is the initial stage of revascularization by "recannulization." In this phase the radiographic findings consist of an increased density of the epiphysis, a smaller ossific nucleus on the affected side, and possibly visible subchondral fracture. When there is a lateral column on scintigraphy, the prognosis is good. In *stage three*, there is gradual filling in of the anterolateral part of the epiphysis that is best visualized in the frog-leg lateral view. This third scintigraphic stage corresponds with the fragmentation stage in the radiograph. The *fourth and final stage* is one of gradual return to normal. Scintigraphy shows there is revascularization via collateral circulation adjacent to the site of the physis (Fig. 3–139). This is referred to as "base filling."

In the bone scan, extrusion of the epiphysis outside the confines of the acetabulum may be seen. Also there may be collapse of the lateral column with avascularity, which again carries a poor prognosis. When the capital femoral physis is healthy, increased uptake at the physis extends across the entire epiphysis and is of the same intensity as in the opposite hip. Decreased activity of the physis indicates growth disturbance. Revascularization and healing of the growth plate by collateral vessels will show increased activity in the physis.

Failure of revascularization of the lateral col-

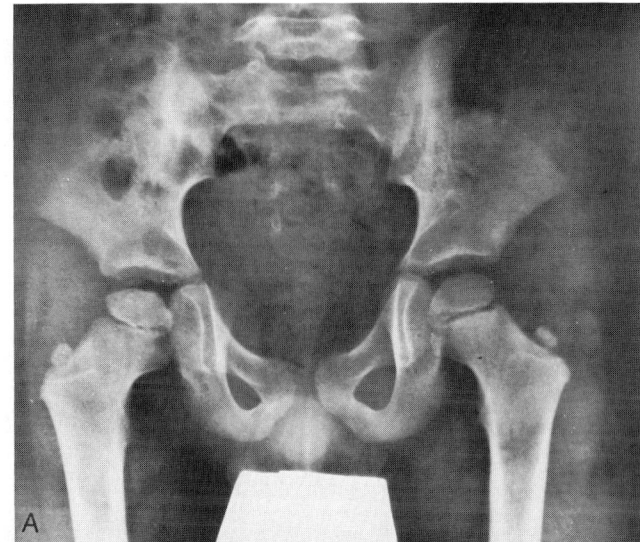
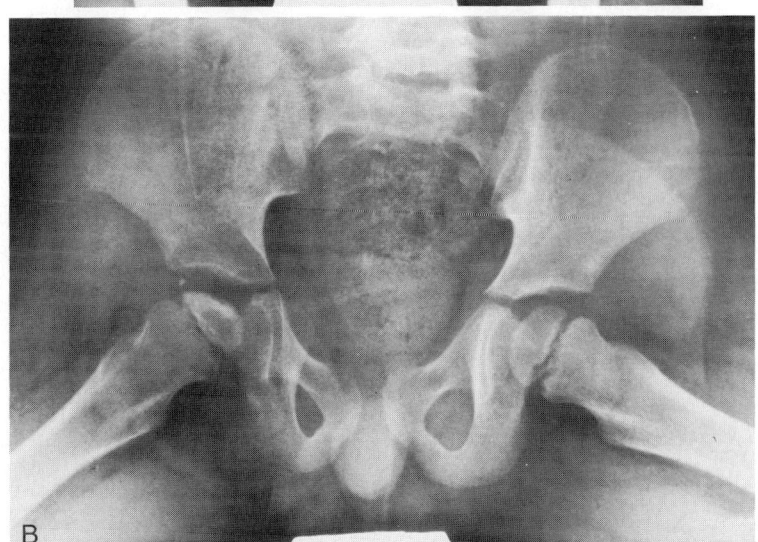

FIGURE 3-134. *Legg-Calvé-Perthes disease of the right hip.*

A and **B.** Anteroposterior and lateral radiograms of both hips. In the lateral projection note the subchondral fracture in the right upper femoral epiphysis.

Table 3-17. *Correlation of Findings of Technetium-99m Scintigraphy With Radiograms in Legg-Calvé-Perthes Disease*

Stage	Bone Scan With Technetium-99m	Radiogram
I	Total lack of uptake	Normal or smaller size of ossific nucleus Increased medial joint space
II	Lateral column	Subchondral fracture Increased density of femoral head Smaller ossific nucleus
III	Gradual filling of anterolateral part of epiphysis	Fragmentation
IV	Base filling in epiphysis adjacent to physis Gradual complete revascularization of femoral head	Reparative—gradual return to normal

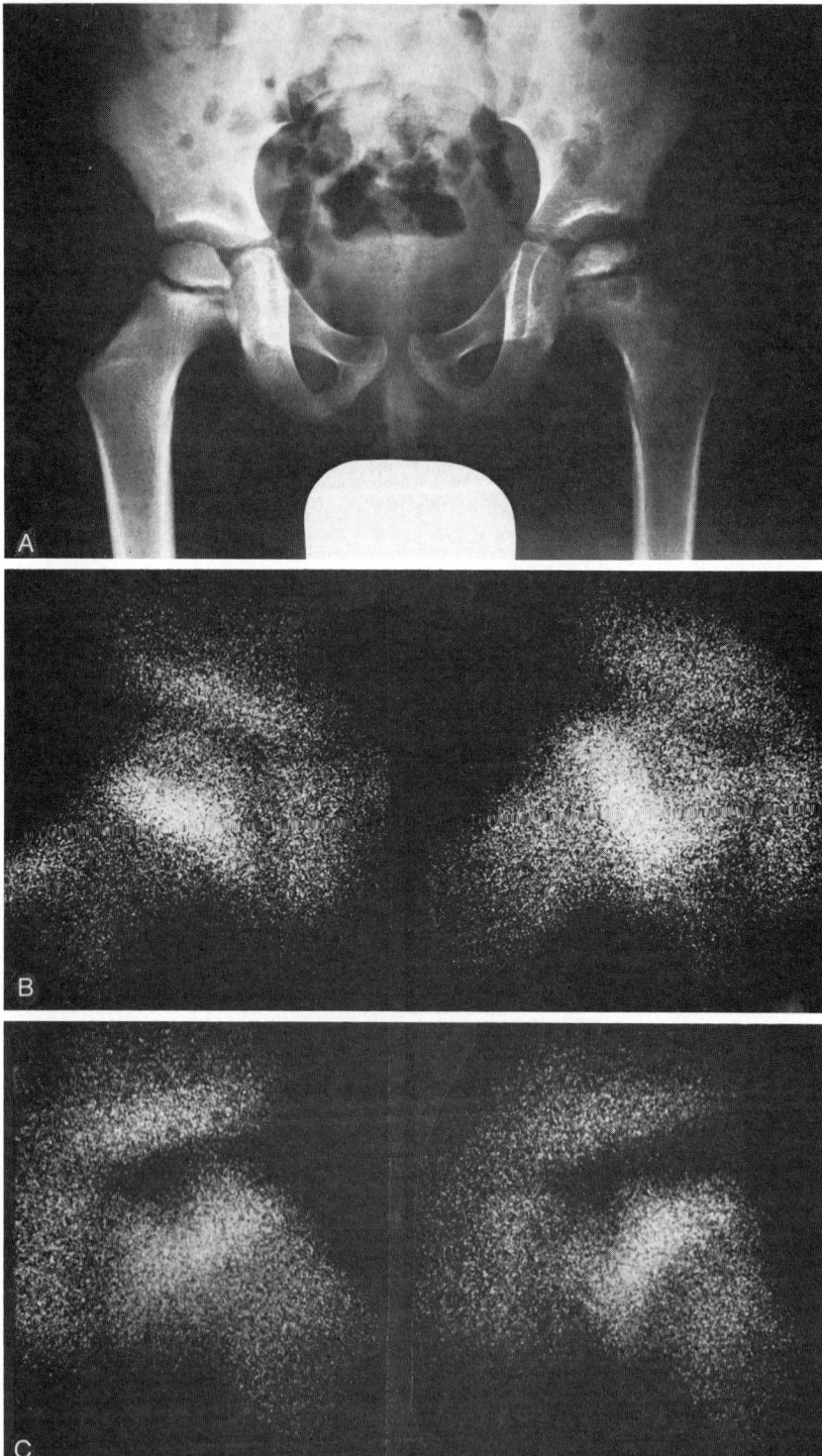

FIGURE 3–135. Bone scan findings with technetium-99m in Legg-Calvé-Perthes disease.

A. Anteroposterior radiogram of both hips showing Legg-Calvé-Perthes disease of the left hip. **B.** Bone scan of the normal right hip showing normal uptake of the nuclide (anteroposterior and "frog" lateral versus pinhole imaging). **C.** Bone scan of the involved left hip showing marked lack of uptake in the femoral head. The capital femoral physis has normal uptake.

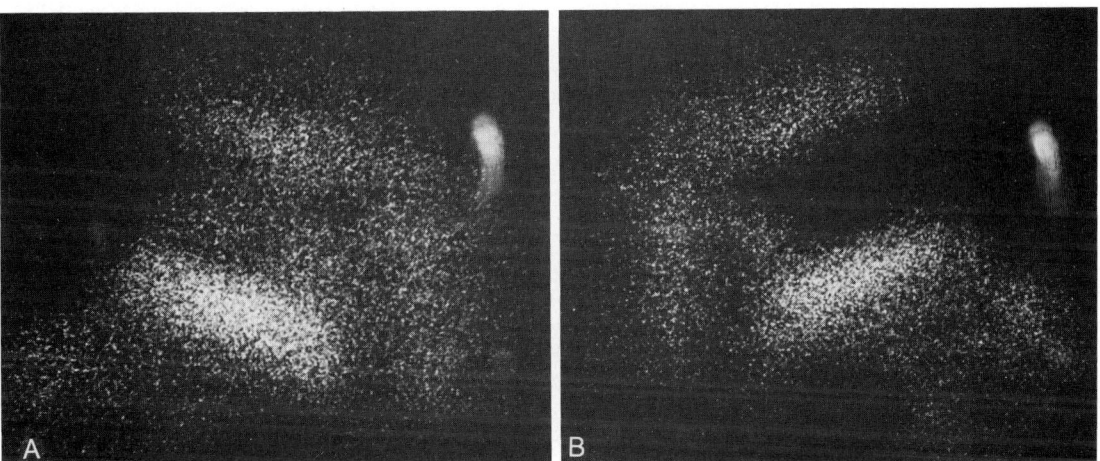

FIGURE 3–136. *First scintigraphic stage in Legg-Calvé-Perthes disease.*

Bone scans with Tc-99m of right and left hips. Note the total lack of uptake of the nuclide in the left femoral head owing to avascular necrosis. **A.** Right hip. **B.** Left hip. (Courtesy of Dr. James Conway, Children's Memorial Hospital, Chicago, Illinois.)

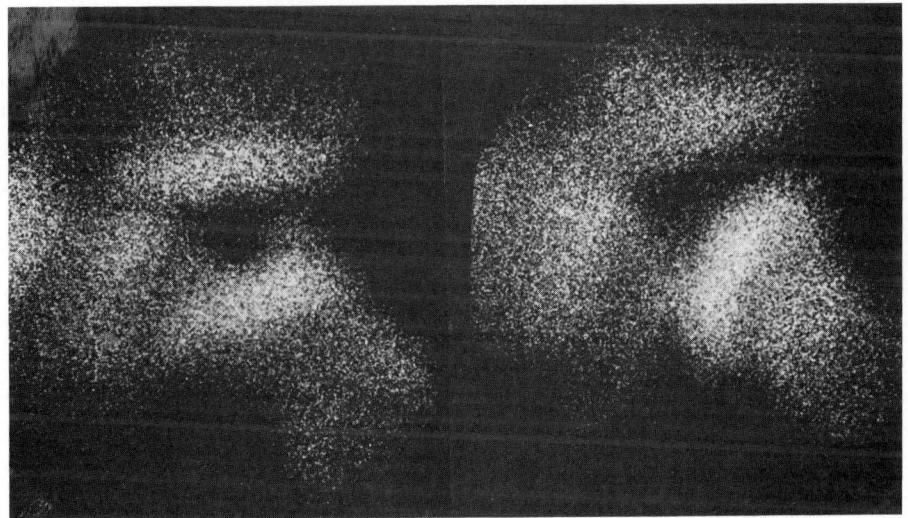

FIGURE 3–137. *Second scintigraphic stage.*

Note the beginning of a lateral column in the anteroposterior projection.

FIGURE 3–138. *Bone scan in Legg-Calvé-Perthes disease.*

Lateral column is well formed and contained within the acetabulum. This is a good prognostic sign.

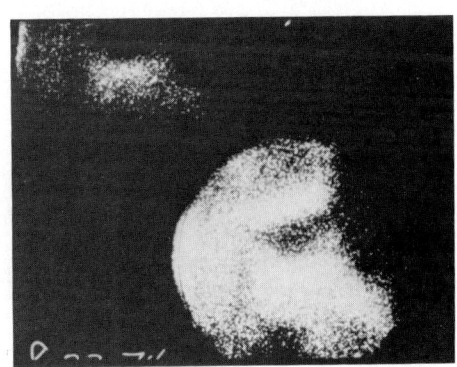

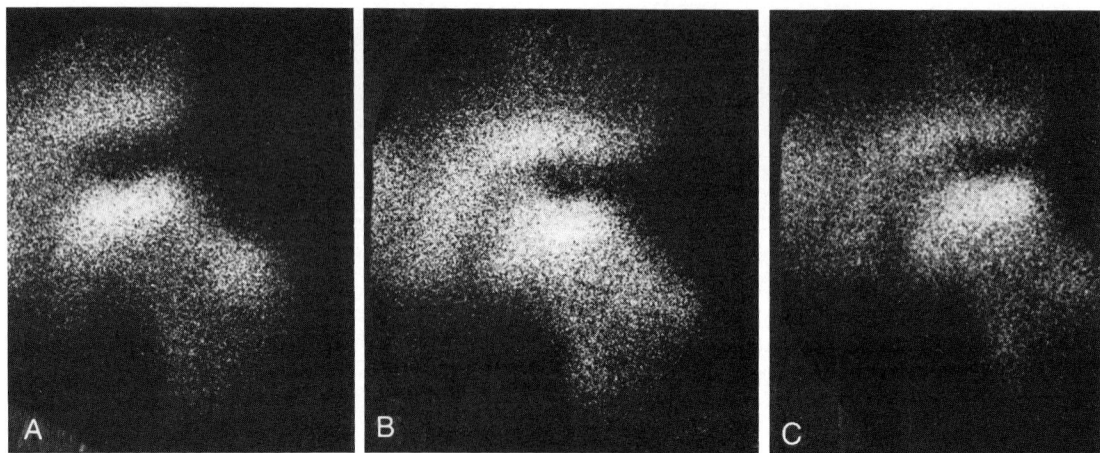

FIGURE 3–139. *Scintigraphic stages in Legg-Calvé-Perthes disease.*

A. Stage I bone scan two weeks after onset of pain and limping. Radiograms showed the smaller size of the ossific nucleus. Scintigraphy shows that the entire head is involved. **B.** Stage III. There is gradual filling in of the anterolateral part of the epiphysis; there is, however, no lateral column, which is a poor prognostic sign. **C.** Stage IV is "base filling," in which there is gradual revascularization via collateral circulation.

umn is a poor prognostic sign (see Fig. 3–139 B). This scintigraphic "head-at-risk" sign precedes Catterall's "radiographic head-at-risk" sign by at least two to three months. Decreased activity of the capital femoral physis heralds growth disturbance; it is an early sign of a poor prognosis, again evident several months prior to the radiographic evidence. Later in the course of the disease the bone scan will show anterolateral extrusion of the epiphysis. A previously present lateral column may disappear, indicating repeated infarct or collapse, signs of a poor prognosis. Areas of metaphyseal rarefaction may show increased activity. Scintigraphic "head at risk" signs are given in Table 3–18.

Magnetic Resonance Imaging (MRI). This technique is still in its early phases of development, with the units available only in selected university medical centers. Recent technologic improvements provide excellent resolution and image reconstitution. Image-acquisition times require that the patient be immobile for approximately one hour; therefore, sedation is necessary in a young child. The cost is another drawback.

Necrotic areas are depicted in the image as regions of low signal intensity (Fig. 3–140). Areas of infarction can be detected prior to radiographic change. The cartilaginous portions of the femoral head and acetabulum can be depicted, producing an arthrogram-like image of the hip without the use of ionizing radiation or the invasive injection of contrast material (which often is performed under general anesthesia). With magnetic resonance imaging the femoral head can be assessed for flattening, irregularity of outline, congruity with the acetabulum, and anterolateral extrusion.[56, 596]

Differential Diagnosis

Toxic Synovitis. In the initial stages of the disease *toxic synovitis of the hip* should be ruled out, especially when the symptoms of irritable hip persist. Clinically, this may be difficult because both Legg-Calvé-Perthes disease and toxic synovitis of the hip have similar features. In general, in toxic synovitis the symptoms are more acute. Proximal thigh atrophy and limb shortening are features of chronic hip disease and are indicative of Legg-Calvé-Perthes disease. Radiograms may be normal in both entities; however, close scrutiny in Legg-Calvé-Perthes disease reveals that the ossific

Table 3–18. Scintigraphic "Head at Risk" Signs in Legg-Calvé-Perthes Disease

Early
  Failure of revascularization of lateral column
  Decreased activity of capital femoral physis, indicating growth disturbance
Late
  Anterolateral extrusion of vascularized capital femoral epiphysis
  Disappearance of previously present lateral column of revascularization on capital femoral epiphysis, indicating repeat infarct, collapse, or both
  Intense metaphyseal activity

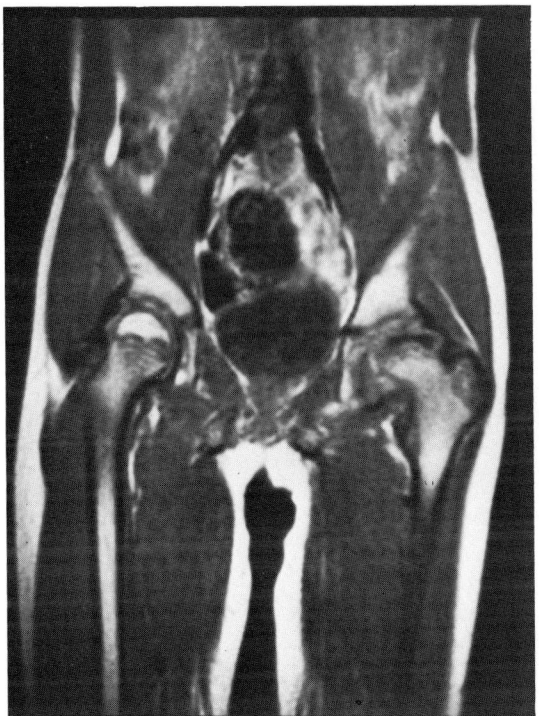

FIGURE 3–140. *Magnetic resonance imaging in Legg-Calvé-Perthes disease of the left hip.*

Note that the necrotic areas are depicted as regions of low signal density. Also note the compression and lateral extrusion of the collapsed femoral head.

nucleus of the affected femoral head is smaller, and a subchondral crescent line may be visible. A bone scan with technetium-99m will make the definite diagnosis; in Legg-Calvé-Perthes disease, uptake will be decreased to a varying extent, whereas in toxic synovitis, the bone scan will be normal or show minimally increased uptake due to inflammatory hypervascularity of the synovium. *Bone scan with technetium-99m should not be performed routinely in toxic synovitis.* It is indicated when symptoms and signs persist and do not respond to an adequate period of bed rest and traction; when there are repeated attacks of toxic synovitis, with each episode longer in duration and becoming more chronic; and when the skeletal age of the child is retarded, stature is short, and there are other constitutional factors indicative of Legg-Calvé-Perthes disease.

Infection. Pyogenic arthritis of the hip or osteomyelitis of the femoral neck should sometimes be considered in the differential diagnosis, especially when the child appears to be sick. In Legg-Calvé-Perthes disease there is no temperature elevation, white blood count is normal, and the erythrocyte sedimentation rate is normal. Gentle palpation will disclose anterior joint tenderness in septic arthritis and posterior tenderness of the metaphysis in osteomyelitis of the femoral neck. The *septic hip joint* assumes a posture of flexion (30 to 50 degrees), lateral rotation (10 to 20 degrees), and abduction (10 to 20 degrees), as this is the position of minimal hydrostatic pressure; passive motion of the infected hip is painful and guarded in all directions. In Legg-Calvé-Perthes disease the hip develops an *adduction contracture*. The radiograms in the septic hip will show capsular distention and a varying degree of lateral displacement of the femoral head. If the findings suggest the possibility of septic arthritis, ultrasonography should be performed, and if there is fluid in the joint, the hip should be aspirated. It is best to perform aspiration in the radiology department under image intensifier control and strict aseptic conditions. If fluid is not aspirated, verification that the joint has been entered is made by injecting a small amount of air or contrast material. The importance of early diagnosis of septic arthritis and immediate drainage cannot be overemphasized.

Juvenile Rheumatoid Arthritis. This disease may involve only or primarily the hip joint. In rheumatoid arthritis the child is usually not acutely ill, and the onset of the symptoms is gradual. Other joints should be diligently examined to rule out arthritic involvement. Tumefaction of the digits is characteristic of rheumatoid disease. Radiograms will show the ossific nucleus of the femoral head to be larger, not smaller, than the contralateral normal hip. The erythrocyte sedimentation rate will be elevated. Other rheumatologic serum studies will assist in making the diagnosis of juvenile rheumatoid disease.

Rheumatic Fever. Occasionally, onset of rheumatic fever may be in the hip joint. It is distinguished from Legg-Calvé-Perthes disease by its migratory, fleeting joint pains, cardiac involvement, and dramatic response to salicylates.

Tuberculosis. Tuberculosis of the hip still exists in North America and in other parts of the world. It is of historic interest to remember that Waldenström, in 1909, described the clinical entity of coxa plana as a benign form of tuberculosis. It is crucial to ask the parents whether there is any family history of tuberculosis and if the child has been exposed to a patient with tuberculosis. This author has seen four children with tuberculosis of the hip being treated by other orthopedic surgeons for Legg-Calvé-Perthes disease during the past decade (Fig. 3–141). A skin test for tuberculosis and

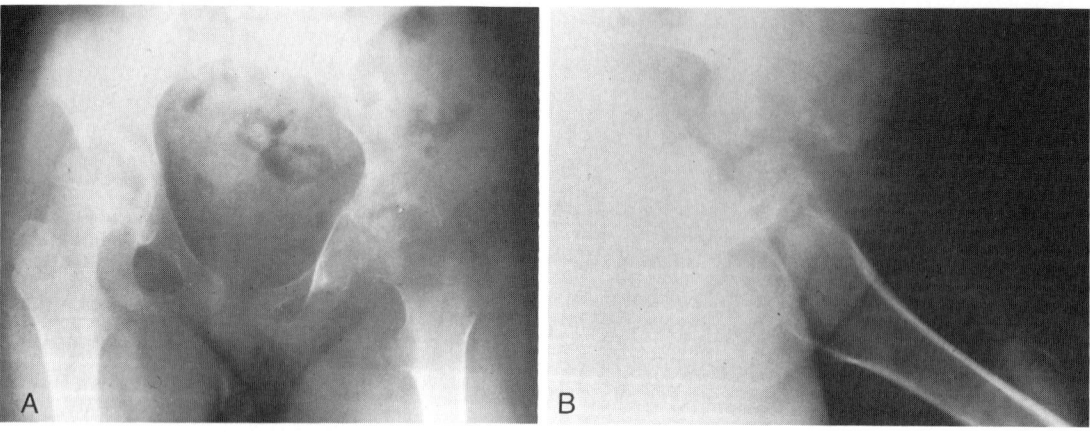

FIGURE 3–141. *Tuberculosis of the left hip in a ten-year-old girl.*

Anteroposterior view (**A**) of both hips and lateral view (**B**) of left hip. For 18 months the disease was misdiagnosed as Legg-Calvé-Perthes disease, and she was treated by containment orthosis.

determination of erythrocyte sedimentation rate should be part of the routine diagnostic workup for Legg-Calvé-Perthes disease.

Tumors. Other conditions to be considered in the differential diagnosis when involvement is unilateral are tumorous lesions involving the femoral head and neck such as eosinophilic granuloma, osteoid osteoma, benign osteoblastoma, chondroblastoma, and lymphoma. These lesions can be readily delineated by appropriate clinical and laboratory studies, bone scan, and computed tomography.

Differential Diagnosis When Both Hips Are Involved. This becomes more difficult. In Legg-Calvé-Perthes disease, involvement is asymmetrical, each femoral head being in a different stage of repair. The cystic changes in the metaphysis, the almost normal appearance of the acetabula and pelvic bones, and the normal spine differentiate Legg-Calvé-Perthes disease from the bone dysplasias. The stature may be short and skeletal maturation may be delayed in relation to chronological age, but the body proportions are normal. The characteristic findings of bone scan with technetium-99m in Legg-Calvé-Perthes disease will establish the diagnosis.

Bone Dysplasia. *Multiple epiphyseal dysplasia* is often mistaken for Legg-Calvé-Perthes disease (Fig. 3–142). This dysplasia is characterized by symmetrical involvement of the femoral heads and affection of other epiphyses, as shown by skeletal survey. The subchondral bony plate of the acetabulum is indistinct and irregular. The progressive changes of the various stages of Legg-Calvé-Perthes disease are absent, another distinguishing feature. There is no lack of radionuclide uptake in the bone scan with technetium-99m in epiphyseal dysplasia (Fig. 3–143). In the *trichorhinophalangeal syndrome*, the femoral heads may be flattened and fragmented, but its diagnosis is readily made by the characteristic clinical features of a pear-shaped nose, sparse hair, and premature fusion of the epiphyses of the phalanges with short, stubby hands. In *spondyloepiphyseal dysplasia*, the epiphyseal changes are associated with platyspondyly and a short trunk. There may be varying degrees of coxa vara.

Hypothyroidism. Epiphyseal changes of hypothyroidism may be confused with Legg-Calvé-Perthes disease. In juvenile cretinism, the ossification of the femoral head is delayed. When it does develop, the ossific nuclei are small and irregular in density; involvement is symmetrical (Fig. 3–144). Laboratory tests will establish the thyroid deficiency. The bone scan is normal in hypothyroidism.

Avascular changes of the femoral head due to *sickle cell disease* or *Gaucher's disease* should always be considered in the differential diagnosis.

Natural History

The radiologic course of the disease is divided by Catterall into the following stages:

1. *Initial phase*, which is subdivided into the phases of onset and fragmentation; this is the period when the femoral head is likely to be deformed.

2. *Healing phase* during which ossification of the biologically deformed head takes place; this phase may last up to two years.

3. *Growing period* during which remodeling occurs.

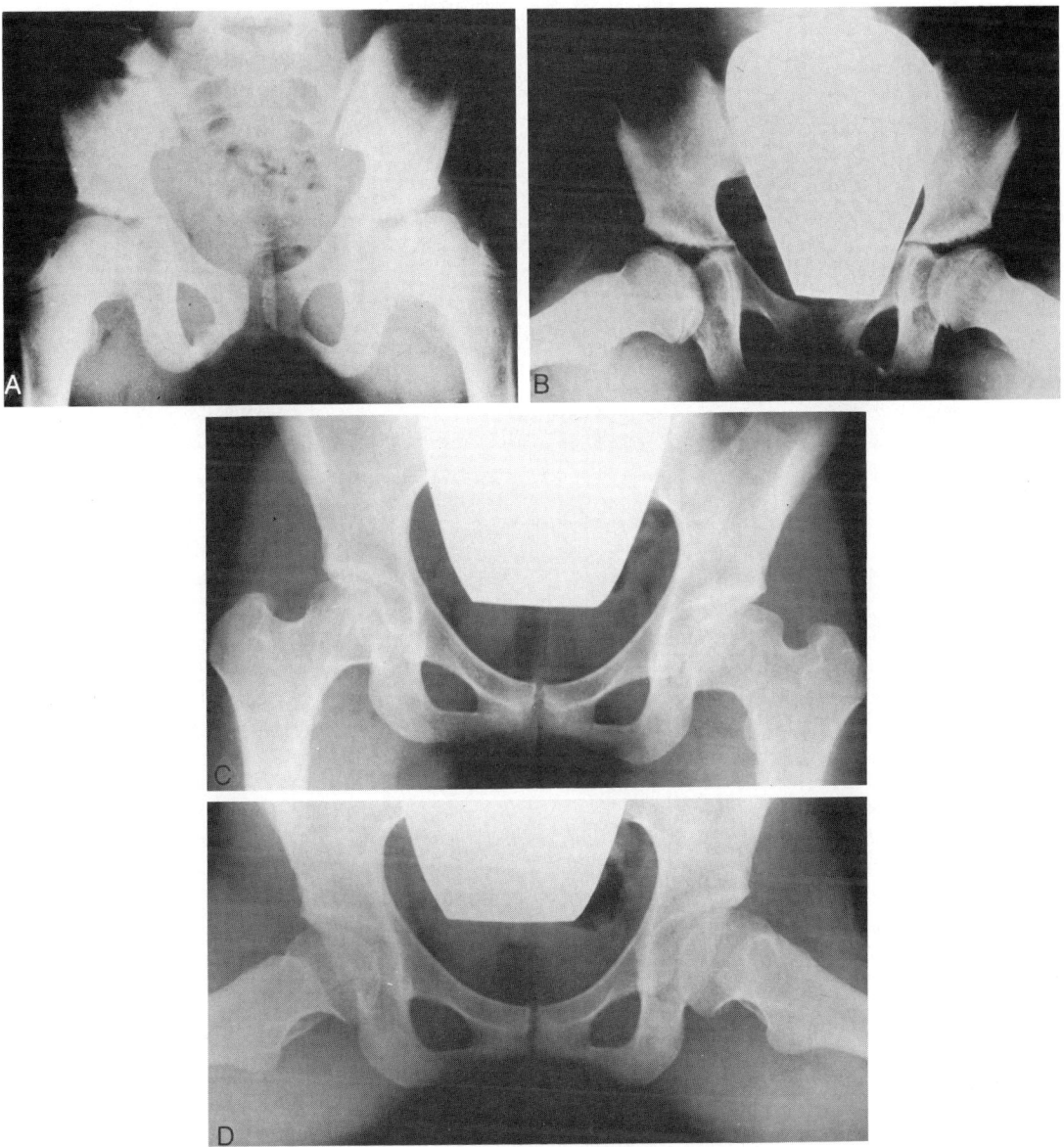

FIGURE 3–142. Multiple epiphyseal dysplasia of both hips.

This is often misdiagnosed as Legg-Calvé-Perthes disease. In epiphyseal dysplasia involvement is symmetrical and the progressive changes of Legg-Calvé-Perthes disease are not present. **A** and **B.** Anteroposterior and lateral radiograms of both hips in an eight-year-old girl with multiple epiphyseal dysplasia. **C** and **D.** Same patient ten years later.

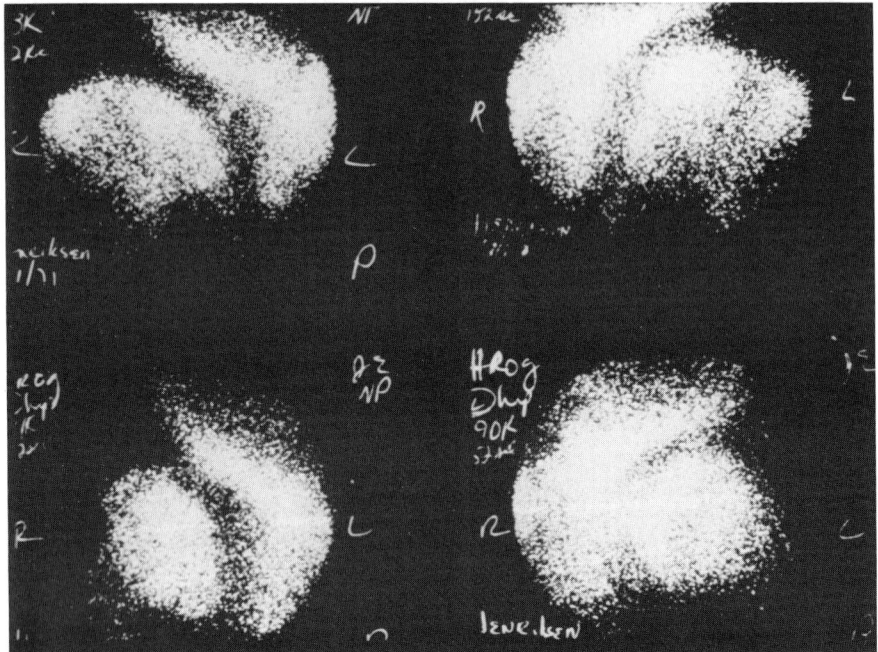

FIGURE 3–143. Bone scan findings with technetium-99m in multiple epiphyseal dysplasia.

Note the scan shows deformity of the femoral heads. The radionuclide uptake is normal.

4. *Definitive period* in which the hip may be normal or may be deformed and show varying degrees of degenerative arthritis.[103]

Prognosis

The outcome in Legg-Calvé-Perthes disease is determined by the following factors:

Patient's Age at Time of Diagnosis. The younger the patient, the better the outcome. The dividing line in prognosis appears to be eight years.[445] This fact is related to three biologic factors: the younger patient has more time to remodel the epiphysis after healing takes place; the acetabulum in the older patient loses its potential to develop; and older patients are heavier and more likely to damage the epiphysis.

Extent of Involvement. The prognosis is proportional to the degree of the radiologic involvement of the epiphysis; the greater the extent the poorer the prognosis.[103] Salter and Thompson compiled the results in four reported series in which Catterall's classification was used.[103, 276, 358, 438, 654] The results were assessed by the Moses concentric circles spaced 2 mm. apart.[578] There was no significant difference in the long-term result between Catterall's Group I and Group II regardless of treatment. The final result was satisfactory in all hips in Group I, whereas it was satisfactory in 93 per cent of those in Group II (94 per cent treated and 92 per cent untreated). The result was definitely different in the hips in Catterall's Group III hips, in which it was satisfactory in 76 per cent of the hips treated by containment methods and in 60 per cent of the hips without treatment. In Group IV the final result was satisfactory in 61 per cent of the hips treated by containment and 41 per cent of the untreated hips.[578] In the radiograms, the most important distinguishing feature between Groups II and III is the presence (Group II) or absence (Group III) of an intact lateral column of the capital femoral epiphysis, which protects the epiphysis from stress and minimizes the possibility of further collapse and subsequent deformity. It should be remembered, however, that lateral displacement and central flattening of the femoral head can occur in Group II—especially in the older age group.

Salter and Thompson have shown that the extent of the subchondral fracture correlates completely with the extent of subsequent maximum resorption. It is an important radiographic sign of prognostic value at an early stage of the disease. They proposed a simple and practical two-group classification of the extent of involvement of the femoral head. In *Group A* the subchondral fracture extends through less

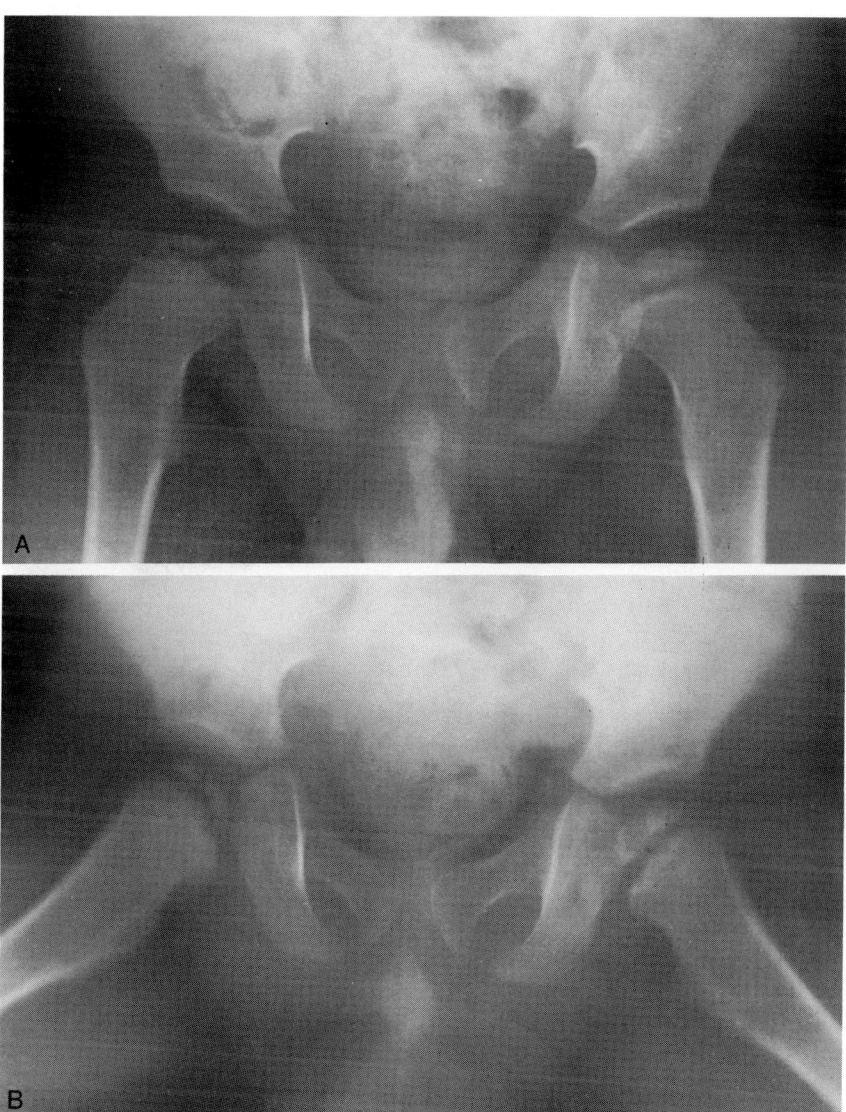

FIGURE 3–144. Epiphyseal changes in hypothyroidism.

These may be mistaken for Legg-Calvé-Perthes disease. **A** and **B.** Anteroposterior and lateral radiograms of both hips of a four-year-old boy with hypothyroidism. Note the delay and irregularity of ossification of the femoral heads.

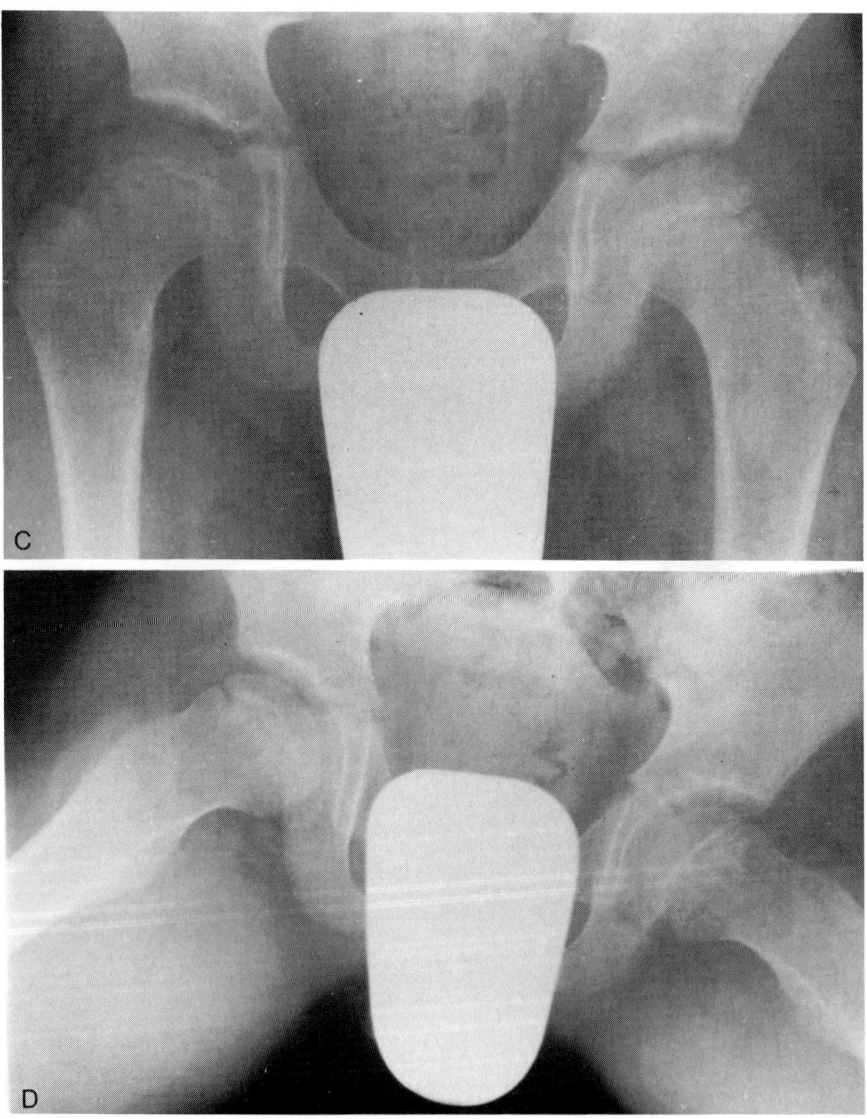

FIGURE 3–144 Continued. Epiphyseal changes in hypothyroidism.

C and D. Two years after treatment with thyroxine. There is complete healing.

than half of the head, and the prognosis is good; whereas in *Group B* more than half of the head is involved, and the outlook is poor.[578]

In general, in the female, involvement is more extensive; therefore, in similar age groups, the prognosis in girls is poorer than in boys.

Protrusion of Femoral Head Beyond Its Normal Confines in the Acetabulum. This is also referred to in the literature as femoral head *extrusion* or *subluxation*. It indicates a poor prognosis and, according to Catterall and Salter, is one of the four major factors in determining whether a femoral head is at risk.[103, 107, 578] The femoral head is uncovered initially because of overgrowth of articular cartilage, especially medially and laterally. Crushing of the trabeculae and flattening of the epiphysis cause the femoral head to be displaced upward and anterolaterally, extruding part of the capital epiphysis out of the acetabulum. The hip subsequently develops adductor spasm and contracture, which further uncovers the femoral head (see Fig. 3–127).[107]

In the radiograph, ossification of the thickened and extruded articular cartilage, lateral to the ossific nucleus, appears as small specks of increased radiopacity (originally described by Catterall as calcification).[103] This is one of the early signs of uncovering of the femoral head. Later on these ossific areas enlarge and coalesce.

Several methods of measuring the epiphyseal extrusion are described in the literature. According to the method of Green and associates, epiphyseal extrusion (EL) is the percentage of the diseased femoral head lateral to Perkins' line (XX_1). It is computed by dividing the amount of the involved femoral head that is uncovered (A–B) by the width of the opposite normal femoral head measured at the physis (C–D): i.e., EL = AB/CD × 100 (Fig. 3–145). Dickens and Menelaus determined the degree of uncovering simply by the amount of the femoral head that is lateral to Perkins' line (Fig. 3–146).

As reported by Green and associates, when the epiphyseal extrusion was more than 20 per cent, the prognosis was poor, but when it was less than 20 per cent, the prognosis was good. In hips in Catterall Group II, when the extrusion was more than 20 per cent, 40 per cent had a good result. When half of the femoral head was involved and the epiphyseal extrusion index was 20 per cent or more, only 8 per cent had a good result. There were no good results in hips in Catterall Group III or Group IV in children over eight years of age with epiphyseal extrusion of more than 20 per cent.[276]

Should one perform arthrography routinely to assess the extent to which the femoral head is uncovered? Gallagher and associates assessed the plain radiograms and arthrograms of 21 patients with Legg-Calvé-Perthes disease. They found that when epiphyseal extrusion is shown by the arthrogram, it could be seen equally well in the plain radiogram.[232] This author believes that arthrography should not be performed routinely.

Growth Disturbance of the Physis. There is a direct relationship between the severity of physeal involvement and the ultimate deformity of the femoral head. In about 90 per cent of cases there is some disturbance of physeal growth in Legg-Calvé-Perthes disease. In the bone scan with technetium-99m this is shown early by the decreased uptake in the physis. Later in the course of the disease, the following radiographic changes will indicate physeal growth disturbance: (1) premature physeal closure, (2) relative overgrowth of the greater trochanter, (3) alteration of physeal shape with

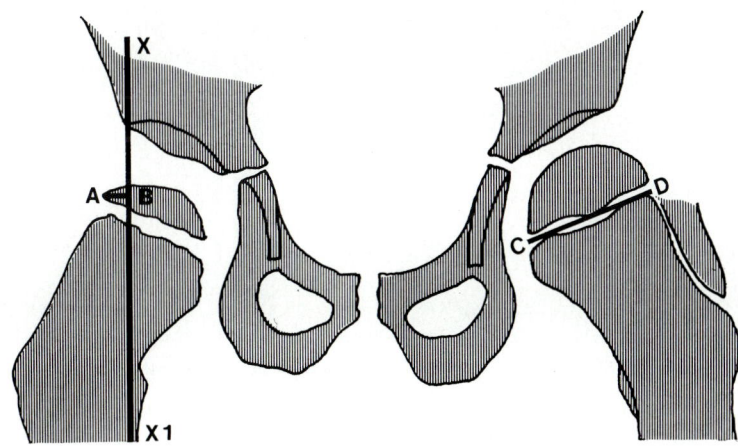

FIGURE 3–145. Method of measuring epiphyseal extrusion index according to Green and associates.

See text for explanation.

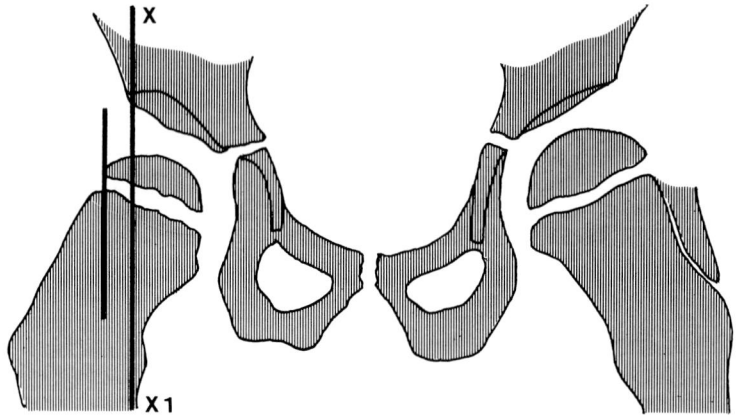

FIGURE 3–146. *Method of determining uncoverage of the femoral head according to Dickens and Menelaus.*

See text for explanation.

convex deformity (growth rate impaired centrally but normal peripherally), (4) lateral extrusion of the capital femoral epiphysis, and (5) medial bowing of the femoral neck (i.e., shortening and increased concavity of the lateral component of Shenton's line) (Fig. 3–147).[390]

Metaphyseal Changes. The presence of diffuse metaphyseal reaction, especially if it involves the anterolateral cortex, adversely influences the prognosis. The metaphyseal changes may become manifest either as an ill-defined juxtaphyseal radiolucent band, as shown in Figure 3–148, or as a localized radiolucent "cystic" defect, which may be single or multiple. On histologic examination these radiolucent areas initially consist of reactive tissue (immature connective tissue, vessels, and a few giant cells). Metaphyseal reaction develops in the initial fragmentation stage and usually heals by ossification in the regenerative stage. The position and size of the metaphyseal radiolucency are important. The larger the metaphyseal lesion, the poorer the prognosis. If the "cystic" area involves the anterolateral cortex of the femoral neck the epiphysis is vulnerable. Ellis studied 126 hips in 100 children with Legg-Calvé-Perthes disease. If the lateral cortex of the upper femoral metaphysis was decalcified, the hips were protected from weight-bearing, and if the metaphyseal rarefaction did not reach the lateral cortex, weight-bearing was allowed, provided the hip was not "irritable." On follow-up the result was good in 52 hips (74 per cent), fair in 14 hips (20 per cent), and poor in 4 hips (6 per cent). The four poor results were associated with weight-bearing when the lateral cortex of the upper femoral metaphysis was involved by the metaphyseal rarefaction, which indicated the hip was vulnerable.[186]

The presence or absence of metaphyseal ex-

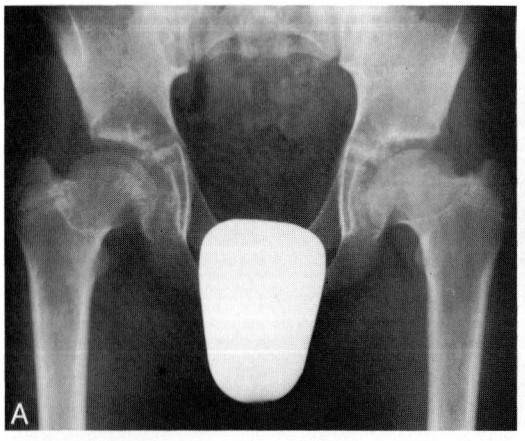
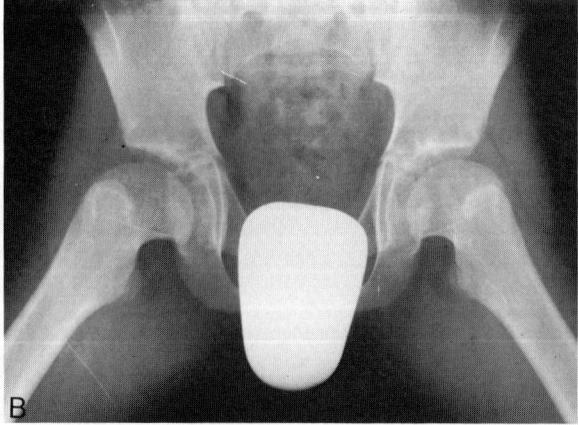

FIGURE 3–147. *Sequelae of premature physeal closure of the capital femoral epiphysis in Legg-Calvé-Perthes disease.*

A and **B.** Anteroposterior and lateral radiograms of both hips. Note the relative overgrowth of the greater trochanter, the lateral extrusion of the femoral head, and the medial bowing of the femoral neck.

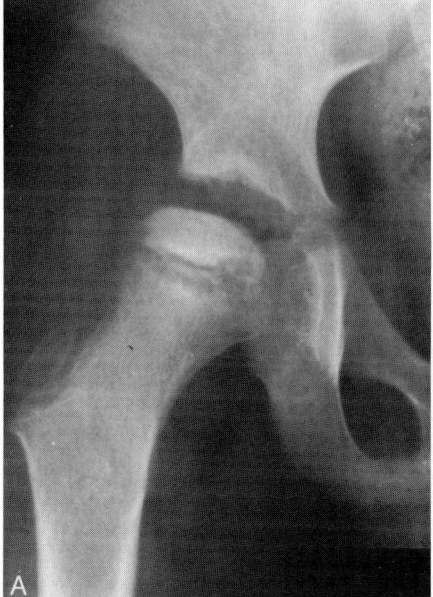 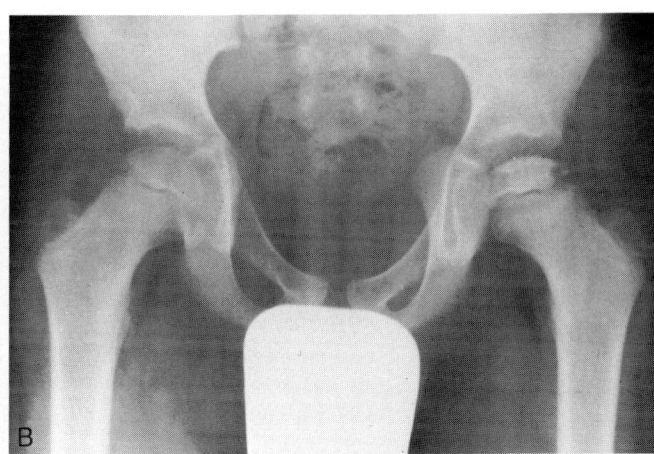

FIGURE 3–148. *Metaphyseal changes in Legg-Calvé-Perthes disease.*

A. Note the ill-defined juxtaepiphyseal radiolucent band in the anteroposterior radiogram of the hips. **B.** Metaphyseal changes associated with Gage's sign, i.e., the area of rarefaction in the lateral part of the capital femoral epiphysis.

pansion should be noted in the anteroposterior radiogram; it is measured in millimeters from the upper lateral corner and the innermost point of its medial convexity and compared with the contralateral normal hip. The absence of metaphyseal expansion means the condition is either early or not extensive. If metaphyseal expansion is present in the first radiogram and the amount does not change, it means the disease process has reached the healing phase and treatment would not alter the ultimate contour of the femoral head.[186]

Stage in the Natural Course of the Disease and the Phase of Progressive Deformation of the Femoral Head. The earlier the stage in the course of the disease in which containment treatment is commenced, the better the prognosis. This is because in the initial stages of Legg-Calvé-Perthes disease, the femoral head is spherical or slightly flattened; by adequate containment and joint mobility, progressive extrusion of the collapsed head may be prevented. Lloyd Roberts and associates have shown that results of femoral osteotomy are frequently poor when the disease is of 20 months' duration or more.[438] The duration of disease is proportional to the severity of the disease.

Persistent Loss of Hip Motion. This is one of the most important clinical signs of poor prognosis. Early in the course of the disease it is due to muscle spasm and soft-tissue contracture. Later in the course of the disease it indicates deformation of the femoral head and hinged abduction. It is vital that treatment restore and maintain full range of motion of the hip.

An Obese Child. Heavy body weight will damage a softened area in the femoral head. Adequate fitting with an orthotic device is very difficult in the obese child. Clinical and radiographic "head at risk" signs are given in Table 3–19.

Table 3–19. *Signs of "Head at Risk" in Legg-Calvé-Perthes Disease According to Catterall*

Clinical
  Loss of hip motion which is persistent and progressive
  Increasing adduction contracture of hip
  The obese child

Radiographic
  Gage's sign: rarefaction in lateral part of epiphysis and subjacent metaphysis
  Calcification lateral to epiphysis
  A diffuse metaphyseal rarefaction
  Lateral extrusion of femoral head
  Growth disturbance of physis

Classification

In Legg-Calvé-Perthes disease the degree of involvement of the femoral head varies; the entire capital femoral epiphysis or only a segment of the anterior part of the femoral head may be affected. Legg described the "cap" and "mushroom" types with their differing prognoses.[420-422] Feuré described "marginal" and "central" forms of coxa plana, and O'Garra distinguished between the "anterior" and "whole head" types (Figs. 3-149 and 3-150).[212, 511] Catterall, in 1971, described and classified four kinds of involvement of the femoral head.[103]

These classifications are based on the extent of maximum radiographic resorption of the capital femoral epiphysis at a later stage in the course of the disease; therefore, the exact degree of involvement is determined in a relatively late phase.

Salter and Thompson gave a simple and practical two-group classification based on the observation that the subchondral crescent-shaped radiolucent line in the radiogram is a pathologic fracture, which initiates the stage of resorption and also heralds the clinical onset of the disease. The extent of subchondral fracture correlates precisely with the subsequent extent of maximum resorption; it is of definite prognostic value in the prediction of the eventual extent of involvement of the femoral head.

Conway and associates gave a biologic classification of Legg-Calvé-Perthes disease based on bone scan findings with technetium-99m. Absence of a lateral column two to three months after the onset of symptoms is a poor prognostic sign. This sign is helpful in deciding whether to treat the disorder several months before the radiographic changes occur.[137]

This author uses all three methods of classification, depending on the stage of the disease when the patient is presented.

Catterall Classification. In a study of the natural history of Legg-Calvé-Perthes disease, Catterall developed his radiographic classification according to the extent of involvement of the femoral head.[103] This classification is made based on good quality anteroposterior and lateral projections. Some of the radiographic findings are present early, whereas others develop late. Often several months of the disease process are required to determine the true amount of involvement. The various radiographic signs are summarized in Table 3-20.

Group I. This is the mildest form, with only the anterior part of the epiphysis involved (Fig. 3-151). In the anteroposterior projections there may be an area of radiolucency in the superior and middle part of the dome of the epiphysis. The epiphyseal height is maintained by viable pillars of bone. The surrounding epiphysis may be slightly sclerotic in appearance. In both the anterior and posterior projections there is a viable tongue of normal trabecular bone extending from the posterior to the anterior margin of the physis. There are no subchondral fracture line, no collapse, and no sequestrum. The physis remains intact. There is no reaction or posterior remodeling in the metaphysis. The prognosis is excellent. During the ensuing several months, the radiolucent area may deepen slightly with growth of the surrounding epiphysis, but soon it reossifies from the periphery. Complete healing takes place without deformity. Treatment is not necessary in Group I.

Table 3-20. Catterall's Classification of Legg-Calvé-Perthes Disease

Epiphyseal Signs	Group I	Group II	Group III	Group IV
Sequestrum	No	Yes	Yes	Yes
Extent of Subchondral fracture line	No	Anterior one third and one half	Anterior two thirds to three fourths	To posterior margin
Junction of involved/ uninvolved segments	Clear	Clear "V" or vertical	Sclerotic in posterior third	Nil
Extent of viable trabecular bone in epiphysis adjacent to physis	Anterior margin	Anterior half	Posterior half	Nil
Capital femoral physis	Intact	Usually intact	Usually involved in its anterolateral part	Involved
Triangular appearance and medial/lateral sides of epiphysis	No	No	Occasional	In early stages
Metaphyseal Signs				
Metaphyseal cystic radiolucency	No	Localized anterolateral	Diffuse or anterior	Diffuse or central
Posterior remodeling	No	No	No	Yes

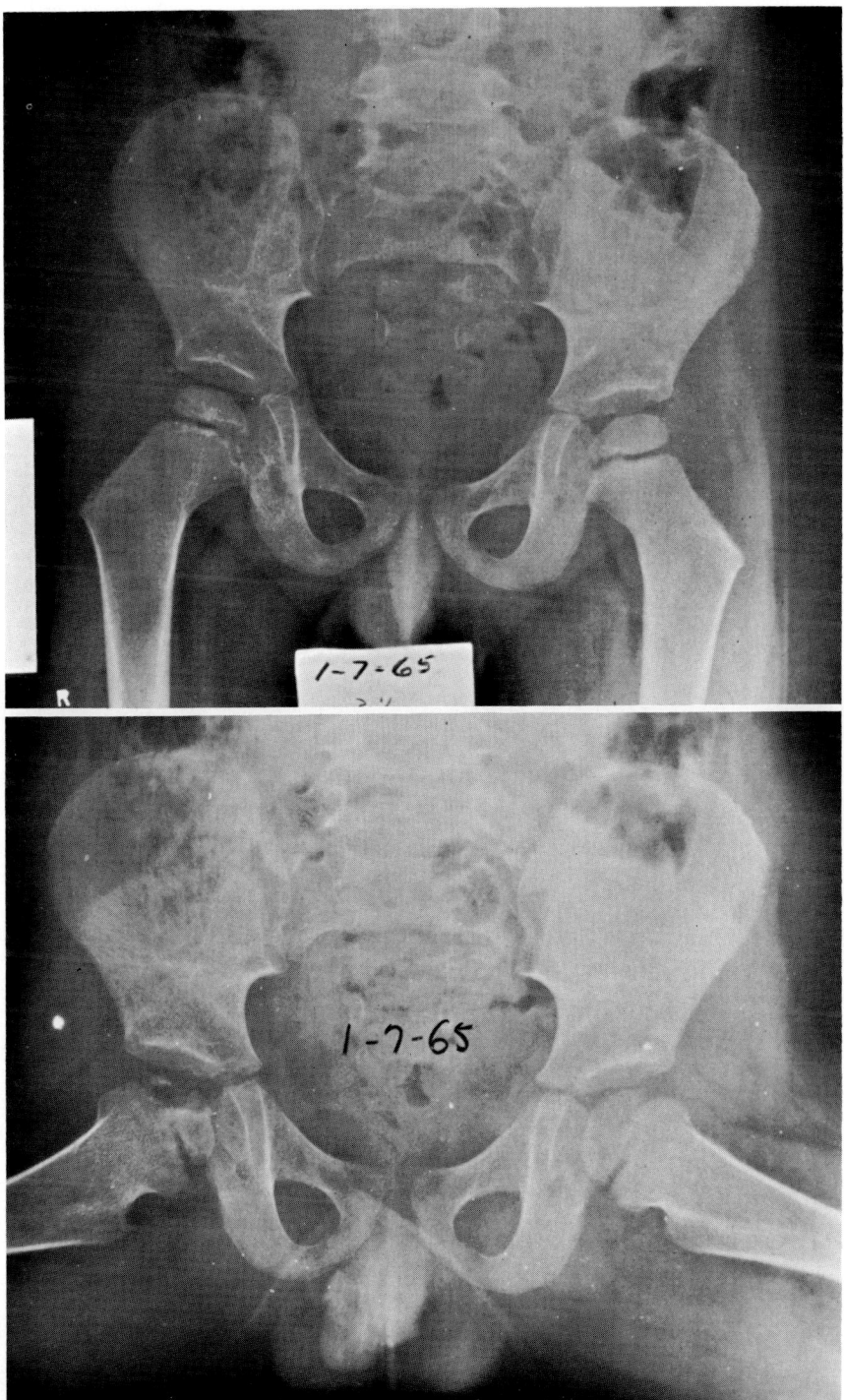

FIGURE 3-149. *Legg-Perthes disease—partial head type.*

Anteroposterior and lateral radiograms of both hips. Note that only the anterior portion of the right femoral head is involved.

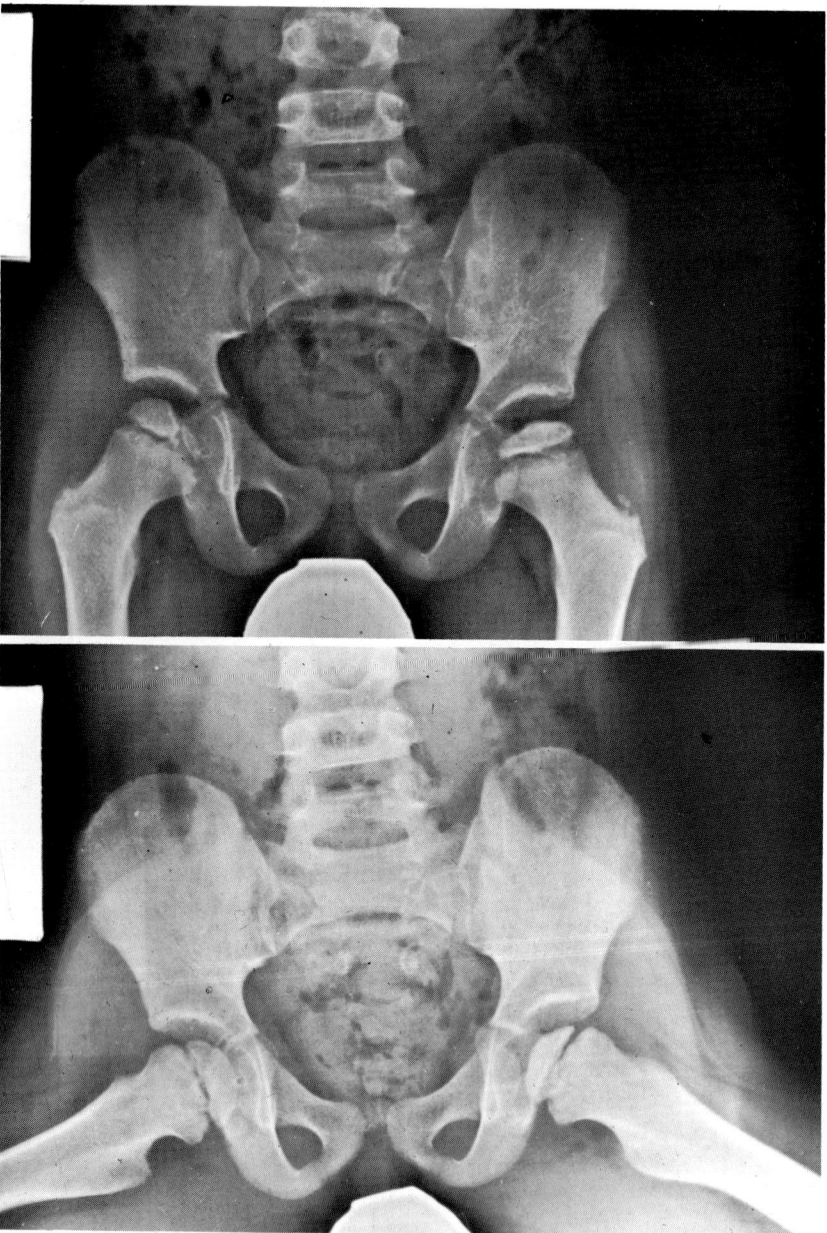

FIGURE 3–150. Legg-Perthes disease—total head type.

Anteroposterior and lateral radiograms of both hips show increased radiopacity of the entire left femoral head (aseptic necrotic stage).

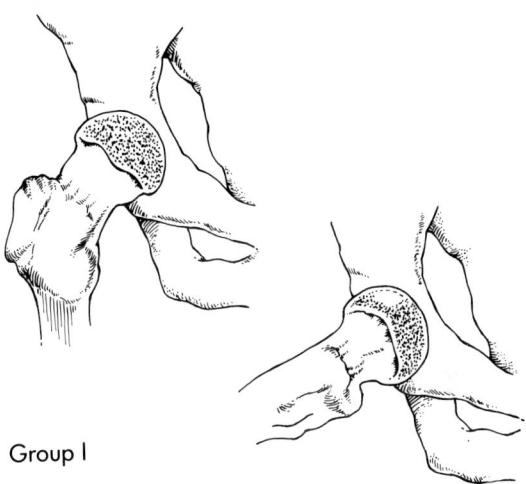

FIGURE 3–151. *Catterall's classification of Legg-Calvé-Perthes disease Group I.*

The disease affects the anterior head of the femur. There is no sequestrum formation, no subchondral fracture line, and no metaphyseal rarefaction.

Group II. Up to half of the femoral head is affected in this variety (Fig. 3–152). The subchondral fracture line extends from the anterior margin to the anterior one third to half of the epiphysis. Following the initial phase of resorption, the involved segment collapses and forms a dense sequestrum. In the anteroposterior radiograms there are medial and lateral pillars of normal bone around the sequestrated segment. These viable bone pillars maintain the height of the epiphysis when collapse of the

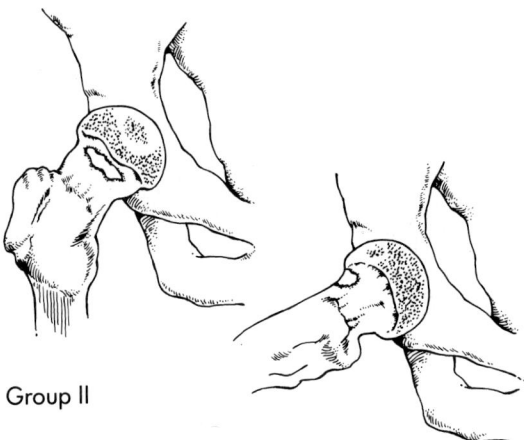

FIGURE 3–152. *Catterall's classification of Legg-Calvé-Perthes disease Group II.*

The disease affects the anterolateral one-third to one-half of the femoral head. There is sequestrum formation—the junction is clear. The subchondral fracture line does not involve the posterior half of the femoral head. There is anterolateral metaphyseal rarefaction, and the lateral pillar is preserved.

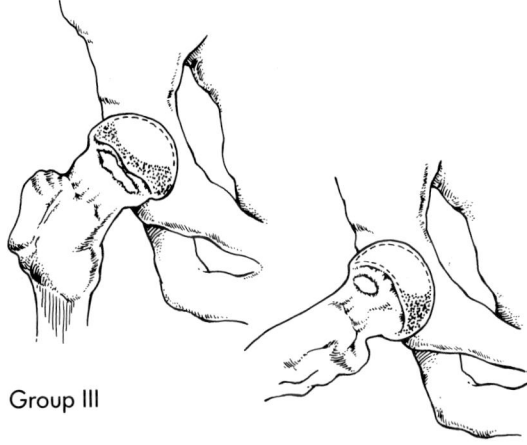

FIGURE 3–153. *Catterall's classification of Legg-Calvé-Perthes disease Group III.*

The disease involves three fourths of the femoral head. The sequestrum is large and the junction sclerotic. The subchondral fracture line extends into the posterior half of the femoral head. There is diffuse metaphyseal rarefaction, and the lateral pillar in the epiphysis is not preserved.

avascular area occurs. In the lateral radiograms the posterior junction of the avascular and viable fragments is separated by a "V" line or a vertical line. The viable tongue of normal bone in the epiphysis adjacent to the physis extends well into the anterior half and third of the physis. Metaphyseal radiolucency is usually small, always located anteriorly in the lateral radiograph; it heals and disappears. There is no posterior remodeling in the metaphyseal region of the femoral neck.

The natural course of Group II is gradual and progressive revascularization and resorption of the collapsed sequestrum from the periphery, giving the appearance of fragmentation followed by segmentation and reossification. The prognosis is good; with skeletal growth remodeling takes place with a good result.

Group III. In this variety, from half to three fourths of the femoral head is involved (Fig. 3–153). The avascular fragment is large; its junction with the posterior viable segment is indefinite, the two blending in one area of sclerosis. The subchondral fracture line, as seen in the lateral projection, extends from the anterior margin of the epiphysis into the posterior three fourths. The physis is unprotected by a viable tongue of bone in the epiphysis; therefore, it may be actively involved in the disease process. Collapse and flattening of the femoral head is usually moderate. In the course of the disease, specks of calcification develop in the anterolateral part of the epiphysis; these are indicative of ossification taking place in the protruded cartilaginous part of the femoral head.

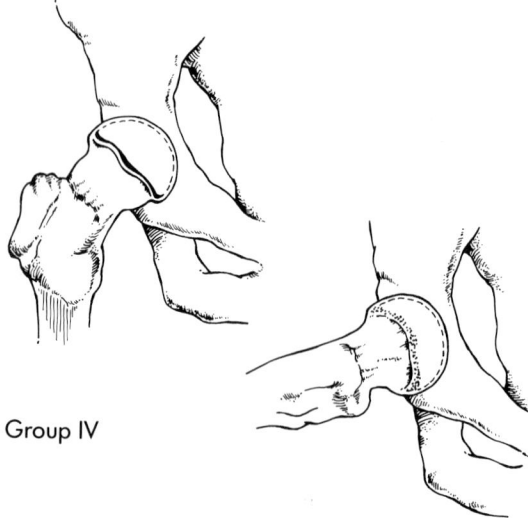

FIGURE 3–154. *Catterall's classification of Legg-Calvé-Perthes disease Group IV.*

The disease involves the entire femoral head. There is sequestrum formation. The subchondral fracture line extends through the entire femoral head, and there is diffuse or central metaphyseal rarefaction.

Metaphyseal rarefaction is marked; it appears in two variations: either as generalized widening of the growth plate, as an anterior large area of radiolucent defect, or as both. As the disease continues, the femoral head collapses. Healing by resorption and reossification takes a much longer time than in Group II. The prognosis is usually poor in the untreated case.

Group IV. The whole epiphysis is involved in this group, which is characterized by early severe collapse of the entire femoral head, producing a dense line in the anteroposterior radiogram (Fig. 3–154). The physis is frequently affected, disturbing growth of the femoral neck and diminishing the potential for remodeling. Metaphyseal rarefaction is marked with posterior remodeling. Resorption of the sequestrum and reossification takes a long time. The prognosis is usually poor; containment may, however, prevent gross deformity of the femoral head.[103]

The significance of Catterall's classification has been assessed by numerous authors.[73, 163, 358, 380, 438, 654, 667] It is of definite value later in the course of the disease in determining the extent of involvement and whether treatment is required.

Salter's Extent of Subchondral Fracture Method.[578] The value of Salter's classification is that it can be used in the early stages of the disease before resorption of the femoral head takes place. Standard anteroposterior and Lowenstein (frog-leg position) lateral radiograms are made. The importance of making a lateral radiogram of the hip cannot be overemphasized; it is imperative to assess all four epiphyseal quadrants (medial, lateral, anterior, and posterior) in order to determine the extent of subchondral fracture and subsequent resorption of underlying bone.

In *Group A* the extent of subchondral fracture is less than half of the femoral head; in *Group B* the extent of subchondral fracture is more than half of the femoral head.

Treatment

The objectives of treatment of Legg-Calvé-Perthes disease are to produce a normal femoral head and neck, a normal acetabulum, a congruous hip joint that is fully mobile, and to prevent degenerative arthritis of the hip later in life. Treatment efforts are directed toward restoration and maintenance of full mobility of the hip, containment of the femoral head in the acetabulum in order to prevent or reduce anterolateral uncovering and extrusion, and resumption of weight-bearing and full activity as soon as possible. Prolonged confinement in bed, either in an institution or at home, is psychosocially unacceptable. The patient should be allowed to be ambulatory and to perform activities of daily living in as nearly normal a manner as possible and with the least discomfort. In treatment planning, the whole child, including his psyche, should be considered.

End result assessments of treated and untreated (control) cases have demonstrated that not all cases of Legg-Calvé-Perthes disease need to be treated. The guidelines for treatment selection are as follows: in all cases in Catterall Group I and in most of those in Catterall Group II in children under seven years of age, the aforementioned goals can be achieved without treatment. Patients in Group II who are eight years of age or older and all those in Catterall Groups III and IV require treatment in order to obtain a satisfactory hip; at the onset it should be made clear to the parents that in spite of all efforts of treatment by containment—orthotic or operative—in a certain percentage of the cases in Catterall Groups III and IV (and Salter's Class B), especially in the child eight years old or older, a normal hip cannot be obtained. This is inherent in the nature of the growth disturbance due to ischemia and the pathobiology of healing of avascular bone in Legg-Calvé-Perthes disease. In these severe cases, the goal of treatment is to improve the result and minimize deformation as much as possible. In such cases, after healing and in the residual stage, reconstructive surgery may be required.

Management of Legg-Calvé-Perthes disease can be divided into various phases. During the *first*, or *initial*, *phase* (irritable period) the hip motion is restored and the hip is assessed (clinically, radiographically, by bone imaging with technetium-99m, and if indicated, by arthrography) to plan strategy for future treatment. The *second phase* (active period) is that of containment (by orthosis or surgery) and maintenance of full mobility of the hip until healing is established. The *third phase* is the *reconstructive phase* (residual period) during which surgical procedures are carried out to correct residual deformities of the upper end of the femur in order to improve the biomechanics and increase the longevity of the hip.

INITIAL PHASE

When there is restriction of its range of motion the first step is to *restore full motion of the hip*; this is imperative before any further treatment is considered. This prerequisite is valid in Catterall Groups I and II as well as in Groups III and IV. One should refrain from overlooking this basic principle in the minimally involved hips. In the initial period, traction is best carried out in the hospital. In the experience of this author, traction at home is often inadequate because discipline and compliance are less than ideal. On rare occasions, the family situation may be conducive to an adequate home traction program. The type of traction recommended is bilateral counterpoised split Russell's traction with a medial rotation strap on the thigh of the involved hip. The traction force should be in line with the deformity. With relief of hip adductor muscle spasm, the range of hip abduction is progressively increased until full range of abduction is obtained. Medial rotation of the hip in extension and flexion must be essentially normal. This may require one to two weeks of traction, depending on the stage in the course of the disease, the severity of involvement, and the deformity of the femoral head. Anti-inflammatory drugs such as salicylates or Naprosyn may be given in selected cases.

Assessment. While the patient is in the hospital appropriate diagnostic studies are performed, and the hip is assessed for extent of involvement, "risk signs," stage in the course of the disease, and degree of deformation of the femoral head. Bone scanning with technetium-99m is performed almost routinely, and hip arthrography is carried out when indicated.

SECOND PHASE—CONTAINMENT AND MAINTENANCE OR RESTORATION OF FULL RANGE OF MOTION OF HIP

The principle of containment is based on the premise that in order to prevent deformation of the necrotic femoral head during its revascularization or resorption phase, it must be placed deeply in the acetabulum where the intra-articular pressure and forces acting on it will be evenly distributed. The vulnerable femoral head is thus prevented from extruding anterolaterally, subjected to the molding action of the acetabulum, and protected from compression by the acetabular rim. Containment strives to provide a congruous hip joint with a spherocentric femoral head concentrically contained in a normally developed acetabulum.

An important factor in the pathogenesis of femoral head deformation, however, is abnormal growth of the thickened articular cartilage of the periphery of the capital epiphysis and of the fibrocartilage formed during absorption and repair of crushed avascular bone trabeculae. This growth disturbance, in part, can be controlled by active motion of the hip with the femoral head concentrically contained within the acetabulum. Motion is life! It enhances synovial nutrition of the epiphyseal growth cartilage. Motion stimulates osteogenesis and subjects the revascularizing and reossifying "biologically plastic" femoral head to the molding effect of the acetabulum. Motion and function minimize muscle atrophy and disuse osteoporosis. The importance of restoration and maintenance of hip motion during this phase of treatment cannot be overemphasized.

Another consideration during this interval is prevention of repeated vascular insults. Such circulatory compromise may result from repeated stress fractures of the partially revascularized femoral head. Repeat infarcts cause patchy areas of revascularization, irregular bone formation, growth disturbance, and deformation of the femoral head. Brotherton and McKibbin have, in a long-term appraisal, given statistical evidence that prolonged recumbency with weight relief on the contained femoral head improves the result of Catterall's Group IV cases (there were no poor results).[73] According to Catterall, in Group III cases "at risk," there is no difference in the incidence of poor results with or without weight relief.[107] The only way to relieve body weight and compressive forces across the hip is to immobilize the joint in a splint with the patient in bed in a recumbent posture. When the hip moves, muscle forces exert greater stress across the hip joint than the static force of body weight. The so-called weight-relieving orthotic devices that allow motion of the hip do not unload the hip, while keeping the hip in a constant fixed position of abduction causes disuse atrophy of the gluteus medius muscle. Prolonged restraint in bed or in a low wheeled platform cart has been tried and has been discarded; it should not be used because of the detrimental psychosocial effect on the whole child.

At present, efforts are directed toward reduction of forces acting on the femoral head; this can be achieved by abducting the hip so that the femoral neck is at an angle of 110 degrees in relation to the longitudinal axis of the body.[308, 529] Weight reduction of the obese child is appropriate. Measures are taken to prevent injury to the hip. Until the exact cause of interruption of blood supply in Legg-Calvé-Perthes disease is known, ischemia cannot be prevented.

Concentric containment of the hip can be obtained by orthosis or by surgery—intertrochanteric varus osteotomy, innominate osteotomy, or a combination of both.

Containment by Orthosis

A number of orthotic devices have been described in the literature, each inventor proclaiming the virtues of his device. This author strongly recommends that the following so-called weight-relieving orthoses *not be used* because they do not contain the femoral head; in fact, they cause de-containment and lateral extrusion of the femoral head. The *obsolete orthoses* are the Sam Browne belt or Snyder sling with crutches, the bent knee brace with crutches, and the patten-bottom caliper orthosis with ischial ring.

The orthoses and cast devices used over the years in treating Legg-Calvé-Perthes disease can be divided into nonambulatory and ambulatory types. The *nonambulatory* devices are: (1) the abduction broomstick plaster cast; (2) the hip spica cast—bivalved; (3) the rolling platform with hips held in abduction in an anterior polypropylene hip splint for daytime prone use and a posterior hip splint for nighttime supine use; and (4) the Milgram hip abduction orthosis, which prevents hip flexion.[168, 473] The *ambulatory* devices may be static (Harrison) or dynamic.[302] The dynamic weight-bearing devices that include both limbs are: (1) the Petrie abduction cast; (2) the Bobechko-Toronto orthosis; (3) the Newington abduction A-frame orthosis; (4) the Roberts abduction-medial rotation, flexion hip-knee orthosis; and (5) the Scottish-Rite orthosis.[51, 52, 146, 529, 557] A *unilateral dynamic containment orthosis* is the trilateral socket hip abduction–flexion–medial rotation orthosis (Table 3–21).[644, 645]

Scottish-Rite Orthosis. Of the numerous types of containment devices available, at present, in North America, the Scottish-Rite orthosis is the most commonly used (Fig. 3–155).[543] It consists of two thigh cuffs (aluminum-reinforced leather), attached to free swivel-type hip joints on an aluminum-reinforced pelvic band. The thigh cuffs are connected by a stainless steel crossbar to a unilateral swivel joint and a contralateral free joint. These joints accommodate the amount of pelvic rotation necessary for walking. The hips are held in 35 to 45 degrees of abduction, and the motion allowed during ambulation is hip flexion and extension. The patient uses the orthosis to walk during the day and, in some cases, sleeps in it during the night. The advantages of the Scottish-Rite orthosis are its simplicity and the great mobility it permits; it does not, however, control hip rotation.

Newington Abduction Orthosis. When, in addition to hip abduction and flexion, medial rotation is required to obtain concentric containment, one has to control hip rotation by extending the orthosis to below the knees. There are two such devices that are in use in the United States. The Newington abduction orthosis consists of a metal A-frame with plastic-reinforced leather cuffs and straps; medial up-

Table 3–21. Containment Orthoses and Plaster Casts Used in Treatment of Legg-Calvé-Perthes Disease

Nonambulatory—recumbent—weight-relieving
  Abduction broomstick plaster cast
  Hip spica cast, bivalved
  Rolling platform with hips held in abduction in polypropylene plaster shells[168]
  Milgram hip abduction orthosis, preventing hip flexion[473]

Ambulatory—static—affected limb only
  Harrison hip containment splint[302]

Ambulatory—dynamic—include both lower limbs
  Petrie abduction cast[529]
  Bobechko-Toronto orthosis[51, 52]
  Newington abduction A-frame orthosis[146]
  Roberts abduction–flexion–medial rotation orthosis[557]
  Scottish-Rite orthosis[543]

Ambulatory unilateral orthosis
  Trilateral socket hip abduction, flexion, medial rotation[644, 645]

rights are attached to foot plates; the hips are held in 45 degrees of abduction and 20 degrees of medial rotation. The only motion allowed is hip flexion and extension. The orthosis is light. The patient walks with Lofstrand crutches (Fig. 3–156). The Newington orthosis, despite its light weight, is cumbersome and difficult to ambulate with; however, it assures concentric containment of the femoral head.

Roberts Orthosis. The Roberts orthosis does control hip rotation by including the knees, which are held in 20 to 30 degrees of flexion. The foot and ankle are free. It is the distal extension of the Scottish-Rite orthosis. If medial

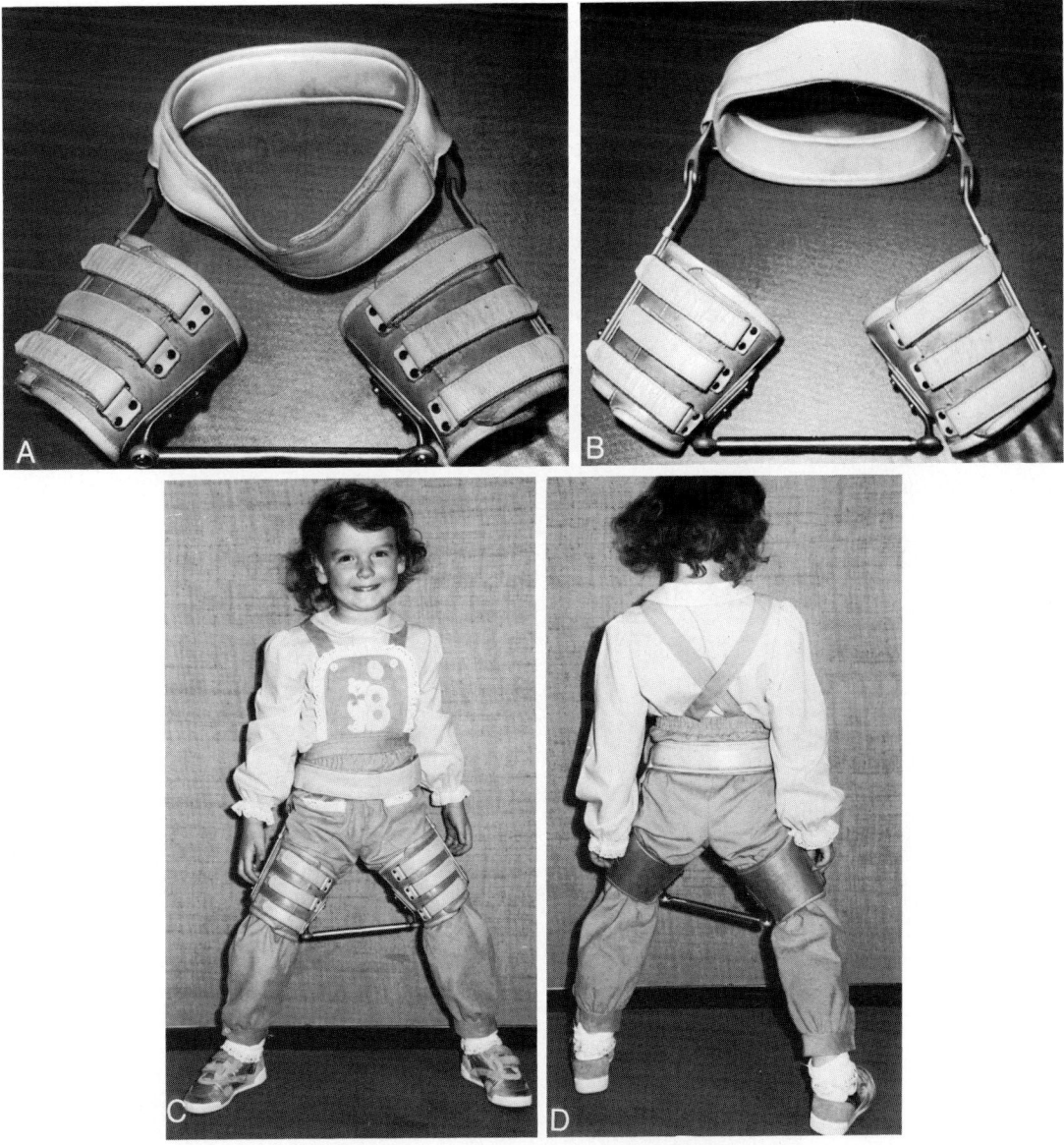

FIGURE 3–155. Scottish-Rite hip orthosis.

A and **B.** Anteroposterior and posteroanterior views of the orthosis. **C** and **D.** Anteroposterior and posteroanterior views of a patient wearing the orthosis.

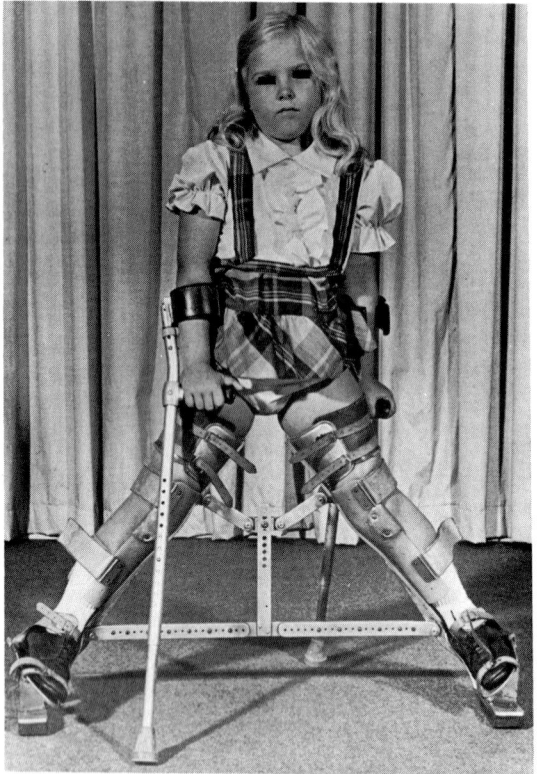

FIGURE 3–156. *The Newington ambulatory hip orthosis.*

Its use is indicated in patients whose arthrogram shows containment of the femoral head when the hip is in abduction–medial rotation. (From Drennan, J. C.: Orthotic management of Legg-Calvé-Perthes disease. *In* Leach, R. E., Hoaglund, F. T., and Riseborough, E. T.: Controversies in Orthopedic Surgery. Philadelphia, W. B. Saunders Co., 1982. Reprinted by permission.)

rotation of the hip is desired, this author favors the Roberts orthosis over the Newington orthosis because the former is less strenuous for the child to get around in.

Trilateral Socket Hip Containment Orthosis. This device keeps the hip in the desired degree of abduction and some flexion and medial rotation (Fig. 3–157). The patient is ambulatory; during gait, the hip motion is abduction–flexion–medial rotation–extension; i.e., concentric mobility of the hip is allowed. In the bilateral limb devices only flexion-extension of the hip in the anteroposterior plane is permitted. In order to mold the "biologically plastic" femoral head to a spherical contour, concentric "around-the-world" mobility is required. Confining hip motion to flexion and extension is like making a hamburger pattie; whereas concentric mobility can be compared to molding a Swedish meatball. The trilateral socket is designed so that the lateral wall is open at and below the greater trochanter and is contoured above the greater trochanter and below the iliac crest to provide lateral stability. This measure also seems to tighten the gluteus medius, causing further hip abduction and anatomic placement of the femoral head in the acetabulum. The absence of a lateral wall also prevents circumferential forces on the thigh that would be transmitted through the femur to the hip. The medial brim of the socket is shaped high enough to cause uncomfortable pressure at the pubic ramus if the hip is adducted. The posterolateral portion of the brim is designed to press into the gluteus maximus causing the extremity to rotate into medial rotation. The cast mold for the ischial socket is made with the hip in the desired degree of abduction, as predetermined from the radiograms. The ischial socket should be custom made, not made commercially. Other components of the orthosis include a medial upright with lengthening adjustment for growth, both above and below the knee joint, a slide guide extension, a shoe attachment slide stirrup, a distal control spring, and a walking heel extension unit. The walking heel is wedged in its posterolateral aspect to increase internal rotation forces. It is also medially placed to reduce the horizontal distance from the floor reaction forces to the vertical weight line from the center of gravity of the body. If the walking heel is placed laterally, a greater effort is required for walking. The shoe for the foot on the uninvolved side requires a lift of adequate height so that the pelvis of the involved side is 1 cm. lower than the contralateral normal side. This pelvic obliquity will place the involved hip in further abduction. A thin cotton cast sock or cotton stockinette should be used to ease the patient into the ischial socket and should be worn at all times with the appliance to prevent friction between the skin and the socket. If this sock remains dry and is regularly cleaned and changed, no skin problems should arise.

Initially, most patients attempt to adduct the involved limb and complain of pubic ramus pressure. The purpose of the high medial brim should be explained to the patient, and he should be instructed to walk with the hip in abduction and medial rotation. Gait training by a physical therapist is important. During the stance phase in the affected lower limb, there should be a negative Trendelenburg sign and further abduction of the involved hip. Standing radiographs of both hips with the brace on should be made to insure that the femoral head is contained in weight-bearing position (Fig. 3–158). Ordinarily it will take five to seven days for a child to become proficient in ambulation.

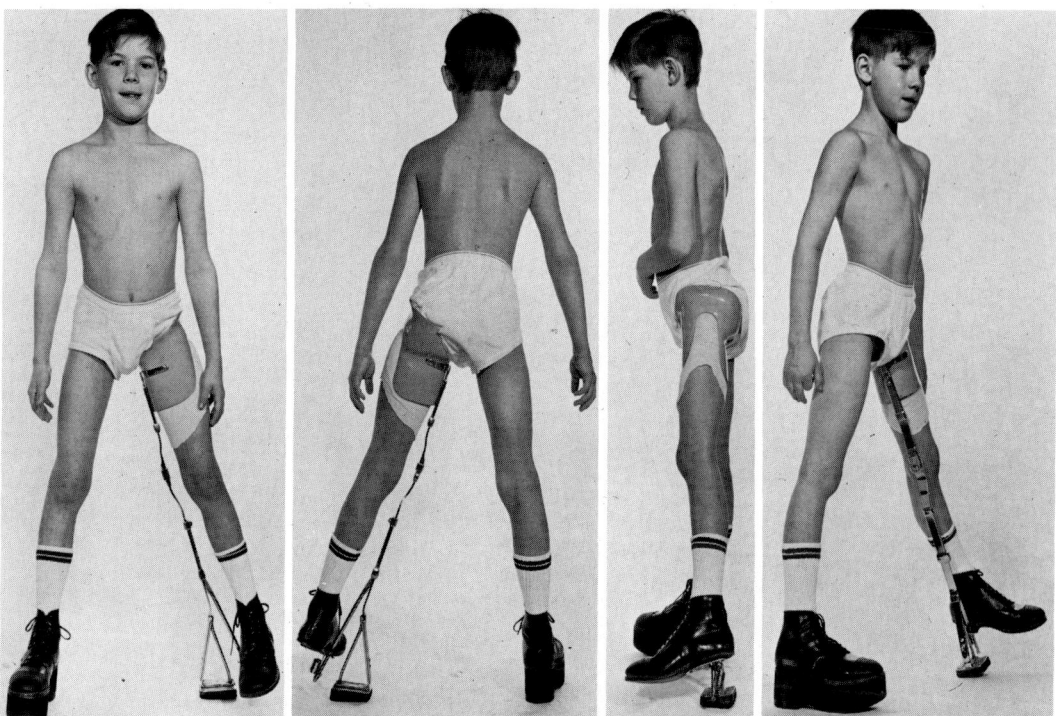

FIGURE 3–157. *Trilateral socket hip abduction orthosis.*

If the patient has been in bed in split Russell's traction up to this time, he will more than likely display some weakness and imbalance.

The parent should encourage the child to pursue all normal activities as long as no weight is borne on the foot and no outside forces are applied to the involved limb.

Patients with bilateral involvement may be treated satisfactorily by this method. Initially, they walk with crutches, but in time they are able to do so independently. It may be more pragmatic and economical to use the Scottish-Rite orthosis in bilateral cases. The fit of the ischial socket should be checked at regular intervals. Reduction of the volume of the proximal thigh owing to disuse atrophy is to be expected. If volume loss is extreme, a new socket may have to be fabricated.

Petrie Abduction Cast. This is used only in the noncompliant patient (one who gets out of the brace frequently or simply does not wear it) or when economic conditions are such that immediate funds are not available for the orthosis. It should be stressed, however, that this method should only be used for short periods. Prolonged immobilization will damage the articular cartilage of the knee. The casts have to be changed every three to four weeks, and each time the child should be admitted to the hospital and receive physical therapy to the knees (active-assisted and gentle passive) until functional range of knee motion is restored. Gluteus medius and quadriceps atrophy can be marked in some cases. The original Petrie cast included the ankles and feet and had a cross bar with which the thigh and leg segments held the hips in the desired degree of abduction and medial rotation. This author utilizes a plastic type rather than the plaster of Paris cast, which makes the Petrie splint much lighter. Also, the feet and ankles are free. The shoes have lateral outside sole and heel wedges of appropriate height so that the feet can be placed on the ground without stress at the subtalar and ankle joints. The Petrie splint should be well padded at the ankles, knees, and upper thighs. Stress on the medial collateral ligament is relieved when the plastic cast fits snugly on the thigh.

The choice of containment device is an individual decision made by the treating orthopedic surgeon. Social, psychologic, and geographic factors are important to consider in making the decision. The local orthotist should be knowledgeable about the type of orthosis. The orthotic device should be inexpensive, lightweight, simple to apply, and need a minimum of repairs.

Prerequisites for Orthotic Containment.

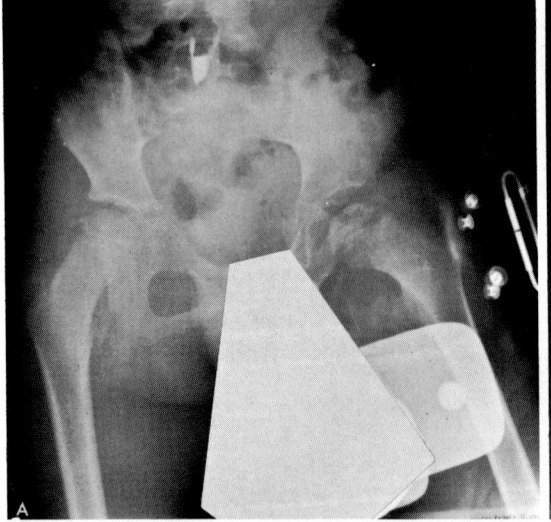
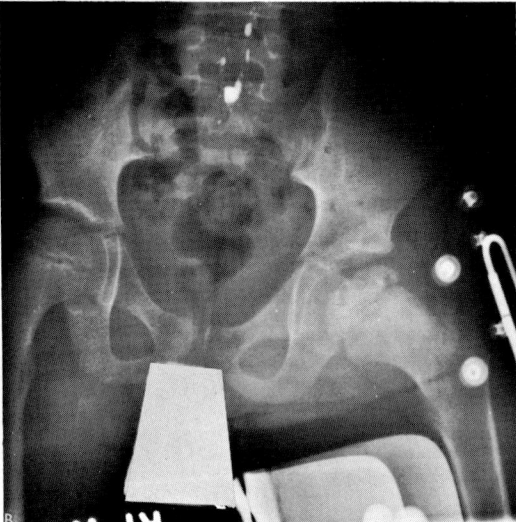
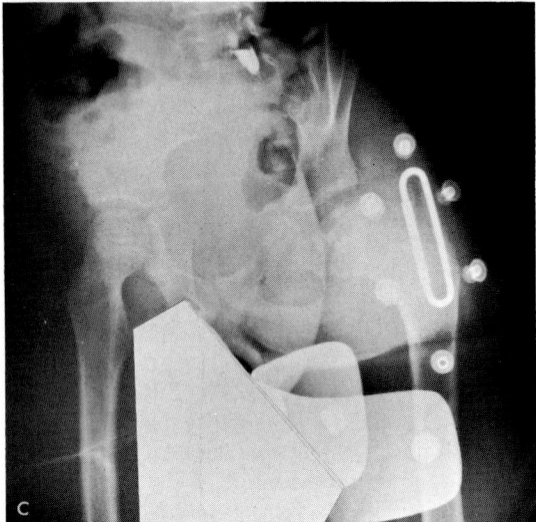

FIGURE 3–158. *Legg-Perthes disease—radiograms of both hips in gait.*

A. Standing on both lower limbs. Note the left hip is in abduction and the avascular femoral head is well seated in the acetabulum. **B.** In stance phase on the left leg. On weight-bearing on the left, there is a negative Trendelenburg sign with further abduction of the affected hip. **C.** Swing phase on left, standing on right leg. The left femoral head is still adequately covered by the acetabulum.

First, there should be full range of motion of the hip with complete relief of muscle spasm *prior* to wearing of the orthosis. When range of motion of the affected hip is lost while walking with the orthosis, the hip is replaced in counterpoised traction; the patient is allowed to be ambulatory in the orthosis again *only when the full range of motion of the hip has been restored.* This vital prerequisite should never be violated.

Second, the *entire femoral head should be concentrically and fully contained within the acetabulum;* this should be documented by anteroposterior radiograms of the hips with the patient standing on both lower limbs with the orthosis. When the hip has full range of motion, and the standing anteroposterior radiogram shows that the lateral edge of the capital femoral physis does not protrude beyond the acteabular rim and Shenton's line is intact (i.e., there is no superior subluxation), routine arthrography to document concentricity of containment is not indicated. If there are superolateral extrusion of the femoral head and persistent restriction of hip motion, however, it is mandatory to perform an arthrogram of the hip. Wearing an orthosis with the hip inadequately abducted does more harm than good. Pressure from the rim of the acetabulum will cause indentation of the femoral head and joint incongruity.

Third, the patient's *motor strength and balance* should be adequate enough to use the orthosis. In general, patients under four years of age have difficulty ambulating with the containment orthosis. Complex orthotic devices should not be prescribed. The young child is best fitted with the Scottish-Rite orthosis.

Every four to eight weeks (initially more

frequent visits are necessary), the patient is reexamined to assess the fit and general comfort of the appliance; the gait pattern—is the child walking with the desired degree of hip abduction and medial rotation?; and the range of motion of the affected hip—full range of motion should be maintained! If the hip motion is restricted, a hip mobilization program should be initiated. Finally, *radiograms of the hips are made*: an anteroposterior view of the hips with the patient standing with the orthosis, an anteroposterior view with the patient standing out of the brace, and a lateral view out of the brace. Proper containment of the femoral head in the acetabulum and extent of healing of the avascular necrosis are assessed. Is the femoral head progressively becoming displaced laterally and superiorly when the child is out of the brace and standing with the hips in neutral weight-bearing position?

Discontinuing Orthotic Treatment. When the course of the disease enters the reparative stage and healing is established, containment treatment can be gradually discontinued because there will be no further deterioration of the overall shape of the femoral head.[106, 210, 654] Establishment of healing is manifested on the radiograms by the appearance of irregular ossification in the capital femoral epiphysis. The increased density of the femoral head should disappear, and there should be no new radiopaque areas. The medial segment of the femoral head should increase in size and height. The metaphyseal rarefaction involving the lateral cortex of the upper femoral metaphysis should ossify. There should be an intact lateral column of normal trabecular bone in the capital epiphysis that supports and shelters the epiphysis from stress and collapse. In addition, there should be normal trabecular bone in the epiphysis across the entire extent of the physis, protecting the growth plate from stress fracture.

In general, the average time for healing to be established after onset is eight months for Catterall Group II, 12 months for Catterall Group III, and 18 months for Catterall Group IV.

Weaning from the orthosis should be a gradual process. The patient is permitted to be out of the brace, initially, for several hours a day at home. In two to three weeks, he should be reassessed to ensure there is no loss of motion. If full range of motion is maintained, periods out of the orthosis are increased during the ensuing six weeks. Then radiograms of the hips are made; if there is no collapse, and if the hip still has full range of motion, the orthosis is totally discontinued. Strenuous activities—jumping, running, and bicycle riding—are avoided until complete healing has taken place. This is shown in the radiogram by complete subchondral ossification and filling-in of the femoral head by normal trabecular bone. The process of complete healing may take from one and a half to a few years, depending on the severity of involvement. Thompson and Westin have demonstrated that it is safe to discontinue orthotic containment early when healing is established. It is not necessary to prolong treatment until complete healing has taken place.[654]

Problems During Treatment With Orthosis. *Persistent or recurrent loss of hip motion* is a common problem. It may be due to repeated infarctions and collapse of the femoral head, or to deformation of the femoral head that blocks hip abduction and medial rotation. In such instances, the child is taken out of the brace and placed in counterpoised split Russell's traction. It is best to readmit the child to the hospital and repeat the bone imaging with technetium-99m to rule out repeat infarctions, which are indicated by the loss of a previously present lateral vascularized column in the bone scan. If full range of motion is not reestablished after traction, arthrography of the hip should be performed to delineate the contour of the femoral head and to rule out "hinged" abduction.

This author strongly recommends the use of the continuous "around-the-world" passive hip motion machine to restore and maintain full range of motion (Fig. 3–159). Initially, while the child is in the hospital, it is used full time. A home program is then set up, with the patient up and around in the orthosis during the day, and in the continuous passive hip motion machine at night. In the experience of this author, this is a biologically sound method of mobilizing the stiff joint in Legg-Calvé-Perthes disease while an attempt is made to control abnormal growth of the capital femoral epiphysis.

Progressive collapse and superolateral extrusion of the femoral head while it is being contained in the orthosis is an ominous sign (Fig. 3–160). These cases require surgical management after appropriate assessment.

Surgical Containment

Surgical containment may be accomplished by femoral osteotomy, innominate osteotomy, or a combination of the two. A definite advantage of surgical containment is that no end point of treatment is required, whereas in containment by orthosis, the surgeon must decide when to discontinue the orthotic treatment. The

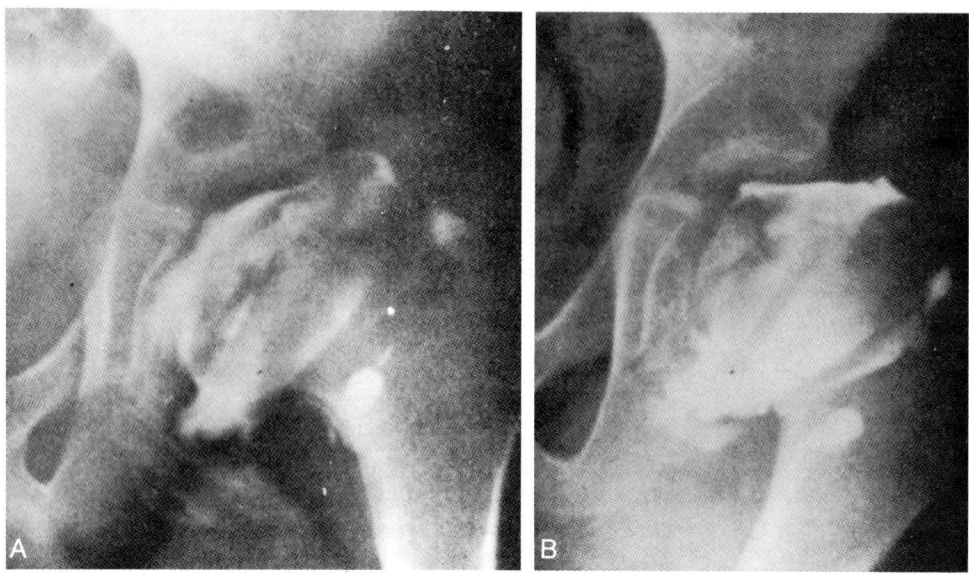

FIGURE 3–163. *Arthrogram of the left hip in Legg-Calvé-Perthes disease.*

The head is collapsed and laterally extruded, causing hinged abduction.

A. Maximal abduction showing the blocking by the extruded anterolateral part of the femoral head and the pooling of the dye medially. **B.** Anteroposterior radiogram of the hip in adduction.

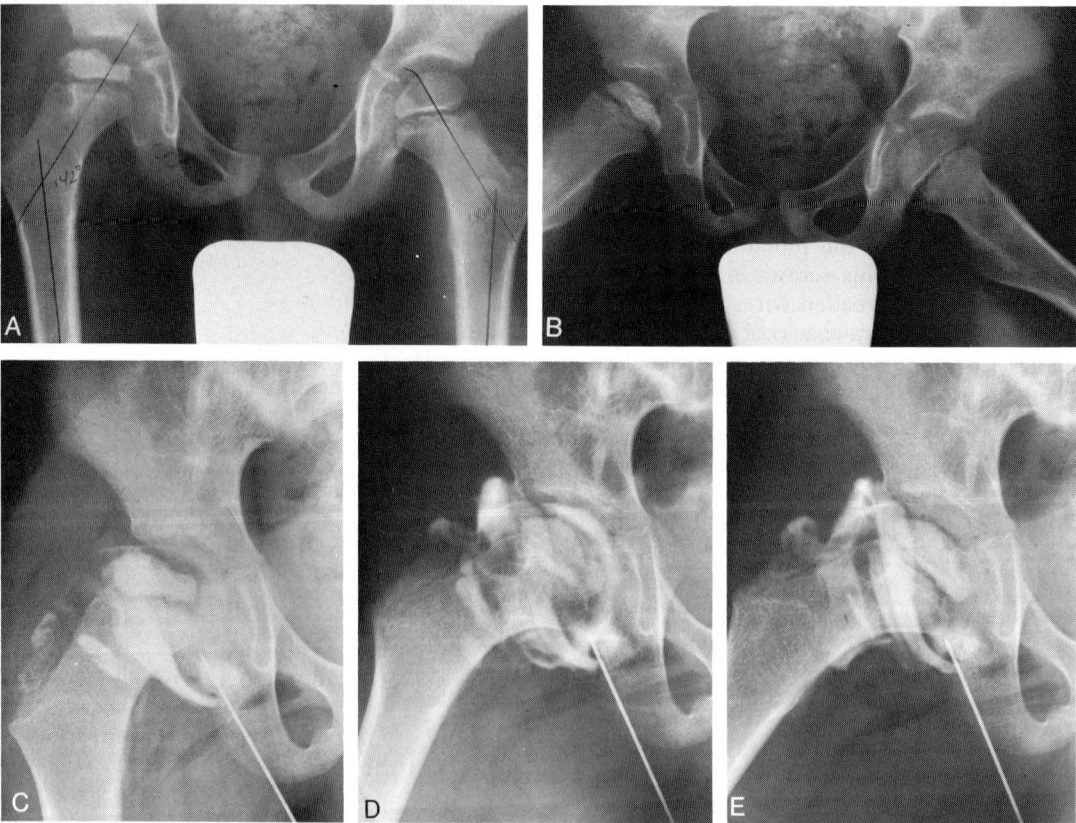

FIGURE 3–164. *Legg-Calvé-Perthes disease of the right hip, contained by Salter's innominate osteotomy, in a six-year-old boy.*

A and **B.** Anteroposterior and lateral radiograms of the hip. Note the superolateral displacement of the collapsed femoral head and the metaphyseal rarefaction that extends anterolaterally. **C, D,** and **E.** Arthrograms of the hip showing that more than 20 per cent of the femoral head is uncovered and it is flattened in its weight-bearing portion. To reduce the femoral head concentrically and to restore Shenton's line, the hip must be abducted 30 degrees, which elevates the tip of the greater trochanter above the joint line. It was therefore decided to perform innominate osteotomy and not an intertrochanteric femoral varus osteotomy.

Salter.[576] *Disadvantages* of Salter's innominate osteotomy are the postoperative stiffness of the hip with prolonged or persistent loss of joint motion, illustrated in Figure 3–164, and its limitation as to the extent of anterolateral coverage that it can provide. Always perform soft-tissue release—hip adductors and iliopsoas. Salter's innominate osteotomy is a derotation osteotomy; it does not enlarge the acetabular capacity. When the femoral head is extruded anterolaterally with an epiphyseal extrusion index of more than 20 per cent, anterolateral coverage by Salter's innominate osteotomy may uncover the femoral head posteriorly. In the initial stage of assessment and after mobilization of the hip, parents may be given the choice between orthotic containment and innominate osteotomy. This author makes it very clear to them, however, that he prefers orthotic containment over innominate osteotomy. In his opinion, innominate osteotomy is indicated when parents do not wish containment because of its psychosocial implications, or when a child is noncompliant. Other surgeons may prefer innominate osteotomy and recommend it as the treatment of choice.[572, 574, 576] It should, however, be performed when there is less than 20 per cent anterolateral epiphyseal extrusion. In the child over eight years of age, there are technical problems if the symphysis pubis is not flexible. It is important to make several vertical incisions in the cartilaginous iliac apophysis and the periosteum on the medial wall of the ilium.

Femoral Osteotomy. According to Catterall, indications for surgical treatment are: all cases at risk, cases in Groups II and III over seven years of age and at risk, and cases in Group IV in which severe flattening has not occurred as demonstrated by arthrography.[107] When concentric containment of the femoral head in the acetabulum is obtained by abduction–medial rotation of the hip, varus lateral derotation

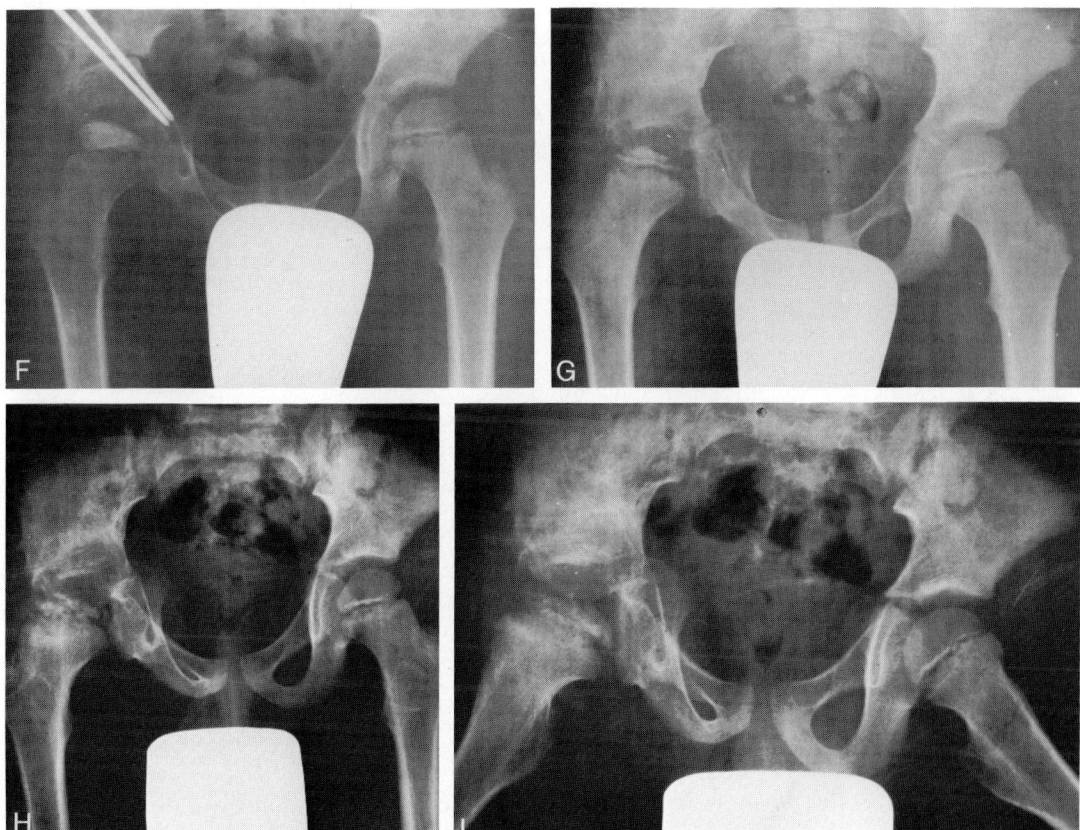

FIGURE 3–164 Continued. *Legg-Calvé-Perthes disease of the right hip, contained by Salter's innominate osteotomy, in a six-year-old boy.*

F. Immediate postoperative radiogram showing coverage of the femoral head with restoration of Shenton's line. G. Six months later, note a deformity of the acetabulum has been created to cover the femoral head. This patient's hip joint was still stiff. H and I. Eighteen months postoperatively. Full range of hip motion has been restored. The acetabulum and femoral head are remodeling.

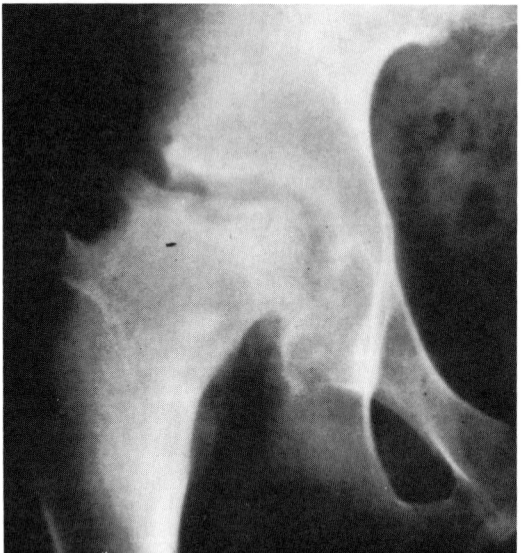

FIGURE 3–165. *Legg-Calvé-Perthes disease of the right hip with collapse and lateral extrusion of the femoral head and hinge abduction.*

Surgery is contraindicated when the femoral head cannot be contained.

osteotomy of the upper femur in the intertrochanteric region is performed. When, in addition to abduction–medial rotation, flexion is required to achieve containment, varus angulation–derotation–extension osteotomy of the upper femur is indicated. This technique is described and illustrated in Plate 15 in Chapter 2.

Containment should be demonstrated preoperatively by arthrography of the hip; when containment cannot be obtained upper femoral osteotomy is contraindicated (Fig. 3–165). Definite advantages of femoral osteotomy are that it decompresses the femoral head, alters stresses across the hip joint, and tends to enhance the remodeling process; there is no acceleration in the *rate* of healing, however. The disadvantage of varus osteotomy of the upper femur lies in the elevation of the greater trochanter and the decrease in the articulotrochanteric distance; this will functionally weaken hip abductor motor strength. Avascular involvement and growth inhibition of the capital femoral physis in Legg-Calvé-Perthes disease will cause shortening of the femoral neck (coxa breva) and relative overgrowth of the greater trochanter. Therefore, the presence of physeal involvement is a relative contraindication to upper femoral osteotomy. The parents should be forewarned that, following varus osteotomy of the femur, a gluteus medius limp and Trendelenburg lurch will develop, and if already present, the limp will be aggravated. The possible necessity of distal-lateral transfer of the greater trochanter to correct the deformity should be discussed with the parents preoperatively.

Another disadvantage of femoral osteotomy is shortening of the femur and the disparity of the lower limb lengths that it produces. This may be significant (2 to 3 cm.) and persist, especially in the older child (over eight years of age). Epiphysiolysis may occur with excessive varization.

Progressive collapse of the femoral head can occur after containment with femoral or innominate osteotomy. Meticulous follow-up care is crucial; the hip should be protected with a three-point partial weight-bearing crutch gait.

Stress fracture, below the plate or through the screw holes after removal of the plate, can occur in femoral osteotomy. This again emphasizes the importance of protecting the hip and restricting the child's participation in contact sports and strenuous physical activities (e.g., jumping from heights or risking falls while bicycle riding).

Combined Femoral and Innominate Osteotomy. Attempts to contain the femoral head should not produce a deformity of the upper femur. Varization should not decrease the neck-shaft angle to less than 120 degrees. If excessive varization is required to contain the femoral head, a combination of intertrochanteric femoral osteotomy and innominate osteotomy is indicated (Fig. 3–166).

THIRD PHASE—RECONSTRUCTIVE SURGERY

Lower Limb Length Inequality. With interruption of the blood supply to the capital femoral epiphysis, varying degrees of ischemia to the growth plate and resultant shortness of the lower limb are almost inevitable in Legg-Calvé-Perthes disease. Subchondral fracture, collapse, and flattening of the capital epiphysis augment the shortening. Varus osteotomy of the proximal femur can further increase the shortening. In a study of 147 patients with unilateral Legg-Calvé-Perthes disease followed by means of orthoradiograms for five years or more, Shapiro found the average total shortening to be 2.14 cm. Four developmental patterns of discrepancy were detected. In *Type A* the discrepancy continually increased with time. In *Type B* the discrepancy increase fell off with time, often reaching a plateau with no subsequent change for several years regardless of skeletal age maturation. In the *Type C* pattern, the discrepancy occurred, reached a plateau for several years,

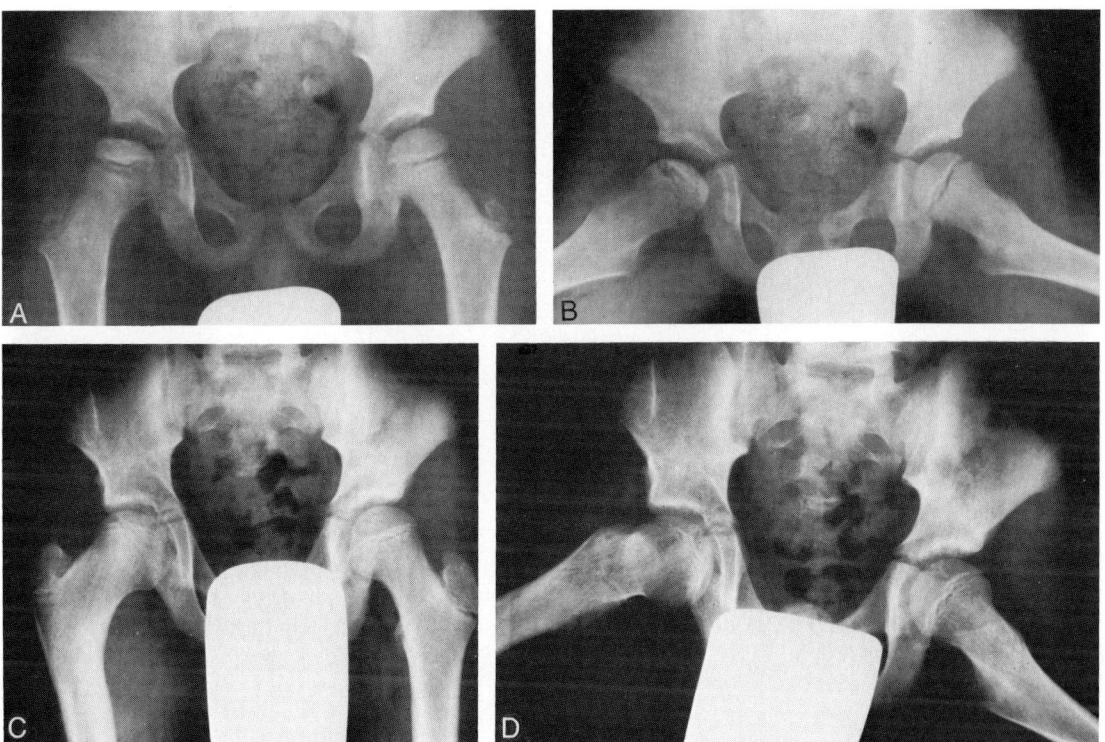

FIGURE 3–166. *Legg-Calvé-Perthes disease of the right hip treated by combination of femoral varization and Salter's innominate osteotomy.*

A and **B.** Preoperative anteroposterior and lateral radiograms of the hips. **C** and **D.** Four years later.

but owing to premature closure of the capital femoral physis, it increased again immediately prior to skeletal maturity. In *Type D* pattern, the discrepancy occurred, reached a plateau, but diminished on its own, correcting itself partially or fully. Epiphysiodesis was performed in 21 per cent of the patients.[601]

It is crucial to follow the limb length inequality in Legg-Calvé-Perthes disease, especially if there is involvement of the proximal femoral physis or if a varization osteotomy of the femur is performed. If the disparity is significant, epiphysiodesis of the contralateral distal femur is performed to equalize limb lengths at the appropriate skeletal age.

Relative Overgrowth of Greater Trochanter and Coxa Breva. Normally the tip of the greater trochanter should be at the level of the center of the femoral head and one and a half times the distance of the radius of the femoral head lateral to the center of the femoral head. With growth disturbance of the capital femoral physis, the femoral neck will be short, and there will be relative overgrowth of the greater trochanter. Deranged biomechanics of the hip will cause gluteus medius limp and Trendelenburg lurch. This is treated by distal and lateral transfer of the greater trochanter (Fig. 3–167).

Hinged Abduction of the Hip. With overgrowth of the articular cartilage on the anterolateral aspect of the femoral head and crushing of the trabeculae within the bony epiphysis there is upward and lateral displacement of the femoral head. The anterolateral portion of the femoral head therefore tends to bulge out from under the lateral rim of the acetabular roof. On attempted hip abduction the extruded enlarged portion of the femoral head impinges against the lateral acetabular rim; at this point of contact, the hip hinges. As a result, the hip is held in the adducted position, and the adductor spasm leads to adduction contracture and functional shortening of the lower limb. The term *hinge abduction* is used to describe the abnormal movement of the hip that occurs when the large uncovered anterolateral part of the deformed femoral head impinges on the lateral lip of the acetabulum and fails to slide within the acetabular socket. Clinically, an attempt to bring the hip into neutral position causes pain and an unpleasant clunking sensation. In time a groove develops on the anterolateral aspect

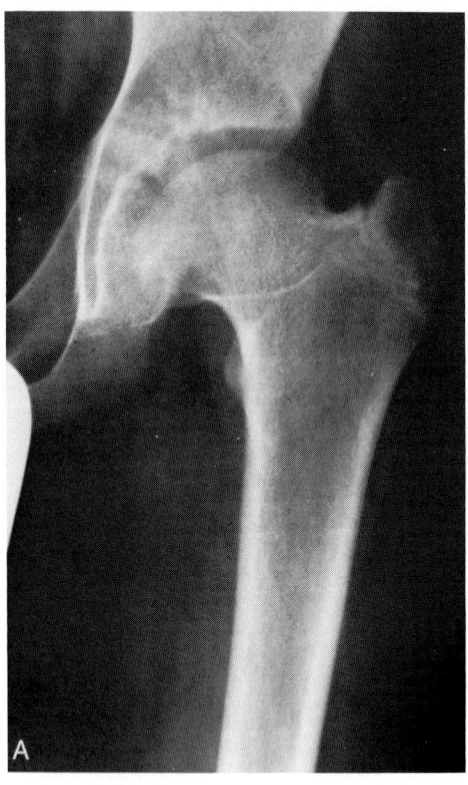
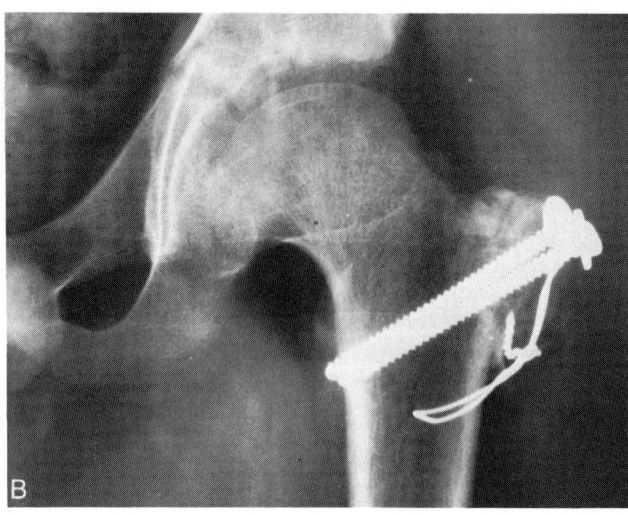

FIGURE 3–167. *Coxa breva and relative overgrowth of the greater trochanter in Perthes' disease treated by distal and lateral transfer of the greater trochanter.*

A. Preoperative radiogram. B. Postoperative radiogram.

of the enlarged femoral head—this dent corresponds to the weight-bearing portion of the femoral head when the hip is positioned in its flexed-adducted posture.

Arthrography of the hip should be performed to delineate the pathologic changes and pathomechanics. Range of hip motion is determined with image intensifier and video recorder.

Treatment. *Abduction-extension intertrochanteric osteotomy* is indicated when these hips are congruent in adduction and some flexion and have a functional range of hip adduction beyond the point of congruity. The point of congruity is usually between 15 and 30 degrees of adduction with 10 to 30 degrees of flexion. Abduction-extension osteotomy of the upper femur will align the lower limb in the middle of the arc of movement, provide a congruent position of the femoral head within the acetabulum in weight-bearing position, relieve the hinging, and improve the remodeling process with rounding of the femoral head. The superior joint space is usually restored to normal width. Following surgery pain is usually relieved. Abduction osteotomy will elongate the lower limb and diminish disparity of limb length. The advantage of abduction-extension osteotomy is that it does not remove bone from the femoral head and thereby derange forces within the hip joint. In the experience of Quain and Catterall, the results were satisfactory in 26 of the 27 hips with hinge abduction treated by abduction-extension osteotomy.[542]

Cheilectomy was used by Garceau and McKay, who surgically excised the protruded portion of the femoral head.[234, 448] Removal of the mechanical block to abduction of the hip improves range of motion. Biomechanically, however, cheilectomy has the serious disadvantage of reducing the load-bearing area of the joint and increasing stress forces across the hip. The procedure, also, does not correct residual shortening or hip abductor muscle weakness. Cheilectomy is recommended by this author if the hip, in adducted position, lacks further functional range of hip adduction. The cheilectomy should be combined with adductor myotomy, iliopsoas lengthening, and the use of the continuous passive concentric hip motion machine to restore range of hip motion (Fig. 3–168).

The Incongruous Hip. In the adolescent, uncovering of the femoral head with incongruity of the hip joint and pain will require a Chiari pelvic osteotomy to cover the femoral head, enlarge the acetabular capacity, and relieve the pain (Fig. 3–169). Often these patients also require distal lateral transfer of the greater trochanter at a later stage to correct gluteus medius lurch.

Van der Heyden and van Tongerloo recommended a shelf procedure to cover the extruded

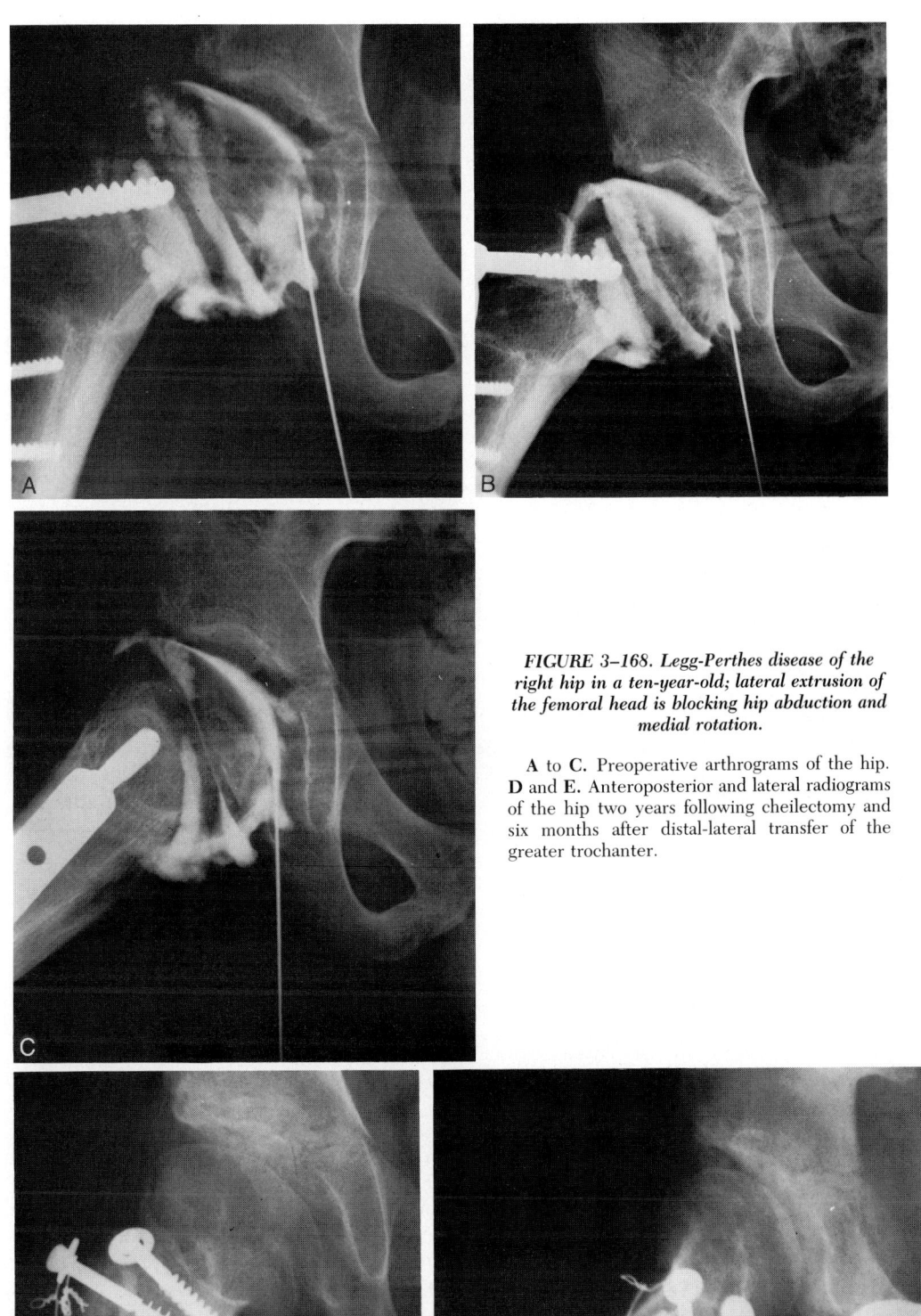

FIGURE 3–168. *Legg-Perthes disease of the right hip in a ten-year-old; lateral extrusion of the femoral head is blocking hip abduction and medial rotation.*

A to **C**. Preoperative arthrograms of the hip. **D** and **E**. Anteroposterior and lateral radiograms of the hip two years following cheilectomy and six months after distal-lateral transfer of the greater trochanter.

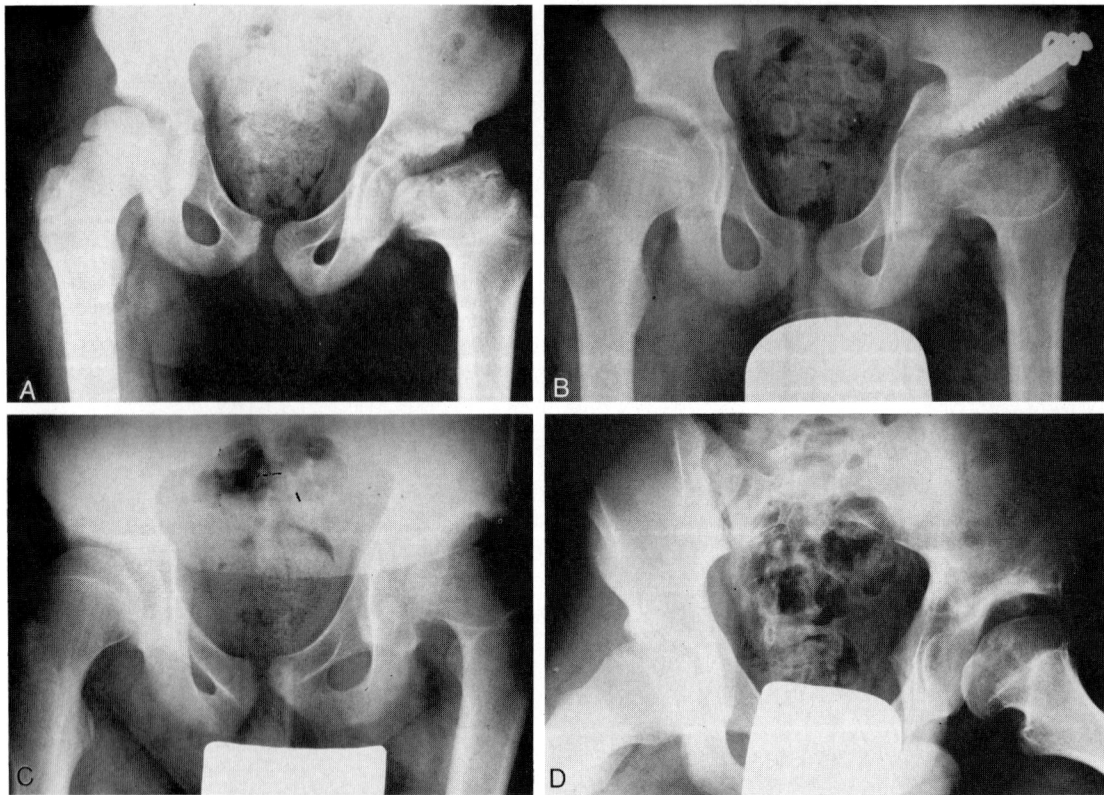

FIGURE 3–169. *Legg-Perthes disease in a 14-year-old boy with collapse of the femoral head and marked incongruity of the hip.*

The patient was treated by Chiari's pelvic osteotomy. **A.** Anteroposterior radiogram of the hip. **B.** Immediately postoperative radiogram. **C** and **D.** Two years later. The patient had complete relief of his pain.

portion of the femoral head; this, however, does not reduce lateral impingement on abduction.[668]

Osteochondritis Dissecans.[*] A rare and late sequela of Legg-Calvé-Perthes disease is osteochondritis dissecans of the femoral head. It occurs primarily in boys. On the average, about nine years after healing of the disease the patient presents with hip pain and limitation of motion. The osteochondritic fragment is located in the superolateral aspect of the dome of the femoral head, a site best depicted in the lateral projection. It appears as a localized area of subchondral bone separated by an area of rarefaction from the remainder of the femoral head (Fig. 3–170).

In surgically explored cases, microscopic examination has shown the osteochondritic fragment is composed of dead bone trabeculae surrounded by living cartilage, fibrocartilage, or fibrous tissue. This observation indicates the persistence of an unhealed necrotic fragment from the time of active disease.[291, 549] There is also evidence that the osteocartilaginous fragment is not necrotic in some cases because it continues to grow, suggesting another possible cause of osteochondritis dissecans in Legg-Calvé-Perthes disease; i.e., some of the living ossification nuclei may have failed to unite with the rest of the femoral head during the healing phase.[291, 358] Linear or computed tomography and magnetic resonance imaging will delineate the pathologic state. Arthrography will show whether the fragment is loose. If the outline of the articular cartilage of the femoral head is smooth with no dissection of the contrast medium deep into the osteochondral fragment, the prognosis is good for spontaneous healing. Treatment consists of protecting the affected hip with a toe-touch three-point crutch gait until symptoms have subsided. If the arthrogram shows that the contrast medium dissects beneath the fragment, however, surgical treatment is indicated if the symptoms justify it and there is evidence of progressive deterioration

---

[*]See References 224, 267, 281, 285, 291, 359, 486, 517, 549, 627, 703.

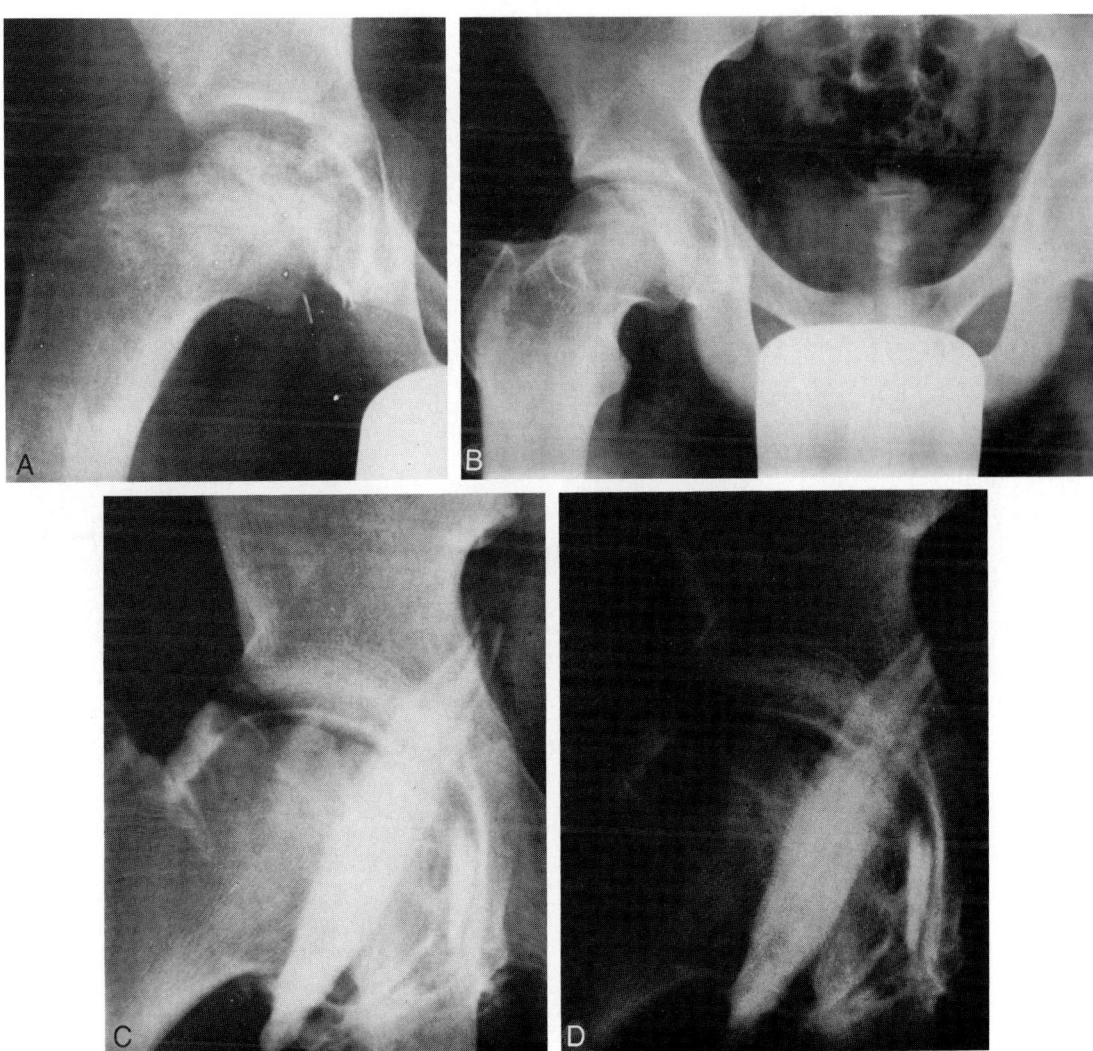

FIGURE 3–170. Osteochondritis dissecans of the right femoral head six years following Legg-Perthes disease.

A and **B.** Radiograms of right hip. **C** and **D.** Arthrograms showing cartilaginous surface is intact—the dye does not penetrate underneath the osteochondral fragment.

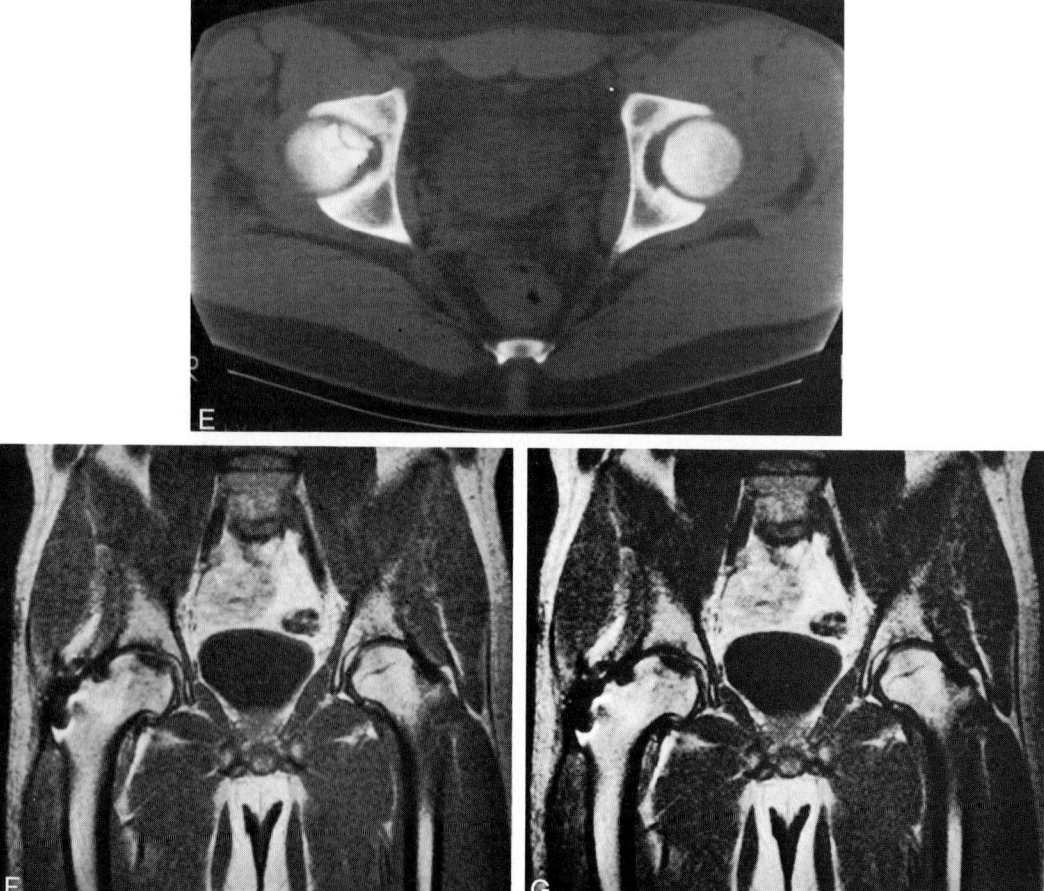

FIGURE 3–170 Continued. *Osteochondritis dissecans of the right femoral head six years following Legg-Perthes disease.*

E. CT scan showing the fragment. F and G. Magnetic resonance imaging scans.

of the hip. During surgery, the femoral head may have to be dislocated gently, preserving the retinacular vessels. If the fragment is small, it is removed and its fibrocartilaginous bed is curetted and drilled. If the fragment is large and loose, it is best to replace and fix it by pins or by bone grafting.[487] Woodward and Decker report a case in which bone grafting of the lesion succeeded in producing union and relieving symptoms.[703] Intertrochanteric derotation and angulation osteotomy may be considered in some cases to remove weight-bearing stress on the osteochondral fragment.

Torn Acetabular Labrum. This is a very rare complication in Legg-Calvé-Perthes disease resulting from abnormal stresses by the femoral head on the lateral aspect of the acetabulum. The stress point may cause a tear in the labrum with resultant pain. In the radiogram there will be a cystic rarefaction in the lateral part of the roof of the acetabulum. Arthrography will demonstrate the torn acetabular labrum. It resembles a bucket-handled tear of the medial meniscus. Treatment consists of excision of the torn labrum and coverage of the femoral head by Chiari's medial displacement osteotomy.[166]

References

1. Allbright, F.: Changes simulating Legg-Perthes disease (osteochondritis deformans juvenilis) due to juvenile myxoedema. J. Bone Joint Surg., *20*:764, 1938.
2. Altan, H., and Geimer, R.: Ueber die interne Zusatztherapie des Morbus Perthes mit dem Angiolytikum Vasculat. Z. Orthop., *104*:68, 1968.
3. Andersen, H.: Histochemical studies on the development of the human hip joint. Acta Anat., *48*:258, 1962.
4. Apley, A. G., and Weintroub, S.: The sagging rope sign in Perthes' disease and allied disorders. J. Bone Joint Surg., *63-B*:43, 1981.
5. Apley, G. A.: Perthes' disease. *In* A System of Orthopaedics and Fractures. New York, Appleton-Century-Crofts, 1968, pp. 273–277.
6. Arct, W. von, Klimek, S., and Oblonczek, G.: Per-

sonal experience with surgical treatment of Legg-Calvé-Waldenström-Perthes. Chir. Narzadow Ruchu Ortop. Pol., 35:357, 1970.
7. Arlet, J., and Ficat, P.: Diagnostic de l'ostéo-nécrose fémoro-capitale primitive au stade I (stade preradiologique). Rev. Chir. Orthop., 54:637, 1968.
8. Arlet, J., Ficat, P., and Durroux, R.: Formes anatomocliniques (radiologiques et étiologiques) des l'ischémie chronique et de l'ostéonécrose, dites primitives. Rev. Rhum. Mal. Ostéoartic., 38:41, 1971.
9. Arlet, J., Ficat, P., Lartigue, G., and Tran, M.: Recherches cliniques sur la pression intra-osseuse dans la métaphyse et l'epiphyse fémorales superiores chez l'homme. Rev. Rhum. Mal. Ostéoartic., 39:717, 1972.
10. Axer, A.: Subtrochanteric osteotomy in the treatment of Perthes' disease. A preliminary report. J. Bone Joint Surg., 47-B:489, 1965.
11. Axer, A., Halperin, N., and Itzchak, Y.: Anteversion of the femur in Legg-Calvé-Perthes syndrome. Isr. J. Med. Sci., 8:1733, 1972.
12. Axer, A., and Schiller, M. G.: The pathogenesis of the early deformity of the capital femoral epiphysis in Legg-Calvé-Perthes syndrome (L.C.P.S.). An arthrographic study. Clin. Orthop., 84:106, 1972.
13. Axer, A., Gershuni, D. H., Hendel, D., and Mirovski, Y.: Indications for femoral osteotomy in Legg-Calvé-Perthes disease. Clin. Orthop., 150:78, 1980.
14. Axer, A., Schiller, M. G., Segal, D., Rzetelny, V., and Gershuni-Gordon, D. H.: Subtrochanteric osteotomy in the treatment of Legg-Calvé-Perthes syndrome (L.C.P.S.). Acta Orthop. Scand., 44:31, 1973.
15. Axer, A., Zaidman, J. L., Gershuni, D. H., Scarf, S., Hartstein, E., and Iaffe, D.: The biochemical response in rabbit hip articular cartilage to induced synovitis (abstract). Clin. Chem., 21:1033, 1975.
16. Axhausen, G.: Der Krankheitsvorgang bei der Köhler'schen Krankheit der Metatarsalkopfchen und bei der Perthes'schen Krankheit des Hüftkopfes. Zentralbl. Chir., 50:553, 1923.
17. Babb, F. S., and Sundberg, A. B.: Legg-Calvé-Perthes disease. Minn. Med., 54:1001, 1971.
18. Bagliani, G. P., and Canale, G.: L'indagnie artrografica nel morbo diperthes. Minerva Ortop., 19:485, 1968.
19. Barbieri, L., and Macchia, P.: Analogie fra la malattia di Legg-Perthes-Calvé e le osteonecrosi primitive della testa del formore nell'adulto. Minerva Orthop., 20:277, 1969.
20. Barbieri, L., and Pietrabissa, G.: Le osteonécrosi della testa del fémore. Minerva Ortop., 20:197, 1969.
21. Barker, D. J. P., Dixon, E., and Taylor, J. F.: Perthes' disease of the hip in three regions of England. J. Bone Joint Surg., 60-B:478, 1978.
22. Barranco, S. D., Traver, R. C., Chiroffe, R. T., and Friedman, E. M.: A comparative study of Legg-Perthes disease. Clin. Orthop., 96:304, 1973.
23. Barta, V. O., Bellyei, A., and Kranicz, J.: Unsere Erfahrungen mit der intertrochanteren Femurosteotomie bei der Perthesschen Krankheit. Beitr. Orthop. Traumatol., 22:610, 1975.
24. Barz, F. -B., and Torklus, D. V.: Morbus Perthes, Folge einer Synovitis? Z. Orthop., 114:116, 1976.
25. Bassett, F. H., Wilson, J. W., Allen, B. L., Jr., and Azuma, H.: Normal vascular anatomy of the head of the femur in puppies with emphasis on the inferior retinacular vessels. J. Bone Joint Surg., 51-A:1139, 1969.
26. Bates, E. H.: The modern approach to Perthes' disease. J. Bone Joint Surg., 59-B:518, 1977.
27. Bauer, R., and Junger, H.: Die Intertrochantare Varisationsosteotomie zur Behandlung des Morbus Perthes. Arch. Orthop. Unfallchir., 79:187, 1974.
28. Bauer, R., and Junger, H.: Intertrochantare Osteotomie beim Morbus Perthes. 63. Kongress der Deutschen Gesellschaft fur Orthopadie und Traumatologie, Sept., 1976. Z. Orthop., 115:494, 1977.
29. Beck, O., and Soukup, P.: Seltene Lokalisationen der invenilen aseptischen Osteochondronekrosen. Beitr. Orthop. Traumatol., 19:592, 1972.
30. Beiler, D. D., and Love, W. H.: Thyroid function in Legg-Perthes disease. J. Bone Joint Surg., 38-A:1320, 1956.
31. Bellyei, V. A., Barta, O., and Kranicz, J.: Die Auswertung der Behandlungsergebnisse der Perthesschen Krankheit. Beitr. Orthop. Traumatol., 22:618, 1975.
32. Beneke, G., and Deutschle, N.: Frühveränderungen in der proximalen Femurepiphyse nach experimenteller Blutkreislaufstörung. Virchows Arch., 344:125, 1967.
33. Bensahel, H., Bok, B., and Flikier, H.: La place de la scintigraphie dans l'ostéochondrite primitive de hanche. Chirurgie, 105:321, 1979.
34. Bensahel, H., Bok, B., Cavailloles, F., and Csukonyi, Z.: Bone scintigraphy in Perthes disease. J. Pediatr. Orthop., 3:302, 1983.
35. Bentzon, P. G. K.: Experimental studies on the pathogenesis of coxa plana. Acta Radiol., 6:155, 1926.
36. Berenyi, P. Z.: Die Beschleunigung der Femurkopfregeneration bei Morbus Perthes durch intraartikulaere Lebertraninjektionen. Z. Orthop., 106:567, 1969.
37. Berenyi, P., Kelemen, J., and Keki, M.: Angiographias vizsgalatok Perthes-es betegeken. Magy. Traumatol. Orthop., 15:176, 1972.
38. Bergmann, E.: Theoretisches, klinisches und experimentelles zur Frage der aseptischen Knochennekrosen. Dtsch. Z. Chir., 206:12, 1927.
39. Bernbeck, R.: Untersuchungen zur Pathologie und Ätiologie der Perthes'schen Krankheit. Verh. Dtsch. Orthop. Ges., 36:241, 1948.
40. Bernbeck, R.: Zur Pathogenese der jugentlichen Hüftkopfnekrose (Perthes-Legg-Calvé). Arch. Orthop. Unfallchir., 421:164, 1950.
41. Bernbeck, R.: Kritisches zum Perthes Problem der Hüfte. Arch. Orthop. Unfallchir., 44:445, 1951.
42. Bernbeck, R.: Perthes-Leiden bei eineiigen Zwillingen. Z. Orthop., 103:299, 1967.
43. Bertrams, J., Schiersmann, P., and Ritgen, G.: HLA antigens in Perthes' disease. Tissue Antigens, 12:157, 1978.
44. Bertrand, P.: Technique de greffe intraépiphysaire dans le traitement de la coxa plana. Rev. Chir. Orthop., 40:116, 1954.
45. Billing, L.: Roentgen examination of the proximal femur end in children and adolescents. Acta Radiol. [Suppl.], 110:1, 1954.
46. Birkeland, I. W., and Zettl, J. H.: A hip-abduction orthosis for Legg-Perthes disease. Orthotics Prosthetics, 28:49, 1974.
47. Bitterauf, H., Mann, M., and Siguda, P.: Die Behandlung der Perthesschen Erkrankung mit eimem Aabspreiz-Innendreh-Apparat. 63. Kongress der Deutschen Gesellschaft fur Orthopadie und Traumatologie, Sept., 1976. Z. Orthop., 115:492, 1977.
48. Bjerkreim, I., and Hauge, M. F.: So-called recurrent Perthes' disease. Acta Orthop. Scand., 47:181, 1976.
49. Blakemore, M. E., and Harrison, M. H. M.: A prospective study of children with untreated Catteral Group I Perthes' disease. J. Bone Joint Surg., 61-B:329, 1979.
50. Bluemm, R. G., Falke, T. H. M., Ziedees des Plantes, B. G. J., and Steiner, R. M.: Early Legg-Perthes disease (ischemic necrosis of the femoral head) demonstrated by magnetic resonance imaging. Skeletal Radiol., 14:95, 1985.

51. Bobechko, W. P.: The Toronto brace for Legg-Perthes disease. Clin. Orthop., *102*:115, 1974.
52. Bobechko, W. P.: The Toronto brace for Legg-Perthes disease. J. Bone Joint Surg., *58-B*:115, 1976.
53. Bobechko, W. P., and Harris, W. R.: The radiographic density of avascular bone. J. Bone Joint Surg., *42-B*:626, 1960.
54. Bohr, H.: Densitometry and 18-F scintigraphy in the study of the revascularization of the femoral head in coxa plana. Acta Orthop. Scand., *44*:417, 1973.
55. Bohr, H.: Skeletal maturation in Legg-Calvé-Perthes disease. Int. Orthop. (S.I.C.O.T.), *2*:277, 1979.
56. Bohr, H.: On the development and course of Legg-Calvé-Perthes disease (LCPD). Clin. Orthop., *150*:30, 1980.
57. Bohr, H., and Larsen, H. E.: On necrosis of the femoral head after fracture of the neck of the femur. J. Bone Joint Surg., *47-B*:330, 1965.
58. Bohr, H., Baadsgaard, K., and Sager, P.: The vascular supply to the femoral head following dislocation of the hip joint. Acta Orthop. Scand., *35*:264, 1965.
59. Bohr, H., Hansen-Leth, C., and Reimann, I.: On the influence of intertrochanteric osteotomies upon the growth and vascularization of the proximal part of the femur in young rabbits. Acta Orthop. Scand., *41*:619, 1970.
60. Borgsmiller, W. K., Whiteside, L. A., Goldsand, E. M., and Lange, D. R.: Effect of hydrostatic pressure in the hip joint on proximal femoral epiphyseal and metaphyseal blood flow. Trans. Orthop. Res. Soc., *5*:23, 1980.
61. Bowen, J. R., and Schmidt, T.: Osteochondroma of the femoral neck in Perthes' disease. J. Pediatr. Orthop., *3*:28, 1983.
62. Bozsan, E. J.: A new treatment of intracapsular fractures of the neck of the femur and Calvé-Legg-Perthes disease. J. Bone Joint Surg., *14*:884, 1932.
63. Branciforti, S., and Montina, S.: Qual'e il destino dell anche osteocondritiche? Minerva Ortop., *5*:404, 1954.
64. Branciforti, S., and Teti, A.: Rapporti anatomo-radiografici e varizaioni goniometriche nel perthes e nelle osteocondriti post-riduttive. Minerva Ortop., *5*:414, 1954.
65. Brezezinski, M., and Ramotowski, W.: Wyniki ambulatoryjnego leczenia choroby Legg-Calvé-Perthesa. Chir. Narzadow Ruchu Ortop. Pol., *37*:85, 1972. (Abstract in Am. Dig. For. Orthop. Lit., 1971, Outpatient treatment of Legg-Calvé-Perthes disease.)
66. Brill, W.: Beitraege zur Aetiologie der Perthes'schen Erkrankung des Hueftgelenkes und der Köehlerschen Metatarsalerkrankung. Arch. Orthop. Unfallchir., *24*:64, 1927.
67. Brindley, H. H.: Disabilities of the hip in children. Am. J. Orthop., *1*:88, 1959.
68. Brizzi, E., Cecchini, M., and Gremigni, D.: La vascolarizzazione arteriosa della testa e del collo del femore dell'uomo. Arch. Ital. Anat. Embriol., *76*:109, 1971.
69. Broder, H.: The late results in Legg-Perthes disease and factors influencing them: A study of one hundred and two cases. Bull. Hosp. Joint Dis., *14*:194, 1953.
70. Broder, H.: Prognosis in Legg-Perthes disease. J. Pediatr., *53*:451, 1958.
71. Brookes, M.: The vascularization of long bones in the human foetus. J. Anat., *92*:261, 1958.
72. Brotherton, B. J.: The long-term results of the treatment of Perthes' disease by recumbency and femoral head containment. J. Bone Joint Surg., *58-B*:131, 1976.
73. Brotherton, B. J., and McKibbin, B.: Perthes' disease treated by prolonged recumbency and femoral head containment: A long-term appraisal. J. Bone Joint Surg., *59-B*:8, 1977.
74. Brown, T. D., and Ferguson, A. B., Jr.: Mechanical property distributions in the cancellous bone of the human proximal femur. Acta Orthop. Scand., *51*:429, 1980.
75. Brown, T. D., and Ferguson, A. B., Jr.: The effects of hip contact aberrations on stress patterns within the human femoral head. Ann. Biomed. Eng., *8*:75, 1980.
76. Brown, T. D., Way, M. E., and Ferguson, A. B., Jr.: Stress transmission anomalies in femoral heads altered by aseptic necrosis. J. Biomech., *13*:687, 1980.
77. Brown, T. D., Way, M. E., Fu, F. H., and Ferguson, A. B., Jr.: Load transmission through the proximal femur of the growing child: A finite element analysis. Internal Publication, Department of Orthopaedic Surgery, University of Pittsburgh, 1980.
78. Bullough, P., Goodfellow, J., and O'Connor, J.: The relationship between degenerative changes and load-bearing in the human hip. J. Bone Joint Surg., *55-B*:746, 1973.
79. Bunch, W. H., and Keagy, R. D.: Application of lower extremity orthoses. In Principles of Orthotic Treatment. St. Louis, Mosby, 1976, pp. 32–47.
80. Burrows, H. J.: Coxa plana with special reference to its pathology and kinship. Br. J. Surg., *29*:23, 1941.
81. Burwell, R. G.: Perthes' disease. J. Bone Joint Surg., *60-B*:1, 1978.
82. Burwell, R. G., Dangerfield, P. H., Hall, D. J., Vernon, C. L., and Harrison, M. H. M.: Perthes' disease: An anthropometric study revealing impaired and disproportionate growth. J. Bone Joint Surg., *60-B*:461, 1978.
83. Burwell, R. G., Coates, C. L., Vernon, C. L., Harrison, M. H. M., Hall, D., Turner, M., Dangerfield, P., and Reeves, B.: Anthropometry and Perthes' disease: A preliminary report. J. Bone Joint Surg., *58-B*:254, 1976.
84. Caffey, J.: The early roentgenographic changes in essential coxa plana: Their significance in pathogenesis. A.J.R., *103*:620, 1968.
85. Caffey, J. P.: Pediatric X-ray Diagnosis. 6th Ed. Vol. II. Chicago, Year Book, 1972, p. 1150.
86. Caldwell, G. A.: End results of coxa plana as related to treatment. South. Med. J., *27*:402, 1934.
87. Calvé, J.: Sur une forme particulière de coxalgie grefée. Sur des déformations caracteristique de l'extremité supérieure du fémur. Rev. Chir. (Paris), *42*:54, 1910.
88. Calvé, J.: A special form of pseudo-coxitis. Practitioner, *89*:59, 1912.
89. Calvé, J., Galland, M., and DeCagny, R.: Pathogenesis of the limp due to coxalgie. J. Bone Joint Surg., *21*:12, 1939.
90. Calver, R., Benugopal, V., Dorgan, J., Bentley, G., and Gimlette, T.: Radionuclide scanning in the early diagnosis of Perthes' disease. J. Bone Joint Surg., *63-B*:379, 1981.
91. Camargo, F. P.: Revascularization of the neck of the femur in Legg-Calvé-Perthes syndrome. Clin. Orthop., *10*:79, 1957.
92. Cameron, J. M., and Izatt, M. M.: Legg-Calvé-Perthes disease. Scott. Med. J., *5*:148, 1960.
93. Canale, S. T.: Legg-Calvé-Perthes disease. In Edmonson, A. S., and Crenshaw, A. H. (eds.): Campbell's Operative Orthopaedics. St. Louis, Mosby, 1980, pp. 1217–1223.
94. Canale, S. T.: Varus derotation osteotomy. In Edmonson, A. S., and Crenshaw, A. H. (eds.): Campbell's Operative Orthopaedics. 6th Ed. St. Louis, Mosby, 1980, pp. 1219–1223.
95. Canale, S. T., D'Anca, A. F., Cotler, J. M., and Snedden, H. E.: Innominate osteotomy in Legg-Calvé-Perthes disease. J. Bone Joint Surg., *54-A*:25, 1972.
96. Canario, A. T., Williams, L., Weintroub, S., Catter-

all, A., and Lloyd Roberts, G. C.: A controlled study of the results of femoral osteotomy in severe Perthes' disease. J. Bone Joint Surg., 62-B:438, 1980.
97. Canestri, G., and Monzali, G. L.: Osteocondrite postriduttiva nella lussazione congenitale dell'anca. Lattante, 28:537, 1957.
98. Carpenter, E. B., and Powell, D. O.: Osteochondrosis of capital epiphysis of femur (Legg-Calvé-Perthes disease). J.A.M.A., 172:525, 1960.
99. Cartier, P., Dagher, F., and Morel, G.: L'ostéotomie de varisation dans la maladie de Legg-Perthes-Calvé. A propos de 50 cas. Rev. Chir. Orthop., 62:27, 1976.
100. Cartier, P., Hautier, S., and Lemoine, A.: L'ostéotomie de varisation dans la nécrose idiopathique de la tête fémorale. Ann. Chir., 16:483, 1972.
101. Castaign, J., Buchet, C., and Delaneau, J.: Problems posés par l'ostéotomie de varisation de Pauwels. Rev. Chir. Orthop., 45:717, 1959.
102. Cathro, A. J. M., and Kirkaldy-Willis, W. H.: Treatment of Perthes' disease of the hip by cancellous bone grafting. Preliminary report. J. Bone Joint Surg., 45-B:284, 1963.
103. Catterall, A.: The natural history of Perthes' disease. J. Bone Joint Surg., 53-B:37, 1971.
104. Catterall, A.: Coxa plana. In Apley, A. G. (ed.): Modern Trends in Orthopaedics. New York, Appleton-Century-Crofts, 1972, pp. 122–147.
105. Catterall, A.: Perthes' disease. Br. Med. J., 1:1145, 1977.
106. Catterall, A.: Legg-Calvé-Perthes syndrome. Clin. Orthop., 158:41, 1981.
107. Catterall, A.: Legg-Calvé-Perthes Disease. Edinburgh, Churchill-Livingstone, 1982.
108. Catterall, A., Lloyd Roberts, G. C., and Wynne-Davies, R.: Association of Perthes' disease with congenital anomalies of genitourinary tract and inguinal region. Lancet, 1:996, 1971.
109. Catterall, A., Pringle, J., Byers, P. D., Fulford, G. E., and Kemp, H. B. S.: Perthes' disease: Is the epiphysial infarction complete? J. Bone Joint Surg., 64-B:276, 1982.
110. Catterall, A., Pringle, J., Byers, P. D., Fulford, G. E., Kemp, H. B. S., Dolman, C. L., Bell, H. M., McKibbin, B., Ralis, Z., Jensen, O. M., Lauritzen, J., Ponseti, I. V., and Ogden, J.: A review of the morphology of Perthes' disease. J. Bone Joint Surg., 64-B:269, 1982.
111. Catto, M.: Pathology of aseptic bone necrosis. In Davidson, J. K. (ed.): Aseptic Necrosis of Bone. Amsterdam, Excerpta Medica, 1976, pp. 3–100.
112. Cavanaugh, L. A., Shelton, E. K., and Sutherland, R.: Metabolic studies in osteochondritis of the capital femoral epiphysis. J. Bone Joint Surg., 18:957, 1936.
113. Cecchini, M., and Gremigni, D.: La vascolarizzazione intraossea dell'epifisi superiore del femore. Arch. Ital. Anat. Embriol., 74:321, 1969.
114. Chapman, E. M.: Thyroid function in Legg-Perthes disease. N. Engl. J. Med., 255:289, 1956.
115. Chiari, K.: International symposium on children's hip problems. Wilmington, Delaware, 1980.
116. Chiari, K., Endler, M., and Hackel, H.: Die Behandlung der Coxa magna bei Morbus Perthes' mit der Beckenosteotomie. 63. Kongress der Deutschen Gesellschaft fur Orthopädie und Traumatologie, Sept., 1976. Z. Orthop., 15:493, 1977.
117. Chiari, K., Endler, M., and Hackel, H.: Die Behandlung der Coxa magna bei M. Perthes' mit der Beckenosteotomie. Arch. Orthop. Trauma Surg., 91:183, 1978.
118. Chicote-Campos, F., Hupfauer, W., and Drerup, S.: Die Konservative Behandlung bei Morbus Perthes. 63. Kongress der Deutschen Gesellschaft für Orthopädie und Traumatologie, Sept., 1976. Z. Orthop., 115:490, 1977.
119. Chigot, P. L.: Kyste "essentiel" de os: Opération ou surveillance? Union Med. Can., 101:71, 1972.
120. Chigot, P. L., and Labbe, G.: Allongements cervicaux après section du grand trochanter chez l'enfant. Rev. Chir. Orthop., 48:199, 1962.
121. Chivabongs, A. Z.: Verlaeuft die perthes'schen Erkrankung einseitig. Z. Orthop., 110:418, 1972.
122. Choyce, C. C.: Traumatic dislocation of the hip in childhood and relation of trauma to pseudocoxalgia. Br. J. Surg., 12:52, 1924.
123. Chuinard, E. G.: Femoral osteotomy in treatment of Legg-Calvé-Perthes syndrome. Orthop. Rev., 8:113, 1979.
124. Chung, S. M.: The arterial supply of the developing proximal end of the human femur. J. Bone Joint Surg., 58-A:961, 1976.
125. Chung, S. M. K., and Moe, J. H.: Legg-Calvé-Perthes disease. Clinical-radiographic correlations. Clin. Orthop., 41:116, 1965.
126. Chung, S. M., and Ralston, E. L.: Necrosis of the femoral head associated with sickle cell anaemia and its genetic variants. J. Bone Joint Surg., 51-A:33, 1969.
127. Clarke, N. M. P., and Harrison, M. H. M.: Painful sequelae of coxa plana. J. Bone Joint Surg., 65-A:13, 1983.
128. Clarke, T. E., Finnegan, T. L., Fisher, R. L., Bunch, W. H., and Gossling, H. R.: Legg-Perthes disease in children less than four years old. J. Bone Joint Surg., 60-A:166, 1978.
129. Cocchiarella, A., Challenor, Y., and Katz, J. F.: Orthosis for use in Legg-Calvé-Perthes disease. Arch. Phys. Med. Rehab., 53:286, 1972.
130. Cockshott, W. P., and Palmer, P. E.: Perthes' disease (letter). Lancet, 1:652, 1960.
131. Coleman, C. R., Slager, R. F., and Smith, W. S.: The effect of environmental influence on acetabular development. Surg. Forum, 9:775, 1958.
132. Coleman, S. S.: Perthes' disease—complications of surgical containment by acetabular osteotomy. Presented at International Symposium on Common Hip Disorders in Children. Wilmington, Delaware, October 20–23, 1980.
133. Colinet, E., Lustygier, M., and de Longree, R.: A propos d'un cas d'ostéonécrose aseptique coxofémorale bilatérale. J. Belg. Rhum. Med. Phys., 22:1, 1967.
134. Compere, C. L., Garrison, M., and Fahey, J. J.: Deformities of the femur resulting from arrestment of growth of the capital and greater trochanteric epiphyses. J. Bone Joint Surg., 22:909, 1940.
135. Conti, R.: La coxometria nella diagnostica e nella terapie dell'artrosi dell'anca. Minerva Radiol., 15:99, 1970.
136. Conway, J. J.: Radionuclide bone imaging in pediatrics. Pediatr. Clin. North Am., 24:701, 1977.
137. Conway, J. J., Weiss, S. C., and Maldonado, V.: Scintigraphic patterns in Legg-Calvés-Perthes disease. Radiology, 102:167, 1983.
138. Cordeiro, E. N.: Femoral osteotomy in Legg-Calvé-Perthes disease. Clin. Orthop., 150:69, 1980.
139. Cotler, J. M.: Surgery in Legg-Calvé-Perthes syndrome. A.A.O.S. Instr. Course Lect., 25:135, 1976.
140. Cotler, J. M., and Donahue, J.: Innominate osteotomy in the treatment of Legg-Calvé-Perthes disease. Clin. Orthop., 150:95, 1980.
141. Craig, W. A., Karmer, W. G., and Watanabe, R.: Etiology and treatment of Legg-Calvé-Perthes syndrome. J. Bone Joint Surg., 45-A:1325, 1963.
142. Crawford, A. H.: Legg-Calvé-Perthes disease coexistent with slipped capital femoral epiphysis. A case report. J. Bone Joint Surg., 57-A:280, 1975.
143. Crock, H. V.: An atlas of the arterial supply of the head and neck of the femur in man. Clin. Orthop., 152:17, 1980.

Akeson, W. H.: The biochemical response of rabbit articular cartilage matrix to an induced talcum synovitis. Acta Orthop. Scand., 52:599, 1981.
243. Gershuni, D. H., Hargens, A. R., Lee, Y., Greenberg, E. N., Zapf, R., and Akeson, W. H.: The questionable significance of hip joint tamponade in producing osteonecrosis in Legg-Calvé-Perthes syndrome. J. Pediatr. Orthop., 3:280, 1983.
244. Gershuni-Gordon, D. H., and Axer, A.: Synovitis of the hip joint. An experimental model in rabbits. J. Bone Joint Surg., 56-B:69, 1974.
245. Giambelli, G., and Lanzetta, A.: Sostituzione con protesi metallica nella necrosi idiopatica della testa femorale. Atti Acad. Med. Lombarda, 22:354, 1967.
246. Giannestras, N.: Legg-Perthes disease in twins. J. Bone Joint Surg., 36-A:149, 1954.
247. Gickler, H.: Furehfaeller der Perthes'schen Erkrankung. Fortschr. Geb. Röentgenstr., 55:441, 1937.
248. Gila, G.: Ereditarieta e osteocondrite dell'anca. Minerva Orthop., 6:79, 1955.
249. Gila, G., and Casto, C.: Revisione statistica delle osteocondriti giovanili. Minerva Ortop., 6:116, 1955.
250. Gilday, P. L., Paul, D., Davidson, J., and Rang, M.: Technetium polyphosphate bone scanning of nonmalignant bone disease in children. J. Bone Joint Surg., 57-B:533, 1975.
251. Gill, A. B.: Legg-Perthes disease of the hip—its early roentgenographic manifestations and its clinical course. J. Bone Joint Surg., 22:1013, 1940.
252. Gill, A. B.: The relationship of Legg-Perthes disease to the function of the thyroid gland. J. Bone Joint Surg., 25:892, 1943.
253. Girdany, B. R., and Osman, M. Z.: Longitudinal growth and skeletal maturation in Perthes' disease. Radiol. Clin. North Am., 6:245, 1968.
254. Girod, G.: Varisizing intertrochanteric derotation osteotomy in Perthes' disease. Beitr. Orthop. Traumatol., 16:419, 1969.
255. Clancy, J.: Lower extremity bracing. Part IV: Lower extremity orthotic components: Applications and indications. A.A.O.S. Instruct. Course Lect., 20:136, 1971.
256. Glasgow, M., Graham-Smith, A., and Catterall, A.: A cause of hip pain following the Smith-Petersen approach. Read at the Royal Society of Medicine, 1978.
257. Glass, R. B. J., Poznanski, A. K., and Fisher, M. R.: Magnetic resonance imaging in Legg-Calvé-Perthes disease. Personal communication, 1988.
258. Gledhill, R. B., and McIntyre, J. M.: Transient synovitis and Legg-Calvé-Perthes disease: A comparative study. Can. Med. Assoc. J., 100:311, 1969.
259. Goff, C. W.: Legg-Calvé-Perthes Syndrome and Related Osteochondroses of Youth. Springfield, Ill. Thomas, 1954.
260. Goff, C. W.: Growth acceleration in Legg-Calvé-Perthes syndrome by complementary feedings of aureomycin. Clin. Orthop., 6:95, 1955.
261. Goff, C. W.: Earlier weight-bearing in Legg-Calvé-Perthes syndrome. J. Bone Joint Surg., 40-A:1200, 1958.
262. Goff, C. W.: Recumbency versus non-recumbency treatment of Legg-Perthes disease. Clin. Orthop., 14:50, 1959.
263. Goff, C. W.: Legg-Calvé-Perthes syndrome. An up-to-date critical review. Clin. Orthop., 22:93, 1962.
264. Goff, C. W.: Influence of small daily doses of tetracycline on the clinical course of Legg-Calvé-Perthes syndrome. Report of a double-blind study. Clin. Orthop., 38:71, 1965.
265. Gold, A. M.: Osteochondritis dissecans of the femoral head. Bull. Hosp. Joint Dis., 1:30, 1940.
266. Goldenberg, R. R.: Traumatic dislocation of the hip followed by Perthes' disease. J. Bone Joint Surg., 20:770, 1938.
267. Goldman, A. B., Hallel, T., Salvati, E. M., and Freiberger, R. H.: Osteochondritis dissecans complicating Legg-Perthes disease. Radiology, 121:561, 1976.
268. Gossling, H. R.: Legg-Perthes disease. Part II. Treatment by recumbency. A.A.O.S. Instruct. Course Lect., 22:296, 1973.
269. Gossling, H. R.: Legg-Perthes disease. Part III. Analysis of poor results. A.A.O.S. Instruct. Course Lect., 22:301, 1973.
270. Gossling, H. R., Gee, R. O., and Pike, M. M.: Legg-Calvé-Perthes disease (abstract). J. Bone Joint Surg., 39-A:691, 1957.
271. Gourdou, J.-F., Danet, A., Guiraud, R., Durroux, R., Ficat, P., and Arlet, J.: Nécrose expérimentale de la tête fémorale d'origine veineuse chez le chien. Rev. Rhumat., 41:739, 1974.
272. Gower, W. E., and Johnston, R. C.: Legg-Perthes disease. Long-term follow-up of thirty-six patients. J. Bone Joint Surg., 53-A:759, 1971.
273. Graham, R. V.: Experimental considerations in Perthes' disease. Med. J. Austr., 1:207, 1930.
274. Gray, I. M., Lowrey, R. B., Renwick, D. H. G.: Incidence and genetics of Legg-Perthes disease (osteochondritis deformans) in British Columbia: Evidence of polygenic determination. J. Med. Genet., 9:197, 1972.
275. Green, N. E., and Griffin, P. P.: Intra-osseous venous pressure in Legg-Perthes disease. J. Bone Joint Surg., 64-A:666, 1982.
276. Green, N. E., Beauchamp, R. D., and Griffin, P. P.: Epiphyseal extrusion as a prognostic index in Legg-Calve-Perthes disease. J. Bone Joint Surg., 63-B:900, 1981.
277. Greenlaw, R. K., Kahn, D. A., and Petrie, J. G.: Experimentally produced changes in rabbit resembling Legg-Calvé-Perthes disease. Surg. Forum, 11:440, 1960.
278. Greenwald, A. S., and Haynes, D. W.: Weight-bearing areas in the human hip joint. J. Bone Joint Surg., 54-B:157, 1972.
279. Grossard, G. D.: Hip pain during adolescence after Perthes' disease. J. Bone Joint Surg., 63-B:572, 1981.
280. Gualtieri, G., and Lanzi, F.: Sul trattamento della osteocondrosi dissecante dell'anca. Minerva Ortop., 16:354, 1965.
281. Guilleminet, M., and Barbier, J. M.: Osteochondritis dissecans of the hip. J. Bone Joint Surg., 39-B:268, 1957.
282. Gunther, S. F., and Gossling, H. R.: Legg-Perthes disease. Part IV. Treatment by abduction ambulation. A.A.O.S. Instruct. Course Lect., 22:305, 1973.
283. Gurd, A. R., and Bobechko, W. P.: Bracing in Legg-Perthes disease. J. Bone Joint Surg., 57-B:533, 1975.
284. Gutezeit, G.: Ossification of femur head granules in infants between the 3rd and 10th month. Beitr. Orthop. Traumatol., 20:638, 1973.
285. Haas, A.: Umbau von Perthes'schen Krankheit in Osteochondritis dissecans. Zentralbl. Chir., 64:2873, 1937.
286. Hagen, W. H.: Coxa plana: Report of two bilateral cases in brothers. J. Bone Joint Surg., 21:1028, 1939.
287. Halkier, E.: The "tear-shaped phenomenon" in Calvé-Perthes disease. Acta Orthop. Scand., 25:287, 1956.
288. Hall, D. J., and Harrison, M. H. M.: An association between congenital abnormalities and Perthes' disease of the hip. J. Bone Joint Surg., 61-B:18, 1979.
289. Hall, G.: Observations on Perthes' disease. (M.D. Thesis.) Manchester, University of Manchester, 1980.
290. Hall, G.: Some observations of Perthes' disease (Robert Jones prize essay of the British Orthopaedic Association 1981). J. Bone Joint Surg., 63-B:631, 1981.
291. Hallel, T., and Salvati, E. A.: Osteochondritis dissecans following Legg-Calvé-Perthes disease. J. Bone Joint Surg., 58-A:708, 1976.
292. Hamsa, W. R., and Campbell, L. S.: Osteochondritis

deformans coxae juvenilis. Familial demonstration. Am. J. Dis. Child., 86:54, 1953.
293. Haraldsson, S.: Derotation varization osteotomy in the treatment of Perthes' disease. Acta Orthop. Scand., 44:105, 1973.
294. Hardcastle, I. H., Ross, R., Hamalainen, M., and Mata, A.: Catterall grouping of Perthes' disease. J. Bone Joint Surg., 62-B:428, 1980.
295. Harino-Zuko, C., and Pietrogrande, V.: Orientations dans le traitement de la maladie de Perthes. In Bailleux, M. A. (ed.), 7th Cong. Intnl. Chir. Orthop. Bruxelles, Im. des Sciences, 1957, pp. 673–680.
296. Harper, P. S., Brotherton, B. J., and Cochlin, D.: Genetic risks in Perthes' disease. Clin. Genet., 10:178, 1976.
297. Harrison, M. H. M.: The "broomstick" treatment of Perthes' disease. J. Bone Joint Surg., 48-B:382, 1966.
298. Harrison, M. H. M., and Bassett, C. A. L.: Use of pulsed electromagnetic fields in Perthes' disease: Report of a pilot study. J. Pediatr. Orthop., 4:579, 1984.
299. Harrison, M. H. M., and Blakemore, M. E.: A study of the "normal" hip in children with unilateral Perthes' disease. J. Bone Joint Surg., 62-B:31, 1980.
300. Harrison, M. H. M., and Burwell, R. G.: Perthes' disease: A concept of pathogenesis. Clin. Orthop., 156:115, 1981.
301. Harrison, M. H. M., and Menon, M. P. A.: Legg-Calvé-Perthes disease. The value of roentgenographic measurement in clinical practice with specific reference to the broomstick plaster method. J. Bone Joint Surg., 48-A:1301, 1966.
302. Harrison, M. H. M., and Turner, M. H.: Containment splintage for Perthes' disease of the hip. J. Bone Joint Surg., 56-B:199, 1974.
303. Harrison, M. H. M., Turner, M. H., and Jacobs, P.: Skeletal immaturity in Perthes' disease. J. Bone Joint Surg., 58-B:37, 1976.
304. Harrison, M. H. M., Turner, M. H., and Nicholson, F. J.: Coxa plana. Results of a new form of splinting. J. Bone Joint Surg., 51-A:1057, 1969.
305. Harrison, M. H. M., Turner, M. H., and Smith, D. N.: Perthes' disease. Treatment with the Birmingham splint. J. Bone Joint Surg., 64-B:3, 1982.
306. Hauge, M. F.: The treatment of coxa plana. A follow-up examination. Acta Orthop. Scand., 26:53, 1957.
307. Haythorn, S. R.: Pathological changes found in material removed at operation in Legg-Calvé-Perthes disease. J. Bone Joint Surg., 31-A:599, 1949.
308. Heikkinen, E., and Puranen, J.: Evaluation of femoral osteotomy in the treatment of Legg-Calvé-Perthes disease. Clin. Orthop., 150:60, 1980.
309. Heikkinen, E. S., Puranen, J., and Suramo, I.: The effect of intertrochanteric osteotomy on the venous drainage of the femoral neck in Perthes' disease. Acta Orthop. Scand., 47:89, 1976.
310. Heikkinen, E., Lanning, P., Suramo, I., and Puranen, J.: The venous drainage of the femoral neck as a prognostic sign in Perthes' disease. Acta Orthop. Scand., 51:501, 1980.
311. Heikkinen, E., Koivisto, E., Lanning, P., Puranen, J., and Suramo, I.: Venous drainage of the femoral neck in various stages of activity in Perthes' disease. Röntgenblätter, 32:46, 1979.
312. Helbo, S.: Morbus Calvé-Perthes. Thesis, Copenhagen. Odense, Fyns Tidendes Bogtrykkeri, 1953.
313. Henard, D. C., and Calandruccio, R. A.: Experimental production of roentgenographic and histological changes in the capital femoral epiphysis following abduction, extension and internal rotation of the hip. J. Bone Joint Surg., 52-A:600, 1970.
314. Henard, D. C., and Calandruccio, R. A.: Experimental production of roentgenographic and histological changes in the capital femoral epiphysis following abduction, extension, and internal rotation of the hip. Surg. Forum, 22:442, 1971.
315. Herndon, C. H., and Aufrank, C. D.: Avascular necrosis of the femoral head in adult. Clin. Orthop., 86:43, 1972.
316. Herndon, C. H., and Heyman, C. H.: Legg-Perthes disease. An evaluation of treatment by traction and ischial weight-bearing brace. J. Bone Joint Surg., 34-A:25, 1952.
317. Herold, H. F.: Avascular necrosis of the femoral head due to malposition in untreated congenital dislocation of the hip. Int. Orthop. (S.I.C.O.T.), 2:293, 1979.
318. Herring, J. A., Lundeen, M., and Wenger, D. R.: Minimal Perthes' disease. J. Bone Joint Surg., 62-B:25, 1980.
319. Herrmann, H. J.: Comparative pathology of epiphyseolysis of the femur head in animals. Beitr. Orthop. Traumatol., 18:26, 1971.
320. Herzog, F. G.: A study of Perthes' disease. Proc. R. Soc. Med., 54:1102, 1961.
321. Heyman, C. H., and Herndon, C. H.: Legg-Perthes disease. A method for the measurement of the roentgenographic results. J. Bone Joint Surg., 32-A:767, 1950.
322. Hirohashi, K., Kanbara, T., Kuroda, K., Okajima, M., Hyashi, M., and Shimazu, A.: Perthes' disease—a classification based on the extent of epiphyseal and metaphyseal involvement. Int. Orthop. (S.I.C.O.T.), 4:47, 1980.
323. Hirotani, H., and Ito, T.: Chondrocyte mitosis in the articular cartilage of femoral heads with various diseases. Acta Orthop. Scand., 46:979, 1975.
324. Hoerdegan, K. M.: Aetiologische Factoren und diagnostische Probleme beime Morbus Perthes. Dtsch. Med. Wochenschr., 98:2087, 1973.
325. Hoerdegan, K. M., and Witt, A. N.: Erfahrungen mit der intertrochanteren Varisierungsosteotomie bei der Legg-Calvé-Perthes'schen Erkrankung. Arch. Orthop. Unfallchir., 70:320, 1971.
326. Hoerdegan, K. M., Kohne, E., and Ludinghausen, M.: Zur aetiologie der Legg-Calvé-Pertheschen Krankheite. Haematologische, genetische und histologische Untersuchungen. Munch. Med. Wochenschr., 113:856, 1971.
327. Holdsworth, F. W.: Epiphyseal growth. Speculations on the nature of Perthes' disease. Ann. R. Coll. Surg., Engl., 39:1, 1966.
328. Horwitz, T.: The deformity in Legg-Calvé-Perthes disease. Bull. Hosp. Joint Dis. (N.Y.), 21:181, 1960.
329. Howard, R. J., and Simmons, R. L.: Viral infection and the surgical patient. Surg., Gynecol. Obstet., 137:1046, 1973.
330. Howe, W. W., Jr., Lacey, T., and Schwartz, R. P.: A study of the gross anatomy of the arteries supplying the proximal portion of the femur and the acetabulum. J. Bone Joint Surg., 32-A:856, 1950.
331. Howorth, M. B.: Coxa plana. J. Bone Joint Surg., 30-A:601, 1948.
332. Howorth, M. B.: Coxa plana. Arch. Pediatr., 76:1, 1959.
333. Hughes, S.: Radionuclides in orthopaedic surgery. J. Bone Joint Surg., 62-B:141, 1980.
334. Huluth, A., Norberg, I., and Olson, S. E.: Coxa plana in the dog. A preliminary report of a clinical, roentgenographic, histological, and microangiographic study. J. Bone Joint Surg., 44-A:918, 1962.
335. Hungerford, D. S.: Early diagnosis of ischemic necrosis of the femoral head. Johns Hopkins Med. J., 137:270, 1975.
336. Hungerford, D. S., and Zizic, T. M.: II. The treatment of ischemic necrosis of bone in systemic lupus erythematosus. Medicine, 59:143, 1980.
337. Hurley, R. M., Steinberg, R. H., Patriquin, H., and

Drummond, K. N.: Avascular necrosis of the femoral head in childhood. Systemic lupus erythematosus. Can. Med. Assoc. J., *111*:781, 1974.
338. Illyes, Z.: Angaben zur Aetiologie de Luzationsperthes. Z. Orthop., *104*:61, 1968.
339. Imhauser, G.: Behandlungen der Pertheschen Erkrankung mit Fixierung in Entlastungs-stellung (17 jaehrige Erfahrungen). Z. Orthop., *107*:553, 1970.
340. Inglis, A.: Genetic implications in coxa plana. J. Bone Joint Surg., *42-A*:711, 1960.
341. Inoue, A., and Ono, K.: A histological study of idiopathic avascular necrosis of the head of the femur. J. Bone Joint Surg., *61-B*:138, 1979.
342. Inoue, A., Freeman, M. A. R., Vernon-Roberts, B., and Mizuno, S.: The pathogenesis of Perthes' disease. J. Bone Joint Surg., *58-B*:453, 1976.
343. Iselin, H.: Über den Zusammenhang von jugentlichem Schenkelkopfschwund und ähnlichen Deformation mit dem Malum senile coxae und Arthritis deformans. Schweiz. Ärzteztg., *48*:1016, 1918.
344. Iwasaki, K., and Mori, Y.: Follow-up study of Perthes' disease. Orthop. Surg. (Tokyo), *21*:94, 1970.
345. Jacchia, G. E., and Faldini, A.: L'evoluzione clinicoradiographica della malattia di Legg-Calvé-Perthes. Arch. Putti Chir. Organi Mov., *22*:135, 1967.
346. Jacobs, B. W.: Early recognition of osteochondrosis of capital epiphysis of femur. J.A.M.A., *172*:527, 1960.
347. Jacobs, B. W.: Synovitis of the hip in children and its significance. Pediatrics, *47*:558, 1971.
348. Jaffe, H. L.: Certain disorders of individual epiphyses, apophyses, and epiphysioid bones. *In* Metabolic, Degenerative, and Inflammatory Diseases of Bones and Joints. Philadelphia, Lea & Febiger, 1972, pp. 565–631.
349. Jani, L.: Die operative Behandlung des Morbus Perthes mit der Variations-Derotations-Osteotomie. Z. Orthop., *108*:406, 1971.
350. Jani, L. F. H., and Dick, W.: Results of three different therapeutic groups in Perthes' disease. Clin. Orthop., *150*:88, 1980.
351. Jansen, M.: On coxa plana and its causation. A theory presented to the American Orthopaedic Association in Washington, D.C., May 2, 1922. J. Bone Joint Surg., *5*:265, 1923.
352. Jensen, O. M., and Lauritzen, J.: Legg-Calvé-Perthes disease. J. Bone Joint Surg., *58-B*:332, 1976.
353. Jequier, M., and Fredenhagen, H.: L'hérédité de la dystrophie épiphysaire des hanches (ostéochondrite déformante juvénile) (Maladie de Legg-Calvé-Perthes). Radiol. Clin. (Paris), *17*:92, 1948.
354. Johnston, R. C., and Smidt, G. L.: Measurement of hip-joint motion during walking. Evaluation of an electrogoniometric method. J. Bone Joint Surg., *51-A*:1083, 1969.
355. Jokisch, H.: Ein Beitrage zur operativen Behandlung des Morbus Perthes. Arch. Orthop. Unfallchir., *56*:664, 1964.
356. Jonsäter, S.: Coxa plana. A histo-pathologic and arthrographic study. Acta Orthop. Scand., Suppl. 12, 1953.
357. Kamhi, E.: Legg-Calvé-Perthes disease. Postgrad. Med., *60*:125, 1976.
358. Kamhi, E., and MacEwen, G. D.: Treatment of Legg-Calvé-Perthes disease. Prognostic value of Catterall's classification. J. Bone Joint Surg., *57-A*:651, 1975.
359. Kamhi, E., and MacEwen, G. D.: Osteochondritis dissecans in Legg-Calvé-Perthes disease. J. Bone Joint Surg., *57-A*:506, 1975.
360. Karadimas, J. E.: Conservative treatment of coxa plana. A comparison of the early results of different methods. J. Bone Joint Surg., *53-B*:315, 1971.
361. Kasperek, H. G., and Schwetlick, W.: Die Behandlung prarthrotischer Hüftdeformitaten. Z. Rheumaforsch., *28*:243, 1969.
362. Katz, J. F.: Protein-bound iodine in Legg-Calvé-Perthes disease. J. Bone Joint Surg., *37-A*:842, 1955.
363. Katz, J. F.: Legg-Calvé-Perthes disease—results of treatment. Clin. Orthop., *10*:61, 1957.
364. Katz, J. F.: "Abortive" Legg-Calvé-Perthes disease or developmental variation in epiphyseogenesis of the upper femur. J. Mt. Sinai Hosp., *32*:651, 1965.
365. Katz, J. F.: Conservative treatment of Legg-Calvé-Perthes disease. J. Bone Joint Surg., *49-A*:1043, 1967.
366. Katz, J. F.: Arthrography in Legg-Calvé-Perthes disease. J. Bone Joint Surg., *50-A*:467, 1968.
367. Katz, J. F.: Femoral torsion in Legg-Calvé-Perthes disease. J. Bone Joint Surg., *50-A*:473, 1968.
368. Katz, J. F.: Minimal Legg-Calvé-Perthes disease. J. Mt. Sinai Hosp., *35*:408, 1968.
369. Katz, J. F.: Legg-Calvé-Perthes disease. The role of distortion of normal growth mechanisms in the production of deformity. Clin. Orthop., *71*:193, 1970.
370. Katz, J. F.: Osteochondroma of the neck of the femur in Legg-Calvé-Perthes disease: Report of two cases. Clin. Orthop., *68*:50, 1970.
371. Katz, J. F.: Legg-Calvé-Perthes disease. A statistical evaluation of 358 cases. Mt. Sinai J. Med., *40*:20, 1973.
372. Katz, J. F.: Recurrent Legg-Calvé-Perthes disease. J. Bone Joint Surg., *55-A*:833, 1973.
373. Katz, J. F.: Legg-Calvé-Perthes disease associated with hereditary multiple exostosis: A case report. Mt. Sinai J. Med., *45*:46, 1978.
374. Katz, J. F.: Nonoperative therapy in Legg-Calvé-Perthes disease. Orthop. Review, *8*:69, 1979.
375. Katz, J. F.: Late modelling changes in Legg-Calvé-Perthes disease (L.C.P.D.) with continuing growth to maturity. Clin. Orthop., *150*:115, 1980.
376. Katz, J. F., and Challenor, Y. B.: Legg-Calvé-Perthes disease. *In* Downey, J. A. (ed.): The Child with Disabling Illness Philadelphia, Saunders, 1974, pp. 319–329.
377. Katz, J. F., and Siffert, R. S.: Skeletal maturity in Legg-Calvé-Perthes disease. Int. Orthop. (S.I.C.O.T.), *1*:227, 1977.
378. Kehl: Kritisches Sammelreferat ueber die "Perthes'-schen Krankheit." (Osteochondritis deformans juvenilis coxae). Dtsch. Med. Wochenschr., *51*:169, 1925.
379. Kelikian, A. S., Tachdjian, M. O., Askew, M. J., and Jasty, M.: Greater trochanteric advancement of the proximal femur: A clinical and biomechanical study. *In* Hungerford, D. S. (ed.): The Hip. St. Louis, C. V. Mosby, 1983, pp. 77–105.
380. Kelly, F. B., Jr., Canale, S. T., and Jones, R. R.: Legg-Calvé-Perthes disease. Long-term evaluation of noncontainment treatment. J. Bone Joint Surg., *62-A*:400, 1980.
381. Kelsey, J. L.: The epidemiology of diseases of the hip: A review of the literature. Int. J. Epidemiol., *6*:269, 1977.
382. Kemp, H. B. S.: Radiological changes in Perthes' disease. Br. J. Radiol., *39*:744, 1966.
383. Kemp, H. B. S.: Perthes' disease: An experimental and clinical study. Ann. R. Coll. Surg. Engl., *52*:18, 1973.
384. Kemp, H. B. S.: Perthes' disease. Nurs. Mirr., March, p. 58, 1975.
385. Kemp, H. B. S.: Perthes' disease—the influence of intracapsular tamponade on the circulation in the hip joint of the dog. Clin. Orthop., *156*:105, 1981.
386. Kemp, H. B. S., and Boldero, J. L.: Radiological changes in Perthes' disease. Br. J. Radiol., *39*:744, 1966.
387. Kemp, H. B. S., and Colmeley, J. A.: Recurrent Perthes' disease. Br. J. Radiol., *44*:6754, 1971.
388. Kempson, G. E.: Mechanical properties of articular cartilage. J. Physiol. (Lond.), *223*:23, 1972.
389. Kenzora, J. E., Steele, R. E., Yosipovitch, Z., Boyd,

R., and Glimcher, M. J.: Tissue biology following experimental infraction of the femur head. Part I. Bone studies. *In* Proc. 36th Ann. Meeting, A.A.O.S., New York, 1969. Abstract in J. Bone Joint Surg., *51-A*:1021, 1969.
390. Keret, D., Harrison, M. H. M., Clarke, N. M. P., and Hall, D. J.: Coxa plana—the fate of the physis. J. Bone Joint Surg., *66-A*:870, 1984.
391. Kidner, F. C.: Causes and treatment of Perthes' disease. Am. J. Orthop. Surg., *14*:339, 1916.
392. Kiepurska, A., and Makuchowa, K.: Osteochondrosis dissecans w nastepstwie choroby Legg-Calvé-Perthesa. Chir. Narzadow Ruchu Orthop. Pol., *38*:79, 1973.
393. Kikuchi, H.: Studies on the conservative therapy of Perthes' disease. J. Kumamoto Med. Soc., *43*:399, 1969.
394. King, E. W., Fisher, R. L., Gage, J. R., and Gossling, H. R.: Ambulation-abduction treatment in Legg-Calvé-Perthes disease (L.C.P.D.). Clin. Orthop., *150*:43, 1980.
395. Kite, J. H., and French, G. O.: The early diagnosis of flatheaded femur. South. Med. J., *45*:581, 1952.
396. Kleinberg, S.: The treatment of early epiphyseolisthesis at the hip by drilling and delayed weight-bearing. Bull. Hosp. Joint Dis., *13*:77, 1952.
397. Kleinman, R. G., and Bleck, E. E.: Increased blood viscosity in patients with Legg-Perthes disease: A preliminary report. J. Pediatr. Orthop., *1*:131, 1981.
398. Klisic, P. J.: Treatment of Perthes' disease in older children. J. Bone Joint Surg., *65-B*:419, 1983.
399. Klisic, P., Blasevic, U., and Seferovic, O.: Approach to treatment of Legg-Calvé-Perthes disease. Clin. Orthop., *150*:54, 1980.
400. Klisic, P., Seferovic, O., and Blazevic, U.: Indications for treatment in coxa plana. Int. Orthop., *1*:33, 1977.
401. Klisic, P., Seferovic, O., and Blazevic, U.: Legg-Calvé-Perthes syndrome: Classification and indications for treatment. Orthop. Rev., *8*:81, 1979.
402. Köhler, R., and Seringe, R.: Ostéochondrite primitive de la hanche ou maladie de Legg-Perthes-Calvé. *In* Cahiers d'enseignement de la Sofcot no. 16. Paris, Expansion Scientifique Française, 1981, pp. 30–96.
403. Konjetzny, G. E.: Zur Pathologie und pathologischen Anatomie der Perthes-Calve'schen Krankheit (Osteochondritis Coxae deformans juvenilis). Acta Chir. Scand., *74*:361, 1934.
404. Korvin, H. G.: Pseudocoxalgia: Calvé-Legg-Perthes disease. Proc. R. Soc. Med., *40*:886, 1947.
405. Kurochkin, I. V.: Orthopedic aid to children with deformities of the talocrural joint following traumatic osteoepiphysiolysis. Orthop. Travmatol. Protez., *34*:81, 1973.
406. LaCroix, P.: Les vaisseaux du ligament rond dans la pathogénie de la coxa plana. Rev. Chir. Orthop., *28*:30, 1942.
407. Lamont, R. L., Muz, J., Heilbronner, D., and Bouwhuis, J. A.: Quantitative assessment of femoral head involvement in Legg-Calvé-Perthes disease. J. Bone Joint Surg., *53-A*:746, 1962.
408. Langenskiöld, A.: Changes on the capital growth plate and the proximal femoral metaphysis in Legg-Calvé-Perthes disease. Clin. Orthop., *150*:110, 1980.
409. Langenskiöld, A., Sarpio, O., and Michelsson, J. E.: Experimental dislocation of the hip in the rabbit. J. Bone Joint Surg., *44-B*:209, 1962.
410. Laron, Z., Axer, A., and Drezner, A.: Growth and development of children with Legg-Calvé-Perthes syndrome in Israel. Isr. J. Med. Sci., *9*:612, 1973.
411. Larsen, E. H., and Reimann, I.: Calvé-Perthes disease. Macro- and microscopic observations (Proc. Scand. Orthop. Soc. - Denmark, 1970). Abstract in Acta Orthop. Scand., *42*:455, 1971.
412. Larsen, E. H., and Reimann, I.: Calvé-Perthes disease. Acta Orthop. Scand., *44*:426, 1973.
413. Larson, C. B.: Rating scale for hip disabilities. Clin. Orthop., *31*:85, 1963.
414. Laurent, L. E., and Poussa, M.: Intertrochanteric varus osteotomy in the treatment of Perthes' disease. Clin. Orthop., *150*:73, 1980.
415. Lauritzen, J.: Resultate af korestolbehandlung ved mb. Calvé-Perthes. Nord. Med., *84*:1599, 1970.
416. Lauritzen, J.: Legg-Calvé-Perthes disease. *In* Proceedings Scand. Orthop. Soc. Denmark, 1970. Abstract in Acta Orthop. Scand., *42*:456, 1971.
417. Lauritzen, J.: The arterial supply to the femoral head in children. Acta Orthop. Scand., *45*:724, 1974.
418. Lauritzen, J.: Legg-Calvé-Perthes disease, a comparative study. Acta Orthop. Scand. Suppl., *159*:1, 1975.
419. Legal, H., and Weseloh, G.: Differentialdiagnose von Hüftkopfnekrosen im Sauglings und Kleinkindesalter. 63. Kongress der Deutschen Gesellschaft fur Orthopädie und Traumatologie, Sept., 1976. Z. Orthop., *115*:487, 1977.
420. Legg, A. T.: An obscure affection of the hip joint. Boston Med. Surg. J., *162*:202, 1910.
421. Legg, A. T.: The end results of coxa plana. J. Bone Joint Surg., *9*:26, 1927.
422. Legg, A. T.: The classic: An obscure affection of the hip joint. Clin. Orthop., *79*:4, 1971.
423. Lehneis, H. R.: Lower extremity bracing. Part III: Principles of orthotic alignment in the lower extremity. A.A.O.S. Instruct. Course Lect., *20*:131, 1971.
424. Lejeune, E., Bouvier, M., Lahneche, B., Ruitton, P., and Queneau, P.: Apport du strontium 87m diagnostic des ostéonécroses aseptiques épiphysaires. Rhumatologie, *24*:83, 1972.
425. Lemoine, A.: Vascular changes after interference with the blood flow of the head of the rabbit. J. Bone Joint Surg., *39-B*:763, 1957.
426. Lemperg, R., Liliequist, B., and Mattsson, S.: Asymmetry of the epiphyseal nucleus in the femoral head in stable and unstable hip joints. Pediatr. Radiol., *1*:191, 1973.
427. Levy, L. J., and Girard, P. M.: Legg-Perthes disease. A comparative study of various methods of treatment. J. Bone Joint Surg., *24*:663, 1942.
428. Lian, G.: Congenital coxa vara and Perthes' disease. Acta Orthop. Scand., *19*:527, 1950.
429. Lilienberg, J.: Femoral head necrosis following overhead extension. Beitr. Orthop. Traumatol., *19*:113, 1972.
430. Lindholm, T. S., Laurent, L. E., Osterman, K., and Snellman, O.: Perthes' disease of a severe type developing after satisfactory closed reduction of congenital dislocation of the hip. J. Bone Joint Surg., *60B*:15, 1978.
431. Lino Ferreira, A. M., and Cortez-Pimentel, J.: Osteonecrose primitiva da cabeca do femur. Na crianca. Rev. Ortop. Traumatol., *13*:3, 1969.
432. Lippert, F. G. III: A long leg brace for comprehensive force measurement design and experimental studies. Acta Orthop. Scand., Suppl. 138, 1971.
433. Lippmann, R. K.: The pathogenesis of Legg-Calvé-Perthes disease. Based upon the pathologic findings in a case. Am. J. Surg., *6*:785, 1929.
434. Ljunggren, G.: Legg-Perthes disease in the dog. Acta Orthop. Scand. Suppl., *95*:1, 1967.
435. Ljunggren, G.: Legg-Perthes disease in the dog. A case report with special reference to initial radiographic changes. Clin. Orthop., *62*:31, 1969.
436. Lloyd Roberts, G. C.: Perthes' disease. Part I: Pathogenesis, classification, and treatment. *In* Lloyd Roberts, G. C. and Ratliff, A. H. C. (eds.): Hip Disorders in Children. London, Butterworth, 1978, pp. 119–149.

437. Lloyd Roberts, G. C.: Editorials and Annotations. The management of Perthes' disease. J. Bone Joint Surg., 64-B:1, 1982.
438. Lloyd Roberts, G. C., Catterall, A., and Salamon, P. B.: A controlled study of the indications and the results of femoral osteotomy in Perthes' disease. J. Bone Joint Surg., 58-B:31, 1976.
439. Lohr, E.: Wesen Ursachen und Verhutungsmoglichkeiten de Kopekernzerfalls. Beitr. Orthop. Traumatol., 12:316, 1965.
440. Louyot, P., Gaucher, A., Pourel, J., Monet, Y., and Tamisier, J. N.: De quelques problémes posé par l'ostoenécrose aseptique de la tête fémorale. Rev. Rhum. Mal. Osteoartic., 38:201, 1971.
441. Lowe, H.: Prognosis of Perthes' disease with special consideration of the problem of early operative treatment. Beitr. Orthop. Traumatol., 16:589, 1969.
442. Lowe, H.: Contribution to the treatment of Calvé-Legg-Perthes disease. Problems of treatment and results of surgical treatment since 1959. Z. Orthop., 106:341, 1969.
443. Lucas, L. S.: Painful hips in children. A.A.O.S. Instruct. Course Lect., 5:144, 1948.
444. Lukins, J. L.: Classification of Perthes' disease and its implications. J. Bone Joint Surg., 57-A:136, 1975.
445. McAndrew, M. P., and Weinstein, S. L.: A long-term follow-up of Legg-Calvé-Perthes disease. J. Bone Joint Surg., 66-A:860, 1984.
446. McComas, E.: Perthes' disease and its occurrence as a familial condition. Med. J. Aust., 2:584, 1946.
447. McCullough, N. C.: Lower extremity bracing. Part I: Introduction to lower extremity orthotics. A.A.O.S. Instruct. Course Lect., 22:116, 1971.
448. McKay, D.: Cheilectomy in Legg-Calvé-Perthes: Indications, technique and results. Orthop. Clin. North Am., 11:141, 1980.
449. McKibbin, B.: Recent advances in Perthes' disease. In McKibbin, B. (ed.): Recent Advances in Orthopaedics. Edinburgh, Churchill-Livingstone, 1975, pp. 173–195.
450. McKibbin, B., and Ralis, Z.: Pathological changes in a case of Perthes' disease. J. Bone Joint Surg., 56-B:438, 1974.
451. Maar, D., Michalickova, J., Filipsky, J., Duhon, J., and Sykora, F.: Niektore nase poznatky pri dlhodobej knozervativnej ustavnej liecbe Legg-Calvé-Perthes choroby. Acta Chir. Orthop. Traumatol., 41:335, 1974.
452. Makuchowa, K., and Rrynkiewicz, K.: Postacie radiologiczne choroby perthesa. Chir. Narzadow Ruchu Ortop. Pol., 38:38, 1973.
453. Makuchowa, K., and Sobipanek, E.: Wiek szkieletowy w chorobie Perthesa. Chir. Narzadow Ruchu Ortop. Pol., 38:73, 1973.
454. Malawski, S., Kiepursk, A., Kurpiwska, D., and Lakomski, M.: Pozne wyniki leczenia choroby Perthesa. Chir. Narzadow Ruchu Ortop. Pol., 38:51, 1973.
455. Mann, M., and Oerke, H. P.: Zur Frage der Position des Hüftkopfes bei der konservativen Perthes-Behandlung. 63. Kongress der Deutschen Gesellschaft fur Orthopädie und Traumatologie. Z. Orthop., 115:491, 1977.
456. Maquet, P.: Traitement biomecanique de la nécrose ischémique de la tête du fémur. Acta Orthop. Belg., 38:526, 1972.
457. Marino-Zuco, C., and Pietrogrande, V.: Orientations dans le traitement de la maladie de Perthes. In Bailleux, M. (ed.): Proc. 7th Cong. Int. Chir. Orthop., Barcelona. Bruxelles, Im. des Sciences, 1957, pp. 673, 680.
458. Markheim, H. R.: Legg-Perthes disease and slipped epiphysis on the same patient. A case report. J. Bone Joint Surg., 31-A:666, 1949.
459. Marklund, T., and Tillberg, B.: Coxa plana: A radiological comparison of the rate of healing with conservative measures and after osteotomy. J. Bone Joint Surg., 58-B:25, 1976.
460. Martin, H. E.: Geometrical-anatomical factors and their significance in early x-ray diagnosis of hip-joint disease in children. Radiology, 56:842, 1951.
461. Matles, A. L.: Reflex sympathetic dystrophy in a child. A case report. Bull. Hosp. Joint Dis., 32:193, 1971.
462. Matsoukas, J. A.: Viral antibody titers to rubella in coxa plana or Perthes' disease. Acta Orthop. Scand., 46:957, 1975.
463. Matsumoto, S.: Studies on positional changes of the circulation of the hip in Legg-Calvé-Perthes disease and allied conditions. J. Jpn. Orthop. Assoc., 43:1013, 1969.
464. Mattner, H. R.: On the hystopathology of Perthes disease. Beitr. Orthop. Traumatol., 15:62, 1968.
465. Matzen, P. F.: Zur operativen Behandlung des genuinen Morbus Perthes. Z. Orthop., 116:867, 1978.
466. Mau, H., and Schmitt, H. W.: Der konstitutinelldysostotische Perthes und die Skelettreifungshemungen beim eigtlichen Perthes. Z. Orthop., 93:515, 1960.
467. Maurer, H. J. and Skandfer, B.: Perthes' disease: A roentgenological clinic study. Z. Orthop., 116:240, 1978.
468. Mayba, I. I.: Legg-Perthes disease. Manit. Med. Rev., 50:16, 1970.
469. Meyer, J.: Dysplasia epiphysealis capitis femoris. A clinical-radiological syndrome and its relationship to Legg-Calvé-Perthes disease. Acta Orthop. Scand., 34:183, 1964.
470. Meyer, J.: Treatment of Legg-Calvé-Perthes disease. Acta Orthop. Scand. Suppl., 86:9, 1966.
471. Meyer, J.: Legg-Calvé-Perthes disease, radiological results of treatment and their late clinical consequences. Acta Orthop. Scand. Suppl., 167:1, 1977.
472. Milch, H.: The brace treatment of epiphysiology. Bull. Hosp. Joint Dis., 13:94, 1952.
473. Milgram, J. E., Norman, A., and Langa, G. A.: Healing of Legg-Calvé-Perthes disease using an abduction brace which prevents hip flexion. J. Bone Joint Surg., 51-A:1240, 1969.
474. Milgram, J. W.: Synovial osteochondromatosis in association with Legg-Calvé-Perthes disease. Clin. Orthop., 145:179, 1979.
475. Mindell, E. R., and Sherman, M. S.: Late results in Legg-Perthes disease. J. Bone Joint Surg., 33-A:1, 1951.
476. Mintowt-Czyz, W., and Tayton, K.: Indication for weight relief and containment in the treatment of Perthes' disease. Acta Orthop. Scand., 54:439, 1983.
477. Mirosky, Y., Axer, A., and Hendel, D.: Residual shortening after osteotomy in Perthes' disease. J. Bone Joint Surg., 66-B:184, 1984.
478. Mizuno, S.: Surgery of the joint capsule for Perthes' disease. Orthop. Surg. (Tokyo), 19:343, 1968.
479. Mizuno, S.: Therapeutic guide for Perthes' disease. Orthop. Surg. (Tokyo), 20:186, 1969.
480. Mizuno, S., Hirayama, M., Kotani, P. T., and Simazu, A.: Pathological histology of Legg-Calvé-Perthes disease with special reference to its experimental production. Med. J. Osaka Univ., 17:177, 1966.
481. Moller, P. F.: The clinical observations after healing of Calvé-Perthes disease compared with the final deformities left by that disease, and the bearing of those final deformities on the ultimate diagnosis. Acta Radiol., 5:1, 1926.
482. Molloy, M. K., and MacMahon, B.: Incidence of Legg-Perthes disease (osteochondritis dissecans). N. Engl. J. Med., 275:988, 1966.
483. Molloy, M. K., and MacMahon, B.: Birth weight and Legg-Perthes disease. J. Bone Joint Surg., 49-A:498, 1967.
484. Monty, C. P.: Familial Perthes' disease resembling

multiple epiphyseal dysplasia. J. Bone Joint Surg., 44-B:565, 1962.
485. Morley, T. R., Short, M. D., and Dowsett, D. J.: Femoral head activity in Perthes' disease: Clinical evaluation of a quantitative technique for estimating tracer uptake. J. Nucl. Med., 19:884, 1978.
486. Morris, M. L., and McGibbon, K. C.: Osteochondritis dissecans following Legg-Calvé-Perthes disease. J. Bone Joint Surg., 44-B:562, 1962.
487. Morrissy, R. T.: Legg-Calvé-Perthes disease. Personal communication, 1986.
488. Mose, K.: Legg-Calvé-Perthes disease. Thesis. Aarhus, Denmark, Universitetsforlaget I Aarhus, 1964.
489. Mose, K.: Legg-Calvé-Perthes Disease; A Comparison Between Three Methods of Conservative Treatment. Aarhus, Universitetsforlaget, 1964.
490. Mose, K.: Methods of measuring in Legg-Calvé-Perthes disease with special regard to the prognosis. Clin. Orthop., 150:103, 1980.
491. Mose, K., Hjorth, L., Ulfeldt, M., Christensen, E. R., and Jensen, A.: Legg-Calvé-Perthes disease: The late occurrence of coxarthrosis. Acta Orthop. Scand., Suppl. 169, 1977.
492. Muirhead-Allwood, W., and Catterall, A.: The treatment of Perthes' disease. J. Bone Joint Surg., 64-B:282, 1982.
493. Muller, V.: Die Epiphysiolysis capitis femoris. Wien. Med. Wochschr., 122:714, 1972.
494. Murphy, R. P., and Marsh, H. O.: Incidence and natural history of "head at risk" factors in Perthes' disease. Clin. Orthop., 132:102, 1978.
495. Murray, R. O., and Jacobson, H. G.: Perthes' disease. In The Radiology of Skeletal Disorders. Congenital Disorders. Baltimore, Williams & Wilkins, 1971, pp. 210–218.
496. Mussbichler, H.: Angiography of the hip region. Comparison between different angiographic modifications. Acta Radiol. (Stockh.), 11:593, 1971.
497. Myhre Jensen, O., and Lauritzen, J.: Legg-Calvé-Perthes disease. J. Bone Joint Surg., 58-B:332, 1976.
498. Nagura, S.: Das Wesen und die Entstehung der Osteochondritis dissecans Konigs (bzw. der Perthes, Köhler II-und ahnlichen Krankheiten und Veranderungen an wachsenden Knocheneden). Zentralbl. Chir., 64:2049, 1937.
499. Nagura, S.: Coxa plana und coxa magna. Arch. Orthop. Unfallchir., 65:264, 1969.
500. Nagura, S.: Die Osteochondritis dissecans des Hüftgelenks und ihre Ätiologie. Arch. Orthop. Unfallchir., 65:371, 1969.
501. Nagura, S.: Ueber die sogenannte idiopathische Hüftkopfnekrose bei Erwachsenen. Arch. Orthop. Unfallchir., 66:138, 1969.
502. Nagura, S., and Kosuge, S.: Die Pathogenese und das Wesen der Perthes'schen Krankheit. Arch. Klin. Chir., 191:347, 1938.
503. Natzler: Ueber deformierende Gelenkerkrankungen des Kindesalters. (21 Orthop. Kongres Gesell.). Verh. Dtsch. Orthop., 21:502, 1927.
504. Nevelos, A. B.: Bilateral Perthes' disease. Acta Orthop. Scand., 51:649, 1980.
505. Nishio, A.: Management of Perthes' disease. Orthop. Surg. (Tokyo), 20:177, 1969.
506. Nishio, A., and Yakushiji, K.: Legg-Calvé-Perthes disease. Hystology and treatment. Yonago Acta Med., 6:1, 1962.
507. Noel, S. M.: Legg-Calvé-Perthes syndrome: Treatment of established deformity. In Proceedings, First International Symposium on Legg-Calvé-Perthes Syndrome. Los Angeles, Orthopedic Hospital, 1977, p. 173–177.
508. Norman, A., and Bullough, P.: The radiolucent crescent line—an early diagnostic sign of avascular necrosis of the femoral head. Bull. Hosp. Joint Dis., 24:99, 1963.
509. Nussbaum, A.: Über Osteochondritis Coxae juvenilis Calvé-Legg-Perthes. Dtsch. Med. Wochenschr., 49:849, 1923.
510. Oestreich, A. E.: Hip pain and its variations: Radiological aspects. J. Natl. Med. Assoc., 66:208, 1974.
511. O'Garra, J. A.: The radiographic changes in Perthes' disease. J. Bone Joint Surg., 41-B:465, 1959.
512. Ogden, J. A.: Changing patterns of proximal femoral vascularity. J. Bone Joint Surg., 56-A:941, 1974.
513. O'Hara, J. P., Davis, N. D., Gage, J. R., Sundberg, A. B., and Winter, R. B.: Long-term follow-up of Perthes' disease treated nonoperatively. Clin. Orthop., 125:49, 1977.
514. Ott, G., and Franke, J.: Co-occurrence of tibia-vara (Blount), Perthes' disease and enchondral dysostosis. Beitr. Orthop. Traumatol., 18:87, 1971.
515. Pacini, D., and Rizzi, G.: Contributo allo studio anatomico del legamento rotondo del femore. Considerazioni sulkla patologia dell'anca. Chir. Organi Mov., 29:196, 1943.
516. Panner, H. J.: A peculiar affection of the capitellum humeri, resembling Calvé-Perthes disease of the hip. Acta Radiol., 10:234, 1929.
517. Pantazopoulos, T., Matsoukas, J., Gavras, M., Nikiforidis, P., and Hartofilakidis-Garofalidis, G.: Osteochondritis dissecans following coxa plana. Acta Orthop. Scand., 43:532, 1972.
518. Papadopoulos, J. S., Agnantis, J., and Popp, W.: Luxationsperthes—gibt es röntgenologische Möglichkeiten für die Voraussage und der Frühdiagnose? Z. Orthop., 115:752, 1977.
519. Pappas, A. M.: The osteochondroses. Pediatr. Clin. North Am., 14:549, 1967.
520. Pauwels, P.: Des affections de la hanche d'origine mechanique et de leur traitement par l'ostéotomie d'adduction. Rev. Chir. Orthop., 37:22, 1951.
521. Pavlansky, R., and Jancova, H.: Certralni kostni step u choroby Calvé-Legg-Perthes. Acta Chir. Orthop. Traumatol. Cech., 38:241, 1971.
522. Pease, C. N.: Avascular necrosis of bone in children. Med. Clin. North Am., 34:165, 1950.
523. Pedersen, H. E., and McCarroll, H. R.: Treatment in Legg-Perthes disease. J. Bone Joint Surg., 33-A:591, 1951.
524. Pemberton, P. A.: Pericapsular iliac osteotomy in treatment of Legg-Calvé-Perthes syndrome. Orthop. Rev., 8:101, 1979.
525. Perpich, M., McBeath, A., and Kruse, D.: Long-term follow-up of Perthes' disease treated with spica casts. J. Pediatr. Orthop., 3:160, 1983.
526. Perry, J.: Kinesiology of lower extremity bracing. Clin. Orthop., 102:18, 1974.
527. Perthes, G. C.: Über Arthrtis deformans juvenilis. Deutsch. Z. Chir., 107:111, 1910.
528. Perthes, G.: Ueber Osteochondritis deformans juvenilis. Arch. Klin. Chir., 101:779, 1913.
529. Petrie, J. G., and Bitenc, I.: The abduction weight-bearing treatment in Legg-Perthes disease. J. Bone Joint Surg., 53-B:54, 1971.
530. Phemister, D. B.: Operation for epiphysitis of the head of the femur (Perthes' disease). Findings and results. Arch. Surg., 2:221, 1921.
531. Phemister, D. B.: Repair of bone in the presence of aseptic necrosis resulting from fractures, transplantations and vascular obstruction. J. Bone Joint Surg., 12:769, 1930.
532. Phillips, K. E.: Evaluation of the hip. Phys. Ther., 55:975, 1975.
533. Pike, M. M.: Legg-Perthes disease, with particular regard to treatment. Conn. Med. J., 4:1, 1940.
534. Pike, M. M.: Legg-Perthes disease. A method of conservative treatment. J. Bone Joint Surg., 32-A:663, 1950.
535. Platt, H.: Pseudo-coxalgia: A clinical and radiographic study. Br. J. Surg., 9:366, 1922.

536. Pohl, J.: Ein Beitrag zur gedeckten Bohrung des Morbus Perthes. Arch. Orthop. Unfallchir., 56:661, 1964.
537. Ponseti, I.: Lesions of the skeleton and of other mesodermal tissues in rats fed sweet-pea (Lathyrus odoratus) seeds. J. Bone Joint Surg., 36-A:1031, 1954.
538. Ponseti, I.: Legg-Perthes disease. Observations on pathological changes in two cases. J. Bone Joint Surg., 38-A:739, 1956.
539. Ponseti, I., and Cotton, R. L.: Legg-Calvé-Perthes disease—pathogenesis and evolution. Failure of treatment with L-triiodothyronine. J. Bone Joint Surg., 43-B:261, 1961.
540. Ponseti, I., Maynard, J. A., Weinstein, S. L., Ippolito, E. O., and Pous, J. G.: Legg-Calvé-Perthes disease. Histochemical and ultrastructural observations of the epiphyseal cartilage and physis. J. Bone Joint Surg., 65-A:797, 1983.
541. Puranen, J., and Heikkinen, E.: Intertrochanteric osteotomy in the treatment of Perthes' disease. Acta Orthop. Scand., 47:79, 1976.
542. Purvis, J. M., Dimon, J. H., Meehan, P. L., and Lovell, W. W.: Preliminary experience with the Scottish Rite Hospital abduction orthosis for Legg-Perthes disease. Clin. Orthop., 150:49, 1980.
543. Quain, S., and Catterall, A.: Hinge abduction of the hip. J. Bone Joint Surg., 68-B:61, 1986.
544. Rab, G. T., DeNatale, J. S., and Herrman, L. R.: Three-dimensional finite element analysis of Legg-Calvé-Perthes disease. J. Pediatr. Orthop., 2:39, 1982.
545. Ralston, E. L.: Legg-Perthes disease and physical development. J. Bone Joint Surg., 37-A:647, 1955.
546. Ralston, E. L.: Legg-Calvé-Perthes disease—factors in healing. J. Bone Joint Surg., 43-A:249, 1961.
547. Ratliff, A. H. C.: Pseudocoxalgia. A study of late results in the adults. J. Bone Joint Surg., 38-B:498, 1956.
548. Ratliff, A. H. C.: Perthes' disease. A study of thirty-four hips observed for thirty years. J. Bone Joint Surg., 49-B:102, 1967.
549. Ratliff, A. H. C.: Osteochondritis dissecans following Legg-Calvé-Perthes disease. J. Bone Joint Surg., 49-B:109, 1967.
550. Ratliff, A. H. C.: Perthes' disease. Part II. The long-term results. In Lloyd Roberts, G. C., and Ratliff, A. H. C. (eds.): Hip Disorders in Children. London, Butterworth, 1978, pp. 150–64.
551. Rauterberg, K.: Biomechanische Aspekte bei der operativen Behandlung des Morbus Perthes. 63. Kongress der Deutschen Gesellschaft fur Orthopädie und Traumatologie. Z. Orthop., 115:493, 1977.
552. Reinker, K. A., and Larson, I. J.: Patterns of progression in Legg-Perthes disease. J. Pediatr. Orthop., 3:455, 1983.
553. Remvig, O., and Mose, H.: Perthes' disease. J. Bone Joint Surg., 43-B:855, 1961.
554. Riedel, G.: Beitrag zur pathologischen Anatomie der Osteochondritis deformans Coxae juvenilis. Zentralbl. Chir., 49:1447, 1922.
555. Riesen, H.: Morbus Perthes. Ther. Umsch., 29:439, 1972.
556. Rigault, P., and Puliquen, J. -C.: Nôtre expérience de l'ostéotomie fémorale dans le traitement de l'ostéochondrite primitive de la hanche (D.P.H.). Rev. Chir. Orthop., 56:635, 1970.
557. Roberts, J. M., Meehan, P., Counts, G., and Counts, W.: Ambulatory abduction brace for Legg-Perthes disease. First International Symposium Legg-Calvé-Perthes syndrome. Los Angeles, 1977, p. 99.
558. Robichon, J., Desjardin, J. P., Koch, M., Hooper, C. E.: The femoral neck in Legg-Perthes disease, its relationship to epiphyseal change and its importance in early prognosis. J. Bone Joint Surg., 56-B:62, 1974.
559. Rokkanen, P.: Role of surgical interventions of the hip joint in the aetiology of aseptic necrosis of the femoral head. Acta Orthop. Scand., 58:1, 1962.
560. Rosch, H., and Stock, D.: Morbus Perthes—Ergebnisse der konservativen Therapie. Z. Orthop., 114:53, 1976.
561. Rosingh, G. E., and James, J.: Early phases of avascular necrosis of the femoral head in rabbits. J. Bone Joint Surg., 51-B:165, 1969.
562. Rostenberg, I., Jimenez, M., and Armendares, S.: Diagnostico deferencial de las osteocondrodisplasias congenitas. Rev. Invest. Clin., 25:261, 1973.
563. Roy-Camille, R., Rogault, P., Pouliquen, J. -C., Rose, B., and Guyonvarch, G.: La hanche douloureuse de l'enfant. Deux problémes actuels: l'ostéochondrite primitive et l'épiphysiolyse. Cah. Med., 12:257, 1971.
564. Ruett, A.: V. Rundtischgesprach Morbus Perthes. 63. Kongress der Deutschen Gesellschaft fur Orthopädie und Traumatologie. Z. Orthop., 115:505, 1977.
565. Ruett, A., and Schmoller, G. von: Zur aetiologie der Perthesschen Erkrankung beim Hund. Z. Orthop., 106:673, 1969.
566. Rybicki, E. F., Simonen, F. A., and Weis, E. B., Jr.: On the mathematical analysis of stress in the human femur. J. Biomech., 5:203, 1972.
567. Rydell, N.: Biomechanics of the hip-joint. Clin. Orthop., 92:6, 1973.
568. Ryder, C. T., Lebourier, J. D., and Kane, R.: Coxa plana. Pediatrics, 19:972, 1957.
569. Salenius, P., and Videman, T.: Growth disturbances of the proximal end of the femur. Acta Orthop. Scand., 41:199, 1970.
570. Salter, R. B.: Experimental and clinical aspects of Perthes' disease. J. Bone Joint Surg., 48-B:393, 1966.
571. Salter, R. B.: Clinical and laboratory research studies on Legg-Perthes disease. In The Hip: Proceedings of the First Open Scientific Meeting of the Hip Society. St. Louis, Mosby, 1973, pp. 4–13.
572. Salter, R. B.: Legg-Perthes disease. Parts III, V. Treatment by innominate osteotomy. A.A.O.S. Instruct. Course Lect. 22:309, 1973.
573. Salter, R. B.: Legg-Perthes diseae. The pathogenesis of deformity and its prevention. Proc. First International Symposium, Legg-Perthes' Syndrome, Los Angeles, 1977.
574. Salter, R. B.: Legg-Perthes disease. The scientific basis for the methods of treatment and their indications. Clin. Orthop., 150:8, 1980.
575. Salter, R. B.: Legg-Perthes disease: Relevant research and its application to treatment. In Leach, R. E., and Hoaglund, F. T. (eds.): Controversies in Orthopaedic Surgery, Chapter 10. Philadelphia, Saunders, 1982.
576. Salter, R. B.: The present status of surgical treatment for Legg-Perthes disease. J. Bone Joint Surg., 66-A:961, 1984.
577. Salter, R. B., and Bell, M.: The pathogenesis of deformity of Legg-Perthes disease: An experimental investigation. J. Bone Joint Surg., 50-B:436, 1968.
578. Salter, R. B., and Thompson, G.: Legg-Calvé-Perthes disease. The prognostic significance of the subchondral fracture and a two-group classification of the femoral head involvement. J. Bone Joint Surg., 66-A:479, 1984.
579. Salter, R. B., Kostuik, J., and Dallas, S.: Avascular necrosis of the femoral head as a complication of treatment for congenital dislocation of the hip in young children: A clinical and experimental investigation. Can. J. Surg., 12:44, 1969.
580. Salter, R. B., Rang, M., and Bell, M.: The scientific basis for innominate osteotomy in the treatment of Legg-Perthes disease. Ann. R. Coll. Phys. Surg. Can., 5:62, 1972.
581. Salter, R. B., Rang, M., Blackstone, I. W., McArthur, R. C., Weighill, F. J., Gygi, A. C., and Stulberg, S. D.: Perthes' disease: The scientific basis of methods of management and their indications. J. Bone Joint Surg., 59-B:127, 1977.
582. Sanchis, M., Zahir, A., and Freeman, M. A. R.: The experimental simulation of Perthes' disease by con-

secutive interruptions of the blood supply to the capital femoral epiphysis in the puppy. J. Bone Joint Surg., 55-A:335, 1973.
583. Sanders, J. A., and MacEwen, G. D.: A long-term follow-up on coxa plana at the Alfred I. duPont Institute. South. Med. J., 62:1042, 1969.
584. Savastano, A. A., and Pizzarello, P. A.: Clinical review of Legg-Perthes disease. Int. Surg., 59:96, 1974.
585. Schaeffer, R. I., Striekroot, F. L., and Purcell, F. F.: The endocrine implication of juvenile chondro-epiphysitis. J.A.M.A., 112:1917, 1939.
586. Schauer, A.: Zur pathologischen Anatomie der spontanen Osteonekrosen. 63. Kongres der Deutschen Gesellschaft für Orthopädie und Traumatologie. Z. Orthop., 115:432, 1977.
587. Scheibner, H.: Die Osteochondritis Coxae juvenilis (Perthessche Erkrankung) nach Reposition angeborener Hüftluxation. Arch. Orthop. Unfallchir., 45:343, 1952.
588. Schepers, A., von Bormann, P. F. B., and Craig, J. J. G.: Coxa magna in Perthes' disease: Treatment by Chiari pelvic osteotomy. J. Bone Joint Surg., 60-B:297, 1978.
589. Schiller, M. G., and Axer, A.: Hypertrophy of the femoral head in Legg-Calvé-Perthes syndrome—L.C.P.S. A study of twenty-nine patients treated by femoral osteotomy. Acta Orthop. Scand., 43:45, 1972.
590. Schiller, M. G., and Axer, A.: Legg-Calvé-Perthes syndrome (L.C.P.S.). A critical analysis of roentgenographic measurements. Clin. Orthop., 86:34, 1972.
591. Schmidt-Wolansky, R.: Perthes' disease: A complication of treated hip dislocation. Beitr. Orthop. Traumatol., 20:81, 1973.
592. Schulitz, K. P.: Morphologische Aspekte des Hüftgelenkes beim Morbus Perthes nach Varisierungsosteotomien. Z. Orthop., 114:377, 1976.
593. Schulitz, K. P., Dustmann, H. O., and Sinn, H.: Gibt es einen Morbus Perthes durch venose Stase? Z. Orthop., 115:299, 1977.
594. Schulitz, K. P., Schööning, B., and Dustmann, H. O.: Zur Indikation der Varisierungsosteotomie beim Morbus Perthes. Z. Orthop., 115:821, 1977.
595. Schulz, P.: Ligamentum teres Luxations Perthes? Beitr. Orthop. Traumatol., 18:584, 1971.
596. Scoles, P. V., Yoon, Y. S., Makley, J. T., and Kalamchi, A.: Nuclear magnetic resonance imaging in Legg-Calvé-Perthes disease. J. Bone Joint. Surg., 66-A:1357, 1984.
597. Seghini, G.: L'autoinnesto cervico-epifisario nella cura della malattia di Perthes. Revisione critica. Minerva Ortop., 6:203, 1955.
598. Sellers, P.: Bilateral Perthes' disease of the hip in a seven-year-old. Nurs. Times, 65:1353, 1969.
599. Seze, S., Mazabraud, A., and Barbot-Lansaman, J.: La nécrose parcellaire de la tête fémorale. Rev. Rhum. Mal. Ostéoartic., 38:1, 1971.
600. Shands, A. R., Raney, R. B., and Brashear, R. H.: Coxa plana. In Handbook of Orthopaedic Surgery. 7th Ed. St. Louis, Mosby, 1967, pp. 336–340.
601. Shapiro, F.: Legg-Calvé-Perthes disease. A study of lower extremity length discrepancies and skeletal maturation. Acta Orthop. Scand., 53:437, 1982.
602. Sharp, I. K.: Acetabular dysplasia. The acetabular angle. J. Bone Joint Surg., 43-B:268, 1961.
603. Shim, S. S., and Foley, T. M.: The limping child: An aid to differential diagnosis. Clin. Proc. Child. Hosp., 18:61, 1962.
604. Shiotsu, T.: Therapy of Perthes' disease. Orthop. Surg. (Tokyo), 20:181, 1969.
605. Siffert, R. S.: Osteochondrosis of the proximal femoral epiphysis. A.A.O.S. Instruct. Course Lect., 22:270, 1973.
606. Singleton, M. C., and LeVeau, B. F.: The hip joint: Structure, stability and stress: A review. Phys. Ther., 55:957, 1975.
607. Singleton, W. B., and Jones, E. L.: The experimental induction of subclinical Perthes' disease in the puppy following arthrotomy and intracapsular tamponade. J. Comp. Pathol., 89:57, 1979.
608. Sjovall, H.: Zř Frage der Behandlung der Coxa plana. Mit besonderer Berücksichtigung der Frimarerfolge bei Konsenquenter Ruhigstellung. Acta Orthop. Scand., 13:324, 1942.
609. Sjovall, H.: Oom Perthes sjukdom dess diagnos och behandlung. Svenska Lakar., 40:214, 1943.
610. Slocum, D. B.: Coxa Plana. Northwest Med., 40:233, 1941.
611. Smith, S. R., Ions, G. K., and Gregg, P. J.: The radiological features of the metaphysis in Perthes' disease. J. Pediatr. Orthop., 2:401, 1982.
612. Smola, E.: L'hypoplasie de l'articulation de hanche chez le nourrisson. Cah. Med. (Paris), 11:1061, 1970.
613. Smola, E.: Theory of Perthes' disease. Z. Orthop., 110:196, 1972.
614. Snyder, C. H.: A sling for use in Legg-Perthes disease. J. Bone Joint Surg., 29:524, 1947.
615. Snyder, C. R.: Legg-Perthes disease in the young hip—does it necessarily do well? J. Bone Joint Surg., 57-A:751, 1975.
616. Soderberg, L.: Simultaneous occurrence of coxa plana enzygotic twins. Acta Orthop. Scand., 27:135, 1957.
617. Somerville, E. W.: Perthes' disease of the hip. J. Bone Joint Surg., 53-B:639, 1971.
618. Somerville, E. W.: Osteotomy in treatment of Perthes' disease of the hip. Orthop. Rev., 8:61, 1979.
619. Soto-Hall, R., Johnson, L. H., and Johnson, R. A.: Variations in the intra-articular pressure of the hip joint in injury and disease—a probable factor in avascular necrosis. J. Bone Joint Surg., 46-A:509, 1964.
620. Spock, A.: Transient synovitis of the hip in children. Pediatrics, 24:1042, 1959.
621. Stahl, F.: Early coxa plana, age studies. Acta Orthop. Scand., 17:180, 1948.
622. Stamp, W. G., and Canales, G.: Late results in osteochondrosis of capital epiphysis of femur (Legg-Calvé-Perthes disease). J.A.M.A., 169:1443, 1959.
623. Steele, P. B.: Further report on the operative treatment of Perthes' disease. A.A.O.S. Instruct. Course Lect. 1:136–143, 1943.
624. Steinhauser, E.: Spaetergebnisse der Perthesschen Erkrankung unter Fixierung in Entlastungsstellung (Imhauser). 17-Jahres-resultate. Z. Orthop., 197:558, 1970.
625. Stephens, F. E., and Kerby, J. P.: Hereditary Legg-Calvé-Perthes disease. J. Hered., 37:153, 1946.
626. Stevens, P. M., Williams, P., and Menelaus, M.: Innominate osteotomy for Perthes' disease. J. Pediatr. Orthop., 1:47, 1981.
627. Stillman, B. C.: Osteochondritis dissecans and coxa plana. J. Bone Joint Surg., 48-B:64, 1966.
628. Stoica, E., and Varna, A.: Experimentelle Forschungen über Necrose des Femurkopfes durch die Methode der gradierten Kapsularen Spannung. Beitr. Orthop. Traumatol., 18:290, 1971.
629. Stulberg, S. D.: Legg-Calvé-Perthes disease: Update. In The Hip: Proceedings of the Sixth Open Scientific Meeting of The Hip Society. St. Louis, Mosby, 1978, pp. 263–269.
630. Stulberg, S. D., and Salter, R. B.: The natural course of Legg-Perthes disease and its relationship to degenerative arthritis of the hip. A long-term follow-up study. Orthop. Trans., 1:105, 1977.
631. Stulberg, S. D., Cooperman, D. R., and Wallenstein, R.: The natural history of Legg-Calvé-Perthes disease. J. Bone Joint Surg., 63-A:1095, 1981.
632. Subramanian, G., and McAfee, J. G.: A new complex of 99mTc for skeletal imaging. Radiology, 99:192, 1971.
633. Subramanian, G., McAfee, J. G., Bell, E. G., Blair, R. J., O'Mara, R. E., and Ralton, P. H.: 99mTc-

labeled polyphosphate as a skeletal imaging agent. Radiology, *102*:701, 1972.
634. Sundt, H.: Malum coxae Calvé-Legg-Perthes. Zentralbl. Chir., *47*:538, 1920.
635. Sundt, H.: Undersokelser over Malum Coxae, Calvé-Legg-Perthes. Kristiania, Norway, 1920.
636. Sundt, H.: Further investigations respecting malum coxae Calvé-Legg-Perthes with special regard to prognosis and treatment. Acta Chir. Scand., Suppl. 148, 1949.
637. Sundt, H.: Malum coxae Calvé-Legg-Perthes. Acta Chir. Scand., Suppl. *148*:1, 1949.
638. Suramo, I., Puranen, J., Heikkinen, E., and Vuorinen, P.: Disturbed patterns of venous drainage of the femoral neck in Perthes' disease. J. Bone Joint Surg., *56-B*:448, 1974.
639. Sutherland, A. D., Savage, J. P., Paterson, D. C., and Foster, B. K.: The nuclide bone-scan in the diagnosis and management of Perthes' disease. J. Bone Joint Surg., *62-B*:300, 1980.
640. Sutro, C. J., and Pomeranz, M. M.: Perthes' disease. Arch. Surg., *34*:360, 1937.
641. Sutter, J.: Isolat et diffusion des mutations chez l'homme. J. Genet. Hum., *13*:108, 1964.
642. Tachdjian, M. O.: Treating Legg-Perthes disease. Postgrad. Med., *45*:197, 1969.
643. Tachdjian, M. O., and Grana, L.: Response of the hip to increased pressure. Clin. Orthop., *61*:199, 1968.
644. Tachdjian, M. O., and Jouett, L. D.: Trilateral socket hip abduction orthosis for the treatment of Legg-Perthes disease. J. Bone Joint Surg., *50-A*:1271, 1968.
645. Tachdjian, M. O., and Jouett, L. D.: Trilateral socket hip abduction orthosis for the treatment of Legg-Perthes disease. Orthol. Prosthet., *22*:49, 1968.
646. Taussig, G.: Réflexions á propos des formes bilatérales d'ostéochondrite primitive de la hanche. Acta Orthop. Belg., *46*:380, 1980.
647. Taussig, G., and Heripret, G.: Maladie de Legg-Perthes-Calvé. A propos de 275 cas. Rev. Chir. Orthop., *55*:305, 1969.
648. Taussig, G., Perves, A., and Heripret, G.: Techniques et résultats des épiphysiodeses dans le traitement des inégalites de longueur des membres inférieurs. Rev. Chir. Orthop., *58*:741, 1972.
649. Taylor, H. L., and Frieder, W.: Quiet hip disease. Am. J. Orthop. Surg., *13*:192, 1915.
650. Teleszynski, Z., Sikora, Z., Gardzinska, E., and Patros, J.: Wyniki zachoawczego leczenia choroby Legg-Calvé-Perthesa. Chir. Narzadow Ruchu Orthop. Pol., *33*:527, 1968.
651. Termansen, N. B., and Okholm, K.: Intraosseous pressure in the femoral head and greater trochanter before and 1–3 years after osteotomy for osteoarthritis of the hip joint. Acta Orthop. Scand., *47*:96, 1976.
652. Theron, J.: Angiography in Legg-Calvé-Perthes disease. Radiology, *135*:81, 1980.
653. Thiers, J., and Normand, D.: L'association ichtyose-épiphysite. Rhumatologie, *23*:159, 1971.
654. Thompson, G. H., and Westin, G. W.: Legg-Calvé-Perthes disease: Results of discontinuing treatment in the early reossification phase. Clin. Orthop., *139*:70, 1979.
655. Thompson, S. K., and Woodrow, J. C.: HLA antigens in Perthes' disease. J. Bone Joint Surg., *63-B*:278, 1981.
656. Tillema, D. A., and Asher, M. A.: Perthes' disease. Current concepts of treatment. J. Kans. Med. Soc., *74*:91, 1973.
657. Tillier, R.: L'ostéochondrite déformante de la hanche. Lyon Chir., *21*:464, 1924.
658. Tracy, H. W.: Coxa plana in siblings. N.C. Med. J., *24*:76, 1963.

659. Trias, A.: Femoral osteotomy in Perthes' disease. Clin. Orthop., *137*:195, 1978.
660. Trueta, J.: La etiologia de la enfermeded de Perthes. Rev. Fac. Med. (Bogata), *24*:743, 1956.
661. Trueta, J.: Perthes' disease. Lancet, *1*:383, 1960.
662. Trueta, J.: The bone growth and development of bones and joints: Orthopaedic aspects. *In* Davis, J. A. (ed.): Scientific Foundations of Paediatrics. Philadelphia, Saunders, 1974, pp. 399–419.
663. Trueta, J., and Pinto de Lina, C. S.: Estudio sobre la osteocondritis de la cabeza femoral o enfermedad de Legg-Calvé-Perthes. Rev. Ortop. Traumatol. Latino-Americana, *4*:115, 1959.
664. Trumble, H. C.: Weight-bearing instruments for walking. Br. Med. J., *1*:1070, 1935.
665. Trusell, J. J.: Nontraumatic avascular necrosis of the femoral head. J. Am. Osteop. Assoc., *71*:51, 1971.
666. Valderrama, J. A. F.: The observation hip syndrome and its late sequalae. J. Bone Joint Surg., *45-B*:462, 1963.
667. Van Dam, B. E., Crider, R. J., Noyes, J. D., and Larsen, L. F.: Determination of the Catterall classification in Legg-Calvé-Perthes disease. J. Bone Joint Surg., *63-A*:906, 1981.
668. Van der Heyden, A. M., van Tongerloo, R. S.: Shelf operation in Perthes' disease. J. Bone Joint Surg., *63-B*:282, 1981.
669. Vestad, E.: Calvé-Legg-Perthes sykdom. Tidsskr. Nor. Laegeforen., *92*:1773, 1972.
670. Voigit, M.: Observation on the coincidence of spondylolysis and spondylolisthesis with Perthes' disease. Beitr. Orthop. Traumatol., *20*:607, 1973.
671. Voiteschuk, M. V.: Experience in the treatment of osteochondropathy of the femoral head in children using cuff traction. Orthop. Travmatol. Protez., *31*:48, 1970.
672. Waldenström, H.: Der obere tuberkulöse Collumherd. Z. Orthop. Chir., *24*:487, 1909.
673. Waldenström, H.: Die Tuberkulose des Collum Femoris im Kindesalter und ihre Beziehunger zur Hüftgelenkenzündung. Stockholm, 1910.
674. Waldenström, H.: The definite form of the coxa plana. Acta Radiol., *1*:384, 1922.
675. Waldenström, H.: On coxa plana. Acta Chir. Scand., *55*:577, 1923.
676. Waldenström, H.: The first stage of coxa plana. Acta Orthop. Scand., *5*:1, 1934.
677. Waldenström, H.: The first stages of coxa plana. J. Bone Joint Surg., *20*:559, 1938.
678. Wamoscher, Z., and Farhi, A.: Hereditary Legg-Calvé-Perthes disease. Am. J. Dis. Child., *106*:97, 1963.
679. Wansborough, R. M., Carrie, A. W., Walker, N. G., and Ruckerbauer, G.: Coxa plana, its genetic aspects and results of treatment with the long Taylor walking caliper. J. Bone Joint Surg., *41-A*:135, 1959.
680. Warren, R. G.: Urinary acid mucopolysaccharides and hydroxyproline in skeletal disorders. Bull. Hosp. Joint Dis., *34*:226, 1973.
681. Watanabe, H.: Treatment of Perthes' disease. Orthop. Surg. (Tokyo), *20*:191, 1969.
682. Watanabe, H., Yonemitsu, H., Shigemoto, H., Okabe, T., and Fukanogi, M.: Brace for Legg-Perthes disease. Kumamoto Med. J., *27*:66, 1974.
683. Watanabe, R. S.: Embryology of the human hip. Clin. Orthop., *98*:8, 1974.
684. Watermann, R.: Zur Gefaessversorgung der distalen Femurepiphyse. Z. Orthop., *101*:247, 1966.
685. Weigert, M., Gronert, H. L., and Klems, H.: Therapie der Hüftkopfnekrose. Z. Orthop., *113*:1070, 1975.
686. Weikel, A. M., and Habal, M. B.: Meralgia paraes-

687. Weiner, D. S., and O'Dell, H. W.: Legg-Calvé-Perthes disease: Observations on skeletal maturity. Clin. Orthop., 68:44, 1970.
688. Weinstein, S. L.: Legg-Calvé-Perthes disease. A.A.O.S. Instruct. Course Lect., 32:275, 1983.
689. Weinstein, S. L.: Improving the prognosis in Legg-Calvé-Perthes. J. Musculoskel. Med., 1:11, 1984.
690. Weissman, S. L., Tadmor, A., Khermosh, O., Michels, C. H., and Chen, R.: Growth of the upper end of the femur. Acta Orthop. Scand., 45:225, 1974.
691. Wenger, D. R.: Selective surgical containment for Legg-Perthes disease. J. Pediatr. Orthop., 1:153, 1981.
692. Wertheimer, L. G., and Lopes, S. de L. F.: Arterial supply of the femoral head. J. Bone Joint Surg., 53-A:545, 1971.
693. Westin, G. W.: The limping child. Pediatr. Clin. North Am., 14:601, 1967.
694. Whitman, R.: Further observtions on the operative treatment of Legg-Perthes disease. Am. J. Surg., 6:791, 1929.
695. Wiberg, G.: Relation between congenital subluxation of the hip and arthritis deformans (a roentgenological study). Acta Orthop. Scand., 10:351, 1939.
696. Wiberg, G.: Shelf operation in congenital dysplasia of the acetabulum and in subluxation and dislocation of the hip. J. Bone Joint Surg., 35-A:65, 1953.
697. Wilk, L. H.: Juvenile osteochondrosis of the hip. J.A.M.A., 192:939, 1965.
698. Willert, H. G.: Pathogenese und Klinik der spontanen Osteonekrosen. 63. Kongress der Deutschen Gesellschaft fur Orthopädie und Traumatologie. Z. Orthop., 115:444, 1977.
699. Williams, L., Wientroub, S., Canario, A. T., and Fixsen, J. A.: Severe Perthes' disease noted 5 years after the successful conservative treatment of congenital dislocation of the hip. J. Pediatr. Orthop., 2:424, 1982.
700. Willner, S.: Difference in leg length in children with coxa plana during and after treatment using unilateral unloading. Acta Orthop. Scand., 46:102, 1975.
701. Wolcott, W. E.: Circulation of the head and neck of the femur. Its relation to nonunion in fractures of the femoral neck. J.A.M.A., 100:27, 1933.
702. Woodhouse, C. F.: Dynamic influences of vascular occlusion affecting the development of avascular necrosis of the femoral head. Clin. Orthop., 32:119, 1964.
703. Woodward, A. H., and Decker, J. S.: Case report: Osteochondritis dissecans following Legg-Perthes' disease. South. Med. J., 69:943, 1976.
704. Wynne-Davies, R.: Some etiologic factors in Perthes' disease. Clin. Orthop., 150:12, 1980.
705. Wynne-Davies, R., and Gormley, J.: The aetiology of Perthes' disease. J. Bone Joint Surg., 60-B:6, 1978.
706. Zahir, A.: Experimental stimulation of Perthes' disease in the puppy. Proc. R. Soc. Med., 64:641, 1971.
707. Zahir, A., and Freeman, M. A. R.: Cartilage changes following a single episode of infraction of the capital femoral epiphysis in the dog. J. Bone Joint Surg., 54-A:125, 1972.
708. Zahir, A., England, J. P. S., and Freeman, M. A. R.: Studies of articular cartilage following infraction of the capital femoral epiphysis in the puppy. Proc. R. Soc. Med., 63:583, 1970.
709. Zemansky, A. P., Jr.: The pathology and pathogenesis of Legg-Calvé-Perthes disease (osteochondritis juvenilis deformans coxae). Am. J. Surg., 4:169, 1928.
710. Zemansky, A. P., and Lippman, R. K.: The importance of the vessels in the round ligament to the head of the femur during the period of growth, and their possible relationship to Perthes' disease. Surg. Gynecol. Obstet., 48:461, 1929.
711. Zenker, H., and Bruns, H.: Die Trochanterversetzung und ihre Ergebnisse. Arch. Orthop. Unfallchir., 77:299, 1973.
712. Zharkov, P. L., Sergeeva, I. A., Saudov, I. D., and Dubrov, E. A.: Early roentgenodiagnosis of osteochondropathy of the head of the femur. Ortop. Travmatol. Protez., 34:30, 1973.
713. Zweymuller, K.: Zur operativen Behandlung des Morbus Perthes. Wien. Med. Wochenschr., 122:440, 1972.
714. Zweymuller, K.: Zur Lateralisation des Oberschenkelkopfesbeim M. Perthes. Arch. Orthop. Unfallchir., 75:239, 1973.

KÖHLER'S DISEASE OF THE TARSAL NAVICULAR

In 1908, Köhler described a self-limited disease of the tarsal navicular characterized by flattening, sclerosis, and irregular rarefaction seen in the radiogram.[13] The condition is uncommon, occurring more frequently in boys (about 75 to 80 per cent) than in girls. The age incidence is related to the sex of the patient, the average age of onset of symptoms being five years for boys and about four years for girls, the disease occurring at least a year earlier in the female. In about one third of cases both feet are involved. Köhler's disease may occur simultaneously with Legg-Perthes disease.[7]

Etiology

There is evidence that Köhler's disease has a mechanical basis, being the result of repetitive compression force. The tarsal navicular is located at the apex of the longitudinal arch of the foot and is subjected to constant strain during locomotion. The navicular, according to Karp, is the last bone of the foot to ossify, the average age of appearance of its ossific nucleus being between 18 and 24 months in girls and between 24 and 30 months in boys. Karp also noted that irregularities of ossification of the navicular bone are not uncommon.[11] Waugh, in a study of serial radiograms of the feet of 52 normal children (26 girls and 26 boys), made the same observation as Karp: that the ossification of the tarsal navicular occurs later in boys than in girls. He also reported that abnormalities of ossification are more frequent in boys and are more common in naviculars that ossify late. Waugh also states that abnormal ossification results from compression of the bony nucleus whose appearance is delayed at a critical phase of the growth of the navicular bone.[27] The same compressional forces occlude the vessels in the spongy osseous tissue and produce aseptic necrosis of bone. Histologic examination of affected bone obtained by biopsy or excision of

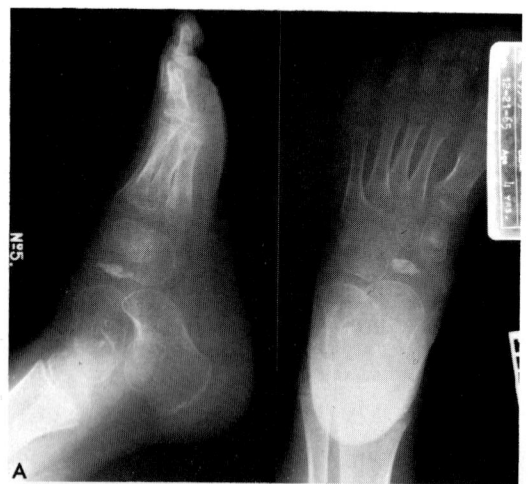
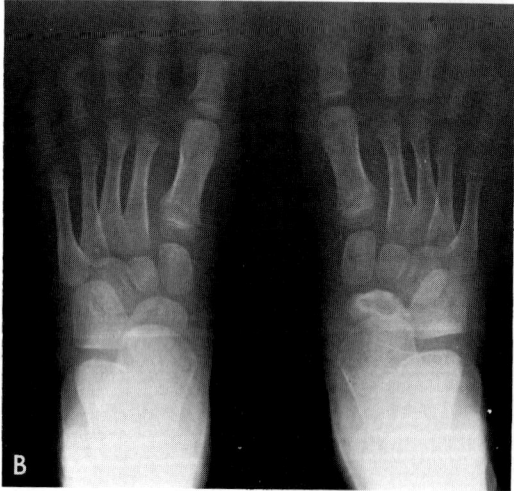
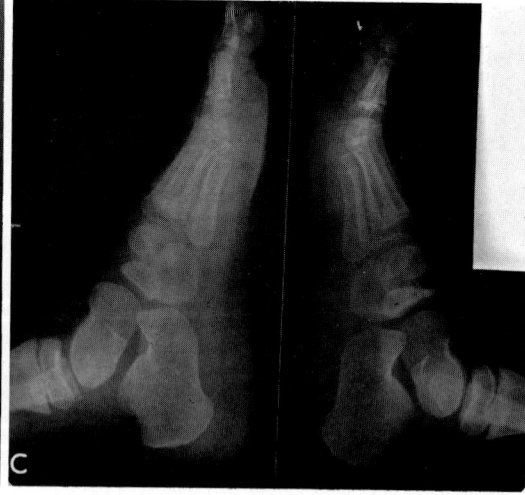

FIGURE 3–171. Köhler's disease of left tarsal navicular.

A. Note the sclerosis and flattening of the tarsal navicular. **B** and **C.** Anteroposterior and lateral radiograms of both feet two years later, showing healing of the left navicular.

the involved navicular has disclosed areas of necrosis, resorption of dead bone, and formation of new bone.[12, 15, 25]

Clinical Features

The child walks with an antalgic limp, bearing his weight on the lateral side of the foot to relieve stress on its medial longitudinal arch. Other clinical manifestations consist of local pain and tenderness over the navicular bone, and not infrequently, reactive thickening and swelling over the affected area. The posterior tibial tendon may be inflamed near its insertion to the scaphoid. On testing, the midtarsal and subtalar joints have full range of motion, an important differential diagnostic point in distinguishing Köhler's disease from rheumatoid or other inflammatory arthritides.

Radiographic Findings

The radiographic picture is characteristic. Diagnostic features are flattening of the tarsal navicular, narrowing in its anteroposterior diameter (as seen in the lateral view), and irregular rarefaction and sclerosis of the affected bone (Fig. 3–171). Irregular ossification of the tarsal navicular is not infrequent in normal feet and should not be mistaken for Köhler's disease. Radiograms of both feet should be made to detect possible bilateral involvement, as, on occasion, equally severe changes may be noted in a totally asymptomatic foot. The diagnosis of Köhler's disease should be made only when symptoms are present.[29]

Scaglietti and associates studied the radiograms of the feet of 100 cases with Köhler's disease of the tarsal navicular and compared them with those of 100 normal children. They found that in 82 per cent the talus projected farther beyond the calcaneus in Köhler's disease. They proposed that the diminution of the anatomic space for the navicular has an etiologic bearing.[21]

Treatment

Treatment varies with the severity of the condition. When there is moderate pain, it is best to protect the foot in a below-knee walking cast with the foot in a 10- to 15-degree varus and 20-degree equinus position for six to eight weeks. During the initial three weeks, it is best to prevent weight-bearing by the use of crutches. Following removal of the plaster cast, strain on the foot is relieved by a soft longitudinal arch support with a ⅛-inch inner heel wedge and a Thomas heel. Strenuous physical activity, such as running, long walks, and active sports, should be avoided. When a foot is asymptomatic or when pain is minimal, a longitudinal arch support is the only necessary treatment. Keeping the child from bearing weight on the foot has no effect on the course of the disease.

In Köhler's disease, the prognosis is very good. The navicular reconstitutes itself in a minimum of six months, but usually between one and a half and three years. Waugh reported normal naviculars in 12 patients who were followed for ten years or more.[27] Most affected navicular bones become normal before the foot has completed its growth, and there is no residual deformity or disability.

Ippolito and associates reviewed 12 patients with Köhler's disease of the tarsal navicular at a follow-up averaging 33 years (minimum of 30 years and maximum of 37 years) after diagnosis. Two types of treatment were used: a weight-bearing cast for three months, which rendered the patients pain free; and longitudinal arch supports, which decreased local pain, for an average of seven months. The tarsal navicular was flattened and fragmented in the active stage of the disease; all the bones were restored to normal shape at the end of skeletal growth. The average time for radiographic restoration to normal was eight months (range 6 to 13 months). None of the patients showed any degenerative change.

References

1. Axhausen, G.: Die Ätiologie der Köhler'schen Erkrankung der Metatarsalkoptchen. Bruns Beitr. Klin. Chir., 126:451, 1922.
2. Axhausen, G.: Die Köhler'schen Erkrankung der Metatarsophalangealgelenke. Med. Klin., 19:561, 1923.
3. Bader, L.: Patologie e clinica del morbo di Köhler, II. Glorizia, Paternelli, 1940.
4. Brailsford, J. F.: Osteochondritis of the adult tarsal navicular. J. Bone Joint Surg., 21:111, 1939.
5. Camerer, J. W.: Zur Ätiologie der Köhlerschen Erkrankung des Os naviculare pedis. Dtsch. Med. Wochenschr., 61:713, 1935.
6. Fournet-Fayard, J., Tran-Minh, V., and Bernard, J.: What is your diagnosis? Köhler's disease. Pediatrie, 36:563, 1981.
7. Froelich, R.: Des apophysites de croissance. Paris Med., 37:430, 1920.
8. Haboush, E. J.: Bilateral disease of the internal cuneiform bone with an associated disease of the right scaphoid bone (Köhler's). J.A.M.A., 100:41, 1933.
9. Hermodsson, I.: Zur Ätiologie der Köhlerschen Krankheit des Os naviculare tarsi. Acta Radiol., 17:68, 1936.
10. Ippolito, E., Pollini, P. T. R., and Falez, F.: Köhler's disease of the tarsal navicular. Long term follow-up of 12 cases. J. Pediatr. Orthop., 4(4):416, 1984.

11. Karp, M.: Köhler's disease of the tarsal scaphoid. J. Bone Joint Surg., 19:84, 1937.
12. Kidner, F. C., and Muro, F.: Köhler's disease of the tarsal scaphoid or os navicular pedis retardatum. J.A.M.A., 83:1, 650, 1924.
13. Köhler, A.: Über eine haufige bisher anscheinend unbekannte Erkrankung einzelner kindlicher Knochen. Munchen. Med. Wochenschr., 55:1923, 1908.
14. Köhler, A.: Eine typische Erkrankung des 2. Metatarsophalangealgelenkes. Munchen. Med. Wochenschr., 67:1289, 1920.
15. Lecene, P., and Mouchet, A.: La scaphoidité tarsienne. Rev. Orthop., 3:serie 11:105, 1928.
16. Lelièvre, J.: Scaphoidite tarsienne de l'enfant (maladie de Köhler-Mouchet). In Pathologie du Pied. 2nd Ed. Paris, Masson, 1961, p. 409.
17. McCauley, G. K., and Kahn, P. C.: Osteochondritis of the tarsal navicula: radioisotopic appearances. Radiology, 123:705, 1977.
18. Martinie-Dubousquet, J.: Scaphoidite tarsienne (première maladie de Köhler). Sem. Hôp. Paris–Ann. Chir., 32:177, 1956.
19. Nagura, S., and Kosuge, S.: Die Entstehung und das Wesen der Köhler'schen Krankheit des Navikulare. Zentralbl. Chir., 66:1186, 1939.
20. O'Donoghue, A. F., Donohue, E. S., and Zimmerman, W. W.: Bilateral osteochondritis of the tarsal navicular and first cuneiform. J. Bone Joint Surg., 30-A:780, 1948.
21. Scaglietti, O., Stringa, G., and Mizzau, M.: Plus-variant of the astragalus and subnormal scaphoid space, two important findings in Köhler's scaphoid necrosis. Acta Orthop. Scand., 32:500, 1962.
22. Schultze, E. O. P.: Das Alb. Köhlersche Knochenbild des Os naviculare pedis bei Kindern. Arch. Klin. Orthop., 100:431, 1913.
23. Sinclair, G. G., Uhlman, R. E., and Zeichner, A. M.: Osteochondrosis of the tarsal navicular bone: Köhler's disease. J. Am. Podiatry Assoc., 71:77, 1981.
24. Smets, W.: La maladie de Köhler du scaphoide tarsien. J. Chir. (Brux.), 33:389, 1936.
25. Speed, K.: Köhler's disease of the tarsal scaphoid bone. Trans. Am. Surg. Assoc., 45:179, 1927.
26. Wagner, A.: Isolated aseptic necrosis of the epiphysis of the first metatarsal bone. Acta Radiol., 11:80, 1930.
27. Waugh, W.: The ossification and vascularization of the tarsal navicular and their relation to Köhler's disease. J. Bone Joint Surg., 40-B:765, 1958.
28. Wiley, J. J., and Brown, D. E.: The bipartite tarsal scaphoid. J. Bone Joint Surg., 63-B:583, 1981.
29. Williams, G. A., and Cowell, H. R.: Köhler's disease of the tarsal navicular. Clin. Orthop., 158:53, 1981.
30. Zeitlin, A.: Some reflections on the etiology of Köhler's disease. Radiology, 24:360, 1935.

FREIBERG'S INFRACTION

Freiberg, in 1914, described a form of anterior metatarsalgia in which the second metatarsal head has a "crushed in" appearance, terming the condition *infraction of the second metatarsal bone*.[11] In the European literature, this entity is also known as Köhler's No. 2 disease, distinguishing it from Köhler's No. 1 disease of the tarsal navicular. Priority should be given to Freiberg, however, as he was the first to report the condition.

This disease is seen in adolescents, usually after 13 years of age. It is more prevalent in the female, with about 75 per cent of the cases occurring in girls. Though the second metatarsal head is the most common site of involvement, other metatarsals may be affected. It may be bilateral.

Etiology

The exact cause of the condition is not definitely known. The general opinion is that it is

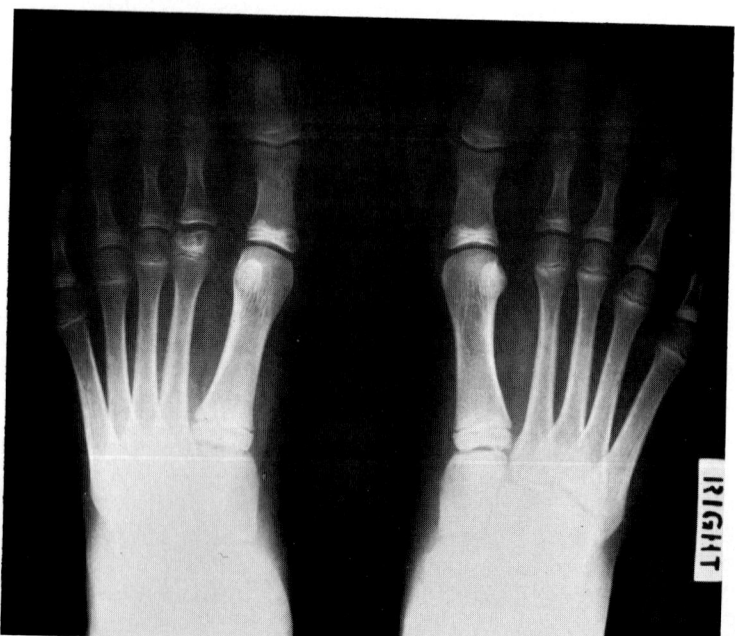

FIGURE 3–172. Freiberg's infraction of the second metatarsal of left foot.

Note the flattening and irregularity of the epiphysis and second metatarsal.

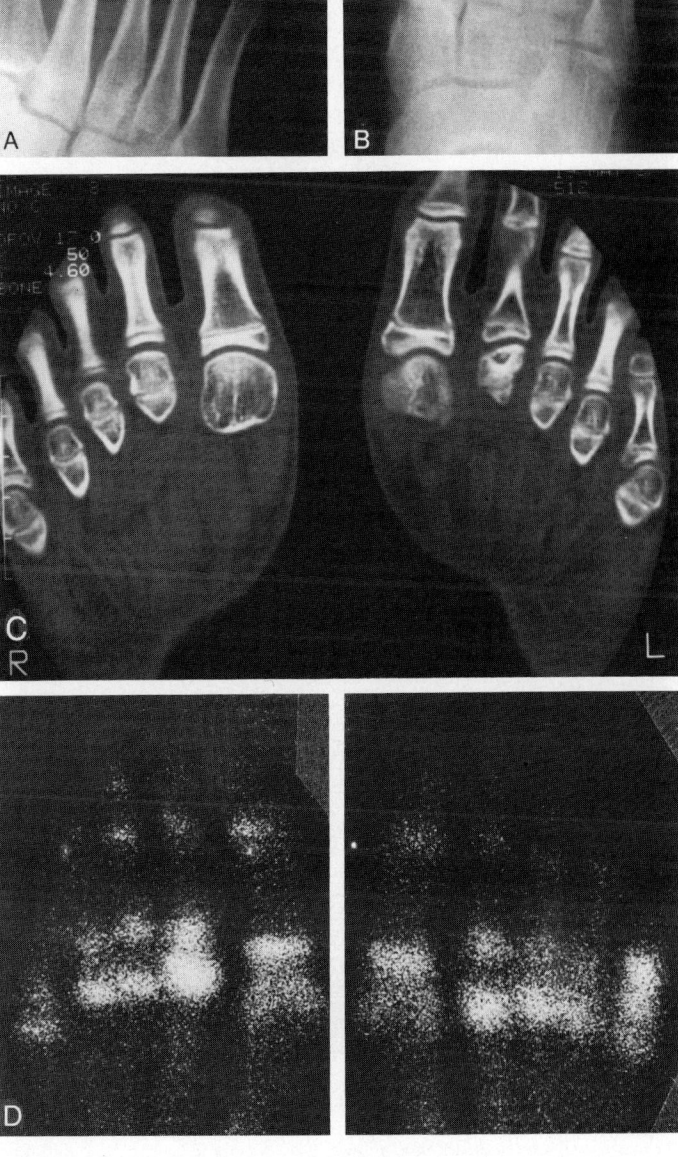

FIGURE 3–173. *Freiberg's infraction of the second metatarsal head in the left foot.*

A and **B.** Oblique and anteroposterior radiograms of the left foot showing the flattening of the second metatarsal head with an area of rarefaction in its center. **C.** CT scan of both feet showing the pathologic changes in greater detail. **D.** Bone scan showing increased uptake in the second metatarsal head.

due to vascular insufficiency and related to aseptic necrosis of other bones. Histologic examination of the affected metatarsal heads has shown areas of necrosis.[1] Smillie thought the process to be traumatic in nature, postulating stress rather than a single injury.[28] Braddock, in his experimental studies of the strength of the second metatarsal and proximal phalanx in various age groups, found that the second metatarsal epiphysis was vulnerable; he believed Freiberg's infraction to be caused by a fracture somewhat modified by its proximity to the physis and articular cartilage.[3]

Clinical and Radiographic Findings

Clinical manifestations consist of pain under the second or any other affected metatarsal head, local swelling, and limitation of motion of the metatarsophalangeal joint. Radiograms of the metatarsal head demonstrate flattening and irregularity (Fig. 3–172). The CT scan will show rarefaction and flattening in the metatarsal head more clearly (Fig. 3–173).

Bone scan with technetium-99m will show increased uptake, indicating it is a stress fracture (Fig. 3–174).

Treatment

Treatment is conservative in the adolescent. In the acute painful stage, the foot is protected in a below-knee walking cast until the symptoms subside, usually in three to four weeks. Then the pressure from the metatarsal head is relieved with a metatarsal pad.

Symptoms may persist despite protection by a cast in some patients. In such rare instances, the avascular bone or the second metatarsal head is curetted under radiographic control. The tendency is not to proceed far enough distally; one must be sure the lesion on the metatarsal head is removed. Do not, however, enter the metatarsal-phalangeal joint! Next, through a separate incision, cancellous bone is removed from the cuboid or lateral cuneiform bone, and the cavity in the metatarsal head is firmly packed with the autogenous bone graft. The foot is protected in a below-knee walking cast for six weeks.

In the adult, if symptoms are disabling and severe, surgical measures consisting of resection of the metatarsal head with a portion of the adjacent shaft are indicated. To prevent recession of the corresponding toe, it is surgically syndactylized with its adjacent normal toe (Fig. 3–175). The silicone elastomer (Silastic) implant prosthesis to replace the head of the metatarsal after resection is not recommended by this author.

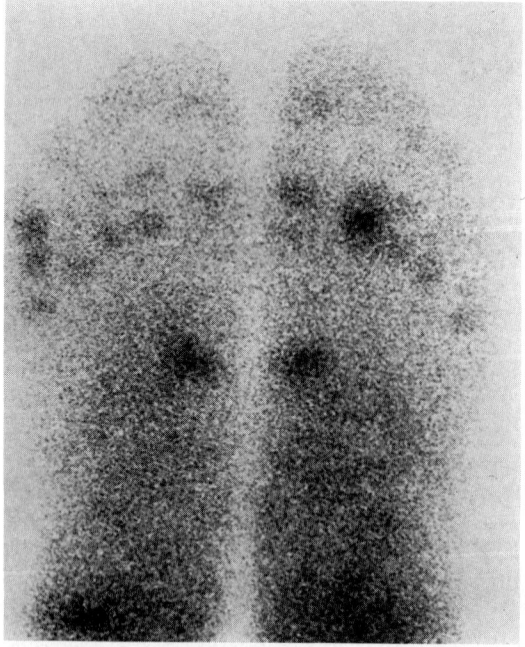

FIGURE 3–174. *Freiberg's infraction of the second metatarsal head of the right foot.*

Bone scan with technetium-99m shows increased uptake.

References

1. Axhausen, G.: Die Köhlersche Erkrankung der Metatarsophalangealgelenke. Med. Klin. Wochenschr., 48:318, 1922.
2. Bordelon, R. L.: Silicone implant for Freiberg's disease. South. Med. J., 70:1002, 1977.
3. Braddock, G. T. F.: Experimental epiphysial injury and Freiberg's disease. J. Bone Joint Surg., 41:154, 1959.
4. Brandes, M., and Ruschenburg, E.: Eine Operative Behandlung der (II.) Koehlerschen Krankheit am Kopfchen des Os Metatarsale. Z. Orthop., 69:353, 1939.
5. Canale, S. T.: Personal communication.
6. Cristallo, V.: Riparazione chirurgica della osteocondrosi di Freiberg Kohler. Minerva Ortop., 17:684, 1966.
7. Derivaux, J.: L'importance de l'ostéonécrose dans la maladie de Köhler II. Ann. Anat. Pathol., 17:394, 1947.
8. Dini, P.: Localizzazioni rae dell'osteocondrite del metatarsi. Arch. Putti, 15:280, 1961.
9. Doub, H. P.: Aseptic necrosis of the epiphyses and short bones; radi studies. J.A.M.A., 127:311, 1945.
10. Fasiani, G. M.: Contributo allo studio della malattia di Köhler del secondo metataseo. Arch. Ital. Chir., 13:741, 1925.
11. Freiberg, A. H.: Infraction of the second metatarsal bone; a typical injury. Surg. Gynecol. Obstet., 19:191, 1914.
12. Freiberg, A. H.: The so-called infraction of the second metatarsal bone. J. Bone Joint Surg., 8:257, 1926.

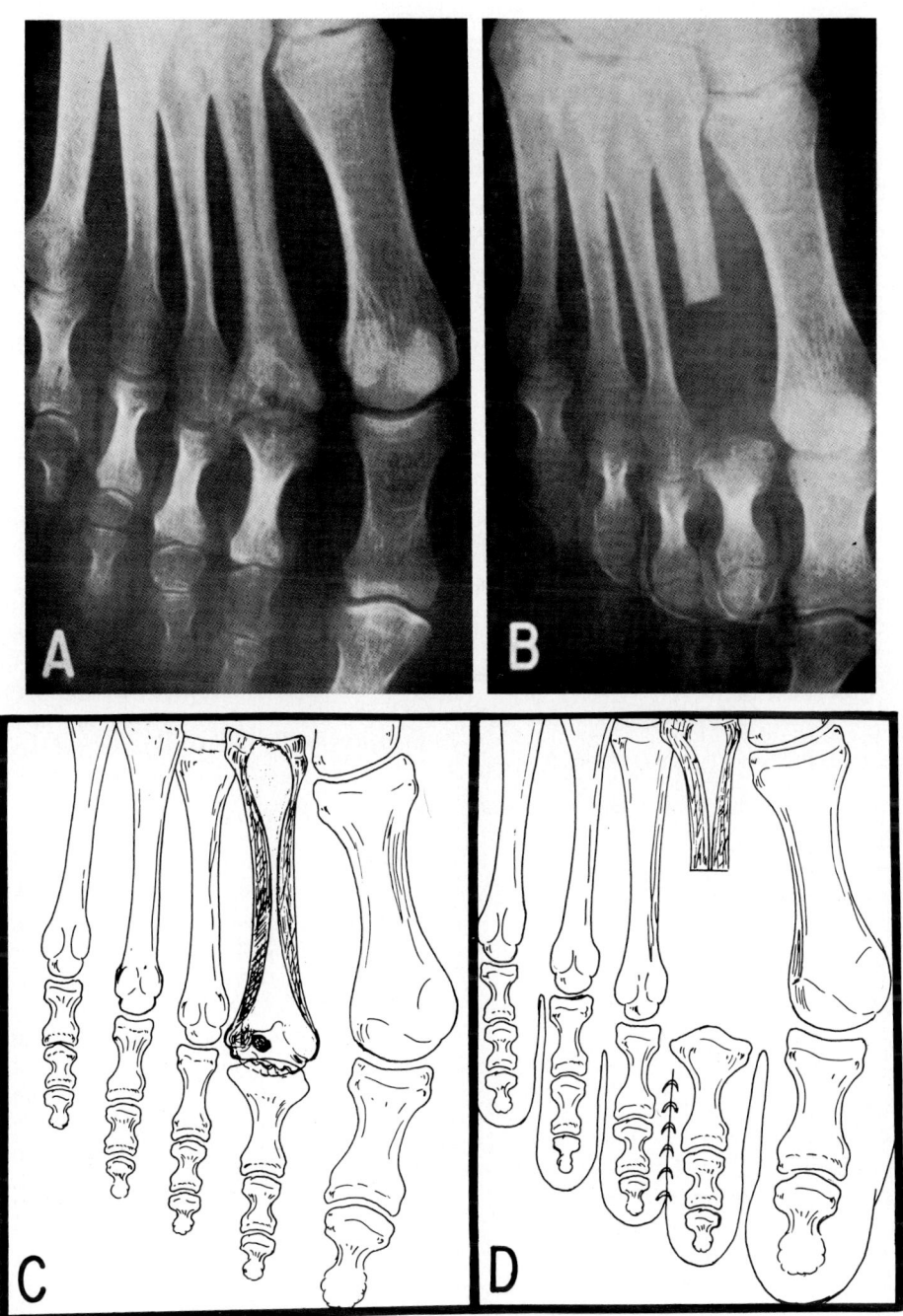

FIGURE 3–175. *Freiberg's infraction of the second metatarsal.*

A. Preoperative radiogram of the foot. **B.** Postoperative radiogram of the foot. A resection of the flattened head and distal shaft was performed, and the second toe was syndactylized to the third toe. **C** and **D.** Line drawings of the radiograms. (From Kelikian, H., Hallux Valgus, Allied Deformities of the Forefoot and Metatarsalgia. Philadelphia, W. B. Saunders Co., 1965, p. 377. Reprinted by permission.)

13. Gauthier, G.: Maladie de Freiberg ou deuxième maladie de Koehler. Proposition d'un traitement de réconstitution a l'état evolué de l'affection (34 cas traités). Rev. Chir. Orthop., 60:Suppl.337, 1974.
14. Hoskinson, J.: Freiberg's disease: A review of the long-term results. Proc. R. Soc. Med., 67:106, 1974.
15. Jewett, E. L.: A case of Freiberg's disease treated by a walking cast. J. Bone Joint Surg., 21:778, 1939.
16. Karp, M. G.: Köhler's disease of the tarsal scaphoid. J. Bone Joint Surg., 29:84, 1937.
17. Kelikian, H.: Hallux Valgus, Allied Deformities of the Forefoot, and Metatarsalgia. Philadelphia, Saunders, 1965, p. 372.
18. Köhler, A.: Eine typische Erkrankung des 2. Metatarsophalangealgelenkes. Munch. Med. Wochenschr., 67:1289, 1920.
19. König, E., and Rauch, H.: Zur Histologie und Ätiologie der Köhler'schen Metatarsalerkrankung. Arch. Klin. Chir., 128:369, 1924.
20. Lawton, J. H.: Early surgical intervention for Freiberg's infraction: Autogenous epiphyseodesis. J. Foot. Surg., 18:68, 1979.
21. Lelièvre, J.: Epiphysite des têtes métatarsiennes (maladie de Freiberg). In Pathologie du Pied. 2nd Ed. Paris, Masson, 1961, pp. 411–413.
22. Lewin, P.: Juvenile deforming metatarsophalangeal osteochondritis. J.A.M.A., 81:189, 1923.
23. Margo, M. K.: Surgical treatment of conditions of the forepart of the foot. J. Bone Joint Surg., 49-A:1667, 1967.
24. Moutier, G.: L'épiphysite métatarsienne. Rev. Orthop., 12:235, 1925.
25. Painter, C. F.: Infraction of the second metatarsal head. Boston Med. Surg. J., 184:533, 1921.
26. Panner, H. J.: A peculiar characteristic metatarsal disease. Acta Radiol., 1:319, 1921–1922.
27. Skillern, P. G., Jr.: Eggshell fracture of head of metatarsal. Ann. Surg., 61:371, 1915.
28. Smillie, I. S.: Freiberg's infraction (Koehler's second disease). J. Bone Joint Surg., 37:580, 1955.
29. Swanson, A. B.: Flexible Implant Resection Arthroplasty in the Hand and Extremities. St. Louis, Mosby, 1973, pp. 1–32, 296–305.
30. Wagner, A.: Isolated aseptic necrosis in the epiphysis of the first metatarsal bone. Acta Radiol., 11:80, 1930.

OSGOOD-SCHLATTER DISEASE

This syndrome is characterized by tenderness and swelling of the patellar tendon and by excessive enlargement of the proximal tibial tubercle. The disease was first described as a separate entity by Osgood, in 1903, and independently a few months later by Schlatter.[30, 32] It is a disease of preadolescence, commonly seen between the ages of 11 and 15 years in boys, and between 8 and 13 years in girls. It is encountered more frequently in the male, three times as often as in the female. There is usually a history of a rapid spurt of growth and active participation in sports—in girls usually figure skating or gymnastics—prior to the onset of symptoms. It is bilateral in about one fourth to half the cases.

Etiology

Osgood-Schlatter disease is caused by traumatic stress from a contracted quadriceps mechanism on the proximal tibial tuberosity in a growth period when the tibial tubercle is very susceptible to strain. The pull of the ligamentum patellae produces detachment of cartilage fragments from a portion of the tibial tuberosity.[6, 10, 24, 39] The tensile force is produced by sudden contracture of the quadriceps femoris in, for example, jumping or running.

Histologic examination of bone excised from the tibial tuberosity and particles of bone embedded in the posterior part of the patellar tendon have disclosed viable cancellous bone surrounded by cartilage, with no evidence of necrosis or inflammation.[7, 31, 41]

The partial loss of continuity of the patellar tendon–cartilage–bone junction at the tibial tubercle sets up an inflammatory and reparative process that results in patellar tendonitis and prominence—swelling of the proximal tibial tubercle.

The stress from the patellar tendon at its point of insertion is the primary cause of the Osgood-Schlatter disease. The irregular ossification within the underlying bone is a secondary change. *The cause is trauma and not avascular necrosis of the proximal tibial tubercle.*

Clinical Picture

Clinically, the presenting complaint is local pain in the anterior aspect of the knee. The discomfort and pain are aggravated on running, going up or down stairs, jumping, or subjecting the knee to direct pressure as by kneeling. With rest, the pain diminishes or disappears. On inspection and palpation, thickening of the patellar tendon and excessive enlargement of the tibial tuberosity are evident. The maximal area of tenderness is at the insertion of the patellar tendon to bone. There is no synovial thickening or effusion in the knee joint. The pain is increased by forced knee extension against resistance or in squatting with the knee in full flexion; both maneuvers put strain on the patellar tendon and the proximal tibial tubercle. The symptoms are aggravated by running and climbing or descending stairs. Associated findings are tautness of the quadriceps mechanism, especially the rectus femoris (as shown by the Ely test), the hamstrings (as shown by straight leg raising), and the triceps surae (as shown by passive dorsiflexion of the ankle).

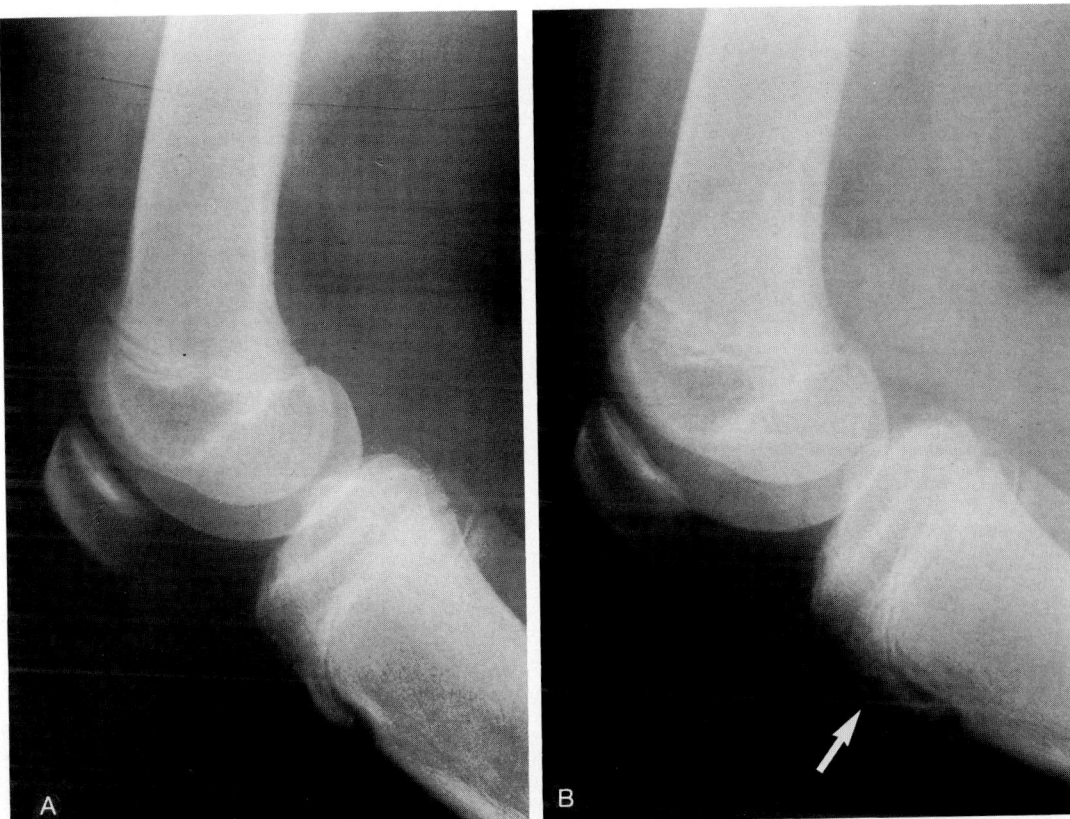

FIGURE 3–176. *Osgood-Schlatter disease of the left proximal tibia with free ossicle lying anterior to the proximal tibial tubercle.*

A. Normal right knee for comparison. **B.** Left knee. Note the arrow pointing to the ossicle.

Radiographic Findings

Radiograms in the acute stage will disclose soft-tissue swelling anterior to the tibial tuberosity and thickening of the ligamentum patellae. These are best visualized in the lateral view. In the male, the ossification center of the proximal tibial tubercle appears at about 11 years of age and fuses at 15 years. Irregularity in its ossification is a normal variation; *fragmentation of the epiphysis is not characteristic of Osgood-Schlatter disease.* In some knees one or more fragments in the tubercle show increased density; this has been the reason in the past for speculation that the cause of Osgood-Schlatter disease is avascular necrosis.

Woolfrey and Chandler have observed three distinct types of radiographic manifestations in the late stages of the disease. In *Type I*, the tibial tuberosity is *prominent* and irregular; in *Type II*, the tibial tuberosity is prominent and irregular, but in addition, there is a small free particle of bone located anterior and superior to the tibial tuberosity; in *Type III*, there is a free bone particle anterior and superior to the tibial tuberosity, but the tuberosity otherwise appears normal (Fig. 3–176 B).[41] Soft-tissue swelling is the only indication of active disease. In the lateral radiogram taken with the knee in full extension with the quadriceps muscle contracted, proximal displacement of the patella may be demonstrated in some cases.

Treatment

The disease is self-limited and ceases when the tibial tubercle fuses to the diaphysis. The type of treatment depends on the severity of the disease. In both mild and severe cases, symptoms will subside following simple restriction of excessive physical activities, such as active sports, running, jumping, basketball, and other impact activities. Participation in these should be limited for three months. The acutely painful knee may require a short period of crutch support. The contracted quadriceps mechanism should be stretched. This is crucial. Elongation of the shortened, hypertrophic, taut quadriceps muscle decreases its constant pull on the proximal tibial tuberosity. The triceps surae and hamstrings muscles are also stretched.

In the severe case or the moderate one that does not respond to the foregoing measures, the treatment consists of immobilization of the knee in a walking above-knee cylinder cast for three weeks, followed by curtailment of strenous exercise or sports for three months. During this period, stretching and muscle strengthening exercises are performed.

Some authors recommend injection of corticosteroids (such as hydrocortisone or prednisone) into the swollen patellar tendon and paraapophyseal soft tissues of the tibial tubercle to provide symptomatic relief. It is not recommended by this author. The local injection of corticosteroids is indicated very occasionally when either acute symptoms persist despite adequate trial of immobilization in a cast or there is a loose ossicle behind the patellar tendon with a surrounding inflamed bursa or both. In such instances, after corticosteroid injection, the quadriceps is protected in a cylinder above-knee walking cast for three weeks. It should be remembered that rupture of a patellar tendon can occur even without its being weakened with corticosteroid injections.

Operative measures are rarely, if ever, indicated. Excision of the prominent tibial tubercle is recommended by Ferciot and Thomson in an adolescent who has had recurring episodes of pain and disability, and in whom conservative measures have failed.[12, 38] In their experience, excision of the tubercle most effectively removes the deformity and cures the discomfort and disability with the shortest convalescence and the least risk. This author strongly recommends conservatism in management of acute Osgood-Schlatter disease; do not operate!

In some patients, an ossicle forms deep in the patellar ligament and anterior to the proximal aspect of the tibial tubercle. This ossicle is usually free from the underlying tibial tubercle and is attached to the distal posterior aspect of the patellar tendon. It is mobile, and a bursa containing viscous fluid may form around it, causing persistence of tenderness and local pain. This condition is called the *unsolved Osgood-Schlatter lesion* by Mital and associates as it does not resolve spontaneously or respond to nonoperative measures.[28] A painful loose ossicle in the patellar tendon is treated by surgical excision.

Both Ferciot and Thomson perform the operation through a longitudinal incision centered over the proximal tibial tubercle. This author recommends a transverse incision because the cosmetic appearance of the scar is more pleasing. The patellar tendon is split longitudinally into halves, and the tuberosity of the tibia is extraperiosteally exposed by elevation and retraction of the tendon medially and laterally. The peripheral and distal portions of the tendon are not detached. Any loose ossicles posterior to the patellar tendon and surrounding thickened bursae are excised. If the proximal tibial tubercle is very prominent it is exposed subperiosteally; cartilage, cortex, and cancellous bone are excised with a sharp osteotome until the bony prominence is completely removed. Tubercle thinning operations should be performed only when the tibial apophyseal and physeal growth plates are closed or near closure; when the tibial tubercle growth plate is open, operative intervention may cause its premature closure and result in genu recurvatum. The two halves of the patellar tendon are sutured together, and the wound is closed in layers. The limb is immobilized in an above-knee walking cylinder cast for three weeks.[12, 38]

Procedures that promote early fusion of the apophysis of the tuberosity to the diaphysis, such as pegging the tubercle to the tibial metaphysis with autogenous bone graft or drilling the tuberosity, are not recommended; they may relieve the symptoms, but the enlarged bony prominence of the tuberosity persists.[3]

Complications

In its residual stage, when the disease is inactive, enlargement of the tibial tuberosity may persist, and the *bony prominence* may become cosmetically deforming, especially in girls. It may also be a source of discomfort on kneeling. A rare complication first reported by Stirling is *premature fusion* of the proximal tibial tubercle and the anterior part of the upper tibial epiphysis. Continued growth of the posterior part of the epiphysis produces *genu recurvatum*.[35] Jeffreys reported such a patient in whom genu recurvatum was severe enough to require correction by osteotomy.[21]

Patella alta is another complication of Osgood-Schlatter disease. Jakob and associates determined the position of the patella in 185 knees with Osgood-Schlatter disease in 125 patients by the Blackburne and Peel method.[2, 20] In the normal person the patellar index is 0.80; they reconfirmed this in 73 control knees. Values over 1.00 represent patella alta. The average patellar index in the knees with Osgood-Schlatter disease measured 1.01 (patella alta) in boys and 0.91 in girls. In the presence of radiographic evidence of a loose ossicle in the patellar tendon, the patellar index is increased to 1.06 in boys. Occasionally the patella may be as much as 2 cm. higher on the involved side than on the normal side, resulting either from the upward pull of the tibial apophysis or from elongation of the patellar tendon. The abnormally high patella may recurrently become dislocated laterally, or it may lead to undue pressure on the lower facet of the patella, with consequent chondromalacia of the patella, and patellofemoral degenerative arthritis.

References

1. Bacon, L. C.: Schlatter's disease. Minn. Med., 19:67, 1936.
2. Blackburne, J. S., and Peel, T. E.: A new method of measuring patellar height. J. Bone Joint Surg., 59-B:241, 1977.
3. Bosworth, D. M.: Autogenous bone pegging for epiphysitis of the tibial tubercle. J. Bone Joint Surg., 16:829, 1934.
4. Bowers, K. D., Jr.: Patellar tendon avulsion as a complication of Osgood-Schlatter's disease. Am. J. Sports Med., 9:356, 1981.
5. Cohen, B., and Wilkinson, R. W.: The Osgood-Schlatter lesion. A radiological and histological study. Am. J. Surg., 95:731, 1958.
6. Cole, J. P.: A study of Osgood-Schlatter disease. Surg. Gynecol. Obstet., 65:55, 1937.
7. Ehrenborg, G.: The Osgood-Schlatter lesion. Acta Chir. Scand., Suppl. 288, 1962.
8. Ehrenborg, G., and Engfeldt, B.: Radiographic changes in the Osgood-Schlatter lesion. Acta Chir. Scand., 121:315, 1961.
9. Ehrenborg, G., and Engfeldt, B.: Histologic changes in the Osgood-Schlatter lesion. Acta Chir. Scand., 121:328, 1961.
10. Ehrenborg, G., and Engfeldt, B.: The insertion of the ligamentum patellae on the tibial tuberosity. Some news in connection with the Osgood-Schlatter lesion. Acta Chir. Scand., 121:491, 1961.
11. Fels, E.: Über die Entwicklung der Tuberositas tibiae und die Genese der Schlatterschen Krankheit. Arch. Klin. Chir., 129:552, 1924.
12. Ferciot, C. F.: Surgical management of anterior tibial epiphysis. Clin. Orthop., 5:204, 1955.
13. Hodgson, E. S., Kaplan, Y. S., and Edmonds, N. R.: Unusual presentation of Osgood-Schlatter's disease. Br. J. Ind. Med., 37:90, 1980.
14. Hogh, J., and Lund, B.: Sequelae of Osgood-Schlatter in adults. Ugeskr. Laeger, 144:1530, 1982.
15. Holstein, E. R., Lewis, G. B., and Schulze, E. R.: Heterotopic ossification of patellar tendon. J. Bone Joint Surg., 45-A:656, 1963.
16. Hughes, E. S. R.: Osgood-Schlatter's disease. Surg. Gynecol. Obstet., 86:323, 1948.
17. Insall, J., and Salvati, E.: Patella position in the normal knee joint. Radiology, 101:101, 1971.
18. Insall, J., Goldberg, V., and Salvati, E.: Recurrent dislocation and the high-riding patella. Clin. Orthop., 88:67, 1972.
19. Jakob, R. P., and Segesser, B.: Quadriceps-Dehnungsubungen—ein neues Konzept in der Behandlung der Tendinosen des Streckapparates am Kniegelenk (jumper's knee). Orthopaede, 9:201, 1980.
20. Jakob, R. P., von Gumppenberg, S., and Engelhardt, P.: Does Osgood-Schlatter disease influence the position of the patella? J. Bone Joint Surg., 63-B:579, 1981.
21. Jeffreys, T. E.: Genu recurvatum after Osgood-Schlatter's disease. Report of a case. J. Bone Joint Surg., 47-B:298, 1965.
22. King, A. G., and Blundell-Jones, G.: A surgical procedure for the Osgood-Schlatter lesion. Am. J. Sports Med., 9:250, 1981.
23. Lancourt, J. E., and Cristini, J. A.: Patella alta and patella infera. J. Bone Joint Surg., 57-A:1112, 1975.
24. LaZerte, G. D., and Rapp, I. H.: Pathogenesis of Osgood-Schlatter's disease. Am. J. Pathol., 34:803, 1958.
25. Levine, J., and Kashyap, S.: A new conservative treatment of Osgood-Schlatter disease. Clin. Orthop., 158:126, 1981.
26. Liselotte, M., and Schott, H. J.: Local hydrocortisone therapy of Schlatter's disease and its local side-effects. Med. Klin., 56:1834, 1961.
27. Mital, M. A., and Matza, R. A.: Osgood-Schlatter's disease: The painful puzzler. Phys. Sports Med., 5:60, 1977.
28. Mital, M. A., Matza, R. A., and Cohen, J.: The so-called unsolved Osgood-Schlatter lesion. A concept based on fifteen surgically treated lesions. J. Bone Joint Surg., 62-A:732, 1980.
29. Ogden, J. A., and Southwick, W. O.: Osgood-Schlatter's disease and tibial tuberosity development. Clin. Orthop., 116:180, 1976.
30. Osgood, R. B.: Lesions of the tibial tubercle occurring during adolescence. Boston Med. Surg., J., 148:114, 1903.
31. Rapp, I. H., and LaZerte, G.: Clinical pathological correlation in Osgood-Schlatter's disease. South. Med. J., 51:909, 1958.
32. Schlatter, C.: Verletzungen des schnabelformigen Forsatzes der oberen Tibiaepiphyse. Beitr. Klin. Chir., 38:874, 1903.
33. Smillie, I. S.: Diseases of the Knee Joint. 2nd Ed. Edinburgh, London, Churchill-Livingstone, 1980.
34. Stinchfield, A. J.: The tenosynovitis of Osgood-Schlatter disease. J. Bone Joint Surg., 45-A:1335, 1963.
35. Stirling, R. I.: Complications of Osgood-Schlatter's disease. J. Bone Joint Surg., 34-B:149, 1952.
36. Straajescu, E., and Bercu, G.: Apophysite rotulienne bilatérale associée à une ostéochondrite tibiale antérieure. Acta Orthop. Belg., 34:879, 1968.
37. Thompson, M. S., and Dickinson, P. H.: Osgood-Schlatter's disease in the Army. J. Int. Coll. Surg., 23:170, 1955.
38. Thomson, J. E. M.: Operative treatment of osteochondritis of the tibial tubercle. J. Bone Joint Surg., 38-A:142, 1956.
39. Uhry, E., Jr.: Osgood-Schlatter's disease. Arch. Surg., 48:406, 1944.
40. Willner, P.: Osgood-Schlatter's disease. Etiology and treatment. Clin. Orthop., 62:178, 1969.
41. Woolfrey, B. F., and Chandler, E. F.: Manifestations of Osgood-Schlatter's disease in late teen age and early adulthood. J. Bone Joint Surg., 42-A:327, 1960.
42. Wray, D. G., and Muddu, B. N.: Operative treatment for longstanding Osgood-Schlatter's disease. J. R. Coll. Surg. Edinb., 27:200, 1982.

PANNER'S DISEASE (OSTEOCHONDRITIS OF THE HUMERAL CAPITELLUM)

Changes in the epiphyses of the humeral capitellum similar to those of Legg-Perthes disease were described by Panner in 1927.[17]

Smith, in 1964, described two patients and reviewed an additional 26 cases recorded in the literature. He concluded that the condition was not related to trauma, was self-limited in its course, and did not require treatment.[23]

Lateral elbow joint damage due to compression forces of the radial head to the capitellum occurs because of repetitive valgus stress while pitching. This has been referred to as "Little League elbow".[2] It occurs primarily in boys between the ages of 11 and 17 years, involving the dominant upper limb. It is also seen in high-performance female gymnasts, in whom involvement may be bilateral.[20]

It is apparent that there are two forms of osteochondrosis of the capitellum of the humerus: one appears to be constitutional and of unknown etiology, occurring in the juvenile period, and possibly nontraumatic in its pathogenesis. This is the form described by Panner. The second form of osteochondrosis of the capitellum of the humerus occurs in the preadolescent and adolescent, and is traumatic in its etiology.

Pathology

In Panner's disease, histologic studies have shown focal avascular necrosis of the subcondral epiphyseal bone with repair and revascularization. The articular cartilage appears normal.

Clinical Features

Pain and stiffness of the elbow are the presenting complaints. On examination, varying degrees of flexion contracture, local tenderness over the capitellum, and minimal synovial thickening and effusion of the elbow joint are found. When there is a loose fragment, the joint will lock.

Radiographic Features

These disclose irregular areas of increased radiolucency with areas of sclerosis in the capitellum (Fig. 3–177). Comparative radiograms of both elbows should be taken. Advanced skeletal maturation of the radial head may result from increased circulation to the part.

Treatment

The type of treatment will depend on whether the osteochondral lesions are attached to the capitellum (Type I), or have become detached and are loose fragments in the elbow joint (Type II).

In Type I lesions, treatment consists of immobilization of the upper limb in an above-elbow cast for three to six weeks until the associated acute synovitis and local tenderness subside. Then the elbow is supported for one to two months in a bivalved cast or a plastic splint, which allows both partial protection and motion to the joint. Stressful elbow activities involving throwing objects should be avoided until radiographically evident healing has taken place.

If after six weeks of protection the osteochondral segment does not heal, drilling of the segment through the arthroscope is indicated. This will enhance the healing process.

When the fragments are detached lesions (Type II), they should be removed by an open arthrotomy, and their base should be drilled. This author has found arthroscopic removal of the bone fragment feasible, but cumbersome and often not thorough. If a loose fragment is left in the elbow joint, the symptoms will persist and there will be permanent residual limitation of range of motion of the elbow.

References

1. Adams, J. E.: Injury to the throwing arm. A study of traumatic changes in the elbow joint of boy baseball players. Calif. Med., 102:127, 1965.
2. Brogdon, B. G., and Crow, N. E.: Little Leaguer's elbow. A.J.R., 83:671, 1960.
3. Busch, E.: Et tilfaelde af Panners Sygdom. Ugeskr. Laeger, 92:720, 1930.
4. Chiroff, R. T., and Cooke, C. P.: Osteochondritis dissecans: A histological and microradiographic analysis of surgically excised lesions. J. Trauma, 15:688, 1975.
5. Elward, J. F.: Epiphysitis of the capitellum of the humerus. J.A.M.A., 112:705, 1939.
6. Haroldsson, S.: On osteochondrosis deformans juvenilis capitoli humeri, including investigation of intra-osseous vasculature in distal humerus. Acta Orthop. Scand., Suppl. 38:1, 1959.
7. Heller, C. J., and Wiltse, L. L.: Avascular necrosis of the capitellum humeri (Panner's disease). J. Bone Joint Surg., 42-A:513, 1960.
8. Klein, E. W.: Osteochondrosis of the capitellum (Panner's disease). Report of a case. A.J.R., 88:466, 1962.
9. Lange, J.: Aseptic necrosis of the capitellum of the humerus: Panner's disease. Acta Chir. Scand., 108:301, 1954.
10. Laurent, L. E., and Lindstrom, B. L.: Osteochondrosis of the capitellum humeri (Panner's disease). Acta Orthop. Scand., 26:111, 1956.
11. Lindholm, T. S., Osterman, K., and Vankka, E.: Osteochondritis dissecans of elbow, ankle and hip: A comparison survey. Clin. Orthop., 148:245, 1980.
12. Lipscomb, A. B.: Baseball pitching injuries in growing athletes. J. Sports Med., 3:25, 1975.
13. March, H. C.: Osteochondritis of the capitellum (Panner's disease). A.J.R., 51:682, 1944.
14. Mitsunagna, M. M., Adishian, D. A., and Bianco, A. J., Jr.: Osteochondritis dissecans of the capitellum. J. Trauma, 22:53, 1981.
15. Nijst, P. M. E. E.: Morbus Panner. Ned. Tijdschr. Geneeskd., 81:1243, 1937.

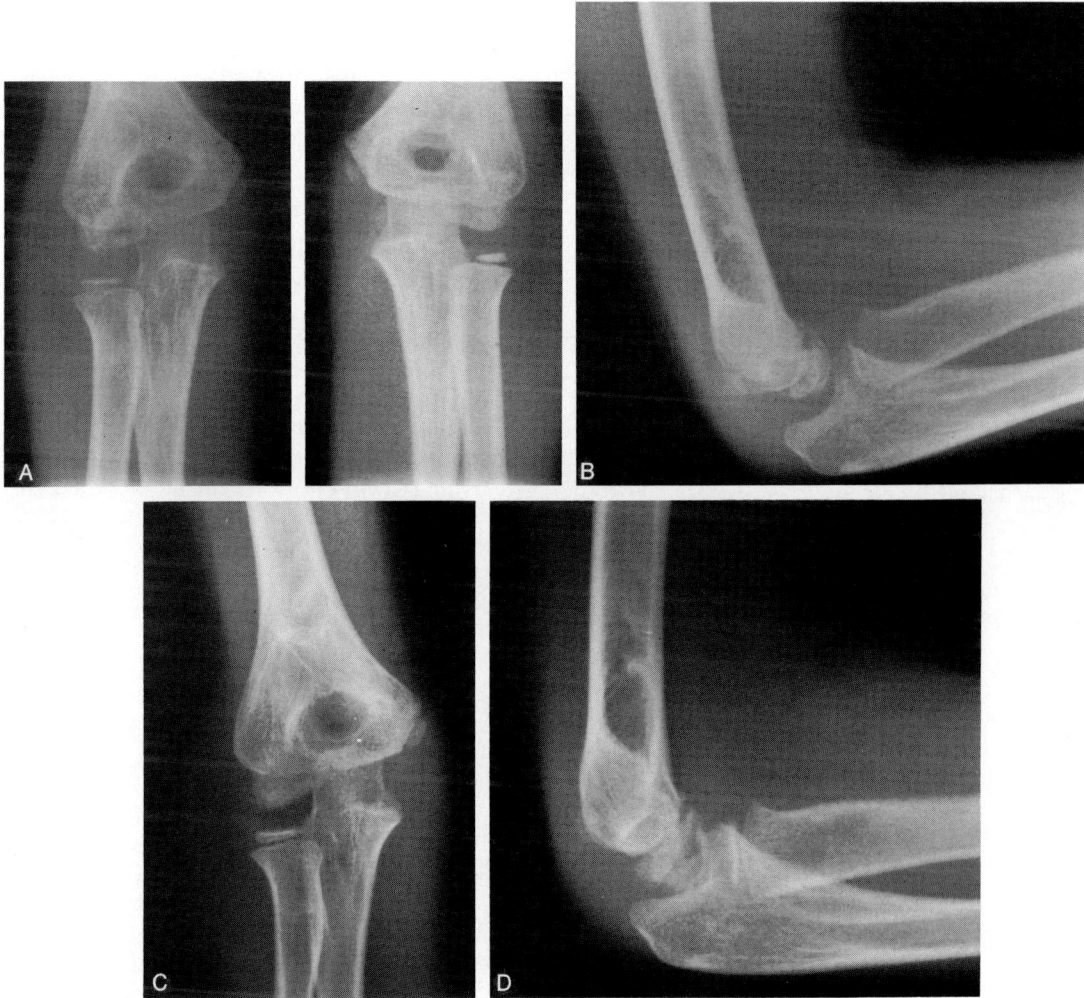

FIGURE 3–177. *Panner's disease of the capitellum of distal right humerus in an eight-year-old boy.*

A. Anteroposterior radiograms of both elbows. **B.** Lateral radiogram of right elbow. Note the irregular area of radiolucency and sclerosis of the capitellum. **C** and **D.** Five months later there is revascularization of the capitellum. Patient was treated by above-elbow cast for two months.

16. Omer, G. E., and Conger, C. C.: Osteochondrosis of the capitulum humeri (Panner's disease). U.S. Armed Forces Med. J., 10:1235, 1959.
17. Panner, H. J.: An affection of the capitulum humeri resembling Calvé-Perthes disease of the hip. Acta Radiol., 8:617, 1927.
18. Panner, H. J.: A peculiar affection of the capitulum humeri, resembling Calvé-Perthes disease of the hip. Acta Radiol., 10:234, 1929.
19. Pritsch, M., Engel, J., and Farin, I.: Panner's disease. Harefuah, 99:171, 1980.
20. Roberts, N., and Hughes, K.: Osteochondritis dissecans of the elbow joint: A clinical study. J. Bone Joint Surg., 32-B:348, 1950.
21. Rokkanen, P.: Osteochondrosis of capitulum humeri (Panner's disease): Report of a case. Ann. Chir. Gynaecol. Fenn., 47:356, 1958.
22. Singer, K. M., and Roy, S. P.: Osteochondrosis of the humerus. Am. J. Sports Med., 12:351, 1984.
23. Smith, M. G. H.: Osteochondritis of the humeral capitulum. J. Bone Joint Surg., 46-B:50, 1964.
24. Suman, R. K., and Miller, J. H.: Panner's disease: Osteochondritis of the capitellum of the humerus. J. R. Coll. Surg. Edinb., 27:62, 1982.
25. Tivnon, M. C., Anzel, S. H., and Waugh, T. R.: Surgical management of osteochondritis dissecans of the capitellum. Am. J. Sports Med., 4:121, 1976.
26. Torg, J. S., Pollack, H., and Sweterlitsch, P.: The effect of competitive pitching on the shoulders and elbows of pre-adolescent baseball players. Pediatrics, 19:267, 1972.
27. Tullos, H. S., and King, J. W.: Lesions of the pitching arm in adolescents. J.A.M.A., 220:264, 1972.
28. Woodward, A. H., and Bianco, A. J., Jr.: Osteochondritis dissecans of the elbow. Clin. Orthop., 110:35, 1975.

MISCELLANEOUS SO-CALLED OSTEOCHONDROSES

Ischiopubic "Osteochondritis"

Irregular rarefaction and swelling of the ischiopubic synchondrosis was thought to be osteochondritis by Van Neck. Further clinical, radiologic, and histopathologic studies, however, do not justify the inclusion of these cases in the group of osteochondritis. Specimens obtained at operation have disclosed normal closing epiphyses. Caffey and Ross found the age of closure of the ischiopubic synchondrosis to be variable, usually between 9 and 11 years of age, but extending from 4 to 12 years. Irregular ossification and swelling of the ischiopubic synchondrosis is a normal finding, occurring at some time in almost all, or perhaps all, children.

Sever's disease, or so-called "apophysitis" of the os calcis, is not an osteochondrosis. Irregularity of ossification and sclerosis of the apophysis is a normal radiographic finding.[1-3]

References

1. Caffey, J., and Ross, S. E.: The ischiopubic synchondrosis in healthy children: Some normal roentgenographic findings. Am. J. Roentgenol., 76:488, 1956.
2. Neck, M. van: Osteochondrite du pubis. Arch. Franco-Belges Chir., 27:238, 1924.
3. Sever, J. W.: Apophysitis of the os calcis. N.Y. Med. J., 95:1025, 1912; Am. J. Orthop., 15:659, 1917.

SLIPPED CAPITAL FEMORAL EPIPHYSIS

During a period of rapid growth in adolescence, weakening of the upper femoral physis and shearing stress from incumbent body weight may cause the femoral head to become displaced from its normal relation to the femoral neck. The usual deformity consists of an upward and anterior movement of the femoral neck on the capital epiphysis, which becomes displaced posteriorly and inferiorly. The femoral head maintains its normal relationship with the acetabulum. Occasionally, however, the slip is outward, i.e., the femoral head is displaced laterally (superiorly) and posteriorly in relation to the femoral neck. During the stance phase of gait the femoral neck tends to move forward, a force that is resisted by the inertia of body weight. Very occasionally in traumatic slip the femoral head may be displaced anteriorly.

Müller is generally recognized as being the first to describe the slipped capital femoral epiphysis as an entity. He coined the term *Schenkelhalsverbiegungen im Jungesalter*, meaning "bending of the femoral neck in adolescence."[269]

Incidence and Epidemiology

The incidence of slipped capital femoral epiphysis varies according to race, sex, and geographic location. There is a greater risk for developing slipped capital femoral epiphysis in the black, the male, and the person residing in the eastern part of the United States. In a study of the incidence and distribution of slipped capital femoral epiphysis in Connecticut and the Southwestern United States, Kelsey and associates reported that the overall annual incidence per 100,000 in the population under 25 years of age in Connecticut was 3.41, whereas in New Mexico it was 0.71, almost a fivefold difference between the two areas. It is lowest in the Mountain and Great Plains states.[189-195]

The male is at greater risk for developing slipped capital femoral epiphysis; the male to female ratio in Connecticut was 2.67 : 1, whereas in the Southwest it was 1.70 : 1. The sex incidence as reported in the literature varies, males being affected two to five times as frequently as females.

There is a definite predilection for the black race. Estimates by Kelsey and associates show the race incidence rates in Connecticut were 7.79 per 100,000 for black males versus 4.74 for Caucasian males; 6.68 for black females versus 1.64 for Caucasian females. The risk among Hispanics appears to be similar to that of Caucasians.[195]

The age of onset is during adolescence—a period of maximal skeletal growth (boys 13 to 15 years and girls 11 to 13). It rarely occurs in girls following menarche. When slipped capital femoral epiphysis occurs in a juvenile (10 years and under) an endocrine diagnostic work-up is in order.

There are no urban-rural gradients; social class does not appear to be of any consequence.

Bilateral involvement of the hips is found in approximately 25 per cent of cases; recently, however, computed tomographic studies have shown the incidence of bilateral involvement to be much higher—up to 50 per cent. The left side is affected somewhat more often than the right.

Classification

Slipping of the upper femoral epiphysis may be classified as *acute* or *chronic*. Acute slip may be further subdivided as acute traumatic and acute on chronic.

The severity of the slipping may be categorized as: *preslip, or Grade I*, in which there is widening and rarefaction of the physis but no actual displacement of the epiphysis; *minimal slip, or Grade II*, in which the extent of maximal displacement of the femoral head is up to one third of the superior metaphyseal width of the femoral neck; *moderate slip, or Grade III*, in which migration of the neck is greater than one third but less than half of the upper metaphyseal diameter of the femoral neck; and *severe, or Grade IV*, in which displacement of the epiphysis is greater than 50 per cent. The degree of displacement of the femoral neck should always be determined in the radiographic view showing the greatest amount of it—almost always the true lateral projection.

Etiology

The cause of slipped capital femoral epiphysis is multifactorial. Four factors may operate in its pathogenesis, namely (1) increased height of the capital femoral physis; (2) changes in the geometry of the capital physis and adjacent bone (i.e., alteration in the inclination angle and planarity of the physis); (3) abnormal loading of the growth plate; and (4) insufficiency of the tensile (collagen) and hydrostatic (proteoglycans) components of the growth plate. It is not essential that all these predisposing factors exist for the slip to occur.

The immediate cause of slipping of the capital femoral epiphysis is mechanical, i.e., the shearing stress exerted on the epiphysis is greater than the resistance provided by the anatomic stability of the physis, and the femoral head is displaced.

In slipped capital femoral epiphysis the displacement of the epiphysis is a gradual process because of the viscoelasticity of the weakened growth plate. The perichondrium is intact. The normal capital femoral epiphysis separates only under the stress of tremendous shearing force; the result is a Salter-Harris Type I epiphyseal fracture separation with disruption of the perichondrium.

The growth plate's anatomic stability against shear stress is provided by the perichondrium, the perichondrial ring, the transphyseal collagen fibers, the mamillary processes, the central and peripheral geometric contour of the physis, the inclination angle of the physis, and the height of the growth plate (Fig. 3–178).[354]

The *perichondrial ring* is a fibrous band that encircles the physis at the cartilage-bone junction. Its shear strength is provided by collagen fibers that run obliquely, vertically, and circumferentially. These collagen fibers span the physis, attaching into the ossification groove on the epiphyseal side and to the subperiosteal bone on the metaphyseal side. The perichondrial ring acts as a limiting membrane, giving mechanical support to the physis. In childhood the perichondrium is thick, accounting for about 75 per cent of the resistance to shear stress. With advancing age it thins and, during the adolescent rapid growth spurts, is further stretched, and its ability to hold the femoral head in place is decreased.

Experimentally it has been demonstrated that the weakest part of the physis is the layer of cartilage cells nearest the metaphysis; once the overlying perichondrium is incised, the epiphysis will be displaced upon application of a shearing force.[196]

The *transphyseal collagen fibers* also provide tensile strength to shearing forces across the growth plate.[62, 133, 362] Under shear stress the transphyseal collagen fibers separate first, indicating that their elastic modulus is higher, plasticity is less, and ultimate strength is less

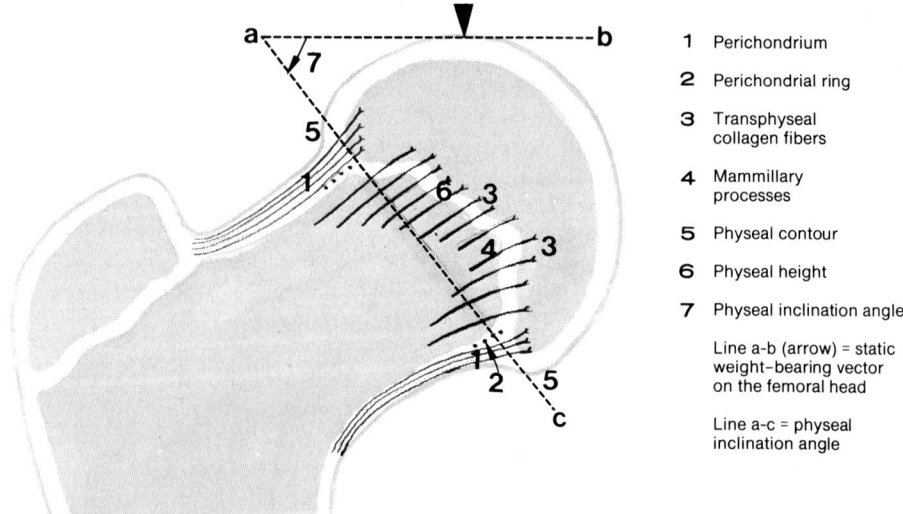

FIGURE 3–178. Anatomic factors that provide stability to the capital femoral epiphysis to shearing stress.

(Redrawn from Speer, D., Experimental epiphysiolysis: etiologic models of slipped capital femoral epiphysis [Fig. 6–2]. Proceedings of the Hip Society. St. Louis, C. V. Mosby Co., 1982, p. 71.)

than that of the perichondrium. This is accounted for by the brittleness of the transphyseal collagen fibers secondary to mineralization.[354] Lathyritic agents influence cross-linking of collagen fiber groups—in osteolathyrism, the decrease in collagen tensile strength causes slipped epiphyses.[4]

The *mammillary processes* at the epiphyseal-metaphyseal interface are interdigitating reciprocal pegs of bone and cartilage that stabilize the growth plate. With skeletal maturation, the load-carrying capacity and the shear resistance of the mammillary processes increase, and the strength of the perichondrial complex decreases.[62]

The *contour of the growth plate* is convex toward the epiphysis, and at the periphery of the physis is undulated. This geometric configuration resists linear and torque shear forces.

The plane of the capital femoral physis in relation to the axis of weight-bearing force, the *physeal inclination angle*, changes its direction in adolescence from horizontal to oblique. This change increases shearing force across the growth plate.

The moment arm through which shear forces act on the soft physis is lengthened by increased *thickness of the growth plate*. The height of the physis is determined by the rates of proliferation and hypertrophy of the cartilage cells, of expansion and calcification of cartilage matrix, and of encroachment of enchondral bone. Increased height of the physis may be caused by (1) increased growth hormone activity (e.g., in pituitary adenoma), exogenous growth hormone, and chorionic gonadotropin; (2) increased somatomedin; (3) hypogonadism; (4) increased testosterone; (5) hypothyroidism; (6) hyperthyroidism (transient); (7) hypopituitarism; (8) decreased vitamin D function (e.g., dietary deficiency, metabolic defect, renal osteodystrophy); (9) hyperparathyroidism (e.g., renal osteodystrophy, parathyroid adenoma); (10) vascular ischemia of the metaphysis; and (11) deficient enchondral ossification.*

Slipped capital femoral epiphysis occurs during a period of accelerated skeletal growth at puberty when significant endocrine changes take place; therefore, the possibility of endocrine dysfunction as a predisposing cause is always raised. Clinically this is supported by the finding that adolescents with slipped capital femoral epiphysis often have adiposogenital syndrome (obesity and underdeveloped genitalia) or, less commonly, are tall and thin, which indicates a very rapid growth spurt.

Growth hormone stimulates the synthesis of somatomedin, which in turn stimulates cartilage cell metabolism, with resultant widening of the hypertrophied cartilage cell layer of the physis.

---

*See references: increased growth hormone, 103, 152, 266, 316; hypogonadism, 136, 285, 301, 348; increased testosterone, 152, 266; hypothyroidism, 106, 136, 144, 151, 181, 259; hypopituitarism, 136, 313; decreased vitamin D, 215, 247, 344; hyperparathyroidism, 61, 215, 247, 344; ischemia, 355, 411.

Discontinuity of the growth plate in slipped capital femoral epiphysis takes place primarily at the hypertrophied cartilage cell layer. The increase in thickness of this layer decreases its shear strength.

Estrogens and androgens depress the proliferation of cartilage cells and cause a decrease in thickness of the growth plate. A comprehensive discussion of the mechanism of action of sex hormones on the physis is presented by Ogden and Southwick.[283] A girl who has had her menarche is almost immune from slipped capital femoral epiphysis.

Harris devised an apparatus to determine the shearing strength of the upper tibial epiphysis in normal rats, in rats receiving growth hormone, and in those receiving estrogen. He demonstrated that, when the epiphyses separate from the diaphysis, the plane of disruption is through the third layer of the physis, and that pituitary growth hormone decreases the shearing strength of the physis while sex hormone increases it.[132] Harris and Hobson further suggested that these findings may be significant in providing an anatomic basis for slipping of the capital femoral epiphysis in man; that slipping in the large obese adolescent may be associated with a deficiency of sex hormone, whereas in the tall thin child, it may be related to an excess of growth hormone. In both circumstances, the physis is subjected to the predominant influence of growth hormone and undergoes a decrease in its shearing strength. This process most probably affects every physis in the body, but the upper femoral epiphyseal plate is particularly subjected to the shearing forces of normal weight-bearing and may slip, perhaps even following trivial unnoticed injury.[133]

Gelberman and associates, in a computed tomographic study in 39 hips, showed that there definitely is a decreased angle of femoral anteversion with the development of slipped capital femoral epiphysis. It appears that the mechanical forces that act across the capital femoral physis are altered by this rotational deformity, which exerts abnormally increased shear stresses and causes anatomic failure of the growth plate.[116]

During puberty, a period of activation of the gonads and the cessation of growth, the structure of the physis varies according to relative levels of growth hormone and sex hormone in the circulation. Surveys of patients with slipped capital femoral epiphysis in the usual age group, however, have failed to demonstrate any endocrine abnormality. Burrows studied 100 cases of slipped capital femoral epiphysis and found normal excretion of urinary ketosteroids. Clinically, however, one quarter of the males and two thirds of the females appeared to have some constitutional abnormality suggesting endocrine dysfunction. He could not demonstrate any relationship between constitutional factors and bilateral affection.[52] Razzano and associates found normal levels of serum growth hormone and urinary estrogens and ketosteroids.[309]

In the literature there are numerous reports of patients with slipped capital femoral epiphysis and concomitant endocrine dysfunction.* There are reported cases of slipped capital femoral epiphysis occurring during the course of treatment for short stature by administration of growth hormones (Fig. 3–179).[103, 316] It seems that a patient receiving growth hormone therapy is at risk for slipped capital femoral epiphysis. In untreated hypothyroidism, slipped capital femoral epiphysis may occur (Fig. 3–180).[26, 96, 259, 283] The weakening of the physis in hypothyroidism is caused by deficiency in the matrix of the cartilage of the growth plate. Slipped capital femoral epiphysis may occur in cretinism (congenital hypothyroidism) or in juvenile myxedema (primary acquired hypothyroidism). In cretinism the upper femoral epiphysis is fragmented, whereas in juvenile myxedema the endocrine disturbance occurs after ossification of the epiphysis is well advanced and, which therefore does not appear stippled in the radiogram. Ossification is delayed, however. The small size of the ossific nucleus of the femoral head should make the orthopedic surgeon suspect hypothyroidism. Radiograms of the left hand should be made for bone age. A short obese child who complains of thigh-knee pain and a limp should have anteroposterior and true lateral radiograms of both hips made to rule out slipped capital femoral epiphysis. A thorough medical history and physical examination are also critical to rule out hypothyroidism. Is the child doing poorly in school? Does he mix up words? Is his recent recall poor? Does he perform calculations slowly? Does he complain of cold and have abnormal diminution of sweating? The hypothyroid child is short and obese with a round fat face. The hair is sparse and coarse. The skin is thick and dry. The tongue is enlarged, and the dentition is often deciduous. The thyroid gland is small or cannot be palpated. There may be pretibial edema. The deep

---

*See references 5, 26, 61, 90, 100, 103, 151, 226, 229, 230, 251, 272, 283, 301, 316, 319, 340, 348, 358, 413.

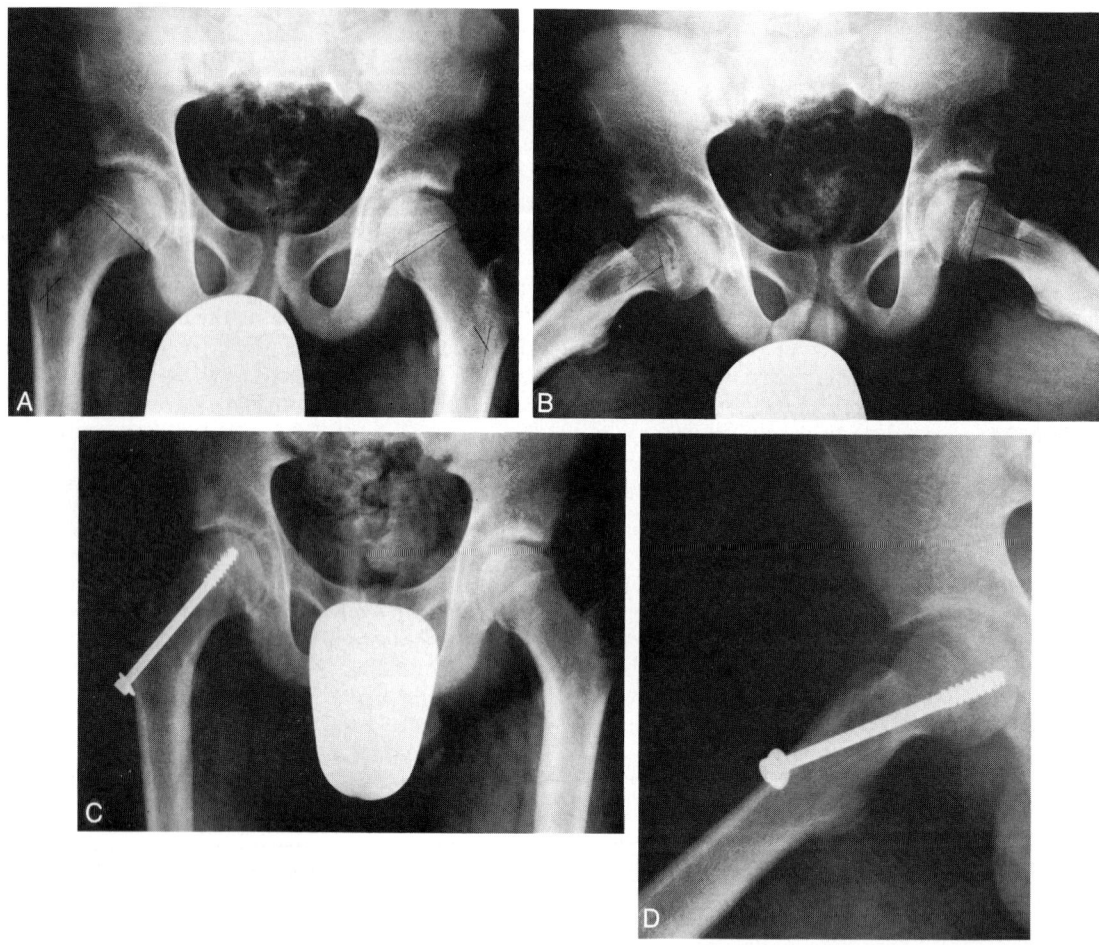

FIGURE 3–179. Slipped capital femoral epiphysis of the right hip in a 12-year-old boy who was receiving growth hormone therapy for short stature.

A and **B.** Initial anteroposterior and frog-leg radiograms of both hips. **C** and **D.** Postoperative radiograms. The right hip was pinned with one Asnis screw.

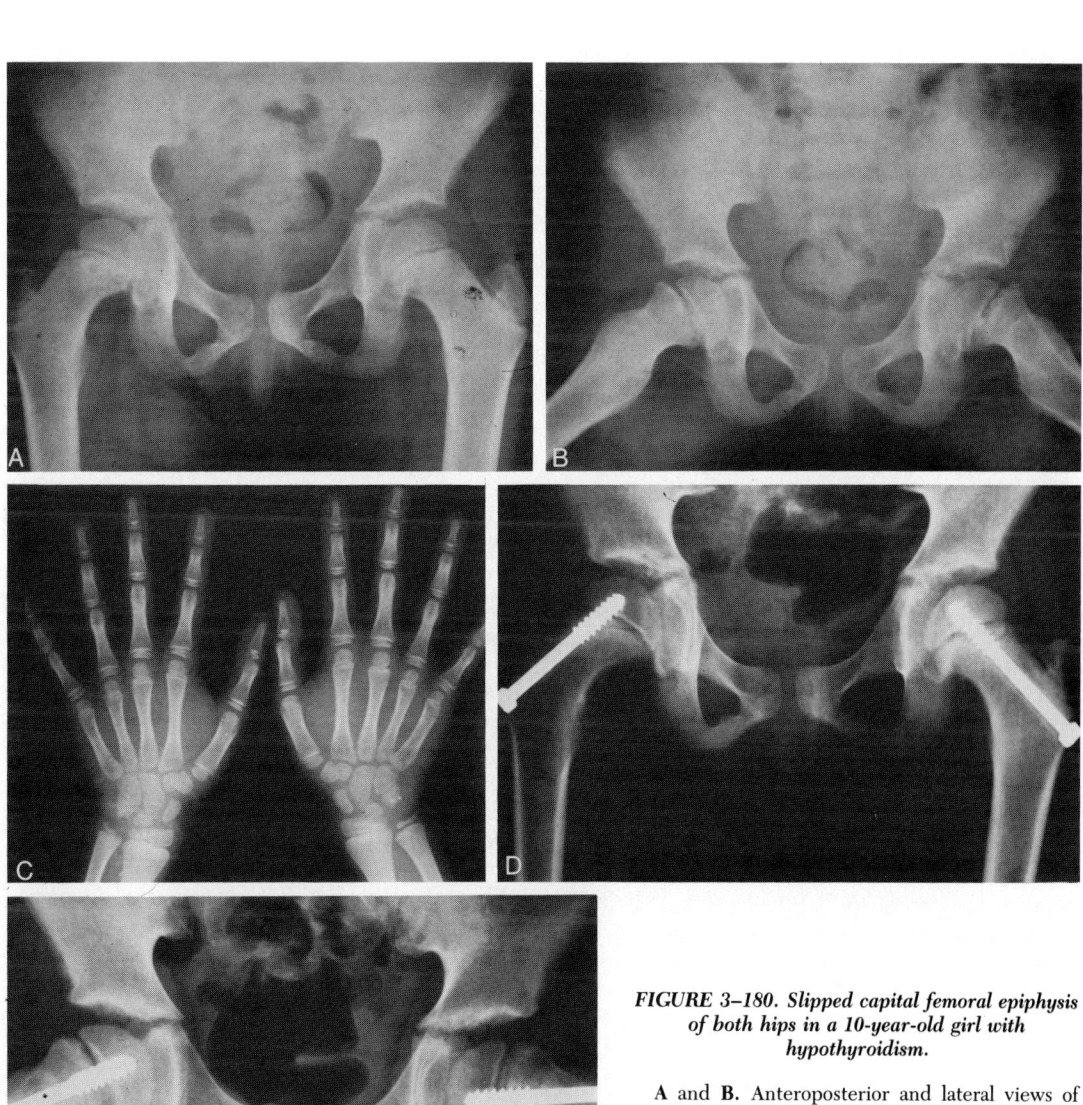

FIGURE 3–180. Slipped capital femoral epiphysis of both hips in a 10-year-old girl with hypothyroidism.

A and **B.** Anteroposterior and lateral views of both hips. **C.** Anteroposterior radiogram of the hands showing marked retardation of bone age. **D** and **E.** Postoperative radiograms of the hips.

tendon reflexes are markedly delayed. Patients suspected of hypothyroidism should have endocrine consultation and laboratory diagnostic studies—low values of T3 and T4 uptake and elevated serum TSH level will substantiate the clinical diagnosis of hypothyroidism. A thyroid scan should also be made. Cardiac and pulmonary function are assessed prior to surgical intervention. Hypothyroid patients tolerate anesthesia poorly, especially because of hypothermia and poor cardiac output. It is preferable to treat them to achieve a euthyroid state prior to operation.

Slipped capital femoral epiphysis can occur during treatment for hypothyroidism. This is owing to the pubertal type of growth spurt following the surge of growth hormone secretion as a result of regeneration of the acidophilic cells in the pituitary as the hypothyroidism is corrected.[413]

Administration of chorionic gonadotropin causes a rapid growth spurt. Hirsch and Hirsch reported slipped capital femoral epiphysis in a boy who was treated with chorionic gonadotropin for "retarded puberty"; in a period of two to three months his height increased 8.9 cm. and he developed right slipped capital femoral epiphysis.[152]

Patients with craniopharyngioma can develop slipped capital femoral epiphysis.[126, 229, 283, 100] Other endocrinopathies in which slipped capital femoral epiphysis has developed are: acromegaly, gigantism, hypopituitarism, hypogonadism, hypogonadism with mosaic (XY/XXY) Kleinfelter's syndrome, and hyperparathyroidism (secondary to adenoma).* It behooves the orthopedic surgeon to suspect and rule out endocrine dysfunction when a patient beyond the usual age range presents with slipped capital femoral epiphysis, and vice versa—patients with endocrinopathy or those receiving growth hormone should be thoroughly checked to rule out slipped capital femoral epiphysis.

The height of the physis will increase in renal osteodystrophy with secondary hyperparathyroidism, and slipped capital femoral epiphysis in association with renal failure has been reported by numerous authors (Fig. 3–181).[45, 107, 200, 247, 278, 344, 363] Pathologic studies of post mortem cases by Krempien and associates have shown that the major changes occurred in the proliferating cartilage cells of the growth plate and in the zone between the metaphysis and the growth plate, the latter change due to hyperparathyroidism.[215] In primary hyperparathyroidism, slipped epiphysis is also noted.[200] Epiphysiolysis in renal failure is due to osteitis fibrosa; the cartilaginous growth plate is separated from the metaphyseal spongiosa by chondroclastic removal of hypertrophic cartilage. The space between the physis and metaphysis is filled with dense fibrous tissue, providing a plane of slippage. The trabeculae of the primary spongiosa consist entirely of woven bone. In the radiogram the wide radiolucent zone between the ossific center and the metaphysis is due to poorly mineralized woven bone and fibrous tissue in the primary spongiosa; the broad radiolucent line does not reflect accumulation of cartilage and chondro-osteoid.[247]

Inheritance

Increased familial incidence of slipped capital femoral epiphysis was reported in 1967 by Rennie, who gave an account of eight families in which more than one case had occurred.[314] In 1982, in a study of the families of 140 patients with slipped capital femoral epiphysis, he found 14 families with more than one case and 23 other families in which the index patient had one or more close relatives with osteoarthritis of the hip, of whom six probably had had slipped capital femoral epiphysis.[315] Ochsner and associates reported ten members of a family with slipped capital femoral epiphysis, and two additional descendants with osteoarthritis probably due to slipped capital femoral epiphysis.[281] Both Rennie and Ochsner believed the mode of inheritance was autosomal and dominant with variable penetrance in the majority.

It should be stressed that the majority of cases of slipped capital femoral epiphysis occur sporadically. It seems, however, that in some families heredity does play a role.

Pathology

The pathologic changes depend on the stage and degree of displacement. They have been well described in the literature.[160, 211, 218, 253, 300, 362, 387]

In the preslipping stage the physis is widened, primarily in the zone of hypertrophy, which is composed of cartilage cells in disarrayed clusters instead of orderly columns. Fibrillated eosinophilic septa separate the cartilage clusters. There are islands of unorganized cartilage dispersed irregularly in the proximal metaphysis. The synovial membrane is engorged, edematous, and swollen. There are no

---

*See references: acromegaly, 229; gigantism, 311, hypopituitarism, 100, 340, 348, 358; hypogonadism, 27, 90, Klinefelter's syndrome, 301; hyperparathyroidism, 61.

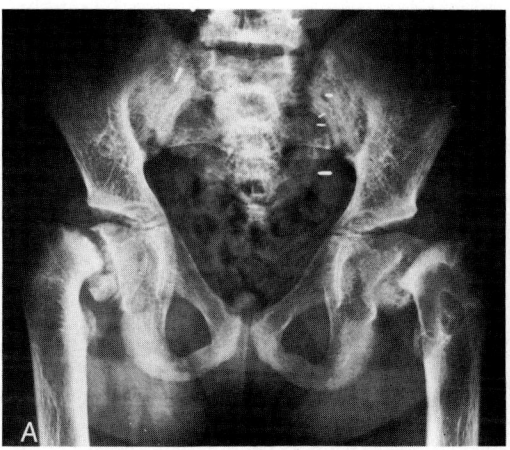 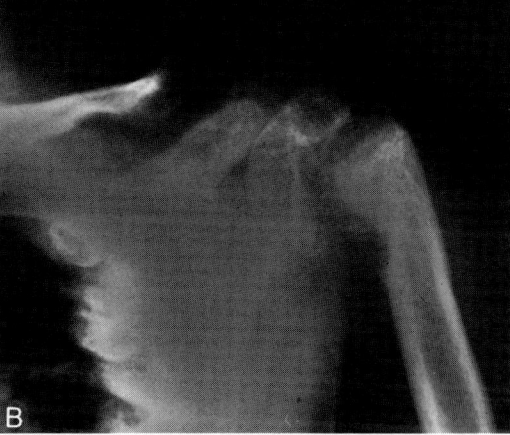

FIGURE 3–181. Bilateral slipped capital femoral epiphysis and slip of the proximal humeral epiphysis in renal osteodystrophy.

A. Anteroposterior view of both hips. B. Anteroposterior view of the left shoulder.

demonstrable changes in the femoral head or acetabulum.

Anatomically the slip takes place in the layer of cartilage cells adjacent to the zone of provisional calcification; the plane of separation, however, is often weaving and irregular; it passes through the different zones of the physis, extending toward the germinal zone or into the metaphysis (Fig. 3–182).[72] This weaving line of separation is due to the irregularity of the contour of the physis in the slip-susceptible age group.[283] A clean cleft through the zone of hypertrophy occurs only in the younger child (under the age of 14 months).[62]

The slipping is usually gradual, and the perichondrium remains attached to the femoral neck, stretching and elongating as the epiphysis migrates. In an acute slip, however, the perichondrium may be stripped from the femoral neck anteriorly and inferiorly. The displacement of the epiphysis is almost always posterior.[6] This is because the physis is an arc in the anteroposterior plane; initially the epiphysis must move posteriorly as it is forced to follow the contour of the physeal arc.[124] There are only a few case reports of acute traumatic slips that are anterior.[187]

As the femoral head becomes displaced posteriorly, it usually also slips inferiorly, and the juxtaepiphyseal portion of the femoral neck projects proximally and anteriorly as a "hump." The synovium will still be engorged and edematous, the synovitis taking several months to subside. Except in cases of acute traumatic slip, there is no hemarthrosis.

The ultrastructure of the growth plate has been reported by Mickelson and associates. In the normal growth plate the chondrocytes in the zone of hypertrophy are arranged in longitudinal columns and separated by thin longitudinal and transverse septa of densely packed parallel collagen fibrils. In the hypertrophied zone of the physis in slipped capital femoral epiphysis, however, the chondrocytes are disorganized; they are disarrayed in clusters and irregular columns (Fig. 3–183).[253]

The cartilage matrix in the zone of hypertrophy in slipped capital femoral epiphysis is definitely abnormal. In the normal human growth plate this cartilage matrix consists of thin bars, longitudinal and transverse septa, that are composed of densely packed, parallel-oriented thin and thick collagen fibrils. This thin bar separates the chondrocytes. In slipped capital femoral epiphysis it is homogeneous and does not contain definite collagenous septa separating the chondrocyte columns. Instead of the normal thin bars, it consists of scattered, irregularly oriented fine fibrils (Fig. 3–184). Seen by light microscopy, it appears as occasional broad eosinophilic bands. The clefts in which slipping takes place are consistently located in the region of the cartilage hypertrophy zone, the weakest portion of the growth plate because it contains no definite longitudinal and transverse septa for structural integrity.

With healing the inferior angle and anterior portion of the neck adjacent to the physis is filled with callus, and when remodeling takes place, the callus becomes incorporated with the femoral neck, and the protruding hump becomes rounded and smooth. If slipping is marked, the bony hump may impinge against the anterior and superior margins of the acetab-

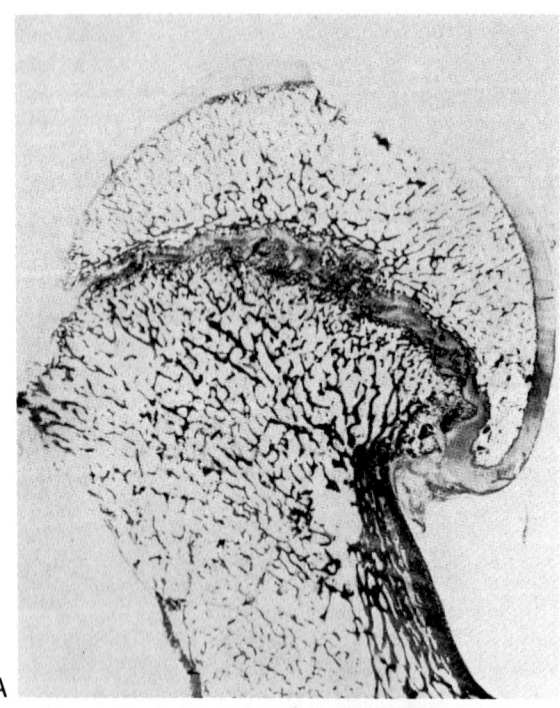
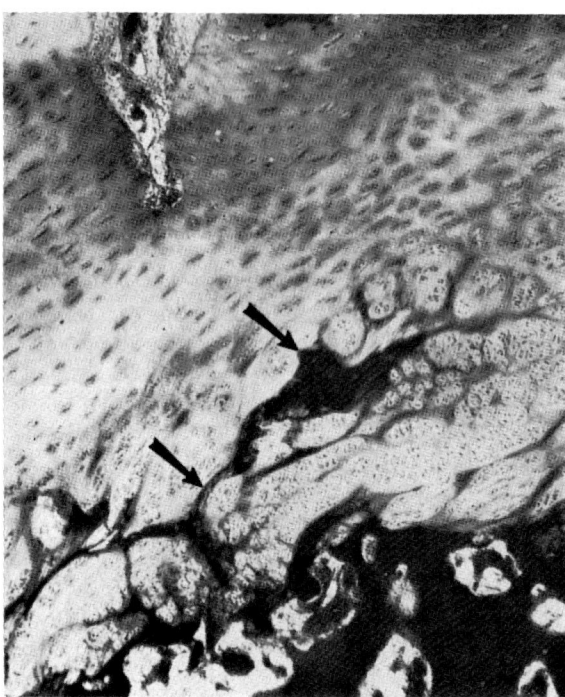
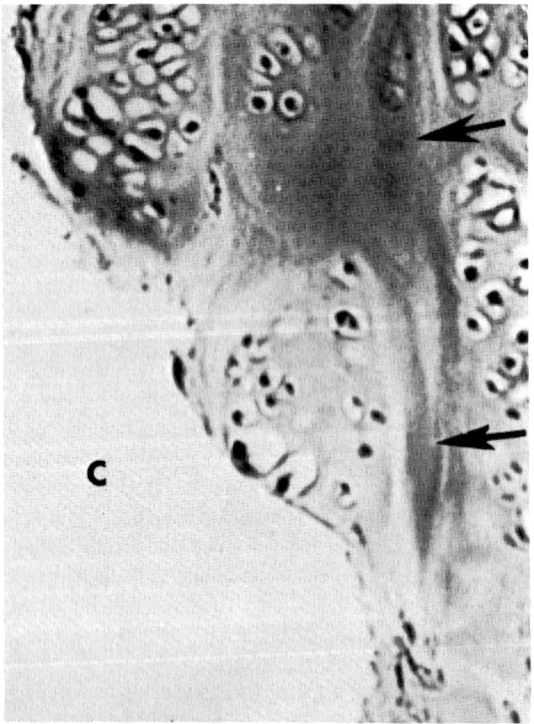

FIGURE 3–182. Photomicrographs of a specimen of slipped capital femoral epiphysis.

A. The entire specimen of the femoral head and neck. Note the slipping has occurred through the hypertrophied zone of the physis. (Hematoxylin and eosin, ×2). **B.** A portion of the growth plate. (Hematoxylin and eosin, ×50). The zone of hypertrophy is widened and composed of chondrocytes in disarrayed clusters instead of orderly columns. Dark-staining eosinophilic bands *(arrows)* separate the cartilage clusters. **C.** Greater magnification of the growth plate. Note the chondrocytes of the hypertrophied zone at the cleft *(C)* region are in disordered clusters and irregular columns. The cartilage cell masses are separated by dark-staining eosinophilic septa *(arrows)*. (Hematoxylin and eosin, ×200.) (From Mickelson, M. R., Ponseti, I. V., Cooper, R. R., and Maynard, J. A.: The ultrastructure of the growth plate in slipped capital femoral epiphysis. J. Bone Joint Surg., 59-A:1076, 1977. Reprinted by permission.)

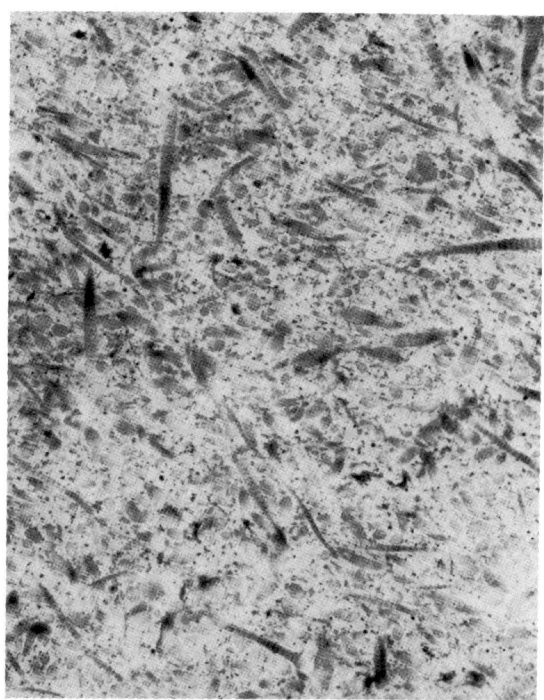

FIGURE 3–183. Cartilage matrix in the zone of hypertrophy of the physis in slipped capital femoral epiphysis.

Note that very fine fibrils are randomly scattered in an amorphous background with electron-dense granules: (×16,100). (From Mickelson, M. R., Ponseti, I. V., Cooper, R. R., and Maynard, J. A.: The ultrastructure of the growth plate in slipped capital femoral epiphysis. J. Bone Joint Surg., 59-A:1076, 1977. Reprinted by permission.)

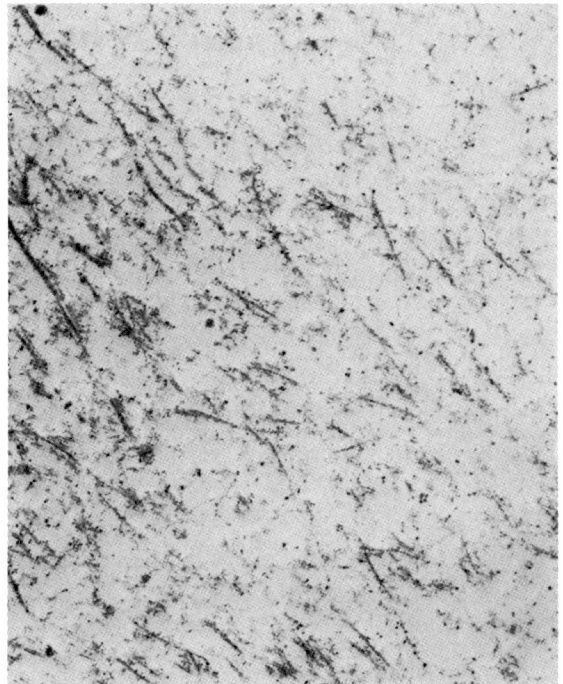

FIGURE 3–184. The ultrastructure of the matrix of the zone of hypertrophic cartilage.

Note the very thin fibrils, scattered at random in an amorphous background with electron-dense granules. (×16,100). (From Mickelson, M. R., Ponseti, I. V., Cooper, R. R., and Maynard, J. A.: The ultrastructure of the growth plate in slipped capital femoral epiphysis. J. Bone Joint Surg., 59-A:1076, 1977. Reprinted by permission.)

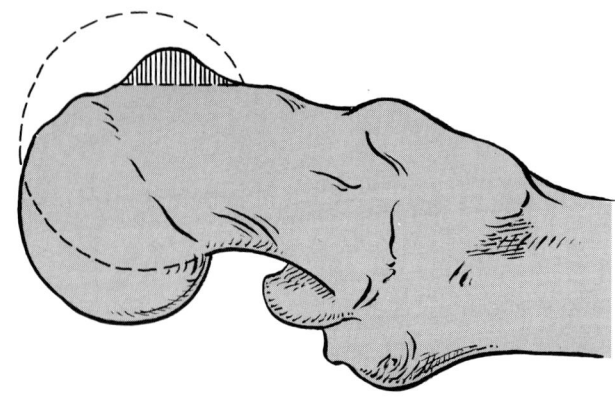
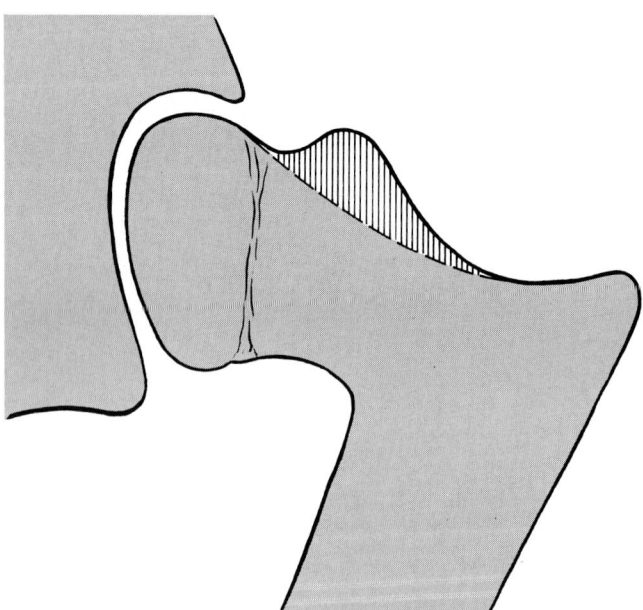

FIGURE 3–185. *Chronic slipped capital femoral epiphysis.*

Note protuberance or "hump" in the anterior and superior margin of the femoral neck. Range of motion of hip will be improved by osteoplasty of the femoral neck.

ulum, causing limited abduction, medial rotation, and maximal flexion (Fig. 3–185). After several months, the edema and swelling of the synovial membrane subside. Within one to three years, the physis ossifies, and bony union takes place between the femoral head and neck.

The findings in the residual stage depend on the integrity of circulation to the femoral head, the viability of the hyaline articular cartilage, and the resulting deformity and faulty joint mechanics.

Degenerative arthritic changes with spurs at the joint margin and narrowing of the joint space may develop later in life, especially if circulation was compromised or there is incongruity of the femoral head in the acetabular socket consequent to deformity. Obesity increases the stress and strain on the mechanically deranged joint.

The pathology of chondrolysis and avascular necrosis is discussed under complications.

Clinical Picture

The symptoms and physical findings vary according to the type of slip, whether it is chronic, acute on chronic, or acute traumatic.

In the *chronic slip* the presenting complaint

is usually pain in the region of the groin and referred to the anteromedial aspect of the thigh and knee. The pain is dull and vague; it may be intermittent or continuous, and is exacerbated by physical activity such as running or sports. The onset of pain may be of several weeks' or months' duration, and it may be related to trivial or significant injury. The patient walks with an antalgic limp and holds the affected lower limb in laterally rotated position. There may be local tenderness anteriorly over the hip joint. The degree of limitation of range of motion depends on the severity of the slip. During the preslipping, or minimal slip, stage medial rotation, abduction, and *flexion* of the hip are slightly limited; when forced these motions are painful. When further slipping occurs, there is greater limitation of motion of the affected hip. A typical finding is that, as the hip is flexed, the thigh tends to ride into lateral rotation and range of maximal hip flexion is restricted—the patient is unable to touch his abdomen with his thigh (Fig. 3–186). In uncomplicated slipped capital femoral epiphysis there is no flexion deformity; instead there is an extension contracture of the hip; i.e., the range of hip flexion is less than normal. The presence of hip flexion deformity should alert the surgeon to the possibility of associated chondrolysis of the hip. A bone scan with technetium-99m should be performed to confirm the diagnosis of chondrolysis.

Actual shortening of 1.2 to 2.0 cm. of the affected limb is common in moderate or severe slip. In chronic slip there will be disuse atrophy of the proximal thigh.

Acute slip is characterized by the sudden onset of severe pain and by the inability to bear weight on the affected lower limb. There are two forms of acute slip: *acute traumatic*, which occurs after significant injury (such as a vehicular accident or a fall from a height), with no previous complaints of pain, and *acute on chronic* slip in which there is sudden onset of severe pain and inability to bear weight in patients who for the past few weeks or months have been experiencing pain in the region of the hip-thigh-knee. The minimal slipped epiphysis becomes further displaced suddenly under the load of body weight after minimal or mod-

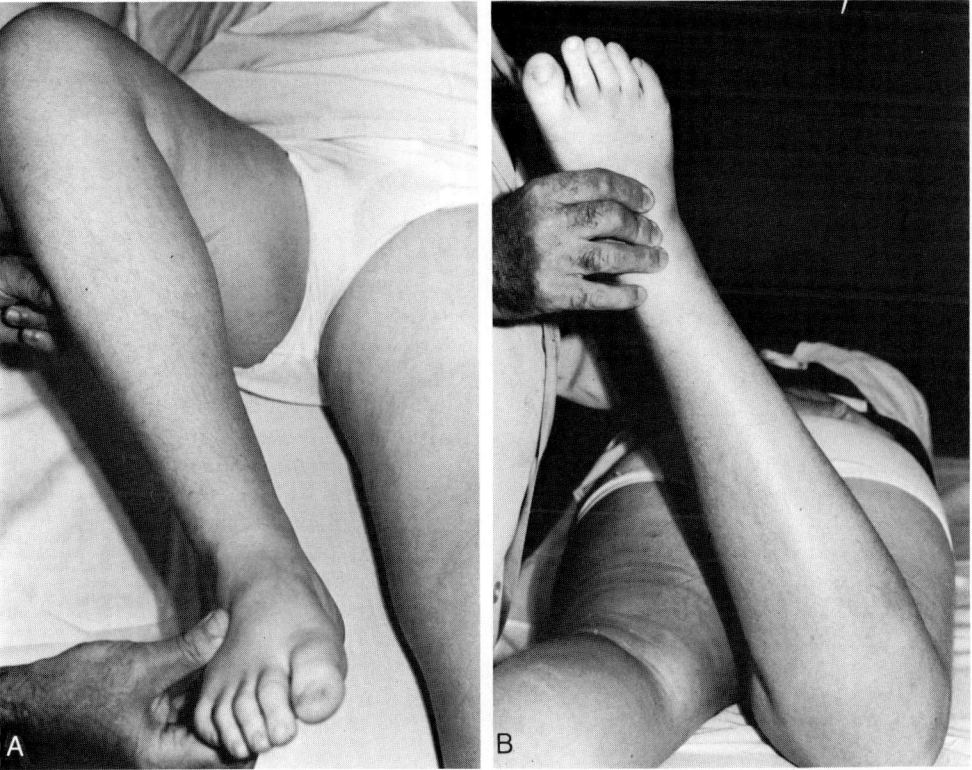

FIGURE 3–186. *Clinical findings in slipped capital femoral epiphysis of the right hip.*

A. Hip flexion is limited, and on flexion the hip rotates laterally. **B.** In prone position with the hips in extension, there is limitation of medial rotation of the right hip.

erate injury. In some cases there is no history of trauma—the patient cannot bear weight because of the severity of pain.

On examination in the acute slip the hip is very painful, the patient guards all ranges of motion. The affected limb is held in marked lateral rotation, and there is obvious shortening. The surgeon should exercise extreme gentleness and should not force the hip to test maximal range of motion; forced movement may aggravate and increase the displacement of the femoral head. Do not ask the patient to walk to inspect his gait abnormality! The patient is immediately taken off his feet, placed in a wheelchair, and after appropriate radiographs have been made (with the x-ray technician instructed to be gentle), he is admitted to hospital and placed in traction; this situation is an emergency.

Radiographic Findings

In the *preslipping, or minimal, stage* the earliest radiographic sign is widening and irregularity of the physis with rarefaction in its juxtaepiphyseal portion. This can be detected readily in the anteroposterior projection in a good quality radiograph. A slip may, however, easily escape notice in the anteroposterior view; it is imperative to take views in the lateral plane also to demonstrate actual slipping, which is always posterior initially. The frog-leg (or Lowenstein) position (in which the hips are flexed, abducted, and laterally rotated, with the knees flexed and the soles of the feet together) is often satisfactory, as it gives a lateral projection of the proximal femur, though not of the acetabulum. When a true lateral projection is possible it will depict the posterior slip best. In both the anteroposterior and lateral radiographs the x-ray beam should be in the same plane as the capital femoral physis; the hip should therefore be in normal medial rotation.[124] In order to compensate for the limitation of medial hip rotation and the degree of femoral retrotorsion, the x-ray tube should be tilted laterally.[169]

The anteroposterior view will reveal medial displacement of the epiphysis and show the upper portion of the femoral neck adjacent to the physis to be bared. In the normal hip, a line along the superior side of the femoral neck transects the overhanging ossified epiphysis (Fig. 3–187 A). In the slipped hip, prolongation of the projection of the superior neck line does not pass through the head or else cuts off less of the head than on the normal side (Trethowan's sign) (Fig. 3–187 B). There will be localized rarefaction in the inferior medial metaphysis of the neck. The so-called "articular portion" of the metaphysis is that part of the juxtaepiphyseal area of the inferior neck that is normally contained within the acetabulum (Fig. 3–187 C). In slipped epiphysis, the articular portion of the metaphysis is excluded from the acetabulum (Fig. 3–187 D).

The metaphyseal blanch sign of Steel is a crescent-shaped area of increased density overlying the metaphysis adjacent to the physis seen on the anteroposterior radiogram. It is an early sign of posterior slipping without medial displacement. Characteristically, the displaced femoral head is superimposed on the area of increased metaphyseal density. The metaphyseal blanch sign is suggestive of slipped capital femoral epiphysis, and a lateral radiogram should be made to confirm or exclude the diagnosis (Fig. 3–188).[356]

When the slip is moderate or severe, the posteriorly slipped femoral head can be visualized through the proximal portion of the neck in the anteroposterior radiogram.

When slipping is recent, as in acute slip, there will be no evidence of healing, but later on, callus will have formed at the inferior and posterior junction of the head and neck. The bared area of the anterior and superior margin of the femoral neck will have been remodeled and become rounded, presenting as a protuberance or "hump."

Measurement of the Amount of Slipping

In the true lateral radiographic view of the normal hip the capital femoral physis and femoral neck lie at right angles to each other—the lower limit of normal is 87 degrees (Fig. 3–189 A). The physeal-neck angle decreases when slipping takes place (Fig. 3–189 B).

In a recent acute slip the distance between the superior edge of the epiphysis and the upper margin of the metaphysis indicates the amount of displacement; this is measured in the true lateral projection, which shows the greatest amount of displacement. In chronic slip remodeling of the femoral neck makes it difficult to measure the amount of displacement of the capital femoral epiphysis.

Southwick recommends measurement of the head-shaft angle in the frog-leg lateral radiogram to record the amount of slipping. A line (X_1) is drawn between the superior and inferior margins of the metaphyseal surface of the capital femoral physis; second, the line Y_1 is drawn

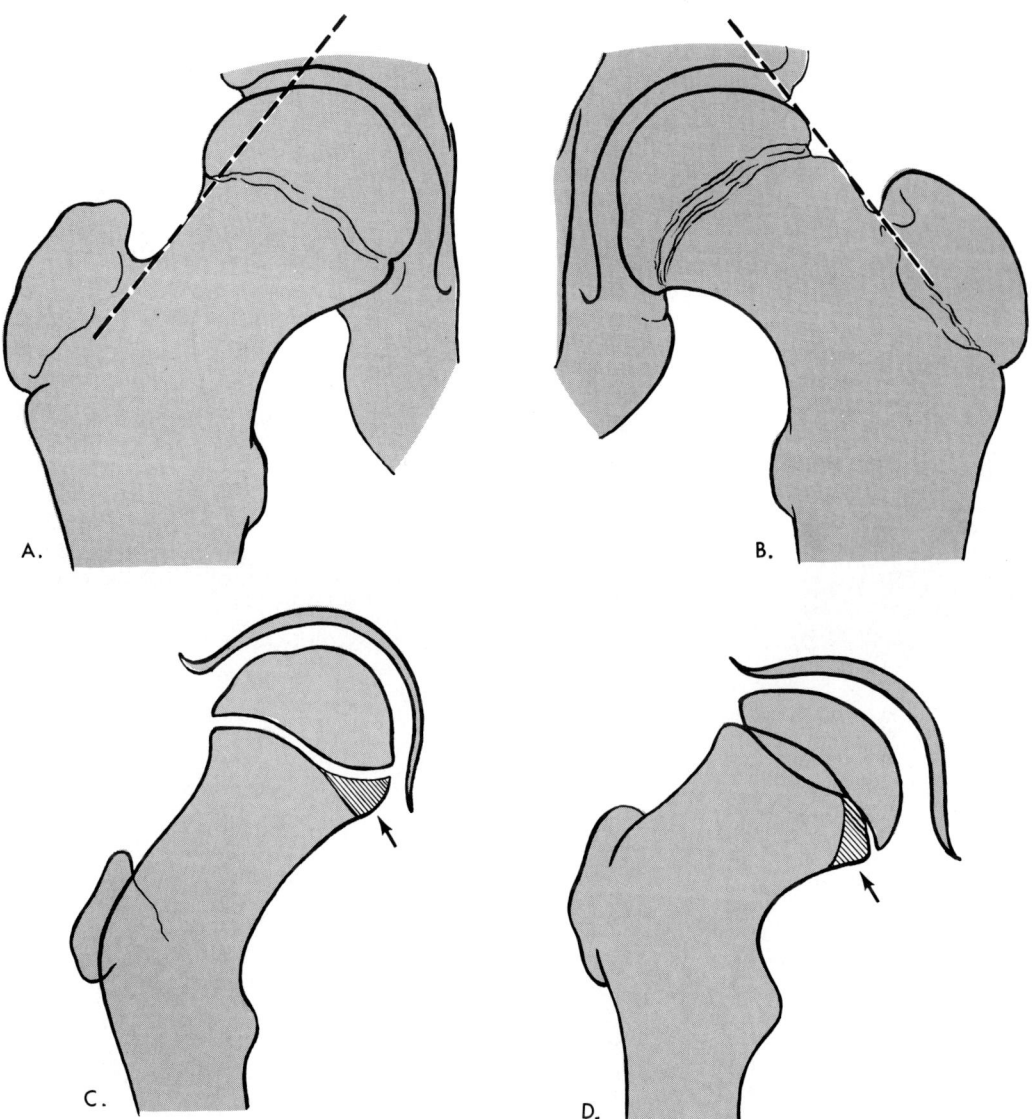

FIGURE 3–187. Radiographic changes of minimal medial slip.

Anteroposterior view of the hips. **A.** In the normal hip, a line along the superior side of the femoral neck transects the overhanging ossified epiphysis; whereas, **B,** in the slipped hip, the projected neck is bared at the epiphyseal plate. Note also the widening and irregularity of the epiphyseal plate. **C.** Normal hip. The "articular portion" of the metaphysis is contained within the acetabulum. **D.** In the slipped hip the "articular portion" of the metaphysis is excluded from the acetabulum.

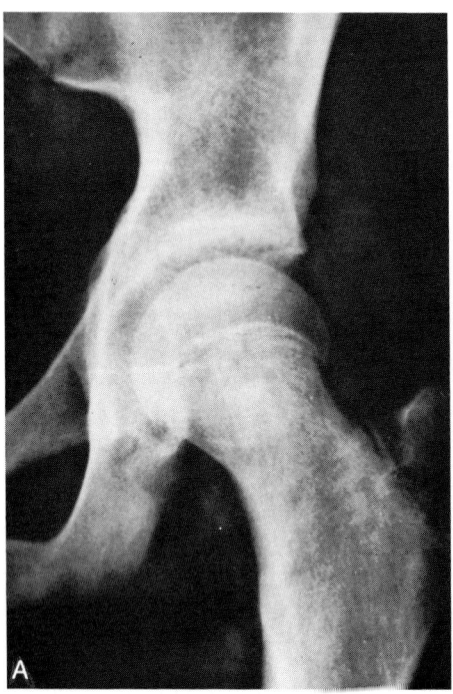
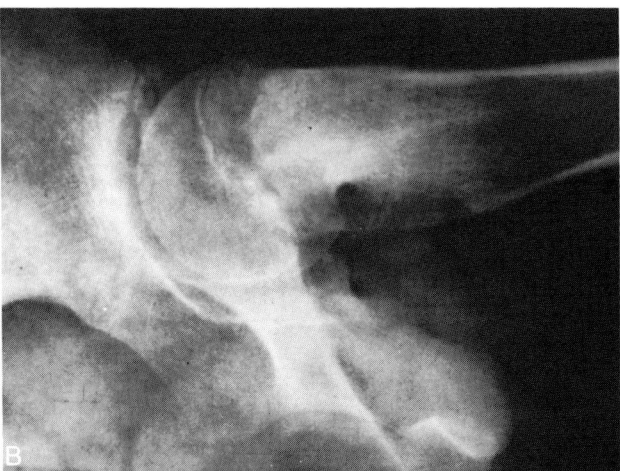

FIGURE 3–188. *Metaphyseal blanch sign of Steel in slipped capital femoral epiphysis.*

A. Anteroposterior view. Note the crescent-shaped area of increased density overlying the metaphysis of the femoral neck adjacent to the physis; this is due to posterior slip. The Kline line, however, is unbroken, i.e., there is no medial displacement. **B.** Lateral view showing the posterior slip. (Courtesy of Howard H. Steel, M.D.)

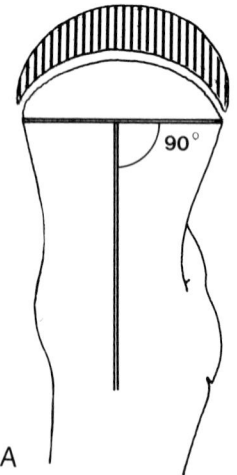
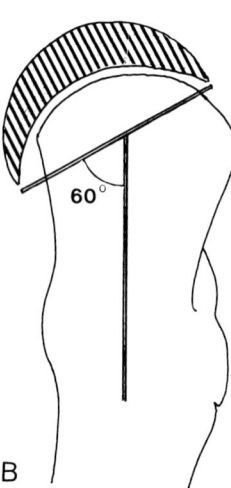

FIGURE 3–189. *The physeal neck–femoral neck angle as measured in the true lateral projection.*

A. Normal hip. The angle is 90 degrees with a lower limit of 87 degrees. **B.** In slipped capital femoral epiphysis the physeal neck angle is decreased—in this instance it is 60 degrees.

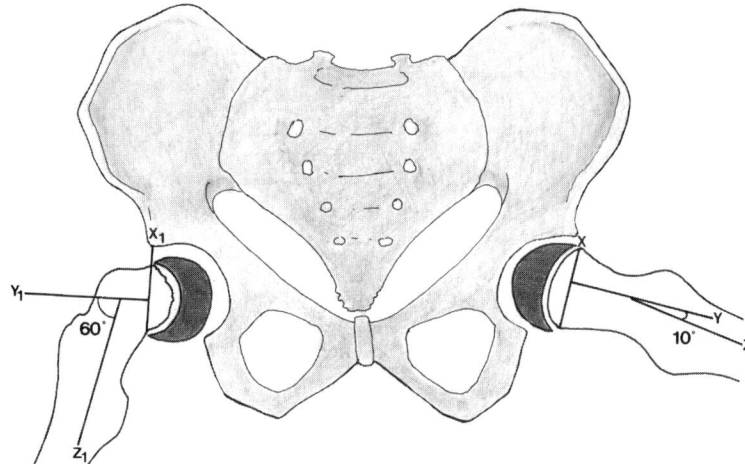

FIGURE 3–190. Southwick method of measuring femoral head–shaft angle.

See text for explanation.

perpendicular to the line X_1; third, the line Z_1 is drawn parallel to the femoral shaft. The lateral head shaft angle is the angle formed by the lines Y_1 and Z_1 (Fig. 3–190).[349]

Computed tomography will depict the exact amount of posterior displacement of the femoral head; it is the most accurate method (Fig. 3–191).

Imaging Findings. Bone imaging with technetium-99m will show increased uptake in the capital femoral physis; this is of special value in unilateral involvement. Other scintigraphic changes in uncomplicated slipped capital femoral epiphysis include apparent widening of the physeal-metaphyseal region in the anterior projection and curvature of the physeal-metaphyseal region in the lateral projection, both due to the posterior slippage, anterior angulation of the femoral neck with the epiphysis in the lateral view, and decreased localization in the physeal-metaphyseal region with severe slippage.

Treatment

Slipped capital femoral epiphysis is an emergency; it is imperative that it be treated immediately, since minor trauma may cause further or complete displacement of the femoral head. As soon as the diagnosis is made, weight-bearing should be forbidden. Resist economic pressures of health maintenance insurance organizations! Do not send the patient home and operate the next day as outpatient surgery! The patient is admitted to the hospital and put in split Russell traction. Medial rotation straps are applied to the thigh and to the leg to correct lateral rotation contracture. With relief of muscle spasm and soft-tissue contracture, one can better evaluate the status of the joint and determine the maximum degree of motion that may be obtained.

The treatment of slipped capital femoral epiphysis is operative, the surgical method depending on the degree of displacement and whether it is acute or chronic.

Conservative means of management such as bed rest and traction only prolong treatment, as several years may be required for the capital epiphysis to fuse, during which period further slipping may occur. The use of a plaster of Paris cast was reported by Wright and King. They applied bilateral below-knee casts with a crossbar in between, holding the hips in abduction and medial rotation. Weight-bearing was not

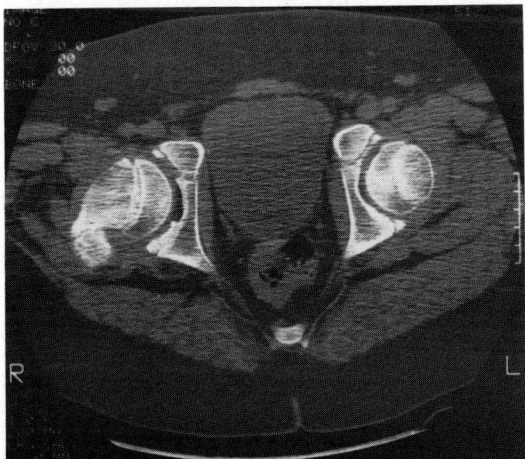

FIGURE 3–191. CT scan of slipped capital femoral epiphysis showing minimal posterior displacement of the right hip.

Left hip had been pinned previously, and the growth plate is closed.

allowed as long as the casts were worn, usually for three to four months. End-result studies showed that the femoral head healed to the neck in situ with no further slipping. They recommended this method of cast treatment for the inexperienced orthopedic surgeon who encounters slipped capital femoral epiphysis very occasionally, as it is safe and devoid of iatrogenic complications.[410] King, however, emphasized the possibility of degenerative arthritis of the hip occurring in adult life when deformity of the femoral head and incongruity of the articular surfaces remained.[199] Moore reported good or excellent results in 88 per cent of 44 cases with cast immobilization.[258] Steel advocates nonoperative treatment.[356] This author does not recommend nonsurgical management, as it is prolonged, further slip may occur, and cast immobilization may cause chondrolysis.

Sex hormones have been tried to induce closure of the physis. As a general principle, it is best not to interfere with the endocrine system of an adolescent. This author will, however, consider sex hormone therapy in the adolescent who is a poor surgical risk, especially near the age at which physeal closure is about to take place, and when definite callus with healing of the slip is beginning to occur.

If the femoral head is displaced less than 65 per cent (according to the Southwick method) or less than two thirds of its diameter, this author recommends internal fixation by pinning in situ. The objective is to stabilize the epiphysis and prevent further slipping until solid bony fusion has occurred. In his opinion, open epiphyseodesis of the capital femoral physis to prevent further slipping is indicated when there is serious risk of the pins' penetrating into the hip joint, specifically in the very obese patient in whom radiographic visualization of the site and depth of pins into the epiphysis is very difficult on the operating table, and in the severe slip in which technically proper placement of the pins is very difficult. Severe valgus slips are very difficult to pin—in such cases open epiphyseodesis is a safe method of treatment.

In Situ Pin Fixation. It is important to choose the proper internal fixation device. The objective of pinning is to lock the epiphysis in place, enhancing physeal closure; it should be simple and cause as little trauma as possible. It should not penetrate the joint. Historically Telson is credited with being the first to report pinning. He used threaded pins.[367] Later the three-flanged Smith-Petersen nail was used by other surgeons because it provided firmer fixation.

The Smith-Petersen nail should not be used, however, because it is bulky, and forceful hammering through the hard femoral neck of an adolescent may cause further trauma and displacement of the epiphysis; the nail may break the subchondral bony plate of the femoral head; it may migrate postoperatively; it can also cause avascular necrosis and subtrochanteric fracture.[89, 128, 183, 324] Wiberg recommends the use of a finer four-flanged nail that is made of Vitallium. He mentions the possibility that the epiphysis may withdraw from the nail because of the growth in length of the neck.[399] Multiple (three or four) Austin Moore pins have been used by Durbin, by Newman, by Schnute, and by other surgeons.[89, 275, 332] These are easily inserted and hold the capital epiphysis securely to the neck. Nuts are applied to the distal threaded portions of the pins to prevent further penetration. Knowles pins, AO hip screws, Hagie pins, or threaded Steinmann pins are preferred by others.

The author designed a special pin (manufactured by Zimmer Mfg. Co., Warsaw, Ind.) that is threaded at each end and has a smooth portion in between. The threaded proximal portion used to grip the femoral head is not as large as that in the Hagie pin. The possibility of penetrating the joint and damaging hyaline articular cartilage is thereby lessened. This method compresses the femoral head and neck together firmly, and closure of the epiphyseal plate takes place in four to six months. Irani and associates graded this author's pin as the best.[175]

At present this author recommends the use of cannulated hip screws for internal fixation of slipped capital femoral epiphysis, either the AO or the Asnis. *Asnis* developed the *guided screw system*, which offers major advantages in the fixation of the slipped capital femoral epiphysis.[12, 13] The guided screw (even though cannulated) is stronger than the 5/32-inch stainless steel Knowles pin (140 per cent to bending and 123 per cent to torque). The shank diameter of the screw is the same as the root diameter of the thread, circumventing potential weakness of this junction. One screw provides excellent fixation in the ordinary chronic slipped capital femoral epiphysis. Two screws are used in acute slip or in the *very* large, obese patient with chronic slip. Unrecognized pin penetration into the hip joint is the single most important iatrogenic factor in causing the dreadful chondrolysis. The risk of pin penetration increases proportionally with the number of pins used.

The proximal femur of the adolescent has

hard bone on both sides of the capital physis. The guided screws are 20 mm. long, and the 6.4 mm. buttress threads provide excellent fixation, causing the growth plate to compress itself as it attempts to grow and enhancing fusion.

Proper positioning and placement of the Asnis screw in the center of the epiphysis is easy to control. Ordinarily this maneuver is difficult because of the hard bone in the adolescent. The guide pin used in the guided screw system is a 9-inch-long 5/32-inch drill driven with power equipment; this neutralizes the increased resistance of the hard bone, rendering accurate placement of the screw relatively easy. The threads are cut by a calibrated tap, which allows the screw to follow easily.

The Asnis screw is cannulated; therefore in doubtful cases Renografin may be injected through an angiocatheter to rule out joint penetration. The presence of radiopaque dye in the joint confirms communication with the joint. Routine injection of Renografin is not recommended, however, because debris left in the screw channel from drilling and tapping may be flushed into the joint. Intra-articular osteocartilaginous debris may cause chondrolysis.

Hagie and Moore pins are difficult to remove. The reverse cutting flutes of threads of the Asnis screws make screw removal very easy.

Recently, AO developed a cannulated screw system with cannulated drills, which appears to be as good as, if not superior to, the Asnis guided screw system.

The technique of hip pinning by the Asnis guided screw system is described and illustrated in Plate 35.

Multiple pin fixation (three or four) should not be used. Brodetti has shown that the arrangement in which the metallic pins are placed (nesting of the pin "tips") may interrupt circulation to the femoral head and result in avascular necrosis (Fig. 3–192).[48] The anterolateral part of the capital femoral epiphysis should be avoided. The point of entry of the screws should be proximal to the lesser trochanter; also it should be anterior. The screw should be directed to the center of the capital femoral physis and epiphysis and not to the center of the femoral neck. One screw is adequate for fixation of chronic slip; and only two screws are used for an acute slip.

Open Epiphysiodesis With Autogenous Bone Graft. The operative technique of open epiphysiodesis is as follows: the anterior capsule of the hip joint is exposed through a limited anterolateral approach. The joint is opened through an "H"-shaped incision into the capsule (Fig. 3–193 A). Two cobra retractors are placed within the capsule, exposing the femoral head and neck and the area of slipping. With a small Kirschner wire or drill point, a rectangular window is fashioned on the anterosuperior aspect of the femoral neck (Fig. 3–193 B). Next, a large hollow mill is inserted through the window and, under image intensifier control, is drilled across the physis into the capital femoral epiphysis (Fig. 3–193 C). The cylindrical core of bone, containing the portions of capital epiphysis, physis, and metaphysis, is removed. An alternative method is to insert progressively larger size drills through the window in the femoral neck and drill the metaphysis, physis, and epiphysis. The drill may be inserted through a separate small incision over the lateral intertrochanteric region. Then a small curet is used to enlarge the cylindrical tunnel, and the capital physis is curetted, removing additional portions of the growth plate (Fig. 3–193 D). From the outer wall of the ilium, corticocancellous strips of bone graft of appropriate size are taken, "sandwiched," and driven as a composite bone peg across the capital physis into the femoral head (Fig. 3–193 E and F). Radiograms are made in the anteroposterior and lateral projections to verify bridging by the graft across the physis and into the epiphysis. The cortical bone removed from the femoral neck is replaced firmly (Fig. 3–193 F). The capsule is closed, and the wound is closed in the usual fashion.

In cases of chronic slipped capital femoral epiphysis, the patient is placed in counterpoised bilateral split Russell traction. Within two to four days—as soon as he is comfortable—he is allowed to be ambulatory with a three-point, toe-touch crutch gait. In cases of acute slip, a bilateral hip spica cast is worn for six weeks, following which the patient is allowed to be ambulatory with a three-point crutch gait. Crutch protection is continued until the radiographic appearance of growth plate closure, which averages two and a half months. Full weight-bearing is then allowed.

Problems and Complications. A definite disadvantage of the open epiphysiodesis is that placing the graft across the capital physis does not check the slipping process. In fact, curetting the growth plate may temporarily decrease the stability, converting a stable situation to an unstable one in which reslipping can occur. An acute slip may occur if the capital physis is reamed or curetted aggressively. Ordinarily, closure of the growth plate takes place rapidly,

Text continued on page 1044

Hip Pinning With the Asnis Guided Screw System

The patient is placed on the fracture table with the involved hip in 10 to 20 degrees of medial rotation. Biplane image intensifier fluoroscopy is set and tested to be certain that the hip (particularly the capital femoral epiphysis) can be adequately visualized. This can sometimes be a problem in the very obese patient.

OPERATIVE TECHNIQUE

A. and **B**. A longitudinal incision is made in muscle on the lateral aspect of the upper thigh, beginning 3 to 4 cm. distal to the prominence of the greater trochanter and extending distally for about 3 to 7 cm. The fascia lata is incised, and the vastus lateralis muscle is split to expose the anterolateral aspect of the upper femoral shaft. A 9-inch long 5/32 inch drill is placed in the pin driver attached to a power drill. The more severe (i.e., the more posterior) the slip, the more anteriorly on the femoral cortex the hole must be drilled. The site of the drill hole should be above the lesser trochanter in the intertrochanteric region; it should not be subtrochanteric. Under image intensifier radiographic control, a hole is drilled through the lateral femoral cortex. The largest smooth Kirschner wire that will easily slide through the cannulated screw (usually .062 mm,) is then drilled through the hole in the lateral femoral cortex, up the center of the femoral neck, across the physis, and into the epiphysis so that it is centered in both the anteroposterior and lateral projections. The hip joint should not be penetrated. To confirm that the tip of the pin is not in the joint, the hip is carefully rotated under image intensifier fluoroscopy to check both anteroposterior and lateral projections.

C. The "blind spot" is the space in the radiographic shadow of the femoral head in which the tip of the pin is projected within the boundaries of the femoral head in the radiogram; the tip of the pin appears to be in the femoral head, but it is not. With one x-ray beam the space of the "blind-spot" is large, but with an increasing number of x-ray views the volume of the "blind spot" becomes progressively smaller.

D. The radiographic projection that shows the tip of the pin in its true position with respect to the articular surface and the subchondral bony plate of the femoral head is the *"critical view."* This is visualized by the "tangential" x-ray beam. The "equator" around the femoral head is delineated by the points on its surface touched by the tangential x-ray beams. The tip of the pin should lie in the plane of this equator in the "critical view."

Plate 35. Hip Pinning With the Asnis Guided Screw System

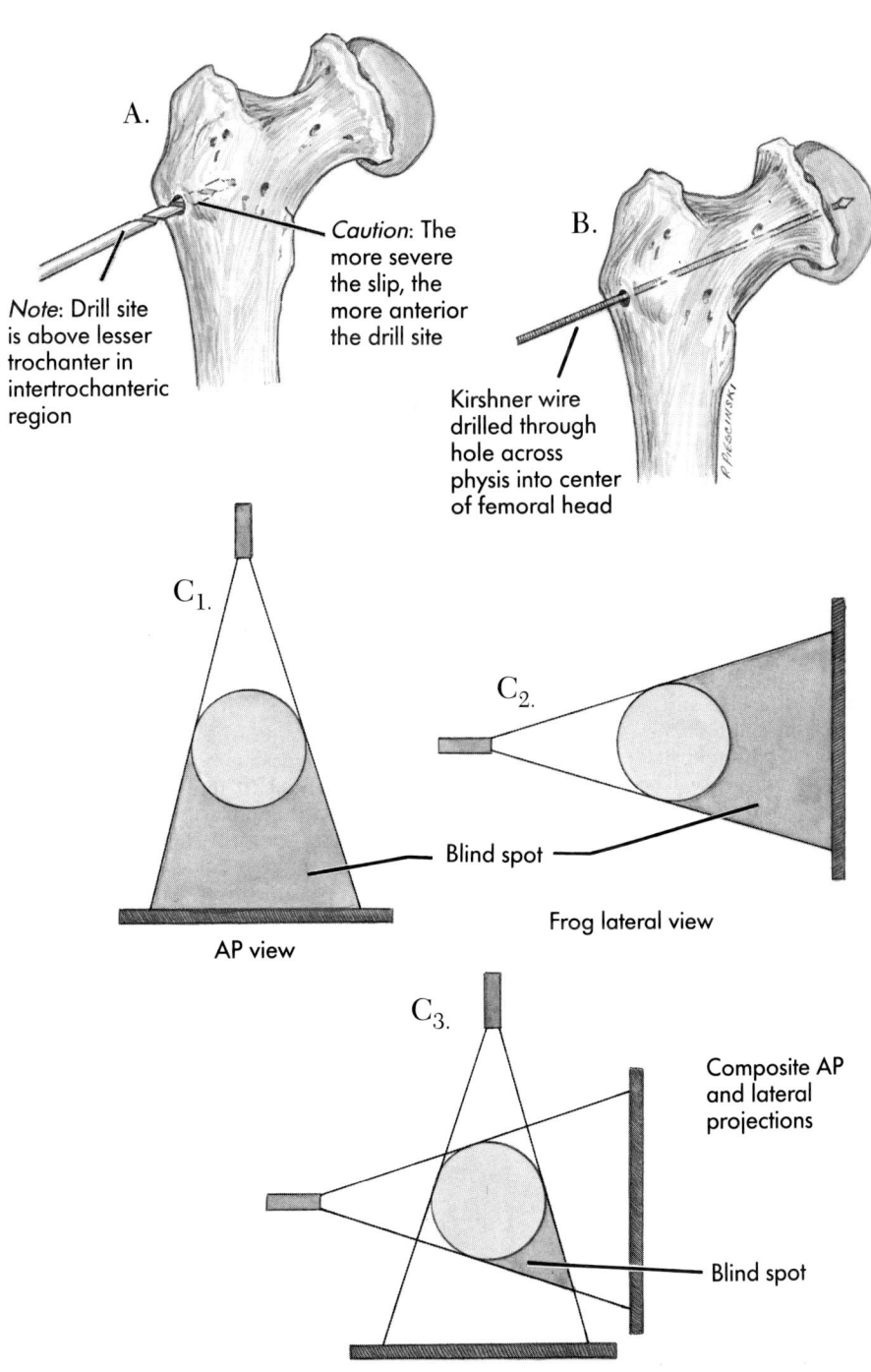

Hip Pinning With the Asnis Guided Screw System (Continued)

F. Abduction-adduction views of the hip are of no assistance, as the hip movement takes place about an axis parallel to and not perpendicular to the x-ray beam. The reliability of the approach-withdraw phenomenon is dependent upon the axis of hip rotation being roughly perpendicular to the central beam of the x-ray.

G. Once verified that the guide pin is in the center of the epiphysis, a $5/32$ inch drill bit is attached to a power drill and, with the pin as a guide, the drill bit is drilled through the lateral femoral cortex, up the center of the neck, across the physis, and into the center of the epiphysis. The tip of the drill bit should be within 0.5 mm. of the subchondral bony plate. In case of doubt, regular radiographs are made under image intensifier fluroscopy, to double check the exact position and depth of the drill. The drill bit is removed.

H1–H2. At this time the surgeon may choose to use either the tap directly or an optional guide pin assembly. Once a hole is drilled, the tap will follow the drill hole even without a guide pin. If the assembly is used a guide pin (which fits in the hole of the cannulated screw) is driven up the predrilled channel, and its position is verified by image intensifier fluroscopy. The inner pin is tapped with a mallet, and the outer component is removed. Next, the cannulated tap is placed over the guide wire and driven through the lateral cortex, the femoral neck, and across the physis into the epiphysis. The shank of the tap is calibrated by shiny and dull etchings. The holes in the tap show the guide pin in the distal hole when the tap is 25 mm. from the end of the pin. Stop when the guide pin is seen in the proximal hole; only 5 mm. is left.

I. The tap is removed, leaving the guide wire in place. A screw of the appropriate length and a washer are selected and placed over the wire, across the physis, and well into the femoral epiphysis.

The guide wire is removed, and if there is any question of joint penetration by the screw, renografin dye may be injected through the cannulated portion of the screw into the epiphysis. If the x-ray shows that any dye enters the hip joint, the screw must be backed out an appropriate distance. A second screw can be placed posterior and inferior to the first in cases of acute slips.

The wound is closed in layers in the usual manner.

POSTOPERATIVE CARE

Immediately after leaving the operating room, the hip is protected by placing the patient in bilateral split Russell traction, with medial rotation straps on the thigh. Active assisted and gentle passive exercises to develop motion in the affected hip are performed while in bed. As soon as the patient is comfortable (usually in two to three days) he is allowed to be ambulatory, protecting the hip by three-point crutch gait, with a gradual increase of weight-bearing on the involved side. When muscle spasm has completely subsided and the hip has functional range of motion, crutch protection is gradually discontinued and full weight-bearing is allowed. In *acute* slip crutch protection is continued with toe-touch gait for a period of six weeks.

Plate 35. Hip Pinning With the Asnis Guided Screw System

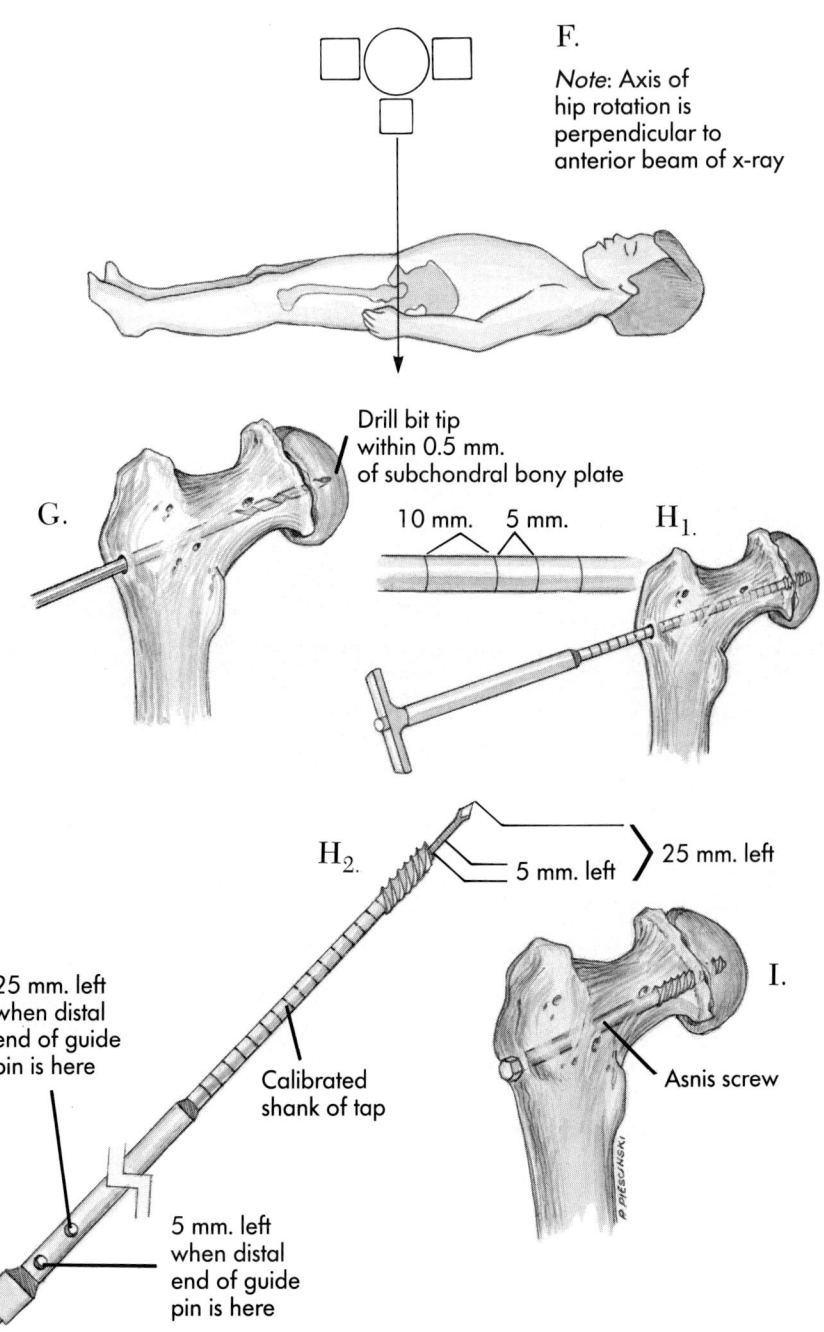

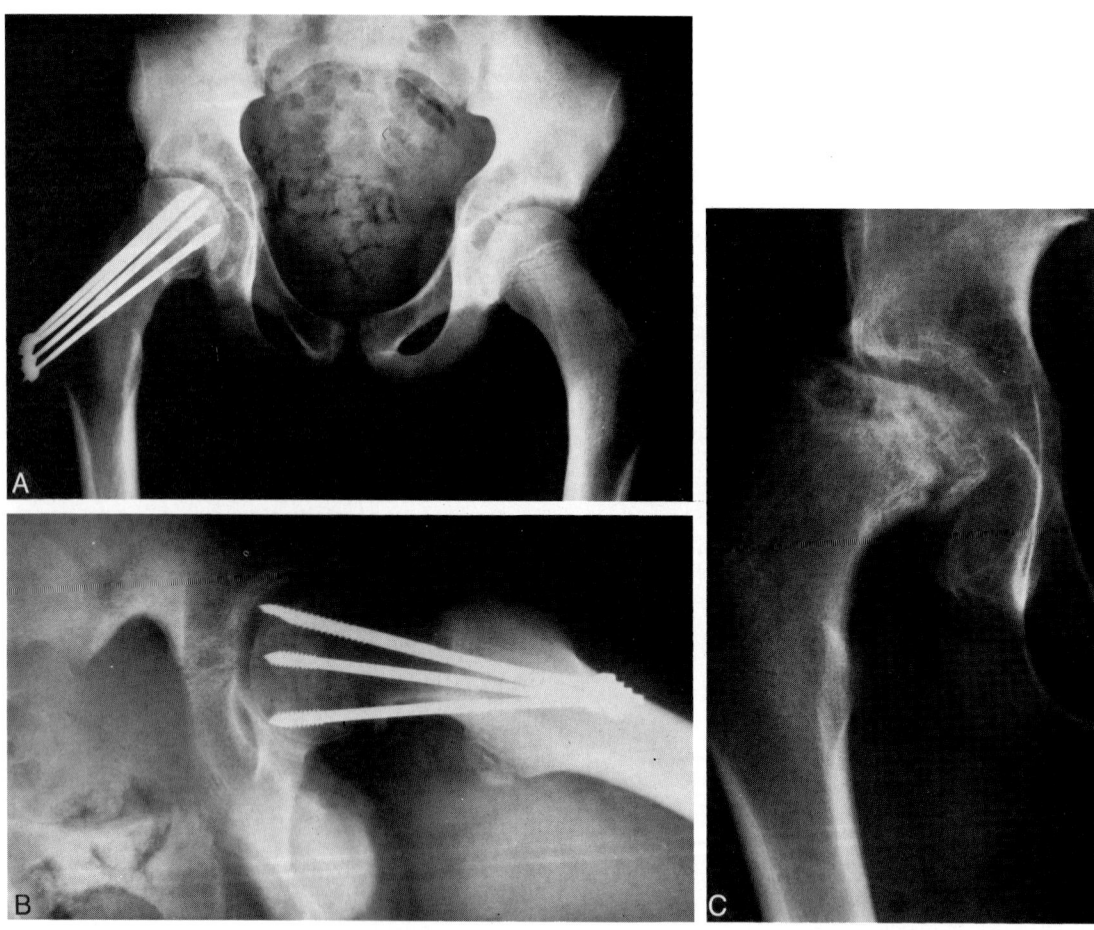

FIGURE 3–192. *Four-pin fixation in slipped capital femoral epiphysis resulting in avascular necrosis of femoral head, collapse, and penetration of pins into hip joint.*

A and **B.** Immediate anteroposterior and lateral radiograms of the hips showing the four-pin fixation and penetration of the anterior and inferior pins into the hip joint. **C.** Following removal of the pins, collapse and superolateral displacement of the femoral head. Use only one screw in chronic slip and two screws in acute slip. Avoid the superolateral quadrant of the capital femoral epiphysis.

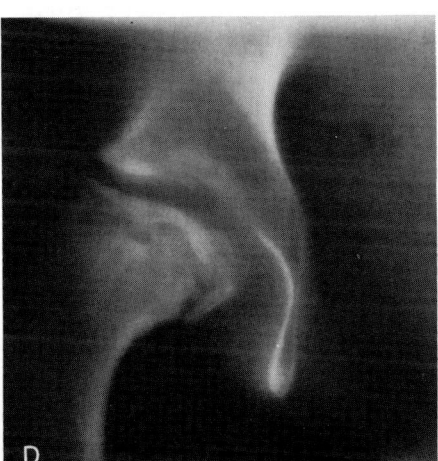
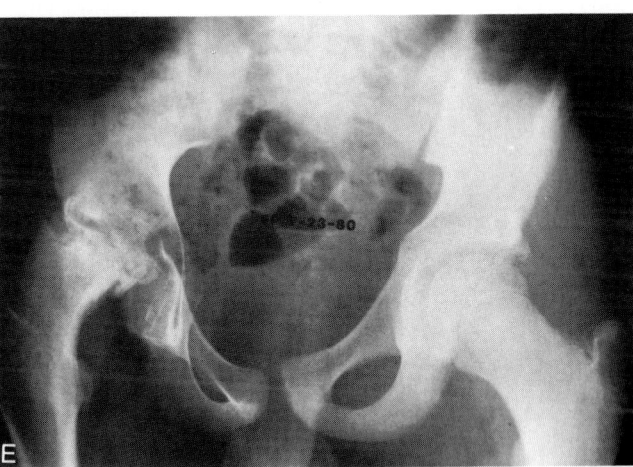
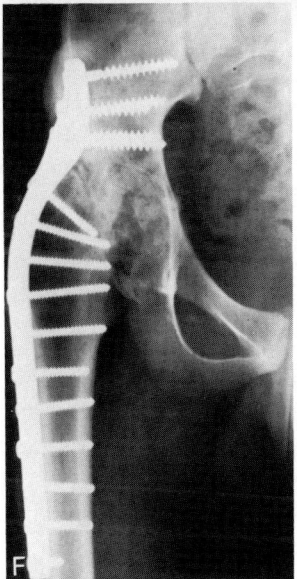

FIGURE 3–192 Continued. Four-pin fixation in slipped capital femoral epiphysis resulting in avascular necrosis of femoral head, collapse, and penetration of pins into hip joint.

D. Linear tomography showing avascular necrosis and collapse of the femoral head. **E.** Anteroposterior view of both hips showing progressive collapse of the femoral head. Hip joint resurfacing was performed without success. **F.** Anteroposterior view of the hip showing hip fusion and internal fixation with a Cobra plate.

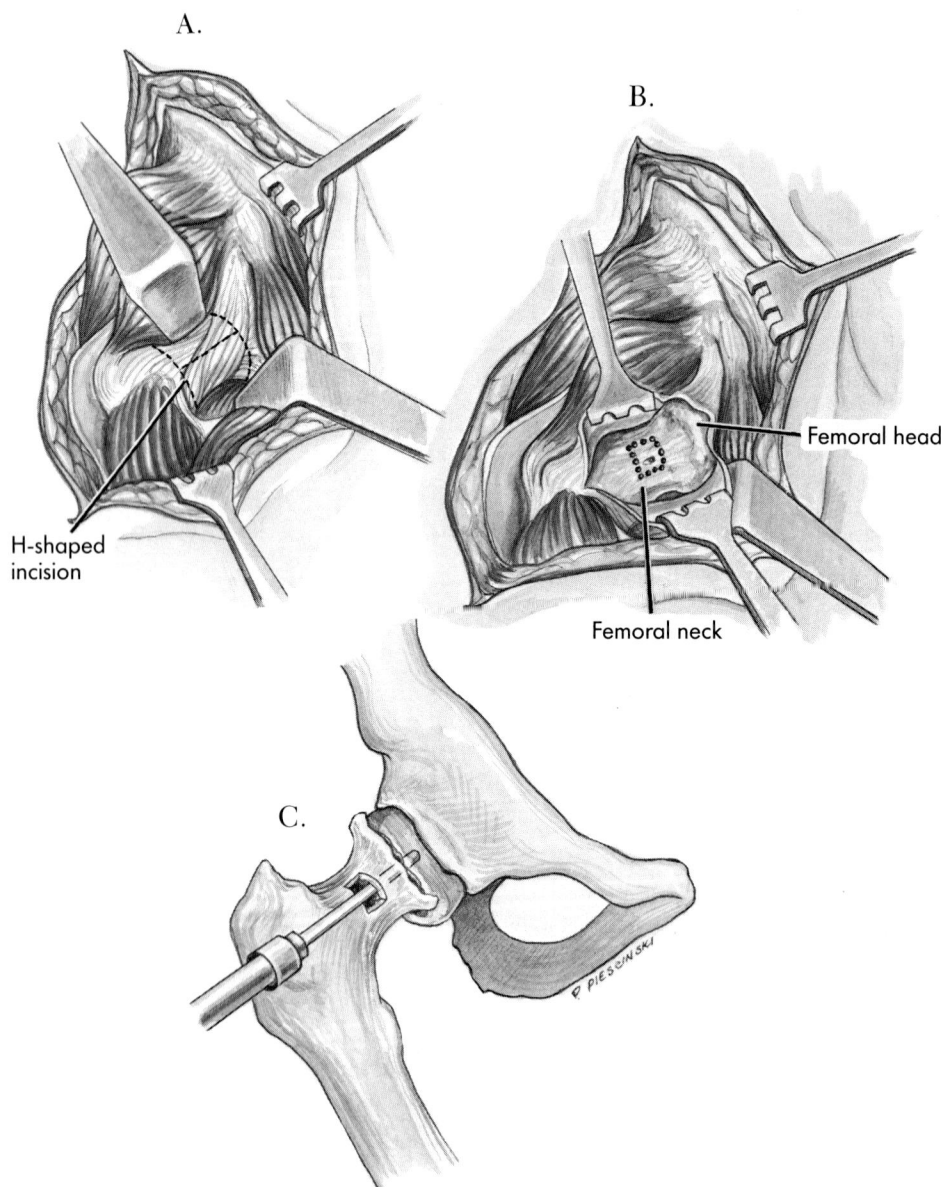

FIGURE 3–193. Open epiphysiodesis with autogenous bone graft.

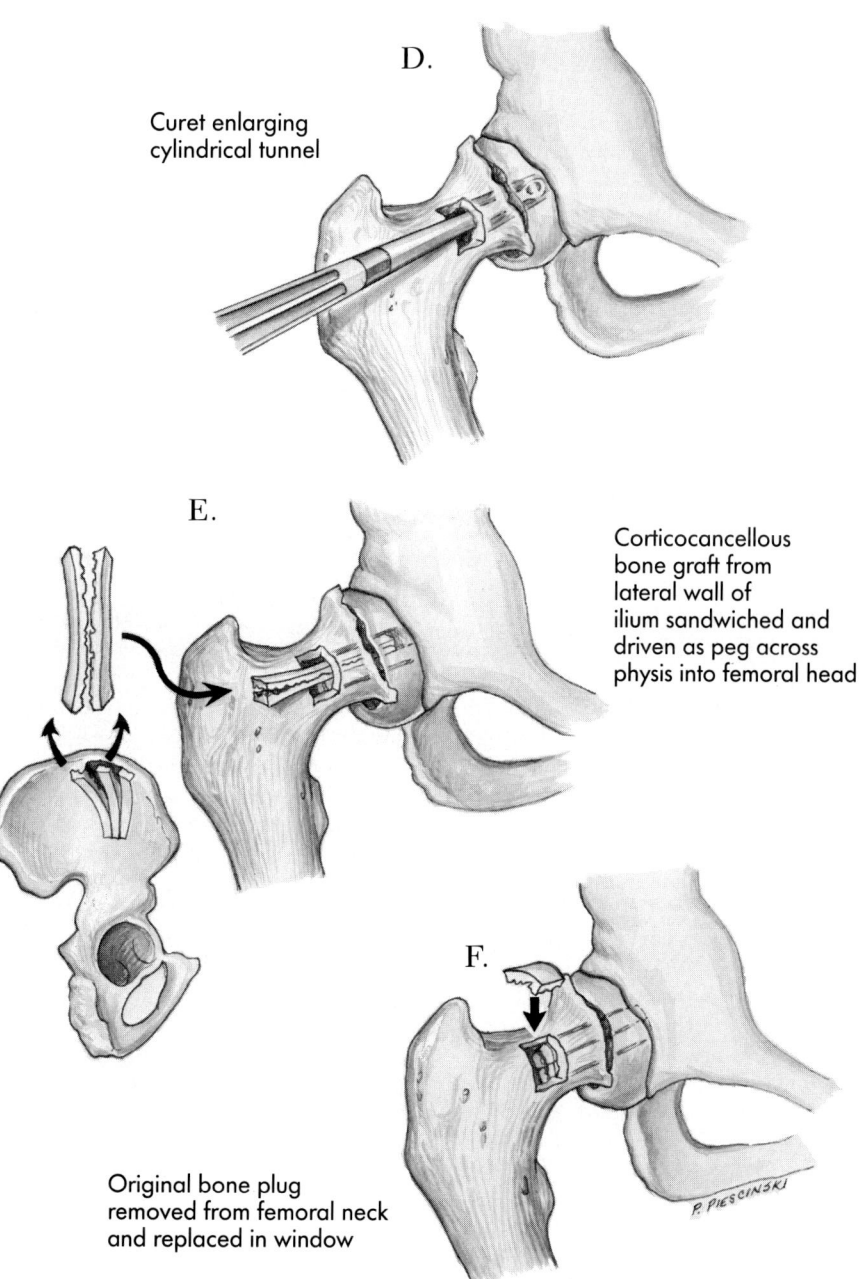

FIGURE 3–193 Continued. *Open epiphysiodesis with autogenous bone graft.*

and once the bone graft bridges epiphyseal to metaphyseal bone, stability is no longer a problem. The importance of protecting the hip following open epiphysiodesis of slipped capital femoral epiphysis, by either hip spica cast or crutches or both, cannot be overemphasized. The graft may resorb, fail to bridge the physis, or undergo stress fracture. Weiner and associates reported four cases of reslipping in 159 hips with chronic slip. One was caused by graft resorption, one was due to placement of the graft short of the capital physis, and two were caused by drilling and curettage of the growth plate.[390]

Other disadvantages of open epiphysiodesis are the magnitude of operative exposure and the amount of blood loss, which is greater than that of simple hip pinning.

Advantages. The incidence of avascular necrosis and acute cartilage necrosis is very low following open epiphysiodesis. In the study of Weiner and associates, of 26 hips with acute slip, there were two cases of avascular necrosis and one case of acute cartilage necrosis. In the group of 159 hips with chronic slip, there was one case of avascular necrosis and not a single case of acute cartilage necrosis. Pin penetration is not a problem in open epiphysiodesis. Another advantage is that a second operation to remove the hardware is avoided.

This author, as stated previously, recommends open epiphysiodesis only when proper placement of the screws is difficult because of technical reasons: (1) in the very obese child in whom adequate visualization of the site and depth of the screw into the epiphysis is difficult; (2) valgus slip; and (3) very severe slips that are difficult to pin.

Remodeling of the Femoral Neck and Adjacent Head. This takes place by new bone formation between the overhanging femoral head and the inferior and posterior surfaces of the femoral neck and by bone resorption and rounding off of the "uncovered" anteroposterior borders of the metaphysis of the femoral neck. The portion of the femoral neck apparently in contact with the acetabulum seems to become part of the articular surface of the femoral head. The new bone formation and resorption are oriented in accordance with stress lines—the biologic processes of nature give the femoral head a more spherical shape and the neck a near-normal contour. Remodeling takes place when the triradiate cartilage is open at the time of in situ pinning. It occurs at a relatively rapid pace, usually within a matter of two to six months. Early weight-bearing enhances the process.

Concomitant with remodeling there is a certain degree of spontaneous correction of the lateral rotation and extension deformity of the hip.

O'Brien and Fahey reported the long-term results of treatment by pinning in situ of 12 hips with moderate to severe slipping. The age of the patients at the time of pinning ranged from 10 years and 8 months to 16 years. The average follow-up was 10 years (with a range from 2 to 17 years). Ten of the twelve patients had excellent remodeling of the femoral neck and head, and were asymptomatic (Fig. 3–194). All ten hips showed spontaneous improvement of limitation of motion, which was essentially normal except in seven hips in which limitation of medial rotation ranging from 5 to 20 degrees persisted. In nine of the ten hips with excellent remodeling, the triradiate cartilage of the acetabulum was open at the time of hip pinning. The two hips with incomplete or no remodeling had no symptoms, and secondary surgery was not performed because it was not indicated. O'Brien and Fahey recommended in situ pinning when the difference between the lateral head-shaft angle (as measured by the Southwick method) between the affected and contralateral normal hip is less than 60 degrees. If remodeling fails to take place, a secondary operation may be indicated to improve function. The anterolateral prominence (the hump), if restricting abduction and medial rotation, may either be excised, or medial rotation flexion osteotomy may be performed at the level of the lesser trochanter to correct lateral rotation-extension deformity of the hip, or both.[280]

Boyer, Mickelson, and Ponseti evaluated long-term results in 149 hips (121 patients) with slipped capital femoral epiphysis. The follow-up period after diagnosis averaged 31 years (range, 21 to 47 years). The mean age of the patients at follow-up was 45 years. The results were very good in most of the 83 hips in which the slip was left unreduced. In the 54 hips treated by surgical procedures to improve the alignment of the slipped capital femoral epiphysis, the results were less favorable and had more complications. In the 12 acute slips the results were good in nine hips; the remaining three developed aseptic necrosis. Femoral neck osteotomy carries a high potential complication rate; if realignment osteotomy is indicated in moderate or severe slips, Boyer and associates recommended it be performed at the subtrochanteric or intertrochanteric level.[44]

Acute Slip. Abrupt displacement of the femoral head is usually precipitated by sudden trauma. In the adolescent it usually takes place

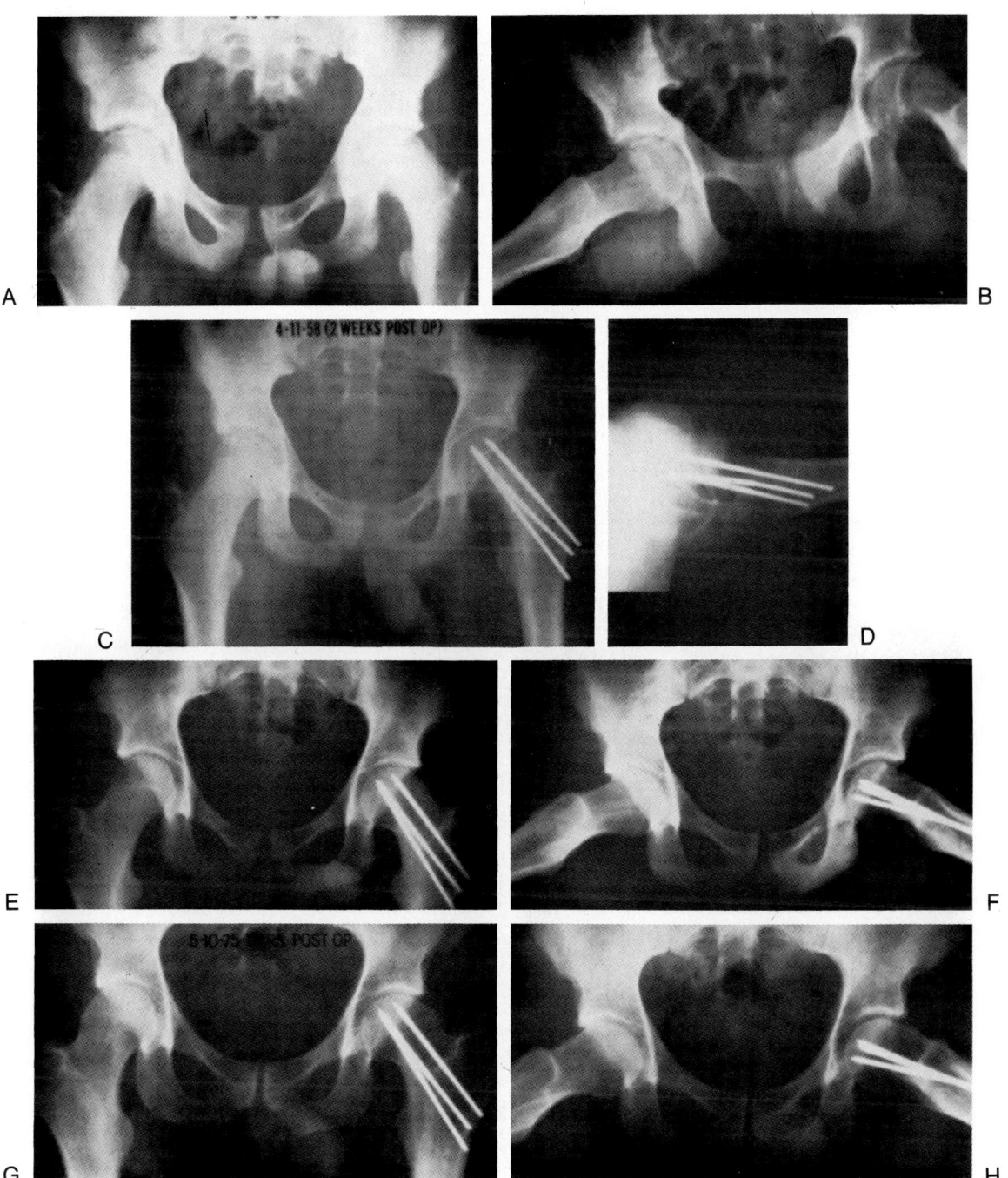

FIGURE 3–194. Moderate slipped capital femoral epiphysis in a 15-year-old boy treated by in situ pinning.

A and **B.** Anteroposterior and lateral radiograms. Note the moderate slip on the left with a 54-degree difference between the lateral head-shaft angles. **C** and **D.** Anteroposterior radiogram of both hips and lateral of left hip after in situ pinning. **E** and **F.** Radiograms two years after hip pinning. Note the rarefaction in the anterior part of the femoral neck where resorption is taking place. **G** and **H.** Seventeen years after hip pinning. Note the remodeling. (From O'Brien, E. T., and Fahey, J. J.: Remodeling of the femoral neck after in situ pinning for slipped capital femoral epiphysis. J. Bone Joint Surg., 59-A:62, 1977. Reprinted by permission.)

through a weakened physis in which there was pre-existing epiphysiolysis; this is demonstrated by the radiographic disclosure of minimal slipping or preslipping, evident in widening of the growth plate and prodromal symptoms (Fig. 3–195). Clinically, acute slipping is characterized by severe pain and by inability to bear weight on the involved limb of less than three weeks' duration. On examination, there is marked limitation of motion of the hip with lateral rotation deformity and shortening. If more than two to three weeks have elapsed since the acute episode, the case should not be classified as an acute slip.

Acute slip can occur in a previously normal capital femoral physis. This is a simple Salter-Harris Type I fracture, usually caused by severe trauma such as an automobile accident or a fall from a height. It can occur at any age. In the younger child it is frequently the result of child abuse. The femoral neck is normal. Displacement of the femoral head is often marked, with avascular necrosis as a frequent complication. The prognosis is poor. Management of Salter-

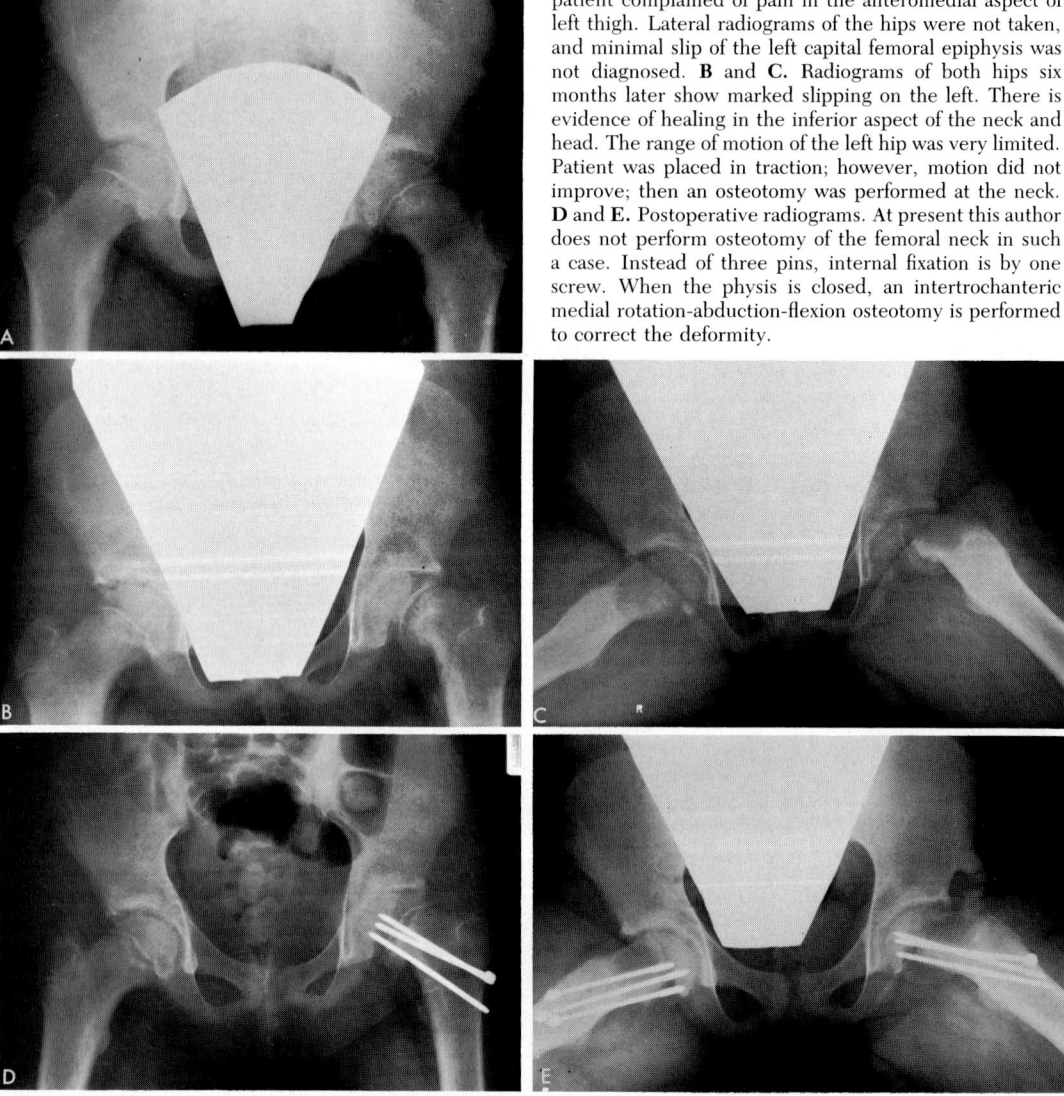

FIGURE 3–195. *Slipped capital femoral epiphysis—the importance of early diagnosis and the value of lateral radiograms of the hips.*

A. Anteroposterior radiogram of both hips. Note the increased width of the epiphyseal plate on the left. The patient complained of pain in the anteromedial aspect of left thigh. Lateral radiograms of the hips were not taken, and minimal slip of the left capital femoral epiphysis was not diagnosed. **B** and **C.** Radiograms of both hips six months later show marked slipping on the left. There is evidence of healing in the inferior aspect of the neck and head. The range of motion of the left hip was very limited. Patient was placed in traction; however, motion did not improve; then an osteotomy was performed at the neck. **D** and **E.** Postoperative radiograms. At present this author does not perform osteotomy of the femoral neck in such a case. Instead of three pins, internal fixation is by one screw. When the physis is closed, an intertrochanteric medial rotation-abduction-flexion osteotomy is performed to correct the deformity.

Harris I fracture of the capital femoral physis is discussed in Chapter 8.

Acute on Chronic Slip. This should be managed as an emergency. Do not send the child home on crutches and pin the hip at a later date. The patient should be admitted to hospital immediately and placed in bilateral split Russell traction with medial rotation straps on the affected thigh and leg. The leg should be carefully handled, as repeated rough manipulation of the limb may cause further slipping. Ordinarily simple skin traction will achieve gradual reduction. Skeletal traction with a pin through the distal femur is not recommended by this author. Within a day or two the patient is taken to the operating room for internal fixation of the displaced femoral head by two cannulated hip screws. If reduction is not achieved by simple skin traction, closed manipulative reduction is carried out under general anesthesia.

Repositioning of the femoral head should be performed in the most gentle manner in order to minimize the risk of vascular damage. Do not attempt repeated closed reductions; only once and a maximum of twice! The Leadbetter maneuver should not be used. The patient is anesthetized on the cart or bed and then gently placed on the fracture table. Longitudinal traction is applied, and the hip is rotated medially. Anteroposterior and lateral radiograms are made to determine the degree of reduction. If this attempt is unsuccessful, the hip is flexed 90 degrees and then extended, while being maintained in neutral rotation. The hip is then placed in longitudinal traction and rotated medially. Do not attempt anatomic reduction, and avoid over-reduction with the femoral head placed in valgus position.

After reduction, the capital epiphysis is internally fixed with two cannulated hip screws (Asnis or AO). When the acute slip is minimal and relatively stable, one screw may be adequate. Do not attempt closed manipulative reduction if more than three weeks have elapsed since the acute episode. Accept the deformity and fix internally in situ. If more than three quarters (or more than 80 per cent) of the femoral head is slipped, open reduction is indicated by the Dunn technique through the transtrochanteric approach and shortening of the femoral neck (see Plate 36).

Postoperatively, the patient with an acute slip is placed in counterpoised bilateral split Russell traction. This author recommends bone imaging with technetium-99m. If the femoral head is alive, the patient is allowed to be ambulatory with crutches (three-point gait with toe-touch on the affected limb) protecting the hip. Partial weight-bearing is gradually increased. If functional range of hip motion is restored, he is then allowed full weight-bearing on the affected limb—it is not necessary to await radiographic evidence of closure of the physis.

Valgus Slip. Posterosuperior (valgus) slip of the capital femoral epiphysis in relation to the femoral neck occurs very rarely; the chronic form is usually associated with marked coxa valga, and the patients are of tall stature—usually in the seventy-fifth percentile or over. In its acute form, the nature of the injury determines the direction of displacement. Adduction–lateral rotation force causes valgus (superoposterior) slip, whereas abduction–lateral rotation force results in varus (posteroinferior) slip. The direction of displacement is almost always posterior because most of the muscles controlling hip movement are inserted distal to the fulcrum of the hip joint, though they spiral off the femoral shaft as lateral rotators of the hip when the capital femoral physis weakens and there is loss of continuity between the femoral head and neck. Active medial rotation of the hip becomes impossible, and the femoral shaft-neck is pulled anteriorly and rotated laterally, exposing the anterior aspect of the upper femoral neck.

The clinical picture of valgus slip is typical; there is limitation of adduction of the hip (abduction contracture) in contrast to varus (posteroinferior) slip in which there is limitation of abduction (i.e., adduction deformity) of the hip. Because the femoral head has become posterior to the femoral neck, there is limitation of hip flexion in both forms.

Radiograms in the anteroposterior projection will show the superior displacement of the femoral head; in the lateral projection the posterior displacement is depicted.

Treatment should be individualized. Internal fixation by hip pinning is difficult; often this author recommends open epiphysiodesis.

Anterior Slip. The direction of slip of the capital femoral epiphysis on the femoral neck is most often (95 per cent of cases) posterior and inferior (varus), very occasionally posterior and superior (valgus), and in the literature there are two case reports of anterior slip. In the case reported by Kampner and Wissinger, there was a history of trauma (sudden medial rotation of the femur while playing baseball), whereas in the case reported by Duncan and Lovell there was no history of injury.[84, 187] The physical findings of anterior slip are different from those

Text continued on page 1062

Dunn Procedure—Open Reduction of Displaced Femoral Head by Shortening Femoral Neck

OPERATIVE TECHNIQUE

A. This procedure is performed with the patient in supine position on a fracture table. The incision begins 2 cm. inferior and lateral to the anterior superior iliac spine and extends toward the greater trochanter and distally along the shaft for a distance of about 10 cm. The subcutaneous tissue is divided in line with the skin incision. The deep fascia is incised. The gluteus maximus fibers are reflected posteriorly, and the tensor fasciae latae and rectus femoris are reflected anteriorly.

B. The vastus lateralis and intermedius muscles are detached from their origin and reflected distally. The anterior and posterior margins of the gluteus medius and minimus muscles are identified, incised and mobilized. The base of the greater trochanter is exposed.

C. With the oscillating saw, the greater trochanter is detached, due care being taken not to injure the vessels in the intertrochanteric fossa. It is important that the superomedial cortex not be cut; rather, a greenstick fracture is produced. A Kirschner wire is used as a guide in making the osteotomy under image intensifier roentgenographic control.

Plate 36. Dunn Procedure—Open Reduction of Displaced Femoral Head by Shortening Femoral Neck

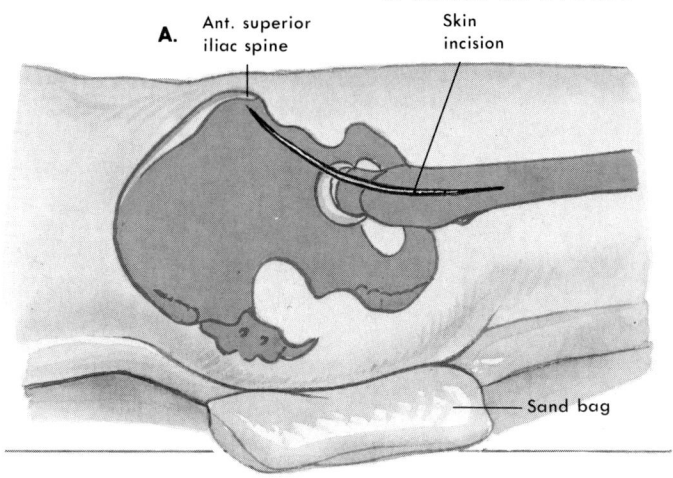

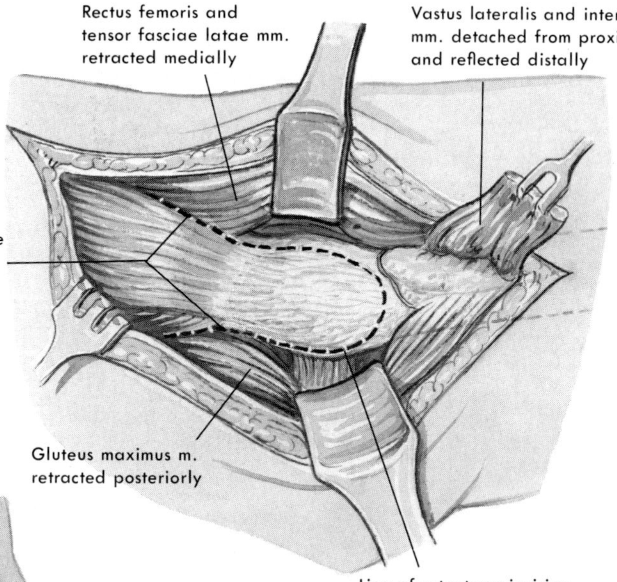

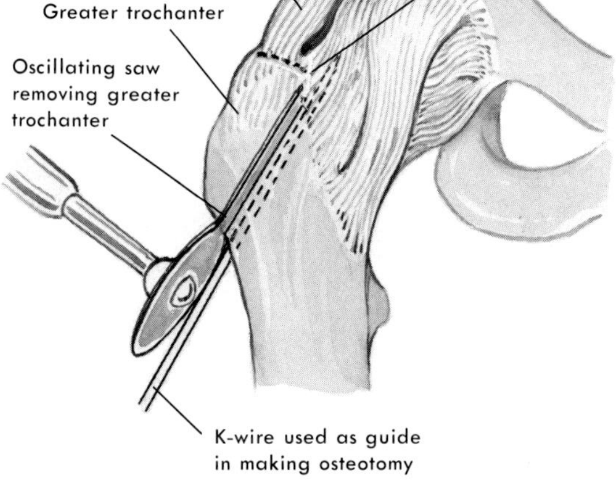

Dunn Procedure—Open Reduction of Displaced Femoral Head by Shortening Femoral Neck *(Continued)*

D. Once the greater trochanter is detached and reflected proximally, a T-shaped incision is made in the capsule around the edge of the acetabulum, down the lateral aspect of the hip joint to the base of the greater trochanter.

E. When the hip joint is open, it is striking to see the dull white covering on the anterior aspect of the femoral neck and the highly vascularized, velvety membrane at the back. In an acute slip there is no callus, but in an acute and chronic slip there will be callus extending from the upper end of the femoral neck from which the capital epiphysis has been displaced. Often it is difficult to determine where the white fibrocartilage ends and where the articular cartilage of the femoral head begins. A longitudinal incision is made on the anterolateral aspect of the femoral neck anterior to the vascular area of the edge and around the anterior margin of the femoral head. The posteroinferior retinacular vessels are shortened.

F. The synovium is gently elevated from the anterior and posterolateral surface of the femoral neck with a periosteal elevator. The retinacular vessels should not be injured.

Plate 36. Dunn Procedure—Open Reduction of Displaced Femoral Head by Shortening Femoral Neck

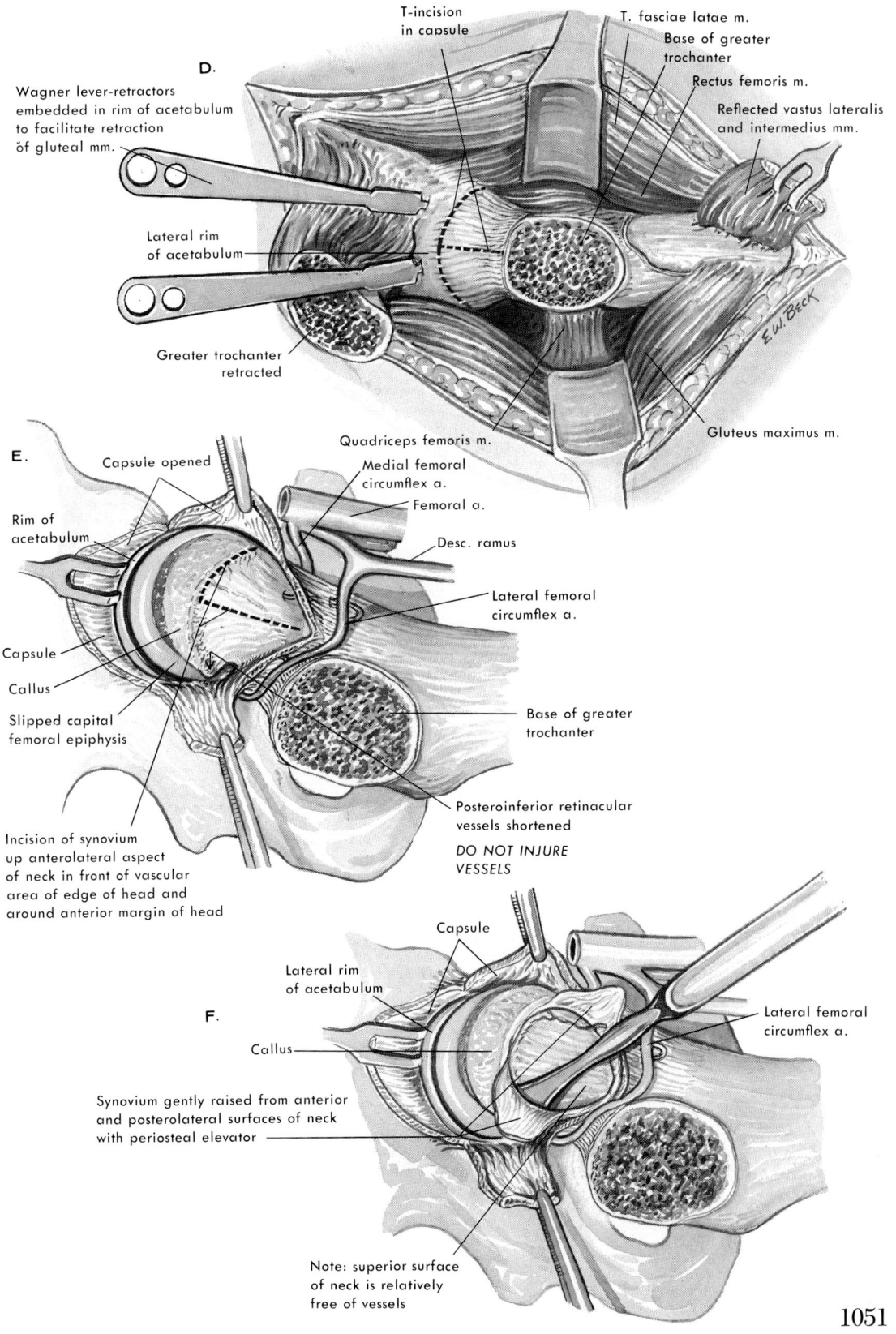

Dunn Procedure—Open Reduction of Displaced Femoral Head by Shortening Femoral Neck *(Continued)*

G. With a gouge, the head is freed of all of the fibrocartilage and callus.

H. The osteotomy line on the upper end of the femoral neck is made for excision of the trapezoid bone segment. The purpose of bone shortening is to prevent stretching of the retinacular vessels when the femoral head is replaced on the femoral neck.

On the back of the femoral neck there will be an osseous beak, which is excised by rongeurs until it is level.

I and J. Next, the head of the femur is replaced on the femoral neck, and three threaded Steinmann pins are used to transfix the shaft, neck, and head of the femur. Two cancellous screws are used to fix the greater trochanter in its normal position.

Plate 36. Dunn Procedure—Open Reduction of Displaced Femoral Head by Shortening Femoral Neck

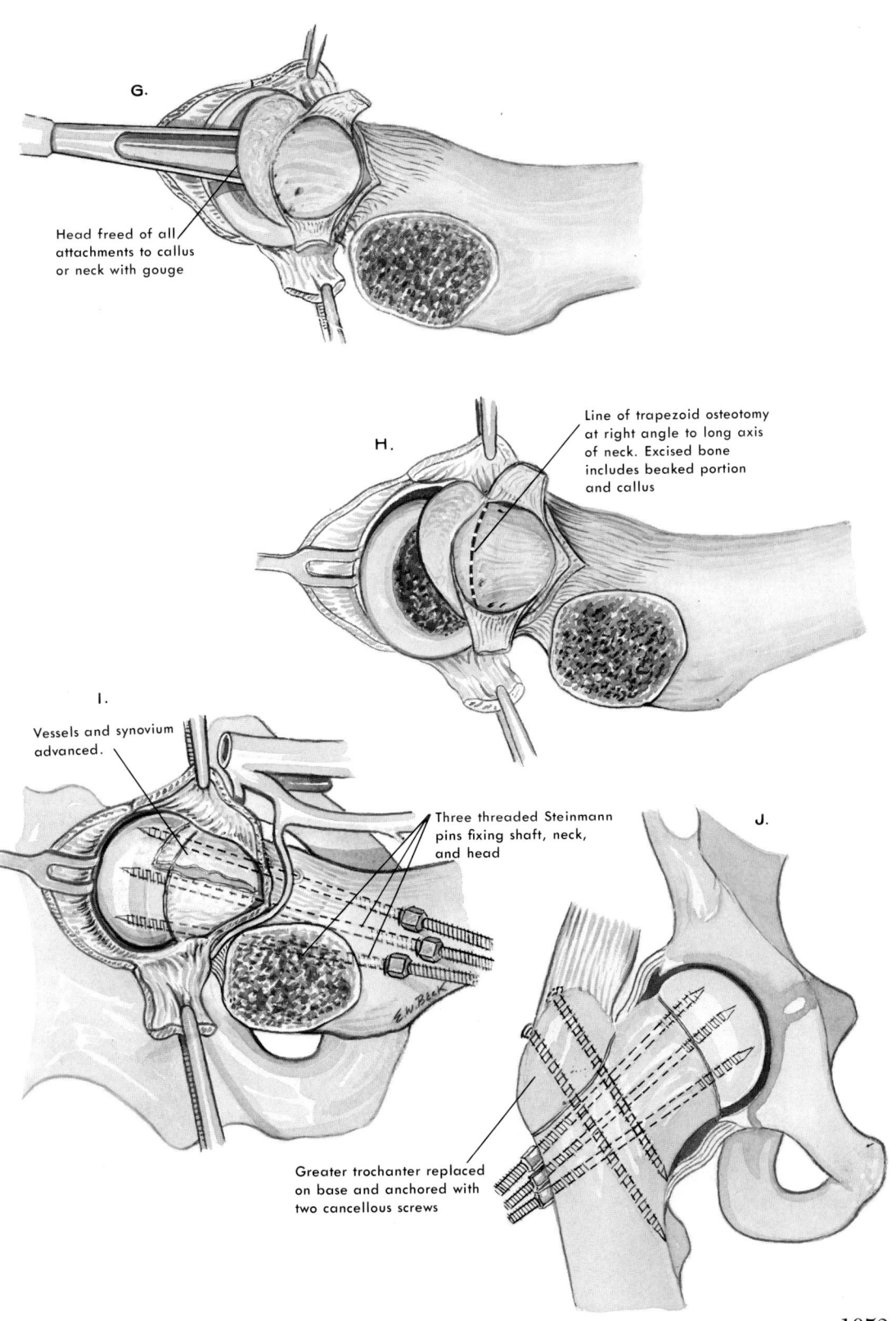

Dunn Procedure—Open Reduction of Displaced Femoral Head by Shortening Femoral Neck (Continued)

K to **Q.** Illustration of the importance of excision of a trapezoid segment of bone from the upper neck of the femur in order to prevent stretching of retinacular vessels.

The wound is closed in layers and the patient placed in split Russell traction. Postoperative rehabilitation and exercise regimen are the same as those following the Kramer osteotomy.

Plate 36. Dunn Procedure—Open Reduction of Displaced Femoral Head by Shortening Femoral Neck

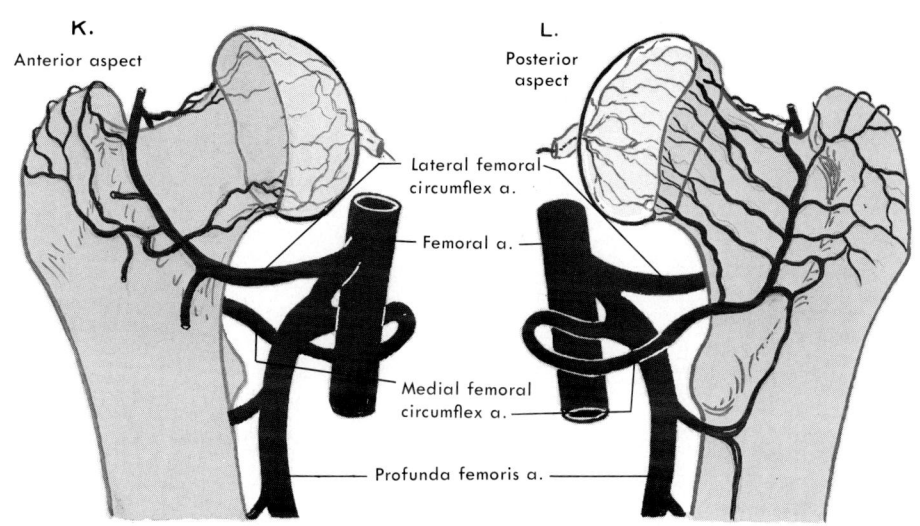

K. Anterior aspect
L. Posterior aspect

- Lateral femoral circumflex a.
- Femoral a.
- Medial femoral circumflex a.
- Profunda femoris a.

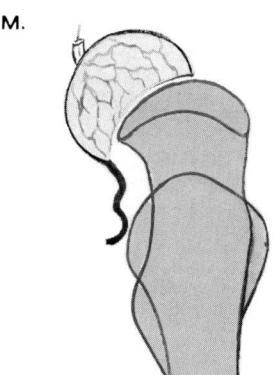

M. Acute on chronic slip. Retinacular vessels shorten after few days

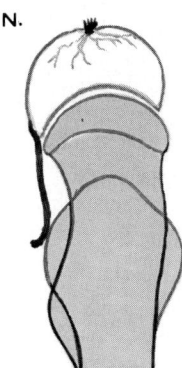

N. Attempted closed reduction will stretch blood vessels. Only blood supply to head is from artery of lig. teres

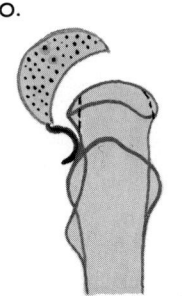

O. Immediate injury

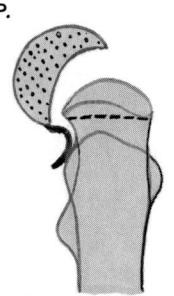

P. Trapezoid osteotomy of neck

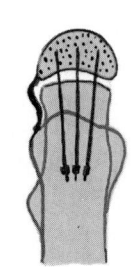

Q. Neck shortened. Retinacular vessels relaxed

Southwick's Biplane Intertrochanteric Osteotomy With Internal Compression Fixation

The patient is placed supine on a radiolucent operating table with the lower limb draped free. The anterior and lateral surfaces of the proximal femur are exposed subperiosteally at the level of the lesser trochanter. Dissection of the posterior surfaces of the femur is not necessary. The psoas tendon is detached at its insertion to the lesser trochanter (see steps E and F).

OPERATIVE TECHNIQUE

A. The junction of the anterior and lateral surfaces of the femur is identified with a longitudinal orientation mark. A transverse mark is made at the level of the lesser trochanter at right angles to the longitudinal orientation mark. This transverse line locates the inferior border of the wedge to be removed. A template composed of adjoining right triangles is placed on the transverse line and the wedge of bone to be resected is outlined on bone.

Next, a 5.5 mm. hole is made with a drill point in the lateral edge of the anterior cortex of the greater trochanter, and with a T-handle chuck a special threaded holding pin, 6.3 mm. in diameter is inserted. The line of insertion is parallel and 6.3 mm. proximal to the hypotenuse (oblique line) of the wedge to be removed from the anterior cortex. The holding pin is directed toward the upper margin of the lesser trochanter.

B. The wedge of bone is removed with a sharp osteotome or an electric saw. The surface on the upper segment is oblique, whereas that of the distal shaft segment is transverse. The osteotomy is completed by continuation of the transverse cut through the lesser trochanter. Avoid injury to the soft tissues posteriorly and medially.

Plate 37. Southwick's Biplane Intertrochanteric Osteotomy With Internal Compression Fixation

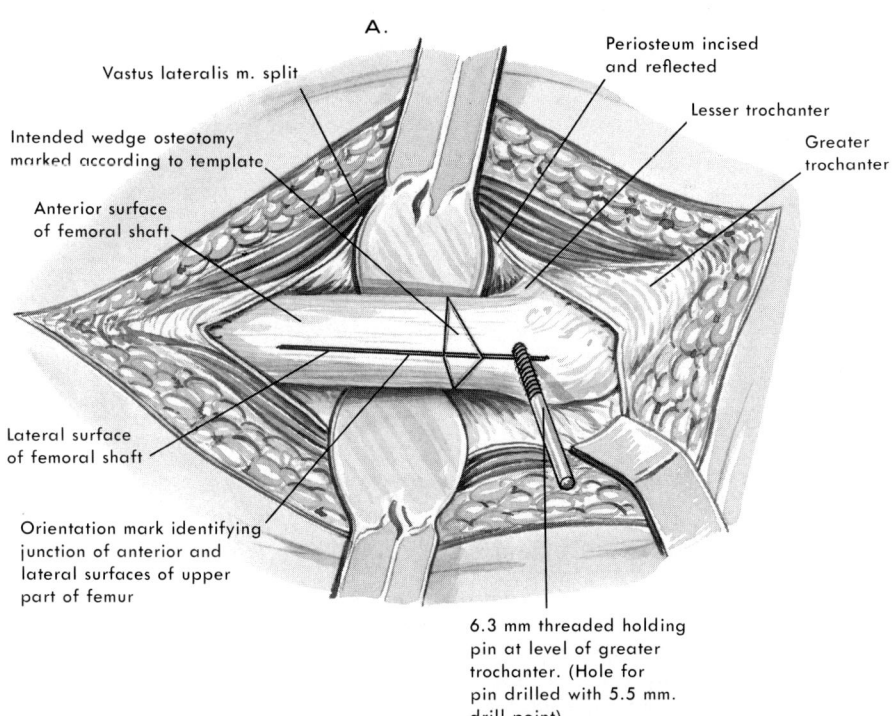
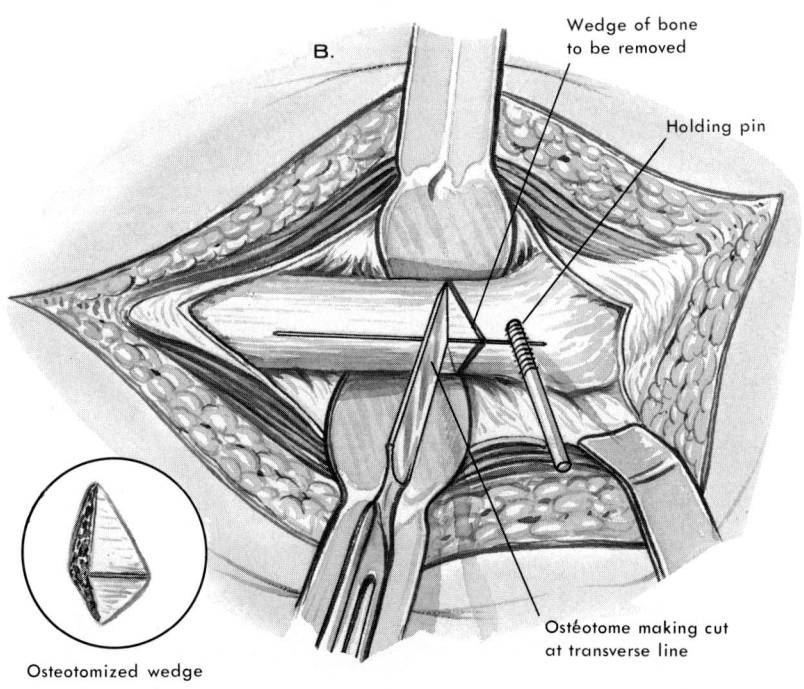

Southwick's Biplane Intertrochanteric Osteotomy With Internal Compression Fixation (Continued)

C. After completion of the osteotomy, the pin in the proximal fragment is used as a handle to fix the proximal segment, and the thigh is abducted and flexed by an assistant until the oblique cut surface of the upper segment fits flush against the transverse cut of the distal segment to correct the lateral rotation deformity to the desired degree. The distal segment is rotated medially the required amount. Once the two fragments are in the desired position, a drill hole, 5.5 mm. in diameter is made in the distal fragment for the second holding pin. Medial displacement of the distal fragment during drilling and insertion of the pin is prevented with a bone hook, which is inserted into the medullary canal of the shaft. It is crucial that the second holding pin be parallel to the pin in the proximal fragment. Its site should be 3 cm. distal to the osteotomy line. The use of the compression block will facilitate placement of the distal pin. If there is any instability of the osteotomized fragments, a third pin may be inserted through a hole in the compression block to control the proximal segment.

D. The knob in the compression block is twisted, compressing the osteotomized segment until the cut surfaces are in stable apposition. All during this procedure, the assistant supports the patient's thigh, preventing slipping or overriding of the osteotomy surfaces.

Plate 37. Southwick's Biplane Intertrochanteric Osteotomy With Internal Compression Fixation

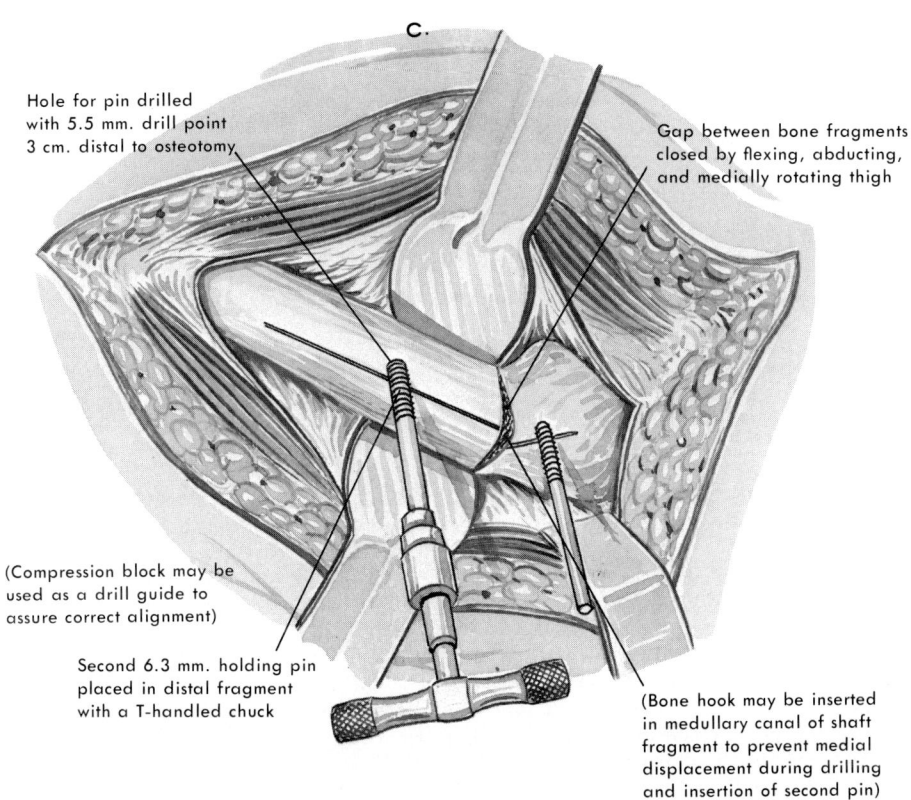

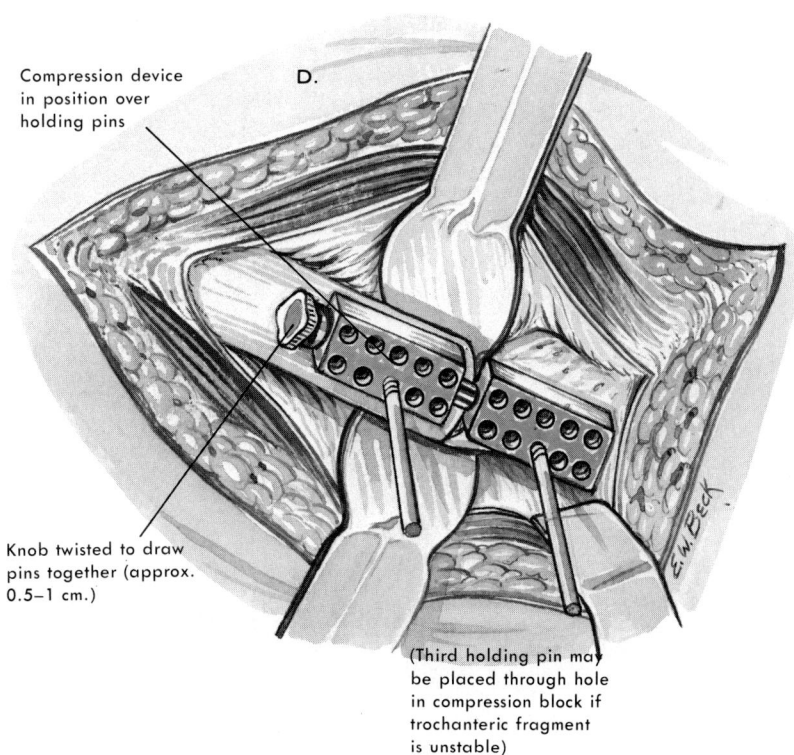

Southwick's Biplane Intertrochanteric Osteotomy With Internal Compression Fixation (Continued)

E. A specially manufactured compression plate is bent to conform to the contour of the femur and fixed with two cancellous bone screws, 5 cm. in length that are inserted in the proximal fragment through predrilled 5.5 mm. holes. One of the screws should cross the neck of the femur into the calcar. The distal fragment is fixed with 4.2 mm. screws.

Sequence of screw placement is important. First, the lower screw in the upper fragment is inserted. Second, the most distal screw in the lower fragment is inserted. Next placed is the screw at the top hole of the proximal fragment. Then the distal screws are inserted in the shaft as marked in the drawing.

F. The compression plate and holding pins are removed, and the adequacy of the fixation plate is double checked. Anteroposterior and frog-leg lateral roentgenograms are made to check the position and adequacy of correction of the deformity.

POSTOPERATIVE CARE

Postoperatively, no hip spica cast is required. The patient is placed in bilateral split Russell's traction with the hip in 30 degrees flexion to relax the capsule. Two to three days postoperatively, as soon as he is comfortable, the patient is allowed to sit at the edge of the bed. As soon as there is adequate muscle strength, he can flex the hip and extend the knee. A three-point crutch gait is permitted with toe touch on the affected side. Crutch protection is continued until bony union has taken place about two to three months postoperatively.

Plate 37. Southwick's Biplane Intertrochanteric Osteotomy With Internal Compression Fixation

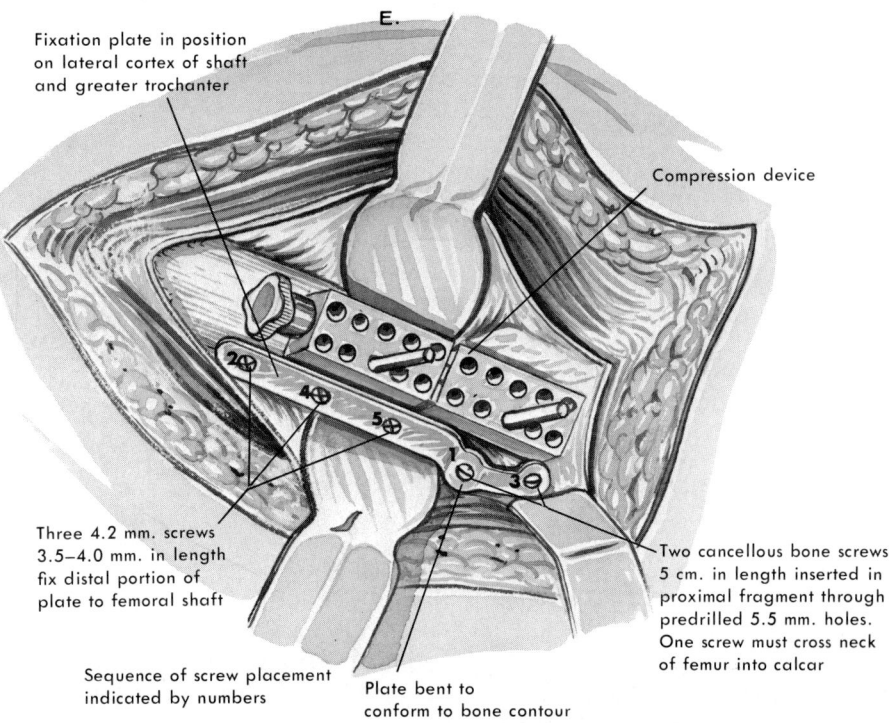

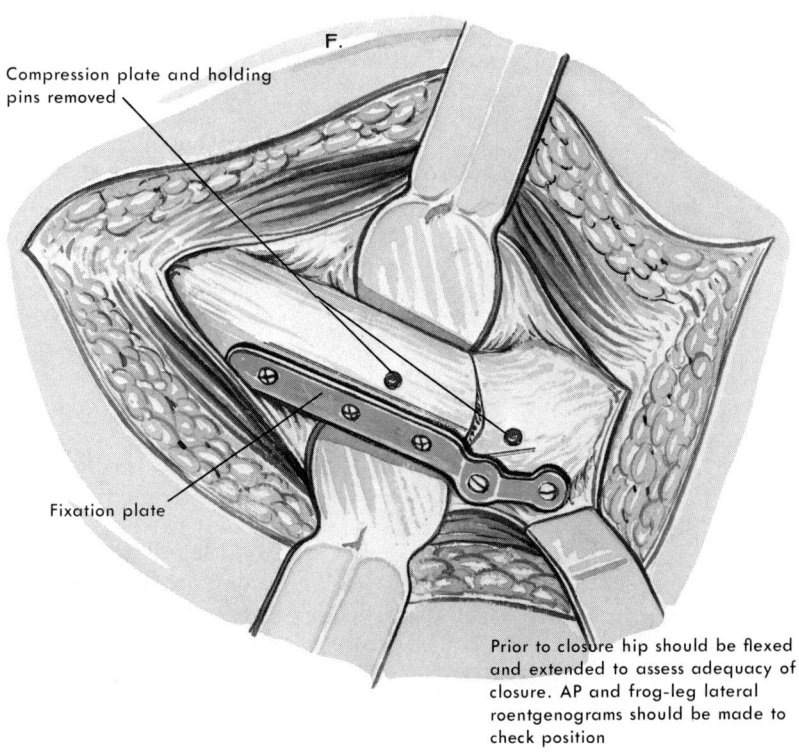

of posterior slip—in anterior slip there is hip flexion deformity and limitation of lateral rotation of the hip. The range of abduction is limited because of inferior displacement of the femoral head.

Treatment consists of open reduction by osteotomy of the femoral neck and internal fixation with one or two cannulated hip screws. Because the posterior-inferior retinacular vessels are intact, the risk of avascular necrosis is not great; however, one should exercise great caution during surgery not to disturb the blood supply to the femoral head.

Osteotomies to Correct the Deformity of Slipped Capital Femoral Epiphysis

When there is a severe slip, more than 70 per cent, an osteotomy is indicated to correct the lateral rotation, extension, and varus deformity. Several options are available. Closing wedge osteotomy through the femoral neck–physeal region corrects the deformity at the pathologic site, but it has a very high incidence of avascular necrosis and chondrolysis and a complication rate of 35 to 40 per cent. Because of such a serious high complication rate, the procedure should seldom be performed.

Dunn Procedure. The only indication to do an osteotomy through the neck of the femur is when the slip is greater than 70 per cent and the severity of joint incongruity is unacceptable; in such an instance the author recommends Dunn's procedure of osteotomy at the neck of the femur with bony shortening through a direct lateral transtrochanteric approach. Its advantages are that the main retinacular blood supply traverses the posterior aspect of the femoral neck. By osteotomizing the greater trochanter and opening the capsule on its superolateral aspect and around the rim of the acetabulum, one can strip the periosteum and its contained vessels under direct vision. By shortening the femoral neck, tension on the retinacular vessels is prevented. The operative technique is described and illustrated in Plate 36.

Among 69 patients (73 hips) Dunn reported 13 cases of chondrolysis and 11 cases of avascular necrosis. Five hips had both chondrolysis and avascular necrosis. The radiographic result was poor in 20 hips, in 15 of them due to avascular necrosis or chondrolysis. The results were less satisfactory in cases of acute on chronic slip, indicating damage to the blood supply to the femoral head at the time of acute displacement. Dunn advises not performing his operation if the growth plate is closed.[87]

Southwick Trochanteric Triplane Osteotomy. Compensatory osteotomies can be performed distal to the site of the deformity by creating a deformity in the opposite direction. The most common procedure is the Southwick trochanteric triplane osteotomy. The technique is described and illustrated in Plate 37. The disadvantages of Southwick osteotomy are that it increases compression forces across the hip joint, with a definite risk for chondrolysis. Rigid internal fixation allows early motion of the hip, thereby decreasing the incidence of chondrolysis.

Osteotomy Through the Base of the Neck of the Femur (Kramer). The correction of deformity is closer to the site of the problem, but has the disadvantage of greater risk of disturbing the blood supply to the femoral head. It corrects lateral rotation deformity adequately. The operative technique is described and illustrated in Plate 38.

Subtrochanteric Osteotomy After Closure of the Growth Plate. This procedure is simple and adequately corrects lateral rotation and extension deformity of the hip. This author finds it the safest way to correct deformity of healed, malunited chronic slipped capital femoral epiphysis. Its disadvantage is the creation of a deformed upper shaft of the femur—this makes total joint replacement difficult when the patient develops degenerative arthritis in adult life.

Problems and Complications

Chondrolysis

Chrondrolysis (or acute necrosis of hyaline articular cartilage) of the hip as a complication of slipped capital femoral epiphysis was first described by Elmslie in 1913.[95] Waldenström, in 1930, established chondrolysis as a definite pathologic entity distinct from avascular necrosis; it has since been reported by numerous authors.*

The etiology of chondrolysis is not exactly known. There are two basic theories of its pathogenesis; Waldenström and later Cruess proposed that it is caused by failure of nutrition of articular cartilage due to lack or paucity of synovial fluid production.[74, 381] Mankin and associates, however, gave scientific evidence that chondrolysis is induced by release of lysosomal enzymes that interfere with the synthetic processes of hyaline cartilage in genetically susceptible individuals; the autolysis of articular car-

---

*See references 36, 85, 91, 92, 120, 173, 184, 268, 381, 391.

tilage is caused by their own degradation products.[241]

The incidence of chondrolysis in association with slipped capital femoral epiphysis has been reported to be 1.1 to 40 per cent, with an average of 8 per cent (Table 3–22).

Factors that determine the prevalence of chondrolysis are race, sex, penetration of pins, prolonged immobilization, valgus osteotomy, and chronic severe slip with joint incongruity (Table 3–23). *Race*—the incidence of chondrolysis is high in the black and Hawaiian. *Sex*—it is more common in the female; the female to male ratio in chondrolysis is 2 : 1 to 5 : 1, whereas in slipped capital femoral epiphysis it is 1 : 2 to 1 : 4. It is obvious that a patient with slipped capital femoral epiphysis who is female and black or Hawaiian is at great risk for developing chondrolysis of the hip. *Penetration of pins into the joint*—introduction of particles of articular cartilage into the joint produces synovitis of the hip; the perpetuating synovitis and presence of cartilage detritus in the joint can elicit an autoimmune response to articular cartilage antigens and result in the destruction of hyaline cartilage. *Prolonged immobilization of the joint*—hip spica cast immobilization or heavy skeletal traction in bed may precipitate or exacerbate cartilage necrosis.[182, 245] *Valgus osteotomy*—an operation such as the Southwick triplane intertrochanteric osteotomy will increase pressure across the joint and predispose to chondrolysis. *Chronic severe slip with incongruity*—hip joint incongruity may be a factor in other cases of chondrolysis. Chondrolysis of the hip may be associated with avascular necrosis and stress fracture of the femoral head. The anatomic integrity of the subchondral bony plate is important in providing mechanical support to the articular cartilage.

Pathology. The anatomic findings vary with the stage of the disease in its natural history.

Table 3–22. Incidence of Chondrolysis in Association With Slipped Capital Femoral Epiphysis

Author	Per Cent	Incidence in Hips
Wiberg	1.1	2 of 185
Hall	1.7	3 of 173
Cruess	2.2	3 of 136
Ponseti and Barta	3.3	3 of 92
Jerre	4.4	9 of 204
Newman	6.7	4 of 60
Durbin	7.4	6 of 81
Lowe	15	15 of 100
Maurer and Larsen	28.2	11 of 39
Orofino et al.	28.4	36 of 127
Tillema and Golding	40	19 of 47

Table 3–23. Patients at High Risk for Chondrolysis in Association With Slipped Capital Femoral Epiphyses

Race—black or Hawaiian
Sex–female
Pin penetration into joint
Valgus osteotomy
Immobilization in spica cast
Heavy skeletal traction
Chronic severe slip

The initial findings are those of a nonspecific inflammatory process—the synovium is thickened with large boggy villous projections; later on the synovial membrane undergoes fibrotic changes. The capsule is thickened. The initial gross appearance of the articular cartilage is normal; however, as the disease process progresses the articular surface becomes thin, attenuated, and soft. The hyaline articular cartilage on both sides of the hip joint—acetabular and femoral—is involved. True pannus formation is not seen. With progression of the disease, gradually granulation tissue invades the articular surfaces and fibrous adhesions form between the capsule, acetabulum, and femoral head. In the chronic stage the articular cartilage may be almost completely disintegrated, exposing raw bone in the femoral head and acetabulum.

Histologic sections in the initial stage show the synovium to be hypertrophied and hypervascularized with perivascular infiltration with round cells consisting of plasma and lymphoid elements. With progression of the chondrolytic process the synovium is gradually replaced by fibrous tissue, and the amount of functioning synovium is progressively diminished. The hyaline cartilage is involved in the necrotic and degenerative process in varying extent and depth.

In the chronic stage of chondrolysis three layers of articular cartilage are noted: an outer fibrous or fibrocartilaginous layer; a middle layer with necrotic chondrocytes and Wexelbaum lacunae; and a deep layer that occasionally appears to be normal but in which the chondrocytes have often undergone varying degrees of necrosis. Electronmicroscopy shows extensive cytolysis of the cartilaginous cells. In some areas cartilage is eroded all the way deep to subchondral bone; in other areas there is a varying degree of repair with fibrocartilage. The collagen content is decreased. The subchondral bone is normal, and the bone trabeculae are viable. There may be fibrosis of bone marrow.

Degenerative arthritic changes with spurs of the joint margin and narrowing or near oblit-
Text continued on page 1066

Kramer's Compensatory Osteotomy of Base of Femoral Neck for Slipped Capital Femoral Epiphysis

OPERATIVE TECHNIQUE

A and **B.** The skin incision begins 2 cm. distal and lateral to the anterior superior iliac spine and curves distally and posteriorly over the lateral aspect of the greater trochanter and the femoral shaft to a point 10 cm. distal to the base of the great trochanter. The subcutaneous tissue and deep fascia are incised longitudinally. The interval between the gluteus medius and tensor fasciae latae is developed. The hip joint capsule is exposed along the anterior superior surface of the femoral neck. The vastus lateralis muscle is detached at its origin and reflected distally. An incision is made in the capsule along the anterior intertrochanteric line. With the hip joint opened, the degree of slip is assessed by inspection. Also, the amount of callus between the cartilage of the femoral head and the normal cortex of the femoral neck is determined. In general, the wedge of bone to be removed is two thirds of the width of the callus as measured directly anteriorly. The inferior osteotomy line is made first, perpendicular to the femoral neck following the anterior intertrochanteric line from above downward. The osteotomies extend posteriorly, leaving the posterior cortex intact. The vessels in the intertrochanteric fossa should be protected from injury.

Next, a threaded Steinmann pin is drilled into the proximal part of the femoral neck to control the upper fragment. The second, or upper, osteotomy line is made with the blade of the osteotome or saw directed obliquely and posteriorly. Again the posterior cortex should be left intact. This will permit making a greenstick fracture in the posterior cortex when the osteotoomy site is closed.

C and **D.** Three threaded Steinmann pins are drilled along the outer cortex of the upper femoral shaft toward the osteotomy site. The osteotomy site is closed by medial rotation and abduction of the distal segment. The three pins are then drilled into the femoral head.

Kramer recommends apophyseodesis of the greater trochanteric growth plate to prevent overgrowth of the greater trochanter. This is done in a child who is relatively young, under 14 years of age in boys and under 12 years of age in girls.

POSTOPERATIVE CARE

The patient is placed in split Russell traction with a medial rotation strap at the thigh. As he is comfortable, he may stand and ambulate with a three-point crutch gait. The pins are removed when the osteotomy is healed and the physis is closed.

Plate 38. Kramer's Compensatory Osteotomy of Base of Femoral Neck for Slipped Capital Femoral Epiphysis

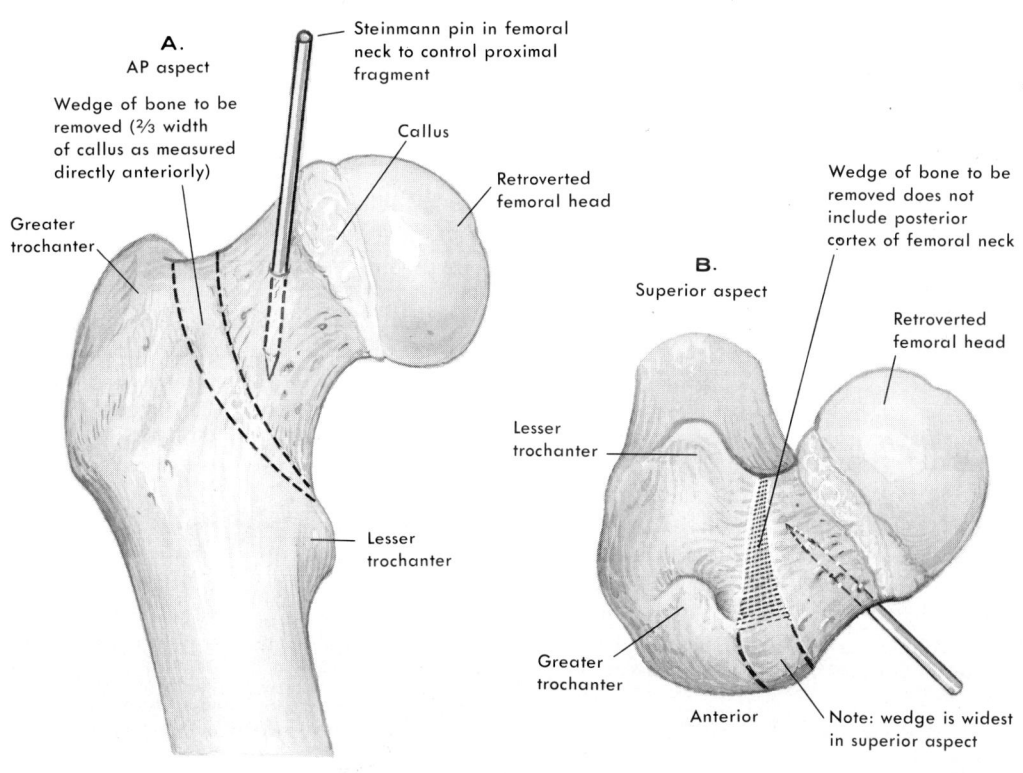

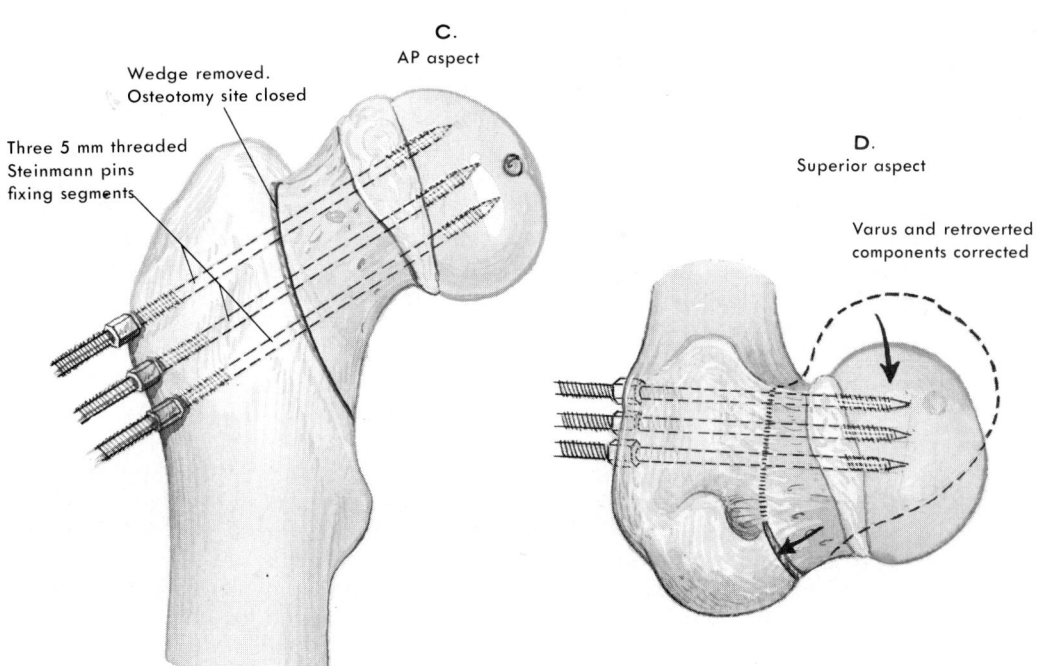

eration of the joint space develop later on in life.

Natural History. Chondrolysis may be subdivided into three stages in the course of the disease: *acute*, the first six weeks; *subacute*, from one and one half to six months, and *chronic*, six months from onset of symptoms and over.

The natural history may follow one of two courses. In the *benign form* there is spontaneous restitution of articular cartilage space with nearly normal return of range of hip motion within 6 to 12 months. In the *recalcitrant form* there is progressive loss of joint space with degenerative arthrosis and fibrous ankylosis of the hip. In the experience of this author, over a third of the cases of chondrolysis associated with slipped capital femoral epiphysis will follow a benign course and almost two thirds a recalcitrant course. It is difficult to predict which hips will do well. Ordinarily failure to respond to conservative treatment with persistent loss of hip motion and progressive narrowing of articular cartilage space are ominous signs. In sequential bone imaging with technetium-99m the recalcitrant form of chondrolysis shows persistent and increasing uptake of the radionuclide, whereas in the benign form the uptake diminishes.

Clinical Picture. Increasing stiffness of the hip with muscle spasm and pain is the presenting complaint. In uncomplicated slipped capital femoral epiphysis the loss of hip motion is in flexion, medial rotation, and abduction, the degree of restriction of joint motion being directly related to the severity of slipping; there is no flexion deformity of the hip. In chondrolysis the loss of hip motion is in all planes and not related to the amount of slipping; also, in chondrolysis there is flexion deformity of the hip. When hip flexion contracture is present one should suspect chondrolysis. In uncomplicated slipped capital femoral epiphysis, some degree of hip motion (the part lost because of muscle spasm and synovitis) returns after bed rest and traction; in chondrolysis loss of hip motion persists with minimal or no response to traction. In the postoperative period of slipped capital femoral epiphysis, other conditions that may cause increasing hip stiffness and pain are postoperative low-grade infection, transient reactive synovitis, and aseptic necrosis. Are the pins penetrating into the joint? In suspicious cases a computed tomographic scan is of great value to rule out pin penetration. If the pins are within the joint, they should be withdrawn and replaced by shorter pins. Appropriate laboratory work (complete blood count and erythrocyte sedimentation rate) is carried out to rule out infection. In chondrolysis the patient is afebrile and has no systemic signs; the erythrocyte sedimentation rate is normal, and there are no laboratory findings to suggest infection.

Radiographic Findings. The initial radiographic change is juxta-articular regional osteoporosis of the acetabulum, femoral head, and neck; it is caused by disuse atrophy and by regional increased blood flow due to hyperemia of the synovium. This osteoporosis is a nonspecific finding.

The next change is narrowing of cartilage space, to less than 50 per cent of the width of the opposite normal hip. If chondrolysis affects both hips the contralateral hip cannot be used for comparison. The normal articular width in the weight-bearing portion of the hip is 4 to 5 mm.; an articular cartilage space of 2 mm. or less is considered to be very suggestive of chondrolysis.

In time there will be premature closure of the growth plates of the femoral head, the triradiate cartilage, and the greater and lesser trochanters. Intrapelvic protrusion of the acetabulum (Otto pelvis) may develop (Fig. 3–196).

Later in the course of chondrolysis there will be irregularity and erosion of subchondral bone. Nuclear magnetic resonance imaging will depict the degree of thinning and erosion of articular cartilage. Arthrography is not recommended by this author because it is difficult to perform because of fibrous adhesions in the joint. Eventually osteoarthritic changes develop consisting of subchondral cysts and osteophytes. In the severe cases of chondrolysis there will be complete fibrous ankylosis.

Bone Scan. In chondrolysis bone imaging with technetium-99m shows increased uptake in both the acetabulum and the femoral head (Fig. 3–197). This is present early, in the acute stage of chondrolysis. In uncomplicated slipped capital femoral epiphysis there is increased uptake only in the capital physis. Early diagnosis of chondrolysis is vital to improve the outcome. When there is hip flexion contracture in slipped capital femoral epiphysis, bone imaging with technetium-99m should be performed. This author was able to diagnose chondrolysis by bone imaging in eight patients with slipped capital femoral epiphysis prior to surgery. Without operative treatment, further slip did not occur in any of these patients. In the opinion of this author, hip pinning or open epiphysiodesis is not indicated in slipped capital femoral epiphysis associated with chondrolysis; the patient, however, should be closely observed.

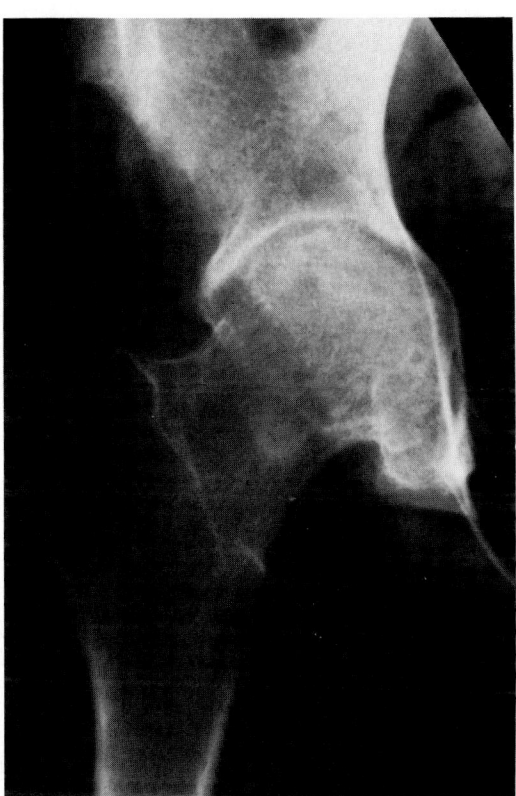

FIGURE 3-196. *Narrowing of the articular cartilage space in chondrolysis of the hip with intrapelvic protrusion of the acetabulum (Otto pelvis).*

Treatment. In the acute stage the patient is placed in bilateral counterpoised split Russell traction. Do not employ unilateral traction because the pelvis on the affected side will tilt distally, and abduction contracture of the hip will develop. This is best carried out in the hospital initially, which allows for an appropriate diagnostic work-up. Active and passive exercises are performed several times a day to increase range of hip motion and correct any contractural deformity. Anti-inflammatory drugs (Naprosyn or salicylates) are administered in the appropriate therapeutic dosage. Vitamin E may be given orally on theoretical grounds, as experimentally it enhances cartilage healing.

When he can tolerate it, the patient is placed in a continuous passive hip motion machine, initially full-time and then part-time. Motion is life! The patient is allowed to be up and around on crutches—three-point gait with partial weight-bearing and protection of the affected lower limb.

Most patients with chondrolysis of the hip are obese; weight reduction by dietary control is crucial.

In six months in the chronic stage of chondrolysis when the hip joint's range of motion is still restricted, or in three months when it does not respond to the foregoing mode of therapy, the patient is taken to the operating room, and under general anesthesia the range of hip motion is assessed. This should be performed very gently in order to avoid stress fractures of the femoral neck. If, under anesthesia, normal range of hip motion is present, treatment by continuous passive hip motion machine, exercise, three-point crutch protection, and anti-inflammatory medication is continued. If, however, under general anesthesia there is marked restriction of hip motion, soft-tissue release is performed. The hip adductors, longus and

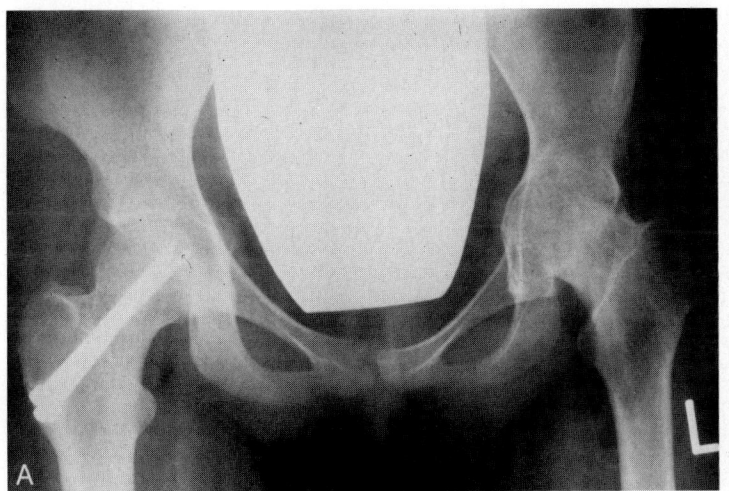 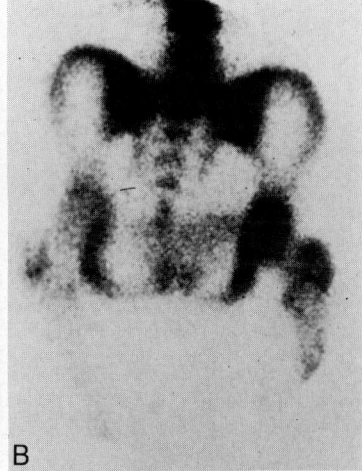

FIGURE 3-197. *Bone imaging with technetium-99m in chondrolysis of the hip.*

A. Radiogram of both hips. Left hip shows marked narrowing of the articular cartilage space. **B.** Bone scan. Note the diffuse increased uptake in both the acetabulum and the femoral head.

brevis, are sectioned, the iliopsoas is lengthened fractionally at its musculotendinous junction, and partial capsulectomy of the hip is carried out. It is crucial to leave the posteroinferior part of the capsule intact; in order to prevent avascular necrosis, do not section the ligamentum teres and do not dislocate the hip. Postoperatively the patient is placed in a continuous passive hip motion machine, and exercises and crutch protection are continued. If at surgery the hyaline articular cartilage appears grossly normal, the hip may be salvaged and functional range of hip motion restored.

Salvage of the hip is impossible if at surgery there are diffuse intra-articular adhesions with marked scarring of the capsule; if the hyaline cartilage is pitted, destroyed, and replaced by fibrous tissue; and if the cartilage necrosis is severe. In such cases, if involvement is unilateral this author recommends hip arthrodesis (Fig. 3–198). The results of hip fusion are very satisfactory. He does not recommend hip joint resurfacing because in his experience the results have been very poor. All cases resulted in failure requiring hip arthrodesis. Severe chondrolysis of both hips can occur occasionally; this poses a very difficult problem of management. There is no satisfactory treatment. One may perform arthrodesis of a hip and total joint replacement of the other hip, or choose total joint replacement of both hips. The long-term results of total joint replacement are poor owing to loosening of the components and stress fracture.

Avascular Necrosis

Avascular necrosis of the femoral head may follow closed reduction of an acute slip, open reduction of a chronic or subacute slip by osteotomy of the femoral neck or, occasionally, compensatory osteotomy at the base of the femoral neck, and pinning of the femoral head-neck by three or four pins (which disturbs the intraosseous blood supply, particularly if they are placed in the anterolateral part of the femoral epiphysis). A markedly displaced acute slip by itself may disturb the blood supply to the femoral head by stretching or tamponading the retinacular vessels.

Avascular necrosis of the femoral head in slipped capital femoral epiphysis is a serious complication. In treating slipped capital femoral epiphysis every effort should be made to prevent it. Open reduction by osteotomy of the femoral neck should not be performed. Utilize a maximum of two cannulated hip screws for internal fixation of acute slip. Pre- and postoperative bone imaging with technetium-99m is very desirable to detect avascular necrosis and is highly recommended by this author. Prior to surgery it is best to maintain the hip in counterpoised bilateral split Russell traction. Inadvertent manipulation and rough handling of the hip may cause further displacement of an acute slip. Initial examination of the hip should be performed very cautiously, and repeated examinations, especially by the house staff, should be avoided. The patient is anesthetized on the cart or bed and then transferred to the fracture table very gently. Do not perform preoperative bone imaging in the department of nuclear medicine. Utilize a portable scanner in the operating room! A cold femoral head is suggestive of avascular necrosis; in such a case, especially when the acute slip is of traumatic origin, the joint capsule is opened during surgery to decompress the hip.

Clinically, in the postoperative period, avascular necrosis is suspected when there is per-

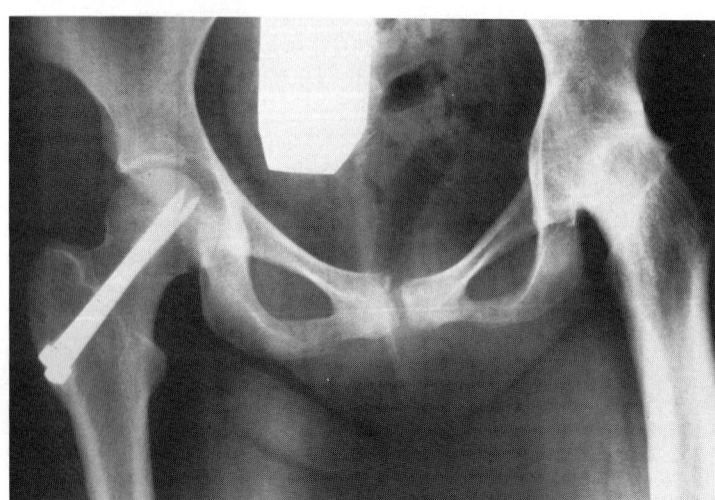

FIGURE 3–198. Severe chondrolysis in slipped capital femoral epiphysis of the left hip treated by hip arthrodesis.

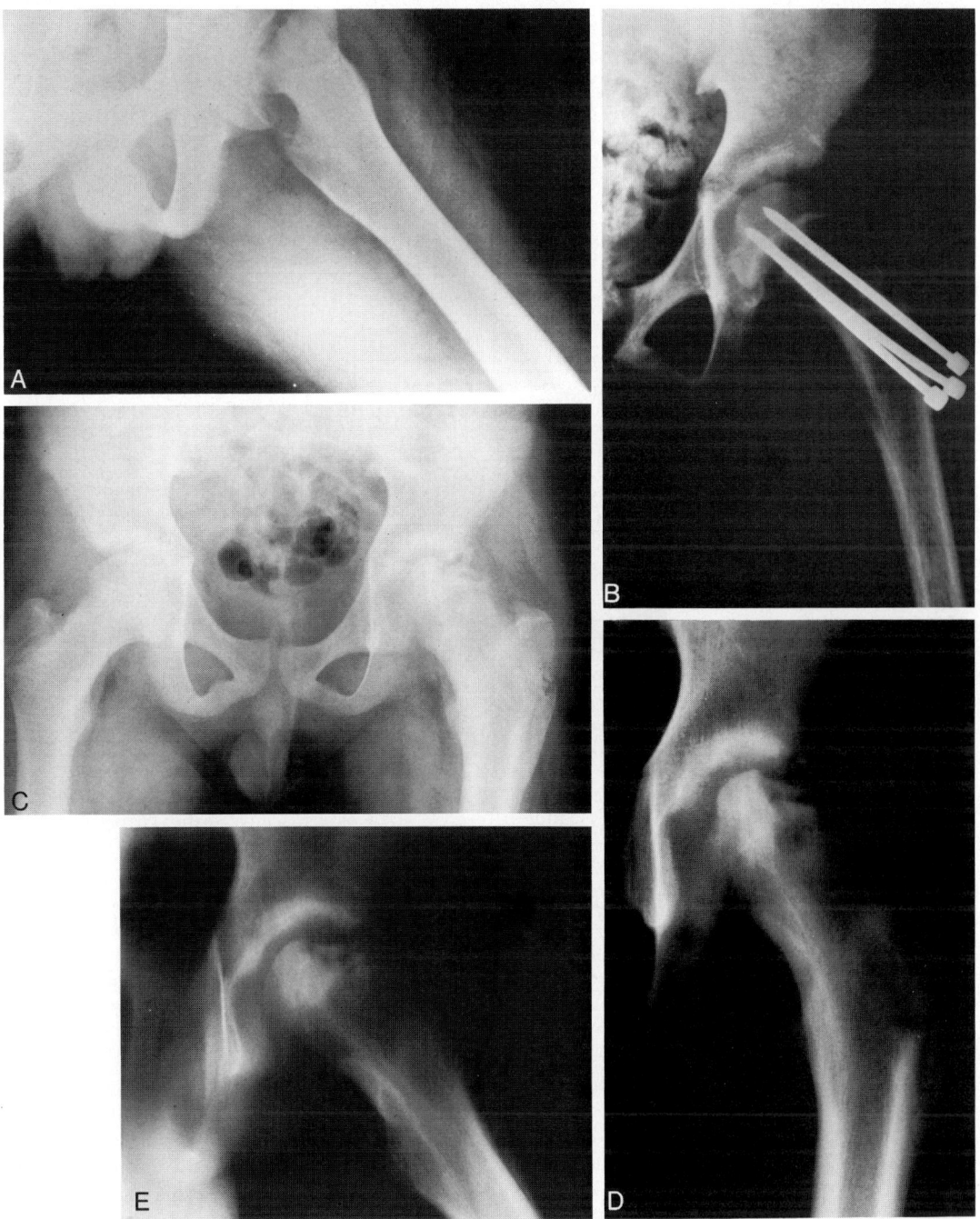

FIGURE 3–199. *Acute slipped capital femoral epiphysis of the left hip complicated by partial avascular necrosis and treated by Sugioka's intertrochanteric osteotomy.*

A. Initial radiogram showing acute slip. **B.** Post reduction and pinning with three screws. **C** to **E.** After removal of the pins, radiograms show segmental avascular necrosis.

Illustration continued on following page

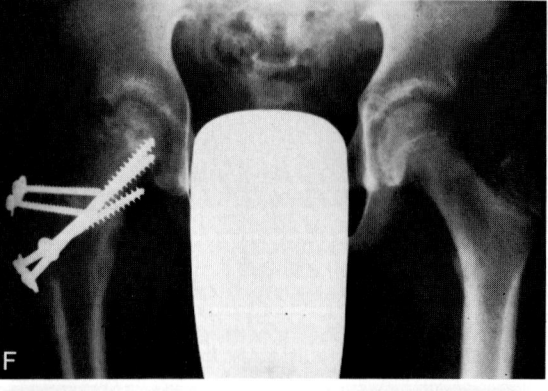
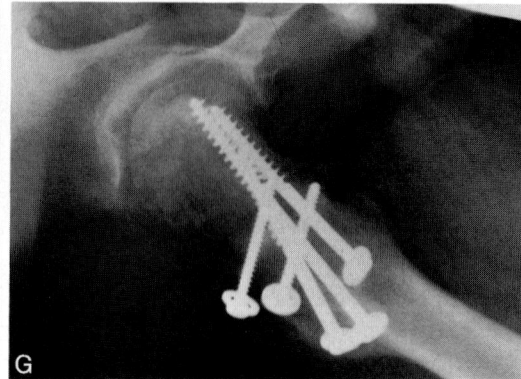
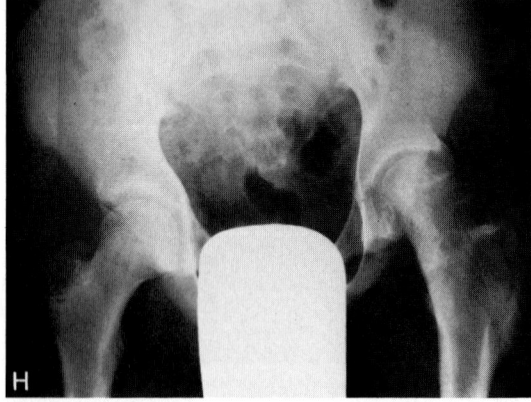

FIGURE 3–199 Continued. *Acute slipped capital femoral epiphysis of the left hip complicated by partial avascular necrosis and treated by Sugioka's introchanteric osteotomy.*

F and G. Following Sugioka's intertrochanteric osteotomy. H. Result two years later. Patient had almost full range of motion of the left hip. No pain and no limp.

sistent pain and limitation of hip motion. Collapse of the femoral head will cause penetration of the pins into the joint, which may cause chondrolysis of the hip; in such an instance, the pins should be removed immediately. When the capital physis is still open there is added danger of further slipping; should one reinsert a smaller size pin? This author recommends open epiphysiodesis. In the presence of total avascular necrosis it is best to utilize viable fibular or iliac bone graft with its vascular supply intact by using microsurgical technique. It will add several hours to the operating time. At present, long-term results are not available. Immediate results are equivocal. It may salvage the hip and avoid hip fusion in the future.

Avascular necrosis of the femoral head may be *total* or *segmental*. The best method to treat segmental avascular necrosis is Sugioka's transtrochanteric derotation osteotomy.[361] Preoperatively computed tomography with torsion studies is carried out to determine the direction and amount of rotation of the femoral head-neck in order to relieve weight-bearing stress on the necrotic fragment. Multiple drilling of the avascular fragment will hasten revascularization; if the fragment is loose it may be stabilized with a single countersunk small screw. In the experience of this author the results of Sugioka's operation in treatment of segmental avascular necrosis have been satisfactory (Fig. 3–199). They are definitely better in the adolescent than in the adult. If the cause of the segmental avascular necrosis is systemic disease, however, e.g., in a patient with kidney transplant or in an alcoholic patient, the results of Sugioka's operation are poor.

When avascular necrosis is total with collapse of the femoral head and involvement is unilateral, the best method of treatment is arthrodesis of the hip. This author utilizes a cobra plate for internal fixation (Fig. 3–200). The position of hip fusion depends on the sex and professional pursuits of the patient; ordinarily the optimum position is 20 degrees of hip flexion, 5 to 10 degrees of hip adduction, and 10 degrees of lateral rotation of the hip. Hip abductor muscle function is preserved by osteotomy of the greater trochanter and reattachment. The goal is preservation of the hip abductor muscle and good bone stock for total joint replacement later in adult life if so desired. The cobra plate is removed once the hip is solidly fused, usually 9 to 12 months postoperatively. When removing the plate and screws it is desirable to curet the screw tracts and pack the holes with autogenous bone graft in order to prevent stress fracture. The hip joint is protected with crutches and

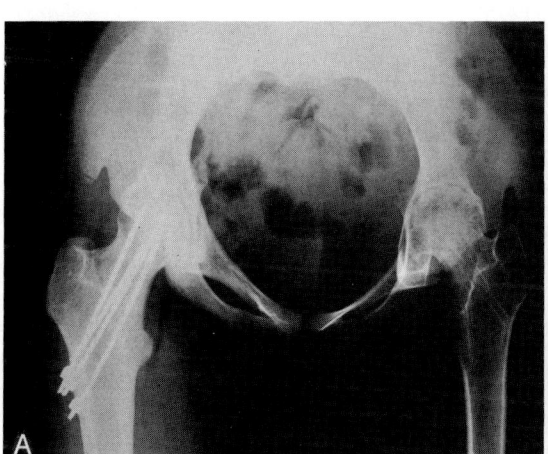
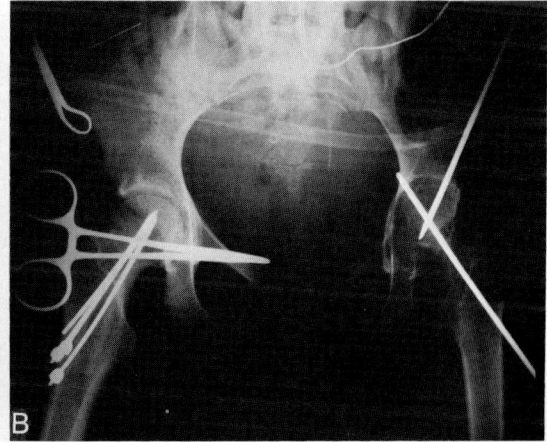
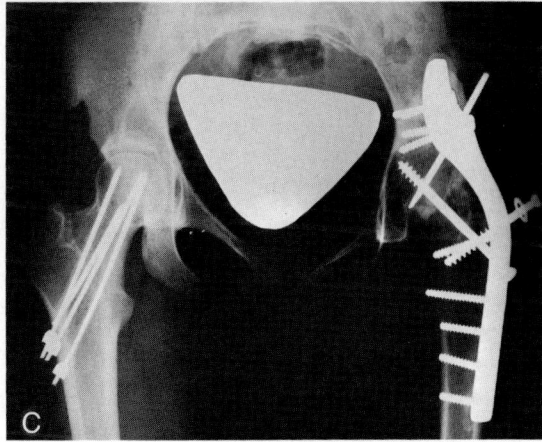

FIGURE 3–200. Avascular necrosis of the left femoral head following open reduction for acute slipped capital femoral epiphysis.

A. Radiogram of both hips showing the avascular necrosis and collapse of the femoral head. **B.** At surgery temporary fixation with crossed threaded Steinmann pins is utilized to check position of the hip prior to plating. **C.** Postoperative view showing the hip fusion with internal fixation with a cobra plate.

three-point partial weight-bearing. An uncooperative patient may have to be placed in a unilateral above-knee walking hip spica cast or plastic orthotic device.

The results of treating total avascular necrosis by hip joint resurfacing have been very poor. The outcome of three cases in which it was performed, in the experience of this author, was three stiff, painful hips; in all three cases the joint resurfacing components had to be removed and the hip fused two to three years postoperatively. Uniform failure of hip joint resurfacing is due to substantial loss of bone substance in the femoral head with eventual collapse and loosening of the components. This author has not performed total joint replacement in total avascular necrosis; it is an option that one must carefully assess in bilateral involvement.

Prior to collapse of the femoral head, vascularized live bone grafting by microsurgical technique may be attempted; fibular bone graft is probably better than iliac, as the thick cortices of the fibula may check collapse of the femoral head. The role of live bone grafting in total avascular necrosis of the femoral head is still

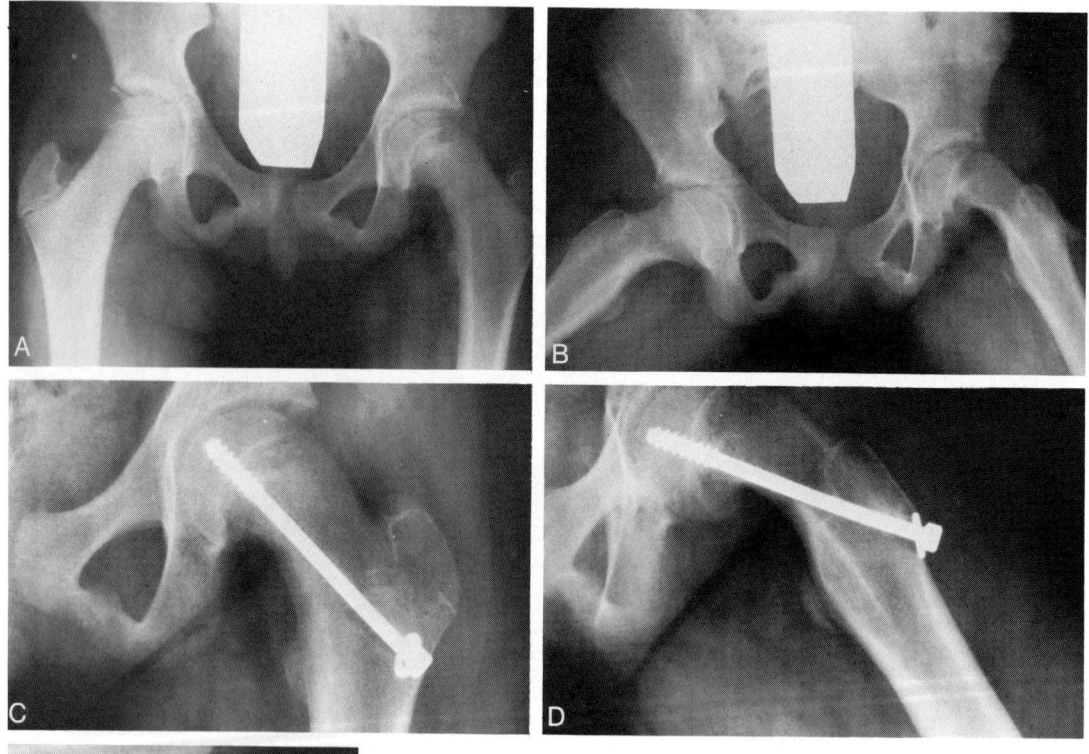

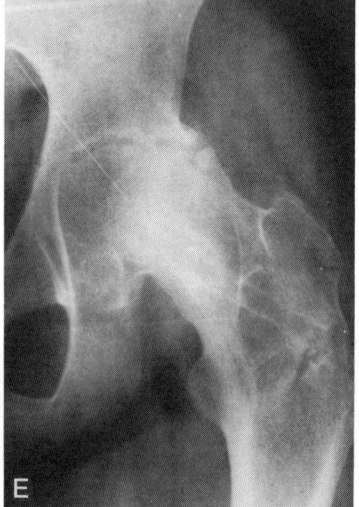

FIGURE 3–201. Stress fracture following removal of the pin fixation for slipped capital femoral epiphysis.

A and **B**. Preoperative anteroposterior and lateral radiographs. **C** and **D**. Following internal fixation with one Asnis screw. **E**. Subtrochanteric fracture following removal of the Asnis screw.

not determined. So far, in the limited experience of this author, the results are not satisfactory, but he will consider the procedure prior to collapse of the femoral head when involvement is bilateral.

Fracture After Pin Removal

A low site of insertion of the hip pins in the subtrochanteric region is a stress point, and there is a possibility of stress fracture (Fig. 3–201).

References

1. Aadalen, R. J., Weiner, D. S., Hoyt, W., and Herndon, C. H.: Acute slipped capital femoral epiphysis. J. Bone Joint Surg., 56-A:1473, 1974.
2. Adams, J. D.: Mechanics and reduction of displaced upper femoral epiphysis. N. Engl. J. Med., 210:178, 1934.
3. Adorjan, I.: On the treatment of advanced slipping of the upper femoral epiphysis. Acta Orthop. Scand., 30:286, 1961.
4. Akiyoshi, M., Oka, M., Suzuki, M., and Nakamura, T.: Histologic manifestations of impaired cross-linking of collagen molecules because of aminoacetonitrile in epiphyseal plates. J. Dent. Res. Suppl., 52:1005, 1973.
5. Al-Aswad, B. I., Weinger, J. M., and Schneider, A. B.: Slipped capital femoral epiphysis in a 35-year-old man. Clin. Orthop., 134:131, 1978.
6. Alexander, C.: The etiology of femoral epiphyseal slipping. J. Bone Joint Surg., 48-B:299, 1966.
7. Altcheck, M.: Acute slipped capital femoral epiphysis. J. Bone Joint Surg., 49-A:1233, 1967.
8. Ambrose, G. B., and McLaughlin, H. L.: Slipped upper femoral epiphysis and trauma. J. Trauma, 1:133, 1961.
9. Anderson, C. E., and Parker, J.: Electron microscopy of the epiphyseal cartilage plate. A critical review of electron microscopic observations on enchondral ossification. Clin. Orthop., 58:225, 1968.
10. Andren, L., and Borgstrom, K. E.: Seasonal variation of epiphysiolysis of the hip and possibility of causal factor. Acta Orthop. Scand., 28:22, 1958.
11. Arkin, A. M., and Katz, J. F.: The effects of pressure on epiphyseal growth. J. Bone Joint Surg., 38-A:1056, 1956.
12. Asnis, S. E.: The guided screw system in intracapsular fractures of the hip. Contemp. Orthop., 10:33, 1985.
13. Asnis, S. E.: The guided screw system in slipped capital femoral epiphysis. Contemp. Orthop., 11:27, 1985.
14. Auckland, C. A.: The etiology of femoral epiphyseal slipping. J. Bone Joint Surg., 48-B:299, 1966.
15. Axhausen, G.: Die Nekrose des proximalen Bruchstucks beim Schenkelhalsbruch und ihre Bedeutung fur das Hüftgelenk. Arch. Klin. Chir., 120:325, 1922.
16. Axhausen, G.: Die Bedeutung der aseptischen Knochennekrose fur die Knochen und Gelenkchirurgie. Z. Orthop. Chir., 47:37, 1926.
17. Badgley, C. E.: Displacement of the upper femoral epiphysis; summary of 27 studied cases. J.A.M.A., 92:355, 1929.
18. Badgley, C. E., Isaacson, A. S., Wolgamot, J. C., and Miller, J. W.: Operative therapy for slipped upper femoral epiphysis. J. Bone Joint Surg., 30-A:19, 1948.
19. Baker, G., and Louis, H.: Treatment of slipped capital femoral epiphysis with pinning. Paper presented at the Western Orthopaedic Association meeting, 1982.
20. Bannister, J.: Slipped femoral capital epiphysis: A review of 49 cases treated at the University of New South Wales Teaching Hospitals over the last ten years. Aust. N.Z. J. Surg., 45:294, 1975.
21. Barmada, R., Bruch, R. F., Gimbel, J. S., and Ray, R. D.: Base of the neck extracapsular osteotomy for correction of deformity in slipped capital femoral epiphysis. Clin. Orthop., 132:98, 1978.
22. Barrett, J., Imrie, D., and Derian, P.: Chondrolysis—a severe complication of slipped capital femoral epiphysis. Paper presented at the American Academy of Orthopaedic Surgeons Research Society Meeting, 1976.
23. Baxter, D. E.: A disease of the hips common in children: Slipped capital femoral epiphysis. St. Joseph Hosp. Med. Surg., 71:31, 1972.
24. Beck, E.: Ein Beitrag zum familiaren Vorkommen der Epiphysiolysis capitis femoris. Z. Orthop., 105:112, 1968.
25. Beck, W.: Die operative Behandlung des jugendlichen Hüftkopfgleitens. Beitr. Klin. Chir., 219:150, 1971.
26. Benjamin, B., and Miler, P. R.: Hypothyroidism as a cause of disease of the hip. Am. J. Dis. Child., 55:1189, 1938.
27. Bennet, G., Koreska, J., and Rang, M.: Pin replacement in slipped capital femoral epiphysis. J. Bone Joint Surg., 63-B:637, 1981.
28. Bennet, G. C., Koreska, J., and Rang, M.: Pin placement in slipped capital femoral epiphysis. J. Pediatr. Orthop., 4:574, 1984.
29. Bentzon, P.: Should reposition of epiphysiolysis capitis femoris not be made? Acta Orthop. Scand., 2:331, 1932.
30. Bernstein, M. A., and Arens, R. A.: Epiphyseolysis. Radiology, 9:497, 1927.
31. Bianco, A. J.: Treatment of mild slipping of the capital femoral epiphysis. J. Bone Joint Surg., 47-A:396, 1965.
32. Bianco, A. J., Jr.: Treatment of slipping of the capital femoral epiphysis. Clin. Orthop., 48:103, 1966.
33. Billing, L.: Roentgen examination of the proximal femur end in children and adolescents. A standardized technique also suitable for determination of the collum-, anteversion-, and epiphyseal angles. A study of slipped epiphysis and coxa plana. Acta Radiol., Suppl. 110, 1954.
34. Billing, L., and Severin, E.: Slipping epiphysis of the hip. A roentgenological and clinical study based on a new roentgen technique. Acta Radiol., Suppl. 174, 1959.
35. Bishop, J., Oley, T., Stephenson, C., and Tullos, H.: Slipped capital femoral epiphysis—a study of fifty cases in black children. Clin. Orthop., 135:93, 1978.
36. Bleck, E.: Idiopathic chondrolysis of the hip. J. Bone Joint Surg., 65-A:1266, 1983.
37. Bobechko, W. P.: Auto-immune reactions of articular cartilage. In Proceedings of the 12th Congress of the International Society of Orthopaedic Surgery and Traumatology, Tel Aviv, Oct. 9–12, 1972. New York, American Elsevier, 1973, pp. 18–26.
38. Bonjour, C.: Offene Reposition bei Epiphysiolysis capitis femoris acuta. Z. Orthop., 110:305, 1972.
39. Borofsky, E., and LaMont, R.: Result of multiple pinning in slipped capital femoral epiphysis. Paper presented at the American Orthopaedic Association Resident's Conference, 1982.
40. Bousseau, M.: Disjonction épiphysaire traumatique de la tête du femur. Bull. Soc. Anatomique de Paris, 42:283, 1867.
41. Boyd, H. B.: Treatment of minimally slipped upper femoral epiphysis. A.A.O.S. Instruct. Course Lect. 21:186, 1972.
42. Boyd, H. B.: Treatment of acute slipped upper femoral epiphysis. A.A.O.S. Instruct. Course Lect. 21:222, 1972.

43. Boyd, H. B., Ingram, A. J., and Bourhard, H. O.: The treatment of slipped femoral epiphysis. South. Med. J., 42:551, 1949.
44. Boyer, D. W., Mickelson, M. R., and Ponseti, I. V.: Slipped capital femoral epiphysis. Long-term follow-up study of one hundred and twenty-one patients. J. Bone Joint Surg., 63-A:83, 1981.
45. Brailsford, J. F.: Slipping of the epiphysis of the head of the femur. Lancet, 1:16, 1933.
46. Bright, R. W., Burstein, A. H., and Elmore, S. M.: Epiphyseal-plate cartilage: A biomechanical and histological analysis of failure modes. J. Bone Joint Surg., 56-A:688, 1974.
47. Brindley, H. H.: Disabilities of the hip in children. Am. J. Orthop., 1:88, 1959.
48. Brodetti, A.: The blood supply of the femoral neck and head in relation to the damaging effects of nails and screws. J. Bone Joint Surg., 42-B:794, 1960.
49. Brogden, W.: Review of the end results of 57 cases of slipped upper femoral epiphysis. J. Bone Joint Surg., 17:179, 1935.
50. Browne, P. S. H., and Wainwright, D.: Severe irreducible slipping of upper femoral epiphysis: A review of 14 cases treated by subtrochanteric osteotomy. Injury, 6:213, 1975.
51. Bruns, D.: Kleine Mitteilungen. Z. Orthop., 92:453, 1960.
52. Burrows, H. J.: Slipped upper femoral epiphysis. Characteristics of a hundred cases. J. Bone Joint Surg., 39-B:641, 1957.
53. Burstein, A. H., Currey, J., Frankel, V. H., Heiple, K. G., Lunseth, P., and Vessely, J. C.: Bone strength. The effect of screw holes. J. Bone Joint Surg., 54-A:1143, 1972.
54. Camero, H. U., Wang, M., and Koreska, J.: Internal fixation of slipped femoral capital epiphysis. Clin. Orthop., 137:148, 1978.
55. Capener, N.: In Platt, H. (ed.): Modern Trends in Orthopedics. (2nd. Series) London, Butterworth, 1956.
56. Carlioz, H., Pous, J. G., and Rey, J. C.: Les épiphysiolyses fémorales supérieures. Rev. Chir. Orthop., 54:388, 1968.
57. Carlioz, H., Vogt, J. C., Barba, L., and Doursounian, L.: Treatment of slipped upper femoral epiphysis: 80 cases operated on over 10 years (1968–1978). J. Pediatr. Orthop., 4:153, 1984.
58. Casey, B. H., Hamilton, H. W., and Bobechko, W. P.: Reduction of acutely slipped upper femoral epiphysis. J. Bone Joint Surg., 54-B:607, 1972.
59. Catterall, A.: Slipped capital femoral epiphysis in hypothyroidism. Paper presented at the Pediatric Orthopedic International Seminar annual meeting, San Francisco, 1986.
60. Chapman, J. A., Deakin, D. P., and Green, J. H.: Slipped upper femoral epiphysis after radiotherapy. J. Bone Joint Surg., 62-B:337, 1980.
61. Chiroff, R. T., Sears, K. A., and Slaughter, W. H., III: Slipped capital femoral epiphyses and parathyroid adenoma: Case report. J. Bone Joint Surg., 56-A:1063, 1974.
62. Chung, S. M. K., Batterman, S. C., and Brighton, C. T.: Shear strength of the human femoral capital epiphyseal plate. J. Bone Joint Surg., 58-A:94, 1976.
63. Clark, N. M. P., and Harrison, M. H. M.: Slipped upper femoral epiphysis. A potential for spontaneous recovery. J. Bone Joint Surg., 68-B:541, 1986.
64. Cleveland, M., Bosworth, D. M., Daly, J. N., and Hess, W. E.: Study of displaced capital femoral epiphyses. J. Bone Joint Surg., 33-A:955, 1951.
65. Colyer, R. A.: Compression external fixation after biplane femoral trochanteric osteotomy for severe slipped capital femoral epiphysis. J. Bone Joint Surg., 62-A:557, 1980.
66. Compere, C. L.: Correction of deformity and prevention of aseptic necrosis in late cases of slipped femoral epiphysis. J. Bone Joint Surg., 32-A:351, 1950.
67. Cordell, L. D.: Slipped capital femoral epiphysis. Postgrad. Med., 60:135, 1976.
68. Cowell, H. R.: The significance of early diagnosis and treatment of slipping of the capital femoral epiphysis. Clin. Orthop., 48:89, 1966.
69. Cozen, L.: Theoretical considerations on the etiology of Legg-Perthes disease and slipped capital femoral epiphysis. Arch. Pediatr., 79:115, 1962.
70. Crawford, A. H.: Legg-Calvé-Perthes disease coexistent with slipped capital femoral epiphysis. J. Bone Joint Surg., 57-A:280, 1975.
71. Crawford, A. H., MacEwen, G. D., and Fonte, D.: Slipped capital femoral epiphysis co-existent with hypothyroidism. Clin. Orthop., 122:135, 1977.
72. Crawford, H. B.: Ten cases of marked slipping of the upper femoral epiphysis. Clin. Orthop., 48:129, 1966.
73. Crider, R. J., Krell, T., McGuire, M., Kummer, F., and Strongwater, A.: Anterolateral approach for moderate to severe slipped capital femoral epiphysis. J. Pediatr. Orthop., 8:661, 1988.
74. Cruess, R. L.: The pathology of acute necrosis of cartilage in slipping of the capital femoral epiphysis. A report of two cases with pathological sections. J. Bone Joint Surg., 45-A:1013, 1963.
75. Culick, R., and Denton, J.: A retrospective study of 125 cases of slipped capital femoral epiphysis. Clin. Orthop., 162:87, 1982.
76. Day, A. J.: Slipped capital femoral epiphysis. I. A device for pinning in situ. II. A method for simultaneous bilateral pinning in situ. Clin. Orthop., 141:181, 1979.
77. Debrunner, A. M.: Prophylaktische Spickung der "gesunden" Seite bei Epiphysiolysis capitis femoris. Arch. Orthop. Unfallchir., 57:243, 1965.
78. D'Epinay, P. L.: Offene Reposition bei akuter Femurkopfepiphysenlosung—Bericht über 21 operierte Falle. Z. Orthop., 110:993, 1972.
79. DePalma, A., Danyo, J., and Stone, W. G.: Slipping of the upper femoral epiphysis. Clin. Orthop., 37:167, 1964.
80. DeRossi, G., Focacci, C., Maini, C. L., and Catino, A.: The particular usefulness of radioisotope methods in some benign bone diseases. Eur. J. Nucl. Med., 4:203, 1973.
81. DeSmet, A. A., Kuhns, L. R., Fayos, J. V., and Holt, J. F.: Effects of radiation therapy on growing long bones. A.J.R., 127:935, 1976.
82. Dickerson, J. D., Newberg, A. H., and Moreland, M. D.: Slipped capital femoral epiphysis (SCFE) following pelvic irradiation for rhabdomyosarcoma. Cancer, 44:480, 1979.
83. Dreizen, S., Snodgrasse, R. M., Webb-Peploe, H., and Spies, T. D.: The effect of prolonged nutritive failure on epiphyseal fusion in the human hand skeleton. A.J.R., 78:461, 1957.
84. Duncan, J. W., and Lovell, W. W.: Anterior slip of the capital femoral epiphysis. Report of a case and discussion. Clin. Orthop., 110:171, 1975.
85. Duncan, J. W., Nasca, R., and Schrantz, J.: Idiopathic chondrolysis of the hip. J. Bone Joint Surg., 61-A:1024, 1979.
86. Duncan, J., Schrantz, J., and Nasca, R.: The bizarre stiff hip. J.A.M.A., 231:382, 1975.
87. Dunn, D. M.: The treatment of adolescent slipping of the upper femoral epiphysis. J. Bone Joint Surg., 46-B:621, 1964.
88. Dunn, D. M., and Angel, J. C.: Replacement of the femoral head by open operation in severe adolescent slipping of the upper femoral epiphysis. J. Bone Joint Surg., 60-B:394, 1978.

89. Durbin, F. C.: The treatment of slipped upper femoral epiphysis. J. Bone Joint Surg., 42-B:289, 1960.
90. Editorial (Section 56): Slipped capital femoral epiphysis (adolescent coxa vara; proximal femoral epiphysiolysis). J.A.M.A., 224:780, 1973.
91. Eisenstein, A., and Rothschild, S.: Biochemical abnormalities in patients with slipped capital femoral epiphysis and chondrolysis. J. Bone Joint Surg., 58-A:459, 1976.
92. El-Khoury, G. Y., and Mickelson, M. R.: Chondrolysis following slipped capital femoral epiphysis. Radiology, 123:327, 1977.
93. Ellis, V. H.: Adolescent coxa vara. Lancet, 1:1440, 1935.
94. Elmslie, R. C.: Erasmus Wilson lecture on injury and deformity of the head of the femur: Coxa vara. Lancet, 1:410, 1907.
95. Elmslie, R. C.: Coxa Vara: Its Pathology and Treatment. London, Frowde, Hodder & Stoughton, 1913.
96. Epps, C. H., Jr., and Martin, E. D.: Slipped capital femoral epiphysis in a sexually mature myxedematous female. J.A.M.A., 183:287, 1963.
97. Fabry, G., MacEwen, G. D., and Shands, A. R., Jr.: Torsion of the femur. J. Bone Joint Surg., 55-A:1726, 1973.
98. Fahey, J. J., and O'Brien, E. T.: Acute slipped capital femoral epiphysis. Review of the literature and report of ten cases. J. Bone Joint Surg., 47-A:1105, 1965.
99. Fairbank, T. J.: Manipulation reduction of slipped femoral epiphysis. J. Bone Joint Surg., 51-B:252, 1969.
100. Falkner, F.: Some physical growth standards for white North American children. Pediatrics, 29:467, 1962.
101. Ferguson, A. B.: Slipped capital femoral epiphysis. In Orthopedic Surgery in Infancy and Childhood. 3rd Ed. Baltimore, Williams & Wilkins, 1968, Chapter 4, pp. 160–170.
102. Ferguson, A. F., and Howorth, M. B.: Slipping of the upper femoral epiphysis. J.A.M.A., 97:1867, 1931.
103. Fidler, M. W., and Brook, C. G. D.: Slipped upper femoral epiphysis following treatment with growth hormone. J. Bone Joint Surg., 56-A:1719, 1974.
104. Fish, J. B.: Cuneiform osteotomy in slipped capital femoral epiphysis. J. Bone Joint Surg., 56-A:1301, 1974.
105. Fish, J. B.: Cuneiform osteotomy of the femoral neck in the treatment of slipped capital femoral epiphysis. J. Bone Joint Surg., 66-A:1153, 1984.
106. Fisher, M., Frogel, M., Raifman, M. A., and Nussbaum, M.: Hypothyroidism and slipped capital femoral epiphysis (letter). J. Pediatr., 96:517, 1980.
107. Floman, Y., Yosipovitch, Z., Licht, A., and Viskoper, R. J.: Bilateral slipped upper femoral epiphysis: A rare manifestation of renal osteodystrophy. Israel J. Med. Sci., 11:15, 1975.
108. Foley, W. B.: Treatment of slipped upper femoral epiphysis. Proc. R. Soc. Med., 39:201, 1946.
109. Forrester-Brown, M.: Slipping of the upper femoral epiphysis. End results after conservative treatment. J. Bone Joint Surg., 23:256, 1941.
110. Francillon, M. R.: Zur Prophylaxe der Arthrosis deformans coxae: Diagnose und Therapie der Epiphysiolysis capitis femoris. Schweiz. Med. Wochenschr., 86:167, 1956.
111. Friberg, S.: Open reduction for slipping of the upper femoral epiphysis. Acta Orthop. Scand., 17:189, 1947.
112. Frymoyer, J.: Chondrolysis of the hip following Southwick osteotomy for severe slipped capital femoral epiphysis. Clin. Orthop., 99:120, 1974.
113. Gage, J. R., Sundberg, A. B., Nolan, D. R., Sletten, R. G., and Winter, R. B.: Complications after cuneiform osteotomy for moderately or severely slipped capital femoral epiphysis. J. Bone Joint Surg., 60-A:157, 1978.

114. Gallanaugh, S.: Traumatic separation of the upper femoral epiphysis in a three-year-old child. Guys Hosp. Rep., 121:211, 1972.
115. Ganz, R.: Die Epiphyseolysis capitis femoris. Ther. Umsch., 29:442, 1972.
116. Gelberman, R. H., Cohen, M. S., Shaw, B. A., Kasser, J. R., Griffin, P. P., and Wilkinson, R. H.: The association of femoral retroversion with slipped capital femoral epiphysis. J. Bone Joint Surg., 68-A:1000, 1986.
117. Ghormley, R. K., and Fairchild, R. D.: Diagnosis and treatment of slipped epiphyses. J.A.M.A., 114:229, 1940.
118. Golding, J. S. R.: Chondrolysis of the hip (abstract). J. Bone Joint Surg., 55-B:214, 1973.
119. Goldman, A. B., Lane, J. M., and Salvati, E.: Slipped capital femoral epiphysis complicating renal osteodystrophy. Radiology, 126:333, 1978.
120. Goldman, A., Schneider, R., and Martel, W.: Acute chondrolysis complicating slipped capital femoral epiphysis. A.J.R., 130:945, 1978.
121. Goldman, J. K., Cahill, G. F., Jr., and Thorn, G. W.: Gigantism with hypopituitarism. Am. J. Med., 34:407, 1963.
122. Grant, I. R.: The treatment of slipped upper femoral epiphysis by fibular grafting. Clin. Orthop., 114:270, 1976.
123. Green, W. T.: Slipping of the upper femoral epiphysis. Arch. Surg., 50:19, 1945.
124. Griffith, M.: Slipping of the capital femoral epiphysis. Ann. R. Coll. Surg. Engl., 58:34, 1976.
125. Griffiths, J. C.: Slipped upper femoral epiphysis in Kenya. E. Afr. Med. J., 46:669, 1969.
126. Gruber, M. A., and Laskin, R. S.: A single stage osteotomy and epiphysiodesis for treatment of moderately displaced femoral capital epiphyses. Clin. Orthop., 107:159, 1975.
127. Haas, S. L.: The localization of the growing point in the epiphyseal cartilage plate of bones. Am. J. Orthop. Surg., 15:563, 1917.
128. Hall, J. E.: The results of treatment of slipped femoral epiphysis. J. Bone Joint Surg., 39-B:659, 1957.
129. Halley, D. K.: Slipped femoral capital epiphysis. Ohio State Med. J., 70:628, 1974.
130. Hansson, L. I.: Sliding nail in treatment of slipped capital femoral epiphysis. IRCS Med. Sci., 3:567, 1975.
131. Hansson, L. I.: Osteosynthesis with the hook-pin in slipped capital epiphysis. Acta Orthop. Scand., 53:87, 1982.
132. Harris, W. R.: The endocrine basis for slipping of the upper femoral epiphysis. An experimental study. J. Bone Joint Surg., 32-B:5, 1950.
133. Harris, W. R., and Hobson, K. W.: Histological changes in experimentally displaced upper femoral epiphysis in rabbits. J. Bone Joint Surg., 38-B:914, 1956.
134. Hartman, J. T., and Gates, D. J.: Recovery from cartilage necrosis following slipped capital femoral epiphysis. A seven-year study of 166 cases. Orthop. Rev., 1:33, 1972.
135. Hauge, M. F.: Wedge ostoetomy in slipped femoral epiphysis with special reference to technique. Acta Orthop. Scand., 28:51, 1959.
136. Heatley, F. W., Greenwood, R. H., and Boase, D. L.: Slipping of the upper femoral epiphyses in patients with intracranial tumours causing hypopituitarism and chiasmal compression. J. Bone Joint Surg., 58-B:169, 1976.
137. Henrikson, B.: The incidence of slipped capital femoral epiphysis. Acta Orthop. Scand., 40:365, 1969.
138. Heppenstall, R. B., Marvel, J. P., Jr., Chung, S. M. K., and Brighton, C. T.: Chondrolysis of the hip. Clin. Orthop., 103:136, 1974.

139. Herndon, C. H.: Treatment of minimally slipped upper femoral epiphysis. A.A.O.S. Instruct. Course Lect., 21:188, 1972.
140. Herndon, C. H.: Treatment of severely slipped upper femoral epiphysis by means of osteoplasty and epiphyseodesis. A.A.O.S. Instruct. Course Lect., 21:214, 1972.
141. Herndon, C. H., Heyman, C. H., and Bell, D. M.: Treatment of slipped capital femoral epiphysis by epiphyseodesis and osteoplasty of the femoral neck. J. Bone Joint Surg., 45-A:999, 1963.
142. Herring, J. A.: Slipped capital femoral epiphysis. J. Pediatr. Orthop., 4:636, 1984.
143. Herrmann, H. J.: Comparative pathology of epiphyseolysis of the femur head in animals. Beitr. Orthop. Traumatol., 18:26, 1971.
144. Heyerman, W., and Weiner, D.: Slipped epiphysis associated with hypothyroidism. J. Pediatr. Orthop., 4:569, 1984.
145. Heyman, C. H.: Treatment of slipping of the upper femoral epiphysis. A study of the results of 42 cases. Surg. Gynecol. Obstet., 89:559, 1949.
146. Heyman, C. H.: The treatment of slipping of the upper femoral epiphysis. A.A.O.S. Instruct. Course Lect., 13:45, 1956.
147. Heyman, C. H., and Herndon, C. H.: Epiphyseodesis for early slipping of the upper femoral epiphysis. J. Bone Joint Surg., 36-A:539, 1954.
148. Heyman, C. H., Herndon, C. H., and Strong, J. M.: Slipped femoral epiphysis with severe displacement. A conservative operative treatment. J. Bone Joint Surg., 39-A:293, 1957.
149. Hiertonn, T.: Wedge osteotomy in advanced femoral epiphysiolysis. Acta Orthop. Scand., 25:44, 1955.
150. Hillman, J. W., Hunter, W. A., and Barrow, J. A.: Experimental epiphysiolysis in rats. Surg. Forum (43rd Clinical Congr.), 8:566, 1957.
151. Hirano, T., Stameloa, S., Harris, V., and Dumbovic, N.: Association of primary hypothyroidism and slipped femoral epiphysis. J. Pediatr., 93:262, 1978.
152. Hirsch, P. J., and Hirsch, S. A.: Slipped capital femoral epiphysis. J.A.M.A., 235:751, 1976.
153. Howorth, M. B.: Slipping of the upper femoral epiphysis. Surg. Gynecol. Obstet., 73:723, 1941.
154. Howorth, M. B.: Slipping of the upper femoral epiphysis. J. Bone Joint Surg., 31-A:734, 1949.
155. Howorth, M. B.: Slipping of the upper femoral epiphysis. A.A.O.S. Instruct. Course Lect. 8:306, 1951.
156. Howorth, M. B.: Treatment of slipping of the upper femoral epiphysis. J. Int. Coll. Surg., 20:716, 1953.
157. Howorth, M. B.: Slipping of the upper femoral epiphysis. Clin. Orthop., 10:148, 1957.
158. Howorth, M. B.: Slipping of the capital femoral epiphysis. Am. J. Orthop., 7:10, 1965.
159. Howorth, M. B.: History of slipping of the capital femoral epiphysis. Clin. Orthop., 48:11, 1966.
160. Howorth, M. B.: Pathology of slipping of the capital femoral epiphysis. Clin. Orthop., 48:33, 1966.
161. Howorth, M. B.: Etiology. Slipping of the capital femoral epiphysis. Clin. Orthop., 48:49, 1966.
162. Howorth, M. B.: Treatment. Slipping of the capital femoral epiphysis. Clin. Orthop., 48:53, 1966.
163. Howorth, M. B.: The bone-pegging operation. For slipping of the capital femoral epiphysis. Clin. Orthop., 48:79, 1966.
164. Howorth, M. B., and Ferguson, A. B.: Slipping of the upper femoral epiphysis. J.A.M.A., 97:1867, 1931.
165. Hulth, A.: The vessel anatomy of the upper femur end with special regard to the mechanism of origin of different vascular disorders. Acta Orthop. Scand., 27:192, 1958.
166. Hummer, C. D.: Avascular necrosis of the capital femoral epiphysis in a child receiving corticosteroids. Clin. Orthop., 125:65, 1977.
167. Humphries, R. E.: Slipped capital femoral epiphysis. J. Med. Soc. N.J., 49:6, 1952.
168. Ilfeld, F. W., and Makin, M.: Damage to the capital femoral epiphysis due to Frejka pillow treatment. J. Bone Joint Surg., 59-A:654, 1977.
169. Imhauser, G.: Zur Frage der operativen und konservativen Behandlung der jugendlichen Hüftkopflosung (Bemerkung zu der gleichnamigen Arbeit von E. Schwenkert). Z. Orthop., 89:547, 1957.
170. Imhauser, G.: Three-dimensional correction osteotomy in severe epiphyseal dislocation. X. SICOT-Kongress, Paris, Les Publications. Acta Med. Belg., 532, 1967.
171. Imhauser, G.: Zur Behandlung der schweren Dislokationen bei der jugendlichen Hüftkopflosung. Z. Orthop., 108:21, 1970.
172. Imhauser, G.: Spätergebnisse der sog. Imhauser-osteotomie bei der Epiphysenlosung. Z. Orthop., 115:716, 1977.
173. Ingram, A., Clarke, M., and Clark, C.: The effect of treatment on the incidence of chondrolysis complicating slipped capital femoral epiphysis. Paper presented at the Pediatric Orthopedic Society meeting, 1976.
174. Ippolito, E., Mickelson, M. R., and Ponseti, I. V.: A histochemical study of slipped capital femoral epiphysis. J. Bone Joint Surg., 63-A:1109, 1981.
175. Irani, R. N., Rosenzweig, A. H., Cotler, H. B., and Schwenther, E. P.: Epiphyseodesis in slipped capital femoral epiphysis. A comparison of various surgical modalities. J. Pediatr. Orthop., 5:661, 1985.
176. Ireland, J., and Newman, P. H.: Triplane osteotomy for severely slipped upper femoral epiphysis. J. Bone Joint Surg., 60-B:390, 1978.
177. Jacobs, B.: Diagnosis and natural history of slipped femoral capital epiphysis. A.A.O.S. Instruct. Course Lect., 21:167, 1972.
178. Jacobs, B.: Treatment of severely slipped upper femoral epiphysis by wedge osteotomy. A.A.O.S. Instruct. Course Lect., 21:197, 1972.
179. Jacobs, P.: A note on the diagnosis of early adolescent coxa vara (slipped epiphysis). Br. J. Radiol., 35:619, 1962.
180. Jahss, S. A.: Slipping of the upper femoral epiphysis. Treatment in the preslipping stage. J. Bone Joint Surg., 15:477, 1933.
181. Jayakumar, S.: Slipped capital femoral epiphysis with hypothyroidism treated by non-operative method. Clin. Orthop., 151:179, 1982.
182. Jerre, T.: A study in slipped upper femoral epiphysis with special reference to the late functional roentgenographic results as to the value of closed reduction. Acta Orthop. Scand., Suppl. 6, 1950.
183. Jerre, T.: Early complications after osteosynthesis with a three-flanged nail in situ for slipped epiphysis. Acta Orthop. Scand., 27:126, 1957.
184. Jones, B.: Adolescent chondrolysis of the hip joint. S. Afr. Med. J., 45:196, 1971.
185. Joplin, R. J.: Slipped capital femoral epiphysis. The still unsolved adolescent hip. J.A.M.A., 188:379, 1964.
186. Judet, J., Judet, R., and Guignard, J.: Coxa-vara des adolescents traitement et resultats. Rev. Chir. Orthop., 47:138, 1961.
187. Kampner, S. L., and Wissinger, H. A.: Anterior slipping of the capital femoral epiphysis. A case report. J. Bone Joint Surg., 54-A:1531, 1972.
188. Kappis, M.: Klinische und roentgenologische Dauergebnisse der Epiphysenlosung am Oberschenkelhals. Zentralbl. Chir., 51:113, 1924.
189. Kelsey, J. L.: An epidemiological study of slipped capital femoral epiphysis. Yale University, Ph.D. Thesis, 1969.
190. Kelsey, J. L.: The incidence and distribution of slipped capital femoral epiphysis in Connecticut. J. Chronic Dis., 23:567, 1971.

191. Kelsey, J. L.: Epidemiology of slipped capital femoral epiphysis: A review of the literature. Pediatrics, 51:1042, 1973.
192. Kelsey, J. L., and Keggi, K. J.: An epidemiological study of the effect of fluorides in drinking water on the frequency of slipped capital femoral epiphysis. Yale J. Biol. Med., 44:274, 1971.
193. Kelsey, J. L., and Southwick, W. O.: Etiology, mechanism, and incidence of slipped capital femoral epiphysis. A.A.O.S. Instruct. Course Lect., 21:182, 1972.
194. Kelsey, J. L., Acheson, M., and Keggi, K. J.: The body build of patients with slipped capital femoral epiphysis. Am. J. Dis. Child., 124:276, 1972.
195. Kelsey, J. L., Keggi, K. J., and Southwick, W. O.: The incidence and distribution of slipped capital femoral epiphysis in Connecticut and Southwestern United States. J. Bone Joint Surg., 52-A:1203, 1970.
196. Key, J. A.: Epiphyseal coxa vara or displacement of capital epiphysis of femur in adolescence. J. Bone Joint Surg., 8:52, 1926.
197. Key, J. A., and Conwell, H. E.: The Management of Fractures, Dislocations, and Sprains. St. Louis, Mosby, 1961.
198. Kiaer, S.: Epiphyseolysis capitis femoris treated with information. Acta Orthop. Scand., 27:81, 1947.
199. King, D.: Slipping capital femoral epiphysis. Clin. Orthop., 48:71, 1966.
200. Kirkwood, J. R., Ozonoff, M. B., and Steinbach, H. L.: Epiphyseal displacement after metaphyseal fracture in renal osteodystrophy. A.J.R., 115:547, 1972.
201. Kirmission, E.: La coxa vara traumatique. Rev. Orthop., 24:89, 1913.
202. Kirmission, E.: Coxa vara et obésité. Bull. Acad. Med. (Paris), 79:183, 1918.
203. Klein, A., Joplin, R. J., and Reidy, J. A.: Treatment of slipped capital femoral epiphysis. J.A.M.A., 136:445, 1948.
204. Klein, A., Joplin, R. J., and Reidy, J.: Slipped Capital Femoral Epiphysis. Springfield, Ill., Thomas, 1953.
205. Klein, A., Joplin, R. J., Reidy, J. A., and Hanelin, J.: Treatment in cases of slipped capital femoral epiphysis at the Massachusetts General Hospital. Arch. Surg., 46:681, 1943.
206. Klein, A., Joplin, R. J., Reidy, J. A., and Hanelin, J.: Roentgenographic changes in nailed slipped capital femoral epiphysis. J. Bone Joint Surg., 31-A:1, 1949.
207. Klein, A., Joplin, R., Reidy, J. A., and Hanelin, J.: Roentgenographic features of slipped capital femoral epiphysis. A.J.R., 66:361, 1951.
208. Klein, A., Joplin, R. J., Reidy, J. A., and Hanelin, J.: Slipped capital femoral epiphysis. J. Bone Joint Surg., 34-A:233, 1952.
209. Klein, A., Joplin, R. J., Reidy, J. A., and Hanelin, J.: Management of the contralateral hip in slipped capital femoral epiphysis. J. Bone Joint Surg., 35-A:81, 1953.
210. Kleinberg, S.: The treatment of early epiphyseolisthesis at the hip by drilling and delayed weight-bearing. Bull. Hosp. Joint Dis., 13:77, 1952.
211. Kleinberg, S., and Buchman, J.: The operative vs. the manipulative treatment of slipped femoral epiphysis. J.A.M.A., 107:1545, 1936.
212. Korn, M. W., and States, J. D.: Slipping capital femoral epiphysis. N.Y. State J. Med., 66:2248, 1966.
213. Korn, M. W., and States, J. D.: Slipping capital femoral epiphysis: A long-term follow-up and review of cases in Rochester, New York. Clin. Orthop., 48:119, 1966.
214. Kramer, W. G., Craig, W. A., and Noel, S.: Compensating osteotomy at the base of the femoral neck for slipped capital femoral epiphysis. J. Bone Joint Surg., 58-A:796, 1976.
215. Krempien, B., Mehls, O., and Ritz, E.: Morphological studies on pathogenesis of epiphyseal slipping in uremic children. Virchows Arch. Pathol. Anat. Histol., 362:129, 1974.
216. Krishnan, S. G., and Shelton, M. L.: Bilateral "reverse" epiphyseolysis of the proximal femoral capital epiphysis. J. Natl. Med. Assoc., 64:437, 1972.
217. Kulick, R., and Denton, J.: A retrospective study of one hundred and twenty-five cases of slipped capital femoral epiphysis. Clin. Orthop., 162:87, 1982.
218. LaCroix, P., and Verbrugge, J.: Slipping of upper femoral epiphysis: A pathological study. J. Bone Joint Surg., 33-A:371, 1951.
219. Lagrange, J., Rigault, P., and Guyonvarch, G.: La reposition sanglante dans les epiphysiolyses de hanche à grand déplacement. Presse Méd., 73:2163, 1965.
220. Lance, D., Carlioz, A., Seringe, R., Postel, M., Lacombe, M. J., and Abelanet, R.: La chondrolyse ou coxite laminaire juvenile après epiphysiolyse fémorale supérieure. Rev. Chir. Orthop., 67:437, 1981.
221. Lang, A. G., and Klassen, R. A.: Cup arthroplasties in teen-agers and children. J. Bone Joint Surg., 59-A:444, 1977.
222. Larson, C. B.: Rating scale for hip disabilities. Clin. Orthop., 31:85, 1963.
223. Leadbetter, G. W.: A treatment for fracture of the neck of the femur. J. Bone Joint Surg., 15:931, 1933.
224. Lehman, W. B., Grant, M. A., Norman, A., and Pugh, J.: The problem of evaluating in situ pinning of slipped capital femoral epiphysis: An experimental model and a review of 63 consecutive cases. J. Pediatr. Orthop., 4:297, 1984.
225. Lenart, G., Veres, I., Bidlo, G., and Kery, L.: Electron diffraction examination of the growth zone of the epiphysis. Acta Orthop. Scand., 44:157, 1973.
226. Lewin, P.: An unusual roentgenographic finding of the hip. A.J.R., 19:290, 1928.
227. Lindstrom, N.: Surgical treatment of epiphyseolysis capitis femoris. Acta Orthop. Scand., 28:131, 1958.
228. Lipscomb, P. R.: Salvage of the poor results of slipped capital femoral epiphysis. Clin. Orthop., 48:153, 1966.
229. Lofgren, L.: Slipping of the upper femoral epiphysis, signs of endocrine disturbance, size of sella turcica and two illustrative cases of simultaneous slipping of the upper femoral epiphysis and tumour of the hypophysis. Acta Chir. Scand., 106:153, 1953.
230. Lovejoy, J. F., and Lovell, W. W.: Adolescent tibia vara associated with slipped capital femoral epiphysis. A report of two cases. J. Bone Joint Surg., 52-A:361, 1970.
231. Lowe, H. G.: Avascular necrosis complicating slipped upper femoral epiphysis. J. Bone Joint Surg., 41-B:618, 1959.
232. Lowe, H. G.: Avascular necrosis after slipping of the upper femoral epiphysis. J. Bone Joint Surg., 43-B:686, 1961.
233. Lowe, H. G.: Necrosis of articular cartilage after slipping of the capital femoral epiphysis. Report of six cases with recovery. J. Bone Joint Surg., 52-B:108, 1970.
234. Lunceford, E. M., Jr.: The use of multiple adjustable Moore nail fixation in slipping of the capital femoral epiphysis. Clin. Orthop., 48:95, 1966.
235. Lutken, P.: Epiphysiolysis capitis femoris (coxa vara epiphysarea) with special reference to bloodless reposition treatment. Acta Orthop. Scand., 10:118, 1939.
236. MacAusland, A. R.: Separation of the capital femoral epiphysis. J. Bone Joint Surg., 17:353, 1935.
237. McAffee, A. L.: Long handled punch for the insertion of Newman's pins in slipped upper femoral epiphysis and intracapsular fractures of the femur. Injury, 13:81, 1981.
238. McCarroll, H. R.: Discussion on open reduction for slipped upper femoral epiphysis. J.A.M.A., 136:449, 1948.
239. McKibbin, B., and Holdsworth, F.: The dual nature of epiphyseal cartilage. J. Bone Joint Surg., 49-B:351, 1967.

240. Mackel, J. L., and Rapp, G. F.: Slipped capital femoral epiphysis. J. Indiana State Med. Assoc., 65:749, 1972.
241. Mankin, H. J., Sledge, C. B., Rothschild, S., and Eisenstein, A.: Chondrolysis of the hip. In The Hip: Proceedings of the Third Open Scientific Meeting of the Hip Society. St. Louis, Mosby, 1975, pp. 127–35.
242. Markheim, H. R.: Legg-Perthes disease and slipped epiphysis in same patient. J. Bone Joint Surg., 31-A:666, 1949.
243. Martin, P. H.: Slipped epiphysis in the adolescent hip. J. Bone Joint Surg., 30-A:9, 1948.
244. Mathiesen, F. R.: Slipping of the proximal femoral epiphysis. Acta Orthop. Scand., 27:115, 1958.
245. Maurer, R. C., and Larsen, I. J.: Acute necrosis of cartilage in slipped capital femoral epiphysis. J. Bone Joint Surg., 52-A:39, 1970.
246. Mayer, L.: The importance of early diagnosis in the treatment of slipping femoral epiphysis. J. Bone Joint Surg., 19:1046, 1937.
247. Mehls, O., Ritz, E., Krempien, B., Gilli, G., Link, K., Willich, E., and Scharer, K.: Slipped epiphysis in renal osteodystrophy. Arch. Dis. Child., 50:545, 1975.
248. Meissner, J.: Rezidiv nach Imhauser-Osteotomie einer Epiphysenabscherung in Kindersalter. Z. Orthop., 110:432, 1972.
249. Melby, A., Hoyt, W. A., and Weiner, D. S.: Treatment of chronic slipped capital femoral epiphysis. J. Bone Joint Surg., 62-A:119, 1980.
250. Menche, D., and Lehman, W.: In-situ pinning of slipped capital femoral epiphysis. Orthop. Rev., 11:129, 1982.
251. Merle d'Aubigne, R., and Mazas, F.: Nouveau Traite de Technique Chirurgicale. Paris, Masson, 1976, pp. 138–150.
252. Meyer, L. C., Stelling, F. H., and Wiese, F.: Slipped capital femoral epiphysis. South. Med. J., 50:543, 1957.
253. Mickelson, M. R., Ponseti, I. V., Cooper, R. R., and Maynard, J. A.: The ultrastructure of the growth plate in slipped capital femoral epiphysis. J. Bone Joint Surg., 59-A:1076, 1977.
254. Milch, H.: Epiphysiolysis or epiphyseal coxa anteverta. J. Bone Joint Surg., 19:97, 1937.
255. Milch, H.: The brace treatment of epiphysiolysis. Bull. Hosp. Joint Dis., 13:94, 1952.
256. Molloy, M. K., and MacMahon, B.: Incidence of Legg-Perthes disease. N. Engl. J. Med., 275:988, 1966.
257. Moore, R. D.: Aseptic necrosis of capital femoral epiphysis following adolescent epiphyseolysis. Surg. Gynecol. Obstet., 80:199, 1945.
258. Moore, R. D.: Conservative management of adolescent slipped capital femoral epiphysis. Surg. Gynecol. Obstet., 80:324, 1945.
259. Moorefield, W. C., Urbaniak, J. R., Ogden, W. S., and Frank, L. J.: Acquired hypothyroidism and slipped capital femoral epiphysis: Report of three cases. J. Bone Joint Surg., 58-A:705, 1976.
260. Morrissy, R. T., Kalderon, A. E., and Gerdes, M. H.: Synovial immunofluorescence in patients with slipped capital femoral epiphysis. J. Pediatr. Orthop., 1:55, 1981.
260a. Morrissy, R. T.: In situ fixation of chronic slipped capital femoral epiphysis. A.A.O.S. Instr. Course Lect., 34:319, 1984.
261. Morrissy, R. T., Steele, R. W., and Gerdes, M. H.: Localized immune complexes and slipped upper femoral epiphysis. J. Bone Joint Surg., 65-B:574, 1983.
262. Morscher, E.: Die operative Therapie der Epiphysiolysis capitis femoris. Z. Orthop., 92:153, 1959.
263. Morscher, E.: Zur Pathogenese der Epiphysiolysis capitis femoris. Arch. Orthop. Unfallchir., 53:331, 1961.
264. Morscher, E.: Resultate der subkapitalen Keilosteotomie bei Epiphysiolysis capitis femoris. Verh. Dtsch. Orthop. Ges., 49. Kongr., S. 256, 1961.
265. Morscher, E.: Strength and morphology of growth cartilage under hormonal influence of puberty. Animal experiments and clinical study on the etiology of local growth disorders during puberty. Reconstr. Surg. Traumatol., 10:3, 1968.
266. Morscher, E., and Schuman, L.: Significance of endocrine factors in etiology of epiphyseal separation of femoral head in juveniles. Orthopäde, 4:70, 1975.
267. Moss, J., Zuelzer, W., and Nogi, J.: Slipped capital femoral epiphysis: A review of treatment and complications (abstract). Orthop. Trans., 7:380, 1982.
268. Moule, N., and Golding, J.: Idiopathic chondrolysis of the hip. Clin. Radiol., 25:247, 1974.
269. Müller, E.: Über die Verbiegung des Schenkelhalses im Wachstumsalter. Beitr. Klin. Chir., 4:137, 1888–1889.
270. Müller, E.: On the deflection of the femoral neck in childhood. Clin. Orthop., 48:7, 1966.
271. Müller, E.: Die Epiphysiolysis capitis femoris. Wein. Med. Wochenschr., 122:714, 1972.
272. Mulli, A.: Zur Therapie der Epiphyseolysis capitis femoris. Schweiz. Med. Wochenschr., 68:346, 1938.
273. Munzenberg, K. J.: Zur Geometrie und Technik der subkapitaen Keilosteotomie bei Epiphyseolysis capitis femoris. Arch. Orthop. Unfallchir., 71:160, 1971.
274. Murray, R. O., and Duncan, C.: Athletic activity in adolescence as an etiological factor in degenerative hip disease. J. Bone Joint Surg., 53-A:406, 1971.
275. Newman, P. H.: The surgical treatment of slipping of the upper femoral epiphysis. J. Bone Joint Surg., 42-B:280, 1960.
276. Nielsen, H. O.: Acute slipped capital femoral epiphysis. Acta Orthop. Scand., 4:987, 1975.
277. Ninomiya, S., Nagasaka, Y., and Tagawa, H.: Slipped capital femoral epiphysis. A study of sixty-eight cases in the eastern half areas of Japan. Clin. Orthop., 119:172, 1976.
278. Nixon, J. R., and Douglas, J. F.: Bilateral slipping of the upper femoral epiphysis in end-stage renal failure. J. Bone Joint Surg., 62-A:18, 1980.
279. Noble, T. P.: Adolescent coxa vara. Ann. Surg., 80:773, 1924.
280. O'Brien, E. T., and Fahey, J. J.: Remodeling of the femoral neck after in situ pinning for slipped capital femoral epiphysis. J. Bone Joint Surg., 59-A:62, 1977.
281. Ochsner, P. E., Razani, R., and Schinzel, A.: Epiphysiolysis capitis femoris mit wahrscheinluch unregelmassig dominantem Erbgang. Z. Orthop., 115:840, 1977.
282. Ogden, J. A.: Changing patterns of proximal femoral vascularity. J. Bone Joint Surg., 56-A:941, 1974.
283. Ogden, J. A., and Southwick, W. O.: Endocrine dysfunction and slipped capital femoral epiphysis. Yale J. Biol. Med., 50:1, 1977.
284. Ogden, J. A., Simon, T. R., and Southwick, W. O.: Cartilage space width in slipped capital femoral epiphysis: The relationship to cartilage necrosis. Yale J. Biol. Med., 50:17, 1977.
285. Oram, V.: Epiphysiolysis of the head of the femur. A follow-up examination with special reference to end results and the social prognosis. Acta Orthop. Scand., 23:100, 1953.
286. Orofino, C., Innis, J. J., and Lowrey, C. W.: Slipped capital femoral epiphysis in Negroes. J. Bone Joint Surg., 42-A:1079, 1960.
287. Osterberg, P. H., and Martin, N. S.: Intracapsular procedures in the treatment of severe slipped upper femoral epiphysis. J. Bone Joint Surg., 53-B:763, 1971.
288. Pare, A.: Cinq Livres de Chirurgie. Paris, 1572.
289. Pearl, A. J., Woodward, B., and Kelly, R. P.: Cunei-

form osteotomy in the treatment of slipped capital femoral epiphysis. J. Bone Joint Surg., 43-A:947, 1961.
290. Perkins, G.: Treatment of adolescent coxa vara. Br. Med. J., 1:55, 1932.
291. Perquis, P., Ferro, R., Gourul, J. C., and Auphan, D.: A propos de deux cas d'epiphysiolyse relevés en deux ans à l'hôpital principal de Dakar. Bull. Soc. Med. Afr. Noire Lang. Fr., 18:45, 1973.
292. Petersen, D.: Ein Fall von Hüftkopfepiphysenlosung mit Abweichung nach vorne-unten. Z. Orthop., 108:206, 1970.
293. Peterson, C. A., and Peterson, H. A.: Analysis of the incidence of injuries to the epiphyseal growth plate. J. Trauma, 12:275, 1972.
294. Phemister, D. B.: Repair of bone in presence of aseptic necrosis resulting from fractures, transplantation, and vascular obstruction. J. Bone Joint Surg., 12:769, 1930.
295. Phemister, D.: Operative arrestment of longitudinal growth of the long bones in the treatment of deformities. J. Bone Joint Surg., 15:1, 1933.
296. Pierce, R., and Mott, W.: Observations on slipped capital femoral epiphysis. Orthop. Trans., 4:335, 1980.
297. Poland, J.: Traumatic Separation of the Epiphysis. London, Smith, Elder, 1898.
298. Pomeranz, M. M., and Sloane, M. F.: Slipping of the proximal femoral epiphysis. Therapeutic results in 101 cases. Arch. Surg., 30:607, 1935.
299. Ponseti, I. V., and Barta, C. K.: Evaluation of treatment of slipping of the capital femoral epiphysis. Surg. Gynecol. Obstet., 86:87, 1948.
300. Ponseti, I. V., and McClintock, R.: The pathology of slipping of the upper femoral epiphysis. J. Bone Joint Surg., 38-A:71, 1956.
301. Primiano, G. A., and Hughston, J. C.: Slipped capital femoral epiphysis in a true hypogonadal male (Klinefelter's mosaic XY/XXY). J. Bone Joint Surg., 53-A:597, 1971.
301a. Pritchett, J. W., and Perdue, K. D.: Mechanical factors in slipped capital femoral epiphysis. J. Pediatr. Orthop., 8:385, 1988.
302. Rabinowitz, M. S.: Slipping of the upper femoral epiphysis. J. Bone Joint Surg., 22:992, 1940.
303. Rainaut, J. J., and Cedard, C.: A propos de la coxa vara des adolescents. Rev. Chir. Orthop., 50:779, 1964.
304. Rang, M.: The Growth Plate and Its Disorders. Baltimore, Williams & Wilkins., 1969, pp. 150–155.
305. Rao, J. P., Francis, A. M., and Siwek, C. W.: The treatment of chronic slipped capital femoral epiphysis by biplane osteotomy. J. Bone Joint Surg., 66-A:1169, 1984.
306. Ratliff, A. H. C.: Pseudocoxalgia. J. Bone Joint Surg., 38-B:498, 1956.
307. Ratliff, A. H. C.: Traumatic separation of the upper femoral epiphysis in young children. J. Bone Joint Surg., 50-B:757, 1968.
308. Rauterberg, K., and Rauterberg, E.: Experimental investigations of the causes of juvenile slipped epiphysis of the head of the femur. Z. Orthop., 112:134, 1974.
309. Razzano, C. D., Nelson, C., and Eversman, J.: Growth hormone levels in slipped capital femoral epiphysis. J. Bone Joint Surg., 54-A:1224, 1972.
310. Rechnagel, K.: Genu recurvatum associated with slipped capital femoral epiphysis. Acta Orthop. Scand., 44:505, 1973.
311. Reeves, G. D., Gibbs, M., Paulshock, B. Z., and Rosenblum, H.: Gigantism with slipped capital femoral epiphysis. Am. J. Dis. Child., 132:529, 1978.
312. Reichelt, A., and Rutt, A.: Untersuchungen zur Ätiologie der Epiphysiolysis bzw. Epiphysiolisthesis capitis femoris. Arch. Orthop. Unfallchir., 67:28, 1969.
313. Rennie, A. M.: The pathology of slipped upper femoral epiphysis. A new concept. J. Bone Joint Surg., 42-B:273, 1960.
314. Rennie, A. M.: Familial slipped upper femoral epiphysis. J. Bone Joint Surg., 49-B:534, 1967.
315. Rennie, A. M.: The inheritance of slipped upper femoral epiphysis. J. Bone Joint Surg., 64-B:180, 1982.
316. Rennie, W., and Mitchell, N.: Slipped capital femoral epiphysis occurring during growth hormone therapy. Report of a case. J. Bone Joint Surg., 56-B:703, 1974.
317. Rey, J. C., and Carlioz, H.: Epiphysiolyses a grand déplacement. Reduction sanglante par la technique de Dunn. Rev. Chir. Orthop., 61:261, 1975.
318. Ridlon, J.: Coxa vara. J.A.M.A., 64:219, 1915.
319. Robb, J. J.: Slipped epiphysis of head of femur. Br. Med. J., 1:643, 1929.
320. Ross, P., Lyne, E., and Morawa, L.: Slipped capital femoral epiphysis long-term results after ten to thirty-eight years. Clin. Orthop., 141:176, 1979.
321. Ruoff, A. C.: The treatment of slipped femoral capital epiphysis utilizing skeletal traction with the Thomson beaded wire. In Delchef, J., de Marneffe, R., and Vander Elst, E. (eds.): Orthopedic Surgery and Traumatology. Amsterdam, Excerpta Medica, 1973, pp. 428–434.
322. Russe, O. A.: Acute and chronic slipped femoral epiphysis. Clin. Orthop., 77:144, 1971.
323. Rutishauser, E., and Taillard, W.: L'ischemie articulaire en pathologie humaine et expérimentale. La notion de pannus vasculaire. Rev. Chir. Orthop., 52:197, 1966.
324. Salenius, P., and Kivilaakso, R.: Results of treatment of slipped upper femoral epiphysis. A survey of 99 treated hips. Acta Orthop. Scand., Suppl. 114, 1968.
325. Salvati, E. A., Robinson, H. J., and O'Dowd, T. J.: Southwick osteotomy for severe chronic slipped capital epiphysis: Results and complications. J. Bone Joint Surg., 62-A:561, 1980.
326. Salzer, M., and Zhuber, K.: Die prophylaktische Operation der "gesunden" Seite bei der Epiphysiolysis capitis femoris. Arch. Orthop. Unfallchir., 72:350, 1972.
327. Scham, S. M.: Capital femoral epiphysiolysis treatment by plugging with cortical beef bone. Acta Orthop. Scand., 39:171, 1968.
328. Scham, S. M.: The triangular sign in the early diagnosis of slipped capital femoral epiphysis. Clin. Orthop., 103:16, 1974.
329. Schecter, L.: Slipped capital femoral epiphysis. An end-result study. J. Bone Joint Surg., 47-A:1128, 1965.
330. Schein, A. J.: Acute severe slipped capital femoral epiphysis. Clin. Orthop., 51:151, 1967.
331. Schmidt, T. L., and Mallo, G. J.: Slipped capital femoral epiphysis in a patient with infantile tibia vara. Orthopedics, 1:471, 1978.
332. Schnute, W.: Slipped capital femoral epiphysis. Clin. Orthop., 11:63, 1958.
333. Schreiber, A.: Epiphysiolysis capitis femoris. Beitrag zür Frage der Beideseitigkeit. Z. Orthop., 97:4, 1963.
334. Schreiber, A., and Dietschi, C.: Nagelung der Epiphysiolysis capitis femoris. Med. Orthop. Technik, 95:122, 1975.
335. Schreiber, A., and Schmied, H. R.: Beitrag zur Kenntnis der Epiphysiolysis capitis femoris; familiar gehauftes Vorkommen. Z. Orthop., 104:368, 1966.
336. Schulitz, K. P., Hamacher, P., and Spier, F.: Beitrag zur Epiphyseolysis capitis femoris. Z. Orthop., 115:133, 1977.
337. Schulitz, K. P., Schoning, B., and Kull, W.: Morphologic and arthrose bei der Epiphyseolysis capitis femoris. Arch. Orthop. Unfallchir., 86:303, 1976.
338. Scott, J. C.: Displacement of the upper epiphysis of femur. In Platt, H. (ed.): Modern Trends in Orthopedics (second series). London, Butterworth, 1956.

339. Scott, W.: Epiphysiolysis of the upper femur. A report of 38 cases. J. Bone Joint Surg., 18:743, 1936.
340. Semple, J. C., and Goldschmidt, R. G.: Epiphyseal maturation and slipping femoral epiphysis in a hypopituitary dwarf. Orthopaedics, Oxford, 2:31, 1969.
341. Severin, E.: Nailing in situ of slipped proximal epiphysis of femur. Acta Orthop. Scand., 24:145, 1954.
342. Shands, A. R.: Slipping of the capital femoral epiphysis (epiphyseal or adolescent coxa vara). In Shands' Handbook of Orthopedic Surgery. 9th Ed. St. Louis, Mosby, 1978, pp. 370–374.
343. Sharrard, W. J. W.: Paediatric Orthopaedics and Fractures. Oxford, Blackwell, 1979, pp. 390–411.
344. Shea, D., and Mankin, H. J.: Slipped capital femoral epiphysis in renal rickets. Report of three cases. J. Bone Joint Surg., 48-A:349, 1966.
345. Singh, S., and Petrie, J. G.: Slipped epiphyses in chondroosteodystrophy. J. Bone Joint Surg., 45-A:1025, 1963.
346. Skinner, S. R., and Berkheimer, G. A.: Valgus of the capital femoral epiphysis. Clin. Orthop., 135:90, 1978.
347. Soeur, R.: Etiology and pathomechanics of slipped upper femoral epiphysis. J. Bone Joint Surg., 41-B:618, 1959.
348. Sorenson, K. H.: Slipped upper femoral epiphysis. Clinical study of aetiology. Acta Orthop. Scand., 39:499, 1968.
349. Southwick, W. O.: Osteotomy through the lesser trochanter for slipped capital femoral epiphysis. J. Bone Joint Surg., 49-A:807, 1967.
350. Southwick, W. O.: Treatment of severely slipped upper femoral epiphysis by trochanteric osteotomy. A.A.O.S. Instruct. Course Lect., 21:200, 1972.
351. Southwick, W. O.: Compression fixation after biplane intertrochanteric osteotomy for slipped capital femoral epiphysis. A technical improvement. J. Bone Joint Surg., 55-A:1218, 1973.
352. Southwick, W. O.: Biplane osteotomy for very severe slipped capital femoral epiphysis. In The Hip. Proceedings of the Hip Society. St. Louis, Mosby, 1975, pp. 105–114.
353. Southwick, W. O.: Editorial. Slipped capital femoral epiphysis. J. Bone Joint Surg., 66-A:1151, 1984.
354. Speer, D. P.: Experimental epiphysiolysis: Etiologic models of slipped capital femoral epiphysis. In The Hip. Proceedings of the Hip Society. St. Louis, Mosby, 1982, pp. 68–88.
355. Stack, R. E., and Peterson, L. F. A.: Slipped capital femoral epiphysis and Down's disease. Clin. Orthop., 28:111, 1966.
356. Steel, H. H.: The metaphyseal blanch sign of slipped capital femoral epiphysis. J. Bone Joint Surg., 68-A:920, 1986.
357. Stewart, J. S. S.: Medullary gonadal dysgenesis (chromatin-positive Klinefelter's syndrome), a genetically determined condition with eunuchoid measurements but early epiphyseal closure. Lancet, 1:1176, 1959.
358. Stovall, S. L.: Separation of the capital femoral epiphysis in the adolescent. Surg. Gynecol. Obstet., Int. Abstr., 88:193, 1949.
359. Strange, F. G.: Slipped upper femoral epiphysis. In The Hip. London, Heinemann, 1965, p. 102.
360. Stulberg, S. D., Cordell, L. D., Harris, W. H., Ramsey, P. L., and MacEwen, G. D.: Unrecognized childhood hip disease: A major cause of idiopathic osteoarthritis of the hip. In The Hip. Proceedings of the Third Open Scientific Meeting of the Hip Society. St. Louis, Mosby, 1975, pp. 212–228.
361. Sugioka, Y., Katsuki, I., and Hotokebuchi, T.: Transtrochanteric rotational osteotomy of the femoral head for the treatment of osteonecrosis. Follow-up statistics. Clin. Orthop., 169:115, 1982.
362. Sutro, C. J.: Slipping of capital epiphysis of femur in adolescence. Arch. Surg., 31:345, 1935.
363. Switzer, P., and Bell, H. M.: Slipping of the capital femoral epiphysis with renal rickets: A case report. Can. J. Surg., 16:330, 1973.
364. Taillard, W., and Grasset, E.: La coxite laminaire juvenile. Rev. Chir. Orthop., 50:159, 1964.
365. Taillard, W., Megevand, A., Scholder, P., and Morscher, H. E.: L'epiphyseolyse de la tête du femur. Doc. Geigy, Acta Rheumatol., no. 21, 1969.
366. Telson, D. R.: Reduction and pinning of slipped femoral epiphysis. N.Y. State J. Med., 53:2647, 1953.
367. Telson, D. R., and Ronsohoff, N. S.: Treatment of fractured neck of femur by axial fixation with steel wires. J. Bone Joint Surg., 17:727, 1935.
368. Theander, G.: Pelvic instability in upper femoral epiphyseolysis. Acta Orthop. Scand., 32:52, 1962.
369. Thrap-Meyer, H.: Epiphysiolysis capitis femoris in two generations: Causistic report. Acta Orthop. Scand., 11:1, 1940.
370. Tillema, D. A., and Golding, J. S. R.: Chondrolysis following slipped capital femoral epiphysis in Jamaica. J. Bone Joint Surg., 53-A:1528, 1971.
371. Towbin, R., and Crawford, A. H.: Neonatal traumatic proximal femoral epiphysiolysis. Pediatrics, 63:456, 1979.
372. Tönnis, D.: Die Epiphyseolysis capitis femoris. Acta Chir., 8:141, 1973.
373. Trueta, J.: The normal vascular anatomy of the human femoral head during growth. J. Bone Joint Surg., 39-B:358, 1957.
374. Trueta, J.: Slipping of the upper femoral epiphysis. In Studies of the Development and Decay of the Human Frame. Philadelphia, Saunders, 1968, p. 298–305.
375. Tschantz, P., Taillard, W., and Ditesheim, P. J.: Epiphyseal tilt produced by experimental overload. Clin. Orthop., 123:271, 1977.
376. Turek, S. L.: Slipped capital femoral epiphysis. In Orthopaedics, Principles and Their Application. 3rd Ed. Philadelphia, Lippincott, 1977, pp. 1081–1096.
377. Ulin, R.: Slipped proximal femoral epiphyses. Clin. Orthop., 41:64, 1965.
378. Vaughn-Jackson, O. J.: Reducibility of slipped femoral capital epiphysis. Proc. R. Soc. Med., 49:812, 1956.
379. Viernstein, K., and Keyl, W.: Die operative Behandlung der Epiphyseolysis capitis femoris. Erfahrungen und Ergebnisse. Z. Orthop., 106:129, 1969.
380. Wagner, L. C., and Donovan, M. M.: Wedge osteotomy of neck of femur in advanced cases of displaced upper femoral epiphysis. A 10 year study. Am. J. Surg., 78:281, 1949.
381. Waldenström, C. H.: On necrosis of the joint cartilage by epiphysolysis capitis femoris. Acta Chir. Scand., 67:936, 1930.
382. Waldenström, C. H.: Necrosis of the femoral epiphysis owing to insufficient nutrition from the ligamentum teres. A clinical study mainly based on experiences with treatment of epiphyseolysis capitis femoris. Acta Chir. Scand., 75:185, 1934.
383. Waldenström, C. H.: Slipping of the upper femoral epiphysis. Surg. Gynecol. Obstet., 71:198, 1940.
384. Walters, R., and Simons, S.: Joint destruction—a sequel of unrecognized pin penetration in patients with slipped capital femoral epiphysis. In The Hip. Proceedings of The Hip Society. St. Louis, Mosby, 1980, pp. 145–157.
385. Wardle, E. N.: Etiology and treatment of slipped epiphysis of head of femur. Br. J. Surg., 21:313, 1933.
386. Watson, E. H., and Lowrey, G. H.: Growth and Development of Children. 4th Ed. Chicago, Year Book, 1962.
387. Wattleworth, A. S., Heiple, K. G., Chase, S. W., and Herndon, C. H.: Pathology of slipped capital femoral epiphysis: A.A.O.S. Instruct. Course Lect., 21:174, 1972.

388. Weiner, D. S.: Hagie pins in acute slipped capital femoral epiphysis (letter to editor; comments by Dr. Raymond Tronzo). J. Bone Joint Surg., 57-A:433, 1976.
389. Weiner, D. S.: Slipped capital femoral epiphysis. Case presentation. Orthopaedic Consultation, 5:Nov.-Dec., 1984.
390. Weiner, D. S., Weiner, S., Melby, A., and Hoyt, W. A.: A 30-year experience with bone graft epiphysiodesis in the treatment of slipped capital femoral epiphysis. J. Pediatr. Orthop., 4:145, 1984.
391. Wenger, D., Mickelson, M., and Ponseti, I.: Idiopathic chondrolysis of the hip. J. Bone Joint Surg., 57:268, 1975.
392. Wertheimer, L. G., and Lopes, S. D. L. F.: Arterial supply of the femoral head. A combined angiographic and histological study. J. Bone Joint Surg., 53-A:545, 1971.
393. Whiteside, L. A., and Schoenecker, P. L.: Combined valgus derotation osteotomy and cervical osteopathy for severely slipped capital femoral epiphysis: Mechanical analysis and report of preliminary results using compression screw fixation and early weight-bearing. Clin. Orthop., 132:88, 1978.
394. Whitman, R.: Further observations on injuries to neck of femur in early life; with reference to distinction between fracture of neck and epiphyseal disjunction as influencing positive treatment. Med. Rec., 1:1, 1909.
395. Whitman, R.: The abduction method considered as the standard routine in the treatment of posture of the neck of the femur. J. Orthop. Surg., 2:547, 1930.
396. Wiberg, G.: Epiphyseolysis capitis femoris. Acta Orthop. Scand., 12:179, 1941.
397. Wiberg, G.: Pinning for slipping of the epiphysis of the femoral head. Acta Orthop. Scand., 18:4, 1948.
398. Wiberg, G.: Wedge osteotomy in serious slipping of the upper femoral epiphysis. Acta Orthop. Scand., 25:63, 1955.
399. Wiberg, G.: Considerations on the surgical treatment of slipped epiphysis with special reference to nail fixation. J. Bone Joint Surg., 41-A:253, 1959.
400. Wiberg, G.: Surgical treatment of slipped epiphysis with special reference to wedge osteotomy of the femoral neck. Clin. Orthop., 48:139, 1966.
401. Willner, P.: Slipped femoral capital epiphysis: Operation and results. J. Int. Coll. Surg., 24:215, 1955.
402. Wilson, P. D.: Displacement of upper epiphysis of the femur treated by open reduction. J.A.M.A., 83:1749, 1924.
403. Wilson, P. D.: Conclusions re treatment of slipping of upper femoral epiphysis. Surg. Clin. North Am., 16:733, 1936.
404. Wilson, P. D.: The treatment of slipping of the upper femoral epiphysis with minimal displacement. J. Bone Joint Surg., 20:379, 1938.
405. Wilson, P. D.: Discussion. J. Bone Joint Surg., 31-A:21, 1949.
406. Wilson, P. D., Jacobs, B., and Schecter, L.: Slipped capital femoral epiphysis. An end-result study. J. Bone Joint Surg., 47-A:1128, 1965.
407. Wojtowycz, M., Starshak, R. J., and Sty, J. R.: Neonatal proximal femoral epiphysiolysis. Radiology, 136:647, 1980.
408. Wolf, E. L., Berdon, W. E., Cassady, J. R., Baker, D. H., Freiberger, R., and Pavlov, H.: Slipped femoral capital epiphysis as a sequela to childhood irradiation for malignant tumors. Radiology, 125:781, 1977.
409. Wolkow, M. W.: Alloplastik von Metallgelenken. Acta Orthop. Scand., 40:571, 1969.
410. Wright, W., and King, D.: The treatment of slipping femoral epiphysis (epiphyseolysis). Am. J. Surg., 91:894, 1956.
411. Zettas, J. P., and Zettas, P.: Abduction contracture: Unusual complication in the treatment of acute capital femoral epiphysiolysis. Clin. Orthop., 146:215, 1980.
412. Zickel, R. E., Hobieka, P., and Ferrer, J. E.: The use of flexion in the radius and fixation of slipped capital femoral epiphysis. J. Bone Joint Surg., 68-A:299, 1986.
413. Zubrow, A. B., Lane, J. M., and Pariss, J. S.: Slipped capital femoral epiphysis occurring during treatment for hypothyroidism. J. Bone Joint Surg., 60-A:256, 1978.

Infections of Bone

PYOGENIC OSTEOMYELITIS

Osteomyelitis is an inflammation of bone, and indicates a pyogenic infection unless the term *osteomyelitis* is otherwise qualified.

Osteomyelitic lesions have been observed in Egyptian mummies dating as far back as four thousand years. Nélaton, in 1844, first coined the name *osteomyelitis* to describe an old disease that was well pictured in the *Corpus Hippocrates*.[282]

The disease most frequently occurs in infants and children, although it may be observed at any age. It is about three to four times as common in males as in females.

Etiology

It is usually a hematogenous infection, but it may occasionally be caused by direct extension of an adjacent infective process or by external introduction of organisms, as in an open fracture.

Occasionally, it is caused by pneumococci, salmonella, or other pyogenic organisms, but the bacterial organism most frequently cultured is *Staphylococcus aureus*. Before the widespread use of penicillin, streptococcus infection was common in infancy.[160] A primary source of infection, such as boils, abscessed teeth, or upper respiratory infection, may often be present. Injury may indirectly cause localization of osteomyelitis, as it establishes a focus of diminished resistance to subsequent infection; it also provides a portal of entry for new infection and may aggravate the severity of an already existing one.

Pathology

Hematogenous osteomyelitis arises in the metaphysis by way of the nutrient vessel.[239] Koch demonstrated that when bacteria are injected intravenously, they tend to localize in the vascular spaces in the metaphysis as early as two hours following inoculation, predisposing the area to be a focus of infection.[219]

The nature of the vascular supply of long bones in children is the underlying reason for localization of the pathogenic bacteria in the metaphyseal sinusoids (Fig. 3–202).

In children, the blood supply of the epiphysis is separate from that of the metaphysis.[189, 389–392] The last ramifications of the nutrient artery to the metaphysis turn down in sharp loops and empty into a system of large sinusoidal veins where the rate of blood flow is decreased.[189] This creates an ideal medium for the proliferation of pathogenic bacteria. Infection originates in the venous side of the loops and spreads to cause secondary thrombosis of the nutrient artery. In the adult this vascular arrangement does not exist, and there is free anastomosis between the metaphyseal and epiphyseal vessels. Osteomyelitis is rare in the adult, but when it does occur it may appear anywhere in the bone.

Inflammation in the bone is characterized by vascular engorgement, edema, cellular response, and formation of an abscess. Irregular decalcification of the infected bone occurs in the early stages, being caused by the resorption of dead bone and, secondarily, by atrophy and disuse. Pyogenic exudate and necrosis in the metaphyseal area are typical histologic findings (Fig. 3–203 A and B).

The infection extends through the haversian system and Volkmann's canals by means of a spreading thrombosis due to the pressure produced by the exudate; this causes interference in circulation (Fig. 3–204). The physis forms a mechanical barrier that prevents spread into the epiphysis, as its blood supply is separate and it does not contain any vascular canals in the growth cartilage. Trueta, in his studies of the changes of the vascular pattern of the human upper femoral epiphysis during growth, has shown that in early infancy vessels do cross the physis. At the age of eight months, however, the physeal cartilage gradually becomes a barrier that is definitely established before the eighteenth month. Trueta states that the infant becomes a child at the age of one year on the basis of development of the blood supply to bone.[390]

Osteomyelitis spreads by way of Volkmann's canals to the subperiosteal space in the meta-

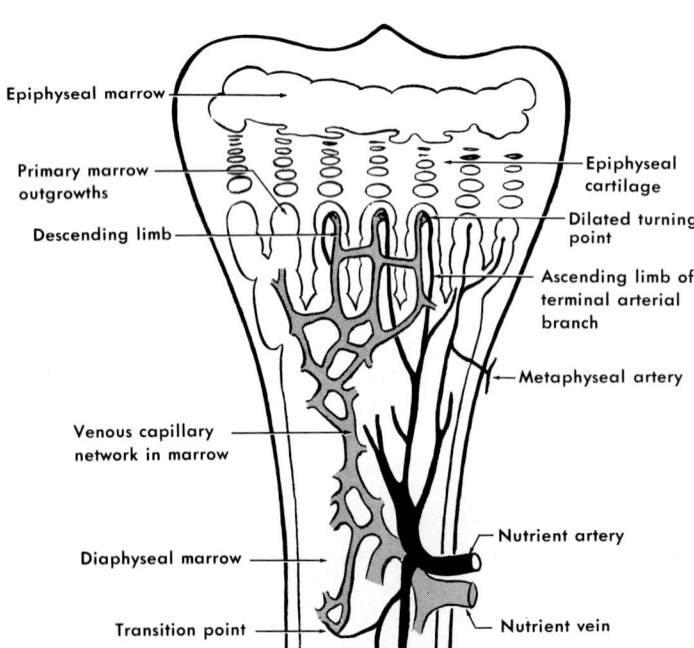

FIGURE 3–202. *Localization of osteomyelitis due to structure of metaphyseal sinusoids.*

Diagram of blood supply of long bones in children showing the structure of metaphyseal sinusoids to be the cause for localization of pathogenic bacteria in the metaphysis. (Redrawn from Trueta, J.: Studies of Development and Decay of the Human Frame. Philadelphia, William Heinemann Medical Books, 1968, p. 258; after T. Hobo. Acta Sch. Med. Univ. Kioto, 4:1, 1921.)

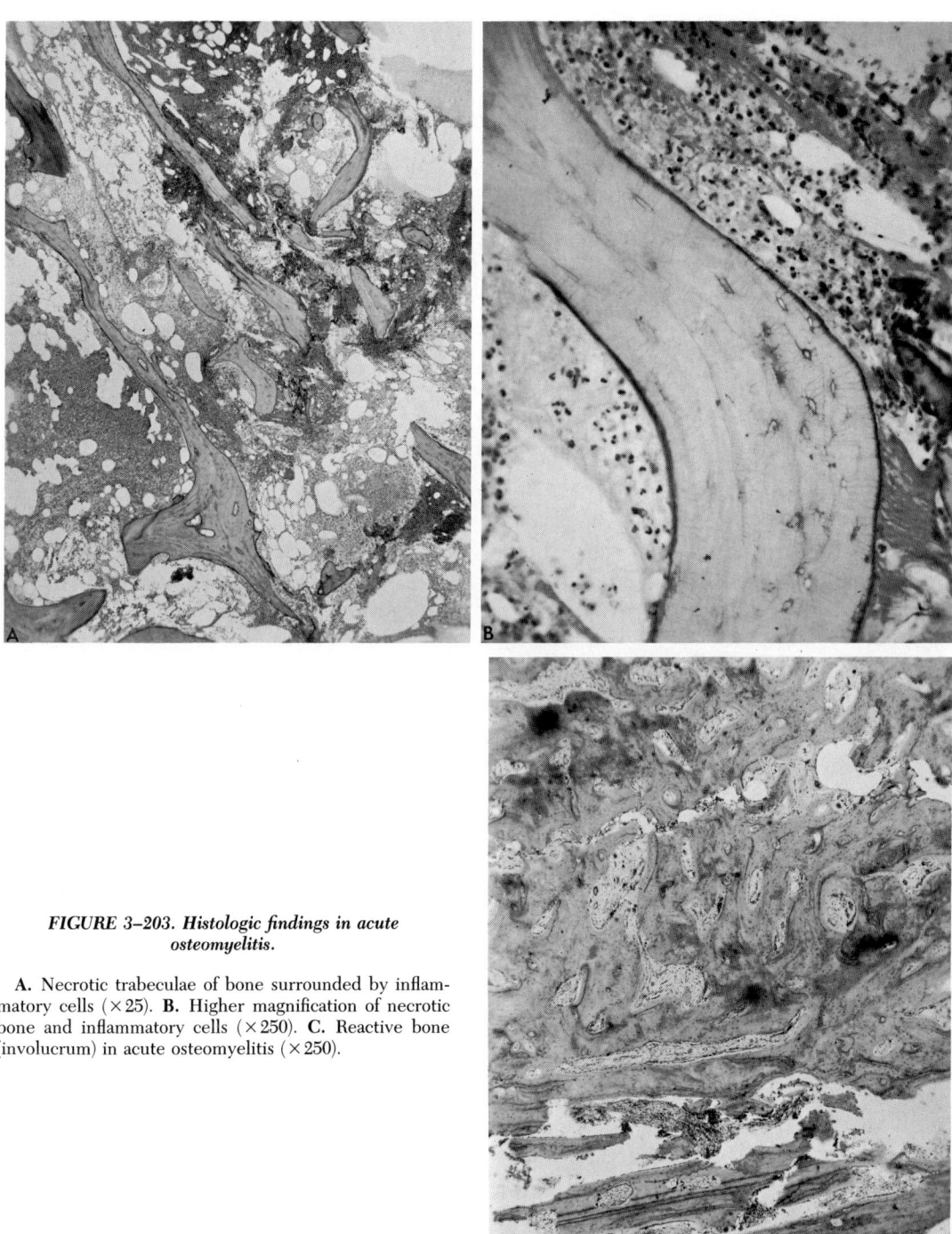

FIGURE 3–203. Histologic findings in acute osteomyelitis.

A. Necrotic trabeculae of bone surrounded by inflammatory cells (×25). **B.** Higher magnification of necrotic bone and inflammatory cells (×250). **C.** Reactive bone (involucrum) in acute osteomyelitis (×250).

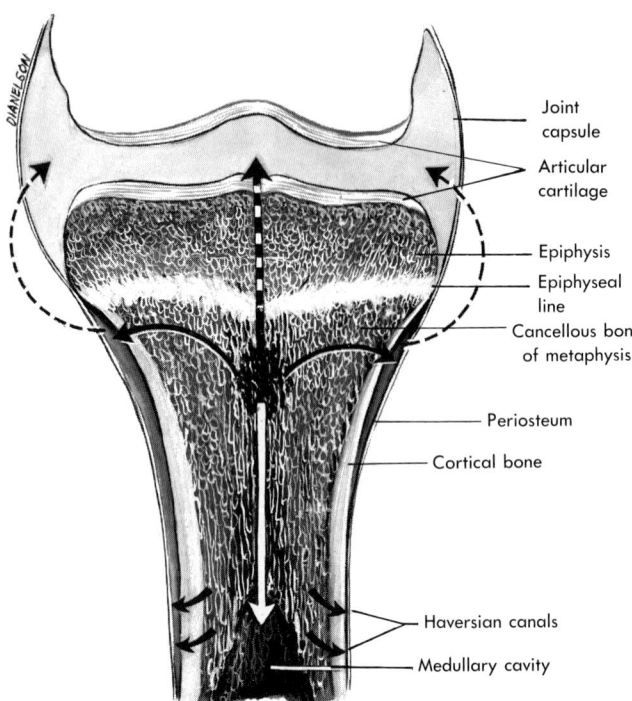

FIGURE 3–204. *Diagram showing spread of acute hematogenous osteomyelitis. The interrupted lines are rare routes.*

physeal area, with elevation of the periosteum. In the child, the periosteum is much more loosely attached than in the adult, and if the infection remains uncontrolled, the periosteum will rupture, allowing the pus to escape into the soft tissues. The purulent material may extend up and down the diaphysis and circumferentially around the bone. If the metaphysis is intra-articular, as in the neck of the femur, the abscess will rupture into the joint, resulting in suppurative arthritis.

In untreated osteomyelitis of childhood, thrombosis of the blood vessels and elevation of the periosteum will deprive the affected denuded cortical bone and the underlying metaphyseal cancellous bone of their blood supply, and the bone dies.

Granulation tissue forms about the dead bone, which becomes separated from the live bone. This separated dead bone, with its surrounding granulation tissue, is called a *sequestrum*. As sequestration occurs, a reparative process is initiated in the periosteum, which forms new live bone around the dead bone. *Involucrum* is the term used to describe the layer of live bone that has formed over the dead bone. The involucrum eventually becomes perforated by sinuses, through which pus escapes. By the process of sequestration and involucrum formation, noncollapsible cavities harboring bacteria, granulation tissue, and dead bone are produced. This constitutes the chronic stage of osteomyelitis, which is characterized by persistent sequestra, and continuous or intermittent drainage of pus from the sinuses.

Sites of Involvement

The most usual sites of involvement are the metaphyses of the lower end of the femur and the upper end of the tibia. Next in frequency are the proximal metaphysis of the femur and the distal metaphyses of the radius and humerus. Any bone may be affected, however. When a flat bone such as the ilium is involved, the presence of infection may not be easily detectable (Fig. 3–205). Some children may have a history of a focus of infection.

Clinical Picture

The symptoms and signs of acute hematogenous osteomyelitis vary with the intensity, location and extent of the infection, the duration of the process, and the age and resistance of the patient. Inadequate antibiotic therapy for fever of unknown origin may mask the acute infection, making diagnosis difficult.

General systemic symptoms are those of acute septicemia, with high fever, chills, vomiting, and dehydration. In the neonatal period and early infancy, there is usually a lack of systemic response. The newborn may be afebrile, but he is irritable, refuses feeding, and

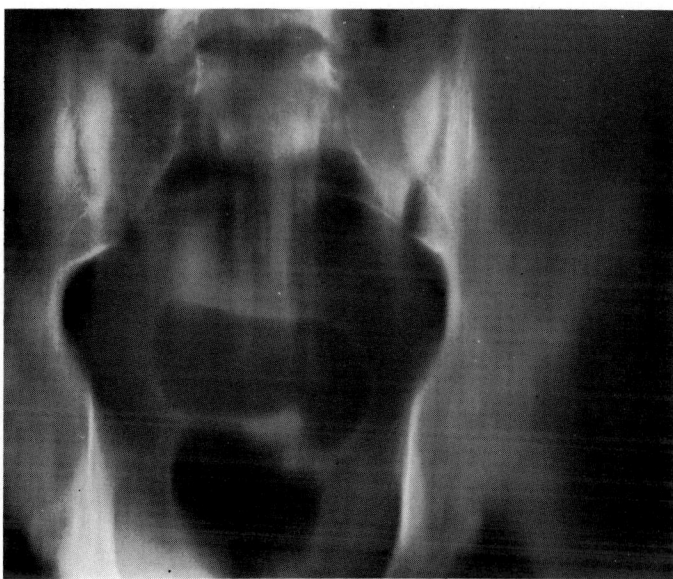

FIGURE 3–205. *Osteomyelitis of left ilium.*

Radiogram of the pelvis shows erosion of the ilium and widening of the sacroiliac joint space. This 14-year-old boy complained of low back pain and low-grade fever of two weeks' duration. On examination, he had a left lumbar scoliosis and marked paravertebral muscle spasm on the left. There was local tenderness over the ilium. X-rays disclosed rarefaction of the inferior portion of the left ilium next to the sacroiliac joint, which was definitely widened. Pus was obtained on aspiration of the bone. It was drained and the hip immobilized in a one and one half hip spica cast.

fails to gain or maintain weight. The paucity of systemic reaction in the premature and newborn infant cannot be overemphasized, since frequently the condition is not recognized, and there is serious delay in diagnosis and treatment.

Pain in the bone is the outstanding local symptom. It is severe and constant, and may be aggravated by the slightest motion. It is caused by tension in the bone produced by the inflammatory exudate and expanding pus. Lack of active motion in the affected limb (pseudoparalysis) may be suggestive of paralytic neuromuscular disease. If a bone in a lower limb is involved, the child will refuse to bear weight on the affected leg or will walk with an antalgic limp. As the disease process becomes more advanced, the periosteum ruptures, the tension in bone is released, and the pain subsides.

On gentle palpation, there is *sharp tenderness over the metaphysis of the affected bone.* The infant will often cry constantly during examination; however, on subtle digital pressure over the point of tenderness, the sudden increase in intensity of the cry is an important clue in localizing the site of infection. Local swelling and heat may be discernible. Redness is unlikely in the early stages, except when the bone affected is close to the skin surface.

The muscles of the adjacent joint are usually in protective spasm, and the joint is held in the most comfortable position, usually in flexion, but to a much lesser degree than is seen in septic arthritis. Occasionally, after several days, there may be sympathetic sterile effusion in the nearby joint, presenting a problem in differential diagnosis.

Radiographic Picture

In the first few days of the disease, after onset of symptoms, the changes in the conventional radiograph are limited to the soft tissues in the form of deep soft-tissue swelling of muscle density at the level of infection, i.e., in the region of the metaphysis in long bones. This soft-tissue swelling is contiguous with the underlying bone. It is the displacement of the lucent deep muscle plane away from the adjacent bone that depicts the localized soft-tissue change. It is paramount to make identical views of the contralateral limb to detect alterations of the lucent planes. The bone structure in the first five to ten days of infection appears to be normal in the conventional radiograph. Soon the muscles swell and the lucent planes between the muscles are obliterated. Initially the deep muscles are involved; then the superficial muscle groups show changes. The last soft-tissue change to take place is edema of subcutaneous tissues. Within five days, the local inflammatory exudate may give a hazy, smoky appearance to the medullary cavity of the metaphysis. Linear and computed tomography will often serve to depict the soft-tissue changes sooner than will regular radiograms; computed tomography will also show increased marrow density prior to conventional radiography.[227]

In 7 to 12 days, irregular spotty areas of rarefaction representing trabeculae absorbed as a result of local hyperemia and necrosis appear in the metaphysis (Figs. 3–206 and 3–207).

Soon subperiosteal new bone formation takes place, indicating the spread of infection through the cortex. With extension of the abscess in the

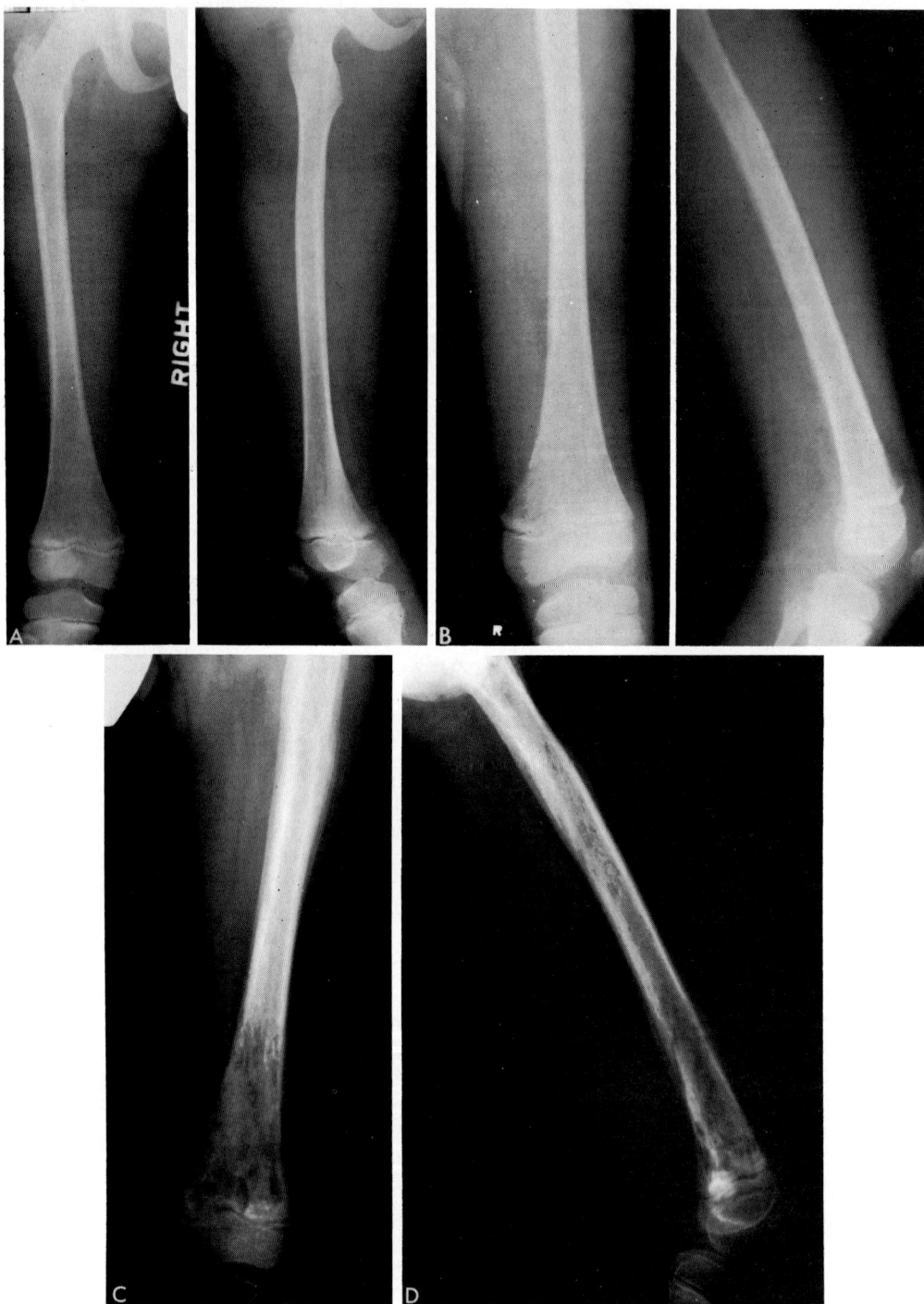

FIGURE 3–206. *Osteomyelitis of distal femur in an eight-year-old boy with extension proximally and complicated by fracture of the femoral neck.*

A. Initial radiograms, anteroposterior and lateral, of right femur failed to show any bone changes. The early radiographic findings are limited to the soft tissues. **B.** Eleven days later. Note the spotty areas of rarefaction in the distal femoral metaphysis. **C** and **D.** Eighteen days after onset of symptoms. There is marked bone destruction of the distal femoral shaft and metaphysis. Note also the extensive new bone formation, extending proximally.

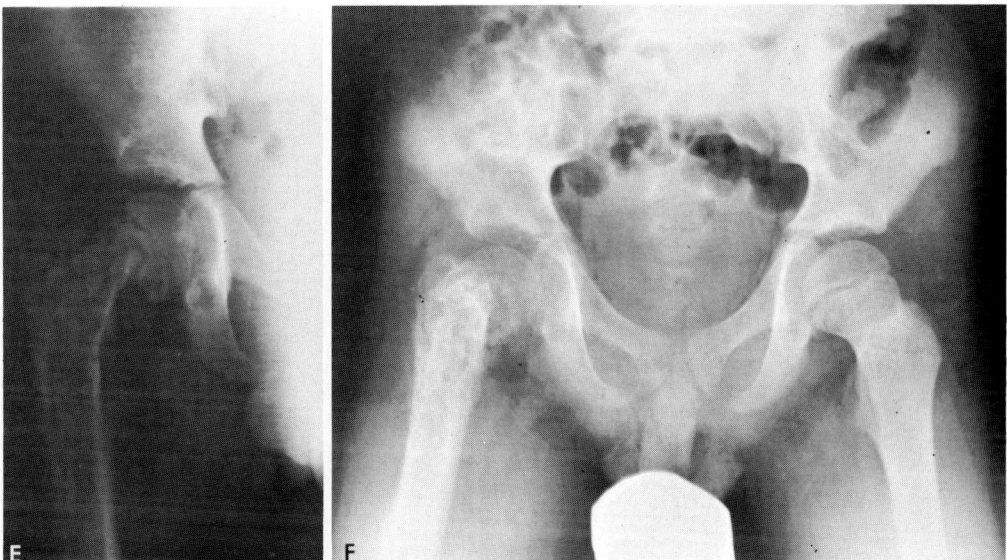

FIGURE 3–206 Continued. *Osteomyelitis of distal femur in an eight-year-old boy.*

E. Radiogram of proximal femur showing extension of osteomyelitis to the femoral neck. **F.** Following minor trauma, the patient sustained a pathologic fracture of the neck of the femur.

medullary canal of the shaft, areas of radiolucency appear and gradually increase in size. The sequestered dead bone appears dense, and its outline is likely to be sharp because of the space created by the surrounding granulation tissue (Fig. 3–208). The relative increase in radiopacity of the sequestrum comes about because it has no blood supply and retains its original mineral content, while the adjacent living bone is decalcified by the hyperemia.

Early and adequate treatment with antibiotics may modify the radiographic manifestations of acute osteomyelitis; in mild infections with immediate control of the osteitis the bone may appear normal, while in severe infections there may be a delay in the radiographic manifestations (Figs. 3–209, 3–210, and 3–211).

Bone Scan*

The diagnosis of acute osteomyelitis can be made during the first 24 to 48 hours by bone imaging with radionuclides, usually 10 to 14 days prior to the development of osseous changes visible in the conventional radiogram. The bone scan will show localized increased uptake of the radionuclide corresponding to the site of acute osteomyelitis, shown in Figure 3–212; this increased radioactivity may persist as long as six months owing to the long period of osteogenesis and repair that takes place in the affected area. A normal bone scan does not rule out acute osteomyelitis, however, because it may be performed prior to local changes in vascular perfusion or bone metabolism. The orthopedic surgeon should be aware of the possibility of false-negative or false-positive bone scans in osteomyelitis. The increased uptake of the radionuclide is nonspecific; it may be found in lesions other than acute osteomyelitis. Bone scanning, however, is noninvasive and dependable, with 90 per cent accuracy in the early detection of acute osteomyelitis before the appearance of radiographic signs. When clinical signs are poorly localized the scan will guide the surgeon to the proper site for aspiration and drainage. It will also detect multiple foci of infection. Bone scanning is performed routinely when a child presents with symptoms and signs of possible osteomyelitis. It should be stressed that before one makes the definitive diagnosis of acute osteomyelitis the bone scan findings should be carefully interpreted in conjunction with clinical history, physical findings, laboratory results (peripheral blood picture, erythrocyte sedimentation rate, recovery of bacterial organism from blood culture or bone aspirate), radiographic findings, and in selected cases CT scan. Occasionally nuclear magnetic resonance imaging is performed to delineate the pathologic changes in difficult cases. It is vital that the orthopedic surgeon assess the

---

*See references 1, 3, 57, 79, 142, 147, 165, 170–173, 183, 192, 238, 242, 253, 255, 323, 336, 337, 340, 397.

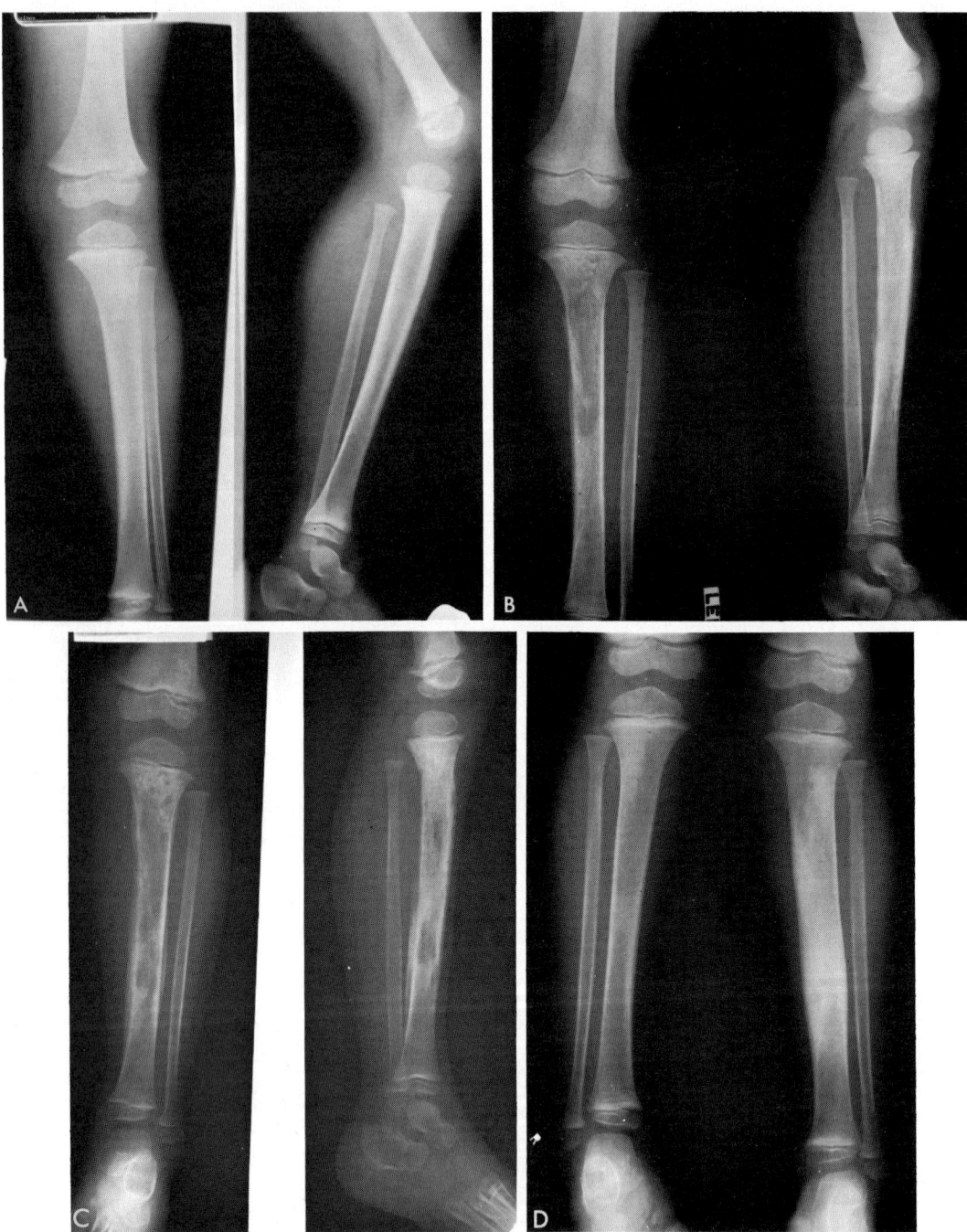

FIGURE 3–207. *Osteomyelitis of proximal tibia in a three-year-old child.*

A. Initial radiograms showing soft tissue swelling. There is a hazy, smoky appearance in the proximal metaphysis of the tibia. **B.** Two weeks later, despite systemic antibiotic therapy, there is extensive bone destruction. The bone was incised and drained. **C.** Postoperative radiograms. **D.** One year later. Note the healing of osteomyelitis and overgrowth of the affected tibia.

FIGURE 3–208. Chronic osteomyelitis of the tibia.

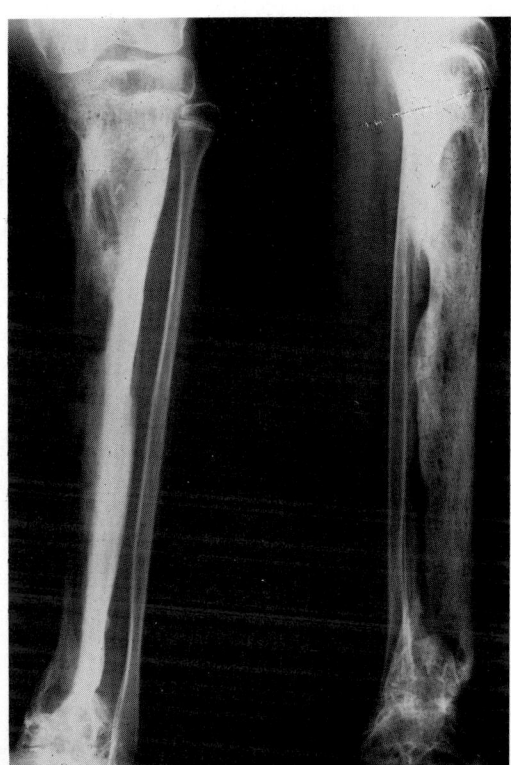

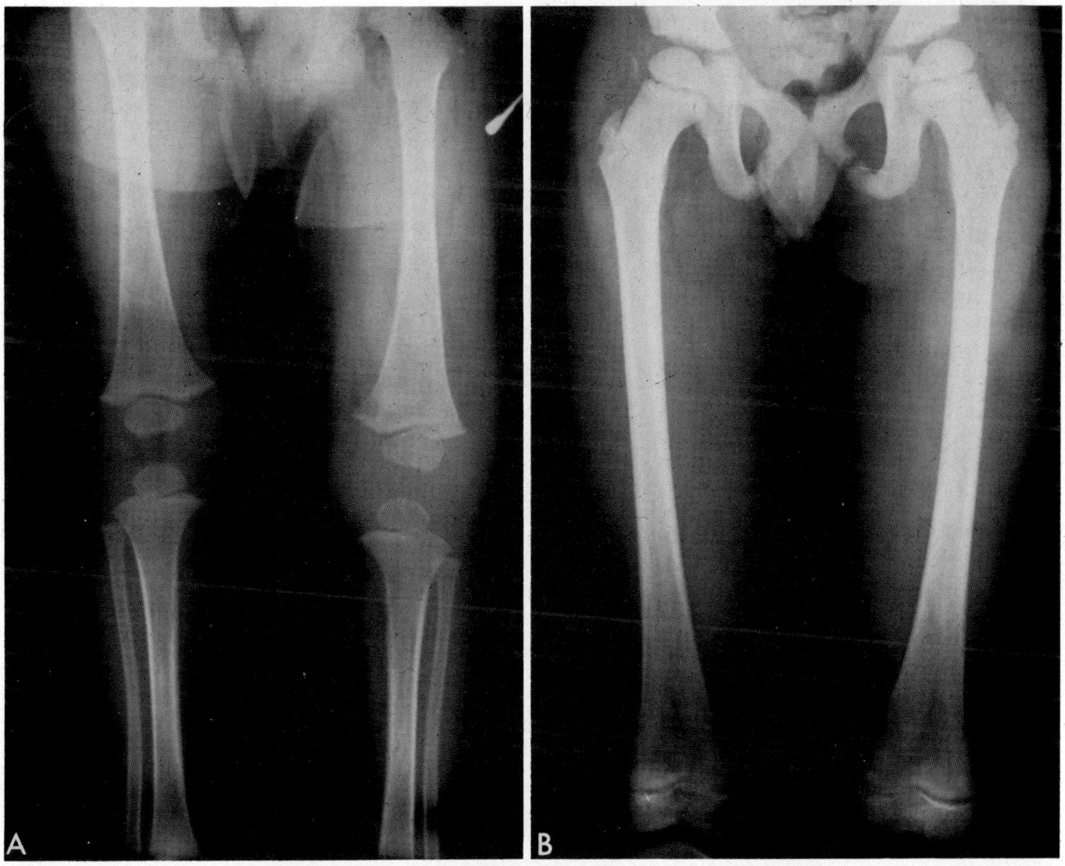

FIGURE 3–209. Osteomyelitis of left distal femoral metaphysis.

A. Note the marked tissue swelling and suggestion of rarefaction in the bone. The pathogenic organism was Streptococcus; the infection responded to systemic penicillin therapy. **B.** Radiogram of femora five years later showing normal bone structure.

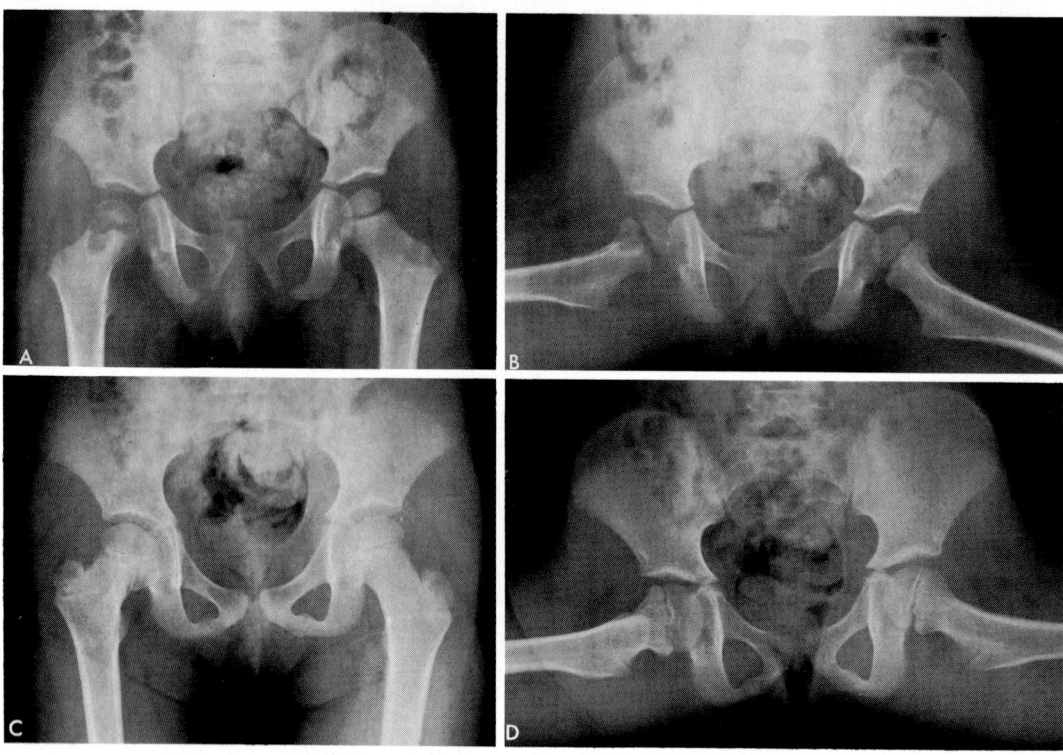

FIGURE 3–210. *Osteomyelitis of right femoral neck.*

Initial radiograms were normal. **A** and **B.** Radiograms taken two weeks following systemic antibiotic therapy. The area of rarefaction in the metaphysis illustrates delayed radiographic changes due to treatment with antibiotics. **C** and **D.** Anteroposterior and lateral radiograms of both hips 18 months later. Note the shortening of the right femoral neck.

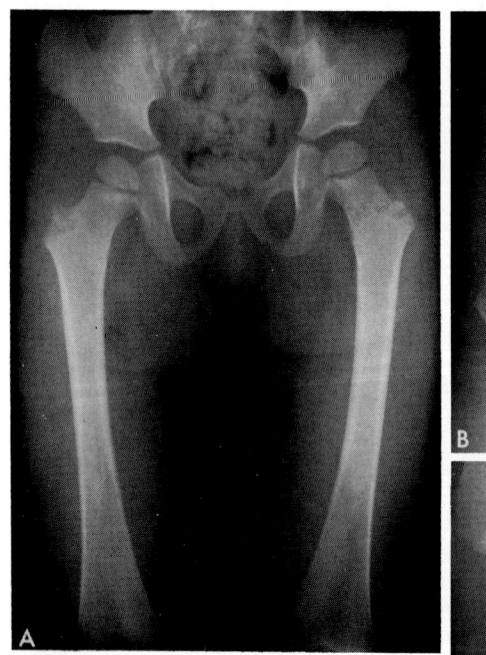

FIGURE 3–211. *Osteomyelitis of the neck of the femur in a two-year-old child.*

A. Initial radiogram of hips. There are no bone changes. She was treated with systemic penicillin. **B** and **C.** Anteroposterior and lateral radiograms of both hips three weeks later. Note the rarefied and sclerotic areas in the right femoral neck.

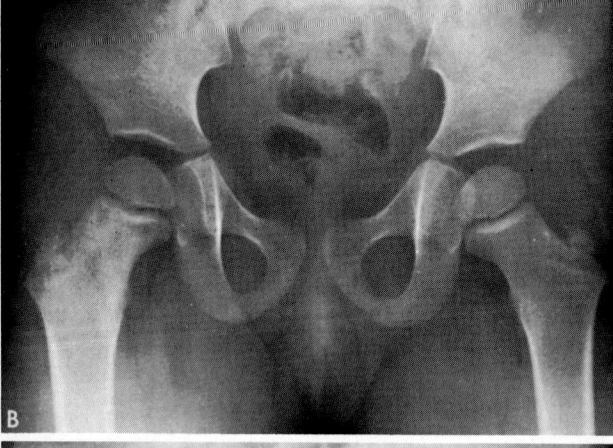

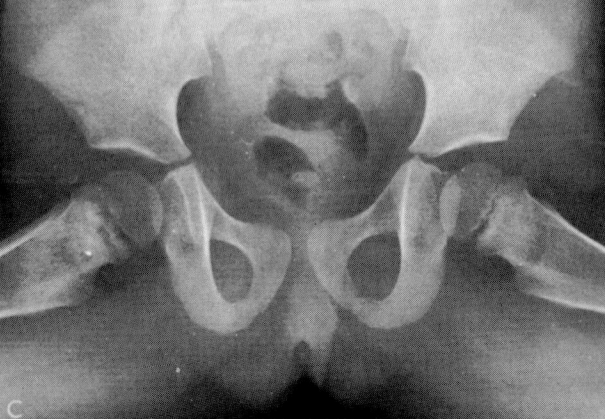

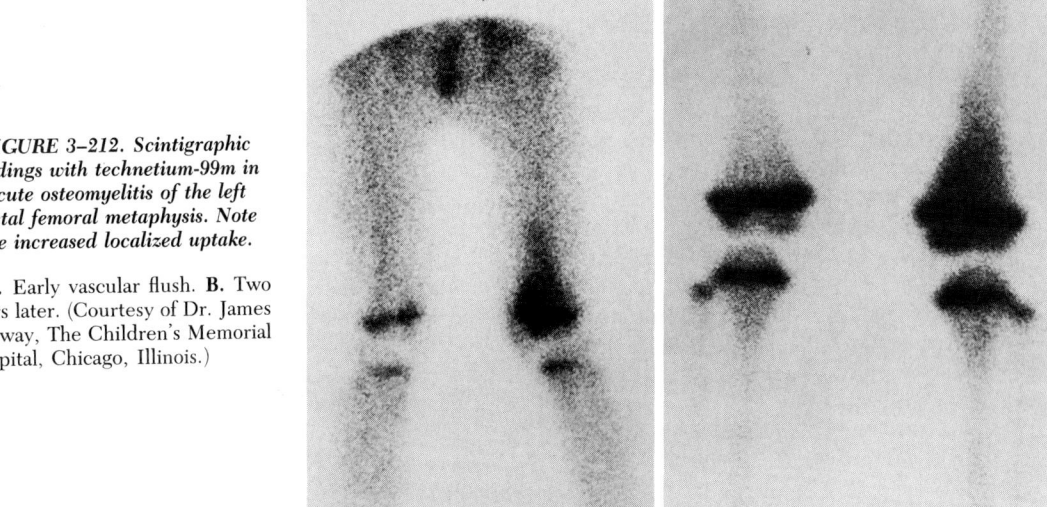

FIGURE 3–212. *Scintigraphic findings with technetium-99m in acute osteomyelitis of the left distal femoral metaphysis. Note the increased localized uptake.*

A. Early vascular flush. **B.** Two years later. (Courtesy of Dr. James Conway, The Children's Memorial Hospital, Chicago, Illinois.)

clinical signs; if they are unequivocal for acute osteomyelitis, do not delay aspiration of the metaphyseal bone because a bone scan or other sophisticated studies cannot be obtained promptly.

The bone scan has its pitfalls. Poor technique is a common problem—improper immobilization of an uncooperative child or abnormal rotation of a limb may give a false-positive or false-negative result. Misinterpretation may be another source of error—not all bone scans are performed or interpreted by experts in pediatric nuclear medicine. False-positive bone scans can occur. For example, in treating tetany in the newborn, calcium gluconate is given intravenously; in such an instance extravasation may result in cellulitis. A bone scan performed to rule out associated osteomyelitis will be false-positive owing to superimposed soft-tissue calcification. Being nonspecific, increased radionuclide uptake may be found in lesions other than acute osteomyelitis, e.g., osteoblastoma and stress fracture. A "cold" (photon-deficient) bone scan may be obtained in acute osteomyelitis as a result of primary medullary thrombosis caused by compression of microcirculation in the medulla by intraosseous abscess or by extrinsic pressure on the nutrient artery by adjacent subperiosteal pus.[15, 33, 74, 140, 152, 380, 385] An initially "cold" bone scan may be "hot" within a few days. There may be another cause of the "cold" scan in a child who presents with a painful limb—it may be due to metastatic bone disease, post-traumatic aseptic necrosis, or sickle cell disease.

The common radionuclide used is technetium-99m; it is always the first choice. When the results are inconclusive gallium-67 citrate is injected. It should be stressed that gallium-67 is not specific for infection; its uptake will be increased in aseptic inflammation and certain tumors. Often imaging is delayed (over 48 hours) because of the slow blood and soft-tissue clearance of the radionuclide and interference from bowel activity. Also, the patient receives a relatively large radiation dose as compared to that of technetium-99m. The advantages of gallium-67 citrate are its greater specificity because it binds to inflamed tissue and, both experimentally and clinically, shows increased uptake shortly after the onset of symptoms and earlier than technetium-99m.[82, 110, 221, 238, 242, 336, 337, 362] False-positives with gallium scan are related to bleeding and bone infarct; false-negatives are related to neutropenia and lesions that are smaller than 1 cm. in diameter.

Indium–WBC imaging is specific in detecting abscesses and acute inflammatory disease. Its disadvantages are that the preparation requires time (about two hours), delayed imaging is necessary (6 to 24 hours as compared with 2 to 3 hours for technetium), and the radiation to spleen and hematopoietic organs is greater than with gallium-67 citrate and much greater than with technetium-99m.

Raptopoulos and associates induced acute osteomyelitis in 18 rabbits by direct injection of a solution of *Staphylococcus aureus* culture in the proximal tibial metaphysis. Over the next four weeks, serial plain radiographs and radionuclide studies with indium-111 oxide–labeled white blood cells and technetium-99m methylene diphosphonate were performed. Visual and quantitative analyses by measuring the isotope activity of indium-111 and technetium-99m over the infected tibiae as compared with the opposite bones revealed that the white blood cell scans were positive in 15 (83 per cent) of the 18 rabbits during the first week after injection of the microorganism. In the same period, the technetium-99m bone scans were positive in only 22 per cent of the animals ($p < 0.005$). In the animals that survived, both white blood cell and bone scans were positive during the second week, and thereafter the bone scans revealed consistently greater activity than was observed with white blood cell scans. Computed tomography performed in six rabbits revealed an increased attenuation coefficient of the medullary cavities of the infected bones of four animals during the first week and of one more during the second week. Plain radiograms became positive after the twelfth day. Results of these studies indicate that in patients with suspected acute osteomyelitis, white blood cell scans and probably computed tomography can detect the disease earlier than technetium-99m bone scans and plain radiograms.[325]

In summary, in practice when clinical signs and symptoms are suggestive of acute osteomyelitis, bone scanning with technetium-99m is preferred. When the results of technetium scanning are equivocal, gallium-67 citrate is preferred; if the lesion is 2 cm. in diameter or greater and there is no marked neutropenia the result will be positive within 48 hours. Routine imaging with indium-WBC is not recommended.

It is important to remember that in neonatal osteomyelitis the bone scan with technetium-99m is not reliable for early diagnosis; its accuracy is only 30 to 40 per cent.[15]

Laboratory Findings

The white blood count is elevated, with a relatively high percentage of neutrophils and a shift to the left of the leukocytes. In the severely ill child, the white blood count may be normal. A positive blood culture may be obtained, particularly if several samples are taken when the fever spikes. The sedimentation rate is elevated and is a general index of activity of the disease.

Diagnosis

The diagnosis of acute osteomyelitis is often overlooked in the first few days of its course because attention is usually focused on the septicemia of the seriously ill child, and other local signs are ignored or misinterpreted. The limbs of any child with clinical findings suggestive of septicemia should be examined for bone infection. Acute osteomyelitis is suspected if there is pain and swelling of the limb with marked tenderness over the metaphyseal region of a long bone. Early diagnosis and immediate treatment are essential to ensure good results. One should not wait for the radiographic changes of bone destruction and periosteal new bone formation before initiating treatment, as by then the diagnosis has been made too late, and bone destruction and chronic osteomyelitis are likely to follow.

There are many disease entities common to infants and children that must be distinguished from acute osteomyelitis, such as acute rheumatic fever, septic arthritis, acute rheumatoid arthritis, cellulitis, acute leukemia, poliomyelitis, infantile cortical hyperostosis, hypervitaminosis A, and malignant bone tumors such as Ewing's sarcoma. Careful and gentle examination of the affected limb is imperative. In *osteomyelitis*, the site of maximal tenderness is localized over the metaphysis, whereas, in *inflammatory joint disease* (e.g., septic or rheumatoid arthritis) the tenderness is found primarily over the joint. Joint motion is another consideration; in arthritis it is painful and limited, despite the gentleness of the examiner, whereas, in osteomyelitis, if the limb is handled delicately, the motion of the adjacent joint is relatively unrestricted and painless. The localization and extent of the swelling must be assessed. In osteomyelitis, sympathetic joint effusion may occur, but usually swelling is maximal over the affected bone and a greater area of the limb is involved, whereas in septic arthritis, it is the joint that is swollen. In inflammatory joint disease a bone scan with technetium-99m shows minimal increased uptake that is periarticular, whereas in osteomyelitis the increased uptake is marked and metaphyseal in location.

In *cellulitis* the skin is red and indurated with a clearly demarcated border; however, if the infected bone is subcutaneous (i.e., the tibia, clavicle, or ulna), some skin changes may be noted later in the course of acute osteomyelitis. In cellulitis there is diffuse increased uptake of technetium-99m in the affected soft tissues with no focal increased activity in the bone. In serial scans the generalized increased activity diminishes rapidly with adequate antibiotic therapy without any localized increased uptake in bone. In osteomyelitis there is increased bony localized uptake that, on serial imaging, remains the same or may increase for up to six months following onset.

The correct management of acute osteomyelitis is to aspirate the affected area of bone to obtain material for bacteriologic examination and to determine whether pus is present. The importance of bone aspiration cannot be overemphasized; it establishes the diagnosis, provides serosanguineous fluid or pus for culture and identification of the pathogenic organism and determination of its antibiotic sensitivity, and assists the surgeon in making the decision whether to drain or not.

The procedure is painful; it is best to perform it with the child appropriately sedated and restrained. Aspirate the site of maximum tenderness, which in long bones is at the metaphysis. Do not explore the wrong place! Utilize image intensifier radiographic control to ensure the proper site and depth of aspiration.

A 16- or 18-gauge lumbar puncture needle with a stylet inside is used. If no subperiosteal pus is found, the needle is advanced to penetrate the cortex, and the intertrabecular spaces in the metaphyseal area are aspirated. In the first few days of the disease, often only serosanguineous fluid or blood will be obtained. The aspirated material is sent to the laboratory for culture and sensitivity studies. Cultures of the blood and material from the nose and throat as well as from any infected skin lesions are made. A smear and Gram stain are also done. Every attempt should be made to isolate the pathogenic organism.

When there is sympathetic effusion in the adjacent joint and there is a problem in differential diagnosis between a septic joint and acute osteomyelitis, the joint is aspirated first through an area of normal skin. The basic consideration is not to contaminate a clean joint.

Treatment

The two important factors in the management of acute osteomyelitis are the stage of the disease and the age of the child. Early diagnosis and immediate treatment are important in order to prevent the development of bone abscess.

ACUTE HEMATOGENOUS OSTEOMYELITIS

Acute osteomyelitis may be subclassified as *early*, without an abscess, or *late*, with abscess. In the former localized pain, tenderness, and swelling are of less than 48 hours duration; in *late acute* osteomyelitis the symptoms have been present three days or longer. It should be emphasized, however, it is the absence or presence of abscess that distinguishes the early from late acute osteomyelitis. Do not make surgical decisions by rigid adherence to a time schedule.

Antibiotic Therapy*

The cornerstone of management of osteomyelitis is antibiotic therapy. Once material has been obtained for culture, it is started promptly. Time is of the essence, and one should not wait for the identification of the organism or its sensitivities. Principles of antibiotic treatment that should be noted are listed in Table 3–24.

Bactericidal antibiotics, that is, those capable of killing the offending pathogen, are preferred to *bacteriostatic antibiotics*, which inhibit bacterial replication but are more dependent upon host defenses to eliminate infection. The specific classes of antibiotics with bactericidal activity include the penicillins and cephalosporins, both of which interfere with cell wall synthesis; aminoglycosides such as gentamicin, tobramycin, and amikacin, which inhibit bacterial protein synthesis; and vancomycin and clindamycin.

In general, the *parenteral* administration of antibiotics is necessary to ensure that optimal concentrations of drug reach the site of infection, as bone represents one of the most difficult organs in which to achieve high antibiotic concentrations. Problems with methods have plagued attempts to assess the degree of penetration of antibiotics into bone accurately because of the almost invariable contamination of bone specimens by serum or blood. It is thought that when clindamycin, penicillins, second- and third-generation cephalosporins, gentamicin, and rifampin are used a substantial fraction of the serum concentration of antibiotics reaches bone and synovial fluid.[124, 333, 382, 398, 419]

Initial antibiotic therapy for bone and joint infection should include agents with a suffi-

---

*Contributed by Ellen Gould Chadwick, M.D., and Stanford T. Shulman, M.D.; Division of Infectious Diseases, Department of Pediatrics, Northwestern University Medical School, the Children's Memorial Medical Center, Chicago, Illinois.

Table 3–24. Antibiotic Therapy of Bone and Joint Infection: General Principles

Bactericidal antibiotics preferred
Large doses needed (usually parenteral administration)*
Broad initial coverage for organisms suspected on basis of patient's age
Change to single best agent when pathogen identified
Adequate length of therapy

*See text for exceptions.

ciently broad spectrum to cover the pathogens most likely for the age of the patient. Clearly, Gram's stain will further define the most likely organism in an aspirate of bone or joint fluid and should, when positive, help guide the choice of antibiotic.

After the causative organism has been identified from cultures of blood, bone, or joint fluid and after antibiotic sensitivities have been determined, the initial broad antibiotic coverage should be modified so that therapy is continued with the single most effective agent with a narrow spectrum. This is important because long-term broad-spectrum antibiotic therapy in a hospital setting can be associated with nosocomial infection by resistant bacteria or fungi; narrow-spectrum drugs are associated with less risk of such complications.

Patients need an antibiotic course long enough to reduce the incidence of recurrent infection or development of chronic infection to the lowest possible level. On the basis of the report of Dich and associates, patients with uncomplicated acute hematogenous osteomyelitis should receive at least 21 days of parenteral antibiotic therapy. In that series, of 87 patients with staphylococcal osteomyelitis, chronic or recurrent osteomyelitis developed in 19 per cent of those who received parenteral antibiotics for 21 or fewer days, but in only 2 per cent of those who were treated parenterally for more than 21 days.[98]

The organisms responsible for acute hematogenous osteomyelitis vary according to the age of the patient (Table 3–25). Therefore, initial antimicrobial therapy must be selected to provide coverage for the most likely organism in each age group.

Neonatal Osteomyelitis. The bacteriology of osteomyelitis in infants less than two months of age is unique because group B beta-hemolytic streptococci *(Streptococcus agalactiae)* and gram-negative enteric bacilli are frequent pathogens. A retrospective study covering the period 1951 to 1976, which included 45 patients less than ten weeks of age with osteomyelitis, describes a shift in the most frequent causative agents during the study period. Prior to 1965, 24 of 25 cases (96 per cent) were caused by *Staphylococcus aureus*, whereas between 1965 and 1976, *S. aureus* was found in only 5 of 16 patients (31 per cent), *Escherichia coli* in 4 of 16 (25 per cent), and group B streptococci in 5 of 16 (31 per cent).[134] This suggests that group B streptococci emerged as a major pathogen in neonatal osteomyelitis during that period. This finding was substantiated by Edwards and associates' series of 21 osteomyelitis patients aged one to seven weeks who were seen between 1965 and 1977. The most common pathogens were group B streptococci (38 per cent), *S. aureus* (28 per cent) and gram-negative enteric bacilli (19 per cent). Two characteristic features of neonatal group B streptococcal osteomyelitis were its subacute indolent course and its predilection for involving a solitary bone, often the proximal humerus.[114] This is in contrast to other types of neonatal osteomyelitis, which frequently present a more acute course and involve multiple bones.

It is vital to treat neonates with suspected osteomyelitis empirically with antibiotics that will eradicate group B streptococcus, *S. aureus*, and gram-negative enteric bacilli. After appropriate diagnostic studies have been performed, initial therapy should include a penicillinase-stable penicillin such as nafcillin (75 to 100 mg./kg./day in divided doses every six to eight hours for patients over seven days of age) for staphylococcal and group B streptococcal coverage, plus an aminoglycoside (such as gentamicin, amikacin, or moxalactam) for the gram-negative organisms. An alternative choice is ceftriaxone or cefuroxime, single agents that are also effective against all the likely pathogens.

Children Between Two Months and Three Years of Age. The most common causes of osteomyelitis in this age group are staphylocci, i.e., *S. aureus* and *S. epidermidis*; streptococci, both alpha- and beta-hemolytic; and *Hemophilus influenzae*, in descending order of frequency.[98, 196] In a 22-year study of osteomyelitis

Table 3–25. Etiology of Osteomyelitis By Age Group

Age Group	Causative Organism		
	Common	Uncommon	Rare
Neonates	S. aureus Group B streptococcus Enteric bacilli	H. influenzae	Candida
1 mo.–3 yr.	S. aureus Streptococci	H. influenzae Pseudomonas species	Candida M. tuberculosis
>3 yr.	S. aureus Streptococci	Pseudomonas species	M. tuberculosis Candida

in 60 infants aged 1 to 24 months, 20 per cent of cases were caused by *H. influenzae* or *S. pneumoniae*.[196] The symptoms of these two infections are identical to those of osteomyelitis of other causes. If the patient displays lethargy or meningismus in conjunction with symptoms of osteomyelitis, however, a lumbar puncture should be performed, because 18 per cent of the patients in the latter series with *H. influenzae* disease had concomitant meningitis. Antibiotics of choice for this age group include those able to penetrate the cerebrospinal fluid and to treat the common causative organisms, i.e., ceftriaxone, cefotaxime, or cefuroxime. Alternatively, the combination of nafcillin and ampicillin is also efficacious, as it displays synergism against ampicillin-resistant (beta-lactamase-positive) strains of *H. influenzae*.[421, 422]

Children Over Three Years of Age. Children older than three years who have acute hematogenous osteomyelitis are usually infected with the same organisms as adults, namely *S. aureus* and streptococci.[98, 196] A semisynthetic penicillin such as nafcillin can be used alone until the results of blood or bone cultures are known. Adolescent patients suspected of having osteomyelitis secondary to intravenous drug abuse should have an aminoglycoside added to the semisynthetic penicillin because of the frequent contamination of needles by pseudomonas species and *Serratia marcescens*. The alternative for initial antibiotic therapy are summarized in Table 3-26.

Sequential Parenteral-Oral Therapy. The role of oral antibiotics in the treatment of osteomyelitis has been investigated in several centers over the past ten years. A total of 61 children with bacteriologically documented osteomyelitis were treated with intravenous antibiotics for an initial 3 to 14 days, at which time oral therapy was substituted to complete a total course of three to six weeks.[221, 285, 319, 382] Patients receiving oral therapy were monitored by weekly or biweekly peak serum bactericidal titers, and all

Table 3–26. Options for Initial Antibiotic Therapy for Acute Bone and Joint Infections in Children

Age	Antibiotics
<2 mo.	Nafcillin + Aminoglycoside
	Nafcillin + Moxalactam
	Ceftriaxone
	Cefuroxime
>2 mo., <3 yr.	Ceftriaxone
	Cefuroxime
	Cefotaxime
	Nafcillin + Ampicillin
>3 yr.	Nafcillin

Table 3–27. Contraindications to Oral Antibiotic Therapy*

Inability to swallow or retain medication
Etiologic agent not established
Inability of laboratory to perform analysis of serum bactericidal activity
Infection with agent for which no effective oral therapy exists (e.g., *Pseudomonas aeruginosa*)
Failure of patient to demonstrate clinical response to parenteral antibiotics

*From Jackson, M. A., and Nelson, J. D.: Etiology and medical management of acute suppurative bone and joint infections in pediatric patients. J. Pediatr. Orthop. 2:313, 1982. Reprinted by permission.

with titers greater than or equal to 1:8 had successful outcomes. Despite an inadequate peak bactericidal titer of less than 1:2 while receiving oral therapy, one patient continued to receive an oral antibiotic for a total of 38 days; he developed chronic osteomyelitis with a draining sinus three weeks after cessation of therapy.[221] All patients tolerated the large doses of the drugs used. Contraindications to oral antibiotic therapy are outlined in Table 3-27.[196]

For staphylococcal or streptococcal infections, dicloxacillin (40 mg./kg./day in divided doses every six hours), cephalexin (100 mg./kg./day in divided doses every six hours), or clindamycin (50 mg./kg./day in divided doses every six hours) should be used. For osteomyelitis caused by *H. influenzae*. Amoxicillin (150 mg./kg./day divided every eight hours) or cefaclor (150 mg./kg./day divided every six hours) should be used. There are no acceptable oral modes of therapy for pseudomonas infections.

The optimal duration of therapy for a sequential parenteral and oral regimen has not been established. It appears that helpful guidelines for determining when to discontinue antibiotics include completion of at least 21 days of therapy, resolution of clinical symptoms and signs of infection, and a normal erythrocyte sedimentation rate. All patients should be monitored closely during oral antibiotic treatment for compliance and maintenance of peak serum bactericidal titers greater than or equal to 1:8. The antibiotic dosages for pediatric bone and joint infections are given in Table 3-28.

Orthopedic Management

The affected limb should be immobilized in a well-padded splint or bivalved cast with the joints in functional position. When the infection is in the upper humerus or proximal femur, counterpoised skin traction (Dunlop for the arm and split Russell for the thigh) is applied for partial immobilization of the part. The patient is much more comfortable, and the rest is good treatment for osteomyelitis. The involved part

Table 3–28. Antibiotic Dosages for Pediatric Bone and Joint Infections

Drug	Dose/Day	Interval	Route
Ampicillin	200 mg./kg.	q 6 hr.	IV, IM
Penicillin	100,000 μ./kg.	q 4–6 hr.	IV, IM
Nafcillin	200 mg./kg.	q 6 hr.	IV
Gentamicin	7.5 mg./kg.	q 8 hr.	IV, IM
Amikacin	15 mg./kg.	q 12 hr.	IV, IM
Moxalactam	225 mg./kg.	q 8 hr.	IV
Ceftriaxone	75 mg./kg.	q 12 hr.	IV, IM
Cefotaxime	150 mg./kg.	q 8 hr.	IV
Cefuroxime	75 mg./kg.	q 8 hr.	IV
Cephalothin	150 mg./kg.	q 4–6 hr.	IV
Carbenicillin	400–600 mg./kg.	q 4–6 hr.	IV
Piperacillin	200–300 mg./kg.	q 4 hr.	IV
Ethambutol	25 mg./kg.	qd	PO
Streptomycin	15 mg./kg.	qd	IM
INH	10–20 mg./kg.	qd	PO
Rifampin	15–20 mg./kg.	bid	PO
Amphotericin B	1 mg./kg.*	over 6 hr.	IV

*Consult pharmacy for initial dosing regimen.

should be accessible for daily inspection to assess the status of local signs in response to antibiotic therapy and to see that the adjacent joint is still not involved. General supportive measures, such as antipyretics, intravenous fluids, transfusion of fresh whole blood or packed cells in the presence of severe anemia, and an adequate high protein diet with supplemental multivitamins, are administered as necessary.

Surgical Drainage. The place of operation continues to be discussed in the literature, with varying degrees of controversy among orthopedic surgeons and pediatricians. With early diagnosis and in the mild forms of acute osteomyelitis with good host resistance or poor bacterial aggressiveness, systemic antibiotics may effect rapid improvement of local and general signs within 24 to 48 hours; in such cases

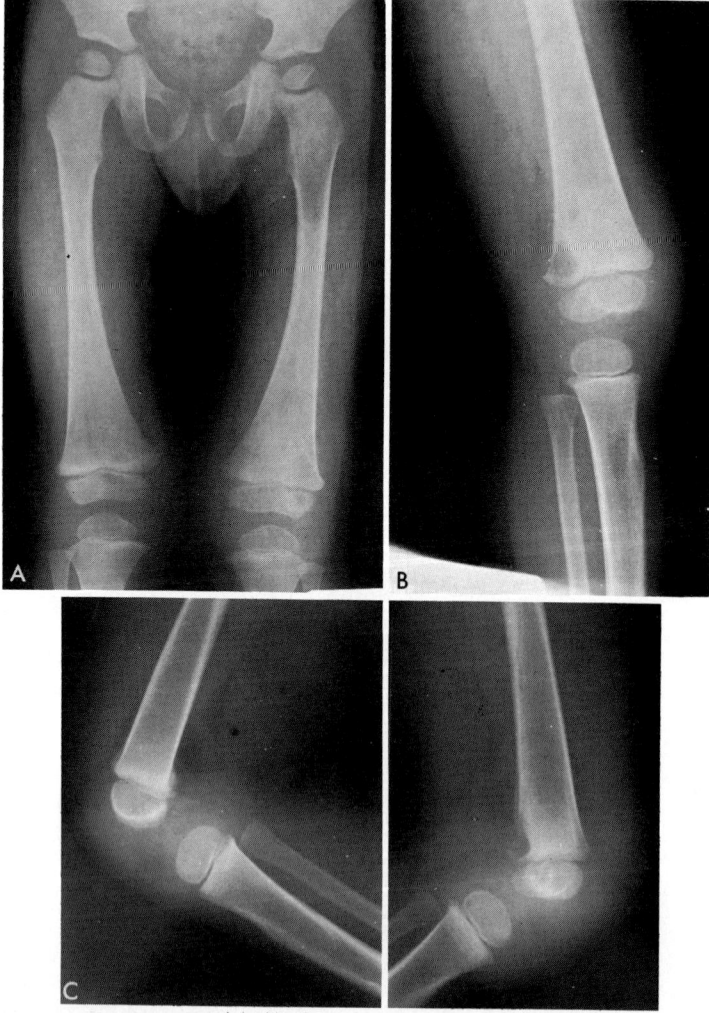

FIGURE 3–213. Osteomyelitis of distal femoral metaphysis and epiphysis on the left.

Occasionally, the epiphysis is involved because of abnormalities in the blood supply. **A** to **C.** Preoperative radiograms. Note the areas of rarefaction.

surgical decompression is unnecessary. The signs of such favorable response are a marked improvement in local tenderness and a decrease of the highly elevated temperature to near normal. Antibiotic therapy should be continued for at least six weeks, the first three weeks parenterally and then orally, provided the patient is compliant and adequate blood levels are maintained.

When there has been a delay in diagnosis and pus is obtained on aspiration of the bone, or the changes indicating bone destruction are already apparent on the radiograph, surgical decompression should be carried out initially. Do not delay operative intervention. The established principle of surgical treatment of any abscess is drainage.

Operative treatment consists of incision and drainage of the pus under pressure in bone, the surgical approach depending on the part affected. Tissue is obtained for histologic examination, and culture specimens are taken. Radiograms are taken in the operating room for accurate localization of the site for drainage (Fig. 3–213). Injury to the physis must be avoided. The periosteum should not be stripped extensively because this will further deprive the underlying cortex of circulation. Decompression is effected through a small window, by removing a 1 by 2 cm. section of wall from the cortex. Large windows weaken the diseased bone, making it more susceptible to pathologic fracture. The affected area is curetted and irrigated copiously with normal saline solution. One or two perforated silicone catheters are placed in the depth of the medullary cavity and attached to Thermovac suction. The wound is closed in a routine manner. The catheters are usually removed in five to seven days, depending on the local and systemic response and findings. Surgical drainage by wide open packing is usually not indicated.

Antibiotics are also administered systemically. This is done initially through the intravenous route, and then orally, as soon as infection is well controlled. Antibiotics are given for a minimum of three weeks and for at least two weeks after subsidence of clinical and laboratory evidence of active osteomyelitis with a normal temperature and sedimentation rate. The limb is immobilized in a splint or bivalved cast for four to six weeks, depending on the degree of bone destruction as shown on the roentgenograms. As soon as acute infection is controlled, the joints of the affected limb are exercised out of the cast for short periods several times a day. The time out of the cast is gradually increased and partial weight-bearing with crutches is permitted. Transition to normal activity is individualized, depending on the integrity of osseous structure as seen in the roentgenograms, the range of joint motion, and muscle function. It is best to be slow in resumption of normal activities in order to avoid stress fractures.

SUBACUTE OSTEOMYELITIS

Osteomyelitis may manifest itself without an acute phase, with an insidious onset, mild pain

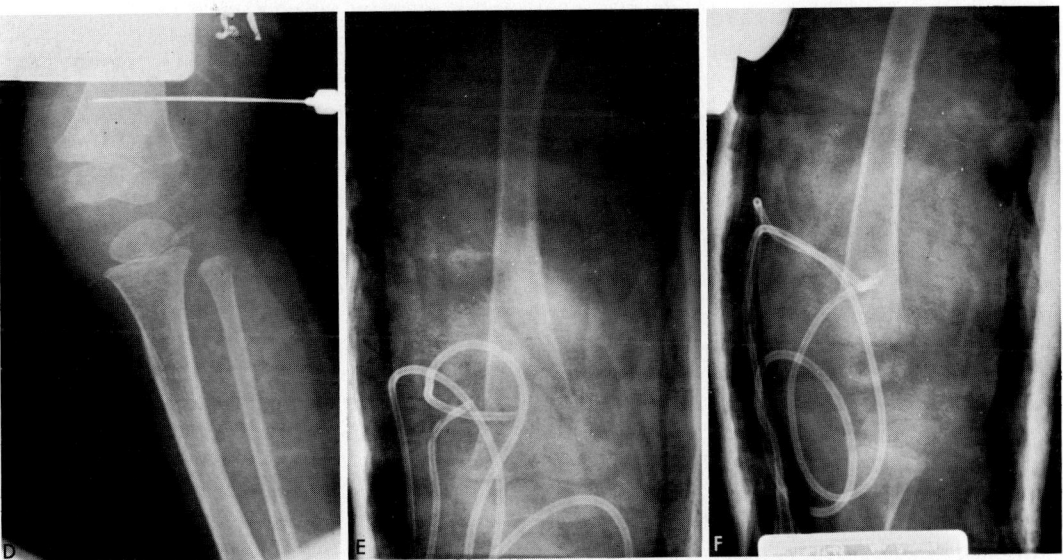

FIGURE 3–213 Continued. Osteomyelitis of distal femoral metaphysis and epiphysis on the left.

D. A lumbar puncture needle is used for accurate localization of the site for drainage. **E** and **F.** Postoperative radiographs through the cast showing drainage tubes.

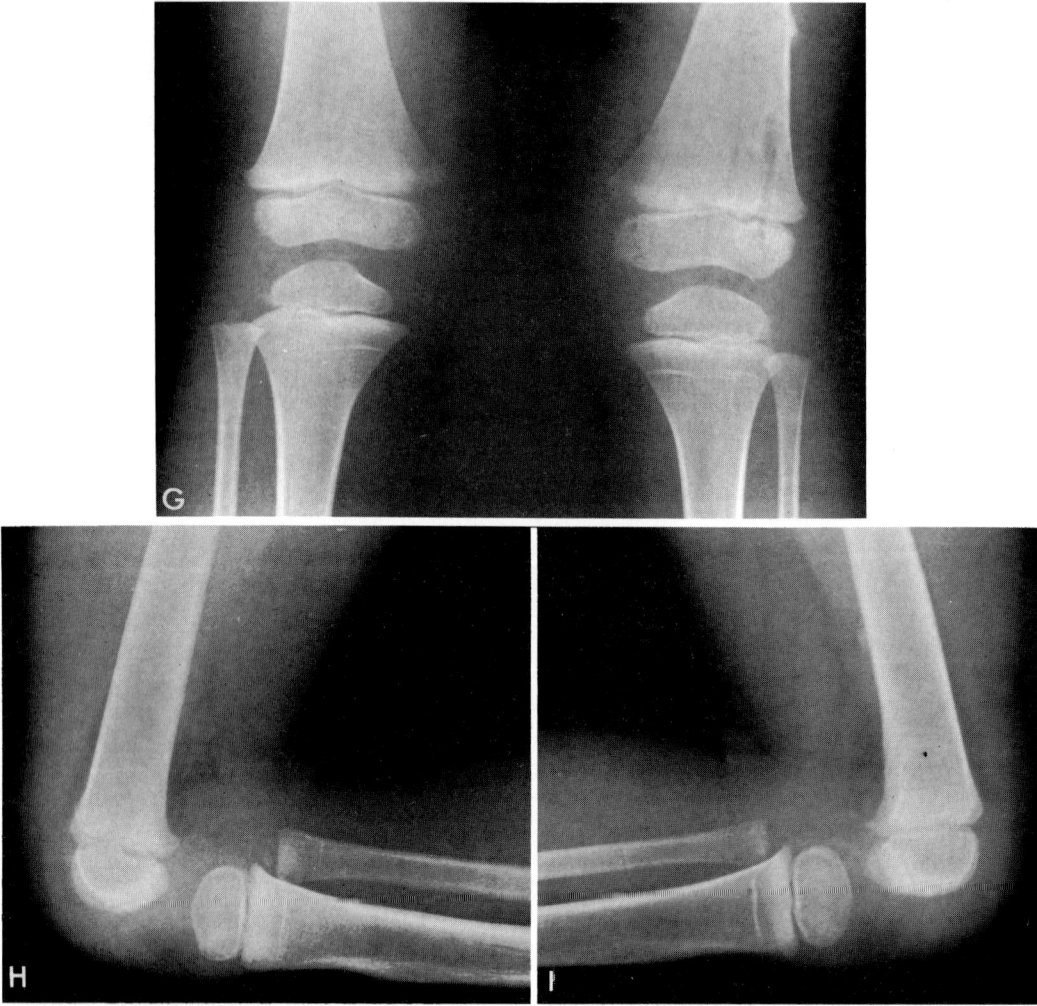

FIGURE 3–213 Continued. Osteomyelitis of distal femoral metaphysis and epiphysis on the left.

G to I. Radiograms of both knees taken a year later. The osteomyelitis has healed and there is no growth disturbance.

with little functional impairment, and few systemic signs and laboratory findings. This *subacute form* of osteomyelitis was first reported in 1836 by Sir Benjamin Brodie as a localized abscess in the tibia without acute symptoms.[46] A low-grade sclerosing nonsuppurative osteomyelitis was described by Garré in 1893.[141] In 1929, Phemister reported primary chronic osteomyelitis.[312] Subsequently several papers on primary subacute osteomyelitis were published. Gledhill, in 1973, gave a radiographic classification of primary subacute osteomyelitis that later was modified by Roberts and associates.[149, 332] Green and colleagues reported primary subacute osteomyelitis presenting in the epiphysis of long bones.[158]

Etiology. Primary subacute osteomyelitis develops because of an altered host-pathogen relationship. Reduced virulence of the pathogenic organism or increased resistance of the host results in a homeostatic balance and bone inflammation without systemic signs and symptoms. *Staphylococcus aureus* is the most frequent pathogenic organism.

Clinical Picture. It is characterized by insidious onset of the symptoms of mild local pain or discomfort, which may be present for several weeks before medical attention is sought. Systemic signs are absent or mild. The child is nontoxic and usually afebrile. Functional disability, if any, is minimal. On examination there is mild to moderate local tenderness at the affected site. There may be minimal or moderate soft-tissue swelling over the lesional area.

Laboratory Findings. They do not support infection. The white blood cell and differential counts are usually normal; the erythrocyte sedimentation rate, however, is frequently elevated. The features differentiating between subacute and acute osteomyelitis are summarized in Table 3-29.

Radiographic Features. The radiographic features vary depending on the anatomic location and the morphology and reaction of the surrounding tissue to the low-grade inflammatory process. The radiographic appearance is highly suggestive of benign or malignant bone tumors. Gledhill originally subdivided the radiographic appearance into four categories.[149] Later, Roberts and associates modified Gledhill's classification into six types (Fig. 3-214).[332] Type I and Type II lesions occur in the metaphysis, whereas Types III and IV are diaphyseal in location. Type V lesions affect the epiphyses of long bones, and Type VI subacute osteomyelitis occurs in the vertebral body. *Type I* has two subtypes: *Type IA* presents as a localized zone of radiolucency of varying size in the metaphysis of a long bone; there is no surrounding reactive bone (Fig. 3-215). The punched out radiographic appearance is very similar to eosinophilic granuloma. *Type IB* is metaphyseal in location; it appears as an area of radiolucency similar to Type IA but is surrounded by sclerotic margins of reactive bone. This is the classic Brodie's abscess. Both categories of Type I subacute osteomyelitis may penetrate the physis.

Type II subacute osteomyelitis occurs in the metaphysis and is characterized by erosion of the regional cortex (Fig. 3-216). The presence of a serpiginous tract extending from the abscess cavity toward the physis or diaphysis is quite characteristic. The aggressive loss of cortical bone gives the radiographic appearance of a malignant bone tumor such as osteogenic sarcoma.

Type III lesions are diaphyseal in location and associated with marked cortical and periosteal reaction. The radiographic appearance simulates osteoid osteoma. The periosteal new bone is often irregular. Linear and computed tomography will show single or intercomminuted zones of radiolucency within the area of hyperostosis.

Type IV lesions are located in the diaphysis of a long bone and are characterized by onion skin layering of subperiosteal new bone, giving a striking similarity to the radiographic findings of early Ewing's sarcoma.

A *Type V* lesion is located in the epiphysis of a long bone, appearing as a concentric area of radiolucency.

Type VI lesions occur in the vertebral body with erosion and collapse of the affected bone.

Diagnosis. Clinical and radiographic diagnosis of subacute osteomyelitis is difficult; often the correct diagnosis is delayed, sometimes as long as three months. In over 50 per cent of cases the disease is misdiagnosed as benign or malignant bone tumor; another misdiagnosis is juvenile rheumatoid arthritis.

Definitive diagnosis is made by culture of bone and the histologic appearance of chronic inflammation of the bone specimen. In about half the cases the bone culture will grow a bacterial organism, which often is staphylococcus coagulase–positive.

Treatment. This consists of surgical curettage and irrigation of the inflamed area, antibiotics, and immobilization of the part. During operative exposure of the metaphyseal lesion injury to the physis should be avoided. Utilize radiographic control. The prognosis is good; following surgery symptoms disappear rapidly, and there is radiographic evidence of healing. A prolonged course of antibiotic therapy for a period of six weeks is recommended.

CHRONIC OSTEOMYELITIS

Chronic osteomyelitis may be considered to be present when symptoms have persisted for longer than three weeks prior to initiation of therapy; when bone infection is evident weeks, months, or years following surgery or trauma; or when infection occurs as a consequence of

Table 3-29. Differential Diagnosis of Subacute and Acute Osteomyelitis

	Subacute	Acute
Localization	Diaphysis, metaphysis, epiphysis, cross physis	Metaphysis
Pain	Mild to moderate	Severe
Systemic illness	No	Fever, malaise
Loss of function	No or minimal	Marked
Prior antibiotics	30–40 per cent	Occasional
Initial x-ray	Frequently abnormal	Bone normal
WBC	Frequently normal	Frequently elevated
ESR	Frequently elevated	Frequently elevated
Blood cultures	Rarely positive	50 per cent positive
Bone cultures	60 per cent positive	90 per cent positive

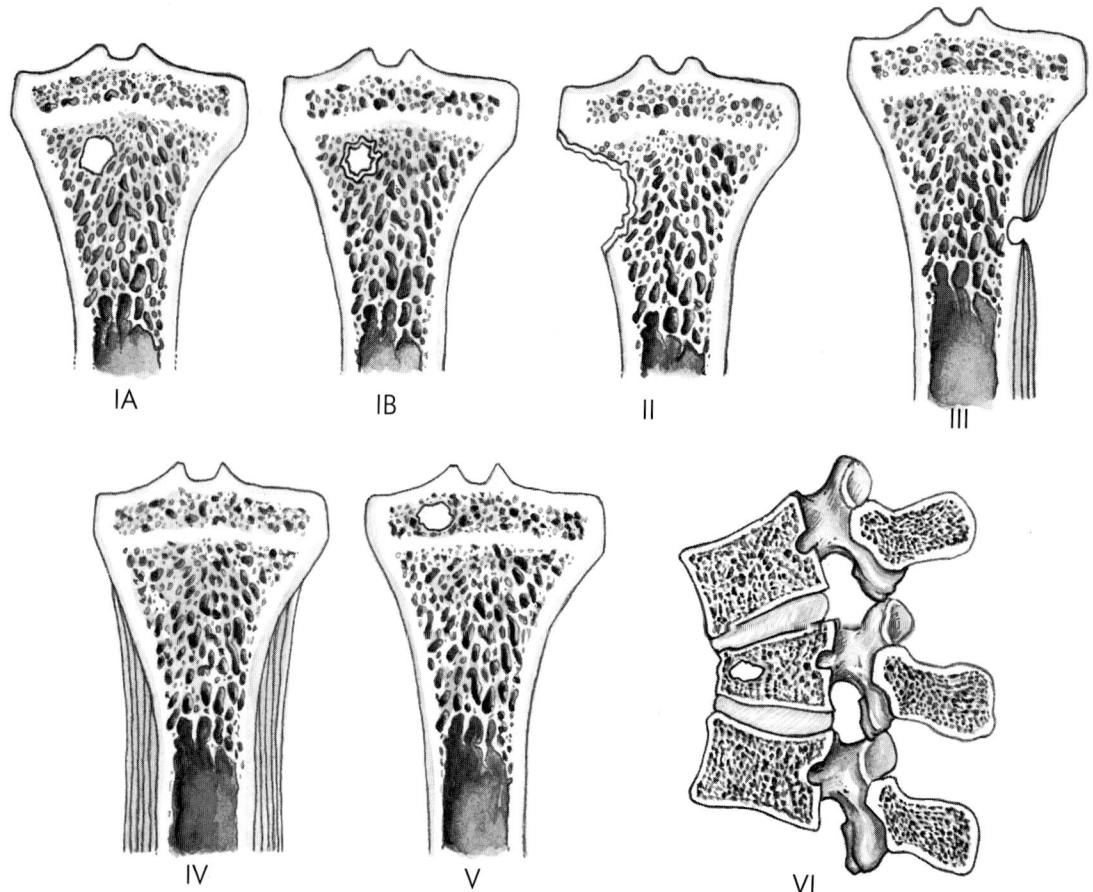

FIGURE 3–214. Radiographic classification of subacute osteomyelitis according to Roberts and associates. It is based on anatomic location, morphology, reaction of the surrounding tissue to the inflammatory lesion, and similarity to benign or malignant bone tumors.

Type I. Metaphyseal area of radiolucency; regional cortex intact. IA. Without marginal sclerosis; simulates eosinophilic granuloma. IB. With surrounding reactive bone—classic Brodie's abscess. **Type II.** Metaphyseal area of radiolucency with erosion of cortex; simulates osteogenic sarcoma. **Type III.** Diaphyseal in location, associated with localized cortical and periosteal reaction. Simulates osteoid osteoma. **Type IV.** Diaphyseal with onion skin subperiosteal new bone formation. Simulates Ewing's sarcoma. **Type V.** Epiphyseal area of radiolucency. **Type VI.** Involves vertebral body with bone destruction. (Redrawn after Roberts, J. M., Drummond, D. S., Breed, A. L., and Chesney, J.: Subacute hematogenous osteomyelitis in children: A retrospective study. J. Pediatr. Orthop., 2:249, 1982.)

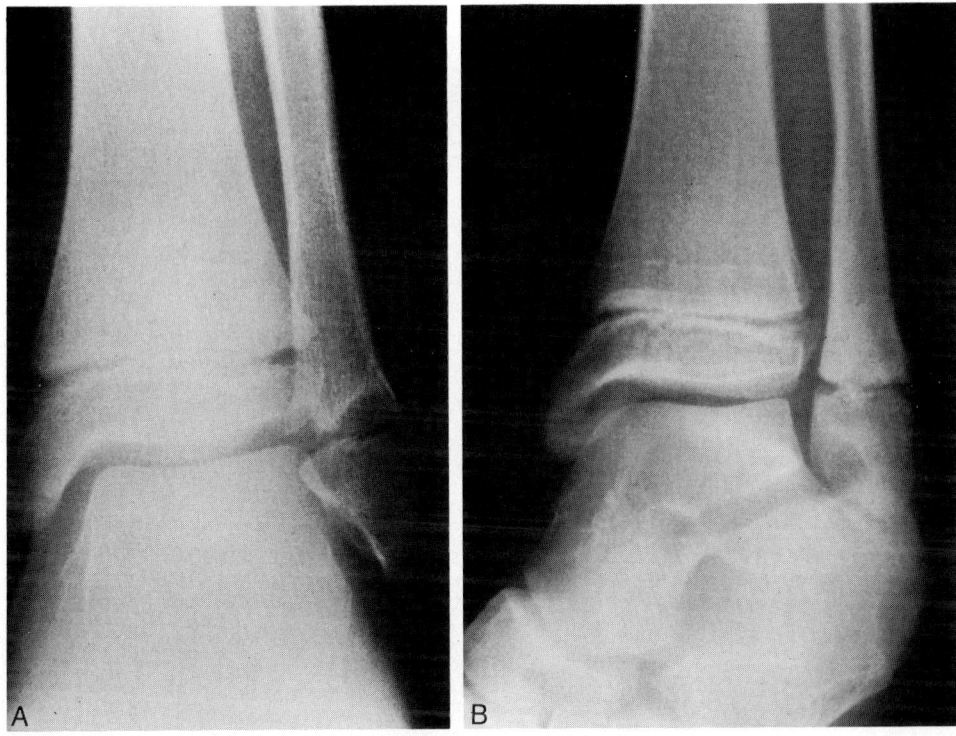

FIGURE 3–215. *Subacute osteomyelitis of distal fibular metaphysis.*

A. Preoperative radiogram showing the area of metaphyseal radiolucency. There is no surrounding reactive bone. **B.** Postoperative radiogram, following curettage and antibiotic therapy, showing complete healing.

incomplete treatment of acute osteomyelitis. Blood cultures are usually negative, and unless the patient is febrile, they are less essential in evaluating the child with chronic osteomyelitis than the one with acute osteomyelitis.

The radiographic features of chronic osteomyelitis are as described under acute osteomyelitis.

Treatment. Because chronic osteomyelitis is so frequently associated with areas of decreased blood flow and consequent compromised antibiotic delivery to the involved site, treatment consists of surgical drainage of the affected area, removal of sequestra of devitalized fibrous tissue, and decompression of cavities with excision of all granulation tissue with a scalpel or sharp curet (Fig. 3–217). Excise a margin of normal-appearing bone adjacent to the involved area in order to eliminate zones of inapparent extension of infection. Premature excision of the sequestrum prior to formation of an adequate involucrum may result in a massive defect of the diaphysis of a long bone. The integrity of the remaining bone and the involucrum should be preserved. Tubes are placed for closed suction irrigation, and the wound is closed primarily. It is necessary to have soft-tissue coverage over the affected bone. On occasion, one may have to resort to skin grafting. In the past, wounds of chronic osteomyelitis were packed with petrolatum and left open for extensive drainage. At present, one has to resort to open packing only occasionally.

For reasons that have not been clarified, the rate of recovery of organisms in chronic osteomyelitis is low, even with optimal specimen handling and excellent bacteriologic technique. Therefore, antibiotic therapy often must be selected empirically. In chronic osteomyelitis that is secondary either to spread from a contiguous focus of infection or to incomplete treatment of acute osteomyelitis, antibiotic therapy should be directed at the organism responsible for the original infection. In postsurgical or de novo chronic osteomyelitis, *Staphylococcus aureus* remains the most common pathogen; therefore, either nafcillin or a first-generation cephalosporin (i.e., cephalothin) is an appropriate antibiotic choice.[182, 221, 285]

The duration of antibiotic therapy for chronic osteomyelitis should be longer than that for acute disease because of the difficulty of effectively delivering antibiotics to affected sites and the propensity for development of very chronic infections with fistula formation unless all bacteria are completely eradicated. Patients should

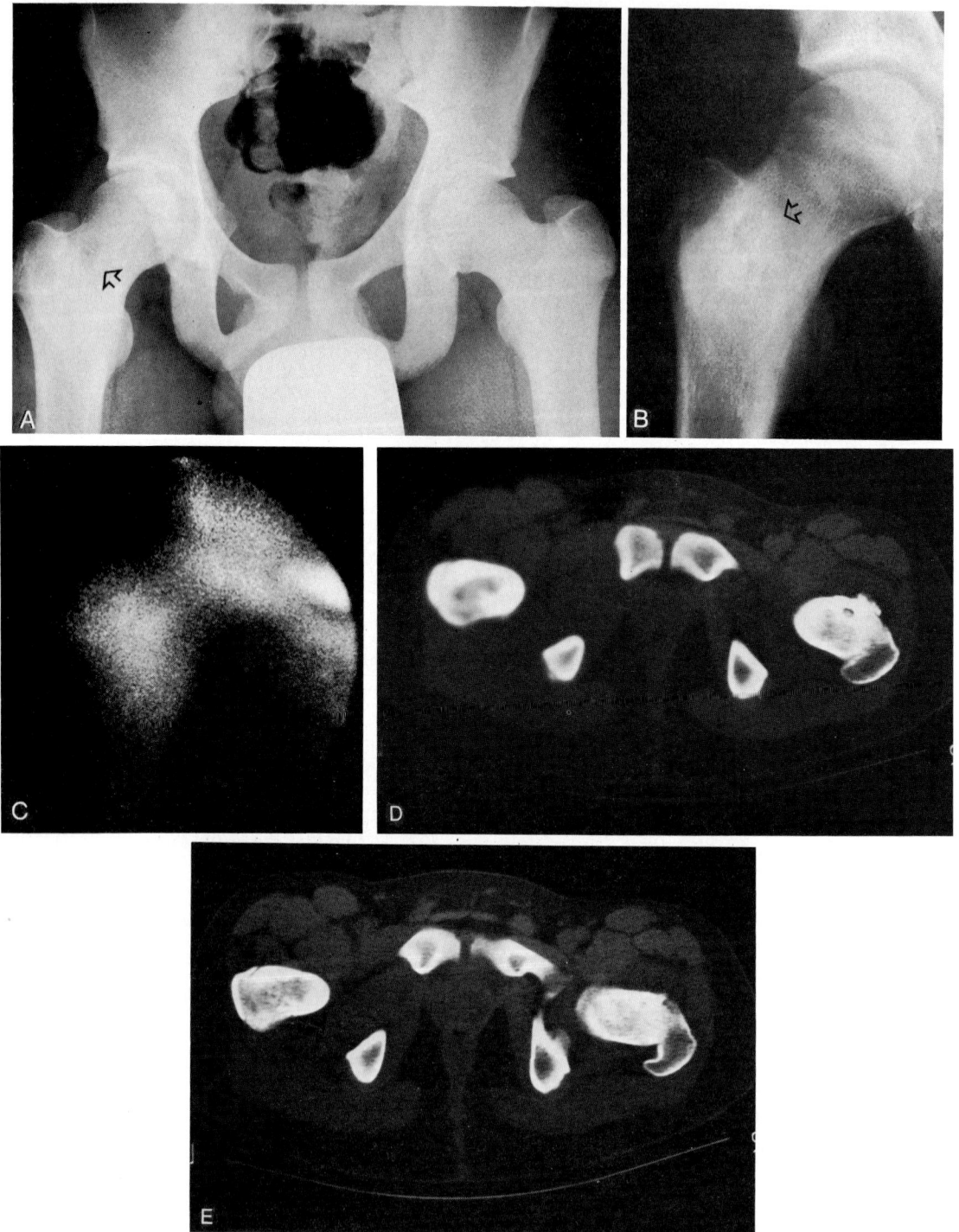

FIGURE 3–216. *Subacute osteomyelitis of the base of the neck of the femur in a 14-year-old boy.*

A and **B.** Plain radiographs of the hip showing the area of radiolucency with an irregular sclerotic border. **C.** The bone scan with technetium-99m showing increased localized uptake. **D** and **E.** CT scans showing the serpiginous sinus extending from the lesion through the cortex.

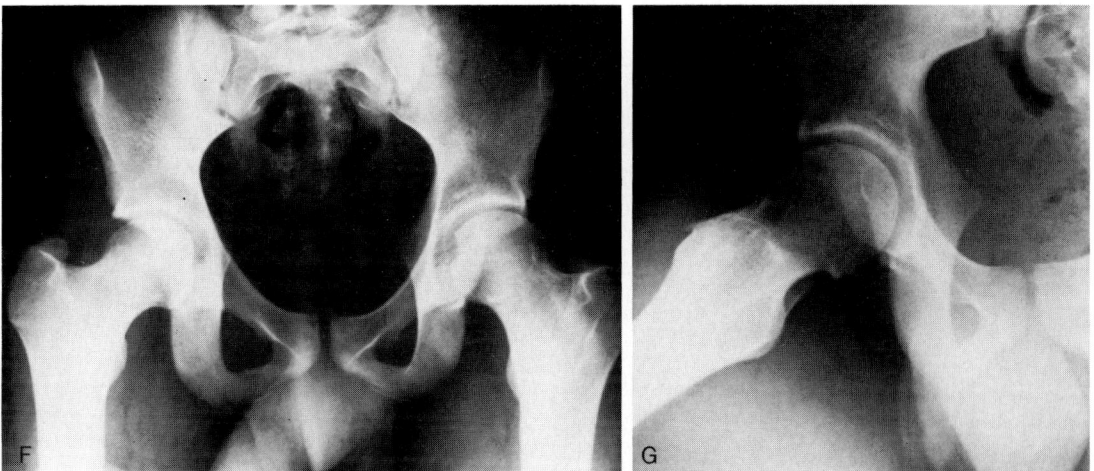

FIGURE 3–216 Continued. *Subacute osteomyelitis of the base of the neck of the femur in a 14-year-old boy.*

F and **G.** Radiograms of the hip two years later showing the normal upper end of the femur.

receive parenteral therapy for at least six weeks to insure that residual organisms not surgically removed have had adequate exposure to bactericidal levels of antibiotic. Subsequently, high-dosage oral therapy should be continued to complete a total of 6 to 12 months of treatment to eliminate any slow-growing organisms. Despite an aggressive combined surgical and medical approach to treatment, it is with distressing frequency that chronic osteomyelitis recurs because of unrecognized sequestra; these recurrent infections require therapy by repeat courses of antibiotics and surgical drainage.

Complications

The prognosis of acute hematogenous osteomyelitis depends on the promptness and adequacy of treatment, the age and general health of the patient, and the type of organism and its virulence. The mortality rate is very low; however, death still occurs in premature and newborn infants with fulminating septicemia associated with osteomyelitis. It results from respiratory failure due to massive pulmonary infection, from heart failure due to cardiac abscess, or from brain abscesses. Immunologically incompetent children are prone to fulminating infections.

Associated *septic arthritis* is the most common complication. It develops particularly in the hip because the proximal femoral metaphysis is intracapsular; with a break in the cortex the suppurative process extends into the joint. The knee, shoulder, and ankle are other sites of septic arthritis secondary to adjacent osteomyelitis. It is imperative not to contaminate the joint during aspiration of a focus of osteomyelitis. Examine the adjacent joints, especially the hip, for early detection of associated septic arthritis, which when it develops as a complication of osteomyelitis should be surgically drained.

Deep thrombophlebitis associated with acute osteomyelitis in children is a very rare complication.

Pathologic fractures of the osteomyelitic bone may occur. The affected limb should be protected postoperatively. If a fracture of the involved bone is sustained it is treated conservatively.

Destruction of the physis may cause shortening as well as various angular deformities such as knock-knees or bowlegs. In the neonate and young infant infection may extend to involve the epiphysis. In the plain radiogram the femoral condyles, the proximal tibial epiphysis, or the proximal femoral metaphysis and capital epiphysis appear to be "missing" (Fig. 3–218). Arthrography is performed to delineate the pathologic anatomy. If the cartilaginous epiphyses are present and the joint is moderately stable, treatment of angular deformities is by corrective osteotomy—closing or open-up wedge. Rotational deformities are corrected simultaneously. If the joint is destroyed and unstable, arthrodesis is the best method of management (Fig. 3–219).

Overgrowth may result from growth stimulation due to increased circulation to the part. This is a sequela and not a complication.

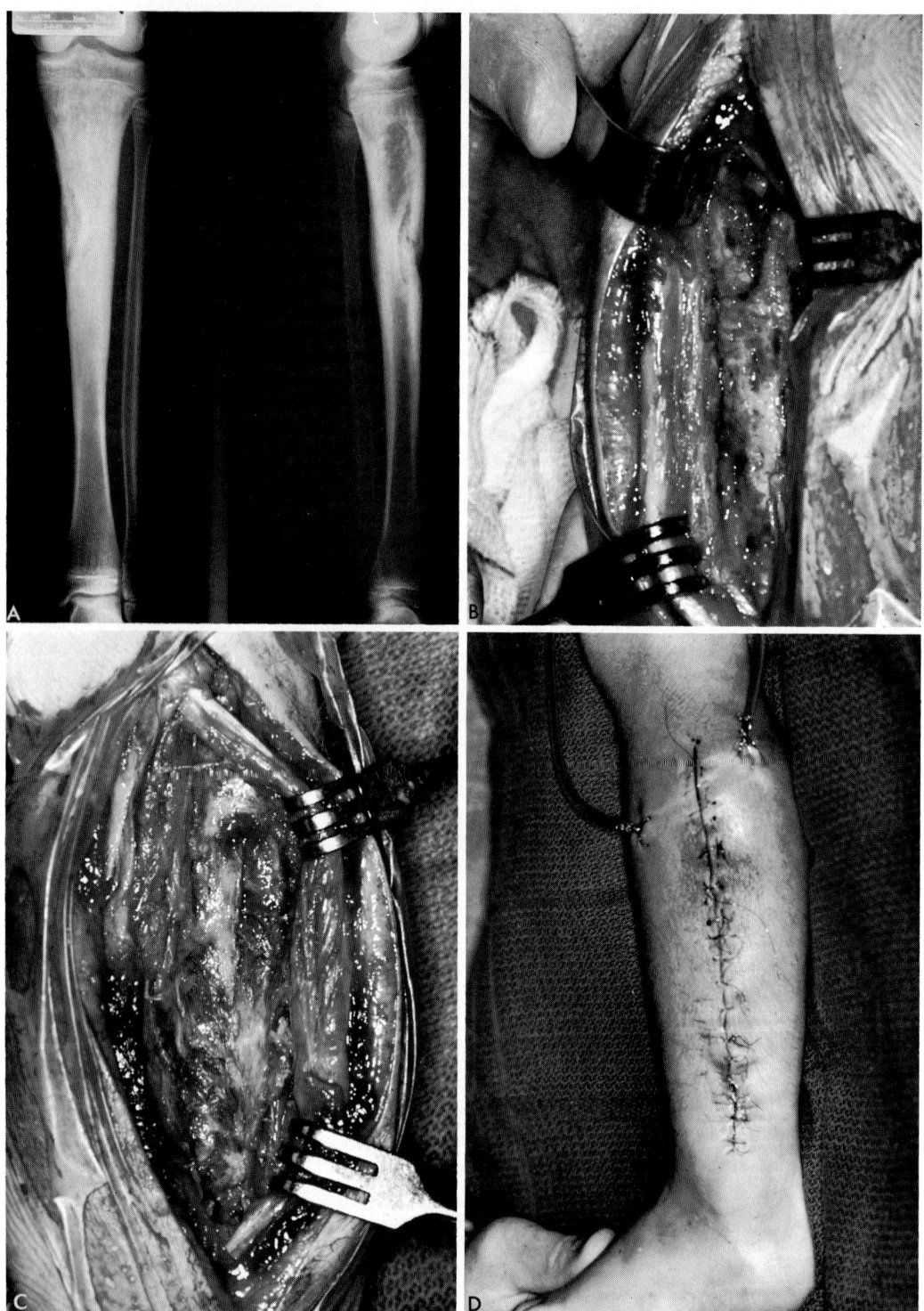

FIGURE 3–217. *Chronic osteomyelitis of the tibia.*

A. Anteroposterior and lateral radiograms. Note the sequestra and the areas of bone destruction. **B** and **C.** Photographs during the operation show the extensive bone destruction. **D.** Postoperative appearance of the leg with the closed suction irrigation tubes in place after primary closure of the wound.

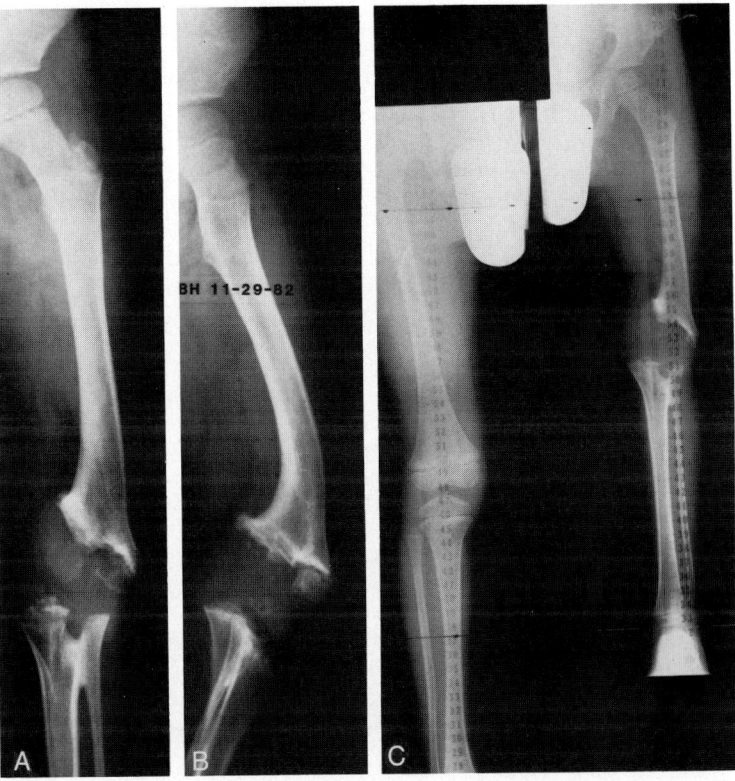

FIGURE 3-218. *Osteomyelitis of the distal femur and proximal tibia in a neonate that extended into the epiphysis.*

Note the marked destruction. The condyles appear to be missing. **A** and **B.** Anteroposterior and lateral radiograms of the femur and proximal tibia at age 18 months. **C.** At age three years showing the marked shortening of the lower limb.

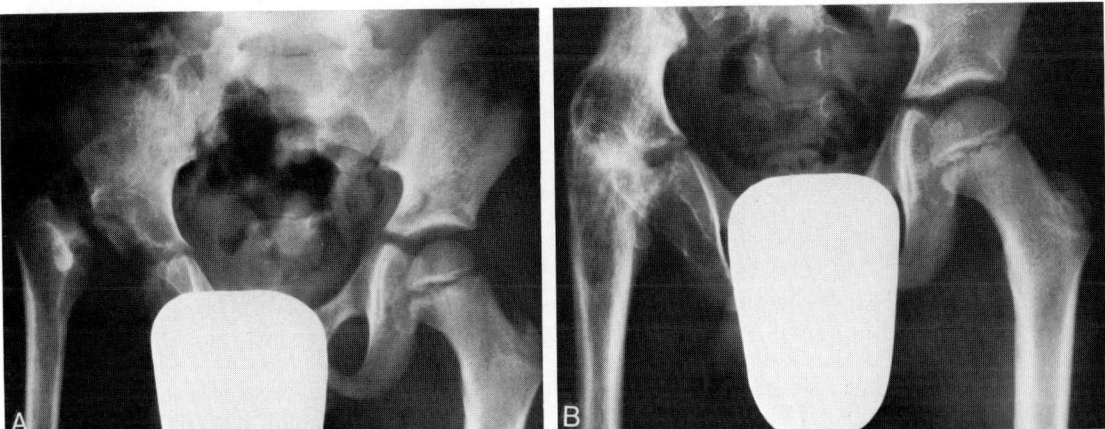

FIGURE 3-219. *Osteomyelitis of the femoral neck in a newborn resulting in marked destruction of the femoral head and neck with dislocation treated by hip fusion.*

A. Preoperative posterior radiogram. **B.** Anteroposterior radiogram of both hips after fusion.

Limb length inequality, if significant, is treated by epiphysiodesis of the contralateral longer limb or limb lengthening.

In treatment of chronic osteomyelitis premature removal of the sequestrum before the formation of the involucrum may result in a massive defect in the diaphysis of a long bone. In the young child the shaft may regenerate spontaneously; the affected limb will, however, be short. Massive defects in the tibia are best treated by a posterior tibiofibular graft or transfer of the ipsilateral fibular diaphysis; the results of surgery are much better than those of spontaneous regeneration.[135]

In persistent chronic osteomyelitis, 0.25 per cent of the cases with sinus tracts develop squamous cell carcinoma or sarcoma in adult life.

Unusual Sites of Involvement

Clavicle. The clavicle is rarely affected; the incidence as reported in the literature varies from 0 to 7 per cent. The diagnosis of acute osteomyelitis of the clavicle is often delayed.[368] The medial part of the bone is the common site of involvement. This is explained by the greater vascular supply and growth at the sternal end than at the acromial end of the clavicle. Initial symptoms and physical findings may be vague, with low-grade systemic signs of fever and elevation of leukocyte count and sedimentation rate; with progression of the infectious process, however, the affected area becomes swollen, warm, and tender. A painful mass in the medial part of the clavicle may be the presenting complaint; this may be mistaken for untreated or ununited fracture. Other entities to consider in the diagnosis are neoplasms and tumorous lesions such as Ewing's sarcoma, eosinophilic granuloma, osteoblastoma, or aneurysmal bone cyst. Sternoclavicular septic arthritis, especially gonorrheal, may mimic acute osteomyelitis of the clavicle. Radiograms will disclose local soft-tissue swelling, an area of radiolucency, and eventually subperiosteal new bone formation and an increasing area of irregular bone destruction. Bone scan with technetium-99m shows increased uptake. Computed or linear tomography is helpful in delineating the lesion. The pediatrician and orthopedic surgeon should be aware of the possibility of acute osteomyelitis of the clavicle and entertain great suspicion of its occurrence. With early diagnosis and appropriate antibiotic therapy the prognosis is excellent. Delayed diagnosis with bone destruction and abscess formation requires surgical incision and drainage. In order to provide a cosmetically acceptable scar the skin incision should be in line with the skin creases in the neck. Chronic osteomyelitis of the clavicle is treated by saucerization of the involved area and drainage, and parenteral antibiotic therapy. Partial or subtotal excision of the clavicle may be required in recalcitrant cases; subperiosteal resection permits a certain degree of regeneration of the bone, and functional disability is not that severe.

Spine. Osteomyelitis of the vertebrae is usually multifocal. It is seen in diabetic children. Onset of symptoms is very acute, and the course fulminating. Clinically when a diabetic child complains of acute back pain with local tenderness, high fever, and leukocytosis, a bone scan with technetium-99m should be performed. It will show increased uptake in the affected vertebrae. A computed tomographic scan will show precisely the extent of the soft-tissue mass, the degree of involvement of bone, and whether a bone abscess is present or not. Later in the course of the disease, radiograms will show destruction of the vertebral bodies.[211] Treatment consists of aspiration and, if pus is obtained, surgical drainage, and antibiotic therapy.

Pelvic Bones. Osteomyelitis of the pelvic bones constitutes 2 to 3 per cent of osteomyelitis of childhood and adolescence. The ilium is by far the most common site of involvement; the ischium and pubis are very rare sites of primary infection. *Staphylococcus aureus*, coagulase-positive, is the common pathogenic organism.

In the *ilium* osteomyelitis usually begins in the area adjacent to the sacroiliac joint. Infection takes place outside the joint, secondary involvement of which is rare, but can occur. Occasionally the acetabulum is the site of primary osteomyelitis. Clinically, depending upon the direction of spread of the inflammation, iliac osteomyelitis in children presents in one of three syndromes: lumbar disc, gluteal, or abdominal.

In the *lumbar disc syndrome*, the inflammatory process extends through the inner cortex of the ilium, deep and inferiorly into the true pelvis, and irritates the upper trunk of the lumbosacral plexus. The presenting complaints are difficulty in walking and pain in the lower back, hip, and thigh. Straight leg raising is limited and painful. Disuse atrophy of the quadriceps femoris may result in diminution or absence of the knee jerk; there is, however, no sensory deficit. On gentle passive manipulation the hip will have relatively free range of rotation; extremes of motion are painful, however. On palpation of the hip anteriorly and the femoral neck region posteriorly there is no pain. On lateral compression of the pelvis and deep palpation of the posterior ilium near the sacroiliac joint, the patient complains of intense pain. These are important findings in the differential diagnosis of iliac osteomyelitis from septic arthritis of the hip.

In the *gluteal syndrome*, the inflammatory process extends toward the outer wall of the ilium; when the cortex is perforated a subgluteal abscess forms. The child complains of pain in the buttock. Manual compression of the pelvis elicits pain in the affected gluteal region. Palpation discloses local tenderness; in the far advanced case a subgluteal soft mass may be palpated. Straight leg raising is restricted, but there are no signs of neurologic deficit.

In the *abdominal syndrome* the inner wall of the ilium is violated by the inflammatory process, which extends anteriorly into the iliac fossa. The symptoms and signs of the abdominal form of iliac osteomyelitis are similar to those of acute appendicitis; some unfortunate children have had appendectomy before the correct diagnosis was made. The signs of iliac osteomyelitis are pain on lateral pelvic compression and localized tenderness over the site of infection near the sacroiliac joint. The importance of diligent systematic physical examination in order to make early diagnosis cannot be overemphasized.

Diagnosis. Radiographs initially appear to be normal; however, bone scan with technetium-99m will show increased localized uptake. Later on in the course of the disease linear and computed tomography will disclose lytic destructive areas in the ilium adjacent to the sacroiliac joint. Differentiating iliac osteomyelitis from Ewing's sarcoma is sometimes difficult. This author strongly recommends computed tomography in suspected cases of iliac osteomyelitis; if there is a lytic lesion, surgical biopsy is indicated. Emperical administration of antibiotics, possibly delaying the diagnosis of Ewing's sarcoma, is not advised. In a suspected case of iliac osteomyelitis when the radiograms (including linear and computed tomography) are normal, but the bone scan is not, an intensive course of intravenous antibiotic therapy can be given with the clinical assumption that the disease is infection and not tumor. In the case of iliac osteomyelitis there will be dramatic improvement within 24 to 48 hours after initiation of antibiotic therapy.

Treatment. It consists of intravenous antibiotics. If a bone abscess has already formed, the infected area should be surgically drained. Appropriate culture is made to identify the etiologic agent. The biopsy material should be sent to the pathology laboratory to confirm the diagnosis of osteomyelitis and to rule out tumor—specifically Ewing's sarcoma.

Tarsal Bones. In about 10 per cent of children with osteomyelitis the primary site of involvement is one of the bones of the foot.[196a] The calcaneus is the most common (6 to 8 per cent), and in order of decreasing frequency, the metatarsals, cuboid, talus, phalanges, and cuneiform bones.

The infection may be of hematogenous origin or caused by external inoculation of organisms, as in puncture wounds.

Pseudomonas osteomyelitis is a serious complication of puncture wounds of the foot.[156] The child may step on a nail, a thorn, a sharp piece of glass, or in the nursery, the heel of a newborn may be infected by a contaminated needle. Mixed infection with more than one organism may occur.

Clinically osteomyelitis of the bones of the foot is an indolent infection with a paucity of systemic manifestations such as pyrexia and leukocytosis. The most constant symptoms are pain and limp. Soon soft-tissue swelling and tenderness develop, and the affected phalanx or metatarsal will appear swollen and be chronically painful.

Early diagnosis is possible before changes become apparent in the radiogram.[387] Bone imaging with radionuclides such as technetium-99m diphosphonate will detect the osteomyelitis very soon after the onset of symptoms. The earliest radiographic findings are loss and distortion of trabecular pattern. Bone resorption and periostitis develop in two to three weeks (Fig. 3–220). Sequestration appears later. Abscess cavities may have marginal sclerosis (Fig. 3–221).

An important aid in diagnosis is aspiration of the site of maximum tenderness. A 16- or 18-gauge lumbar puncture needle with a stylet inside is used; it is imperative to prepare the skin thoroughly for asepsis. If subperiosteal pus is not found, the needle is advanced to penetrate the cortex and the intertrabecular spaces. Often, in the first few days of the disease only serosanguineous fluid or blood will be obtained. The aspirated material is sent to the laboratory for culture and sensitivity studies. A smear and Gram stain are also done. Every attempt should be made to isolate the pathogenic organism.

Immediate treatment is vital. Once material

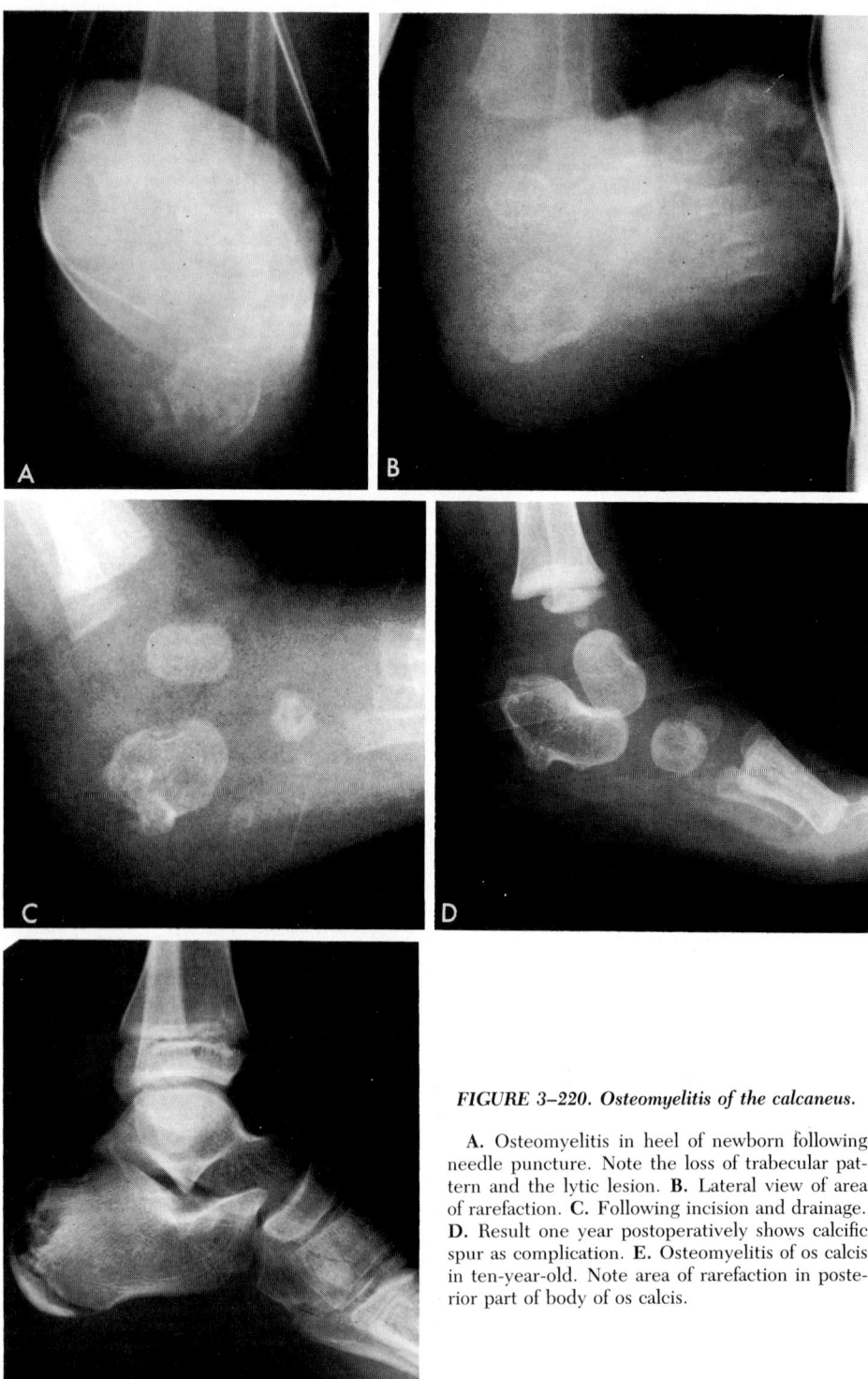

FIGURE 3–220. *Osteomyelitis of the calcaneus.*

A. Osteomyelitis in heel of newborn following needle puncture. Note the loss of trabecular pattern and the lytic lesion. **B.** Lateral view of area of rarefaction. **C.** Following incision and drainage. **D.** Result one year postoperatively shows calcific spur as complication. **E.** Osteomyelitis of os calcis in ten-year-old. Note area of rarefaction in posterior part of body of os calcis.

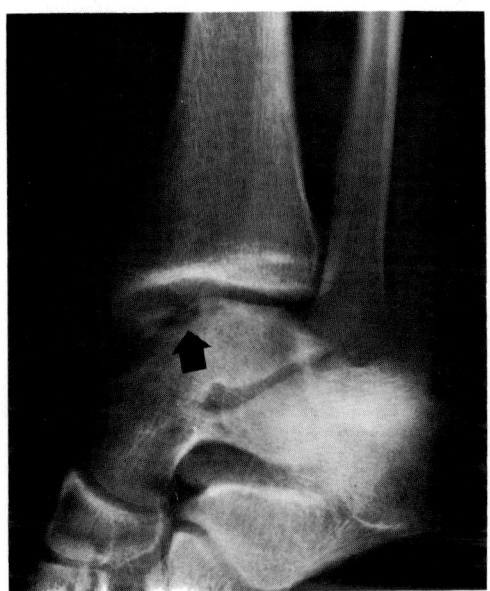

FIGURE 3–221. Osteomyelitis of the talus.

Note the area of radiolucency surrounded by marginal sclerosis (*arrow*).

has been obtained for culture, antibiotic therapy is started promptly. If Gram's stain discloses gram-negative bacteria, *Pseudomonas aeruginosa* is the probable organism. In the case of Pseudomonas osteomyelitis, the antibiotics given are penicillin (carbenicillin or piperacillin) and an aminoglycoside (gentamicin). If the smear shows gram-positive cocci, aqueous penicillin or sodium methicillin is given intravenously in appropriate dosage. As soon as the pathogenic organism and its sensitivities are determined, the antibiotic is changed to the most effective one.

Three weeks of parenteral therapy in conjunction with surgical debridement is generally adequate to cure this disease. In the series of Jacobs and associates, however, a mean of 10.8 days of antimicrobial therapy with surgical debridement was adequate.[197]

The affected foot and leg are immobilized in a well-padded splint with the ankle in functional position. The foot is inspected daily to assess the status of the local signs in response to antibiotic therapy and to see that the adjacent joints are not involved.

If pus is aspirated or if the systemic antibiotic therapy does not effect rapid improvement within 24 to 48 hours, surgical decompression in the form of incision and drainage is carried out.

In adults, partial or complete resection of the calcaneus has been advocated for osteomyelitis. The split-heel technique of Gaenslen is favored by most surgeons.[138a] In children a more conservative surgical approach is preferable. Broudy, Scott, and Watts reported 16 cases of calcaneal osteomyelitis, 14 of which required surgical treatment; in 11, administration of appropriate antibiotics, debridement, and curettage through medial and lateral incisions resulted in cure. A split-heel technique is used when extensive debridement of the calcaneus is required in cases of chronic osteomyelitis or those in which less extensive debridement has failed.[46a] The growth of the apophysis of the calcaneus should be preserved when possible. In children, excision of the calcaneus for chronic osteomyelitis is not recommended.

The scar after the Gaenslen approach is deeply located and painless; the tissues on each side of the incision curl in and form thick cushions for weight-bearing. This author, however, objects to the cosmetic appearance of the hindfoot after the Gaenslen incision; he finds the surgical approach described by Banks and Laufman to be very satisfactory. The patient is placed in prone position. The skin incision is made along the posterior aspect of the heel in line with one of the skin creases; it extends as far as necessary on the medial and lateral aspects of the hindfoot to facilitate exposure. The skin flaps are undermined and elevated, the periosteum is incised in line with the skin incision, and the plantar soft tissues are stripped from their origin on the os calcis. The body of the calcaneus is exposed medially, laterally, and inferiorly (Fig. 3–222).[19a]

Antoniou and Conner reported seven cases of osteomyelitis of the talus (five children and two adults). The characteristic finding was formation of an abscess in the body of the talus. In three of the five children the cavity was apparent on the initial radiograms. The pus from three of the abscesses contained coagulase-negative micrococci; from one abscess, the organism cultured was penicillin-resistant *Staphylococcus*, and the other abscess was sterile. The osteomyelitis responded to curettage and antibiotic therapy.[12]

Sesamoid Bones. The sesamoid bones of the first metatarsophalangeal joint are occasionally the site of hematogenous osteomyelitis. These bones are named after the seeds of *Sesamum indicum* because of their configuration. Their cartilaginous anlage develop at the third month of fetal life, and ossification begins at the age of eight years. Normally the sesamoid bones may ossify from one, two, or more centers of ossification. Bipartite or multipartite sesamoids are present in 7 to 10 per cent of feet, most

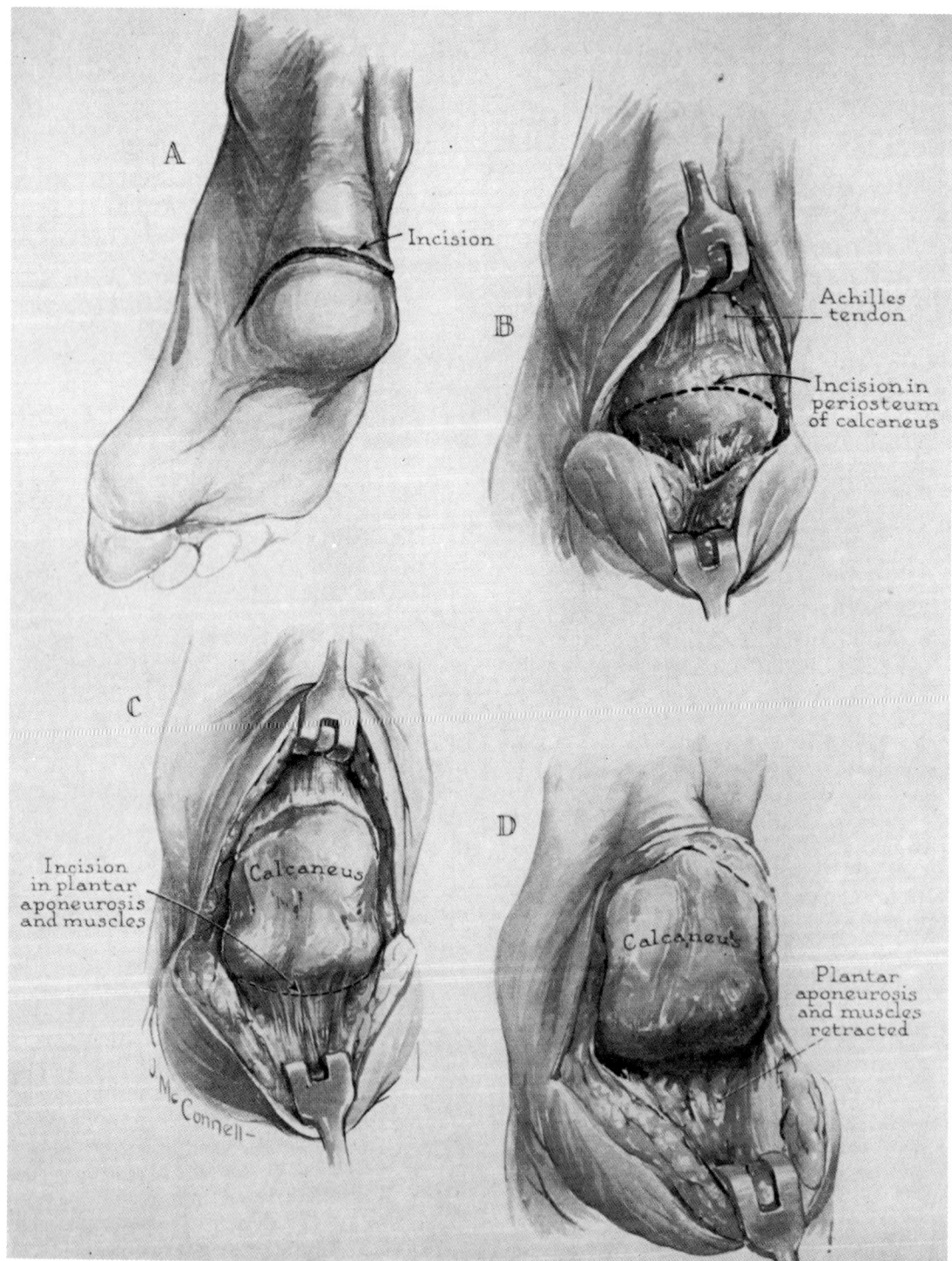

FIGURE 3–222. *Surgical exposure of the calcaneus through a circumferential heel incision.*

(From Banks, S. W., and Laufman, H.: An Atlas of Surgical Exposures of the Extremities. Philadelphia, W. B. Saunders Co., 1953, p. 379. Reprinted by permission.)

commonly occurring in the medial sesamoid (90 per cent). Normal partition of the sesamoids is unilateral in about 75 per cent of cases; therefore, comparison radiograms of the other foot are not reliably helpful.[28a]

The sesamoid bones of the hallux are almost always located in the tendon of the flexor hallucis brevis; on their plantar aspect lies the thick fibrous pad of the ball of the foot, and dorsally they articulate with the articular surface of the first metatarsal head.

In the dorsoplantar projection of the radiogram of the foot, the medial (tibial) sesamoid lies within the outline of the first metatarsal head and is larger than the lateral (fibular) sesamoid, which extends beyond the lateral margin of the first metatarsal head. For better visualization of the sesamoid, axial views in the anteroposterior and lateral planes are necessary. Occasionally tomography may be helpful.

Osteomyelitis of the sesamoids usually occurs in children over eight years of age and in young adults. Occasionally it may be seen in adults. Often there is no history of recent acute injury. The presenting complaint is pain in the forepart of the foot. In the early stages of the disease there is little local or systemic evidence of infection. The diagnosis is frequently delayed or overlooked because the symptoms are thought to be due to foot strain or cellulitis. In the adult male the condition may be misdiagnosed as gout. On examination there are local tenderness of the affected sesamoid and swelling and redness in the region of the first metatarsophalangeal joint.

The initial radiograms are normal, but within 10 to 14 days the sesamoid appears to be irregular and fragmented (Fig. 3–223). This stage is followed by relatively increased density and sequestration and migration of the dead bone fragments.

Eventually an abscess develops on the medial and dorsal aspects of the head of the first metatarsal; the abscess does not extend into the thick plantar surface under the sesamoid bone. Periostitis of the first metatarsal shaft may develop.

Treatment consists of incision, drainage, and removal of the sesamoid bone, combined with chemotherapy. The prognosis is good, with permanent healing as a rule.

References

1. Adatepe, M. H., Powell, O. M., Isaacs, G. H., Nichols, K., and Cefola, R.: Hematogenous pyogenic vertebral osteomyelitis: Diagnostic value of radionuclide bone imaging. J. Nucl. Med., 27:1680, 1986.
2. Agerholm, M., and Trueta, M.: Acute hematogenous osteomyelitis treated with penicillin. Lancet, 1:877, 1946.
3. Ailsby, R., and Staheli, L.: Pyogenic infection of the sacroiliac joint in children, radioisotope bone scanning as a diagnostic tool. Clin. Orthop., 100:96, 1974.
4. Akhmedov, M. A., and Rakhimov, A. U.: Pathological fractures and dislocations in hematogenic osteomyelitis in children. Ortop. Travmatol. Protez, 7:50, 1981.
5. Alperin, L. J., and Bender, M. J.: Osteitis pubis. Am. J. Dis. Child., 88:227, 1954.
6. Altemeier, W. A., and Largen, T.: Antibiotics and chemotherapeutic agents in infections of the skeletal system. J.A.M.A., 150:1462, 1952.
7. Altemeier, W. A., and Reinecke, M. D.: Roentgenographic interpretation of acute hematogenous osteomyelitis treated with penicillin. A.J.R., 54:437, 1945.
8. Altemeier, W. A., and Wadsworth, C. L.: An evaluation of penicillin therapy in acute hematogenous osteomyelitis. J. Bone Joint Surg., 30-A:657, 1948.
9. Ambrose, G. B., and Neers, C. S.: Vertebral osteomyelitis. A diagnostic problem. J.A.M.A., 197:101, 1966.
10. Anderson, J. R., Scobie, W. G., and Watt, B.: The treatment of acute osteomyelitis in children: A 10-year experience. J. Antimicrob. Chemother., 7-A:43, 1981.
11. Anderson, J. R., Orr, J. D., MacLean, D. A., and Scobie, W. G.: Acute haematogenous osteitis. Arch. Dis. Child., 55:953, 1980.
12. Antoniou, D., and Conner, A. N.: Osteomyelitis of the calcaneus and talus. J. Bone Joint Surg., 56-A:338, 1974.
13. Apell, R. G., and Willich, E.: Roentgen diagnosis of structural changes in the pubic area in children and adolescents. Personal case reports, differential diagnosis and literature review. Radiology, 23-2:66, 1983.
14. Asmar, B. I., and Dajani, A. S.: Ampicillin-chloramphenicol interaction against enteric Gram-negative organisms. Pediatr. Infect. Dis., 2:39, 1983.

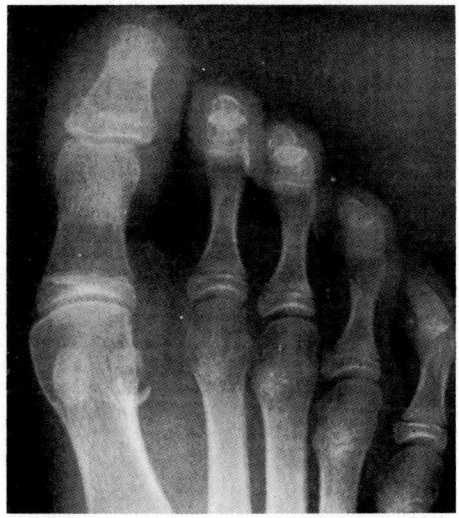

FIGURE 3–223. *Osteomyelitis of the lateral sesamoid bone of the first metatarsophalangeal joint of the right foot.*

The anteroposterior radiogram shows definite fragmentation of the lateral seramoid bone with increased density of the proximal fragment. (From Torgerson, W. R., and Hammond, G.: Osteomyelitis of the sesamoid bones of the first metatarsophalangeal joint. J. Bone Joint Surg., 51-A:1421, 1969. Reprinted by permission.)

15. Ash, J. M., and Gilday, D. L.: The futility of bone scanning in neonatal osteomyelitis: Concise communication. J. Nucl. Med., 21:417, 1980.
16. Avila, L.: Primary pyogenic infection of the sacro-iliac articulation. J. Bone Joint Surg., 23-A:922, 1941.
17. Badgley, C. E.: Osteomyelitis of the ileum. Arch. Surg., 28:83, 1934.
18. Baker, L. R. I., Brian, M. D., Miller, J. K., and Raphael, M. J.: Osteomyelitis: An unusual sequel to neutropenia. Br. Med. J., 1:722, 1967.
19. Balsam, D., Farruggia, S., Goldfarb, C. R., and Stringer, B.: Bone scintigraphy for neonatal osteomyelitis: Simulation by extravasation of intravenous calcium. Radiology, 135:185, 1980.
19a. Banks, S. W., and Laufman, H.: Surgical Exposure of the Extremities. Philadelphia, Saunders, 1953, p. 378.
20. Banks, A. J., and Menon, J.: The changing face of osteomyelitis. Lancet, 2:858, 1980.
21. Bannatyne, R. M., and Karmali, M. A.: Meningococcal osteomyelitis. Can. Med. Assoc. J., 125:1313, 1981.
22. Barson, W. J.: Group C streptococcal osteomyelitis. J. Pediatr. Orthop., 6:346, 1986.
23. Baylin, G. J., and Glenn, J. C., Jr.: Soft tissue changes early in acute osteomyelitis. A.J.R., 58:142, 1947.
24. Bearse, C.: Osteomyelitis of the ilium in children. J.A.M.A., 80:991, 1923.
25. Beaupre, A., and Carroll, N.: The three syndromes of iliac osteomyelitis in children. J. Bone Joint Surg., 61-A:1087, 1979.
26. Beerman, C. A.: The treatment of acute hematogenous osteomyelitis of the long bones in infants and children. J. Pediatr., 33:378, 1948.
27. Benedict, E. B.: Carcinoma in osteomyelitis. Surg. Gynecol. Obstet., 53:1, 1931.
28. Benner, E. J.: The use and abuse of antibiotics. J. Bone Joint Surg., 49-A:977, 1967.
28a. Bennet, K.: Septische Osteomyelitis als Ätiologie der sog. Typischen Erkrangung der Serambeine des metatarsal knochens. Acta Chir. Scand., 76:103, 1935.
29. Berard, J., Chauvot, P., and Michel, C. R.: Negative bone scintigraphy in osteomyelitis in children. Difficulties in interpretation. Rev. Chir. Orthop., 68:475, 1982.
30. Bergdahl, S., Ekengren, K., and Eriksson, M.: Neonatal hematogenous osteomyelitis: Risk factors for long-term sequelae. J. Pediatr. Orthop., 5:564, 1985.
31. Bergdahl S., Elinder, G., and Eriksson, M.: Treatment of neonatal osteomyelitis with cloxacillin in combination with fusidic acid. Scand. J. Infect. Dis., 13:281, 1981.
32. Berges, O., Berger, J. P., Boccon-Gibod, L., and Faure, C.: Case report 165: BCG-osteomyelitis of the proximal end of the humerus with an abscess dissecting into the deltoid muscle. Skeletal Radiol., 7:75, 1981.
33. Berkowitz, I. D., and Wenzel, W.: "Normal" technetium bone scans in patients with acute osteomyelitis. Am. J. Dis. Child, 134:828, 1980.
34. Berquist, T. H., Brown, M. L., Fitzgerald, R. H., Jr., and May, G. R.: Magnetic resonance imaging: Application in musculoskeletal infection. Magn. Reson. Imaging, 3:219, 1985.
35. Berry, D. D., Box, Q. T., and Brouhard, B. H.: Adverse reactions to parenteral lincomycin. Pediatrics, 67:389, 1981.
36. Blanche, D. A.: Osteomyelitis in infants. J. Bone Joint Surg., 34-A:71, 1952.
37. Blockey, N. J.: Chronic osteomyelitis. An unusual variant. J. Bone Joint Surg., 65-B:120, 1983.
38. Blockey, N. J., and McAllister, T. A.: Antibiotics in acute osteomyelitis in children. J. Bone Joint Surg., 54-B:299, 1972.
39. Blockey, N. J., and Watson, J. T.: Acute osteomyelitis in children. J. Bone Joint Surg., 52-B:77, 1970.
40. Boland, A. I., Jr.: Acute hematogenous osteomyelitis. Orthop. Clin. North Am., 3:225, 1972.
41. Bonakdar-pour, A., and Gaines, V. D.: The radiology of osteomyelitis. Orthop. Clin. North Am., 14:21, 1983.
42. Bonkfiglio, M., Kim, Y. M., and Lange, I. A.: Pyogenic vertebral osteomyelitis. Disc space infections. Clin. Orthop., 96:234, 1973.
43. Borovik, P. I., Borovik, G. A., Konovart, B. N., and Troshkov, A. A.: Treatment of septicopyemic forms of acute hematogenous osteomyelitis using dimexide and hyperbaric oxygenation. Vestn. Khir. 127:94, 1981.
44. Borris, L. C., and Helleland, H.: Growth disturbance of the hind part of the foot following osteomyelitis of the calcaneus in the newborn. A report of two cases. J. Bone Joint Surg., 68-A:302, 1986.
45. Bose, K. S.: Observations on changes of pattern of chronic pyogenic osteomyelitis following inadequate administration of penicillin: Their similarity with other bone diseases. J. Indian Med. Assoc., 32:271, 1959.
46. Brodie, B.: Pathological and Surgical Observations of the Diseases of the Joints. 4th Ed. London, Longman, 1836.
46a. Broudy, A. S., Scott, R. D., and Watts, H. G.: The split-heel technique in the management of calcaneal osteomyelitis in children. Report of three cases. Clin. Orthop., 119:202, 1976.
47. Broughton, R. A., Edwards, M. S., Haffer, A., and Baker, C. J.: Unusual manifestations of neonatal group B streptococcal osteomyelitis. Pediatr. Infect. Dis., 1:410, 1982.
48. Bruschwein, D. A., Brown, M. L., and McLeod, R. A.: Gallium scintigraphy in the evaluation of disk-space infections. J. Nucl. Med., 21:925, 1980.
49. Bryson, A. F., and Mandell, R. B.: Primary closure after operative treatment of gross chronic osteomyelitis. Lancet, 1:1179, 1964.
50. Bryson, Y. J., Connor, J. D., LeClere, M., et al.: High dose oral dicloxacillin treatment of acute staphylococcal osteomyelitis in children. J. Pediatr., 94:673, 1979.
51. Buchman, J.: The rationale of the treatment of chronic osteomyelitis. Bull. Hosp. Joint Dis., 9:177, 1948.
52. Buchman, J.: A survey of progress in the understanding of the osteomyelitic lesion and its therapy. Bull. Hosp. Joint Dis., 18:60, 1957.
53. Buchman, J.: Osteomyelitis. A.A.O.S. Instruct. Course Lect., 16:232, 1959.
54. Buchman, J., and Fenton, R. L.: The role of the surgical approach in the treatment of acute hematogenous osteomyelitis with antibiotic agents. N.Y. State J. Med., 53:2632, 1953.
55. Burleson, R. L., Johnson, M. C., and Head, H.: Scintigraphic demonstration of experimental abscesses with intravenous Ga citrate and Ga labeled blood leucocytes. Ann. Surg., 178:446, 1973.
56. Burman, M., Weinkle, I. N., and Langsam, M. J.: Adolescent osteochondritis of the symphysis pubis with considerations of normal radiographic changes in symphysis pubis. J. Bone Joint Surg., 16:649, 1934.
57. Burrows, P. E., Greenberg, I. D., and Reed, M. H.: The distal femoral defect: Technetium-99m pyrophosphate bone scan results. J. Can. Assoc. Radiol., 33:91, 1982.
58. Butler, E. C. B.: The treatment, complications and late results of acute hematogenous osteomyelitis. Br. J. Surg., 28:261, 1940.
59 Cabanela, M. E., Sim, F., Beabout, J. W., and

Dahlin, M. D.: Osteomyelitis appearing as neoplasms. Arch. Surg., *109*:68, 1974.
60. Caldwell, G. A., and Wickstrom, J.: The closed treatment of acute hematogenous osteomyelitis. Results in 67 cases. Ann. Surg., *131*:734, 1950.
61. Campagne, D., Goumy, P., Raynaud, E. J., and Veyre, A.: Scintigraphy in infectious bone pathology in children. Value and limitations. Arch. Fr. Pediatr., *39*:49, 1982.
62. Canale, S. T., and Manugian, A. H.: Neonatal osteomyelitis of the os calcis: A complication of repeated heel punctures. Clin. Orthop., *156*:178, 1981.
63. Capener, M., and Pierce, K. C.: Pathological fractures in osteomyelitis. J. Bone Joint Surg., *14-A*:501, 1932.
64. Capitanio, M. A., and Kirkpatrick, J. A.: Early radi observations in acute osteomyelitis. A.J.R., *108*:488, 1970.
65. Cass, J. M.: Staphylococcus aureus infections of the long bones in the newly born infant. Arch. Dis. Child., *15*:55, 1940.
66. Chilton, S. J., Aftimos, S. F., and White, P. R.: Diffuse skeletal involvement of streptococcal osteomyelitis in a neonate. Radiology, *134*:390, 1980.
67. Chung, S. M. K., and Borns, P.: Acute osteomyelitis adjacent to the sacro-iliac joint in children. Report of two cases. J. Bone Joint Surg., *55-A*:630, 1973.
68. Chusid, M. J., and Sty, J. R.: Pneumococcal arthritis and osteomyelitis in children. Clin. Pediatr., *20*:105, 1981.
69. Clarke, A. M.: Neonatal osteomyelitis: A disease different from osteomyelitis of older children. Med. J. Aust., *1*:237, 1958.
70. Clawson, D. K., and Dunn, A. W.: Management of common bacterial infections of bones and joints. J. Bone Joint Surg., *49-A*:164, 1967.
71. Clawson, D. K., and Stevenson, J. K.: Treatment of chronic osteomyelitis. Surg. Gynecol. Obstet., *120*:59, 1965.
72. Clinefelter, E. W.: Osteitis pubis. Review of the literature and report of a case. A.J.R., *63*:368, 1950.
73. Cole, W. G., Dalziel, R. E., and Leitl, S.: Treatment of acute osteomyelitis in childhood. J. Bone Joint Surg., *64-A*:218, 1982.
74. Coletti, R. B., Moreland, M. S., Peters, R. F., and Young, P. C.: Primary sternal osteomyelitis with a negative bone scan. Orthopedics, *3*:209, 1980.
75. Collert, S.: Osteomyelitis of the spine. Acta Orthop. Scand., *48*:283, 1977.
76. Compere, E. L.: Treatment of osteomyelitis and infected wounds by closed irrigation with a detergent-antibiotic solution. Acta Orthop. Scand., *32*:324, 1962.
77. Compere, E. L., Metzger, W. I., and Mitra, R. N.: The treatment of pyogenic bone and joint infections by closed irrigation (circulation) with a non-toxic detergent and one or more antibiotics. J. Bone Joint Surg., *49-A*:614, 1967.
78. Compere, E. L., Schnute, A. J., and Catell, L. M.: The use of penicillin in the treatment of acute hematogenous osteomyelitis. Report of twelve cases. Ann. Surg., *122*:954, 1945.
79. Conway, J. J.: Radionuclide bone imaging in pediatrics. Pediatr. Clin. North Am., *24*:701, 1977.
80. Cooppan, R., D'Elia, J., Friedberg, S. and Schoenbaum, S.: Vertebral osteomyelitis in insulin-dependent diabetics. South Afr. Med. J., *50*:1993, 1976.
81. Cottington, G. M., Ferguson, A. B., Jr., and Riden, J. M.: Osteomyelitis since the advent of antibiotics: A study of infants and children. Clin. Orthop., *14*:97, 1959.
82. Cox, F., and Hughes, W. T.: Gallium 67 scanning for the diagnosis of infection in children. Am. J. Dis. Child., *133*:1171, 1979.
83. Crane, L. R., Kapdi, C. C., Lerner, A. M., Silberberg, B. K., and Wolfe, J. N.: Xeroradiographic, bacteriologic, and pathologic studies in experimental staphylococcus osteomyelitis. Proc. Soc. Exp. Biol. Med., *156*:303, 1977.
84. Crock, H. V., Kame, S. K., and Yoshzava, H.: Observations on the venous drainage of the human vertebral body. J. Bone Joint Surg., *55-B*:528, 1973.
85. Cunningham, R. J.: Osteomyelitis of the ribs. Br. Med. J., *5365*:1128, 1963.
86. Curtiss, P. H., Jr.: Some uncommon forms of osteomyelitis. Clin. Orthop., *96*:84, 1973.
87. Das De, S., and McAllister, T. A.: Pseudomonas osteomyelitis following puncture wounds of the foot in children. Injury, *12*:334, 1981.
88. D'Avanzo, M., D'Ascoli, C., Di Lena, C., Gaudino, E., and Esposito, V.: Clinical and etiopathogenetical remarks about some cases of neonatal osteoarthritis. Pediatria, *90*:269, 1982.
89. Davis, J. C., Heckman, J. D., DeLee, J. C., and Buckwold, F. J.: Chronic non-hematogenous osteomyelitis treated with adjuvant hyperbaric oxygen. J. Bone Joint Surg., *68-A*:1210, 1986.
90. Delbarre, F., Rondier, J., Delrieu, F., Evrard, J., Cayla, J., Menkes, C. J., and Amor, B.: Pyogenic infection of the sacroiliac joint. J. Bone Joint Surg., *57-A*:819, 1975.
91. Dennison, W. M.: Haematogenous osteitis in children. Preliminary report on treatment with penicillin. J. Bone Joint Surg., *30-B*:110, 1948.
92. Dennison, W. M.: Osteomyelitis—an historical survey. Glasgow Med. J., *32*:121, 1951.
93. Dennison, W. M.: Unilateral limb lengthening associated with hematogenous osteitis in childhood. Arch. Dis. Child., *27*:54, 1952.
94. Dennison, W. M.: Haematogenous osteitis in the newborn. Lancet, *2*:474, 1955.
95. Devas, M. B.: Malignant change in chronic osteomyelitis. Br. J. Surg., *40*:140, 1952.
96. Deysine, M., Rosario, E., and Isenberg, H. D.: Acute hematogenous osteomyelitis: An experimental model. Surgery, *79*:97, 1976.
97. Deysine, M., Rafkin, H., Teicher, I., et al.: Diagnosis of chronic and postoperative osteomyelitis with gallium 67 citrate scans. Am. J. Surg., *129*:632, 1975.
98. Dich, V. Q., Nelson, J. D., and Haltalin, K. C.: Osteomyelitis in infants and children. A review of 163 cases. Am. J. Dis. Child., *129*:1278, 1975.
99. Dickson, F. D.: The clinical diagnosis, prognosis, and treatment of acute hematogenous osteomyelitis. J.A.M.A., *127*:212, 1945.
100. Dickson, F. D., Diveley, R. L., and Kiene, R. H.: Subacute and chronic osteomyelitis. Treatment with use of chemotherapeutic agents, antibiotics, and primary closure: Follow-up report. Arch. Surg., *66*:60, 1953.
101. Digby, J. M., and Kersley, J. B.: Pyogenic nontuberculous spinal infection. An analysis of thirty cases. J. Bone Joint Surg., *61-B*:47, 1979.
102. Dillehunt, R. B.: Osteomyelitis in infants. Surg. Gynecol. Obstet., *61*:96, 1935.
103. Dilmaghani, A., Close, R., and Rhinelander, F. W.: A method for closed irrigation and suction therapy in deep wound infections. J. Bone Joint Surg., *51-A*:323, 1969.
104. Dombrowski, E. T., and Dunn, A. W.: Treatment of osteomyelitis by debridement and closed wound irrigation-suction. Clin. Orthop., *43*:215, 1965.
105. Donovan, R. M., and Shah, K. J.: Unusual sites of acute osteomyelitis in childhood. Clin. Radiol., *33*:222, 1982.
106. Donowitz, L. G., Cole, W. Q., and Lohr, J. A.: Acute spinal epidural abscess presenting as hip pain. Pediatr. Infect. Dis., *2*:44, 1983.
107. Dunkle, L. M., and Brock, N.: Long-term follow-up of ambulatory management of osteomyelitis. Clin. Pediatr., *21*:650, 1982.
108. Dunn, E. J., Bryan, D. M., Nugent, J. T., and

Robinson, R. A.: Pyogenic infections of the sacro-iliac joint. Clin. Orthop., *118*:113, 1976.
109. Duszynski, D. O., Kuhn, J. P., Afshani, E., and Riddlesperger, M. M., Jr.: Early radionuclide diagnosis of acute osteomyelitis. Radiology, *117*:337, 1975.
110. Dye, S. F., Lull, R. J., McAuley, R. J., Van Dam, E. B., and Young, W.: Time sequence of bone and gallium scan changes in acute osteomyelitis: An animal model (abstr.). J. Nucl. Med., *20*:647, 1979.
111. Ebong, W. W.: Bilateral pelvic osteomyelitis in children with sickle-cell anemia. Report of four cases. J. Bone Joint Surg., *64-A*:945, 1982.
112. Ebong, W. W.: Pathological fracture complicating long bone osteomyelitis in patients with sickle cell disease. J. Pediatr. Orthop., *6*:177, 1986.
113. Edwards, J. E., Jr., Lehrer, R. I., Stiehm, E. R., Fischer, T. J., and Young, L. S.: Severe candidal infections. Clinical perspective, immune defense mechanisms and current concepts of therapy. Ann. Intern. Med., *89*:91, 1978.
114. Edwards, M. S., Baker, C. J., Granberry, W. M., and Barrett, F. F.: Pelvic osteomyelitis in children. Pediatrics, *61*:62, 1978.
115. Eid, A. M., Issa, H., and Deif, A. I.: Some immunological aspects of staphylococcal haematogenous osteomyelitis. Arch. Orthop. Trauma Surg., *96*:221, 1980.
116. Eismont, F. J., Bohlman, H. H., Soni, P. L., Goldberg, V. M., and Freehafer, A. A.: Vertebral osteomyelitis in infants. J. Bone Joint Surg., *64-B*:32, 1982.
117. Eismont, F. J., Bohlman, H. H., Soni, P. L., Goldberg, V. M., and Freehafer, A. A.: Pyogenic and fungal vertebral osteomyelitis with paralysis. J. Bone Joint Surg., *65-A*:19, 1983.
118. Ekengren, K., Bergdahl, S., and Eriksson, M.: Neonatal osteomyelitis. Radiographic findings and prognosis in relation to site of involvement. Acta Radiol., *23*:305, 1982.
119. Engler, H. S., Fernandez, A., Bliven, F. E., and Novetz, W. H.: Cancer arising in scars of old burns and in chronic osteomyelitis, ulcers, and drainage sites. Surgery, *55*:654, 1964.
120. Epremian, B. E., and Perez, L. A.: Imaging strategy in osteomyelitis. Clin. Nucl. Med., *2*:218, 1977.
121. Erasmie, U., and Hirsch, G.: Acute haematogenous osteomyelitis in children—the reliability of skeletal scintigraphy. Z. Kinderchir., *32*:360, 1981.
122. Evans, E. M., and Daires, D. M.: The treatment of chronic osteomyelitis by saucerization and secondary skin grafting. J. Bone Joint Surg., *51-B*:454, 1969.
123. Fedotov, V. K., Mozgove'i, I. V., Pedder, V. V., and Nikulin, V. I.: Determination of the borders of osteomyelitic focus in the long tubular bones. Vestn. Khir., *127*:103, 1981.
124. Feigin, R. D., McAlister, W. H., San Joaguin, V. H., and Middlekamp, J. N.: Osteomyelitis of the calcaneus. Am. J. Dis. Child., *119*:61, 1970.
125. Fellander, M.: Paraplegia in spondylitis: Results of operative treatment. Paraplegia, *13*:75, 1975.
126. Fernandez-Ulloa, M., Vasavada, P. J., Hanslits, M. L., Volarich, D. T., and Elgazzar, A. H.: Diagnosis of vertebral osteomyelitis: Clinical, radiological and scintigraphic features. Orthopedics, *8*:1144, 1985.
127. Filipe, G., and Samson, B.: Les arthrites sacro-iliaques à pyogenes de l'enfant. Chir. Pediatr., *19*:101, 1978.
128. Fitzgerald, R. H., Jr.: Orthopaedic Sepsis and Osteomyelitis. Part 1. Antimicrobial therapy for the musculoskeletal system. A.A.O.S. Instruct. Course Lect. *31*:1, 1982.
129. Fitzgerald, R. H., Jr.: Experimental osteomyelitis: Description of a canine model and the role of depot administration of antibiotics in the prevention and treatment of sepsis. J. Bone Joint Surg., *65-A*:371, 1983.

130. Fleisher, G. R., Paradise, J. E., Plotkin, S. A., and Borden, S., IV: Falsely normal radionuclide scans for osteomyelitis. Am. J. Dis. Child., *134*:499, 1980.
131. Flores, A.: Severe disability of the hand caused by sequelae of osteomyelitis of the forearm during childhood. Analysis of 10 cases. Bol. Med. Hosp. Infant. Mex., *37*:1161, 1980.
132. Fotter, R., and Hollwarth, M.: Importance of bone scanning of osteoscintimetry for assessing development of acute haematogenous childhood osteomyelitis. Z. Orthop., *118*:15, 1980.
133. Fountain, S. S.: A single-stage combined surgical approach for vertebral resections. J. Bone Joint Surg., *61-A*:1101, 1979.
134. Fraser, J.: Acute osteomyelitis. Br. Med. J., *2*:605, 1924.
135. Fox, L., and Sprung, K.: Neonatal osteomyelitis. Pediatrics, *62*:535, 1978.
136. Frazier, J. K., and Anzel, S. H.: Osteomyelitis of the greater trochanter in children. Report of three cases. J. Bone Joint Surg., *63-A*:833, 1981.
137. Frederickson, B., Yuan, H., and Olans, R.: Management and outcome of pyogenic vertebral osteomyelitis. Clin. Orthop., *131*:160, 1978.
138. Fuselier, H. A., Jr., and Busby, J.: Osteomyelitis of the pubis. South. Med. J., *73*:1649, 1980.
138a. Gaenslen, F. J.: Split heel approach in osteomyelitis of the os calcis. J. Bone Joint Surg., *13*:759, 1931.
139. Garcia, A., Jr., and Grantham, S. A.: Hematogenous pyogenic vertebral osteomyelitis. J. Bone Joint Surg., *42-A*:429, 1960.
140. Garnett, E. S., Cockshott, W. P., and Jacobs, J.: Classical acute osteomyelitis with a negative bone scan. Br. J. Radiol., *50*:757, 1977.
141. Garre, C.: Über besondere Formen und Folgezustande der akuten infektiosen Osteomyelitis. Beitr. Klin. Chir., *10*:241, 1893.
142. Gelfand, M. J., and Silverstein, E. B.: Radionuclide imaging. Use in diagnosis of osteomyelitis in children. J.A.M.A., *237*:245, 1977.
143. Gersten, E., Allison, M. S., and Dalton, H. C.: An epidemiologic study of 100 consecutive cases of osteomyelitis. South. Med. J., *63*:365, 1970.
144. Giedion, A., Holthusen, W., Masel, L. F., and Vischer, D.: Subacute and chronic "symmetrical" osteomyelitis. Ann. Radiol., *15*:329, 1972.
145. Gilday, D. L.: Problems in the scintigraphic detection of osteomyelitis. Radiology, *135*:791, 1980.
146. Gilday, D. L., and Paul, D. J.: Differentiation of osteomyelitis and cellulitis in children using combined blood pool and bone scan (abstr.). J. Nucl. Med., *15*:494, 1974.
147. Gilday, D. L., Paul, D. J., and Paterson, J.: Diagnosis of osteomyelitis in children by combined blood pool and bone imaging. Radiology, *117*:331, 1975.
148. Gilmour, W. N.: Acute hematogenous osteomyelitis. J. Bone Joint Surg., *44-B*:841, 1962.
149. Gledhill, R. B.: Subacute osteomyelitis in children. Clin. Orthop., *96*:57, 1973.
150. Gledhill, R. B.: Various phases of pediatric osteomyelitis. A.A.O.S. Instr. Course Lect., *22*:245, 1973.
151. Glover, S. C., and Geddes, A. M.: Treatment of pyogenic osteomyelitis. J. Antimicrob. Chemother., *8*:347, 1981.
152. Goergen, T. G., Alazraki, N. P., Halpern, S. E., Heath, V., and Ashburn, W. L.: "Cold" bone lesions: A newly recognized phenomenon of bone imaging. J. Nucl. Med., *15*:1120, 1974.
153. Goforth, W. P., Karlin, J. M., Scurran, B. L., and Silani, S. H.: Hematogenous osteomyelitis of the fifth metatarsal: A case report. J. Am. Podiatry Assoc. *72*:285, 1982.
154. Goldberg, I., Shauer, L., Klier, I., and Seelenfreund, M.: Neonatal osteomyelitis of the calcaneus following

a heel pad puncture: A case report. Clin. Orthop., 158:195, 1981.
155. Goldstein, E. J., Ahonkhai, V. I., Cristofaro, R. L., Pringle, G. F., and Sierra, M. F.: Source of pseudomonas in osteomyelitis of heels. J. Clin. Microbiol., 12:711, 1980.
156. Gordon, S. L., Evans, C., and Greer, R. B.: Pseudomonas osteomyelitis of the metatarsal sesamoid of the great toe. Clin. Orthop., 99:188, 1974.
157. Green, M., Nyhan, W. L., Jr., and Fousek, M. D.: Acute hematogenous osteomyelitis. Pediatrics, 17:368, 1956.
158. Green, N. E., Beauchamp, R. D., and Griffin, P. P.: Primary subacute epiphyseal osteomyelitis. J. Bone Joint Surg., 63-A:107, 1981.
159. Green, W. T.: Osteomyelitis in infancy. J.A.M.A., 105:1835, 1935.
160. Green, W. T., and Shannon, M. A.: Osteomyelitis of infants. A disease different from osteomyelitis of older children. Arch. Surg., 32:462, 1936.
161. Greengard, J.: Acute hematogenous osteomyelitis in infancy. Med. Clin. North Am., 30:135, 1946.
162. Greenstone, G., and Greensides, R.: Osteomyelitis of the pelvis. A diagnostic problem. Am. J. Dis. Child., 132:581, 1978.
163. Griffin, P. P.: Bone and joint infections in children. Pediatr. Clin. North Am., 14:533, 1967.
164. Griffiths, H. E. D., and Jones, D. M.: Pyogenic infection of the spine. A review of twenty-eight cases. J. Bone Joint Surg., 53-B:383, 1971.
165. Haase, D., Martin, R., and Marrie, T.: Radionuclide imaging in pyogenic vertebral osteomyelitis. Clin. Nucl. Med., 5:533, 1980.
166. Hald, J. D., Jr., and Sudmann, E.: Acute hematogenous osteomyelitis: Early diagnosis with computed tomography. Acta Radiol., 23:55, 1982.
167. Haldeman, K. A.: Acute osteomyelitis. A clinical and experimental study. Surg. Gynecol. Obstet., 59:25, 1934.
168. Hall, B. B., and Fitzgerald, R. H.: The pharmacokinetics of penicillin in osteomyelitis canine bone. J. Bone Joint Surg., 65-A:526, 1983.
169. Hall, J. E., and Silverstein, E. A.: Acute hematogenous osteomyelitis. Pediatrics, 31:1033, 1963.
170. Hamilton, S., and Hurley, G. D.: Radio-isotope bone scanning in suspected osteomyelitis in children. Eur. J. Nucl. Med., 4:325, 1976.
171. Handmaker, H.: Combined imaging in osteomyelitis. J. Nucl. Med., 19:697, 1978.
172. Handmaker, H.: Acute hematogenous osteomyelitis: Has the bone scan betrayed us? Radiology, 135:787, 1980.
173. Handmaker, H., and Leonards, R.: The bone scan in inflammatory osseous disease. Semin. Nucl. Med., 6:95, 1976.
174. Handmaker, H., and O'Mara, E. R.: Gallium imaging in pediatrics. J. Nucl. Med., 18:1057, 1977.
175. Haque, I. U.: The production of a one-bone forearm as a salvage procedure after haematogenous osteomyelitis. A case report. J. Bone Joint Surg., 64-A:454, 1982.
176. Harris, N. H.: Some problems in the diagnosis and treatment of acute osteomyelitis. J. Bone Joint Surg., 42-B:535, 1960.
177. Harris, N. H., and Kirkaldy-Willis, W. H.: Primary subacute pyogenic osteomyelitis. J. Bone Joint Surg., 47-B:526, 1965.
178. Harsha, W. N.: The natural history of acute hematogenous osteomyelitis. South. Med. J., 57:370, 1964.
179. Hart, V. L.: Acute hematogenous osteomyelitis in children. J.A.M.A., 108:524, 1937.
180. Hartrampf, C. R., Scheflan, M., and Bostwick, J., III: The flexor digitorum brevis muscle island pedicle flap: A new dimension in heel reconstruction. Plast. Reconstr. Surg., 66:264, 1980.

181. Hayden, C. K., Jr., and Swischuk, L. E.: Paraarticular soft tissue changes in infections and trauma of the lower extremity in children. A.J.R., 134:307, 1980.
182. Hedstrom, S. A.: The prognosis of chronic staphylococcal osteomyelitis after long-term antibiotic treatment. Scand. J. Infect. Dis., 6:33, 1974.
183. Hemingway, D. L., and Lieberman, C. M.: Bone scan findings with radiographic clinical and surgical correlation in extensive osteomyelitis: A case report. Clin. Nucl. Med., 5:29, 1980.
184. Henderson, K. C., Roberts, R. S., and Dorsey, S. B.: Group B beta-hemolytic streptococcal osteomyelitis in a neonate. Pediatrics, 59:Suppl.:1053, 1977.
185. Henson, S. W., Jr., and Coventry, M. B.: Osteomyelitis of the vertebrae as the result of infection of the urinary tract. Surg. Gynecol. Obstet., 102:207, 1956.
186. Higgins, T. T., Browne, D., and Bodian, M.: A penicillin-treated series of cases of osteomyelitis in childhood. Br. Med. J., 1:757, 1947.
187. Higham, M.: Infection in a puncture wound after it "healed." Hosp. Pract., 18:47, 1983.
188. Highland, T. R., and LaMont, R. L.: Osteomyelitis of the pelvis in children. J. Bone Joint Surg., 65-A:230, 1983.
189. Hobo, T.: Zur Pathogenese der akuten haematogenen Osteomyelitis. Acta Sch. Med. Univ. Kioto, 4:1, 1921.
190. Holloway, W. J.: Treatment of osteomyelitis and infectious arthritis. Del. Med. J., 53:347, 1981.
191. Horsky, I., Huraj, E., Sr., Huraj, E., Jr., and Dudakova, M.: Preliminary experience with treatment of osteomyelitis with gentamycin PMMA balls and chains. Acta Chir. Orthop. Traumatol. Cech., 48:451, 1981.
192. Howie, D. W., Savage, J. P., Wilson, T. G., and Paterson, D.: The technetium phosphate bone scan in the diagnosis of osteomyelitis in childhood. J. Bone Joint Surg., 65-A:431, 1983.
193. Hutto, J. H., and Ayoub, E. M.: Streptococcal osteomyelitis and arthritis in a neonate. Am. J. Dis. Child., 129:1449, 1975.
194. Isaacs, D., Bower, B. D., and Moxon, E. R.: Neonatal osteomyelitis presenting as nerve palsy. Br. Med. J. (Clin. Res.), 292:1071, 1986.
195. Iudin, I. B., Zhirova, L. F., Prokopenko, I. D., and Klepikov, I. I.: Septic shock in the clinical picture of acute hematogenous osteomyelitis in children. Klin. Khir., 1:38, 1983.
196. Jackson, M. A., and Nelson, J. D.: Etiology and medical management of acute suppurative bone and joint infections in pediatric patients. J. Pediatr. Orthop., 2:313, 1982.
196a. Jacobs, J. C.: Acute osteomyelitis. N.Y. State J. Med., 5:90, 1978.
197. Jacobs, N. M., and Rice, T. W.: Puncture wound osteomyelitis (letter). J. Pediatr., 107:645, 1985.
198. James, T.: Acute osteomyelitis in infancy and early childhood. Br. J. Surg., 41:87, 1953.
199. Jensen, T. M., and Jensen, H. P.: Shortening of the extremities after neonatal osteomyelitis (English abstract). Ugeskr. Laeger, 148:2030, 1986.
200. Jergesen, F., and Jawetz, E.: Pyogenic infections in orthopedic surgery, combined antibiotic and closed wound treatment. Am. J. Surg., 106:152, 1963.
201. Johannsen, A., Jepsen, O. L., and Winge, J.: Radiological and scintigraphic examination of the sacroiliac joints in the diagnosis of sacroiliitis. Dan. Med. Bull., 21:246, 1974.
202. Jones, D. C., and Cady, R. B.: "Cold" bone scans in acute osteomyelitis. J. Bone Joint Surg., 63-B:376, 1981.
203. Jones, G. B.: Place of surgery in treatment of acute haematogenous osteomyelitis. Proc. R. Soc. Med., 64:1200, 1971.
204. Jordan, M. C., and Kirby, W. M. M.: Pyogenic vertebral osteomyelitis; treatment with antimicrobial

agents and bed rest. Arch. Intern. Med., *128*:405, 1971.
205. Jupiter, J. B., Ehrlich, M. G., Novelline, R. A., Leeds, H. C., and Keim, D.: The association of septic thrombophlebitis with subperiosteal abscesses in children. J. Pediatr., *101*:690, 1982.
206. Kahn, D. S., and Pritzker, K. P., II.: The pathophysiology of bone infection. Clin. Orthop., *96*:12, 1973.
207. Kamran, D., Muller, W., Peter, H. H., and Rieger, C. L.: Clinical and immunologic findings in BCG osteomyelitis. Monatsschr. Kinderheilkd., *130*:899, 1982.
208. Kandel, S. N., and Mankin, H. J.: Pyogenic abscesses of the long bones in children. Clin. Orthop., *96*:108, 1973.
209. Kaplan, S. L.: Osteomyelitis in children. Compr. Ther., *8*:69, 1982.
210. Kaplan, S. L., Mason, E. O., Jr., and Feigin, R. D.: Clindamycin versus nafcillin or methicillin in the treatment of staphylococcus aureus osteomyelitis in children. South. Med. J., *75*:138, 1982.
211. Kattapuram, S. V., Phillips, W. C., and Boyd, R.: CT in pyogenic osteomyelitis of the spine. A.J.R., *140*:1199, 1983.
212. Kelly, P. J., Martin, W. J., and Coventry, M. B.: Chronic osteomyelitis. II. Treatment with closed irrigation and suction. J.A.M.A., *213*:1843, 1970.
213. Kemp, H. B. S., Jackson, J. W., and Shaw, N. C.: Laminectomy in paraplegia due to infective spondylosis. Br. J. Surg., *61*:66, 1974.
214. Kemp, H. B. S., Jackson, J. W., Jeremiah, M. D., and Hall, A. J.: Pyogenic infections occurring primarily in intervertebral discs. J. Bone Joint Surg., *55-B*:698, 1973.
215. Kessel, A. W. L.: Acute osteomyelitis. Br. Med. J., *1*:352, 1956.
216. Kienitz, M.: Cephalosporin antibiotics in the treatment of acute osteomyelitis in children. Postgrad. Med. J., *47*:S87, 1971.
217. King, D. M., and Mayo, K. M.: Subacute haematogenous osteomyelitis. J. Bone Joint Surg., *51-B*:458, 1969.
218. King, D. M., and Mayo, K. M.: Infective lesions of the vertebral column. Clin. Orthop., *96*:248, 1973.
219. Koch, J.: Untersuchengen über die Lokalisation der Bakterien das Verhalten des Knochen markes und die Veranderungen der Knochen, ins besondere der Epiphysen, bei Infektionskrankheiten. Z. Hyg. Infektionskr., *69*:436, 1911.
220. Kochhar, V. L., and Srivastava, K. K.: Unusual lesions of the clavicle. Int. Surg., *61*:51, 1976.
221. Kolyvas, E., Rosenthal, L., Ahronheim, G. A., Lisbona, R., and Marks, M. I.: Serial Ga-citrate imaging during treatment of acute osteomyelitis in childhood. Clin. Nucl. Med., *3*:461, 1978.
222. Komolafe, F.: Pyogenic osteomyelitis of the rib in children. Pediatr. Radiol., *12*:245, 1982.
223. Kozlowski, K.: Brodie's abscess in the first decade of life. Report of eleven cases. Pediatr. Radiol., *10*:33, 1980.
224. Kozlowski, K., Masel, J., Harbison, S., and Yu, J.: Multifocal chronic osteomyelitis of unknown etiology. Report of five cases. Pediatr. Radiol., *13*:130, 1983.
225. Kramer, S. J., Post, J., and Sussman, M.: Acute hematogenous osteomyelitis of the epiphysis. J. Pediatr. Orthop., *6*:493, 1986.
226. Kudriavtsev, V. A., Udal'tsova, G. A., and Vorypin, D. M.: Acute hematogenous osteomyelitis of the spine in children. Vestn. Khir., *128*:93, 1982.
227. Kuhn, J. P., and Berger, P. E.: Computed tomographic diagnosis of osteomyelitis. Radiology, *130*:503, 1979.
228. Kulowski, J.: Pyogenic osteomyelitis of the spine. J. Bone Joint Surg., *18*:343, 1936.
229. Kulowski, J.: Management of hematogenous pyogenic osteomyelitis. Surgery, *40*:1094, 1956.
230. Kunze, W., Gunther, E., and Bauer, I.: Neonatal osteomyelitis and arthritis caused by group B streptococcus. Acta Paediatr. Acad. Sci. Hung., *21*:227, 1980.
231. Lai, T. K., Hingston, J., and Scheifele, D.: Streptococcal neonatal osteomyelitis. Am. J. Dis. Child., *134*:711, 1980.
232. Lardé, D., Mathieu, D., Frija, J., Gaston, A., and Vasile, N.: Vertebral osteomyelitis: Disk hypodensity on CT. A.J.R., *139*:963, 1982.
233. Langenskiöld, A.: Femur remodelled during growth after osteomyelitis causing coxa vara and shaft necrosis. J. Pediatr. Orthop., *2*:289, 1982.
234. Leeson, M., Weiner, D., and Klein, L.: Osteomyelitis of the clavicle in children. Orthopedics, *5*:428, 1982.
235. Leftridge, C. A., Jr.: Osteomyelitis of the calcaneus secondary to heel pad puncture. A case report. J.A.M.A., *69*:507, 1977.
236. Lehey, E. B.: Primary closure in chronic (non-tuberculous) osteomyelitis. N.Y. J. Med., *52*:1045, 1952.
237. Letts, R. M., Afifi, A., and Sutherland, J. B.: Technetium bone scanning as an aid of atypical acute osteomyelitis in children. Surg. Gynecol. Obstet., *140*:899, 1975.
238. Lewin, J. S., Rosenfield, N. S., Hoffer, P. B., and Downing, D.: Acute osteomyelitis in children: Combined Tc-99m and Ga-67 imaging. Radiology, *158*:795, 1986.
239. Lexer, E.: Experiment über osteomyelitis. Arch. Klin. Chir., *53*:266, 1896.
240. Lilien, L. E., Harris, V. J., Ramaurthy, R. S., and Pildes, R. S.: Neonatal osteomyelitis of the calcaneus: Complication of heel puncture. J. Pediatr., *88*:478, 1976.
241. Lim, M. O., Gresham, E. L., Franken, E. A., Jr., and Leake, R. D.: Osteomyelitis as a complication of umbilical artery catherization. Am. J. Dis. Child., *131*:142, 1977.
242. Lisbona, R., and Rosenthall, L.: Observations on the sequential use of 99M Tc-phosphate complex and 67Ga imaging in osteomyelitis, cellulitis, and septic arthritis. Radiology, *123*:123, 1977.
243. Louw, J. H., and Shandling, B.: Acute haematogenous osteomyelitis with special reference to osteitis of the neck of the femur. Arch. Dis. Child., *36*:117, 1961.
244. Lovell, W. W., King, R. E., and Alldredge, R.: Carcinoma in skin, sinuses, and bone following chronic osteomyelitis. South. Med. J., *50*:266, 1957.
245. McAdam, J. W.: Penicillin treatment of acute hematogenous osteomyelitis. Br. J. Surg., *33*:167, 1945.
246. McElvenny, R. T.: The use of closed circulation and suction in the treatment of chronically infected, acutely infected, and potentially infected wounds. Am. J. Orthop., *3*:86, 1961.
247. McHenry, M. C., Alfidi, R. J., Wilde, A. H., and Hawk, W. A.: Hematogenous osteomyelitis. Clev. Clin. Q., *42*:125, 1975.
248. McKellar-Hall, R. D.: A short note on the changing outlook in osteomyelitis brought about by the introduction of penicillin. Med. J. Aust., *1*:401, 1946.
249. Mader, J. T., and Wilson, K. J.: Comparative evaluation of cefamandole and cephalothin in the treatment of experimental staphylococcus aureus osteomyelitis in rabbits. J. Bone Joint Surg., *65-A*:507, 1983.
250. Mader, J. T., Guckian, J. C., Glass, D. L., and Reinarz, F. A.: Therapy with hyperbaric oxygen for experimental osteomyelitis due to staphylococcus aureus in rabbits. J. Infect. Dis., *138*:312, 1978.

251. Mader, J. T., Brown, G. L., Guckian, J. C., Wells, C. H., and Reinarz, J. A.: A mechanism for the amelioration by hyperbaric oxygen of experimental staphylococcal osteomyelitis in rabbits. J.Infect. Dis., 142:915, 1980.
252. Mahboubi, S.: CT appearance of nidus in osteoid osteoma versus sequestration in osteomyelitis. J. Comput. Assist. Tomogr., 10:457, 1986.
253. Majd, M.: Radionuclide imaging in early detection of childhood osteomyelitis and its differentiation from cellulitis and bone infarction. Ann. Radiol., 20:9, 1977.
254. Majd, M., and Frankel, R. S.: Bone scanning in osteomyelitis, cellulitis, and bone infarcts in children. J. Nucl. Med., 16:547, 1975.
255. Majd, M., and Frankel, R. S.: Radionuclide imaging in skeletal inflammatory and ischemic disease in children. A.J.R., 126:832, 1976.
256. Makins, G. H., and Abbott, F. L.: On acute primary osteomyelitis of the vertebrae. Ann. Surg., 23:510, 1896.
257. Marandian, M. H., Mortazavi, H., Behvad, A., Haghigat, H., Lessani, M., and Youssefian, B.: Bone scan in the diagnosis of infectious osteoarthritis. Sem. Hôp. Paris, 56:873, 1980.
258. Markestad, T.: Hematogenous osteomyelitis in children. Tidsskr. Nor. Laegenforen, 100:212, 1980.
259. Marks, M. I.: Haemophilus influenzae type B and pyogenic osteomyelitis. J. Antimicrob. Chemother., 9:495, 1982.
260. Marks, K. L., and Turner, W. L.: Carcinoma occurring in the sinuses of chronic osteomyelitis. Br. J. Surg., 38:206, 1950.
261. Mathieson, A. J.: Primary pyogenic osteomyelitis of the ribs. Br. Med. J., 5358:668, 1963.
262. Meyer, T. L., Kregler, A. B., and Smith, W. S.: Antibiotic management of staphylococcal osteomyelitis. J. Bone Joint Surg., 47-A:285, 1967.
263. Meyers, B. R., Berson, B. L., Gilbert, M., and Hirschman, S. Z.: Clinical patterns of osteomyelitis due to gram-negative bacteria. Arch. Intern. Med., 131:228, 1973.
264. Miller, J. I. I., and Gates, G. F.: Scintigraphy of sacroiliac pyarthrosis in children. J.A.M.A., 238:2701, 1977.
265. Miller, W. B., Murphy, W. A., and Gilula, L. A.: Brodie abscess: Reappraisal. Radiology, 132:15, 1979.
266. Miskew, D. B., Block, R. A., and Witt, P. F.: Aspiration of infected sacroiliac joints. J. Bone Joint Surg., 61-A:1071, 1979.
267. Mitra, R. N.: Experimental osteomyelitis in rabbits. J. Int. Coll. Surg., 41:171, 1964.
268. Mok, P. M., Reilly, B. J., and Ash, J. M.: Osteomyelitis in the neonate. Clinical aspects and the role of radiography and scintigraphy in diagnosis and management. Radiology, 145:677, 1982.
269. Mollan, R. A. B., and Piggot, J.: Acute osteomyelitis in children. J. Bone Joint Surg., 59-B:2, 1977.
270. Morgan, A., and Yates, A. K.: The diagnosis of acute osteomyelitis of the pelvis. Postgrad. Med. J., 42:74, 1966.
271. Morrey, B. F., and Bianco, A. S.: Hematogenous osteomyelitis of the clavicle in children. Clin. Orthop., 125:24, 1977.
272. Morrey, B. F., and Peterson, H. A.: Hematogenous pyogenic osteomyelitis in children. Orthop. Clin. North Am., 6:935, 1975.
273. Morrey, B. F., Bianco, A. J., and Rhodes, K. H.: Hematogenous osteomyelitis at uncommon sites in children. Mayo Clin. Proc., 53:707, 1978.
274. Morrissy, R. T.: Bone and joint sepsis in children. A.A.O.S. Instr. Course Lect., 31:49, 1982.
275. Morse, T. S., and Pryles, C. V.: Infections of the bones and joints in children. N. Engl. J. Med., 262:846, 1960.
276. Murphy, J., Anderson, N., and White, M.: Early diagnosis of acute osteomyelitis in childhood using radionuclide bone scanning. Ir. Med. J., 73:166, 1980.
277. Murphy, M. E.: Primary pyogenic infection of sacroiliac joint. N.Y. State J. Med., 77:1309, 1977.
278. Murray, R. A.: Importance of soft tissue to treatment of chronic osteomyelitis. J.A.M.A., 180:198, 1962.
279. Musher, D. M., Thorsteinsson, S. B., Minuth, J. N., and Luchi, R. J.: Vertebral osteomyelitis; still a diagnostic pitfall. Arch. Intern. Med., 136:105, 1976.
280. Nachlas, I. W., and Markheim, H. R.: Acute hematogenous osteomyelitis. A study of treatment. J. Bone Joint Surg., 30-A:673, 1948.
281. Nade, S.: Acute haematogenous osteomyelitis in infancy and childhood. J. Bone Joint Surg., 65-B:109, 1983.
282. Nélaton, A.: Eléments de Pathologie Chirurgicale. Paris, Gerner-Baillière, 1844.
283. Nelson, D. L., Hable, K. A., and Matsen, J. M.: Proteus mirabilis osteomyelitis in two neonates following heel puncture. Am. J. Dis. Child., 125:109, 1973.
284. Nelson, H. T., and Taylor, A.: Bone scanning in the diagnosis of osteomyelitis. J. Nucl. Med., 19:696, 1978.
285. Nelson, J. D., Bucholz, R. W., Kusmiesz, H., and Shelton, S.: Benefits and risks of sequential parenteral-oral cephalosporin therapy for suppurative bone and joint infections. J. Pediatr. Orthop., 2:255, 1982.
286. Nerdrum, H. J., and Karlsen, R. L.: Isotope-examination with Tc-diphosphonate in inflammatory skeletal diseases. Tidsskr. Nor. Laegeforen., 100:572, 1980.
287. Nersesiants, I. V., and Zakharova, L. B.: Early morphological changes in acute hematogenic osteomyelitis. Vestn. Khir., 126:85, 1981.
288. Neu, H. C., Meropol, N. J., and Fu, K. P.: Antibacterial activity of ceftriaxone (Ro 13-9904), a β-lactamase–stable cephalosporin. Antimicrob. Agents Chemother., 19:414, 1981.
289. Nguyen, V. D., London, J., and Cone, R. O., 3rd: Ring sequestrum: Radiographic characteristics of skeletal fixation pin-tract osteomyelitis. Radiology, 158:129, 1986.
290. Niebauer, J. J.: Development of squamous-cell carcinomata in the sinus tracts of chronic osteomyelitis. J. Bone Joint Surg., 28:280, 1946.
291. Nixon, G. W.: Hematogenous osteomyelitis of metaphyseal-equivalent locations. A.J.R., 130:123, 1978.
292. Nixon, G. W.: Problems and complications of acute hematogenous osteomyelitis. Personal communication, 1986.
293. Norden, C. W.: Experimental osteomyelitis. IV. Therapeutic trials with rifampin alone and in combination with gentamicin, sisomicin, and cephalothin. J. Infect. Dis., 132:493, 1975.
294. Norden, C. W.: Experimental osteomyelitis. V. Therapeutic trials with oxacillin and sisomicin alone and in combination. J. Infect. Dis., 137:155, 1978.
295. Norden, C. W., and Dickens, D. R.: Experimental osteomyelitis. III. Treatment with cephaloridine. J. Infect. Dis., 127:525, 1973.
296. Norden, C. W., and Kennedy, E.: Experimental osteomyelitis. I. A description of the model. J. Infect. Dis., 122:410, 1970.
297. Norden, C. W., and Kennedy, E.: Experimental osteomyelitis. II. Therapeutic trials and measurement of antibiotic levels in bone. J. Infect. Dis., 124:565, 1971.
298. Norden, C. W., Niedereiter, K., and Shinners, E. M.: Treatment of experimental chronic osteomyelitis due to Staphylococcus aureus with teicoplanin. Infection, 14:136, 1986.
299. O'Brien, T., McManus, F., MacAuley, P. H., and Ennis, J. T.: Acute haematogenous osteomyelitis. J. Bone Joint Surg., 64-B:450, 1982.

300. O'Connell, C. J., Chery, A. V., and Zoll, J. G.: Osteomyelitis of the cervical spine: Candida guilliermondi. Ann. Intern. Med., 79:748, 1973.
301. Ogden, J. A., and Lister, G.: The pathology of neonatal osteomyelitis. Pediatrics, 55:474, 1975.
302. Orr, H. W.: The treatment of acute osteomyelitis by drainage and rest. J. Bone Joint Surg., 9:733, 1927.
303. Orr, H. W.: The treatment of osteomyelitis and other infected wounds by drainage and rest. Surg. Gynecol. Obstet., 45:446, 1927.
304. Orr, H. W.: Osteomyelitis and Compound Fractures and Other Infected Wounds. St. Louis, Mosby, 1929.
305. Ottolenghi, C. E.: Aspiration biopsy of the spine. J. Bone Joint Surg., 51-A:1531, 1969.
306. Pachlau, G.: Die Besonderheiten des Osteomyelitis im frühen Kindesalter. Monatschr. Kinderheilkd., 55:280, 1932.
307. Painter, C. F.: Brodie's abscess in pelvic bone. N. Engl. J. Med., 202:585, 1930.
308. Paley, D., Moseley, C. F., Armstrong, P., and Prober, C. G.: Primary osteomyelitis caused by coagulase-negative staphylococci. J. Pediatr. Orthop., 6:622, 1986.
309. Park, C. H., Kapadia, D., and O'Hara, A. E.: Three phase bone scan findings in stress fracture. Clin. Nucl. Med., 6:587, 1981.
310. Peirson, E. L., Jr.: Osteochondritis of symphysis pubis. Surg. Gynecol. Obstet., 49:834, 1929.
311. Peterson, S., Knudsen, F. U., Andersen, E. A., and Egeblad, M.: Acute haematogenous osteomyelitis and septic arthritis in childhood. A 10-year review and follow-up. Acta Orthop. Scand., 51:451, 1980.
312. Phemister, D. P.: Chronic fibrous osteomyelitis. Ann. Surg., 90:756, 1929.
313. Pope, T. L., Teague, W. G., Kossack, R., Bray, S. T., and Flannery, D. B.: Pseudomonas sacroiliac osteomyelitis: Diagnosis by gallium citrate Ga 67 scan. Am. J. Dis. Child., 136:649, 1982.
314. Potter, C. M. C.: Osteomyelitis in the newborn. J. Bone Joint Surg., 36-B:578, 1954.
315. Price, C. T., and Mills, W. L.: Radial lengthening for septic growth arrest. J. Pediatr. Orthop., 3:88, 1983.
316. Prigg, E. K.: The treatment of chronic osteomyelitis with the use of muscle transplant or iliac graft. J. Bone Joint Surg., 28:576, 1946.
317. Pritchard, A. E., and Robinson, M. P.: Staphylococcal infection of the spine. Lancet, 2:1165, 1961.
318. Prober, C. G.: Oral antibiotic therapy for bone and joint infections. Pediatr. Infect. Dis., 1:8, 1982.
319. Prober, C. G., and Yeager, A. S.: Use of the serum bactericidal titer to assess the adequacy of oral antibiotic therapy in the treatment of acute hematologenous osteomyelitis. J. Pediatr., 95:131, 1979.
320. Probst, F. P., Björksten, B., and Gustavson, K. H.: Radiological aspects of chronic recurrent multifocal osteomyelitis. Ann. Radiol., 21:115, 1978.
321. Prokopova, L. V., Aleksiuk, K. P., Nikolaeva, N. G., and Bugaeva, T. L.: Metaepiphyseal osteomyelitis in children. (English abstract.) Khirurgiia (Mosk.), 8:122, 1986.
322. Puig, G. J.: Pyogenic osteomyelitis of the spine: Differential diagnosis through clincial and roentgenographic observations. J. Bone Joint Surg., 28:29, 1946.
323. Rao, B. R., Winebright, J. W., and Bartow, J.: Value of total-body bone scan in a child with osteomyelitis. Clin. Nucl. Med., 5:559, 1980.
324. Rao, S., Solomon, N., Miller, S., and Dunn, E.: Scintigraphic differentiation of bone infarction from osteomyelitis in children with sickle cell disease. J. Pediatr., 107:685, 1985.
325. Raptopoulos, V., Doherty, P. W., Goss, T. P., King, M. A., Johnson, K., and Gantz, N. M.: Acute osteomyelitis: Advantage of white cell scans in early detection. A.J.R., 139:1077, 1982.
326. Ray, M. K., and Ruckley, R. W.: Osteomyelitis of the clavicle. Br. J. Clin. Pract., 36:329, 1982.
327. Razinkov, A. G., and Kosiakov, G. A.: Treatment of acute hematogenic osteomyelitis in children taking into account the immunological reactivity and coagulation properties of the blood. Klin. Khir., 6:45, 1980.
328. Rendle-Short, A.: Acute osteomyelitis of the ilium. Br. Med. J., 2:97, 1931.
329. Resnick, D., Pineda, C. J., Weisman, M. H., and Kerr, R.: Osteomyelitis and septic arthritis of the hand following human bites. Skeletal Radiol., 14:263, 1985.
330. Rhodes, K. H.: Antibiotic management of acute osteomyelitis and septic arthritis in children. Orthop. Clin. North Am., 6:915, 1975.
331. Rinsky, L., Goris, M. L., Shurman, D. J., and Nagel, D. A.: 99 Technetium bone scanning in experimental osteomyelitis. Clin. Orthop., 128:361, 1979.
332. Roberts, J. M., Drummond, D. S., Breed, A. L., and Chesney, J.: Subacute hematogenous osteomyelitis in children: A retrospective study. J. Pediatr. Orthop., 2:249, 1982.
333. Rodriguez, W., Ross, S., Khan, W., McKay, D., and Moskowitz, P.: Clindamycin in the treatment of osteomyelitis in children. Am. J. Dis. Child., 131:1088, 1977.
334. Rolan, E., Couceiro, J. M., Rodriguez Blanco, R., Ruza, J., Hernandez, M. S., and Vicente, R.: A case of neonatal infection with osteomyelitis of the sternum and its partial destruction. An. Esp. Pediatr., 13:1043, 1980.
335. Rosenthal, R. E., Spickard, W., Anderson, M., Douglas, R., and Rhamy, R. K.: Osteomyelitis of the symphysis pubis: A separate disease from osteitis pubis. J. Bone Joint Surg., 64-A:123, 1982.
336. Rosenthall, L., Kloiber, R., Damtew, B., and Al-Majid, H.: Sequential use of radiophosphate and radiogallium imaging in the differential diagnosis of bone, joint, and soft tissue infection. Quantitative analysis. Diagn. Imaging, 51:249, 1982.
337. Rosenthall, L., Lisbon, R., Hernandez, M., and Hadjipavlou, A.: 99m Tc PP and 67 Ga imaging following insertion of orthopedic devices. Radiology, 133:717, 1979.
338. Ross, P. M., and Flemming, J. L.: Vertebral body osteomyelitis; spectrum and natural history. Clin. Orthop., 118:190, 1976.
339. Rowling, D. E.: The positive approach to chronic osteomyelitis. J. Bone Joint Surg., 41-B:681, 1959.
340. Russin, L. D., and Staab, E. V.: Unusual bone scan findings in acute osteomyelitis: Case report. J. Nucl. Med., 17:617, 1976.
341. Sachs, W.: Radionuclide scanning in osteomyelitis. J. Foot Surg., 25:311, 1986.
342. Sankarankutty, M.: Pyogenic osteomyelitis of the clavicle (a report of two cases and review of the literature). Br. J. Clin. Pract., 35:116, 1981.
343. Sapico, F. L., and Mongomerie, J. Z.: Pyogenic vertebral osteomyelitis: Report of nine cases and review of the literature. Rev. Infect. Dis., 1:754, 1979.
344. Savoini, E., Capanna, R., Mercuri, M., Stilli, S., and Calderoni, P.: Results in the immunotherapeutic and surgical treatment of hematogenous chronic osteomyelitis in children. Chir. Organi Mov., 67:397, 1981.
345. Schaad, O. B., McCracken, G. H., and Nelson, J. D.: Pyogenic arthritis of the sacroiliac joint in pediatric patients. Pediatrics, 66:375, 1980.
346. Scheman, L., Janota, M., and Lewin, P.: The production of experimental osteomyelitis. Preliminary report. J.A.M.A., 117:1525, 1941.
347. Schmidt, D., Murbarak, S., and Gelbeman, R.: Septic shoulders in children. J. Pediatr. Orthop., 1:67, 1981.
348. Schopfer, K., Matter, L., Brunner, C., Pagon, S., Stanisic, M., and Baerlocher, K.: BCG osteomyelitis.

Case report and review. Helv. Paediatr. Acta, 37:73, 1982.
349. Schroeder, S. A., Catino, D., Toala, P., and Finland, M.: Chronic pseudomonas osteomyelitis. Report on the use of gentamycin sulphate in three cases. J. Bone Joint Surg., 52-A:1611, 1970.
350. Schubiner, H., Letourneau, M., and Murray, D. L.: Pyogenic osteomyelitis versus pseudo-osteomyelitis in Gaucher's disease. Report of a case and review of the literature. Clin. Pediatr., 20:667, 1981.
351. Schwartz, R. H., and Reing, C. M.: Acute hematogenous osteomyelitis secondary to Hemophilus influenzae. J. Pediatr. Orthop., 1:385, 1981.
352. Scoles, P. V., Hilty, M. D., and Sfakianakis, G. N.: Bone scan patterns in acute osteomyelitis. Clin. Orthop., 153:210, 1980.
353. Season, E. H., and Miller, P. R.: Multifocal subacute pyogenic osteomyelitis in a child, a case report. Clin. Orthop., 116:76, 1976.
354. Season, E. H., and Miller, P. R.: Primary subacute pyogenic osteomyelitis in long bones of children. J. Pediatr. Surg., 11:347, 1976.
355. Sefton, G. K.: Osteomyelitis after closed femoral fracture in a child. J. R. Coll. Surg. Edinb., 27:113, 1982.
356. Shahar, E., Frand, M., and Rotem, Y.: Ewing sarcoma simulating acute osteomyelitis. Harefuah, 98:167, 1980.
357. Shandling, B.: Acute hematogenous osteomyelitis: A review of 300 cases treated during 1952–1959. S. Afr. Med. J., 34:520, 1960.
358. Shannon, J. G., and Woolhouse, F. M.: Treatment of chronic bone infection. J. Bone Joint Surg., 36-A:841, 1954.
359. Siagailo, P. T., and Nosar', A. E.: Primary chronic osteomyelitis in children. Klin. Khir., 12:48, 1981.
360. Siemsen, J. K., and Waxman, A. D.: Early diagnosis of hematogenous osteomyelitis. J. Nucl. Med., 15:533, 1974.
361. Siffert, R. S.: The effect of juxta-epiphyseal pyogenic infection on epiphyseal growth. Clin. Orthop., 10:131, 1957.
362. Silva, J., Jr., and Harvey, W. C.: Detection of infections with gallium-67 and scintigraphic imaging. J. Infect. Dis., 130:125, 1974.
363. Simms, R. G., Brown, B. S., Hyndman, J. C., and Goldbloom, R. B.: Osteomyelitis of the pubis in childhood. Can. Med. Assoc. J., 124:1028, 1981.
364. Singson, R. D., Berdon, W. E., Feldman, F., Denton, J. R., Abramson, S., and Baker, D. H.: "Missing" femoral condyle: An unusual sequela to neonatal osteomyelitis and septic arthritis. Radiology, 161:359, 1986.
365. Sitarz, A. L., Bedon, W. E., Wolff, J. A., and Baker, D. H.: Acute lymphocytic leukemia masquerading as acute osteomyelitis. A report of two cases. Pediatr. Radiol., 9:33, 1980.
366. Solheim, L. F., Paus, G., Liverud, K., and Stoen, E.: Chronic recurrent multifocal osteomyelitis. A new clinical-radiological syndrome. Acta Orthop. Scand., 51:37, 1980.
367. Speed, K.: Growth problems following osteomyelitis of adolescent long bones. Surg. Gynecol. Obstet., 34:469, 1922.
368. Srivastava, K. K., Garg, L. D., and Kochhar, V. L.: Osteomyelitis of the clavicle. Acta Orthop. Scand., 45:662, 1974.
369. Staab, E. V., and McCartney, W. H.: Role of gallium 67 in inflammatory disease. Semin. Nucl. Med., 8:219, 1978.
370. Staheli, L. T., Nelp, W. B., and Marty, R.: Strontium 87m scanning: Early diagnosis of bone and joint infections in children. J.A.M.A., 221:1159, 1972.

371. Starr, C. L.: Acute hematogenous osteomyelitis. Arch. Surg., 4:567, 1922.
372. Stauffer, R. N.: Pyogenic vertebral osteomyelitis. Orthop. Clin. North Am., 6:1015, 1975.
373. Stevens, D. B.: Experimental osteomyelitis. Surg. Forum, 14:450, 1963.
374. Stone, D. B., and Bonfiglio, M.: Pyogenic vertebral osteomyelitis. Arch. Intern. Med., 112:491, 1963.
375. Sullivan, D. C., Rosenfield, N. S., Ogden, J., and Gottschalk, A.: Problems in the scintigraphic detection of osteomyelitis in children. Radiology, 135:731, 1980.
376. Sullivan, J. A., Vasileff, T., and Leonard, J. C.: An evaluation of nuclear scanning in orthopaedic infections. J. Pediatr. Orthop., 1:73, 1981.
377. Sultanvaev, T. Z.: Errors in the diagnosis and treatment of acute hematogenic osteomyelitis in children. Khirurgiia, 4:92, 1982.
378. Suzuki, Y., Hisada, K., and Takeda, M.: Demonstration of myositis ossificans by 99m-technetium-pyrophosphate bone scanning. Radiology, 11:663, 1974.
379. Swartzendruber, D. C., Nelson, G., and Hayes, R. L.: Gallium 67 localization in lysosomal-like granules of leukemic and nonleukemic murine tissues. J. Natl. Cancer Inst., 46:941, 1971.
380. Sy, M. W., Westring, D. W., and Weinberger, G.: "Cold" lesions on bone imaging. J. Nucl. Med., 16:1013, 1975.
381. Teates, C. D., and Williamson, B. R. J.: "Hot and cold" bone lesion in acute osteomyelitis. A.J.R., 129:157, 1977.
382. Tetzlaff, T. R., McCracken, G. H., and Nelson, J. D.: Oral antibiotic therapy for skeletal infections of children. J. Pediatr., 92:485, 1978.
383. Thompson, J., and Lewis, I. C.: Osteomyelitis in the newborn. Arch. Dis. Child., 25:273, 1950.
384. Thompson, R. H. S., and Dubos, R. J.: Production of experimental osteomyelitis in rabbits by intravenous injection of Staphylococcus aureus. J. Exp. Med., 68:191, 1938.
385. Trackler, R. T., Miller, K. E., Sutherland, D. H., and Chadwick, D. L.: Childhood pelvic osteomyelitis presenting as a "cold" lesion on bone scan: Case report. J. Nucl. Med., 17:620, 1976.
386. Trauner, D. A., and Connor, J. A.: Radioactive scanning in diagnosis of acute sacroiliac osteomyelitis. Pediatrics, 87:751, 1975.
387. Treves, S., Khettry, J., Broker, F. H., Wilkinson, R. H., and Watts, H.: Osteomyelitis: Early scintigraphic detection in children. Pediatrics, 57:173, 1976.
388. Tronzo, R. G., and Dowling, J. J.: Acute hematogenous osteomyelitis of children in era of broad-spectrum antibiotics. A comprehensive review. Clin. Orthop., 22:108, 1962.
389. Trueta, J.: Acute hematogenous osteomyelitis: Its pathology and treatment. Bull. Hosp. Joint Dis., 14:5, 1953.
390. Trueta, J.: The normal vascular anatomy of the human femoral head during growth. J. Bone Joint Surg., 39-B:358, 1957.
391. Trueta, J.: Acute hematogenous osteomyelitis: Its pathology and treatment. Bull. N.Y. Acad. Med. 35:25, 1959.
392. Trueta, J.: The three types of acute hematogenous osteomyelitis. A clinical and vascular study. J. Bone Joint Surg., 41-B:671, 1959.
393. Trueta, J., and Morgan, J. D.: Late results in the treatment of 100 cases of acute haematogenous osteomyelitis. Br. J. Surg., 41:449, 1954.
394. Tumeh, S. S., Aliabadi, P., Weissman, B. N., and McNeil, B. J.: Chronic osteomyelitis: Bone and gallium scan patterns associated with active disease. Radiology, 158:685, 1986.

395. Uhren, R., and Curtis, P.: Calcaneal osteomyelitis of the newborn: A case report. J. Fam. Pract., *11*:809, 1980.
396. Visudhiphan, P., Chiemchanya, S., Somburanasin, R., and Dheandhanoo, D.: Torticollis as the presenting sign in cervical spine infection and tumor. Clin. Pediatr., *21*:71, 1982.
397. Wald, E. R., Mirro, R., and Gartner, J. C.: Pitfalls in the diagnosis of acute osteomyelitis by bone scan. Clin. Pediatr., *19*:597, 1980.
398. Waldvogel, F. A., and Vasey, H.: Osteomyelitis: The past decade. N. Engl. J. Med., *303*:360, 1980.
399. Waldvogel, F. A., Medoff, G., and Swartz, M. N.: Osteomyelitis: A review of clinical features, therapeutic considerations, and unusual aspects. N. Engl. J. Med., *282*:198, 260, 316, 1970.
400. Waldvogel, F. A., Medoff, G., and Swartz, M. N.: Osteomyelitis: Clinical Features, Therapeutic Considerations and Unusual Aspects. Springfield, Ill., Thomas, 1971.
401. Waugh, W.: Fibrosarcoma occurring in a chronic bone sinus. J. Bone Joint Surg., *34-B*:642, 1952.
402. Wedge, J. H., Oryschak, A. F., Robertson, D. E., and Kirkaldy-Willis, W. H.: Atypical manifestations of spinal infections. Clin. Orthop., *123*:155, 1977.
403. Weeks, J. L., Garcia-Prats, J. A., and Baker, C. J.: Methicillin-resistant Staphylococcus aureus osteomyelitis in a neonate. J.A.M.A., *245*:1662, 1981.
404. Weinstein, A. J.: Selection of antimicrobial therapy. Instr. Course Lect., *31*:14, 1982.
405. Weinstein, J. M.: Hyperbaric medicine. N.I.T.A., *5*:126, 1982.
406. Weissberg, E. D., Smith, A. L., and Smith, D. H.: Clinical features of neonatal osteomyelitis. Pediatrics, *53*:505, 1974.
407. Weld, P. W.: Osteomyelitis of the ilium masquerading as acute appendicitis. J.A.M.A., *173*:634, 1960.
408. Wenger, D. R., Bobechke, W. P., and Gilday, D. L.: The spectrum of intervertebral disc-space infection in children. J. Bone Joint Surg., *60 A*:100, 1978.
409. Wheeler, R. D., Rinsky, L. A., Bleck, E. E., and Gouis, M.: False-negative bone scans in osteomyelitis: A clinical and experimental study. Orthop. Trans., *4*:102, 1980.
410. White, M., and Dennison, W. M.: Acute haematogenous osteitis in childhood. J. Bone Joint Surg., *34-B*:608, 1952.
411. White, R. G., Davidson, D. C., and Paterson, D.: Acute haematogenous osteomyelitis. Rec. Adelaide Child. Hosp., *1*:509, 1977.
412. Wilensky, A. O.: Osteomyelitis of the vertebrae. Ann. Surg., *89*:561, 1929.
413. Wilensky, A. O.: Osteomyelitis: Its Pathogenesis, Symptomatology and Treatment. New York, Macmillan, 1934.
414. Wilkinson, F. R.: Diagnosis and early treatment of acute hematogenous osteomyelitis in children. Pediatrics, *1*:796, 1948.
415. Wilson, J. C., and McKeever, F. M.: Bone growth disturbance following hematogenous acute osteomyelitis. J.A.M.A., *107*:1188, 1936.
416. Wilson, J. C., and McKeever, F. M.: Hematogenous acute osteomyelitis in children. J. Bone Joint Surg., *18*:328, 1936.
417. Winters, J. L., and Cahen, I.: Acute hematogenous osteomyelitis. A review of 66 cases. J. Bone Joint Surg., *42-A*:691, 1960.
418. Wittmann, D. H., and Schassan, H. H.: Distribution of moxalactam in serum, bone, tissue fluid, and peritoneal fluid. Rev. Infect. Dis., *4*:Suppl.:S610, 1982.
419. Wolf, C. R., and Brower, T.: Primary pyogenic arthritis of the sacro-iliac joint. Clin. Orthop., *70*:239, 1970.
420. Wolman, B.: Acute osteomyelitis in infancy. Acta Paediatr., *45*:595, 1956.
421. Yogev, R., Burkholder, E., and Davis, A. T.: Synergistic action of ampicillin and nafcillin against ampicillin-resistant Haemophilis influenzae. Antimicrob. Agents Chemother., *17*:461, 1980.
422. Yogev, R., and Kabat, W. J.: Synergistic action of nafcillin and ampicillin against ampicillin-resistant Haemophilus influenza type b bacteremia and meningitis in infant rats. Antimicrob. Agents Chemother., *18*:122, 1980.
423. Young, F.: Acute osteomyelitis of the ilium. Surg. Gynecol. Obstet., *58*:986, 1934.

SALMONELLA OSTEOMYELITIS

Bone infection due to salmonella organisms is rare. During the era before antibiotics, when typhoid fever was prevalent, Murphy reported an incidence of 0.84 per cent of osteomyelitis among 18,840 patients with typhoid fever.[26] The incidence is lower for paratyphoid fever and other salmonella infections.[13, 31]

In typhoid osteomyelitis, the lesions appear in the late convalescent stage of the disease as chronic abscesses in bone; they may point subcutaneously. Fibrosis and calcification of surrounding soft tissues tend to localize the infection. The vertebrae, ribs, and long bones may be involved. Food poisoning salmonellae, such as *Salmonella dublin*, have on occasion been cultured from osteomyelitic lesions.[24]

Salmonella Bone Infection in Hemoglobinopathies

In children with sickle cell disease, i.e., hemoglobinopathies SS, SC, or S-thalassemia, salmonella-caused osteomyelitis is not uncommon.[1–3, 8, 9, 11, 17, 18, 21, 36–38]

While *Staphylococcus aureus* is a common agent of osteomyelitis in these patients, the incidence of salmonella osteomyelitis is several hundredfold higher than that of the general population.[3] This higher incidence is accounted for by three factors. First, the local thrombosis in small vessels of the intestinal mucosa may lead to disruption of the mucosal integrity, facilitating bloodstream invasion by intraluminal bacteria. Second, the duration of bacteremia may be prolonged by the hyposplenic state of the patient with sickle cell disease, allowing bacteria greater opportunity to establish infection.[12] Finally, the marrow hyperplasia and multiple infarctions of bone are foci of hypoxia and aseptic necrosis; these act as points of lowered resistance that favor the localization and spread of salmonella organisms. The long bones and

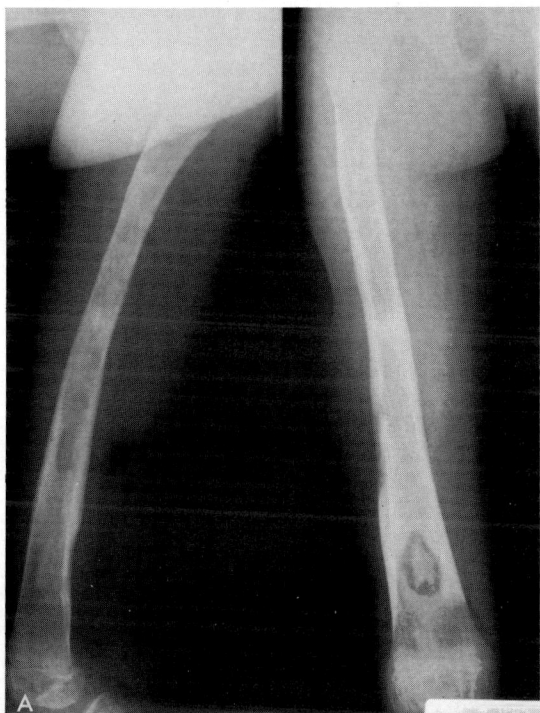
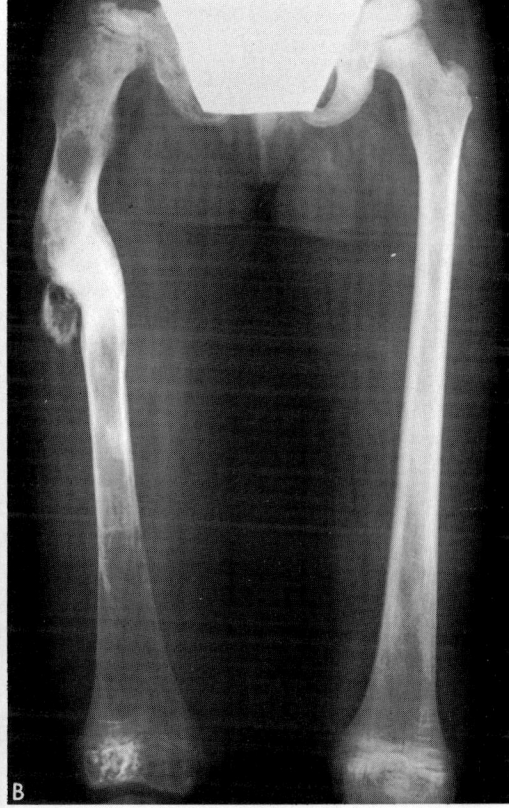
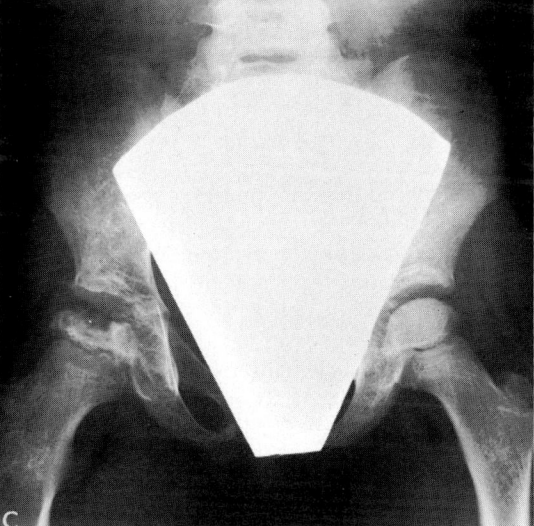

FIGURE 3–224. Salmonella-caused osteomyelitis of the femur in a child with sickle cell disease.

A. Anteroposterior and lateral views of the femur showing destructive lesion in the distal shaft. Note the sequestrum. **B.** Postoperative radiograms of both femora. The sequestrum was removed and the infected femur was thoroughly curetted. **C.** Anteroposterior radiogram of hips of same patient. Note the avascular changes in both femoral heads.

Illustration continued on following page

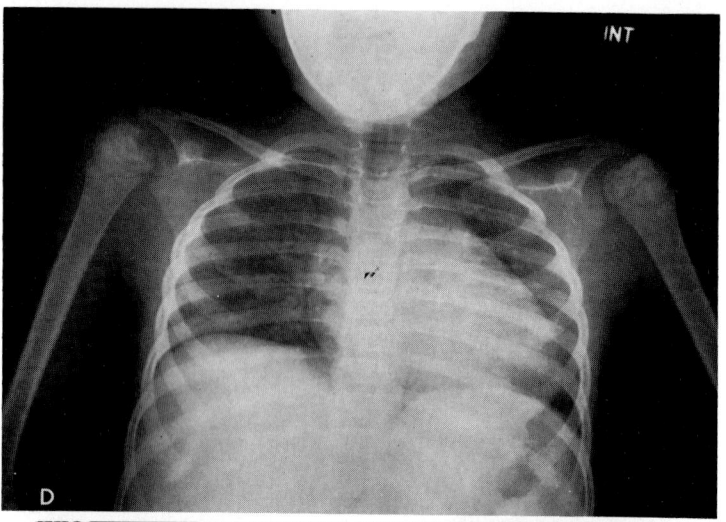
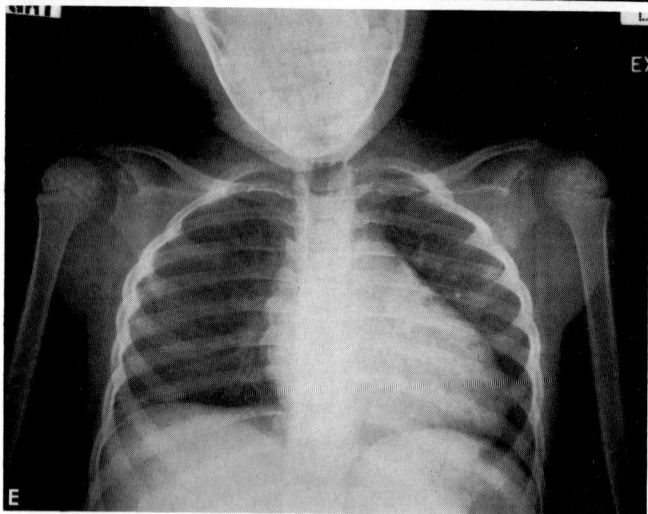

FIGURE 3–224 Continued. *Salmonella*-caused osteomyelitis of the femur in a child with sickle cell disease.

D and **E.** Anteroposterior radiograms of both shoulders taken in internal and external rotation when the child was younger. Note the aseptic necrotic changes in the humeral heads.

vertebrae are common sites. Salmonella osteomyelitis is characterized by frequent involvement of multiple sites.

The onset of the disease is insidious, with low-grade fever and local bone pain and swelling. Within 7 to 12 days, the radiograms will disclose multiple punched-out destructive lesions throughout the metaphysis and diaphysis with extensive subperiosteal new bone formation and irregular sclerosis (Fig. 3–224). The undermined and widened haversian canals in sickle cell anemia enhance the spread of infection through the medulla as well as the cortex.

Treatment

Salmonellae are considerably more sensitive to third-generation cephalosporins such as moxalactam, cefotaxime, and ceftriaxone than to the more traditional drugs used for salmonellosis, such as ampicillin or chloramphenicol.[27] Surgical drainage of the bone abscess and closed suction–irrigation are often indicated. Whole blood is transfused to correct the anemia as necessary. The recurrence rate is high. In resistant chronic cases, it is best to pack the wound wide open for extensive drainage and close it secondarily when the infection is under control. The use of hyperbaric oxygenation should also be considered.[15, 19, 23, 28, 33]

References

1. Adeyokunnu, A. A., and Hendrickse, R. G.: Salmonella osteomyelitis in childhood. A report of 63 cases seen in Nigerian children of whom 57 had sickle cell anaemia. Arch. Dis. Child., 55:175, 1980.
2. Annotation: Sickle cells and salmonella. Br. Med. J., 2:537, 1957.
3. Barrett-Connor, E.: Bacterial infection and sickle cell anemia. Medicine, 50:97, 1971.

4. Beaupre, A., and Carroll, N.: The three syndromes of iliac osteomyelitis in children. J. Bone Joint Surg., 61-A:1087, 1979.
5. Chari, P. R., Choudary, H. R., Dutt, K. P., and Naidu, M. L.: Typhoid osteomyelitis: Report of a case. Aust. N.Z. J. Surg., 41:174, 1971.
6. Charosky, C. B., and Marcove, R. C.: Salmonella paratyphi osteomyelitis. Report of a case simulating a giant cell tumor. Clin. Orthop., 99:190, 1974.
7. Cherubin, C. E., Neu, H. C., Imperato, P. J., Harvey, R. P., and Bellen, N.: Septicemia with non-typhoid Salmonella. Medicine (Baltimore), 53:365, 1974.
8. deTorregrosa, M. V., Dapena, R. B., Hernandez, H., and Ortiz, A.: Association of salmonella-caused osteomyelitis and sickle-cell disease. J.A.M.A., 174:354, 1960.
9. Ebong, W. W.: Bilateral pelvic osteomyelitis in children with sickle-cell anemia. Report of four cases. J. Bone Joint Surg. 64-A:945, 1982.
10. Ebrahim, G. J., and Grech, P.: Salmonella osteomyelitis in infants. J. Bone Joint Surg., 48-B:350, 1966.
11. Engh, C. A., Hughes, J. L., Abrams, R. C., and Bowerman, J. W.: Osteomyelitis in the patient with sickle-cell disease. Diagnosis and management. J. Bone Joint Surg., 53-A:1, 1971.
12. Feigin, R. D., and Cherry, J. D.: Textbook of Pediatric Infectious Disease. Philadelphia, Saunders, 1981, p. 558.
13. Giaccai, L., and Idriss, H.: Osteomyelitis due to salmonella infection. J. Pediatr., 41:73, 1952.
14. Gupta, J. C.: Unusual local manifestations of salmonella infections. J. Indian Med. Assoc., 42:31, 1964.
15. Hamblen, D. L.: Hyperbaric oxygenation. J. Bone Joint Surg., 50-A:1129, 1968.
16. Harris, N. H.: Salmonella typhi osteomyelitis. Proc. R. Soc. Med., 59:709, 1966.
17. Hendricksee, R. G., and Collard, P.: Salmonella osteomyelitis in Nigerian children. Lancet, 1:80, 1960.
18. Hook, E. W.: Salmonella osteomyelitis in patients with sickle-cell anemia. N. Engl. J. Med., 257:403, 1957.
19. Hopkinson, W. L., and Towers, A. G.: Effects of hyperbaric oxygen on some common pathogenic bacteria. Lancet, 2:1361, 1963.
20. Hughes, J. G., and Carroll, D. S.: Salmonella osteomyelitis complicating sickle-cell disease. Pediatrics, 19:184, 1957.
21. Landesman, S. H., Rao, S. P., and Ahonkhai, V. I.: Infections in children with sickle cell anemia. Special reference to pneumococcal and salmonella infections. Am. J. Pediatr. Hematol. Oncol., 4:407, 1982.
22. L'e, C. T.: Salmonella vertebral osteomyelitis: A case report with literature review. Am. J. Dis. Child., 136:722, 1982.
23. McAllister, T. A., Stark, J. N., Norman, J. N., and Ross, R. M.: Inhibitory effects of hyperbaric oxygen on bacteria and fungi. Lancet, 2:1040, 1963.
24. Miller, A. A.: Salmonella dublin osteomyelitis of the spine. Report of a fatal case. Br. Med. J., 1:194, 1954.
25. Mills, K. L.: Osteomyelitis of the spine due to Salmonella muenchen. J. Bone Joint Surg., 46-B:697, 1964.
26. Murphy, J. B.: Bone and joint disease in relation to typhoid fever. Surg. Gynecol. Obstet., 23:119, 1916.
27. Neu, H. C., Meropol, N. J., and Fu, K. P.: Antibacterial activity of ceftriaxone (ro 13–9904), a β-lactamase-stable cephalosporin. Antimicrob. Agents Chemother., 19:414, 1981.
28. Ollodart, R. M., Seitz, C. R., Blair, E., Henning, G., and Buxton, R. W.: Effect of hyperbaric oxygen on gram-negative bacilli. Clin. Res., 12:37, 1964.
29. Ortiz-Neu, C., Marr, J. S., Cherubin, C. E., and Neu, H. C.: Bone and joint infections due to salmonella. J. Infect. Dis., 138:820, 1978.
30. Roberts, A. H., and Hillburg, L. E.: Sickle-cell disease with salmonella osteomyelitis. J. Pediatr., 52:170, 1958.
31. Rozansky, R., Ehrenfield, E. N., and Matoth, Y.: Paratyphoid osteomyelitis. Report of two cases. Br. Med. J. 2:297, 1948.
32. Simon, S. D., and Silver, C. M.: Salmonella osteomyelitis. Report of three cases, one with fatal outcome and autopsy. J. Int. Coll. Surg., 28:197, 1957.
33. Slack, W. K., Thomas, D. A., and Perkins, D.: Hyperbaric oxygenation in chronic osteomyelitis. Lancet, 1:1093, 1965.
34. Smilack, J. D., and Goldberg, M. A.: Bone and joint involvement with Arizona hinshawii. Report of a case and review of the literature. Am. J. Med. Sci., 270:503, 1975.
35. Specht, E. E.: Hemoglobinopathic salmonella osteomyelitis. Orthopedic aspects. Clin. Orthop., 79:110, 1971.
36. Walker, G. F.: Typhoid spine in a Nigerian with sickle haemoglobin. J. Bone Joint Surg., 45-B:683, 1963.
37. Widen, A. L., and Cordon, L.: Salmonella typhimurium osteomyelitis with sickle-cell hemoglobin E disease. A review and case report. Ann. Intern. Med., 54:510, 1961.
38. Wigh, R., and Thompson, H. J.: Cortical fissuring in osteomyelitis complicating sickle cell anemia. Radiology, 55:553, 1950.

BRUCELLAR OSTEOMYELITIS

Brucellar osteomyelitis is caused by several of the brucella species, including *B. abortus*, *B. melitensis*, and *B. suis*. The condition is most commonly observed in farmers, meat packers, or persons who drink unpasteurized milk. It rarely occurs in children.

Brucellosis due to *B. abortus* is the most common type seen in the United States and Europe, and is the type most likely to be complicated by bone infection.

Vertebrae, usually lumbar, are the most common sites of involvement, accounting for about three quarters of all cases of brucellar osteomyelitis.[9] The long tubular bones of the limbs, the hip, the knee joint, and the flat trunk bones may be affected.[10, 14, 15] Other joints and bursae may also be involved.[3, 5]

Pain and tenderness are present at the site of localization. Other clinical symptoms are those of systemic brucellosis, such as loss of weight, leukocytosis, fever, and malaise.

Radiographic findings may show simultaneous destructive and regenerative osseous changes. Bony projections on the anterior surfaces of the vertebrae may give a characteristic "parrot beak" appearance.

Diagnosis is usually made by a positive reaction to intradermal injection of Brucellergen and the finding of a high titer of agglutinating antibodies in the patient's serum. A positive blood culture is difficult to obtain, but should be attempted when the patient is febrile.

Treatment consists of administration of tetracycline combined with streptomycin.[11] Recurrence rate of the diesase is high, and it may be secondarily complicated by a staphylococcus infection.

Chronic brucellar osteomyelitis is recalcitrant to treatment. It will require wide saucerization and secondary closure.[6]

References

1. Bonfiglio, M., Mickelson, M. R., and El-Khoury, G. Y.: Brucellar osteomyelitis. Case report 221. Skeletal Radiol., 9:208, 1983.
2. Bullock, W. E., Tobian, L. G., and Arnesen, P. M.: An unusual case of brucellar osteomyelitis associated with serum blocking antibody activity. Ann. Intern. Med., 61:938, 1964.
3. Coventry, M. B., Ivins, J. C., Nichols, D. R., and Weed, L. A.: Infection of the hip by Brucella suis. J.A.M.A., 141:320, 1949.
4. Henderson, R. J., and Hill, D. M.: Subclinical brucella infection in man. Br. Med. J., 3:154, 1972.
5. Johnson, E. W., Jr., and Weed, L. A.: Brucellar bursitis. J. Bone Joint Surg., 36-A:133, 1954.
6. Kelly, P. J., Martin, W., Schirger, A., and Weed, L. A.: Brucellosis of the bones and joints. J.A.M.A., 174:347, 1960.
7. Kulowski, J., and Vinke, T. H.: Undulant (Malta) fever spondylitis. Report of a case, due to Brucella melitensis, bovine variety, surgically treated. J.A.M.A., 99:1656, 1932.
8. Lal, S., Modawal, K. K., Fowle, A. S. E., Peach, B., and Popham, R. D.: Acute brucellosis treated with trimethoprim and sulphamethoxazole. Br. Med. J., 3:256, 1970.
9. Lowbeer, L.: Brucellotic osteomyelitis of the spinal column in man. Am. J. Pathol., 24:723, 1948.
10. Lowe, G. H., Jr., and Lipscomb, P. R.: Brucellosis osteomyelitis. Report of two cases in which shafts of long bones were involved. Surgery, 22:525, 1947.
11. Magill, G. B., and Killough, J. H.: Oxytetracycline-streptomycin therapy in brucellosis due to Brucella melitensis. Arch. Intern. Med., 91:204, 1953.
12. Mantle, J. A.: Brucellar spondylitis. J. Bone Joint Surg., 37-B:456, 1955.
13. Seal, P. V., and Morris, C. A.: Brucellosis of the carpus. Report of a case. J. Bone Joint Surg., 56-B:327, 1974.
14. Spink, W. W.: Pathogenesis of human brucellosis with respect to prevention and treatment. Ann. Intern. Med., 29:238, 1948.
15. Spink, W. W.: The Nature of Brucellosis. Minneapolis, University of Minnesota Press, 1956.
16. Steindler, A.: Orthopedic complications of brucellosis. J. Iowa Med. Soc., 30:256, 1940.
17. Young, E. J.: Human brucellosis. Clin. Med., 83:8, 1976.
18. Zammit, F.: Undulant fever spondylitis. Br. J. Radiol., 31:683, 1958.

SYPHILIS OF BONE

Bone syphilis may be *congenital* (infected in utero) or *acquired* (infected in postnatal life). Since the advent of antibiotics the incidence of syphilis has markedly diminished. The *Treponema pallidum* reaches bone through the he-

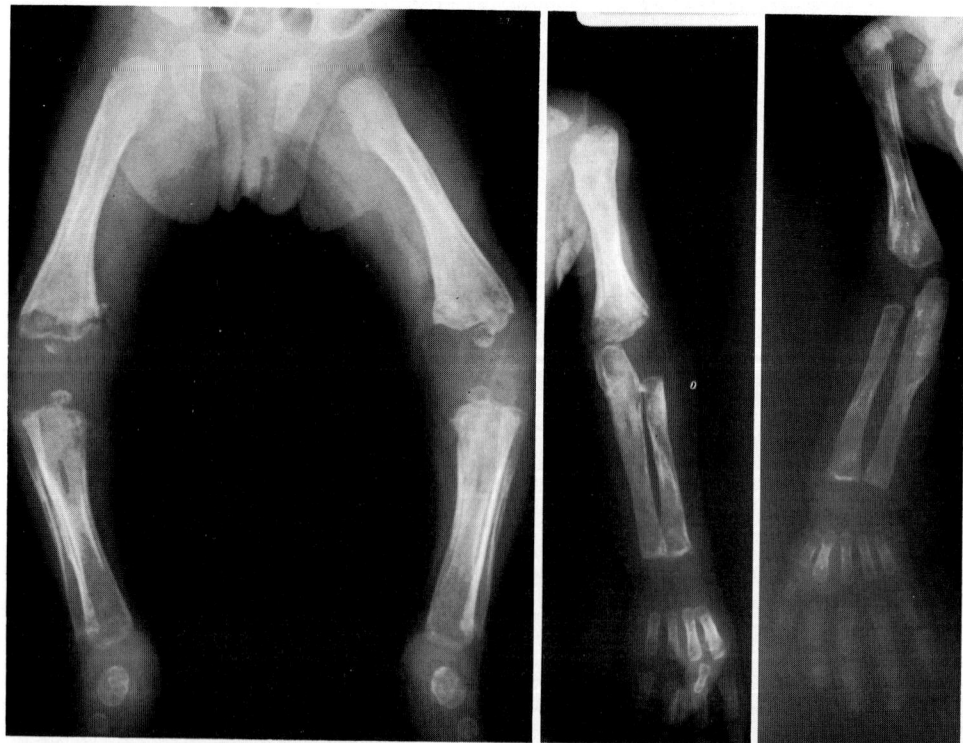

FIGURE 3–225. Congenital syphilis in a three-month-old girl.

Radiograms of both lower and upper limbs. Note the metaphysitis with areas of rarefaction and the marked symmetrical new bone formation.

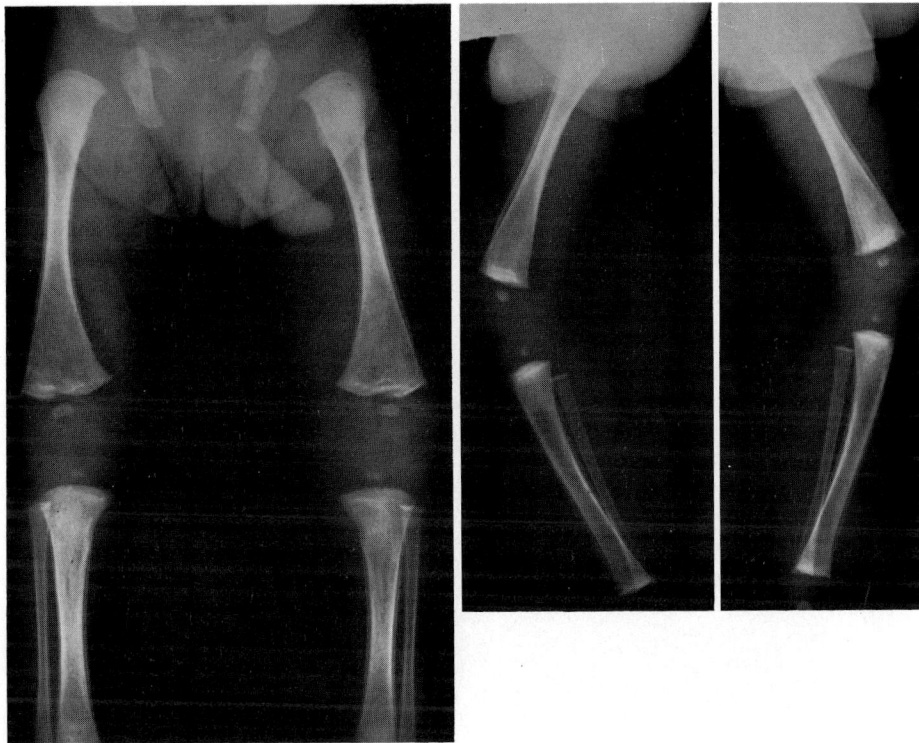

FIGURE 3–226. *A three-month-old child with congenital syphilis.*

Anteroposterior and lateral views of both lower limbs. Note the periostitis affecting both femora and tibiae.

matogenous route, and as early as 36 hours following infection, it can be demonstrated in the bone marrow. The organisms tend to localize in the metaphysis and diaphysis, and do not spread to joints, as do tubercle bacilli. The tibia, femur, humerus, and cranial bones are the most common sites of involvement; however, any bone may be affected.

The patient may be stillborn with stigma of lues; or he may be born alive with evidence of lues. Some infected infants appear healthy, the evidence of syphilis developing one to two months postnatally.

In early infancy the usual finding is syphilitic metaphysitis (Fig. 3–225). Symmetrical involvement of multiple bones is characteristic. The normal osseous tissue is replaced by infected granulation tissue. Osteoid production is poor or absent. The physis becomes widened, irregular, and ill-defined because of abnormal transformation of cartilage into bone. The epiphyses are usually not involved. In the radiogram the acute metaphysitis shows as erosions and infarctions in the zones of provisional calcifications, which may be dense or absent, as transverse metaphyseal radiolucent zones. Tiny prongs in the juxtaepiphyseal area give a serrated, sawtooth appearance. Areas of bone destruction are represented as foci of rarefaction in the corners between the physis and metaphysis. With proper staining techniques, spirochetes can be demonstrated in the histologic sections. Pathologic fracture may occur through the weakened metaphyseal area. Necrosis may develop, and frank pus can form if the disease process is not arrested.

The infection spreads up and down the medullary canal, extending through the cortex to the periosteum. Marked subperiosteal osteogenesis takes place, the new bone surrounding the original cortex along the entire length of the diaphysis (Fig. 3–226). The intervening space between the two layers of bone may be filled with cancellous bone or granulation tissue. In later childhood or adolescence syphilitic osteoperiostitis produces a dense, circumscribed swelling over the convex side of the bone. In the tibia the subperiosteal apposition of bone on the anterior cortical surface produces the so-called "saber shin" of congenital syphilis (Fig. 3–227).

Periostitis and osteoperiostitis are seen in the acute form in the late stage of syphilis. Absence of pain differentiates it from pyogenic osteomyelitis. Bone syphilis responds to treatment with penicillin.

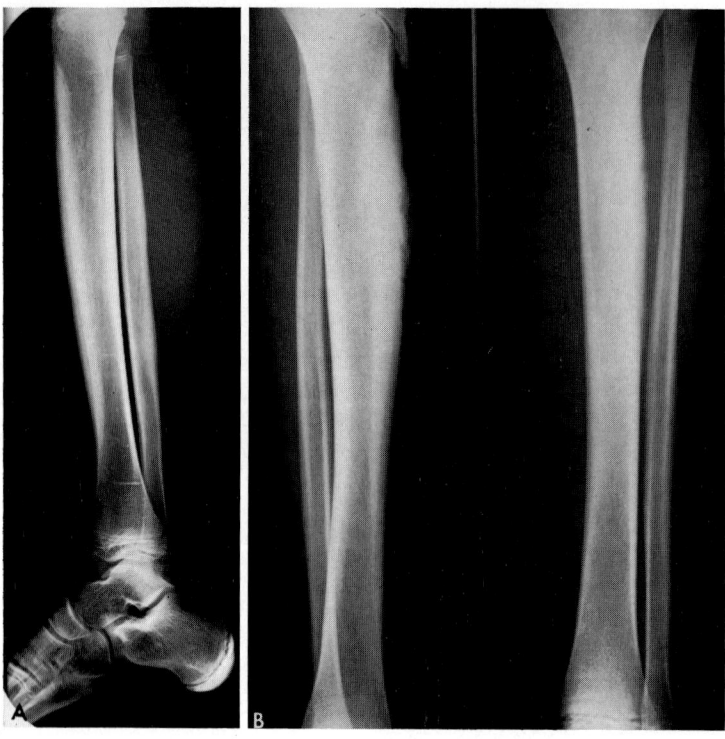

FIGURE 3–227. "Saber shin" in congenital lues.

A. Note the periostitis on the anterior surface of the tibia. **B.** Anteroposterior and lateral views of the tibia of an older patient show more marked involvement.

References

1. Bauer, M. F., and Caravati, C. M.: Osteolytic lesions in early syphilis. Br. J. Vener. Dis., 43:175, 1967.
2. Caffey, J.: Syphilis of the skeleton in early infancy: The non-specificity of many of the roentgenographic changes. A.J.R., 42:637, 1939.
3. Caffey, J.: Some traumatic lesions in growing bones other than fractures and dislocations: Clinical and radiological features. Br. J. Radiol., 30:25, 1957.
4. Coblentz, D. R., Cimini, R., Mikity, V. G., and Rosen, R.: Roentgenographic diagnosis of congenital syphilis in the newborn. J.A.M.A., 212:1063, 1970.
5. Cremen, B. J., and Fisher, M. B.: The lesions of congenital syphilis. Br. J. Radiol., 43:333, 1970.
6. Dzebolo, N. N.: Congenital syphilis: Unusual presentation. Radiology, 136:372, 1980.
7. Fiumara, N. J.: Syphilis in newborn children. Clin. Obstet. Gynecol., 18:183, 1975.
8. Ingraham, N. R. J.: Lag phase in early congenital osseous syphilis; roentgenographic study. Am. J. Med. Sci., 191:819, 1936.
9. Lawson, T. L.: Chronic bone infections in Africans. Ten cases from Nigeria. J. Bone Joint Surg., 33-B:584, 1951.
10. Levin, E. J.: Healing in congenital osteosyphilis. A.J.R., 110:591, 1970.
11. McCracken, G. H., and Kaplan, J. M.: Penicillin treatment for congenital syphilis. J.A.M.A., 228:855, 1974.
12. McGladdery, H.: Osteolytic bone syphilis. Five case reports. J. Bone Joint Surg., 32-B:226, 1950.
13. McLean, S.: Roentgenographic and pathologic aspects of congenital osseous syphilis. Am. J. Dis. Child., 41:130, 1931.
14. McLean, S.: Correlation of roentgenographic and pathologic aspects of congenital osseous syphilis, with particular reference to the first months of life. Am. J. Dis. Child., 41:363, 1931.
15. McLean, S.: Correlation of roentgenologic picture with gross and microscopic examination of pathologic material in congenital osseous syphilis. Am. J. Dis. Child., 41:607, 1931.
16. McLean, S.: Correlation of clinical picture with osseous lesions of congenital syphilis as shown by x-rays. Am. J. Dis. Child., 41:887, 1931.
17. McLean, S.: Osseous lesions of congenital syphilis: Summary and conclusions in 102 cases. Am. J. Dis. Child., 41:1411, 1931.
18. Morton, J. J.: Syphilis of bone. Urol. Cutan. Rev., 43:72, 1939.
19. Park, E. A., and Jackson, D. A.: The irregular extensions of the end of the shaft in the x-ray photograph in congenital syphilis, with pertinent observations. J. Pediatr., 13:748, 1938.
20. Pick, L.: Angeborene Knochensyphilis. In Handbuch der speziellen path. Anatomie und Histologie. Berlin, Springer, 1920, p. 240.
21. Reiter, S., and Oigaard, A.: The unusual case: Persistence of metaphyseal changes in penicillin treated congenital syphilis. Pediatr. Radiol., 7:229, 1978.
22. Robinson, R. C. V.: Congenital syphilis. Arch. Dermatol., 99:559, 1969.
23. Rosenfeld, S. R., Weinert, C. R., and Kahn, B.: Congenital syphilis, a case report. J. Bone Joint Surg., 65-A:115, 1983.
24. Skapinker, S., and De Villiers Minaar, A. B.: Syphilitic disease of the long bones in the Bantu. J. Bone Joint Surg., 33-B:578, 1951.
25. Solomon, A., and Rosen, E.: Aspect of trauma and the bone changes of congenital lues. Pediatr. Radiol., 3:176, 1975.

26. Tan, K. L.: The re-emergence of early congenital syphilis. Acta Paediatr. Scand., 22:203, 1940.
27. Thomason, H. A., and Mayoral, A.: Syphilitic osteomyelitis. J. Bone Joint Surg., 22:203, 1940.
28. Toohey, J. S.: Skeletal presentation of congenital syphilis: Case report and review of the literature. J. Pediatr. Orthop., 5:104, 1985.
29. Wilkinson, R. H., and Heller, R. M.: Congenital syphilis; resurgence of an old problem. Pediatrics, 47:27, 1971.

TUBERCULOSIS OF BONE

Tubercle bacilli often lodge in the metaphyses or epiphyses of long bones and frequently involve the adjacent joint (Fig. 3–228). Occasionally, the tuberculous infection may affect the diaphysis. Bone tuberculosis is discussed in detail in the section on tuberculous arthritis.

Tuberculous dactylitis or *spina ventosa* occurs in children usually under five year of age.[7] The majority of cases are in black children. The metacarpals, metatarsals, or phalanges may be affected, more frequently in the hand than in the foot. The disease may involve several digits, which become swollen and fusiform or spindle-shaped. There is little if any pain, and disability is minimal. Shortening and contracture of the affected digit will result. Radiograms disclose expansion by cystlike rarefaction of the infected

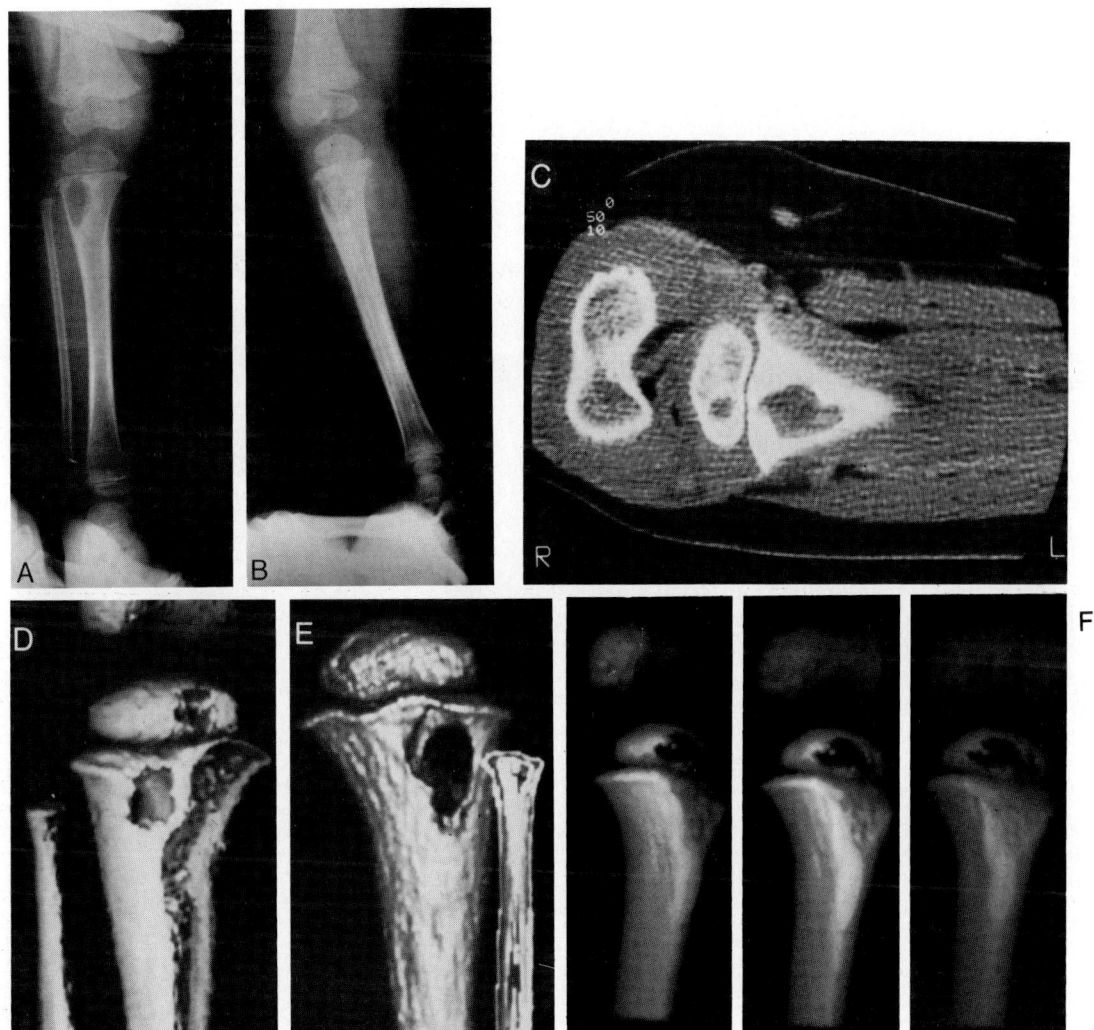

FIGURE 3–228. *Tuberculosis of the proximal metaphysis of the tibia with extension into the epiphysis. Note the erosion of the regional cortex.*

A and B. Original radiograms.
C to E. CT scan and three-dimensional reconstruction.
F. Three-dimensional reconstruction one year after antituberculosis drug therapy. The lesion in the metaphysis is almost healed, but the rarefaction in the epiphysis is still present.

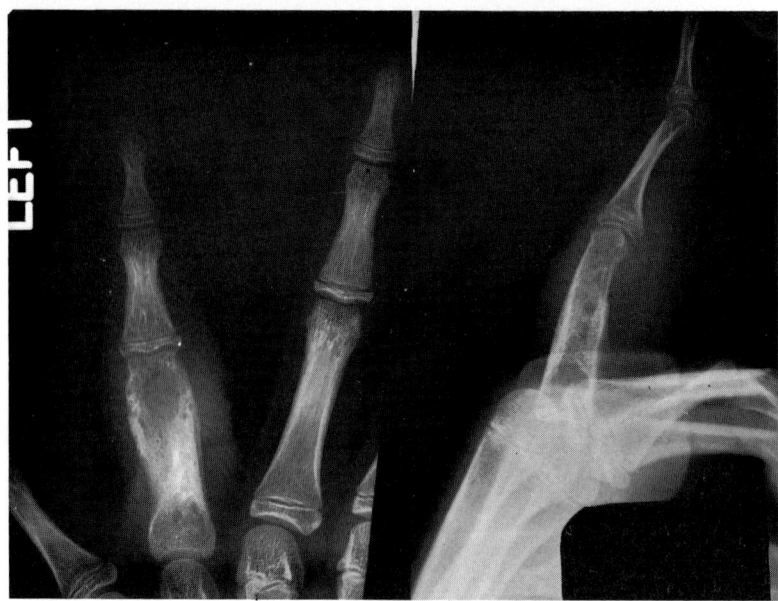

FIGURE 3–229. *Tuberculous dactylitis–spina ventosa.*

Note the cystic rarefaction of the proximal phalanx of left ring finger and minimal subperiosteal new bone formation.

short tubular bone with some subperiosteal new bone formation (Fig. 3–229). The condition should be distinguished from solitary enchondroma or multiple enchondromatosis, in which periosteal reaction is minimal or absent unless complicated by a fracture; the fusiform enlargement of fingers seen in pauciarticular arthritis, in which there is no cystlike rarefaction of bone; and syphilitic dactylitis, in which there is marked subperiosteal new bone formation and the serologic test for syphilis is positive.

The course of tuberculous osteomyelitis is characteristically insidious, with symptoms present for many months to years prior to establishment of the diagnosis. Clues that should lead to further evaluation for tuberculous osteomyelitis include a positive intermediate-strength (5 T.U.) tuberculin skin test, evidence of past or current tuberculosis, or a history of tuberculosis in the family. Biopsy of the bone in osseous tuberculosis reveals granulomatous inflammation with or without the presence of acid-fast organisms. Every attempt should be made to obtain a culture from the diseased bone in order to confirm the diagnosis and to perform susceptibility tests.

The treatment of skeletal tuberculosis should be initiated with isoniazid and another antituberculous drug such as ethambutol, streptomycin, or rifampin. If the patient is known to be infected with a resistant strain of *M. tuberculosis* or comes from an area endemic for resistant strains, e.g., the Far East, a third drug should be added. The affected part should be splinted in functional position. Prognosis is good.

References

1. Alexander, C. H., and Mansuy, M. M.: Disseminated bone tuberculosis (so-called multiple cystic tuberculosis). Radiology, 55:839, 1950.
2. Bergdahl, S., Fellander, M., and Robertson, B.: BCG osteomyelitis. Experience in the Stockholm region over the years 1961–1974. J. Bone Joint Surg., 58-B:212, 1976.
3. Elphick, H. R., and Turnbill, H. M.: Problems in the diagnosis and management of skeletal tuberculosis. Med. J. Aust. 2:943, 1970.
4. Erikson, U., and Hjelmstedt, A.: Roentgenologic aspects of BCG-osteomyelitis. Radiology, 101:575, 1971.
5. Foucard, T., and Hjelmstedt, A.: BCG-osteomyelitis and -osteoarthritis as a complication following BCG-vaccination. Acta Orthop. Scand., 42:142, 1971.
6. Friedman, B., and Kapur, V. N.: Newer knowledge of chemotherapy in the treatment of tuberculosis of bones and joints. Clin. Orthop., 97:5, 1973.
7. Hardy, J. B., and Hartman, J. R.: Tuberculous dactylitis in childhood. J. Pediatr., 30:146, 1947.
8. Komins, C.: Multiple cystic tuberculosis. A review and a revised nomenclature. Br. J. Radiol., 25:1, 1952.
9. Lynch, A. F.: Tuberculosis of the great trochanter. A report of 8 cases. J. Bone Joint Surg., 64-B:185, 1982.
10. Manzella, J. P., Vanvoris, L. P., and Hruska, J. F.: Isolated calcaneal tuberculous osteomyelitis. A case report. J. Bone Joint Surg., 61-A:946, 1979.
11. Martini, M., Adjrad, A., and Boudjemaa, A.: Tuberculous osteomyelitis. Int. Orthop., 10:201, 1986.
12. Paus, B.: The changed pattern of bone and joint tuberculosis in Norway. Acta Orthop. Scand., 48:277, 1977.
13. Roaf, R., Kirkaldy-Willis, W. H., and Cathro, A. J. H.: Surgical Treatment of Bone and Joint Tuberculosis. Edinburgh-London, Livingstone, 1959.
14. Shanmugasundaram, T. K.: Bone and Joint Tuberculosis. Madras (India), Kothandram, 1983.

15. Silva, J. F.: A review of patients with skeletal tuberculosis treated at the University Hospital, Kuala Lumpar. Int. Orthop., 4:79, 1980.
16. Sorrel, E., and Sorrel Deperine, Mme.: Tuberculose Osseuse et Ostéo-articulaire. Paris, Masson, 1932.
17. Stuart, D.: Local osteo-articular tuberculosis complicating closed fractures. Report of two cases. J. Bone Joint Surg., 58-B:248, 1976.
18. Tuli, S. M., and Kumar, S.: Early results of treatment of spinal tuberculosis by triple drug therapy. Clin. Orthop., 81:56, 1971.
19. Tuli, S. M., Kumar, K., and Sen, P. C.: Penetration of antituberculous drugs in clinical osteoarticular tubercular lesions. Acta Orthop. Scand., 48:362, 1977.
20. Tuli, S. M., Brighton, C. T., Morton, H. E., and Clark, L. W.: The experimental induction of localised skeletal tuberculous lesions and their accessibility to streptomycin. J. Bone Joint Surg., 56-B:551, 1974.

FUNGUS INFECTIONS OF BONE

Mycotic osteomyelitis is a general term referring to several rare diseases caused by fungus infection within bone. Actinomycosis, blastomycosis, coccidioidomycosis, and sporotrichosis occur the most frequently. Usually the primary infection originates in the soft tissues and later extends directly to bone. Fungal infections of bone, tuberculosis, and pyogenic osteomyelitis are quite similar in their radiographic appearance.[44] The possibility of mycosis should be remembered in chronic osteomyelitis so that a fungal etiology is not overlooked.

Actinomycosis

Actinomycosis is a chronic infection that usually involves the soft tissues of the head and neck.[9, 22, 37, 40, 46] It may spread to the lungs and large intestine. Bone becomes affected from the adjacent infected tissue by direct extension; in the oral cavity and neck, the mandible is involved; the infection extends to the dorsal spine and ribs from the lungs, and to the pelvic bones and lumbosacral spine from the colon and appendix. In bone, multiple abscesses are formed and connected by sinuses composed of granulomatous inflammatory tissue in the periphery and of purulent exudate in the center. The fungal colonies found in the abscesses appear as amorphous yellow granules (the so-called "sulfur granules").

In the human the pathogenic organism is *Actinomycosis israeli*, and in animals *Actinomycosis bovis*. Occasionally men are infected by *bovis* strains. In North America, actinomycosis is prevalent in Mississippi, North Carolina, and the northeastern United States.

Radiographically, the affected bone has a moth-eaten appearance with some reactive new bone formation. In the vertebral column certain features distinguish actinomycosis of the spine from tuberculosis. Actinomycosis spares the intervertebral discs but often involves the transverse processes and heads of neighboring ribs; collapse of vertebral bodies and kyphosis are rare; sclerosis is generally mixed with rarefaction with a lattice pattern in the radiogram.[17, 37]

Treatment. It consists of administration of penicillin; one can have recourse to streptomycin, chlortetracycline and chloramphenicol. Antibiotics should be administered in large doses and for a prolonged period, at least four to six weeks, and usually for several months.

Recurrence due to reactivation of latent fungi is common. Antibiotics should not be discontinued until there is definite radiographic evidence of healing. When there is bone involvement with multiple abscesses, surgical excision of the lesion is indicated.

Blastomycosis of Bone

North American blastomycosis is predominantly a disease of the skin and lungs; however, bones and joints may be involved, either from direct extension of an adjacent soft-tissue infection or as a result of hematogenous spread. It is a very rare condition and is well covered in the literature.[2, 5, 21, 31, 35] In the United States, blastomycosis is endemic to a zone that extends from Wisconsin to Louisiana and across Kentucky to the Carolinas.

In blastomycosis, a suppurative pseudotuberculous granulomatous reaction is produced, which causes destructive chronic osteomyelitis of the vertebrae, ribs, skull, and sometimes long bones.

Diagnosis is made by direct smear, culture, skin testing, and serology. Amphotericin B and 2-hydroxystilbamidine have proved to be two potent drugs that effect cure. Amphotericin B is nephrotoxic, however, and kidney function should be followed closely.

Coccidioidomycosis

A fungus infection caused by *Coccidioides immitis*, coccidioidomycosis is endemic to the southwestern parts of the United States, especially the San Joaquin Valley of California. The infection usually stems from inhalation of dust containing fragments of the fungal mycelium. The lungs are the primary site of pathologic involvement. Dissemination is rare, but it does produce bone lesions, some of which are multiple. The spine, the pelvis, the bones of the hands and feet, and those around the knees and ankles are most often involved. The coccidioides found produces a granulomatous tuberculoid type of tissue reaction with caseation. Clinically, transient pleuritic chest pain is the most constant symptom; it may be accompanied by a cough and fever.

If the infection is suspected, serial x-rays of the chest should be taken. Initially, a small round lesion will be found, which rapidly progresses to a diffuse infiltrate, and then resolves within approximately 20 days. Skeletal lesions are depicted in the radiograph as osteolytic areas of radiolucency with periosteal new bone formation.[25] They are difficult to differentiate from pyogenic osteomyelitis. Diagnosis is made by identification of *C. immitis* spores under the microscope. Serologic and skin tests are not sufficiently specific for diagnosis. For years, the bone lesions may remain latent and inactive, with some surrounding reactive sclerosis.

Treatment is by systemic amphotericin B for six weeks. The value of adjunctive agents such as 5-fluorocystosine or ketoconazole remains unclear. The bone and synovial lesions are excised when feasible.

Sporotrichosis

Sporotrichosis is an occupational disease of florists and gardeners, as the pathogenic organism *Sporotrichum schenckii* is universally found in soil.[24] In this chronic granulomatous infection skin and subcutaneous tissues are the most common site. Few pulmonary cases have been reported. Bone may be involved by direct extension from a skin lesion or secondarily, with spread of the infection via the blood stream, with formation of focal abscesses, and with periosteal reactive osteogenesis. Sporotrichosis is sometimes found in association with sarcoidosis or tuberculosis. Chemotherapy with amphotericin B and iodide is effective. Pulmonary resection and excision of the lesions may be indicated.

Other fungal infections that may involve bone are histoplasmosis, maduromycosis and cryptococcosis.

Cryptococcus Neoformans (Torula Histolytica).[11, 29, 34, 40] Parasitic disease of bone in the human is usually caused by *Taenia echinococcus* (hydatid disease of bone). It is extremely rare in North America.

References

1. Adler, S., Randall, J., and Plotkin, S.: Candida osteomyelitis and arthritis in a neonate. Am. J. Dis. Child., 123:595, 1972.
2. Alfred, K. S., and Harbin, M.: Blastomycosis of bone. Report of a case. J. Bone Joint Surg., 32-A:887, 1950.
3. Anderson, P. L., and Stenderup, A.: Candida albicans antibodies in candidiasis. Scand. J. Infect. Dis., 6:63, 1974.
4. Banks, D. C., Yates, D. B., Cawdrey, H. M., Harries, M. G., and Kidner, P. H.: Infection from intravenous catheters. Lancet, 1:443, 1970.
5. Baylin, G. J., and Wear, J. M.: Blastomycosis and actinomycosis of the spine. A.J.R., 69:395, 1953.
6. Bennett, J. E.: Chemotherapy of systemic mycoses (first of two parts). N. Engl. J. Med., 290:30, 1974.
7. Birsner, J. W., and Smart, J.: Osseous coccidioidomycosis. A.J.R., 76:1052, 1956.
8. Boeckman, C. R., and Krill, C. E., Jr.: Bacterial and fungal infections complicating parenteral alimentation in infants and children. J. Pediatr. Surg., 5:117, 1970.
9. Brett, M. S.: Advanced actinomycosis of the spine treated with penicillin and streptomycin. Report of a case. J. Bone Joint Surg., 33-B:215, 1951.
10. Bujak, J. S., Kwon-Chung, K. J., and Chusid, M. J.: Osteomyelitis and pneumonia in a boy with chronic granulomatous disease of childhood caused by a mutant strain of Aspergillus nidulans. Am. J. Clin. Pathol., 61:361, 1974.
11. Carter, R. A.: Coccidioidal granuloma: Roentgen diagnosis. A.J.R., 25:715, 1931.
12. Chmel, H., Grieco, M. H., and Zickel, R.: Candida osteomyelitis. Report of a case. Am. J. Med. Sci., 266:299, 1973.
13. Cohen, R., and Bos, J.: Two new fungicides for Coccidiodes immitsi (Stilbamidine and Rimacidin). Arch. Pediatr., 69:33, 1952.
14. Cohen, R., and Gifford, M. A.: Proven case of cured disseminated coccidioidomycosis. Arch. Pediatr., 70:81, 1953.
15. Cohen, R., and O'Connor, R.: Para-aminobenzoic acid as a fungicide for Coccidiodes immitis. Arch. Pediatr., 70:404, 1953.
16. Collins, V. P.: Bone involvement in cryptococcosis (torulosis). A.J.R., 63:102, 1950.
17. Cope, V. Z.: Actinomycosis of bone with special reference to the infection of the vertebral column. J. Bone Joint Surg., 33-B:205, 1951.
18. Cox, L. B., and Tolhurst, J. C.: Human torulosis. A clinical, pathological, and microbiological study, with a report of 13 cases. Melbourne University Press, 1946.
19. Cramblett, H. G.: Less common systemic and visceral mycotic infections. *In* Shirkey, H. C. (ed.), Pediatric Therapy. St. Louis, Mosby, 1972, p. 487.
20. Curry, C. R., and Quie, P. G.: Fungal septicemia in patients receiving parenteral hyperalimentation. N. Engl. J. Med., 285:1221, 1971.
21. Cushard, W. G., Jr., Kohanim, M., and Lantis, L. R.: Blastomycosis of bone. Treatment with intramedullary amphotericin B. J. Bone Joint Surg., 51-A:704, 1969.
22. Davies, A. B.: Actinomycosis involving a long bone. Br. Med. J., 1:705, 1932.
23. Diament, M. J., Weller, M., and Bernstein, R.: Candida infection in a premature infant presenting as discitis. Pediatr. Radiol., 12:96, 1982.
24. Duran, R. J., Coventry, M. B., Weed, L. A., and Kierland, R. R.: Sporotrichosis. A report of twenty-three cases in the upper extremity. J. Bone Joint Surg., 39-A:1332, 1957.
25. Dykes, J., Segesman, J. K., and Birsner, J. W.: Coccidioidomycosis of bone in children. Am. J. Dis. Child., 85:34, 1953.
26. Edwards, J. E., Jr., Turkel, S. B., Elder, H. A., Rand, R. W., and Guze, L. B.: Hematogenous candida osteomyelitis. Report of three cases and review of the literature. Am. J. Med., 59:89, 1975.
27. Freeman, J. B., Wienke, J. W., and Soper, R. T.: Candida osteomyelitis associated with intravenous alimentation. J. Pediatr. Surg., 9:783, 1974.

28. Gill, J. A., and Gerald, B.: Blastomycosis in childhood. Radiology, 91:965, 1968.
29. Gosling, H. R., and Gilmer, W. S., Jr.: Skeletal cryptococcosis (torulosis). Report of a case and review of the literature. J. Bone Joint Surg., 38-A:660, 1956.
30. Grebe, A. A.: Monostotic coccidioidal infection. Report of a case, successfully treated with 2-hydroxystilbamidine. J. Bone Joint Surg., 36-A:859, 1954.
31. Hall, R. H., and Medeloff, J.: Blastomycotic osteomyelitis. J. Bone Joint Surg., 34-A:977, 1952.
32. Klingberg, W. G.: Generalized histoplasmosis in infants and children: Review of 10 cases with apparent recovery. J. Pediatr., 36:728, 1950.
33. Krick, J. A., and Remington, J. S.: Treatment of fungal infections. Arch. Intern. Med., 135:344, 1975.
34. Kulowski, J., and Stovall, S.: Maduromycosis of tibia in a native American. J.A.M.A., 135:429, 1947.
35. Levitas, J. R., and Baum, G. L.: Surgical aspects of blastomycosis. Surgery, 33:93, 1953.
36. Lindstrom, F. D., and Lindholm, T.: Candida albicans arthritis treated with flucytosine. Ann. Intern. Med., 79:131, 1973.
37. Lubert, M.: Actinomycosis of the vertebrae. A.J.R., 51:669, 1944.
38. Maki, D. G., Goldman, D. A., and Rhame, F. S.: Infection control in intravenous therapy. Ann. Intern. Med., 79:867, 1973.
39. Mazet, R., Jr.: Skeletal lesions in coccidioidomycosis. Arch. Surg., 70:633, 1955.
40. McCormack, L. J., Dickson, J. A., and Reich, A. R.: Actinomycosis of the humerus. Case report. J. Bone Joint Surg., 36-A:1255, 1954.
41. Mendelsohn, B. G.: Actinomycosis of a metacarpal bone. J. Bone Joint Surg., 47-B:739, 1965.
42. O'Connell, C. J., Cherry, A. V., and Zoll, J. G.: Osteomyelitis of cervical spine: Candida guilliermondii. Ann. Intern. Med., 79:748, 1973.
43. Oyston, J. K.: Madura foot. A study of twenty cases. J. Bone Joint Surg., 43-B:259, 1961.
44. Reeves, R. J., and Pedersen, R.: Fungus infection of bone. Radiology, 62:55, 1954.
45. Svirsky-Fein, S., Langer, L., Milbauer, B., Khermosh, O., and Rubinstein, E.: Neonatal osteomyelitis caused by Candida tropicalis. J. Bone Joint Surg., 61-A:455, 1979.
46. Tarreus, J. A., and Wood, M. M. W.: Streptomycin in the treatment of actinomycosis. Lancet, 1:1091, 1949.
47. Winter, W. G., Jr., and Larson, R. K.: Disseminated coccidioidomycosis in a child (letter). Am. J. Dis. Child., 129:1237, 1975.

VIRAL OSTEOMYELITIS

Osteomyelitis Variolosa

Now eradicated in the United States and Europe, smallpox is still endemic in other parts of the world. Two to five per cent of the children affected by smallpox virus also contract viral osteomyelitis.

The first reference to osteomyelitis variolosa was made by Bidder, in 1873.[2] Detailed reviews of the subject were given by Cockshott and MacGregor, as well as by Davidson and Palmer.[4, 8]

The severity of the initial smallpox infection and the degree of the bones changes cannot be correlated, as extensive osteomyelitis occurs in cases of relatively mild smallpox. The age distribution is between 9 months and 14 years. There is no definite sex predilection.

Bone changes are often symmetrical. Common sites of involvement include the bones about the elbow, the tibiae, and the fibulae. The hands and feet may be affected. The spine, pelvis, and ribs are usually not involved.

Clinically, the bone disease manifests itself 5 to 28 days after the onset of the rash. Local findings consist of periarticular swelling, and limited and painful motion of the adjacent joint. A varying degree of local pain and tenderness is present, but usually it is not marked. The bone lesions may be obvious in some cases, the radiograph depicting the typical changes of osteomyelitis; there is a lack of correlation between the radiographic findings and the clinical picture. The general well-being of the patient and the paucity of a systemic response are striking. Infection may extend to the nearby joint, which will be distended with effusion and will drain spontaneously through sinuses if not aspirated.

Radiograms in the early stages disclose soft-tissue swelling around joints with a band of rarefaction in the metaphysis. Soon subperiosteal new bone forms around the shaft, usually extending throughout its entire length (Fig. 3–230). The cortex beneath the subperiosteal new bone remains visible in its normal position and gradually merges with the periosteal reactive bone. Epiphyseal separation may result from the transverse metaphysitis. The small bones of the wrists, hands, and feet show patchy areas of rarefaction and distention with expansion of the bone itself.

The disease is self-limiting, but it has a slow course resulting in multiple deformities, ankylosis of the joints, and growth disturbance. There is no treatment. Antibiotics and chemotherapy do not prevent the development of osteomyelitis and in no way affect its outcome.[12] Surgery is not indicated. It is important to diagnose the condition in order to prevent unnecessary treatment.

Vaccinial Osteomyelitis

Bone lesions following vaccination against smallpox in a three-week-old boy were reported by Cochran, Connolly, and Thompson.[3] The clinical and radiographic picture resembled Caffey's infantile cortical hyperostosis. The scapula and mandible were involved, with transient local soft-tissue swelling. Radiograms disclosed subperiosteal new bone formation. Chronic in-

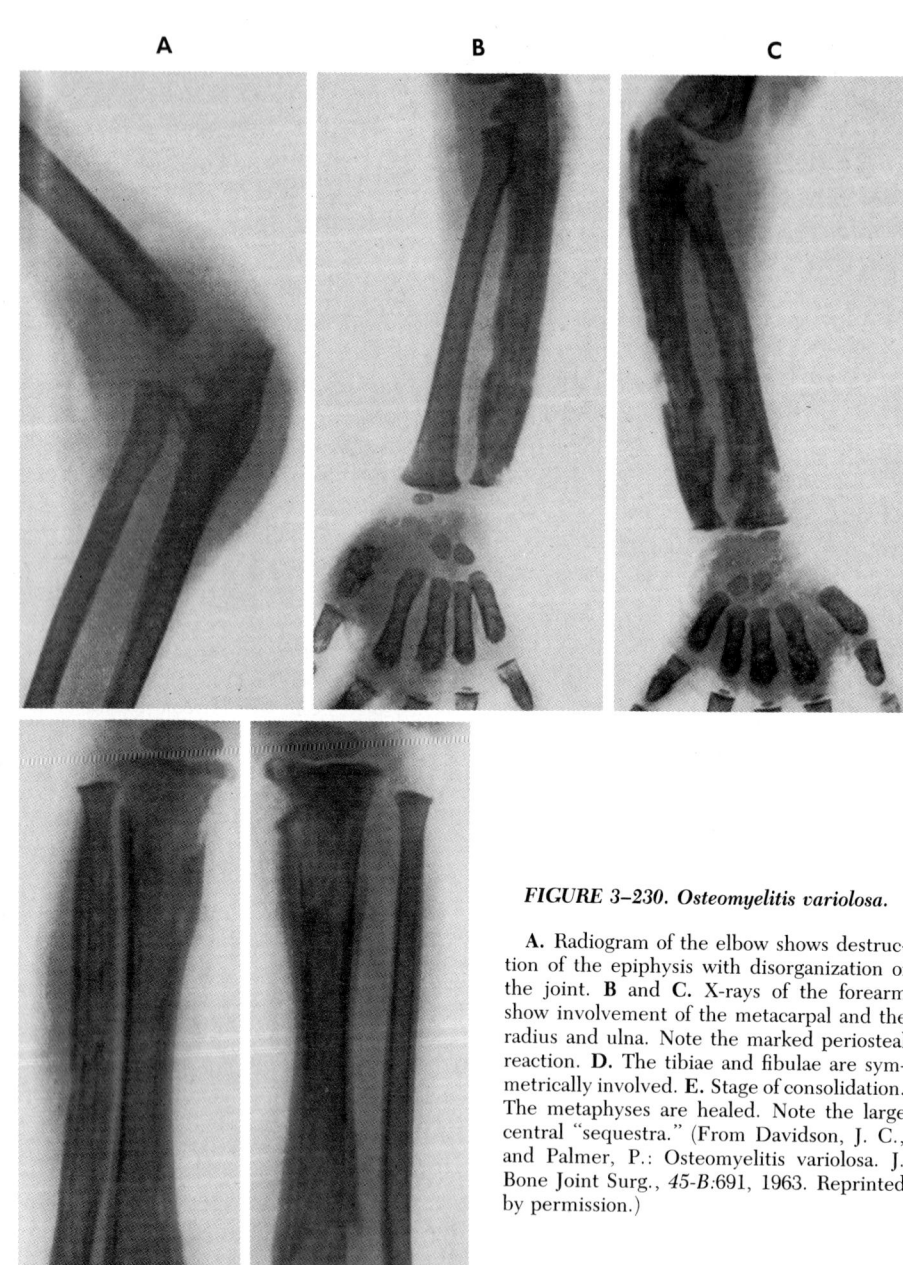

FIGURE 3–230. *Osteomyelitis variolosa.*

A. Radiogram of the elbow shows destruction of the epiphysis with disorganization of the joint. **B** and **C.** X-rays of the forearm show involvement of the metacarpal and the radius and ulna. Note the marked periosteal reaction. **D.** The tibiae and fibulae are symmetrically involved. **E.** Stage of consolidation. The metaphyses are healed. Note the large central "sequestra." (From Davidson, J. C., and Palmer, P.: Osteomyelitis variolosa. J. Bone Joint Surg., *45-B*:691, 1963. Reprinted by permission.)

flammatory change was found on histologic examination of biopsied tissue, and vaccinia virus was cultured from the lesion.

Cat-Scratch Fever

Cat-scratch fever may be complicated by osteomyelitis. Adams and Hindman reported lesions in the iliac bone in a five-year-old boy, and Collipp and Koch reported findings in the femoral neck in a four-year-old boy.[1, 6]

References

1. Adams, W. C., and Hindman, S. M.: Cat-scratch disease associated with osteolytic lesion. J. Pediatr., 44:665, 1954.
2. Bidder, A.: Zur Kenntniss der eitrigen Gelenktzundungen bei Variola. Deutsch. Z. Chir., 2:453, 1873.
3. Cochran, W., Connolly, J. H., and Thompson, I. D.: Bone involvement after vaccination against smallpox. Br. Med. J., 2:285, 1963.
4. Cockshott, P., and MacGregor, M.: Osteomyelitis variolosa. Q. J. Med., N.S., 27:369, 1958.
5. Cockshott, P., and MacGregor, M.: The natural history of osteomyelitis variolosa. J. Fac. Radiol., 10:57, 1959.
6. Collipp, P. J., and Koch, R.: Cat-scratch fever associated with an osteolytic lesion. N. Engl. J. Med., 260:278, 1959.
7. Davidson, J. C.: Sickle cell anaemia in an African child from Nyasaland. Cent. Afr. J. Med., 7:402, 1961.
8. Davidson, J. C., and Palmer, P. E. S.: Osteomyelitis variolosa. J. Bone Joint Surg., 45-B:687, 1963.
9. Middlemiss, H.: Tropical Radiology. London, Heinemann, 1962, pp. 11–13.
10. Neve, A.: Cases of bone disease after smallpox in young children. Lancet, 2:609, 1887.
11. Sharma, R.: Osteomyelitis variolosa during corticosteroid therapy. J. Indian Med. Assoc., 41:202, 1963.
12. Sword, J. M.: Smallpox in Central Province, Nyasaland. Br. Med. J., 5245:165, 1961.

CHRONIC GRANULOMATOUS DISEASE OF CHILDHOOD

Chronic granulomatous disease of childhood is a hereditary condition characterized by purulent granulomatous and eczematoid skin lesions, granulomatous lymphadenitis with suppuration, hepatosplenomegaly, recurrent slowly resolving pneumonias, and chronic osteomyelitis. The syndrome occurs in males and is transmitted as a sex-linked recessive trait. It is caused by an inability of the polymorphonuclear leukocytes and monocytes to destroy the pathogenic organisms adequately, although phagocytosis by the leukocytes is normal.

The primary concern of the orthopedist is with the bone manifestations of this syndrome.[29] The granulomatous infectious process involves the lungs, pleura, liver, spleen, lymph nodes, pericardium, genitourinary tract, and skeleton. The pathogenic bacteria are of relatively low-grade virulence; the common organisms are *Staphylococcus epidermidis, Staphylococcus aureus, Serratia marcescens,* and *Candida.* In the early stages of bone involvement, the usual clinical findings of osteomyelitis, such as pain, fever, erythema, local tenderness, and other signs of inflammation are absent. It is only during the late stages, when radiograms disclose extensive bone destruction, that the typical signs of osteomyelitis develop. Early in the course of the disease scintigraphy with gallium-67 will localize the inflammatory sites.

Small bones of the hands and feet are predilected sites of primary involvement, though infection may originate in the metaphysis of any long bone. Being of relatively low-grade virulence, the pathogenic organisms cause a granulomatous infection similar to tuberculous osteomyelitis.

In the radiogram, extensive bone destruction with widening of the affected bone and minimal reactive sclerosis is evident (Fig. 3–231). During continuous antibiotic therapy, osteomyelitis may continue to progress, and new areas of involvement may develop.

Long-term antibiotic therapy may eventually cure the osteomyelitic lesions. Surgical measures in the form of incision and drainage are indicated in some cases. The disease, however, is characterized by a protracted course with frequent recurrences and a poor prognosis, and progresses to eventual death in about 40 per cent of the affected children.

References

1. Baehner, R. L.: Disorders of leukocytosis leading to recurrent infection. Pediatr. Clin. North Am., 19:935, 1972.
2. Baehner, R. L.: Neutrophil dysfunction associated with states of chronic and recurrent infection. Pediatr. Clin. North Am., 2:377, 1980.
3. Bassani, F., Capsoni, F., Lazzarin, A., and Rossi, A.: Chronic granulomatous disease. Pediatr. Radiol., 11:105, 1981.
4. Berendes, H., Bridges, R. A., and Good, R. A.: A fatal granulomatosis of childhood. The clinical study of a new syndrome. Minn. Med., 40:309, 1957.
5. Bridges, R. A., Berendes, H., and Good, R. A.: A fatal granulomatosis disease of childhood. Am. J. Dis. Child., 97:387, 1959.
6. Buescher, E. S., and Gallin, J. I.: Leukocyte transfusions in chronic granulomatous disease: Persistence of transfused leukocytes in sputum. N. Engl. J. Med., 307:800, 1982.
7. Bujak, J. S., Kwon-Chung, K. J., and Chusid, M. J.: Osteomyelitis and pneumonia in a boy with chronic granulomatous disease of childhood caused by a mutant strain of Aspergillus nidulans. Am. J. Clin. Pathol., 61:361, 1974.

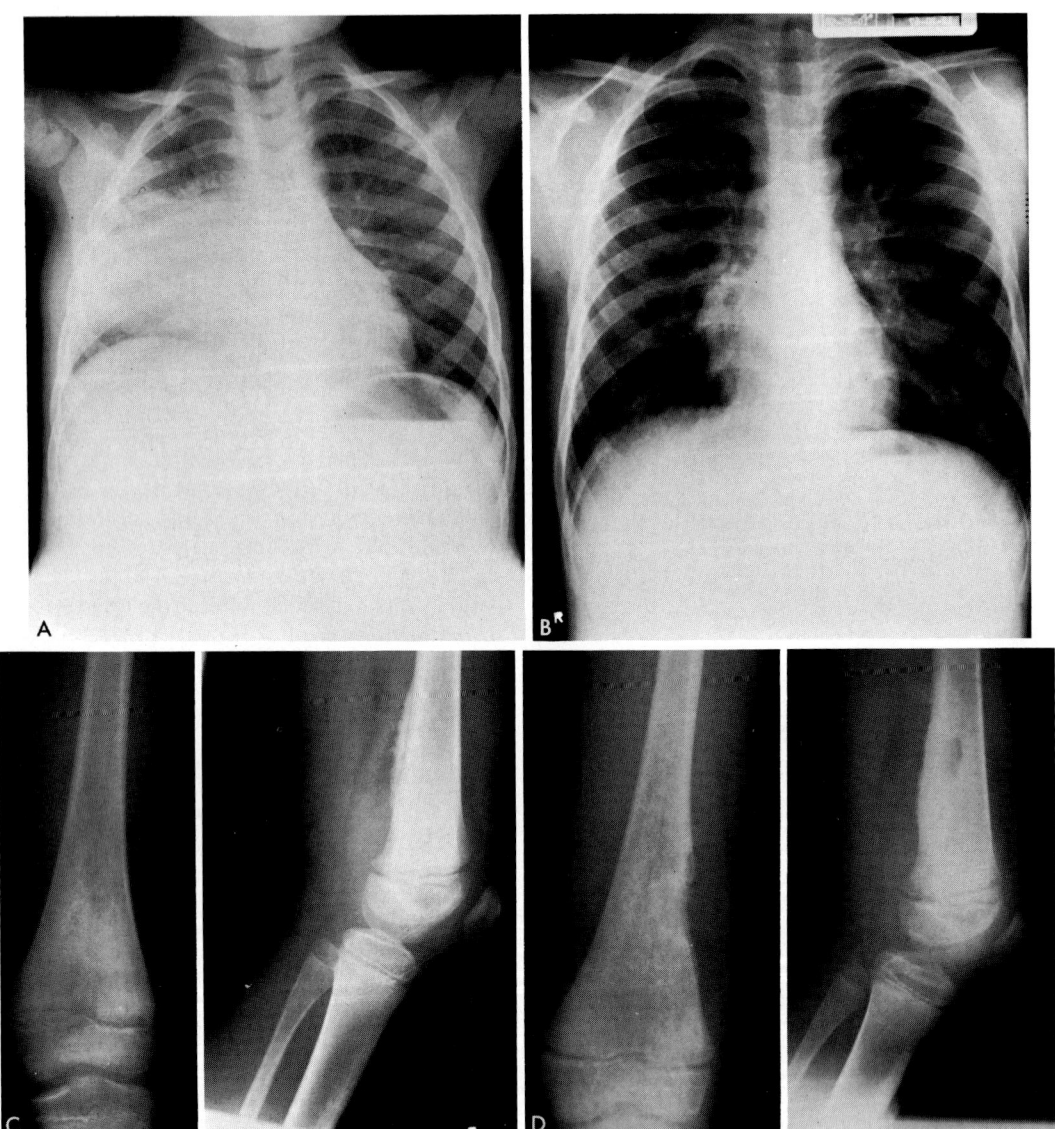

FIGURE 3–231. Chronic granulomatous disease of childhood in a five-year-old boy.

A. Radiogram of chest. There is pneumonia of right middle lobe, which was treated with antibiotics. **B.** Radiogram of chest at nine years of age shows that lung lesions have resolved; however, he complained of pain in right thigh and knee. There was inguinal lymphadenopathy and hepatosplenomegaly. **C.** Anteroposterior and lateral radiograms of right knee and distal femur disclose areas of rarefaction and sclerosis in the femoral shaft and metaphyses, with periosteal new bone formation. Granulomatous tissue was found on biopsy of the lesion. **D.** Postoperative radiograms four months later.

8. Carson, J. J., Chadwick, D. L., Brubaker, D. A., Cleland, R. A., and Landing, B. H.: Thirteen boys with progressive septic granulomatosis. Pediatrics, 35:405, 1965.
9. Davis, W. C., Huber, H., Douglas, S. D., and Fudenburg, H. H.: A defect in circulating mononuclear phagocytes in chronic granulomatous disease in childhood. J. Immunol., 101:1093, 1968.
10. Foroozanfar, N., Lucas, C. F., Joss, D. V., Hugh-Jones, K., and Hobbs, J. R.: Ascorbate (1 g/day) does not help the phagocyte killing defect of X-linked chronic granulomatous disease. Clin. Exp. Immunol., 51:99, 1983.
11. Good, R. A., Quie, P. G., Windhorst, D. B., Page, A. R., Rodey, G. E., White, J., Wolfson, J. J., and Holmes, D. B.: Fatal granulomatous disease of childhood. A hereditary defect of leukocyte function. Semin Hematol., 5:215, 1968.
12. Hartenberg, M. A., and Kodroff, M. B.: Chronic granulomatous disease of childhood. Probable diffuse gastric involvement. Pediatr. Radiol., 14:57, 1984.
13. Holmes, B., Quie, P. G., Windhorst, D. B., and Good, R. A.: Fatal granulomatous disease of childhood. An inborn abnormality of phagocytic function. Lancet, 1:1225, 1966.
14. Holmes, B., Page, A. R., Windhorst, D. B., Quie, P. G., and Good, R. A.: The metabolic pattern and phagocytic function of leukocytes from children with chronic granulomatous disease. Ann. N.Y. Acad. Sci., 155:888, 1968.
15. Johnston, R. B., Jr., and Baehner, R. L.: Chronic granulomatous disease: Correlation between pathogenesis and clinical findings. Pediatrics, 48:730, 1971.
16. Johnston, R. B., Jr., and McMurray, J. S.: Chronic familial granulomatosis. Am. J. Dis. Child., 114:370, 1967.
17. McFarland, P. S., Speirs, A. L., and Sommerville, R. G.: Fatal granulomatous disease of childhood and benign lymphocytic infiltration of the skin (congenital dysphagocytosis). Lancet, 1:408, 1967.
18. Matamoros, N., North, M. E., Ciria, L., and Webster, A. D.: Chronic granulomatous disease with normal neutrophil glutathione peroxidase activity in a brother and sister. Acta Paediatr. Scand., 71:327, 1982.
19. Mendelsohn, H. B., and Berant, M.: Chronic granulomatous disease: A new clinical variant. Acta Paediatr. Scand., 71:869, 1982.
20. Papanicolaou, N., Curnutto, J. T., Nathan, D. G., Treves, S.: Gallium-67 scintigraphy in children with chronic granulomatous disease. Pediatr. Radiol., 13:137, 1983.
21. Payne, N. R., Hays, N. T., Regelmann, W. E., Sorenson, M., Mills, E. L., and Quie, P. G.: Growth in patients with chronic granulomatous disease. J. Pediatr., 102:397, 1983.
22. Quie, P. G., White, J. G., Holmes, B., and Good, R. A.: Decreased bacteriocidal activity in polymorphonuclear leukocytes in children with chronic granulomatous disease (abstr.). J. Clin. Invest., 45:1058, 1966.
23. Quie, P. G., White, J. G., Holmes, B., and Good, R. A.: In vitro bacteriocidal capacity of human polymorphonuclear leukocytes: Diminished activity in chronic granulomatous disease of childhood. J. Clin. Invest., 46:668, 1967.
24. Quie, P. G., Kaplan, E. L., Page, A. R., Gruskay, F. L., and Malawista, S. E.: Defective polymorphonuclear leukocyte function and chronic granulomatous disease in two female children. N. Engl. J. Med., 278:976, 1968.
25. Robinson, M. F., McGregor, R., Collins, R., and Cheung, K.: Combined neutrophil and T-cell deficiency: Initial report of a kindred with features of the hyper-IgE syndrome and chronic granulomatous disease. Am. J. Med., 73:63, 1982.
26. Schmidt, W. F., III, Poncz, M., Russell, M. O., and Schwartz, E.: Unusual manifestations of chronic granulomatous disease. Am. J. Dis. Child., 135:376, 1981.
27. Windhorst, D. B., Page, A. R., Holmes, B., Quie, P. G., and Good, R. A.: The pattern of genetic transmission of the leukocyte defect in fatal granulomatous disease of childhood. J. Clin. Invest., 47:1026, 1968.
28. Wolfson, J. J., Quie, P. G., Laxdal, S. D., and Good, R. A.: Roentgenologic manifestations in children with a genetic defect of polymorphonuclear leukocyte function. Chronic granulomatous disease of childhood. Radiology, 91:37, 1968.
29. Wolfson, J. J., Kane, W. J., Laxdal, S. D., Good, R. A., and Quie, P. G.: Bone findings in chronic granulomatous disease of childhood. J. Bone Joint Surg., 51-A:1573, 1969.

Bone Manifestations of Hematologic Disorders

ANEMIA

Fanconi's Anemia

Congenital aplastic anemia in association with multiple deformities was reported by Fanconi in 1927.[2] This rare condition is familial and is most probably inherited as an autosomal recessive trait. The skeletal deformities are common, with aplasia or hypoplasia of the radius, first metacarpal, and thumb being the most consistent associated anomalies. Congenital dislocation of the hip, syndactyly, and angular deformities or shortening of long bones may also occur. Nonskeletal anomalies include hyperpigmentation of the skin, microcephaly, mental retardation, congenital strabismus, deafness, hypogonadism, and malformations of the urinary tract.[2, 9]

The erythropoietic failure is usually not recognized at birth. It manifests itself during the first years of life by the symptoms of easy bleeding and recurrent infection. Hematologic studies will disclose the severe anemia, granulocytopenia, and thrombocytopenia. Not infrequently, the orthopedic surgeon is consulted initially because of the skeletal deformities. Anomalies of the thumb, first metacarpal, or radius should arouse suspicion of Fanconi's aplastic anemia.[8]

Treatment consists of transfusion of whole blood and antibiotics. Corticosteroids have been shown to have no effect. The prognosis is poor, with death occurring from uncontrolled infection or from intracerebral or gastrointestinal bleeding. On occasion, some affected children with hypoplastic anemia do well, requiring orthopedic treatment of their skeletal deformities.

References

1. Dawson, J. P.: Congenital pancytopenia associated with multiple congenital anomalies (Fanconi type): Review of the literature and report of a twenty-year-old female with a 10-year follow-up and apparently good response to splenectomy. Pediatrics, 15:325, 1955.
2. Fanconi, G.: Familiäre infantile pernizöseähnliche Anämie (Perniziöses Blutbild und Konstitution). Jahrb. Kinderheilkd., 117:257, 1927.
3. Juhl, H., Wesenberg, R. L., and Gwinn, J. L.: Roentgenographic findings in Fanconi's anemia. Radiology, 89:646, 1967.
4. Kwee, M. L., Poll, E. H., van de Kamp, J. J., deKoenig, H., Eriksson, A. W., and Joenje, H.: Unusual response to bifunctional alkylating agents in a case of Fanconi's anaemia. Hum. Genet., 64:384, 1983.
5. Lazzaroni Fossati, F., de Toni, T., Cavaliere, G., Gastaldi, R., and Balzarini, C.: Caratteristiche fentipiche della'anemia di Fanconi. Presentazione di un caso e revisione della letteratura. Minerva Pediatr., 35:943, 1983.
6. McDonald, R., and Goldschmidt, B.: Pancytopenia with congenital defects (Fanconi's anemia). Arch. Dis. Child., 35:367, 1960.
7. Minagi, H., and Steinbach, H. L.: Roentgen appearance of anomalies associated with hypoplastic anemias of childhood: Fanconi's anemia and congenital hypoplastic anemia (erythrogenesis imperfecta). A.J.R., 97:100, 1966.
8. Moseley, J. E.: Bone Changes in Hematologic Disorders. New York, Grune & Stratton, 1963.
9. Silver, H. K., Blair, W. C., and Kempe, C. H.: Fanconi syndrome: Multiple congenital anomalies with hypoplastic anemia. Am. J. Dis. Child., 83:14, 1952.

Hemoglobinopathies

The principal abnormal hemoglobins that cause clinical manifestations of interest to the orthopedic surgeon are hemoglobin S, hemoglobin C, and the beta-thalassemia type. In this section only sickle cell disease and thalassemia are discussed.

Thalassemias (Cooley's Anemia or Mediterranean Anemia)

The thalassemias, first reported by Cooley in 1927, are a group of familial chronic microcytic hemolytic anemias that result from impaired production of adult hemoglobin (Hgb. A).[10] Beta-thalassemia, the most common form, is caused by deficient synthesis of beta-polypeptide chains. Initially, the disease was found only in natives of the Mediterranean area, particularly Greece, Italy, and Sicily. In the past three decades, however, it has been described in persons of Negro, Jewish, Oriental, and various European origins. The exact mechanism of its inheritance has not yet been delineated.[25] Thalassemia major, however, is most probably inherited as a recessive trait.[24]

The disease occurs in two forms, thalassemia major and minor, corresponding to the homozygous and heterozygous genotypes. Recently, a third type, thalassemia intermedia, has been described, the clinical manifestations of which are between those of thalassemia major and thalassemia minor.

Thalassemia Minor. In this heterozygous form the condition is asymptomatic, and the affected children have normal longevity. The only findings are a mild anemia (the average hemoglobin concentration being 2 to 3 gm. per 100 ml. lower than normal), with moderate hypochromia, anisocytosis, poikilocytosis, and at times, slight splenomegaly.

Thalassemia Major. The homozygous type is characterized by severe progressive hemolytic anemia and jaundice that manifests itself between 6 and 12 months of age. The skin is muddy yellow initially, owing to anemia and jaundice, but later on, it takes on a greenish-brown color. Splenomegaly and hepatomegaly result from extramedullary hematopoiesis and hemosiderosis. The facies is mongoloid, owing to intramedullary expansion and enlargement of the facial bones. Malocclusion of the teeth and jaw develops from expansion of the upper and lower maxillae. Growth is impaired. Thinning of the bones may lead to pathologic fractures.

The hematologic findings consist of severe hypochromia, marked microcytosis, and the presence of numerous bizarre, fragmented poikilocytes and target cells. The hemoglobin level in the untreated case progressively decreases to less than 5 gm. per 100 ml. There are large amounts of fetal hemoglobin in the red cells.

The characteristic changes become manifest in the radiograms during the second year of life and become more clearly defined with increasing age. The entire skeleton is affected. The long and short tubular bones are distended and dilated by the hyperplastic marrow. The trabeculae in the spongiosa are irregular and coarse. The cortex is thinned from internal resorption and may bulge outward (Fig. 3–232). In the skull, the diploic space is widened, the outer table is thinned, and the trabeculae are aligned in a radial pattern in the spongiosa, giving the "hair-on-end" appearance shown in Figure 3–232. Premature fusion of the epiphyseal ossification centers, particularly those of the proximal humerus and distal femur, has been reported by Currarino and Erlandson.[11]

During adolescence the bone lesions in the ribs begin to regress, whereas, in the trunk, they persist because of physiologic changes in the marrow of the skeleton that occur with advancing age.

Transfusion is the only method of treatment.

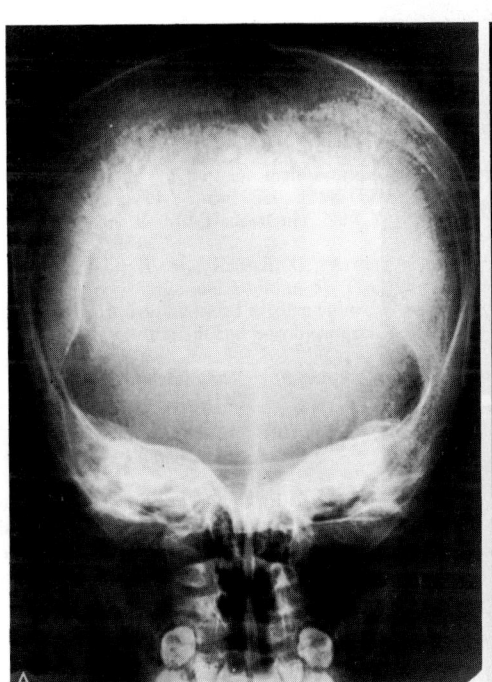
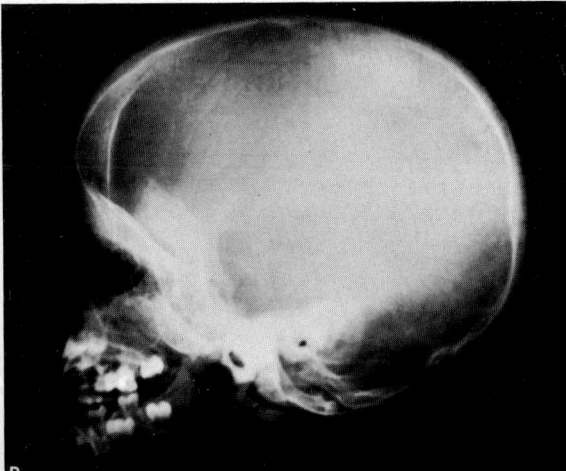
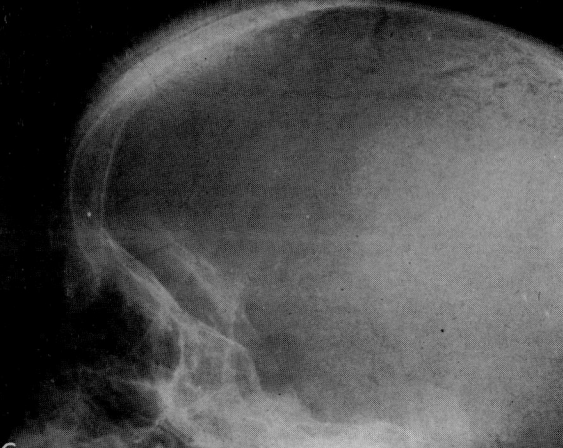

FIGURE 3–232. Skeletal changes in Cooley's anemia.

A to C. Radiograms of the skull. The diploic spaces are widened and the outer table is thinned. Note the "hair-on-end" appearance.

Illustration continued on following page

The term *sickle cell disease* also includes conditions in which the abnormal hemoglobin-S is combined with other types of abnormal hemoglobin, such as C, D, and E. These are referred to as mixed hemoglobinopathies. Hemoglobin-S may be associated with other types of hereditary diseases such as thalassemia (sickle cell thalassemia disease), spherocytosis, or ovalocytosis.

SKELETAL MANIFESTATIONS

The osseous manifestations caused by sickle cell disease may be divided into the following five groups.[26, 55]

Changes Due to Marrow Hyperplasia. Erythroid hyperplasia results from hypoxia caused by the extensive hemolysis of the abnormal and fragile sickle cells. Resorption of the bone trabeculae in the spongiosa takes place, the cortex thins, the medullary cavity widens, with sparse trabecular pattern, and the bones have an increased radiolucency. Reactive new bone formation may cause coarsening of the trabeculae.

In children, these changes are found where there is active marrow, i.e., the skull, vertebral column, pelvis, and long and short tubular bones. In the older adolescent and adult, the changes in the limbs become less pronounced as the marrow undergoes fatty change with increasing age.

In the skull, a "ground glass" appearance is given by the loss of trabecular pattern, the diploic space is widened, and the outer table is thinned. The so-called "hair-on-end" appearance of the skull, so typical of Cooley's anemia, is less common in sickle cell disease.

The height of the vertebrae becomes reduced, and the intervertebral discs bulge into the bodies (Fig. 3–233 A). Widening of the trabecular pattern, osteoporosis, and cortical thinning are also seen in the ribs, pelvis, and other flat bones, as well as in the metacarpals and metatarsals.

Changes Due to Infarction. Accumulation of the sequestered sickle cells in the vascular channels causes anoxia and aseptic necrosis. Any bone may be affected. The femoral head is most often involved, and the avascular changes resemble Legg-Perthes disease (Fig. 3–233 B to E). In sickle cell disease, however, the avascular changes are less extensive, sparing the lateral third of the head and occurring just prior to closure of the capital epiphysis, in contrast to Legg-Perthes disease, which is encountered in the four to ten age group. The head of the humerus may also be affected. Vertebral bodies may collapse partially or totally following avascular necrosis.

The shafts of long bones, particularly the femur, may undergo necrosis. Clinically, there may be localized soft-tissue swelling and tenderness, with systemic reactions of fever and leukocytosis. The radiograms disclose patchy areas of bone destruction and periosteal new bone formation resembling osteomyelitis. Laboratory findings will differentiate the two conditions. With repair, the regional cortex will thicken, and the medullary cavity will be occupied by new bone, which will give a chalky appearance in the radiogram.

In infants between 6 and 12 months of age, the short tubular bones of the hands and feet may be involved, a condition that has been termed "the hand-foot syndrome."[42, 48, 76, 77] The hands and feet are painful and swollen. The symptoms, usually precipitated by cold weather, last for one to two weeks. Initially, radiograms may be normal, but within two or three weeks, patchy areas of bone destruction and periosteal reaction are evident. Involvement is often multiple and diffuse (Fig. 3–234 and 3–235). Soon repair processes take place by "creeping substitution," and within four to six months the radiograms will appear to be normal. Attacks may recur. The hands and feet are spared after the sixth year of life, and the long bones become affected.

Changes Due to Disturbance of Growth. Retardation of growth is common in patients with sickle cell disease. Skeletal age is retarded, sexual maturation is delayed, and stature is short. This may be due to the chronic anemia, infarction of the epiphyses, or osteomyelitis. Golding and associates reported 48 of 51 patients with sickle cell disease to have diminished stature.[26] Kyphosis due to compression of vertebrae is another factor causing shortening of the trunk.[7, 45, 73, 78]

Changes Due to Osteomyelitis. Bone infection due to salmonella and related strains is not uncommon in sickle cell disease. It should be differentiated from the sickle cell crisis, in which the affected part is hot and swollen and there are associated fever and leukocytosis. Bone infarction should also be distinguished from osteomyelitis. In infection there is often a symmetrical intracortical longitudinal fissuring. There is evidence of sequestration and involucrum formation. There may be the soft-tissue change of subperiosteal elevation. Scintigraphy with technetium-99m or gallium-47 does not distinguish the two conditions. Technetium-99m will show focal areas of diminished activity at sites of bone infarct. In the early phases, however, there may be increased activity due to the hyperemic response as a result of the

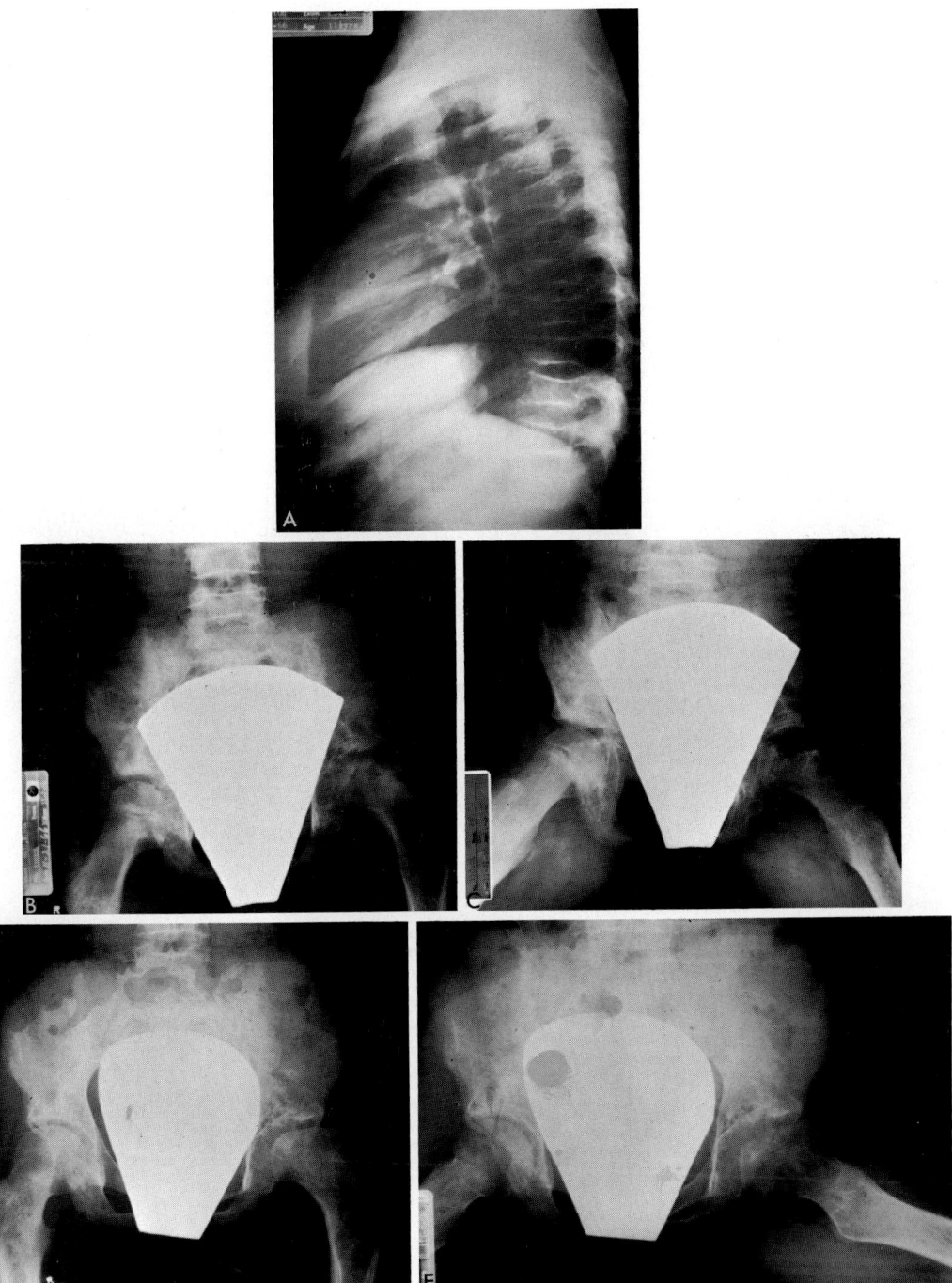

FIGURE 3–233. *Sickle cell disease in an 11-year-old girl.*

A. Lateral radiogram of the spine showing reduction in the height of the vertebrae. **B** and **C.** Anteroposterior and lateral radiograms of the hips. Note the avascular changes in the left femoral head. **D** and **E.** Three years later, radiograms show healing of left capital femoral epiphysis. The coxa magna deformity is evident.

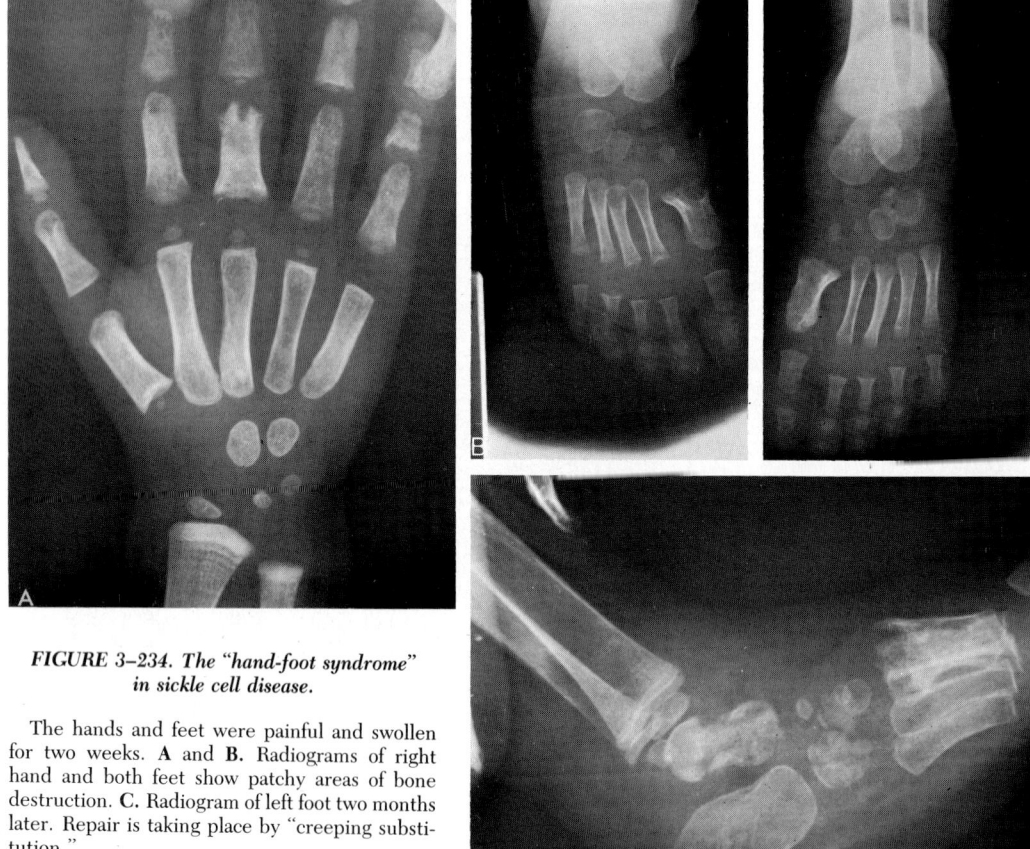

FIGURE 3-234. The "hand-foot syndrome" in sickle cell disease.

The hands and feet were painful and swollen for two weeks. **A** and **B**. Radiograms of right hand and both feet show patchy areas of bone destruction. **C**. Radiogram of left foot two months later. Repair is taking place by "creeping substitution."

FIGURE 3–235. The "hand-foot syndrome" in sickle cell disease in an eight-month-old infant.

Radiograms of hands and feet reveal diffuse involvement of the short tubular bones with patchy areas of destruction and some periosteal reaction.

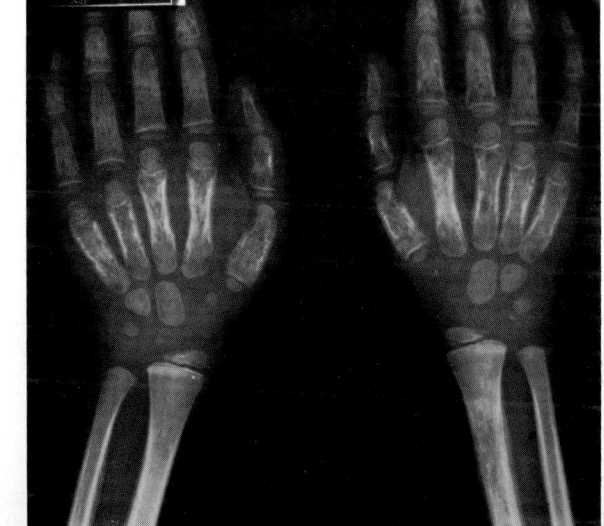

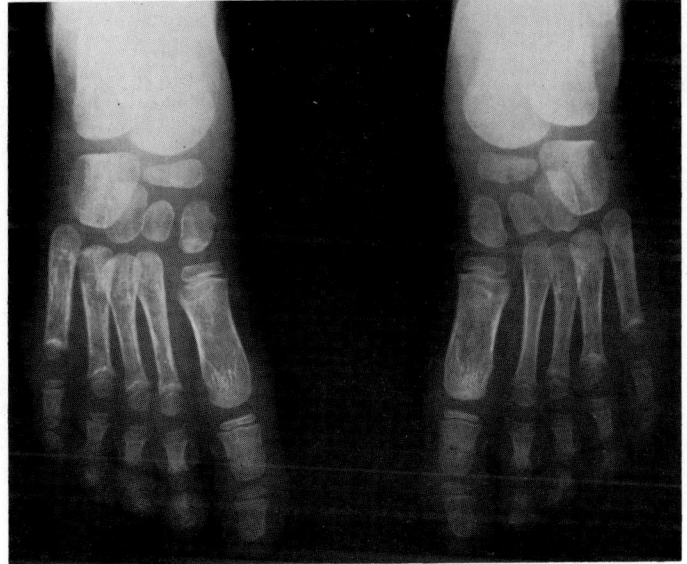

establishment of pathways for collateral circulation. This revascularization of the infarct will manifest itself on the bone scan as patchy areas of increased activity and will obscure focal areas of hyperactivity when the infarct is complicated by osteomyelitis. Therefore, bone scan with technetium-99m is of dubious value in the diagnosis of osteomyelitis in sickle cell disease.[2, 39, 46] CT scanning and magnetic resonance imaging may assist in detecting the involucrum and bone abscess.

Pathologic Fractures. These may occur spontaneously or following minimal injury in the long bones and vertebrae, being caused by diminished strength of the osteoporotic bone. On occasion, however, fracture may occur through an infarcted area.

TREATMENT

Because of the high incidence in the black population, a sickle cell preparation should be performed before any surgical procedure is undertaken. If the preparation demonstrates the presence of the sickling trait, a hemoglobin electrophoresis should be performed preoperatively.

This varies according to the bone manifestation. *Hand-foot syndrome* (sickle-cell dactylitis) is managed conservatively. Use of antibiotics is of doubtful value. Operative intervention is not indicated.

Avascular necrosis, especially of the femoral head, presents a very difficult problem. One may follow the same principles of containment as outlined for Legg-Perthes disease, but in such a chronic condition its value is doubtful. Surgical measures for containment, such as varus derotation osteotomy of the femur or innominate osteotomy, should be undertaken with trepidation. The painful incongruous hip in the adolescent may be treated by Chiari's pelvic osteotomy as a temporizing measure. Often, in these hips, the disease will progress to severe stiff degenerative arthritis, and total joint replacement may be required. It is recommended that the surgeon assess all factors and be very selective.

Osteomyelitis is treated by the appropriate antibiotic therapy, chloramphenicol being the most effective drug. Occasionally, incision and drainage is required, in which case primary closure is recommended. The wounds should not be left open for drainage. Septic arthritis, especially of the hip, should be operated on and decompressed immediately. *Acute polyarthritis* may occur without bacterial infection. The joint is aspirated to rule out sepsis. If the problem is nonspecific synovitis, treatment is nonoperative with splinting, exercise, and protection from weight-bearing.

In general, tourniquet ischemia during surgery should be avoided. Other measures to minimize the chance of sickling during surgery are maintaining a high oxygen level in the blood, adequate hydration, blood volume, and normal body temperature during the operation. Transfusions of packed normal erythrocytes are of great value; it is desirable that the percentage of hemoglobin-S be less than 45 per cent.

References

1. Almklov, J. R., Hansen, A. E., and Schneider, M.: Long bone involvement in sickle-cell anemia. Pediatrics, 5:204, 1950.
2. Amundsen, T. R., Siegel, M. J., and Siegel, B. A.: Osteomyelitis and infarction in sickle cell hemoglobinopathies; differentiation by combined technetium and gallium scintigraphy. J. Nucl. Med., 22:322, 1981.
3. Bentley, P. G., and Howard, E. R.: Surgery in children with homozygous sickle cell anemia. Ann. R. Coll. Surg. Engl., 61:55, 1979.
4. Black, P. H., Kunz, L. J., and Schwartz, M. N.: Salmonellosis—a review of some unusual aspects. N. Engl. J. Med., 262:811, 1960.
5. Bohrer, S. P.: Acute long bone diaphyseal infarcts in sickle cell disease. Br. J. Radiol., 43:685, 1970.
6. Bohrer, S. P.: Fracture complicating bone infarcts and/or osteomyelitis in sickle-cell disease. Clin. Radiol., 22:83, 1971.
7. Bohrer, S. P.: Growth disturbance of the distal femur following sickle cell bone infarcts and/or osteomyelitis. Clin. Radiol., 25:221, 1974.
8. Buchman, J.: Sickle cell disease simulating osteomyelitis. Bull. Hosp. Joint Dis., 10:239, 1949.
9. Carrington, H. T., Ferguson, A. P., and Scott, R. B.: Studies in sickle-cell anemia—bone involvement simulating aseptic necrosis. A.M.A.J. Dis. Child., 95:157, 1958.
10. Carroll, D. S., and Evans, J. W.: Roentgen findings in sickle-cell anemia. Radiology, 53:834, 1949.
11. Carroll, D. S.: Roentgen manifestations of sickle cell disease. South. Med. J., 50:1486, 1957.
12. Chavhan, P. M., Kondlapoodi, P., and Natta, C. L.: Pathology of sickle cell disorders. Pathol. Annu., 2:253, 1983.
13. Chung, S. M. K., and Ralston, E. L.: Necrosis of the femoral head associated with sickle-cell anemia and its genetic variants. A review of the literature and study of thirteen cases. J. Bone Joint Surg., 51-A:33, 1969.
14. Chung, S. M., Alavi, A., and Russell, M. O.: Management of osteonecrosis in sickle cell anemia and its growth variants. Clin. Orthop., 130:158, 1978.
15. Cockshott, W. P.: Dactylitis and growth disorders. Br. J. Radiol., 36:19, 1963.
16. Constant, E., Green, R. L., Wagner, D. K.: Salmonella osteomyelitis of both hands and the hand-foot syndrome. Arch. Surg., 102:148, 1971.
17. Danford, E. A., Marr, R., and Elsey, E. C.: Sickle cell anemia. With unusual bone changes. A.J.R., 45:223, 1941.
18. DeTorregrosa, M. V., Dapena, R. B., Hernandez, H., and Ortiz, A.: Association of salmonella-caused osteomyelitis and sickle-cell disease. J.A.M.A., 174:354, 1960.
19. Diggs, L. W.: Sickle cell crises. Am. J. Clin. Pathol., 44:1, 1965.

20. Diggs, L. W., Pullman, H. N., and King, J. C.: The bone changes in sickle-cell anemia. South. Med. J., 30:249, 1937.
21. Ebing, W. W.: The treatment of severely ill patients with sickle cell anemia and associated septic arthritis. Clin. Orthop., 149:145, 1980.
22. Ebing, W. W.: The treatment of chronic osteomyelitis in sickle cell anemia. Int. Surg., 67:361, 1982.
23. Engh, C. A., Hughes, H., Abrams, R. C., and Bowerman, J. C.: Osteomyelitis in the patient with sickle cell disease. J. Bone Joint Surg., 53-A:1, 1971.
24. Gelpi, A. P., and Perrine, R. P.: Sickle cell disease and trait in white population. J.A.M.A., 224:605, 1973.
25. Golding, J. S. R.: Conditions of the hip associated with hemoglobinopathies. Clin. Orthop., 90:22, 1973.
26. Golding, J. S. R., MacIver, J. E., and Went, L. N.: The bone changes in sickle-cell anaemia and its genetic variants. J. Bone Joint Surg., 41-B:711, 1959.
27. Gunderson, C., D'Ambrosia, R. D., and Shoji, H.: Total hip replacement in patients with sickle-cell disease. J. Bone Joint Surg., 59-A:760, 1976.
28. Hamburg, A. E.: Skeletal changes in sickle-cell anemia. J. Bone Joint Surg., 32-A:893, 1950.
29. Hanissian, A. S., and Silverman, A.: Arthritis of sickle cell anemia. South. Med. J., 67:28, 1974.
30. Harcke, H. T., Capitanio, M. A., and Naiman, J. L.: Sternal infarction in sickle-cell anemia: Concise communication. J. Nucl. Med., 22:322, 1981.
31. Henkin, W. A.: Collapse of the vertebral bodies in sickle cell anemia. A.J.R., 62:395, 1949.
32. Hook, E. W., Campbell, C. G., Weens, H. S., and Cooper, G. R.: Salmonella osteomyelitis in patients with sickle-cell anemia. N. Engl. J. Med., 257:403, 1957.
33. Hughes, J. G., and Carroll, D. S.: Salmonella osteomyelitis complicating sickle cell disease. Pediatrics, 19:184, 1957.
34. Huisman, T. H.: Sickle cell anemia: A review of diagnosis features. Am. J. Hematol., 6:173, 1979.
35. Ivy, R. E., and Howard, F. H.: Sickle cell anemia with unusual bone changes. Pediatrics, 43:312, 1953.
36. Janik, J., and Seeler, R. A.: Perioperative management of children with sickle hemoglobinopathy. J. Pediatr. Surg., 15:117, 1980.
37. Keeley, K., and Buchanan, G. R.: Acute infarction of long bones in children with sickle cell anemia. J. Pediatr., 101:170, 1982.
38. Kimmelstiel, P.: Vascular occlusion and ischemia infarction in sickle cell disease. Am. J. Med. Sci., 216:11, 1948.
39. Koren, A., Fedchteyn, S., and Katsuni, E.: Early diagnosis of bone infarction in children with sickle cell anemia by MDP 99m Tc scanning. Harefuah, 102:182, 1982.
40. Koren, A., Garty, I., and Katzuni, E.: Bone infarction in children with sickle-cell disease: Early diagnosis and differentiation from osteomyelitis. Eur. J. Pediatr., 142:93, 1984.
41. Kramer, M. S., Rooks, Y., and Pearson, H. A.: Growth and development in children with sickle cell trait. A prospective study of matched pairs. N. Engl. J. Med., 299:686, 1978.
42. Lambotte, C.: Hand-foot syndrome in sickle cell disease (letter). Am. J. Dis. Child., 104:200, 1962.
43. Landesman, S. H., Rao, S. P., and Ahonkhai, V. I.: Infections in children with sickle cell anemia. Special reference to pneumococcal and salmonella infections. Am. J. Pediatr. Hematol. Oncol., 4:407, 1982.
44. Legant, O., and Ball, R. P.: Sickle-cell anemia in adults. Roentgenographic findings. Radiology, 51:665, 1948.
45. Luban, N. L., Leikin, S. L., and August, G. A.: Growth and development in sickle cell anemia. Preliminary report. Am. J. Pediatr. Hematol. Oncol., 4:61, 1982.
46. Lutzker, L. J., and Alavi, A.: Bone imaging in sickle cell disease. Semin. Nucl. Med., 6:83, 1976.
47. McIntosh, S., Rooks, Y., Ritchey, A. K., and Pearson, H. A.: Fever in young children with sickle cell disease. J. Pediatr., 96:199, 1980.
48. Macht, S. H., and Roman, P. W.: The radiological changes in sickle cell anemia. Radiology, 51:697, 1948.
49. Middlemiss, J. H., and Raper, A. B.: Skeletal changes in haemoglobinopathies. J. Bone Joint Surg., 48-B:693, 1966.
50. Morrison, J. C., Whybrew, W. D., and Bucovaz, E. T.: Use of partial exchange transfusion preoperatively in patients with sickle cell hemoglobinopathies. Am. J. Obstet. Gynecol., 132:59, 1978.
51. Moseley, J. E.: Patterns of bone change in the sickle cell states. J. Mt. Sinai Hosp., 26:424, 1959.
52. Moseley, J. E., and Manley, J. B.: Aseptic necrosis of bone in sickle cell disease. Radiology, 60:656, 1953.
53. Nachamie, B. A., and Dorfman, H. D.: Ischemic necrosis of bone in sickle cell trait. Mt. Sinai J. Med. N.Y., 41:527, 1974.
54. Nachamie, B. A., and Neel, J. V.: The inheritance of sickle cell anemia. Science, 110:64, 1949.
55. O'Hara, A. E.: Roentgenographic osseous manifestations of the anemias and the leukemias. Clin. Orthop., 52:63, 1967.
56. Pauling, L., Itano, H. A., Singer, S. J., and Wells, I. C.: Sickle cell anemia, a molecular disease. Science, 110:543, 1949.
57. Phebus, C. K., Gloninger, M. F., and Maciak, B. J.: Growth patterns by age and sex in children with sickle cell disease. J. Pediatr., 105:28, 1984.
58. Porter, F. S., and Thurman, W. G.: Studies of sickle cell disease. Diagnosis in infancy. Am. J. Dis. Child., 106:35, 1963.
59. Reynolds, J.: The Roentgenological Features of Sickle Cell Disease and Related Hemoglobinopathies. Springfield, Ill., Thomas, 1965.
60. Reynolds, J. Pritchard, J. A., Tudders, D., and Mason, R. A.: Roentgenographic and clinical appraisal of sickle cell beta-thalassemia disease. A.J.R., 118:378, 1973.
61. Rothchild, B. M., and Sebes, J. I.: Calcaneal abnormalities and erosive bone disease associated with sickle cell anemia. Am. J. Med., 71:427, 1981.
62. Rowe, C. W., and Haggar, M. E.: Bone infarcts in sickle cell anemia. Radiology, 68:661, 1957.
63. Sain, A., Sham, R., and Silver, L.: Bone scan in sickle cell crisis. Clin. Nucl. Med., 3:85, 1978.
64. Schuer, H. K., Swan, J. L., and Clement, D. H.: Salmonella osteomyelitis and abnormal haemoglobin disease. Pediatrics, 20:439, 1957.
65. Scott, R. B.: Sickle cell anemia—pathogenesis and treatment. Pediatr. Clin. North Am., 9:649, 1962.
66. Sebes, J. I., and Brown, D. L.: Terminal phalangeal sclerosis in sickle cell disease. A.J.R., 140:763, 1983.
67. Sergeant, G. R., Ashcroft, M. T., and Miller, P. F.: The clinical features of hemoglobin S.C. disease in Jamaica. Br. J. Haematol., 24:491, 1973.
68. Smith, C. H.: Blood Disease of Infancy and Childhood. St. Louis, Mosby, 1960, p. 256.
69. Smith, E. W., and Conley, C. L.: Clinical features of the genetic variants or sickle cell disease. Bull. Johns Hopkins Hosp., 94:289, 1954.
70. Smith, J. A.: Management of sickle cell disease: Progress during the past 10 years. Am. J. Pediatr. Hematol. Oncol., 5:360, 1983.
71. Specht, E. E.: Hemoglobinopathic salmonella osteomyelitis. Orthopedic aspects. Clin. Orthop., 79:110, 1971.
72. Stein, R. E., and Urbaniak, J.: Use of the tourniquet during surgery in patients with sickle cell hemoglobinopathies. Clin. Orthop., 151:231, 1980.
73. Stevens, M. C., Padwick, M., and Sergeant, G. R.: Observations on the natural history of dactylitis in

homozygous sickle cell disease. Clin. Pediatr., 20:311, 1981.
74. Trowell, H. C., Raper, A. B., and Welbourn, H. F.: The natural history of homozygous sickle-cell anemia in central Africa. Q. J. Med., N.S.: 26:401, 1956.
75. Victor, A. B., and Imperiale, L. E.: The pulmonary and small bone changes in infants with sickle cell anemia. N.Y. State J. Med., 57:1403, 1957.
76. Watson, R. J., Burko, H., Megas, H., and Robinson, M.: The hand-foot syndrome in sickle cell disease in young children. Pediatrics, 31:975, 1963.
77. Weinberg, A. G., and Curiano, G.: Sickle cell dactylitis: Histopathologic observations. Am. J. Clin. Pathol., 58:518, 1972.
78. Whitten, C. F.: Growth status of children with sickle cell anemia. Am. J. Dis. Child., 102:355, 1961.
79. Wigh, R., and Thompson, H. J., Jr.: Cortical fissuring in osteomyelitis complicating sickle cell anemia. Radiology, 55:553, 1950.
80. Worrall, V. T., and Butera, V.: Sickle-cell dactylitis. J. Bone Joint Surg., 58-A:1161, 1976.

RETICULOENDOTHELIAL NEOPLASIA

Leukemia

Leukemia is the most common cancer in children. All organ systems are eventually involved; in the acute disease skeletal manifestations are common. Initially, it is difficult to make the diagnosis because of the diffuse symptoms. Bone and joint pain is the most common presenting complaint, often misdiagnosed as rheumatic fever, septic arthritis, osteomyelitis, internal derangement of the knee, rheumatoid arthritis, or polymyositis. When a child presents with obscure bone or joint pain the orthopedic surgeon should be highly suspicious of leukemia.[23]

Bone pain is diffuse, nonspecific, and may extend to adjacent joints. It results from distention of the medullary cavities by the massive proliferation of hemapoietic tissue. Frequent sites are the long bones and spinal column. There may or may not be associated radiographic changes. Low-grade fever may be present.

On laboratory examination the white blood count may be elevated, depressed, or normal. Severe anemia is common; when the hemoglobin is 9 gm. per 100 ml., leukemia should be ruled out. Often the erythrocyte sedimentation rate is elevated.

In the radiogram, at sites of active enchondral bone growth (usually the distal end of the femur and the proximal end of the tibia), transverse and narrow radiolucent areas appear (Fig. 3–236).[2, 8] These juxtaepiphyseal radiolucent zones are caused by destruction of bone trabeculae by the proliferation of tumor tissue. Depression of enchondral bone formation due to the child's

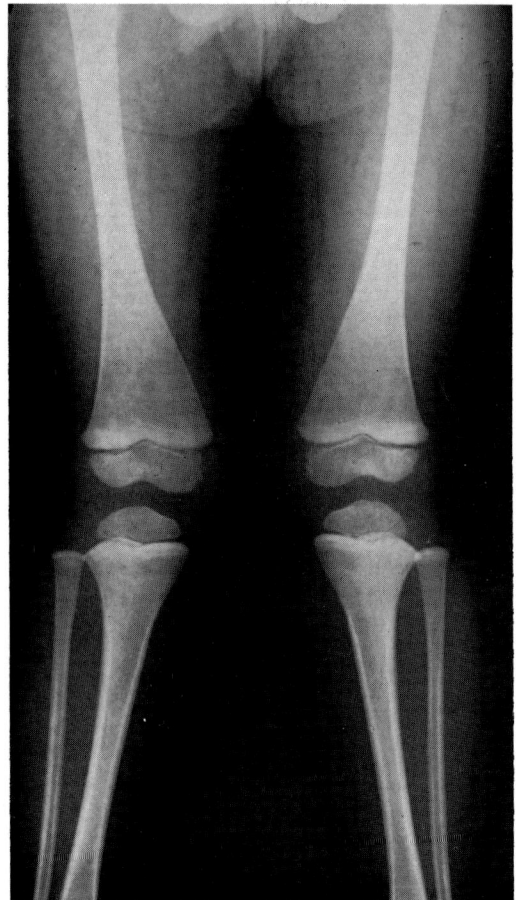

FIGURE 3–236. Bone manifestations of acute leukemia.

Radiogram of both lower limbs. Note the transverse and narrow areas of radiolucency in the metaphyses of distal femora and proximal tibiae.

general debility may be another factor. These areas of rarefaction are not pathognomonic for leukemia, as they are also commonly observed in a variety of chronic disorders.[27]

Osteopenia is generalized. With progression of the disease lytic areas develop: they manifest themselves as lucent areas that may be demarcated or moth-eaten in appearance. There may be associated cortical thinning and eventual erosion. The lytic lesions may involve the metaphysis of long bones, skull, pelvis, and tubular bones of the hands and feet; there may be associated subperiosteal new bone formation, suggesting acute osteomyelitis. These lesions, however, are nonspecific and not pathognomonic of leukemia. In a rare instance, the reaction of bone to leukemic infiltration may be almost exclusively osteoblastic with no evidence of radiolucent osteolytic lesions.

Occasionally pathologic fracture may be the presenting symptom.

Scintigraphic findings with technetium-99m are unreliable in leukemia; there may be increased uptake in asymptomatic areas and normal uptake in obvious lytic lesions.[7] When there is such a dichotomy between clinical and radiographic or radionuclide findings, one should be suspicious of leukemia, particularly if there are associated anemia and leukopenia.

Final diagnosis is made by bone marrow studies. Treatment is administered by the hematologist. In a terminal case, when pathologic fracture or a complicated osteomyelitis due to a lowered resistance to infection occurs, orthopedic attention will be required.

References

1. Armas, R., Neumann, R., and Goldsmith, S. J.: Differential skeletal uptake of TC-99m-tagged pyrophosphate and methylene diphosphonate in leukemia. J. Nucl. Med., 24:799, 1983.
2. Baty, J. M., and Vogt, E. C.: Bone changes of leukemia in children. A.J.R., 34:310, 1935.
3. Bedwell, C. A., and Dawson, A. M.: Chronic myeloid leukemia in a child presenting as acute polyarthritis. Arch. Dis. Child., 29:78, 1954.
4. Benoit, Y., Delbeke, M. J., and Eggesbo, E. S.: Skeletal changes in children with acute lymphoblastic leukemia. Tijdschr. Kindergeneeskd., 49:153, 1981.
5. Bos, G. D., Simon, M. A., Spiegel, P. G., and Moohr, J. W.: Childhood leukemia presenting as a diaphyseal radiolucency. Clin. Orthop., 135:66, 1978.
6. Chan, K. W., Miller, D. R., and Tan, C. T.: Osteosarcoma and acute myeloblastic leukemia after therapy for childhood Hodgkin disease—a case report. Med. Pediatr. Oncol., 8:143, 1980.
7. Clausen, N., Gøtze, H., Pedersen, A., Riis-Petersen, J., and Tjalve, E.: Skeletal scintigraphy and radiography at onset of acute lymphocytic leukemia in children. Med. Pediatr. Oncol., 11:291, 1983.
8. D'Astous, J., Corrigan, M., and Wiley, J.: The musculo-skeletal manifestations of acute lymphatic leukemia in childhood. Orthop. Trans., 8:460, 1984.
9. Dulac, O., Fromange, A., and Arthuis, M.: Neurologic complications of acute leukemia. Arch. Fr. Pediatr., 38:189, 1981.
10. Follis, R. H., Jr., and Park, E. A.: Some observations on the morphologic basis for the roentgenographic changes in childhood leukemia. Bull. Hosp. Joint Dis., 12:67, 1951.
11. Gibson, J., Joshua, D. E., Collis, D., and Kronenberg, H.: Chronic myeloid leukaemia presenting as femoral head necrosis. Scand. J. Haematol., 32:376, 1984.
12. Hann, I. M., Gupta, S., Palmer, M. K., and Morris-Jones, P. H.: The prognostic significance of radiological and symptomatic bone involvement in childhood acute lymphoblastic leukaemia. Med. Pediatr. Oncol., 6:51, 1979.
13. Hughes, R. G., and Kay, H. E.: Major bone lesions in acute lymphoblastic leukaemia. Med. Pediatr. Oncol., 10:67, 1982.
14. Jaffe, H. L.: Skeletal manifestations of leukemia and malignant lymphoma. Bull. Hosp. Joint Dis., 13:217, 1952.
15. Jaffe, H. L.: Tumors and Tumorous Conditions of the Bones and Joints. Philadelphia, Lea & Febiger, 1958, pp. 398-401.
16. Kalayjian, B. S., Herbut, P. A., and Erf, L. A.: The bone changes of leukemia in children. Radiology, 47:223, 1946.
17. Masera, G., Carnelli, V., Ferrari, M., Recchia, M., and Bellini, F.: Prognostic significance of radiological bone involvement in childhood acute lymphoblastic leukaemia. Arch. Dis. Child., 52:530, 1977.
18. Moseley, J. E.: Bone Changes in Hematologic Disorders. New York, Grune & Stratton, 1963, pp. 78–92.
19. Newman, A. J., and Melhorn, D. L.: Vertebral compression in childhood leukemia. Am. J. Dis. Child., 125:863, 1973.
20. Nies, B. A., Kundel, D. W., Thomas, L. B., and Freireich, E. J.: Leukopenia, bone pain, and bone necrosis in patients with acute leukemia. A clinicopathologic complex. Ann. Intern. Med., 62:698, 1965.
21. Nixon, G. W., and Gwinn, J. L.: The roentgenographic manifestations of leukemia in infancy. Radiology, 107:603, 1973.
22. Pear, B. L.: Skeletal manifestations of the lymphomas and leukemias. Semin. Roentgenol., 9:229, 1974.
23. Rogalsky, R. J., Black, G. B., and Reed, M. H.: Orthopaedic manifestations of leukemia in children. J. Bone Joint Surg., 68-A:494, 1986.
24. Rosenfield, N. S., and McIntosh, S.: Prospective analysis of bone changes in treated childhood leukemia. Radiology, 123:413, 1977.
25. Silberstein, M. J., Tangshewinsirikul, P., Chu, J. -Y., and Graviss, E. R.: Bone changes in a neonate with congenital leukemia. Radiology, 131:370, 1979.
26. Silverman, F. N.: Skeletal lesions in leukemia: Clinical and roentgen observations in infants and children with review of the literature. A.J.R., 59:819, 1948.
27. Silverstein, M. N., and Kelly, P. J.: Leukemia with osteoarticular symptoms and signs. Ann. Intern. Med., 59:637, 1963.
28. Simmons, C. R., Harle, T. S., and Singleton, E. B.: The osseous manifestations of leukemia in children. Radiol. Clin. North Am., 6:115, 1968.
29. Sullivan, M. P.: Intracranial complications of leukemia in children. Pediatrics, 20:757, 1957.
30. Thomas, L. B., Forhner, C. E., Frei, E., III, Besse, B. E., and Stabenau, J. R.: The skeletal lesions of acute leukemia. Cancer, 14:609, 1961.
31. Van Slyck, E. J.: The bony changes in two malignant hematologic diseases. Orthop. Clin. North Am., 3:733, 1972.

Lymphoma, Lymphosarcoma, and Hodgkin's Disease

These three entities are very rare in children. Enlarged lymph nodes in the neck, or in the inguinal or axillary regions, are the common initial findings. With invasion of the bone marrow, adjacent bones may be secondarily involved and present a mottled appearance in the radiograms (Fig. 3–237). Diganosis is made by histologic examination of tissue obtained at biopsy. Treatment consists of radiation and chemotherapy.

References

1. Appell, R. G., Oppermann, H. C., and Brandeis, W. E.: Skeletal lesions in Hodgkin's disease. Review of literature and case reports. Pediatr. Radiol., 11:61, 1981.
2. Appell, R. G., Buhler, T., Willich, E., and Brandeis, W. E.: Absence of prognostic significance of skeletal involvement in acute lymphocytic leukemia and non-Hodgkin lymphoma in children. Pediatr. Radiol., 15:245, 1985.

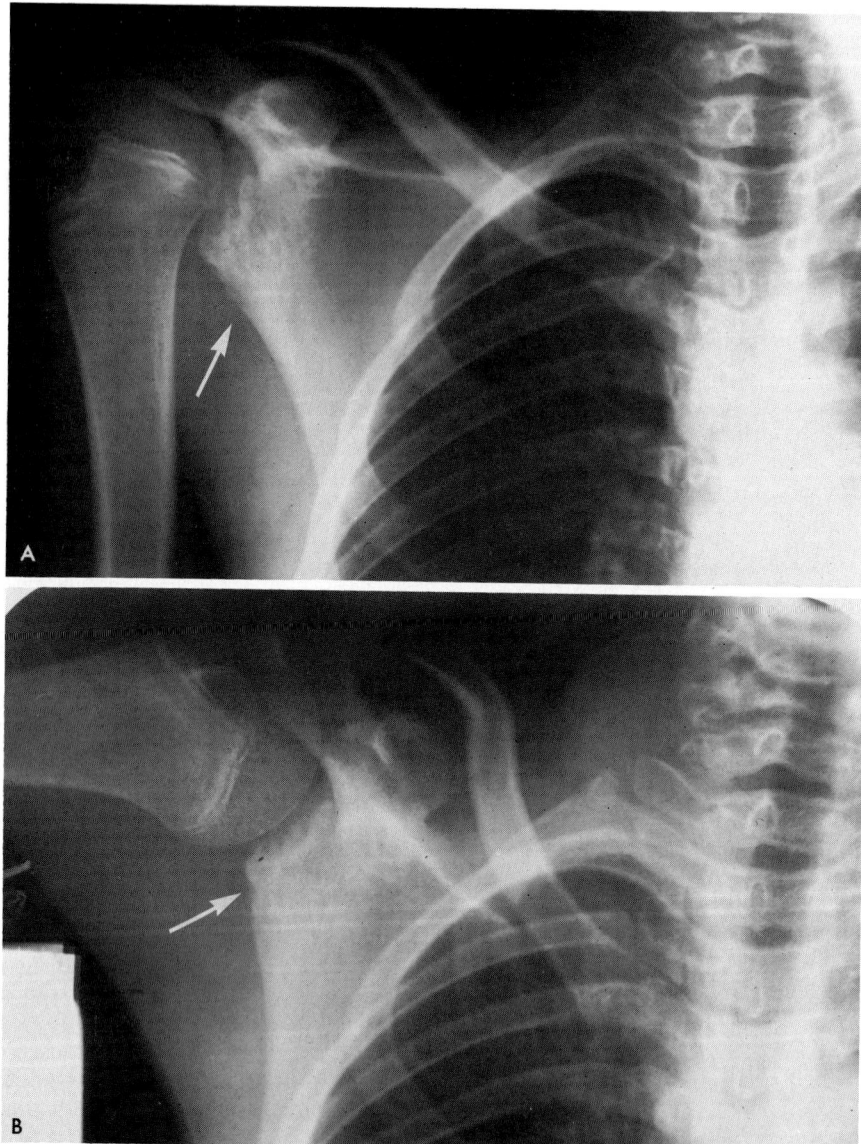

FIGURE 3–237. *Hodgkin's disease of the scapula. Note the mottled areas of rarefaction.*

3. Aprin, H., Calandra, J., Mir, R., and Lee, J. Y.: Radiation-induced chondrosarcoma of the clavicle complicating Hodgkin's disease. Clin. Orthop., 209:189, 1986.
4. Baccarini, M., Bosi, A., and Papa, G.: Second malignancy in patients treated for Hodgkin disease. Cancer, 46:1735, 1980.
5. Berman, B. W., McIntosh, S., Goldenring, H., and Prosnitz, L. R.: Hodgkin's disease as epitrochlear adenopathy. Am. J. Dis. Child., 134:319, 1980.
6. Bessler, W., Egloff, B., and Sulser, H.: Case report 267. Post radiation osteosarcoma left innominate bone with pulmonary metastasis arising from irradiated site of a previously diagnosed and treated lymphoma of bone (left innominate bone). Skeletal Radiol., 11:216, 1984.
7. Brandeis, W. E., Tan, C., Wang, Y., Good, R. A., and Day, N. K.: Circulating immune complexes, complement and complement component levels in childhood Hodgkin's disease. Clin. Exp. Immunol., 39:551, 1980.
8. Braunstein, E. M.: Hodgkin disease of bone: Radiographic correlation with the histological classification. Radiology, 137:643, 1980.
9. Braunstein, E. M., and White, S. J.: Non-Hodgkin lymphoma of bone. Radiology, 135:59, 1980.
10. Brody, R. S., and Schottenfield, D.: Multiple primary cancers in Hodgkin disease. Semin. Oncol., 7:187, 1980.
11. Burkhardt, R., Frisch, B., and Bartl, R.: Bone biopsy in haematological disorders. J. Clin. Pathol., 35:257, 1982.
12. Cancellos, G. P., DeVita, V., Arseneau, J. C., Whang-Peng, J., and Johnson, R. E. C.: Second malignancies complicating Hodgkin disease in remission. Lancet, 26:947, 1975.
13. Coles, W. C., and Schulz, M. D.: Bone involvement in malignant lymphoma. Radiology, 50:458, 1948.
14. Coltman, C. A., and Dixon, D. O.: Second malignancies complicating Hodgkin disease. A southwest oncology group 10-year-follow-up. Cancer Treat. Rep., 66:1023, 1982.
15. Dearth, J. C., Gilchrist, G. S., Burgert, E. O., Jr., Telander, R. L., and Cupps, R. E.: Management of stages I to III Hodgkin's disease in children. J. Pediatr., 96:829, 1980.
16. Derek, R., Jenkin, T., and Berry, M. P.: Hodgkin's disease in children. Semin. Oncol., 7:202, 1980.
17. Durkovsky, J., Michalikova, B., and Petrik, P.: Results of radiotherapy in Hodgkin's disease. Neoplasma, 27:723, 1980.
18. Farrell, C., Perry, M. C., Bourgeois, C. H., Abernathie, D. L., and Hakami, N.: Osteosarcoma—a complication of chemotherapy for Hodgkin's disease in children. Am. J. Clin. Oncol., 6:75, 1983.
19. Gill, P. G., Souter, R. G., and Morris, P. G.: Results of surgical staging in Hodgkin's disease. Br. J. Surg., 67:478, 1980.
20. Glicksman, A. S., Pajak, T. F., Gottlieb, A., Nissen, N., Stutzman, L., and Cooper, M.: Second malignant neoplasms in patients successfully treated for Hodgkin disease. A cancer and leukemia group B study. Cancer Treat. Rep., 66:1035, 1982.
21. Granger, W., and Witaker, R.: Hodgkin's disease in bone, with special reference to periosteal reaction. Br. J. Radiol., 40:939, 1967.
22. Halperin, E., Greenberg, M. S., and Suit, H. D.: Sarcoma of bone and soft tissue following treatment of Hodgkin disease. Cancer, 53:232, 1984.
23. Horan, F. T.: Bone involvement in Hodgkin's disease: A survey of 201 cases. Br. J. Surg., 56:277, 1969.
24. Hustu, H. O., and Pinkel, D.: Lymphosarcoma, Hodgkin's disease and leukemia in bone. Clin. Orthop., 52:83, 1967.
25. Jacquillat, C., Khayat, D., Desprez-Curely, J. P., and Weil, M.: Non-Hodgkin lymphoma occurring after Hodgkin disease. 4 new cases and a review of the literature. Cancer, 53:459, 1984.
26. Jones, B., and Klinberg, W. G.: Lymphosarcoma in children—a report of 43 cases and a review of the recent literature. J. Pediatr., 63:11, 1963.
27. Klein, R. M., Thelmo, W., Dorf, D., and Ambinder, J.: Case report 269. Malignant lymphoma (large cell immunoblastic type) with wide spread dissemination in the skeleton as well as lymph nodes and probably the liver and spleen. Skeletal Radiol., 11:224, 1984.
28. Krikorian, J. G., Burke, J. S., Rosenberg, S. A., and Kaplan, H. S.: Occurrence of non-Hodgkin lymphoma after therapy for Hodgkin disease. N. Engl. J. Med., 300:452, 1979.
29. Lange, B., and Littman, P.: Management of Hodgkin's disease in children and adolescents. Cancer, 51:1371, 1983.
30. Lumb, G., and MacKenzie, D. H.: Round-cell tumours of bone. Br. J. Surg., 43:380, 1956.
31. Malpas, J. S.: Lymphomas in children. Semin. Hematol., 19:301, 1982.
32. Meher-Honji, D. R., De Souza, L. J., and Culcuttawalla, T. F.: Unusual sternal mass in Hodgkin's disease. J. Bone Joint Surg., 54-A:402, 1972.
33. Meyer, J. E., Longgood, E. M., and Lindfors, K. K.: Impact of thoracic computed tomography on radiation therapy planning in Hodgkin disease. J. Comput. Assist. Tomogr., 8:892, 1984.
34. Mills, S. E., Sloop, F. B., Jr., Thiele, A. L., Miller, C. W., and Zazakos, C. P., Jr.: Case report 251. Hodgkin's disease, nodular sclerosing variant, primary form. Skeletal Radiol., 10:287, 1983.
35. National Cancer Institute sponsored study of classification of non-Hodgkin lymphoma, summary and description of a working formula for clinical usage. Cancer, 49:2112, 1982.
36. Nelson, D. F., Cooper, S., Weston, M. G., and Rubin, P.: Second malignant neoplasms in patients treated for Hodgkin disease with radiotherapy or radiotherapy and chemotherapy. Cancer, 48:2386, 1981.
37. Niebrugge, D., Monzon, C., Perry, M. C., and Hakami, N.: Osteogenic sarcoma following Hodgkin's disease. Cancer, 48:416, 1981.
38. Parker, B. R., Marglin, S., and Castellino, R. N.: Skeletal manifestations of leukemia, Hodgkin disease and non-Hodgkin lymphoma. Semin. Roentgenol., 15(4):302, 1980.
39. Pear, B. L.: Skeletal manifestations of the lymphoma and leukemias. Semin. Roentgenol., 10:229, 1974.
40. Phillips, W. C., Kattapuram, S. V., and Doseretz, D. E.: Primary lymphoma of bone: Relationship of radiographic appearance and prognosis. Radiology, 144:285, 1982.
41. Poppema, S., and Lennert, K.: Hodgkin's disease in childhood: Histopathologic classification in relation to age and sex. Cancer, 45:1443, 1980.
42. Samuels, T. S., Howard, B. A., Rubenstein, J. D., and Srigley, J.: Case report 409. Non Hodgkin lymphoma (diffuse histiocytic or malignant lymphoma, diffuse, large cell B-cell immunophenotype). Skeletal Radiol., 16:78, 1987.
43. Skovby, F., and Sullivan, M. P.: Herpes zoster and varicella in children with Hodgkin's disease. Acta Paediatr. Scand., 71:269, 1982.
44. Stuhlbarg, J., and Ellis, F. W.: Hodgkin's disease of bone: Favorable prognostic significance? A.J.R., 93:568, 1965.
45. Sullivan, D. M., and Solonick, D. M.: Case report 414. Nodular sclerosing Hodgkin disease involving sternum and chest wall. Skeletal Radiol., 16:166, 1987.

46. Tawil, E., and Mercier, J. P.: Second malignancy complicating Hodgkin disease. C.A.R., *34*:108, 1983.
47. Tester, W. J., Kinsella, T. J., and Waller, B.: Second malignant neoplasms complicating Hodgkin disease: The national cancer institute experience. J. Clin. Oncol., 2:762, 1984.
48. Zolezzi, P., Caorsi, I., Albornoz, C., and Niada, P.: Hodgkin's lymphoma in children. Correlation of histopathology and survival time (1969–1979). Rev. Chir. Pediatr., 52:7, 1981.

Tumors and Tumorous Conditions of Bone

BONE TUMORS

All components of bone are derived from the mesoderm; therefore, bone tumors are potentially composed of any of its four stem cell types; namely, the fibroblast, the chondroblast and the osteoblast (mesenchymal cell series), and the reticulomyelogenic series.

Classification

A classification of bone tumors cannot be totally comprehensive, as there is a great range of variation and the origin of some tumors is, as yet, obscure; the one in Table 3–30, however, may serve as a general framework for discussion.

Clinical Picture

The complaints that lead a patient with a bone tumor to seek medical advice are pain, the presence of an unusual mass, or a pathologic fracture; or a lesion may be discovered incidentally when a radiogram is made for other reasons. Pain is the most common presenting symptom. A benign tumor is likely to be painless unless its presence causes some mechanical difficulty or results in a pathologic fracture, whereas a malignant tumor is more likely to be painful. The pain is insidious in its onset, at first transient, but gradually becoming persistent. Initially, simple analgesics will relieve the pain, but they become progressively ineffective. The fast-growing malignant lesions have rapid

Table 3–30. Classification of Primary Tumors of Bone

Tissue Origin	Benign Neoplasm	Malignant Neoplasm
Bone	Osteoma Osteochondroma? Osteoid osteoma Osteoblastoma	Osteogenic sarcoma Parosteal osteosarcoma

Cartilage	Enchondroma
	Chondroblastoma
	Chondromyxoid fibroma
	Juxtacortical chondroma
	Osteochondroma
		Chondrosarcoma
		  Primary
		  Secondary

Fibrous	Nonossifying fibroma Multiple nonossifying fibroma Desmoplastic fibroma Fibrous dysplasia Osteofibrous dysplasia (Campanacci)	Fibrosarcoma
Uncertain	Giant cell tumor Fibrous histiocytoma	Malignant giant cell tumor Malignant fibrous histiocytoma Adamantinoma
Marrow elements Hematopoietic	— Histiocytosis X	Malignant lymphoma Reticulum cell sarcoma Lymphosarcoma Hodgkin's disease Leukemia
Fat	Lipoma	Liposarcoma
Vascular	Hemangioma Glomus tumor Hemangiopericytoma	Angiosarcoma Hemangioendothelioma Malignant hemangiopericytoma
Notochord	—	Chordoma
Undifferentiated cell (mesenchyme)	—	Mesenchymal sarcoma

onset of pain that is more disturbing at night. It may be extremely severe, especially when it is located in an areas where there is little room for expansion of the tumor. Rapid growth and hemorrhage of the tumor increase the intensity of pain. When a pathologic fracture takes place, it is characterized by a sudden increase in the intensity of pain.

The presence of a palpable mass is an important finding on physical examination. One should determine its size, consistency, mobility, and whether it is painful on palpation. A rapidly growing lesion is more likely to be malignant than benign. In taking the history, it is helpful to compare the size of the mass to a dime, a nickel, a quarter, or a half dollar, and if the tumor is larger, to a tennis ball, a football, and so on. It is important to measure and record the size of the tumor as accurately as possible for comparison in subsequent examinations. The consistency of the mass is determined next. Is it firm or soft? Does it feel cystic or bony and hard? A cystic or fluid-filled mass should be examined with a flashlight to determine whether it transilluminates. In general fluid-filled lesions are commonly benign, whereas large hard masses are more likely to be malignant. Is there a distinct change from normal to abnormal at the margins of the mass? Is the mass of the same consistency as the surrounding normal tissue? Malignant swellings usually invade the adjacent tissues. An increase in local temperature is more suggestive of a malignant than a benign lesion.

Mobility of a mass is of great help in ascertaining its nature. When the mass is fixed, it is either attached to bone or is intraosseous. An osseous tumor is unaffected by muscle contraction. Intramuscular tumors are usually mobile when the muscle is relaxed and become fixed when the muscle is contracted. Deep, mobile lesions that are unaffected by muscle action are beneath the deep fascia and extramuscular. Tumors that are superficial and that can be moved about have not invaded deep fascia and are not indicative of malignancy.

Tenderness to palpation indicates an active process and is due to inflammatory response. An abscess or infection is very painful and usually accompanied by other signs of inflammation such as erythema, edema, lymphangitis, and adenopathy, whereas moderate tenderness is indicative of an active neoplastic process, and the absence of tenderness suggests a quiescent lesion. One should, however, beware because rapid growth and necrosis of a malignant tumor may mimic infection—as, for example, in the differential diagnosis between Ewing's sarcoma and osteomyelitis. When a rapidly growing malignant tumor is subcutaneous, it may cause vascular dilatation, increased local heat, and skin turgor; such a tumor may be mistaken for thrombophlebitis or an infectious process. Neoplastic inflammatory response, however, is characterized by a firmer feeling and lack of local pitting edema, and the cutaneous tissue is not as red as with infection. Point tenderness is indicative of lesions such as an osteoid osteoma, a neural lesion, or a glomus tumor.

The range of motion of joints may be limited because of muscle spasm or mechanical interference. There may be reactive synovitis when the lesion is adjacent to a joint or if the joint is directly involved. Muscle atrophy is not uncommon; and an antalgic limp may be present.

A vascular tumor is suspected if elevation or steady firm pressure causes a diminution in its size, if the size is increased by the use of a venous tourniquet, or if a thrill or palpable pulsation is present. A pathologic fracture may occur in primary or metastatic malignant tumors, or one may complicate a benign process such as a unicameral bone cyst.

Invasion of a nerve will cause neurologic symptoms and signs such as stabbing pain, paresthesia, hypoesthesia, or motor weakness. Pathologically, the nerve may be encased by the lesion or trapped against bone or rigid fascia. Neurologic dysfunction is uncommon except when tumors are in anatomic areas where nerves are unable to move freely, such as the sciatic notch or neural foramina.

Radiographic Features

When a bone tumor is suspected, conventional radiographic examinations should be made of the affected part. A great deal can be learned by the radiographic appearance. First, the anatomic location of the lesion; second, the effect on the local bone, a suggestion as to its histogenic type by the specific radiographic characteristics, and whether it is aggressive; and third, the reaction of surrounding tissue in the zone of transition between the lesion and the host bone. Often one can distinguish a tumor that is malignant from one that is benign, although sometimes differential diagnosis may be difficult or even impossible. A conventional radiogram is the most cost effective tool in musculoskeletal oncology; it is noninvasive, is low-cost, and depicts the gross pathologic image of the tumor.

Anatomic Site of the Tumor. This is of great

diagnostic assistance. Is the tumor located in the axial skeleton or in the long bones? In a specific bone, is the lesion intraosseous, has it broken through the cortex? Is it subperiosteal or intracortical? For example, a tumor in the body of a child's vertebra is usually eosinophilic granuloma, whereas in the posterior elements of the spine, it is usually an osteoblastoma or an aneurysmal bone cyst. In the pelvis, Ewing's sarcoma is common in the child, and in the adult both Ewing's sarcoma and chondrosarcoma are common. In the ribs, one should consider fibrous dysplasia or Ewing's sarcoma. In the long bones, the anatomic site of a tumor provides a diagnostic clue. A lesion in the epiphysis when the physis is still open is most probably chondroblastoma; other possibilities are eosinophilic granuloma or epiphyseal osteomyelitis. Giant cell tumor is the most common tumor in the epiphysis when the growth plate is closed. When the physis is open, giant cell tumor in an adolescent may involve the metaphysis. The diaphysis is a common site for Ewing's sarcoma, histiocytosis X, fibrous dysplasia, osteofibrous dysplasia (Campanacci syndrome), and adamantinoma. The metaphysis of the long bones is the site for a multitude of tumors, including benign tumors such as unicameral bone cyst. Osteogenic sarcoma is commonly located in the metaphysis. In Table 3–31, the common anatomic sites for primary bone tumors are shown.

Internal Radiographic Appearance of the Lesion. If the bone trabeculae are destroyed, it

Table 3–31. Common Anatomic Sites of Primary Bone Tumors

Location	Bone Tumor
Spine	
Posterior elements (spinous process, lamina, pedicles)	Aneurysmal bone cyst Osteoma Osteoblastoma

Anterior elements (vertebral body)	In a child
	  Histiocytosis X ("vertebra plana")
	  Hemangioma

	In an adult
	  Metastases
	  Multiple myeloma
	  Paget's disease
	  Hemangioma
	  Chordoma

Long bones	

Epiphysis	Physis open
	  Chondroblastoma
	  Eosinophilic granuloma (epiphyseal osteomyelitis)*

Metaphysis	Multitude of benign lesions such as unicameral bone cyst Common site for osteogenic sarcoma
Diaphysis	Fibrous dysplasia Histiocytosis X Ewing's sarcoma Osteoblastoma Adamantinoma Lymphoma
Parosteal	Myositis ossificans* Osteosarcoma Chondrosarcoma Enchondroma

Ribs	In children and adolescents
	  Fibrous dysplasia
	  Ewing's sarcoma
	  Metastases

	In adults
	  Ewing's sarcoma
	  Chondrosarcoma
	  Fibrous dysplasia
	  Multiple myeloma
	  Metastases

*Not a tumor

Table 3–31. *Common Anatomic Sites of Primary Bone Tumors* Continued

Location	Bone Tumor

Pelvis	In children
	  Ewing's sarcoma
	  Fibrous dysplasia
	  Aneurysmal bone cyst
	  Osteoblastoma
	
	In adults
	  Ewing's sarcoma
	  Chondrosarcoma
	  Paget's disease
	  Multiple myeloma
	  Metastases

Scapula	Ewing's sarcoma Osteoblastoma Aneurysmal bone cyst

Multiple lesions	In children
	  Multiple hereditary exostoses
	  Fibrous dysplasia (Albright's)
	  Histiocytosis X
	  Enchondroma (Ollier's)
	  Multiple hemangiomatosis
	  Metastases-neuroblastoma, hypernephroma
	  Lymphoma
	
	In adults
	  Multiple myeloma

indicates an aggressive lesion. Often bone destruction is accompanied by new bone or cartilage formation. One should distinguish between ossification and calcification. Ossification is the mineralization of a bone matrix, which may be normal or tumorous bone; for example, osteogenic sarcoma is characterized by tumor bone formation. Calcification is unstructured mineralization that appears in the radiogram as more haphazard and denser than ossification. Calcification is indicative of a cartilaginous process such as that seen in chondrosarcoma or enchondroma.

Zone of Transition Between the Lesion and the Host Bone. If it is clearly demarcated and narrow with an area of surrounding sclerosis, the lesion is probably benign. If the zone of transition is wide with an irregular contour and unclear outline, it indicates an aggressive permeative process in which the host bone did not have time to respond to the neoplasm. Aggressive is a nonspecific term indicating a rapidly growing tumor that may be malignant or an acute infection.

A tumor may invade the cortex and elicit periosteal new bone formation. Reactive bone under the elevated periosteum at the margin of the tumor is referred to as "Codman's triangle." This is suggestive of an aggressive process. Onion skin and sunburst appearances are nonspecific. A soft-tissue mass is usually visible in the radiogram if a malignant tumor is of considerable duration. In Ewing's sarcoma, for example, there is a mottled rarefaction of the spongiosa and overlying cortex reflecting bone destruction. Periosteal new bone formation, often of the laminated onion peel form is common, and a soft-tissue mass overlying the area of bone destruction is frequently found, indicating perforation of the cortex and spread into the adjacent soft tissues by the neoplasm.

Expansion and thinning of the cortex without destruction can be caused by a tumor; this is indicative of a benign lesion such as enchondroma, fibrous dysplasia, or an aneurysmal bone cyst. The significance of the host tissue response to the lesion is summarized in Table 3–32.

Isotope Scans*

Scintigraphic bone imaging for changes in the uptake of technetium polyphosphonate (Tc-99m) or gallium citrate is a very sensitive but nonspecific tool in the diagnosis and staging of bone tumors.

---

*See references 13, 16, 32, 34, 42, 47, 48, 75, 89.

Table 3–32. Response to Lesion—Its Diagnostic Significance

Zone of transition
  Narrow and geographic—slow growing
  Wide and permeative—aggressive
Response of cortex
  Containment—slow growing
  Expanded but contained
    Aneurysmal bone cyst
    Fibrous dysplasia
    Enchondroma
  Destroyed—aggressive
Response of periosteum
  Elevation—aggressive (not specific)
Special features
  Calcification—indicates cartilage producing process
  Ossification—bone producing process

Techniques of scintigraphy are total body imaging, spot films, magnification imaging (spot Con-Electronic) and single photon emission computed tomography (SPECT).

Scintigraphy in bone tumors is of value in early detection, in delineation of pattern of disease, and in localization of the disease. Intensity of uptake is variable, and it does not differentiate benign from malignant lesions. Hot bone tumors on isotope scan are fibrous dysplasia, osteoid osteoma, osteoblastoma, aneurysmal bone cyst, giant cell tumor, adamantinoma, osteogenic sarcoma, Ewing's sarcoma, and neuroblastoma. Cold lesions are eosinophilic granuloma, multiple myeloma, and anaplastic sarcoma. With extension of the tumorous process there may be peripheral increase (extension pattern). Radiotherapy will decrease the increased uptake, whereas in some tumors with healing there will be an increase in intensity of localization (flare response).

Technetium Polyphosphonate (Tc-99m). A greater uptake of technetium-99m may be due either to increased blood flow to the part or to active mineralization. Six hours is the functional half-life of Tc-99m, and about three hours after injection, the intravascular phase of increased uptake fades rapidly as the nonfixed isotope is collected and excreted by the urinary tract. Therefore, any increased activity due to hypervascularlity in osseous or soft tissue will disappear after three hours, whereas increased activity due to incorporation in the mineral crystals in any tissue, normal or neoplastic, will persist up to six hours. It is possible to distinguish between increased activity due to hypervascularity and that due to active mineralization by sequential imaging.

Scanning with Tc-99m provides an overview of the skeleton much more effectively than a radiographic skeletal survey. It involves less radiation and is more sensitive. An increased uptake on the bone image should be correlated with conventional radiograms, as false-positives are possible. The bone scan will detect additional sites of involvement in benign bone tumors when multiple lesions are present as in fibrous dysplasia, multiple hereditary exostoses, multiple enchondromatosis, hemangiomas, and histiocytosis X. Scintigraphy with technetium-99m (portable) in the operating room will assist in determining whether a lesion such as an osteoid osteoma has been totally excised.

A bone scan will provide information on the presence of skeletal metastases, and therefore, is of great value in the initial surgical staging of a primary malignant tumor. It should be stressed, however, that scintigraphic bone imaging is a *nonspecific tool* and is not of value in differentiating benign from malignant lesions. Another disadvantage of the bone scan is that in malignant bone tumors, because of the increase in blood flow in the surrounding tissues, it will not reliably determine the local extent of the lesion. Nor can an intraosseous extension be determined accurately because of increased local uptake. The value of bone imaging in soft-tissue tumors is very limited except in the detection of skeletal metastases. Vascular soft tissue tumors will, however, show increased local uptake.

Bone-forming lesions are "hotter" than fibrous or cartilaginous lesions, but the degree of intensity of uptake does not correlate with the grade of malignancy. Scintigraphy will detect occult microextensions and satellite lesions in malignant bone sarcoma; therefore, the bone image will be "hot" beyond the radiographic margins of the tumor. Sites of necrosis or hemorrhage within a lesion will be depicted as "cold" areas in the bone scan.

By serial scanning, one can detect changes in activity of a lesion. For example, a "cold" osteochondroma that becomes "hot" indicates activity, and further immediate investigations are warranted to rule out chondrosarcomatous changes.

Gallium-67 Citrate.[36, 60] The main value of a gallium scan is in the diagnosis of soft-tissue tumors. Noninflammatory benign tumors usually appear normal, whereas soft-tissue sarcomas and infections of bone and soft tissues show increased uptake. When a gallium scan is normal, one can feel quite comfortable that a tumor is benign. Because the gallium scan does not elicit the increased blood flow phenomenon, delineation of the intra- and extraosseous extent of primary bone tumors is better than with technetium-99m. Iodine-131 meta-iodobenzylguanidine (MIGB) is of definite value in the diagnosis of and determination of the effect of therapy on neuroblastoma and metastatic pheochromocytoma in the limbs and axial skeleton.[46, 84]

Computed Tomography*

Computed tomography (CT scanning) provides a cross-sectional display of the limbs and the trunk, and allows differentiation of bone, muscle, fat, and major neurovascular structures by tissue density quantitation. It clearly visualizes anatomically difficult areas such as pelvis, sacrum, subscapular region, and spine. The greater amount of fat in the extracompartmental areolar tissue differentiates it from intracompartmental tissues, delineating the various compartments; the fascial septa are relatively radiodense and outlined by the radiolucency of the fat. It is of great value in staging to know whether a lesion is intra- or extracompartmental. The CT scan clearly indicates the intraosseous extent of the primary bone tumor in the transverse plane, but it is, however, best to combine it with a conventional tomogram for longitudinal visualization. It will show the anatomic site of a soft-tissue tumor and its relationship to adjacent neurovascular and osseous structures. It can also depict an intracortical lesion as small as 5 mm. in diameter.

Magnetic Resonance Imaging†

This is a noninvasive imaging technique in which great advances are being made at present. It produces images of superior contrast without exposing the patient to ionizing radiation. There is no risk of infection from contrast agents. It allows three-dimensional imaging in the transverse, coronal, and sagittal planes. It is superior to computed tomography in delineating the margins of most soft-tissue tumors and the margins of bone tumors in fat and adjacent normal bone and muscle. Spin echo pulse sequences with short repetition times provide excellent anatomic detail, bone tumors being best shown by spin echo 1000/30 images or inversion recover images.

Angiography

Angiography is invasive and painful for the patient, and in pediatric patients, general anesthesia is almost always necessary. Computed tomography, more sensitive and noninvasive, has become the method of choice for detecting the extraosseous extent of bone tumors. The principal indication for angiography is when limb salvage versus amputation of the limb is in question; in such instances, visualization of the vascular tree by angiography is crucial. Also, angiography is performed preoperatively when vascular tumors such as cavernous hemangioma are to be excised.[20, 41, 45, 51, 54]

Ancillary Studies

Lymphangiography will detect regional lymph node metastases, but many false-positive findings in the inguinal and femoral lymph nodes are common; therefore, it is not recommended in primary sarcoma of the limbs.

Intravenous pyelography and *cystography* should be performed if a tumor is located in the pelvis or sacrum. It will delineate the relationship of the lesion to the ureter, bladder, and urethra. In intrapelvic tumors, a *barium enema* also is indicated to verify the relationship of the pelvic tumor to the large bowel. In vertebral column tumors, *myelography* will depict the relationship of the tumor to the spinal cord and nerve roots; nuclear magnetic resonance imaging is noninvasive, however, and should be performed before myelography.

Soft-tissue sarcomas may spread to the liver and spleen, and *liver-spleen scans* are indicated in such cases. Metastases to the lungs should also be ruled out. Plain anteroposterior and lateral radiograms of the chest are made, but resolution is only 1 cm., and nodules may be hidden behind a rib. Dual anteroposterior and single lateral views have a resolution of 5 mm. If there is any question of pulmonary metastases a CT scan has a resolution of 2 mm. and is of great value in transverse localization.

Laboratory Tests

These are usually nonspecific and of no diagnostic value. The *erythrocyte sedimentation rate* is elevated in Ewing's sarcoma, lymphoma of bone, leukemia, and other metastatic bone tumors; it is also elevated in osteomyelitis. In Ewing's sarcoma, a highly elevated erythrocyte sedimentation rate carries a poor prognosis.

The *alkaline phosphatase level* is elevated in osteosarcoma. Its value is much in question, however, in the presence of extremely high values, one should rule out multicentric osteogenic sarcoma. Immunologic laboratory studies have not proved to be of any value at present.

---

*See references 5, 18, 40, 50, 53, 63, 82.
†See references 7–9, 14, 49, 52, 69.

The clinical approach for diagnosis and staging of bone tumors is presented in Figure 3–238, and that for soft-tissue tumors in Figure 3–239.

Staging

The natural history of an untreated malignant tumor is divided into progressive stages, each subsequent stage implying a more ominous outcome. The stages are subdivided by prognostic factors: the histologic grade (G), the anatomic setting (T), and the presence or absence of metastases (M). Grades are referred to as low (G_1) and high (G_2). *Low-grade lesions* (G_1) are well differentiated, show few mitotic figures, few or no atypical cells, minimal or no necrosis, and no vascular invasion; they produce a fair amount of mature matrix. In general, the chances of local recurrence or metastasis is slight, and low-grade lesions can be adequately treated with relatively conservative surgical measures. *High-grade lesions* (G_2) are poorly differentiated, have frequent mitoses, a considerable number of atypical cells, necrosis, little and immature matrix, and show vascular invasion. Because the staging system serves as a guide to treatment it is best to call the grades surgical and not histologic (Table 3–33).

The second factor in prognosis is the accessibility of the lesion to surgical eradication. Therefore, the anatomic site of a lesion (T) can be subdivided into compartments by its relationship to the natural barriers to extension, i.e., intracompartmental (T_1) and extracompart-

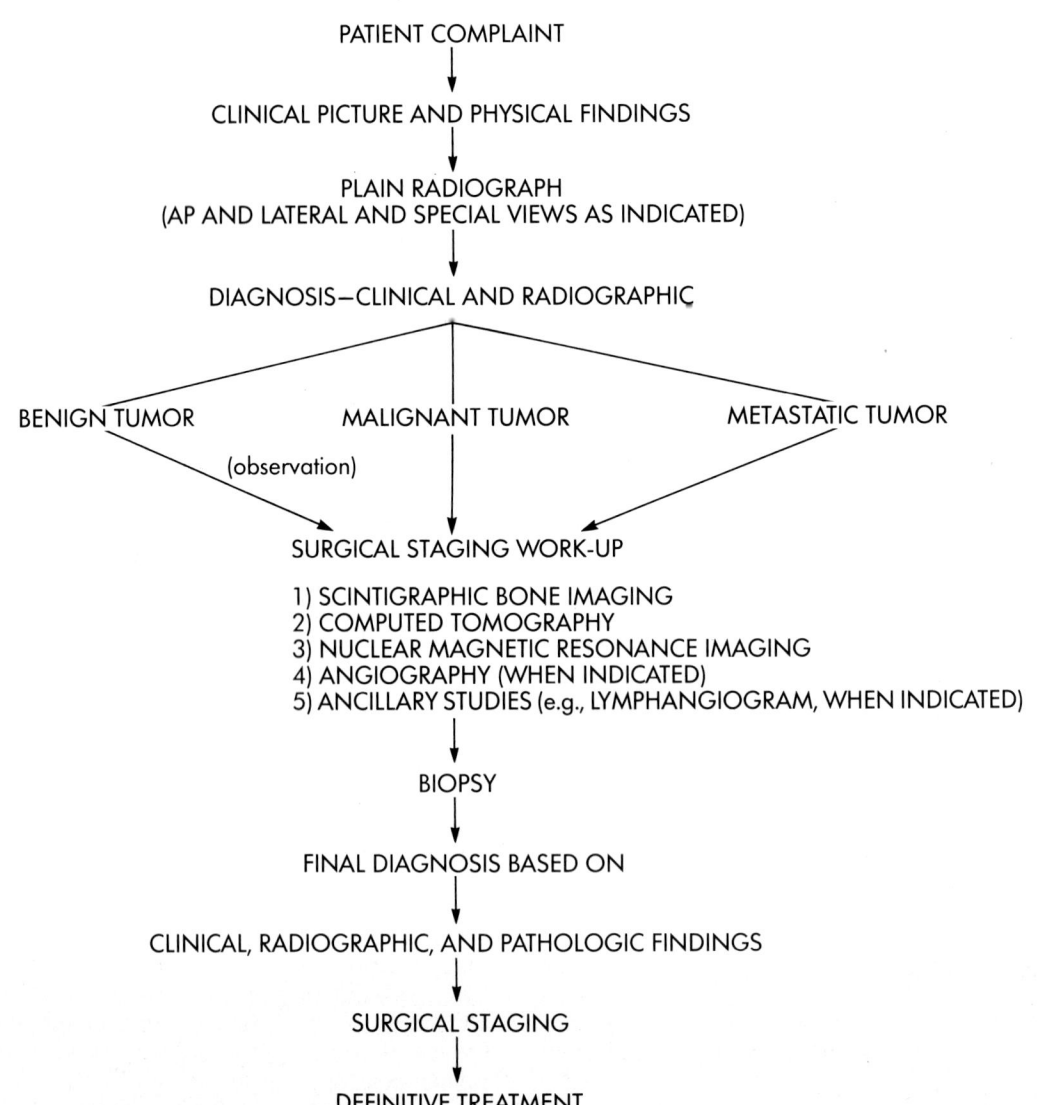

FIGURE 3–238. Approach for diagnosis and staging of bone tumors. (Courtesy of M. Simon, M.D.)

Table 3–33. Surgical Stages of Malignant Tumors*

Surgical Stage	Surgical Grade (G)	Surgical Site (T)	Metastases (M)
I A	Low (G_1)	Intracompartmental (T_1)	M_0
B	Low (G_1)	Extracompartmental (T_2)†	M_0
II A	High (G_2)	Intracompartmental (T_1)	M_0
B	High (G_2)	Extracompartmental (T_2)†	M_0
III	Any G	Any T	M_1

*From Enneking, W. J.: Musculoskeletal Tumor Surgery. New York, Churchill-Livingstone, 1983. Reprinted by permission.

†Extracompartmental (T_2) may occur either as a primary site or by extension of an intracompartmental lesion.

mental (T_2). An *entire bone* is a compartment; when the tumor is confined to the bone, it is intracompartmental (T_1); when an intraosseous lesion breaks the cortex and extends into the soft tissues it becomes extracompartmental (T_2). A *joint* is a compartment; when an intra-articular lesion invades the capsule and extends into the soft tissues, its surgical site (T) graduates from intracompartmental (T_1) to extracompartmental (T_2). A specific *muscle group* that is encased by fasciae is a compartment; when a lesion within a muscle extends into the fascia and encroaches on adjacent tissues it becomes extracompartmental (T_2). The interfascial planes containing major vessels and nerves have no proximal or distal barriers; therefore, they are not compartments. The *skin and subcutaneous fat* are compartments because they are bounded by the deep fascia, which acts as a barrier to deeper invasion. *Parosseous potential spaces* are compartments because they are bounded by the periosteum externally and by the bony cortex deeply. A lesion arising on the external surface of a bone is intracompartmental (T_1); it becomes extracompartmental (T_2) when it invades and breaks the periosteum. In the hand

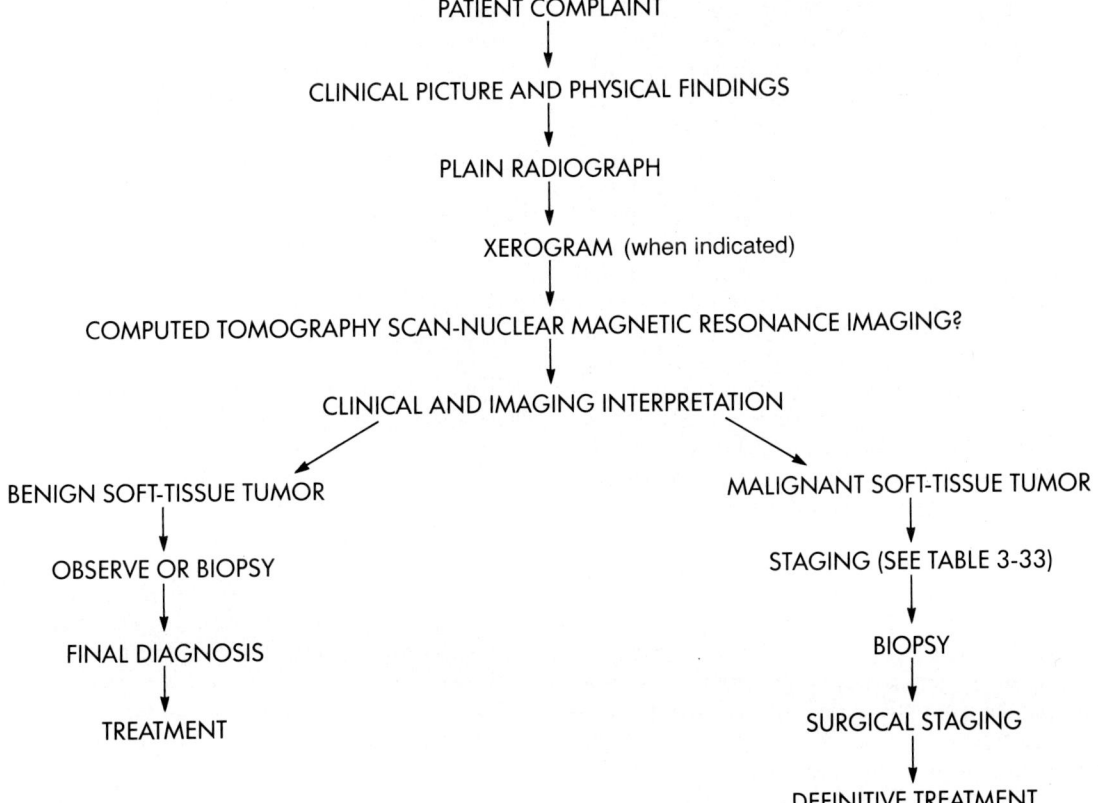

FIGURE 3–239. Approach for diagnosis and staging of soft-tissue tumors. (Courtesy of M. Simon, M.D.)

Table 3–34. Subdivision of Surgical Sites by Relationship of Tumor to Natural Barriers to Extension

Surgical Sites (T)	
Intracompartmental (T_1)	Extracompartmental (T_2)
Intraosseous →	Soft-tissue extension
Parosseous →	Extracompartmental extension
Intraarticular →	Soft-tissue extension
Superficial to deep fascia →	Deep fascial extension

Primary Intracompartmental
  Ray of hand or foot
  Posterior calf
  Anterolateral leg
  Anterior thigh
  Medial thigh
  Posterior thigh
  Buttocks
  Volar forearm
  Dorsal forearm
  Anterior arm
  Posterior arm
  Periscapular (posterior)
Intramuscular compartment →
	Primary extracompartmental
	  Mid and hind foot
	  Popliteal space
	  Groin—femoral triangle
	  Intrapelvic
	  Mid-hand
	  Antecubital fossae
	  Axilla
	  Periclavicular
	  Paraspinal
	  Head and neck
	  Chest wall
	  Subscapular (anterior)
	Intercompartmental, bicompartmental, or extracompartmental extension

and foot the rays rather than the digits are bounded by natural barriers; other intrafascial compartments are the posterior calf, anterolateral leg, anterolateral thigh, medial thigh, posterior thigh, buttocks, volar forearm, dorsal forearm, anterior arm, posterior arm, and periscapular region. Extrafascial planes or spaces are extracompartmental (T_2); these include the midfoot and hindfoot, popliteal space, groin-femoral triangle, intrapelvic region, midhand, antecubital fossa, axilla, periclavicular and paraspinal regions, and head and neck.[22] It should be noted that a space confined by fasciae in the transverse plane, but not bounded proximally or distally, has incomplete barriers to extension and therefore is extracompartmental (Table 3–34.) An intracompartmental lesions (T_1) may become extracompartmental (T_2) when the lesion extends beyond the barriers of its original anatomic site; a lesion that originates in extracompartmental tissues is also extracompartmental (T_2). It is also vital to realize that sarcomas may have satellite lesions in the extracapsular reactive zone; therefore, the entire tumor, capsule (or pseudocapsule), and reactive zone should be within the compartment for the lesion to be classified as intracompartmental. Iatrogenically an inadequate operation may convert an intracompartmental lesion to a recurrent extracompartmental lesion. The prognosis is worse in deeper lesions than superficial ones, and also when the reactive zone abuts or encircles major neurovascular structures.

The presence of metastases (M_1) in sarcoma makes the outlook for survival gloomy. When there is no metastasis (M_0), the prognosis is much better (see Table 3–33).

Benign lesions, on the basis of their natural history and behavior, can be staged. Arabic numerals are used to designate the various stages: *Stage 1*—benign, latent; *Stage 2*—benign, active; and *Stage 3*—benign and aggressive with malignant potential. Anatomic setting, whether intracompartmental or extracompartmental, is not of prognostic value and, therefore, is not utilized.

Principles of Surgical Management

There are two principal types of surgery, conservative resection and radical amputation. Adjunctive management with chemotherapy and irradiation has altered the indications for aggressive ablation of limbs and swayed the pendulum toward salvaging of limbs. This has raised many questions: how much surgery is adequate, what is the best adjunctive method of management, and what are the best methods of reconstruction in limb salvage surgery? Determinants of the type of surgical treatment are the pathologic status (general surgical margins); the anatomy (the specific surgical margins for the extent of the tumor, whether it is intracompartmental, extracompartmental, or bicompartmental, and the site of the tumor—whether it

Table 3–35. Surgical Margins as Correlated With Pathology

Surgical Margins	Pathology
Intralesional	Benign self-healing bone tumors
Marginal	Benign soft-tissue tumors
	Locally aggressive benign bone tumors
	Locally aggressive bone tumors
Wide	Low-grade sarcomas
Radical	High-grade sarcomas

is appendicular or in axial bones and whether it involves expandable or nonexpandable bone); and other factors such as whether surgery is an adjuvant and whether the tumor is recurrent.

Surgical margins should be defined in making the decision. In general, there are four types of oncologic wound margins: intracapsular, marginal, wide, and radical (Table 3–35).

Intracapsular margin. When a tumor is removed piecemeal from within the capsule or pseudocapsule, leaving behind parts of the lesion and a reactive zone containing satellites and skips in the surrounding tissue, the wound margin is intracapsular. Examples are curettage of bone tumors and debulking in soft-tissue lesions.

Marginal Margin. In this type, the plane of dissection is extracapsular, and the tumor is removed en bloc between the capsule and the reactive zone or within the reactive zone. Left behind are portions of reactive zone containing satellites and skips.

Wide Margin. The plane of dissection is outside the reactive zone through normal tissue. The tumor is removed en bloc within the compartment of origin with no natural barriers between the lesion and the margin. Skipped lesions may be left even though the lesion is intracompartmental.

Radical Margin. When the lesion is removed en bloc with the entire compartment, with natural barriers between the margin of the wound and the lesion in all dimensions, it is referred to as a radical margin.

Surgical procedures may be classified according to the margin of the wound. They may be local excision or ablation of a part (Figs. 3–240 and 3–241) (Table 3–36).

An intralesional procedure leaves behind macroscopic disease (e.g., debulking of a soft-tissue tumor or curettage of a bone lesion). A marginal procedure leaves microscopic disease; examples are pericapsular excision of a soft-tissue tumor and excision of a bone tumor through the reactive zone. A wide excision may leave "skip" or "satellite" disease. An example is ablation of a tumor with a normal cuff or surrounding tissue (intracompartmental). A radical procedure leaves no residual tumor behind. The procedure is extracompartmental, ablating the bone or muscle outside the compartment.

Treatment

As a general rule, the definitive treatment of benign tumors is as follows. *Stage 1 (benign, latent)* lesions can be adequately treated by intralesional excisions; in some cases marginal local excision may be desirable. *Stage 2 (benign, active)* lesions are well encapsulated without satellites and can be definitively treated by marginal local excision. A wide margin is not necessary. Inadvertent contamination during the procedure should be avoided, as transplanted active cells may cause recurrence. Intralesional excision will result in local recurrence in about a third of cases. In some Stage 2 benign lesions extracapsular marginal excision may be too hazardous because of the anatomic location (such as aneurysmal bone cyst or osteoblastoma in the cervical spine invading the vertebral bodies and neural foramina); in such instances intralesional excision (curettage) is supplemented by adjunctive therapy (irradiation) to control the tumor.

Stage 3 *(benign, aggressive)* lesions are controlled by wide excision. A marginal excision will result in recurrence in about half the cases. In some anatomic situations a wide excision is undesirable or cannot be accomplished; in such

Table 3–36. Types of Excision of Tumor as Related to Surgical Margins*

Type	Plane of Dissection	Result
Intralesional	Debulking or curettage	Leaves macroscopic disease
Marginal	Pericapsular reactive zone	Likely to leave microscopic disease
Wide	Normal cuff of tissue (intracompartmental)	May leave "skip" or "satellite" disease
Radical	Whole bone or muscle outside compartment (extracompartmental)	No residual

*Needs surgical *and* pathologic verification.

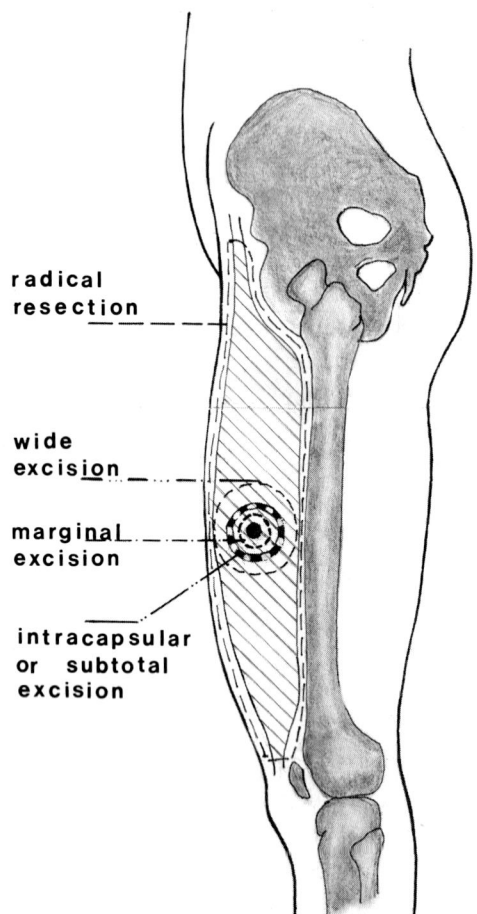

FIGURE 3–240. *Diagram of the four types of local procedures.*

The solid circle is the tumor and the hatched areas are the reactive zone. Intracapsular, or intralesional, excision in soft-tissue tumors is subtotal piecemeal removal and leaves behind tumorous tissue in the margins of the wound. In bone (curettage) it will also leave behind residual tumor. In marginal local excision the dissection is to the reactive zone peripheral to the pseudocapsule. In wide local excision dissection is through grossly normal tissue in all directions. It is sometimes referred to as resection. Radical local excision is extracompartmental removal of the tumor.

instances marginal excision is preferable to intralesional excision, because it carries less risk of recurrence.

Definitive treatment of malignant tumors is as follows: *Stage 1A (malignant, low-grade, intracompartmental with no metastases)* should be treated by wide surgical procedures. *Stage 1B (malignant, low-grade, extracompartmental with no metastases)* tumors are best treated by amputation. Salvage attempts by wide local excision will result in a high rate or recurrence. This should be made clear to a patient who selects a local excision for preservation of function. *Stage 2A (malignant, high-grade, intracompartmental, no metastases)* tumors are excised with a radical margin to remove satellites and skips. *Stage 2B (malignant, high-grade, extracompartmental, no metastases)* tumors are best treated by amputation. In some instances disarticulation should be the procedure of choice.

The treatment of *Stage 3 lesions (malignant, low-grade, intra- or extracompartmental, with metastases)* should be individualized. Adjuvant therapy is given in an attempt to control the tumor. Ablation of the limb may be indicated, and also surgical excision of metastases to the lungs may be carried out. This is described

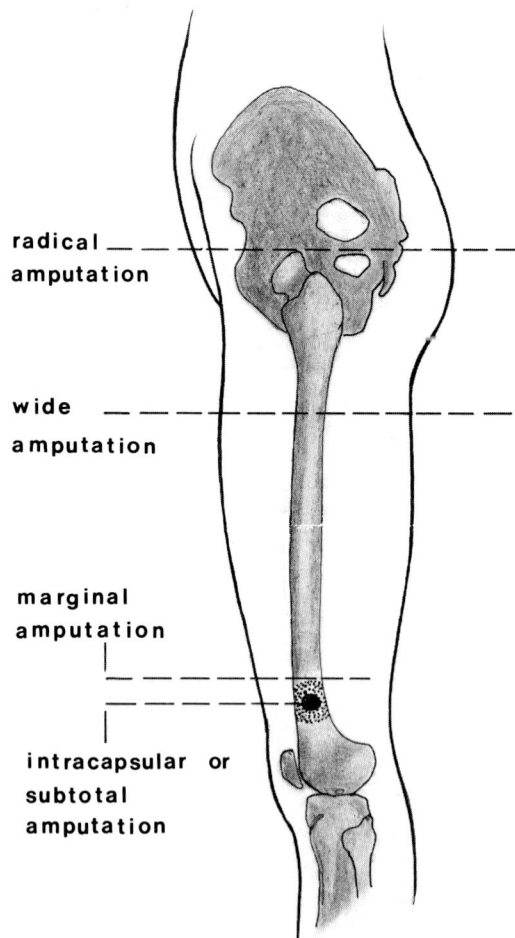

FIGURE 3–241. *Diagram of various types of amputation.*

The tumor is a solid circle and the hatched area is the reactive zone. Intracapsular amputation is subtotal removal—it leaves tumor behind. In marginal amputation the plane of ablation is in the reactive zone. In wide amputation the level of ablation is through normal tissue proximal to the reactive zone, but it is intracompartmental. The procedure may leave residual skipped lesions. Radical amputation, or disarticulation, is an extracompartmental ablation of the part. It leaves no tumor behind.

further in the text dealing with the various malignant tumors.

The different types of adjuvant therapeutic agents utilized for musculoskeletal tumors are chemotherapy, radiation therapy, and immunotherapy. In the past local physical or chemical agents such as carbolic acid and hypertonic saline have been tried and have been shown to be of no value.

In children, *cryosurgery* is not indicated because of damage to the growth plate due to the inability to control the penetration of the freeze and to excessive necrosis of normal tissues such as nerves, skin, and vessels with consequent gangrene of articular cartilage leading to subsequent degenerative arthritis and a high incidence of pathologic fracture of necrotic bone. The use of methylmethacrylate is indicated to bind and stabilize pathologic fractures and to pack large cavities. It should be understood, however, that methylmethacrylate cement will prevent the healing of the cavity in the bone. The advantage of methylmethacrylate is that it extends the margins of subtotal curettage with few problems and complications.

Chemotherapy is the definitive modality of treatment for marrow cell tumors and lymphomas, and surgery is an adjunct. The primary decisions are made and treatment administered by the oncologist, and the role of the surgeon is seondary—to provide orthopedic care for pathologic fractures and biomechanical problems and growth disturbances.

Radiation therapy is sometimes a surgical adjunct, and in other circumstances it is the definitive method of therapy. The decision whether it is an adjunctive or definitive modality of treatment depends on staging, location, and presence or absence of metastases. The radiotherapist and surgeon should communicate, but the planning decisions are made by the oncologist, who should be the captain of the team.

Immunotherapy is another adjunctive therapy that is going through trials. At present its role has not been delineated.

Operative Procedural Considerations

Biopsy.[2, 19, 31, 40, 43, 70, 76] The definitive diagnosis of all tumors is made by biopsy and study of the histologic picture. Staging should always precede biopsy; this sequence provides better clinical, radiologic, and pathologic correlation and facilitates immediate surgery. Also, postoperative infection, increased probability of pathologic fracture, and a larger hematoma are avoided. In general, this author recommends an open biopsy when the lesion is surgically accessible because it allows the surgeon to obtain representative tissue and verify the extent of the lesion by direct visualization. The disadvantages of open biopsy are that there is a greater chance of tumor spillage, and accuracy of imaging decreases after biopsy. In malignant lesions, an incisional biopsy is performed, whereas in benign lesions, a marginal excisional biopsy is carried out.

When a malignant tumor is suspected, the part is not exsanguinated prior to application of a tourniquet. Placement of the biopsy incision is important. It should be in line with future incisions for a definitive procedure; under no circumstance should it be perpendicular to the definitive incision. The circulation to an amputation flap should always be borne in mind. In general, longitudinal incisions are preferred over transverse ones. Avoid neurovascular structures and traverse as few compartments as possible. Be cautious around limb girdles.

Intraoperative radiographic verification of the site of biopsy of bone tumors is always necessary. The bone biopsy should be made through a circular hole or an oblong window to prevent pathologic fracture. Specimens should be marked with a suture for the orientation of the pathologist. Frozen sections are made when possible to ensure that adequate tissue is obtained for diagnosis. The tourniquet is then released and complete hemostasis obtained. The biopsy site is coagulated, and bone wax is used if bone bleeding cannot be controlled. The wound is tightly closed in layers with closely placed sutures. Suction drains should be close to the wound margin. The limb that has been operated on may require splinting for comfort and to prevent a pathologic fracture. This author recommends the use of closed biopsy by either trocar or needle when the site of the lesion is surgically inaccessible or difficult, as in a vertebral body. It should be borne in mind, however, that there is a great risk of sampling error. After closed biopsy, frozen sections are mandatory.

Details of other surgical techniques are discussed in the management of individual tumors.

References

1. Ackerman, L. V., and Spjut, H. J.: Tumors of Bone and Cartilage. Washington, D.C.: Armed Forces Institute of Pathology, 1962.
2. Adler, O., and Rosenberger, A.: Fine needle aspiration biopsy of osteolytic metastatic lesions. A.J.R., *133*:15, 1979.

3. Aegerter, E., and Kirkpatrick, J. A.: Orthopedic Diseases. Philadelphia, Saunders, 1975.
4. Altman, A. J., and Schwartz, A. D.: Malignant Diseases of Infancy, Childhood and Adolescence. Philadelphia, Saunders, 1978.
5. Berger, P. E., and Kuhn, J. P.: Computed tomography of tumors of the musculoskeletal system in children. Radiology, 127:171, 1978.
6. Bernardino, M. E., Jing, B. S., Thomas, J. L., Lindell, M. M., Jr., and Zornoza, J.: The extremity soft tissue lesion: A comparative study of ultrasound, computed tomography and xeroradiography. Radiology, 139:53, 1981.
7. Berquist, T. H.: Magnetic resonance imaging: Preliminary experience in orthopedic radiology. Magn. Res. Imaging, 2:41, 1984.
8. Brady, T. J., Rosen, B. R., Pykett, I. L., McGuire, M. H., Mankin, H. J., and Rosenthal, D. I.: NMR imaging of leg tumors. Radiology, 149:181, 1984.
9. Brady, T. J., Gebhardt, M. C., Pykett, I. L., Buonanno, F. S., Newhouse, J. H., Burt, C. T., Smith, R. J., Mankin, H. J., Kistler, J. P., Goldman, M. R., Hinshaw, W. S., and Pohost, G. M.: NMR imaging of forearms in healthy volunteers and patients with giant cell tumor of bone. Radiology, 144:549, 1982.
10. Bogumil, G. P., and Schwamm, H. A.: Orthopaedic Pathology—A Synopsis with Clinical and Radiographic Correlation. Philadelphia, Saunders, 1985.
11. Caffey, J.: Pediatric X-ray Diagnosis. 7th Ed. Chicago, Year Book, 1979.
12. Campbell, C. J., Roach, J. F., and Jabbur, M.: Xeroroentgenography: Evaluation of its use in diseases of the bone and joints of the extremities. J. Bone Joint Surg., 41-A:271, 1959.
13. Chew, F. S., and Hudson, T. M.: Radionuclide bone scanning of osteosarcoma: Falsely extended uptake patterns. A.J.R., 139:49, 1982.
14. Cohen, M. D., Klatte, E. C., Baehner, R., Smith, J. A., Martin Simmerman, P., Carr, B. E., Provisor, A. J., Weetman, R. M., Coates, T., Sidduqui, A., Weisman, S. J., Berkow, R., McKenna, S., and McGuire, W. A.: Magnetic resonance imaging of bone marrow diseases in children. Radiology, 151:715, 1984.
15. Coley, B. L.: Neoplasms of Bone and Related Conditions. 2nd Ed. New York, Hoeber, 1960.
16. Corcoran, R. J., Thrall, J. H., Kyle, R. W., et al.: Solitary abnormalities in bone scans of patients with extraosseous malignancies. Radiology, 121:663, 1976.
17. Dahlin, D. C.: Bone Tumors—General Aspects and Data on 6221 Cases. 3rd Ed. Springfield, Ill., Thomas, 1978.
18. DeSantos, L. A., Goldstein, H. M., Murray, J. A., and Wallace, S.: Computed tomography in the evaluation of musculoskeletal neoplasms. Radiology, 128:89, 1978.
19. DeSantos, L. A., Murray, J. A., and Ayala, A. G.: The value of percutaneous needle biopsy in the management of primary bone tumors. Cancer, 43:735, 1979.
20. Dos Santos, R.: Arteriography in bone tumours. J. Bone Joint Surg., 32-B:17, 1950.
21. Edeiken, J., and Hodes, P. J.: Roentgen Diagnosis of Diseases of Bone. 2nd Ed. Baltimore, Williams & Wilkins, 1975.
22. Enneking, W. F.: Musculoskeletal Tumor Surgery. New York, Churchill-Livingstone, 1983.
23. Enneking, W. F., Spanier, S. S., and Goodman, M. A.: A system for the surgical staging of musculoskeletal sarcoma. Clin. Orthop., 153:106, 1980.
24. Enneking, W. F., Spanier, S. S., and Goodman, M. A.: The surgical staging of musculoskeletal sarcoma. J. Bone Joint Surg., 62-A:1027, 1980.
25. Enneking, W. F., Spanier, S. S., and Malawer, M. M.: The effect of the anatomic setting on the results of surgical procedures for soft parts sarcoma of the thigh. Cancer, 47:1005, 1981.
26. Enneking, W. F., Chew, F. S., Springfield, D. S., Hudson, T. M., and Spanier, S. S.: The role of radionuclide bone-scanning in determining the resectability of soft tissue sarcomas. J. Bone Joint Surg., 62-A:249, 1981.
27. Ewing, J.: The classification and treatment of bone sarcoma. Report of the International Conference on Cancer. London, 1928.
28. Ewing, J.: A review of the classification of bone tumors. Surg. Gynecol. Obstet., 68:971, 1939.
29. Farinas, P. L.: Differential diagnosis of bone tumors of extremities by arteriography. Radiology, 29:29, 1937.
30. Ferguson, A. B.: Roentgen Diagnosis of the Extremities and Spine. New York, Hoeber, 1941.
31. Frankel, C. J.: Aspiration biopsy of the spine. J. Bone Joint Surg., 36-A:69, 1954.
32. Galasko, C. S. B.: The pathological basis for skeletal scintigraphy. J. Bone Joint Surg., 57-B:353, 1975.
33. Geschickter, C. F., and Copeland, M. M.: Tumors of Bone. 3rd Ed. Philadelphia, Lippincott, 1949.
34. Gilday, D. L., Ash, J. M., and Reilly, B. J.: Radionuclide skeletal survey for pediatric neoplasms. Radiology, 123:399, 1977.
35. Gilmer, W. S., Jr., Higley, G. B., Jr., and Kilgore, W. E.: Atlas of Bone Tumors: Including Tumor-Like Lesions. St. Louis, Mosby, 1963.
36. Glass, R. B., Fernbach, S. K., Conway, J. J., and Shkolnik, A.: Gallium scintigraphy in American Burkitt lymphoma: Accurate assessment of tumor load and prognosis. A.J.R., 145:671, 1985.
37. Graham, W. D.: Bone Tumors. London, Butterworth, 1966.
38. Greenfield, G. B.: Radiology of Bone Diseases. 2nd Ed. Philadelphia, Lippincott, 1975.
39. Grundmann, E.: Malignant Bone Tumors. New York, Springer-Verlag, 1976.
40. Hajdu, S. I., and Melamed, M. R.: Needle biopsy of primary malignant bone tumors. Surg. Gynecol. Obstet., 133:829, 1971.
41. Halpern, M., and Freiberger, R. H.: Arteriography in orthopedics. A.J.R., 94:194, 1965.
42. Harcke, H. T., Conway, J. J., Tachdjian, M. O., et al.: Scintigraphic localization of bone lesions during surgery. Skeletal Radiol., 13:211, 1985.
43. Hartman, J. T., and Phalen, G. S.: Needle biopsy of bone. J.A.M.A., 200:201, 1967.
44. Hermann, G., and Rose, J. S.: Computed tomography in bone and soft tissue pathology of the extremities. J. Comput. Assist. Tomogr., 3:58, 1979.
45. Herzberg, D. L., and Schreiber, M. H.: Angiography in mass lesions of the extremities. A.J.R., 111:541, 1971.
46. Hoefnagel, C. A., Voute, P. A., deKraker, J., and Marcuse, H. R.: Radionuclide diagnosis and therapy of neural crest tumors using iodine-131 metaiodobenzylguanidine. J. Nucl. Med., 28:308, 1987.
47. Hudson, T. M.: Scintigraphy of aneurysmal bone cyst. A.J.R., 142:761, 1984.
48. Hudson, T. M., and Chew, F. S.: Radionuclide bone scanning of osteosarcoma: Falsely extended uptake patterns. A.J.R., 139:49, 1982.
49. Hudson, T. M., Hamlin, D. J., and Fitzsimmons, J. R.: Magnetic resonance imaging of fluid levels in an aneurysmal bone cyst and in anticoagulated human blood. Skeletal Radiol., 13:267, 1985.
50. Hudson, T. M., Schakel, M., II, and Springfield, D. S.: Limitations of computed tomography following excisional biopsy of soft tissue sarcomas. Skeletal Radiol., 13:49, 1985.
51. Hudson, T. M., Haas, G., Enneking, W. F., and Hawkins, I. F., Jr.: Angiography in the management of musculoskeletal tumors. Surg. Gynecol. Obstet., 141:11, 1975.
52. Hudson, T. M., Hamlin, D. J., Enneking, W. F., and Pettersson, H.: Magnetic resonance imaging of bone

and soft tissue tumors: Early experience in 31 patients compared with computed tomography. Skeletal Radiol., 13:134, 1985.
53. Hudson, T. M., Springfield, D. S., Spanier, S. S., Enneking, W. F., and Hamlin, D. J.: Computed tomography of benign exostosis and exostotic chondrosarcoma: Difficulty in evaluating cartilage thickness. Radiology, in press.
54. Hudson, T. M., Scheibler, M., Springfield, D. S., Hawkins, I. R., Jr., Enneking, W. F., and Spanier, S. S.: Radiologic imaging of osteosarcoma: Role in planning surgical treatment. Skeletal Radiol., 10:137, 1983.
55. Hudson, T. M., Schiebler, M., Springfield, D. S., Enneking, W. F., Hawkins, I. F., Jr., and Spanier, S. S.: Radiology of giant cell tumors of bone. Computed tomography, arthro-tomography and scintigraphy. Skeletal Radiol., 11:85, 1984.
56. Huvos, A. G.: Bone Tumors. Philadelphia, Saunders, 1979.
57. Jaffe, H. L.: Tumors and Tumorous Conditions of the Bones and Joints. Philadelphia, Lea & Febiger, 1958.
58. Keats, T. E.: An Atlas of Normal Roentgen Variants That May Simulate Disease. Chicago, Year Book, 1973.
59. Kerns, L. L., and Simon, M. A.: Surgical theory, staging, definitions, and treatment of musculoskeletal tumors. Surg. Clin. North Am., 63:671, 1983.
60. Kirchner, P. T., and Simon, M. A.: The clinical value of bone and gallium scintigraphy for soft-tissue sarcomas of the extremities. J. Bone Joint Surg., 66-A:319, 1984.
61. Koehler, A., and Zimmer, E. A.: Borderlands of the Normal and Early Pathologic in Skeletal Roentgenography. New York, Grune & Stratton, 1968.
62. Lange, T. A., Austin, C. W., Seibert, J. J., Angtuaco, T. L., and Yandow, D. R.: Ultrasound imaging as a screening study for malignant soft-tissue tumors. J. Bone Joint Surg., 69-A:100, 1987.
63. Levine, E., Lee, K. R., Neff, J. R., Maklad, N. F., Robinson, R. G., and Preston, D. F.: Comparison of tomography and other imaging modalities in the evaluation of musculoskeletal tumors. Radiology, 131:431, 1979.
64. Lichtenstein, L.: Bone Tumors. 5th Ed. St. Louis, Mosby, 1979.
65. Lodwick, G. S.: Atlas of Tumor Radiology. The Bones and Joints. Chicago, Year Book, 1971, pp. 65–79.
66. Luck, J. V.: Bone and Joint Diseases. Pathology Correlated with Roentgenological and Clinical Features. Springfield, Ill., Thomas, 1950, pp. 439–440, 484–485.
67. Marcove, R. C., and Miller, T. R.: Treatment of primary and metastatic bone tumors by cryosurgery. J.A.M.A., 207:1890, 1969.
68. Moon, K. L., Genant, H. K., Helms, C. A., Chafetz, N. I., Crooks, L. E., and Kaufman, D. L.: Musculoskeletal applications of nuclear magnetic resonance. Radiology, 147:161, 1983.
69. Moon, K. L., Davis, P. L., Kaufman, D. L., Crooks, L. E., Sheldon, P. E., Miller, T., Brito, A. C., and Watts, J. C.: Nuclear magnetic resonance imaging of a fibrosarcoma tumor implanted in the rat. Radiology, 148:177, 1984.
70. Moore, T. M., Meyers, M. H., Patzakis, M. J., Terry, R., and Harvey, J. P.: Closed biopsy of musculoskeletal lesions. J. Bone Joint Surg., 61-A:375, 1979.
71. Murray, R. O., and Jacobson, H. G.: The Radiology of Skeletal Disorders. 2nd Ed. London, Churchill-Livingstone, 1977.
72. Nelson, S. W.: Some fundamentals in the radiologic differential diagnosis of solitary bone lesions. Semin. Roentgenol., 1:244, 1966.
73. Nessi, R., and Coopmans de Yoldi, G.: Xeroradiography of bone tumors. Skeletal Radiol., 2:143, 1978.
74. The Netherlands Committee on Bone Tumors: Radiological Atlas of Bone Tumors. Baltimore, Williams & Wilkins, 1973.
75. Nostrand, D. V., Madewell, J. E., McNiesh, L. M., et al.: Radionuclide bone scanning in giant tumor cell. J. Nucl. Med., 27:329, 1986.
76. Ottolenghi, C. E.: Diagnosis of orthopedic lesions by aspiration biopsy: Results of 1,061 punctures. J. Bone Joint Surg., 37-A:443, 1955.
77. Phemister, D.: Panel on Bone Tumors. Proc. First Natl. Cancer Conference, 1949.
78. Pistenma, D. A., McDougall, I. R., and Kriss, J. P.: Screening for bone metastases. J.A.M.A., 231:46, 1975.
79. Pollen, J. J., Witztum, K. F., and Ashburn, W. L.: The flare phenomenon on radionuclide bone scan in metastatic prostate cancer. A.J.R., 142:773, 1984.
80. Price, C. H. G., and Ross, F. G. M. (eds.): Bone—Certain Aspects of Neoplasia. London, Butterworth, 1973.
81. Pugh, D. G.: Roentgenological Diagnosis of Diseases of Bone. Baltimore, Williams & Wilkins, 1960.
82. Rosenthal, D. I.: Computed tomography in bone and soft tissue neoplasms: Application and pathologic correlation. CRC Crit. Rev. Diagn. Imaging, 18:243, 1983.
83. Schajowicz, F.: Tumors and Tumor-like Lesions of Bones and Joints. New York, Springer-Verlag, 1981.
84. Shulkin, B. L., Schen, S. W., Sisson, J. C., and Shapiro, B.: Iodine-131 MIBG scintigraphy of the extremities in metastatic pheochromocytoma and neuroblastoma. J. Nucl. Med., 28:315, 1987.
85. Simon, M. A.: Biopsy of musculoskeletal tumors. J. Bone Joint Surg., 64-A:188, 1982.
86. Simon, M. A.: Diagnostic and staging strategy for musculoskeletal tumors. In Evarts, C. M., (ed.): Surgery of the Musculoskeletal System. Vol. 4. Chap. 11. New York, Churchill-Livingstone, 1983, pp. 5–38.
87. Simon, M. A.: Causes of increased survival of patients with osteosarcoma: Current controversies. J. Bone Joint Surg., 66-A:306, 1984.
88. Simon, M. A., and Enneking, W. F.: The management of soft-tissue sarcomas of the extremities. J. Bone Joint Surg., 58-A:317, 1976.
89. Simon, M. A., and Kirchner, P. T.: Scintigraphic evaluation of primary bone tumors. J. Bone Joint Surg., 62-A:758, 1980.
90. Simon, M. A., Spanier, S. S., and Enneking, W. F.: Management of adult soft tissue sarcomas of the extremities. Surg. Annu., 11:363, 1979.
91. Wahner, H. W., Kyle, R. A., and Beabout, J. W.: Scintigraphic evaluation of the skeleton in multiple myeloma. Mayo Clin. Proc., 55:739, 1980.
92. Willis, R. A.: Pathology of Tumours. London, Butterworth, 1948, p. 670.
93. Wilner, D.: Radiology of Bone Tumors and Allied Disorders. Philadelphia, Saunders, 1982.
94. Young, J. L., Jr., and Miller, R. W.: Incidence of malignant tumors in U.S. children. J. Pediatr., 86:254, 1975.

OSTEOCHONDROMA

Osteochondroma, or solitary osteocartilaginous exostosis, is characterized by a cartilage-capped, osseous projection protruding from the surface of the affected bone. It is not a true neoplasm because the osseous tissue produced is normal in every respect. It should be considered rather as a developmental defect in which there is a disturbance in the location and direction of enchondral cartilaginous growth. The exostosis is produced by progressive enchondral ossification of the hood of the hyaline cartilaginous cap, which acts as an enchondral plate.

Etiology

Two theories have been proposed to explain the pathogenesis of osteochondroma. Virchow, in 1891, postulated the physeal theory—that a portion of the physeal cartilage becomes separated from the parent tissue, rotates 90 degrees, and grows in a direction transverse to the long axis of the bone. He could not provide reasons for the separation and rotation of the detached physeal cartilage.[60] In 1920 Keith proposed that a defect in the perichondral ring surrounding the physis is the cause of osteochondroma.[34] Müller's periosteal theory states that exostoses are produced by small nests of cartilage derived from the cambium layer of the periosteum.[46]

D'Ambrosia and Ferguson, by producing osteochondroma by physeal cartilage transplantation, provided support to the developmental physeal plate defect theory.[16] It seems that the most plausible cause of osteochondroma is a perversion in the direction of growth of the physis with lateral protrusions of portions of the growth plate causing the development of eccentric, cartilage-capped bone prominences.

Incidence and Anatomic Site

It is, by far, the most common of the benign tumorous bone conditions. It occurs in adolescents or young children, the lesion being discovered between 10 and 20 years of age in about 80 per cent of cases. Both sexes are equally affected.

Any bone preformed in cartilage may be subject to this condition; however, about half the cases involve the long tubular bones of the limbs, with the lower metaphysis of the femur and the upper metaphyses of the tibia and humerus being the most common locations. Other areas of predilection are the distal radius, distal tibia, and proximal and distal fibula. The lesion is usually located in the metaphyseal area, and with growth it moves away from the physis.

An exostosis may occasionally develop in a flat bone—the scapula, ilium, rib, or skull. Isolated cases are reported in the cervical spine.[19, 32, 47, 62]

Pathology

The lesion may be sessile or pedunculated, varying in diameter from 1 to 10 cm. Its surface is rather knobby (Fig. 3–242 B). The exostosis may appear plateau-like, roughly hemispheric, cauliflower-like, or tubular in contour with a pronged end. It is covered by either thin or comparatively thick perichondrium, which is adherent to the underlying irregular surface and is continuous with that of the adjacent bony cortex. When the perichondrium is stripped, the bluish-white hyaline cartilage of the cap will be exposed. The cartilaginous cap may be 1 to 3 mm. in thickness, as shown on perpendicular section of the tumor. The younger the patient, the greater the size and thickness of the cap.

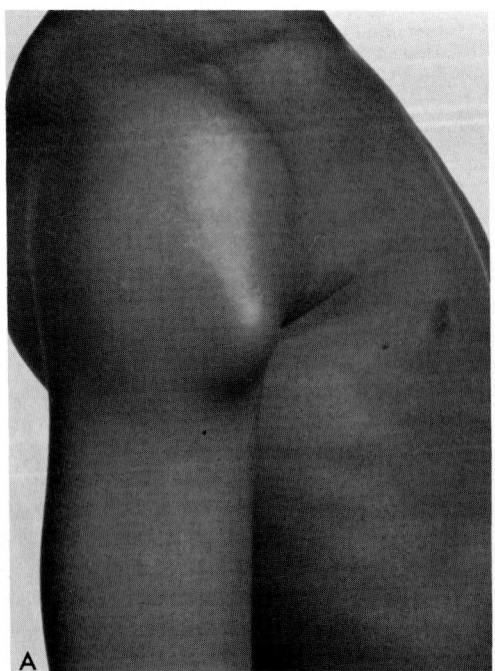
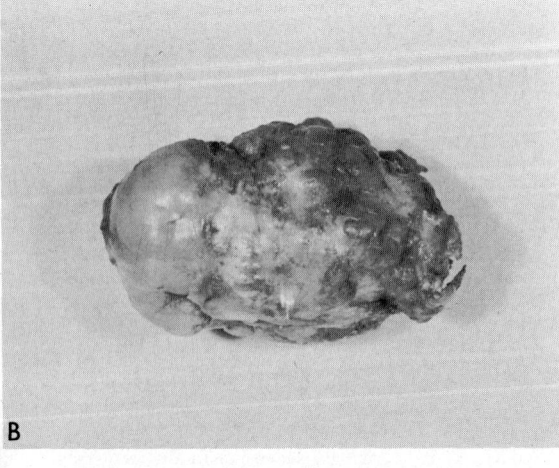

FIGURE 3–242. *Osteochondroma of proximal humerus.*

A. Clinical appearance is that of a local protruding mass. B. Gross appearance of excised lesion. Note its knobby cartilaginous surface.

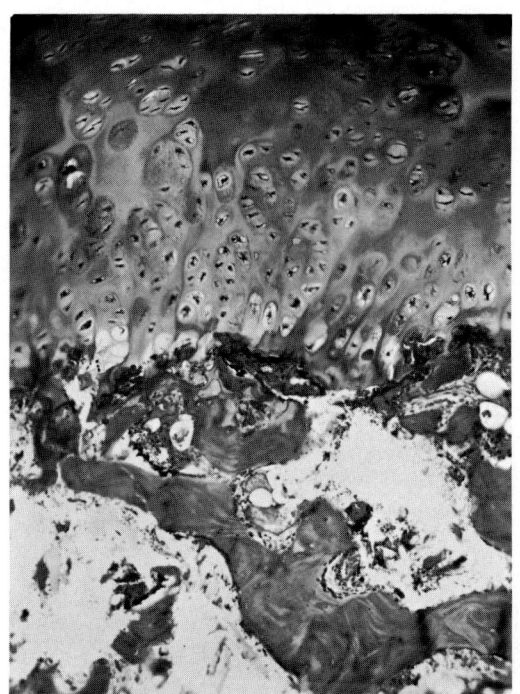

FIGURE 3–243. Osteochondroma.

Histologic appearance of osteocartilaginous junction (× 100). Note the enchondral ossification and the foci of proliferating cartilage cells in its deep layers.

The interior of the exostosis consists of normal spongiosa that is continuous with that of the affected bone, with a defect in the cortex at the site of the exostosis.

A bursa may develop over the osteochondroma, especially if the lesion is large and is irritated by the movement of adjacent muscles and tendons. This bursal sac has been termed "exostosis bursata."[54] The bursal sac may contain mucinous fluid and fibrinous rice bodies, which may sometimes be calcified.

On microscopic examination of osteochondroma in a child, normal enchondral ossification is seen at the cartilage-bone junction (Fig. 3–243). Foci of proliferating cartilage cells are found in its deep layers. There are areas of cartilage cores within the subchondral spongiosa next to the growth zone; these usually gradually resorb, but on occasion, may persist. One may observe fibrosed marrow impregnated by calcium detritus and calcified cartilage. The marrow in the interior of the exostosis is predominantly fatty. Growth of the exostosis is by enchondral ossification on the deep surface of the cartilage cap, with growth generally ceasing at maturity and sometimes earlier.

The appearance of the cartilaginous cap depends on the stage of growth. It undergoes regressive changes and tends to involute and gradually disappear in the older adult. Remnants of quiescent cartilage can persist far into adult life, however, and very occasionally may reactivate and undergo chondrosarcomatous change.

Clinical Picture

The lesion is usually discovered incidentally on radiographic examination or on palpation of a protruding mass in the affected area (see Fig. 3–242 A). The osteochondroma often is not tender, but pain will result following direct injury to the tumor or a fracture through the stalk of a pedunculated lesion. It may impinge upon nerves, especially if it is large. Compression of the cauda equina may result from a lesion in the lumbar spine, and one involving the ankle or foot may cause difficulty in walking or in wearing shoes.

Radiographic Findings

Its radiographic appearance is characterized by a bony protuberance that is juxtaphyseal in location, directed toward the shaft, and has the cortex and spongiosa continuous with that of the affected bone (Fig. 3–244). There may be slight metaphyseal widening at the site of the exostosis. The cartilaginous cap is not visible; masses of calcified cartilage may, however, be represented as blotches of radiopacity.

In the long bones the exostosis is usually pedunculated; the sessile type may take a broad-based form, a cauliflower form, or be circumferential in appearance. In the flat bones, such as the ilium, exostoses are usually sessile in type, and usually located near the cartilaginous ends of the bone. In the sternum the exostosis may grow to a very large size and press on mediastinal structures. Osteochondromas rarely develop in the carpal and tarsal bones, despite the fact that these bones are preformed in cartilage (Fig. 3–245).[26]

Ultrasonography will be helpful in delineating the extent of a painful swollen bursa over the exostosis and the thickness of the cartilaginous cap.

Treatment

Surgical excision of a solitary exostosis is indicated (1) when it presses on peripheral nerves and vessels such as the popliteal artery or peroneal nerve at the knee, or in the vertebral column, the spinal cord, or spinal nerves; (2) when it interferes with joint motion and

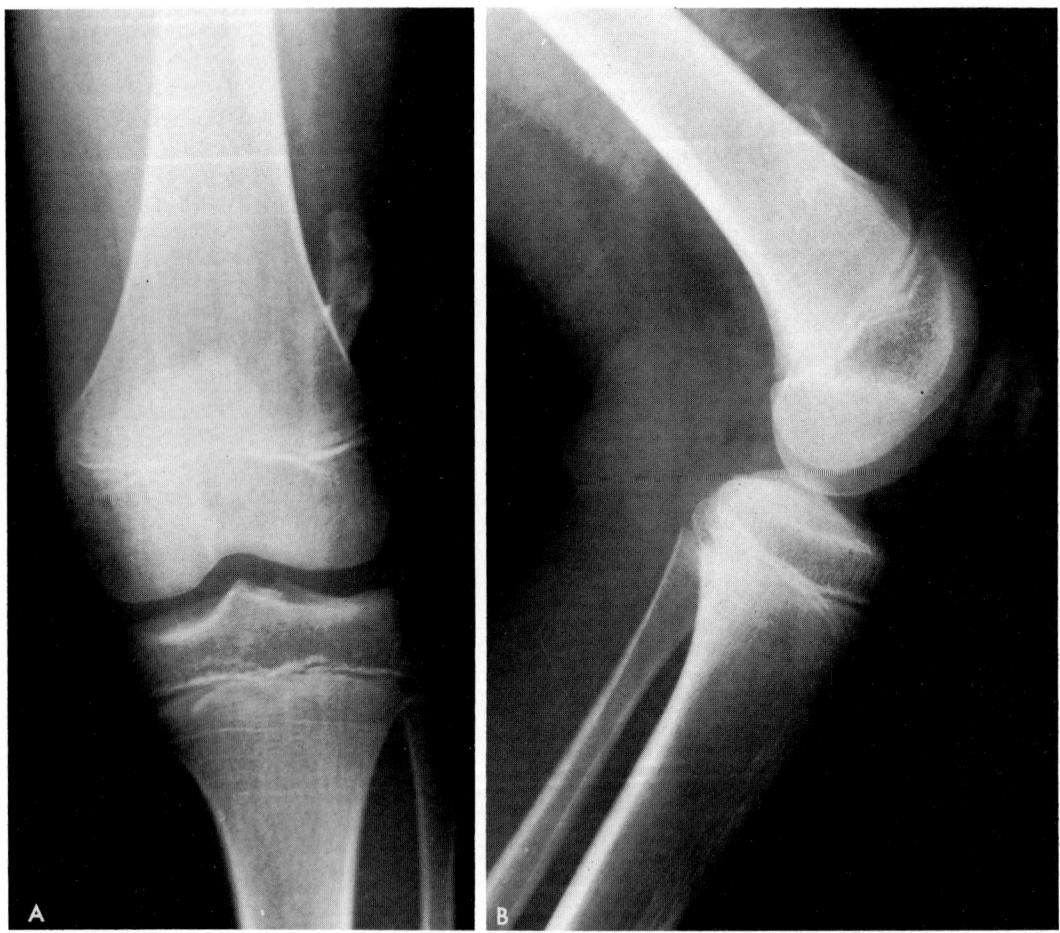
FIGURE 3–244. Radiographic appearance of osteochondroma of distal femur in an 11-year-old boy.

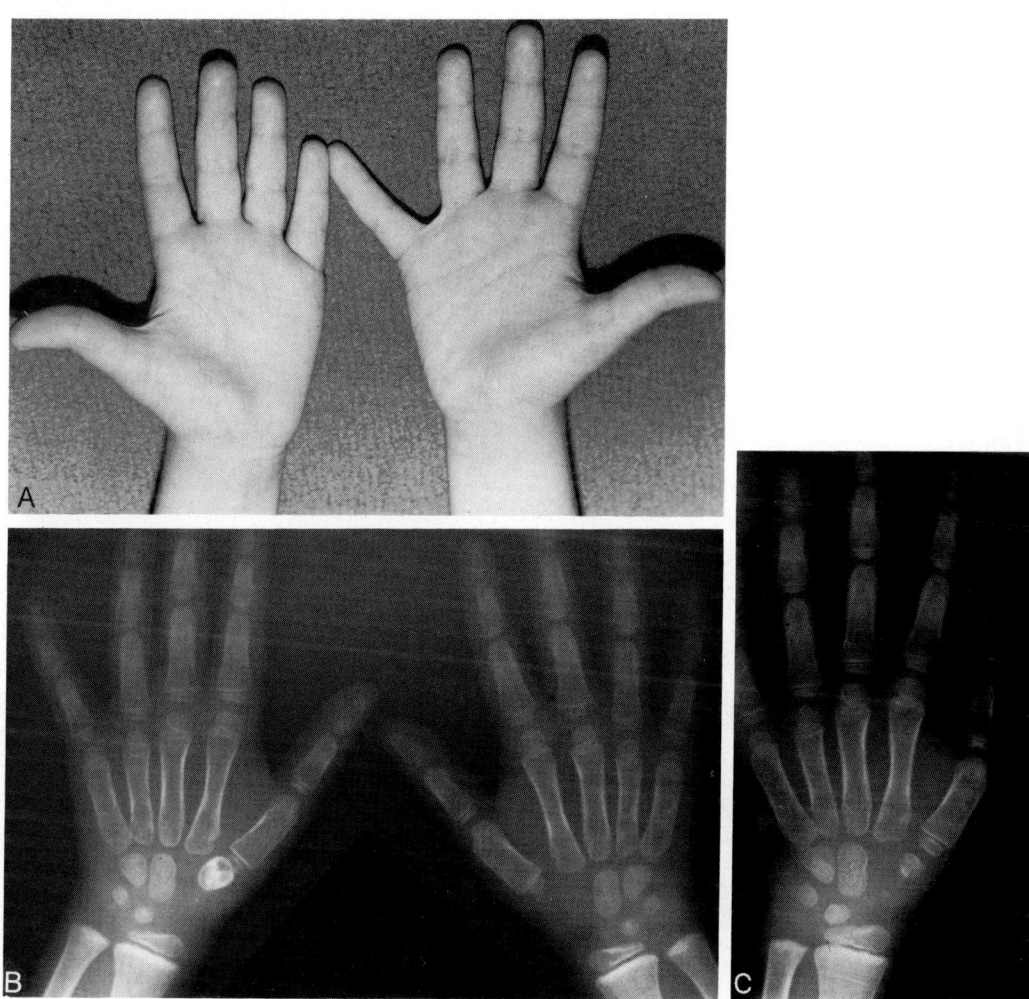

FIGURE 3-245. *Osteochondroma of the carpal pisiform of the right hand.*

A. Preoperative photograph of the hand shows the mass at the base of the thenar eminence. **B.** Preoperative radiogram shows the increased radiopacity at the pisiform bone. **C.** Postoperative radiogram; note that the osteochondroma is excised.

mechanics by compromising adjacent structures; (3) when it is at a site that subjects the exostosis to frequent injury; (4) when a pedunculated osteochondroma fractures at its base following trauma; (5) or when a painful bursa develops because of irritation, necessitating removal of the lesion. Likewise, when the deformity of the bony protuberence is cosmetically unacceptable, or there is clinical and radiographic suspicion of malignant change, the exostosis is excised. Sometimes even when there are no bothersome symptoms, the author recommends removal of the tumor, the decision depending in part on the location and accessibility of the lesion and in part on future problems that it may cause.

The surgical technique is illustrated in Plate 39. At operation, the periosteum, perichondrium, and cartilaginous cap of the tumor should not be disturbed; they should be removed together with the tumor in order to prevent recurrence of the lesion. It is imperative that the adjacent growth plate not be injured.

Problems and Complications

Pseudoaneurysm. A rare complication of osteochondroma of the femur is pseudoaneurysm of the femoral artery in the adductor canal or the popliteal fossa.* The wall of a pseudoaneurysm consists of an intimal layer that lines the inner surface of the hematoma and in turn is surrounded by a fibrous capsule. The wall of a true aneurysm contains the layers of a normal

---

*See references 1, 8, 9, 11, 17, 20, 23–25, 28, 29, 36, 39, 40, 45, 51, 52, 55, 57.

Excision of Osteochondroma from Medial Aspect of Distal Femoral Metaphysis

A. A longitudinal incision is made over the protruding mass. Subcutaneous tissue and deep fascia are divided.

B. The vastus medialis muscle is split in the direction of its fibers.

C. By blunt dissection, the tumor is exposed, leaving the bursal sac and the perichondrium attached to the osteochondroma undisturbed.

D. The periosteum is incised around the base of the tumor. Next, drill holes are made at its base, and with a curved osteotome, the tumor is excised.

E. The vastus medialis muscle and fascia are sutured. The skin is closed in routine manner. A compression dressing or an above-knee cylinder cast is applied.

Plate 39. Excision of Osteochondroma from Medial Aspect of Distal Femoral Metaphysis

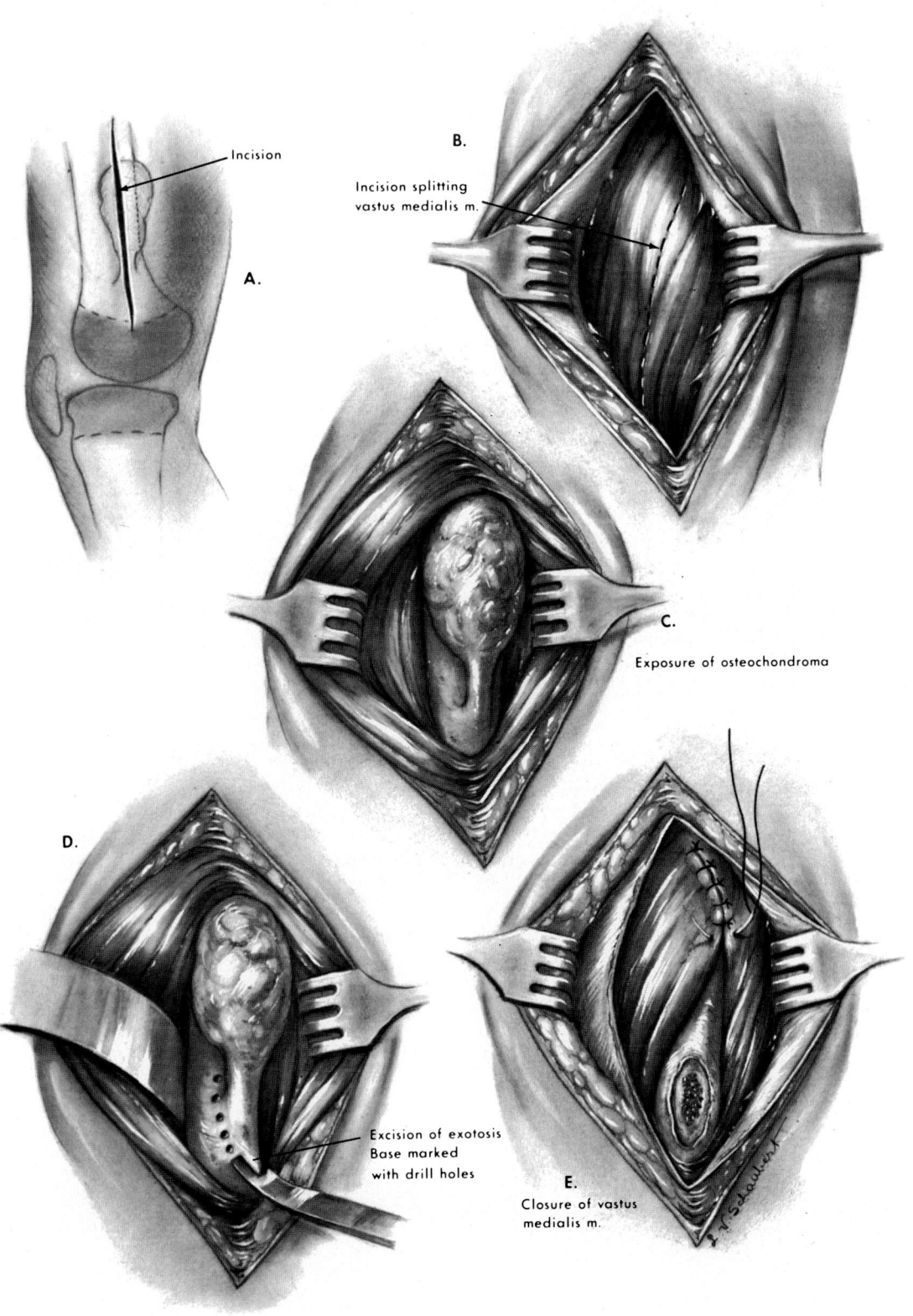

1169

arterial wall, i.e., intimal, medial, and adventitial layers. The cause of a pseudoaneurysm may be acute fracture of the cartilaginous cap that is displaced, leaving spikes of bone to puncture the artery.[39] Often, however, the perforations of the vessel wall are due to gradual erosion rather than acute laceration. The artery is gradually abraded by repeated flexion-extension of the knee as in bicycling. This complication usually occurs in the skeletally mature patient. In the young, the vessel is better protected by the cartilaginous cover of the exostosis. Clinically, the pseudoaneurysm presents as an enlarging mass, which may be warm and pulsatile. A systolic bruit may be audible. A CT scan and an angiogram will establish the diagnosis. Treatment consists of excision of the pseudoaneurysm and the osteochondroma. The perforation in the arterial wall is repaired.

Secondary Sarcomatous Change. Chondrosarcomatous change occurs very rarely in solitary osteochondroma, probably less than 0.25 per cent. Jaffe stated that 1 per cent undergo malignant change, and Dahlin reported an incidence of 4.1 per cent in the solitary osteochondromas surgically treated at the Mayo Clinic—but these figures represent selected cases referred to oncology centers.[15, 33] Malignant change evolves very slowly, usually occurring in adult life; Garrison and associates reported 30.7 years as the average age of the patient with a range of 10 to 72 years.[21] It should be suspected when an osteochondroma begins to grow rapidly and the patient complains of recent onset of pain. Frequent sites of secondary sarcoma developing in solitary osteochondroma are the proximal femur and humerus, whereas in multiple hereditary exostoses they are the pelvis and scapula. Early radiographic findings of sarcomatous change are loss of fine line demarcation on the external surface of the exostosis, which becomes fuzzy and granular in appearance. Later on, the cortex of the exostosis loses its continuity with that of the parent bone. Small areas of radiolucency and calcification develop in the medullary cavity of the exostosis; further on during the growth of chondrosarcoma blotchy areas of increased radiopacity develop in the center of the tumor, which tends to obscure and destroy the exostosis from which it arose. Still later, the tumor extends into soft tissues. Clusters of disorganized calcification, a dense inhomogeneous center, and a thick (greater than 3 cm.) cartilaginous cap that is lobulated are the definite radiographic findings indicating chondrosarcoma.

Nuclear magnetic resonance (NMR) imaging is of great value in early diagnosis of malignant transformation in osteochondroma; it depicts changes not visualized in the plain radiograms and delineates extension of the tumor mass into adjacent soft tissues, thereby assisting in surgical staging and planning of treatment.[35] When NMR is not available, computed axial tomography is utilized to delineate the thickness of the cartilaginous cap and extension of the tumor.

Scintigraphic imaging with technetium-99m methylene diphosphonate does not qualitatively differentiate the benign active exostosis from chondrosarcoma.[30] Lange and associates correlated the radiographic, scintigraphic, and histologic findings in 24 patients with solitary or multiple exostosis; they studied 25 excised tumors, of which two were exostotic chondrosarcoma. Bone scan reflected the level of active enchondral ossification of an exostosis, indicating the activity of its growth. Two patterns of activity were present in both skeletally immature and mature patients; first was the *inactive scan*, seen in quiescent lesions with no histo-

*Table 3–37. Criteria Differentiating Osteochondroma from Chondrosarcoma**

Criterion	Osteochondroma	Chondrosarcoma
Relation to parent bone	Continuity of cortex and medullary cavity with parent bone	Gradual loss of continuity of cortex
External surface of tumor	Distinct, well demarcated	Fuzzy and indistinct
Cartilaginous cap (best visualized on NMR)	Thin, less than 1 cm.	Thick, greater than 3 cm., lobulated, extending into soft tissues
Matrix pattern	Dense at periphery with solid cortex Normal cancellous bone centrally	Periphery granular in appearance with small areas of rarefaction and disorganized calcification
		Later, blotchy areas of calcification within center of tumor with streaky densities extending peripherally
Adjacent soft tissue	Normal	Large soft-tissue mass containing disorganized areas of calcification

*Modified from Kenney, P. J., et al.: The use of computed tomography to distinguish osteochondroma and chondrosarcoma. Radiology, *1139*:129, 1981.

logic evidence of enchondral bone formation, and second, was the scan with *increased uptake*, seen in *active* osteochondroma with active enchondral bone formation. They could demonstrate active enchondral growth of benign exostosis in adults, well beyond the time of skeletal maturity.[37] Both Lange and associates and Hudson and associates reported two cases of intrapelvic chondrosarcoma that were definitely malignant but showed no increased uptake on bone scan, indicating lack of enchondral bone formation and minimum vascularity.[30, 37] Experience with gallium scans has shown similar results.[53] It is evident that bone scintigraphy alone cannot satisfactorily differentiate a benign from a malignant exostosis. Imaging criteria differentiating osteochondroma from chondrosarcoma are given in Table 3–37. When clinical, plain radiographic, and NMR imaging or CT scan findings are suggestive of malignant changes, biopsy should be performed to rule out chondrosarcoma. The chondrosarcoma is of the peripheral type and usually does not metastasize. The prognosis after excision is excellent.

References

1. Anastasi, G. W., Wertheimer, H. M., and Brown, J. R.: Aneurysm with osteochondromas of the femur. Arch. Surg., 87:636, 1963.
2. Anderson, R. L., Popowitz, L., and Li, J. K. H.: An unusual sarcoma arising in a solitary osteochondroma. J. Bone Joint Surg., 51-A:1199, 1969.
3. Bennett, G. E., and Berkheimer, G. A.: Malignant degeneration in a case of benign exostosis. Surgery, 10:781, 1941.
4. Bennett, R. G., and Gammer, S.: Painful callus of the thumb due to phalangeal exostosis. Arch. Dermatol., 108:826, 1973.
5. Blesham, M. H., and Levy, R. M.: An unusual location of an osteochondroma. Radiology, 127:456, 1978.
6. Bowmen, J. R., and Schmidt, T.: Osteochondroma of the femoral neck in Perthes' disease. J. Pediatr. Orthop., 3:28, 1983.
7. Callan, J. E., and Wood, V. E.: Spontaneous resolution of an osteochondroma. J. Bone Joint Surg., 57-A:723, 1975.
8. Cassie, G. F., Dawson, A. S., and Sheville, E.: False aneurysm of femoral artery from cancellous exostosis of femur. Report of a case in a boy of fourteen. J. Bone Joint Surg., 57-B:379, 1975.
9. Chirls, M., Lichtman, H., and Grant, A. D.: Osteochondroma of the femur involving the popliteal artery—Case report. Bull. Hosp. Joint Dis., 22:150, 1961.
10. Chrisman, O. D., and Goldenberg, R. R.: Untreated solitary osteochondroma. Report of two cases. J. Bone Joint Surg., 50-A:508, 1968.
11. Clark, P. M., and Keokarn, T.: Popliteal aneurysm complicating benign osteocartilaginous exostosis. Review of the literature and report of one case. J. Bone Joint Surg., 47-A:1386, 1965.
12. Cole, A. R. C., and Darte, J. M. M.: Osteochondromata following irradiation in children. Pediatrics, 32:285, 1963.
13. Cooley, L. H., and Torg, J. S.: "Pseudowinging" of the scapula secondary to subscapular osteochondroma. Clin. Orthop., 162:119, 1982.
14. Copeland, R. L., Meehan, P. L., and Morrissy, R. T.: Spontaneous regression of osteochondromas. Two case reports. J. Bone Joint Surg., 67-A:971, 1985.
15. Dahlin, D. C.: Bone Tumors. 3rd Ed. Springfield, Ill., Thomas, 1978, p. 18.
16. D'Ambrosia, R., and Ferguson, A. B. R.: The formation of osteochondroma by epiphyseal cartilage transplantation. Clin. Orthop., 61:103, 1968.
17. Denman, F. R., Schindler, T. O., Hampton, J., and Hanson, L.: Aneurysm of the popliteal artery caused by an osteochondroma of the femur. J. Bone Joint Surg., 41-A:1526, 1959.
18. El-Khoury, G. Y., and Bassett, G. S.: Symptomatic bursa formation with osteochondromas. A.J.R., 133:895, 1979.
19. Fielding, J. W., and Ratzan, S.: Osteochondroma of the spine. J. Bone Joint Surg., 55-A:640, 1973.
20. Fischer, K. A., and Jackson, B. B.: Traumatic aneurysm of the popliteal artery from perforation by an osteochondroma. J. Trauma, 4:339, 1964.
21. Garrison, R. C., Unni, K. K., McLeod, R. A., Pritchard, D. J., and Dahlin, D. C.: Chondrosarcoma arising in osteochondroma. Cancer, 49:1890, 1982.
22. Ghormley, R. K., Meyerding, H. W., Mussey, R. D., Jr., and Luckey, C. A.: Osteochondromata of the pelvic bones. J. Bone Joint Surg., 28:40, 1946.
23. Gomez-Reino, J. J., Radin, A., and Gorevic, P. D.: Pseudoaneurysm of the popliteal artery as a complication of osteochondroma. Skeletal Radiol., 4:26, 1979.
24. Greenway, G., Resnick, D., and Bookstein, J. J.: Popliteal pseudoaneurysm as a complication of an adjacent osteochondroma. Angiographic diagnosis. A.J.R., 132:294, 1979.
25. Han, S. K., Henein, M. H., Novin, N., and Giargiand, F. A., Jr.: An unusual arterial complication seen with a solitary osteochondroma. Am. Surg., 43:471, 1977.
26. Heiple, K. G.: Carpal osteochondroma. J. Bone Joint Surg., 43-A:861, 1961.
27. Hensinger, R. N., Cowell, H. R., Ramsey, P. L., and Leopold, R. G.: Familial dysplasia epiphysealis hemimelica associated with chondromas and osteochondromas. J. Bone Joint Surg., 56-A:1513, 1974.
28. Hershey, S. L., and Lansden, F. T.: Osteochondromas as a cause of false popliteal aneurysms. Review of the literature and report of two cases. J. Bone Joint Surg., 54-A:1765, 1972.
29. Hudson, O. C.: Traumatic aneurysm of the popliteal artery due to an osteochondroma. Am. J. Surg., 90:528, 1955.
30. Hudson, T. M., Chew, F. S., and Manaster, B. J.: Scintigraphy of benign exostosis and exostotic chondrosarcoma. A.J.R., 140:581, 1983.
31. Hunter, J.: The Works of John Hunter, with Notes. Vol. 1. J. F. Palmer (ed.). London, Longmans, 1835, pp. 533–534.
32. Inglis, A. E., Rubin, R. M., Lewis, R. J., and Villacin, A.: Osteochondroma of the cervical spine. Case report. Clin. Orthop., 126:127, 1977.
33. Jaffe, H. L.: Tumors and Tumorous Conditions of Bones and Joints. Philadelphia, Lea & Febiger, 1958, p. 143.
34. Keith, A.: Studies on the anatomical changes which accompany certain growth disorders of the human body. J. Anat., 54:101, 1920.
35. Kenney, P. J., Gilula, L. A., and Murphy, W. A.: The use of computed tomography to distinguish osteochondroma and chondrosarcoma. Radiology, 139:129, 1981.
36. Kover, J. H., Schwalbe, N., and Levowitz, B. S.: Popliteal aneurysm due to osteochondroma in athletic injury. N.Y. State J. Med., 70:3001, 1970.
37. Lange, R. H., Lange, T. A., and Rao, B. K.: Correlative radiographic, scintigraphic, and histological evaluation of exostosis. J. Bone Joint Surg., 66-A:1454, 1984.
38. Lee, F. A.: Solitary cartilaginous exostosis of the ilium

presenting as an abdominal mass. Am. J. Dis. Child., *114*:195, 1967.
39. Lesser, A. J., and Greeley, L. E.: Femoropopliteal arteriovenous aneurysm caused by fractured osteochondroma of the femur. J.A.M.A., *167*:1830, 1958.
40. Manner, R., and Makinen, E.: Angiographic findings in a false popliteal aneurysm due to osteochondroma of the femur. Pediatr. Radiol., *3*:244, 1975.
41. Masson, A. F., and Pullan, J. M.: Aneurysm complicating exostosis. Br. J. Surg., *53*:929, 1966.
42. Milch, R. A.: Osteochondroma of the talus. Am. J. Surg., *87*:145, 1954.
43. Milgram, J. W.: The origins of osteochondromas and enchondromas. A histopathologic study. Clin. Orthop., *174*:264, 1983.
44. Moore, J. R., Curtis, R. M., and Shaw Wilgis, E. F.: Osteocartilaginous lesions of the digits in children. An experience with 10 cases. J. Hand Surg., *8*:309, 1983.
45. Mukerjea, S. K.: Traumatic aneurysm of the popliteal artery due to osteochondroma. Br. J. Surg., *54*:810, 1967.
46. Müller, E.: Über hereditäre multiple cartilaginäre Exostosen und Ecchondrosen. Beitr. Pathol. Anat., *57*:232, 1913.
47. Novick, G. S., Pavlov, H., and Bullough, P. G.: Osteochondroma of the cervical spine: Report of two cases in preadolescent males. Skeletal Radiol., *8*:13, 1982.
48. Padua, S., and Mizzau, M.: Evoluzione maligna delle esostosi. Arch. Putti., *20*:296, 1965.
49. Paling, M. R.: The "disappearing" osteochondroma. Skeletal Radiol., *10*:40, 1983.
50. Parsons, T. A.: The snapping scapula and subscapular exostosis. J. Bone Joint Surg., *55-B*:345, 1973.
51. Paul, M.: Aneurysm of the popliteal artery from perforation by a cancellous exostosis of the femur. Report of a case. J. Bone Joint Surg., *35-B*:270, 1953.
52. Schoene, H. R., Berthelsen, S., and Ahn, C.: Aneurysm of femoral artery secondary to osteochondroma. J. Bone Joint Surg., *55-A*:847, 1973.
53. Simon, M. A., and Kirschner, P. T.: Scintigraphic evaluation of primary bone tumors. Comparison of technetium 99m phosphonate and gallium citrate imaging. J. Bone Joint Surg., *62-A*:758, 1980.
54. Smithius, T.: Exostosis bursata. Report of a case. J. Bone Joint Surg., *46-B*:544, 1964.
55. Solhaugh, J. H., and Olerud, S. E.: Pseudoaneurysm of the femoral artery caused by osteochondroma of the femur. J. Bone Joint Surg., *57-A*:867, 1975.
56. Solomon, L.: Bone growth in dysplasial aclasis. J. Bone Joint Surg., *43-B*:700, 1961.
57. Stevenson, C. A., and Zuska, J. J.: Aneurysm of the popliteal artery from perforation by a solitary exostosis of the femur. J. Bone Joint Surg., *39-A*:431, 1957.
58. Trotter, D., Zindrick, M., and Ibrahim, K.: An unusual presentation of an osteochondroma: Report of a case. J. Bone Joint Surg., *66-A*:299, 1984.
59. Van Winkle, G. N., and Mazur, J. M.: Iatrogenic exostosis in a patient treated for osteomyelitis. J. Pediatr. Orthop., *3*:610, 1983.
60. Virchow, R.: Ueber multiple Exostosen, mit Vorlegung von Präparaten. Berl. Klin. Wochenschr., *28*:1082, 1891.
61. Wilner, D.: Solitary exostosis. *In* Radiology of Bone Tumors and Allied Disorders. Philadelphia, Saunders, 1982, pp. 272–355.
62. Wu, K. K., and Guise, E. R.: Osteochondroma of the atlas: A case report. Clin. Orthop., *136*:160, 1978.

MULTIPLE CARTILAGINOUS EXOSTOSIS

This relatively uncommon, but by no means rare, generalized hereditary developmental affection of the skeleton is characterized by the presence of multiple cartilaginous and bony exostoses protruding from bones preformed in cartilage. Keith coined the term *diaphyseal aclasis* (stressing abnormality of the modeling process).[13] *Hereditary deforming chondrodysplasia* was the name proposed by Ehrenfried, but its use was subsequently discouraged because of confusion with Ollier's dyschondroplasia (multiple enchondromatosis.[5, 6] Jaffe, in 1943, proposed the now popular term *hereditary multiple exostoses*.[12]

Genetics and Sex Incidence

The disorder is of autosomal dominant inheritance. There is a definite predilection for the male in the ratio of approximately 7:3.

Localization

Any bone preformed in cartilage may be the site of the lesion. Bones of intramembranous formation are not involved. The long bones of the limbs are more severely affected than the ribs, spine, scapula, and pelvis. The exostoses are most frequent in the metaphyseal areas of the proximal and distal femur, proximal and distal tibia, proximal humerus, and distal radius and ulna; lesions of the proximal ends of the radius and ulna are relatively infrequent as are those at the distal end of the humerus.

In the scapula the exostoses arise along the growth areas of the body and adjacent to the epiphyses of the coracoid process and acromion. Those in the ribs are broad-based and flat, usually developing near the anterior cartilaginous ends. In the pelvis the apophyseal region of the ilium is a common site; occasionally an exostosis may develop in the region of the ischiopubic synchondrosis.

The metatarsals, metacarpals, and phalanges may be involved; in the short tubular bones the exostoses appear as small flat tumefactions. Growth disturbance with shortening of a metatarsal or metacarpal (usually the fourth and fifth) is not uncommon. The calcaneus is occasionally involved; the other tarsal and carpal bones, however, are usually not affected. In the vertebral column the exostoses develop adjacent to secondary centers of ossification such as that of a transverse process or spinous process.

Pathology

The pathologic picture of a single lesion in multiple exotosis is similar to that of a solitary osteochondroma, but the cartilage cap is usually thicker. If it exceeds 1 cm. in thickness, one should be suspicious of chondrosarcomatous change. On the under surface of the cartilage cap, the zone of enchondral ossification is irregular, with proliferation of cartilage cells. With maturation of the osteochondroma, this growth zone narrows and eventually closes as a thin plate of subchondral bone.

Clinical Features

Multiple exostosis usually manifests itself during childhood, but is not evident at birth. Diagnosis is rarely made before two years of age. Clinical complaints are absent or minimal. The children are usually brought for orthopedic examination because of the presence of hard "bumps" in the bones or because the parents themselves are affected.

Early in childhood, lumps appear about the knees, ankles, or shoulders in the metaphyseal region of the long bones (Fig. 3–246 A). Protuberances will be seen on the scapula or the rib cage (Fig. 3–247 A and B). The knobby appearance of the child is so characteristic that one can easily make a diagnosis merely by clinical inspection. There is definite shortness of the upper and lower limbs in relation to the length of the trunk; the shortness of stature is usually mild, but it is disproportionate, the limbs being involved to a greater degree than the spine.

Clinically the more significant deformities are in the region of the forearm and leg—where two bones are in close longitudinal relationship. The disparate longitudinal growth rate of the two bones and the tethering effect of the interosseous membranes are factors in the pathogenesis of deformity.

In the upper limb the ulna is shorter than the radius; therefore, the radius is bowed laterally, with its concavity toward the short ulna. Normally four fifths of the longitudinal growth of the ulna takes place distally, whereas only about three fourths of that of the radius occurs at its distal epiphysis. The distal end of the ulna is more severely affected than that of the radius. Progressive posterolateral dislocation of the radial head is a common deformity (Fig. 3–248). Flexion deformity of the elbow is usually present. At the wrist, radial deviation is restricted and ulnar deviation is increased. Range of rotation of the forearm may be limited owing to blocking by an exostosis or bowing of the radius or both; pronation is more frequently restricted than supination. The humerus may be shortened.

In the lower limb, *tibia valga* is frequently present. The valgus deformity is usually at the proximal metaphyseal-diaphyseal region but can occur in the midshaft (Fig. 3–249). It is usually entirely within the tibia and not at the knee, i.e., there is no abnormal femoral-tibial lateral angulation. The degree of tibia valga is measured by the angle formed between the proximal tibial physis and the longitudinal axis of the medial cortical surface of the tibia or the center of the tibial diaphysis. In the normal tibia, this measures about 90 degrees (Fig. 3–250).

At the ankle joint the lateral half of the distal tibial epiphysis is deficient, while the medial part is normal in its ossification. The lateral part therefore slants proximally and laterally. The superior articular surface of the talus is oblique. The degree of ankle valgus deviation varies. Shapiro and associates classified abnormality of the distal tibial epiphysis into three grades of severity. In *Type I* (mild deformity) the subchondral surface of the distal tibial epiphysis angles upward and laterally from its central portion, but the lateral margin of the subchondral bone remains well within the epiphyseal side of the physis. In Type II (moderate deformity), the distal subchondral bone slopes into the lateral margin of the distal tibial physis. In Type III (severe deformity), the subchondral bone slants into the distal tibial physis in the lateral third rather than to its lateral edge (Fig. 3–251).[23]

The fibula may be short in relation to the tibia, altering the normal relationship of the distal tibial and fibular malleoli, and producing valgus ankle. In the normal adolescent the distal fibular physis is at the level of the tibiotalar articular space, and the tip of the lateral malleolus is distal to that of the medial malleolus. In hereditary multiple exostosis with valgus ankle and relative fibular shortening, the distal fibular physis progressively rises in relation to the tibiotalar articular space; the fibular malleolus may be at the same level as the medial malleolus or proximal to it (Figs. 3–252 and 3–253).

At the hip, coxa valga is present in about one fourth of the patients (Figs. 3–254 and 3–255). This may be associated with acetabular dysplasia. The distal femur may develop a varus tilt. Disparity of lower limb length is not uncommon—it may be as great as 4 cm. The pattern of growth of the tibiae and femora is variable; frequently the discrepancy in length increases at a slow or moderate rate; it may remain unchanged in some cases, however, and very occasionally it may decrease spontaneously. There is no correlation between the degree of

Text continued on page 1180

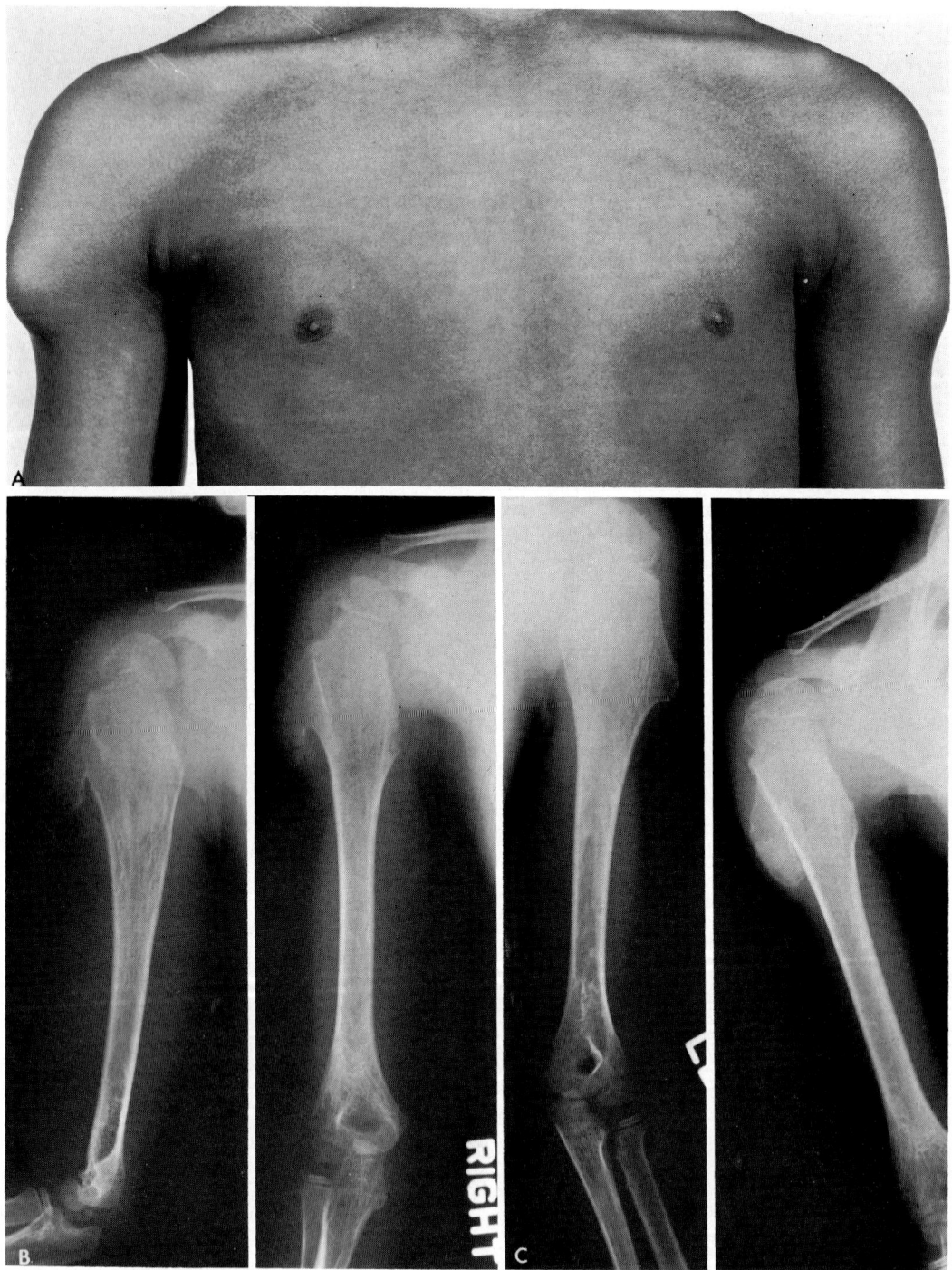

FIGURE 3–246. Multiple hereditary exostosis.

A. Clinical appearance of the protuberances in the proximal upper limbs. **B** and **C.** Radiograms of both humeri. Note the pedunculated exostoses arising in the metaphyseal area and directed distally toward the shaft. The affected metaphyseal area is broadened.

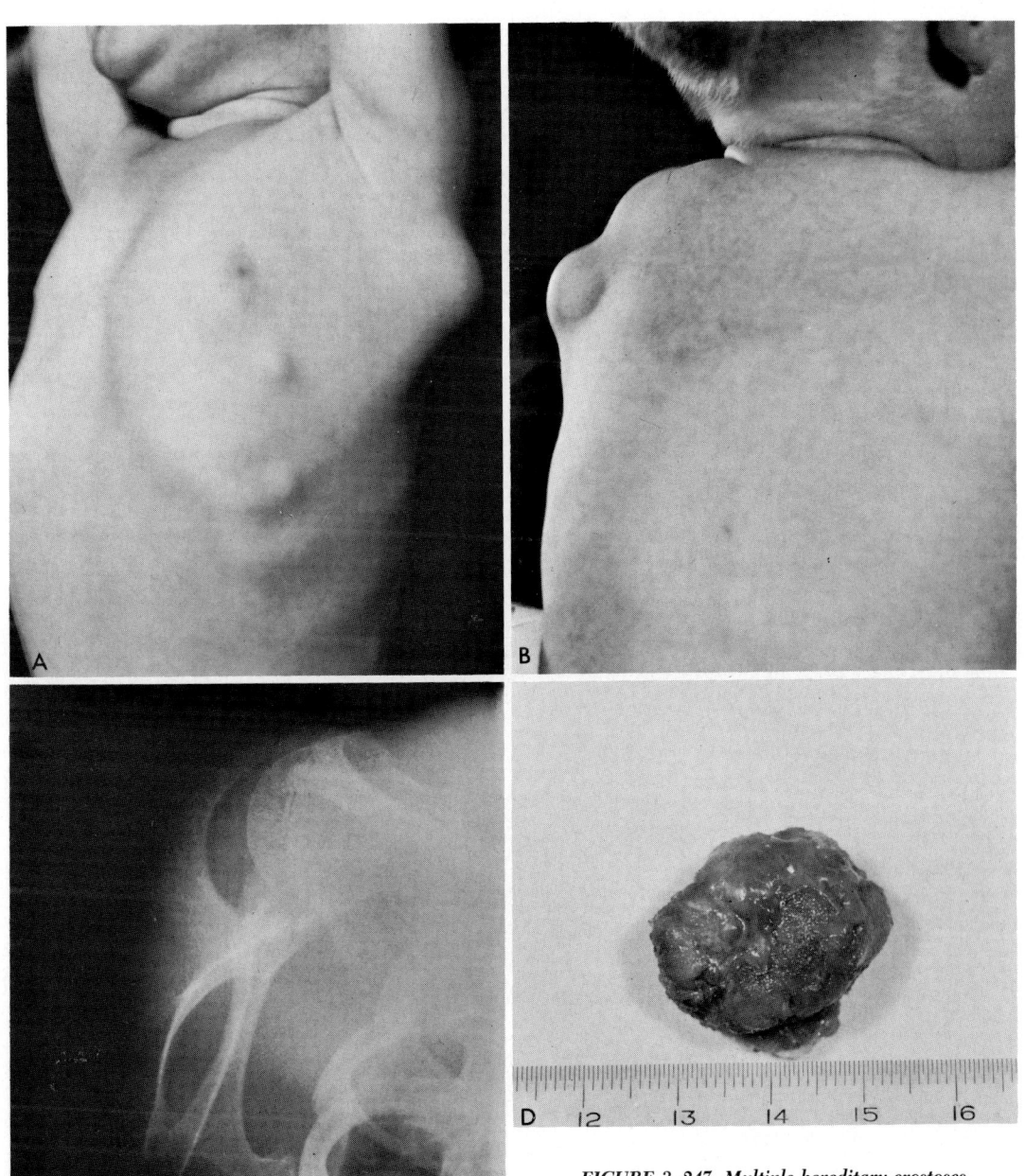

FIGURE 3-247. Multiple hereditary exostoses.

A and **B.** Photographs of child show the bony "lumps" on the rib cage and left scapula. **C.** Radiogram of scapula. Note the exostosis on its deep surface. **D.** Gross appearance of excised exostosis from scapula.

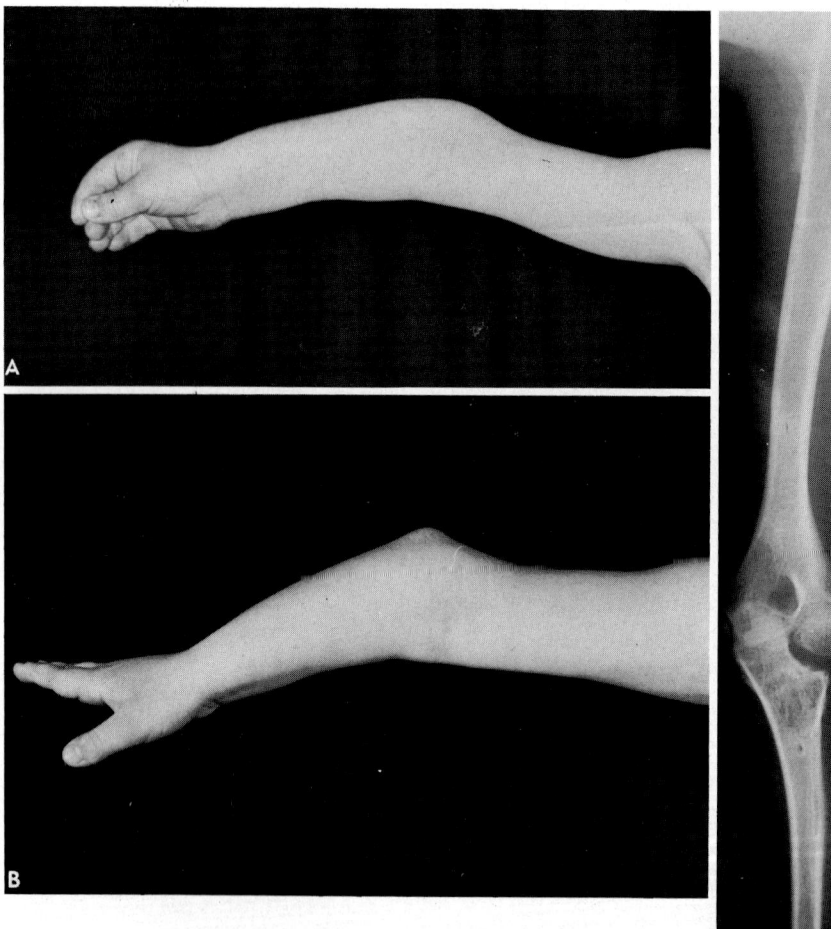

FIGURE 3-248. Multiple hereditary exostosis.

A and **B.** Photographs of forearm showing typical deformity. The radius is externally bowed. **C.** Radiograms of upper limb. Note the posterolateral dislocation of the radial head.

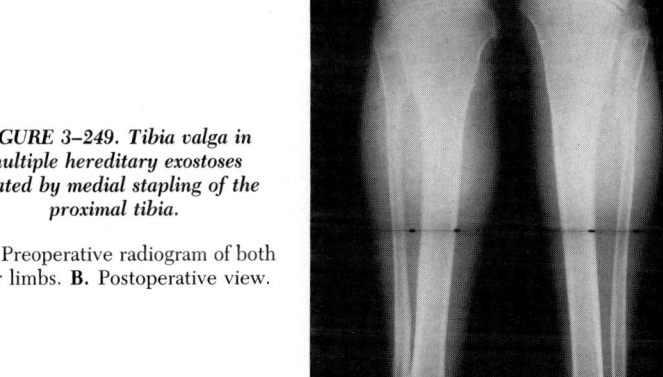
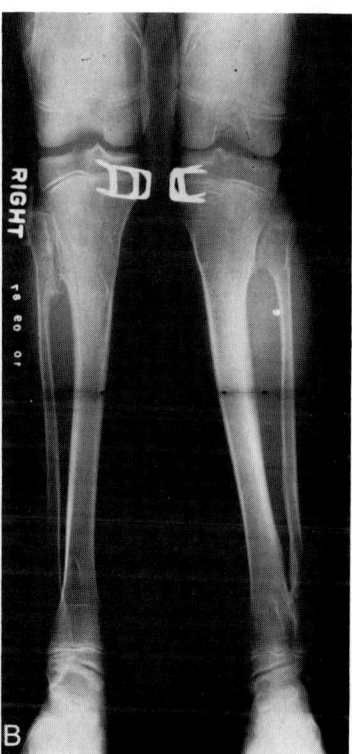

FIGURE 3–249. *Tibia valga in multiple hereditary exostoses treated by medial stapling of the proximal tibia.*

A. Preoperative radiogram of both lower limbs. **B.** Postoperative view.

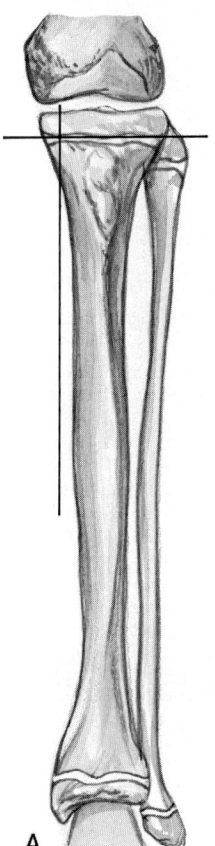
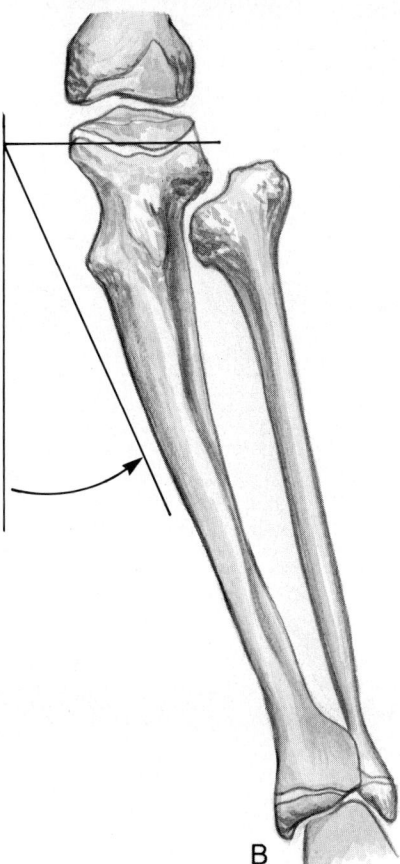

FIGURE 3–250. *Tibia valga in multiple hereditary exostoses.*

Relationship of the proximal tibial physis to the longitudinal axis of the tibia: **A.** Normal. The longitudinal axis of the medial tibial cortex is perpendicular to a line drawn parallel to the proximal tibial physis. **B.** In multiple hereditary exostosis the angle between the medial tibial cortex and a line drawn perpendicular to the proximal tibial physis is 25 degrees. Note the valgus deformity is within the tibia and not in the knee joint. The apex of the deformity is in the tibial metaphysis.

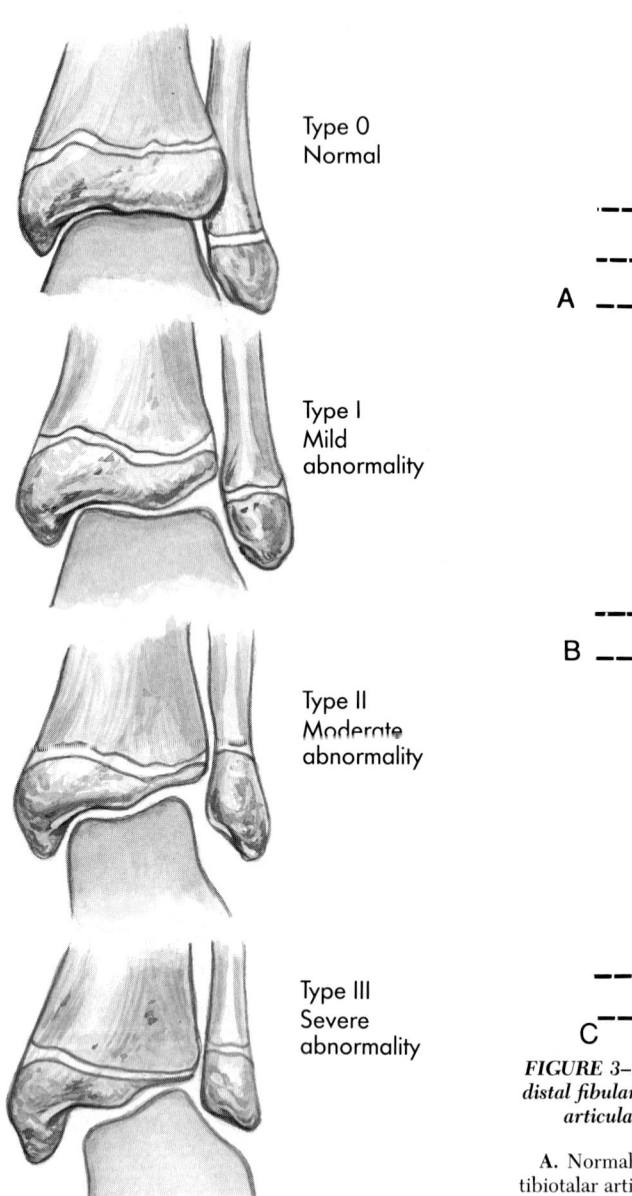

FIGURE 3–251. *Classification of severity of deformity of the distal tibial epiphysis in hereditary multiple exostoses. (See text for explanation.)*

(Redrawn after Shapiro, F., Simon, S., and Glimcher, M. J.: Hereditary multiple exostoses. Anthropometric, roentgenographic and clinical aspects. J. Bone Joint Surg., 61-A:815, 1979.)

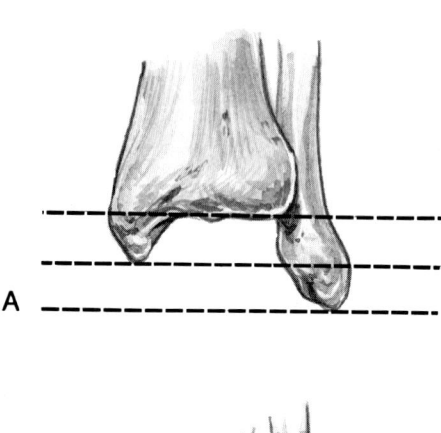

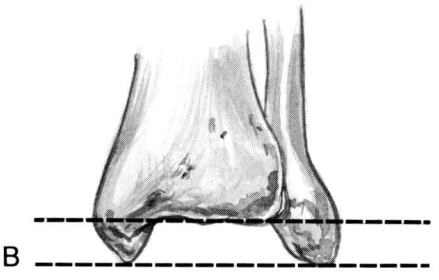

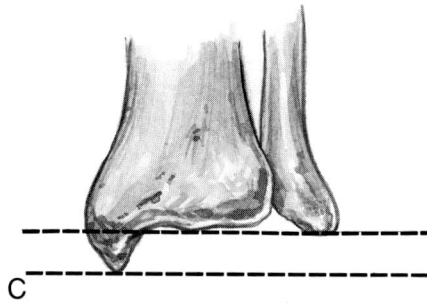

FIGURE 3–252. *Relationship of the lateral malleolus and distal fibular physis to the medial malleolus and tibiotalar articular spaces in multiple hereditary exostoses.*

A. Normal. The distal fibular physis is at the level of the tibiotalar articular space, and the tip of the lateral malleolus is distal to that of the tibia. **B.** In moderate valgus ankle, note the relative shortening of the fibula. With elevation of the distal fibular physis proximal to the tibiotalar joint space, the tips of the lateral and medial malleolus are level. **C.** In severe valgus ankle the tip of the lateral malleolus is proximal to that of the medial malleolus. (Redrawn after Shapiro F., Simon, S., and Glimcher, M. J.: Hereditary multiple exostoses. Anthropometric, roentgenographic, and clinical aspects. J. Bone Joint Surg., 61-A:81, 1979.)

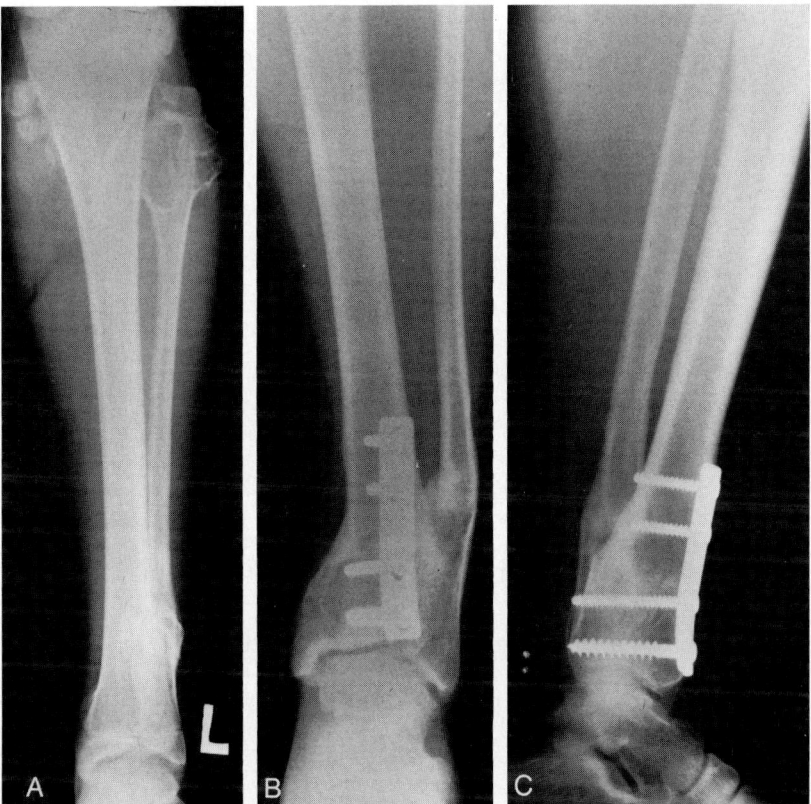

FIGURE 3–253. *Abnormality of the ankle joint in multiple hereditary exostosis.*

A. Anteroposterior view of the ankle. Ossification in the medial part of the distal tibial epiphysis is normal, whereas in the lateral half it is deficient; the subchondral bony plate of the distal tibial epiphysis slants proximally and laterally, producing valgus ankle. The tip of the fibular malleolus is elevated to the level of the ankle joint. **B** and **C.** Postoperative radiogram following varus osteotomy.

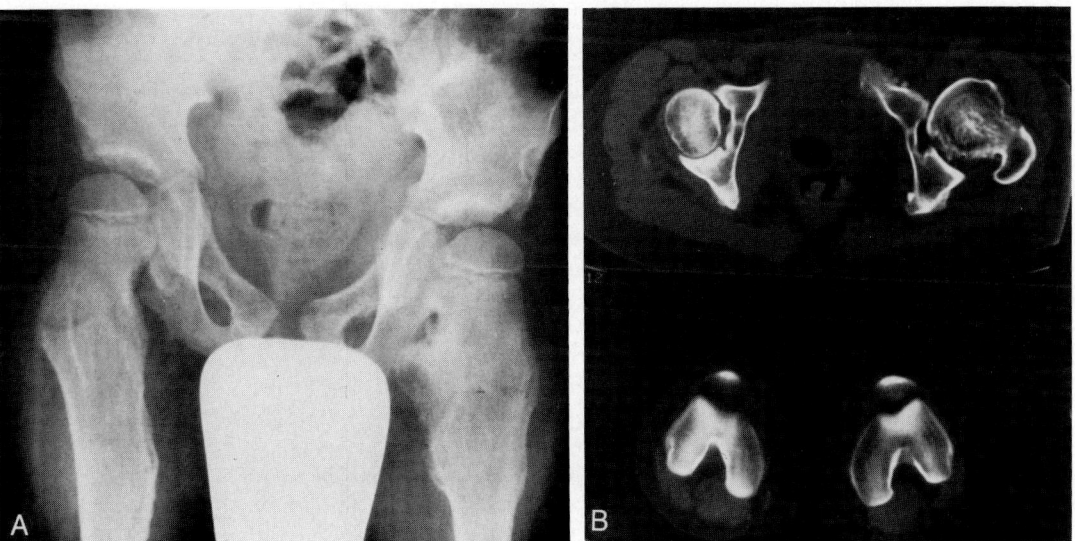

FIGURE 3–254. *Severe coxa valga with subluxation of the left hip in multiple hereditary exostoses.*

A. Anteroposterior view of both hips and proximal femora. **B.** CT scan showing lateral subluxation of the left hip.

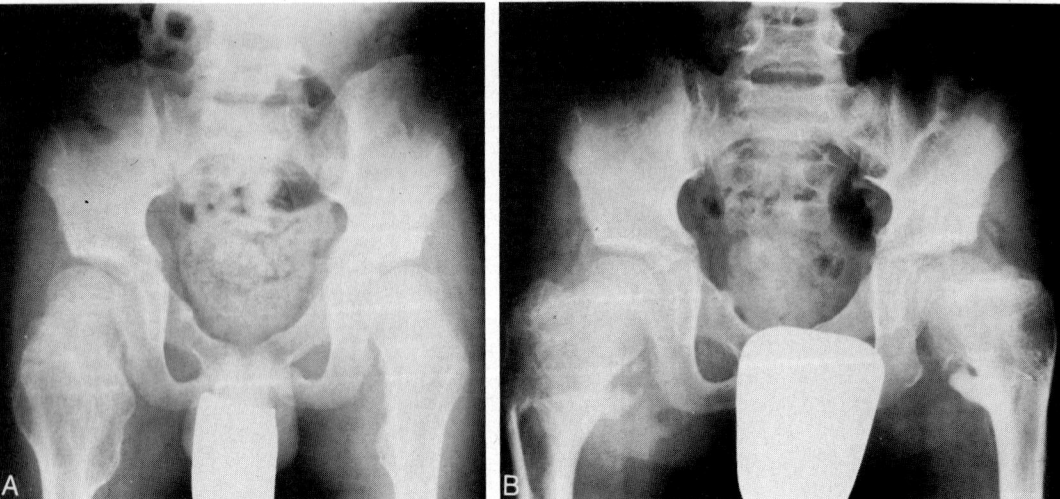

FIGURE 3–255. *Severe coxa valga in multiple hereditary exostoses treated by intertrochanteric varization osteotomy.*
A. Preoperative radiograms of both hips. B. Postoperative radiograms.

shortening of a long bone and the number and size of the exostoses.

Stature of patients with hereditary multiple exostoses tends to be short with mild disproportion, as the degree of involvement of the limbs is greater than that of the spine. Occasionally the stature may be above the mean; true dwarfism is rare.[23]

Radiographic Findings

In multiple exostosis, the bone area is involved to a much greater extent than in solitary osteochondroma. The affected metaphyeal area is broadened, indicating defective modeling of the bone (Fig. 3–256). Otherwise, the radiographic findings for an individual exostosis are similar to those of osteochondroma. The exostoses vary in size and number. Initially they appear as excrescences arising from the metaphyseal cortex in close proximity to the physis. With skeletal growth they grow away from the physis. The configuration of the exostoses varies—they may be hooked or pointed, sessile or pedunculated, or cauliflower-like (see Fig. 3–246 B and C). The exostoses almost always point away from the physis. The metaphyseal region of affected long bones is widened, creating the so-called trumpet-shaped deformity. In the lower limb the region of the knee is markedly involved. In the forearm (radius and ulna) and in the leg (tibia and fibula) the exostoses may impinge on the adjacent bone, producing pressure deformation and diastasis of the adjacent joints. Occasionally two exostoses may interlock, producing synostosis.

Treatment

One should be conservative in considering surgical intervention in cases of multiple hereditary exostosis. Exostoses are multiple; restraint should be exercised in excision of individual lesions. The mere presence of an osteochondroma is not an indication for surgery in multiple hereditary exostoses. Removal of the tumor is indiated when it is painful, when it interferes with joint or muscle function, when it presses on nerves or vessels, or when it is causing deformity. Children with multiple hereditary exostoses undergo numerous operations for removal of the exostoses and correction of deformities, and the psychologic effect of multiple procedures on the growing child should be considered. These patients have a normal life expectancy except when malignant transformation of the exostoses is a complication.

Surgery is indicated to correct deformities in the upper limb; those that require close observation and treatment are the relatively short ulna, the laterally bowed radius leading to progressive posterolateral dislocation of the radial head, and ulnar deviation and subluxation of the radiocarpal articulation (Figs. 3–257 and 3–258). Deformities, once present, do not improve with growth.

Ulnar Drift of the Wrist. If the carpus is not subluxated this can be simply treated by asymmetrical arrest of the radial half of the distal radial physis. This is usually performed around 10 to 11 years of skeletal age. If preservation of the length of the forearm is a consideration, the

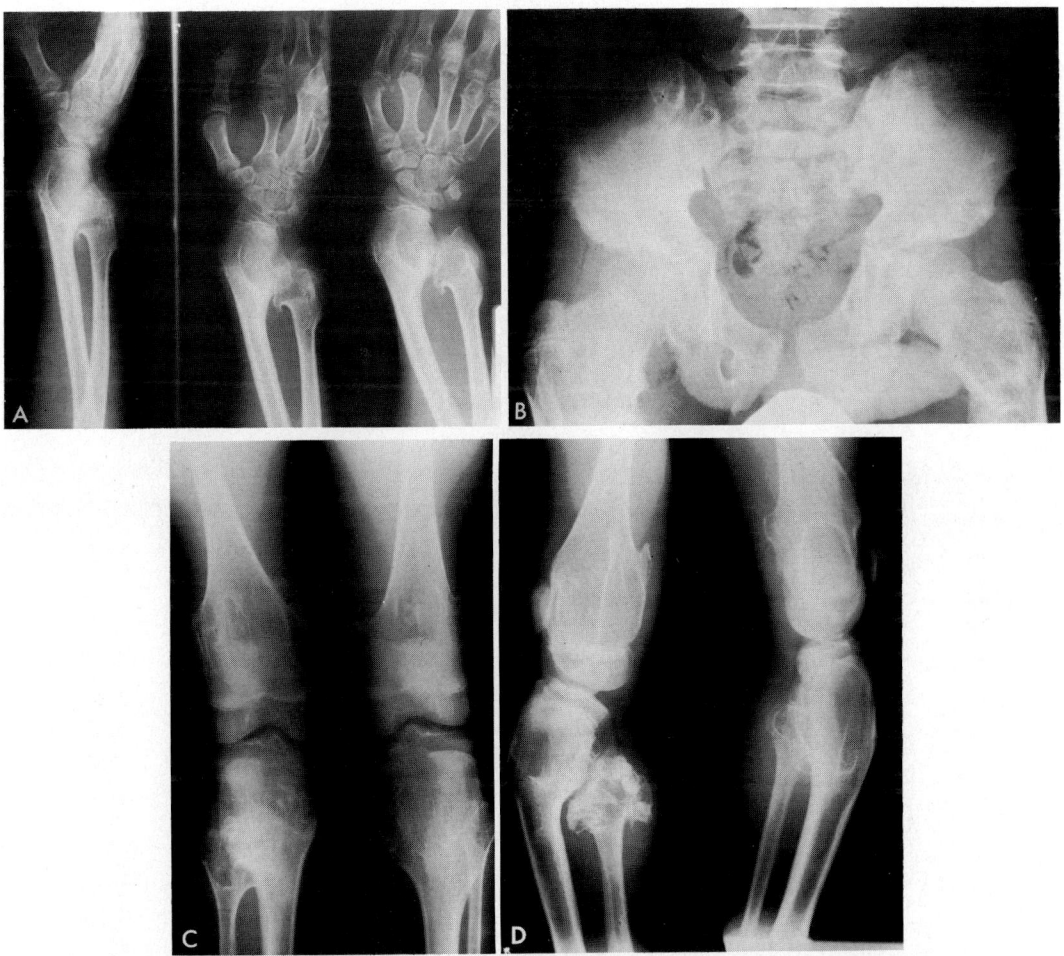

FIGURE 3–256. Multiple hereditary exostoses in an 11-year-old boy.

A. Views of wrist. Note the shortened ulna, the exostoses, and the widened metaphyses. **B.** Anteroposterior radiogram of pelvis. **C** and **D.** Anteroposterior and lateral radiograms of knees. The massively enlarged exostosis of right proximal fibula caused paresis of peroneal nerve. The whole proximal third of the fibula was excised.

Illustration continued on following page

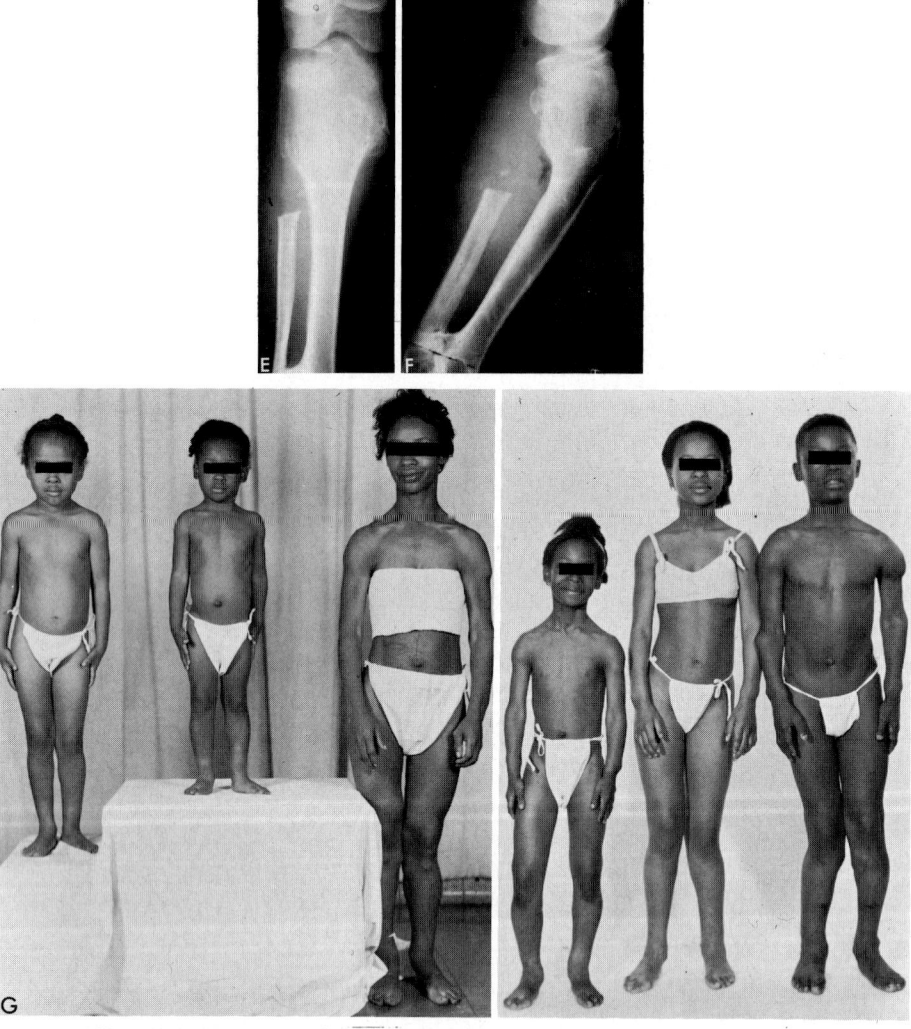

FIGURE 3–256 Continued. Multiple hereditary exostoses in an 11-year-old boy.

E and **F.** Postoperative radiograms. **G.** The entire family. The mother and five offspring have multiple hereditary exostosis. The condition is transmitted as a dominant trait.

The small AO or Orthofix or Wagner lengthening device is applied. The osteotomy is performed with a small oscillating saw. The ulna is lengthened slowly. Sometimes soft tissues, especially the flexor carpi ulnaris and extensor carpi ulnaris muscles, require fractional lengthening at their musculotendinous junctions. The osteotomized fragments are fixed with small cortical screws, a plate, or both. An autogenous bone graft from the ilium is often indicated to enhance osteogenesis. If the shortened ulna is slender, a Z-lengthening may be undesirable because of the risk of stress fracture. In such an instance, a transverse osteotomy is performed, and a fibular graft is interposed; internal fixation is by an intramedullary device such as a Steinmann pin or a Rush nail. The ulna may be lengthened gradually by the Wagner diaphyseal technique or De Bastiani callostasis or the Ilizarov technique.

If there is an exostosis between the upper part of the radius and ulna, and it is a factor in

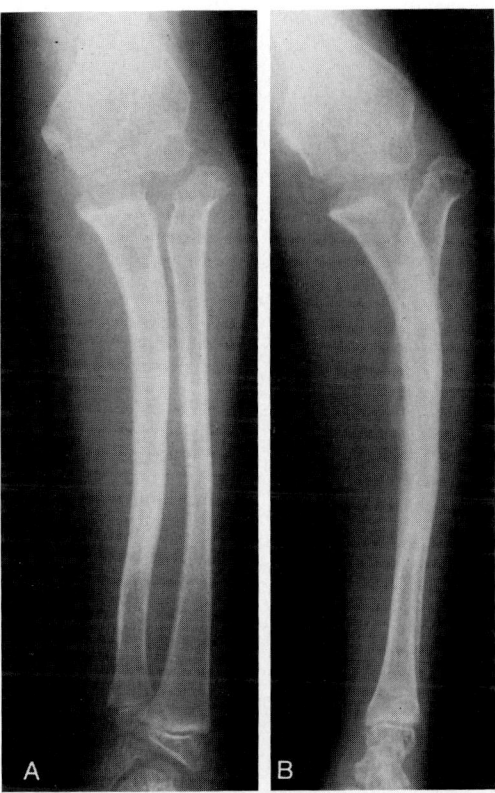

FIGURE 3-257. *Dislocation of the radial head in multiple congenital hereditary exostoses.*

A and **B.** Anteroposterior and lateral views of the forearm including the elbow and wrist.

short ulna may be lengthened. If the radius is bowed laterally the bowing is corrected by a closing-wedge osteotomy at the same time. Caution! Do not produce radioulnar synostosis!

If the radial head is subluxating the ulna should be lengthened. Restoration of ulnar length and the normal longitudinal relationship between the radius and ulna will reduce the subluxated radial head (Fig. 3-259).

Operative Technique of Z-Step Cut Lengthening of the Ulna. The posterolateral aspect of the ulna is exposed subperiosteally through a posterior incision that begins at the lower end of the shortened ulna and extends proximally along its subcutaneous margin for a distance of 8 to 12 cm. The deep fascia is incised, the periosteum is divided longitudinally, and the ulnar shaft is exposed subperiosteally. The extensor carpi ulnaris with its tendon is retracted anteriorly. With a small Kirschner wire, the Z-step cut osteotomy line is drilled in the ulna. Two threaded pins are inserted into the proximal shaft, and two pins are inserted distally.

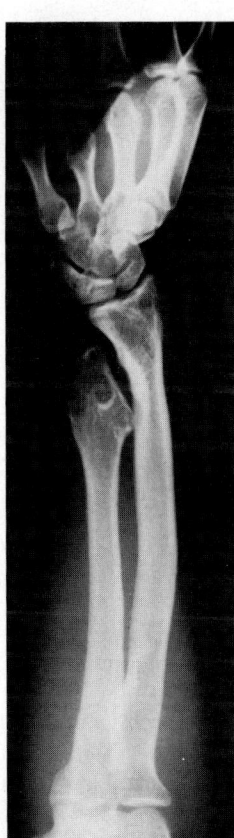

FIGURE 3-258. *The wrist joint in multiple hereditary exostoses.*

Note the short ulna and ulnar subluxation of the radial carpal articulation.

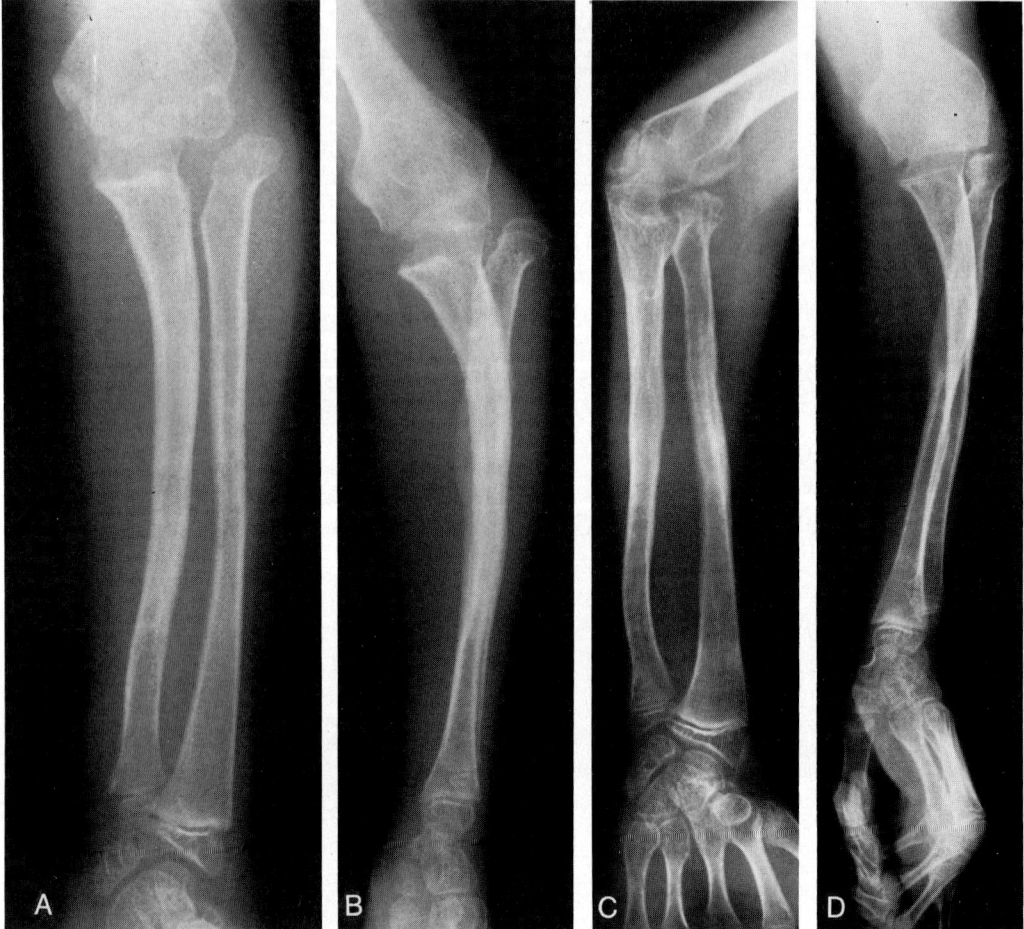

FIGURE 3–259. *Dislocation of the radial head in multiple hereditary exostoses reduced by lengthening the ulna and shortening the radius.*

A and **B.** Preoperative anteroposterior and lateral radiogram of the forearm showing wrist and elbow joints. **C** and **D.** Postoperative views showing the reduction of the dislocated radial head.

lateral subluxation of the radial head, the exostosis should be excised. Posterolateral tilting of the radial head can be corrected by closing-wedge osteotomy at its neck. When there is marked disparity between the length of the ulna and the length of the radius, a simultaneous elongation of the ulna and shortening of the radius is indicated (Fig. 3–260).

Marked shortening of the humerus may result from growth disturbance by an exostosis. In such an instance, the humerus may be lengthened by the Wagner diaphyseal lengthening or Ilizarov or De Bastiani callostasis technique (Fig. 3–261).

In the lower limbs, progressive coxa valga may cause instability of the hip and require varization osteotomy to contain the femoral head in the acetabulum (see Fig. 3–255). An exostosis on the medial part of the femoral neck and in the intertrochanteric region may cause subluxation and progressive limitation of motion of the hip joint; this requires excision. In the leg, the upper end of the fibula may have to be excised if the peroneal nerve is entrapped in the osteochondroma (Plate 40). Tibia valga and valgus ankle are corrected by osteotomy. At the appropriate skeletal age, tibia valga can be corrected by stapling the medial upper tibial physis (see Fig. 3–249) and ankle valgus by stapling the medial distal tibial physis.

Sarcomatous Transformation

Reliable statistics concerning chondrosarcomatous change in multiple hereditary exostoses

Text continued on page 1190

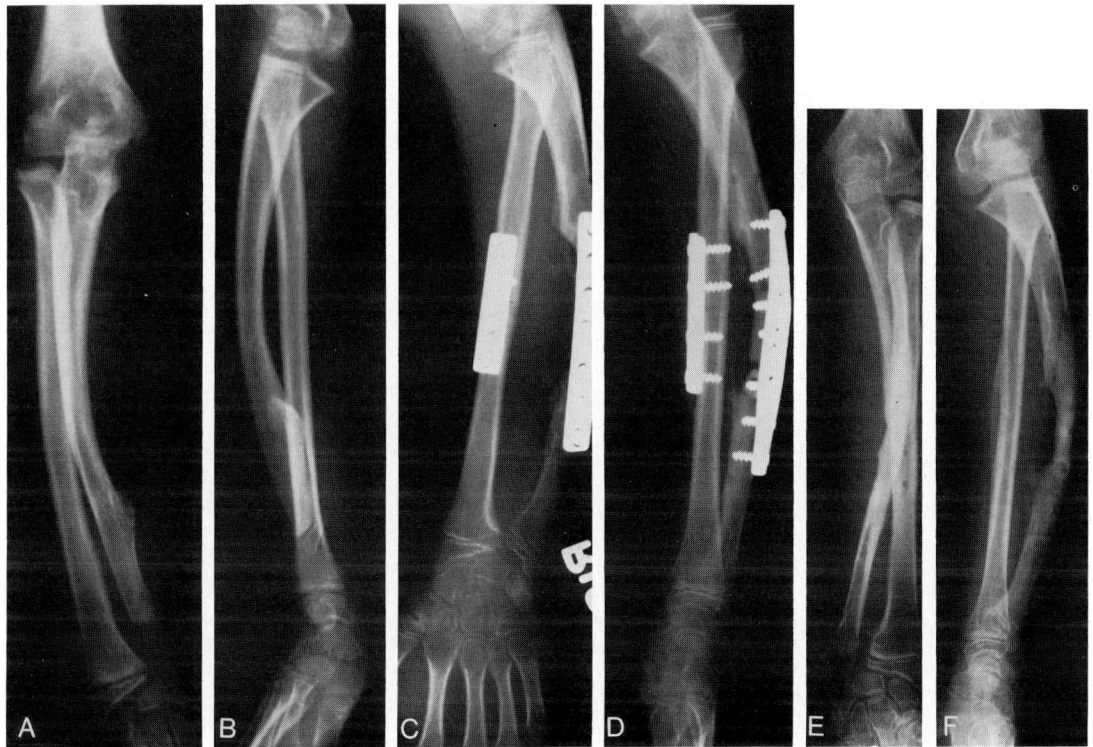

FIGURE 3-260. *Short ulna and ulnar drift of the carpus in multiple hereditary exostoses.*

The ulna was lengthened and the radius shortened simultaneously. The normal longitudinal relationship between the radius and ulna was restored, and stability of the wrist was provided. **A** and **B.** Preoperative anteroposterior and lateral radiograms of the forearm including wrist and elbow. Note the marked shortening of the ulna and the ulnar drift of the carpus. **C** and **D.** Immediate postoperative radiograms. **E** and **F.** Radiographs of the forearm one year later after removal of the plaster.

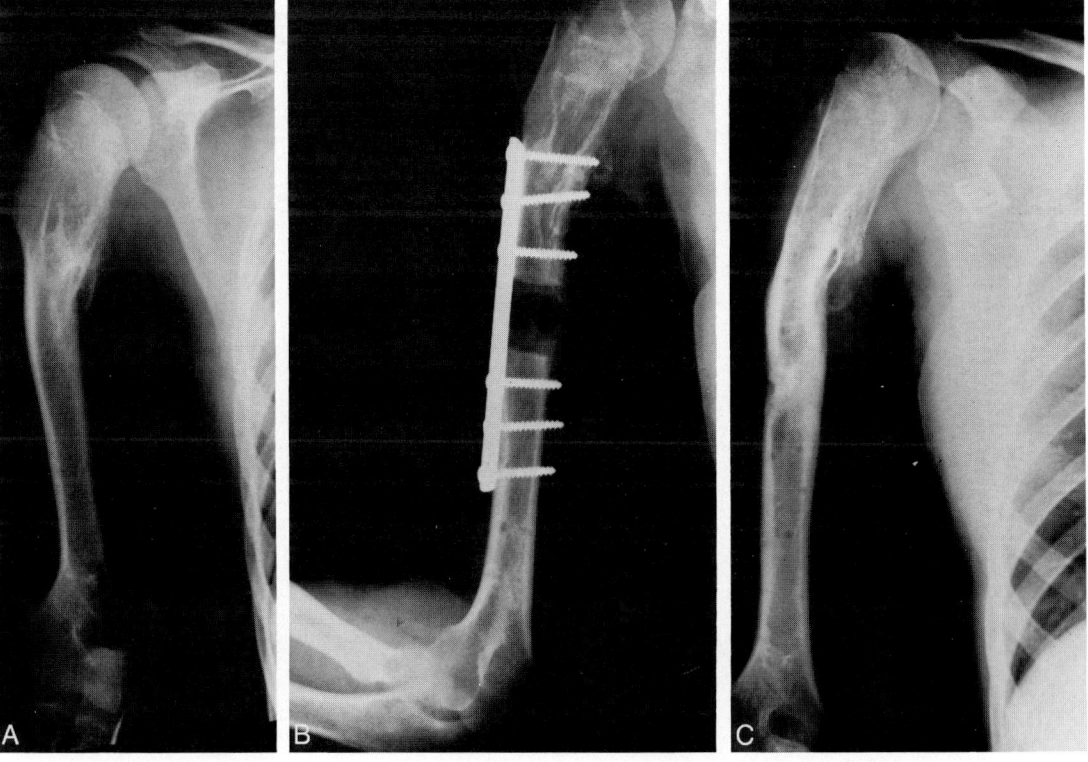

FIGURE 3-261. *Short humerus in multiple hereditary exostoses lengthened by Wagner diaphyseal lengthening.*

A. Preoperative radiogram. **B** and **C.** Postoperative radiograms.

Excision of Proximal Fibula with Multiple Exostoses

OPERATIVE TECHNIQUE

A. The patient is placed in semilateral decubitus position. With a pneumatic tourniquet on the proximal thigh the lower limb is prepared and draped in the usual fashion. The incision begins 5 to 7 cm. above the knee joint line, in line with the biceps femoris tendon, and extends distally and laterally to the head of the fibula, where it curves forward for a distance of 5 to 7 cm. The subcutaneous tissue is divided in line with the skin incision, and the deep fascia is sectioned.

B. The iliotibial band is retracted anteriorly, and the long head of the biceps femoris is carefully exposed by blunt dissection. The common peroneal nerve is identified along its medial border and is retracted distally. Great care is exercised not to injure the common peroneal nerve by too vigorous retraction.

C. The fibular collateral ligament is sectioned near its insertion and tagged with 2-0 nonabsorbable sutures. The upper end and proximal shaft of the fibula with the multiple exostosis is exposed. The biceps femoris tendon is sectioned at its insertion to the head of the fibula and reflected proximally. The peroneus longus and brevis muscles are elevated subperiosteally and deviated distally; stay anterior and do not damage nerve supply to peroneal muscles. The gastrocnemius and soleus muscles are retracted posteriorly. The level of section of the fibular shaft is determined.

Plate 40. Excision of Proximal Fibula with Multiple Exostoses

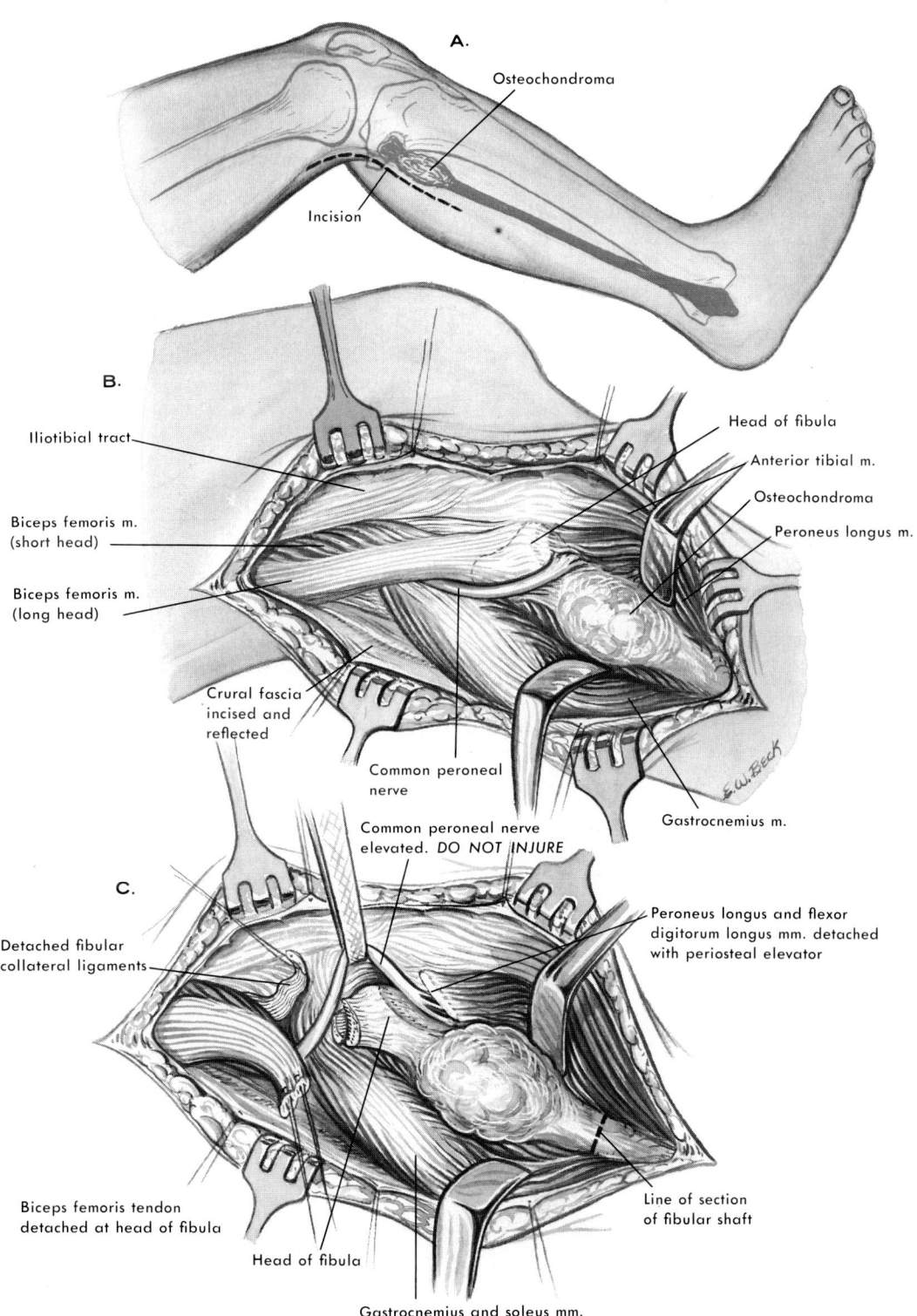

Excision of Proximal Fibula with Multiple Exostoses

OPERATIVE TECHNIQUE *(Continued)*

D. The shaft of the fibula is sectioned with an electric saw, and the proximal fibular segment is pulled laterally and proximally. By extraperichondrial and extraperiosteal dissection it is completely excised. The tourniquet is released, and complete hemostasis is achieved.

E. The biceps femoris tendon and the fibular collateral ligament are firmly reattached to the lateral condyle of the tibia; drill holes in the tibia and anchor the tendon and ligament securely to bone with nonabsorbable suture. The extensor digitorum longus and peroneus longus muscles are sutured to overlying soleus and gastrocnemius muscles. The wound is closed in layers in the usual fashion. An above-knee cast is applied with the knee in about 30 degrees of flexion and the foot and knee in neutral position.

POSTOPERATIVE CARE

The cast is removed six weeks postoperatively, and graduated active and passive exercises are performed to obtain full extension and flexion of the knee and to restore normal motor strength of the muscles controlling the knee.

Plate 40. Excision of Proximal Fibula with Multiple Exostoses

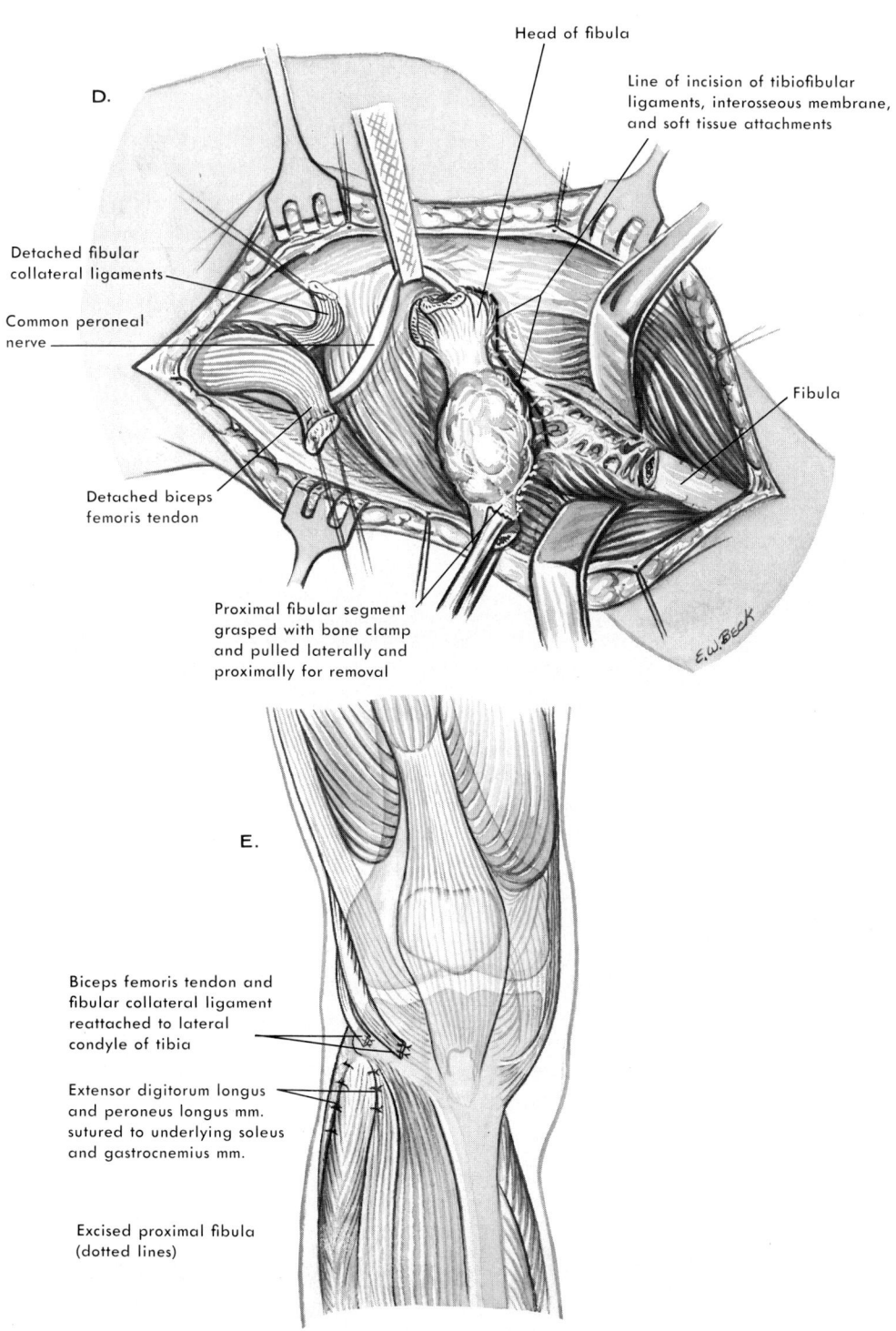

are not available. Jaffe reports the incidence as 11 per cent, but states that it may be as high as 20 per cent, a figure that seems too high and one that probably reflects statistics from a nonrepresentative, artificial group.[12] Occurrence of malignant transformation in 2 per cent of patients is perhaps a more accurate estimate; per lesion, however, the incidence of chondrosarcomatous change in multiple exostosis is no higher than that of solitary osteochondroma. Sarcomatous change is more common in the severe cases, usually occurring in an exostosis of the axial skeleton late in adult life. For diagnosis and treatment, see the section on osteochondroma.

References

1. Bessel Hagen, F.: Ueber Knochen- und Gelenkanomalien, insbesondere bei partiellem Riesenwuchs und bei multiplen cartilaginaren Exostosen. Arch. Klin. Chir., 41:420–466, 505–552, 749–823, 969–970, 1891.
2. Bethge, J. F. J.: Hereditäre, multiple Exostoses und ihre pathogenetische Deutung. Arch. Orthop. Unfallchir., 54:667, 1963.
3. Brown, I. D., and San, D. G.: Multiple osteochondroses of the feet in a West Indian family. J. Bone Joint Surg., 55-B:864, 1973.
4. Conheim, J.: Ein Fall von multiplen Exostosen. Virchows Arch. Pathol. Anat., 38:561, 1867.
5. Ehrenfried, A.: Multiple cartilaginous exostoses—hereditary deforming chondrodysplasia. A brief report on a little known disease. J.A.M.A., 64:1642, 1915.
6. Ehrenfried, A.: Hereditary deforming chondrodysplasia—multiple cartilaginous exostoses. A review of the American literature and report of twelve cases. J.A.M.A., 68:502, 1917.
7. Epstein, D. A., and Levin, E. J.: Bone scintigraphy in hereditary multiple exostoses. A.J.R., 130:331, 1978.
8. Fairbank, H. A. T.: Diaphyseal aclasia. J. Bone Joint Surg., 31-B:105, 1949.
9. Gibney, V. P.: Hereditary multiple exostoses. Four cases with results. Am. J. Med. Sci., 72:73, 1876.
10. Hale, K.: Hereditary deforming chondrodysplasia or multiple exostoses. Ann. Surg., 92:92, 1930.
11. Jaffe, H. L.: Hereditary multiple exostoses. Ann. Pathol., 36:335, 1943.
12. Jaffe, H. L.: Tumors and Tumorous Conditions of the Bones and Joints. Philadelphia, Lea & Febiger, 1958, p. 143.
13. Keith, A.: Studies on the anatomical changes which accompany certain growth-disorders of the human body. I. The nature of the structural alterations in the disorder known as multiple exostoses. J. Anat., 54:101, 1920.
14. Larson, N. E., Dodge, H. W., Jr., Rushton, J. G., and Dahlin, D. C.: Hereditary multiple exostoses with compression of the spinal cord. Proc. Staff Meet. Mayo Clin., 32:729, 1957.
15. Leveuf, J.: Le problème de la croissance de l'os en longueur étudié à la lumière de la maladie exostosique. Rev. Orthop. Chir., 32:5, 1946.
16. McCormack, E. B.: The surgical management of hereditary multiple exostoses. Orthop. Rev., 10:57, 1981.
17. Madigan, R., Worrall, T., and McClain, E.: Cervical cord compression in hereditary multiple exostosis. Review of the literature and report of a case. J. Bone Joint Surg., 56-A:410, 1974.
18. Morgan, J. P., Carlson, W. D., and Adams, O. R.: Hereditary multiple exostosis in the horse. J. Am. Vet. Med. Assoc., 140:1320, 1962.
19. Müller, E.: Über hereditäre multiple cartilaginäre Exostosen und Ecchondrosen. Beitr. Pathol. Anat., 57:232, 1913–14.
20. Ogden, J. A.: Multiple hereditary oteochondroma. Clin. Orthop., 116:48, 1976.
21. von Recklinghausen, F.: Ein Fall von multiplen Exostosen. Virchows Arch. Pathol. Anat., 35:203, 1866.
22. Roman, G.: Hereditary multiple exostosis. A rare cause of spinal cord compression. Spine, 3:230, 1978.
23. Shapiro, F., Simon, S., and Glimcher, M. J.: Hereditary multiple exostoses. Anthropometric, roentgenographic, and clinical aspects. J. Bone Joint Surg., 61-A:815, 1979.
24. Siffert, R. S., and Levy, R. N.: Correction of wrist deformity in diaphyseal aclasia by stapling. Report of a case. J. Bone Joint Surg., 47-A:1378, 1965.
25. Slepian, A., and Hamby, W. B.: Neurologic complications associated with hereditary deforming chondrodysplasia. J. Neurosurg., 8:529, 1951.
26. Solomon, L.: Bone growth in diaphyseal aclasia. J. Bone Joint Surg., 43-B:700, 1961.
27. Solomon, L.: Hereditary multiple exostosis. J. Bone Joint Surg., 45-B:292, 1963.
28. Solomon, L.: Hereditary multiple exostosis. Am. J. Hum. Genet., 16:351, 1964.
29. Solomon, L.: Carpal and tarsal exostoses in hereditary multiple exostoses. Clin. Radiol., 18:412, 1967.
30. Solomon, L.: Chondrosarcoma in hereditary multiple exostoses. South Afr. Med. J., 48:671, 1974.
31. Stark, J. D., Adler, N. N., and Robinson, W. H.: Hereditary multiple exostoses. Radiology, 59:212, 1952.
32. Todd, J. N., III, Hill, S. R., Jr., Nickerson, J. F., and Tingley, J. O.: Hereditary multiple exostoses, pseudohypoparathyroidism and other genetic defects of bone, calcium and phosphorous metabolism. Am. J. Med., 30:289, 1961; Abst., Radiology, 78:155, 1962.
33. Vanzant, B. T., and Vanzant, F. R.: Hereditary deforming chondrodysplasia. J.A.M.A., 119:786, 1942.
34. Virchow, R.: Ueber multiple Exostosen, mit Vorlegung von Präparaten. Berl. Klin. Wochenschr., 28:1082, 1891.
35. Yenikomshian, H. A., and Blake, H. K.: Familial bony dystrophy with multiple exostoses. Radiology, 24:623, 1935.

SOLITARY ENCHONDROMA AND MULTIPLE ENCHONDROMATOSIS

Enchondromas are benign cartilaginous growths in the interior of a bone. When an enchondroma affects a single bone, it is termed *solitary*. The term *multiple enchondromatosis* is used when these growths are found in several bones; it is then a manifestation of extensive bone dysplasia. In solitary enchondroma, the cartilaginous lesion always develops in the medullary cavity of the bone, whereas in multiple enchondromatosis, some of the cartilage may be formed by the periosteum as well and then penetrate into the interior of the bone.

Solitary Enchondroma

This relatively uncommon lesion is a dysplastic mass of cartilage in the medulla of the metaphysis or diaphysis of a long bone or a bone preformed in cartilage. There is no sex predilection, and it appears in an age group ranging from 5 to 50 years.

It is often found in the bones of the limbs, particularly in the phalanges and metacarpals of the hand and in the phalanges and metatarsals of the foot. Of the long tubular bones, the femur and humerus are frequent sites of localization. On occasion, the ribs, sternum, innominate bones, and vertebral column may also be affected. In the hand or foot, solitary enchondroma is usually located near an epiphysis and may extend into it if the physis is closed (Fig. 3–262).

Clinical Picture. In the phalanges, metatarsals, and metacarpals, the presence of an enchondroma is usually discovered following a pathologic fracture sustained in local trauma. On palpation, there will be considerable local tenderness if there is a recent fracture. Some patients, however, present a firm local swelling in the region of the affected phalanx or metacarpal without fracture or local pain. The flexor profundus longus tendon may be avulsed by an enchondroma in the phalanx.[7, 16] When the lesion is in one of the long tubular bones, it is usually quiescent, with no clinical signs evident until adulthood; it is usually found incidentally when a radiogram is made for another reason.

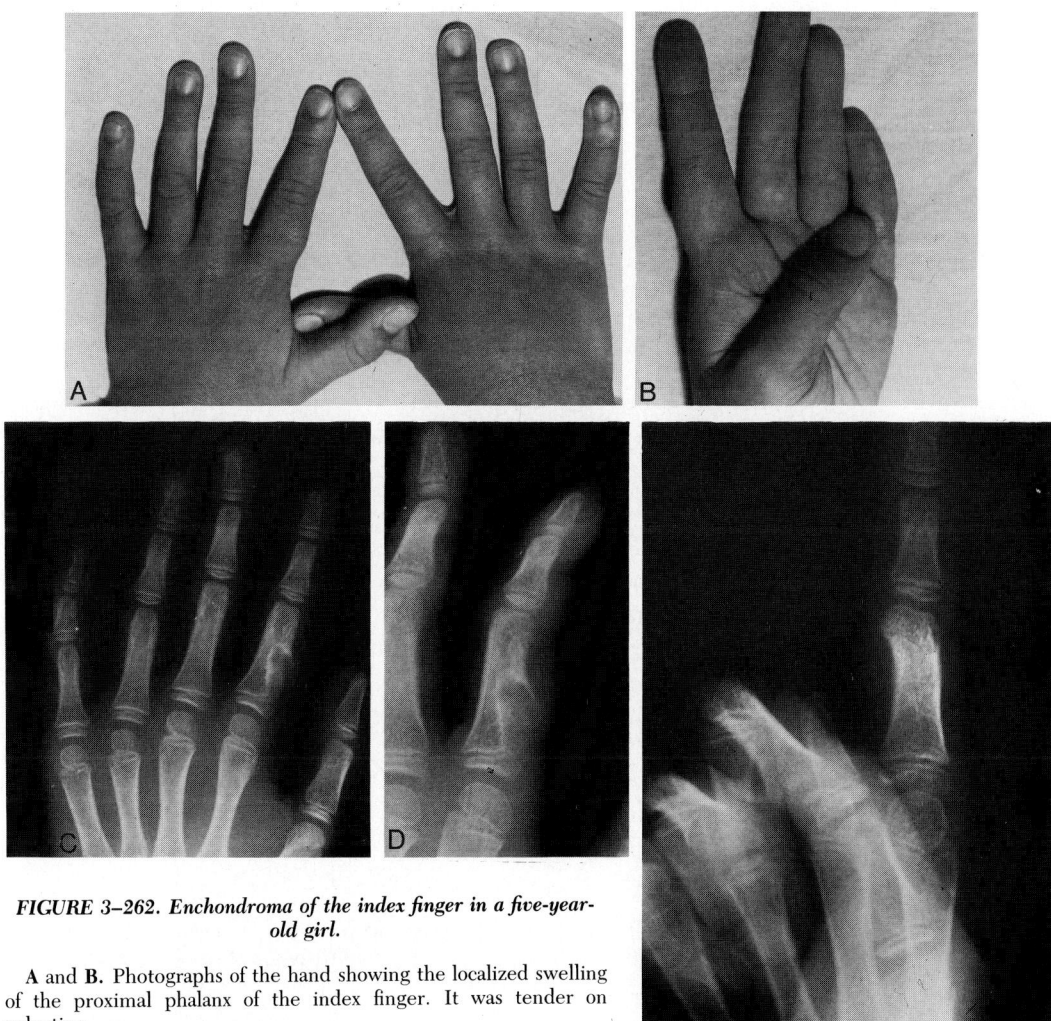

FIGURE 3–262. Enchondroma of the index finger in a five-year-old girl.

A and B. Photographs of the hand showing the localized swelling of the proximal phalanx of the index finger. It was tender on palpation.
C and D. Anteroposterior and oblique, lateral radiograms of the hand including the index finger. Note the rarefaction in the lesional area with bulging and thinning of the regional cortex. E. Postoperative radiogram. The enchondroma was excised and the bone was grafted with autogenous bone. Note the physis is open and not disturbed.

Radiographic and Imaging Findings. Radiograms disclose an ovoid area of rarefaction with bulging and thinning of the cortex (Fig. 3-263). Pathologic fractures or infractions, if present, will be evident. The cartilaginous lesion and surrounding bone are sharply demarcated with minimal or no periosteal reactive response. These radiographic features are characteristic of enchondroma. In the flat bones and vertebral column, computed tomography will delineate the intrinsic details of the lesion. The presence of a reactive rim of calcification is typical of enchondroma. Computed tomography is particularly indicated in radiographically obscure areas.

Scintigraphy with technetium-99m will reveal increased uptake, particularly in the more peripheral areas of the active lesion. Sudden marked increase in the uptake of the isotope may indicate malignant transformation. With bone growth the enchondroma slowly increases in size; after skeletal maturity it remains static. In its latent stage the enchondroma calcifies; in the radiogram the calcified enchondroma is

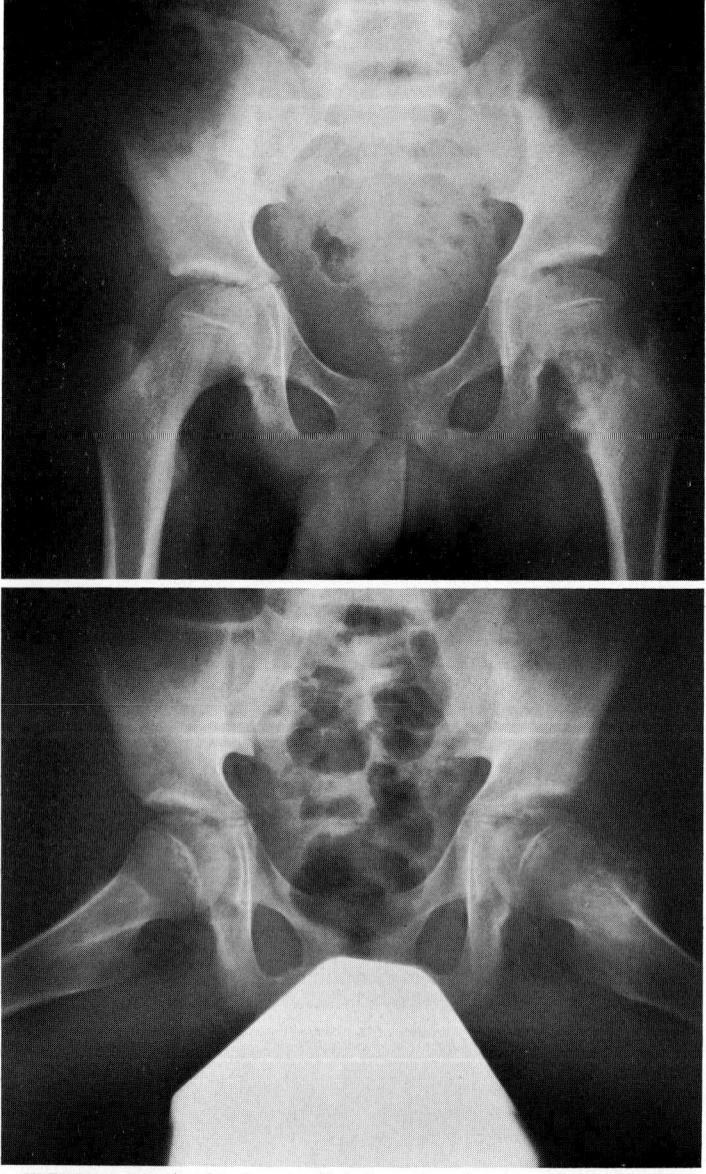

FIGURE 3–263. *Enchondroma of left femoral neck in a 14-year-old boy.*

Radiograms of hips. Note the ovoid area of rarefaction, which has bulged and thinned the anteroinferior cortex of the femoral neck.

distinctly punctate or stippled with a uniform distribution throughout the lesion.

Staging. In the growing skeleton, enchondromas are active Stage 2 benign lesions. After skeletal maturity they become latent Stage 1. In adult life malignant transformation occurs very rarely, in which case they become Stage 1 A or B secondary chondrosarcoma.

Differential Diagnosis. Solitary enchondroma of the short tubular bones must be differentiated from epithelial inclusion cysts, which affect the distal half of the terminal phalanges. A solitary focus of fibrous dysplasia, a nonossifying fibroma, or a unicameral bone cyst in a metacarpal may produce a similar radiographic picture. Rarefied punched-out lesions in the phalanges are also produced by Boeck's sarcoid and by gout.

Surgical Pathology. On gross inspection enchondroma appears as a glistening white, grayish-white, or pearly tissue that has a gritty feel on palpation due to intrinsic calcification. The tumor cuts readily with a knife, as if it were a piece of chalk. Degenerating areas of enchondroma may be soft. The histologic picture is that of small, predominantly uninuclear cartilage cells arranged in lobular masses (Fig. 3–264). The intercellular substance is partially or wholly hyaline cartilage. The ground substance may undergo calcification.

In children with active Stage 2 enchondroma there may be an occasional double nuclei in a

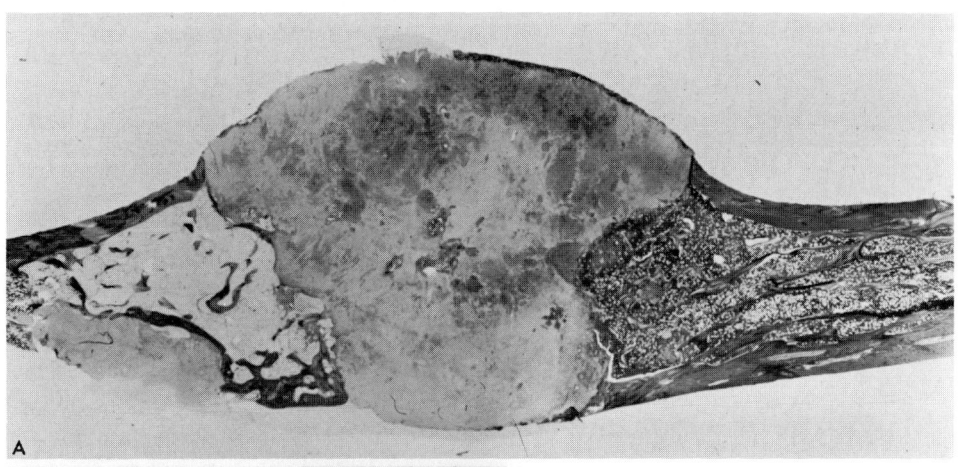

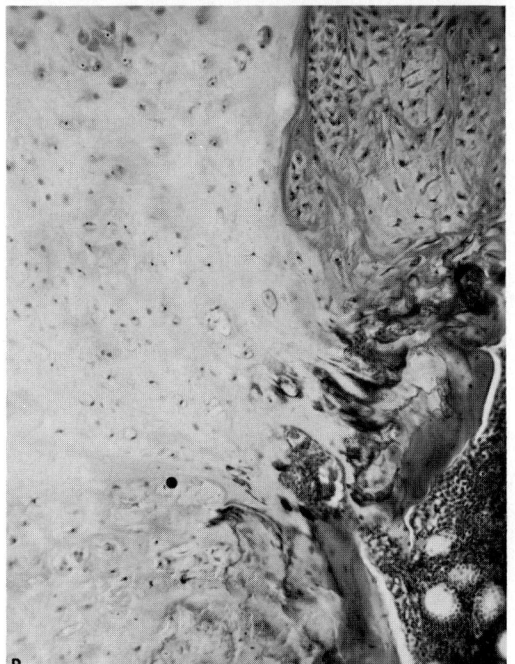

FIGURE 3–264. Enchondroma of rib— histologic findings.

A. Section of whole specimen. **B.** Photomicrograph of higher magnification (× 100). The chondrocytes are small, predominantly unicellular, and are arranged in lobular masses.

single lacuna and areas consisting of cartilaginous cells with no matrix; there may be one or two mitotic figures. In the growing child these sporadic findings indicate activity of the dysplastic cartilaginous lesion; they should not be misinterpreted as signs of malignancy.

Malignant change of a solitary enchondroma in the phalanx, metacarpal, or metatarsal bone is extremely rare. In the long tubular bones, there is some likelihood of malignant transformation, however, though this is usually a very slow process. Histologically, the possibility of chondrosarcoma is suggested when the tissue is hypercellular, when the nuclei are generally plumper, and when there are several binuclear cartilage cells or giant cartilage cells. Malignant change of an enchondroma in childhood and adolescence is unknown.

Treatment. The common form of treatment of solitary enchondroma of a short or long tubular bone consists of complete intracapsular excision by curettage down to normal bone and filling of the defect with matchsticks and chips of autogenous bone graft. Collapse of the distended cortical wall may be indicated if the lesional area is large, as in a long bone. There is a definite recurrence rate after intracapsular excision by curettage. Recurrence rate after surgical excision is very low and after en bloc wide excision it is nil; the latter, however, results in an unacceptable functional deficit, and because of the benign nature of the tumorous process it is not indicated.

The clinically asymptomatic active Stage 2 enchondroma in a growing child is best observed. One should wait until it matures into a Stage 1 latent lesion. Malignant transformation of enchondroma into chondrosarcoma does not occur in children, and "preventive" excision should not be performed. A calcified enchondroma in a long bone of the mature skeleton is also observed when it is asymptomatic, has no features of malignant change, and scintigraphic activity is minimal or modest. It must be borne in mind, however, that enchondroma in the pelvis, scapula, sternum, vertebrae, and proximal areas of the large long bones (upper femur and humerus) have greater likelihood of malignant transformation. In such instances the patient should be followed closely. Hallmarks of malignancy are the development of pain in a previously asymptomatic lesion, the radiographic findings of radiolucent bone destruction beyond the periphery of calcification, scalloped erosion of the endosteum of the overlying cortex, and erosion of "buttresses" of reactive bone in the medullary canal by the aggressive cartilaginous radiolucent tumor.[2, 5, 17, 19]

A recurrence warrants wide surgical excision. Sarcoma, if it occurs, metastasizes late, increasing the possibility of cure if the lesion is widely excised. Amputation may be indicated in selected cases. Radiation or chemotherapy is not indicated.

References

1. Adler, C. P., Klumper, A., and Wenz, W.: Enchondroma—radiology and pathology. Radiologe, *19*:341, 1979.
2. Bonfiglio, M., and Platz, C. E.: Case report 141: Malignant fibrous histiocytoma associated with enchondroma of bone. Skeletal Radiol., *6*:127, 1981.
3. Caballes, R. L.: Enchondroma protuberans masquerading as osteochondroma. Hum. Pathol., *13*:734, 1982.
4. Campanacci, M., Leonessa, C., and Boni, A.: Cartilaginous tumors in the hand bones: Report of 112 cases. Chir. Organi Mov., *62*:483, 1975.
5. Dohler, R., Heinemann, G., Busanny-Caspari, W., et al.: Chondrosarcoma of the first metatarsal—primary or secondary to enchondroma? Arch. Orthop. Trauma Surg., *95*:221, 1979.
6. Feldman, F. G.: Cartilaginous tumors and cartilage-forming tumor-like conditions of the bones and soft tissues. *In* Ranniger, K. (ed.): Handbuch Medizinische Radiology, Band 6. Berlin, Springer, 1977.
7. Froimson, A. I., and Shall, L.: Flexor digitorum profundus avulsions through enchondroma. J. Hand Surg., *9-B*:343, 1984.
8. Gilmer, W. S., Jr., Kilgore, W., and Smith, H.: Central cartilage tumors of bone. Clin. Orthop., *26*:81, 1963.
9. Hamlin, J. A., Adler, L., and Greenbaum, E. I.: Central enchondroma—a precursor to chondrosarcoma? J. Can. Assoc. Radiol., *22*:206, 1971.
10. Jaffe, H. L., and Lichtenstein, L.: Solitary benign enchondroma of bone. Arch. Surg., *46*:480, 1943.
11. Keating, R. B., Wright, P. W., and Staple, T. W.: Enchondroma protuberans of the rib. Skeletal Radiol., *13*:55, 1985.
12. Laurence, W., and Franklin, E. L.: Calcifying enchondroma of long bones. J. Bone Joint Surg., *35-B*:224, 1953.
13. McCrea, E. S., and Johnston, G. S.: Enchondroma on bone scan in a patient with breast cancer. South. Med. J., *77*:1059, 1984.
14. Mason, M. L.: Tumors of the hand. Surg. Gynecol. Obstet., *64*:129, 1937.
15. Milgram, J. W.: The origins of osteochondromas and enchondromas. A histopathologic study. Clin. Orthop., *174*:264, 1983.
16. Ogunro, O.: Avulsion of flexor profundus, secondary to enchondroma of the distal phalanx. J. Hand Surg., *8*:315, 1983.
17. Remagen, W., Nidecker, A., and Dolanc, B.: Case report 368: Enchondroma of the tibia with extension degeneration, recurrence with secondary and malignant transformation to highly differentiated chondrosarcoma. Skeletal Radiol., *15*:330, 1986.
18. Schultz, R. G., and Kearns, R. J.: Tumors in the hand. J. Hand Surg., *8*:803, 1983.
19. Wu, K. K., Frost, H. M., and Guise, E. E.: A chondrosarcoma of the hand arising from an asymptomatic benign solitary enchondroma of 40 years' duration. J. Hand Surg., *8*:317, 1983.
20. Wynne-Davies, R., and Fairbank, T. J.: Fairbank's Atlas of General Affections of the Skeleton. Edinburgh, Churchill-Livingstone, 1976, p. 130.
21. Zimny, M. L., and Redler, I.: Ultrastructure of solitary enchondromas. J. Hand Surg., *9-B*:95, 1984.

Multiple Enchondromatosis or Ollier's Disease

This is a rare nonhereditary developmental defect characterized by the presence of circumscribed masses of cartilage arranged in linear fashion in the interior of bones. The eponym *Ollier's disease* is used to refer to the condition in which distribution of the enchondromata is predominantly unilateral.* It is also referred to as *dyschondroplasia*, a term that implies that this is a developmental affection rather than a neoplastic disease.[22] Multiple enchondromatosis in association with multiple hemangiomas of the skin is designated *Maffucci's syndrome*.

Multiple enchondromatosis seems to be due to hamartomatous proliferation of cartilage cells that originate within the bone as well as from the cambium layer of the periosteum.

There is great variation in the distribution and extent of the lesions. They may be limited to the bones of one or both hands or to those of a single limb, usually a lower one. When the condition is more extensive, both the upper and lower limbs may be involved, in which instance there is a definite tendency to be predominant on one side.

Pathologic examination discloses an affected long bone to be shortened and bowed, with a widened and broadened metaphyseal region. When the affected bone is sectioned longitudinally, the masses of cartilage are disclosed as numerous small rounded or ovoid grayish-white areas separated by bony septa. Histologic findings are similar to those of solitary enchondroma with the exception that the lesional tissue is hypercellular, and there is less likelihood of calcium impregnation of the intercellular matrix.

Clinically, the signs of enchondromatosis are manifested early in childhood. When the hand is affected, increasing swelling of the fingers may be the initial complaint. The digits may be so enlarged and deformed that the hand appears grotesque and its functional use is impaired. Genu valgum is another deformity that may be present when the femur or tibia is affected. Because of asymmetrical involvement of the lower limbs, lower limb length disparity is a frequent finding; it may be as much as 2 to 4 cm. at three years of age and increase up to 10 to 25 cm. at maturity. The child may present with a short-leg limp. Deformity of the forearm is common, with bowing, limitation of pronation, and ulnar deviation of the hand.

Hemangiomas of the skin and subcutaneous tissues are the most common extraskeletal abnormality found in association with multiple enchondromatosis. They may be associated with superficial phlebectasia. Hemangiomas have been noted in internal organs. Multiple pigmented nevi and vitiligo are other occasional nonskeletal manifestations.

Radiographic findings usually are more extensive than those found clinically. The radiographic picture is quite typical (Figs. 3–265 and 3–266). In the long bones, the lesion is manifested as elongated, longitudinal, radiolucent streaks that involve the metaphysis and extend down the shaft. The epiphyses usually are not involved in the young child; after closure of the physis, however, the lesion may extend into the epiphysis. The cortex may be thin over the growing cartilaginous tumor, as a consequence of which pathologic fractures may result. Spotty calcification is often found within the tumorous tissue. The short tubular bones of the hands and feet are commonly expanded by the lesion and assume a globular shape (Fig. 3–267).

Treatment involves procedures such as epiphysiodesis or limb lengthening to correct unequal limb lengths and measures such as osteotomy to correct knock-knees and other angular deformities.

Sarcomatous change may develop during adult life; the real incidence of this is unknown. Increased localized growth and pain are hallmarks of possible malignancy.[6, 15, 17] In such an instance, biopsy of the lesion is usually indicated.

References

1. Anderson, I. F.: Maffucci's syndrome. Report of a case with a review of the literature. S. Afr. Med. J., 39:1066, 1965.
2. Andren, L., Dymling, J. F., Elner, A., et al.: Maffucci's syndrome: Report of four cases. Acta Chir. Scand., 126:397, 1963.
3. Armstrong, E. A., McLennan, J. E., Benton, C., Chambers, A. A., Perlman, A. W., and Conners, J. W.: Maffucci's syndrome complicated by an intracranial chondrosarcoma and a carotid body tumor: Case report. J. Neurosurg., 55:479, 1981.
4. Bean, W. B.: Dyschondroplasia and hemangiomata (Maffucci's syndrome). Arch. Intern. Med., 95:767, 1955.
5. Beranbaum, S. L., and Tzamouranis, G.: Maffucci's syndrome; dyschondroplasia with hemangiomatosis: Report of a case. A.J.R., 80:479, 1958.
6. Braddock, G. T. F., and Hadlow, V. D.: Osteosarcoma in enchondromatosis (Ollier's disease). Report of a case. J. Bone Joint Surg., 48-B:145, 1966.
7. Bromer, R. S., and John, R. L.: Ollier's disease, unilateral chondrodysplasia. Report of a case with a review of the literature. A.J.R. 26:428, 1931.
8. Cameron, A. H., and McMillan, D. H.: Lipomatosis

---

*See references 7, 10, 14, 19, 20, 22, 23, 26, 35, 45, 61.

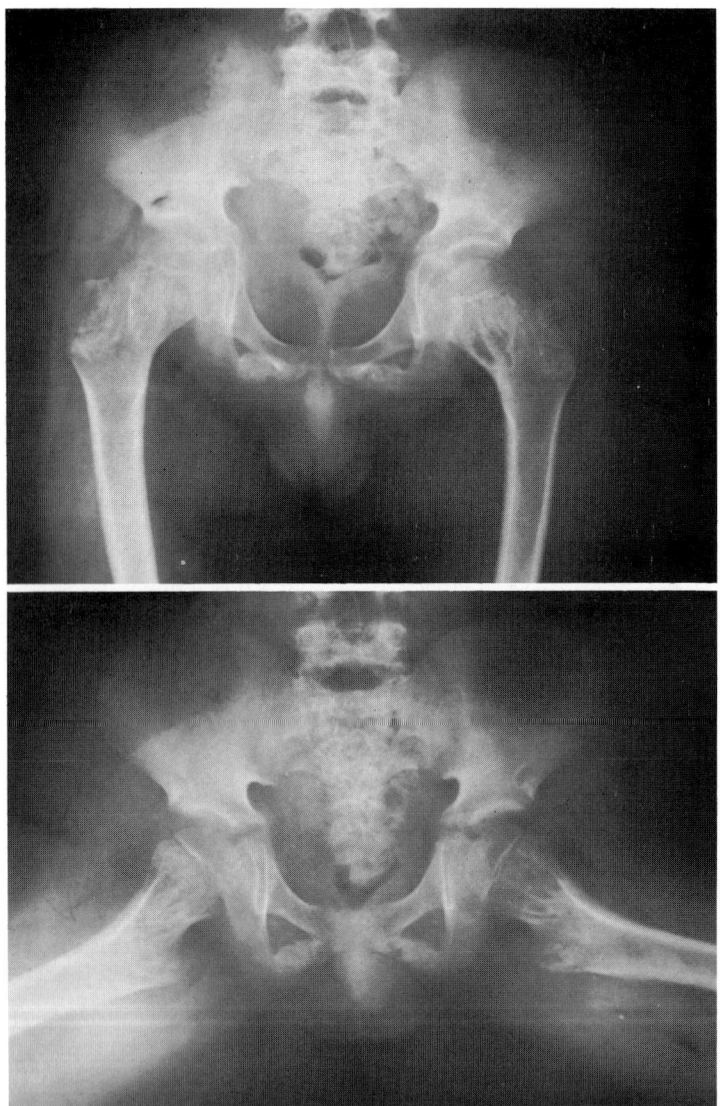

FIGURE 3–265. Multiple enchondromata limited to the femoral necks.

Anteroposterior and lateral views of the hips. Note the longitudinal radiolucent streaks.

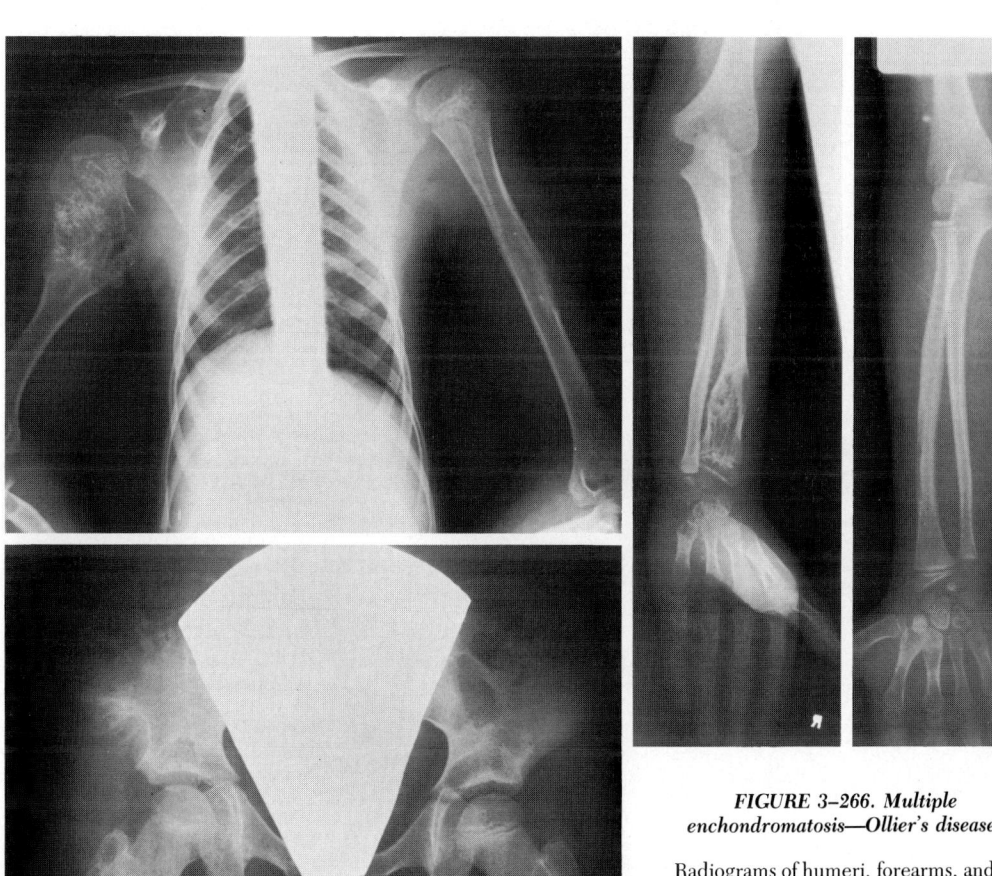

FIGURE 3–266. Multiple enchondromatosis—Ollier's disease.

Radiograms of humeri, forearms, and hips of an 11-year-old girl with predominant involvement of the right side.

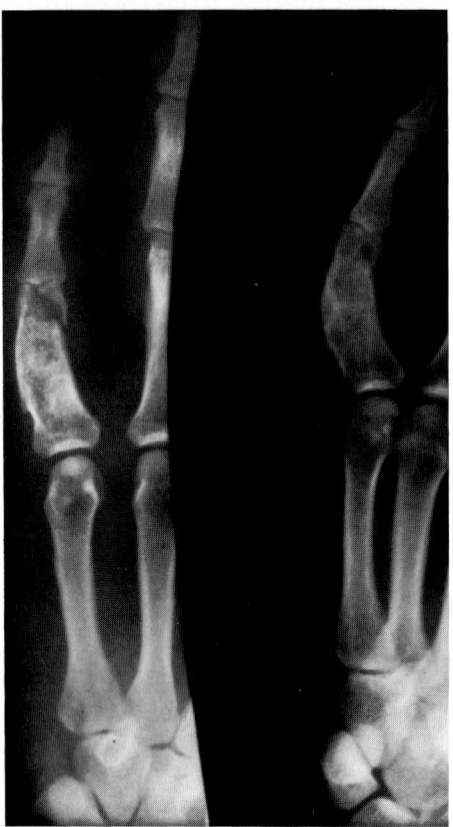

FIGURE 3-267. Multiple enchondromatosis.
Anteroposterior and oblique views of left hand. Note the globular shape of the area of rarefaction of the proximal phalanx of the little finger. (Courtesy of Dr. Andrew K. Poznanski.)

of skeletal muscle in Maffucci's syndrome (dyschondroplasia with hemangiomata). J. Bone Joint Surg., 38-B:692, 1956.
9. Carleton, A., Elkington, J. S. C., Greenfield, J. G., and Robb-Smith, A. H. T.: Maffucci's syndrome (dyschondroplasia with haemangiomata). Q. J. Med., 11:203, 1942.
10. Carter, R. M.: Ollier's dyschondroplasia; report of a case. J. Bone Joint Surg., 22:1063, 1940.
11. Cauble, W. G., and Bowman, H. S.: Dyschondroplasia and hemangiomas (Maffucci's syndrome). Presentation of one case. Arch. Surg., 97:678, 1968.
12. Chen, V. T., and Harrison, D. A.: Maffucci's syndrome. Hand, 10:292, 1978.
13. Cleveland, M.: Chondrodysplasia. Surg. Gynecol. Obstet., 47:338, 1928.
14. Cleveland, M., and Fielding, W.: Chondrodysplasia (Ollier's disease). Report of a case with a thirty-eight year follow-up. J. Bone Joint Surg., 41-A:1341, 1959.
15. Cook, P. L., and Evans, P. G.: Chondrosarcoma of the skull in Maffucci's syndrome. Br. J. Radiol., 50:833, 1977.
16. Cording, R., and Rutt, A.: Maffucci's syndrome (Dyschondro-Dysplasie in Verbindung mit Hämagiomen). Z. Orthop., 120:662, 1982.
17. Cowan, W. K.: Malignant change and multiple mitoses in Ollier's disease. J. Clin. Pathol., 18:650, 1965.
18. Cremer, H., Gullotta, F., and Wolf, L.: The Maffucci-Kast syndrome. Dyschondroplasia with hemangiomas and frontal lobe astrocytoma. J. Cancer Res. Clin. Oncol., 101:231, 1981.
19. Dahle, M.: Chondrodysplasia (Ollier's disease). Multiple enchondromatosis? Acta Chir. Scand., 83:329, 1940.
20. de Groot, J. W. C.: Two atypical cases of chondrodysplasia. J. Pediatr., 39:715, 1951.
21. Elmore, S. M., and Cantrell, W. D.: Maffucci's syndrome; case report with a normal karyotype. J. Bone Joint Surg., 48-A:1607, 1966.
22. Fairbank, H. A. T.: Dyschondroplasia. Synonyms: Ollier's disease, multiple enchondromata. J. Bone Joint Surg., 30-B:689, 1948.
23. Fevre, M., and Alptekin: Maladie d'Ollier. Syndrome de Kast. Rev. Chir. Orthop., 40:15, 1954.
24. Gutman, E., McCutcheon, S., and Garber, P.: Enchondromatosis with hemangiomas (Maffucci's syndrome). South. Med. J., 71:466, 1978.
25. Halper, H., and Wedlick, L.: Maffucci's syndrome with report of a case. Med. J. Aust., 1:936, 1951.
26. Heckman, J. A.: Ollier's disease. Arch. Surg., 63:861, 1951.
27. Ikram-ul-Haq, and Tait, G. B.: Maffucci's syndrome. J. Int. Coll. Surg., 43:133, 1965.
28. Indra, K. J., Bery, K., and Chawla, S.: Dyschondroplasia with multiple haemangiomata—Maffucci's syndrome. Br. J. Radiol., 36:697, 1963.
29. Johnson, J. L., Webster, J. R., Jr., and Sipply, I.: Maffucci's syndrome (dyschondroplasia with hemangiomas). Am. J. Med., 28:864, 1960.
30. Kaibara, N., Mitsuyasu, M., Katsuki, I., Hotokebuchi, T., and Takagishi, K.: Generalized enchondromatosis with unusual complications of soft tissue calcifications and hemangiomas. Skeletal Radiol., 8:43, 1982.
31. Kast, A., and von Recklinghausen, F.: Ein Fall von Enchondrodrom mit ungewohnlicher Multiplication. Virchow. Arch. Pathol. Anat., 118:1, 1889.
32. Kolar, J., Schwank, R., and Dobrkovsky, M.: Maffucci syndrome. Fortschr. Geb. Rontgenstr., 97:226, 1962; Abst. Radiology, 80:1020, 1963.
33. Krause, G. R.: Dyschondroplasia with hemangiomata (Maffucci's syndrome): Case report. A.J.R., 52:620, 1944.
34. Kuzma, J. F., and King, M.: Dyschondroplasia with hemangiomatosis (Maffucci's syndrome) and teratoid tumor of ovary. Arch. Pathol., 46:74, 1948.
35. Langenskiöld, A.: Ollier's disease and its relation to other forms of chondrodysplasia. Acta Orthop. Scand., 17:93, 1947.
36. Lewis, R. J., and Ketcham, A. S.: Maffucci's syndrome: Functional and neoplastic significance. Case report and review of the literature. J. Bone Joint Surg., 55-A:1465, 1973.
37. Lichtenstein, L.: Bone Tumors. 5th Ed. St. Louis, Mosby, 1977, p. 30.
38. Loewinger, R. J., Lichtenstein, J. R., Dodson, W. E., et al.: Maffucci's syndrome: A mesenchymal dysplasia and multiple tumor syndrome. Br. J. Dermatol., 96:317, 1977.
39. Lowell, S. H., and Mathog, R. H.: Head and neck manifestations of Maffucci's syndrome. Arch. Otolaryngol., 105:427, 1979.
40. MacPherson, R. I., and Letts, R. M.: Skeletal disease associated with angiomatosis. J. Can. Assoc. Radiol., 29:90, 1978.
41. McWilliams, H. L., and Bonovich, K. P.: Maffucci's syndrome, an unusual manifestation. Am. Surg., 45:756, 1979.
42. Maffucci, A.: Di un caso di encondroma ed angioma multiplo. Mov. Med. Chir. Napoli, 25:399, 1881.
43. Mainzer, F., Minagi, H., and Steinbach, H. L.: The variable manifestations of multiple enchondromatosis. Radiology, 99:377, 1971.
44. Marberg, K., Dalith, F., and Bank, H.: Dyschondroplasia with multiple hemangiomata (Maffucci's syndrome). Ann. Intern. Med., 49:1216, 1958.
45. Margolis, J.: Ollier's disease. Arch. Intern. Med., 103:279, 1959.

46. Marmor, L.: Chondrodysplasia. Case report of Ollier's disease. Am. J. Surg., *108*:733, 1964.
47. Meckler, L. C.: Dyschondroplasia and hemangiomata. A case report of Maffucci's syndrome. Ohio State Med. J., *60*:672, 1964.
48. Montagne, A., Jr., and Ubilluz, H.: Maffucci's syndrome. South. Med. J., 76:264, 1983.
49. Niechajev, I. A., and Hansson, L. I.: Maffucci's syndrome: Case report. Scand. J. Plast. Reconstr. Surg., *16*:215, 1982.
50. Resnick, D., and Niwayama, G.: Diagnosis of Bone and Joint Disorders, with Emphasis on Articular Abnormalities. Vol. 3. Philadelphia, Saunders, 1981.
51. Richardson, J. A., Jr., and Diddams, A. C.: Maffucci's syndrome. Arch. Intern. Med., *109*:186, 1962.
52. Rimoin, D. L.: International nomenclature of constitutional diseases of bone. Revision—May, 1977. Birth Defects, *14*:39, 1978.
53. Sanerkin, M. G., and Woods, C. G.: Fibrosarcomata and malignant fibrous histiocytomata arising in relation to enchondromata. J. Bone Joint Surg., *61-B*:366, 1979.
54. Schajowicz, F.: Tumors and Tumorlike Lesions of Bone and Joints. New York, Springer, 1981.
55. Schnall, A. M., and Genuth, S. M.: Multiple endocrine adenomas in a patient with the Maffucci syndrome. Am. J. Med., *61*:952, 1976.
56. Spranger, J., Kemperdieck, H., Bakowski, H., and Opitz, J. M.: Two peculiar types of enchondromatosis. Pediatr. Radiol., 7:215, 1978.
57. Strang, C., and Ranie, I.: Dyschondroplasia with haemangiomata (Maffucci's syndrome). J. Bone Joint Surg., *32-B*:376, 1950.
58. Sun, T. C., Swee, R. G., Shives, T. C., and Unni, K. K.: Chondrosarcoma in Maffucci's syndrome. J. Bone Joint Surg., *67-A*:1214, 1985.
59. Tiwisina, T.: Dyschondroplasie (Ollier) mit multiplen Haemangiomen und ortlicher maligner Entartung (Chondrosarkom) Beitr. Klin. Chir., *188*:8, 1954.
60. Umansky, A. L.: Dyschondroplasia with hemangiomata (Maffucci's syndrome): Report of early case with mild osseous manifestations. Bull. Hosp. Joint Dis., 7:59, 1946.
61. Wynne-Davies, R., and Fairbank, T. J.: Fairbank's Atlas of General Affections of the Skeleton. Edinburgh, Churchill-Livingstone, 1976, p. 130.
62. Zocchi, D., Innas, V., and Calderoni, P.: Maffucci's syndrome. Report of 3 cases and review of the literature. Ital. J. Orthop. Traumatol., 9:263, 1983.

PERIOSTEAL CHONDROMA

This is a rare lesion that presents beneath the periosteum as a protruding mass of unossified mature cartilage. Deep it is limited by the underlying bony cortex, and superficially by the overlying fibrous layer of periosteum. The tumor seems to arise from the multipotential cells in the deep layer of the periosteum; the developing cells differentiate into chondroblasts instead of osteoblasts. Periosteal chondroma is a true neoplasm instead of a developmental lesion; it continues to increase in size after skeletal maturity.

Pathology

The tumor is hard, encapsulated, protruding from underlying bone as a hemisphere. On its deep surface there is a thin calcified layer of reactive tissue. Histologically it consists of mature cartilage cells with no evidence of malignancy.

Clinical Features

Ordinarily periosteal chondroma is asymptomatic; it presents as a painless nontender mass that is discovered incidentally in a radiograph or clinically by palpation. Any bone preformed in cartilage may be affected; however, it has definite predilection for the proximal metaphysis of the humerus immediately above the insertion of the deltoid muscle. The proximal femoral metaphysis in the region of the neck is another frequent site.

Radiographic and Imaging Findings

It manifests as a shallow craterlike cortical defect in the diaphysis or metaphysis of a long bone. A thin rim of reactive bone separates the tumor from the underlying cortex; at the upper and lower limits of the chondroma this reactive bone may appear as small Codman's triangles. The cartilaginous nature of the lesion is suggested by the presence of faint calcification.

Computed tomography will show the depth of the crater. Nuclear magnetic resonance imaging will depict the cartilaginous tumor and its extent. Scintigraphy with technetium-99m will show increased uptake about the reactive zone. Periosteal chondroma is an active Stage 2 benign lesion that remains so after cessation of skeletal growth for a long time. Very occasionally it becomes a locally aggressive Stage 3 benign lesion.

Treatment

En bloc marginal extracapsular excision is the treatment of choice. The margins of the tumor are best delineated by magnetic resonance imaging.

Sarcomatous transformation of periosteal chondroma is reported in the literature.[26] In such an instance wide excision is an effective method of treatment.

References

1. Alcott, D. L., and Dubansky, M.: Periosteal chondroma. A report of a case. Am. J. Pathol., *26*:294, 1956.
2. Bertoni, F., Boriani, S., Laus, M., and Campanacci, M.: Periosteal chondrosarcoma and periosteal osteosarcoma. Two distinct entities. J. Bone Joint Surg., *64-B*:370, 1982.
3. Boriani, S., Bacchini, P., Bertoni, F., and Campanacci, M.: Periosteal chondroma. A review of twenty cases. J. Bone Joint Surg., *65-A*:205, 1983.

4. Cary, G. R.: Juxtacortical chondroma. J. Bone Joint Surg., 47-A:1405, 1965.
5. Cooke, G. M., and Pearce, J. G.: Periosteal chondroma. Report of two cases with atypical radiologic features. J. Can. Assoc. Radiol., 27:301, 1976.
6. Cooper, R. R.: Juxtacortical chondrosarcoma. A case report. J. Bone Joint Surg., 47-A:524, 1965.
7. deSantos, L. A., and Spjut, H. J.: Periosteal chondroma. A radiographic spectrum. Skeletal Radiol., 6:15, 1981.
8. Enneking, W. F., Spanier, S. S., and Goodman, M. A.: Current concepts review. The surgical staging of musculoskeletal sarcoma. J. Bone Joint Surg., 62-A:1027, 1980.
9. Feinberg, S. B., and Wilber, M. C.: Periosteal chondroma. A report of two cases. Radiology, 66:383, 1956.
10. Jacobson, S. A.: Epichondroma. A supraosseous benign tumor of cartilage. Bull. Hosp. Joint Dis., 26:93, 1965.
11. Jaffe, H. L.: Juxtacortical chondroma. Bull. Hosp. Joint Dis., 17:20, 1956.
12. Jaffe, H. L.: Tumors and Tumorous Conditions of the Bones and Joints. Philadelphia, Lea & Febiger, 1958, pp. 196–202.
13. Keiller, V. H.: Cartilaginous tumors of bone. Surg. Gynecol. Obstet., 40:512, 1925.
14. Kirchner, S. G., Pavlov, H., Heller, R. M., and Kaye, J. J.: Periosteal chondromas of the anterior tibial tubercle: Two cases. A.J.R., 131:1088, 1978.
15. Lichtenstein, L.: Tumors of periosteal origin. Cancer, 8:1060, 1955.
16. Lichtenstein, L.: Bone Tumors. 2nd Ed. St. Louis, Mosby, 1965, pp. 345–346.
17. Lichtenstein, L., and Hall, J. E.: Periosteal chondroma. A distinctive benign cartilage tumor. J. Bone Joint Surg., 34-A:691, 1952.
18. McWorter, G. L.: Chondromata of the thumb. Surg. Clin. North Am., 4:629, 1920.
19. Mason, M. L.: Tumors of the hand. Surg. Gynecol. Obstet., 64:129, 1937.
20. Merlino, A. F., and Nixon, J. E.: Periosteal chondroma. Report of an atypical case and review of the literature. Am. J. Surg., 107:773, 1964.
21. Meyer, R.: Juxtacortical chondroma. Br. J. Radiol., 31:106, 1958.
22. Nosanchuk, J. S., and Kaufer, H.: Recurrent periosteal chondroma. Report of two cases and a review of the literature. J. Bone Joint Surg., 51-A:375, 1969.
23. Pazzaglia, U. F., and Ceciliani, L.: Periosteal chondroma of the humerus leading to shortening. A case report. J. Bone Joint Surg., 67-B:290, 1985.
24. Roberts, R. E.: Some observations on osteochondromata, chondromata and cystic diseases of bone. Br. J. Radiol., 10:196, 1937.
25. Rockwell, M. A., Saiter, E. T., and Enneking, W. F.: Periosteal chondroma. J. Bone Joint Surg., 54-A:102, 1972.
26. Scaglietti, O., and Stringa, G.: Periosteal myxoma of infancy and periosteal chondroma of adolescence with local malignancy. Clin. Orthop., 9:147, 1957.
27. Unni, K. K., Dahlin, D. C., and Beabout, J. W.: Periosteal osteogenic sarcoma. Cancer, 37:2476, 1976.

BENIGN CHONDROBLASTOMA

This is a rare benign tumor that was originally described by Codman in 1931.[16] In the literature it is also referred to as benign epiphyseal chondroblastoma, benign chondroblastoma, and Codman's tumor. It occurs in late adolescence, usually between the ages of 10 and 17 years. It is more common in the male. Ordinarily epiphyseal in location, it has a predilection for the proximal humerus, distal femur, and proximal tibia. It has, however, been reported to occur in the skull, maxilla, vertebral column, rib, pelvis, fingers and hand (capitate), patella, talus, and calcaneus.* Multifocal benign chondroblastoma has been reported by Roberts and Taylor.[80]

The histologic appearance is very typical, characterized by polyhedral cells, which are closely compacted with focal areas of calcification and necrosis (Fig. 3–268). The latter findings will be best visualized if lesional tissue is processed without decalcification. Those not familiar with the tumor may suspect malignancy, but mitotic figures are absent.

Clinical complaints are mild. Pain is usually the presenting symptom and is relieved by salicylates; this is similar to osteoid osteoma. Because the lesion is in close relation to it, the adjacent joint may be somewhat swollen and limited in its range of motion. On palpation the lesion may be locally tender. If the tumor is in a lower limb, an antalgic limp may be encountered.

---

*See references: skull, 13, 26, 39; maxilla, 3; spine, 11; rib, 7; pelvis, 63, 68; fingers, 72; hand, 65; patella, 16; talus, 10, 69; calcaneus, 52, 56.

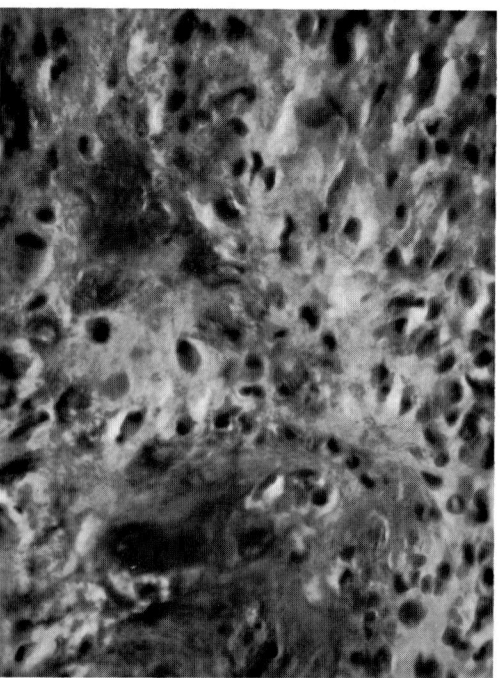

FIGURE 3–268. Benign chondroblastoma.

Photomicrograph showing the characteristic polyhedral cells, which are closely packed with focal areas of calcification and necrosis ($\times$ 450).

In the radiograms, an oval or round radiolucent area, usually between 1 and 4 cm. in diameter, is present. It is often delimited by a rim of mature reactive bone. Rarefaction in the lesional area is fuzzy and somewhat mottled owing to fine punctate areas of calcification. The regional cortex may be bulged, and there may be some periosteal new bone deposition. The lesion is eccentrically located in the epiphysis and may extend into the adjacent metaphysis. Linear and computed tomography will depict the fine intrinsic calcification and the extent of the tumor.

In the differential diagnosis, giant cell tumor, enchondroma, and eosinophilic granuloma should be considered.

Treatment usually consists of complete curettage and excision of the lesion (with an attempt to avoid interfering with the joint and disturbing growth of the physis in the immature skeleton). The defect is filled with bone grafts. There is definite risk of recurrence after intracapsular curettage. Marginal intracapsular excision often results in cure, but this is performed only when the tumor has recurred. Intracapsular excision with wide surgical margin is carried out when the lesion is aggressive Stage 3.[47, 53, 68, 78, 101] Secondary chondrosarcoma has been seen to develop, especially after irradiation, but it is extremely rare.

References

1. Abdul-Karim, F. W., Ayala, A. G., and Spjut, H. J.: Case report 321: Extraosseous chondroblastoma in the subcutaneous tissue of the right shoulder. Skeletal Radiol., 14:73, 1985.
2. Aegerter, E., and Kirpatrick, J. A., Jr.: Orthopedic Diseases. 4th Ed. Philadelphia, Saunders, 1975, p. 539.
3. Al-Dewachi, H. S., Al-Naib, N., and Sangal, B. L.: Benign chondroblastoma of the maxilla: A case report and review of chondroblastomas in cranial bones. Br. J. Oral Surg., 18:150, 1980.
4. Alexander, C.: Case report 5: Chondroblastoma of tibia. Skeletal Radiol., 1:63, 1976.
5. Aprin, H.: Benign chondroblastoma. Orthopaedics, 4:1134, 1981.
6. Aronsohn, R. S., Hart, W. R., and Martel, W.: Metaphyseal chondroblastoma of bone. A.J.R., 127:686, 1976.
7. Assor, D.: Brief notes. Chondroblastoma of the rib. J. Bone Joint Surg., 55-A:208, 1973.
8. Bloem, J. L., and Mulder, J. D.: Chondroblastoma: A clinical and radiological study of 104 cases. Skeletal Radiol., 14:1, 1985.
9. Braunstein, E., Martel, W., and Weatherbee, L.: Periosteal bone apposition in chondroblastoma. Skeletal Radiol., 4:34, 1979.
10. Breck, L. W., and Emmett, J. E.: Chondroblastoma of the talus: A case report. Clin. Orthop., 7:132, 1956.
11. Buraczewski, J., Lyaskowska, J., and Rudowski, W.: Chondroblastoma (Codman's tumour) of the thoracic spine. J. Bone Joint Surg., 39-B:705, 1957.
12. Campanacci, M., Ginnti, A., Martucci, E., and Trentani, C.: Epiphyseal chondroblastoma (a study of 39 cases). Ital. J. Orthop. Traumatol., 3:67, 1977.
13. Cares, H. L., and Terplan, K.: Chondroblastoma of the skull: A case report. J. Neurosurg., 35:614, 1971.
14. Castleman, B.: Case records of the Massachusetts General Hospital (case 33-1964). N. Engl. J. Med., 271:94, 1964.
15. Castleman, B., and McNeill, J. M., (eds.): Bone and Joint Clinicopathological Conferences of the Massachusetts General Hospital. Boston, Little, Brown, 1966, p. 220.
16. Codman, E. A.: Epiphyseal chondromatous giant cell tumors of the upper end of the humerus. Surg. Gynecol. Obstet., 52:543, 1931.
17. Cohen, J., and Cahen, I.: Benign chondroblastoma of the patella. J. Bone Joint Surg., 45-A:824, 1963.
18. Coleman, S. S.: Benign chondroblastoma with recurrent soft-tissue and intra-articular lesions—report of a case. J. Bone Joint Surg., 48-A:1554, 1966.
19. Coley, B. L., and Higinbotham, N. L.: The significance of cartilage in abnormal locations. Cancer, 2:777, 1949.
20. Coley, B. L., and Santoro, A. J.: Benign central cartilaginous tumors of bone. Surgery, 22:411, 1947.
21. Copeland, M. M., and Geschickter, C. F.: Chondroblastic tumors of bone, benign and malignant. Ann. Surg., 129:724, 1949.
22. Dahlin, D. C.: Chondromyxoid fibroma of bone with emphasis on its morphological relationship to benign chondroblastoma. Cancer, 9:195, 1956.
23. Dahlin, D. C., and Ivins, J. C.: Benign chondroblastoma. A study of 125 cases. Cancer, 30:401, 1972.
24. Dahlin, D. C., and Salvador, A. H.: Cartilaginous tumors of the soft tissues of the hands and feet. Mayo Clin. Proc., 49:721, 1974.
25. Dahlin, D. C., and Thomas, C. L.: Benign chondroblastoma. In Bone Tumors. General Aspects and Data on 6,221 cases. Springfield, Ill., Thomas, 1978, p. 43.
26. Denko, J. V., and Krauel, L. H.: Benign chondroblastoma of bone: An unusual localization in temporal bone. Arch. Pathol., 59:710, 1955.
27. Ewing, J.: Neoplastic Diseases. A Treatise on Tumors. 3rd Ed. Philadelphia, Saunders, 1928, pp. 293–334.
28. Fechner, R. E., and Wilde, H. D.: Chondroblastoma in the metaphysis of the femoral neck. J. Bone Joint Surg., 56-A:413, 1974.
29. Firtel, S. L.: Benign chondroblastoma of bone. Report of a case. Newark Beth Israel Hosp. J., 4:117, 1953.
30. Fobben, E. S., Dalinka, M. K., and Schiebler, M. L.: Magnetic resonance imaging: appearance at 1.5 tesla of cartilaginous tumors involving the epiphysis. Skeletal Radiol., 16:647, 1987.
31. France, W. G.: Benign chondroblastoma of bone. Br. J. Surg., 39:357, 1952.
32. Geschickter, C. F., and Copeland, M. M.: Tumors of Bone. 3rd Ed. Philadelphia, Lippincott, 1949, p. 164.
33. Gilmer, W. S., Higley, G. B., and Kilgore, W. E.: Atlas of Bone Tumors. St. Louis, Mosby, 1963.
34. Goodsell, J. O., and Hubinger, H. L.: Benign chondroblastoma of mandibular condyle: Report of a case. J. Oral Surg., 22:355, 1964.
35. Gravanis, M. B., and Giansanti, J. S.: Benign chondroblastoma: Report of four cases with a discussion of the presence of ossification. Am. J. Clin. Pathol., 55:624, 1971.
36. Green, P., and Whittaker, R. P.: Benign chondroblastoma: Case report with pulmonary metastases. J. Bone Joint Surg., 57-A:418, 1975.
37. Hadders, H. N., Donner, R., and Van Rijssel, T. G.: Chondroblastoma benignum. Ned. Tijdschr. Geneeskd., 100:2648, 1956.
38. Hammarstrom, S.: Ein Fall von chondroblastischem Sarkom. Acta Radiol., 15:608, 1934.

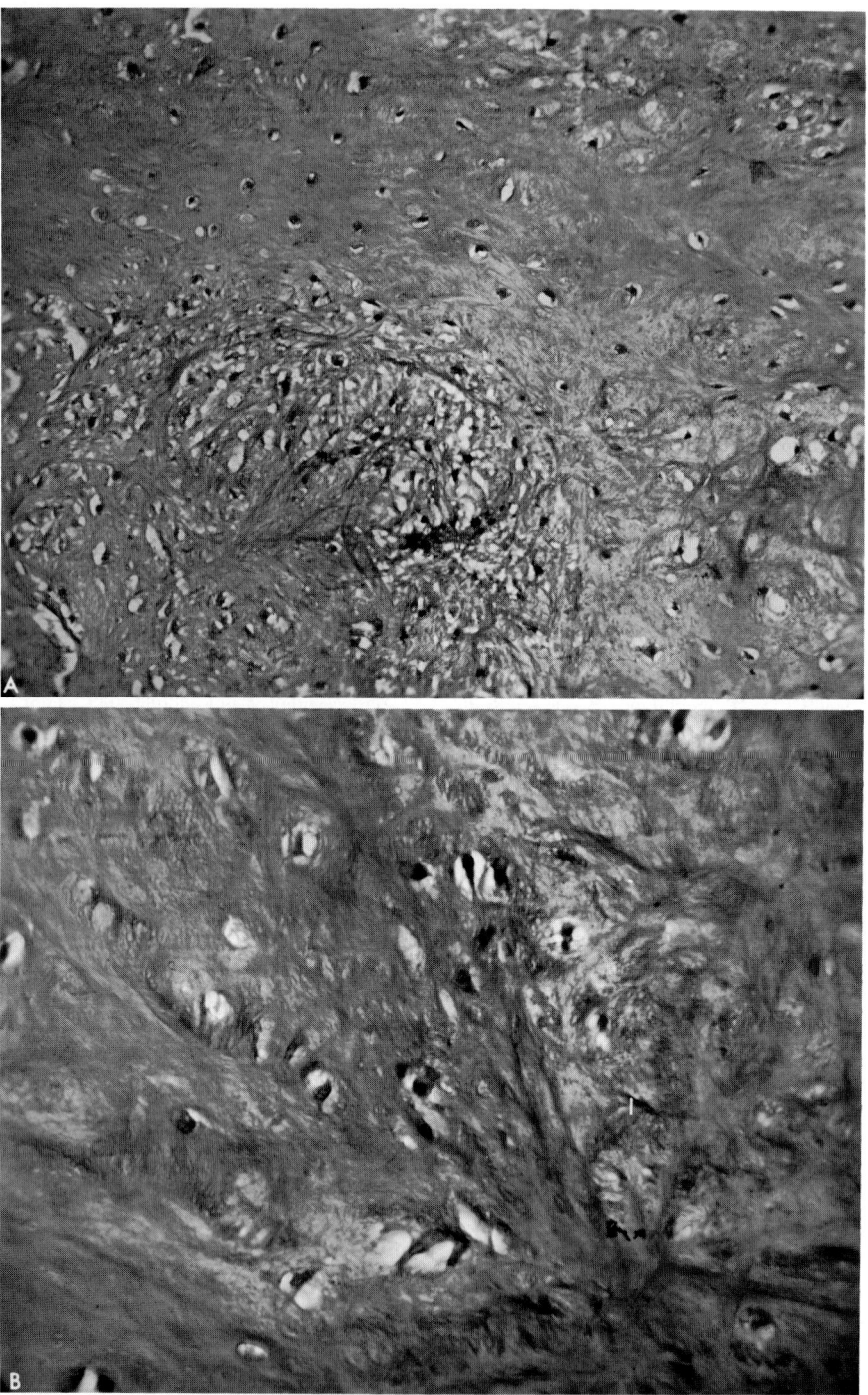

FIGURE 3–269. Chondromyxoid fibroma of neck of right femur.

A and **B.** Photomicrographs (× 100 and × 250) showing the characteristic histologic picture. Note the ovoid and moderate-sized nuclei of the cells which are widely separated by myxoid and chondroid matrix.

mors; very occasionally they may be active Stage 3.

Treatment

Extracapsular marginal excision is the treatment; the resultant defect, if large, is grafted with autogenous cancellous and cortical bone. If the lesion is close to the physis it is best to delay surgical intervention until the tumor has grown away from the growth plate and a safe zone of normal cancellous bone is present between the two. There is no place for radiation therapy or chemotherapy in the management of chondromyxoid fibroma.

References

1. Adler, C. P.: Fibromyxoma of the femoral neck. J. Cancer Res. Clin. Oncol., 101:183, 1981.
2. Adler, C. P.: Case report 338: Chondromyxoid fibroma (CMF) of the radius associated with an aneurysmal bone cyst (ABC). Skeletal Radiol., 14:305, 1985.
3. Aegerter, E., and Kirkpatrick, J. A., Jr.: Orthopedic Diseases. 4th Ed. Philadelphia, Saunders, 1975, p. 545.
4. Andrew, T., Kenwright, J., and Woods, C.: Periosteal chondromyxoid fibroma of the tibia. Acta Orthop. Scand., 53:467, 1982.
5. Attar, S.: Myxoma: Clinicopathologic study. Am. J. Surg., 91:755, 1956.
6. Bauer, T. W., Dorfman, H. D., and Latham, J. T.: Periosteal chondroma. A clinicopathologic study of 23 cases. Am. J. Surg. Pathol., 6:631, 1982.
7. Bauer, W. H., and Harell, A.: Myxoma of bone. J. Bone Joint Surg., 36-A:263, 1954.
8. Benedetti, G. B., Canepa, G., and Garcia, M.: Il fibroma condromixoide dell'osso. Arch. Putti Chir. Organi Mov. 17:44, 1962.
9. Benson, W. R., and Bass, S., Jr.: Chondromyxoid fibroma: First report of occurrence of this tumor in vertebral column. Am J. Clin. Pathol., 25:1290, 1955.
10. Besse, B. E., Jr., Dahlin, D. C., Pugh, D. G., and Ghormley, R. K.: Aneurysmal bone cysts: Additional considerations. Clin. Orthop., 7:93, 1956.
11. Bialik, V., Kedar, A., Ben-Arie, Y., Kleinhaus, U., and Fishman, J.: Case report 315: Parosteal (periosteal juxtacortical) chondromyxoid fibroma of the upper end of the femur. Skeletal Radiol., 13:323, 1985.
12. Bloodgood, J. C.: Bone tumors: Myxoma. Ann. Surg., 80:817, 1924.
13. Boriani, S., Bacchini, P., Bertoni, F., and Campanacci, M.: Periosteal chondroma, a review of twenty cases. J. Bone Joint Surg., 65-A:205, 1981.
14. Bruce, K. W., and Royer, R. Q.: Central fibromyxoma of maxilla. Oral Surg., 5:1277, 1952.
15. Chacha, P. B., and Tan, K. K.: Periosteal myxoma of the femur. J. Bone Joint Surg., 54-A:1091, 1972.
16. Coley, B. L.: Neoplasms of Bone. 2nd Ed. New York, Hoeber, 1960, p. 139.
17. Coley, B. L., and Santoro, A. J.: Benign central cartilaginous tumors of bone. Surgery, 22:411, 1947.
18. Conaty, J. P., Biddle, M., and McKeever, F. M.: Osseous coccidioidal granuloma. J. Bone Joint Surg., 41-A:1109, 1959.
19. Copello, O.: Mixoma del metatarsiano. Bol. Trab. Soc. Cir. Buenos Aires, 19:1151, 1935.
20. Crabbe, W. A.: Chondromyxoid fibroma of bone. Proc. R. Soc. Med., 55:353, 1962.
21. Dabska, M., Rudowski, W., and Loth, F.: Fibroma chondromyxoides. Nowotwory, 9:275, 1959.
22. Dahlin, D. C.: Chondromyxoid fibroma of bone with emphasis on its morphological relationship to benign chondroblastoma. Cancer, 9:195, 1956.
23. Dahlin, D. C.: Bone Tumors. 3rd Ed. Springfield, Ill., Thomas, 1978.
24. Dahlin, D. C., and Beabout, J. W.: Differentiation of lowgrade chondrosarcomas. Cancer, 28:461, 1971.
25. Dahlin, D. C., Wells, A. H., and Henderson, E. D.: Chondromyxoid fibroma of bone; report of two cases. J. Bone Joint Surg., 35-A:831, 1953.
26. De Santos, L. A., and Spjut, H. J.: Periosteal chondroma: Radiographic spectrum. Skeletal Radiol., 6:15, 1981.
27. Dutz, W., and Stout, A. P.: The myxoma in childhood. Cancer, 14:629, 1961.
28. Edmunds, L. H., and Jones, H.: CMF of bone. Bull. Mason Clin., 10:1, 1956.
29. Feldman, F., Hecht, H. L., and Johnston, A. D.: Chondromyxoid fibroma of bone. Radiology, 94:249, 1970.
30. Fery, A., Schmitt, D., and Lefakis, P.: Malignant degeneration of a recurrent chondromyxoid fibroma. Ann. Chir., 31:719, 1977.
31. Fillippone, M. J.: Malignant chondromyxofibroma. Case report. J. Am. Podiatry Assoc., 56:237, 1966.
32. Frank, M. W. E., and Rockwood, C. A.: Chondromyxoid fibroma: Review of the literature and report of four cases. South. Med. J., 62:1248, 1969.
33. Freund, E.: Unusual cartilaginous tumor formation of the skeleton. Arch. Surg., 33:1054, 1936.
34. Gerard-Marchant, P.: Un cas de fibrome chondromyxoide. Mém. Acad. Chir., 84:126, 1958.
35. Gilmer, W. S., Highley, G. B., Jr., and Kilgore, W. E. (eds.): Atlas of Bone Tumors. St. Louis, Mosby, 1963, pp. 36–39.
36. Gilmer, W. S., Jr., Kilgore, W., and Smith, H.: Central cartilaginous tumors of bone. Clin. Orthop., 26:81, 1963.
37. Goorwitch, J.: Chondromyxoid fibroma of rib: Report of an unusual benign primary tumor. Dis. Chest, 20:186, 1951.
38. Hadders, H. N., and Osterdoom, H. J.: Chondromyxoid fibroma of bone: Case. Ned. Tijdschr. Geneeskd., 98:555, 1954.
39. Harbert, F., Gerry, R. G., and Dimmette, R. M.: Myxoma of maxilla. Oral Surg., 2:1414, 1949.
40. Herfarth, H.: Ein zentrales Myxom der Tibia. Arch. Klin. Chir., 170:283, 1932.
41. Hill, J. A., Victor, T. A., Dawson, W. J., and Milgram, J. W.: Myxoma of the toe. J. Bone Joint Surg., 60-A:128, 1978.
42. Hovnanian, A. P.: Myxoma of maxilla, report of two cases. Oral Surg., 6:927, 1953.
43. Hutchison, J., and Park, W. W.: Chondromyxoid fibroma of bone. Report of a case. J. Bone Joint Surg., 42-B:542, 1960.
44. Iwata, S., and Coley, B. L.: Report of six cases of chondromyxoid fibroma of bone. Surg. Gynecol. Obstet., 107:571, 1958.
45. Jaffe, H. J.: Tumors and Tumorous Conditions of Bones and Joints. Philadelphia, Lea & Febiger, 1958, p. 203.
46. Jaffe, H. L., and Lichtenstein, L.: Chondromyxoid fibroma of bone: A distinctive benign tumor likely to be mistaken especially for chondrosarcoma. Arch. Pathol., 45:541, 1948.
47. Lamb, H. D.: Myxoma of orbit, with case report and anatomical findings. Arch. Ophthalmol., 57:425, 1928.
48. Lawson, J. P., and Barwick, K. W.: Case report 209: Chondromyxoid fibroma of the left first rib. Skeletal Radiol., 9:53, 1982.
49. Lettin, A. W. F.: Unusual case of chondromyxoid fibroma of bone. Proc. R. Soc. Med., 56:10, 1963.

50. Levy, W., Aegerter, E., and Kirkpatrick, J.: The nature of cartilaginous tumors. Radiol. Clin. North Am., 2:327, 1964.
51. Lichtenstein, L.: Bone Tumors. 4th Ed. St. Louis, Mosby, 1972, p. 57.
52. Lichtenstein, L., and Bernstein, D.: Unusual benign and malignant chondroid tumors of bone. Cancer, 12:1142, 1959.
53. Lichtenstein, L., and Kaplan, L.: Benign chondroblastoma of bone: Unusual localization in femoral capital epiphysis. Cancer, 2:793, 1949.
54. Lipkin, S. I.: Malignant chondromyxoid fibroma of humerus. Vopr. Onkol., 12:61, 1966. (In Russian).
55. Lodwick, G. S.: The Bones and Joints. Chicago, Year Book, 1971, pp. 168–183.
56. Marcove, R. C., Kambolis, C., Bullough, P. G., and Jaffe, H. L.: Fibromyxoma of bone. Cancer, 17:1209, 1964.
57. Mauck, R. H., and Carpenter, E. B.: Chondromyxoid fibroma of bone. Report of case. Virginia Med. Monthly, 86:210, 1959.
58. McClur, D. K., and Dahlin, D. C.: Myxoma of bone. Report of three cases. Mayo Clin. Proc., 52:249, 1977.
59. Mayer, B. S.: Chondromyxoid fibroma of lumbar spine. J. Can. Assoc. Radiol., 29:271, 1978.
60. Murphy, N. B., and Price, C. H. G.: The radiological aspects of chondromyxoid fibroma. Clin. Radiol., 22:261, 1971.
61. Norman, A., and Steiner, G. C.: Case report 38. Skeletal Radiol., 2:105, 1978.
62. Norman, A., and Steiner, G. C.: Case report 66. Skeletal Radiol., 3:115, 1979.
63. Ottolenghi, C. E., and Petracchi, L. J.: Chondromyxosarcoma of the calcaneus. J. Bone Joint Surg., 35-A:211, 1953.
64. Perou, M. L., Kolis, J. A., Zaeske, E. V., and Borja, S. R.: Myxoma of the toe. Cancer, 20:1030, 1967.
65. Plum, F. G., and Pugh, D. G.: Roentgenographic aspects of benign chondroblastoma of bone. A.J.R., 79:584, 1958.
66. Prichard, R. W., Stoy, R. P., and Barwick, J. T. F.: Chondromyxoid fibroma of the scapula. J. Bone Joint Surg., 46-A:1759, 1964.
67. Rahimi, A., Beabout, J. W., Ivins, J. C., and Dahlin, D. C.: Chondromyxoid fibroma: A clinicopathological study of 76 cases. Cancer, 30:726, 1972.
68. Ralph, L. L.: Chondromyxoid fibroma of bone. J. Bone Joint Surg., 44-B:7, 1962.
69. Ryall, R. D.: Chondromyxoid fibroma of bone. Br. J. Radiol., 43:71, 1970.
70. Salzer, M., and Salzer-Kuntschik, M.: Das chondromyxoid Fibrom. Langenbecks Arch. Klin. Chir., 312:216, 1965.
71. Scaglietti, O., and Stringa, G.: Myxoma of bone in childhood. J. Bone Joint Surg., 43-A:67, 1961.
72. Schajowicz, F.: Tumors and Tumorlike Lesions of Bone and Joints. New York, Springer-Verlag, 1981.
73. Schajowicz, F., and Gallardo, H.: Chondromyxoid fibroma (fibromyxoid chondroma) of bone. J. Bone Joint Surg., 53-B:198, 1971.
74. Schayik, S., and Rosman, M. A.: Malignant degeneration of a chondromyxoid fibroma in a child. Can. J. Surg., 18:354, 1975.
75. Seth, H. N., and Rao, B. D. P.: Chondromyxoid fibroma of bone: Report on three cases. Indian J. Pathol. Bacteriol., 7:112, 1964.
76. Shlapoberskii, V. I., and Zatsepin, S. T.: Clinical observations of chondromyxoid fibroma of bone. Vopr. Onkol., 10:15, 1964.
77. Siderman, S., Sarrafian, S., and Topouzian, L. K.: Chondromyxoid fibroma of bone: Report of a case with a pathological fracture. Northwest. Univ. Med. School Q. Bull., 34–35:346, 1960.
78. Spjut, H. J., Dorfman, H. D., Fechner, R. E., and Ackerman, L. V.: Atlas of Tumor Pathology. Second Series, Fascicle 5, Tumors of Bones and Cartilage. Washington, D. C., Armed Forces Institute of Pathology, 1971, p. 50.
79. Sponsel, K. H., McDonald, J. R., and Ghormley, R. K.: Myxoma and myxosarcoma of soft tissue of extremities. J. Bone Joint Surg., 34-A:820, 1952.
80. Stout, A. P.: Myxoma, tumor of primitive mesenchyme. Ann. Surg., 127:706, 1948.
81. Stradford, H. T.: Chondromyxoid fibroma of bone. Bull. Charlotte Mem. Hosp., 3:71, 1948.
82. Teitelbaum, S. L., and Bessone, L.: Resection of a large chondromyxoid fibroma of the sternum. Report of the first case and review of the literature. J. Thorac. Cardiovasc. Surg., 57:333, 1969.
83. Turcotte, B., Pugh, D. G., and Dahlin, D. C.: The roentgenographic aspects of chondromyxoid fibroma of bone. A.J.R., 87:1085, 1962.
84. Uehlinger, E.: Die pathologische Anatomie der Knochengeschwulste. Helv. Chir. Acta, 26:597, 1959.
85. Uematsu, A., Coy, J. T., III, Hodges, S. O., Goodman, R. P., and Brower, T. D.: Malignant chondromyxoid fibroma of the scapula. South. Med. J., 70:1469, 1977.
86. Vix, V. A., and Fahmy, A.: Unusual appearance of a chondromyxoid fibroma. Radiology, 92:365, 1969.
87. Wrenn, R. N., and Smith, A. G.: Chondromyxoid fibroma. South. Med. J., 47:848, 1954.
88. Zeman, S. C., and Hurley, E. J.: Chondromyxoid fibroma of the rib initially seen as a pulmonary lesion. J.A.M.A., 242:2588, 1979.

OSTEOID OSTEOMA

Osteoid osteoma is a bone lesion characterized by the formation of a small nidus of variably calcified osteoid tissue in a stroma of relatively loose vascular connective tissue surrounded by a margin of dense sclerotic bone; the lesion is typically painful. It was described as a distinct entity by Jaffe in 1935.[72] Prior reports of apparent examples of this lesion can, however, be found in the literature, referred to by such names as "sclerosing nonsuppurative osteomyelitis," osteomyelitis of Garré, or "localized or cortical bone abscess." The condition should be differentiated from benign osteoblastoma or "giant osteoid osteoma"; the latter does resemble osteoid osteoma histologically. The distinction between the two is one of size (osteoblastoma is larger), degree of sclerosis (osteoid osteoma in general has a greater degree of surrounding dense sclerotic bone), and natural course (osteoblastoma can be more aggressive).

Age and Sex Predilection

Osteoid osteoma occurs mainly in children and young adults from approximately 10 to 25 years of age, and is twice as prevalent in the male as in the female. The lesion is not rare.

Sites of Involvement

Any bone may be affected, the most common locations being the femur and the tibia, though the lesion is sometimes found in the fibula, humerus, vertebrae, talus, and calcaneus. In extremely rare cases, a rib, iliac bone, patella, metatarsal, or phalanx may be the site of the tumor.

Pathology

The lesion is believed to be a neoformation. It is not inflammatory or infectious in its pathogenesis, and it does not represent a reparative phenomenon.

Characteristically, there is a nidus composed of a highly vascular connective tissue matrix in which there are varying degrees of osteoid tissue and irregular trabeculae of immature bone (Fig. 3–270). The lesional cells are osteoblasts, distinct from the proliferating mesenchymal cells in the surrounding reactive rows. Over a period of months or years, the nidus stimulates the production of dense bone, which surrounds it and extends some distance from it. If the lesion is intracortical, the reactive cortical hyperostosis will be marked. As a rule the reactive bone is more vascular than normal bone, and the overlying periosteum is thickened. At surgery, when the nidus is exposed, it stands out as a reddish-blue vascular soft tissue in contrast to the dense surrounding reactive bone. With maturation the nidus undergoes a variable degree of calcification.

Clinical Findings

Osteoid osteoma may present a wide range of symptoms and, in some cases, neurologic phenomena, depending on the area that is affected.

Pain is the initial complaint; it is mild at first, then tends to increase to the point at which it interferes with sleep. The pain may be intermittent, but it usually is continuous. The patient will usually volunteer the information that aspirin relieves the pain dramatically, but temporarily. Athletic activities aggravate the pain. Occasionally, ingestion of alcoholic beverages will precipitate intense pain. On examination, excruciating point tenderness at the site of the lesion is characteristic. A local smooth, hard swelling may be palpable in superficially located lesions. The swelling is due to sclerotic periosteal reaction; there is usually acute local tenderness over its apex.

When the tumor occurs in a bone in the lower limb, the patient may limp slightly; when it is in a joint, he may complain of stiffness. "Sympathetic synovitis" may be caused by a lesion under the articular cartilage. Disuse atrophy is also common. When a vertebra or a rib is affected there may be paravertebral muscle spasm and spinal deformity. When a patient presents with painful scoliosis, osteoid osteoma should be ruled out by bone scan with technetium-99m. Neurologic disorders may be mimicked; for example, excessive perspiration and pain in the hand may be found when the lesion is located in the upper humerus or cervical spine. Symptoms may suggest sciatica when it is in the proximal femur or the pelvis. Quadriceps atrophy and absence or diminution of knee reflex may suggest spinal cord tumor; occasionally neurosurgeons have performed myelography to rule out intraspinal lesions, and later the diagnosis of osteoid osteoma of the femur has been made.

Often, in its early stages, the lesion is not recognized, the discomfort having been ascribed to psychologic causes.

Radiographic and Imaging Findings

The radiographic picture is typical and diagnostic. The nidus characteristically appears as a small radiolucent area with surrounding sclerosis of bone that may extend some distance from it (Figs. 3–271 to 3–276). An intense reactive zone many times the size of the primary lesion is typical of osteoid osteoma. The dense cortical bone, however, often obscures the radiolucency of the small nidus, necessitating overexposure and "coning down" views from various angles to demonstrate the nidus. A radiologically occult nidus is readily shown and delineated from the surrounding bony sclerosis by linear and computed tomography (Fig. 3–277 D). Calcification in the central portion of the nidus will be depicted as a radiopaque fleck in the radiogram. In magnetic nuclear resonance studies the nidus is silent (Fig. 3–278).

Bone imaging with technetium-99m shows an intense increase in uptake in the nidus (Fig. 3–277 C). Activity in the surrounding sclerotic area is immense but less than that of the nidus. Isotopic scanning is of great value in identification of the area of the lesion; particularly in the spine and pelvis, which may be radiographically obscure areas. Computed tomography will locate the nidus within the sclerotic area of bone.

When osteoid osteoma is suspected the sequential diagnostic work-up for identification of the lesion should be as follows: first, conventional radiographs; second, isotopic scanning; and third, computed tomography with or with-

Text continued on page 1215

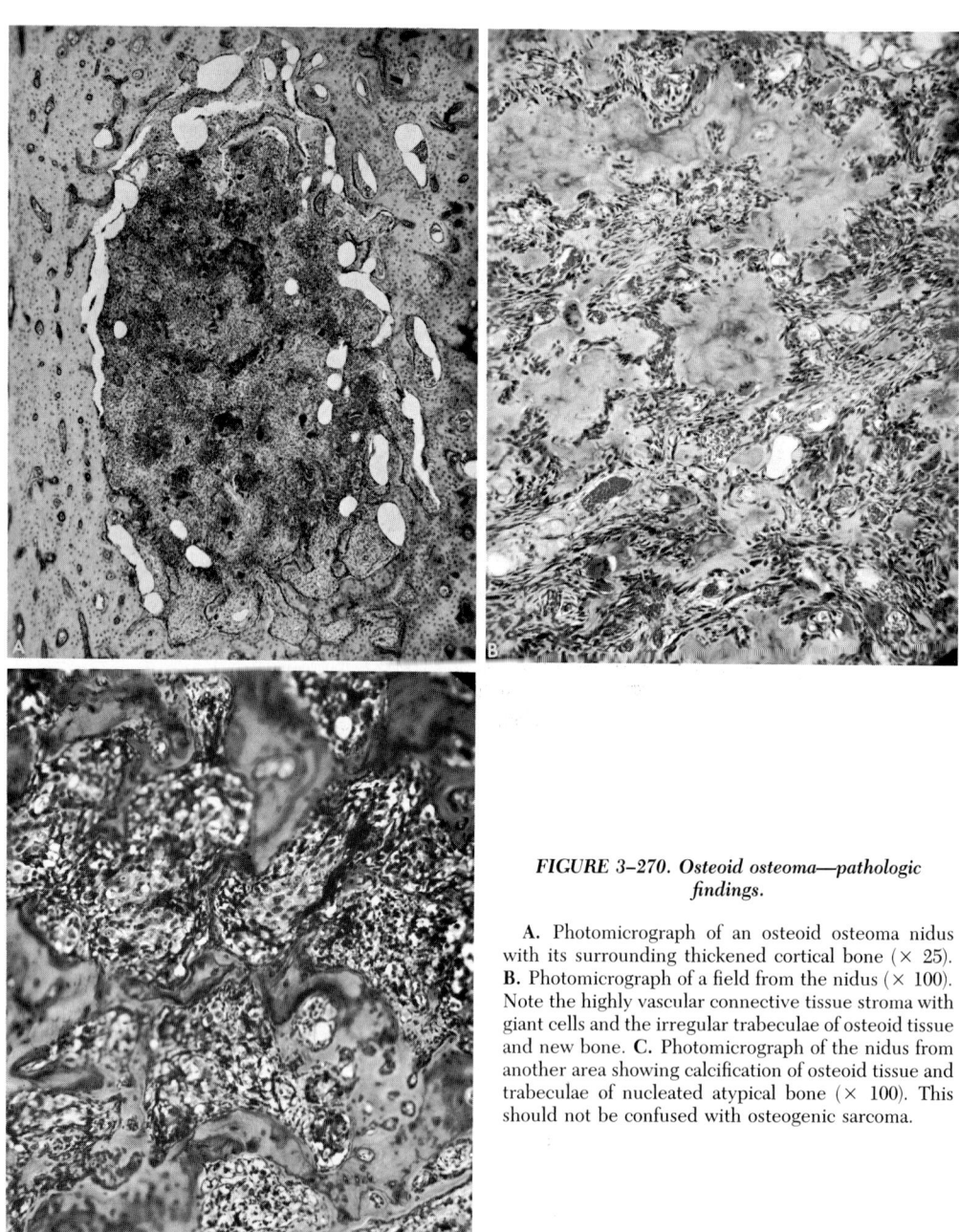

FIGURE 3–270. *Osteoid osteoma—pathologic findings.*

A. Photomicrograph of an osteoid osteoma nidus with its surrounding thickened cortical bone (× 25). **B.** Photomicrograph of a field from the nidus (× 100). Note the highly vascular connective tissue stroma with giant cells and the irregular trabeculae of osteoid tissue and new bone. **C.** Photomicrograph of the nidus from another area showing calcification of osteoid tissue and trabeculae of nucleated atypical bone (× 100). This should not be confused with osteogenic sarcoma.

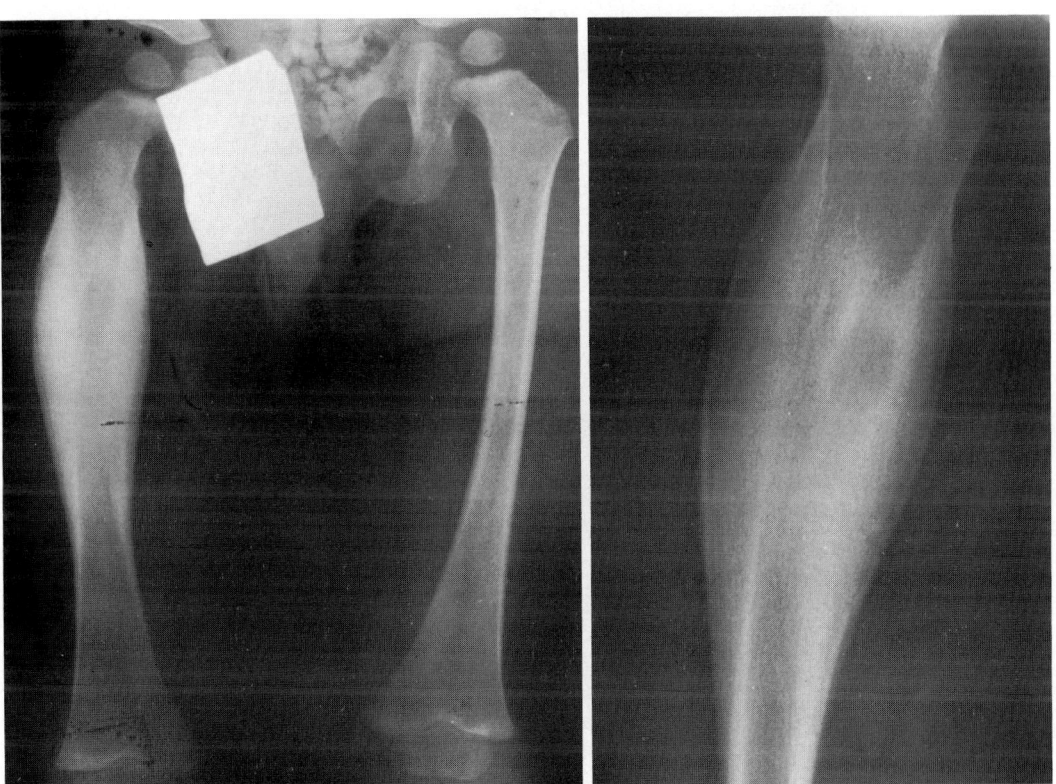

FIGURE 3-271. Osteoid osteoma of femur.

Radiograms showing the nidus and the marked reactive cortical thickening.

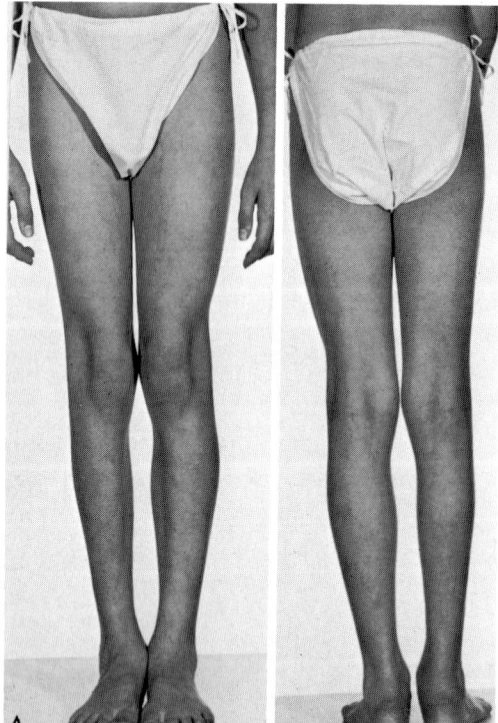

FIGURE 3–272. Osteoma of talus.

A 12-year-old girl presented with a right antalgic limp of one year's duration. **A.** Photographs of the patient show disuse atrophy of the right leg. **B** and **C.** Radiograms of ankle. Note the radiolucent lesion in the superomedial area of the talus. Clinically, there was excruciating local tenderness on palpation.

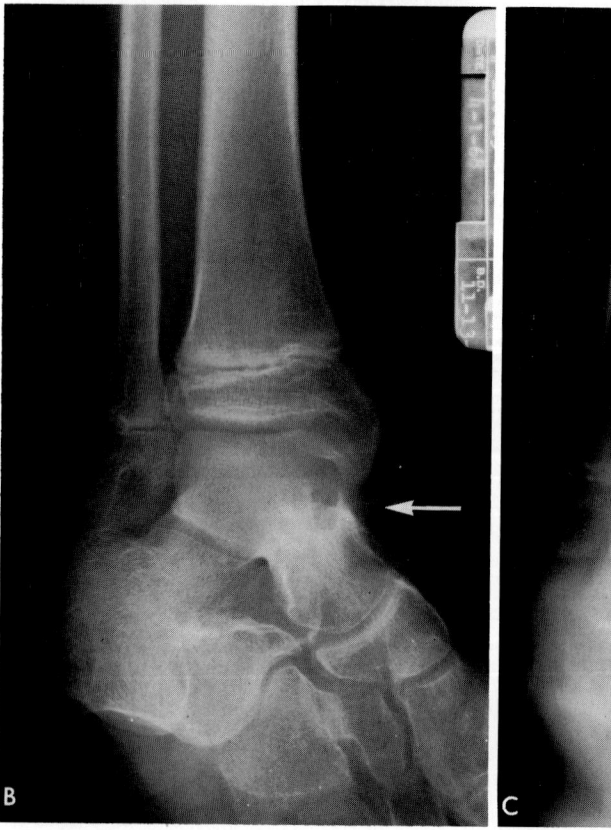
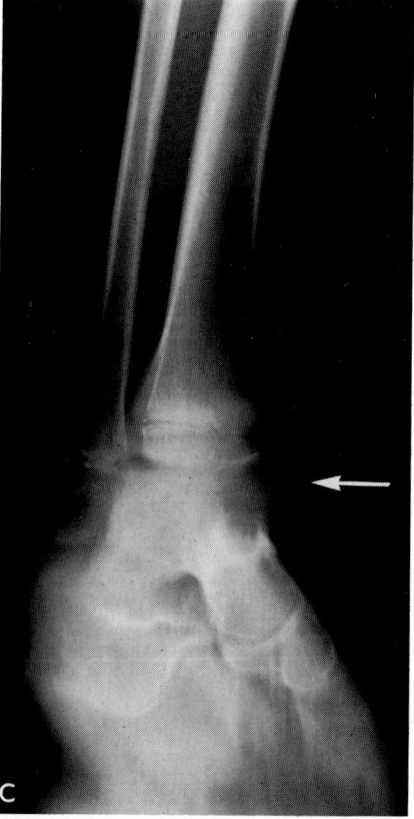

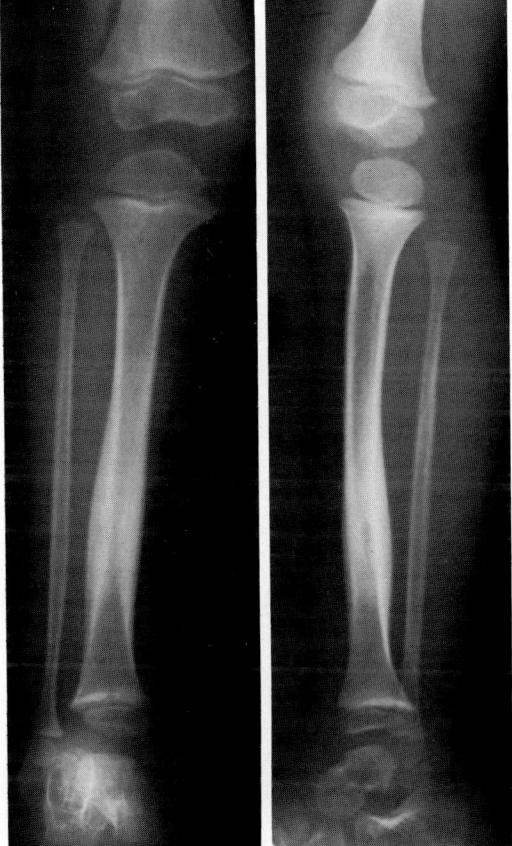

FIGURE 3–273. *Osteoid osteoma of the tibia.*

Radiograms show the extensive cortical hyperostosis, which is obscuring the intracortical nidus at the junction of the middle and distal third of the diaphysis.

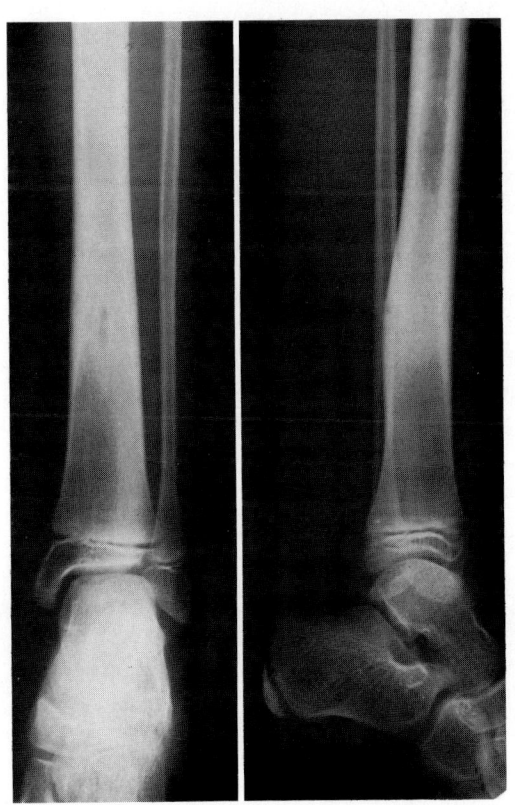

FIGURE 3–274. *Osteoid osteoma of the tibia.*

The reactive cortical thickening is not as marked as that shown in Figure 3–273, but the nidus is well seen.

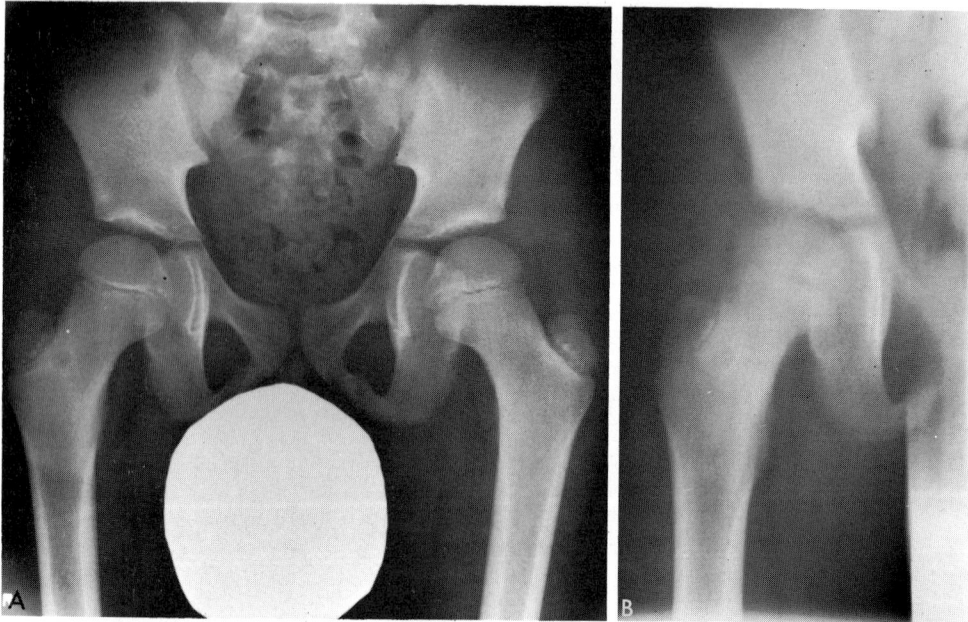

FIGURE 3–275. *Osteoid osteoma of intertrochanteric region of right femur.*

A. Radiogram and, **B,** laminagram showing the radiolucent nidus.

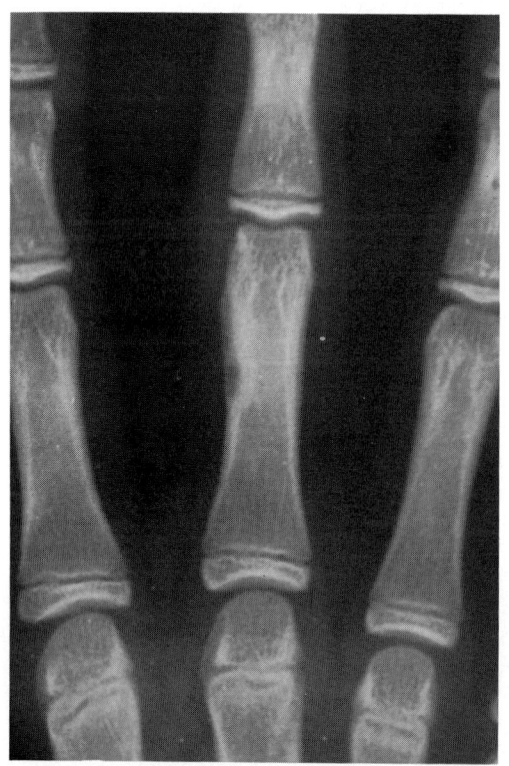

FIGURE 3–276. *Osteoid osteoma of the proximal phalanx of long finger.*

Note the radiolucent nidus in the cortex.

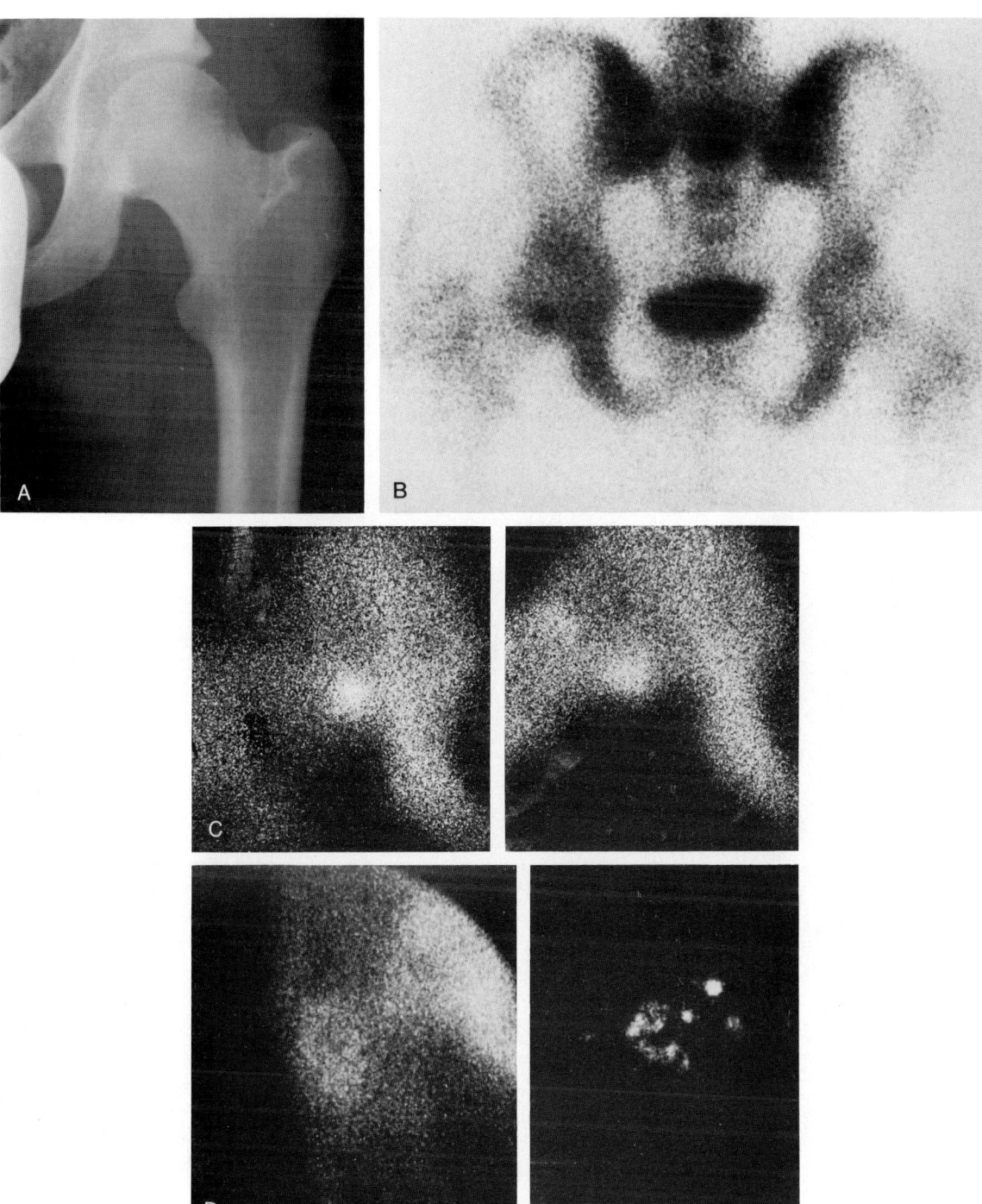

FIGURE 3–277. Osteoid osteoma of the femoral head in an 18-year-old boy.

A. Anteroposterior radiogram of the left hip. There is a suggestion of increased radiopacity of the inferior medial part of the femoral head. **B** and **C.** Scintigraphy with technetium-99m pinhole imaging showing increased local uptake. Note the slight increased radiopacity with a small zone of radiolucency in its periphery. These findings were not diagnostic. **D.** Localization of the nidus by intraoperative technetium-99m bone scanning. **E.** Scan of the excised nidus showing intense uptake.

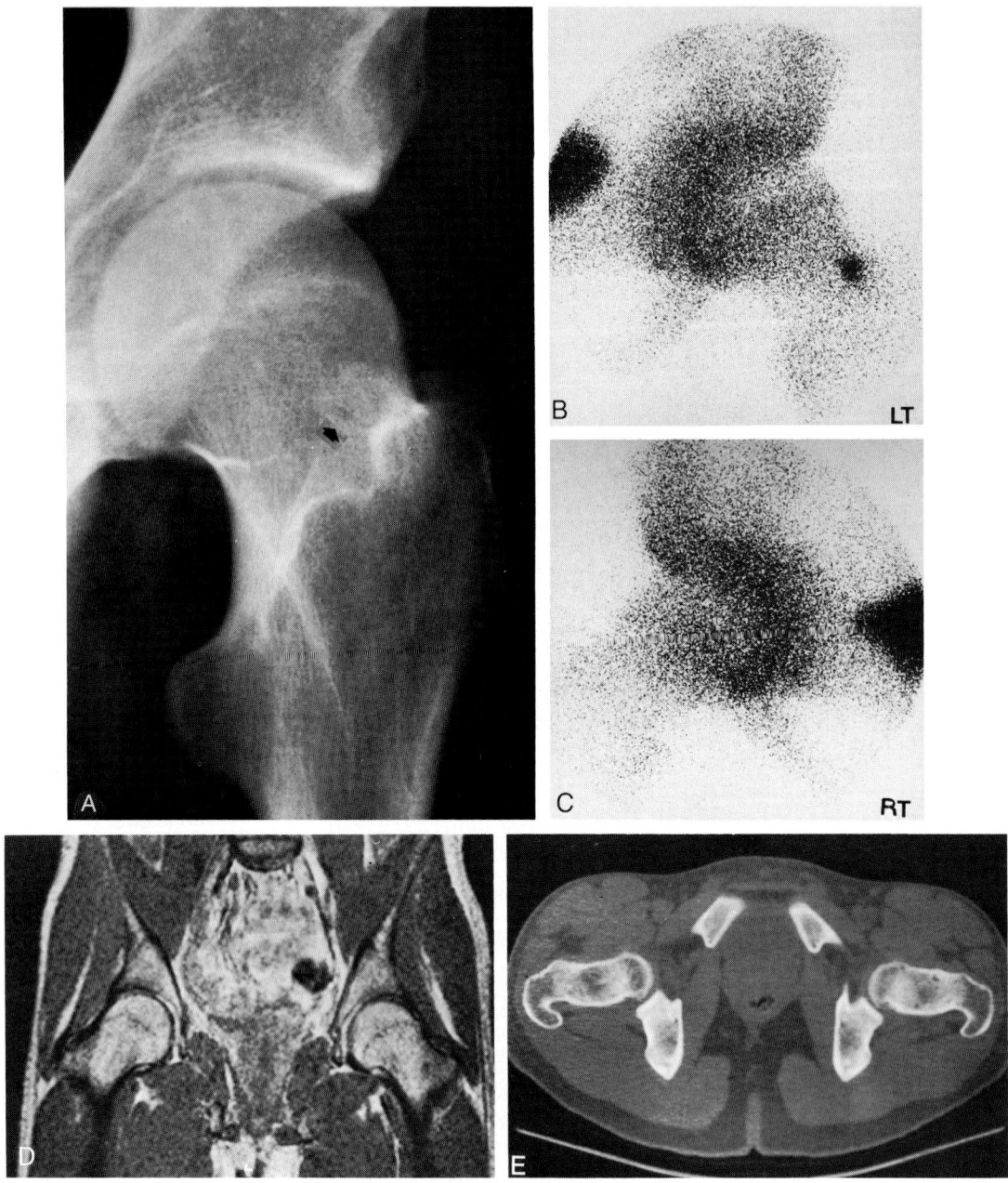

FIGURE 3-278. Osteoid osteoma of the femoral neck.

A. Anteroposterior radiogram of the left hip. Note the slight increased radiopacity with a small zone of radiolucency in its periphery. **B.** Technetium-99m scintigraphy shows increased local uptake superiorly at the base of the left femoral head. **C.** Scintigraphy showing the normal right hip. **D.** On magnetic resonance imaging, the site of the nidus is silent. **E.** CT scan of both hips showing the area of radiolucency in the left femoral neck.

out linear tomography. Magnetic resonance imaging may be obtained in selected cases.

In the differential diagnosis one should consider subacute osteomyelitis because a bone abscess is depicted on the radiogram in much the same way as the nidus of osteoid osteoma. A small bone abscess usually is round and has irregular channels extending into the sclerotic reactive bone, whereas the nidus of an osteoid osteoma is oval in configuration and does not have irregular extensions into the surrounding reactive bone. Clinically, the pain pattern of the two conditions is dissimilar, and local heat and swelling are more prominent in bone abscess. Local aspiration of the lesion (if superficial) done under image intensifier control or open biopsy will establish the diagnosis.

Solitary enostosis, commonly encountered in the neck of the femur, represents a mass of compacted trabeculae of mature lamellar bone; it should not be mistaken for osteoid osteoma, as it does not contain a nidus and is asymptomatic.

Osteoblastoma is much larger than the small nidus of osteoid osteoma.

Natural History

Osteoid osteoma is a self-limited lesion that tends to mature spontaneously in two to five years. The nidus gradually calcifies and ossifies, blending into the surrounding sclerotic bone. With maturation of the lesion the local pain gradually diminishes, the patient becoming symptom-free in several years. The usual trend is gradual conversion of a Stage 2 tumor into a Stage 1 latent process. Following ossification of the nidus the sclerosis of surrounding bone may persist indefinitely and continue to show increased activity on isotopic scanning.

Treatment

Salicylates are usually effective in providing relief of the symptoms. If the patient's disability is not marked, a period of observation with salicylate analgesia may be the preferred method of treatment. There is a possibility of spontaneous arrest after three to five years. If a nonoperative method of management is chosen, it will require two to three years of salicylate therapy. It should be explained to the patient and family, however, that it is impossible to forecast the natural history of the untreated lesion.

The painful lesion that causes muscle atrophy, limp, and functional disability is best treated surgically. The desire of the patient and his parents should be considered in making the decision. The surgical options are intracapsular curettage or marginal en bloc excision. The objective of surgery is to *excise the nidus*. Removal of the surrounding sclerotic bone is not necessary, as it will recede after removal of the nidus. The relief from pain is immediate, dramatic, and permanent. Recurrence of the pain is due to failure to excise the nidus completely.

En bloc excision ensures removal of the nidus, but it weakens the anatomic integrity of the part, causing a definite risk of pathologic fracture. In the neck of the femur this complication may be more disastrous than the disability of the original lesion. This author recommends restraint from wide marginal en bloc excision; it is best, if marginal excision is necessary, to remove only a limited margin of reactive bone about the nidus.

Incomplete excision will be followed by the prompt return of pain, requiring a second operation; therefore, it is crucial to localize the nidus at surgery in order to excise it totally with minimal removal of the surrounding reactive bone. The following technical details are recommended, particularly if the nidus is intracortical or surrounded by reactive sclerosis: First, preoperative computed tomography and, if indicated, conventional linear tomography are performed. Second, the use of intraoperative radioisotope scanning; prior to surgery, technetium-99m methylene diphosphonate is injected intravenously in a dose of 200 mCi./kg. (500 mEq./kg.) of body weight. This author recommends the use of a portable scanner with a gamma camera equipped with pinhole collimation. Before making the skin incision, the site of the lesion is determined by the scanner. The anatomic area is then exposed by the appropriate surgical approach. Next, conventional radiograms are made in several projections with a radiopaque marker to ensure that the correct anatomic site will be excised. A sterile needle containing one drop of the radioisotope is utilized to verify the site of most intense radioisotope uptake. Next, the nidus with minimal surrounding reactive bone is excised. With the portable scanner, anteroposterior, lateral, and oblique views of the lesion are obtained. The nidus will be visualized as a focal area of intense uptake surrounded by a zone of much less intense uptake (see Fig. 3–277 E). Rescanning will verify that the nidus is no longer present and the previously intense area of radioisotope uptake has disappeared. This technique confirms the complete removal of the nidus while the patient is still under anesthesia and the operative field is still open.

Following excision of the nidus, the size and location of the local defect may require autogenous cancellous-cortical bone grafting. In the femoral neck internal fixation by screw plate may be necessary to prevent pathologic fracture.

Irradiation and chemotherapy are ineffective; they should not be given.

In the vertebral column, the surgical approach for excision of the nidus presents special technical problems. The majority of osteoid osteomas of the spine are located in the pedicle at the base of the transverse process; there may be a varying degree of extension into the posterolateral aspect of the vertebral body or into the lamina.[86] It is only very occasionally that the nidus of an osteoid osteoma may be in the base of the spinous process or in the posterolateral part of the vertebral body.[179, 187] When there is no clinical or laboratory evidence of nerve root compression, exploration of the spinal canal is not indicated.

Kirwan and associates described a surgical approach to expose the pedicle without entering the spinal canal. Under general endotracheal anesthesia with the patient prone, a posterior midline incision is made at the appropriate level, and with a Cobb elevator the posterior vertebral elements are exposed in the usual fashion. On the side of the lesion, the tip of the transverse process is exposed by stripping the soft tissues subperiosteally as far laterally as possible. The anterior surface of the transverse process is exposed by detaching the soft tissues with an elevator. Hemostasis is obtained by electrothermy. Often the apophyseal facet joint will be swollen. Excise the transverse process—this gives direct access to the junction of the pedicle, lamina, and pars interarticularis (Fig. 3–279). With rongeurs and curets, the nidus is removed. Preservation of the apophyseal joint and pars interarticularis leaves the stability of the vertebral column undisturbed, and spinal fusion is not required.[86]

References

1. Ackerman, L. V.: Extra-osseous localized non-neoplastic bone and cartilage formation (so-called myositis ossificans). Clinical and pathological confusion with malignant neoplasms. J. Bone Joint Surg., 40-A:279, 1958.
2. Aegerter, E., and Kirkpatrick, J. A.: Orthopedic Diseases. 3rd Ed. Philadelphia, Saunders, 1968, p. 556.
3. Apple, D. F., Jr., and Loughlin, E. C., Jr.: Osteoid osteoma of the ankle in an athlete, Am. J. Sports Med., 9:254, 1981.
4. Barnes, R.: Osteoid osteoma. J. R. Coll. Surg., 2:144, 1956.
5. Beerman, P. J., Crowe, J. E., Sumner, T. E., and Roberts, J. E.: Case report 164. Osteoid osteoma of ossification center of tibia. Skeletal Radiol., 7:71, 1981.
6. Bleifield, C.: Osteoid osteoma; articular communication and minimal pain. N.Y. State J. Med., 81:1371, 1981.
7. Blery, M., and Le Roux, B.: Ostéome ostéoïde vertébral. A propos de six cas. Ann. Radiol., 21:59, 1978.
8. Bordelon, R. L., Cracco, A., and Book, M. K.: Osteoid-osteoma producing premature fusion of the epiphysis of the distal phalanx of the big toe. A case report. J. Bone Joint Surg., 57-A:120, 1975.
9. Braun, S., Chevrot, A., Tomeno, B., Delbarre, F., Pallardy, G., Mountounet, J., and Kulas-Durand, R.: A propos des ostéomes ostéoïdes phalangiens (13 cas personnels). Rev. Rhum., 46:225, 1979.
10. Bussiere, J. -L., Sauvezie, B., Lopitaux, R., Prin, P., Valentin, P., and Rampon, S.: Ostéome ostéoïde avec synovite d'allure rhumatoïde. Rev. Rhum., 43:651, 1976.
11. Byers, P. D.: Solitary benign osteoblastic lesions of bone: Osteoid osteoma and benign osteoblastoma. Cancer, 22:43, 1968.
12. Calandriello, B.: Sul granuloma osteoide. Arch. Putti, 7:263, 1965.
13. Caldicott, W. J. H.: Diagnosis of spinal osteoid osteoma. Radiology, 92:1192, 1969.
14. Cameron, B. M., and Friend, L. F.: Osteoid osteoma of sacrum: Report of a case. J. Bone Joint Surg., 36-A:876, 1954.
15. Carroll, R. E.: Osteoid osteoma in the hand. J. Bone Joint Surg., 35-A:888, 1953.
16. Chandler, F. A., and Kaell, I. I.: Osteoid-osteoma. Arch. Surg., 60:294, 1950.
17. Chaquat, Y., Kanovitch, B., Boscher, D., and Paquet,

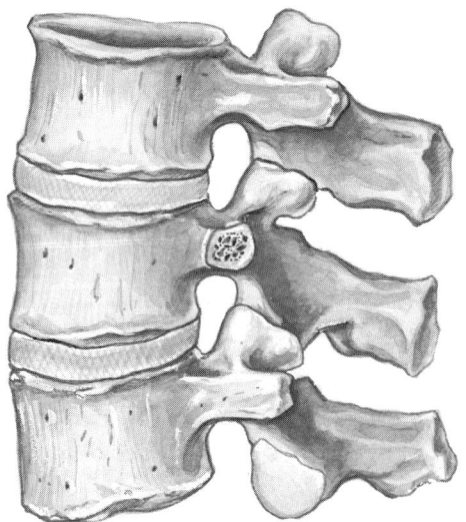

FIGURE 3–279. *Surgical approach for excision of osteoid osteoma of the spine with preservation of integrity of the facet joint.*

Excising the transverse process permits direct access to the junction of the pedicle, lamina, and pars interarticularis. (Redrawn after Kirwan, E. O'G., Hutton, P. A. N., Pozo, J. L., and Ransford, A. O.: Osteoid osteoma and benign osteoblastoma of the spine. J. Bone Joint Surg., 66-B:21, 1984.)

J.: L'ostéome ostéoïde. A propos de cinq observations. Rev. Rhum., *43*:297, 1976.
18. Clark, C. R., Ozonoff, M. B., and Drennan, J. C.: Case report 157. Osteoid osteoma of the femoral neck with localized synovitis. Skeletal Radiol., *6*:286, 1981.
19. Cohen, M. D., Harrington, T. M., and Ginsberg, W. W.: Osteoid osteoma: 95 cases and a review of the literature. Semin. Arthritis Rheum., *12*:265, 1983.
20. Coley, B. L., and Lenson, N.: Osteoid osteoma. Am. J. Surg., *77*:3, 1949.
21. Colton, C. L., and Hardy, J. G.: Evaluation of a sterilizable radiation probe as an aid to the surgical treatment of osteoid osteoma. Technical note. J. Bone Joint Surg., *65-A*:1019, 1983.
22. Corbett, J. M., Wilde, A. H., McCormack, L. J., and Evarts, C. M.: Intra-articular osteoid osteoma. A diagnostic problem. Clin. Orthop., *98*:225, 1974.
23. Cronemeyer, R. L., Kirchmer, N. A., De Smet, A. A., and Neff, J. R.: Intra-articular osteoid-osteoma of the humerus simulating synovitis of the elbow. A case report. J. Bone Joint Surg., *63-A*:1172, 1981.
24. Dahlin, D. C.: Bone Tumors: General Aspects and Data on 6,221 Cases. 3rd Ed. Springfield, Ill., Thomas, 1978, pp. 75–85.
25. Dahlin, D. C., and Johnson, E. W., Jr.: Giant osteoid osteoma. J. Bone Joint Surg., *36-A*:559, 1964.
26. Daly, J. G.: Case report. Osteoid osteoma of the skull. Br. J. Radiol., *46*:392, 1973.
27. Davison, W. R.: Osteoid osteoma: Report of atypical cases. Clin. Orthop., *7*:113, 1956.
28. Delrieu, F., Amor, B., Oradia, J. P., and Levy, P.: L'ostéome ostéoïde de l'astragale (2 cas). J. Radiol., *53*:437, 1972.
29. De Wet, I. S.: Osteoid osteomata. Review of the literature with a report of five cases. South Afr. J. Surg., *5*:13, 1967.
30. Didier, A.: Osteoma osteoide de cuello de femur. An. Cir., *14*:1, 1949.
31. Dockerty, M. B., Ghormley, R. K., and Jackson, A. E.: Osteoid osteoma, a clinicopathologic study of 20 cases. Ann. Surg., *133*:77, 1951.
32. Dreznik, I., Grunebaum, M., and Horodniceanu, C.: Radiographic aspects of osteoid osteoma in childhood and adolescence. Harefuah, *99*:349, 1980.
33. Dunlop, J. A. Y., Morton, K. S., and Elliott, G. B.: Recurrent osteoid osteoma. Report of a case with a review of the literature. J. Bone Joint Surg., *52-B*:128, 1970.
34. Edeiken, J., DePalma, A. F., and Hodes, P. J.: Osteoid osteoma (roentgenographic emphasis). Clin. Orthop., *49*:201, 1966.
35. Estersohn, H. S., and Day, J. C., Jr.: Osteoid osteoma: Benign osteoblastic lesion of bone. J. Am. Podiatry Assoc., *71*:568, 1981.
36. Fagerberg, S., and Rudstrom, P.: Osteoid osteoma of vertebral arch; case report. Acta Radiol., *40*:383, 1953.
37. Fehring, T. K., and Green, N. E.: Negative radionuclide scan in osteoid osteoma. A case report. Clin. Orthop., *185*:245, 1984.
38. Ferrer, J. M.: Osteoid osteoma of the vertebral column. Rev. Clin. Esp., *77*:10, 1960.
39. Flaherty, R. A., Pugh, D. G., and Dockerty, M. B.: Osteoid osteoma. A.J.R., *76*:1041, 1956.
40. Fontaine, R., Muller, J. N., Warter, P., Wuyts, J. L., and Juillier, B.: L'ostéome ostéoïde (à propos de 5 cas). J. Radiol. Electrol., *49*:118, 1968.
41. Foss, E. I., Dockerty, M. B., and Good, C. A.: Osteoid osteoma of mandible; report of case. Cancer, *8*:592, 1955.
42. Fountain, E. M., and Burge, C. H.: Osteoid osteoma of the cervical spine. A review and case report. J. Neurosurg., *18*:380, 1961.
43. Freiberger, R. H.: Osteoid osteoma of the spine. A cause of backache and scoliosis in children and young adults. Radiology, *75*:232, 1960.
44. Freiberger, R. H., Loitman, B. S., Helpern, M., and Thompson, T. C.: Osteoid osteoma. A report on 80 cases. A.J.R., *82*:194, 1959.
45. Gamba, J. L., Martinez, S., Apple, J., Harrelson, J. M., and Nunley, J. A.: Computed tomography of axial skeletal osteoid osteomas: A.J.R., *142*:769, 1984.
46. Garcia, G., Lance, J. F., and Lin, J. J.: Osteoid osteoma: An unusual presentation. Clin. Orthop., *156*:216, 1981.
47. Geshickter, C. F., and Copeland, M. M.: Tumors of Bone. 3rd Ed. Philadelphia, Lippincott, 1949, p. 366.
48. Ghelman, B., and Vigorita, V. J.: Postoperative radionuclide evaluation of osteoid osteomas. Radiology, *146*:509, 1983.
49. Ghelman, B., Thompson, F. M., and Arnold, W. D.: Intraoperative radioactive localization of an osteoid osteoma. J. Bone Joint Surg., *63-A*:826, 1981.
50. Gilday, D. L.: Diagnosis of obscure childhood osteoid osteomas with the bone scan (abstract). J. Nucl. Med., *15*:494, 1974.
51. Giustra, P. E., and Freiberger, R. H.: Severe growth disturbance with osteoid osteoma. A report of two cases involving the femoral neck. Radiology, *96*:285, 1970.
52. Glynn, J. J., and Lichtenstein, L.: Osteoid-osteoma with multicentric nidus. A report of two cases. J. Bone Joint Surg., *55-A*:855, 1973.
53. Goldberg, V. M., and Jacobs, B.: Osteoid osteoma of the hip in children. Clin. Orthop., *106*:41, 1975.
54. Golding, J. S. R.: The natural history of osteoid-osteoma; with a report of twenty cases. J. Bone Joint Surg., *36-B*:218, 1954.
55. Goldstein, G. S., Dawson, E. G., and Batzdorg, U.: Cervical osteoid osteoma: A cause of chronic upper back pain. Clin. Orthop., *129*:177, 1977.
56. Gore, D. R., and Mueller, H. A.: Osteoid-osteoma of the spine with localization aided by 99mTc-polyphosphate bone scan. A case report. Clin. Orthop., *113*:132, 1975.
57. Gould, N.: Articular osteoid osteoma of the talus: A case report. Foot Ankle, *1*:284, 1981.
58. Granieri, U., Maiuri, F., Colantuono, C., and Maiuri, L.: Vertebral osteoid osteoma, rare cause of nerve root compression and scoliosis in childhood. Riv. Neurol., *50*:278, 1980.
59. Habermann, E. T., and Stern, R. E.: Osteoid-osteoma of the tibia in an eight month old boy. A case report. J. Bone Joint Surg., *56-A*:633, 1974.
60. Halperin, N., Gadoth, N., Reif, R., and Axer, A.: Osteoid osteoma of the proximal femur simulating spinal root compression. Clin. Orthop., *162*:191, 1982.
61. Hamilton, J. F.: Osteoid osteoma. Surg. Gynecol. Obstet., *81*:465, 1945.
62. Haskel, L., Progrund, H., and Rosenmann, E.: Osteoid osteoma presenting as an osteocartilaginous exostosis. Isr. J. Med. Sci., *17*:380, 1981.
63. Heiman, M. L., Cooley, C. J., and Bradford, D. S.: Osteoid osteoma of a vertebral body. Report of a case with extension across the intervertebral disk. Clin. Orthop., *118*:159, 1976.
64. Helms, C. A., Hattner, R. S., and Vogler, J. B. III.: Osteoid osteoma: Radionuclide diagnosis. Radiology, *151*:779, 1984.
65. Hermann, R. M., and Blount, W. P.: Osteoid osteoma of the lumbar spine. J. Bone Joint Surg., *43-A*:568, 1961.
66. Herrlin, K., Ekelund, L., Lovdahl, R., and Persson, B.: Computed tomography in suspected osteoid osteomas of tubular bones. Skeletal Radiol., *9*:92, 1982.
67. Horwitz, T.: Osteoid osteoma of the astragalus. Radiology, *39*:226, 1942.
68. Huguenin, P., and Bensahel, H.: Reflexions à propos de l'ostéome ostéoïde chez l'enfant. Chir. Pediatr., *19*:83, 1978.
69. Jackson, A. E., Dockerty, M. B., and Ghormley, R.

K.: Osteoid osteoma: Clinical study of 20 cases. Proc. Staff Meet. Mayo Clin. 24:380, 1949.
70. Jackson, I. J.: Osteoid osteoma of the lamina and its treatment. Am. Surg., 19:17, 1953.
71. Jackson, R. P., Reckling, F. W., and Mantz, F. A.: Osteoid osteoma and osteoblastoma. Similar histologic lesions with different natural histories. Clin. Orthop., 128:303, 1977.
72. Jaffe, H. L.: Osteoid-osteoma: A benign osteoblastic tumor composed of osteoid and atypical bone. Arch. Surg., 31:709, 1935.
73. Jaffe, H. L.: Osteoid-osteoma of bone. Radiology, 45:319, 1945.
74. Jaffe, H. L.: Primary bone tumors. Chicago Med. Soc. Bull., 50:10, 1947.
75. Jaffe, H. L.: Osteoid-osteoma. Proc. R. Soc. Med., 46:1007, 1953.
76. Jaffe, H. L.: Tumors and Tumorous Conditions of the Bones. Philadelphia, Lea & Febiger, 1958, pp. 98–104.
77. Jaffe, H. L., and Lichtenstein, L.: Osteoid-osteoma: Further experience with its benign tumor of bone, with special reference to cases showing the lesion in relation to shaft cortices and commonly misclassified as instances of sclerosing non-suppurative osteomyelitis or cortical-bone abscess. J. Bone Joint Surg., 22:645, 1940.
78. Jaffe, H. L., and Mayer, L.: An osteoblastic osteoid tissue-forming tumor of metacarpal bone. Arch. Surg., 24:550, 1932.
79. Johnson, G. F.: Osteoid osteoma of femoral neck: Report of three cases. A.J.R., 74:65, 1955.
80. Karlsberg, P. C., and Kittelson, A. C.: Osteoid osteoma. Radiol. Clin. North Am., 2:337, 1964.
81. Kattapuram, S. V., Kushner, D. C., Phillips, W. C., and Rosenthal, D. I.: Osteoid osteoma: An unusual cause of articular pain. Radiology, 147:383, 1983.
82. Kehl, D. K., Alonso, J. E., and Lovell, W. W.: Scoliosis secondary to an osteoid-osteoma of the rib. A case report. J. Bone Joint Surg., 65-A:701, 1983.
83. Keim, H. A., and Reina, E. G.: Osteoid-osteoma as a cause of scoliosis. J. Bone Joint Surg., 57-A:159, 1975.
84. Kendrick, J. I., and Evarts, C. M.: Osteoid-osteoma. A critical analysis of 40 tumors. Clin. Orthop., 54:51, 1967.
85. Kenzora, J. E., and Abrams, R. C.: Problems encountered in the diagnosis and treatment of osteoid osteoma of the talus. Foot Ankle, 2:172, 1981.
86. Kirwan, E. O'G., Hutton, P. A. N., Pozo, J. L., and Ransford, A. O.: Osteoid osteoma and benign osteoblastoma of the spine. Clinical presentation and treatment. J. Bone Joint Surg., 66-B:21, 1984.
87. Klein, M. J., Lusskin, R., Becker, M. H., and Antopol, S. C.: Osteoid osteoma of the clavicle. Clin. Orthop., 143:162, 1979.
88. Kleinberg, S.: Osteoid osteoma of femur: Report of a case. Am. J. Surg., 53:168, 1941.
89. Kleinberg, S.: Osteoid-osteoma: Report of five cases. N.Y. State J. Med., 43:332, 1943.
90. Kleinberg, S.: Osteoid osteoma. Am. J. Surg., 66:396, 1944.
91. Knotsson, F.: Roentgenographic appearance of osteoid osteoma in children. Acta Radiol., 45:125, 1956.
92. Kozlowski, K.: Osteoid osteoma (some diagnostic problems). Radiol. Diagn. (Berl.), 23:317, 1982.
93. Kruger, G. D., and Rock, M. G.: Osteoid osteoma of the distal femoral epiphysis. A case report. Clin. Orthop., 222:203, 1987.
94. Lapidus, P. W., and Salem, E. P.: Osteoid osteoma. Report of a case with probable double lesion. Arch. Surg., 58:318, 1949.
95. Lapidus, P. W., and Wilson, M. J.: Osteoid osteoma: Report of three cases. Bull. New York Med. Coll., 10:37, 1947.
96. Lawrie, T. R., Aterman, K., Path, F. C., and Sinclair, A. M.: Painless osteoid osteoma, a report of two cases. J. Bone Joint Surg., 52-A:1357, 1970.
97. Lejeune, E., Dejour, H., Bouvier, M., Llorca, G., and Andre-Fouet, A.: L'ostéome ostéoïde du pied. A propos de quatre observations. Rev. Rhum., 46:711, 1979.
98. Leroy, V., Couturaud, M., Lathelize, H., Valette, C., Beck, C., Dunoyer, J., Treves, R., and Desproges-Gotteron, R.: La scintigraphie osséuse est-elle si fiable dans la recherche de l'ostéome ostéoïde? Rev. Rhum., 47:53, 1980.
99. Levine, E., and Neff, J. R.: Dynamic computed tomography scanning of benign bone lesions: Preliminary results. Skeletal Radiol., 9:238, 1983.
100. Levi-Valensin, G., Bernageau, J., Guerin, C., and Bard, M.: Ostéome ostéoïde. Problèmes actuels. J. Radiol. Electrol., 57:640, 1976.
101. Levy, J. M., Hubbard, J. O., and Crowe, J. K.: Computed tomography—guided removal of an osteoid osteoma: A case report. Cardiovasc. Intervent. Radiol., 5:14, 1982.
102. Levy, Y., Rosenheck, S., Torok, G., and Torok, G.: Osteoid osteoma of the distal phalanx of the thumb. Acta Orthop. Scand., 50:667, 1979.
103. Lewis, R. W.: Osteoid osteoma. A review of portions of the literature and presentation of cases. A.J.R., 52:70, 1944.
104. Lichtenstein, L.: Benign osteoblastoma. A category of osteoid- and bone-forming tumors other than classical osteoid osteoma, which may be mistaken for giant-cell tumor or osteogenic sarcoma. Cancer, 9:1044, 1956.
105. Lichtenstein, L.: Bone Tumors. 5th Ed. St. Louis, Mosby, 1977, pp. 78–91.
106. Lindbom, A., Lindvall, N., Soderberg, G., and Spjut, H.: Angiography in osteoid osteoma. Acta Radiol., 54:327, 1960.
107. Lisbona, R., and Rosenthall, L.: Role of radionuclide imaging in osteoid osteoma. A.J.R., 132:77, 1979.
108. Lofgren, L.: Osteoid osteoma. Acta Chir. Scand., 104:383, 1953.
109. Logroscino, D.: L'osteome osteide. Arch. Putti, 4:275, 1954.
110. Lundeen, M. A., and Herring, J. A.: Osteoid-osteoma of the spine: Sclerosis in two levels. A case report. J. Bone Joint Surg., 62-A:476, 1980.
111. MacLellan, D. I., and Wilson, F. C.: Osteoid osteoma of the spine. J. Bone Joint Surg., 49-A:111, 1967.
112. McCombs, R. K., and Olson, W. H.: Positive 18F bone scan in a case of osteoid osteoma. J. Nucl. Med., 16:465, 1975.
113. McGuire, M. H., and Mankin, H. J.: Osteoid osteoma: An unusual presentation as a rib lesion. A case report. Orthopedics, 7:305, 1984.
114. McKeever, F. M.: Osteoid osteoma. West. J. Surg., 58:213, 1950.
115. Mallens, W. M., Pauwells, E. K., and Tetteroo, Q. F.: Bone scintigraphy as a guide to the diagnosis of osteoid osteoma. Radiol. Clin. (Basel), 46:300, 1977.
116. Marcove, R. C., and Freiberger, R. H.: Osteoid osteoma of the elbow—a diagnostic problem. J. Bone Joint Surg., 48-A:1185, 1966.
117. Mau, H.: Osteoid osteoma of the vertebral column. Z. Orthop., 120:761, 1982.
118. Mayer, L.: The surgery of osteoid osteoma. Bull. Hosp. Joint Dis., 12:174, 1951.
119. Meissner, P. J., Jr., and Mauro, G.: Osteoid osteoma: A literature review and case report. J. Foot Surg., 20:25, 1981.
120. Mitnick, J. S., Braunstein, P., and Genieser, N. B.: Osteoid osteoma of the hip: Unusual isotopic appearance. A.J.R., 133:322, 1979.
121. Moberg, E.: The natural course of osteoid osteoma. J. Bone Joint Surg., 33-A:166, 1951.
122. Moberg, E.: Further observations on "corticalisos-

teoide" or "osteoid osteoma." Acta Radiol. (Stockh.), 38:279, 1952.
123. Morrison, G. M., Hawes, L. E., and Sacco, J. J.: Incomplete removal of osteoid osteoma. Am. J. Surg., 80:476, 1950.
124. Morton, K. S., and Bartlett, L. H.: Benign osteoblastic change resembling osteoid osteoma. J. Bone Joint Surg., 48-B:478, 1966.
125. Morton, K. S., Vassar, P. S., and Knickerbocker, W. J.: Osteoid osteoma and osteoblastoma: Reclassification of 43 cases using Schajowicz's classification. Can. J. Surg., 18:148, 1975.
126. Munk, J., Peyser, E., and Gellei, B.: Osteoid osteoma of the frontal bone. Br. J. Radiol., 33:328, 1960.
127. Mustard, W. T., and DuVal, F. W.: Osteoid osteoma of vertebrae. J. Bone Joint Surg., 41-B:132, 1959.
128. Nelson, O. A., and Greer, R. B.: Localization of osteoid osteoma of the spine using computerized tomography. A case report. J. Bone Joint Surg., 65-A:263, 1983.
129. Nikitin, M. N., and Ermolaev, I. U. F.: Osteoid osteoma of the pedicle of the third cervical vertebral arch. Ortop. Travmatol. Protez., 7:60, 1983.
130. Norman, A., and Dorfman, H. D.: Osteoid-osteoma inducing pronounced overgrowth and deformity of bone. Clin. Orthop., 110:233, 1975.
131. O'Brien, T. M., Murray, T. E., Malone, L. A., Dervan, P., Walsh, M., McManus, F., and Ennis, J. T.: Osteoid osteoma: Excision with scintimetric guidance. Radiology, 153:543, 1984.
132. O'Hara, J. P., Tegtmeyer, C., Sweet, D. E., and McCue, F. C.: Angiography in the diagnosis of osteoid-osteoma of the hand. J. Bone Joint Surg., 57-A:165, 1975.
133. Omojola, M. F., Cockshott, W. P., and Beatty, E. G.: Osteoid osteoma: An evaluation of diagnostic modalities. Clin. Radiol., 32:199, 1981.
134. Orlowski, J. P., and Mercer, R. D.: Osteoid osteoma in young children and adults. Pediatrics, 59:526, 1977.
135. Ottolenghi, C.: Osteoma osteoide del calcáneo. Bol. Trab. Acad. Argentina Cir., 24:533, 1940.
136. Papanicolaou, N., and Treves, S.: Bone scintigraphy in the preoperative evaluation of osteoid osteoma and osteoblastoma of the spine. Ann. Radiol., 27:104, 1984.
137. Papassotiriou, V., Weyrauch, U., and Heinze, D.: Osteoid osteoma of the spine: A cause of scoliosis and hip and lumbar spine stiffness in childhood. R.O.F.O., 135:238, 1981.
138. Paus, B. C., and Kim, T. K.: Osteoid osteoma of the spine. Acta Orthop. Scand., 33:24, 1963.
139. Phelan, J. T.: Osteoid osteoma. Surgery, 121:112, 1965.
140. Phelip, X., Mouries, D., Blanc, D., Delpy, B., and Cabanel, G.: Les manifestations articulaires de l'ostéome ostéoïde. Rhumatologie, 30:219, 1978.
141. Pieterse, A. S., Vernon-Roberts, B., Paterson, D. C., Cornish, B. L., and Lewis, P. R.: Osteoid osteoma transforming to aggressive (low grade malignant) osteoblastoma: A case report and literature review. Histopathology, 7:799, 1983.
142. Pines, B., Lavine, L., and Grayzel, D.: Osteoid osteoma. J. Int. Coll. Surg., 13:249, 1950.
143. Ponseti, I., and Barta, C. K.: Osteoid osteoma. J. Bone Joint Surg., 29:767, 1947.
144. Posternikova, T. T., and Frolov, V. K.: Osteoid osteoma of the proximal portion of the femur in children. Ortop. Travmatol. Protez., 4:57, 1981.
145. Prabhakar, B., Raja Reddy, D. R., Dayananda, B., and Raghava Rao, G. R.: Osteoid osteoma of the skull. J. Bone Joint Surg., 54-B:146, 1972.
146. Pritchard, J. E., and McKay, J. W.: Osteoid osteoma. Can. Med. Assoc. J., 58:567, 1948.
147. Purcell, H. M., Mills, S. D., and Lipscomb, P. R.: Osteoid osteoma. Pediatrics, 9:295, 1952.

148. Rand, J. A., Sim, F. H., and Unni, K. K.: Two osteoid-osteomas in one patient. A case report. J. Bone Joint Surg., 64-A:1243, 1978.
149. Ransford, A. O., Pozo, J. L., Hutton, P. A. N., and Kirwan, E. O. G.: The behavior pattern of the scoliosis associated with osteoid osteoma or osteoblastoma of the spine. J. Bone Joint Surg., 66-B:16, 1984.
150. Reed, R. J.: Fibrous dysplasia of bone. Arch. Pathol., 75:480, 1963.
151. Rinsky, L. A., Goris, M., Bleck, E. E., Halpern, A., and Hirshman, P.: Intraoperative skeletal scintigraphy for localization of osteoid-osteoma in the spine. Case report. J. Bone Joint Surg., 62-A:143, 1980.
152. Rivero, S., and Catolla Cavalcanti, G. F.: Varieta articolare del granuloma osteoide di Jaffe. Minerva Ortop., 17:32, 1966.
153. Rivero, S., and Catolla Cavalcanti, G. F.: Osteoma osteoide e coxalgia sintomatica nell'eta infanto-giovanile. Considerazioni su 4 casi. Minerva Ortop., 28:1, 1977.
154. Rosborough, D.: Osteoid osteoma. Report of a lesion in the terminal phalanx of a finger. J. Bone Joint Surg., 48-B:485, 1966.
155. Rushton, M. A.: Osteoid-osteoma of mandibular alveolus. Oral Surg., 4:86, 1951.
156. Rushton, J. G., Mulder, D. W., and Lipscomb, P. R.: Neurologic symptoms with osteoid osteoma. Neurology, 5:794, 1955.
157. Sabanas, A. O., Bickel, W. H., and Moe, J. H.: Natural history of osteoid osteoma of the spine. Am. J. Surg., 91:880, 1956.
158. Sacks, S.: Osteoid osteoma. Report of a case with pain in the arm for ten years. South Afr. Med. J., 28:766, 1954.
159. Samoilova, L. I., Beliaeva, A. A., and Posternikova, T. T.: Painless osteoid osteoma. Ortop. Travmatol. Protez., 5:47, 1981.
160. Sankaron, B.: Osteoid osteoma. Surg. Gynecol. Obstet., 99:193, 1954.
161. Savitz, M. H., Rothschild, E. J., Chang, T., Worcester, D., and Peck, H. M.: Primary vertebral tumor in an adolescent girl. Mt. Sinai J. Med. (N.Y.), 48:84, 1981.
162. Scaglietti, O., and Calandriello, B.: Sulla varieta articolare del "granuloma osteoide." Arch. Putti, 12:9, 1959.
163. Schajowicz, F., and Lemos, C.: Osteoid osteoma and osteoblastoma. Closely related entities of osteoblastic derivation. Acta Orthop. Scand., 41:272, 1970.
164. Schulman, L., and Dorfman, H. D.: Nerve fibers in osteoid osteoma. J. Bone Joint Surg., 52-A:1351, 1970.
165. Seitz, W. H., Jr., and Dick, H. M.: Intraepiphyseal osteoid osteoma of the distal femur in an 8-year-old girl. J. Pediatr. Orthop., 3:505, 1983.
166. Seruzier, E., Simonin, J. -L., Ducastelle, C., Hemet, J., Biga, N., Thomine, J. -M., and Deshayes, P.: Ostéome ostéoïde avec synovite. A propos de deux observations. Rev. Rhum., 43:521, 1976.
167. Sevitt, S., and Horn, J. S.: A painless and calcified osteoid osteoma of the little finger. J. Pathol. Bacteriol., 67:571, 1954.
168. Seze, de S., Debeyre, J., Ordonneau, P., Djian, A., and Mazabraud, A.: L'ostéome ostéoïde à propos de 6 observations personnelles. Rev. Rhum., 22:191, 1955.
169. Shereff, M. J., Cullivan, W. T., and Johnson, K. A.: Osteoid osteoma of the foot. J. Bone Joint Surg., 65-A:638, 1983.
170. Sherman, M. S.: Osteoid osteoma associated with changes in adjacent joint. Report of two cases. J. Bone Joint Surg., 29:483, 1947.
171. Sherman, M. S.: Osteoid osteoma. Review of the literature and report of thirty cases. J. Bone Joint Surg., 29:918, 1947.
172. Sherman, M. S., and McFarland, G., Jr.: Mechanism

of pain in osteoid osteoma. South. Med. J., 58:163, 1965.
173. Sim, F. H., Dahlin, D. C., and Beabout, J. W.: Osteoid-osteoma: Diagnostic problems. J. Bone Joint Surg., 57-A:154, 1975.
174. Simons, G. W., and Sty, J.: Intraoperative bone imaging in the treatment of osteoid osteoma of the femoral neck. J. Pediatr. Orthop., 3:399, 1983.
175. Smith, F. W., and Gilday, D. L.: Scintigraphic appearances of osteoid osteoma. Radiology, 137:191, 1980.
176. Snarr, J. W., Abell, M. R., and Martel, W.: Lymphofollicular synovitis with osteoid osteoma. Radiology, 106:557, 1973.
177. Sorensen, S., and Mathiasen, M. S.: Osteoid osteoma. Ugeskr. Laeger., 143:3395, 1981.
178. Spence, A. J., and Lloyd Roberts, G. C.: Regional osteoporosis in osteoid osteoma. J. Bone Joint Surg., 43-B:501, 1961.
179. Spjut, H. J., Dorfman, H. D., Fechner, R. E., and Ackerman, L. V.: Atlas of Tumours of Bone and Cartilage. Washington, D.C., Armed Forces Institute of Pathology, 1970, pp. 120–140.
180. Stojanovic, J., Papa, J., and Cicin-Sain, T. B.: Computer tomography and angiographic pictures of an osteoid osteoma of the spine. R.O.F.O., 137:226, 1982.
181. Strach, E. H.: Osteoid osteoma. Br. Med. J., 1:1031, 1953.
182. Swee, R. G., McLeod, R. A., and Beabout, J. W.: Osteoid osteoma: Detection, diagnosis, and localization. Radiology, 130:117, 1979.
183. Symeonides, P. P.: Osteoid osteoma of the lumbar spine. South. Med. J., 63:975, 1970.
184. Tavernier, L., Guilleminet, M., and Faysse, R.: Sur une forme speciale d'ostéome-ostéoïde à point de depart cortical et à evolution para-osséuse: L'ostéome-ostéoïde à forme exostosante. Lyon Chir., 45:133, 1950.
185. Vauzelle, J. L., and Caille, J. P.: Paraosseous osteoid osteoma. Anatomo-pathological study of a case. Arch. Anat. Cytol. Pathol., 30:307, 1982.
186. Vickers, C. W., Pugh, C. D., and Ivins, J. C.: Osteoid osteoma. A fifteen-year follow-up of an untreated patient. J. Bone Joint Surg., 41-A:357, 1959.
187. Walker, J. W.: Experiences with benign bone tumours in paediatric practice. Radiology, 58:662, 1952.
188. Wallace, G. T.: Some surgical aspects of osteoid osteoma. J. Bone Joint Surg., 29:777, 1947.
189. Wedge, J. H., Chang, S., and MacFadyen, D. J.: Computed tomography in localization of spinal osteoid osteoma. Spine, 6:423, 1981.
190. William, H., Simon, M. D., and Bellier, M. L.: Intracapsular epiphyseal osteoid osteoma of the ankle joint. A case report. Clin. Orthop., 108:200, 1975.
191. Winter, P. F., Johnson, P. M., Hilal, S. K., and Feklldman, F.: Scintigraphic detection of osteoid osteoma. Radiology, 122:177, 1977.
192. Worland, R. L., Ryder, C. T., and Johnston, A. D.: Recurrent osteoid-osteoma. Report of a case. J. Bone Joint Surg., 57-A:277, 1975.

BENIGN OSTEOBLASTOMA

This rather rare osteoblastic bone lesion is benign; it may, however, be locally aggressive in its biologic performance. It is characterized histologically by an abundant number of osteoblasts and by the presence of a large amount of osteoid tissue in a highly vascular matrix. The name *benign osteoblastoma* was given by Lichtenstein and Jaffe.[48, 60] Prior to that, terms used to denote the condition were *giant osteoid osteoma* and *osteogenic fibroma of bone*.[26, 40, 55]

Age and Sex Predilection

The lesion is frequently encountered in children and adolescents, with 70 per cent of the cases occurring in the first two decades of life. The peak age incidence is between 10 and 20 years of age. There is a significant sex prevalence in the male, with a male to female ratio of 2:1.

Location

The neural arches of the vertebral column are a very common site of involvement. The short tubular bones of the feet and hands, the long tubular bones of a limb (particularly the femur and tibia), and the calvarium are other frequent locations. It occasionally may occur in a rib, scapula, innominate bone, or patella. Lichtenstein and Sawyer, in their series of 31 cases, report that the large limb bones and the vertebral column account for 60 per cent; the calvarium for 20 per cent; and the bones of the hands and feet for about 18 per cent.[62]

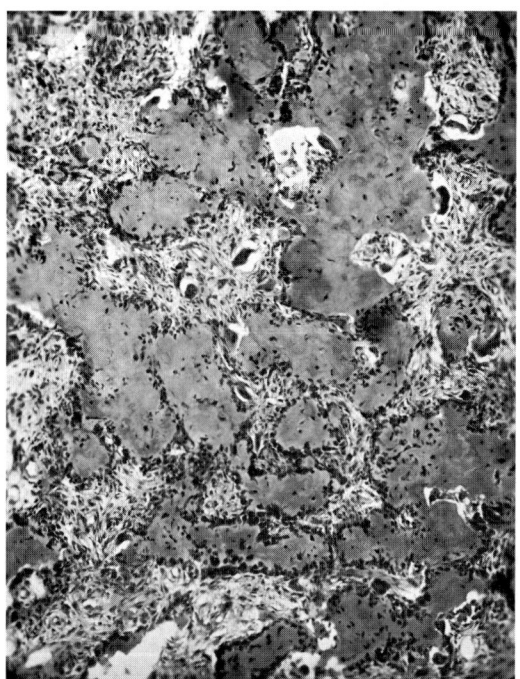

FIGURE 3–280. *Benign osteoblastoma.*

Histologic findings as shown in photomicrograph ($\times$ 100). Note the highly vascularized connective tissue matrix and the trabeculae of osteoid and new bone with layers of osteoblasts lined against them.

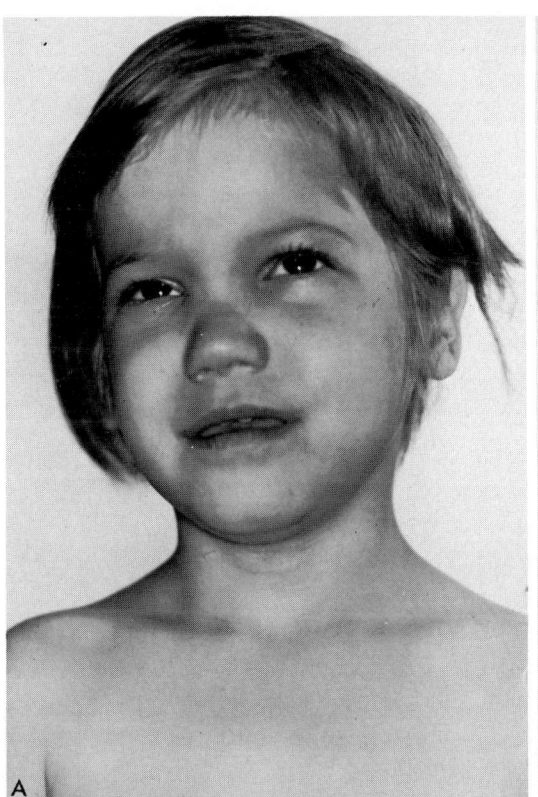
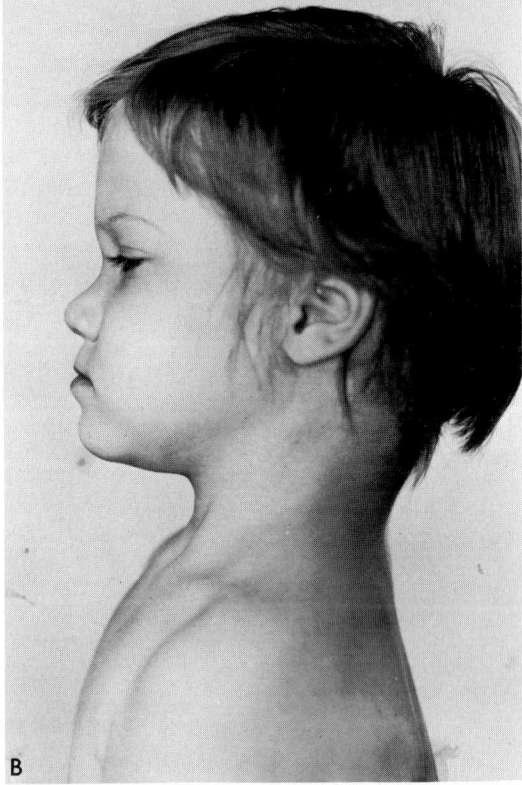
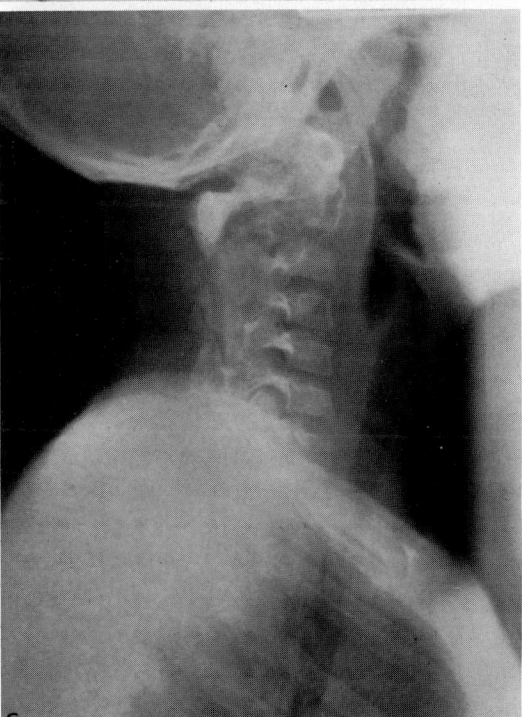

FIGURE 3–281. *Benign osteoblastoma of cervical spine in a six-year-old girl.*

A and **B.** Clinical appearance. Patient presented with a painful torticollis and tender swelling in left upper neck. **C.** Lateral radiogram of cervical spine showing the mottled radiolucency of the expanded vertebral bodies of the second and part of the third cervical vertebrae. The posterior processes are also involved. The lesion was surgically excised and bone grafted to fuse the vertebrae from C1 to C4.

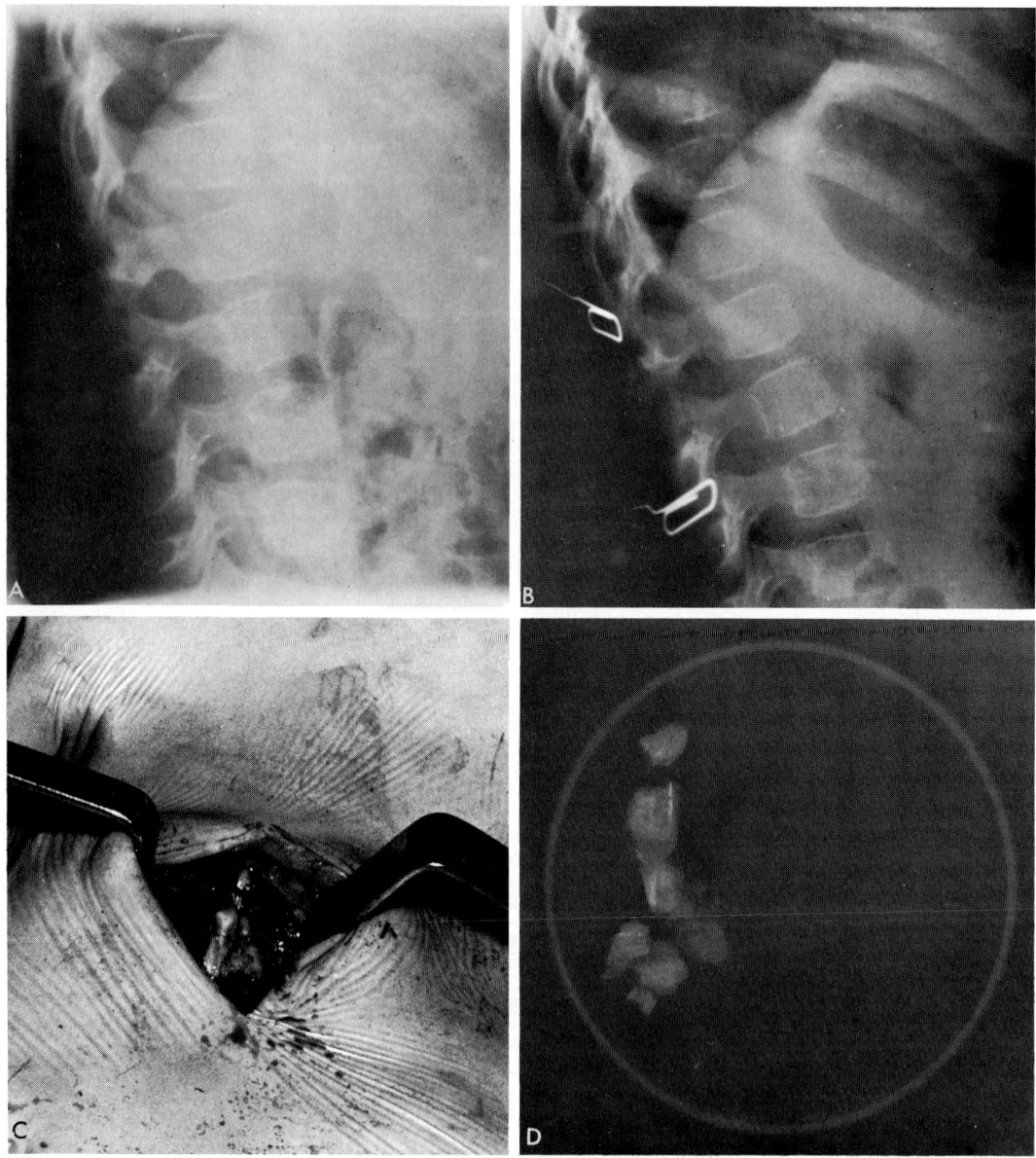

FIGURE 3–282. *Benign osteoblastoma of spinous process and laminae of first lumbar vertebra in a four-year-old girl.*

The patient complained of acute back pain of two months' duration. **A** and **B.** Lateral radiograms of upper lumbar spine showing mottled rarefaction of the spinous process and lamina of first lumbar vertebra. **C.** Gross appearance at operation. The affected spinous process is dark in color. **D.** Radiograms of excised lesional tissue.

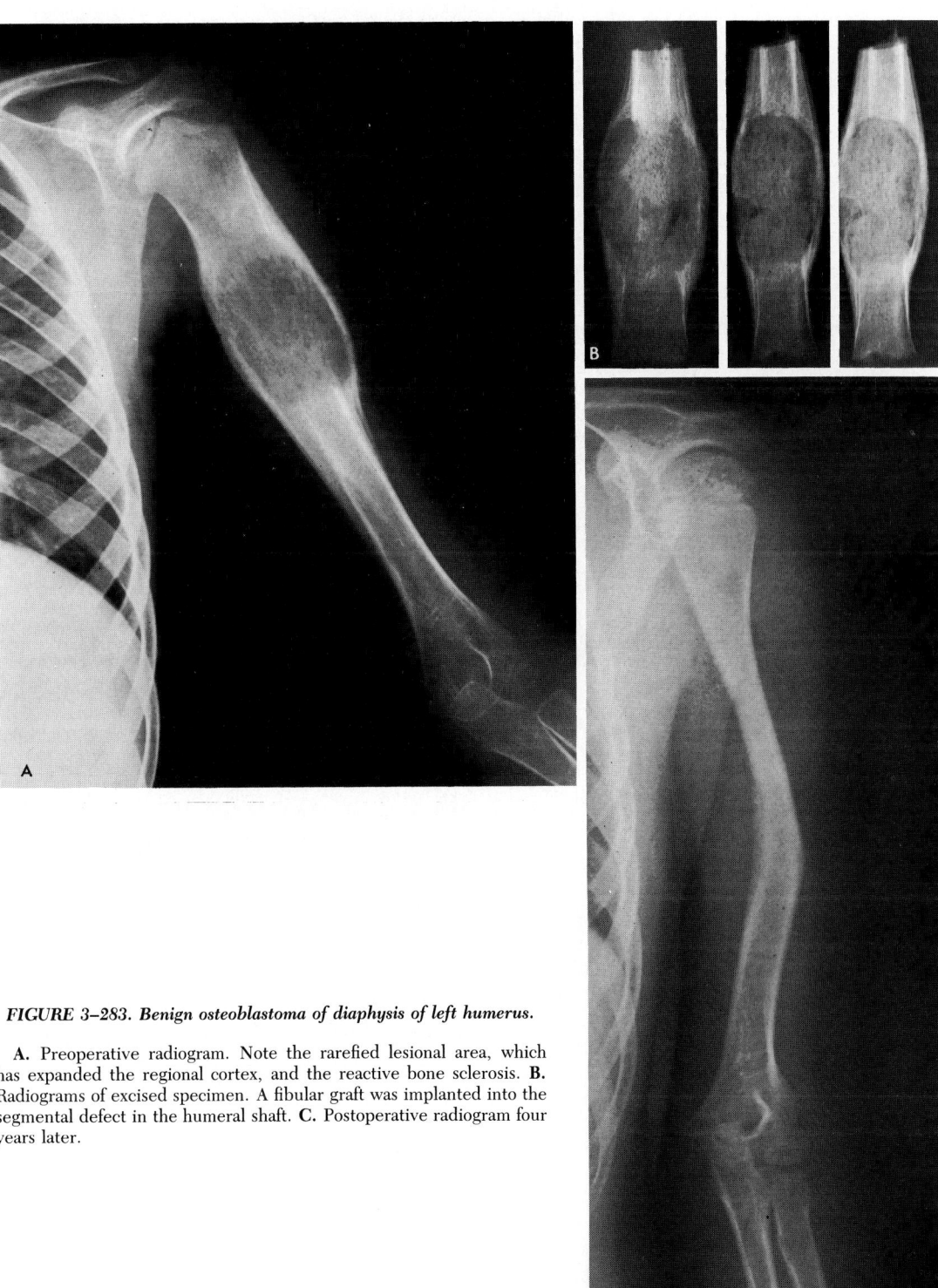

FIGURE 3–283. Benign osteoblastoma of diaphysis of left humerus.

A. Preoperative radiogram. Note the rarefied lesional area, which has expanded the regional cortex, and the reactive bone sclerosis. **B.** Radiograms of excised specimen. A fibular graft was implanted into the segmental defect in the humeral shaft. **C.** Postoperative radiogram four years later.

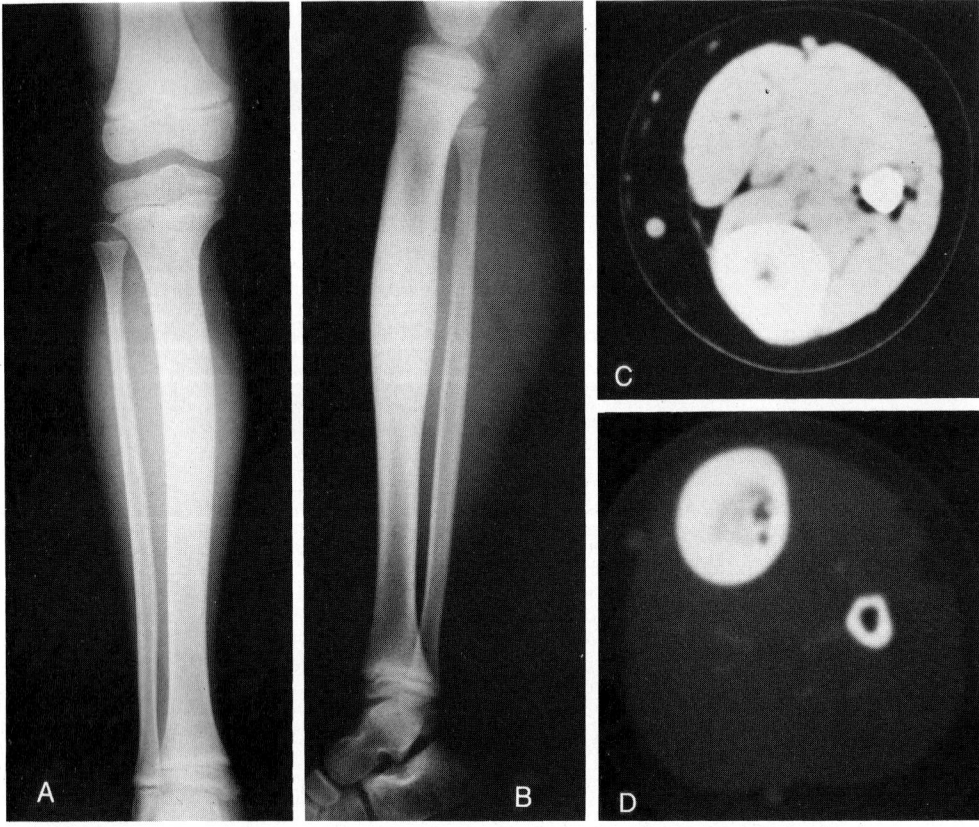

FIGURE 3–281. Benign osteoblastoma of the tibial diaphysis in an eight year old treated by segmental resection.

A and B. Initial anteroposterior and lateral radiographs of the tibia. Note the increased radiopacity of reactive bone obscuring the area of radiolucency. C and D. CT scan showing the periosteal and endosteal new bone formation and the area of radiolucency.

Pathology

Benign osteoblastoma is a larger tumor than osteoid osteoma and may measure up to 10 cm. at its greatest diameter. It destroys and expands the affected bone; it is, however, delimited by thickened periosteal connective tissue or by a shell of cortical new bone, suggesting the benign nature of the lesion. It may, on occasion, perforate the cortex and produce a soft-tissue tumor mass.

On gross pathologic examination, the lesional tissue has a more or less gritty consistency and is reddish in color. It is a vascular tumor that bleeds easily, consequently causing difficulty with hemostasis at the time of operation.

The microscopic picture varies, depending on the maturity of the lesion. The characteristic finding is the excessive abundance of osteoblasts, which may be found in focal nodular or solid aggregates or lined up in layers against the surface of an osteoid or bone spicule. Dense sheets of osteoid tissue and irregular calcified new bone may be seen. As a rule, the connective tissue stroma is very vascular (Fig. 3–280).

Clinical Findings

Local pain is the major complaint, but in contrast to osteoid osteoma, it is more of a dull ache and not severe, does not awaken the patient at night, and does not respond to salicylates. If the affected bone is one that is readily palpable, like the tibia or metacarpal, a local swelling may be detected. Lesions in the neural arch of the spinal column may extend into the intraspinal canal, compress the spinal nerves or the cord, and cause neurologic signs. Benign osteoblastoma should always be considered in the differential diagnosis when an adolescent or a child is presented with backache, sciatica or brachalgia, or acquired paraplegia.

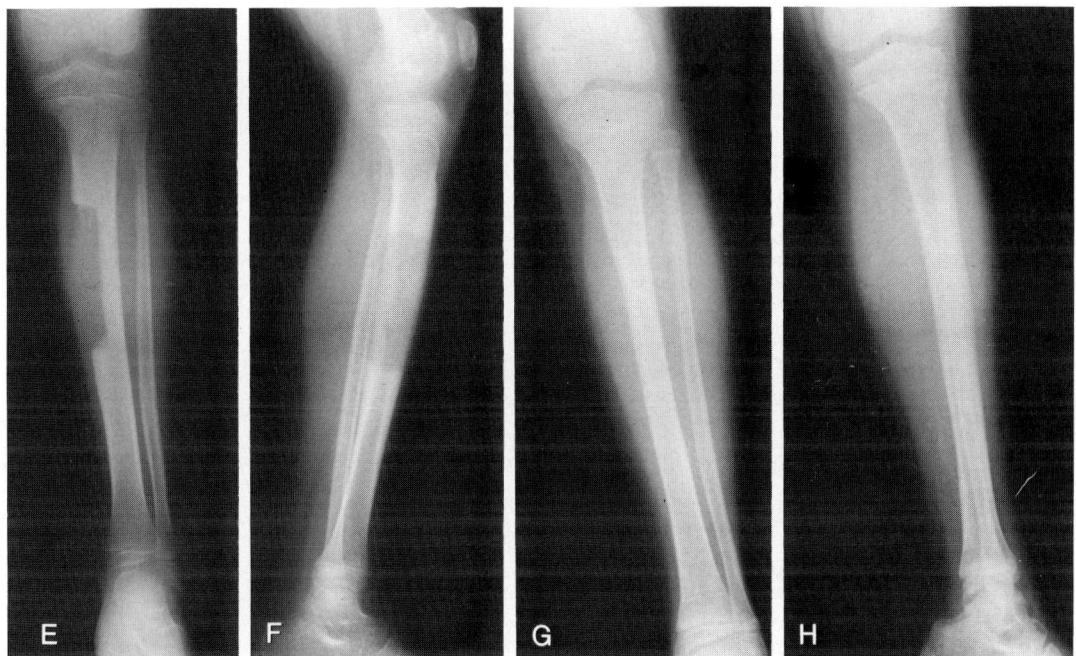

FIGURE 3–284 Continued. Benign osteoblastoma of the tibial diaphysis in an eight-year-old treated by segmental resection.

E and F. Immediate postoperative radiograms. G and H. One year later there are filling in of the defect and remodeling of bone.

Radiographic and Imaging Findings

The lesion is radiolucent, usually more than 2 cm. in diameter, possibly measuring up to 7 to 10 cm. (Figs. 3–281 to 3–283). If the lesion is mature and calcified, a varying degree of opacity may be found in the radiolucent shadow. The affected area of bone is usually expanded. On occasion, the regional cortex may be perforated by a soft-tissue mass. A delicate shell of periosteal new bone usually delimits the tumor.

Scintigraphy with technetium-99m shows intense increased uptake (Fig. 3–284).

Benign osteoblastoma is a Stage 1A lesion.

Differential Diagnosis

Differentiation between an aneurysmal bone cyst and benign osteoblastoma in the vertebral column may be especially difficult.

Osteogenic sarcoma may be histologically confused with the condition, owing to the presence of a great number of osteoblasts and sheets of osteoid tissue. In benign osteoblastoma, however, there is absence of sarcomatous large, plump connective tissue stromal cells, sarcoma giant cells, and tumor cartilage and bone.

The histologic pictures of benign osteoblastoma and osteoid osteoma are quite similar; however, the differentiating features of benign osteoblastoma are the larger size, progressive bone destruction, and lack of sharply defined boundaries.

Treatment

Treatment should be conservative because of the benign nature of the lesion and consists of local excision of the lesional tissue. When the neural arches of the vertebral column are involved and the tumor impinges on the spinal cord or its nerve roots, the area should be decompressed. When it is located in a surgically inaccessible site, moderate doses of radiation therapy may be administered, as this mode of treatment will provoke ossification and healing of the lesion.

Complications

Malignant transformation of benign osteoblastoma has been reported in the literature.[44,]

[67, 71, 86] The biologic behavior of the so-called benign osteoblastoma may be very aggressive locally; perhaps it is best to use the term *benign* with restraint.

References

1. Abdelwahab, I. F., Frankel, V. H., and Klein, M. J.: Case report 351: Aggressive osteoblastoma of the third lumbar vertebra. Skeletal Radiol., 15:164, 1986.
2. Acquaviva, R., et al.: Vertebral osteoblastoma. Report of a case. J. Med. Maroc, 4:265, 1968.
3. Adler, C. P.: Einteilung und Morphologie der Knochentumoren. Langenbecks Arch. Chir. (Kongressber), 358:359, 1982.
4. Adler, C. P.: Röntgenologische und pathologisch-anatomische Diagnostik von Knochentumoren. Röntgenpraxis, 36:37, 1983.
5. Adler, C. P.: Morphologie der Knochenkrankheiten. Stuttgart, Thieme, 1983.
6. Adler, C. P.: Case report 255: Osteoblastoma of the lesser trochanter of the left femur. Skeletal Radiol., 11:65, 1984.
7. Aegerter, E., and Kirkpatrick, J. A., Jr.: Orthopedic Diseases. 4th Ed. Philadelphia, Saunders, 1975, p. 487.
8. Akbarnia, B. A., and Rooholamini, S. A.: Scoliosis caused by benign osteoblastoma of the thoracic or lumbar spine. J. Bone Joint Surg., 63-A:1146, 1981.
9. Belgrano, M.: Raro caso di osteoblastoma della rotula. Minerva Ortop., 12:206, 1961.
10. Berciano, J., Perex-Lopez, J. L., Fernandez, F., Val, F., and Leno, C.: Voluminous benign osteoblastoma of the skull. Surg. Neurol., 20:383, 1983.
11. Bertoni, F., Unni, K. K., McLeod, R. A., and Dahlin, D. C.: Osteosarcoma resembling osteoblastoma. Cancer, 55:416, 1985.
12. Bethge, J. F. J.: Benignes Osteoblastom. Chirurg, 34:121, 1963.
13. Borghi, A., and D'Ettorre, A.: The benign osteoblastoma. Riv. Radiol., 13:47, 1973.
14. Byers, P. D.: Solitary benign osteoblastic lesions of bone. Osteoid osteoma and benign osteoblastoma. Cancer, 22:43, 1968.
15. Calcagni, V., and Tos, L.: L'Osteoblastoma del tarso. Chir. Organi Mov., 52:228, 1963.
16. Canepa, G., and Defabiani, F.: Osteoblastoma del radio. Minerva Ortop., 16:645, 1965.
17. Capanna, R. M., Van Horn, J. R., Ayala, A., Picci, P., and Bettelli, G.: Osteoid osteoma and osteoblastoma of the talus. A report of 40 cases. Skeletal Radiol., 15:360, 1986.
18. Case presentation: 72–1961. Osteoblastoma. N. Engl. J. Med., 265:700, 1961.
19. Castleman, B., and McNeill, J. M. (eds.): Bone and Joint Clinicopathological Conference of the Massachusetts General Hospital. Boston, Little, Brown, 1966, p. 172.
20. Chaise, F., and Witvoet, J.: Benign osteoblastoma of the hand. Sem. Hôp. Paris, 60:49, 1984.
21. Ciaramella, G., and Gualtieri, G.: Sull'osteoblastoma benigno (nota di casistica). Arch. Ortop., 77:217, 1964.
22. Clutter, D. J., Leopold, D. A., and Gould, L. V.: Benign osteoblastoma. Report of a case and review of the literature. Arch. Otolaryngol., 110:334, 1984.
23. Cohen, D. M., Dahlin, D. C., and MacCarty, C. S.: Vertebral giant-cell tumor and variants. Cancer, 17:461, 1964.
24. Crabbe, W. A., and Wardill, J. C.: Benign osteoblastoma of the spine. Br. J. Surg., 50:571, 1963.
25. Dahlin, D. C.: Bone Tumors. 3rd Ed. Springfield, Ill., Thomas, 1978, p. 70.
26. Dahlin, D. C., and Johnson, E. W., Jr.: Giant osteoid osteoma. J. Bone Joint Surg., 36-A:559, 1954.
27. Dias, L., and Frost, H. M.: Osteoblastoma of the spine. A review and report of eight new cases. Clin. Orthop., 91:141, 1973.
28. DiGiglia, J. W., Bradford, J. K., Leonard, G. L., and McFarland, G. B.: Benign osteoblastoma of the rib. South. Med. J., 64:624, 1971.
29. Dominok, G. W., and Knoch, H. G.: Knochengeschwulste und geschwulstahnliche Knochenerkrankungen. Stuttgart, Fisher, 1982.
30. Dorfman, H. D., and Weiss, S. W.: Borderline osteoblastic tumors: Problems in the differential diagnosis of aggressive osteoblastoma and low-grade osteosarcoma. Semin. Diagn. Pathol., 1:215, 1984.
31. Doron, Y., and Gruszkiewicz, J.: Benign osteoblastoma of vertebral column and skull. Surg. Neurol., 7:86, 1977.
32. Eisenbrey, A. B., Huber, P. J., and Rachmaninoff, N.: Benign osteoblastoma of the spine with multiple recurrences. J. Neurosurg., 31:468, 1969.
33. Epstein, B. S.: The Vertebral Column. Chicago, Year Book, 1974, p. 24.
34. Gelberman, R., and Olson, C. O.: Benign osteoblastoma of the atlas. A case report. J. Bone Joint Surg., 56-A:808, 1974.
35. Gertzbein, S. D., Cruickshank, B., Hoffman, H., Taylor, G. A., and Cooper, P. W.: Recurrent benign osteoblastoma of the second thoracic vertebra. A case report. J. Bone Joint Surg., 55-B:841, 1973.
36. Giannestras, N. J., and Diamond, J. R.: Benign osteoblastoma of the talus. A review of the literature and report of a case. J. Bone Joint Surg., 40-A:469, 1958.
37. Gibbons, J. M., Jr., and Hammond, G.: Benign osteoblastoma. Lahey Clin. Bull., 13:97, 1963.
38. Goidanich, I. F., and Battaglia, L.: Osteoblastoma (fibroma osteogenetica). Chir. Organi Mov., 46:353, 1958.
39. Goidanich, I. F., and Zanasi, R.: Osteoma osteoide ed osteomielite sclerosante due entita cliniche definite e distinte. Chir. Organi Mov., 43:427, 1956.
40. Golding, J. S. R., and Sissons, H. A.: Osteogenic fibroma of bone. Report of two cases. J. Bone Joint Surg., 36-A:428, 1954.
41. Goldman, R. L.: The periosteal counterpart of benign osteoblastoma. Am. J. Clin. Pathol., 56:73, 1971.
42. Guy, R., Lafond, G., Gagnon, P. A., Raymond, O., and Bourgeois, J.: L'ostéoblastoma bénin (fibroma ostéogénique l'ostéome ostéoïde geant). Union Med. Can., 88:666, 1959.
43. Ikawa, T., Kamizaki, Y., and Ishikawa, T.: Benign osteoblastoma of the maxillary sinus. Rhinology, 21:373, 1983.
44. Jackson, J. R., and Bell, M. E. A.: Spurious "benign osteoblastoma." A case report. J. Bone Joint Surg., 59-A:397, 1977.
45. Jackson, R. O.: Recurrent osteoblastoma: A review. Clin. Orthop., 131:229, 1978.
46. Jackson, R. O., Reckling, F. W., and Mantz, F. A.: Osteoid osteoma and osteoblastoma: Similar histologic lesions with different natural histories. Clin. Orthop., 128:303, 1977.
47. Jaffe, H. L.: Osteoid osteoma. A benign osteoblastic tumor composed of osteoid and atypical bone. Arch. Surg., 31:709, 1935.
48. Jaffe, H. L.: Benign osteoblastoma. Bull. Hosp. Joint Dis., 17:141, 1956.
49. Jaffe, H. L.: Tumors and Tumorous Conditions of the Bones and Joints. Philadelphia, Lea & Febiger, 1958, p. 107.
50. Jaffe, H. L., and Mayer, L.: An osteoblastic osteoid tissue-forming tumor of a metacarpal bone. Arch. Surg., 24:550, 1932.

51. Janin, Y., Epstein, J. A., Carras, R., and Khan, A.: Osteoid osteoma and osteoblastomas of the spine. Neurosurgery, 8:31, 1981.
52. Kawamoto, T., Kitaoka, K., Abe, H., and Nakamura, N.: Benign osteoblastoma of the atlas. Case report. Neurol. Med. Chir. (Tokyo), 25:223, 1985.
53. Kenan, S., Floman, Y., Robin, G. C., and Laufer, A.: Aggressive osteoblastoma. A case report and review of the literature. Clin. Orthop., 195:294, 1985.
54. Kent, J. N., Castro, H. F., and Girotti, W. R.: Benign osteoblastoma of the maxilla. Case report and review of the literature. Oral Surg., 27:209, 1969.
55. Kirkpatrick, H. J. R., and Murray, R. C.: Osteogenic fibroma of bone: Report of a case. J. Bone Joint Surg., 37-B:606, 1955.
56. Kirwan, E. O., Hutton, P. A., Pozo, J. L., and Ransford, A. O.: Osteoid osteoma and benign osteoblastoma of the spine. Clinical presentation and treatment. J. Bone Joint Surg., 66-B:21, 1984.
57. Kopp, W. K.: Benign osteoblatoma of the coronoid process of the mandible: Report of a case. J. Oral Surg., 27:653, 1969.
58. Kumar, S., Prakash, B., Singh, A. K., Naviakha, R. K., and Malhotra, V.: Benign osteoblastoma of the lumbar spine. Indian Pediatr., 20:942, 1983.
59. Lepage, J., Rigault, P., Nezelof, C., Padovani, J. P., Pierre-Kahn, A., and Guyanvarch, G.: Benign osteoblastoma in children. Apropos of 8 cases, 4 with spinal localization. Rev. Chir. Orthop., 70:117, 1984.
60. Lichtenstein, L.: Benign osteoblastoma. A category of osteoid- and bone-forming tumors other than classical osteoid osteoma, which may be mistaken for giant-cell tumor or osteogenic sarcoma. Cancer, 9:1044, 1956.
61. Lichtenstein, L.: Bone Tumors, 5th Ed. St. Louis, Mosby, 1977, p. 92.
62. Lichtenstein, L., and Sawyer, W. R.: Benign osteoblastoma: Further observations and report of twenty additional cases. J. Bone Joint Surg., 46-A:755, 1964.
63. Lodwick, G. S.: The Bones and Joints. Chicago, Year Book, 1971, pp. 316–327.
64. McLeod, R. A., Dahlin, D. C., and Beabout, J. W.: The spectrum of osteoblastoma. A.J.R., 126:321, 1976.
65. McNeill, J. M., and Robbins, L. L.: X-ray Seminar Cases of the Massachusetts General Hospital. Boston, Little, Brown, 1971, p. 174.
66. Marsh, B. W., Bonfiglio, M., Brady, L. P., and Enneking, W. F.: Benign osteoblastoma: Range of manifestations. J. Bone Joint Surg., 57-A:1, 1975.
67. Mayer, L.: Malignant degeneration of so-called benign osteoblastoma. Bull. Hosp. Joint Dis., 28:4, 1967.
68. Mayer, L.: Letter to the editor. Benign (?) osteoblastoma. Bull. Hosp. Joint Dis., 29:236, 1968.
69. Meary, R., D'Aubigne, R. M., and Mazabraud, A.: Ostéoblastomes bénins. Mem. Acad. Chir., 91:911, 1965.
70. Merryweather, R., Middlemiss, J. H., and Sanerkin, N. G.: Malignant transformation of osteoblastoma. J. Bone Joint Surg., 62-B:381, 1980.
71. Mirra, J. M., Kendrick, R. A., and Kendrick, R. E.: Pseudomalignant osteoblastoma versus arrested osteosarcoma. Cancer, 37:2005, 1976.
72. Mitchell, M. L., and Ackerman, L. V.: Metastatic and pseudomalignant osteoblastoma: A report of two unusual cases. Skeletal Radiol., 15:213, 1986.
73. Ossuthorre, J. D., and Hungerford, G. D.: Benign osteoblastoma of the maxillary sinus. Head Neck Surg., 6:605, 1983.
74. Pettine, K. A., and Klassen, R. A.: Osteoid-osteoma and osteoblastoma of the spine. J. Bone Joint Surg., 68-A:354, 1986.
75. Pieterse, A. S., Vernon-Roberts, B., Paterson, D. C., Cornish, B. L., and Lewis, P. R.: Osteoid osteoma transform to aggressive (low grade malignant) osteoblastoma: A case report and literature review. Histopathology, 7:789, 1983.
76. Pochaczevsky, R., Yen, Y. M., and Sherman, R. S.: The roentgen appearance of benign osteoblastoma. Radiology, 75:429, 1960.
77. Potter, C., Conner, G. H., and Sharkey, F. E.: Benign osteoblastoma of the temporal bone. Am. J. Otol., 4:318, 1983.
78. Rand, R. W., and Rand, C. W.: Intraspinal Tumors of Childhood. Springfield, Ill., Thomas, 1960, pp. 330–339.
79. Ransford, A. O., Pozo, J. L., Hutton, P. A. N., and Kirwan, E. O'G.: The behavior pattern of scoliosis associated with osteoid osteoma or osteoblastoma of the spine. J. Bone Joint Surg., 66-B:16, 1984.
80. Revell, P. A., and Scholtz, C. L.: Aggressive osteoblastoma. J. Pathol., 127:195, 1979.
81. Roessner, M., Metze, K., and Heymer, B.: Aggressive osteoblastoma. Pathol. Res. Pract., 179:433, 1985.
82. Rosensweig, J., Pintar, K., Mikail, M., and Mayman, A.: Benign osteoblastoma (giant osteoid osteoma). Report of an unusual rib tumor and review of the literature. Can. Med. Assoc. J., 89:1189, 1963.
83. Salzer, M., and Salzer-Kuntschik, M.: Das benigne Osteoblastom. Langenbecks Arch. Klin. Chir., 302:755, 1963.
84. Sanchis Olmos, V., Torrelles, M. F., and Criado, M. F.: Osteoma parostal de clavicula. Acta Ortop. Traumatol. Iberica., 4:471, 1956.
85. Schajowicz, F., and Lemos, C.: Osteoid osteoma and osteoblastoma. Closely related entities of osteoblastic derivation. Acta Orthop. Scand., 41:272, 1970.
86. Schajowicz, F., and Lemos, C.: Malignant osteoblastoma. J. Bone Joint Surg., 58-B:202, 1976.
87. Schein, A. J.: Osteoblastoma of the scapula. A case report. J. Bone Joint Surg., 41-A:359, 1959.
88. Seki, T., Fukada, H., Ishii, Y., Hanaoka, H., Yatabe, S., Takano, M., and Koide, O.: Malignant transformation of benign osteoblastoma. A case report. J. Bone Joint Surg., 57-A:424, 1975.
89. Shatz, A., Calderon, S., and Mintz, S.: Benign osteoblastoma of the mandible. Oral Surg., 61:189, 1986.
90. Sollazzo, M.: Su di un caso di osteoblastoma benigno dell'astragalo. Chir. Organi Mov., 63:89, 1974.
91. Sooknundun, M., Kacker, S. K., and Kapila, K.: Benign osteoblastoma of the nasal bones (a case report). J. Laryngol. Otol., 100:229, 1986.
92. Spjut, H. F., Dorfman, H. D., Fechner, R. E., and Ackerman, L. V.: Atlas of Tumor Pathology, Second Series, Fascicle 5, Tumors of Bone and Cartilage. Washington, D.C., Armed Forces Institute of Pathology, 1971, p. 132.
93. Stutch, R.: Osteoblastoma—a benign entity? Orthopaed. Rev., 4:27, 1975.
94. Tehranzadeh, J., Jenkins, J. J., and Horton, J. A.: Case report 249: Osteoblastoma with secondary aneurysmal bone cyst of the frontal bone. Skeletal Radiol., 10:276, 1983.
95. Trifaud, A., Payan, H., Bureau, H., and Argenson, C.: Les ostéoblastomes bénins. A propos de cinq observations. Mem. Acad. Chir., 91:890, 1965.
96. Tulloh, H. P., and Denys, H.: Osteoblastoma in a rib in childhood. Clin. Radiol., 20:337, 1969.
97. van der Waal, I., Greebe, R. B., and Elias, E. A.: Benign osteoblastoma of the maxilla. Report of a case. Int. J. Oral Surg., 12:355, 1983.
98. von Ronnen, J. R.: Case report 2. Osteoblastoma of petrous pyramid of skull. Skeletal Radiol., 1:57, 1976.
99. von Ronnen, J. R.: Case report 4. Osteoblastoma of spinous process of C2. Skeletal Radiol., 1:61, 1976.
100. Weatherly, C. R., Jaffray, D., and O'Brien, J. P.: Radical excision of an osteoblastoma of the cervical spine. A combined anterior and posterior approach. J. Bone Joint Surg., 68-B:325, 1986.
101. Wilner, D.: Radiology of Bone Tumors and Allied Disorders. Philadelphia, Saunders, 1982, p. 217.
102. Yllanes, H., and Compere, E. L.: Benign osteoblas-

toma. A rare tumor involving the humerus of a 5-year-old boy. Clin. Orthop., 42:147, 1965.
103. Yoshikawa, S., Nakamura, T., Takagi, M., Imamura, T., Okano, K., and Sasaki, S.: Benign osteoblastoma as a cause of osteomalacia. J. Bone Joint Surg., 59-B:279, 1977.

FIBROUS DYSPLASIA

Fibrous dysplasia is a term coined by Lichtenstein and Jaffe to describe a disorder that primarily involves bone but is occasionally associated with extraskeletal abnormalities.[56-58, 67, 68] The condition is characterized by the presence of expanding fibro-osseous tissue in the interior of the affected bones. It is primarily a lesion of the growing skeleton.

It may be classified into three groups: The *monostotic* type, in which only one bone is affected; a *polyostotic* form, in which multiple bones are involved; and a *polyostotic* form in association with *endocrine abnormalities* such as precocious puberty, premature skeletal maturation, or hyperthyroidism—commonly known as Albright's disease.

Etiology

The exact cause and fundamental nature of the condition remain obscure. It appears to be a developmental abnormality of bone-forming mesenchyme. The primitive fibrous tissue proliferates within the bony medulla, encroaching on the cortex from within and producing expansion.

A possible congenital basis is suggested by unilateral involvement in the polyostotic form of the disease. The pathologic picture indicates that monostotic and polyostotic forms are manifestations of the same biologic process. Existing evidence negates an endocrine malfunction as a cause of the skeletal lesions.

The disorder is not hereditary. All reported cases are sporadic. Two cases in a mother and her daughter were reported by Firat and Stutzman.[36] Lemli reported female monozygotic twins, one with McCune-Albright syndrome and the other with only sporadic evidence of fibrous dysplasia in the skull. It seems that the phenotypic expression can vary in spite of identical genotype and the occurrence of fibrous dysplasia in monozygotic twins suggests the possibility of genetic origin.[63]

Incidence

The exact incidence of fibrous dysplasia is unknown. It is not a rare disorder. The monostotic form is much more common than the polyostotic form. There is no sex predilection in monostotic fibrous dysplasia, but the polyostotic form is much more common in the female, with a female to male ratio of 3:1.

Skeletal lesions most probably have a congenital basis, but the condition is usually discovered in childhood or adolescence because of deformity or fracture due to weakening of the structural integrity of the affected bone. In the mandible it is often detected in early adult life. Occasionally, particularly in the rib, it may be diagnosed for the first time in an adult, because it is asymptomatic at that site.

Localization

Almost any bone may be affected by fibrous dysplasia. The monostotic type often involves the femur, tibia, humerus, rib, or a facial bone. It has been reported in the calvarium, vertebrae, pelvis, scapula, tarsus, carpus, metatarsals, metacarpals, and phalanges.

In the polyostotic type, there is a tendency for segmental distribution in the bones of one limb, usually the lower one; in such an instance, the femur, tibia, fibula, some of the bones of the foot, and a portion of the innominate bone are usually involved. This segmental distribution of the lesions in a single limb is a hallmark of polyostotic fibrous dysplasia. Skull bones may be affected along with an upper limb. In about half these patients the craniofacial bone is involved. In some, skeletal involvement is very diffuse, and more than half the skeleton is involved at the time of initial examination.[48] Occasionally the entire skeleton seems to be affected.

Ordinarily in the long bones fibrous dysplasia involves the diaphysis and metaphysis; however, epiphyseal involvement prior to closure of the physis has been reported.[78]

Clinical Findings

In monostotic fibrous dysplasia, clinical findings depend on the site of the lesion. The patient with an affected rib may be asymptomatic; the lesion is discovered incidentally in a chest radiogram. There may be pain and a limp when the neck of the femur is involved, or local swelling when the lesion is in a superficial bone such as the tibia or mandible.

In polyostotic fibrous dysplasia the skeletal changes are usually more severe, giving rise to symptoms and signs such as pain, a limp, shortening or bowing, and other deformities. Disability may be serious. A "shepherd's crook deformity" with outward bowing of the femoral

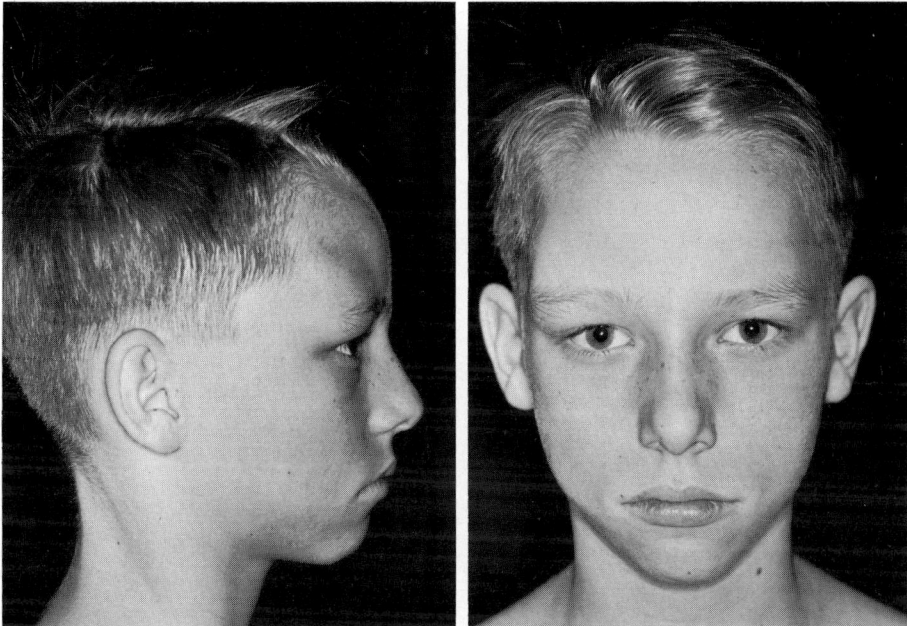

FIGURE 3–285. *Fibrous dysplasia of right orbital bones. Note the deformity of the face.*

shaft and varus deformity of the femoral neck will cause a short-leg gluteus medius limp. There is increased susceptibility to pathologic fracture. In the series reported by Harris and associates 85 per cent of the patients sustained fractures and 40 per cent had three or more fractures.[47]

When the mandible or the orbital bones are the site of fibrous dysplasia, progressive grotesque deformity of the face may be the presenting complaint (Fig. 3–285).

Involvement of the spine is quite rare; when it occurs the lumbar spine is commonly affected. Vertebral collapse, angular deformity, and spinal cord compression can result. In some cases spinal cord compression is caused by the posteriorly expanding fibrous tumor.[76]

Nonskeletal Manifestations

Of these, the most common is *abnormal cutaneous pigmentation*, caused by the presence of an unusual amount of melanin, especially in the basal epidermal cells. This results in yellow-brown blotches on the skin, which have been called café-au-lait spots. These pigmented areas are clearly demarcated, with irregular dented margins and a texture similar to that of the surrounding skin. The café-au-lait spots may be very extensive, involving large areas of the trunk, face, or limbs, and have a tendency to distribute themselves parallel to the skeletal lesions. A possible biologic relationship of skin pigmentation to various features of polyostotic fibrous dysplasia and Albright's syndrome is undetermined. Polyostotic fibrous dysplasia and precocious puberty (or other endocrine disorders) can coexist without café-au-lait spots of the skin; and these changes in skin pigmentation can coexist with polyostotic fibrous dysplasia without endocrine changes or precocious puberty. Monostotic fibrous dysplasia is not ordinarily associated with café-au-lait spots.

Pigmented skin changes do occur in neurofibromatosis. Albright distinguished them from those of polyostotic fibrous dysplasia. In fibrous dysplasia the indented irregular margins are similiar to the coast of Maine, whereas those in neurofibromatosis are irregular and smooth, resembling the coast of California.[3, 4, 16]

Sexual precocity is most often seen in the female with premature ovarian stimulation. Secondary sex characteristics appear early, with development of large breasts, prominent areoli, and growth of pubic and axillary hair. Menstruation may begin at an age as early as three months. The clinical syndrome of sexual precocity with cutaneous pigmentation and polyostotic fibrous dysplasia was first described by McCune in 1936 and by Albright and co-workers in 1937.[4, 72] Most cases of Albright's syndrome are in girls.[1, 13, 31, 111]

Acceleration of maturation in which the skeletal age is much further advanced than chronologic age may be observed. In such a child, abnormally rapid growth may result in a height that is excessive for his age. Eventually, however, the epiphysis will fuse prematurely, and the ultimate stature will usually be below average.

Sexual precocity in boys in association with polyostotic fibrous dysplasia may also occur but is very rare.[9] Other endocrinopathies associated with polyostotic fibrous dysplasia are hyperthyroidism, Cushing's syndrome, acromegaly, hyperparathyroidism, and hypophosphatemic rickets.* The pathogenesis of association of polyostotic fibrous dysplasia with endocrine disorders is not known. The possible role of hypersecretion of hypothalamic releasing hormone was proposed by Hall and Warwick.[46] Lightner and associates described a boy, aged five years and five months, with gigantism (due to growth hormone excess) and sexual precocity; the accumulation of estradiol suppressed the secretion of follicle-stimulating hormone and had an apparent positive feedback effect on release of luteinizing hormone. They interpreted these findings as compatible with abnormal hypothalamic function and as the mechanism for the endocrinopathies associated with the McCune-Albright syndrome.[70] Danon and associates described a six-month-old girl with McCune-Albright syndrome and congenital Cushing's syndrome, and proposed the possible cause of associated endocrinopathies as autonomous hyperfunction of the peripheral endocrine glands.[24] This hypothesis is supported by D'Armiento and associates.[25]

The orthopedic surgeon treating a patient with polyostotic fibrous dysplasia should be aware of its possible association with endocrinopathies and obtain an endocrine consultation prior to surgical intervention.

Myositis ossificans progressiva and intramuscular myxoma may be associated with polyostotic fibrous dysplasia.[37, 71] Visual disturbances may result from pressure atrophy of the optic nerve.

Pathology

At operation the affected area of the bone will be found distended with a smooth external surface. The lesional tissue is grayish white in color or, at times, reddish gray if it is vascular. It is of firm consistency and feels gritty on palpation—a sensation that has been likened to rubbing sandpaper. The mass of tissue is solid except for small degenerative cystic areas due to cellular necrosis. Islands of hyaline cartilage may be found (Fig. 3–286).

Histologically, the lesion is fibrous tissue

---

*See references: hyperthyroidism, 5, 32, 52, 87, 90, 106; Cushing's syndrome, 10, 29; acromegaly, 18; hyperparathyroidism, 32; and hypophosphatemic rickets, 6, 65.

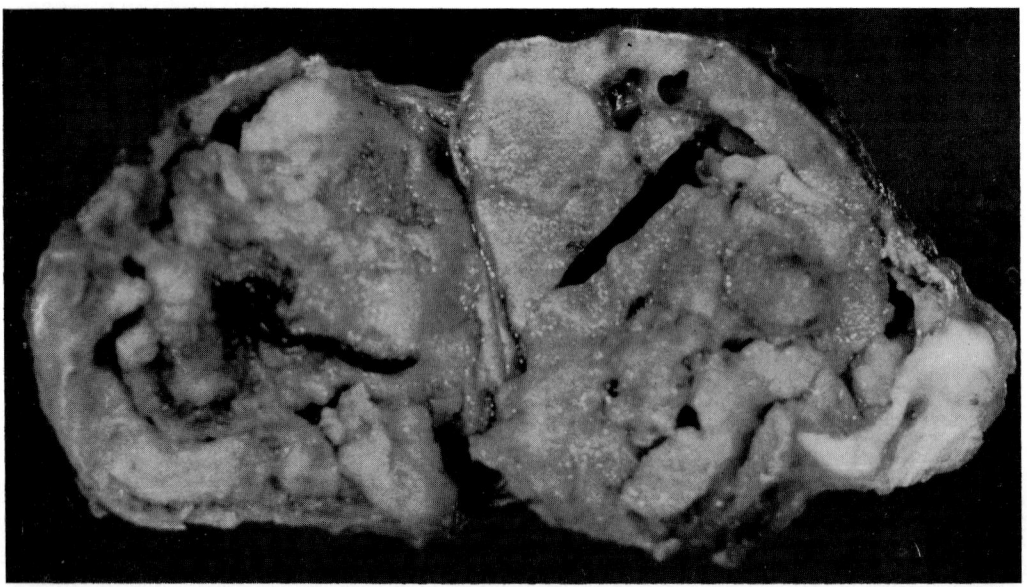

FIGURE 3–286. Fibrous dysplasia—gross appearance of a specimen.

The lesional tissue is grayish white in color, of firm consistency, and gritty on palpation. Note the small cysts and islands of hyaline cartilage.

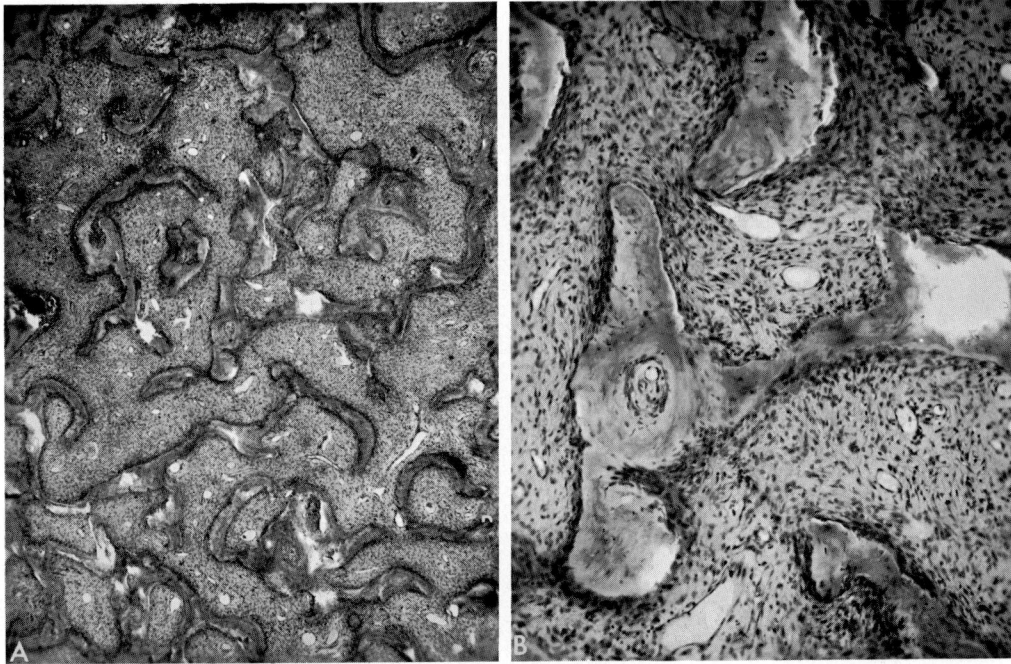

FIGURE 3–287. *Fibrous dysplasia—histologic findings.*

A. Photomicrograph showing the delicate, spindly connective tissue stroma in which are scattered thin spicules of fiber bone with wide osteoid seams (× 25). **B.** Greater magnification showing same pathologic picture in detail (× 100).

composed of collagen fibers arranged rather loosely or whorled in which are dispersed fiber-bone trabeculae formed through osseous metaplasia of fibrous tissue (Fig. 3–287). The connective tissue cells are rich in alkaline phosphatase.[17] The newly formed bone trabeculae are thin with wide osteoid seams. They are not oriented along lines of stress. Multinuclear giant cells and nests of foam cells can be seen, particularly within areas undergoing focal degeneration. Fluid-filled cysts lined by hyalinized fibrous tissue may be observed. In the polyostotic form, islands of hyaline cartilage may be present. Periosteal reaction to fracture is normal, but endosteal reaction and internal callus formation are usually poor.

Radiographic and Imaging Findings

The changes in the radiograms are produced by the solid fibro-osseous mass in the interior of the affected bone and the response of the regional cortical bone to this tumorous tissue. The rather radiolucent shadow cast in the radiogram suggests a cystic structure, but the word *cyst* should not be used, as it implies a fluid-filled cavity. The myriad, thin calcified trabeculae of the lesion give a ground-glass appearance to the area of radiolucency (Figs. 3–288 and 3–289).

The cortex of the affected bone may be thinned by endosteal erosion, which creates a scalloped pattern and gives a "multilocular" appearance to the lesion. This is an optical illusion, however, due to bony ridges on its inner surface. The lesion is unicameral. The radiolucent and multilocular radiographic appearance is not typical of fibrous dysplasia, but is seen in other lesions, such as solitary bone cyst. Sequestra have been reported in fibrous dysplasia.[83]

In the long bones, the lesions are usually metaphyseal in location, extending into the middiaphysis. When the skull is affected there is increased radiopacity and marked thickening of the frontal, sphenoid, ethmoid, and maxillary bones. The capacity of the orbits is reduced, and the paranasal sinuses are obliterated.

Periosteal reaction is absent, except when a pathologic fracture has occurred through the lesion. Fractures heal with a collar of callus, ordinarily within the normal period. Other deformities will be revealed in the radiograms, e.g., coxa vara, "shepherd's crook" deformity of the proximal femur, and genu varum or valgum.

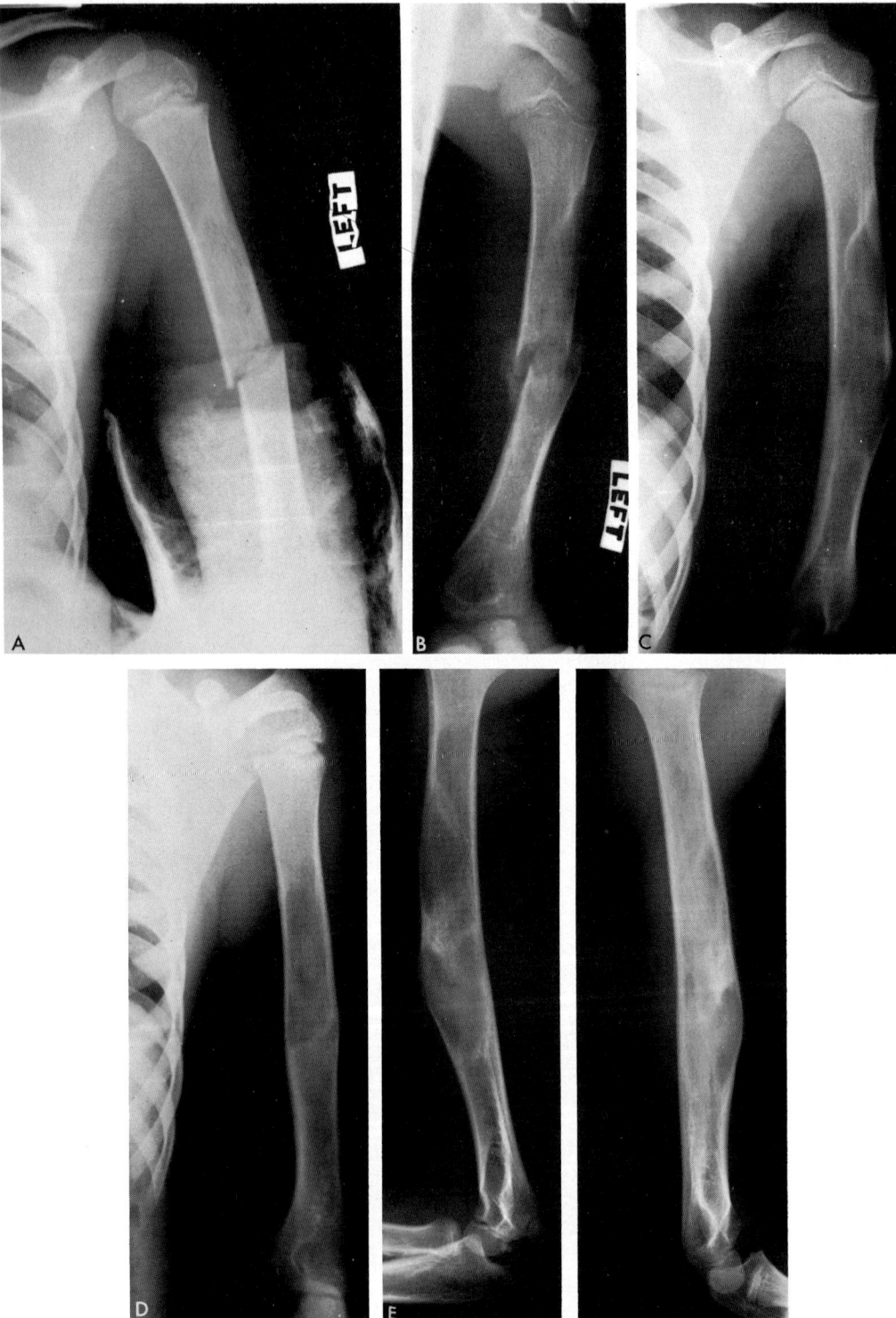

FIGURE 3–288. Fibrous dysplasia of left humerus.

A. A pathologic fracture through the lesion in the midshaft of the humerus was sustained in a fall. It was treated in a hanging cast. **B.** Anteroposterior radiogram of the humerus six weeks later shows healing of the fracture and the cystlike lesion. **C** and **D.** Anteroposterior and lateral radiograms of the humerus one year later. The "ground glass" appearance of the area of radiolucency is characteristic of fibrous dysplasia. Note the outward bowing of the humerus and thinning of the cortex. The lesion was curetted and a bone graft performed. **E.** Radiograms of humerus two years later. The lesion has recurred.

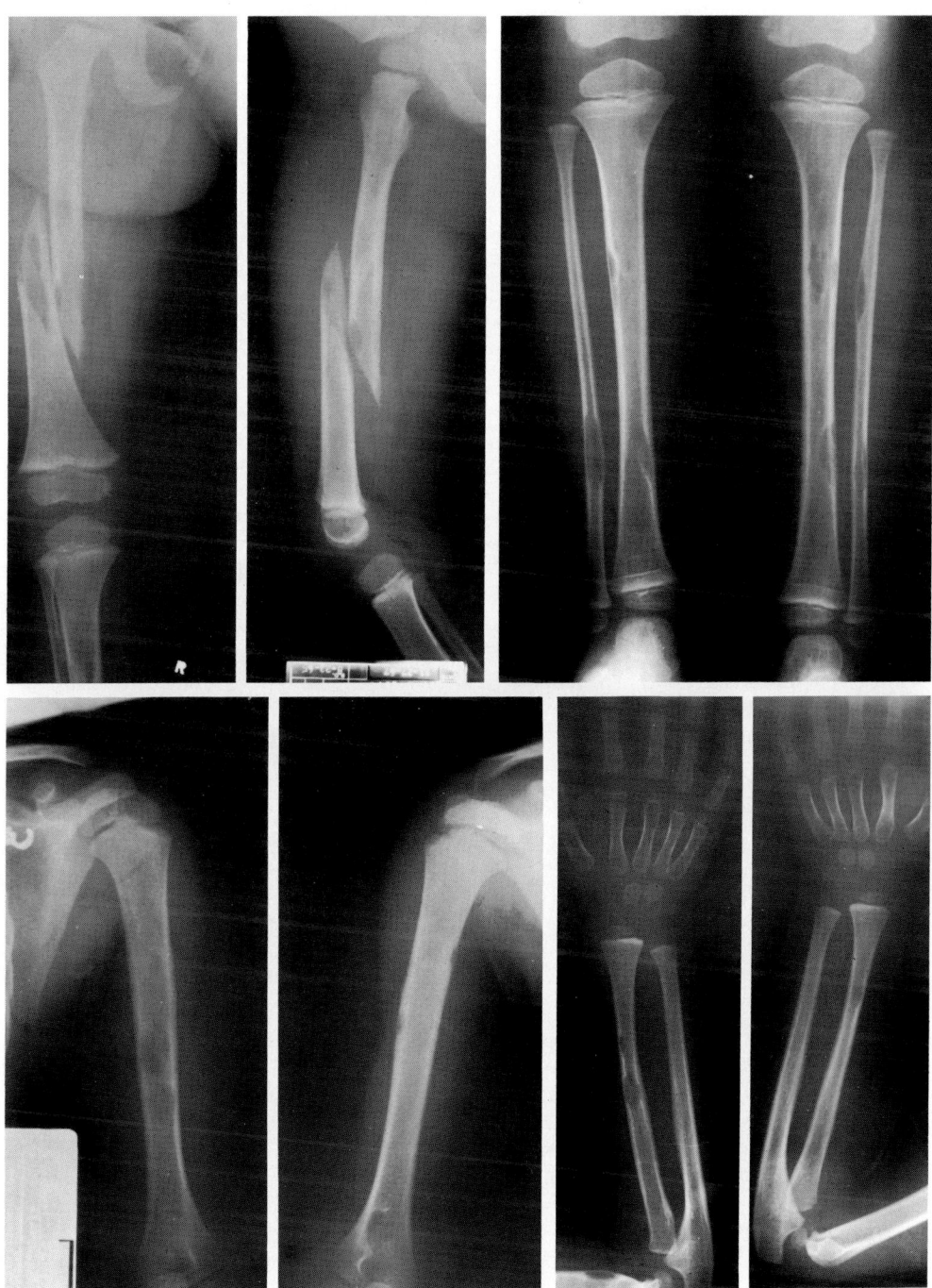

FIGURE 3–289. Polyostotic fibrous dysplasia in a two-year-old girl.

Diagnosis was made when she sustained a fracture of the right femur in a fall.

Bone scan with technetium-99m will show increased uptake (Fig. 3–290C). This can present difficulties in differentiating fibrous dysplasia from infection or malignant tumor. The bone scan is, however, of great value in assessing the extent and multiplicity of involvement and the activity of the disease.

Computed tomography will demonstrate the amorphous "ground-glass" appearance of the lesion in fibrous dysplasia (Fig. 3–291).[22] Osteomyelitis and eosinophilic granuloma are low-density tumors (in CT numbers the range is 20 to 40 Hounsfield units [H]); whereas the lesions of fibrous dysplasia have much higher numbers (70 to 130H)—due to the greater density of the primitive bone trabeculae.[49, 104] Because of their fluid content, unicameral bone cysts have a much lower density than fibrous dysplasia. One of the unique values of computed tomography lies in the assessment of craniofacial lesions, particularly in the orbital region. Soft-tissue extension out of bone, particularly in the spine and orbitofacial region, is also well demonstrated by CT scan. In the very rare case of malignant transformation of fibrous dysplasia, the CT scan is of value in delineating the extent of the tumor and thereby assisting in the strategy of management.

The differential diagnosis should consider primary or secondary hyperthyroidism, solitary bone cyst, solitary or multiple enchondromas, aclasial fibrous defects, eosinophilic granuloma, and neurofibromatosis. In monostotic fibrous dysplasia, biopsy is often required for accurate diagnosis. In the polyostotic form diagnosis may frequently be made from the radiographic, bone scintigraphic, and computed tomographic studies alone.

Natural Course

The histologic evolution of fibrous dysplasia has been studied by Harris and associates by repeated biopsy examination of tissues at various intervals. Changes with time were minimal—they included a decrease in cellularity, an increased deposit of collagen, and a slight decrease in the amount of bone in relation to fibrous tissue. The woven bone trabeculae were not converted into a lamellar bone pattern. There was no concentration of the trabeculae along stress lines, despite resorption and accretion of bone. The lesions did not become sclerotic with skeletal maturation.[47]

In children, the skeletal lesions are likely to progress. New lesions may appear in areas that previously appeared to be normal on the radiograms. There may be extension of existing lesions, and the involved bones may show increasing deformity. Following maturity, the lesions tend to be stabilized; progression has, however, been noted in some adult patients.[47] Pregnancy may stimulate activity of the fibrous dysplasia.

Treatment

Surgical intervention is indicated when lesions are complicated by fractures, cause significant or progressive deformity that jeopardizes the integrity of the shaft or is cosmetically disfiguring, or are symptomatic, causing pain. The mere presence of fibrous dysplasia in bone is not an indication for operation. Surgical overtreatment should be avoided.

The radiographic changes of monostotic fibrous dysplasia are not distinctive, histologic examination of the lesion is required to make the definitive diagnosis. At operation for biopsy the lesional tissue is excised and bone grafting is performed. It may, however, be impossible to eradicate extensive lesions; therefore, diagnostic biopsy should *not* always be synonymous with thorough curettage and massive bone grafting. The problems attendant on such an extensive procedure are pathologic fracture and recurrence. Factors affecting the decision for or against complete excision of the fibrous tissue are the location and size of the tumor, the age of the patient, and the biologic behavior of the lesion. A more conservative approach and restraint from aggresive surgery should be exercised in the young child, especially with the polyostotic form. In such an instance postoperative recurrence is common. In contrast, an expanding lesion in the femoral neck that is thinning the cortex warrants a more radical excision of the lesion to prevent progressive coxa vara deformity. If the tumor recurs another operation is performed.

The choice of bone graft material depends on the size of the lesion, age of the patient, and the surgeon's individual preference. When possible this author recommends autogenous corticocancellous graft. In the young child and in the polyostotic form the sources of autogenous graft are limited; therefore, one has to resort to freeze-dried corticocancellous homograft or even allograft. Cortical bone provides structural support; in addition, it does not resorb as readily as cancellous bone. Allografts also require a longer period for resorption; hence, the appearance of recurrence is delayed. Eventually, however, the type of graft utilized probably does not affect the rate of recurrence. When all

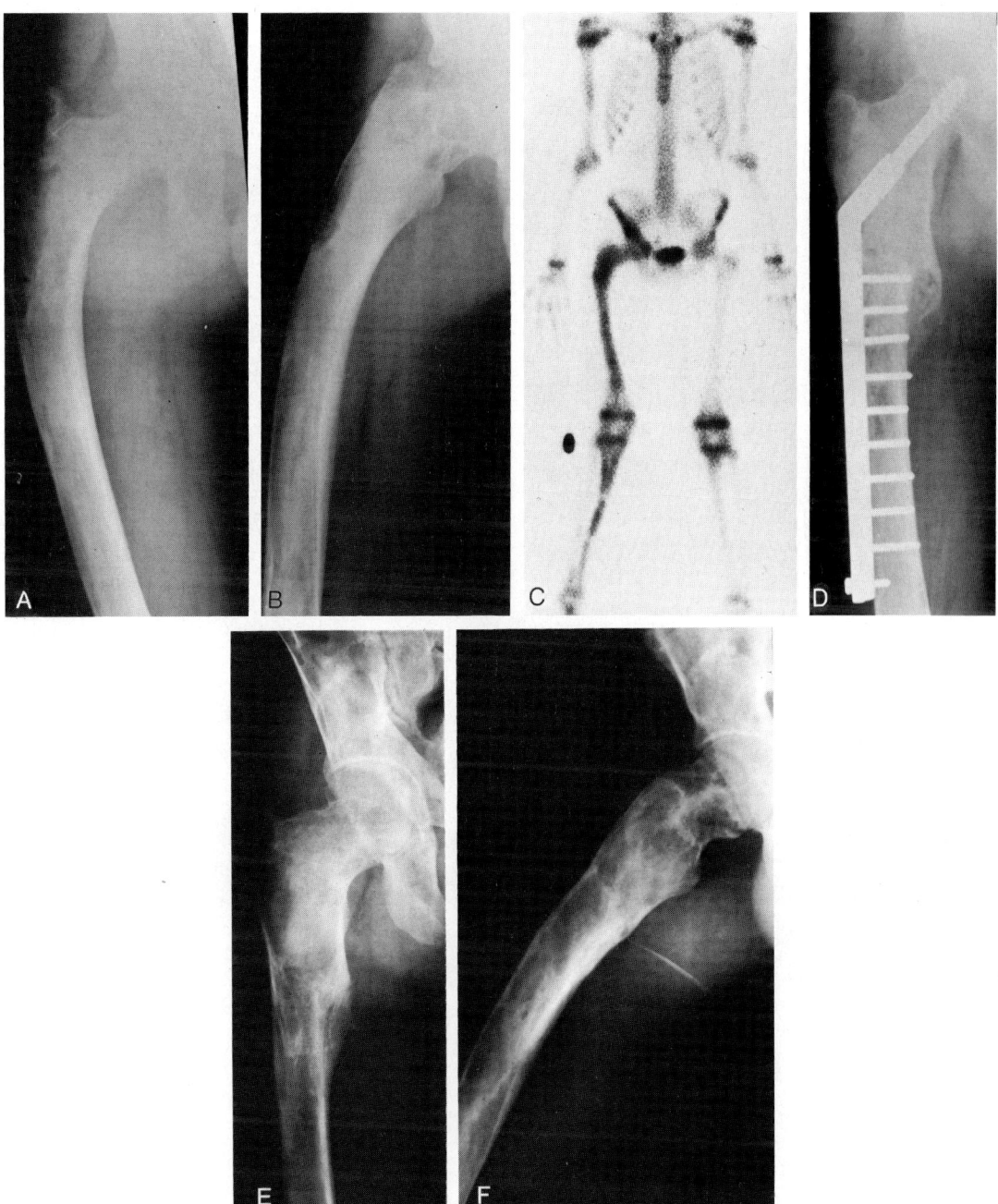

FIGURE 3–290. *Fibrous dysplasia with lateral bowing of the proximal femur in a 16-year-old boy.*

A and **B.** Anteroposterior and lateral radiograms showing area of radiolucency and thinning and erosion of the lateral cortex of the bowed proximal femur. **C.** Scintigraphy with technetium-99m showing increased uptake. **D.** Postoperative anteroposterior radiogram of the hip and upper third of the femur. The lesion was curetted, a graft with autogenous bone was performed, and a plate was applied. **E** and **F.** Anteroposterior and lateral radiograms of upper half of the femur showing the plate and screws removed and the osteotomy healed. Patient is asymptomatic.

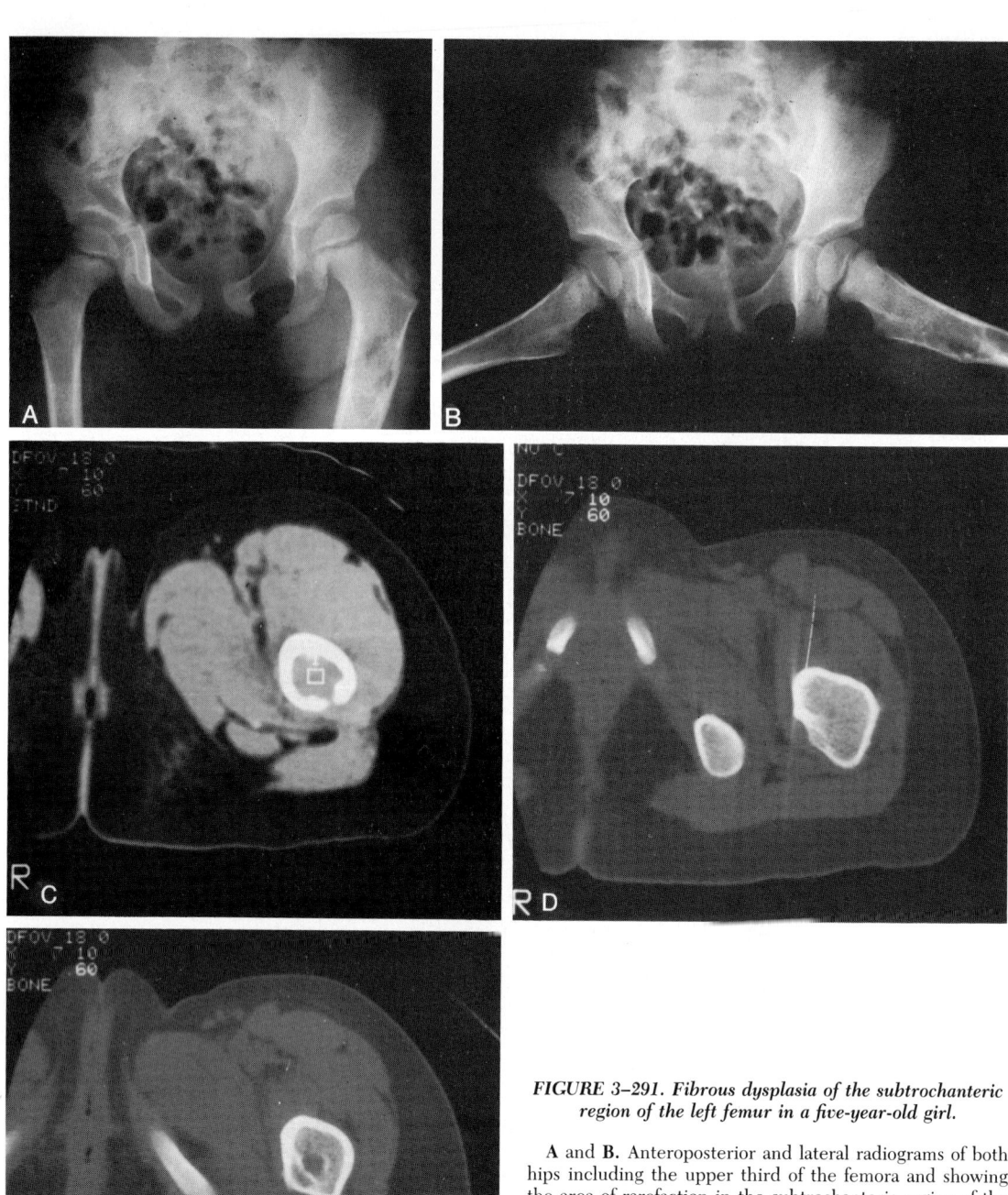

FIGURE 3–291. Fibrous dysplasia of the subtrochanteric region of the left femur in a five-year-old girl.

A and **B**. Anteroposterior and lateral radiograms of both hips including the upper third of the femora and showing the area of rarefaction in the subtrochanteric region of the left femur. **C** to **E**. CT study showing the "ground glass" appearance of the lesion.

abnormal tissue is not excised the lesion may recur by absorption of the graft by the active dysplastic fibrous tissue.

Fibrous dysplasia of the rib is best treated by excision. A lesion in the phalanx, metacarpal, or metatarsal may be subperiosteally excised and augmented by a bone graft.

Pathologic Fracture. Weakening of the involved bone and deformity of the fragile bone under stress lead to pathologic fracture, a disabling problem in fibrous dysplasia. These fractures are sustained following minimal trauma; they are minimally displaced and heal at a normal rate. Delayed union or nonunion are not problems. In the series of 125 fractures reported by Harris and associates there were only two cases with delayed union.[47] The fractures are managed by standard methods of treatment according to the site of fracture. The principles are the same as for a fracture of a normal bone. In the growing skeleton conservative measures are recommended. The emphasis is on restoration of alignment and an early return to normal function. Following the initial period of traction, the cast-brace technique is utilized. This functional method has diminished the duration of rigid immobilization, shortened the period of hospitalization, and permitted an early return to normal function at home and school.

Recurrent fractures of the long bones require internal fixation with intramedullary rods, especially in the adolescent nearing skeletal maturity (Fig. 3–292). A common pitfall with femoral shaft fractures is failure to assess the femoral neck region thoroughly. The possible development of progressive coxa vara should not be overlooked.

Fractures of the proximal femur—particularly of the intertrochanteric and neck regions—pose tremendous problems of management. Technical problems are not yet solved. Coxa vara and "shepherd's crook" deformity should be prevented. Lesions in the proximal femur should be closely observed. Is there progressive expansion of the intramedullary lesion? The integrity of the cortices of the femoral neck, especially the inferior, should be carefully assessed. Is there infraction? Is the lesional tissue encroaching on the capital femoral physis? One cannot overemphasize the importance of using computed tomography and bone imaging with technetium-99m to delineate the extent of the lesion. Experience with nuclear magnetic resonance imaging is limited at present, but the technique appears to be very promising for staging fibrous dysplasia.

If there is progressive Coxa vara deformity, early surgery by curettage and bone grafting is highly recommended. In certain cases one or two screws with a side plate are used for internal fixation to provide additional support. Injury to the growth plate of the femoral head should be avoided if possible. "Shepherd's crook" deformity and coxa vara are treated by valgus–medial displacement osteotomy combined with excision of the lesional tissue, bone grafting, and internal fixation. The level of the osteotomy should preferably be intertrochanteric. On occasion, when the intertrochanteric region is extensively involved and weak, the osteotomy may have to be carried out at the subtrochanteric level. In fragile bones with extensive involvement there is a tendency to settle for less than anatomic correction. The goal is to achieve overcorrection. Sometimes surgical correction should be carried out in stages—i.e., first, excise the lesion and perform the bone graft; and second, correct the deformity by osteotomy. Each case should be individualized.

Internal fixation should be stable. One may use a long AO plate with two cancellous screws into the femoral neck.[28, 59] The plate should extend below the involved area of the bone; otherwise the bone will fracture below the plate. The thin cortices do not allow stable screw fixation, and one may have to resort to a nut and bolt combination. Any disorder involving fragile bone has additional problems with rigid plate fixation. The bone underneath the plate becomes softer, and the screw holes, after removal of the plate, are stress areas with potential for recurring fracture. After the plate and screws have been removed local bone grafting of the screw holes may be indicated.

Internal fixation with an intramedullary rod (Huckstap nail) with two cancellous screws into the femoral neck or a Zickel nail may be preferable. The intramedullary nail alleviates some of the problems of the side plate, but technically it is more difficult, especially if the bone is bowed at various levels because of previous malunited fractures.

Severe angular deformities, such as genu valgum or varum, are treated by closing-wedge osteotomies, bone grafting, and internal fixation. Asymmetrical growth arrest by stapling may be considered in skeletally immature patients. Lower limb length disparity may require epiphysiodesis of the contralateral limb at the appropriate skeletal age.

Malignant transformation is treated by aggressive local resection or amputation. Radiation therapy is contraindicated, as it is of no

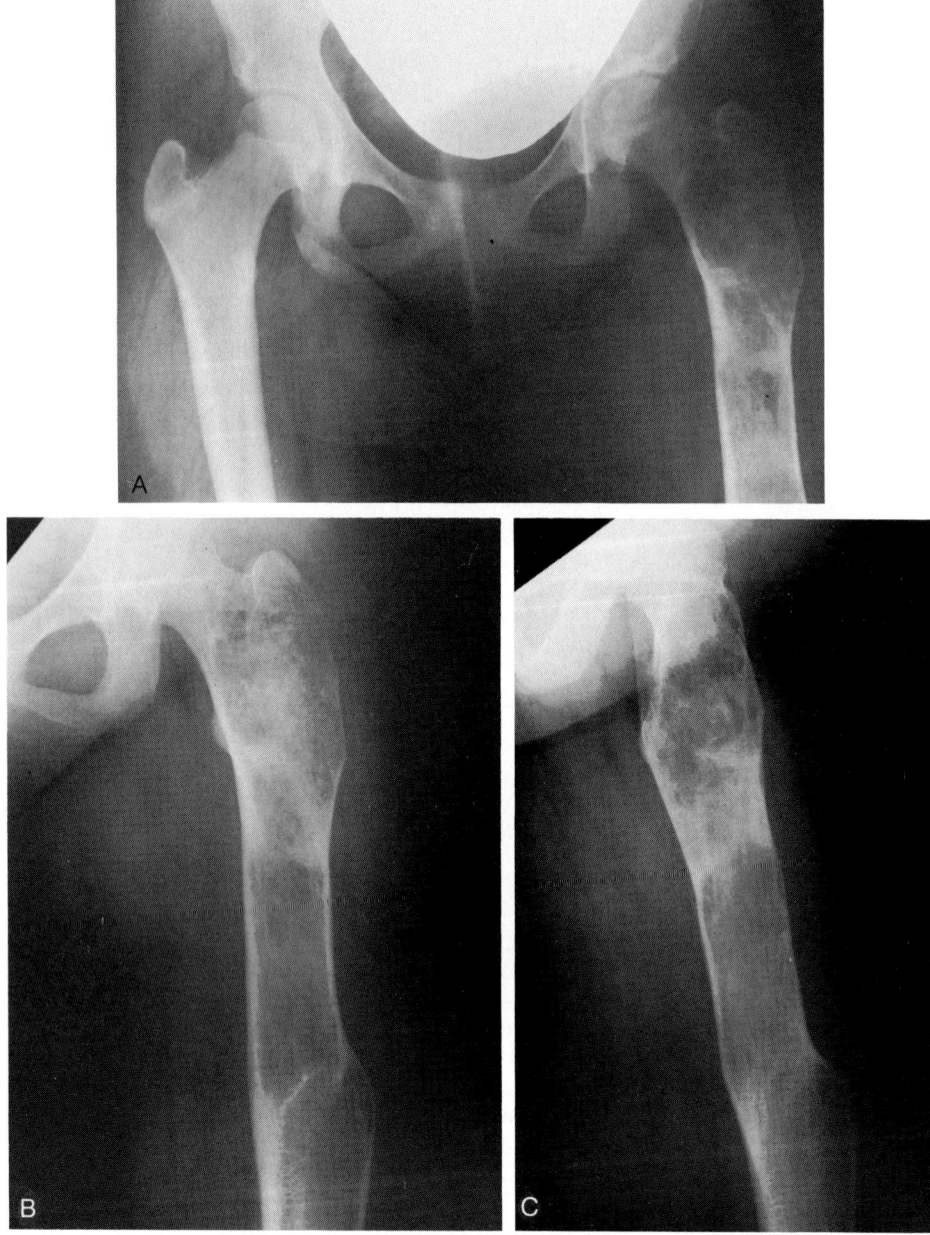

FIGURE 3–292. Multiple fibrous dysplasia of the left femur in a 13-year-old girl with pathologic fracture at the junction of the middle and distal thirds of the femoral shaft.

A to C. Preoperative radiograms.

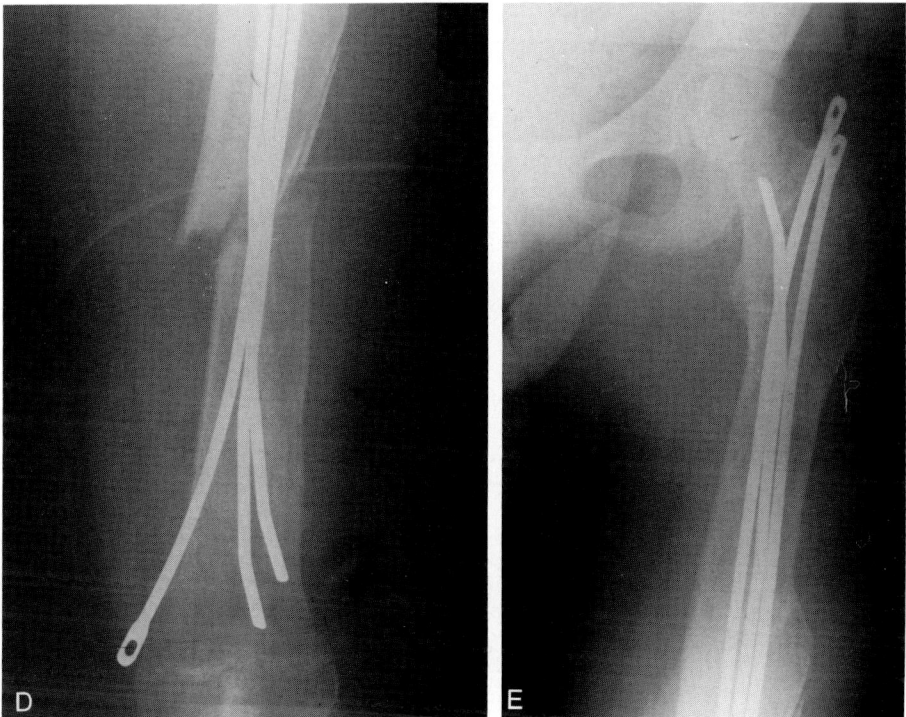

FIGURE 3–292 Continued. *Multiple fibrous dysplasia of the left femur in a 13-year-old girl with pathologic fracture at the junction of the middle and distal thirds of the femoral shaft.*

D and E. Postoperative views of the intramedullary fixation with Ender's rods.

help and may provoke malignant transformation.[2, 20, 33, 80, 86, 95, 97, 98, 105]

At present there are no drugs available to arrest the progression of the lesions in polyostotic fibrous dysplasia. The hormonal abnormalities in Albright's disease are managed by the endocrinologist.

Malignant Transformation

Sarcomatous degeneration may take place spontaneously in an exceedingly rare case, probably less than 0.5 per cent.* Atypical patterns of fibrous tissue have been reported by Cohen.[19] Persistent pain and rapid changes in the radiograms are the danger signals and should be pursued further by appropriate bone scintigraphy, computed tomography, and biopsy. Osteosarcoma is the most common neoplasm developing in fibrous dysplasia. Other malignant tumors include fibrosarcoma, chondrosarcoma, adamantinoma, and giant cell tumor.

---

*See references 2, 20, 33, 42, 52, 80, 86, 95, 97, 98, 105.

References

1. Aarskog, D., and Tveteraas, E.: McCune-Albright's syndrome following adrenalectomy for Cushing's syndrome in infancy. J. Pediatr., 73:89, 1968.
2. Abelanet, R., Forest, M., Meary, R., Languepin, A., and Tomeno, B.: Sarcomes sur dysplasie fibreuse des os. A propos d'une forme complexe hémimélique et revue de la litterature. Rev. Chir. Orthop., 61:179, 1975.
3. Albright, F.: Polyostotic fibrous dysplasia: A defense of the entity. J. Clin. Endocrinol., 7:307, 1947.
4. Albright, F., Butler, A. M., Hampton, A. O., and Smith, P.: Syndrome characterized by osteitis fibrosa disseminata, areas of pigmentation and endocrine dysfunction with precocious puberty in females. N. Engl. J. Med., 216:727, 1937.
5. Andrews, B. S., and Podolsky, S.: Thyrotrophin in Albright's syndrome with hyperthyroidism. Ann. Intern. Med., 81:561, 1974.
6. Badgley, C. E., O'Connor, S. J., and Kudner, D. F.: Congenital kyphoscoliotic tibia. J. Bone Joint Surg., 34-A:349, 1952.
7. Bamatter, F.: Dysplasie polyostotique fibreuse de Jaffe-Lichtenstein et diathèse hémorragique. Ann. Paediatr., 159:249, 1942.
8. Benedict, P. H.: Endocrine features in Albright's syndrome (fibrous dysplasia). Metabolism, 11:30, 1962.
9. Benedict, P. H.: Sex precocity and polyostotic fibrous dysplasia. Report of a case in a boy with testicular biopsy. Am. J. Dis. Child., 111:426, 1966.
10. Benjamin, D. R., and McRoberts, J. W.: Polyostotic

fibrous dysplasia associated with Cushing's syndrome. Arch. Pathol., 96:175, 1973.
11. Bonduelle, M., and Claisse, R.: Dysplasie fibreuse des os et syndrome d'Albright. Leur place nosologique. Sem. Hôp. Paris, 24:514, 1948.
12. Braunwarth, K.: Gleichzeitiges Auftreten von fibrosen Dysplasie (Jaffe-Lichtenstein) und extraossalen Fibromyxomen. Fortschr. Geb. Rontgenstr., 78:589, 1953.
13. Breck, L.: Treatment of fibrous dysplasia of bone by total femoral plating and hip nailing. A case report. Clin. Orthop., 82:82, 1972.
14. Buttner, A., and Eysholdt, K. G.: Die angeborenen Verbiegungen und Pseudoarthrosen des Unterschenkels. Ergeb. Chir. Orthop., 36:165, 1950.
15. Campanacci, M., Giunti, A., Leonossa, C., Pagni, P., and Trentani, C.: Pathological fractures in osteopathies and bony dysplasias. Ital. J. Orthop. Traumatol., 1:7, 1975.
16. Case Records of the Massachusetts General Hospital. Case 4. N. Engl. J. Med., 292:199, 1979.
17. Changus, G. W.: Osteoblastic hyperplasia of bone: Histochemical appraisal of fibrous dysplasia of bone. Cancer, 10:1157, 1957.
18. Chung, K. F., Alaghband-Zadeh, J., and Guz, A.: Acromegaly and hyperprolactinemia in McCune-Albright syndrome. Evidence of hypothalamic dysfunction. Am. J. Dis. Child., 137:134, 1983.
19. Cohen, J.: Fibrous dysplasia: Histologic study of two unusual cases. J. Bone Joint Surg., 38-A:337, 1956.
20. Coley, B. L., and Stewart, F. W.: Bone sarcoma in polyostotic fibrous dysplasia. Ann. Surg., 121:872, 1945.
21. Dabaoka, M., and Buraczewski, J.: On malignant transformation in fibrous dysplasia. Oncology, 26:369, 1956.
22. Daffner, R. H., Kirks, D. R., Gehweiler, J. A., Jr., and Heaston, D. K.: Computed tomography of fibrous dysplasia. A.J.R., 139:943, 1982.
23. Dahlin, D. C.: Bone Tumors. Springfield, Ill., Thomas, 1978.
24. Danon, M., Robboy, S. J., Kim, S., Scully, R., and Crawford, J. D.: Cushing syndrome, sexual precocity, and polyostotic fibrous dysplasia (Albright syndrome) in infancy. J. Pediatr., 87:917, 1975.
25. D'Armiento, M., Reda, G., Camagna, A., and Tardella, L.: McCune-Albright syndrome: Evidence for autonomous multi-endocrine hyperfunction. J. Pediatr., 102:584, 1983.
26. Dent, G. E., and Gertner, J. M.: Hypophosphatemic osteomalacia in fibrous dysplasia. Q. J. Med., 45:411, 1976.
27. DePalma, A., and Almad, I.: Fibrous dysplasia associated with shepherd's crook deformity of the humerus. Clin. Orthop., 97:38, 1973.
28. DePalma, A., and Dodp, P.: Reconstructive surgery in fibrous dysplasia of bone. Clin. Orthop., 19:132, 1962.
29. DePalma, A., and Smythe, U.: Recurrent fibrous dysplasia in a cortical bone graft. A case report. Clin. Orthop., 26:136, 1963.
30. Dockerty, M. B., Ghormley, R. K., Kennedy, R. L. J., and Pugh, D. G.: Albright's syndrome (polyostotic fibrous dysplasia with cutaneous pigmentation in both sexes and gonadal dysfunction in females). Arch. Intern. Med., 75:357, 1945.
31. Ehrig, U., and Wilson, D. R.: Fibrous dysplasia of bone and primary hyperparathyroidism. Ann. Intern. Med., 77:234, 1972.
32. Falconer, M. A., Cope, C. L., and Robb-Smith, A. H. T.: Fibrous dysplasia of bone with endocrine disorders and cutaneous pigmentation (Albright's disease). Q. J. Med., 11:121, 1947.
33. Feintuch, T.: Chondrosarcoma arising in a cartilaginous area of previously irradiated fibrous dysplasia. Cancer, 31:877, 1973.
34. Fevre, M.: Les pseudarthroses de jambe du nouveauné secondaires aux dystrophies kystiques congénitales. Rev. Chir. Orthop., 40:305, 1954.
35. Figarella, J.: Sur le traitement de la dysplasie fibreuse des os. Rev. Chir. Orthop., 58:Suppl. I:253, 1972.
36. Firat, D., and Stutzman, L.: Fibrous dysplasia of bone. Review of twenty-four cases. Am. J. Med., 44:421, 1968.
37. Frame, B., Azad, N., Reynolds, W. A., and Saeed, S. M.: Polyostotic fibrous dysplasia and myositis ossificans progressiva. A report of coexistence. Am. J. Dis. Child., 124:120, 1972.
38. Franghenheim, P.: Angeborene Ostitis fibrosa als Ursache einer intrauterinen Unterschenkelfraktur. Arch. Klin. Chir., 117:22, 1921.
39. Funk, F. J., and Wells, R.: Hip problems in fibrous dysplasia. Clin. Orthop., 90:77, 1973.
40. Georgiade, N., Masters, F., Horton, C., and Pickrell, K.: Ossifying fibromas (fibrous dysplasia) of the facial bones in children and adolescents. J. Pediatr., 46:36, 1955.
41. Gibson, M. J., and Middlemiss, J. H.: Fibrous dysplasia of bone. Br. J. Radiol., 44:1, 1971.
42. Gimes, B.: Malignant degeneration of fibrous dysplasia. Fortschr. Geb. Roentgenstr., 113:11, 1970.
43. Gordon, I. R. S.: Fibrous lesions of bone in childhood. Br. J. Radiol., 37:253, 1964.
44. Grabias, S. L., and Campbell, C. J.: Fibrous dysplasia. Orthop. Clin. North Am., 8:771, 1977.
45. Hackett, L. J., Jr., and Christopherson, W.: Polyostotic fibrous dysplasia. J. Pediatr., 35:767, 1949.
46. Hall, R., and Warwick, C.: Hypersecretion of hypothalamic releasing hormone: A possible explanation of the endocrine manifestation of polyostotic fibrous dysplasia (Albright's syndrome). Lancet, 1:1313, 1972.
47. Harris, W. H., Dudley, H. R., Jr., and Barry, R. J.: The natural history of fibrous dysplasia. J. Bone Joint Surg., 44-A:207, 1962.
48. Henry, A.: Monostotic fibrous dysplasia. J. Bone Joint Surg., 51-B:300, 1969.
49. Higashi, T., Iguchi, M., Shimura, A., and Kruglik, G. D.: Computed tomography and bone scintigraphy in polyostotic fibrous dysplasia. Oral Surg., 50:580, 1980.
50. Hu, L. B.: Case report 455. Polyostotic fibrous dysplasia (disseminated). Skeletal Radiol., 16:679, 1987.
51. Husband, P., and Snodgrass, G. J. A. I.: McCune-Albright syndrome with endocrinological investigations. Report of a case. Am. J. Dis. Child., 119:164, 1970.
52. Huvos, A. G.: Bone Tumors. Diagnosis, Treatment and Prognosis. Philadelphia, Saunders, 1979, pp. 9–17.
53. Huvos, A. G., Higinbotham, N. L., and Miller, T. R.: Bone sarcomas arising in fibrous dysplasia. J. Bone Joint Surg., 54-A:1047, 1972.
54. Immerkamp, M.: Die maligne Entartung bei fibroser Dysplasie. Z. Orthop., 113:331, 1975.
55. Ireland, D. C. R., Soule, E. H., and Ivins, J. C.: Myxoma of somatic soft tissues. A report of 58 patients, 3 with multiple tumors and fibrous dysplasia of bone. Mayo Clin. Proc., 48:401, 1973.
56. Jaffe, H. L.: Fibrous dysplasia of bone. A disease entity and specifically not an expression of neurofibromatosis. J. Mt. Sinai Hosp., 12:364, 1945.
57. Jaffe, H. L.: Fibrous dysplasia of bone. Bull. N.Y. Acad. Med., 22:588, 1946.
58. Jaffe, H. L.: Tumors and Tumorous Conditions of the Bones and Joints. Philadelphia, Lea & Febiger, 1958, pp. 117–142.
59. Joishy, S. K., and Morrow, L. B.: McCune-Albright

syndrome associated with a functioning pituitary chromophobe adenoma. J. Pediatr., 89:73, 1976.
60. Keyl, W.: Korrectur osteotomien an den unteren Extremitäten bei fibröser Knochendysplasie. Z. Orthop., 109:73, 1971.
61. Krogius, A.: Ein Fall von Ostitis fibrosa mit multiplen fibromyxomatosen Muskeltumoren. Acta Chir. Scand., 64:465, 1929.
62. Laporte, F., Leger, H., and Malchair, G.: Le syndrome d'Albright. J. Chir., 82:457, 1961.
63. Lemli, L.: Fibrous dysplasia of bone. Report of female monozygotic twins with and without the McCune-Albright syndrome. J. Pediatr., 91:947, 1977.
64. Lennon, D., and Houghton, N.: The McCune-Albright syndrome. Aust. Radiol., 21:69, 1977.
65. Lever, E. G., and Pettingale, K. W.: Albright's syndrome associated with a soft-tissue myxoma and hypophosphatemic osteomalacia. Report of a case and review of the literature. J. Bone Joint Surg., 65-B:621, 1983.
66. Lewin, M. L.: Fibrous dysplasia of the mandible in children. Plast. Reconstr. Surg., 25:161, 1960.
67. Lichtenstein, L.: Polyostotic fibrous dysplasia. Arch. Surg., 36:874, 1938.
68. Lichtenstein, L., and Jaffe, H. L.: Fibrous dysplasia of bone. A condition affecting one, several, or many bones, the graver cases of which may present abnormal pigmentation of skin, premature sexual development, or still other extraskeletal abnormalities. Arch. Pathol., 33:777, 1942.
69. Lick, R. F., and Viehweger, G.: Ein Beitrag zur Diagnose der fibrosen Dysplasia des Knochensystems. Fortschr. Geb. Röntgenstr., 97:33, 1962.
70. Lightner, E. S., Penny, R., and Frasier, S. D.: Growth hormone excess and sexual precocity in polyostotic fibrous dysplasia (McCune-Albright syndrome): Evidence for abnormal hypothalamic function. J. Pediatr., 87:922, 1975.
71. Logel, R. J.: Recurrent intramuscular myxoma associated with Albright's syndrome. J. Bone Joint Surg., 58-A:565, 1976.
72. McCune, D. J.: Osteitis fibrosa cystica: The case of a nine year old girl who exhibits precocious puberty, multiple pigmentation of the skin and hyperthyroidism. Am. J. Dis. Child., 52:743, 1936.
73. Mazabraud, A., and Girard, J.: Un cas particulier de dysplasie fibreuse à localisations osséuses et tendineuses. Rev. Rhum., 34:652, 1957.
74. Mazabraud, A., Semat, P., and Rose, P.: A propos de l'association de fibromyxomes des tissus mous à la dysplasie fibreuse des os. Presse Mèd., 75:2223, 1967.
75. Milgram, J. W.: Malignant transformation of polyostotic fibrous dysplasia of bone. Bull. Hosp. Joint Dis., 36:137, 1975.
76. Montoya, G., Evarts, C., and Dohn, D.: Polyostotic fibrous dysplasia and spinal cord compression. J. Neurosurg., 29:102, 1968.
77. Mouterde, P., Rigault, P., Padovani, J. P., Finidori, G., Beneux, J., Pouliquen, J. C., Jaubert, F., and Guyonvarch, G.: Les problèmes orthopédiques de la dysplasie fibreuse des os chez l'enfant. A propos de 23 observations. Chir. Pediatr., 19:169, 1978.
78. Nixon, G. W., and Condon, V. R.: Epiphyseal involvement in polyostotic fibrous dysplasia. A report of two cases. Radiology, 106:167, 1973.
79. Peck, F. B., and Sage, C. U.: Diabetes mellitus associated with Albright's syndrome. Am. J. Med. Sci., 208:35, 1944.
80. Perkinson, N. B., and Higinbotham, N. L.: Osteogenic sarcoma arising in polyostotic fibrous dysplasia. Report of a case. Cancer, 8:396, 1955.
81. Phemister, D. B., and Grimson, K. S.: Fibrous osteoma of the jaws. Ann. Surg., 105:564, 1937.
82. Pouyanne, L., Honton, J. L., Gourdon, A., and Planes, A.: Dysplasie fibreuse de l'extrémité du femur avec deformation en "houlette de berger." Bordeux Chir., 4:234, 1962.
83. Pratt, A. D., Felson, B., Wiot, J. F., and Paige, M.: Sequestrum formation in fibrous dysplasia. A.J.R., 106:162, 1969.
84. Pritchard, J. E.: Fibrous dysplasia of the bones. Am. J. Med. Sci., 222:313, 1951.
85. Reed, R. J.: Fibrous dysplasia of bone. A review of 25 cases. Arch. Pathol., 75:480, 1963.
86. Riddel, D. U.: Malignant change in fibrous dysplasia. J. Bone Joint Surg., 46-B:251, 1964.
87. Rieth, K. G., Comite, F., Shawker, T. H., and Cutler, G. B.: Pituitary and ovarian abnormalities demonstrated by CT and ultrasound in children with features of the McCune-Albright syndrome. Radiology, 153:389, 1984.
88. Rosencrantz, M.: A case of fibrous dysplasia (Jaffe-Lichtenstein) with vertebral fracture and compression of the spinal cord. Acta Orthop. Scand., 36:435, 1965.
89. Russell, L. W., and Chandler, F. A.: Fibrous dysplasia of bone. J. Bone Joint Surg., 32-A:323, 1950.
90. Samuel, S., Gilman, S., Maurer, H. S., and Rosenthal, I. M.: Hyperthyroidism in an infant with McCune-Albright syndrome: Report of a case with myeloid metaplasia. J. Pediatr., 80:275, 1972.
91. Sasen, J., and Rosenberg, R.: Neurologic complications of fibrous dysplasia of the skull. Arch. Neurol., 18:363, 1968.
92. Savage, P. E., and Stoker, D. J.: Fibrous dysplasia of the femoral neck. Skeletal Radiol., 11:119, 1984.
93. Schlumberger, H. G.: Fibrous dysplasia of single bones (monostotic fibrous dysplasia). Milit. Surg., 99:504, 1946.
94. Schlumberger, H. G.: Fibrous dysplasia (ossifying fibroma) of the maxilla and mandible. Am. J. Orthodont. and Oral Surg., 32:579, 1946.
95. Schwartz, D. T., and Alpert, M.: The malignant transformation of fibrous dysplasia. Am. J. Med. Sci., 247:350, 1964.
96. Semian, D. W., Willis, J. B., and Bove, K. E.: Congenital fibrous defect of the tibia mimicking fibrous dysplasia. A case report. J. Bone Joint Surg., 57-A:854, 1975.
97. Seth, R. S.: Fibrous dysplasia of the rib with sarcomatous change. J. Bone Joint Surg., 44-A:183, 1962.
98. Slow, I. N.: Osteogenic sarcoma arising in pre-existing fibrous dysplasia. J. Oral Surg., 29:126, 1971.
99. Spjut, H., Dorfman, H., Fechner, K., and Ackerman, L.: Tumors of Bone and Cartilage. Washington, D.C., Armed Forces Institute of Pathology, 1971, pp. 270–280.
100. Stauffer, H. M., Arbuckle, R. K., and Aegerter, E. E.: Polyostotic fibrous dysplasia with cutaneous pigmentation and congenital arteriovenous aneurysms. J. Bone Joint Surg., 23:323, 1941.
101. Sternberg, W. H., and Joseph, V.: Osteodystrophia fibrosa combined with precocious puberty and exophthalmic goiter. Am. J. Dis. Child., 63:748, 1942.
102. Stewart, M. J., Gilmer, W. S., and Edmonson, A. S.: Fibrous dysplasia of bone. J. Bone Joint Surg., 44-B:302, 1962.
103. Strasburger, P., Garber, G. S., and Hallock, H.: Fibrous dysplasia of bone. J. Bone Joint Surg., 33-A:407, 1951.
104. Stuhler, T., Brocker, W., Kaiser, G., and Poppe, H.: Fibrous dysplasia in the light of new diagnostic methods. Arch. Orthop. Trauma Surg., 94:254, 1979.
105. Sutro, C. J.: Osteogenic sarcoma of the tibia in a limb affected with fibrous dysplasia. Bull. Hosp. Joint Dis., 12:217, 1951.
106. Tanaka, T., and Suwa, S.: A case of McCune-Albright

107. Turner, A. F., Mikity, V. G., and Meyers, H. I.: Neonatal fibrous dysplasia. J. Pediatr., 62:936, 1963.
108. Uehlinger, E.: Osteofibrosis deformans juvenilis. (Polyostotische fibrose Dysplasie Jaffe-Lichtenstein.) Virchows Arch. Pathol. Anat., 306:255, 1940.
109. Valls, J., Polak, M., and Schajowicz, F.: Fibrous dysplasia of bone. J. Bone Joint Surg., 32-A:311, 1950.
110. Vines, R. H.: Polyostotic fibrous dysplasia. Arch. Dis. Child., 27:351, 1952.
111. Warrick, C. K.: Polyostotic fibrous dysplasia—Albright's syndrome. J. Bone Joint Surg., 31-B:175, 1949.
112. Warrick, C. K.: Some aspects of polyostotic fibrous dysplasia. Possible hypothesis to account for the associated endocrinological changes. Clin. Radiol., 24:125, 1973.
113. Wirth, W. A., Leavitt, D., and Enzinger, F. M.: Multiple intramuscular myxomas. Another extraskeletal manifestation of fibrous dysplasia. Cancer, 27:1167, 1971.
114. Zangeneh, F., Lulejian, G. A., and Steiner, M. M.: McCune-Albright syndrome with hyperthyroidism. Am. J. Dis. Child., 111:644, 1966.
115. Zimmer, J. F., Dahlin, D. C., Pugh, D. G., and Clagett, O. T.: Fibrous dysplasia of bone: Analysis of 15 cases of surgically verified costal fibrous dysplasia. J. Thorac. Surg., 31:488, 1956.

OSTEOFIBROUS DYSPLASIA OF THE TIBIA AND FIBULA (CAMPANACCI SYNDROME)

Osteofibrous dysplasia of the tibia and fibula is a definite pathologic entity that is exclusively confined to the tibia and fibula. It differs from fibrous dysplasia with regard to age distribution, site of occurrence, radiographic features, histology, and clinical course. It was first reported in the literature in 1921 by Frangenheim, who used the name *congenital osteitis fibrosa*.[5] Other terms used in the literature for this distinct entity are *congenital fibrous dysplasia*, *congenital fibrous defect of the tibia*, and *ossifying fibroma*.[6, 7, 9] Many cases are reported as simple fibrous dysplasia. The term *osteofibrous dysplasia* of the tibia and fibula was proposed by Campanacci because of the congenital origin of the lesion, histologic resemblance to fibrous dysplasia, and exclusive occurrence in the tibia and fibula.[1]

Age and Sex Predilection

The lesion is slightly more common in boys. It is almost always discovered in the first decade of life, before five years of age in about two thirds of the cases. Sometimes osteofibrous dysplasia is present at or shortly after birth.

Localization

The tibia is almost always involved; the ipsilateral fibula may also be affected. Very occasionally the lesion may be restricted to the fibula. Bilateral involvement is rare. The site of involvement is diaphyseal with encroachment on the metaphysis. In the tibia, it is often localized in the middle third, but proximal and distal extensions are found. Sometimes the lesion in the tibia does arise in the distal or proximal third. On rare occasions there is diffuse involvement of the entire shaft of the tibia by multiple dysplastic lesions. When osteofibrous dysplasia is limited to the fibula, the distal third of the fibular shaft is affected.

Clinical Features

The presenting complaint is localized hard swelling of the tibia, which is bowed anteriorly or anterolaterally to a varying degree. The lesion is painless when not complicated by pathologic fracture.

Radiographic Features

The characteristic finding is eccentric intracortical osteolysis with moderate or marked expansion of the external surface of the cortex, which may be very thin or eroded in places. The inner surface of the rarefied cortex is marginated by a band of sclerosis, which encroaches and narrows the medullary canal. The areas of rarefaction may be multiple, giving a "bubble" appearance, or they may be confluent (Figs. 3-293 and 3-294). In some places the rarefied osteolytic areas have a ground-glass appearance. The tibia may be bowed anteriorly or anterolaterally. Pathologic fracture may be present. In the fibula the lesion involves the whole circumference of the shaft, whereas in the tibia involvement is eccentric.

Pathology

On gross inspection at surgery the periosteum is intact. The affected cortex is thinned and may be perforated at some places. The lesional tissue is whitish-yellow or reddish in color, of soft-tissue consistency, and often slightly granular.

The histologic findings are characterized by fibrous tissue surrounding bone trabeculae bordered by active osteoblasts and zonal architecture that is best depicted when the biopsy specimen is a full-thickness wedge of tissue from the periosteum to the deep center of the lesion. Proceeding from the center of the medullary cavity toward the external surface of the cortex, the lesional tissue at the center is exclusively or predominantly fibrous with scanty, thin, and immature trabeculae of woven bone.

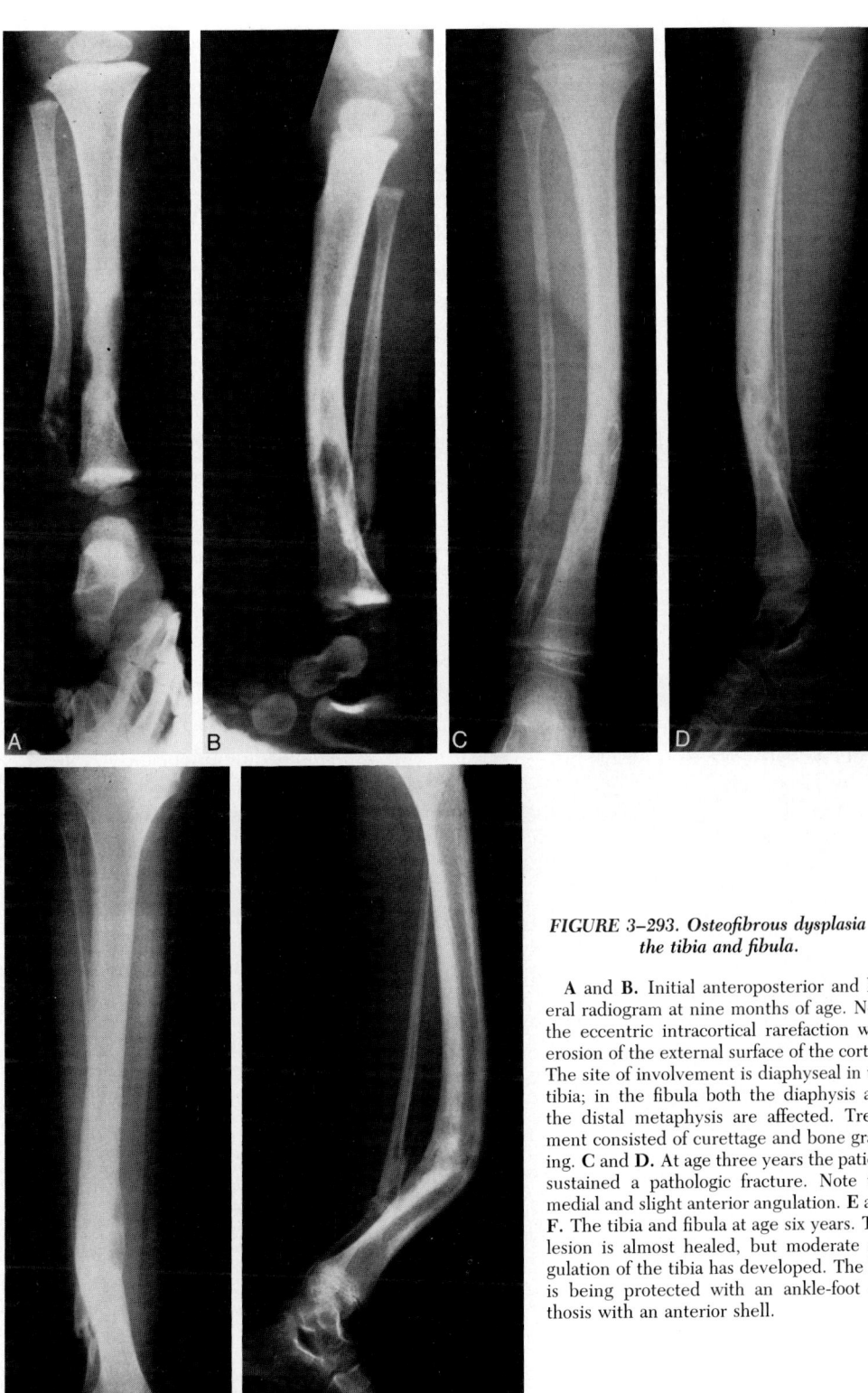

FIGURE 3-293. Osteofibrous dysplasia of the tibia and fibula.

A and **B.** Initial anteroposterior and lateral radiogram at nine months of age. Note the eccentric intracortical rarefaction with erosion of the external surface of the cortex. The site of involvement is diaphyseal in the tibia; in the fibula both the diaphysis and the distal metaphysis are affected. Treatment consisted of curettage and bone grafting. **C** and **D.** At age three years the patient sustained a pathologic fracture. Note the medial and slight anterior angulation. **E** and **F.** The tibia and fibula at age six years. The lesion is almost healed, but moderate angulation of the tibia has developed. The leg is being protected with an ankle-foot orthosis with an anterior shell.

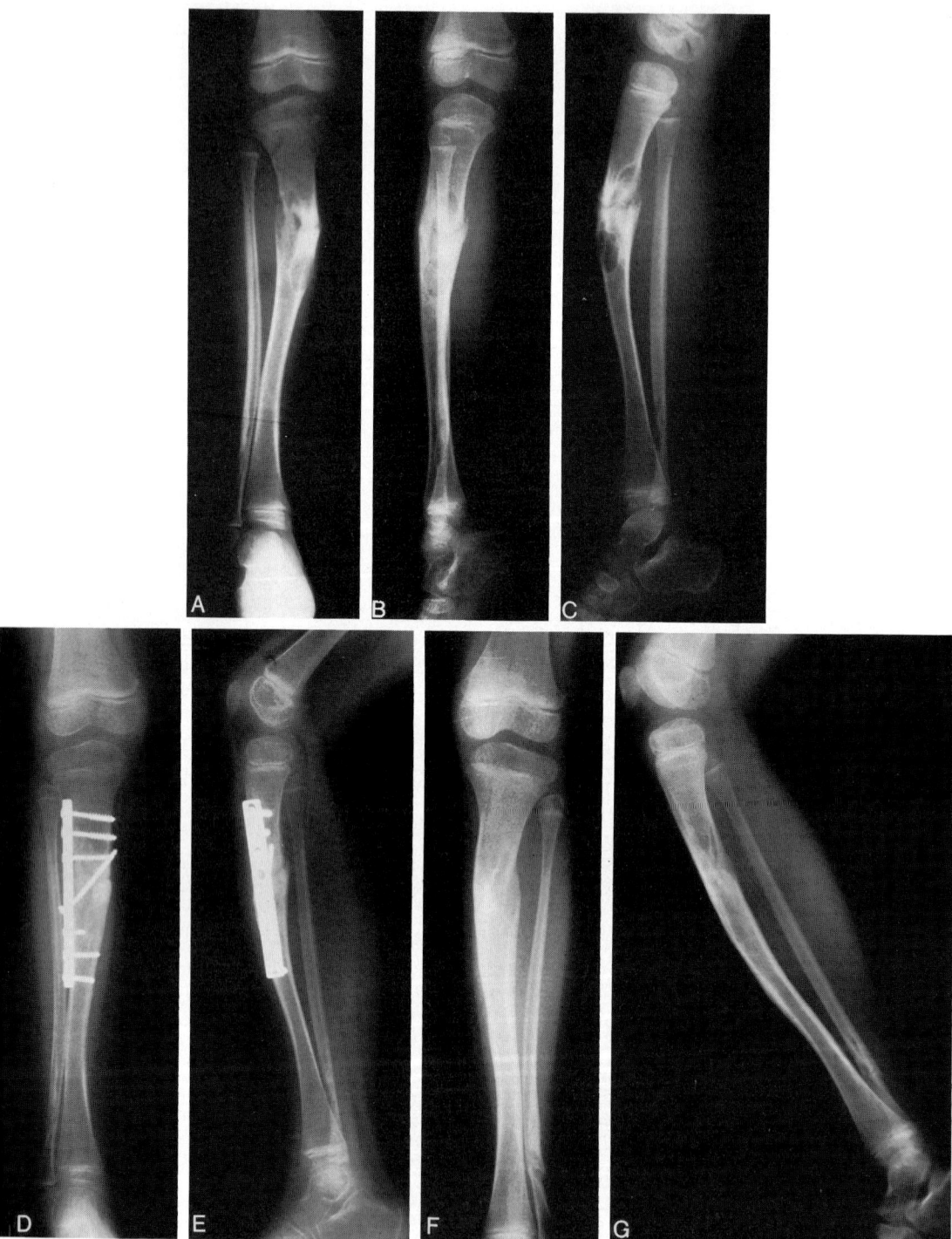

FIGURE 3–294. *Osteofibrous dysplasia of the tibia and fibula in a three-year-old girl.*

A to **C.** Anteroposterior, oblique, and lateral radiograms of the tibia and fibula. Note the typical localization of the lesion in the diaphysis of the tibia in its middle third. There is a stress fracture through the lesion of the tibia with valgus deformity. Note also the lesion in the lower third of the fibular shaft. **D** and **E.** Anteroposterior and lateral radiograms of the tibia and fibula after treatment consisting of excision of the lesional tissue by curettage, autogenous iliac bone grafting, and internal fixation. **F** and **G.** Anteroposterior and lateral radiograms of the tibia two years later showing the healed fracture. There is a small area of radiolucency in the posterior upper diaphysis of the tibia. The patient is asymptomatic.

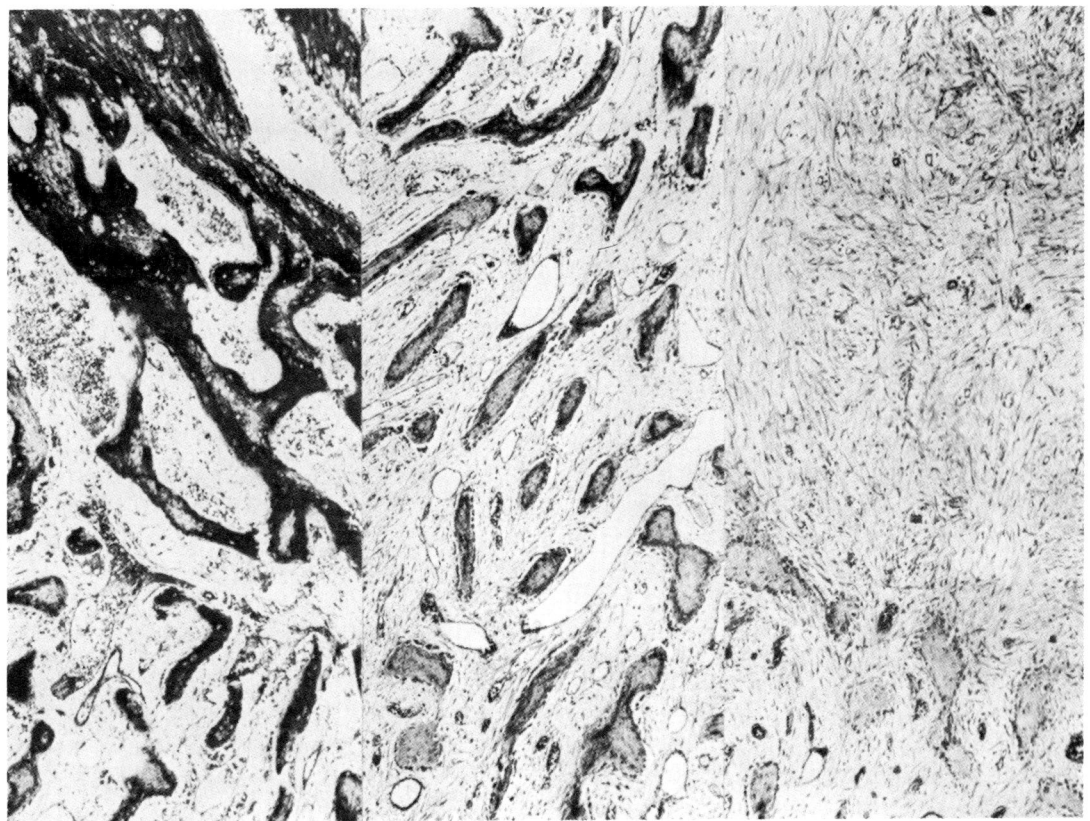

FIGURE 3–295. *Histologic findings of osteofibrous dysplasia of the tibia and fibula (Campanacci syndrome).*

Note the zonal architecture with gradual change from a loose fibrous zone in the center to cancellous cortex to the periphery (× 50). (From Campanacci, M., and Lans, M.: Osteofibrous dysplasia of the tibia and fibula. J. Bone Joint Surg., 63-A:367, 1981. Reprinted by permission.)

Toward the periphery the bone trabeculae become progressively wider, more numerous, lamellar, mature, and anastomotic (Fig. 3–295). The fibrous tissue is variably cellular, rather loose, with delicate collagen fibers, and often has a storiform pattern. There may be areas of packed collagen fibers. The fibroblasts are well differentiated. There may be numerous multinuclear giant cells, particularly at sites of hemorrhage and bone resorption. The newly formed bone trabeculae are always bordered by active osteoblasts—this is the most obvious feature distinguishing osteofibrous dysplasia from fibrous dysplasia (Fig. 3–295).

Differential Diagnosis

Monostotic fibrous dysplasia does occur in the tibia and fibula, and it should be differentiated from osteofibrous dysplasia. The two are separate distinct entities and are distinguished by the age of the patient and the clinical characteristics, radiographic features, its histology, and its clinical course.

Age. Monostotic fibrous dysplasia is usually detected after the age of ten years, whereas osteofibrous dysplasia is detected before the first decade of life, usually during the first five years.

Clinical Characteristics. In osteofibrous dysplasia the tibia is more swollen and is bowed anteriorly, whereas in monostotic fibrous dysplasia, anterior or anterolateral bowing of the tibia is rarely seen.

Radiographic Features. Osteofibrous dysplasia is characterized by its eccentric expansion, intracortical osteolysis, and deeper margin of osteosclerosis, which encroach on the medulla. Conversely, fibrous dysplasia is intramedullary in its site with a ground-glass appearance of the area of rarefaction.

Histology. In fibrous dysplasia the lesional tissue is more cellular and less mature; the bone trabeculae are woven bone and rarely ringed with osteoblasts, whereas in osteofibrous dysplasia they are characteristically bordered by active osteoblasts. Also, the bone trabeculae in osteofibrous dysplasia are a mixture of woven and lamellar bone with a zonal architectural distribution.

Clinical Course. Osteofibrous dysplasia may regress spontaneously, or continue to grow slowly or rapidly to spread to almost the entire diaphysis. Its course is difficult to predict. In fibrous dysplasia spontaneous regression rarely, if ever, takes place.[2]

Adamantinoma of the tibia may mimic osteofibrous dysplasia, but usually occurs in patients over ten years of age. The lesion contains epithelioid components seen on thorough histologic examination, its biologic performance is aggressive, running a long, indolent course, and at times it can be malignant and metastasize.

Treatment

The natural course of osteofibrous dysplasia varies; it may grow slowly or it may rapidly extend to involve the entire diaphysis, or on occasion it may regress spontaneously. Its biologic performance displays a wide spectrum of growth; the common course is one of steady moderate growth and expansion during the first five to ten years of life. Then it slows down and stops expanding after completion of skeletal growth.

Marginal subperiosteal resection or curettage in the young child is often followed by recurrence of the lesion. A wide extraperiosteal en bloc resection will presumably achieve a cure, but such a radical and disabling procedure is rarely if ever indicated. Therefore, a conservative approach is recommended.

Despite the characteristic clinical and radiographic features of osteofibrous dysplasia, after appropriate staging this author recommends open biopsy to make a definitive diagnosis. It should be noted, however, 4 of the 35 patients of Campanacci were not operated on.[2] There was no histologic confirmation of the radiographic diagnosis. After biopsy, the leg is protected in a knee-ankle-foot orthosis (KAFO) with a free ankle, drop-lock knee, and anterior shell on the anterior convexity of the leg. Pathologic fractures are treated by closed methods or by open reduction with bone grafting. This author recommends internal fixation in extensive lesions, particularly when angular deformity of the tibia is corrected at the same time. In his personal experience, delayed healing can be a problem (see Fig. 3–293).

Marginal excision of the tumor is successful in the skeletally mature patient. In the growing child, if surgical removal has to be performed because of rapid expansion of the lesion and bone destruction, it is recommended that a wide excision be performed.

References

1. Campanacci, M.: Osteofibrous dysplasia of long bones. A new clinical entity. Ital. J. Orthop. Traumatol., 2:221, 1976.
2. Campanacci, M., and Laus, M.: Osteofibrous dysplasia of the tibia and fibula. J. Bone Joint Surg., 63-A:367, 1981.
3. Campanacci, M., and Leonessa, C.: Displasia fibrosa dello scheletro. Chir. Organi Mov., 59:195, 1970.
4. Campanacci, M., Giunti, A., Leonessa, C., Pagnani, P., and Trentani, C.: Pathological fractures in osteopathies and bony dysplasias. Ital. J. Orthop. Traumatol., Suppl. 1, 1975.
5. Frangenheim, P.: Angeborene Ostitis fibrosa als Ursache einer intrauterinen Unterschenkelfraktur. Arch. Klin. Chir., 117:22, 1921.
6. Goergen, T. G., Dickman, P. S., Resnick, D., Saltzstein, S. L., O'Dell, C. W., and Akeson, S. H.: Long bone ossifying fibromas. Cancer, 39:2067, 1977.
7. Kempson, R. L.: Ossifying fibroma of the long bones. A light and electron microscopic study. Arch. Pathol., 82:218, 1966.
8. McFarland, B.: "Birth fracture" of the tibia. Br. J. Surg., 27:706, 1940.
9. Semian, D. W., Willis, J. B., and Bove, K. E.: Congenital fibrous defect of the tibia mimicking fibrous dysplasia. A case report. J. Bone Joint Surg., 57-A:854, 1975.

FIBROUS DEFECTS OF BONE

Fibrous defects of bone are common lesions in childhood, consisting of focal areas of nonspecific stroma of whorled bundles of connective tissue with a few multinuclear giant cells (Fig. 3–296). They are commonly found in the metaphyseal areas of long bones, particularly the femur and tibia. Often they are cortical in location, but can be found in cancellous bone. These fibrous lesions of bone are developmental defects due to localized disturbance of bone growth and not true neoplasms.

In the literature there is confusion as to terminology; they are referred to as fibrous cortical defects, fibrous metaphyseal defects, fibrous endosteal defects, and nonossifying or nonosteogenic fibromas.[10, 24, 44] The histologic appearance of all these lesions is similar; the difference is in their size and radiographic appearance, which reflect the varying phases of development of the same lesion. Lichtenstein proposed that small, circular or ovoid areas in the metaphysis of long bones that tend to disappear spontaneously with skeletal growth are developmental defects of ossification (i.e., fibrous defects in bone, whereas fibrous medul-

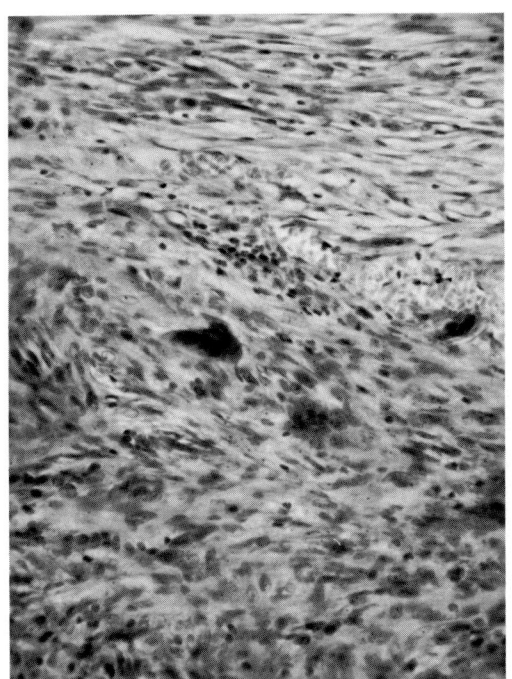

FIGURE 3–296. *Fibrocortical defect—histologic features.*

Photomicrograph showing the spindle-shaped connective tissue cells with an occasional multinucleated giant cell (× 250).

lary lesions that persist and sometimes increase in size are nonossifying fibroma.[31]

Wilner provided the following radiographic classification of fibrous lesions in bone:
Fibrous metaphyseal defect
  Fibrous cortical defect
  Fibrous endosteal defect
Fibrous metaphyseal-diaphyseal defect
  Fibrous medullary defect
    Peripheral (nonossifying or nonosteogenic fibroma)
    Central[44]

Fibrous Metaphyseal Defect

These lesions may be cortical or endosteal in their location. Their radiographic appearance is distinctive. The *fibrous metaphyseal cortical defect* presents as a sharply defined area of radiolucency eccentrically located in the metaphyseal cortex of a long bone, usually oval, its longitudinal axis lying parallel to that of the bone, and measuring 1 to 2 cm. in diameter. The inner border of the radiolucent area is sclerotic and radiopaque, and may be smooth or scalloped; the overlying cortex is thin and expanded (Fig. 3–297).

The *fibrous metaphyseal endosteal defect* is essentially a later stage in the development of a fibrous cortical defect that has persisted and grown away from the physis, measuring 2 to 4 cm. in diameter.

Historically, fibrous metaphyseal defect was first recognized by Sontag and Pyle; in their serial radiographic study of skeletal growth of 200 children they observed "cyst-like" areas of rarefaction in the distal femoral metaphysis, frequently on the medial side. Involvement was often bilateral.[43] Subsequently other radiographic and clinical studies were made by Caffey in 1955 and Selby in 1961.[10, 40]

The incidence of fibrous metaphyseal cortical defect is about 30 per cent (it was 22 per cent in girls and 53 per cent in boys in Sontag and Pyle's series of 200 children, 36.4 per cent in Caffey's series of 1000 children, and 27 per cent in Selby's study of 151 children.).[10, 40, 43]

Location. The great majority of lesions occur in the distal metaphysis of the femur, about 90 per cent of them along its medial and posterior aspect and about 10 per cent in the lateral cortex; very occasionally both medial and lateral walls of the distal femoral metaphysis are involved. The tibia is the next site of predilection (10 per cent of cases, with the proximal metaphysis of the tibia being more often affected than its distal metaphysis). Fibrous cortical defects of the tibia may be anterior, posterior, medial, or lateral in their location. In decreasing order of frequency other long bones involved are the fibula, upper femur, upper humerus, ribs, and other long bones.

Age. Fibrous metaphyseal *cortical* defect is usually found between the ages of two and eight years. Fibrous metaphyseal *endosteal* defect is detected usually in older children—between six and ten years.

Natural History. This developmental lesion usually appears near the physis, then migrates away from it with enchondral growth. In most cases it undergoes spontaneous regression, becoming smaller and indistinct and eventually disappearing within two to five years. Occasionally instead of regression the fibrous lesion may proliferate and increase in size; in such an instance it may be primarily located in the cortex and bulge into the endosteum (fibrous endosteal cortical defect), or it may extend into the medullary cavity, involving a greater portion of the width of the bone (fibrous medullary defect or nonossifying fibroma).[24]

Clinical Picture. Fibrous metaphyseal cortical defect is asymptomatic; it is an incidental finding on a radiogram taken for some other purpose. Fibrous metaphyseal endosteal defect

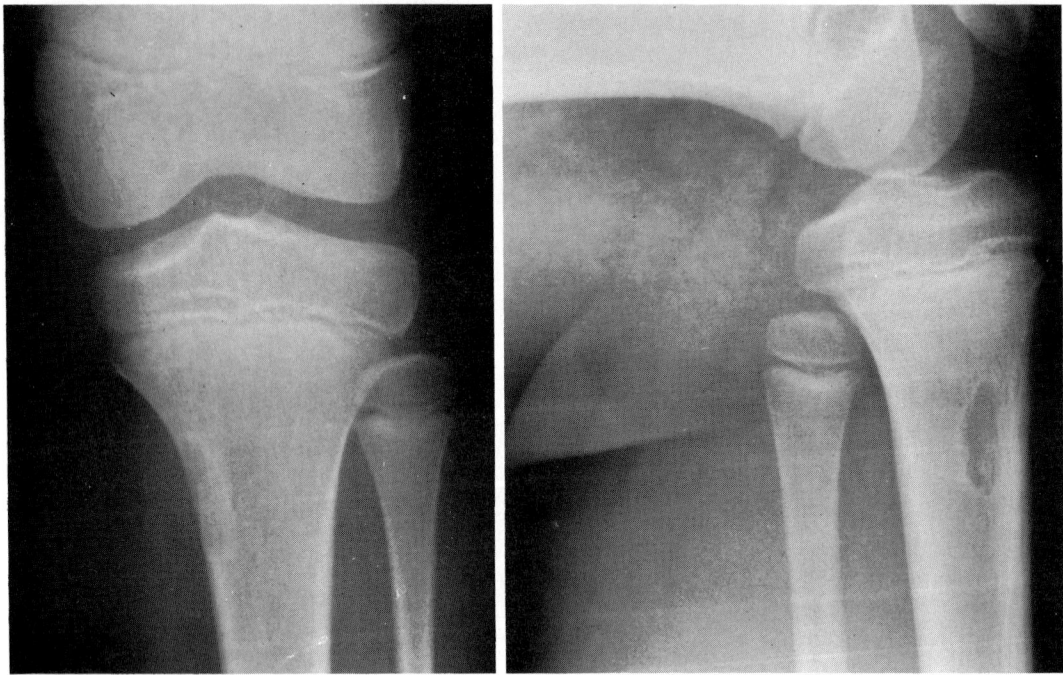

FIGURE 3-297. Fibrocortical defect of proximal tibia.

Radiograms show an oval-shaped radiolucency that is sharply defined and eccentrically located with its longitudinal axis parallel to that of the bone. The radiographic features are distinctive and a diagnostic biopsy should not be performed.

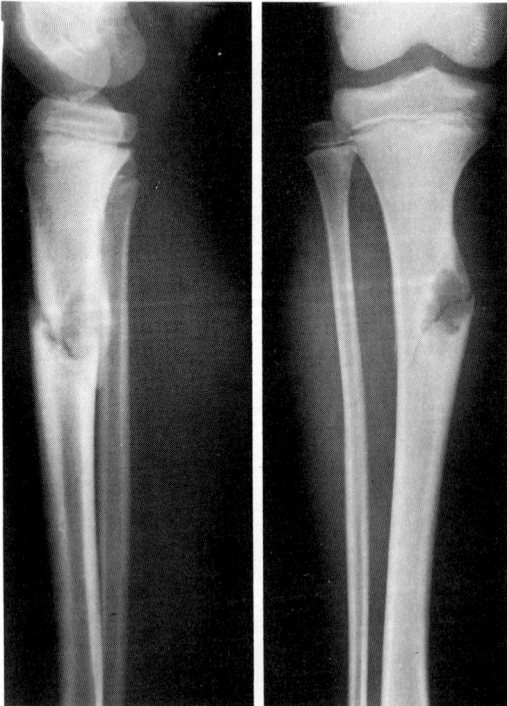

FIGURE 3-298. Pathologic fracture through a nonossifying fibroma of proximal tibia.

is usually clinically silent, occasionally it may be symptomatic, causing mild local pain and tenderness.

Fibrous Medullary Defect

Fibrous medullary defect may be symptomatic, particularly if at the site of infraction or a pathologic fracture (Fig. 3–298).

Differential Diagnosis. Fibrous metaphyseal cortical or endosteal defects have a characteristic and distinctive radiographic appearance, therefore diagnostic biopsy should not be performed. On rare occasions one should consider in the differential diagnosis juxtacortical chondroma, periosteal neurofibroma or ganglion, chronic cortical abscesses, or osteoid osteoma.

Fibrous medullary defects may mimic monostotic fibrous dysplasia, unicameral bone cyst, chondromyxoid fibroma, juxtacortical chondroma, Brodie's abscess, neurofibromatosis, and bone lesions of hyperparathyroidism.

The bone scan with technetium-99m may show a mild increase in uptake in fibrous defect of bone; in fibrous dysplasia, the uptake of the radionuclide is much more intense.

Treatment. Fibrous metaphyseal defects do not usually require treatment. The natural history of large lesions is followed by sequential radiographs. When the diagnosis is in doubt, or when there is a complication of pathologic fracture, or when the lesion is large enough to weaken the anatomic integrity of the affected bone, intralesional excision by curettage down to normal bone and filling of the defect with autogenous bone graft is indicated.

References

1. Adams, J. P., and Goldner, J. L.: Fibrous lesions of bone. South. Med. J., *46*:529, 1953.
2. Allen, D. H.: A variation of diaphyseal development which simulates the roentgen appearance of primary neoplasms of bone. A.J.R., *69*:940, 1953.
3. Barnes, G. R., Jr., and Gwinn, J. L.: Distal irregularities of the femur simulating malignancy. A.J.R., *122*:180, 1974.
4. Bhagwandeen, S.: Malignant transformation of a non-osteogenic fibroma of bone. J. Pathol. Bacteriol., *93*:562, 1966.
5. Brenner, R. J., Hattner, R. S., and Lilien, D. L.: Scintigraphic features of nonosteogenic fibroma. Radiology, *131*:727, 1979.
6. Brower, A. C.: Cortical defect of the humerus at the insertion of the pectoralis major. A.J.R., *128*:677, 1977.
7. Brower, A. C., Culver, J. E., Jr., and Keats, T. E.: Histological nature of the cortical irregularity of the medial posterior distal femoral metaphysis in children. Radiology, *99*:389, 1971.
8. Bullough, P. G., and Walley, J.: Fibrous cortical defect and non-ossifying fibroma. Postgrad. Med. J., *41*:672, 1965.
9. Burrows, H. J.: Metaphyseal fibrous defect. *In* Platt, H. S., (ed.): Modern Trends in Orthopaedics. London, Butterworth, 1950, p. 425.
10. Caffey, J.: On fibrous defects in cortical walls of growing tubular bones. Adv. Pediatr., 7:13, 1955.
11. Campbell, C. J., and Harkess, J.: Fibrous metaphyseal defect of bone. Surg. Gynecol. Obstet., *104*:329, 1957.
12. Cappell, D. F.: Endosteal fibroma of the fibula. Br. J. Surg., *22*:891, 1935.
13. Compere, C. L., and Coleman, S. S.: Nonosteogenic fibroma of bone. Surg. Gynecol. Obstet., *105*:588, 1957.
14. Cunningham, J. B., and Ackerman, L. V.: Metaphyseal fibrous defects. J. Bone Joint Surg., *38-A*:797, 1956.
15. Devlin, J. A., Bowman, H. E., and Mitchell, C. L.: Non-osteogenic fibroma of bone. J. Bone Joint Surg., *37-A*:472, 1955.
16. Evans, G. A., and Park, W. M.: Familial multiple non-osteogenic fibromata. J. Bone Joint Surg., *60-B*:416, 1978.
17. Fabris, D., Candiotto, S., Mammano, S., Ferraro, C., and Agostini, S.: Antalgic scoliosis due to nonosteogenic fibroma of the L1 neural arch: Report of a case. J. Pediatr. Orthop., *6*:103, 1986.
18. Farrow, R.: Non-osteogenic fibroma of bone. Postgrad. Med. J., *30*:206, 1954.
19. Fisette, J.: Metaphyseal fibrous cortical defect and nonossifying fibroma. J. Belge. Radiol., *43*:317, 1960.
20. Golding, C.: Radiology and orthopaedic surgery. Nonosteogenic fibroma. J. Bone Joint Surg., *48-B*:321, 1966.
21. Gordon, I. R. S.: Fibrous lesions of bone in childhood. Br. J. Radiol., *37*:253, 1964.
22. Hastrup, J., and Skov Jensen, T.: Osteogenic sarcoma arising in a nonosteogenic fibroma of bone. Acta Pathol. Microbiol. Scand., *63*:493, 1965.
23. Hatcher, C. H.: The pathogenesis of localized fibrous lesions in the metaphyses of long bones. Ann. Surg., *122*:1016, 1945.
24. Jaffe, H. L., and Lichtenstein, L.: Non-osteogenic fibroma of bone. Am. J. Pathol., *18*:205, 1942.
25. Keats, T.: The distal anterior femoral metaphyseal defect: An anatomic variant that may simulate disease. A.J.R., *121*:101, 1974.
26. Keats, T. E., Smith, T. H., and Sweet, D. E.: Craniofacial dysostosis with fibrous metaphyseal defects. A.J.R., *124*:271, 1975.
27. Kimmelstiel, P., and Rapp, I.: Cortical defect due to periosteal desmoids. Bull. Hosp. Joint Dis., *12*:286, 1951.
28. Kirkpatrick, J. A., and Wilkinson, R. H.: Post-traumatic fibrous tissue lesion distal end of femur. Parosteal (juxtacortical) desmoid. Skeletal Radiol., *2*:189, 1978.
29. Kyriakos, M., and Murphy, W. A.: Concurrence of metaphyseal fibrous defect and osteosarcoma. Report of a case and review of the literature. Skeletal Radiol., *6*:179, 1981.
30. Leonard, M. H., Hart, M. S., and Eckfeldt, R. W.: Nonossifying fibroma of bone: Successive lesions in the same tibial metaphysis. Radiology, *70*:582, 1958.
31. Lichtenstein, L.: Bone Tumors. 5th Ed. St. Louis, Mosby, 1977, p. 1942.
32. Magliato, H. J., and Nastasi, A.: Non-osteogenic fibroma occurring in the ilium. Report of a case. J. Bone Joint Surg., *49-A*:384, 1967.
33. Marek, F. M.: Fibrous cortical defect. Bull. Hosp. Joint Dis., *16*:77, 1955.
34. Maudsley, R. H., and Stansfeld, A. G.: Non-osteogenic fibroma of bone (fibrous metaphyseal defect). J. Bone Joint Surg., *38-B*:714, 1956.
35. Morton, K. S.: Bone production in non-osteogenic fibroma. An attempt to clarify nomenclature in fibrous lesions. J. Bone Joint Surg., *46-B*:233, 1964.
36. Phelan, J. T.: Fibrous cortical defect and nonosseous fibroma of bone. Surg. Gynecol. Obstet., *119*:807, 1964.

the development of a dilated and engorged vascular bed within the affected area in bone.[77-79] The possibility of an arteriovenous shunt mechanism in the causation of the vascular spaces is supported by Jaffe.[60, 62] The process is nonneoplastic–this is supported by the microscopic appearance of the lesion and the resolution of some incompletely removed cysts.[6, 31]

Age and Sex Distribution

The "cyst" occurs in older children, adolescents, and young adults; about 80 per cent of the patients are less than 20 years of age. It is very rare in children under four years of age, but can occur in infancy. There is no sex predilection.

Sites of Involvement

Aneurysmal bone cyst occurs throughout the skeleton, with the most common site being one of the long tubular bones of the limbs (about 50 per cent of reported cases); next in frequency is the vertebral column (about 20 per cent).[112] Other reported areas of involvement are the clavicle, pubic bone, innominate bone, ischium, phalanges, carpal bones, metatarsals, calcaneus talus, patella, mandible, and maxilla.*

In the long tubular bones aneurysmal bone cyst commonly involves the metaphyseal region; occasionally the diaphysis may be the location. A rapidly expanding lesion may extend into the epiphysis.[38, 58, 84]

In the spine, the lesion may be situated in the vertebral body or the posterior neural elements—pedicles, laminae, and spinous processes. The tumorous lesion may affect parts of two adjacent vertebrae. The neighboring ribs may show signs of erosion. Multiple vertebrae are involved in about 40 per cent of spinal lesions, the tumor occurring in the cervical, dorsal, or lumbar parts of the vertebral column. In the series reported by Tillman and associates four adjacent vertebrae were affected, with the presenting complaint of severe motor weakness of all four limbs.[112]

Pathology

The primary form of aneurysmal bone cyst consists of a well-limited, usually encapsulated mass of soft, friable tissue; blood may exude from a mesh of honeycomb spaces. The size of the lesion varies; it may be as large as 12 by 8 by 4 cm. or as small as 2 by 2 by 1.5 cm. The ratio of tissue to spaces varies. The lesion is usually contained within a thin subperiosteal shell of new bone. On curetting the "cyst" wall, one obtains reddish-brown soft tissue.

On microscopic examination there are variable numbers of small or large anastomosing channels or spaces, lined by delicate or thick fibrous walls that lack the elastic lamina and muscle layer found in blood vessels (Fig. 3–299). The channel walls may have a complete or incomplete lining of endothelial cells. The fibrous walls contain foreign-body giant cells, granules of hemosiderin, and long thin strips of osteoid tissue or immature bone trabeculae.

Some of the cavernomatous spaces may envelop lakes of blood, which may be under pressure; other spaces may contain blood-tinged fluid or even clear fluid. Focal organizing blood clots may be present.

The secondary aneurysmal bone cyst shows the same histologic features and findings as the primary form; however, on thorough examination of the lesion the presence of another entity coexisting with aneurysmal bone cyst is found.

Clinical Features

Local pain of several weeks' or months' duration is the presenting complaint. If the affected bone is superficial a tender swelling may be palpable. A bruit may be transmitted from a large aneurysmal bone cyst. When the lesion is near the end of a long bone, some degree of stiffness and pain in the adjacent joint is common. With progressive enlargement of an aneurysmal bone cyst in the vertebral column, compression of the cord or nerve roots may cause neurologic deficit, such as motor weakness and sensory disturbance in the limbs. If the lesion is in the lumbar region, there may be loss of bladder and bowel control.

Radiographic and Imaging Findings

The radiographic findings vary with the maturity and location of the lesion. Radiographically aneurysmal bone cyst develops through the following three progressive stages: first it begins in the cancellous portion of the medullary bone and is confined by the cortex. In this initial stage the radiographic appearance is that of an ovoid or round area of increased radiolu-

---

*See references: clavicle, 96; pubic bone, 48; innominate bone, 53; ischium, 15; phalanges, 24, 40, 43; carpal bones, 80; metatarsals, 16, 42; calcaneus, 57; talus, 108; patella, 109; mandible, 9, 35, 72; maxilla, 41, 75.

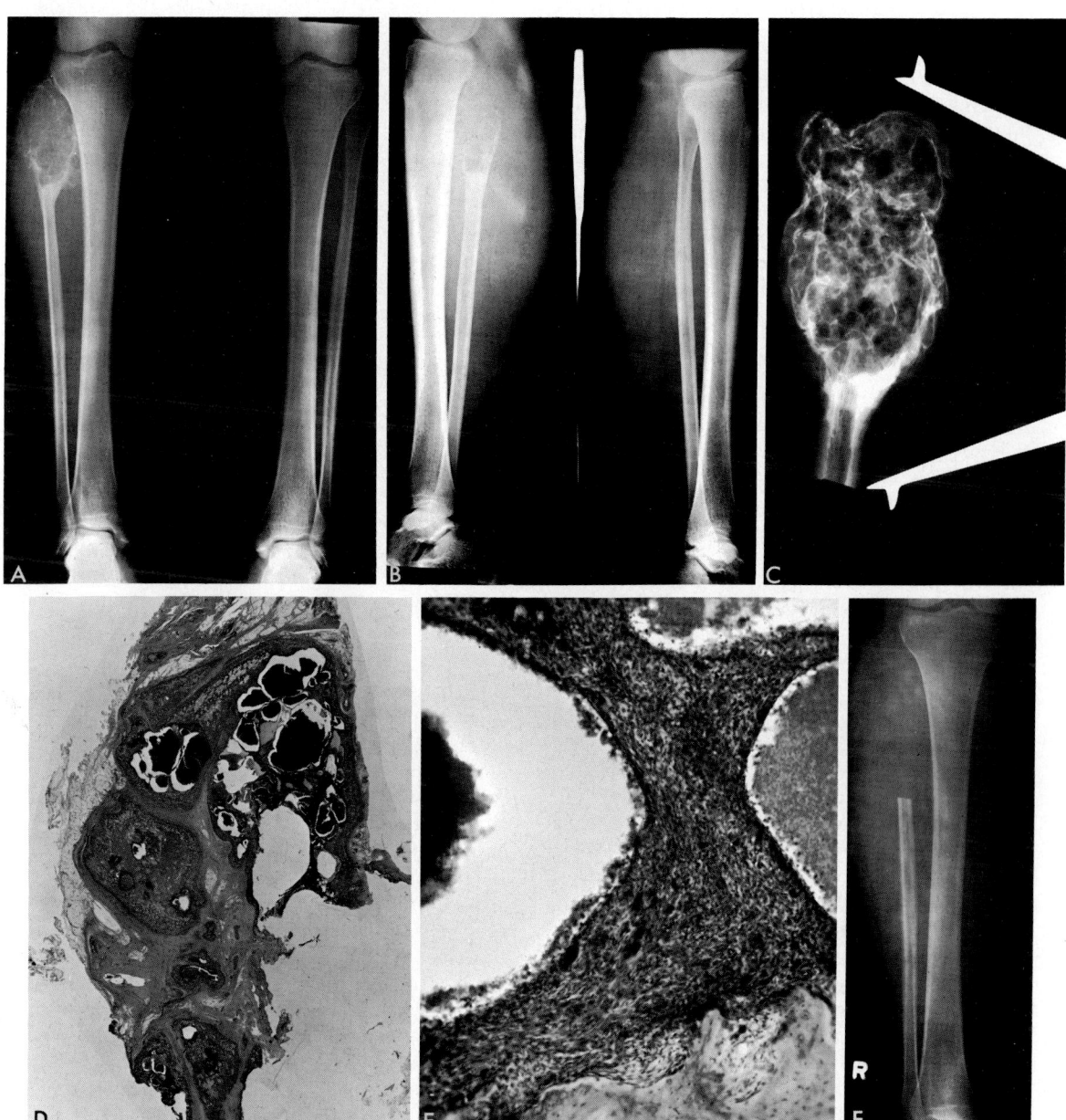

FIGURE 3-299. Aneurysmal bone cyst of proximal fibula.

A and **B**. Radiograms showing "blown-out" radiolucency of upper end of fibula involving epiphyseal and metaphyseal areas. **C**. Radiogram of resected specimen. **D**. Photomicrograph of gross specimen showing the large multilocular blood spaces lined with fibrous wall tissue, which contain collections of multinuclear giant cells, hemosiderin, xanthomatous cells, and trabeculae of osteoid tissue ($\times$ 10). **E**. Photomicrograph of a part of the fibrous wall ($\times$ 100). Note the fibroblasts, giant cells, hemosiderin, and newly-formed bone trabeculae. **F**. Postoperative radiogram showing that about one third of the proximal fibula has been resected.

cency with varying degrees of expansion and thinning of the regional cortex from within. Second, the aneurysmal bone cyst becomes eccentric, raises the periosteum, and shows the characteristic expansile "soap-bubble" or "blown-out" area of radiolucency. The distended area is contained within an "eggshell" covering of subperiosteal bone with an ill-defined inner margin and usually without marginal sclerosis. Within the lesion there is no significant mineralization, but multiple fine irregular septa may be found. The elevation of the periosteum may result in laminated layers of subperiosteal new bone formation (Codman's triangle) at the junction of the cyst with the diaphyseal side of the long bone. Finally, with progressive expansion the lesion seems to explode, the continuity of its shell of subperiosteal bone is lost, and it extends into soft tissue. Infractions or fractures are not uncommon.

Radiographically, the activity of aneurysmal bone cyst is, according to Capanna and associates, classified as *inactive*—complete periosteal shell with the intraosseous margin defined by a sclerotic rim of reactive bone; *active*—incomplete periosteal shell and a sharply defined intraosseous border, or *aggressive*—no evidence of reparative osteogenesis, no periosteal shell, and an ill-defined endosteal margin.[20, 21]

The location of the lesion may produce certain radiographic changes. In the long bones it appears as an area of eccentric radiolucency in the metaphysis, which gradually enlarges into a ballooned extracortical mass outlined by subperiosteal new bone formation, often with a raised triangle of layered subperiosteal new bone (Codman's triangle). Aggressive aneurysmal bone cysts have the potential for crossing the growth plate and disturbing growth.[20, 22, 39, 84] Physeal cartilage is a relative but not absolute barrier to tumor extension. Such invasion of the physis is more common in adolescents near completion of growth. Capanna and associates studied 198 cases of aneurysmal bone cyst in the files of the Istituto Orthopedico Rizzoli, Bologna, Italy. In this series 39 cases were juxtaepiphyseal, i.e., the aneurysmal bone cyst occurred in a long bone adjacent to an open growth plate. Of these 39 cases, ten patients were 13 or more years of age, and seven of these ten cases (70 per cent) showed obvious invasion of the growth plate on the plain radiograph. Of the 29 patients who were less than 13 years of age, only 2 (7 per cent) had invasion of the physis.[20]

In the short *tubular bones* the lesion is more central, and it extends into the diaphysis and

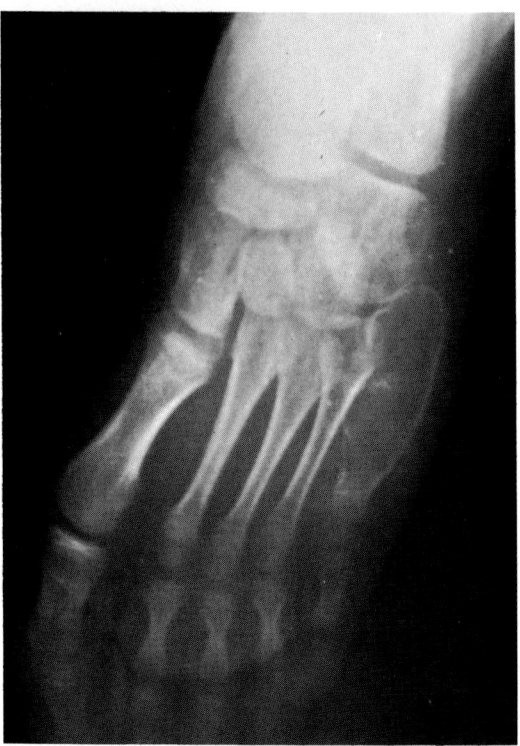

FIGURE 3–300. *Aneurysmal bone cyst of the fifth metatarsal.*

subarticular region—this is explained by the small size of the bones and its occurrence in older patients near completion of growth (Fig. 3–300). Fractures were frequently seen in the short tubular bones. In *flat bones* the bone and its cortices are thin—therefore, cortical erosion and soft-tissue extension are commonly found. In the *spine* the lesion appears to be quite aggressive, frequently with expansion and osteolysis of adjacent vertebrae and sometimes of the ribs; the spinal cord and nerve roots may be compressed. Although there is a definite predilection for the lumbar spine, any level of the spinal column may be affected.[55] The posterior elements of a vertebra (the pedicles, transverse process, laminae, and spinous process) are more frequently involved than the vertebral body. Linear tomography and computed tomography are of particular value in delineating the extent of vertebral involvement. When there is evidence of cord compression, nuclear magnetic resonance imaging should be carried out. Angiography will show staining and pooling of the dye within the cystic area. Arteriography is of no value in differential diagnosis, but it is helpful in delineating the extent of the lesion. The indistinct pools of contrast medium reflect the sinusoidal distribution of the thin-walled vascular spaces. Selective arterial catheterization may be employed to determine the blood supply to the spinal cord and the extent of the mass.[81]

Scintigraphy. Bone imaging with technetium-99m shows increased activity associated with aneurysmal bone cyst, predominantly around the periphery of the cyst; it is less in the center. Some scintigrams disclose diffuse, more or less homogenous increased uptake throughout the lesion. In a study of scintigrams of 25 aneurysmal bone cysts, Hudson found increased activity in every case. In 22 of them, the activity was correlated with the true pathologic extent of the lesions; in these 22 cases the pattern of uptake extended beyond the true tumor margins. Scintigraphy is recommended prior to biopsy when the diagnosis of a lesion is still unknown; it is of limited value in delineating the extent of a known aneurysmal bone cyst; in such instances computed and linear tomography and nuclear magnetic resonance imaging are of more value.[59]

Diagnosis

Diagnosis of aneurysmal bone cyst should be made *by open, not closed, biopsy*. It is crucial to rule out underlying lesions and secondary aneurysmal bone cyst by careful pathologic studies of adequate tissue.

In the differential diagnosis one should consider the following *benign* lesions: histiocytosis (eosinophilic granuloma), osteoblastoma, simple or unicameral bone cyst, fibrous dysplasia, and unusual giant cell tumors. Because of the aggressive features of aneurysmal bone cyst, one often suspects *malignant tumors*: these include telangectic osteosarcoma, fibrosarcoma, fibrous histiocytoma, and secondary metastases such as neuroblastoma. *Infections* in bone such as hydatic disease, tuberculosis, and fungal lesions may simulate aneurysmal bone cyst in the radiogram.

Treatment

Surgical excision or curettage of the lesion and packing of the defects with bone graft, preferably autogenous, are the best treatment. Total excision or resection of the lesion may be performed in selected sites such as the rib, fibula, patella, or a carpal bone. In the spine when the lesion involves only the transverse or spinous process, resection is the procedure of choice; curettage is recommended for more central lesions. When aneurysmal bone cyst threatens the integrity of the spinal cord, decompression is performed as an emergency measure. Vertebral body lesions are best approached through an anterior approach. In unstable lesions stabilization of the spine may be indicated.

Radiation alone is not recommended because of the possible development of postirradiation sarcoma. Tillman and associates reported six cases of aneurysmal bone cyst developing postirradiation sarcoma, three of which were in the spine.[112] Radiation myelopathy is another complication that may occur at a rate as high as 2.9 per cent after radiotherapy of the spine.[94] In aggressive lesions that are surgically inaccessible or when complete curettage of the lesion is too risky one may consider a combination of surgery with low-dosage irradiation therapy (cobalt)—less than 1500 rads; the parents and patient should be informed of its potential for provoking malignant transformation and the complication of postirradiation myelopathy.

In biopsy and curettage of aneurysmal bone cyst of the long and short tubular bones, the growth plate is identified radiographically to avoid injury, growth arrest, and premature fusion. Without surgical trauma to the growth plate, risk of subsequent growth disturbance is 10 per cent in cases with no preoperative physeal extension. An important technical detail is to pack the bone graft subperiosteally.

Complications. These include the development of sarcomatous change, especially after irradiation therapy; structural deformation of the affected area (kyphosis or scoliosis in the spine, varus, valgus, or recurvatus deformity around joints; growth arrest (partial or complete) with resultant limb length disparity; and infection.

Recurrence occurs in 10 to 20 per cent of cases of aneurysmal bone cyst. The chance of recurrence diminishes with increasing age of affected patients and aggressive surgical removal. When there is persistent radiolucency of a lesion that is asymptomatic and not increasing in size, it is observed without surgical intervention. Some of these incompletely removed lesions resolve in time. One should not jump into surgery or radiation therapy. If the radiolucent areas increase in size and show aggressive activity, repeat curettage and bone grafting are recommended. Cortical in addition to cancellous bone graft should be used. On the whole, the prognosis of aneurysmal bone cyst is excellent, with cure in 90 to 95 per cent of cases.

References

1. Aegerter, E., and Kirkpatrick, J.: Orthopedic Diseases. 4th Ed. Philadelphia; Saunders, 1975, pp. 424–433.
2. Agrillo, U., Vangelista, S., and Chiappetta, F.: Cervical aneurysmal bone cyst. Case report. J. Neurosurg. Sci., 25:235, 1981.
3. Amidio, C., De Serio, N., Monastero, A., and Sensale, F.: Personal studies on ionizing radiotherapy and topical intracavitary corticosteroid treatment of aneurysmatic bone cysts. Minerva Med., 73:2829, 1982.
4. Angerpointer, T., Engert, J., Konrad, E., and Meister, P.: Malignant degeneration of aneurysmal bone cysts in childhood. Z. Kinderchir., 26:143, 1979.
5. Barbier, C. H.: Aneurysmal bone cyst of the hand. An unusual situation. J. Hand Surg., 9-B:89, 1984.
6. Barnes, R.: Aneurysmal bone cyst. J. Bone Joint Surg., 38-B:301, 1956.
7. Beeler, J. W., Helman, C. H., and Campbell, J. A.: Aneurysmal bone cyst of the spine. J.A.M.A., 163:914, 1957.
8. Benoit, B.: Les kystes osseux anévrysmal du rachis. J. Med. Lyon, 44:330, 1961.
9. Berry, M., Krishan, A., and Bhargava, S.: An aneurysmal bone cyst of the mandible. A case report. Aust. Radiol., 17:196, 1973.
10. Besse, B. E., Dahlin, D. C., Pugh, D. G., and Ghormley, R. K.: Aneurysmal bone cyst: Additional considerations. Clin. Orthop., 7:93, 1956.
11. Bieder, C.: Le kyste anévrysmal des os. Paris, Thèse, 1961, p. 642.
12. Biesecker, J. L., Marcove, R. C., Huvos, A. G., and Mike, V.: Aneurysmal bone cysts. A clinicopathologic study of 66 cases. Cancer, 26:615, 1970.
13. Billings, K. J., and Werner, L. G.: Aneurysmal bone cyst of the first lumbar vertebra. Radiology, 104:19, 1972.
14. Bloodgood, J. C.: Benign bone cysts, ostitis fibrosa, giant-cell sarcoma, and bone aneurysm of the long pipe bones. Ann. Surg., 52:145, 1910.
15. Bonakdarpour, A., Levy, W. M., and Aogerter, E.: Primary and secondary aneurysmal bone cyst: A radiological study of 75 cases. Radiology, 126:75, 1978.
16. Booher, R. J.: Aneurysmal bone cyst of a metatarsal. J. Bone Joint Surg., 39-A:435, 1957.
17. Buraczewski, J., and Dabska, M.: Pathogenesis of aneurysmal bone cyst. Relationship between the aneurysmal bone cyst and fibrous dysplasia of bone. Cancer, 28:597, 1971.
18. Burkhalter, W. C., Schroeder, F. C., and Eversmann, W. W., Jr.: Aneurysmal bone cysts occurring in the metacarpals. A report of three cases. J. Hand Surg., 3:579, 1978.
19. Canlorbe, P.: Kyste anévrysmal de l'atlas. Arch. Fr. Pediatr., 18:809, 1961.
20. Capanna, R., Springfield, D. S., Biagini, R., Ruggieri, P., and Giunti, A.: Juxtaepiphyseal aneurysmal bone cyst. Skeletal. Radiol., 13:21, 1985.
21. Capanna, R., Albisinni, U., Picci, P., Calderoni, P., Campanacci, M., and Springfield, D. S.: Aneurysmal bone cyst of the spine. J. Bone Joint Surg., 67-A:527, 1985.
22. Carlson, D. H., Wilkinson, R. H., and Bhakkaviziam, A.: Aneurysmal bone cysts in children. A.J.R., 116:644, 1972.
23. Cedar, C., Rainaut, J. -J.: Le kyste anévrysmal de l'os. Ann. Chir., 19:1104, 1965.
24. Chalmers, J.: Aneurysmal bone cysts of the phalanges. A report of three cases. Hand, 3:296, 1981.
25. Chateau, R., Fau, R., Groslambert, R., and Perret, J.: A propos d'un cas de kyste anévrysmal de la 4 vertèbre cervicale. Rev. Neurol., 11:468, 1964.
26. Clough, J. R., and Price, C. H. G.: Aneurysmal bone cysts. Review of twelve cases. J. Bone Joint Surg., 50-B:116, 1968.
27. Clough, J. R., and Price, C. H. G.: Aneurysmal bone cysts: Pathogenesis and long term results of treatment. Clin. Orthop., 97:52, 1973.
28. Cremer, H., and Munzenberg, K. J.: Aneurysmatic osseous cyst with malignant course (author's transl.). Z. Orthop., 118:225, 1980.
29. Cruz, M., and Coley, B. L.: Aneurysmal bone cyst. Surgery, 103:67, 1956.
30. Dabezias, E. J., D'Ambrosia, R. D., Chuinard, R. G., and Ferguson, A. B.: Aneurysmal bone cyst after fracture. J. Bone Joint Surg., 64-A:617, 1982.
31. Dabska, M., and Buraczewski, J.: Aneurysmal bone cyst. Pathology, clinical course and radiological appearances. Cancer, 23:371, 1969.
32. Dahlin, D. C.: Bone Tumors. 3rd Ed. Springfield, Ill., Thomas, 1978. p. 370.
33. Dahlin, D. C., and McLeod, R. A.: Aneurysmal bone cyst and other nonneoplastic conditions. Skeletal. Radiol., 8:243, 1982.
34. Dahlin, D. C., Besse, B. E., Pugh, D. G., and Ghormley, R. K.: Aneurysmal bone cysts. Radiology, 64:56, 1955.
35. Daugherty, J. W., and Eversole, L. R.: Aneurysmal bone cyst of the mandible: Report of a case. J. Oral Surg., 29:737, 1971.
36. DeSantos, L. A., and Murray, J. A.: The value of arteriography in the management of aneurysmal bone cysts. Skeletal. Radiol., 2:137, 1978.
37. Donaldson, W. F., Jr.: Aneurysmal bone cyst. J. Bone Joint Surg., 44-A:25, 1962.
38. Dyer, R., Stelling, C. B., and Fechner, R. E.: Epiphyseal extension of an aneurysmal bone cyst. A.J.R., 137:172, 1981.
39. Edling, N. P.: Is the aneurysmal bone cyst a true pathologic entity? Cancer, 18:1127, 1965.
40. El-Khoury, G., and Seaman, R. W.: Case report 125; Aneurysmal bone cyst terminal phalanx of the first toe. Skeletal Radiol., 5:201, 1980.
41. Ellis, D. J., and Walters, P. J.: Aneurysmal bone cyst of the maxilla. Oral Surg., 34:26, 1972.
42. Erseven, A., Garti, A., and Weigl, K.: Aneurysmal bone cyst of the first metatarsal bone minicking malignant tumor. Clin. Orthop., 181:171, 1983.
43. Ewald, F. C.: Bone cyst in a phalanx of a two-and-a-half-year-old child. Case report and discussion. J. Bone Joint Surg., 54-A:399, 1972.
44. Faris, W. F., Rubin, B. D., and Fielding, J. W.: Aneurysmal bone cyst of the patella. A case report. J. Bone Joint Surg., 60-A:711, 1978.
45. Faure, C., Boccon-Gibod, L., Herve, J., and Pernin, P.: Case report 154. Aneurysmal bone cyst of L2. Skeletal Radiol., 6:229, 1981.
46. Fry, V. G., and van Dellen, J. R.: Aneurysmal bone cysts of the spine. S. Afr. Med. J., 58:211, 1980.
47. Fuhs, S. E., and Herndon, J. H.: Aneurysmal bone cyst involving the hand. A review and report of two cases. J. Hand Surg., 4:152, 1979.
48. Garnjobst, W., and Hopkins, R.: Aneurysmal bone cyst of pubis. Report of a case presenting as an abdominal mass. J. Bone Joint Surg., 49-A:971, 1967.
49. Ginsberg, L. D.: Congenital aneurysmal bone cyst. Case report with comments on the role of trauma in the pathogenesis. Radiology, 110:175, 1974.
50. Godfrey, L. W., and Gresham, G. A.: The natural history of aneurysmal bone cyst. Proc. R. Soc. Med., 52:900, 1959.
51. Gunterberg, B., Kindblom, L. -G., and Laurin, S.: Giant cell tumor of bone and aneurysmal bone cyst: A correlated histologic and angiographic study. Skeletal Radiol., 2:65, 1977.
52. Guy, R., Raymond, O., and Samson, R., et al.:

Aneurysmal bone cyst. J. Can. Assoc. Radiol., 7:40, 1956.
53. Haberman, E. T., Cabot, W., and Smith, H. S.: Aneurysmal bone cyst of the pelvis. An unusual case presentation. Bull. Hosp. Joint Dis., 35:151, 1974.
54. Hadders, H. N., and Oterdoom, H. J.: The identification of aneurysmal bone cyst with hemangioma of the skeleton. J. Pathol. Bacteriol., 71:193, 1956.
55. Hay, M. C., Paterson, D., and Taylor, T. K. F.: Aneurysmal bone cysts of the spine. J. Bone Joint Surg., 60-B:406, 1978.
56. Henley, F. T., and Ricketts, G. L.: Aneurysmal bone cyst presenting as a chest mass. Radiology, 92:1103, 1969.
57. Hertzanu, Y., Mendelsohn, D. B., and Gottschalk, F.: Aneurysmal bone cyst of the calcaneus. Radiology, 151:51, 1984.
58. Hooper, J. C.: Aneurysmal bone cyst penetrating the tibial epiphysis after curettage. Med. J. Aust., 1:200, 1971.
59. Hudson, T. M.: Scintigraphy of aneurysmal bone cysts. A.J.R., 142:761, 1984.
60. Jaffe, H. L.: Aneurysmal bone cyst. Bull. Hosp. Joint Dis., 11:3, 1950.
61. Jaffe, H. L.: Tumors and Tumorous Conditions of the Bones and Joints. Philadelphia; Lea & Febiger, 1958, pp. 54–62.
62. Jaffe, H. L., and Lichtenstein, L.: Solitary unicameral bone cyst with emphasis on the roentgen picture, the pathologic appearance and the pathogenesis. Arch. Surg., 44:1004, 1942.
63. Jereb, B., and Smith, J.: Giant aneurysmal bone cyst of the innominate bone treated with irradiation. Br. J. Radiol., 53:489, 1980.
64. Kaernbach, A., Strecker, E. P., and Schafer, J. H.: Aggressive aneurysmale Knochencyste der Wirbelsaule im Kindesalter. Radiologe, 18:279, 1978.
65. Kagan, E. M., and Klimova, M. K.: Anevrizmaticheskie kisty kostei. Vestn. Rentgenol. Radiol., 40:3, 1965.
66. Kaufman, R. A., and Towbin, R. B.: Telangiectatic osteosarcoma simulating the appearance of an aneurysmal bone cyst. Pediatr. Radiol., 11:102, 1981.
67. Kimmelman, C. P., Potsic, W. P., and Schut, L.: Aneurysmal bone cyst of the sphenoid in a child. Ann. Otol. Rhinol. Laryngol., 91:339, 1982.
68. Klumper, A. von: Differentialdiagnose aneurysmatische Knochenzyste und nicht ossifizierendes Fibrom. Fortschr. Geb. Röntgenstr., 127:261, 1977.
69. Kokino, M. J., Baskir, O., Cakmak, M., and Domanic, U.: Resection of a giant aneurysmal bone cyst and replacement by a massive autogenous bone graft (author's transl.). Rev. Chir. Orthop., 66:467, 1980.
70. Koskinen, E. V. S., Visuri, T. I., Holmstrom, T., and Roukkula, M. A.: Aneurysmal bone cyst: Evaluation of resection and of curettage in 20 cases. Clin. Orthop., 118:136, 1976.
71. Kozlowski, K., and Middleton, R. W.: Aneurysmal bone cysts—review of 10 cases. Aust. Radiol., 24:170, 1980.
72. Kozlowski, K., Masel, J., Sprague, P., Tamaela, L., Kan, A., and Middleton, R.: Mandibular and paramandibular tumors in children. Report of 16 cases. Pediatr. Radiol., 11:183, 1981.
73. Kubicz, S.: Aspect radiologique du kyste osseux anévrysmal chez l'enfant. Ann. Radiol., 13:211, 1970.
74. Lapeyrie, M., Picard, J. J., and Pous, J. G.: Le kyste anévrysmal des os. Problèmes diagnostiques et thérapeutiques. A propos de 6 observations. Rev. Chir. Orthop., 6:375, 1951.
75. Le Jeune, F. E., and Bordelon, J. P.: Aneurysmal bone cyst of the maxillary antrum. Eye Ear Nose Throat Mon., 49:216, 1970.
76. Levy, W. M., Miller, A. S., Bonakdarpour, A., and Aegerter, E.: Aneurysmal bone cyst secondary to other osseous lesions. Report of 57 cases. Am. J. Clin. Pathol., 63:1, 1975.
77. Lichtenstein, L.: Aneurysmal bone cyst. A pathological entity commonly mistaken for giant cell tumor and occasionally for hemangioma and osteogenic sarcoma. Cancer, 3:279, 1950.
78. Lichtenstein, L.: Aneurysmal bone cyst. Further observations. Cancer, 6:1228, 1953.
79. Lichtenstein, L.: Aneurysmal bone cyst. Observations on 50 cases, J. Bone Joint Surg., 39-A:873, 1957.
80. Lin, E., Engel, J., Bubis, J. J., and Herman, O.: Aneurysmal bone cyst of the hamate bone. J. Hand Surg., 9-A:847, 1984.
81. Lindblom, A., Soderberg, G., Spjut, H. J., and Sundquist, O.: Angiography of aneurysmal bone cyst. Acta Radiol., 55:12, 1961.
82. MacCarthy, O. S., Dahlin, D. C., Doyle, J. B., Jr., Lipscomb, P. R., and Pugh, D. G.: Kystes osseux anévysmal du rachis. J. Neurosurg., 18:671, 1961.
83. MacPherson, R. I.: Aneurysmal bone cyst of spine diagnosed by percutaneous opacification. J. Can. Assoc. Radiol., 31:210, 1980.
84. McCarthy, S. M., and Ogden, J. A.: Epiphyseal extension of an aneurysmal bone cyst. J. Pediatr. Orthop., 2:171, 1982.
85. McQueen, M. M., Chalmers, J., and Smith, G. D.: Spontaneous healing of aneurysmal bone cysts. J. Bone Joint Surg., 67-B:310, 1985.
86. Makhija, M. C.: Bone scanning in aneurysmal bone cyst. Clin. Nucl. Med., 6:500, 1981.
87. Malta, de Schott, P. C.: Cisto osseo aneurismatico. Treatise, University of Rio de Janeiro, 1970.
88. Marks, R. D., Jr., Scruggs, H. J., Wallace, K. M., and Fenn, J. O.: Megavoltage therapy in patients with aneurysmal bone cysts. Radiology, 118:421, 1976.
89. Mayer, L., and Kestler, O. C.: Aneurysmal bone cyst of spine. Bull. Hosp. Joint Dis., 5:16, 1944.
90. Mole, L., Beugnet, O., Peter, R., and Forster, E.: Kyste anévrysmal de l'os. A propos de deux observations. J. Radiol. Electrol., 43:921, 1962.
91. Murphy, W. A., Strecker, E. B., and Schoenecker, P. L.: Transcatheter embolisation therapy of an ischial aneurysmal bone cyst. J. Bone Joint Surg., 64-B:166, 1982.
92. Nezelof, C., Michel, J., and D'Amato, J.: Le kyste anévrysmal de l'os. Ses principaux caractères anatomoradiologiques. A propos de 6 observations personelles. Rev. Chir. Orthop., 46:369, 1960.
93. Nobler, M. P., Higinbotham, N. L., and Phillips, R. F.: The cure of aneurysmal bone cyst. Irradiation superior to surgery in an analysis of 33 cases. Radiology, 90:1185, 1968.
94. Palmer, J. J.: Radiation myelopathy. Brain, 95:109, 1972.
95. Parrish, F. F., and Pevey, J. K.: Surgical management of aneurysmal bone cyst of the vertebral column. A report of three cases. J. Bone Joint Surg., 49-A:1597, 1967.
96. Pointu, J., Kehr, P., Sejourne, P., Mathevon, H., Destree, G., and Lang, G.: Aneurysmal cyst of the clavicle: An uncommon lesion and a difficult diagnosis (author's transl.). Sem. Hôp. Paris, 58:1141, 1982.
97. Poolos, P. N., and White, R. J.: Aneurysmal bone cyst of the cervical spine: A twelve-year follow-up after surgical treatment. Surg. Neurol., 14:259, 1980.
98. Prakash, B., Banerji, A. K., and Tandon, P. N.: Aneurysmal bone cyst of the spine. J. Neurol. Neurosurg. Psychiatry, 36:112, 1973.
99. Pullan, C. R., Alexander, F. W., and Halse, P. C.: Aneurysmal bone cyst. A report of three cases. Arch. Dis. Child., 53:899, 1978.
100. Reed, R. J., and Rothenberg, M.: Lesions of bone that may be confused with aneurysmal bone cyst. Clin. Orthop., 35:150, 1964.

101. Rigault, P., Beneux, J., and Desvignes, P.: Le kyste anévrysmal des os chez l'enfant. A propos de 16 cas. Ann. Pediatr., 19:223, 1972.
102. Ring, S. M., Beranbaum, E. R., Madayag, M. A., et al.: Angiography of aneurysmal bone cyst. Bull. Hosp. Joint Dis., 33:1, 1972.
103. Roukkula, M., and Salovaara, E.: Aneurysmal bone cyst of the fourth thoracic vertebra with compression of the spinal cord. Acta Radiol., 57:373, 1962.
104. Ruiter, D. J., Russel, T. G., and Van Der Velde, E. A.: Aneurysmal bone cysts. A clinicopathological study of 105 cases. Cancer, 39:2231, 1977.
105. Sapexa, P. S.: Aneurysmal bone cyst. J. Indian Med. Assoc., 63:95, 1974.
106. Sherman, R. S., and Soong, K. Y.: Aneurysmal bone cyst: Its roentgen diagnosis. Radiology, 68:54, 1957.
107. Slowick, F. A., Jr., Campbell, C. J., and Kettelkamp, D. B.: Aneurysmal bone cyst. An analysis of thirteen cases. J. Bone Joint Surg., 50-A:1142, 1968.
108. Soreff, J.: Aneurysmal bone cyst of the talus. Acta Orthop. Scand., 47:358, 1976.
109. Srivastava, K. K., Ahuja, S. C., and Kochhar, V. L.: Aneurysmal bone cyst of the patella. Aust. N.Z. J. Surg., 43:54, 1973.
110. Taylor, F. W.: Aneurysmal bone cyst. J. Bone Joint Surg., 38-B:293, 1956.
111. Thompson, P. C.: Subperiosteal giant-cell tumor. Ossifying subperiosteal hematoma. Aneurysmal bone cyst. J. Bone Joint Surg., 36-A:281, 1954.
112. Tillman, B. P., Dahlin, D. C., Lipscomb, P. R., and Stewart, J. R.: Aneurysmal bone cyst: An analysis of ninety-five cases. Mayo Clin. Proc., 43:478, 1968.
113. Verbiest, H.: Giant-cell tumours and aneurysmal bone cysts of the spine with special reference to the problems related to removal of the vertebral body. J. Bone Joint Surg., 47-B:699, 1965.
114. Vicenzi, G.: Familial incidence in two cases of aneurysmal bone cyst. Ital. J. Orthop. Traumatol., 7:251, 1981.
115. Volkov, M. V., and Berszhnoi, A. P.: Aneurysmal spinal cysts in children. Ortop. Travmatol. Protez., 8:54, 1982.
116. West, A., and Polito, M. A.: Aneurysmal bone cyst in the foot. Report of a case and review. J. Am. Podiatry Assoc., 71:446, 1981.
117. Winter, A., and Firtel, S.: Aneurysmal bone cyst of vertebra with compression symptoms. A case report. J.A.M.A., 177:870, 1961.
118. Yadav, S. S., Aurora, A. L., Sharma, S., Thomas, S., and Rajagopal, N.: Multicentric aneurysmal bone cyst (report of a case). Indian J. Cancer, 19:116, 1982.

UNICAMERAL BONE CYST

This not uncommon benign lesion is a true bone cyst consisting of a single cavity (unicameral) lined with a thin membrane and containing straw-colored fluid. A disease of the growing skeleton, it occurs at an age between early childhood and adolescence and is predominant in males with a 2:1 male to female ratio.

Sites of Involvement

In about 50 per cent of cases the unicameral bone cyst is located in the proximal metaphyseal region of the humerus. The next most common site is the femur (frequently the upper part); more than 75 per cent of all unicameral bone cysts occur in the proximal humerus and femur. In the younger patient the humerus is a more common location than the femur. Next in frequency of involvement are the proximal tibia and the upper or lower end of the fibula. Occasionally it is encountered in the calcaneus, rib, scapula, patella, radius, ulna, metacarpal, or metatarsal.* These rare sites of involvement are usually in the older age group. In patients over 17 years of age, 52 per cent of unicameral bone cysts have a predilection for the calcaneus and the pelvis.

The lesion is characteristically solitary. Two unicameral bone cysts in the same patient, one in the proximal humerus and one in the distal tibia, are reported by Sadler and Rosenhain.[84]

Etiology

Since Bloodgood's classic article on cystic lesions in bone, extensive literature has been published on the subject, but the exact cause is yet undetermined.[7] Several theories have been proposed. Pommer postulated that intramedullary hemorrhage produces the solitary cyst. A fibrous wall encapsulates the blood, acting as a semipermeable membrane as it draws the fluid into the cavity. The increasing pressure causes erosion of the surrounding cancellous osseous tissue and thinning of the cortex.[76]

Von Mikulicz proposed that the cyst results from a hiatus in the physeal plate produced by mechanical injury.[104]

Jaffe and Lichtenstein postulated that the unicameral bone cyst seems to stem from a localized failure of ossification in the metaphyseal area during periods of rapid growth.[42]

Johnson and Kindred pointed out in their study of the anatomy of bone cysts that the lining of the cyst wall is composed of various primitive mesenchymal elements, and they suggested that the cysts originate from dysplastic tumorlike tissue.[44]

Cohen proposed that the cause of the cyst is blockage of the circulation and drainage of the interstitial fluid in rapidly growing bone. He based this theory of the pathogenic mechanism on the finding that the chemical constituents of the fluid in simple bone cysts were similiar to those of serum.[16, 17] Further evidence of venous obstruction was obtained by Cohen by injecting contrast medium into unicameral bone cysts in two patients. The contrast medium exuded

---

*See references: calcaneus, 1, 3, 21, 47, 56, 96, 97, 103; rib, 94; scapula, 27, 28; radius, 50, 71; ulna, 101.

through the walls of the cyst when low injection pressure was used.[17] It seems that the most probable etiology of unicameral bone cyst is venous obstruction caused by a developmental abnormality.

Cohen's hypothesis is further supported by the reports of three cases in which unicameral bone cysts were inadvertently discovered while under development.[9, 105] The cysts developed within a period of two to four years at sites of benign lesions that had the radiographic appearance of calcified cartilage rests or nonossifying fibromas. They occurred during growth periods at sites of extensive bone remodeling. Thus three stages of cyst development may be postulated: first, formation of a form of fibrous tissue in an area of rapid resorption of bone; second, blockage of sinusoidal vessels with subsequent accumulation of interstitial fluid in the fibrous tissue; and third, equilibration of the cyst fluid with that in the unblocked vessels, giving it characteristics similar to those of serum plasma. Once the process of cyst formation begins, the cystic cavity enlarges.

Chigira and associates measured the internal pressure of sample bone cysts and found it to be higher than the normal pressure of the bone marrow in the contralateral limb. The oxygen tension of the cyst fluid was markedly lower than that of either venous or arterial blood measured simultaneously. The cysts were treated by multiple drilling. The pressure within them gradually decreased as the number of drill holes increased. The clinical outcome in seven cases treated by the multiple drilling method was excellent;[14] Kuboyama and associates also reported that repeated percutaneous drilling was highly effective in the treatment of unicameral bone cysts. These results give further evidence that venous obstruction is the most probable primary cause of the unicameral bone cyst.[52]

Pathology

At operation, on exposure of the cyst, the cortex of the tumor will be found to be "eggshell" thin, the wall having a bluish sheen due to the color of the contained fluid seen through the translucent cortex. When the cortex is opened, a straw-colored fluid will escape. If there has been a recent fracture, this fluid may be hemorrhagic or serosanguineous. The cystic cavity is unilocular unless, disturbed by repeated pathologic fractures, it will be partitioned by fibrous septa. The walls of the cyst may have bony ridges. The cavity is lined by a thin connective tissue membrane that is usually several millimeters in thickness and reddish-brown in color.

The histologic appearance is not pathognomonic. The membrane consists of connective tissue in which are dispersed macrophages, giant cells, a granular yellowish-brown pigment of hemosiderin, and xanthoma cells (Fig. 3–301). Lipid is manifest under the microscope as fusiform, sharp-pointed crystals. One may also encounter reactive bone tissue or spicules of immature bone from a healing fracture in the wall of the cyst.

Clinical Findings

The cyst may be asymptomatic and discovered incidentally when radiograms are made for some other reason, such as a chest x-ray. Occasionally, there may be complaints of vague discomfort.

Often the cyst is discovered incidentally following trauma with resultant infraction or fracture through it. Usually there is little noticeable evidence of local pain until this occurs. An antalgic limp when the lesion is present in the upper portion of the femoral shaft may serve to draw attention to it.

Radiographic and Imaging Findings

Radiograms disclose an expanding radiolucent lesion that is vaguely trabeculated (Figs. 3–302 and 3–303); it may be ridged, however, giving an appearance of pseudoloculation. The cyst is located centrally in the proximal or distal metaphyseal-diaphyseal region of a long bone, adjacent to or abutting the metaphyseal side of the physis and extending for about 3 to 5 cm. A band of cancellous bone is usually present between the growth plate and the cyst. The cyst enlarges in the long axis of the bone. Depending on its duration and the extent of its growth, the cyst's distance from the physis varies. The growth plate is usually not violated; occasionally, however, the physis may be traversed, and the cyst may extend into the epiphysis (Fig. 3–304).

The cortex of the cystic area is thinned from its inner surface. In the humerus cortical thinning is symmetrical, whereas in the upper end of the femur it is lateral and the calcar is often spared.

If a fracture has occurred, its line is either transverse or oblique, but usually there is no great displacement at the fracture site even if continuity is disrupted. Periosteal reaction

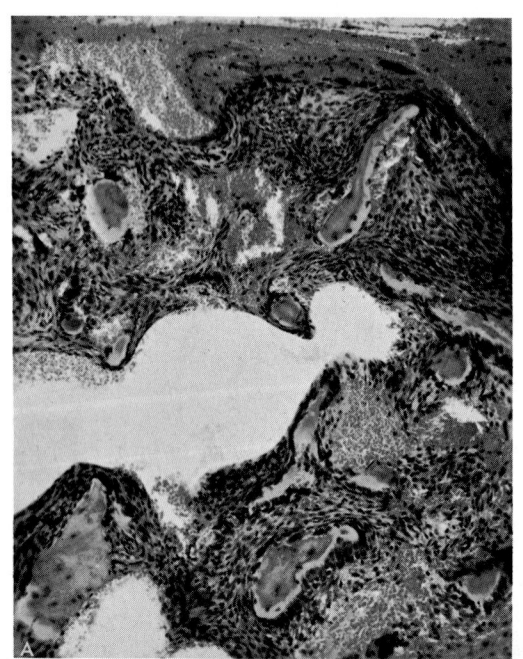
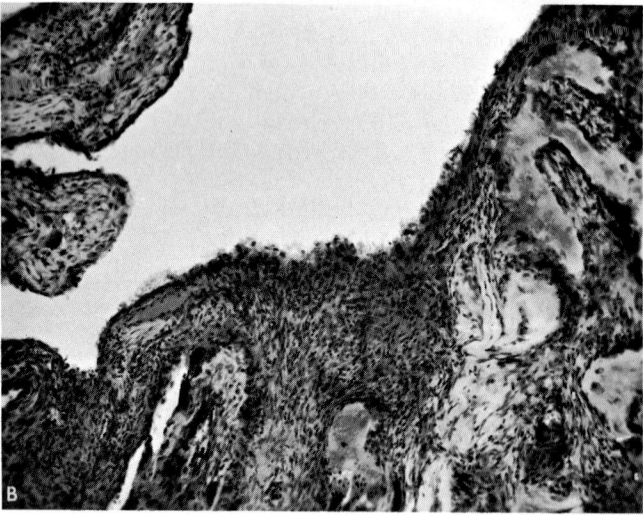

FIGURE 3–301. Histologic appearance of unicameral bone cyst.

Photomicrograph of section through the wall. **A.** × 100. **B.** × 250. Note the living membrane consisting of granulating connective tissue with macrophages, giant cells, and spicules of reactive bone. On top of the section there is a layer of fibrin and old blood.

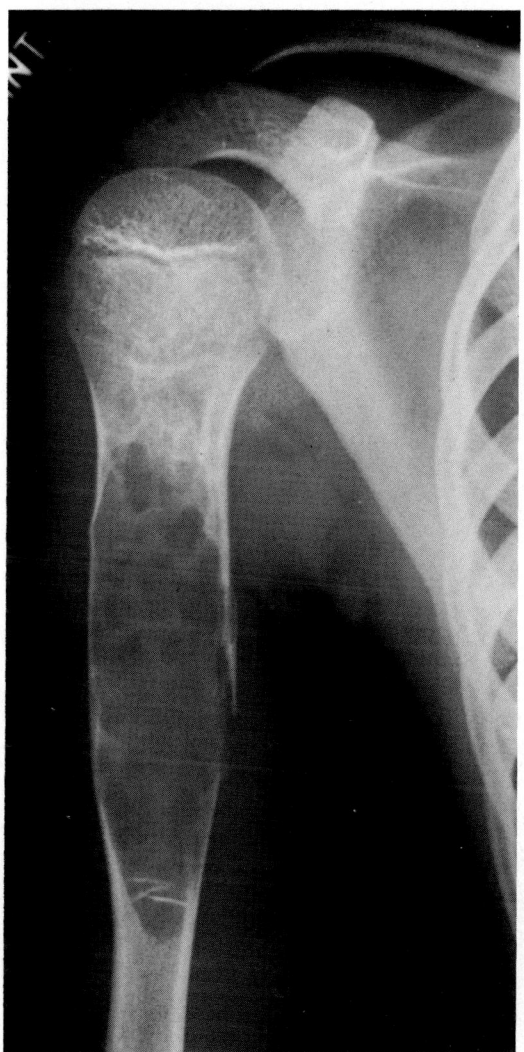

FIGURE 3–302. *A large unicameral bone cyst of proximal right humerus.*

The cortex is thinned from its intramedullary surface. There is an infraction of its medial cortex.

forms layers of new bone. Cysts of long standing partly fill in through a process of osteofibrosis. Occasionally complete spontaneous reconstitution occurs, particularly after repeated fractures.

The "fallen fragment sign" described by Reynolds may assist in the radiographic diagnosis of unicameral bone cyst. Following a pathologic fracture a fragment of the bony cortex may be dislodged and fall to the dependent portion of the fluid-filled cystic cavity. The fluid contained in the cyst permits gravitational displacement of the cortical fragment. In solid lesions gravitational migration of such fragments is prevented.[80]

Computed tomography is of great value in distinguishing the density of fluid from that of solid tumors. This author uses the CT scan routinely and highly recommends it for radiographic differential diagnosis.

In uncomplicated unicameral bone cyst the bone scan with technetium-99m will be normal or show minimal diminution of uptake. When a pathologic fracture occurs, it will, during its healing stage, show increased uptake of the radionuclide.

Cysts that abut the physis are classified as *active*, retaining growth potential. Cysts that have "migrated" away from the metaphysis with skeletal growth are classified as *latent*. Active cysts are considered more likely to recur.[32, 35, 42, 100] Norman and Schiffman found the recurrence rate to be 32 per cent for children under ten years of age, but only 10 per cent for patients over ten years old. In their series, of the 11 cysts that recurred, only 6 were within 1 cm. of or abutted the physis, the remaining 5 were in the diaphysis.[72] Spence and associates reported 8.3 years as the mean age of patients who had recurrences.[98, 99] It is evident that the age of the patient (over or under ten years) is a factor to be considered in predicting recurrence.

Differential Diagnosis

The principal radiographic finding that confirms the clinical picture is the large centrally located radiolucent area in the affected shaft. The regional cortex is thinned, and there is a slight increase in the bony contour. Radiographic appearance and clinical observations are usually adequate for definitive diagnosis; the following possibilities should be considered, however, and can be differentiated by such factors as location, age of the patient, and pathologic findings.

If the "blowout" distention typical of *aneurysmal bone cyst* is not present in the x-ray picture, its possibility can most probably be eliminated. Furthermore, the solitary bone cyst is centrally located, in contrast to the eccentrically located aneurysmal bone cyst. Confusion may arise when a blood clot or large spaces filled with blood or both are found on histologic examination of a solitary bone cyst that has sustained a recent fracture.

Eosinophilic granuloma may be distinguished by the clinical presence of pain; its location, which is more likely to be near the middle of the shaft than near the end; its size, as it is usually not as large as a solitary bone cyst; the presence of a large amount of subperiosteal new

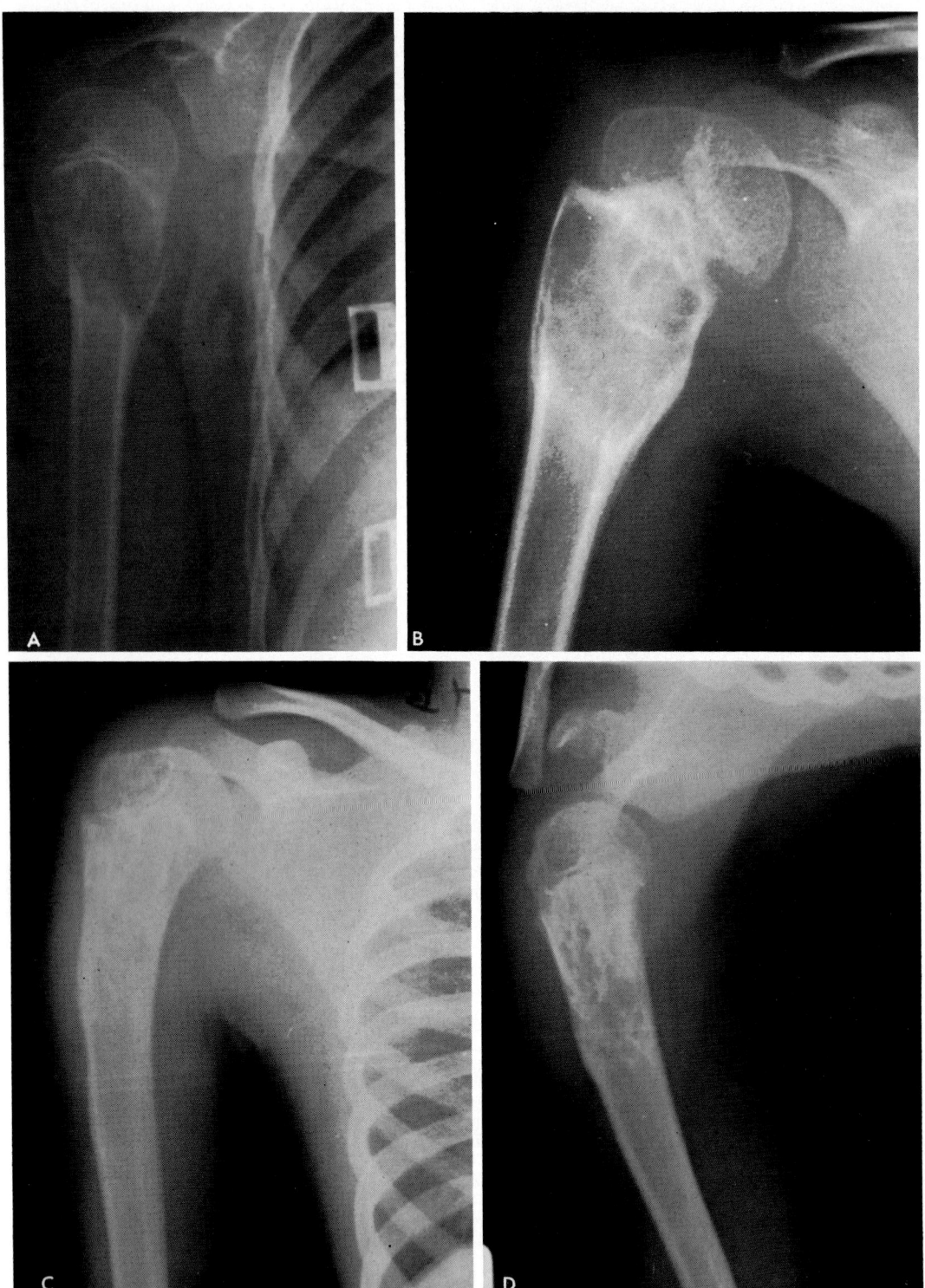

FIGURE 3–303. Unicameral bone cyst in proximal humerus.

A and **B.** Preoperative radiograms showing healing of pathologic fracture. **C** and **D.** Postoperative radiograms. The lesion has healed following curettage and bone grafting.

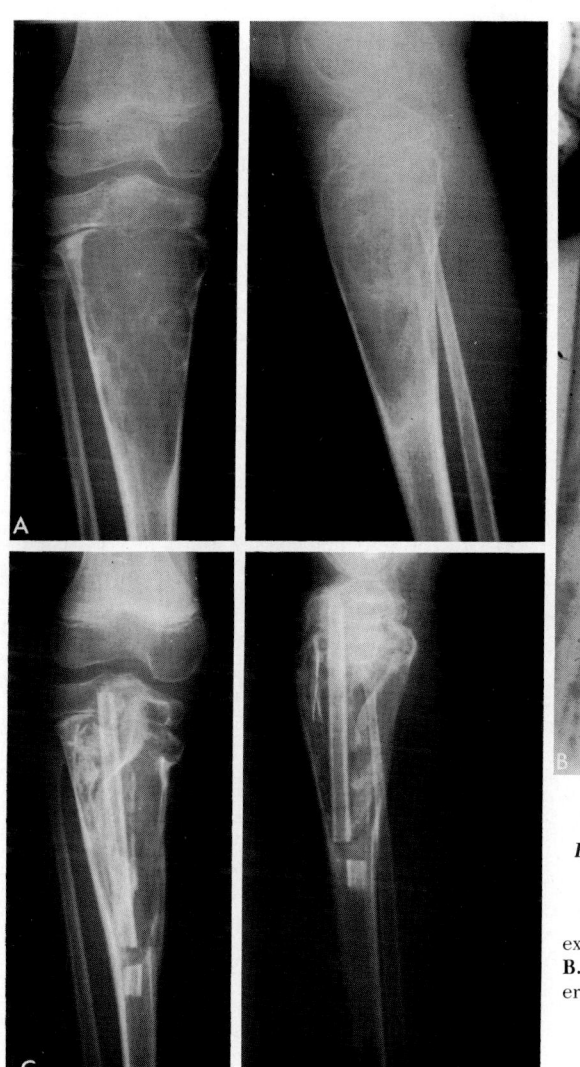
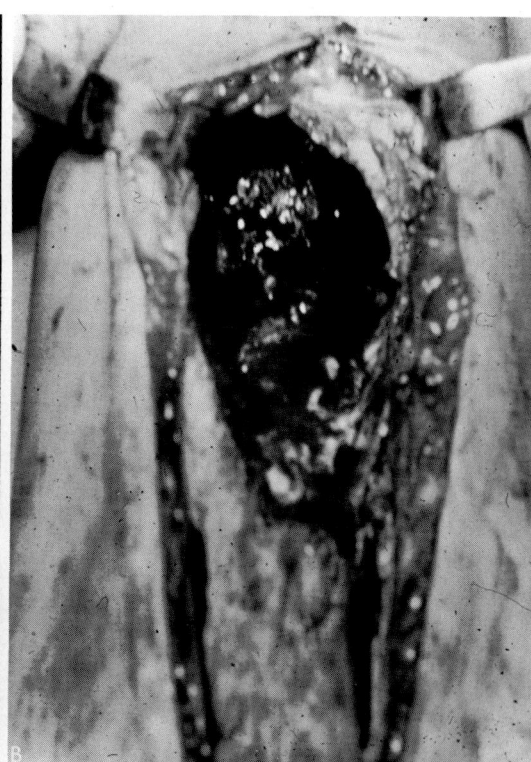

FIGURE 3–304. Unicameral bone cyst of the proximal tibia.

The physis has been transgressed and the cyst has extended into the epiphysis. **A.** Preoperative radiograms. **B.** Gross appearance at operation. **C.** Immediate postoperative radiograms.

bone extending beyond the radiolucent area; and the finding of histiocytes and eosinophilic leukocytes on the histologic examination.

In *enchondroma*, location is an important clue in diagnosis, as this lesion commonly lies within the diaphysis of a short tubular bone, the *rarest* location for a solitary bone cyst. The presence of punctate radiopacities indicates calcification and ossification within a cartilaginous tumor. In some rare cases, however, in which differentiation cannot be made on the basis of radiographic findings alone, the cartilaginous nature of the lesion seen on histologic examination will point to enchondroma.

Radiograms alone are not usually sufficient for definitive diagnosis of *solitary fibrous dysplasia*, as a radiolucent shadow similar to that of a solitary bone cyst is seen. The "ground glass" shadow cast by the fine trabeculae of the fibro-osseous lesion of fibrous dysplasia is quite characteristic and may be demonstrated clearly by a magnifying lens. Bone scan with technetium-99m shows diffuse increased uptake in fibrous dysplasia, whereas in unicameral bone cyst it may show diminished or normal uptake. Computed tomography will show solid density in fibrous dysplasia and fluid density in unicameral bone cyst. Pathologic examination will confirm the diagnosis.

There should not be much confusion of a solitary bone cyst with a *giant cell tumor*. The latter almost always involves the actual epiphyseal end of the bone and is most often found in adults; in children, however, giant cell tumor may be metaphyseal in its location. The cells of this tumor are typically spindle-shaped or ovoid stromal cells in which are dispersed many giant multinuclear cells. In the case of a unicameral bone cyst, these giant cells may be seen, but the stromal cells are absent.

Treatment

Factors to consider in deciding on the treatment of unicameral bone cyst are: (1) the site of involvement, whether it is non–weight-bearing (e.g., the proximal humerus); or weight-bearing (the upper end of the femur); (2) the location within the affected bone—is it juxtaphyseal or growing away from the physis?; (3) the size of the cyst and its activity—is it progressively increasing in size and weakening the bone with risk of repeated fractures?; (4) the degree of septation or loculation within the cyst due to previous pathologic fractures or treatment; and (5) whether it is complicated by a recent fracture. Sometimes the psychologic trauma to a physically active child who is prohibited from or afraid of partaking in normal activities and sports becomes an additional factor in the timing of treatment.

Ordinarily there is no urgency in instituting definitive treatment. The benign nature of the lesion is explained to the parents. Aspiration or biopsy or both are recommended when there is a doubt about the radiographic diagnosis. CT and bone scans are of great value in the differential diagnosis and delineation. In the rare dubious case when biopsy is performed, it should be coordinated with definitive treatment.

Inordinate delay should be avoided, particularly in the weight-bearing bones; such delays increase the hazards of repeated fractures, shortening, deformity, and growth retardation due to physeal involvement.

Often, unicameral bone cysts present with pathologic fracture. Should one wait for the initial spontaneous fracture to heal or proceed with immediate definitive treatment? In a non–weight-bearing bone, it is best to observe while the fracture is healing and assess the rate of growth of the cyst. Occasionally a cyst may heal completely after a fracture, but often it persists.

A cyst may stay stationary, grow at a slow rate, or enlarge at a fast rate. Its proximity to the physis and the age of the patient are important prognostic factors. Definitive treatment may be deferred in a slowly growing or stationary cyst located in the diaphysis in a patient over ten years of age, whereas a rapidly enlarging cyst should be treated soon in order to prevent repeated fractures, extensive surgery, and possible growth plate involvement. Healing fractures may produce septa and result in a multicameral cyst that is difficult to treat with corticosteroid injections. Pathologic fractures in a weight-bearing bone, particularly the proximal femur, require immediate definitive treatment.

Modalities of definitive treatment available are: injection into the cyst of corticosteroids; multiple drilling and drainage of the cystic cavity; curettage of the membranous wall and bone grafting; subtotal resection with bone grafting; subtotal resection without bone grafting; and total resection (diaphysectomy) and bone grafting.*

Corticosteroid Injection

Direct injection of methylprednisone acetate

---

*See references: corticosteroids, 10, 25, 30, 47, 87–91; multiple drilling and drainage, 14, 52; subtotal resection and bone grafting, 2, 29, 58; total resection and bone grafting, 33, 61, 102.

into the cystic cavity was introduced by Scaglietti. The fluid in the cyst is a transudate, and steroids are effective in preventing transudate formation in inflammatory synovial processes. Scaglietti and associates postulated that the membranous wall of the cyst degenerates after injection of corticosteroids, production of transudate ceases, and osteoblastic activity commences.[87–91] Scaglietti and Campanacci and their associates reported overall good results in 96 per cent of their cases. The cyst was considered healed when the regional cortex thickened and the cystic cavity showed increased density with calcification of the central radiolucent area. Thirty-six per cent of their cases required multiple injections.[10, 90, 91] Oppenheim and Galleno reported the results in 20 patients treated by steroid injection. Initial response was positive in 40 per cent; with further injections, good results were achieved in 75 per cent.[73] The results of injections were good in 80 per cent of 10 cases reported by Kohler and 67 per cent of 12 cases reported by Fernbach and associates.[30, 49]

Operative Technique of Corticosteroid Injections. It is performed under general anesthesia as an outpatient procedure under strict aseptic technique. The cystic area is prepared and draped as in a formal surgical procedure. Craig biopsy needles or 16-gauge needles with stylets are used to puncture the cyst under image intensifier radiographic control. If thin, the cortex may be punctured with manual pressure. Do not break the point of the needle! When the cortex is thick, a drill guide and an electric drill are used to make a hole in the cortex. Keep the drill guide in place to assist in locating the hole for insertion of the needle with the stylet inside. Do not fracture the cortex and collapse the cystic cavity! The contents of the cavity are aspirated, and the volume of aspirated fluid is measured. A contrast examination with Renografin diluted 1:1 with normal saline is performed next to demonstrate the presence of intracystic fibrous or osseous septa and loculation. The presence of these septa is not necessarily related to previous fractures or surgical procedures. They prevent distribution of the injected methylprednisone, and the incidence of failure of healing increases.[12, 13] Therefore it is important to inject the corticosteroid into each cystic cavity individually in multicameral bone cysts. The cystic cavity is thoroughly flushed with normal saline solution. The methylprednisone acetate (Depo-Medrol), 40 mg. per milliliter, is then instilled into the cystic cavity as a milliliter per milliliter replacement of the aspirate, but never exceeding 3 ml. (120 mg.). A simple compression dressing is applied. Immobilization of the limb is usually not required. Weight-bearing long bones of the lower limb are protected by the use of crutches. When the humerus is aspirated, partial support is provided by a sling for a period of two to three weeks. In the lower limb the duration of crutch protection depends upon the integrity of the regional cortex.

Radiographic changes usually are not noted in the first two to three months; therefore, barring the complication of a pathologic fracture, radiographic studies in this immediate postinjection period are generally not necessary. Radiograms to assess healing are made at two-month intervals. Radiographic signs of healing include diminution in the size of the cyst, cortical thickening, remodeling of the surrounding bone, and increased internal density due to calcification or new bone trabeculation. If, in six months, there is no evidence of healing, the injection is repeated, utilizing the same technique. Ordinarily two or three injections of corticosteroids are sufficient; Scaglietti, however, recommends up to four injections, if necessary, to obtain healing.[88–91]

The advantages of corticosteroid injection are evident: the procedure is relatively simple; leaves no operative scar; entails very little morbidity, allowing a prompt return to normal activity; and the results are almost as good as those of open surgery. Steroid injection is highly recommended as the method of choice in the initial treatment of unicameral bone cysts.

Complications of steroid injection: Steroid flush was seen in one patient in the series of Oppenheim and Galleno.[73] This author has observed two cases of Cushing's syndrome that developed after steroid injection in a unicameral bone cyst; both cases resolved spontaneously within six months. Preoperatively, the possibility of such a complication should be explained to the parents. Overdosage should be avoided. It is best not to exceed a total of 120 mg. of methylprednisone acetate.

Decompression of Cyst by Multiple Drilling

Kuboyama and Chigira and their associates have shown that multiple percutaneous drilling is highly effective in the treatment of unicameral bone cyst. The fluid escapes through the drill holes, the internal pressure in the cyst diminishes and the deranged hydrodynamics are restored to normal. Kuboyama removes the Kirschner wires after drilling; whereas Chigira and associates leave two or three Kirschner

Text continued on page 1270

Curettage and Bone Grafting of Unicameral Bone Cyst
OPERATIVE TECHNIQUE

A. The skin incision begins just below and 1 cm. medial to the superolateral corner of the axillary fold and extends distally for a distance of 10 to 12 cm. The subcutaneous tissue and deep fascia are divided along the line of the skin incision. The skin flap is developed and retracted laterally.

B. The cephalic vein is identified in the deltopectoral groove and retracted medially with a thin strip of deltoid muscle. Ramifications of the cephalic vein from the deltoid muscle are ligated or coagulated.

C. The upper portion of the humerus and the tendon of the pectoralis major muscle are exposed by lateral retraction of the deltoid muscle. The long head of the biceps and the deltoid branches of the thoracoacromial artery are identified. It is best to ligate the vessels. The arm is medially rotated, and the periosteum is incised lateral to the long head of the biceps and the tendon of the pectoralis major muscle.

D. Gently the periosteum is elevated, exposing the thinned "eggshell" cortical wall of the bone cyst.

Plate 41. Curettage and Bone Grafting of Unicameral Bone Cyst

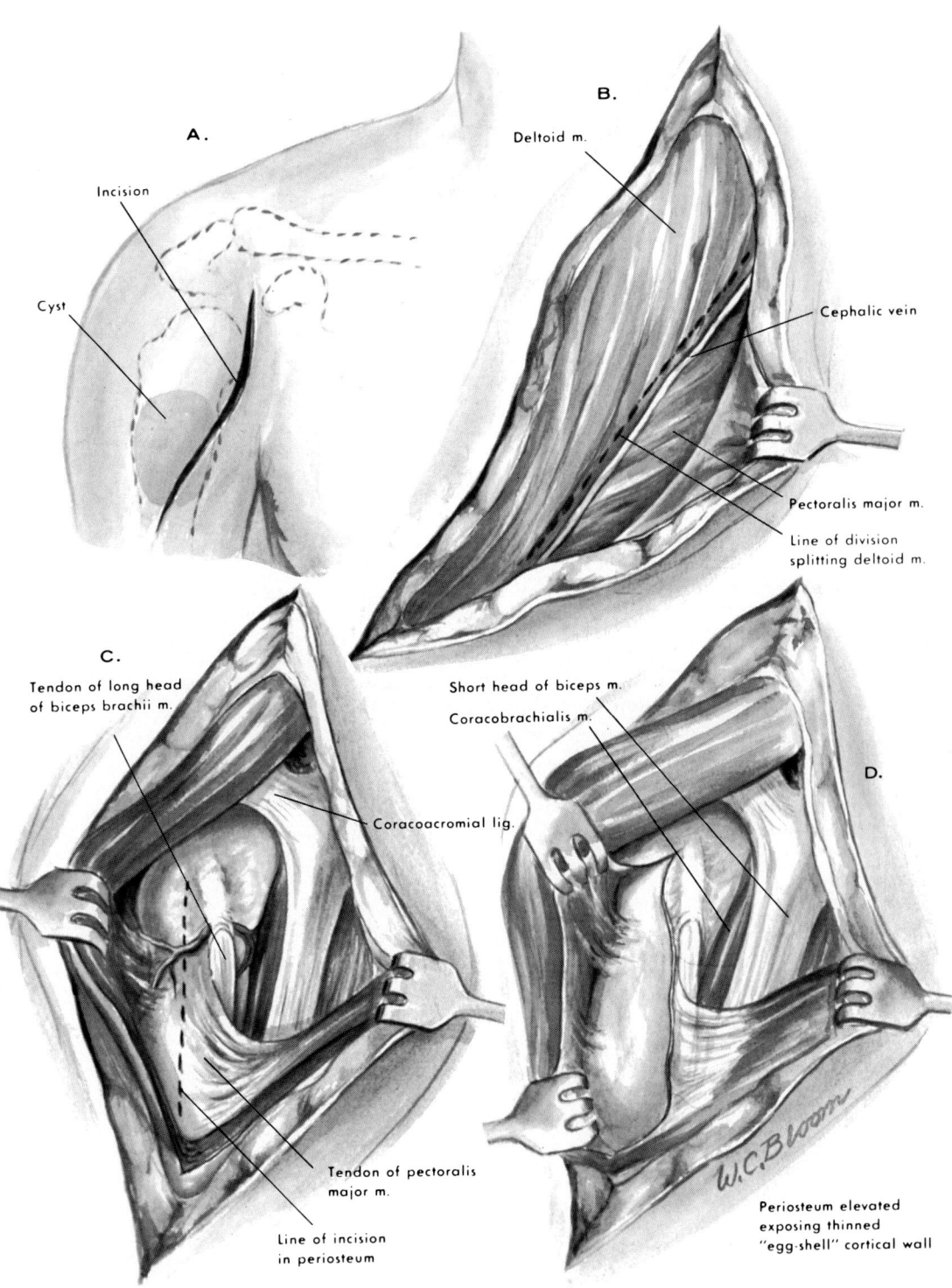

Curettage and Bone Grafting of Unicameral Bone Cyst (Continued)

E. The cyst is aspirated. A straw-colored or amber fluid is usually obtained; however, if there has been a recent fracture, the fluid may be hemorrhagic or serosanguineous.

F. Next, with drill holes and osteotomes, a large rectangular window is made by removing the cyst wall.

G. Connective tissue membrane is thoroughly curretted from the wall of the cyst. The proximal humeral physis should not be injured.

H. Next, the cavity is tightly packed with autogenous bone grafts. If in doubt, it is best to take radiograms in the operating room to determine the extent of the cyst. Usually it is unilocular; however, repeated fractures may cause partition of the cavity by fibrous septa.

I. The window is closed with an outer plate of iliac bone graft.

J. The periosteum and the wound are closed in layers in the usual manner. A Velpeau bandage reinforced with a few layers of plaster of Paris cast is applied.

POSTOPERATIVE MANAGEMENT

Sutures are removed in about two weeks, but immobilization in a cast-reinforced Velpeau bandage is continued for eight weeks until there is radiographic evidence of healing with incorporation of the grafts and obliteration of the cystic cavity.

Plate 41. Curettage and Bone Grafting of Unicameral Bone Cyst

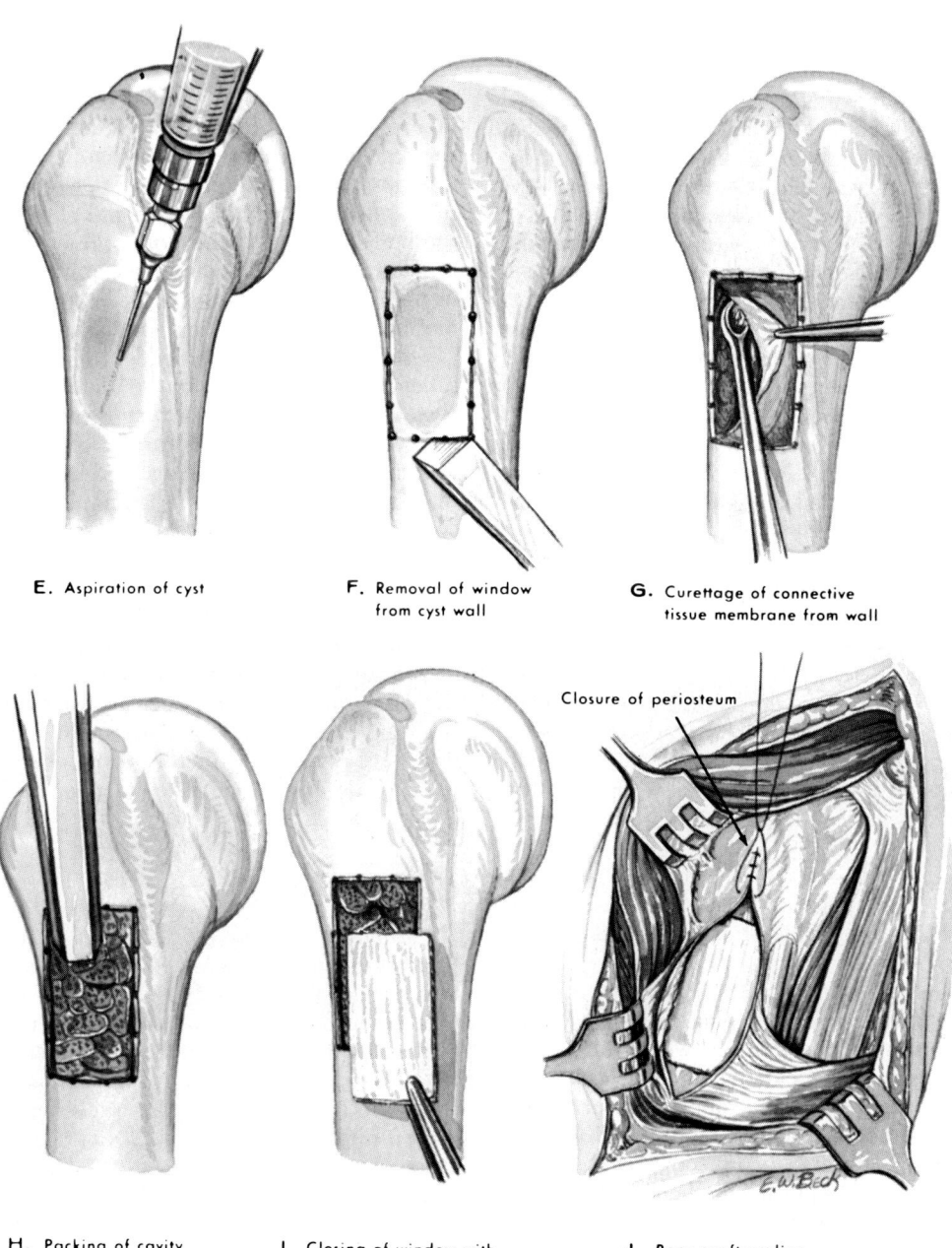

E. Aspiration of cyst

F. Removal of window from cyst wall

G. Curettage of connective tissue membrane from wall

H. Packing of cavity with bone grafts

I. Closing of window with outer plate of iliac bone

J. Bone graft sealing tightly packed cavity

rare in both skeletally immature and mature patients. Reports in the literature include cysts in the proximal part of the tibia, femur, and humerus.[18, 39, 71] An illustrative case is shown in Figure 3–304. These cases are treated by local injection of corticosteroids and protection in a cast to prevent or minimize damage to the growth plate violated by the cyst.

References

1. Abe, M.: Solitary bone cyst of the calcaneus. J. Jpn. Orthop. Assoc., 51:171, 1977.
2. Agerholn, J. C., and Goodfellow, J. W.: Simple cysts of the humerus treated by radical excision. J. Bone Joint Surg., 47-B:714, 1965.
3. Ayers, W. W., and Cameron, B. M.: Cysts of the os calcis. U.S. Armed Forces Med. J., 8:1102, 1957.
4. Badgley, C. E.: Unicameral cysts of the long bones. Treatment by crushing cystic walls and onlay grafts. J. Bone Joint Surg., 39-A:1429, 1957.
5. Baker, D. M.: Benign unicameral bone cyst. A study of forty-five cases with long-term follow-up. Clin. Orthop., 71:140, 1970.
6. Bensahel, H., and Baum, C.: Traitement des kystes osseux solitaires du col du fémur chez l'enfant. J. Chir., 107:61, 1974.
7. Bloodgood, J. C.: Benign bone cysts, ostitis fibrosa, giant-cell sarcoma and bone aneurysm of the long pipe bones. Ann. Surg., 52:145, 1910.
8. Boseker, E. H., Bickel, W. H., and Dahlin, D. C.: A clinicopathologic study of simple unicameral bone cysts. Surg. Gynecol. Obstet., 127:550, 1968.
9. Broder, H. M.: Possible precursor of unicameral bone cysts. J. Bone Joint Surg., 50-A:503, 1968.
10. Campanacci, M., De Sessa, L., and Bellando Randone, P.: Cisti ossea (rivisione di 275 osservazioni; risultati della cura chirurgica e primi risultati della cura incruenta con metilprednisolone acetato). Chir. Organi Mov., 62:471, 1975.
11. Campos, O. P.: Treatment of bone cyst by intracavity injection of methylprednisolone acetate. A message to orthopedic surgeons. Clin. Orthop., 165:43, 1982.
12. Capanna, R., Albisinni, U., Caroli, G. C., and Campanacci, M.: Contrast examination as a prognostic factor in the treatment of solitary bone cyst by cortisone injection. Skeletal Radiol., 12:97, 1984.
13. Capanna, R., Dal Monte, A., Gitelis, S., and Campanacci, M.: The natural history of unicameral bone cyst after steroid injection. Clin. Orthop., 166:204, 1982.
14. Chigira, M., Maehara, S., Arita, S., and Udagawa, E.: The aetiology and treatment of simple bone cysts. J. Bone Joint Surg., 65-B:633, 1983.
15. Clark, L.: The influence of trauma on the unicameral bone cyst. Clin. Orthop., 22:209, 1962.
16. Cohen, J.: Simple bone cysts. Studies of cyst fluid in six cases with a theory of pathogenesis. J. Bone Joint Surg., 42-A:609, 1960.
17. Cohen, J.: Etiology of simple bone cysts. J. Bone Joint Surg., 52-A:1493, 1970.
18. Cohen, J.: Unicameral bone cysts. A current synthesis of reported cases. Orthop. Clin. North Am., 8:715, 1977.
19. Coleman, B., Vidoli, M. F., and Crimmings, F. J.: Solitary cyst. Radiology, 47:142, 1946.
20. Conrado, F. M., and Passaretti, U.: Prime esperienze terapeutiche con cortisouier nelle cisti ossee giovanilli. Chir. Organi Mov., 63:239, 1976.
21. Coues, W. P.: Case of bone cyst of os calcis. Boston Med. Surg. J., 170:611, 1914.
22. Creyssel, J.: Sur le pronostic éloigné et le traitement des kystes solitaires des os. Lyon Chir., 50:98, 1955.
23. Czitrom, A. A., and Pritzker, K. P. H.: Simple bone cyst causing collapse of the articular surface of the femoral head and incongruity of the hip joint. A case report. J. Bone Joint Surg., 62-A:842, 1980.
24. Daum, R., Buhr, H., and Pflugfelder, H.: Chirurgische Therapie und Ergebnisse von juvenilen Knochenzysten. Klin. Pädiat, 187:518, 1976.
25. De Palma, L.: L'impiego dell'acetato di metilprednisolone nel trattamento delle cisti ossee solitarie. Arch. Putti Chir. Organi Mov., 29:341, 1978.
26. Eder, H., and Spranger, M.: Zur Problematik der operativen Therapie von Knochenzysten am coxalen Femurende. Z. Orthop., 116:214, 1978.
27. Ehrlich, M., and Chaglassian, J.: Unicameral bone cyst in the scapula. Clin. Orthop., 103:80, 1974.
28. Esteve, P.: Plombage des kystes solitaires des os par un lambeau musculaire. Mem. Acad. Chir., 88:585, 1962.
29. Fahey, J. J., and O'Brien, E. T.: Subtotal resection and grafting in selected cases of solitary unicameral bone cyst. J. Bone Joint Surg., 55-A:59, 1973.
30. Fernbach, S. K., Blumenthal, D. H., Poznanski, A. K., Dias, L. S., and Tachdjian, M. O.: Radiographic changes in unicameral bone cysts following direct injection of steroids: A report of 12 cases. Radiology, 140:689, 1981.
31. Galasko, C. S. B.: The fate of simple bone cysts with fracture. Clin. Orthop., 101:302, 1974.
32. Garceau, G. J., and Gregory, C. F.: Solitary unicameral bone cyst. J. Bone Joint Surg., 36-A:267, 1954.
33. Gartland, J. J., and Cole, F. L.: Modern concepts in the treatment of unicameral bone cysts of the proximal humerus. Orthop. Clin. North Am., 6:487, 1975.
34. Grabias, S., and Mankin, H. J.: Chondrosarcoma arising in histologically proved unicameral bone cyst. J. Bone Joint Surg., 56-A:1501, 1974.
35. Graham, J. J.: Solitary unicameral bone cyst. A follow-up study of 31 cases with proven pathological diagnosis. Bull. Hosp. Joint Dis., 13:106, 1952.
36. Gualtieri, I., Gualtieri, G., and Montfusco, E.: Risultati ottenuti nel trattemanto delle cisti ossee mediante infiltrazioni con acetato di metilprednisolone. Osp. Ital. Chir., 29:155, 1976.
37. Hagberg, S., and Mansfield, L.: The solitary bone cyst. A follow-up study of 24 cases. Acta Chir. Scand., 133:25, 1967.
38. Harms, J., and Groth, P.: Ergebnisse der Resektion, autologen Spanplastik und Überbruckungsosteosynthese juveniler Knochenzysten. Arch. Orthop. Trauma. Surg., 92:285, 1978.
39. Hutter, C. G.: Unicameral bone cyst. Report of an unusual case. J. Bone Joint Surg., 32-A:430, 1950.
40. Imhauser, G.: Zur Therapie der grossen jugendlichen Knochzysten im oberen Femurbereich. Chirurg, 34:226, 1963.
41. Jaffe, H. L.: Tumors and Tumorous Conditions of the Bones and Joints. Philadelphia, Lea & Febiger, 1958, pp. 63–75.
42. Jaffe, H. L., and Lichtenstein, L.: Solitary unicameral bone cyst: With emphasis on the roentgen picture, the pathologic appearance and the pathogenesis. Arch. Surg., 44:1004, 1942.
43. James, A. G., Coley, B. L., and Higinbotham, N. L.: Solitary (unicameral) bone cyst. Arch. Surg., 57:137, 1948.
44. Johnson, L. C., and Kindred, R. G.: The anatomy of bone cysts. J. Bone Joint Surg., 40-A:1440, 1958.
45. Johnson, L. C., Vetter, H., and Puschar, W. G. J.: Sarcoma arising in bone cysts. Virchows Arch. Pathol. Anat., 335:428, 1962.
46. Khermosh, O., and Weissman, S. L.: Coxa vara, avascular necrosis and osteochondritis dissecans com-

plicating solitary bone cysts of the proximal femur. Clin. Orthop., 126:143, 1977.
47. Kingsberry, L. B.: Solitary cyst of the os calcis in adults and children. Report of eight cases. J. Int. Coll. Surg., 27:83, 1957.
48. Kleiger, B.: Unicameral bone cyst, 15 year follow-up. Bull. Hosp. Joint Dis., 30:53, 1969.
49. Kohler, R.: Traitement des kystes essentiels des os par l'injection de corticoides. Lyon Chir., 78:158, 1982.
50. Kozlowski, K., and Masel, J.: Simple bone cysts. (Report of two unusual cases). Aust. Radiol., 26:269, 1982.
51. Kruls, H. J. A.: Pathologic fractures in children due to solitary bone cysts. Reconstr. Surg. Traumatatol., 17:113, 1979.
52. Kuboyama, K., Shido, T., Harada, A., and Yokoe, S.: Therapy of solitary unicameral bone cyst with percutaneous trepination. Rinsho Seikei. Geka (Japanese), 16:288, 1981.
53. Lefranc, J.: Résultats éloingés du traitement des kystes osseux essentiels de l'enfant et l'adolescent (d'après 62 observations). Thèse Méd., Paris, 1955, No. 542.
54. Lefranc, J., and Nezelof, C.: Les kystes essentiels des os longs. Etude anatomo-pathologique et traitement chirurgical. Rev. Chir. Orthop., 43:385, 1957.
55. Linthhoudt, D. van, and Lagier, R.: Calcaneal cysts. A radiological and anatomico-pathological study. Acta Orthop. Scand., 49:310, 1978.
56. Lodwick, G. S.: Juvenile unicameral bone cyst. A roentgen reappraisal. A.J.R., 80:495, 1958.
57. McGlynn, F. J., Mickelson, M. R., and El-Khoury, G. Y.: The fallen fragment sign in unicameral bone cyst. Clin. Orthop., 156:157, 1981.
58. McKay, D. W., and Nason, S. S.: Treatment of unicameral bone cysts by subtotal resection without grafts. J. Bone Joint Surg., 59-A:515, 1977.
59. McNamee, W. B., Gartland, J. J., and Irani, R.: Diaphysectomy for unicameral bone cyst. J. Bone Joint Surg., 55-A:1311, 1973.
60. Maeda, F.: A consideration on the pathogenesis of solitary bone cysts. J. Jpn. Orthop. Assoc., 37:529, 1963.
61. Matthrass, H. H., and Immenkamp, M.: Surgical treatment of solitary unicameral bone cyst. In Grundman, E. (ed.): Malignant Bone Tumors. Berlin, Springer-Verlag, 1976, pp. 231–238.
62. Meary, R., Tomeno, B., Mechin, J. F., and Languepin, A.: Images kystiques bénignes de nature indéterminée de l'extrémité supérieure du fémur chez l'adolescent et l'adulte. Ann. Radiol., 19:751, 1976.
63. Miles, J. E., and Degenshein, G. A.: Solitary bone cysts. Am. J. Surg., 91:170, 1956.
64. Mirra, J. M., Bernard, G. W., Bullough, P. G., Johnston, W., and Mink, G.: Cementum-like bone production in solitary bone cysts. (So-called "cementoma" of long bones.) Report of three cases. Electron microscopic observations supporting a synovial origin to the simple bone cyst. Clin. Orthop., 135:295, 1978.
65. Mittelmeier, H.: Resektion und freie Spanplastik zur Behandlung rezidivierender Knochenzysten des Humerus. Langenbecks Arch. Klin. Chir., 309:122, 1965.
66. Moed, B. R., and LaMont, R. L.: Unicameral bone cyst complicated by growth retardation. Report of three cases. J. Bone Joint Surg., 64-A:1379, 1982.
67. Morchoisne, P., and Masse, P.: Evolution radiologique des kystes essentiels des os. Ann. Radiol., 13:811, 1970.
68. Morton, K. S.: The pathogenesis of unicameral bone cyst. Can. J. Surg., 7:140, 1964.
69. Neer, C., Francis, K., Johnston, A., and Kiermnan, H.: Current concepts in the treatment of solitary unicameral bone cyst. Clin. Orthop., 97:40, 1973.
70. Neer, C. S., Francis, K. C., Marcove, R. C., Terz, J., and Carbonara, P. N.: Treatment of unicameral bone cyst. J. Bone Joint Surg., 48-A:731, 1966.
71. Nelson, J. P., and Foster, R. J.: Solitary bone cyst with epiphyseal involvement. A case report. Clin. Orthop., 118:147, 1976.
72. Norman, A., and Schiffman, M.: Simple bone cysts: Factors of age dependency. Radiology, 124:779, 1977.
73. Oppenheim, W. L., and Galleno, H.: Operative treatment versus steroid injection in the management of unicameral bone cysts. J. Pediatr. Orthop., 4:1, 1984.
74. Ottolenghi, C. E., Schajowicz, F., and Raffa, J.: Le kyste osseux essential uniloculaire: étude clinique et anatomopathologique de 123 cas. Rev. Chir. Orthop., 55:287, 1969.
75. Peltier, L. F., and Jones, R. H.: Treatment of unicameral bone cysts by curettage and packing with plaster of paris pellets. J. Bone Joint Surg., 60-A:820, 1978.
76. Pommer, G.: Zur Kenntnis der progressiven Hamatomund Phlegmasieverandungen der Rohrenkochen. Arch. Orthop. Unfallchir., 17:17, 1920.
77. Porat, S., Lowe, J., and Rousso, M.: Solitary bone cyst in the infant radius. A case report. Clin. Orthop., 135:131, 1978.
78. Prietto, C., Orofino, C. F., and Waugh, T. R.: Unicameral bone cyst in the scapula. Clin. Orthop., 125:183, 1976.
79. Ravaglia, M.: La resezione sottoperiostale nelle cisti ossee solitarie del bambino. Scapello, 2:51, 1973.
80. Reynolds, J.: The "fallen fragment sign" in the diagnosis of unicameral bone cysts. J. Radiol., 92:949, 1969.
81. Rigault, P., Alain, J. L., Padovani, J. P., and Plumerault, J.: Les kystes osseux essentiels se l'extrémité supérieure du fémur chez l'enfant. Notre expérience de 12 cas. Rev. Chir. Orthop., 61:221, 1975.
82. Robins, P. R., and Peterson, H. A.: Management of pathologic fractures through unicameral bone cysts. J.A.M.A., 222:80, 1972.
83. Roth, F. -J., Daum, R., and Pflugfelder, H.: Das Schicksal der operierten juvenilen Knochenzyste im Röntgenbild. Fortschr. Geb. Rontgenstr., 117:52, 1972.
84. Sadler, A. H., and Rosenhain, F.: Occurrence of two unicameral bone cysts in the same patient. J. Bone Joint Surg., 46-A:1551, 1964.
85. Sanguinetti, C.: Una particolare tecnica operativa per le cisti ossee solitarie. Ital. J. Orthop. Traumatol., 1:353, 1975.
86. Savastano, A. A.: The treatment of bone cysts with intracyst injections of steroids: Injection of steroids will largely replace surgery in the treatment of benign bone cysts. R.I. Med. J., 62:93, 1979.
87. Scaglietti, O.: L'azione osteogenetica dell'acetato di metilprednisone. Bull. Sci. Med., (Bologna), 146:159, 1974.
88. Scaglietti, O., Marchetti, P. G., and Bartolizzi, P.: Sulla azione topica del corticosteroid in microcristalli in alcuni lesioni dello scheletro. Arch. Putti Chir. Organi Mov., 27:9, 1976.
89. Scaglietti, O., Marchetti, P. G., and Bartolozzi, P.: Risultati a distanza dell'azione topica dell'acetato di metilprednisolone in microcristalli in alcuni lesioni dello scheletro. Arch. Putti Chir. Organi Mov., 29:11, 1978.
90. Scaglietti, O., Marchetti, P. G., and Bartolozzi, P.: The effects of methylprednisolone acetate in the treatment of bone cysts: Results of three years follow-up. J. Bone Joint Surg., 61-B:200, 1979.
91. Scaglietti, P. G., Marchetti, P. G., and Bartolozzi, P.: Final results obtained in the treatment of bone cysts with methylprednisolone acetate (Depo-Medrol) and a discussion of results achieved in other bone lesions. Clin. Orthop., 165:33, 1982.

92. Schnepp, J., and Marchetti, P. G.: Table ronde: Les kystes essentiels osseux (Venise, 1978). Rev. Chir. Orthop., 65:3, 1979.
93. Siegel, I. M.: Brisement forcé with controlled collapse in treatment of solitary unicameral bone cyst. Arch. Surg., 92:109, 1966.
94. Shulman, H. S., Wilson, S. R., Harvie, J. N., and Cruickshank, B.: Unicameral bone cyst in a rib of a child. A.J.R., 128:1058, 1977.
95. Sirry, A.: The pseudocystic triangle in the normal os calcis. Acta Radiol., 36:516, 1951.
96. Smith, N. R.: Cyst of the os calcis. J. Bone Joint Surg., 12:416, 1930.
97. Smith, R. W., and Smith, C. F.: Solitary unicameral bone cyst of the calcaneus. A review of twenty cases. J. Bone Joint Surg., 56-A:49, 1974.
98. Spence, K. F., Sell, K. W., and Brown, R. H.: Solitary unicameral bone cyst: Treatment with freeze-dried cancellous bone allograft. J. Bone Joint Surg., 51-A:87, 1969.
99. Spence, K. F., Bright, R. W., Fitzgerald, S. P., and Sell, K. W.: Solitary unicameral bone cyst: Treatment with freeze-dried crushed cortical-bone allograft. J. Bone Joint Surg., 58-A:636, 1976.
100. Stewart, M. J., and Hamel, H. A.: Solitary bone cyst. South. Med. J., 43:927, 1950.
101. Sturz, H., and Witt, A. N.: Juvenile Knochenzysten der Ulna. Verlaufsbeobachtungen bei seltener Lokalisation. Arch. Orthop. Trauma. Surg., 94:105, 1979.
102. Sturz, H., Zenker, H., and Buckl, H.: Total subperiosteal resection treatment of solitary bone cysts of the humerus. Arch. Orthop. Trauma. Surg., 93:231, 1979.
103. Verstandig, C. C.: Clinical note: Solitary unicameral bone cyst of the os calcis. N. Engl. J. Med., 237:21, 1947.
104. Von Mikulicz, J.: Über cystische Degeneration der Knochen. Verh. Gesellsch. Deutsch. Naturforsch. Arzte. 76th Meeting, 2nd Half. Part II., 1905, p. 107.
105. Weisel, A., and Hecht, H.: Development of unicameral bone cyst. Case report. J. Bone Joint Surg., 62-A:664, 1980.
106. Wilber, M. C., and Hyatt, G. W.: Bone cysts: Results of surgical treatment in 200 cases (abstract). J. Bone Joint Surg., 42-A:820, 1960.
107. Witt, A. N., Walcher, K., and Zenker, H.: Die Resektionsbehandlung rezidivierender juveniler Knochenzysten. Arch. Orthop. Unfallchir., 74:105, 1972.

HISTIOCYTOSIS X

Histiocytosis X, a term coined by Lichtenstein, is a syndrome consisting of a group of conditions that are characterized by the presence of granulomatous lesions with histiocytic proliferation.[86, 87] It includes eosinophilic granuloma of bone, Hand-Schüller-Christian disease, and Letterer-Siwe disease.

Eosinophilic granuloma of bone was described as an entity by Lichtenstein and Jaffe, and by Otani and Ehrlich.[89, 111] The disseminated forms of the disease were described earlier. Christian first reported the triad of multiple focal areas of bone destruction, exophthalmos, and diabetes insipidus.[32] The fulminating form of histiocytosis X was originally reported by Letterer, and later by Siwe.[85, 126] In 1941, Farber and associates made the plausible proposition that eosinophilic granuloma of bone, Hand-Schüller-Christian disease, and Letterer-Siwe disease are all variants of the same disease process, and Green, Farber, and McDermott reported a series of cases that supported this contention.[46, 61] A recent review by Lichtenstein substantiated the integrated concept of histiocytosis X as a nosologic entity embracing all these conditions.[88] Because the basic cause of this granulomatous histiocytic process is still unknown, the preceding traditional eponyms are still in use.

Lichtenstein gave the following classification of histiocytosis X:

A. Histiocytosis X, localized to bone (eosinophilic granuloma, solitary or multiple)

B. Histiocytosis X, disseminated, acute or subacute (Letterer-Siwe syndrome)

1. With destructive skeletal lesions (eosinophilic granuloma)

2. With transition to chronic phase (Schüller-Christian syndrome)

C. Histiocytosis, disseminated, chronic (Schüller-Christian syndrome)

1. With destructive skeletal lesions (eosinophilic granuloma)

2. With early extraskeletal lesions (indicate sites) resembling eosinophilic granuloma

3. With acute or subacute exacerbation (Letterer-Siwe syndrome)

4. With involvement predominantly of bones, lungs, pituitary or brain or both, skin, mucous membranes (oral, anal, genital), liver, or lymph nodes (in varying combinations, as the case may be).[88]

There is debate as to whether these disparate clinical syndromes should be grouped together as a single nosologic entity. Daneshbod and Kissane, on the basis of pathologic findings, clinical features, and prognosis, proposed that histiocytosis X is at least two different disease entities.[38] The first is *progressive disseminated histiocytosis* (Letterer-Siwe disease): it involves two or more organ systems, occurs in children less than three years of age and has an extremely poor prognosis for survival irrespective of therapy. The histologic appearance in this group is characterized by generalized "pure" infiltrate of histiocytes with well-defined cytoplasmic borders. These "malignant" histiocytes involve the reticuloendothelial system and other tissues. Eosinophils, giant cells, and mitosis are usually not found.[105] The second form of histiocytosis is benign in its clinical course, and occurs in older children (usually over three years of age); the patients are not systemically ill. The cytologic picture consists of histiocytes with ill-defined borders giving a syncytial appearance, eosinophils, giant cells, and necrosis or fibrosis. The prognosis is good; extensive systemic therapy is not required. The lesions may regress spontaneously. The natural outcome is resolution. The lesion in this second form heals regardless of the type of treatment—excision, curettage, a small dose of radiation, or biopsy alone.[94]

Etiology

The exact cause of histiocytosis is unknown. It most probably represents a reaction to an exogenous agent with a response that resembles both a neoplasm and an inflammation. The Langerhans histiocyte is the cell of origin in the lesion of histiocytosis X. It has been suggested that histiocytosis X should be considered as proliferation of abnormal Langerhans epidermal cells.[106] A causative microorganism has not been isolated from the lesions by bacteriologic, fungal, or viral cultural techniques. The nature of the disease makes the viral etiology an attractive hypothesis. Attempts to transplant the lesion to animals have been unsuccessful. It is not a disorder of lipid metabolism. There is no hereditary pattern.

Pathologic Features

The histologic picture consists of a reticulated mass of histiocytes infiltrated with eosinophilic leukocytes (Fig. 3–306). The histiocyte is a large macrophage with a central indented nucleus and regular chromatin with one or two nucleoli. The cytoplasm is filled with many lipid vacuoles. A loose syncytial appearance is imparted to the cells when they occur in sheets. There may be other reactive elements such as neutrophils, lymphocytes, and plasma cells. With maturation of the lesion the histiocytes may show giant cell formation, and a greater amount of lipid material may accumulate in their cytoplasm. Upon healing, fibrosis gradu-

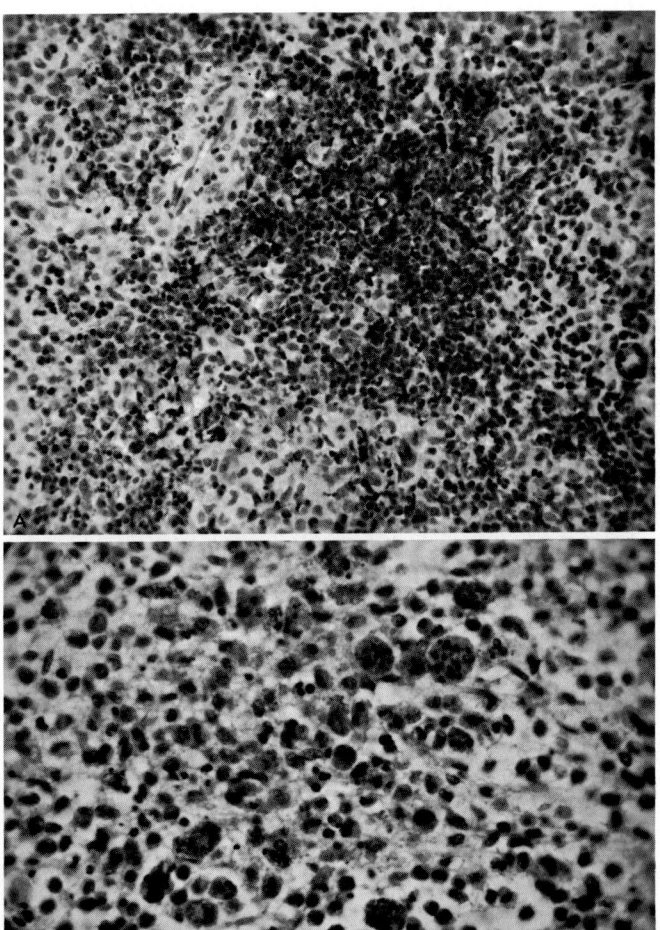

FIGURE 3–306. Eosinophilic granuloma—histologic findings.

A. Photomicrograph showing the larger pale histiocytes intermingled with the darker eosinophilic leukocytes (× 250). **B.** Greater magnification (× 450). The histiocytes and eosinophilic leukocytes are shown in more detail.

ally replaces the lesion. In the disseminated and acute forms the tumorous tissue is primarily histiocytic. The granulomatous histiocytic process not only develops within bone, but may appear in the skin, lymph nodes, liver, lungs, kidneys, oral cavity, female genitalia, and central nervous system. The ultrastructure of the histiocyte in all three forms (eosinophilic granuloma, Hand-Schüller-Christian disease, and Letterer-Siwe disease) is characterized by the presence in the cytoplasm of Langerhans granules (Birbeck bodies). These inclusions (150 to 1500 μm. in length) are located throughout the histiocyte—adjacent to the cell membranes, centrally in the cytoplasm, or close to the nucleus. The inclusion body may be dilated at one end, appearing racket-shaped. The total width of the inclusion body is 400 to 450 Å, and it contains parallel membranes 60 to 70 Å thick (Fig. 3–307). The giant cells ultrastructurally exhibit features similar to the nuclear and cytoplasmic components of the histiocytes.

The presence of Langerhans, or Birbeck, granules is highly characteristic but not pathognomonic of histiocytosis X. They are also seen in monocytic leukemia, reticulohistiocytoma, reactive histiocytosis in various tumors, and in the Langerhans cells of the epidermis. Clinical, radiographic, and pathologic features should be correlated to make the appropriate diagnosis.[71]

The clinical features and management of the various categories of histiocytosis X are described separately. Although the majority of the patients fall into one of the three syndromes, in certain cases no clear-cut syndrome exists and the treatment plan should be individualized.

Letterer-Siwe Disease

This is the acute (or subacute) disseminated progressive form of histiocytosis that characteristically occurs during the first year of life. Visceral involvement is diffuse and severe. The patient is presented with fever and debilitating infection due to marrow failure. Hepatomegaly, splenomegaly, and lymphadenopathy are marked. A granular appearance of the pulmonary parenchyma, as seen in the chest radiogram, is due to the widespread infiltration of the lungs (Fig. 3–308). The infant is pale and has petechial and macular hemorrhages in the

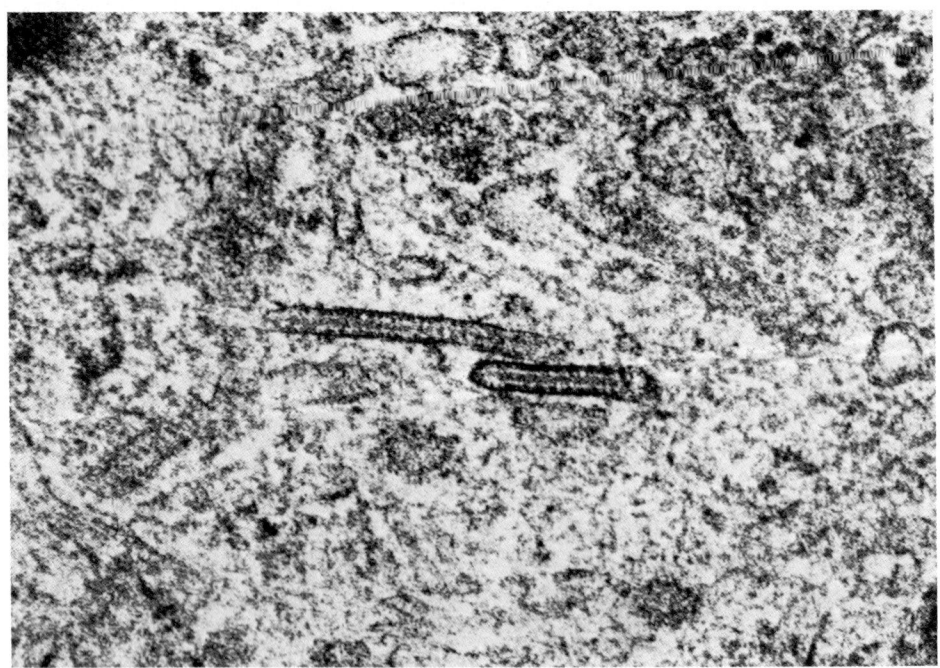

FIGURE 3–307. Tubular inclusion body within the cytoplasm of a typical histiocyte of eosinophilic granuloma (× 140,000).

(From Katz, R. L., Silva, E. G., DeSantos, L. A., and Lukeman, J. M.: Diagnosis of eosinophilic granuloma of bone by cytology, histology, and electron microscopy of transcutaneous bone-aspiration biopsy. J. Bone Joint Surg., 62-A:1280, 1980. Reprinted by permission.)

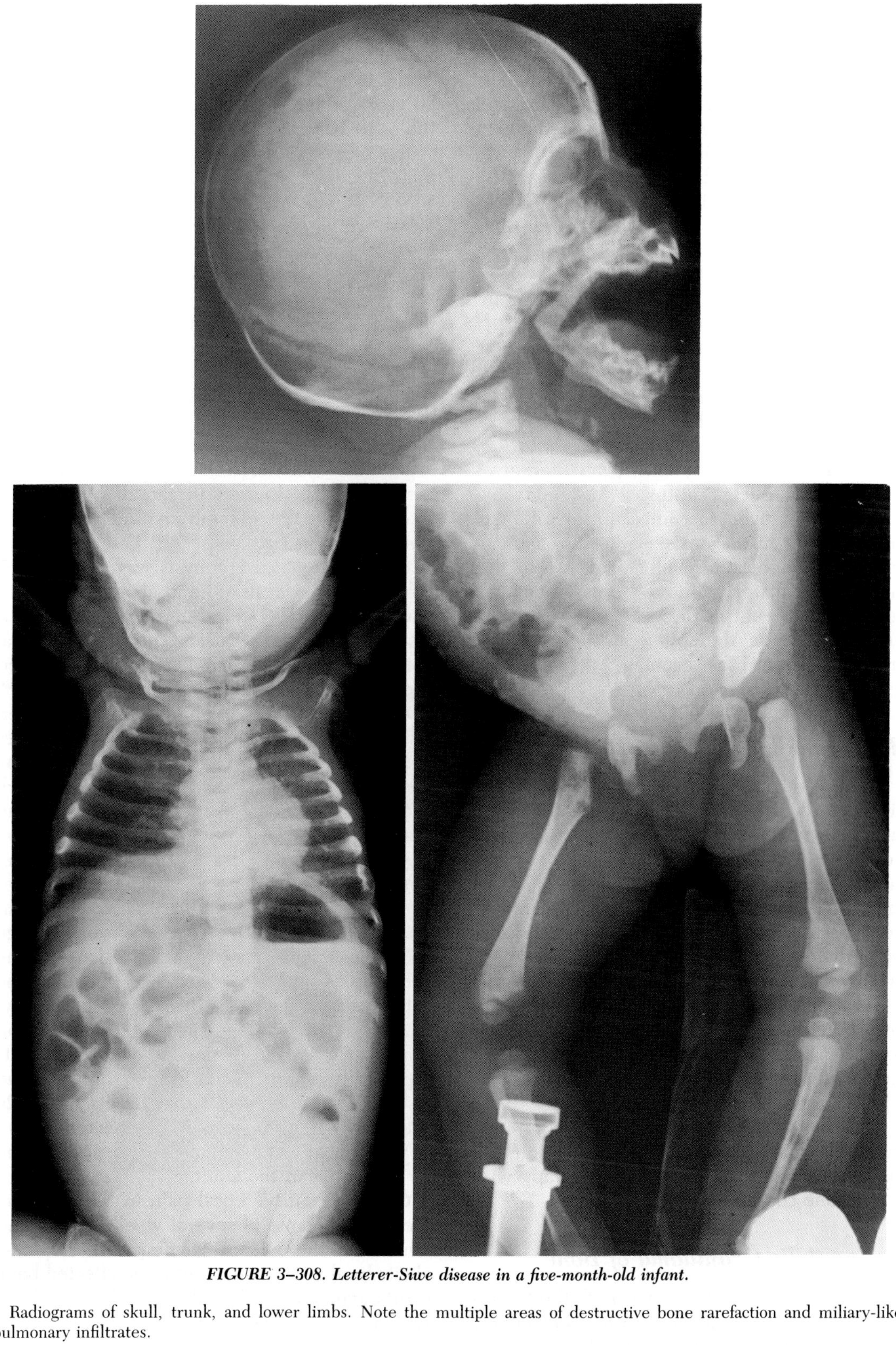

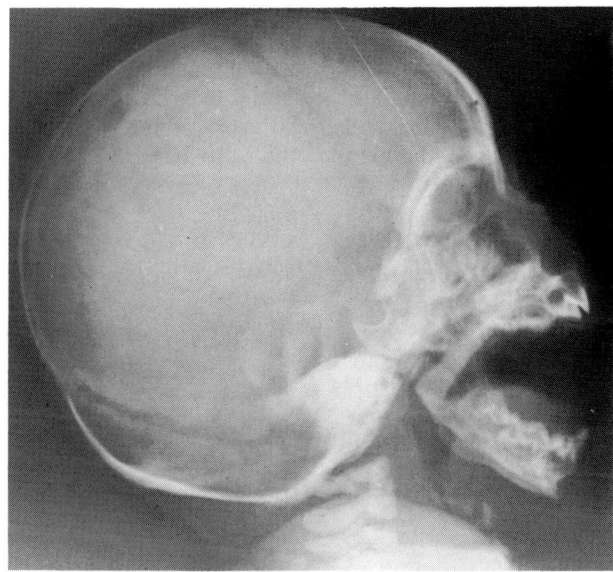

FIGURE 3–308. *Letterer-Siwe disease in a five-month-old infant.*

Radiograms of skull, trunk, and lower limbs. Note the multiple areas of destructive bone rarefaction and miliary-like pulmonary infiltrates.

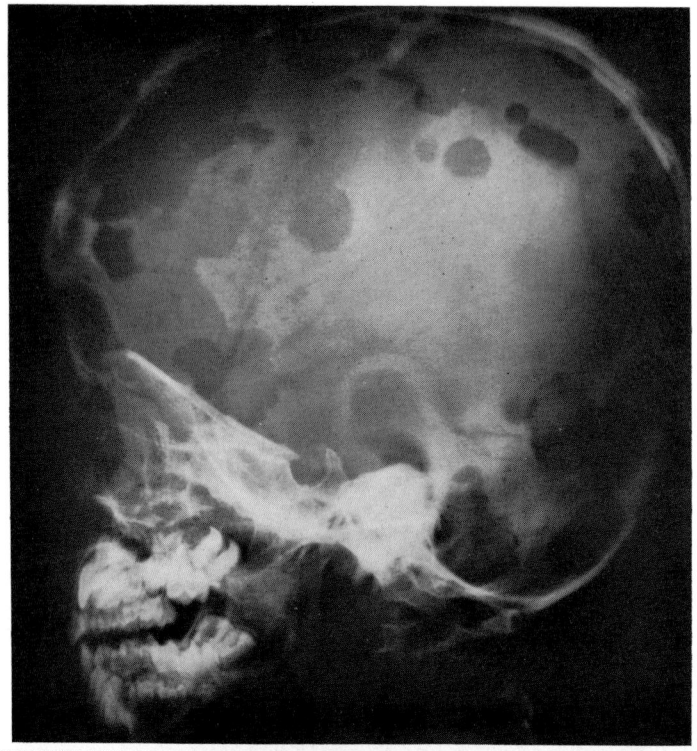
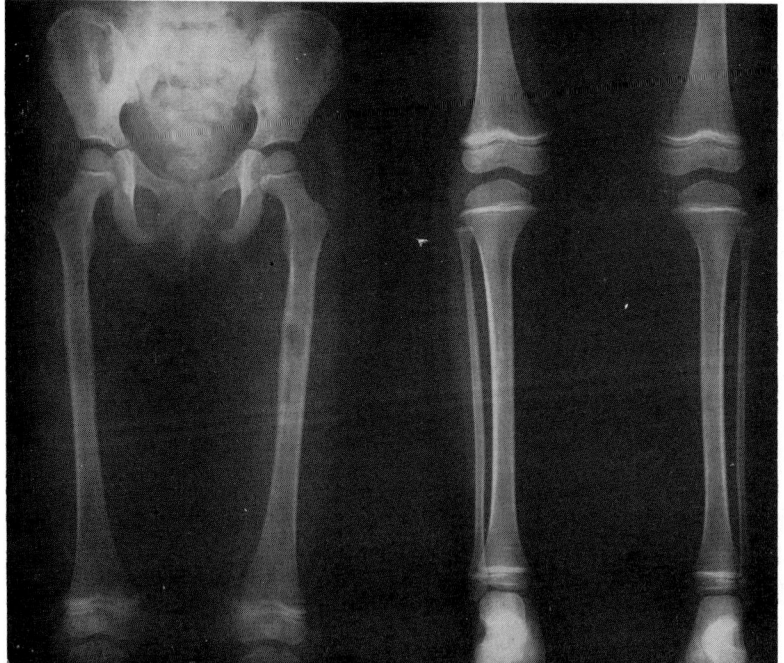

FIGURE 3–310. Hand-Schüller-Christian disease.

Radiograms of skull and lower limbs. Note multiple sharply defined radiolucent defects.

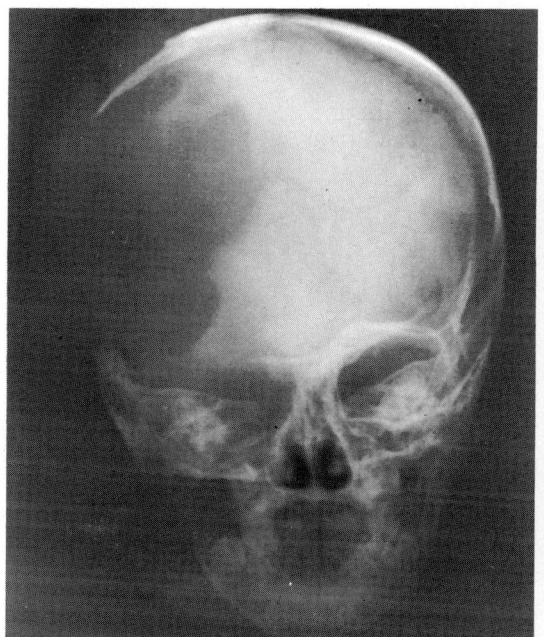 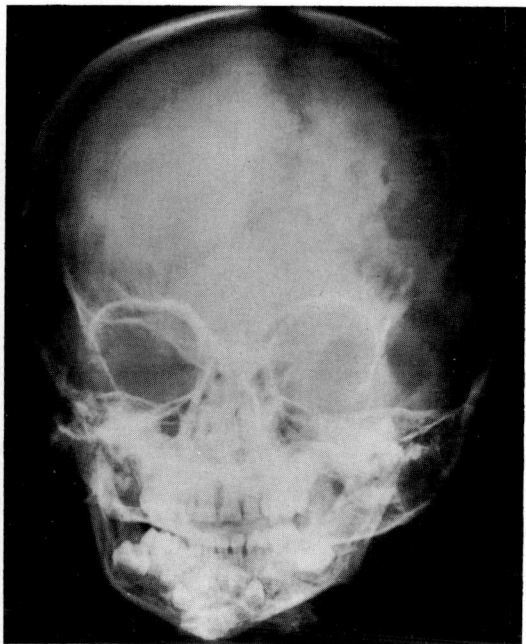

FIGURE 3–311. *Hand-Schüller-Christian disease.*
Radiograms of skull showing the large sharply outlined rarefactions.

may be a variable degree of atrophy of the thigh or the calf and an antalgic limp. Pathologic fracture may occur through the lesion with consequent increase in the size of the swelling and the intensity of pain. Some patients may present with a pathologic fracture. Headache, stiff neck, proptosis, and low-grade fever are other less frequent symptoms and signs.

Radiographic and Imaging Findings. Histiocytosis X produces a rapidly destructive lytic process in bone, giving a "punched out" appearance in the radiogram (Fig. 3–312). Other radiographic manifestations vary according to the site of the lesion. In some cases the radiographic picture is very characteristic, whereas in others malignant or infectious processes must be considered in the differential diagnosis. In such instances it is mandatory to perform biopsy and histologic examination of tissues for definitive diagnosis.

In flat bones, such as the skull and pelvis, the lesions appear "punched out," sharply circumscribed, usually with no periosteal or endosteal reaction. The area of radiolucency is sharply marginated by normal looking bone. A beveled appearance may result from differential destruction of the inner and outer tables of the skull or medial and lateral walls of the ilium. In the skull the lesion is oval or round in shape, but sometimes satellite lesions may coalesce with the main lesion, giving a "map-like" picture that is referred to as the geographic skull (see Fig. 3–310). The radiographic appearance of eosinophilic granuloma of the skull is almost pathognomonic; one can be certain of the diagnosis. In the ilium or scapula, the large bony trabeculae may be less involved or spared by the destructive process, causing the lesion to appear loculated. Occasionally in the skull a central nidus of bone, described by Wells as a *"button sequestrum,"* may be present within the sharply demarcated radiolucent lesion.[139] This is not pathognomonic of histiocytosis X, as other entities may produce the "button sequestrum" in the skull, e.g., osteomyelitis, dermoid cyst, radiation necrosis, hemangioma, metastatic carcinoma, and healing of a surgical defect.[102] Periosteal new bone formation usually does not occur in the flat bones. Marginal sclerosis due to healing can be secondary to treatment or occur spontaneously.

The second site where diagnosis of eosinophilic granuloma is almost certain is in the spine when *vertebra plana* is present.[21, 34, 35] The common level of spinal involvement is thoracic, less frequently lumbar, and rarely cervical. Here the radiographic appearance is characteristic; initially there is a purely lytic lesion without collapse; later on compression fracture occurs, the degree of collapse varying from partial to complete. In severe cases a dense white wafer of bone, 1 or 2 mm. in height, is all that

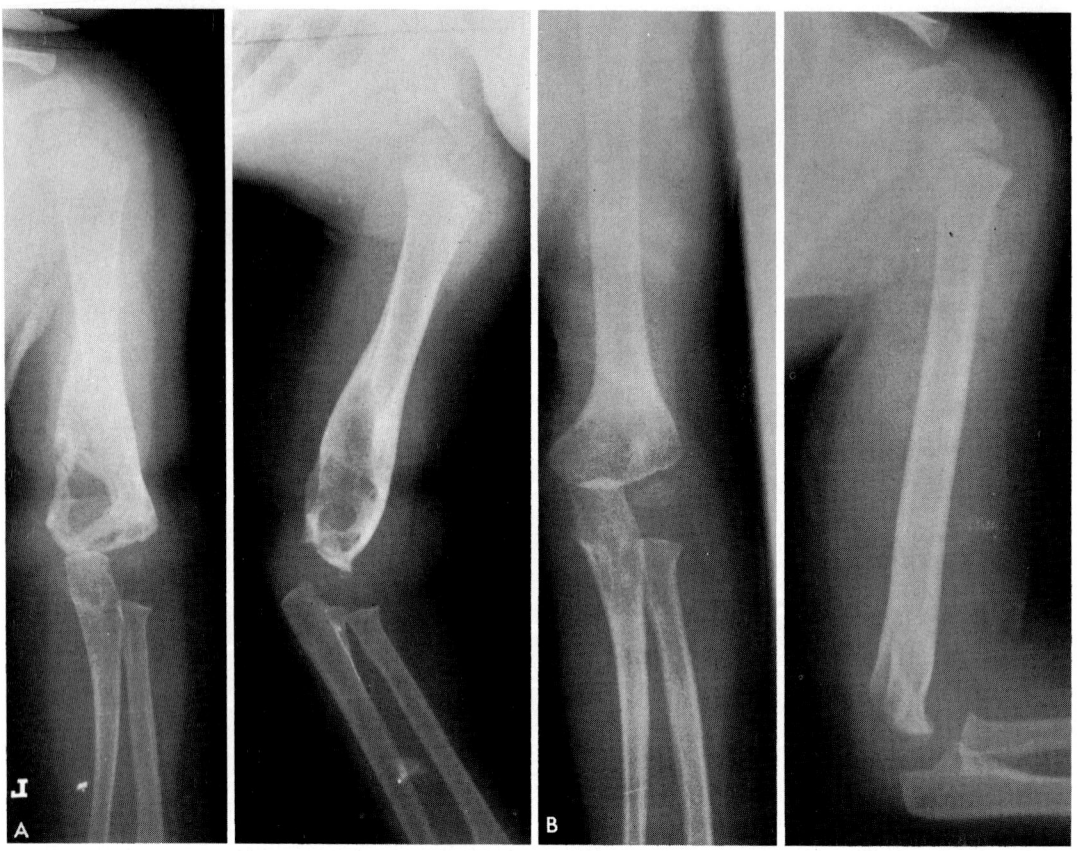

FIGURE 3-312. *Eosinophilic granuloma of distal left humerus.*

A. Radiograms showing the large area of rarefaction involving the distal metaphyses and shaft of humerus. Treatment consisted of 800 r irradiation. **B.** Radiograms of same patient 18 months later. The lesion has healed.

is left of the area previously occupied by the vertebral body ("silver dollar vertebra") (Fig. 3–313). This was described by Calvé as an osteochondrosis analogous to Legg-Perthes disease.[21] Compere and associates, in 1954, demonstrated in four cases proved by biopsy that vertebra plana is the result of eosinophilic granuloma and is not due to avascular necrosis.[35] According to Compere, the radiographic features of vertebra plana that are characteristic of eosinophilic granuloma are involvement of only one vertebral body, intact and widened disc interspaces above and below the collapsed vertebra, and homogenous density of the collapsed vertebral body.[34, 35] In the lateral radiogram the sclerotic disclike vertebra is elongated, projecting 1 to 2 cm. anterior and posterior to the margins of the adjacent uninvolved vertebrae. The intact pedicles provide some support posteriorly, thus the degree of posterior protrusion into the spinal canal is less than anterior protrusion. It is very rare that severe collapse causes paraplegia.[53, 142] Nerve root compression may cause varying degrees of neurologic deficit, which is transient; following treatment and healing of the vertebral lesion neurologic function is returned to normal.[40, 91, 123] The end plates of the vertebral body are usually intact; with healing, a variable degree of vertebral height is restored.[73, 103] The trabecular pattern does not return to normal, but remains coarsened or sclerotic. Kyphosis may be present.

More than one vertebra may be involved. The characteristic appearance of vertebra plana is not always present. Of the 14 cases reported by Enriquez and associates 9 had more than one level affected, and only 3 developed typical vertebra plana.[45]

Inflammatory processes such as pyogenic infection or tuberculosis may involve the vertebral bodies. Histiocytosis X is differentiated from inflammatory lesions by the absence of disc interspace narrowing and by the lack of an associated paravertebral soft-tissue mass. The most common proven cases of vertebra plana are caused by histiocytosis, but by no means is it the only etiology. Other entities are Gaucher's disease, lymphoma, undifferentiated sar-

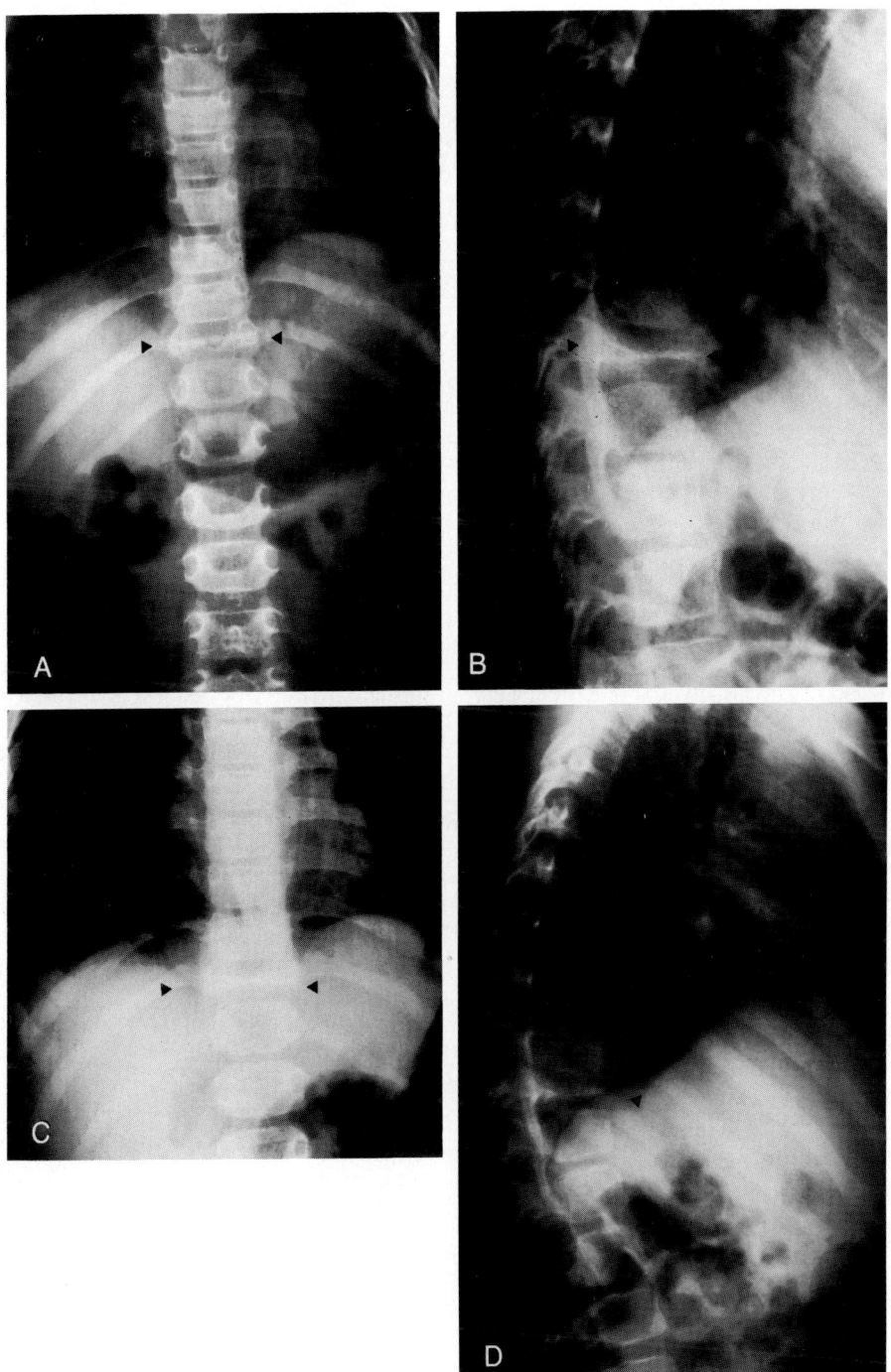

FIGURE 3–313. Eosinophilic granuloma of the eleventh thoracic vertebra (vertebra plana).

A and **B.** Anteroposterior and lateral views of the thoracolumbar spine—note the collapse of the body of the eleventh thoracic vertebra (*arrow*). **C** and **D.** Anteroposterior and lateral views of the spine six years later. There is partial restoration of the height of the collapsed vertebral body.

coma, metastatic carcinoma, and osteogenesis imperfecta. Computed tomography and nuclear magnetic resonance imaging are of great value in delineating the pathologic changes in the vertebral column.

In the *long bones* the destructive process begins in the medulla. In its very initial stage it manifests itself as localized osteoporosis, giving a "washed out" appearance. Soon an irregular lytic area of variable size develops in the medulla of the diaphysis or metaphysis, usually with endosteal erosion. Medullary rarefaction may be accompanied by expansion of the involved bone, particularly in the clavicle or ulna. Rapidly developing lytic lesions may cause complete dissolution of the regional cortex. A soft-tissue mass may be discerned in the radiogram. Ordinarily the destructive erosion of the cortex is slower in its course, resulting in excessive periosteal new bone formation—the "onion peel" appearance. This is most often seen in diaphyseal lesions. Such a radiographic picture is also seen in Ewing's sarcoma and osteomyelitis. It is mandatory to perform biopsy and histologic examination of tissue for definitive diagnosis. With healing and organization of periosteal new bone the involved bone thickens. Pathologic fracture of long bones may be the presenting radiographic feature.

A chest radiogram should be made to rule out pulmonary infiltration. Computed tomography (CT scan) is of great value in delineating the nature of the lytic lesion, particularly in the pelvis, spine, and skull.

Scintigraphic findings with technetium-99m vary. Osteolytic lesions identified in the plain radiogram may not always be detected by scintigraphy.[37] The percentage of false negatives varies. Siddiqui and associates studied the skeletal lesions in 21 children with histocytosis X (3 cases of the bone and bone marrow) with technetium-99m as well as gallium-67 citrate. Seven of the twenty bone scans were completely normal in patients with extensive radiographic evidence of bone involvement. In only one case did the bone scan show change earlier than the plain radiograph. There were no "cold" lesions on the bone scan. Also, technetium-99m–sulfur colloid bone marrow scans and gallium-67 citrate whole body scans proved of no value.[124] Parker and associates, in a study of 18 cases found that only 35 per cent of the individual lesions visible on radiographs were seen on radionuclide studies.[113] The radiographic skeletal survey is far superior to scintigraphy.

Diagnosis. Percutaneous biopsy is performed to obtain bone tissue and aspirations for cytologic diagnosis. It is simple and fast; in easily accessible lesions it can be performed as an outpatient procedure. The exact location of the lesion is precisely determined by appropriate radiography, linear tomography, and computed tomography. It is vital to plan the surgical approach to the lesion preoperatively. Inadvertent injury to adjacent neurovascular structures and organs should be avoided. In children it is best to perform the procedure under general anesthesia. In the cooperative adult or older adolescent, local anesthesia with appropriate sedation may be used.

The procedure is performed under image intensifier fluoroscopic guidance. First use a guide pin to localize the position of the lesion accurately. Then, with an Ackerman needle (a 12- or 13-gauge saw-toothed trocar), obtain a core of bone. An aspirating needle (18 to 23 gauge) is then introduced within the core biopsy trocar into the destructive lytic area of radiolucency. The tissue is aspirated and collected in a heparinized syringe. Plain radiograms are made in the anteroposterior and lateral projections for permanent recording of the site of biopsy. The core biopsy specimen for routine histologic examination is fixed in 10 per cent formaldehyde, whereas the specimen for electronmicroscopy is placed in 2 per cent glutaraldehyde. The pathologist should be available in the operating room suite to process the fine needle aspirate. The cytologic smear discloses excellent detail of cellular morphology, providing more adequate diagnostic material than the corresponding histologic sections.

Open biopsy is performed when lesions are not easily accessible for percutaneous needle biopsy or when results of closed biopsy are equivocal. The shape of the biopsy should be circular, not rectangular; this will prevent stress concentration on the square corners and pathologic fracture.

In the differential diagnosis of eosinophilic granuloma, one should consider osteomyelitis, Ewing's sarcoma, malignant lymphoma, osteosarcoma of bone, metastatic carcinoma, and aneurysmal bone cyst. It is crucial to perform a biopsy for final diagnosis of the lesion. In osteomyelitis, frank pus may be aspirated; neutrophils are abundant on histologic examination, and bacterial organisms may be cultured. Granulomatous inflammatory lesions, such as those due to atypical mycobacteria, may closely mimic eosinophilic granuloma; the etiology is determined by appropriate bacteriologic and laboratory studies. The histologic finding will differentiate Ewing's sarcoma, lymphoma, and osteogenic sarcoma from eosinophilic granuloma.

Treatment

Eosinophilic granuloma of bone is a benign lesion that occasionally is self-limited, healing spontaneously.[25, 66, 94] Often, however, treatment is indicated because of pain, tenderness, and progressive expansion of the lesion. The goals of therapy are to stop the growth of the lesion, promote healing, provide relief of pain, and prevent complications such as fracture or involvement of the physis and consequent growth arrest. Modalities of treatment available are: intralesional injection of steroids; surgical excision of the lesion by curettage, with or without bone grafting; support of the involved part to prevent pathologic fracture and deformity; and occasionally low-dosage radiotherapy for lesions that are not easily accessible surgically. The choice of method of treatment depends on the location and size of the lesion, the patient's age, and the natural course of the disease. Eosinophilic granuloma of bone is not an aggressive process; it has an excellent prognosis for healing, regardless of the method of treatment utilized.[94]

Percutaneous intralesional injection of methylprednisone sodium succinate. This was first described by Cohen and associates in 1980.[33] Prednisone appears to have a direct suppressive effect on the cells of the lesion or antigens contained within it; its exact mechanism of action is unknown, however. Nauert and associates reported the results of intralesional injection of methylprednisone sodium succinate in 14 cases—healing was achieved in every lesion without complications.[102] In 9 of the 14 cases the period of follow-up ranged from 25 to 48 months. The dosage of methylprednisone sodium succinate injected was 125 to 150 mg.

Technique. The procedure is painful owing to marrow expansion; therefore, it is best performed under general anesthesia in children. A superficial lesion in a cooperative mature adolescent or an adult may be done under local anesthesia. The percutaneous injection may be combined with percutaneous biopsy for the pathologic diagnosis by frozen section and cytologic smear. If the regional cortex is destroyed a 19-gauge hypodermic needle with a stylet inside is used to penetrate the center of the lesion; when the cortex is intact an Ackerman-Turkel biopsy needle is utilized to create a tunnel, the hypodermic needle is inserted through the hole of the Ackerman needle, and the steroid is injected. One should be cautious, however, that the hole made in the bone is no larger than the needle gauge because if it is the injected steroid will leak out around the needle. The steroid should be retained within the lesion to promote healing. The involved part is appropriately supported in a splint or sling for comfort. The procedure can be performed as outpatient surgery if the lesion is superficial.

Within the first two weeks postinjection the pain rapidly subsides. Significant radiographic improvement, however, is not seen until three months following injection. Initially a sclerotic margin forms around the sharply defined borders of the lytic lesion. Laminated periosteal reaction, if present, gradually solidifies, and the cortical thickening decreases. Then the lytic areas gradually fill in with trabeculated bone. In the early stages of healing the newly formed bone trabeculae are thick, but gradually they assume a normal structure. Complete healing of the lesion usually takes place within 18 to 24 months postinjection. Radiographic follow-up examinations are made at three-month intervals the first year and then at yearly intervals. If there is no clinical response the injection is repeated; one must, however, wait for a minimum of six months before considering reinjection.

It is evident that percutaneous injection of methylprednisone is the preferable way to treat eosinophilic granuloma localized to one or two bones, especially if their location is easily accessible anatomically. The procedure is effective, safe, cost effective, can usually be performed as outpatient surgery, and obviates surgical scars and therapeutic levels of ionizing radiation.

Surgical Curettage. This procedure is indicated when intralesional injection of the methylprednisone fails or when an open biopsy is performed, at which time one may proceed with curetting the lesion. The importance of preventing fracture should be emphasized. Simultaneous autogenous bone grafting is performed to support the structural integrity of the remaining tissue. When the spine is affected a Milwaukee brace is used for support; it will unload the anterior vertebral bodies and allow remodeling and restoration of normal spinal alignment. In the lower limbs, following an initial period of immobilization in a cast, support is given by a light orthosis, applying principles of fracture bracing.[19] Subperiosteal resection of an involved rib, clavicle, or fibula may be performed; however, it is not recommended by this author. Eosinophilic granuloma has an excellent prognosis; it heals without resorting to such aggressive surgical measures.

In multiple radiographic lesions the symptomatic lesion only is curetted. The asymptomatic lesions are observed for up to one year, as they may spontaneously regress and heal.

and Begg, C. F.: A reappraisal of eosinophilic granuloma of bone. Medicine (Baltimore), 48:375, 1969.
91. Lindenbaum, B., and Gettes, N. I.: Solitary eosinophilic granuloma of the cervical region. Clin. Orthop., 68:112, 1970.
92. Lucaya, J.: Histiocytosis X. Am. J. Dis. Child., 121:289, 1971.
93. McCullough, C. J.: Eosinophilic granuloma of bone. Acta Orthop. Scand., 51:389, 1980.
94. McGavran, M. H., and Spady, H. A.: Eosinophilic granuloma of bone. A study of twenty-eight cases. J. Bone Joint Surg., 42-A:979, 1960.
95. Melhem, R. E., Hajjar, J. J., and Balassanian, N.: Histiocytosis X. A report of 15 cases in the pediatric age group. Br. J. Radiol., 37:898, 1964.
96. Mickelson, M. R., and Bonfiglio, M.: Eosinophilic granuloma and its variations. Orthop. Clin. North Am., 8:933, 1977.
97. Mierau, G. W., Favara, B. E., and Brenman, J. M.: Electron microscopy in histiocytosis X. Ultrastruct. Pathol., 3:137, 1982.
98. Miller, D. R.: Familial reticuloendotheliosis: Concurrence of disease in five siblings. Pediatrics, 38:986, 1966.
99. Moe, P. J.: Letterer-Siwe's disease (acute disseminated histiocytosis X), disseminated I-V coagulation, and hemolytic-uremic syndrome. Pediatrics, 48:491, 1971.
100. Moe, P. J., and Hansen, A. E.: Reticuloendothelial granuloma. Am. J. Dis. Child., 99:175, 1960.
101. Myers, D. A., Strandjord, S. E., Marcus, R. B., Jr., Pierson, K. K., and Walker, R. D., 3rd: Histiocytosis X presenting as a primary penile lesion. J. Urol., 126:268, 1981.
102. Nauert, C., Zornoza, J., Ayala, A., and Harle, T. S.: Eosinophilic granuloma of bone: Diagnosis and management. Skeletal Radiol., 10:227, 1983.
103. Nesbit, M. E., Kieffer, S., and D'Angio, G. J.: Reconstitution of vertebral height in histiocytosis X. J. Bone Joint Surg., 51-A:1360, 1969.
104. Nesbit, M. E., Jr., O'Leary, M., Dehner, L. P., and Ramsay, N. K.: The immune system and the histiocytosis syndromes. Am. J. Pediatr. Hematol. Oncol., 3:141, 1981.
105. Newton, W. A., Jr., and Hamoudi, A. B.: Histiocytosis: A histologic classification with clinical correlation. In Rosenberg, H. S. and Bolande, R. P. (eds.): Perspectives in Pediatric Pathology. Vol. 1. Chicago, Year Book, 1973, pp. 251–283.
106. Nezelof, C., Basset, F., and Rousseau, M. F.: Histiocytosis X. Histogenetic arguments for a Langerhans cell origin. Biomedicine, 18:365, 1973.
107. Nitter, L.: Three cases of eosinophilic granuloma of the pelvis in children. Acta Radiol., 46:731, 1956.
108. Oberman, H.: Idiopathic histiocytosis: A clinicopathological study of 40 cases and review of the literature on eosinophilic granuloma of bone. Hand-Schüller-Christian disease and Letterer-Siwe disease. Pediatrics, 28:307, 1961.
109. Ochsner, S. F.: Eosinophilic granuloma of bone. Experience with 20 cases. A.J.R., 57:719, 1966.
110. Osband, M. E., Lipton, J. M., Lavin, P., Levey, R., Vawter, G., Greenberger, J. S., McCaffrey, R. P., and Parkman, R.: Histiocytosis-X. N. Engl. J. Med., 304:146, 1981.
111. Otani, S., and Ehrlich, J. C.: Solitary granuloma of bone simulating primary neoplasm. Am. J. Pathol., 16:479, 1940.
112. Parker, B. R., and Castellino, R. A.: Pediatric Oncologic Radiology. St. Louis, Mosby, 1977, p. 209.
113. Parker, B. R., Pickney, L., and Etcubanas, E.: Relative efficacy of radiographic and radionuclide bone surveys in the detection of the skeletal lesions of histiocytosis X. Radiology, 134:377, 1980.
114. Ponseti, I. V.: Bone lesions in eosinophilic granuloma. Hand-Schüller-Christian disease and Letterer-Siwe disease. J. Bone Joint Surg., 39-A:811, 1948.
115. Poulsen, J. O., and Thommesen, P.: An unusual case of histiocytosis of the spine. Acta Orthop. Scand., 47:59, 1976.
116. Pouyanne, L.: La vertebra-plana. Localisation rachidienne du granulome éosinophilique. Rev. Chir. Orthop., 40:25, 1954.
117. Richter, M. P., and D'Angio, G. J.: The role of radiation therapy in the management of children with histiocytosis X. Am. J. Pediatr. Hematol. Oncol., 3:161, 1981.
118. Rigault, P., and Finidori, G.: Les localisations vertébrales de histiocytose X. Aspect orthopaedique. Rev. Chir. Orthop., Suppl. 2, 63:190, 1977.
119. Ruff, S., Chapman, G. K., Taylor, T. K. F., and Ryan, M. D.: The evolution of eosinophilic granuloma of bone: A case report. Skeletal Radiol., 10:37, 1983.
120. Sbarbaro, J. L., and Francis, K. C.: Eosinophilic granuloma of bone. J.A.M.A., 178:706, 1961.
121. Schajowicz, F., and Slullitel, J.: Eosinophilic granuloma of bone and its relationship to Hand-Schüller-Christian and Letterer-Siwe syndromes. J. Bone Joint Surg., 55-B:545, 1973.
122. Schüller, A.: Über eigenartige Schädeldefkte im Jugendalter. Fortschr. Rontgenstr., 23:12, 1915.
123. Sherk, H. H., Nicholson, J., and Nixon, J. E.: Vertebra plana and eosinophilic granuloma of the cervical spine in children. Spine, 3:116, 1978.
124. Siddiqui, A. R., Tashjian, J. H., Lazarus, K., Wellman, H. N., and Baehner, R. L.: Nuclear medicine studies in evaluation of skeletal lesions in children with histiocytosis X. Radiology, 140:787, 1981.
125. Sims, D. O.: Histiocytosis X. Follow-up of 43 cases. Arch. Dis. Child., 52:433, 1977.
126. Siwe, S.: The reticulo-endothelioses in children. Adv. Pediatr., 4:117, 1949.
127. Slater, J. M., and Swarm, O. J.: Eosinophilic granuloma of bone. Med. Pediatr. Oncol., 8:151, 1980.
128. Smith, D. G., Nesbit, M. E., D'Angio, G. J., and Levitt, S. H.: Histiocytosis X: Role of radiation therapy in management with special reference to dose levels employed. Radiology, 106:419, 1973.
129. Starling, K. A.: Chemotherapy of histiocytosis. Am. J. Pediatr. Hematol. Oncol., 3:157, 1981.
130. Starling, K. A., Iyer, R., Silva-Sosa, M., Komp, D., Herson, J., and Trueworthy, R. C.: Chlorambucil in histiocytosis X: A Southwest oncology group study. J. Pediatr., 96:266, 1980.
131. Stern, M. B., Cassidy, R., and Mirra, J.: Eosinophilic granuloma of the proximal tibial epiphysis. Clin. Orthop., 118:153, 1976.
132. Stormby, N., and Akerman, M.: Cytodiagnosis of bone lesions by means of fine-needle aspiration biopsy. Acta Cytol., 17:166, 1973.
133. Takahashi, M., Martel, W., and Oberman, H. A.: The variable roentgenographic appearance of idiopathic histiocytosis. Clin. Radiol., 17:48, 1966.
134. Teja, K., Sabio, H., Langdon, D. R., and Johanson, A. J.: Involvement of the thyroid gland in histiocytosis X. Hum. Pathol., 12:1137, 1981.
135. Teplick, J. G., and Broder, H.: Eosinophilic granuloma of bone. A.J.R., 78:502, 1957.
136. Usui, M., Matsuno, T., Kobayashi, M., Yagi, T., Sasaki, T., and Ishii, S.: eosinophilic granuloma of the growing epiphysis. A case report and review of the literature. Clin. Orthop., 176:201, 1983.
137. Vogel, J. M., and Vogel, P.: Idiopathic histiocytosis. Semin. Hematol., 9:349, 1972.
138. Wallgren, A.: Systemic reticuloendothelial granuloma; nonlipoid reticuloendotheliosis and Schüller-Christian disease. Am. J. Dis. Child., 60:471, 1940.

139. Wells, P. O.: The button sequestrum of eosinophilic granuloma of the skull. Radiology, 67:746, 1956.
140. West, W. O.: Velban as treatment for diffuse eosinophilic granuloma of the bone. Report of a case. J. Bone Joint Surg., 55-A:1755, 1973.
141. Weston, W. J., and Goodson, G. M.: Vertebra plana (Calvé). J. Bone Joint Surg., 41-B:477, 1959.
142. Yabsley, R. H., and Harris, W. R.: Solitary eosinophilic granuloma of a vertebral body causing paraplegia. Report of a case. J. Bone Joint Surg., 48-A:1570, 1966.
143. Zinkham, W. H.: Multifocal eosinophilic granuloma. Am. J. Med., 60:457, 1976.

NEUROFIBROMATOSIS (VON RECKLINGHAUSEN'S DISEASE)

This is a multisystemic hereditary disorder characterized by a basic aberration of the supportive tissue of the central and peripheral nervous systems and associated with variable abnormalities of the skeleton, skin, and soft tissues.

Historically, cases of neurofibromatosis were reported by Tilesius, Smith, Virchow, and Kolliker prior to von Recklinghausen's book in 1882.[55, 147, 163, 172, 181] It was, however, von Recklinghausen who coined the term *neurofibroma*, demonstrated nerve elements in the fibrous tissue tumors, and correlated the nervous and dermal lesions. Therefore, the eponym *von Recklinghausen's disease* remains.

Etiology

The etiology is unknown. Many theories have been proposed. The suggested infectious and endocrine origins have been disproved. At present the dysontogenic theory is in favor, which proposes that neurofibromatosis is a congenital defect leading to dysplasia of ectodermal and mesodermal tissues. In the neurogenic theory, deviation in the development of the primitive neuroblast is purported to be the pathogenic factor.[46] It is considered a hamartomatous disorder of neural crest origin involving the neuroectoderm, mesoderm, and endoderm with the potential of affecting almost any organ system.[90]

Heredity

Inheritance is by autosomal dominant transmission. There may be variable penetrance and expressivity in some cases. Mutations do occur. It is difficult to estimate the frequency of neurofibromatosis because of its marked clinical variability. According to Wynne-Davies and associates, the frequency may be as high as one in 2000 to 3000 births with a possible prevalence of 22 per million population of index patients or 28 per million including affected relatives.[193]

Pathology

The proliferating cells of neurofibromatosis originate in either or both the Schwann sheath cells and the supportive cells.[5, 133] Histologically, neurofibromas are made up of masses of spindle cells that may contain aggregates of palisaded nuclei (Fig. 3–314). Bone lesions reveal poorly delineated masses of spindle cells rather resembling fibrocytes with a tendency to palisading in some areas. Grossly, neurofibromas are pale, moderately firm masses that involve a small portion or a longer segment of peripheral nerve. They may also be located in branches of the autonomic system or meninges. The nerve trunks are usually increased in diameter and are twisted in their normal course; they may be tender to pressure on the contiguous nerve fibers. Paraplegia may occur.[125] Occasionally tuberous sclerosis and gliomas of the central nervous system may be noted, and endocrine disturbance may be caused by an enlarging neurofibroma.

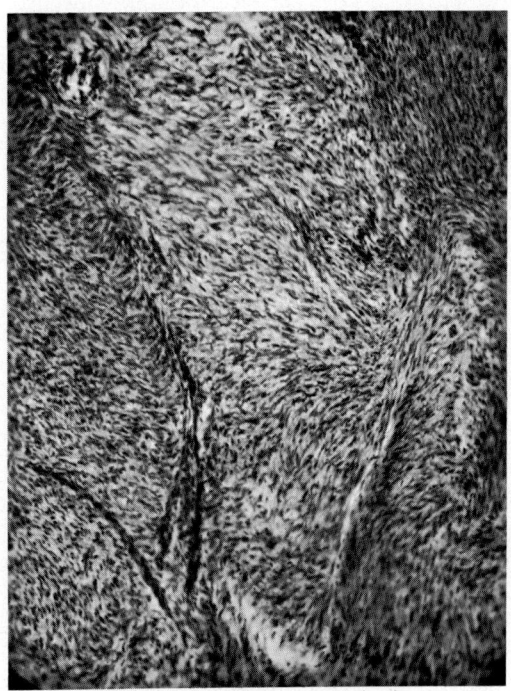

FIGURE 3–314. Neurofibromatosis.

Photomicrograph of tissue curetted from lesion in tibia (× 100). Note the spindle-shaped stroma with "palisading" of the nuclei.

Clinical Features

There are three clinical forms of neurofibromatosis: first, the *peripheral form* with café au lait spots and neurofibromas, second, the *central form* with multiple neoplasms in the central nervous system, and third the *mixed form* with both peripheral lesions and neurofibromas and tumors of the central nervous system.[196]

Soft-tissue findings are the following: 1. *Café au lait spots* are pigmentations that are tan and macular; they are melanotic in origin and located in and around the basal layer of the epidermis (Fig. 3–315). The café au lait spots of neurofibromatosis have smooth edges in contrast to the jagged edges of those in fibrous dysplasia. The melanocytes of the café au lait spots of neurofibromatosis contain giant melanosomes, whereas in fibrous dysplasia, such giant melanosomes are not usually present.[96] The spots are usually found in areas of skin not exposed to sun; they vary in shape, size, and number. Five or more with a diameter of at least 0.5 cm. are required for diagnosis of neurofibromatosis. They may not be present in infancy, but usually appear by nine years of age. A café au lait spot may be present in a normal person. 2. *Nodules* (fibroma molluscum) are dermal neurofibromas that contain axons and Schwann cells on electromicroscopy (Fig. 3–316). They usually develop after puberty. Dermal neurofibromas are rarely associated with central nervous system lesions. There may be subcutaneous neurofibromatous tumors (see Fig. 3–320 E to G). 3. *Nevi* are dark brown hyperpigmented areas of skin that tend to overlie plexiform neurofibromas (Fig. 3–317). The underlying plexiform neurofibroma may be very sensitive and have a "ropey," "bag of worms" feeling to palpation. They have a 10 per cent incidence of malignant degeneration. This risk dictates that surgical treatment be carried out early for pigmented nevi. 4. *Elephantiasis*, or *pachydermatocele*, are raised hypertrophic villi of the skin that have a typical appearance (Fig. 3–318). There may be dysplasia of the underlying bone. 5. *Verrucous hyperplasia* is an overgrowth of the skin with thickening and a velvety soft feel (Fig. 3–319). Surface infection of verrucous hyperplasia is common. Often it is unilateral; the appearance is very grotesque, and it may be associated with elongation of the ipsilateral limb. 6. *Axillary freckles* are diffuse hyperpigmented spots 1 to 3 mm. in diameter usually located in the axillary region.

Skeletal Findings. There is a high incidence of skeletal involvement, the bone deformities resulting either directly from the destructive neurofibromatous tissue or from localized or systemic aberrations of skeletal growth and de-

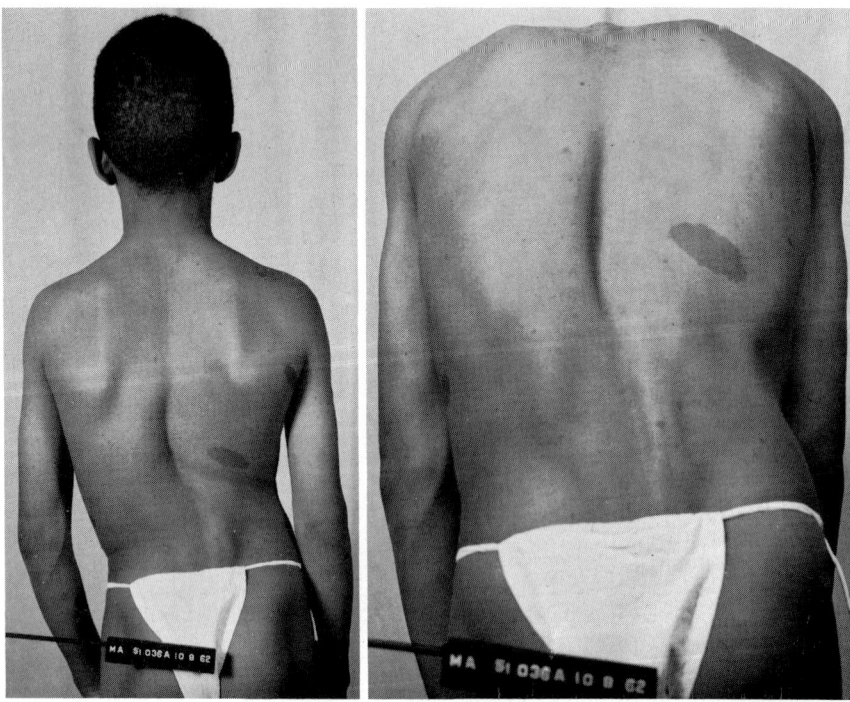

FIGURE 3–315. *Neurofibromatosis with scoliosis.*

Note the café-au-lait spots on right side of trunk.

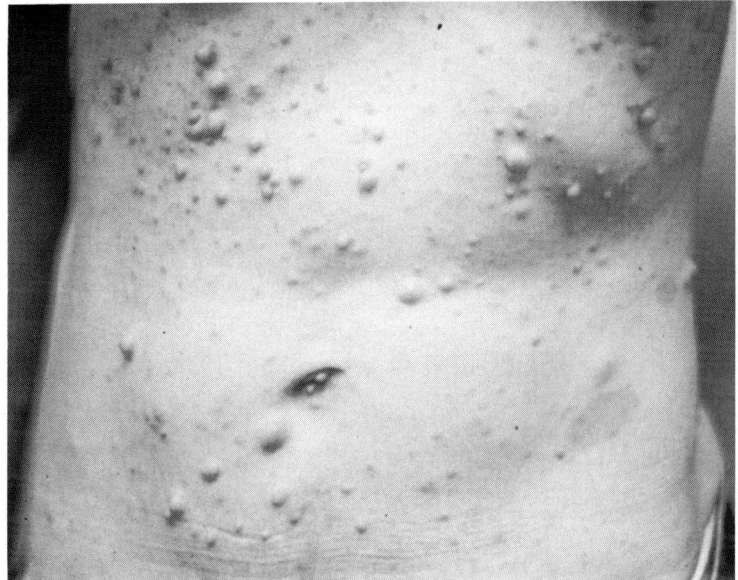

FIGURE 3–316. *Fibroma molluscum (multiple dermal neurofibroma in neurofibromatosis).*

(From Crawford, A. H.: Neurofibromatosis in children. Acta Orthop. Scand., Suppl. 57:218, 1986. Reprinted by permission.)

velopment. The most unusual and striking of these irregularities is focal gigantism, the result of hypertrophy of a single bone, digit, or entire limb. Other bone lesions may include defects of the cortices of bones (caused by irritation of the periosteum by the neurofibromatous tissue), cystlike rarefactions (due to growth of the proliferating tissue within the medullary cavity), bowing, unusual lengthening or shortening, and a change in the internal structure (Fig. 3–320). Pseudarthrosis of the tibia or fibula is common; this is discussed in detail in Chapter 2.

Scoliosis is a deformity frequently associated with neurofibromatosis (see Figs. 3–315 and 3–

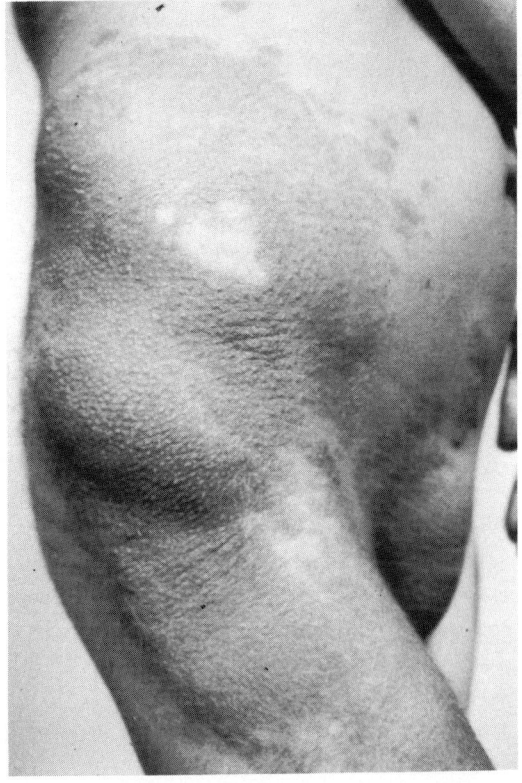

FIGURE 3–317. *A large nevus overlying a plexiform neurofibroma.*

(From Crawford, A. H.: Neurofibromatosis in children. Acta Orthop. Scand., 57:Suppl. 218, 1986. Reprinted by permission.)

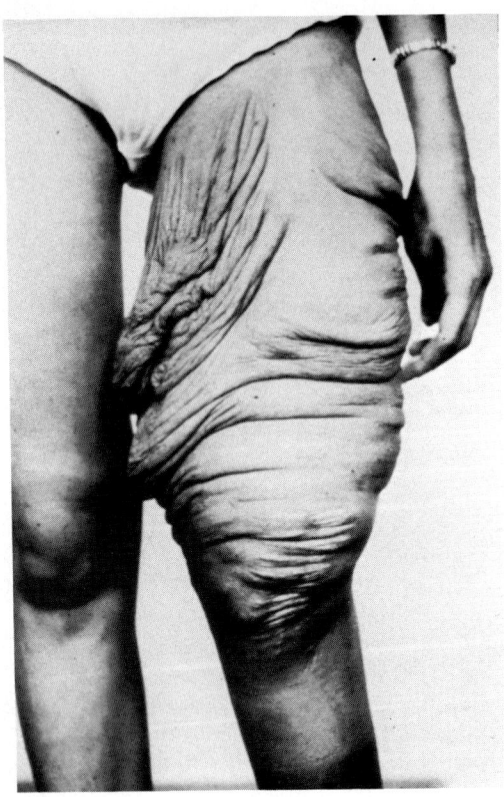

FIGURE 3–318. *Elephantiasis in neurofibromatosis.*

Note the thickening of the skin with redundant folds. (From Crawford, A. H.: Neurofibromatosis in children. Acta Orthop. Scand., 57: Suppl. 218, 1986. Reprinted by permission.)

FIGURE 3–319. *Verrucous hyperplasia over the left buttock in neurofibromatosis.*

(From Crawford, A. H.: Neurofibromatosis in children. Acta Orthop. Scand., 57:Suppl. 218, 1986. Reprinted by permission.)

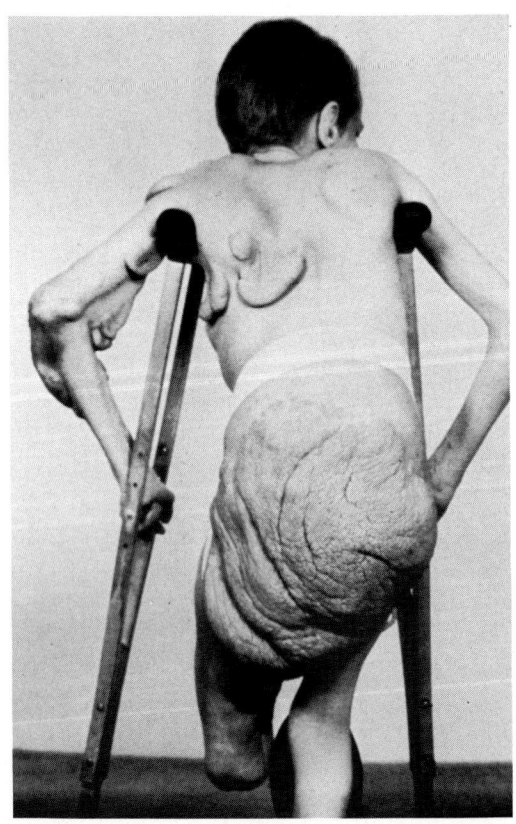

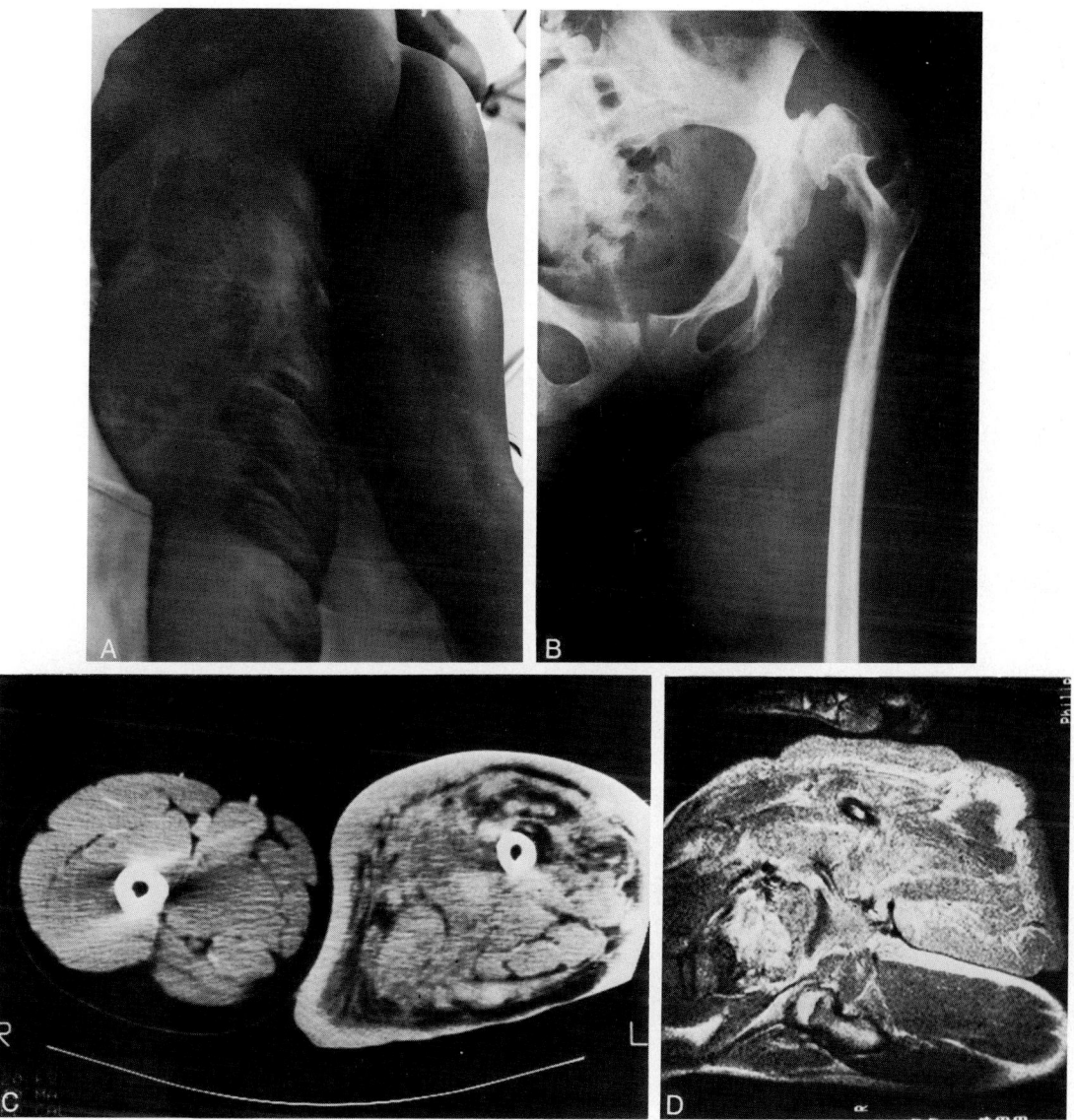

FIGURE 3–320. *Neurofibromatosis in a 12-year-old girl.*

A. Clinical appearance of her thighs and hips. Note the elephantiasis. **B.** Anteroposterior radiogram of the left hip and upper two thirds of the femur. The hip is dislocated with marked dysplasia of the acetabulum and attenuation of the femoral neck. **C** and **D.** CT scans of upper thigh and hip region showing marked soft-tissue changes.

Illustration continued on following page

321). It varies in its degree of severity. Its cause is unknown; there is no consistent pattern. The curve may be short with severe wedging of the affected vertebrae (see Chapter 6). It may be accompanied by kyphosis (Fig. 3–322). The cervical and dorsolumbar spine may show scalloping of the vertebral bodies with deformity of the pedicles and widening of the intervertebral foramina. A dumbbell neurofibroma may be present. Rarely, there may be intrathoracic meningocele. Computed tomography and myelography are required for accurate delineation of the pathologic situation.

Neoplasms. There is a 5 per cent incidence of associated neoplasms in neurofibromatosis. In the central nervous system these include acoustic neuroma, glioma, neurosarcoma, and ganglioneuroblastoma. In the peripheral soft tissues they are fibrosarcoma, neurofibrosarcoma, and neurogenic sarcoma. The incidence of malignancy increases with maturity, reaching to more than 20 per cent in the adult. The

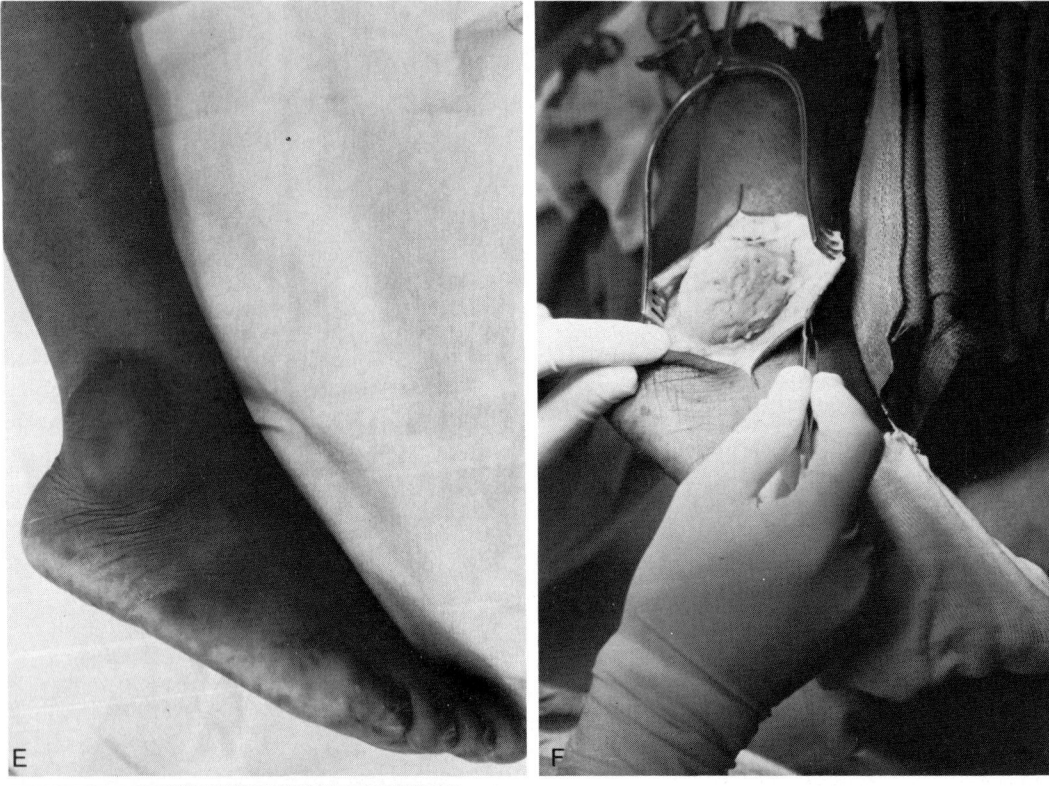
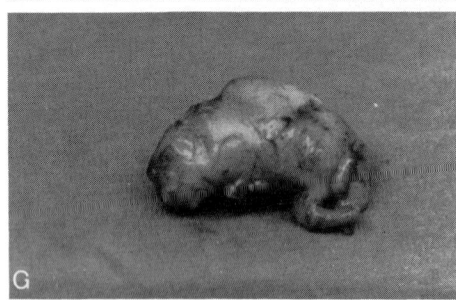

FIGURE 3–320 Continued. Neurofibromatosis in a 12-year-old girl.

E to G. Neurofibromatosis of ankle in same patient. Clinical appearance, findings at surgery, and gross specimen.

more severely involved the patient, the higher the incidence of malignant change.

To make a conclusive diagnosis of neurofibromatosis, there should be two of the four most commonly occurring findings: café au lait spots, positive family history, histologic diagnosis of neurofibroma, and characteristic bony lesions.

Treatment

Treatment is dependent on the nature of the presenting deformity. Excision of the hypertrophied soft tissue and nodular masses may be indicated. Amputation of grotesque or gigantic digits serves to improve appearance and function. If scoliosis is present, early spinal fusion may be indicated, as the curve may progress very rapidly (see Chapter 6). Painful lesions in bone are excised and, if necessary, repaired by bone grafting. Treatment of congenital pseudarthrosis of the tibia associated with neurofibromatosis is described in Chapter 2.

References

1. Abdel-Dayem, H. M., and Papademetriou, T.: Subperiosteal hemorrhage in neurofibromatosis: Appear-

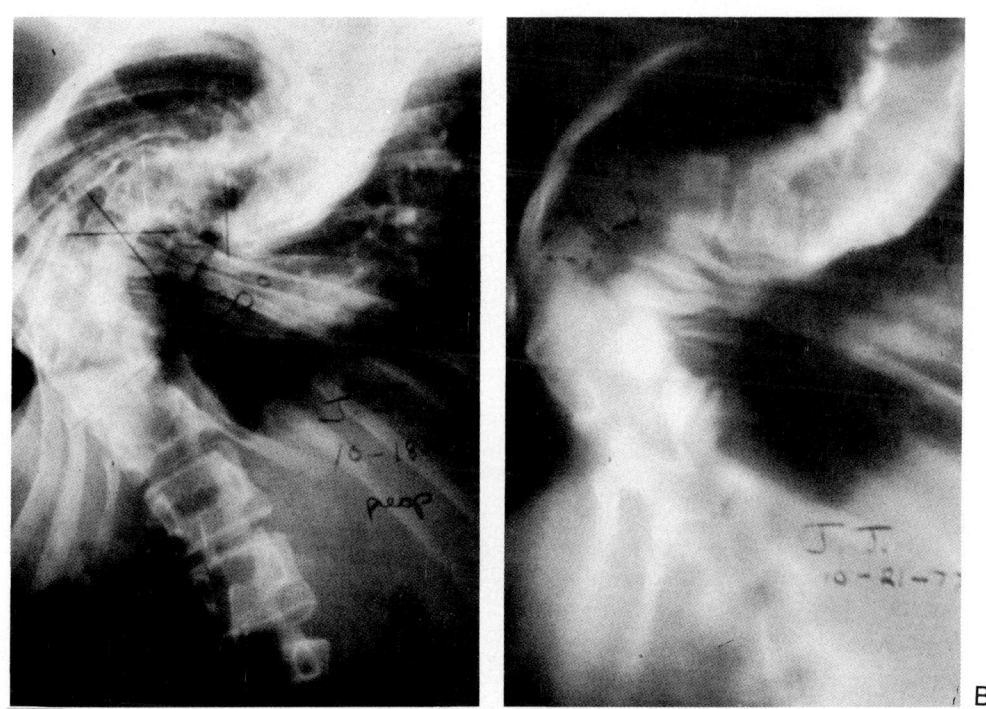

FIGURE 3–321. *Short segmented angulated "kinky" scoliosis in neurofibromatosis.*

A. Anteroposterior radiogram of the spine. **B.** Plain tomography. (From Crawford, A. H.: Neurofibromatosis in children. Acta Orthop. Scand., 57[Suppl.]:218, 1986. Reprinted by permission.)

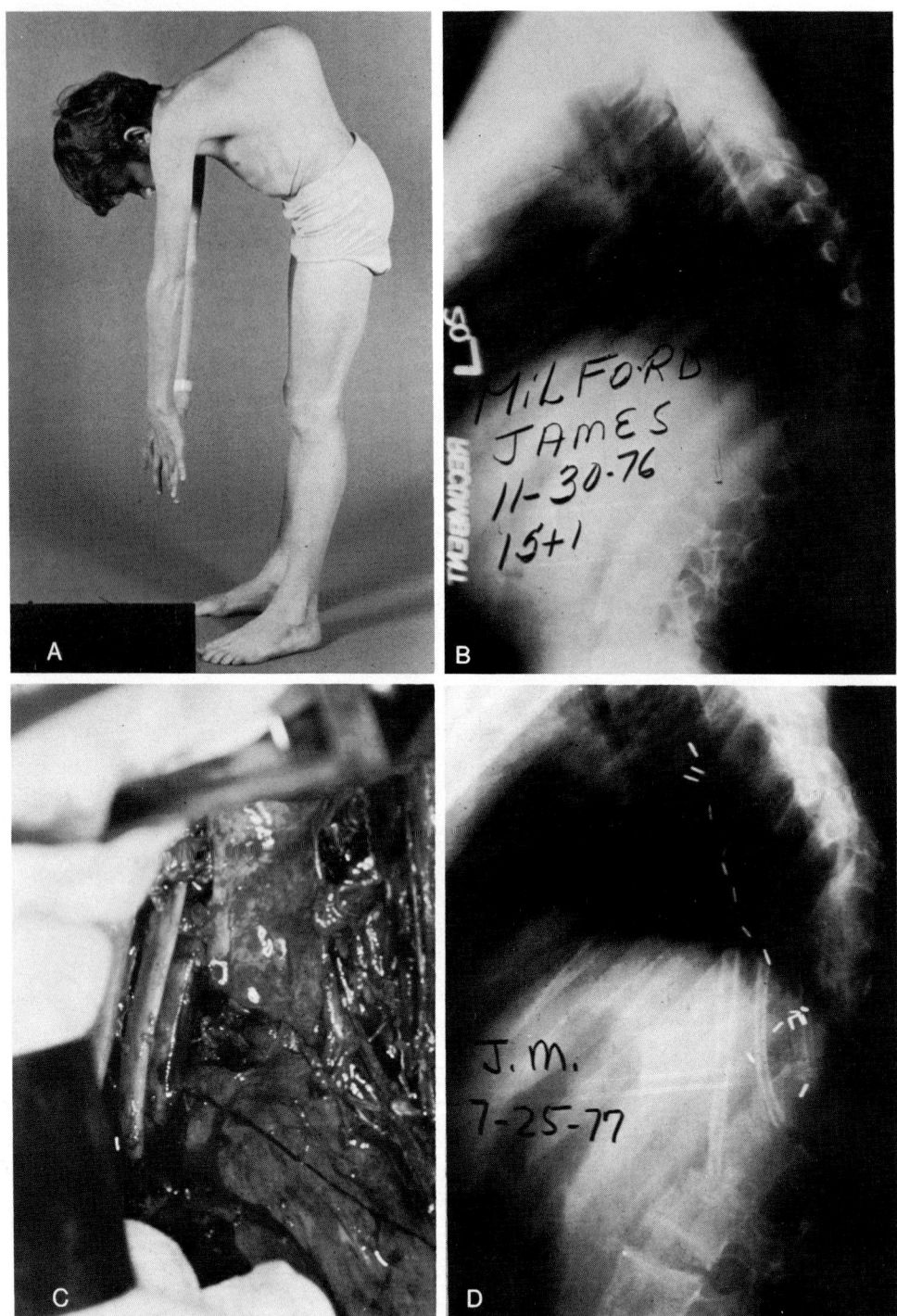

FIGURE 3–322. *Severe kyphosis of thoracic spine in neurofibromatosis.*

A. Clinical appearance. **B.** Preoperative lateral radiograph of spine. **C.** Operative photograph. Note the fibular and rib grafts across the apex of the kyphus. **D.** Lateral of the spine six months postoperatively showing the position of the fibula and rib grafts.

ance in bone scintigraphy. Clin. Nucl. Med., 6:272, 1981.
2. Adkins, J. C., and Ratvich, M. D.: Children's Hospital of Pittsburgh, The operative management of von Recklinghausen's neurofibromatosis in children, with special reference to lesions of the head and neck. Surgery, 82:343, 1977.
3. Adrian, C.: Ueber Neurofibromatose und ihre Komplikationen. Beitr. Klin. Chir., 31:1, 1901.
4. Aegerter, E. E.: The possible relationship of neurofibromatosis, congenital pseudarthrosis and fibrous dysplasia. J. Bone Joint Surg., 32-A:618, 1950.
5. Aegerter, E., and Kirkpatrick, J. A., Jr.: Orthopedic Diseases. 3rd Ed. Philadelphia, Saunders, 1968.
6. Albright, F., Butler, A. M., Hampton, A. O., and Smith, P.: Syndrome characterized by osteitis fibrosa disseminata, areas of pigmentation and endocrine dysfunction, with precocious puberty in females. N. Engl. J. Med., 216:727, 1937.
7. Alldred, A. J.: Congenital pseudarthrosis of the clavicle. J. Bone Joint Surg., 45-B:312, 1963.
8. Allibone, E. C., Illingworth, R. S., and Wright, T.: Neurofibromatosis (von Recklinghausen's disease) of the vertebral column. Arch. Dis. Child., 35:153, 1960.
9. Andersen, K. S.: Congenital pseudarthrosis of the leg. J. Bone Joint Surg., 58-A:657, 1976.
10. Andersen, K. S.: Congenital pseudarthrosis of the tibia and neurofibromatosis. Acta Orthop. Scand., 47:108, 1976.
11. Bader, J. L., and Miller, R. W.: Neurofibromatosis and childhood leukemia. J. Pediatr., 92:925, 1978.
12. Baldwin, D. M., and Weiner, D. S.: Congenital bowing and intraosseous neurofibroma of the ulna. J. Bone Joint Surg., 56-A:803, 1974.
13. Barber, C. G.: Congenital bowing and pseudarthrosis of the lower leg. Manifestations of von Recklinghausen's neurofibromatosis. Surg. Gynecol. Obstet., 69:618, 1939.
14. Barone, D. A.: Neurofibromatoses: A clinical overview. Postgrad. Med., 66(2):73,79, 1979.
15. Bartlett, R., Otis, R. D., and Laakso, A. O.: Multiple congenital neoplasm of soft tissues. Cancer, 14:913, 1961.
16. Basset, C. A. L., Caulo, N. P., and Dort, J. S.: Congenital pseudarthrosis of the tibia: Treatment with pulsating electromagnetic field. Presented at the American Academy of Orthopaedic Surgeons, Las Vegas, Nevada, 1981.
17. Bauer, J. W., and Radowski, M. A.: Congenital multiple fibromatosis. A.J.R., 118:200, 1973.
18. Beatty, E. C., Jr.: Congenital generalized fibromatosis in infancy. Am. J. Dis. Child., 103:602, 1962.
19. Berk, L., and Mankin, H. J.: Spontaneous pseudarthrosis of the tibia occurring in a patient with neurofibromatosis. Report of a case in a man 41 years old. J. Bone Joint Surg., 46-A:619, 1964.
20. Biot, B., Fauchet, R., and Stagnara, P.: Les lésions vertébrales de la neurofibromatose. Rev. Chir. Orthop., 60:607, 1974.
21. Bolande, R. P.: Neurofibromatosis—the quintessential neurocristopathy: Pathogenetic concepts and relationships. Adv. Neurol., 29:67, 1981.
22. Booher, F. J., and McPeak, C. J.: Juvenile aponeurotic fibromas. Surgery, 46:924, 1959.
23. Boyd, H. B., and Sage, F. P.: Congenital pseudarthrosis of the tibia. J. Bone Joint Surg., 40-A:1245, 1958.
24. Bradford, D. S.: Neurofibromatosis in children. A.A.O.S. Instruct. Course Lect., Las Vegas, Nevada, 1976.
25. Brasfield, R. D., and Das Gupta, T. K.: von Recklinghausen's disease: A clinicopathologic study. Ann. Surg., 175:86, 1972.
26. Breig, A.: Biomechanics of the Central Nervous System: Some Basic and Normal Pathologic Phenomena Concerning Spine, Disk, and Cord. Stockholm, Almquist & Wiskel, 1960.
27. Brighton, C. T., Friedenberg, Z. B., Zemski, L. M., and Pollis, B. R.: Direct current stimulation of nonunion and congenital pseudarthrosis. Exploration of its clinical application. J. Bone Joint Surg., 57-A:368, 1975.
28. Briner, J., and Yunis, E.: Ultrastructure of congenital pseudarthrosis of the tibia. Arch. Pathol., 95:97, 1973.
29. Brooks, B., and Lehman, E. P.: The bone changes in Recklinghausen's neurofibromatosis. Surg. Gynecol. Obstet., 38:587, 1924.
30. Bruwer, A. J., and Kierland, R. R.: Neurofibromatosis and congenital unilateral pulsating and nonpulsating exophthalmos. Arch. Ophthalmol., 53:2, 1955.
31. Casselman, E. S., and Mandell, G. A.: Vertebral scalloping in neurofibromatosis. Pediatr. Radiol., 131:89, 1979.
32. Chaglassian, J. H., Riseborough, E. J., and Hall, J. E.: Neurofibromatous scoliosis. Natural history and results of treatment in thirty-seven cases. J. Bone Joint Surg., 58-A:695, 1976.
33. Chao, D. H.: Congenital neurocutaneous syndromes in childhood. Neurofibromatosis. J. Pediatr., 55:189, 1959.
34. Charache, H.: Multiple neurofibroma with sarcomatous transformation and skeletal involvement. Arch. Dermatol. Syph., 40:185, 1939.
35. Charnley, J.: Congenital pseudarthrosis of the tibia treated by intramedullary nail. J. Bone Joint Surg., 38-A:238, 1956.
36. Chu, J. Y., O'Connor, D. M., and Danis, R. K.: Neurofibrosarcoma at irradiation sites in a patient with neurofibromatosis and Wilms' tumor. CA, 131:333, 1981.
37. Clemis, J. D.: The coexistence of acoustic neuroma and otosclerosis. Laryngoscope, 83:1959, 1973.
38. Cobb, J. N.: Outline for the study of scoliosis. A.A.O.S. Instruct. Course Lect., 5:261, 1948.
39. Cobb, N.: Neurofibromatosis and pseudarthrosis of the ulna: A case report. J. Bone Joint Surg., 50-B:146, 1968.
40. Cole, W. G., and Meyers, N. A.: Neurofibromatosis in childhood. Aust. N.Z. J. Surg., 48:360, 1978.
41. Condon, V. R., and Allen, R. P.: Congenital generalized fibromatosis. Radiology, 76:444, 1961.
42. Couselo Sanchez, J. M., Fuster Siebert, M., de Miguel Zaragoza, R., Cabanas Gancedo, R., and Monasterio Corral, L.: Juvenile chronic myeloid leukemia associated with familial neurofibromatosis. An. Esp. Pediatr., 14:287, 1981.
43. Cowell, H. R., Hall, J. N., and MacEwen, G. D.: Genetic aspects of idiopathic scoliosis: A Nicholas Andry Award Essay, 1970. Clin. Orthop., 86:121, 1972.
44. Crawford, A. H.: Neurofibromatosis in the pediatric patient. Orthop. Clin. North Am., 9:11, 1978.
45. Crawford, A. H.: Neurofibromatosis in childhood. A.A.O.S. Instruct. Course Lect., 19:56–74, 1981.
46. Crawford, A. H.: Neurofibromatosis in children. Acta Orthop. Scand., 57:Suppl. 218, 1986.
47. Crowe, F. W., Schull, W. J., and Neil, J. V.: A Clinical, Pathologic, and Genetic Study of Multiple Neurofibromatosis. Springfield, Ill, Thomas, 1956.
48. Crowe, F. W., and Schull, W. J.: Diagnostic importance of café-au-lait spot in neurofibromatosis. Arch. Intern. Med., 91:758, 1953.
49. Curtis, B. L., Fisher, R. L., Butterfield, W. L., and Saunders, F. P.: Neurofibromatosis with paraple-

gia. A report of 8 cases. J. Bone Joint Surg., 51-A:843, 1969.
50. Drescher, E., Woyke, S., Markiewicz, C., and Tegi, S.: Juvenile fibromatosis in siblings. J. Pediatr. Surg., 2:427, 1967.
51. Ducatman, B. S., Scheithaur, B. W., and Dahlin, D. C.: Malignant bone tumors associated with neurofibromatosis. Mayo Clin. Proc., 58:578, 1983.
52. Ducroquet, R.: A propos des pseudarthroses et inflexions congénitales du tibia. Mém. Acad. Chir., 63:863, 1937.
53. Dunn, A. W.: Case of overgrowth of leg and anterolateral bowing of tibia in neurofibromatosis. Am. J. Orthop., 7:120, 1965.
54. Edvardsen, P.: Resection osteosynthesis and Boyd amputation of congenital pseudarthrosis of the tibia. J. Bone Joint Surg., 55-B:179, 1973.
55. Ewing, J.: Neoplastic Diseases. A Treatise on Tumors. 3rd Ed. Philadelphia, Saunders, 1928, p. 166.
56. Eyre-Brook, A. L., Baily, R. A. J., and Price, C. H. G.: Infantile pseudarthrosis of the tibia. J. Bone Joint Surg., 51-B:604, 1969.
57. Fairbank, H. A. T.: Neurofibromatosis: Atlas of general infections of the skeleton. J. Bone Joint Surg., 32-B:266, 1950.
58. Fiaklow, P. J., Sagebeil, R. W., Gartler, S. M., and Rimoin, D. L.: Multiple cell origin or hereditary neurofibromatosis. N. Engl. J. Med., 284:298, 1971.
59. Fienman, N. L.: Comprehensive therapy. Pediatric neurofibromatosis: Review. Front. Med., 7:66, 1981.
60. Fienman, N. L.: Pediatric neurofibromatosis: Review. Compr. Ther., 7:66, 1981.
61. Fienman, N. L., and Yakovac, W. C.: Neurofibromatosis in childhood. J. Pediatr., 76:339, 1970.
62. Fishchenko, V. I., Uleshchenko, V. A., and Vovk, N. N.: Scoliosis on a background of neurofibromatosis. Ortop. Travmatol. Protez., 12:23, 1981.
63. Fisher, E. R., and Vuzevski, V. D.: Cytogenesis of schwannoma (neurilemmoma), neurofibroma, dermatofibrosarcoma as revealed by electron microscopy. Am. J. Clin. Pathol., 49:141, 1968.
64. Fleming, M. P., and Miller, W. E.: Renovascular hypertension due to neurofibromatosis. A.J.R., 113:452, 1971.
65. Ford, F. R.: Paraplegia due to severe scoliosis. In Ford, F. R. (ed.): Diseases of the Nervous System in Infancy, Childhood and Adolescence. 3rd Ed. Springfield, Ill., Thomas, 1952.
66. Frank, L.: Von Recklinghausen disease traced through five generations. Arch. Dermatol. Syph., 55:109, 1947.
67. Frenk, N.: Ultrastructure of the pigment with Albright's syndrome. Dermatologica, 143:12, 1971.
68. Friedman, M. M.: Neurofibromatosis of bone. A.J.R., 51:623, 1944.
69. Fulton, J. F.: Robert W. Smith's description of generalized neurofobromatosis (1849). N. Engl. J. Med., 200:1315, 1929.
70. Garland, A.: Four brothers with neurofibromatosis. Br. Med. J., 2:120, 1941.
71. Goel, M. K.: Osseous lesions in neurofibromatosis. Unpublished data.
72. Goldman, I. R.: Congenital malformation of vertebrae (hemivertebrae) with aplasia of corresponding ribs. Associated with lateral meningomyelocele: Report of a case. Arch. Pathol., 47:153, 1949.
73. Gould, E. P.: The bone changes occurring in von Recklinghausen's disease. Q. J. Med., 11:221, 1918.
74. Green, W. T., and Rudo, N.: Pseudoarthrosis and neurofibromatosis. Arch. Surg., 46:639, 1943.
75. Gregg, P. J., Price, B. A., Ellis, H. A., and Stevens, J.: Pseudarthrosis of the radius associated with neurofibromatosis. Clin. Orthop., 171:175, 1982.
76. Gross, P., Bailey, F. R., and Jacox, H. W.: Primary intramedullary neurofibroma of the humerus. Arch. Pathol., 28:716, 1939.
77. Guthrie, G. P., Jr., Tibbs, P. A., McAllister, R. G., Jr., Stevens, R. K., and Clark, D. B.: Hypertension and neurofibromatosis. Case report. Hypertension, 4:894, 1982.
78. Hagelstrom, L.: Deformities of the spine and multiple neurofibromatoses (von Recklinghausen). Acta Chir. Scand., 93:169, 1946.
79. Hall, B. D., and Spranger, J. W.: Familial congenital bowing with short bones. Radiology, 132:611, 1979.
80. Hallock, H.: The cause of multiple small bone transplants in the treatment of pseudarthrosis of the tibia of congenital origin or following osteotomy for the correction of congenital deformity. J. Bone Joint Surg., 20-A:646, 1938.
81. Harding, E. K.: Congenital anterior bowing of the tibia. The significance of the different types in relation to pseudarthrosis. Ann. R. Coll. Surg. (English translation), 51:817, 1972.
82. Harkin, J. C., and Reed, R. J.: Tumors of the peripheral nervous system. Second series, Fascicle 3. Washington D.C., Armed Forces Institute of Pathology, 1969.
83. Harris, W. C., Jr., Alpert, W. J., and Marcinko, D. E.: Elephantiasis neuromatosa in von Recklinghausen's disease. A review and case report. J. Am. Podiatry Assoc., 72:70, 1982.
84. Heard, G. E., Holt, J. F., and Naylor, B.: Cervical vertebral deformity in von Recklinghausen's disease of the nervous system. A review with necropsy findings. J. Bone Joint Surg., 44-B:880, 1962.
85. Hecht, F., and McCaw, B. K.: Neurofibromatosis and malignancy (letter to the editor) J. Pediatr., 91:1010, 1979.
86. Heiple, K. G., Perrin, E., and Aikawa, M.: Congenital generalized fibromatosis. J. Bone Joint Surg., 54-A:663, 1972.
87. Henderson, M. S.: Congenital pseudarthrosis of the tibia. J. Bone Joint Surg., 10:483, 1978.
88. Hensley, C. D.: The rapid development of a "subperiosteal bone cyst" in multiple neurofibromatosis. J. Bone Joint Surg., 35-A:197, 1953.
89. Holt, J. F.: Neurofibromatosis in children. A.J.R., 130:615, 1978.
90. Holt, J. F., and Wright, E. M.: The radiologic features of neurofibromatosis. Radiology, 51:647, 1948.
91. Hosoi, K.: Multiple neurofibromatosis (von Recklinghausen's disease) with special reference to malignant transformation. Arch. Surg., 22:258, 1931.
92. Hunt, J. C., and Pugh, D. C.: Skeletal lesions in neurofibromatosis. Radiology, 76:1, 1961.
93. Inglis, K.: The nature of neurofibromatosis and related lesions, with special reference to certain lesions of bones. J. Pathol. Bacteriol., 62:519, 1950.
94. Jacobsen, S. T., Crawford, A. H., Millar, E. A., and Steel, H. H.: The Syme amputation in patients with congenital pseudarthrosis of the tibia. J. Bone Joint Surg., 65-A:533, 1983.
95. Johnson, B. L., and Charneco, D. R.: Café-au-lait spots in neurofibromatosis and in normal individuals. Arch. Dermatol., 102:442, 1970.
96. Kaplan, J., Cushing, B., Chang, C. H., Poland, R., Roscamp, J., Perrin, E., and Bhaya, N.: Familial T-cell lymphoblastic lymphoma: Association with von Recklinghausen neurofibromatosis and Gardner syndrome. Am. J. Hematol., 12:247, 1982.
97. Kessel, A. W. L.: Intrathoracic meningocele, spinal deformity, and multiple neurofibromatosis. J. Bone Joint Surg., 33-B:87, 1951.
98. Kite, J. H.: Congenital pseudarthrosis of the tibia, fibula. Report of 15 cases. South. Med. J., 34:1021, 1941.
99. Klatte, E. C., Franken, E. A., and Smith, J. A.: The

radiographic spectrum in neurofibromatosis. Semin. Roentgenol., *11*:17, 1976.
100. Klose: Recklinghausensche Neurofibromatose mit schwerer Deformierung der Halswirbelsaule. Klin. Wochenschr., 5:817, 1926.
101. Knight, W. A., Murphy, W. K., and Gottlieb, J. A.: Neurofibromatosis associated with malignant neurofibromas. Arch. Dermatol., *107*:747, 1973.
102. Kort, J. S.: Congenital pseudarthrosis of the tibia: Treatment with pulsating electromagnetic field. A.A.O.S. Instruct. Course Lect., Las Vegas, Nevada, 1981.
103. Kullman, L., and Wouters, H. W.: Neurofibromatosis, gigantism, and subperiosteal hematoma: Report of two children with extensive subperiosteal bone formation. J. Bone Joint Surg., *54-B*:130, 1977.
104. Langenskiöld, A.: Pseudarthrosis of the fibula and progressive valgus deformity of the ankle in children: Treatment by fusion of the distal tibial and fibular metaphyses: Review of three cases. J. Bone Joint Surg., *49-A*:436, 1967.
105. Lavine, L. S., Lustrin, I., Shamos, M. H., Rinald, R. A., and Liboff, A. R.: Electric enhancement of bone healing. Science, *175*:118, 1972.
106. Laws, J. W., and Pallis, C.: Spinal deformities in neurofibromatosis. J. Bone Joint Surg., *45-B*:674, 1963.
107. Lehman, E. P.: Recklinghausen's neurofibromatosis and the skeleton. A plea for complete study of the disease. Arch. Dermatol. Syph., *14*:178, 1926.
108. Leung, P. C.: Congenital pseudarthrosis of the tibia. Three cases treated by free vascularized iliac crest graft. Clin. Orthop., *175*:4550, 1983.
109. Levine, D. B.: Spondylolisthesis, neurofibromatosis, and thoracic meningocele: A case report. J. Bone Joint Surg., *52-A*:403, 1970.
110. Lin, J. T., Hsieh, B. S., Yen, T. G., Chen, W. Y., Hsieh, Y. F., and How, S. W.: Extrarenal fibromuscular hyperplasia in neurofibromatosis—a case report. Taiwan I. Hsueh Hui Tsa Chih., *81*:1454, 1982.
111. Lloyd Roberts, G. C., and Shaw, N. E.: The prevention of pseudarthrosis in congenital kyphosis of the tibia. J. Bone Joint Surg., *51-B*:100, 1969.
112. Locht, R. C., Huebert, H. T., and McFarland, D. F.: Subperiosteal hemorrhage in cyst formation in neurofibromatosis. Clin. Orthop., *155*:141, 1981.
113. Lonstein, J. E., Winter, R. B., Moe, J. H., Bradford, D. S., Chou, S. N., and Pinto, W. C.: Neurologic deficits secondary to spinal deformity. Spine, 5:331, 1980.
114. Loop, J. W., Akeson, W. H., and Clawson, D. K.: Acquired thoracic abnormalities in neurofibromatosis. A.J.R., 93:416, 1965.
115. McCarroll, H. R.: Clinical manifestations of congenital neurofibromatosis. J. Bone Joint Surg., *32-A*:601, 1950.
116. McFarland, B.: Pseudarthrosis of the tibia in childhood. J. Bone Joint Surg., *33-B*:36, 1951.
117. McKeen, E. A., Bodurtha, J., Meadows, A. T., Douglass, E. C., and Mulvihill, J. J.: Rhabdomyosarcoma complicating multiple neurofibromatosis. J. Pediatr., 93:992, 1978.
118. McKellar, C. C.: Congenital pseudarthrosis of the tibia: Treatment by tibial lengthening and corrective osteotomy seven years after successful bone graft: A case report. J. Bone Joint Surg., *55-A*:195, 1973.
119. Mandell, G. A.: The pedicle in neurofibromatosis. A.J.R., *130*:675, 1978.
120. Manske, P. R.: Forearm pseudarthrosis and neurofibromatosis. Clin. Orthop., *139*:125, 1979.
121. Masihuz, Z.: Pseudarthrosis of the radius associated with neurofibromatosis. J. Bone Joint Surg., *59-A*:977, 1977.
122. Masserman, R. L., Peterson, H. A., and Bianco, A.: Congenital pseudarthrosis of the tibia: A review of the literature and 52 cases from the Mayo Clinic. Clin. Orthop., 99:140, 1974.
123. Meszaros, W. T., Guzzo, F., and Schorsh, H.: Neurofibromatosis. A.J.R., 98:557, 1966.
124. Merten, D. F., Gooding, C. A., Newton, T. H., and Malamud, N.: Meningiomas of childhood and adolescence. J. Pediatr., *84*:696, 1974.
125. Miller, A.: Neurofibromatosis with reference to skeletal changes, compression myelitis, and malignant degeneration. Arch. Surg., 32:109, 1936.
126. Moe, J. H.: Neurofibromatosis. *In* Hardy, J. H. (ed.): Spinal Deformity in Neurological and Muscular Disorders. St. Louis, Mosby, 1974.
127. Moe, J. H.: Scoliosis and Other Spinal Deformities. Philadelphia, Saunders, 1978.
128. Moore, B. H.: Some orthopedic relationships of neurofibromatosis. J. Bone Joint Surg., 23:109, 1941.
129. Moore, J. R.: Delayed autogenous bone graft in the treatment of congenital pseudarthrosis. J. Bone Joint Surg., *31*:23, 1949.
130. Moore, J. R.: Congenital pseudarthrosis of the tibia. A.A.O.S. Instruct. Course Lect., 6:222, 1957.
131. Morrissey, R. T.: Congenital pseudarthrosis of the tibia. A long-term follow-up study. Clin. Orthop., *166*:14, 1982.
132. Morrisey, R. T., Riseborough, E. J., and Hall, J. E.: Congenital pseudarthrosis of the tibia. J. Bone Joint Surg., *63-B*:367, 1981.
133. Murray, M. R., Stout, A. P., and Bradley, C. F.: Schwann cell versus fibroblast as the origin of the specific nerve sheath tumor; observations upon normal nerve sheaths and neurilemmomas in vitro. Am. J. Pathol., 16:41, 1940.
134. National Neurofibromatosis Foundation, Inc.: Newsletter: Neurofibromatosis: A historical perspective. 6(1):8, 1983.
135. Nogaard, F.: Osseous changes in Recklinghausen's neurofibromatosis. Acta Radiol., *18*:460, 1937.
136. Ormsby, O. S., and Montgomery, H.: Diseases of the Skin. 8th Ed. Philadelphia, Lea & Febiger, 1954.
137. Payne, J. F.: Multiple neuro-fibromata in connection with molluscum fibrosum. Trans. Pathol. Soc. London, 38:59, 1887.
138. Pellock, J. M., Kleinman, P. K., McDonald, B. M., and Wixson, D.: Childhood hypertensive stroke with neurofibromatosis. Neurology, 30:656, 1980.
139. Penfield, W., and Young, A. W.: The nature of von Recklinghausen's disease and the tumors associated with it. Arch. Neurol. Psychiatry, 23:320, 1930.
140. Pitt, M., Mosher, J. F., and Ediken, J.: Abnormal periosteum in bone in neurofibromatosis. Radiology, *103*:143, 1972.
141. Pless, J., Roed-Peterson, K., and Nielson, K.: Microglossia neurofibromatosis. Ugeskr. Laeger., *139*:655, 1977.
142. Pohl, R.: Meningocele im Brustraum unter dem Bilde cine intrathorakelen Rundschattens. Röntgenpraxis, 5:747, 1933.
143. Pollnitz, R.: Neurofibromatosis in childhood: A review of 25 cases. Med. J. Aust., 2:49, 1976.
144. Preiser, S. A., and Davenport, C. B.: Multiple neurofibromatosis (von Recklinghausen's disease and its inheritance). Am. J. Med. Sci., *156*:507, 1918.
145. Radhakrishnar, S., Varadarajan, V., and Narenden, S.: Neurofibromatosis of the transverse colon and omentum. J. Indian Med. Assoc., 71:287, 1978.
146. Rankin, E.: Neurofibromatosis in the radius of a 9-year-old. Personal communication, 1975.
147. Recklinghausen, F. von: Ueber die multiplen Fibrome der Haut ihre Beziehung zu den multiplen Neuromen. August Hirschwald, 1882.
148. Rezian, S. M.: The incidence of scoliosis due to neurofibromatosis. Acta Orthop. Scand., *47*:534, 1976.

149. Riccardi, V. M.: Neurofibromatosis. *In* Riccardi, V. M., and Mulvihill, J. J., (eds.).: Advances in Neurology, Vol. 29. New York, Raven Press, 1981.
150. Riccardi, V. M., and Kleiner, B.: Neurofibromatosis: A neoplastic birth defect with two age peaks of severe problems. Birth Defects, *13*:131, 1977.
151. Robin, G. C.: Scoliosis and neurologic disease. Isr. J. Med. Sci., *9*:578, 1973.
152. Rockower, S., McKay, D., and Nason, S.: Dislocation of the spine in neurofibromatosis. A report of two cases. J. Bone Joint Surg., *64-A*:1240, 1982.
153. Saggese, G., Ziccardi, D., and Biagioni, M.: A case of von Recklinghausen's neurofibromatosis with precocious puberty. Minerva Pediatr., *33*:847, 1981.
154. Sammons, B. P., and Thomas, D. F.: Extensive lumbar meningocele associated with neurofibromatosis. A.J.R., *81*:1021, 1959.
155. Samuelson, B.: Neurofibromatosis (von Recklinghausen's disease). A Clinical, Psychiatric, and Genetic Study. Goteborg, Sweden, University Press, 1981.
156. Sane, S., Yunis, E., and Greer, R.: Subperiosteal or cortical cyst and intramedullary neurofibromatosis: Uncommon manifestations of neurofibromatosis. A case report. J. Bone Joint Surg., *53-A*:1194, 1971.
157. Savini, R., and Vicenzi, G.: Le deformita del rachide nella neurofibromatosi. Studio clinico-radiografico di 46 casi. Gior. Ital. J. Orthop. Traumatol., *2*:37, 1976.
158. Schenkein, I., Buerker, E. D., Helson, L., Axelrod, F., and Dancer, J.: Increased nerve growth stimulating activity in disseminated neurofibromatosis. N. Engl. J. Med., *290*:613, 1974.
159. Schwartz, A. M., and Ramos, R. M.: Neurofibromatosis and multiple nonossifying fibromas. A.J.R., *135*:617, 1980.
160. Scott, J. C.: Scoliosis and neurofibromatosis. J. Bone Joint Surg., *47-B*:240, 1965.
161. Sharp, J. C., and Young, R. H.: Recklinghausen's neurofibromatosis. Clinical manifestations in thirty-one cases. Arch. Intern. Med., *59*:299, 1937.
162. Sheklakov, N. D.: A case of neurofibromatosis with 9242 tumors. Vestn. Venerol. Dermatol., *3*:51, 1950.
163. Smith, R. W.: A Treatise on the Pathology, Diagnosis, and Treatment of Neuroma. Dublin, Hodges & Smith, 1849.
164. Sofield, H. A., and Millar, E. A.: Fragmentation, realignment, and intramedullary rod fixation of deformities of the long bones in children. A 10-year appraisal. J. Bone Joint Surg., *41-A*:1371, 1959.
165. Speed, K.: Malignant degeneration of neurofibromata of peripheral nerve trunks (von Recklinghausen's disease). Ann. Surg., *116*:81, 1942.
166. Stagnara, P., Biot, B., and Fauchet, R.: Evaluation critique du traitement chirurgical des lésions vertébrales de la neurofibromatose. Rev. Chir. Orthop., *61*:17, 1975.
167. Stay, E. J., and Vawter, G.: The relationship between nephroblastoma and neurofibromatosis (von Recklinghausen's). Cancer, *39*:2550, 1977.
168. Steg, N. L., Wong, A. K. C., Wang, C. C., and Casey, P. A.: The potential of computerized dermatoglyphia analysis as demonstrated through studies of patients with myelomeningoceles and neurofibromatosis. *In* Bergsma, D., and Lawry, R. B. (eds).: Numerical Taxonomy of Birth Defects and Polygenic Disorders. New York, Allan R. Liss Series, March of Dimes 13, *3-A*:158–159, 1977.
169. Stout, A. P.: Tumors of the peripheral nervous system. *In* Atlas of Tumor Pathology. Washington, D.C., Armed Forces Institute of Pathology, 1949.
170. Suziki, M., Tamura, E., Kamoshita, S., and Saito, M.: Clinical observations of phacomatosis in infancy and childhood. I. von Recklinghausen's disease. Paediatr. Univ. Tokyo, *9*:23, 1963.

171. Takahashi, M.: Studies in neurofibromatosis and pigmented macules of nevus spilus. Tohoku J. Exp. Med., *118*:255, 1976.
172. Tilesius von Tilenau, W. G.: Historia Pathologica Singularis Cutis Turpitudinus. Leipzig, Crusius, 1793.
173. Treves, F.: Congenital deformity. Br. Med. J., *2*:1140, 1884.
174. Treves, F.: Congenital deformity. Br. Med. J., *1*:595, 1885.
175. Treves, F.: A case of congenital deformity. Trans. Pathol. Soc. London, *36*:494, 1895.
176. Treves, F.: Elephant Man and Other Reminiscences. New York, Holt, 1924.
177. Thannhauser, S. J.: Neurofibromatosis (von Recklinghausen) and osteitis fibrosa cystica localisata et disseminata (von Recklinghausen): A study of a common pathogenesis of both diseases. Medicine (Baltimore), *23*:105, 1944.
178. Uhlmann, E., and Grossman, A.: von Recklinghausen's neurofibromatosis with bone manifestations. Ann. Intern. Med., *14*:225, 1940.
179. Vannes, C. P.: Congenital pseudarthrosis of the leg. J. Bone Joint Surg., *48-A*:1467, 1966.
180. Veliskakis, K. P., Wilson, P. D., Jr., and Levone, D. B.: Neurofibromatosis and scoliosis: Significance of the short angular spine curvature. J. Bone Joint Surg., *52-A*:883, 1970.
181. Virchow, R.: Ueber de Reform der pathologischen und therapeutischen Anschauungen durch die mikroskopischen Untersuchungen. Arch. Pathol. Anat. Phys. Klin. Med., *1*:207, 1847.
182. Waggener, J. D.: Ultrastructure of benign peripheral nerve sheath tumors. Cancer, *19*:699, 1966.
183. Weber, F. P. I.: Cutaneous pigmentation as an incomplete form of Recklinghausen's disease, with remarks on the classification of incomplete and anomalous forms of Recklinghausen's disease. Br. J. Dermatol., *21*:49, 1909.
184. Weber, F. P.: Periosteal neurofibromatosis with a short consideration of the whole subject of neurofibromatosis. Q. J. Med., *23*:151, 1930.
185. Wehbe, M. A., and Mickelson, M. R.: Malignant schwannoma in neurofibromatosis elephantiasis of the upper extremity. Clin. Orthop., *167*:164, 1982.
186. Weichert, K. A., Ding, M. S., Benton, C., and Silverman, F. N.: Macrocranium and neurofibromatosis. Radiology, *107*:163, 1973.
187. Weiland, A. J., and Daniel, R. K.: Congenital pseudarthrosis tibia: Treatment with vascularized autogenous fibular grafts. A preliminary report. Johns Hopkins Med. J., *147*:89, 1980.
188. Weiss, R. S.: (A) von Recklinghausen's disease in the Negro; (B) Curvature of the tibia in siblings with neurofibromatosis. J. Bone Joint Surg., *53-B*:314, 1971.
189. Well, J. M., Bulmar, J. A., and Graff, D. J. C.: Congenital defects of the tibia in siblings with neurofibromatosis. J. Bone Joint Surg., *53-B*:314, 1971.
190. Whitehouse, D.: Diagnostic value of the café-au-lait spot in children. Arch. Dis. Child., *41*:316, 1966.
191. Winter, R. B., and Edwards, W. C.: Case report. Neurofibromatosis with lumbosacral spondylolisthesis. J. Pediatr. Orthop., *1*:91, 1981.
192. Winter, R. B., Moe, J. H., Bradford, D. S., Lonstein, J. E., Pedras, C. V., and Weber, A. H.: Spine deformity in neurofibromatosis. J. Bone Joint Surg., *61-A*:677, 1979.
193. Wynne-Davies, R., Hall, C. M., and Apley, A. G.: Atlas of Skeletal Dysplasias. Edinburgh, Churchill-Livingstone, 1985, pp. 566–575.
194. Yaghmai, I., and Tafazoli, M.: Massive subperiosteal hemorrhage in neurofibromatosis. Radiology, *122*:439, 1977.

195. Yong-Hing, K., Kalamchi, A., and MacEwen, G. D.: Cervical spine abnormalities in neurofibromatosis. J. Bone Joint Surg., 61-A:695, 1979.
196. Young, D. F., Eldridge, R., and Gardner, W. J.: Bilateral acoustic neuroma in a large kindred. J.A.M.A., 214:347, 1970.

ADAMANTINOMA

A rare primary tumor of long bones was so named by Fischer because of its resemblance to ameloblastoma (adamantinoma) of the mandible.[25]

Localization

The lesion has a strong predilection for the tibia (about 90 per cent of cases); it has, however, been found in other long bones, such as the ulna, humerus, femur, and fibula, and in the capitate. Multifocal involvement of the tibia and fibula has been reported; in one patient in addition to the tibia and fibula the femur was also affected.[65]

Age and Sex Predilection

With no sex predilection, adamantinoma is a tumor of adult life with a median age occurrence of the mid-thirties. It does occur, however, in adolescence and, rarely, in childhood. This author has treated a case in a three-year-old boy.

Clinical Features

The presenting complaint is local pain with an insidious onset, developing over a period of several months to years. There may be a history of trauma. On palpation there is localized hard swelling and tenderness of a varying degree.

Radiographic and Imaging Findings

The lesion is commonly located in the middle third of the diaphysis of a long bone; it may, however, extend to either end to involve the metaphyses. On rare occasions, with aggressive adamantinomas, the epiphysis may be affected. Primary location in the epiphysis has not been reported.

The radiographic appearance depends on the site of origin of the tumor—whether intracortical or intramedullary. When the lesions begin *in the cortex*, as shown in Figure 3–323, the internal radiographic pattern may be one of several types: a solitary area of irregular rarefaction in the cortex, which is expanded on its outer surface (penetration of the cortex will result in loss of cortical outlines); *bubbled locules* in which multiple areas of expanded cortical rarefaction are separated by delicate septa; *sawtoothed lysis* caused by external subperiosteal bone erosion; and *fibrosclerosis*, which consists of numerous small areas of cortical rarefaction with sclerotic margins. Ordinarily there is little if any periosteal rarefaction. In intracortical lesions there may be marginal buttressing. In the *intramedullary types* of adamantinoma the radiographic pattern may be circumscribed lytic, multilocular expansile, or satellite sclerotic; on rare occasions intramedullary lesions may resemble reticulated honeycomb or be frankly destructive. The radiographic appearance is suggestive but not diagnostic of adamantinoma.[69]

Scintigraphy with technetium-99m will show increased uptake in the lesional area. The periphery of the area of increased uptake on the scan corresponds to the rim of the reactive zone about the lesion.

Computed tomography will clearly delineate the area of bone destruction—cortical or intramedullary, the nature of the reactive areas in the transition zone, and whether there is soft-tissue extension.

Arteriography shows marked increased vascularity with abnormal vascular channels in the area of bone destruction.

Adamantinoma is usually a Stage 1A lesion when seen initially and untreated.

Differential Diagnosis

Multiple areas of radiolucency with an admixture of sclerosis of the diaphyseal and metaphyseal regions of a long bone may be seen in a number of other bone tumors. *Benign lesions* to consider in the differential diagnosis are fibrous dysplasia, nonossifying fibroma, desmoplastic fibroma, osteoblastoma, osteofibrous dysplasia (Campanacci syndrome), periosteal fibroma, and aneurysmal bone cyst. Brown tumor in hyperparathyroidism should be ruled out. Hemophilic pseudotumor may give a similar radiographic appearance. Hydatid bone cyst should be considered in certain third-world countries. In the adult, the lytic phase of Paget's disease may be mistaken for adamantinoma in the radiograph. *Malignant lesions* to consider in the differential diagnosis are myosarcoma, fibrosarcoma, reticulum-cell sarcoma, osteogenic sarcoma, and metastatic carcinoma.

Pathologic Findings

On gross inspection the lesional tissue is grayish white, firm in consistency, with scattered cystic areas of hemorrhage.

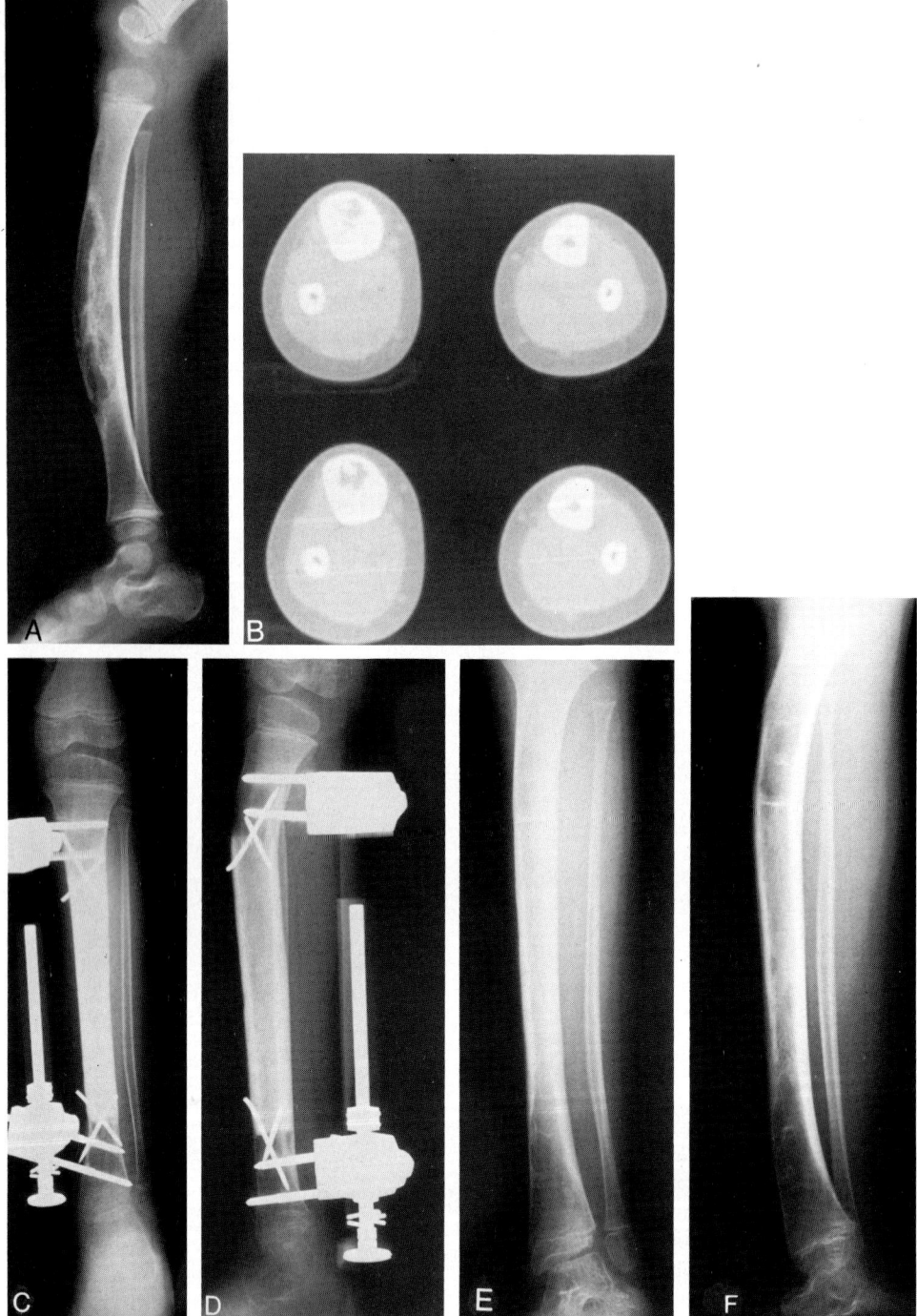

FIGURE 3–323. *Adamantinoma of tibia in a three-year-old boy.*

A and **B.** Preoperative radiogram showing the irregular area of cortical erosion and bubble appearance. **B.** Computerized axial tomography showing the cortical tumor encroaching on the medullary cavity. **C** and **D.** Anteroposterior and lateral radiograms of the tibia after excision and allografting with a cadaveric humerus. **E** and **F.** Three years after surgery. Note the reconstitution of the allograft. Patient is asymptomatic and walking with no protection.

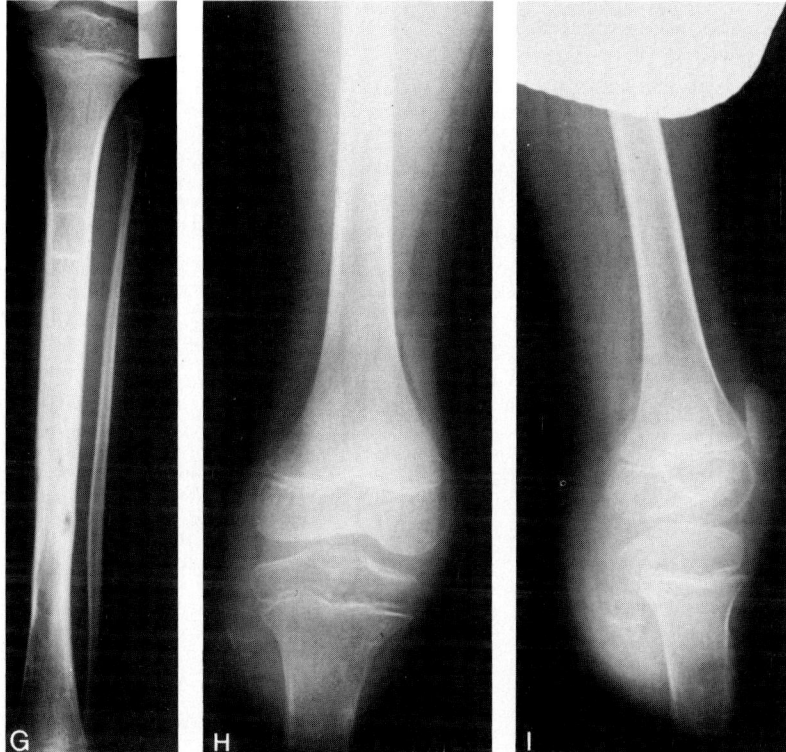

FIGURE 3–323 Continued. *Adamantinoma of tibia in a three-year-old boy.* **G.** One year later showing recurrence of tumor in the center of the allograft. **H** and **I.** Below-knee amputation was performed.

The histologic picture varies in different areas of the same specimen and from tumor to tumor. In general there are three basic patterns: *first*, masses of epithelial cells forming islets and surrounded by columnar cells that are arranged in palisade fashion. In the center of the lesion the stellate cells are arranged in anastomosing elongated masses supported by dense fibrous tissue stroma. In the center of the reticulum there are cystic areas. This pattern of histologic appearance could easily be metastatic adenocarcinoma.[4, 31] The *second* pattern consists of islands of cells resembling basal cells that are dispersed in a fibrous stroma. There are cystic areas in the epithelial masses. The peripheral cells show palisading. The *third* histologic pattern consists of squamous epithelial islands scattered throughout a fibrous stroma with evidence of pearl formation. This epidermal appearance resembles squamous cell carcinoma.[36]

Enamel tissue and teeth have not been noted in any of the cases reported to date. There is some controversy as to pathogenesis of adamantinoma; it has been proposed by various authors that the cell of origin is the angioblast, the synovial cell, and the epithelioid cell. The *angioblastic derivation* of the tumor from the primitive vascular mesenchymal cells is supported by the histochemical presence of alkaline phosphatase in the endothelial angioblasts of the lesional tissue but its absence in true adamantinoma of the mandible.[12] Also, tissue culture studies of adamantinoma have shown formation of precollagen fibers, supporting the mesenchymal origin of the tumor.[31] Dahlin favors the mesenchymal angioblastic genesis of adamantinoma.[15] It has been proposed to name the lesion *malignant angioblastoma* instead of adamantinoma.[6, 12, 22, 26, 35, 38, 58]

The *synovial origin* of the tumor is suggested by its biphasic (glandular and fibrous) histologic pattern. It has been suggested that adamantinoma is an undifferentiated sarcoma, similar to synovial sarcoma.[30]

The *epithelial origin* of adamantinoma and its development from misplaced embryonal nests of epithelium was originally proposed by Fischer and later supported by Lichtenstein.[25, 36] Because of its common location in the tibia, traumatic implantation of the basal cells of the skin into bone has been postulated.

Treatment

Marginal excision often results in recurrence; therefore it is recommended that the tumor be excised by a wide surgical margin. In the tibia, if the tumor has penetrated the medullary canal, a full segmental resection is performed in order to achieve a wide surgical margin; an allograft is utilized for reconstruction. If the tumor is well marginated and intracortical, involving the anterior cortex only, an attempt may be made to preserve the posterior cortex to facilitate reconstruction; it should, however, be understood that it carries a greater risk of recurrence. When adamantinoma is aggressive, extending into soft tissues, or when attempted segmental resection has failed and there is aggressive recurrence, a below-knee amputation or knee disarticulation is performed. If pulmonary metastases develop they are removed by wide excision.

References

1. Albores Saavedra, J., Diaz Gutierrez, D., and Altamirano Dimas, M.: Adamantinoma de la tibia. Observaciones ultrastructurales. Rev. Med. Hosp. Gral. Mex., 31:241, 1968.
2. Anderson, C. E., and Saunders, J. B. deC. M.: Primary adamantinoma of the ulna. Surg. Gynecol. Obstet., 75:351, 1942.
3. Baker, A. H., and Hawksley, L. M.: A case of primary adamantinoma of the tibia. Br. J. Surg., 18:415, 1931.
4. Baker, P. L., Dockerty, M. B., and Coventry, M. B.: Adamantinoma (so-called) of the long bones. J. Bone Joint Surg., 36-A:704, 1954.
5. Bell, A. L.: A case of adamantinoma of the femur. Br. J. Surg., 30:81, 1942.
6. Besemann, E. F., and Perez, M. A.: Malignant angioblastoma, so-called adamantinoma, involving the humerus. A case report. A J R., 100:538, 1967.
7. Bishop, E. L.: Adamantinoma of the tibia. South. Med. J., 30:571, 1937.
8. Braidwood, A. S., and McDougall, A.: Adamantinoma of the tibia. J. Bone Joint Surg., 56-B:735, 1974.
9. Bullough, P. G., and Goldberg, V. M.: Multicentric origin of adamantinoma of the tibia. A case report. Rev. Hosp. Spec. Surg., 1:71, 1971.
10. Campanacci, M., Giunti, A., and Leonessa, C.: Adamantinoma delle ossa lunghi. Chir. Organi Mov., 58:385, 1969.
11. Campanacci, M., Giunti, A., Bertoni, F., Laus, M., and Gitelis, S.: Adamantinoma of the long bones. The experience at the Istituto Ortopedico Rizzoli. Am. J. Surg. Pathol., 5:533, 1981.
12. Changus, G. W., Speed, J. S., and Stewart, F. W.: Malignant angioblastoma of bone. A reappraisal of adamantinoma of long bone. Cancer, 10:540, 1957.
13. Cohen, D. M., Dahlin, D. C., and Pugh, D. G.: Fibrous dysplasia associated with adamantinoma of the long bones. Cancer, 15:515, 1962.
14. Cohn, B. T., Brahms, M. A., and Froimson, A. I.: Metastasis of adamantinoma sixteen years after knee disarticulation. J. Bone Joint Surg., 68-A:772, 1986.
15. Dahlin, D. C.: Bone Tumors. 3rd Ed. Springfield, Ill., Thomas, 1978, pp. 296–306.
16. Dameron, T. B., Jr.: Adamantinoma of the appendicular skeleton. Johns Hopkins Med. J., 145:107, 1979.
17. Delarue, J., Chomette, G., and Brocheriou, C.: Adamantinome du tibia et "dysplasie fibreuse." Ann. Anat. Pathol., 9:373, 1964.
18. Diepeveen, W. P., Hjort, G. H., and Pock-Steen, O. C.: Adamantinoma of the capitate bone. Acta Radiol., 53:377, 1960.
19. Dockerty, M. B., and Myerding, H. W.: Adamantinoma of tibia: Report of two new cases. J.A.M.A., 119:932, 1942.
20. Donna, R., and Dickland, V.: Adamantinoma of the tibia. J. Bone Joint Surg., 48-B:138, 1966.
21. Dunne, R. E.: Primary adamantinoma of the tibia. N. Engl. J. Med., 218:634, 1938.
22. Elliott, G. B.: Malignant angioblastoma of long bone. So-called tibial adamantinoma. J. Bone Joint Surg., 44-B:25, 1962.
23. Enneking, W. F.: Surgical considerations in specific tumors. Adamantinoma. In Musculoskeletal Tumor Surgery. Vol. 2. New York, Churchill-Livingstone, 1983, pp. 1488–1492.
24. Ewing, J.: Neoplastic Diseases. 3rd Ed. Philadelphia, Saunders, 1926, p. 752.
25. Fischer, B.: Über ein primäres Adamantinoma der Tibia. Frankfurter Z. Pathol., 12:422, 1913.
26. Gikas, P. W., and Headington, J. T.: Angioblastic tumors of bone and skin. Report of a case. J. Bone Joint Surg., 45-A:554, 1963.
27. Halpert, B., and Dohn, H. P.: Adamantinoma in the tibia. Arch. Pathol., 43:313, 1947.
28. Hebbel, R.: Adamantinoma of the tibia. Surgery, 7:860, 1940.
29. Hertz, J.: Adamantinoma of the long bones. Acta Orthop. Scand., 22:64, 1952.
30. Hicks, J. D.: Synovial sarcoma of the tibia. J. Pathol. Bacteriol., 67:151, 1954.
31. Huvos, A. G., and Marcove, R. C.: Adamantinoma of long bones. A clinicopathological study of fourteen cases with vascular origin suggested. J. Bone Joint Surg., 57-A:148, 1975.
32. Jaffe, H. J.: Tumors and Tumorous Conditions of the Bones and Joints. Philadelphia, Lea & Febiger, 1958, p. 213.
33. Johnson, L. C.: Congenital pseudarthrosis, adamantinoma of long bone and intracortical fibrous dysplasia of the tibia. J. Bone Joint Surg., 54-A:1355, 1972.
34. King, E. S. J.: Tissue differentiation in malignant synovial tumours. J. Bone Joint Surg., 34-B:97, 1952.
35. Lederer, H., and Sinclair, A. J.: Malignant synovioma simulating "adamantinoma of the tibia." J. Pathol. Bacteriol., 67:163, 1954.
36. Lichtenstein, L.: Bone Tumors. 5th Ed. St. Louis, Mosby, 1977, pp. 355–362.
37. Lipper, S., and Kahn, L. B.: Case Report 235. Diagnosis: Ewing-like adamantinoma of the left radial head and neck. Skeletal Radiol., 10:61, 1983.
38. Llombart-Bosch, A., and Ortuno-Pacheko, G.: Ultrastructural findings supporting the angioblastic nature of the so-called adamantinoma of the tibia. Histopathology, 2:189, 1978.
39. Lodwick, G. S.: Atlas of Tumor Radiology. The Bones and Joints. Chicago, Year Book, 1971, pp. 414–419.
40. Mandard, J. C., LeGal, Y., and Fievez, M.: L'adamantinome des os longs. Ann. Anat. Pathol., 16:483, 1971.
41. Mangalik, V. S., and Mehrotra, R. M. L.: Adamantinoma of the tibia. Report of a case. Br. J. Surg., 39:429, 1952.
42. Markel, S. F.: Ossifying fibroma of long bone. Its distinction from fibrous dysplasia and its association with adamantinoma of long bone. Am. J. Clin. Pathol., 69:91, 1978.
43. Meffley, W. H., and Northrup, S. W.: Adamantinoma of the tibia. J. Int. Coll. Surg., 10:291, 1947.
44. Meister, E. K., Konrad, E., and Huber, G.: Malignant tumor of humerus with features of "adamantinoma" and Ewing's sarcoma. Pathol. Res. Pract., 166:112, 1979.
45. Milgram, J. W.: Adamantinoma. A case report. Bull. Hosp. Joint Dis., 35:55, 1974.

46. Moon, N. F.: Adamantinoma of the appendicular skeleton. A statistical review of reported cases and inclusion of 10 new cases. Clin. Orthop., 43:189, 1965.
47. Morgan, A. D., and Mackenzie, D. H.: A metastasizing adamantinoma of the tibia. J. Bone Joint Surg., 38-B:892, 1956.
48. Naji, A. F., Murphy, J. A., Stasney, R. J., Neville, W. E., and Chrenka, P.: So-called adamantinoma of long bones. Report of case with massive pulmonary metastases. J. Bone Joint Surg., 46-A:151, 1964.
49. Netherlands Committee on Bone Tumours: Radiological Atlas of Bone Tumours. Vol. 1. Baltimore, Williams & Wilkins, 1966, pp. 213–221.
50. Rankin, J. O.: Adamantinoma of the tibia. J. Bone Joint Surg., 21:425, 1939.
51. Rehbock, D. J., and Barber, C. G.: Adamantinoma of the tibia. Report of a case. J. Bone Joint Surg., 20-A:187, 1938.
52. Rosai, J.: Adamantinoma of the tibia—electron microscopic evidence of its epithelial origin. Am. J. Clin. Pathol., 51:786, 1969.
53. Rosen, R. S., and Schwinn, C. P.: Adamantinoma of limb bone. Malignant angioblastoma. A.J.R., 97:727, 1966.
54. Ryrie, B. J.: Adamantinoma of the tibia: Aetiology and pathogenesis. Br. Med. J., 2:1000, 1932.
55. Schajowicz, F.: Adamantinoma of long bones. In Tumors and Tumorlike Lesions of Bones and Joints, New York, Springer-Verlag, 1981, pp. 383–389.
56. Schneider, H., and Enderle, A.: Zur Differentialdiagnoze eines metastasierenden Adamantinoma der Tibia und Fibula. Arch. Orthop. Traumatol. Surg., 94:143, 1979.
57. Schulenburg, C. A. R.: Adamantinoma. Ann. R. Coll. Surg., 8:329, 1951.
58. Shah, I. C., Castro, F. B., Miller, T. R., and Gerson, G. N.: Malignant angioblastoma (so-called adamantinoma) of humerus. Int. Surg., 57:753, 1972.
59. Sowa, D. T., and Dorfman, H. D.: Unusual localization of adamantinoma of long bones. Report of a case of isolated fibular involvement. J. Bone Joint Surg., 68-A:293, 1986.
60. Spjut, H. J., Dorfman, H. D., Fechner, R. E., and Ackerman, L. V.: Tumors of bone and cartilage. In Atlas of Tumor Pathology. Fascicle 5. Washington, D.C., Armed Forces Institute of Pathology, 1971.
61. Stetsula, V. I.: On the problem of histogenesis of "adamantinoma" of long tubular bones. Vopr. Onkol., 9:73, 1963.
62. Stoker, D. J.: Case report. Adamantinoma of tibia. Skeletal Radiol., 1:187, 1977.
63. Theros, E. G., and Ishak, B. W.: An exercise in radiologic-pathologic correlation. Radiology, 89:747, 1967.
64. Thomas, R. G.: Adamantinoma of the tibia. Br. J. Surg., 26:547, 1939.
65. Unni, K. K., Dahlin, D. C., Beabout, J. W., and Ivins, J. C.: Adamantinomas of long bones. Cancer, 34:1796, 1974.
66. van Haelst, U. J. G. M., and de Haas van Dorsser, A. M.: A perplexing malignant bone tumor. Highly malignant so-called adamantinoma or non-typical Ewing's sarcoma. Virchows Arch., 365:63, 1975.
67. Weiss, S. W., and Dorfman, H. D.: Adamantinoma of long bone. An analysis of nine new cases with emphasis on metastasizing lesions and fibrous dysplasia-like changes. Hum. Pathol., 8:141, 1977.
68. Willis, R. A.: Pathology of Tumours. London, Butterworth, 1948, p. 280.
69. Wilner, D.: Radiology of Bone Tumors and Allied Disorders. Philadelphia, Saunders, 1982, p. 2391.
70. Wolfort, B., and Sloane, D.: Adamantinoma of the tibia. A report of two cases. Bull. Hosp. Joint Dis., 20:1011, 1938.
71. Yoneyama, T., Winter, W. G., and Milsow, L.: Tibial adamantinoma: Its histogenesis from ultrastructural studies. Cancer, 40:1138, 1977.
72. Zand, A., Chambers, G. H., and Street, D. M.: So-called "adamantinoma of long bone." Clin. Orthop., 86:178, 1972.

OSTEOGENIC SARCOMA

Probably the most common of the malignant bone tumors, osteogenic sarcoma develops from cells of the mesenchymal series, which form neoplastic osteoid and osseous tissue either directly or indirectly by rapid growth of the tumor through a cartilaginous stage of development.

The *classic osteogenic sarcoma* develops in the interior of a bone. A related entity, but yet one distinct from the central lesion, is *juxtacortical osteogenic sarcoma*, which develops in relation to the periosteum and immediate parosteal connective tissue; it is less common, but has a much better prognosis. *Endosteal osteosarcoma* is a variant of parosteal osteosarcoma that arises within bone from the endosteum; it is a *low-grade* malignant tumor that grows slowly and metastasizes late. *Telangiectatic osteosarcoma* is a *high-grade* malignant lesion that shows little evidence of ossification, undergoing cystic and necrotic changes due to its rapid growth; pathologic fracture of the bone weakened by the rapid destructive osteolytic process is common.[58, 75, 126] *Paget's sarcoma* is not encountered in children.[69, 70, 109, 141] In this section the *classic osteogenic sarcoma* is discussed.

Classic Osteogenic Sarcoma

Generally, the tumor occurs in the age group of 10 to 25 years, though it has been found at ages as young as 5 years and as old as 50. When osteogenic sarcoma develops in an older person, the possibility of malignant transformation of a pre-existing benign bone disease such as Paget's disease of bone or fibrous dysplasia should be considered.[80, 130, 145]

Incidence in the male is almost equal to that in females.

The tumor is usually located near the metaphyseal region of a long bone, but on occasion, may be diaphyseal in its site. The most common sites are the lower end of the femur and the upper end of the tibia, accounting for over 50 per cent of cases. The upper ends of the humerus and the femur are next in frequency of localization. On a rare occasion, it may be encountered in the fibula, pelvic bones, or in the vertebral column.[56, 57, 60, 102, 123, 136] Occurrence in the distal part of a limb (hand or foot) is extremely rare.[46] The tumor has, however, been described in every bone in the body. In the literature there are numerous reports of multiple or multicentric osteogenic sarcoma.*

Pathologic Findings. The tumor ordinarily begins its development in the medullary cavity of a long bone near the metaphysis, but by the time it is recognized, it has already penetrated and extended through the cortex, raising the periosteum (Fig. 3–324). In more advanced cases, the periosteal barrier may be broken, and one finds a soft-tissue tumor mass invading the contiguous muscle tissue. In general, the central portion of the neoplasm displays heavier ossification than do the peripheral areas. The ossified portions are of a gritty consistency and have a yellowish appearance; the more cellular areas are elastic and whitish in color. In a sagittal section of an amputated specimen, the boundaries of the epiphyseal end of the tumor are not clearly distinguishable. The physis is less readily violated than the cortical wall, and it remains unbroken until later in the course of the disease, when the articular hyaline cartilage serves to block the extension of the neoplasm into the joint. Transepiphyseal extension has been reported.[52, 167] Toward the diaphyseal end, the advancing tumor presents as a conical plug that marks the limit of growth of the lesion lengthwise along the shaft. Skip extension may occasionally occur, a fact that must be borne in mind in determining the optimum level for amputation.

Histologic diagnosis of osteogenic sarcoma is simple if microscopic examination shows the presence of a frankly sarcomatous stroma and direct formation of neoplastic osteoid and bone (Fig. 3–325). In some pathologic specimens, however, tumor osteoid bone cannot be demonstrated, only collagen strands that are being interwoven with the tumor cells. In anaplastic areas the neoplasm will consist of pleomorphic cells with little intercellular substance. In other tumors neoplastic cartilage and atypical spindle-shaped cells may be the predominant feature.

The microscopic picture of osteogenic sarcoma has been divided into four types by Aegerter. In the first form, osteoid production is the predominant finding; in the second type, both osteoid and cartilage are formed; in the

---

*See references 4, 16, 31, 61, 62, 68, 101, 106, 128, 146, 164.

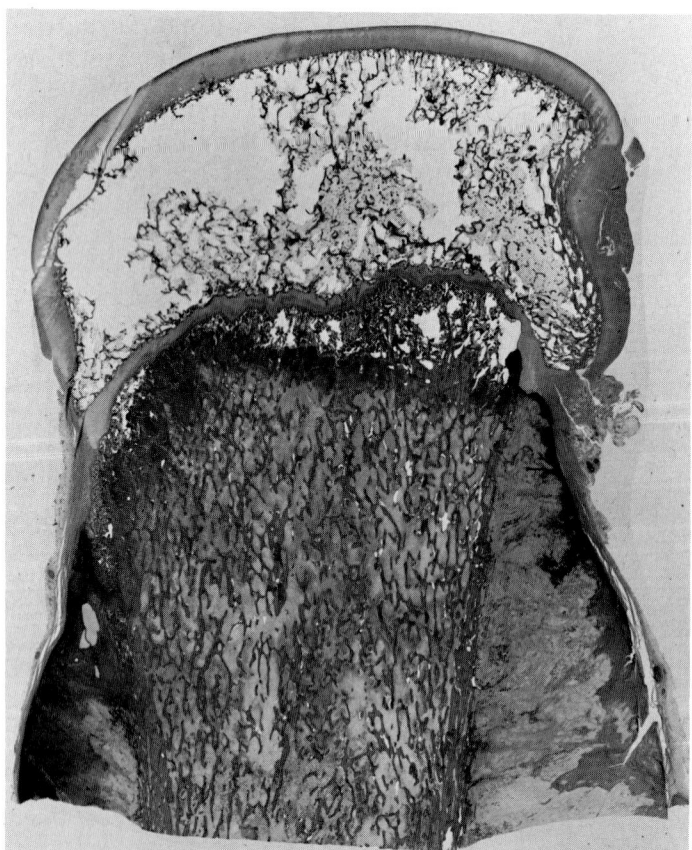

FIGURE 3–324. Osteogenic sarcoma of proximal humerus.

Photomicrograph of sagittal section of amputated specimen. The neoplasm is metaphyseal in location; it has perforated the cortex and raised the periosteum. The physis is unbroken; it does not become violated until later in the course of the disease (× 10).

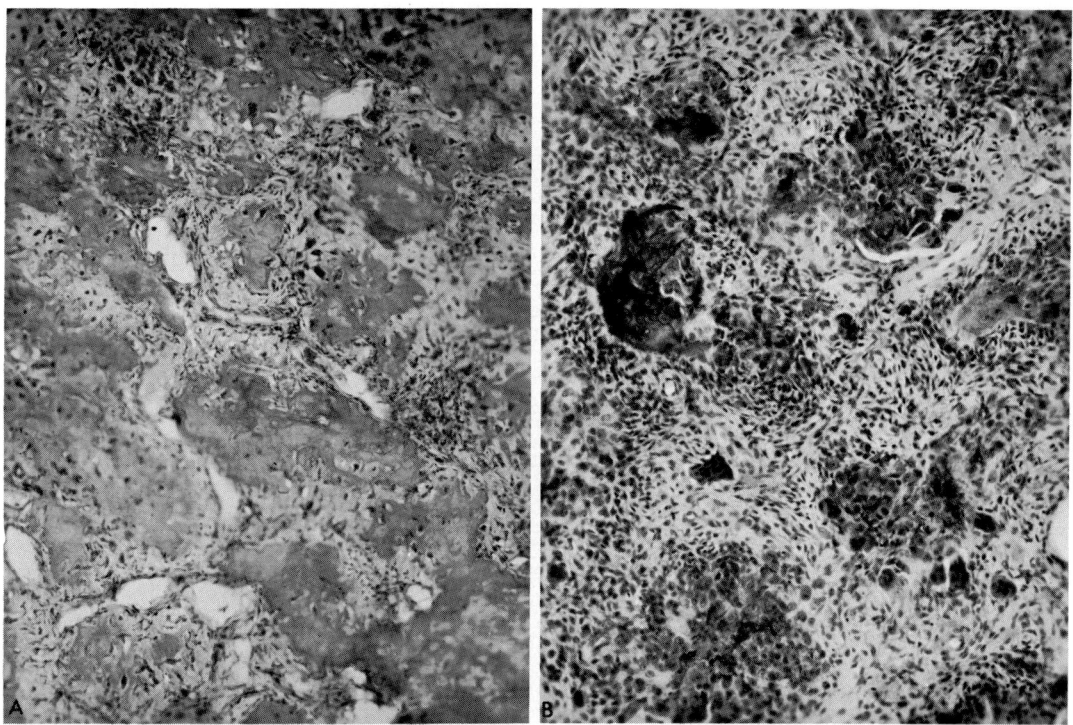

FIGURE 3–325. *Osteogenic sarcoma—histologic findings.*

A. Photomicrograph showing the sarcomatous stroma and the direct formation of neoplastic osteoid and bone (× 100).
B. Greater magnification (× 250).

third type, neither osteoid nor cartilage is produced, but collagen is formed; in the fourth, there is little or no indication of the presence of these intercellular substances.[2] Attempts to correlate the four histologic types with the clinical performance of osteogenic sarcoma have been futile. On the basis of histologic findings alone, one cannot predict the rate of growth, the advent of metastasis, or the duration of survival. The prognostic significance of the number of mitotic figures is uncertain; at best, it is an index of the rate of growth.

Clinical Findings. Local pain in the affected part is the presenting complaint; initially, the pain is intermittent, but within a matter of weeks, becomes severe and constant. There may be a history of trauma that has precipitated discomfort from the tumor. When a lower limb is affected, an antalgic limp may develop. As the condition progresses, local swelling that is hard and fixed may be palpated. There may also be increased local heat and sensitivity to pressure. Its firmness varies, depending on the extent of ossification. The tumor may become visible as it increases in size. Limitation of joint motion and disuse atrophy of the muscles are other findings.

At the time of diagnosis, the general health of the child is usually fair; on occasion, however, in an instance of rapidly growing neoplasm, pulmonary metastases may have already occurred in the early stages, and the general condition will be very poor. A pathologic fracture through the lesion may be the presenting condition.

Radiographic and Imaging Findings. Osteogenic sarcoma presents a typical radiographic picture characterized by destructive and osteoblastic changes (Figs. 3–325 to 3–329).[47, 72, 78, 79, 94] The neoplasm usually begins eccentrically in the metaphyseal region of a long bone. Bone destruction manifests itself as a loss of normal trabecular pattern and the appearance of irregular ill-defined, poorly marginated, ragged radiolucent defects. New bone formation may be neoplastic or reactive and appears in the form of areas of increased radiopacity.

The cortex is seen to be invaded by the growing tumor, as evidenced by destruction of the cortical wall and raising of the periosteum. The "sunburst" appearance is produced by the formation of spicules of new bone laid down perpendicularly to the shaft along the vessels passing from the periosteum to the cortex.

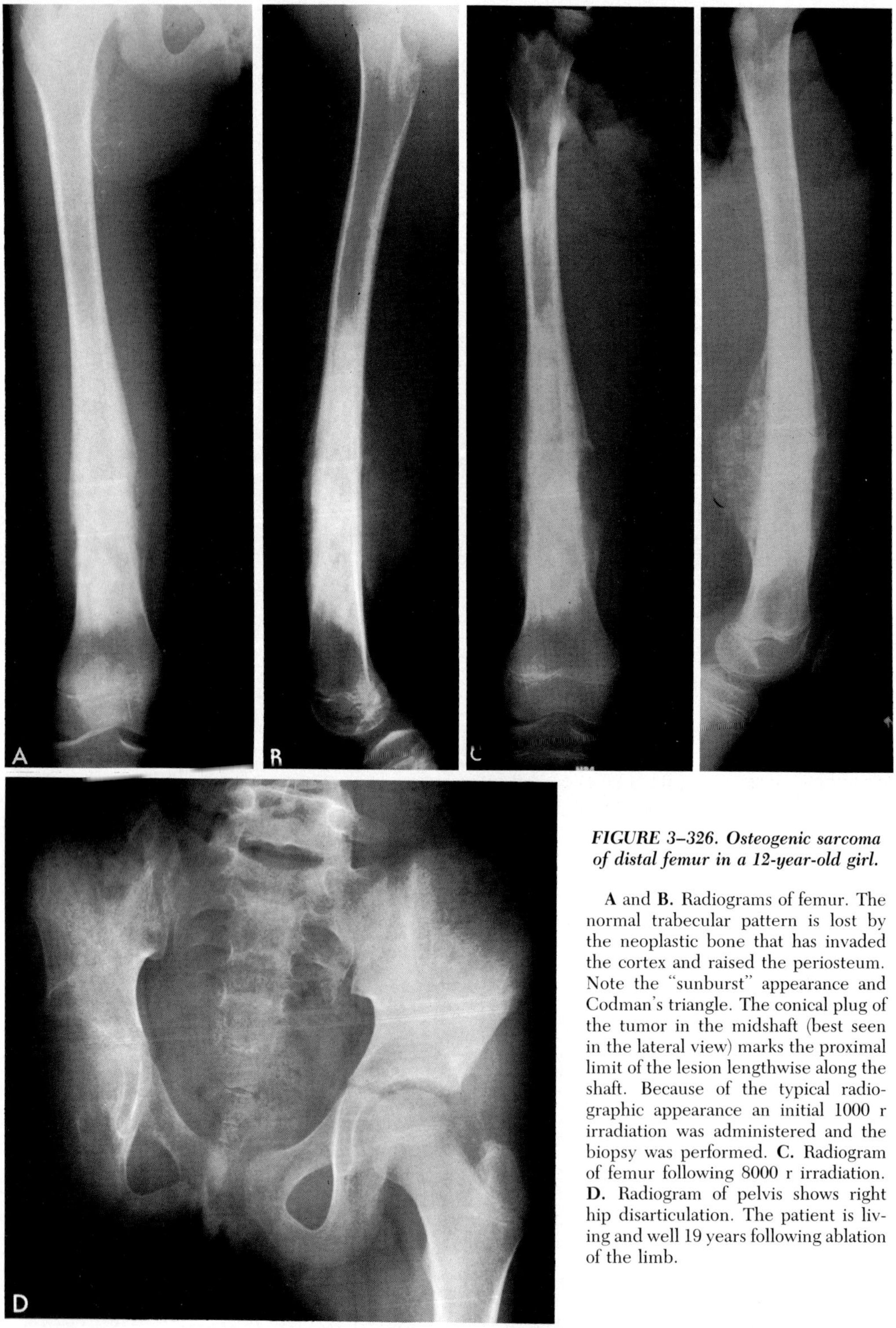

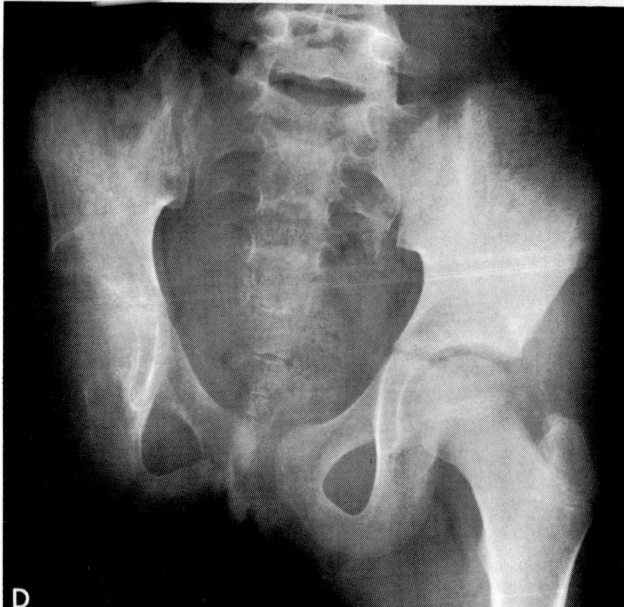

FIGURE 3–326. Osteogenic sarcoma of distal femur in a 12-year-old girl.

A and **B.** Radiograms of femur. The normal trabecular pattern is lost by the neoplastic bone that has invaded the cortex and raised the periosteum. Note the "sunburst" appearance and Codman's triangle. The conical plug of the tumor in the midshaft (best seen in the lateral view) marks the proximal limit of the lesion lengthwise along the shaft. Because of the typical radiographic appearance an initial 1000 r irradiation was administered and the biopsy was performed. **C.** Radiogram of femur following 8000 r irradiation. **D.** Radiogram of pelvis shows right hip disarticulation. The patient is living and well 19 years following ablation of the limb.

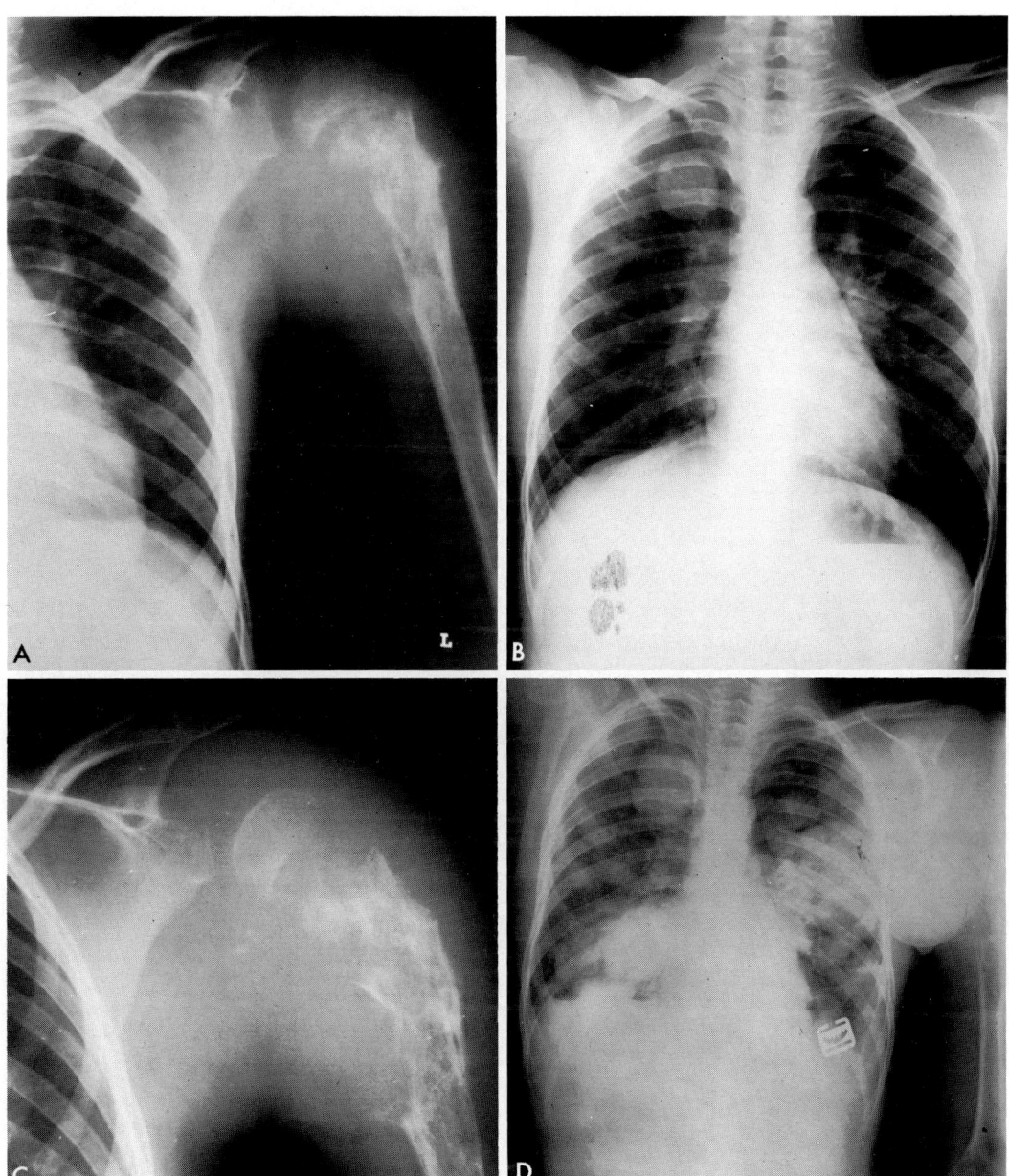

FIGURE 3–327. *Osteogenic sarcoma of left proximal humerus in a 12-year-old boy.*

The patient complained of pain in the left arm and shoulder of one month's duration. **A.** Radiogram of left humerus showing the malignant lesion. **B.** Chest radiogram showing metastasis in right upper lobe. Palliative irradiation and chemotherapy were administered. **C.** Two months later, radiogram of left humerus. **D.** Chest radiogram, three months after initial radiogram, shows diffuse metastasis to lungs. The patient died a few days later.

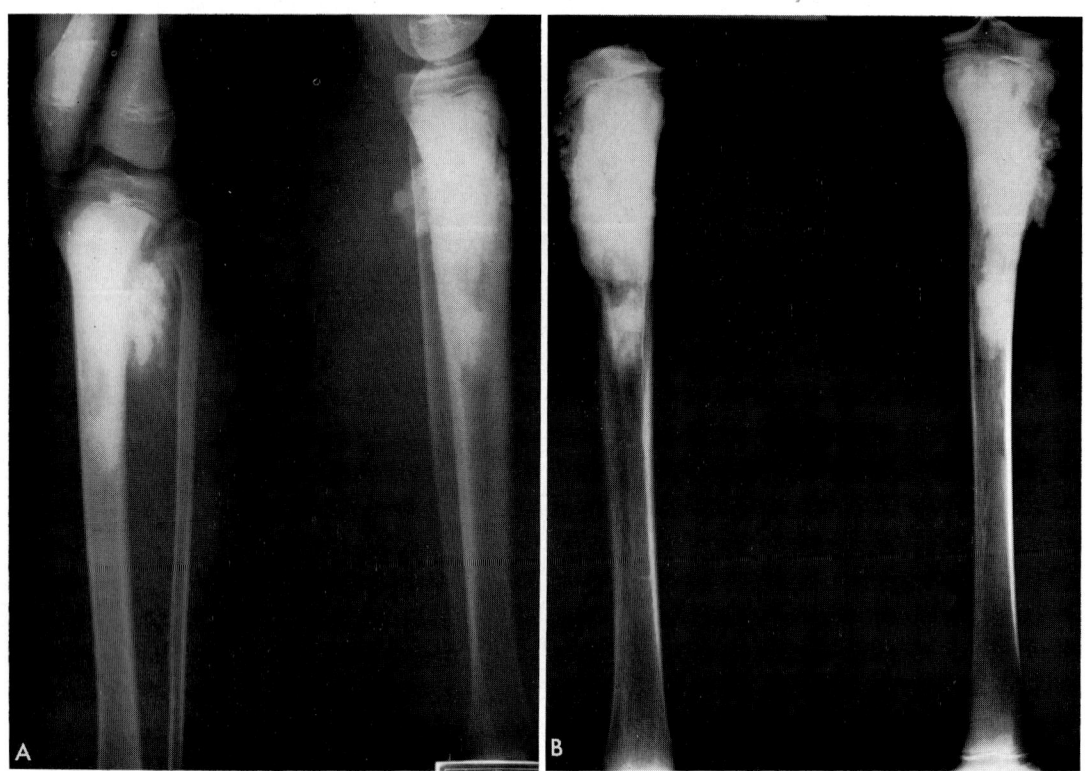

FIGURE 3–328. Osteogenic sarcoma of proximal tibia.

A. Initial radiograms. A knee disarticulation was performed. **B.** Radiograms of amputated tibia.

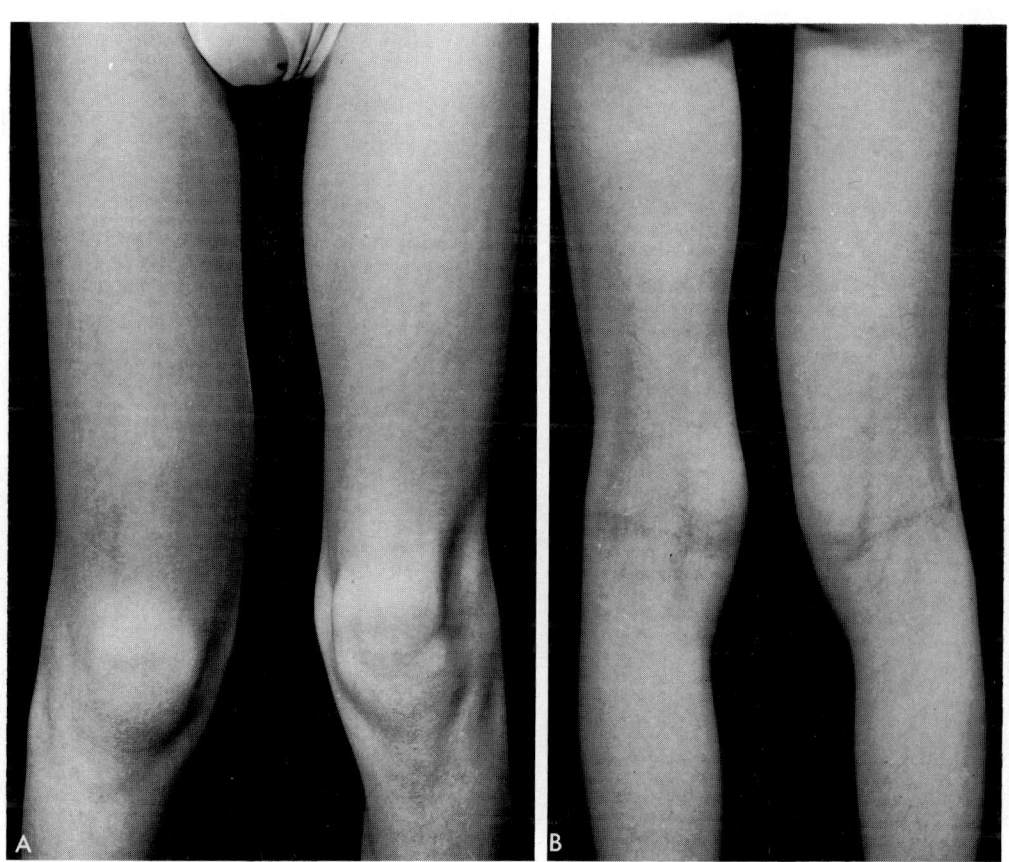

FIGURE 3–329. Osteogenic sarcoma of right distal femur.

A and **B.** Photographs of patient show the swelling of lower right thigh.

Illustration continued on following page

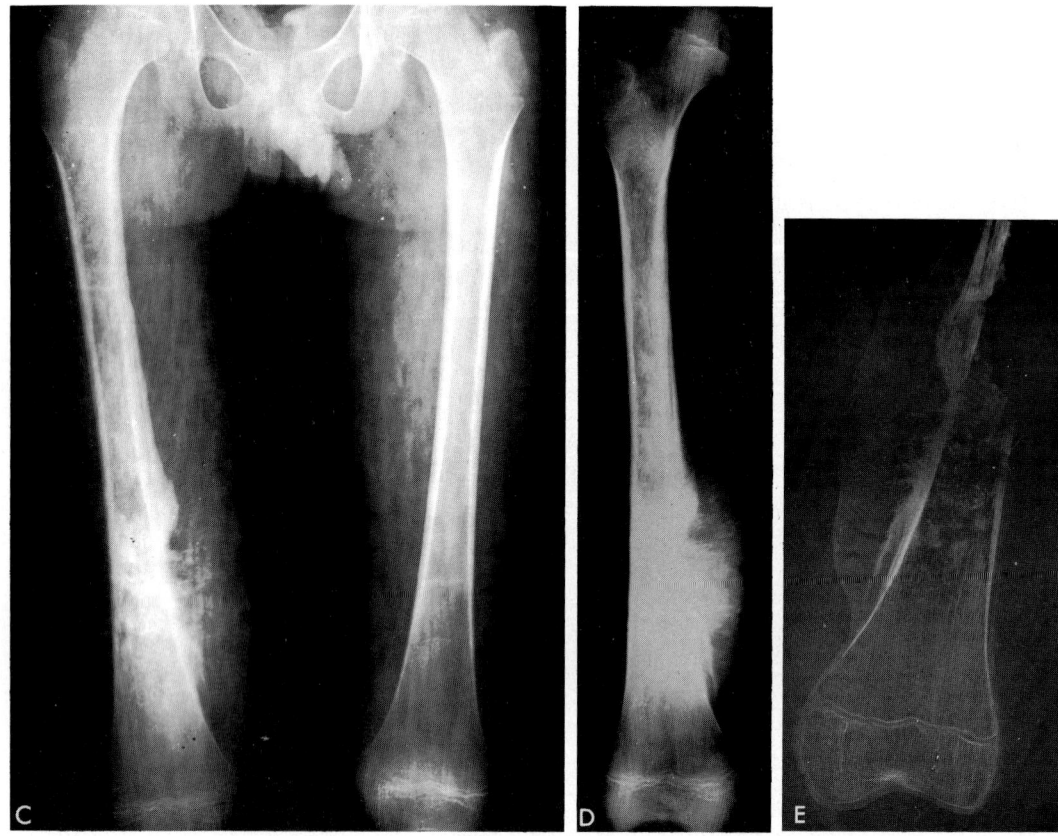

FIGURE 3–329 Continued. Osteogenic sarcoma of right distal femur.

C and **D.** Radiograms of femora. Note the "sunburst" appearance and the areas of increased radiopacity (neoplastic bone) and that of radiolucency (bone destruction). **E.** Radiogram of sectional specimen.

Codman's triangle has its base perpendicular to the shaft and is created by the subperiosteal reactive new bone; it is not characteristic of osteogenic sarcoma, as it is also seen in osteomyelitis and Ewing's sarcoma. A soft-tissue mass will be discernible in the radiograms as the tumor advances further, transgressing the cortex. Pathologic fracture may occur.

Linear tomography and computed tomography are of great value in depicting the details of bone destruction and tumor bone production within the lesion. The neoplastic bone is amorphous and not stress oriented (Fig. 3–330). The areas of cortical erosion by the tumor tissue are well delineated. The degree of soft-tissue extension and the relationship of the extra-compartmental tumor to fascial planes is clearly demonstrated by the CT scan. Occult skip metastases of 2 mm. or more in long bones are also well visualized by CT scan. Pulmonary metastases of 3 mm. or more in diameter are identified by CT scan. It should be noted that conventional radiograph of the chest (dual inspiration and expiration views) will detect metastatic nodules 10 mm. or greater in diameter; ordinary tomography will demonstrate metastatic lesions between 5 and 10 mm. The importance of pulmonary CT scan in staging of osteosarcoma cannot be overemphasized.[27, 40, 41, 44, 76, 91, 162] Experience with nuclear magnetic resonance imaging is very promising; it seems to be at least as valuable as computed tomography.[14] This author recommends the use of both CT scan and magnetic resonance imaging in the preoperative staging of osteosarcoma.

Bone scan with technetium-99m will show marked increase in the uptake of the radionuclide; this is due to active formation of new tumor bone (Fig. 3–331). The vascularity of the lesion augments the intensity of the uptake. Ordinarily the margins of the increased isotope activity mark the extent of the osteosarcoma; this is not absolute, however, as the tumor may extend beyond the margin of increased radioisotope uptake.

Angiography is of great value in delineating the extent of soft-tissue extension and its relationship to adjacent neurovascular structures. The early arterial phase demonstrates the reactive neovasculature about the tumor extending into the soft tissues, whereas the late venous phase shows the intrinsic vascularity as a "tumor blush."[26, 96, 137, 186] Angiography is of particular value when limb salvage is being combined with radical ablation of osteogenic sarcoma.

Laboratory Findings. The serum alkaline phosphatase level is elevated in osteosarcoma reflecting osteogenesis in the neoplastic tissue. The degree of elevation of this enzyme is commensurate with the activity of the neoplastic osteoblasts within the lesion and the size of the tumor. The course of osteosarcoma can be monitored by serial determination of levels of serum alkaline phosphatase; following ablation of the tumor the enzyme level falls to near normal; it rises with development of metatases and recurrence. Clinically sequential determinations of serum alkaline phosphatase levels are utilized to assess response to chemotherapy.

An immunologic finding in osteogenic sarcoma is the presence of antisarcoma antibody in the serum, as determined by hemagglutinins or by precipitins against extracts of osteosarcoma. With ablation of the tumor the level of identifiable antisarcoma antibody increases, and with the development of metastases and recurrence it falls.[113, 124] The drawbacks of this immunologic method of monitoring the biologic performance of osteosarcoma are its technical difficulty and lack of sufficient tumor material.

Staging, Biopsy, and Treatment

Osteogenic sarcoma is treated by radical excision and adjuvant chemotherapy. Its clinical and radiographic diagnosis should always be confirmed by histologic examination of adequate tissue obtained by open biopsy prior to definitive treatment. Exuberant callus of a stress fracture, subacute osteomyelitis, active myositis ossificans, aneurysmal bone cyst, and eosinophilic granuloma are some of the benign conditions that can easily be mistaken for osteogenic sarcoma. Ewing's sarcoma, fibrosarcoma, and metastatic carcinoma are some of the malignant lesions that must be considered in the differential diagnosis.

Staging. Carefully planned staging of the lesion should precede open biopsy. The objectives of staging are to establish the final tissue diagnosis, to delineate the local extent of the tumor, and to discover any distant metastasis. Both staging and open biopsy should be carried out by the surgeon who will perform the definitive operation. Determination of local extent of disease after biopsy performed elsewhere is difficult and inaccurate because of the disruption of tissue planes, hematoma formation, and wound healing. In choosing the proper surgical procedure it is vital to know whether there are natural barriers to tumor extension. Is the lesion intracompartmental (bounded by natural barriers to tumor extension) or extracompartmental (with no proximal, distal, or peripheral barriers to tumor extension)? During staging one should meticulously assess the muscle compartment and tumor proximity to neurovascular structure. Is limb salvage feasible?

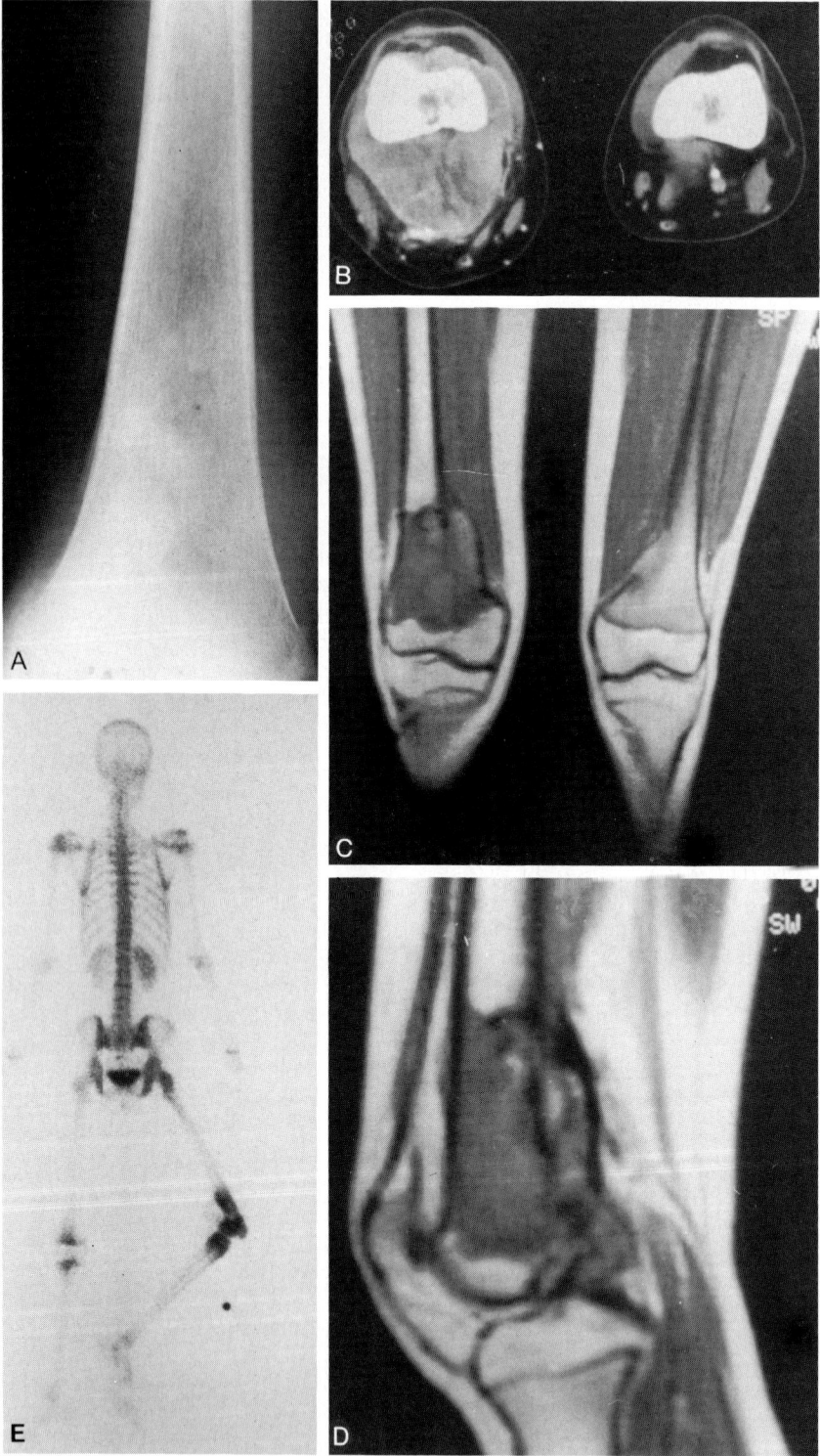

FIGURE 3–330. Osteogenic sarcoma of left distal femur.

A. Plain anteroposterior radiogram. Note the distal metaphyseal and lower diaphyseal sclerotic lesion. **B.** The CT scan showing bone forming tumor. **C** and **D.** Magnetic resonance imaging shows the extent of the tumor and its relationship to popliteal soft tissue. **E.** Bone scan with technetium-99m showing increased uptake in the distal femoral metaphyseal region.

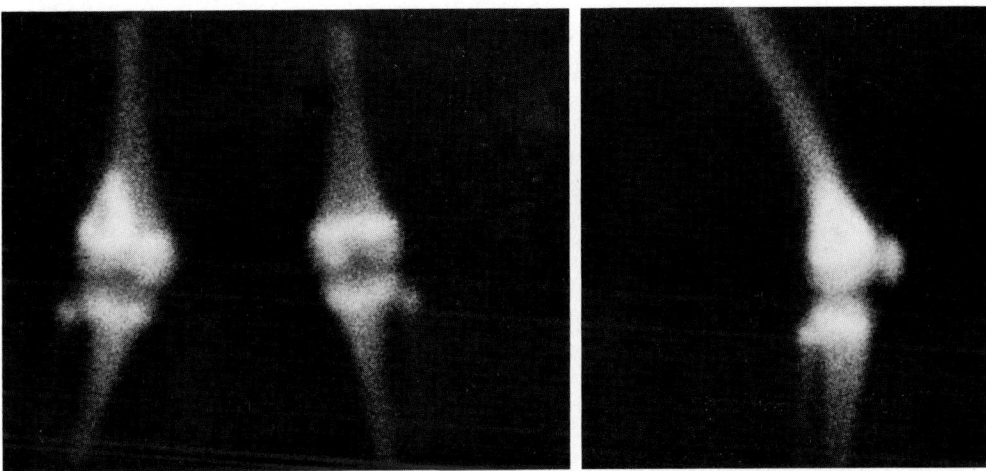

FIGURE 3–331. *Osteogenic sarcoma of right distal femoral metaphysis.*

Bone scan findings with technetium-99m. Note the intense increased uptake in the lesional area.

In preoperative staging of osteogenic sarcoma the following diagnostic tests are performed: (1) complete history and physical examination; (2) complete blood count with differential, erythrocyte sedimentation rate, and serum levels of calcium, phosphates, and alkaline phosphatase; (3) conventional radiograph of the part and the chest; (4) scintigraphy with technetium-99m and in selected cases also with gallium-67 citrate, (5) linear tomography to assess longitudinal intraosseous extent, (6) computed tomography of the part involved by the primary tumor and of the chest (to rule out metastases); (7) nuclear magnetic resonance imaging; and (8) biplanar peripheral angiography in selected cases, especially if limb salvage is contemplated.

A pediatric oncologist, radiologist, and pathologist should be consulted from the beginning; they should be involved in the staging and decision-making process. If the staging, open biopsy, and histologic examination of frozen sections indicate the tumor is osteogenic sarcoma, the pediatric oncolgist (who is also a hematologist) should perform a bone marrow examination when the patient is under general anesthesia. Management of osteogenic sarcoma is by a multidisciplinary approach. The patients should be treated in medical centers specializing in pediatric oncology.

Biopsy. Prior to performing an open biopsy the surgeon should be knowledgeable in the differential diagnosis and local extent of the lesion; before placing the incision, he should be cognizant of the principles of limb-salvage surgery and amputation flaps. Technical details of biopsy are presented elsewhere (p. 1161). It is crucial to verify the site of biopsy by radiograph in the operating room. Always obtain frozen sections to ensure you have diagnostic tissue. Take cultures of the tissue specimen. Consult the pathologist prior to biopsy as to special stains, cytology, electron microscopy, and immunocytochemistry.

There is always danger of the tumor spreading as a result of open biopsy. To prevent spilling neoplastic cells into vascular channels, it is advisable to use a coagulation diathermy knife at biopsy. Proponents of immediate ablation argue that biopsy delays radical therapy. Immediate definitive wide excision of osteogenic sarcoma requires a thorough clinical, radiologic, and pathologic correlation. An experienced pathologist might make a correct diagnosis on the basis of a frozen section, but amputation of a limb with a benign lesion as a result of an overdiagnosis of malignancy is never justified. It is always best to rely on permanent sections for final diagnosis. In case of uncertainty and doubt, it is best to obtain expert consultation.

The techniques used in immediate amputation are: application of double tourniquets and performance of amputation at a chosen level between the two tourniquets; repreparation and redraping of the patient and use of new surgical attire and instruments; and meticulous closure of the primary site of the tumor. At present this author does not recommend immediate amputation in treatment of osteogenic sarcoma because the results of such therapy have been most disappointing with only about a 10 to 15 per cent five-year survival rate. It is evident that tumor cells may enter the circulation in the beginning and lodge in the lungs and other areas as micrometastases. Immediate amputation does not stop the development and growth of these metastatic foci. In the past Ferguson recommended delaying amputation until a "quiet period," and further advised the use of radiation.[59] Cade recommended delaying amputation for six months; if, at the end of the time, pulmonary metastases were not manifest, the affected limb was ablated.[17] Green advocated the following plan: First, prebiopsy radiation of short duration: 1000 to 2000 r over five or six days with open biopsy on the same day as the last exposure (administration of this amount of radiation ordinarily did not affect histologic interpretation but would injure the tumor cells that might be escaping into the circulation at the time of biopsy); second, adequate open biopsy; third, postbiopsy radiation to the extent of 6000 to 8000 r, given in divided doses; and fourth, prompt amputation at the end of this radiation course.[71]

In those days there were no chemotherapeutic agents that were effective against osteogenic sarcoma. The advent of newer agents has changed the protocol of treatment of this tumor. The prognosis is much improved; other factors in improvement of the five-year survival rate are early diagnosis, thorough surgical staging, and meticulous planning of operative treatment. In the past the natural history of classic osteogenic sarcoma treated by amputation alone or by amputation and radiotherapy was pulmonary metastasis in eight to ten months and death from disseminated metastases within two years of diagnosis. At present with early diagnosis, accurate staging, and appropriate radical excision with pre- and post-surgery chemotherapy the outlook is much brighter. Rosen and associates projected 80 per cent of the cases to be disease free at five year follow-up.[152] At present the chemotherapeutic agents administered are high-dosage methotrexate (HD MTX); citrovorum factor rescue (CFR), Adriamycin, and a combination of bleomycin, cyclophosphamide and dactinomycin (BCD). With intense research, newer and more effective drugs may develop in the future. Chemotherapy is administered by the pediatric oncologist. It is the practice of this author to have a patient with osteogenic sarcoma or other malignant musculoskeletal tumor admitted to the hospital on the joint orthopedic and oncology services. After the immediate period of definitive surgery, the patient is transferred to the oncology service.

The term *osteogenic sarcoma* includes a wide spectrum of neoplastic cell types with varying severity of malignancy. The response to chemotherapy, i.e., high-dosage methotraxate and citrovorum factor rescue varies; the osteoblastic, telangiectatic, fibrous histiocytomatous and fibrosarcomatous types of osteogenic sarcoma show very good response to chemotherapy; whereas, the small-cell type show poor response. The small-cell type of osteogenic sarcoma is more sensitive to Adriamycin and the combination of bleomycin, cyclophosphamide and dactinomycin.[152]

Treatment Plan. The treatment plan for osteogenic sarcoma is as follows: *first*, open biopsy to make definitive diagnosis, *second*, preoperative adjuvant chemotherapy for four to six weeks. Its advantages are: that it reduces edema and decreases the size of the primary tumor, rendering limb salvage surgery feasible; it assesses the drugs used by determining the response of the primary tumor to a specific chemotherapeutic agent or agents in the individual patient, and thereby it allows the administration of the optimally effective chemotherapeutic agents postoperatively. In the patient who does not respond, the agent or agents are replaced by other effective drugs. Early administration of chemotherapeutic agents, if effective, will destroy occult micrometastases and occult microextensions and will improve the overall prognosis for survival. *Third* is definitive surgery followed by additional adjuvant chemotherapy for 12 months. The choice of adjuvant chemotherapy following definitive surgery depends upon assessment of the extent of tumor cell destruction as shown by histologic examination of the resected primary tumor.

In Grade I there is minimal or no effect;

In Grade II the response is partial with 50 to 90 per cent tumor necrosis;

In Grade III there is greater than 90 per cent tumor necrosis, but definite foci of viable tumor are seen in some histologic sections; and

In Grade IV there are no viable tumor cells noted in any of the histologic sections.

In Grades I and II responses the chemotherapeutic agents are changed. Such individualization of adjuvant chemotherapy has definitely improved the prognosis.[152]

The potential for metastasis of osteogenic sarcoma varies with its type: parosteal osteogenic sarcoma and endosteal osteogenic sarcoma are low grade (G_1) with less than 10 per cent metastatic potential, whereas classic osteosarcoma, radiation osteogenic sarcoma, and osteogenic sarcoma developing in Paget's disease are high grade (G_2), having a greater than 10 per cent metastatic potential. There is uniformity of opinion that the part involved by osteogenic sarcoma should be ablated; there is, however, controversy whether the operative local control of the malignant tissue should be by wide local resection (supported by the limb salvage enthusiasts) or by amputation of the limb—wide resection by transmedullary ablation or radical resection by disarticulation.

Before surgical ablation of the primary tumor it is essential to rule out the presence of metastases. Osteogenic sarcoma spreads to the lungs early; therefore in addition to conventional radiography, one should make linear tomographic and computed tomographic studies of the chest. Also scintigraphic studies should be performed. It may be several months before metastases attain sufficient size to become discernible in conventional radiograms.

Limb Salvage. This course of action is based on the principle that a part of a limb that can be used should be preserved, provided it does not adversely affect survival. Surgical adjuvant chemotherapy (ordinarily high-dosage methotrexate for osteogenic sarcoma) has made limb salvage feasible when diagnosis is made early, the tumor is intracompartmental, and neurovascular structures are not involved. Other surgical adjuvants to limb salvage are radiotherapy and immunotherapy. Proximity to vital structures is a more important consideration than tumor size. The objective of limb salvage is to preserve and to provide maximal function.[134]

In the lower limb, stability and limb length are the primary considerations, whereas in the upper limb, the goal is provision of dexterity and sensation. The drawbacks of limb salvage are that the preserved limb may be disfigured (e.g., after Van Nes rotationplasty), there is increased risk of local recurrence, and there is the possibility of skip lesions.

In the treatment of osteogenic sarcoma, measures by which the limb may be spared are resection of the entire involved bone—such as the fibula, radius or ulna (converting to a one-bone forearm), clavicle, scapula, or hemi-pelvis; and local resection and replacement of the ablated part by a "spacer." A resected en bloc segment of diaphysis of a long bone can be replaced by an autograft (such as vascularized fibula, massive bone graft, or sliding autograft) or by an allograft. When local resection includes the entire epiphyseal end of a long bone, one may replace it with an internal prosthesis or allograft.[91] An alternative is to fuse the joint by sliding arthrodesis or allograft arthrodesis.[53] When an internal prosthesis is inserted in a growing child, limb length inequality becomes a problem until skeletal maturity; this can be managed by exchanging the prosthesis for a longer and larger one or having an adjustable prosthesis that can be lengthened. Another problem with prosthetic replacement in a child is durability, because of his overactive, vigorous, and irresponsible performance. Other problems of bone replacement with "spacers" are the large size of tumors, extracompartmental involvement of fascia and skin, and failure of primary resection with recurrent lesions and recurrence of primary tumor. In such instances, when the tumor involves the distal or proximal femur and is extracompartmental with involvement of vessels or skin, and in cases of failure of primary treatment *Van Nes rotationplasty* is an alternative method of partial preservation of a limb.[83, 95, 153, 167] When rotationplasty is performed it is essential to assess the remaining growth in the lower limbs so that at skeletal maturity the turnabout ankle is level with the opposite normal knee (See Plate 29 in Chapter 2).

Amputation. The level of amputation is determined by close scrutiny of the conventional radiographs, bone imaging with technetium-99m and galium-67 citrate, linear and computed tomography, and nuclear magnetic resonance imaging. These surgical staging studies should be performed immediately prior to definitive surgery after completion of preoperative adjuvant chemotherapy. Skip metastases and recurrence of osteogenic sarcoma in the amputation stump are definite problems.[51, 52, 116] This author tends to incline more toward radical than wide excision if in doubt. The operative techniques of amputation and disarticulation at various levels in the upper and lower limbs are described and illustrated in Plates 42 to 50.

The patient and the parents need psychologic support; initially there will be tremendous emotional resistance to ablation of a limb. It is further complicated by the potential gloomy outlook. It is vital that these patients see other children with amputations and prostheses during the four to six weeks of preoperative adjuvant chemotherapy. Treatment of these children and adolescents in a children's hospital with a specialized multidisciplinary oncology clinic is of great value. The supportive services of an oncology nurse clinician are crucial. The stump of the lower limb amputation can be fitted immediately with a temporary prosthesis.

If pulmonary metastasis has already taken place at the time of initial diagnosis, the decision whether to amputate depends on factors such as the amount of disability of the affected limb caused by local pain and tremendous size of the tumor, which may be so large and painful that the only means of controlling the misery is

Text continued on page 1382

Hemipelvectomy (Banks and Coleman)

The patient lies on his unaffected side and is maintained in position by sandbags and kidney rests, which are placed well above the iliac crests. The underneath normal limb is flexed at the hip and knee and fastened to the table by wide adhesive straps. The uppermost arm is supported on a rest. The perineal area and, in the male, the scrotum and penis are shielded away from the operative field by sterile self-adhering skin drapes. The operative area is prepared and draped so that the proximal thigh, the inguinal and gluteal regions, and the abdomen are sterile. It should be possible to turn the patient on his back and side without contaminating the surgical field.

A. The outlines of the skin flaps, consisting of ilioinguinal, iliogluteal, and posterior incisions, are marked with methylene blue. With the patient placed on his back, the ilioinguinal incision is made first. It begins at the pubic tubercle and passes upward and backward parallel to Poupart's ligament to the anterior superior iliac spine and then posteriorly on the iliac crest. Its posterior limit depends upon the desired level of section of the innominate bone.

B. The subcutaneous tissue and fascia are divided along the line of the skin incision. The periosteum over the iliac crest is incised between the attachments of the abdominal muscles superiorly and the tensor fasciae and the gluteus medius inferiorly.

C. The abdominal muscles are detached from the iliac crest and medial wall of the ilium. The tributaries of deep circumflex vessels are ligated.

D. Next the inguinal ligament is divided and along with the spermatic cord and abdominal muscles is retracted superiorly. The lower skin flap is retracted inferiorly, and by blunt dissection the inner pelvis is freed. The inferior epigastric artery and lumboinguinal nerve are exposed, ligated, and divided.

Plate 42. Hemipelvectomy (Banks and Coleman)

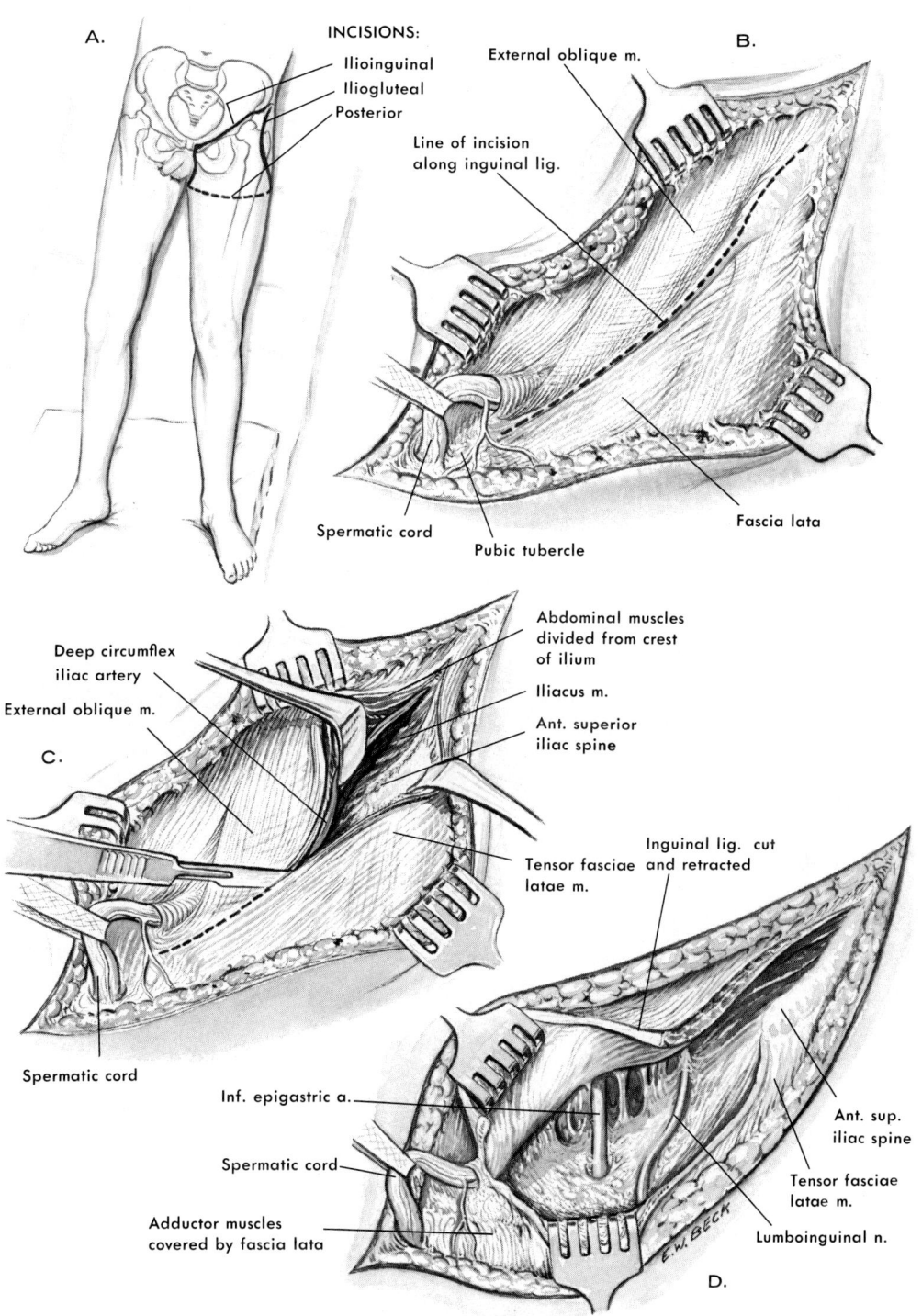

Hemipelvectomy (Banks and Coleman) (Continued)

E. In the loose areolar tissue the external iliac vessels and femoral nerve are gently dissected out. The external iliac artery and vein are individually clamped, severed, and doubly ligated with needle suture 0 silk.

F. The rectus abdominis and adductor muscles are detached from the pubic bone, which is subperiosteally exposed. The bladder is retracted superiorly. The pubic bone is osteotomized 1.5 cm. lateral to the symphysis. Depending upon the proximity of the tumor, the osteotomy may have to be at the symphysis pubis. Injury to the bladder or urethra should be avoided. Any bleeding from the retropubic venous plexus is controlled by coagulation and packing with warm laparotomy pads.

Plate 42. Hemipelvectomy (Banks and Coleman)

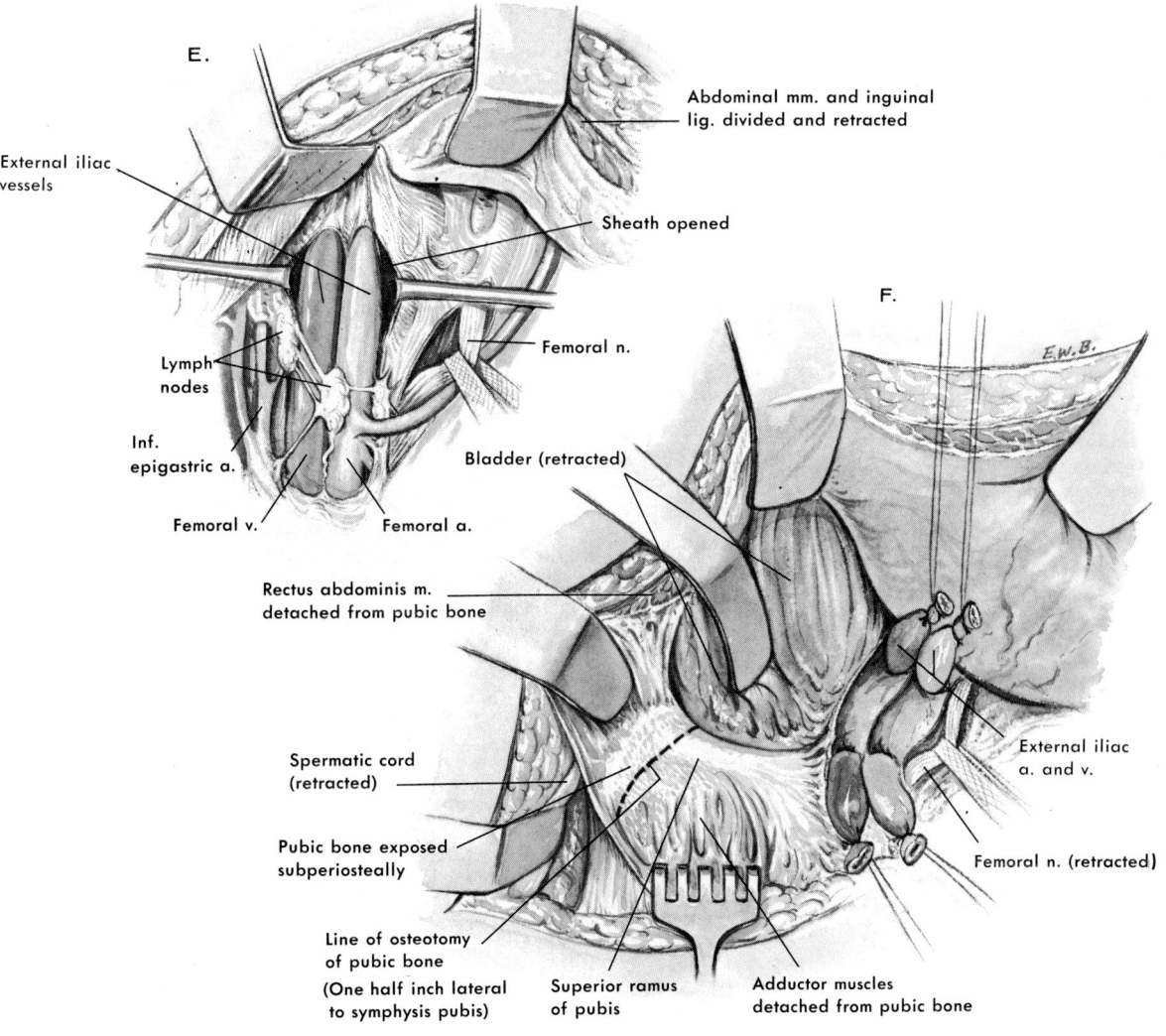

Hemipelvectomy (Banks and Coleman) (Continued)

G. The patient is then turned to his side. The drapes are adjusted and reinforced to ensure sterility of the operative field. First, the anterior incision is extended posteriorly to the posterior superior iliac spine. From the upper end of the anterior incision, the second or iliogluteal incision is started. It extends to the thigh, curving forward to an area about 5 cm. distal to the greater trochanter. It then passes backward around the posterior aspect of the thigh to meet the anterior incision. The subcutaneous tissue and fascia are divided in line with the skin incision.

H. By blunt and sharp dissection the gluteus maximus is separated from the gluteus medius and tensor fasciae latae to the depth of the greater trochanter. The gluteus maximus is transected at its insertion, mobilized by blunt dissection, and retracted posteriorly. Vessels and nerves to the gluteus maximus muscle are preserved. (Inferior gluteal nerve and artery emerge distal to the piriformis muscle, and the superior gluteal artery proximal to it.)

I. The sciatic nerve is clamped, ligated, and sharply divided distal to the origin of the inferior gluteal nerve. The piriformis, gemelli, and obturator internus muscles are transected near their insertion.

Plate 42. Hemipelvectomy (Banks and Coleman)

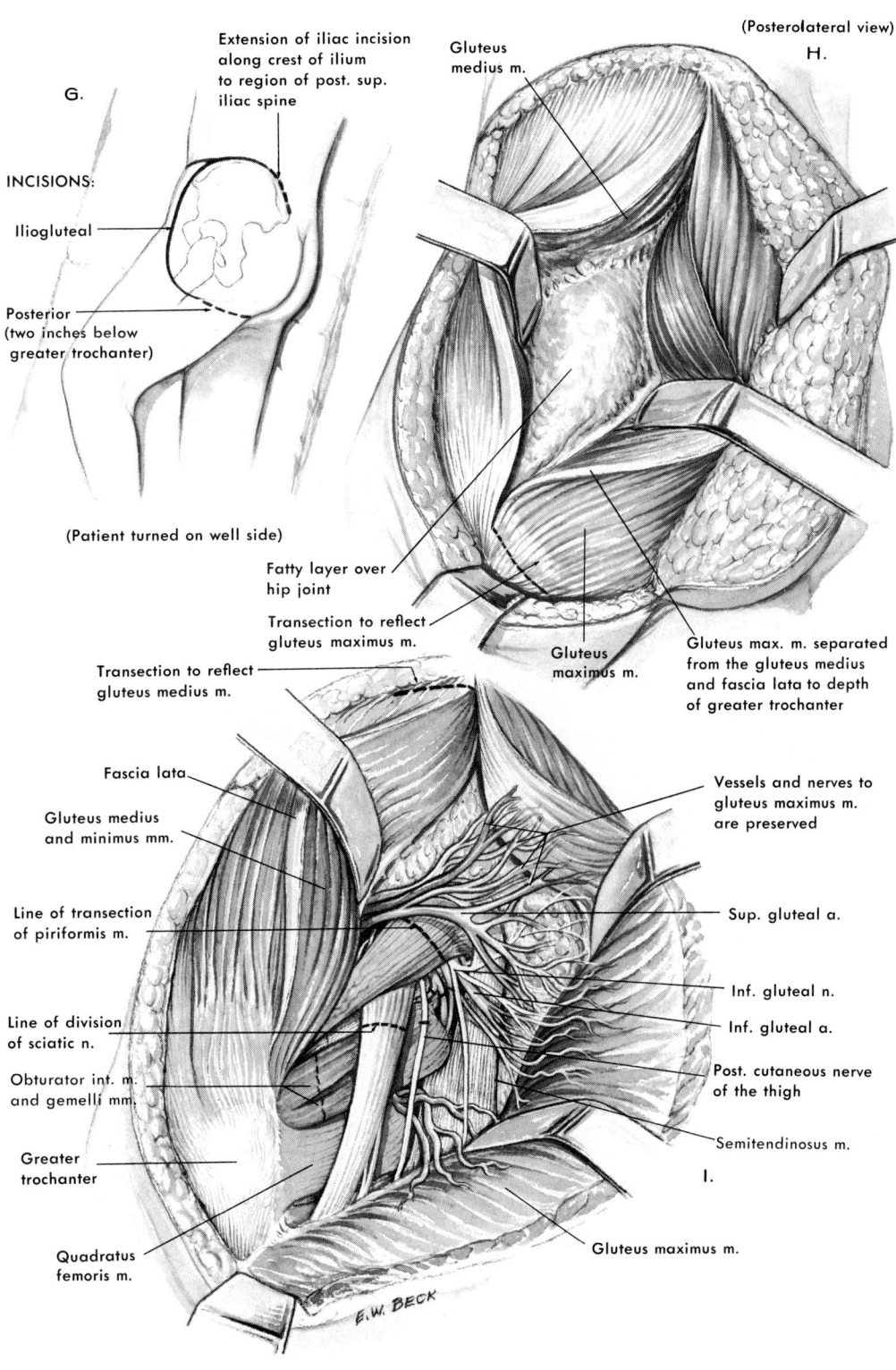

Hemipelvectomy (Banks and Coleman) (Continued)

J. The ilium is subperiosteally exposed by elevation and detachment of the latissimus dorsi and sacrospinalis muscles, the posterior portion of the gluteus medius, and the anterior fibers of the gluteus maximus. The inner wall of the ilium is also subperiosteally exposed anteriorly to the sacroiliac joint. Chandler retractors are placed in the sciatic notch, and with a Gigli saw the ilium is osteotomized about 5 cm. anterior to the posterior gluteal line. The site of osteotomy of the ilium depends upon the location of the tumor; it is carried out further posteriorly if the neoplasm is adjacent to the gluteal line.

K. Next, the patient is repositioned on his back, and the hip is maximally flexed in some abduction. The posterior incision is completed.

L. Then the hip is manipulated into maximal abduction and external rotation, laying open the pelvic area and giving wide exposure to the remaining intrapelvic structures to be severed.

M. From above downward, the femoral nerve, iliopsoas muscle, obturator vessels, obturator nerve, levator ani, and coccygeus muscles are sectioned. The vessels are doubly ligated prior to division to prevent troublesome bleeding.

N. The gluteus maximus muscle is sutured to the divided margin of the external oblique muscle and lateral abdominal wall. A couple of perforated silicone catheters are inserted and connected to Hemovac suction.

O. Fascia, subcutaneous tissue, and skin are closed in layers in the usual manner. A pressure dressing is applied.

Plate 42. Hemipelvectomy (Banks and Coleman)

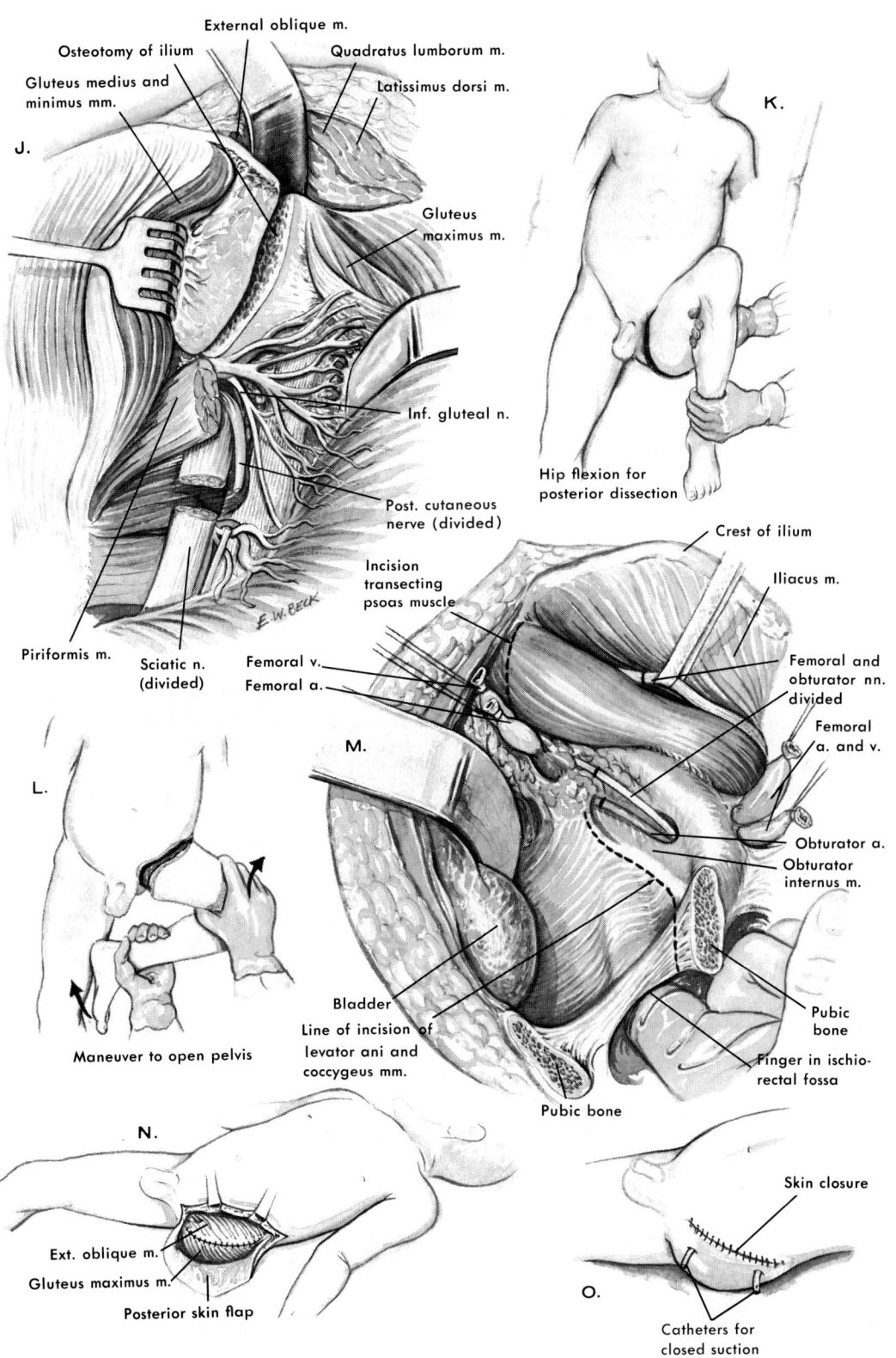

Hip Disarticulation

A. An anterior racquet type of incision is made, starting at the anterior superior iliac spine and extending medially and distally, parallel with Poupart's ligament, to the middle of the inner aspect of the thigh about 2 inches distal to the origin of the adductor muscles; and then it is continued around the back of the thigh at a level about 2 inches distal to the ischial tuberosity. Next, the incision is carried along the lateral aspect of the thigh about 3 inches distal to the base of the greater trochanter and is curved proximally and medially to join the first incision at the anterior superior iliac spine.

B. The subcutaneous tissue and the fascia are divided in line with the skin incision. The long saphenous vein is exposed and ligated, after tracing to its junction with the femoral vein. If lymph node dissection is indicated, it can be performed at this stage. The sartorius muscle is divided at its origin from the anterior superior iliac spine and is reflected distally. The origins of the two heads of the rectus femoris, one from the anterior inferior iliac spine and the other from the superior margin of the acetabulum, are detached and reflected distally. The femoral nerve is isolated, ligated with 00 silk sutures, and divided on a tongue blade with a sharp scalpel or razor blade just distal to the ligature. The femoral artery and vein are isolated, doubly ligated with 00 silk sutures proximally and distally and severed in between.

C. Next, the hip is abducted to expose its medial aspect, and the adductor longus is detached at its origin from the pubis and reflected distally. The anterior branch of the obturator nerve is exposed deep to the adductor longus and is traced proximally.

D. The adductor brevis is retracted posteriorly. The posterior branch of the obturator nerve is isolated and dissected proximally to the main trunk of the obturator nerve, which is sharply divided. Next, the obturator vessels are isolated and ligated. One should be careful not to sever the obturator artery inadvertently as it will retract into the pelvis and cause bleeding that is difficult to control.

Plate 43. Hip Disarticulation

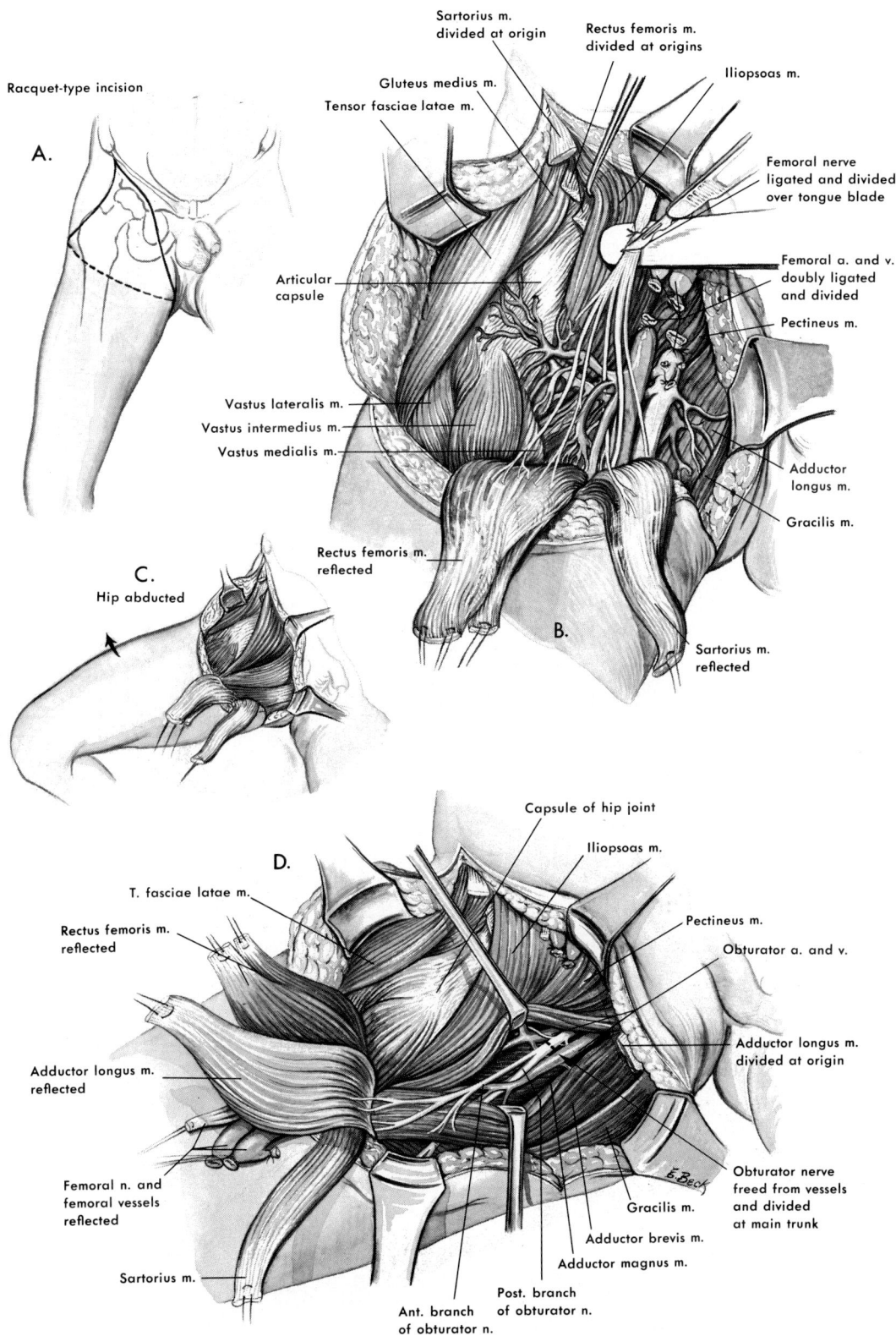

Hip Disarticulation *(Continued)*

E. The pectineus, adductor brevis, gracilis, and adductor magnus are severed near their origin. It is best to use a coagulation knife.

F. The hip is then flexed, externally rotated, and abducted, bringing into view the lesser trochanter. The iliopsoas tendon is exposed, isolated, and divided at its insertion and reflected proximally.

Plate 43. Hip Disarticulation

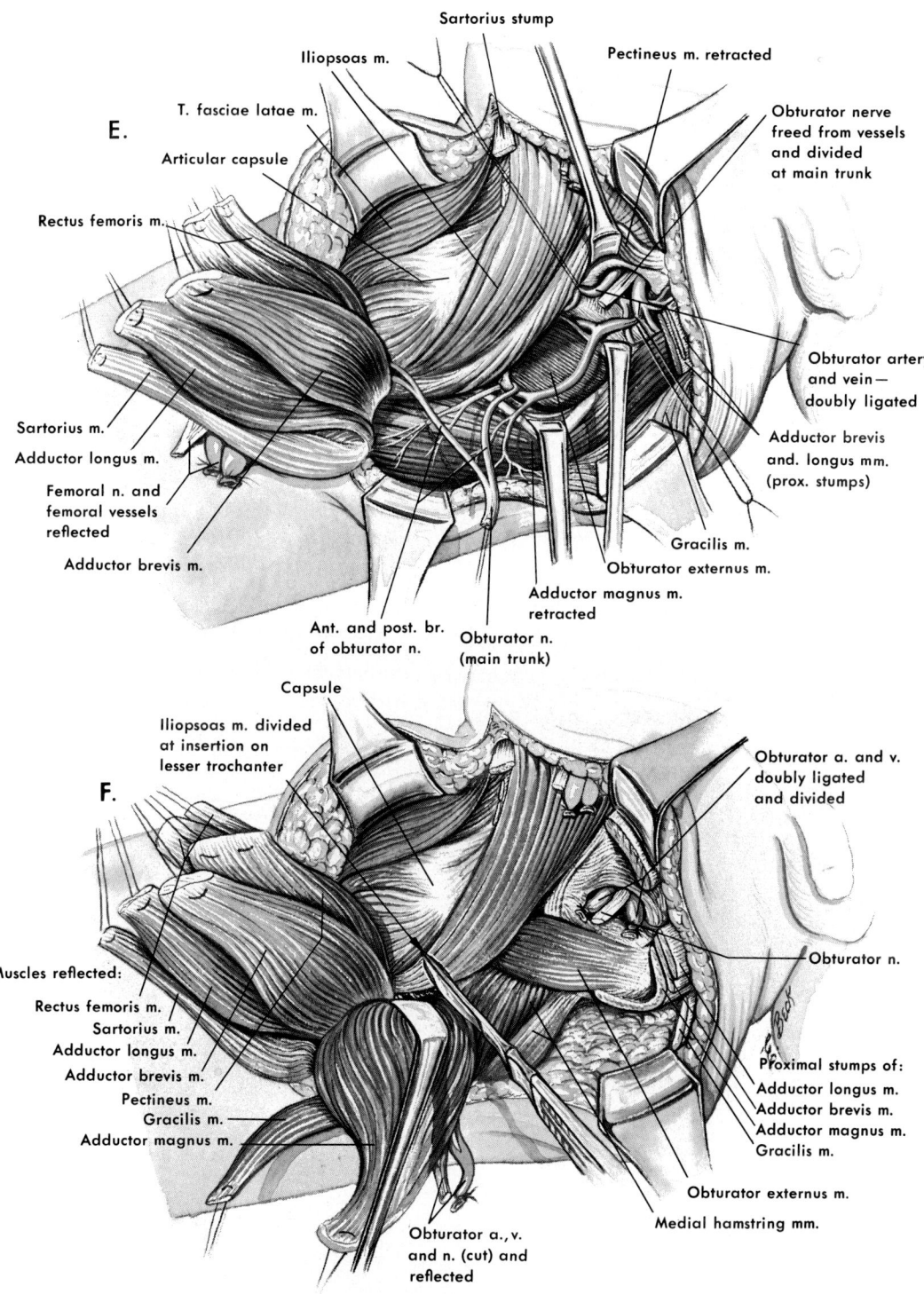

Hip Disarticulation (Continued)

G. Next, to facilitate surgical exposure, a sterile sandbag is placed under the pelvis, and the patient is turned onto the side away from the site of operation. The hip is internally rotated.

H. The gluteus medius and gluteus minimus muscles are divided at their insertion into the greater trochanter and, together with the tensor fasciae latae muscle, are reflected proximally. The gluteus maximus muscle is detached at its insertion and retracted upward. The free ends of the gluteus maximus, medius, and minimus muscles and the tensor fasciae latae muscle are marked with 0 silk suture for reattachment.

I. The muscles to be detached at their insertion through the posterior incision are shown. The short rotators of the hip, i.e., quadratus femoris, obturator externus, gemelli, and obturator internus, are detached from their insertion into the femur.

J. Next the sciatic nerve is identified, dissected free, pulled distally, and crushed with a Kocher hemostat at a level 2 inches proximal to the ischial tuberosity, and is ligated with 00 silk suture to prevent hemorrhage from its accompanying vessels. Then it is sharply divided just distal to the ligature.

Plate 43. Hip Disarticulation

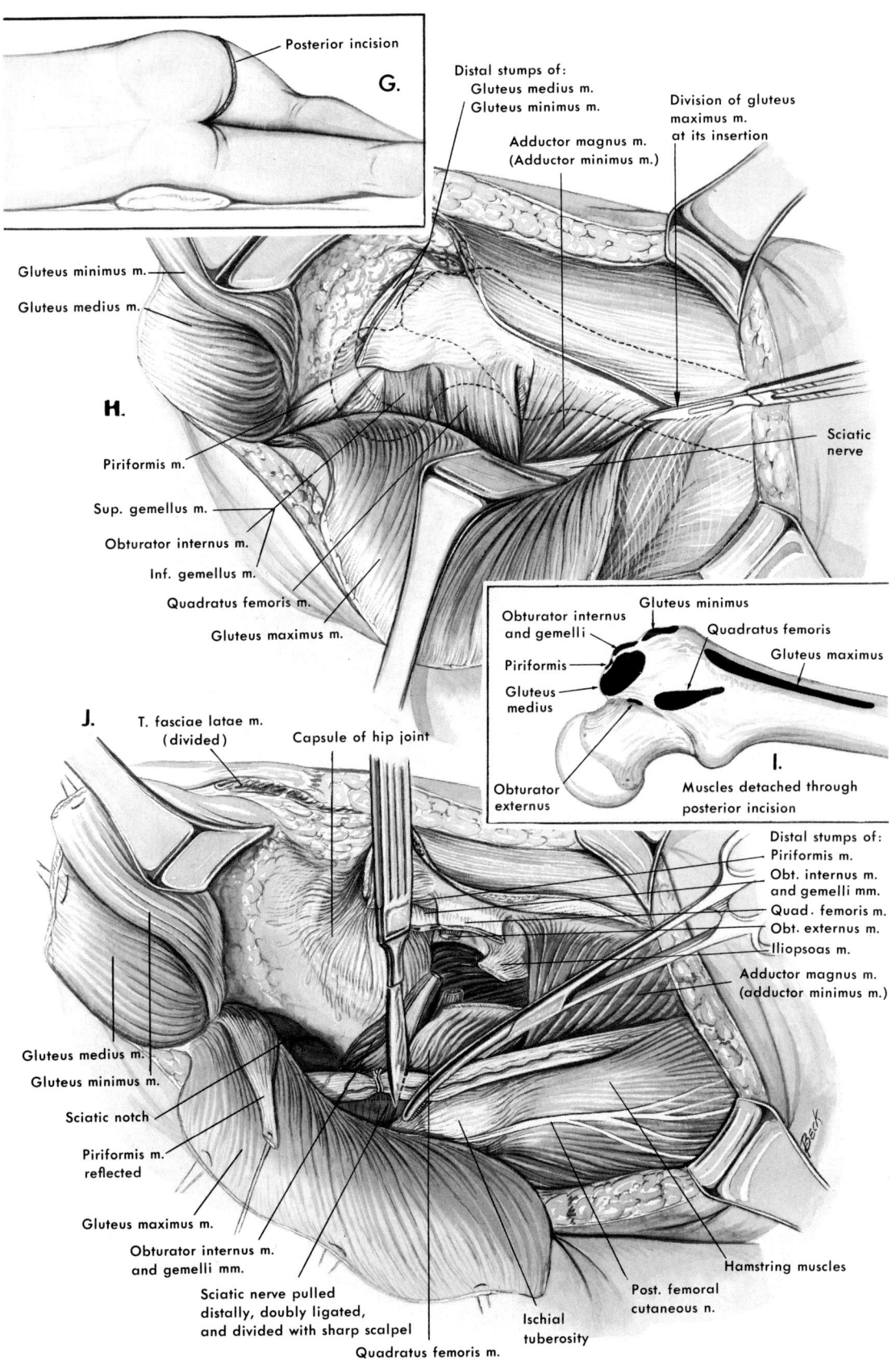

Hip Disarticulation (Continued)

K. The hamstring muscles are detached at their origin from the ischial tuberosity.

L. The capsule of the hip joint is divided near the acetabulum, and the ligamentum teres is severed, completing the disarticulation.

Plate 44. Ischial-Bearing Above-Knee Amputation (Mid-Thigh Amputation)

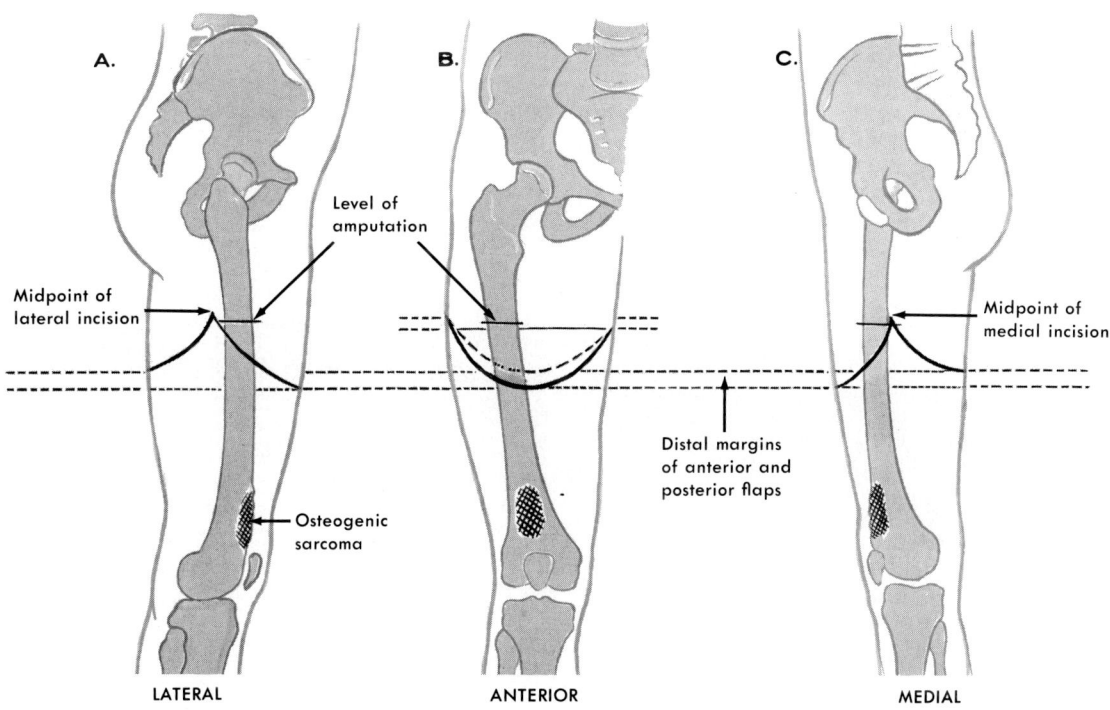

Ischial-Bearing Above-Knee Amputation (Mid-Thigh Amputation) (Continued)

D. The subcutaneous tissue and deep fascia are divided in line with the skin incision, and the anterior and posterior flaps are reflected proximally to the amputation level.

E to G. Next, the femoral vessels and saphenous nerve are identified. They are located deep to the sartorius muscle, between the adductor longus and the vastus medialis muscles. The *deep femoral vessels* are found adjacent to the femur in the interval between the adductor magnus, adductor longus, and the vastus medialis muscles. There are variations in the origin of the deep femoral artery, as shown in G. The femoral artery and vein are isolated, doubly ligated with heavy silk sutures, and divided. The saphenous nerve is pulled distally and divided with a sharp scalpel. If the amputation level is high, the deep femoral vessels may be ligated and divided through this anteromedial approach.

Plate 44. Ischial Bearing Above-Knee Amputation (Mid-Thigh Amputation)

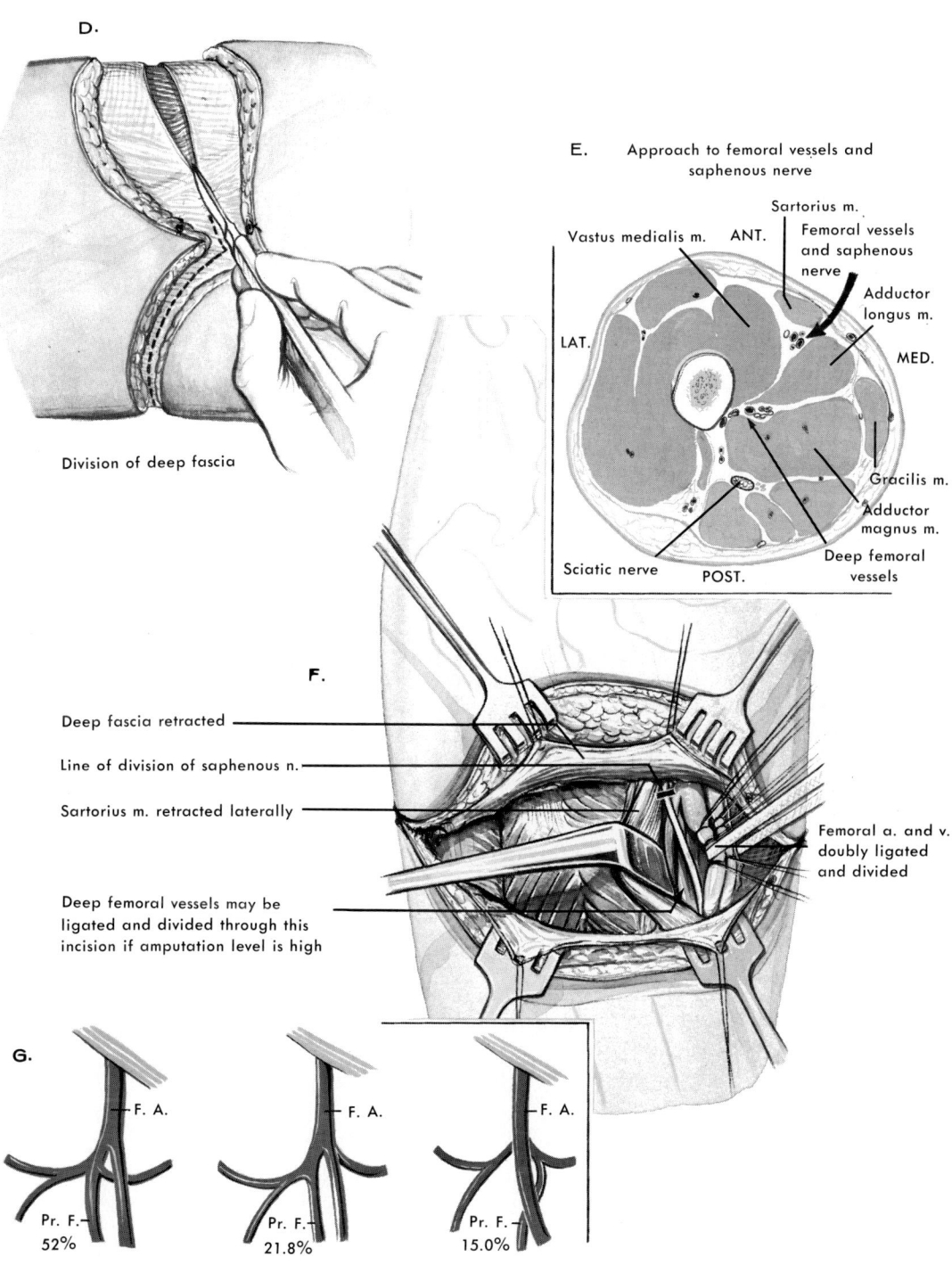

Ischial-Bearing Above-Knee Amputation (Mid-Thigh Amputation) (Continued)

H and **I.** Next, the hip is acutely flexed for approach to the posterior structures. The sciatic nerve is exposed in the interval between the medial hamstrings medially and the long head of the biceps femoris laterally. With a Kocher forceps, it is pulled distally, doubly ligated, and sharply divided over a tongue blade.

J and **K.** The posterior approach to the deep femoral vessels when the level of amputation is distal.

Plate 44. Ischial Bearing Above-Knee Amputation (Mid-Thigh Amputation)

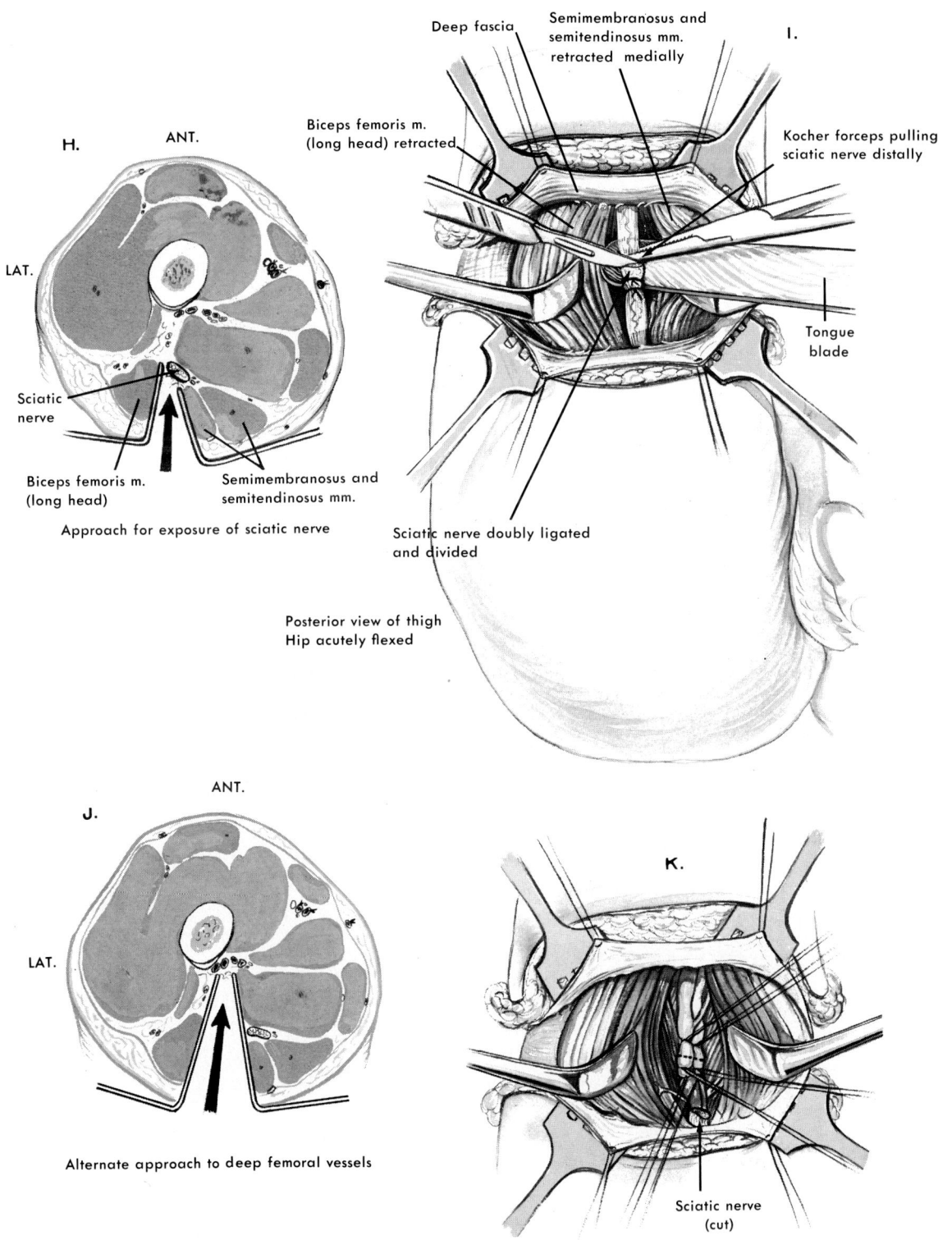

Ischial-Bearing Above-Knee Amputation (Mid-Thigh Amputation) (Continued)

L. With an amputation knife, the quadriceps and adductor muscles are sectioned and beveled upward to the site of bone division so that the anterior myofascial flap is approximately 1.5 cm. in thickness. The posterior muscles are divided transversely. Muscular branches of the femoral vessels are clamped and ligated, as necessary.

M. The proximal muscles are retracted upward with an amputation shield, and the periosteum is incised circumferentially.

N. Next, the femur is sectioned with a saw immediately distally to the periosteal incision.

O. With a rongeur, the prominence of the linea aspera is excised and the bone end is made smooth with a file. The wound is irrigated with normal saline solution to wash away all loose fragments of bone.

Plate 44. Ischial Bearing Above-Knee Amputation (Mid-Thigh Amputation)

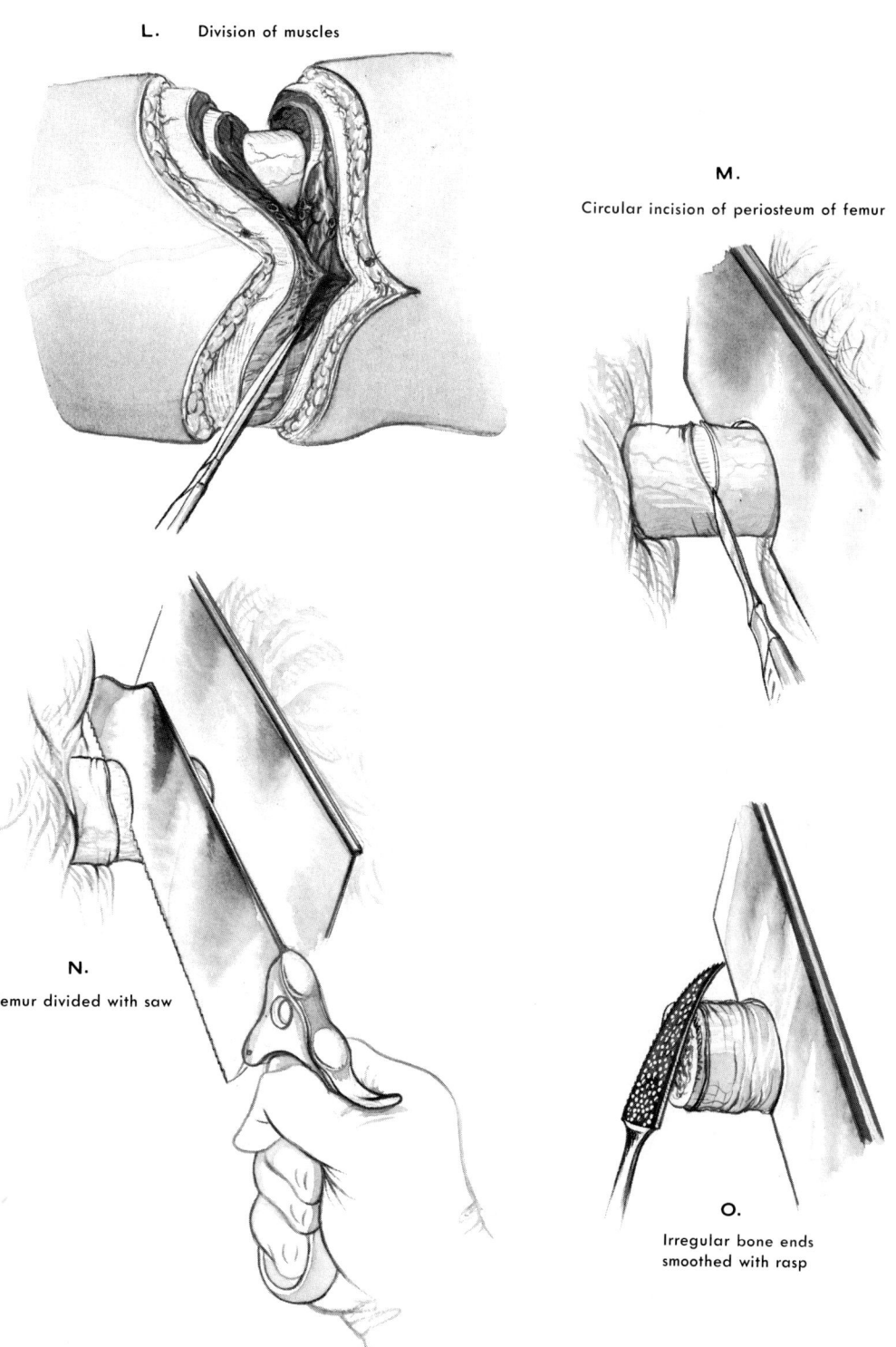

L. Division of muscles

M. Circular incision of periosteum of femur

N. Femur divided with saw

O. Irregular bone ends smoothed with rasp

Ischial-Bearing Above-Knee Amputation (Mid-Thigh Amputation) (Continued)

P. Hot packs are applied over the wound and the tourniquet is released. After five minutes the stump is inspected for any bleeders.

Q. The anterior and posterior myofascial flaps are pulled distally and approximated with interrupted sutures through their fascial layer. Suction catheters are placed in the wound and connected to a Hemovac evacuator.

R. The subcutaneous tissue and skin are closed in the usual manner. Immediate prosthetic fitting in the operating room is employed by the author, and the patient is allowed to be ambulatory on the first postoperative day.

Plate 44. Ischial Bearing Above-Knee Amputation (Mid-Thigh Amputation)

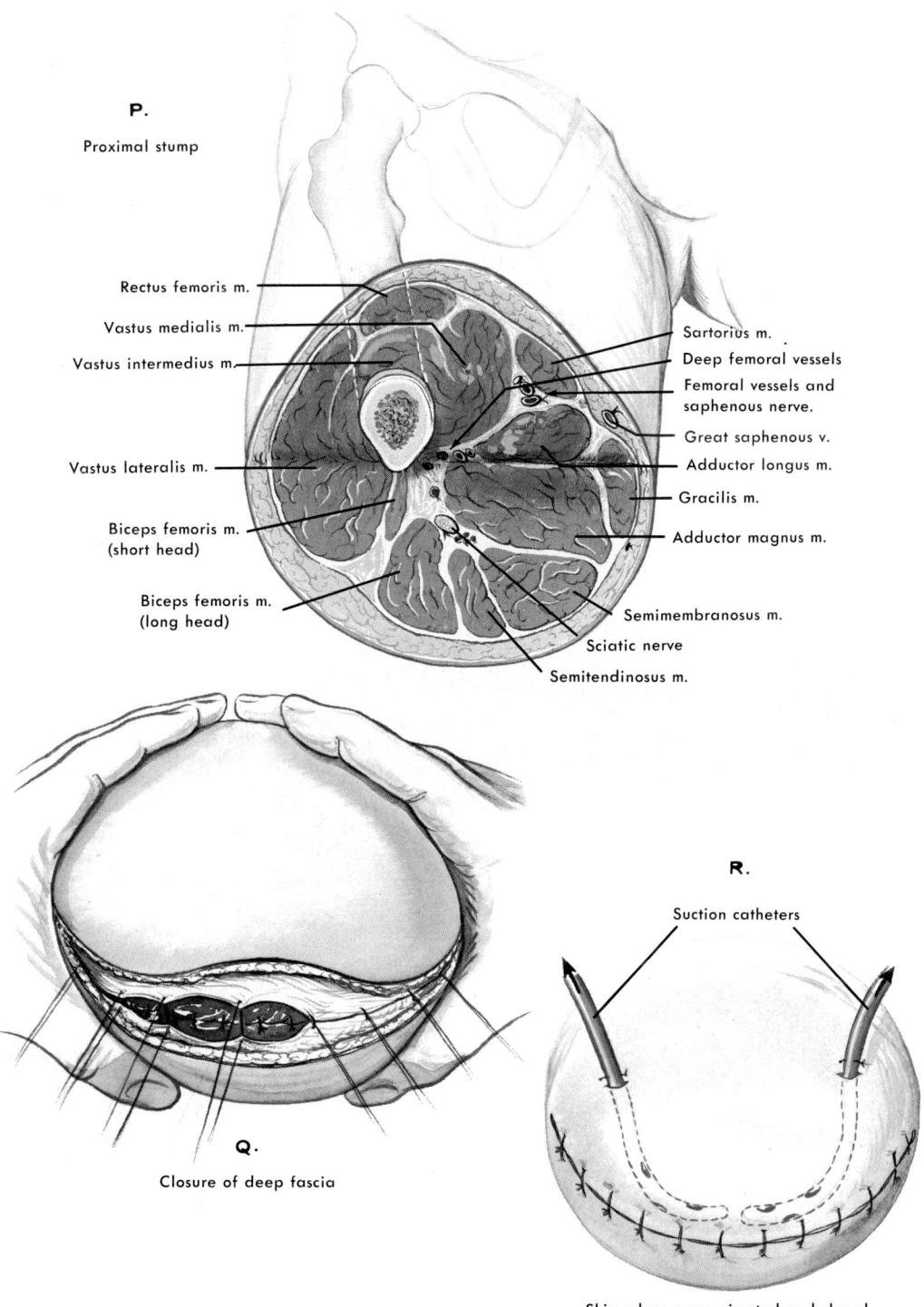

Disarticulation at the Knee Joint

The patient is placed in lateral position so that he can easily be turned into a supine, prone, or semilateral posture. The operation is performed under pneumatic tourniquet ischemia.

A. The skin incisions are placed in such a manner that a long anterior and a short posterior flap are provided; thus, the operative scar is posterior and away from the weight-bearing skin. Measuring from the distal pole of the patella to the distal border, the length of the anterior flap is equal to the anteroposterior diameter of the knee, whereas the posterior flap is half the length of the anterior flap. The medial and lateral proximal points of the incisions are at the joint line at the junction of the anterior two thirds and posterior one third of the diameter of the knee. The anterior and posterior wound flaps are raised, including the subcutaneous tissue and the deep fascia.

B. The medial aspects of the knee joint and the proximal tibia are exposed. Tendons of the sartorius, gracilis, semimembranosus, and semitendinosus muscles are identified and marked with 00 silk whip sutures, then sectioned near their insertions on the tibia. The ligamentum patellae is detached at the proximal tibial tubercle. The anterior and medial joint capsule and synovial membrane are divided proximally near the femoral condyles.

C. Next, the lateral aspect of the knee joint is exposed. The iliotibial tract is divided and the biceps femoris tendon is sectioned from its attachment to the head of the fibula. The lateral part of the joint capsule and synovial membrane is divided above the joint line.

Plate 45. Disarticulation at the Knee Joint

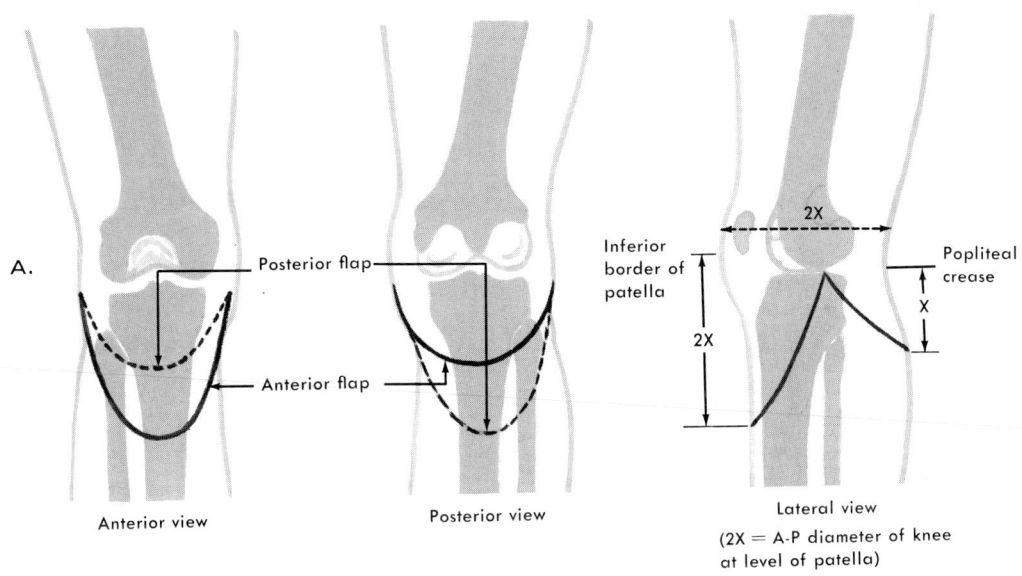

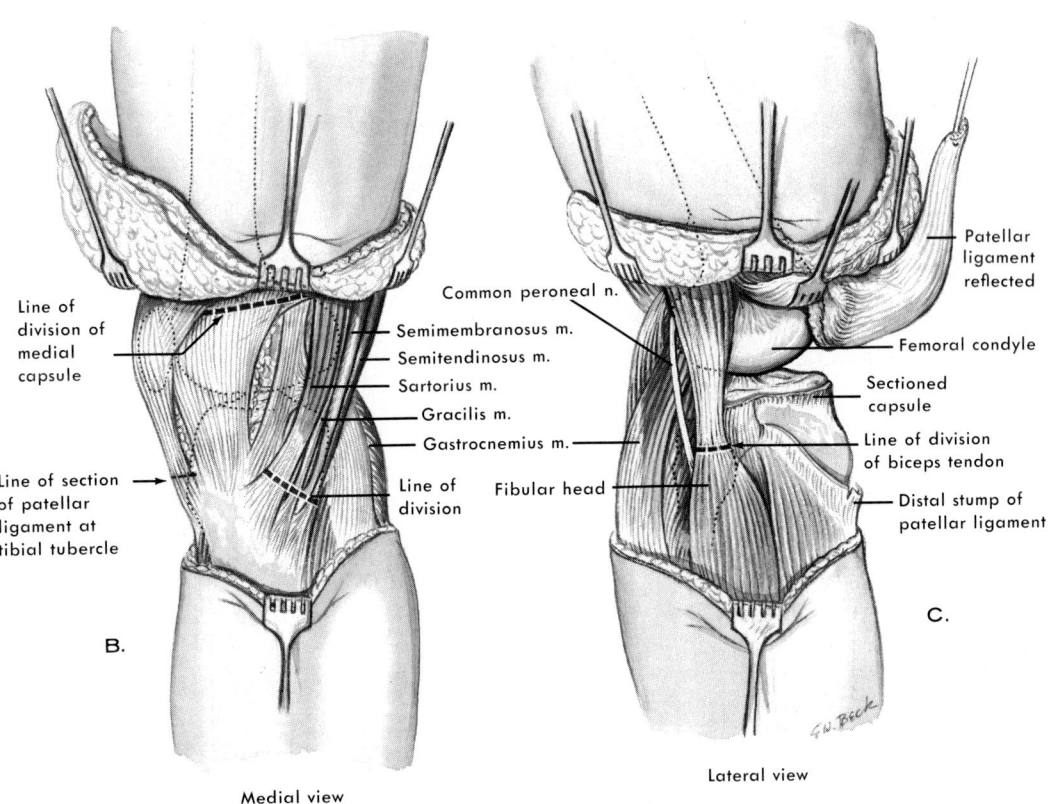

Disarticulation at the Knee Joint (Continued)

D. Now the patient is turned into semiprone position and the popliteal fossa is exposed. By blunt dissection the popliteal vessels are identified; the popliteal artery and vein are separately doubly ligated distal to the origin of the superior genicular branches and divided. The tibial nerve and common peroneal nerve are pulled distally, sharply divided with a scalpel, and allowed to retract proximally. The medial and lateral heads of the gastrocnemius are extraperiosteally elevated and stripped from the posterior aspect of the femoral condyles. The distal femoral epiphyseal plate should not be damaged. The plantaris and popliteus muscles, the oblique popliteal ligament, the posterior part of the capsule of the knee joint, and the meniscofemoral ligaments are completely divided.

E. Next, the patient is turned into semisupine position and the knee is acutely flexed. The cruciate ligaments are identified and sectioned, completing the amputation. The pneumatic tourniquet is released and complete hemostasis is secured.

F. The patellar ligament is sutured to the medial and lateral hamstrings in the intercondylar notch. In children, the patella is usually not removed and reshaping of the femoral condyles should not be performed because of the danger of damage to the growth plate. Synovectomy is not indicated.

G. Two catheters are placed in the wound for closed suction. The deep fascia and subcutaneous tissue of the anterior and posterior flaps are approximated with interrupted sutures, and the skin is closed in routine fashion.

Plate 45. Disarticulation at the Knee Joint

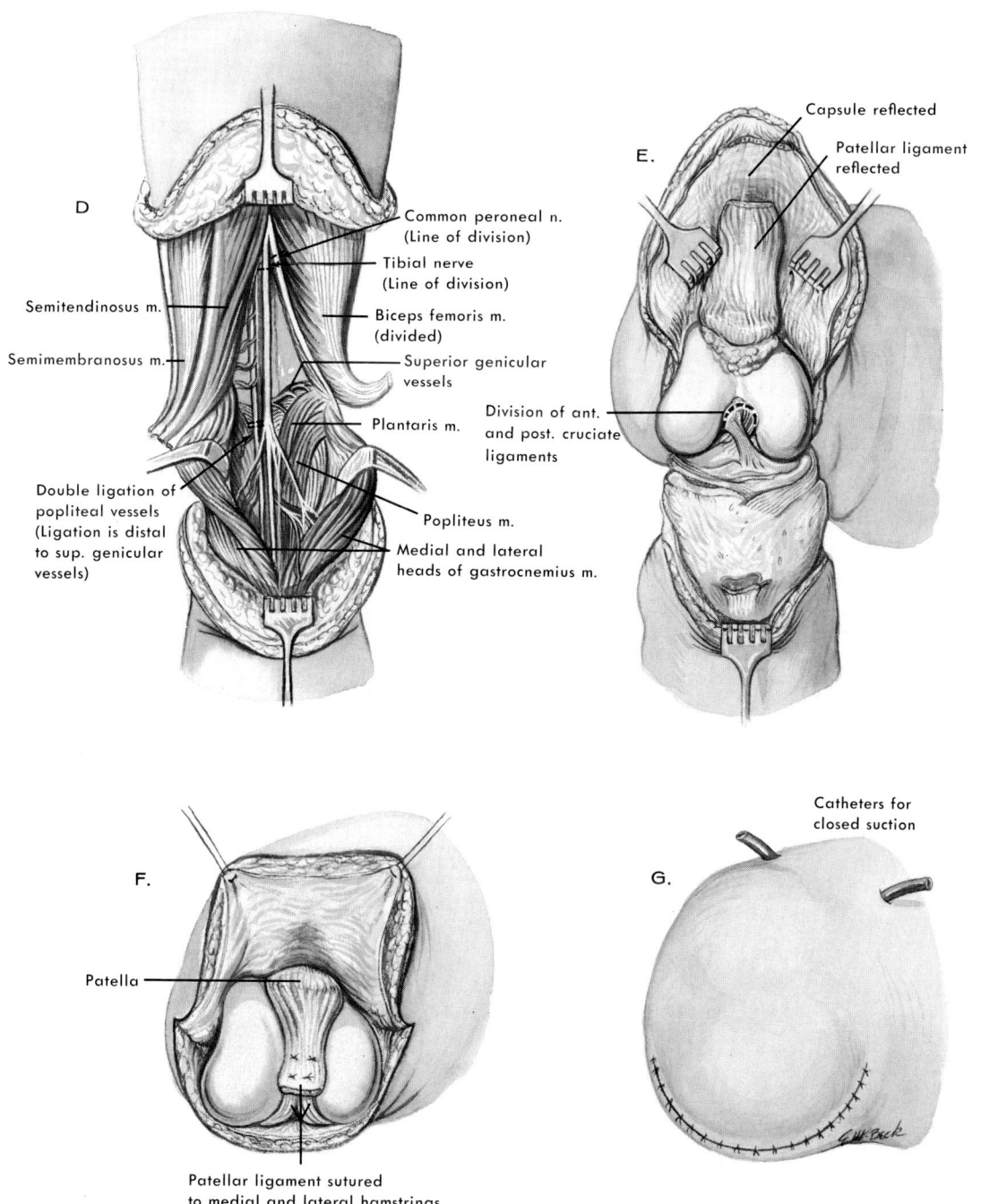

Below-Knee Amputation

The level of amputation is determined preoperatively. With the patient in supine position, a pneumatic tourniquet is applied on the proximal thigh.

A and B. The line of incision for the anterior and posterior flaps is marked on the skin, and the anteroposterior diameter of the leg at the level of bone section is measured. The anterior flap can be fashioned slightly longer than the posterior flap, or they may be made of equal length, as the position of the scar is not especially important in prosthetic fitting. The length of each flap is half the anteroposterior diameter of the leg.

C and D. The incisions are deepened to the deep fascia, which is divided in line with the skin incision. The anterior and posterior flaps are raised proximally in one layer, including skin, subcutaneous tissue, and deep fascia. Over the anteromedial surface of the tibia, the periosteum is incised with the deep fascia, and both are elevated as a continuous layer to the intended level of amputation.

In the interval between the extensor digitorum longus and peroneus brevis muscles, the superficial peroneal nerve is identified; the nerve is pulled distally, is sharply divided, and is allowed to retract proximally well above the end of the stump.

The anterior tibial vessels and deep peroneal nerve are identified, doubly ligated, and divided.

Plate 46. Below-Knee Amputation

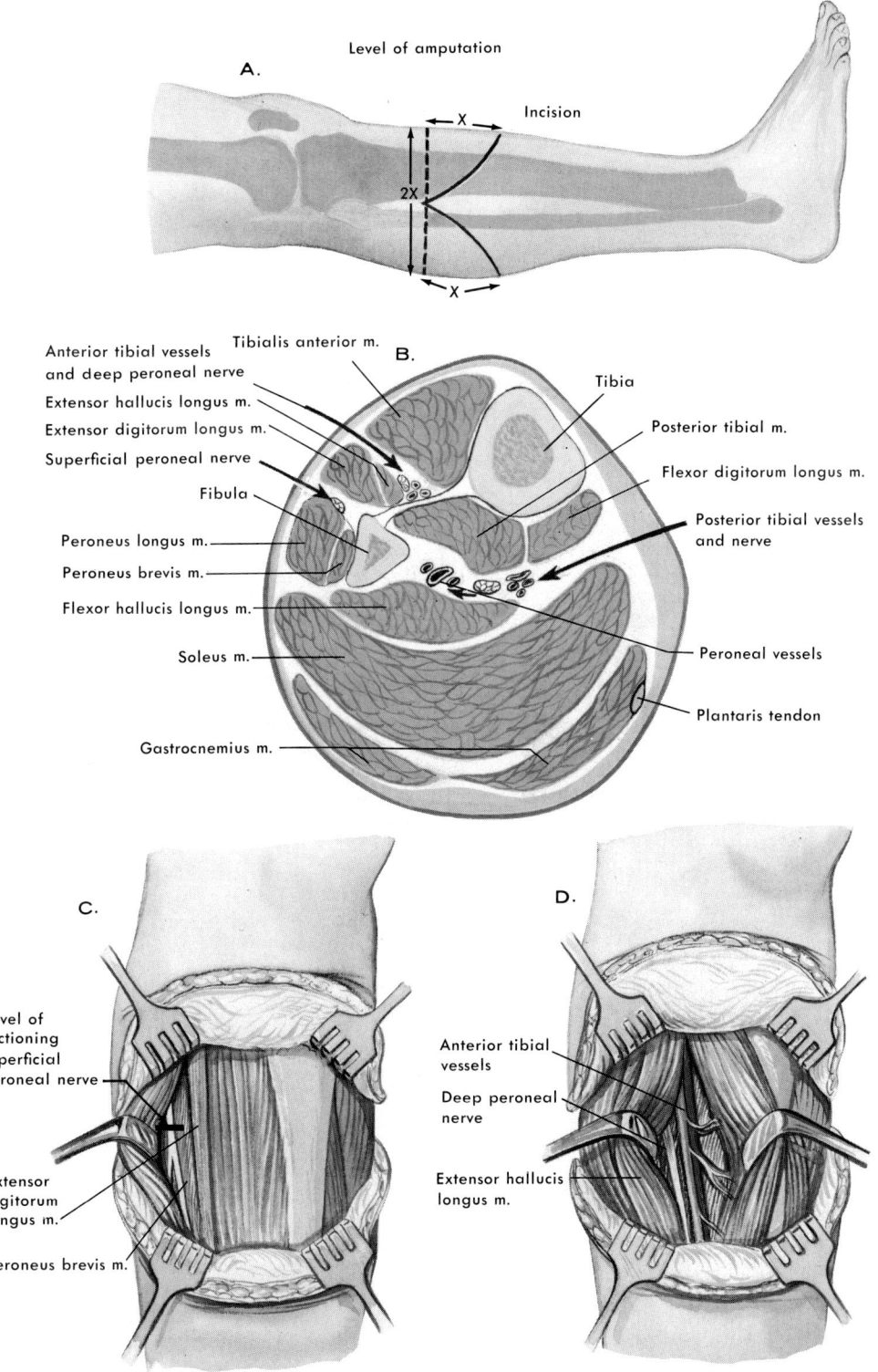

Below-Knee Amputation (Continued)

E and F. The muscles in the anterior tibial compartment are sectioned about 0.75 cm. distal to the level of bone section. The tibial crest is beveled as follows: Beginning 2 cm. proximal to the level of amputation, a 45-degree distal oblique cut is made, ending 0.5 cm. anterior to the medullary cavity.

G. Then the tibia is transversely sectioned. The angle of division should be at right angles to the axis of the bone.

H. The fibula is cleared of surrounding muscle and, with a Gigli saw, it is sectioned 2 to 3 cm. proximal to the distal end of the tibia. The bone ends are smoothed and rounded with a rasp. All periosteal fringes are excised and the wound is irrigated with normal saline to remove bone dust.

Next the posterior muscles in the leg are sectioned. The posterior tibial and peroneal vessels are carefully identified, doubly ligated, and then divided. The tibial nerve is pulled distally and divided with a sharp knife. A fascial flap is developed from the gastrocnemius aponeurosis so that it can be brought forward to cover the end of the stump.

I and J. The tourniquet is released following application of hot laparotomy pads and pressure over the cut surfaces of the muscles and bones. After five minutes the pads are removed and complete hemostasis is secured. The wound should be completely dry. The fascia of the gastrocnemius muscle is brought anteriorly and sutured to the fascia. Muscles may be partially excised if they are bulky at the side of the stump. Hemovac suction drainage catheters are placed deep to the triceps surae fascia. The subcutaneous tissue and skin are closed with interrupted sutures. A nonadherent dressing and a plaster of Paris cylinder are applied for immediate prosthetic fitting.

Plate 46. Below-Knee Amputation

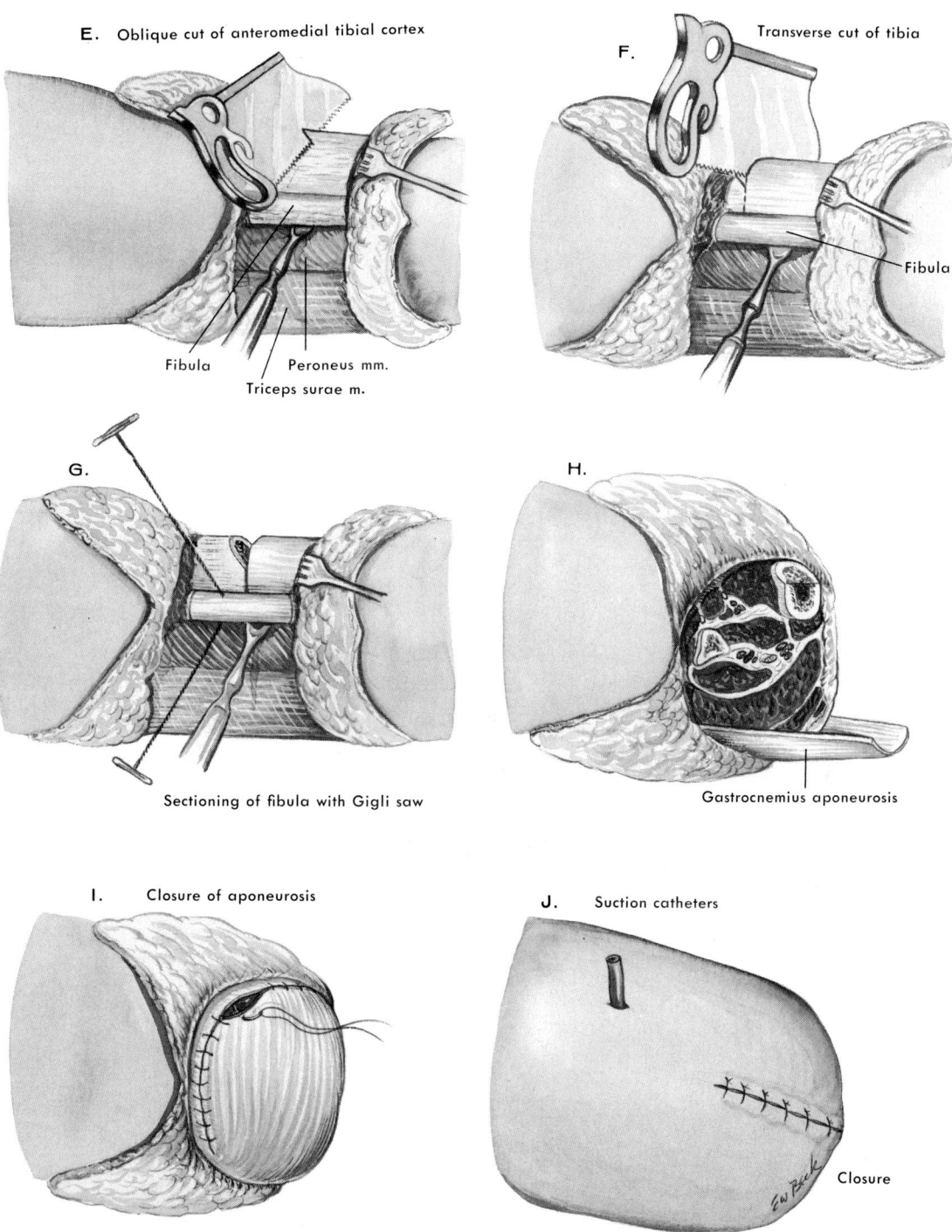

Forequarter Amputation from Posterior Approach (Littlewood Technique)

The patient is placed in lateral position and his neck, chest, and whole upper limb are prepared and draped. Blood loss is minimal, but adequate whole blood should be available for transfusion if necessary.

A to C. The cervicothoracic incision begins at the medial end of the clavicle and extends laterally along the anteroinferior border of the clavicle to the lateral protuberance of the acromion, where it curves posteriorly; then it is continued along the lateral border of the scapula to its inferior angle, where it curves medially to terminate 3 to 4 cm. lateral to the midline of the spine.

The pectoroaxillary incision begins at the center of the clavicle and extends inferolaterally along the deltopectoral groove; it then crosses the anterior axillary fold and joins the posterior incision at the lower third of the lateral border of the scapula. The subcutaneous tissue and fascia are divided in line with the skin incision and the wound flaps are mobilized to expose the underlying muscles.

Plate 47. Forequarter Amputation from Posterior Approach (Littlewood Technique)

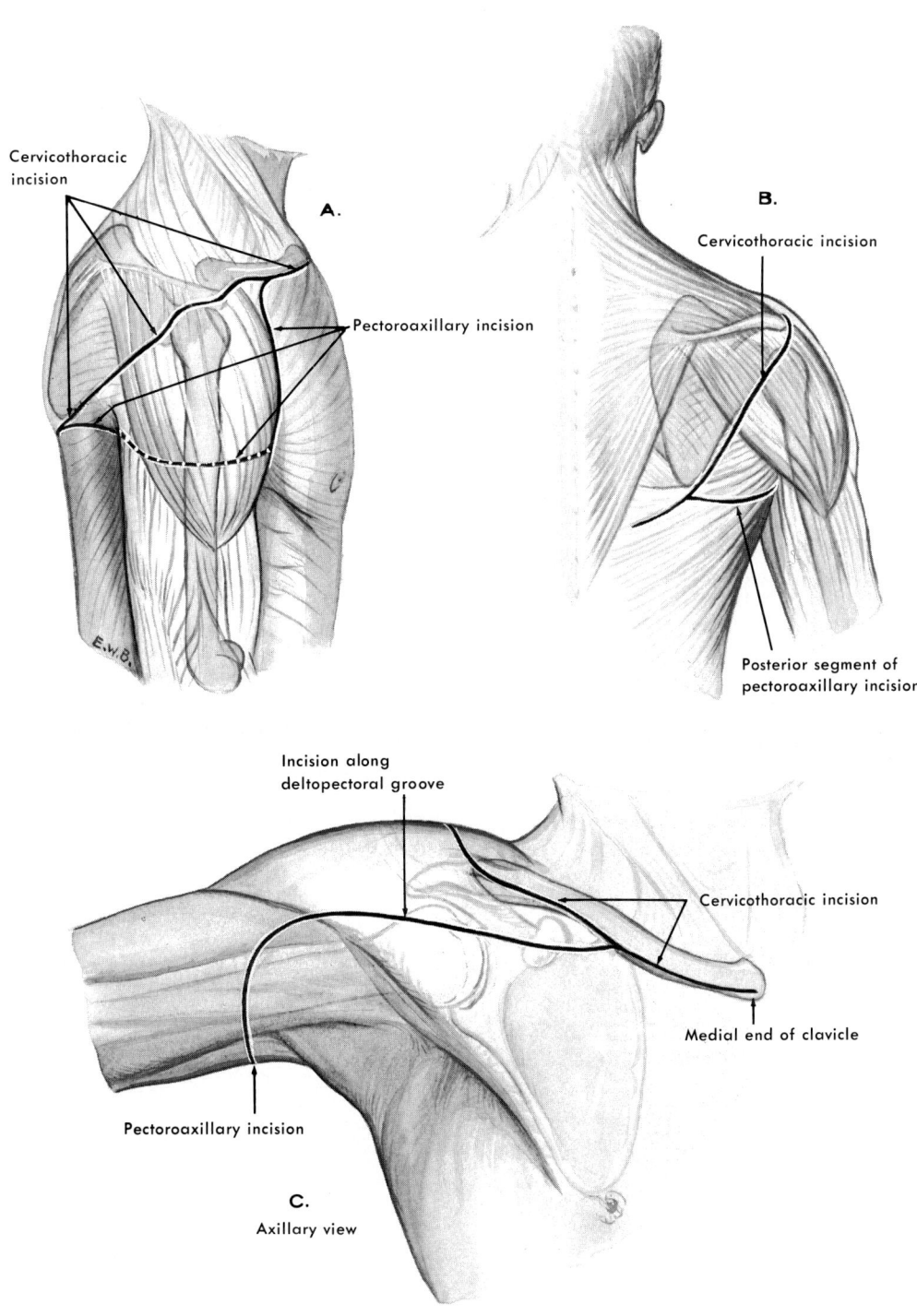

Forequarter Amputation from Posterior Approach (Littlewood Technique) (Continued)

D and **E.** Then the muscles connecting the scapula to the trunk are detached from the scapula in layers and marked with "whip" silk sutures. First, the trapezius and latissimus dorsi are divided.

Plate 47. Forequarter Amputation from Posterior Approach (Littlewood Technique)

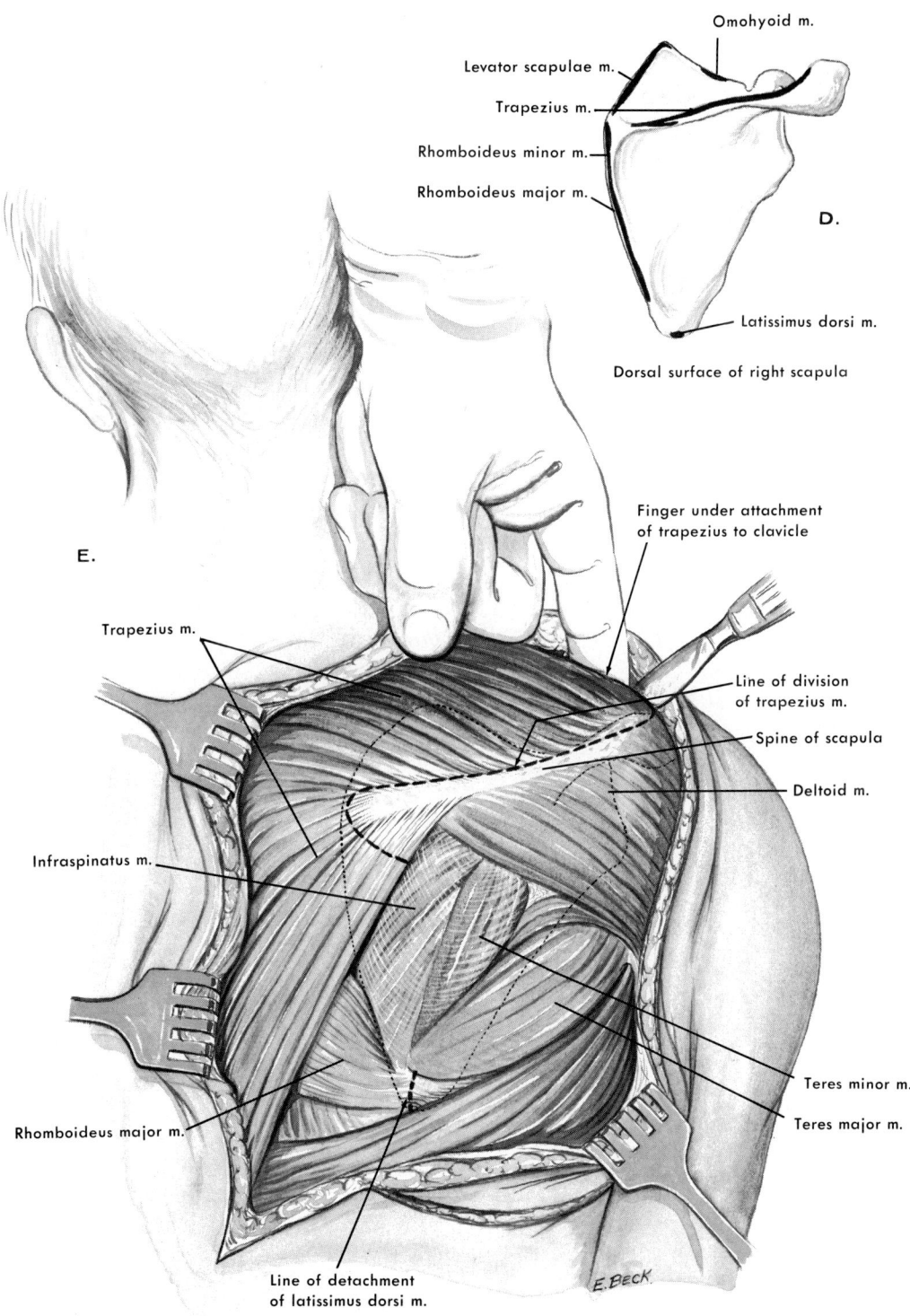

1357

Forequarter Amputation from Posterior Approach (Littlewood Technique) (Continued)

F. Next, the omohyoid, levator scapulae, and rhomboid muscles are detached. Transverse cervical and transverse scapular vessels are ligated and divided as dissection proceeds. The cords of the brachial plexus are sectioned with a very sharp scalpel near their origin.

Plate 47. Forequarter Amputation from Posterior Approach (Littlewood Technique)

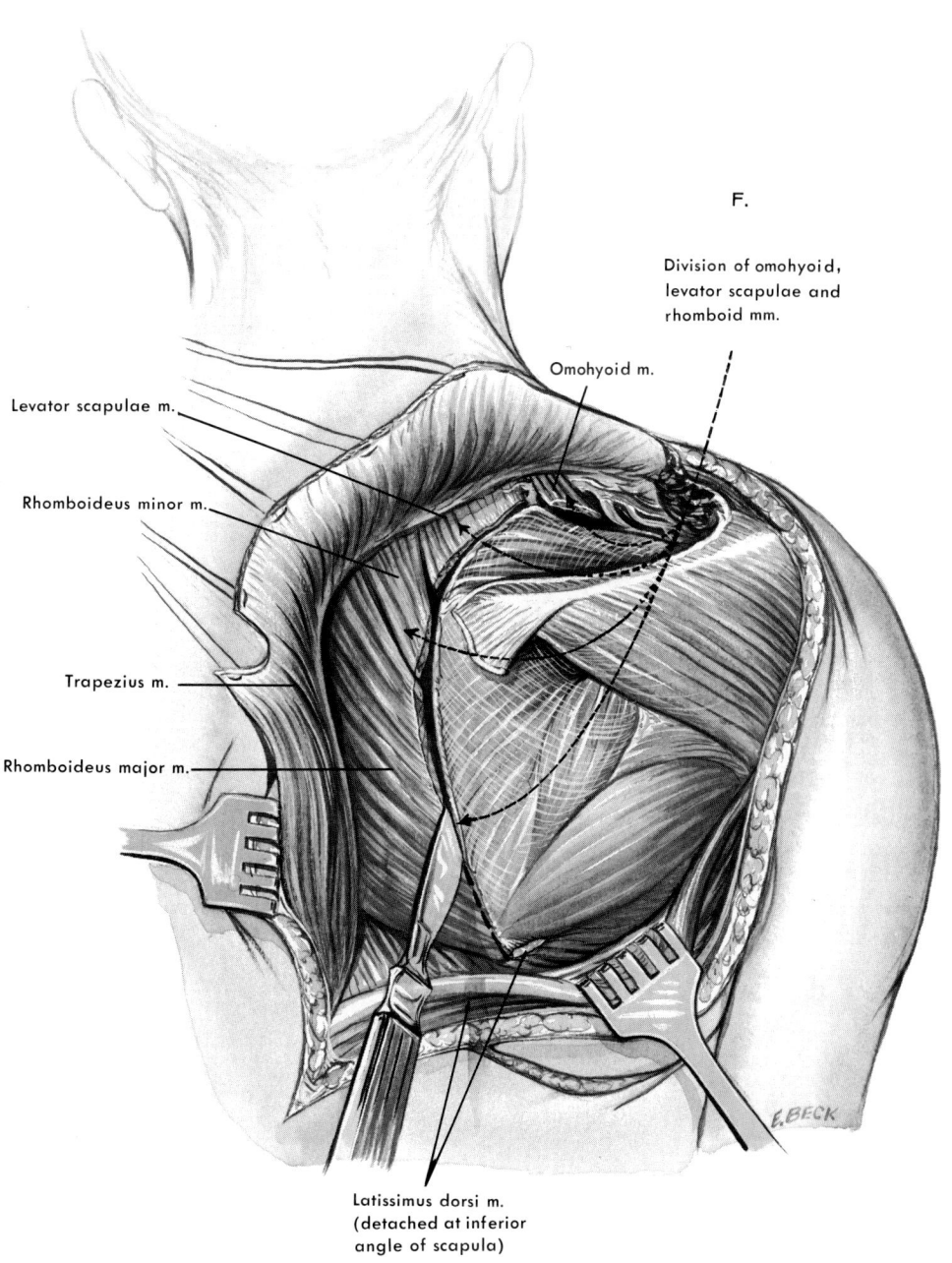

Forequarter Amputation from Posterior Approach (Littlewood Technique) (Continued)

L to N. The subclavian vessels and brachial plexus are exposed by allowing the upper limb to fall anteriorly. The subclavian artery and vein are isolated, individually clamped, doubly ligated with sutures, and divided

Plate 47. Forequarter Amputation from Posterior Approach (Littlewood Technique)

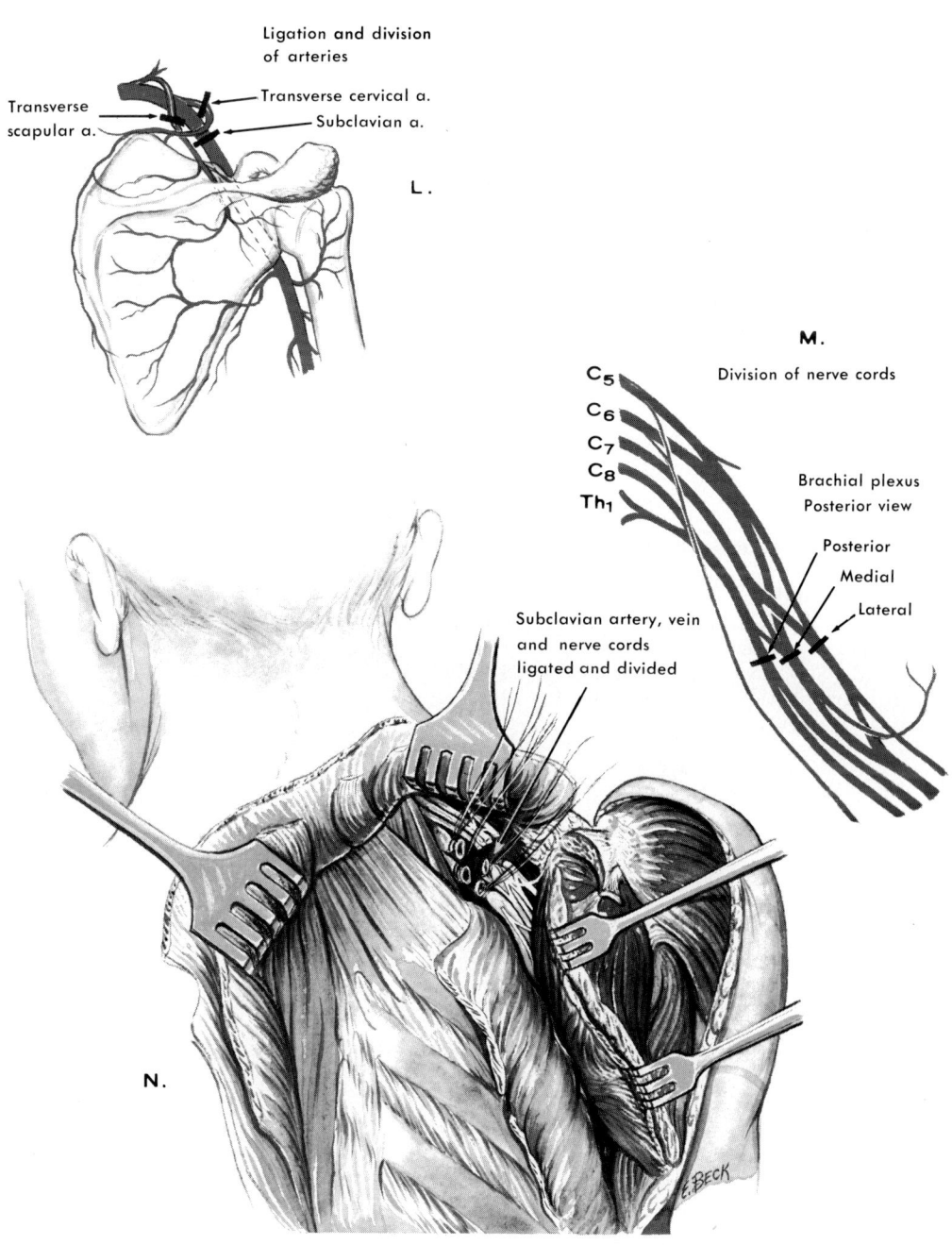

Forequarter Amputation from Posterior Approach (Littlewood Technique) (Continued)

O to **Q.** Then the pectoralis major and minor, the short head of the biceps, coracobrachialis and latissimus dorsi are sectioned, completing ablation of the limb.

R. The wound flaps are approximated and sutured together. Closed suction catheters are inserted and connected to the Hemovac evacuator. A firm compression dressing is applied.

Plate 47. Forequarter Amputation from Posterior Approach (Littlewood Technique)

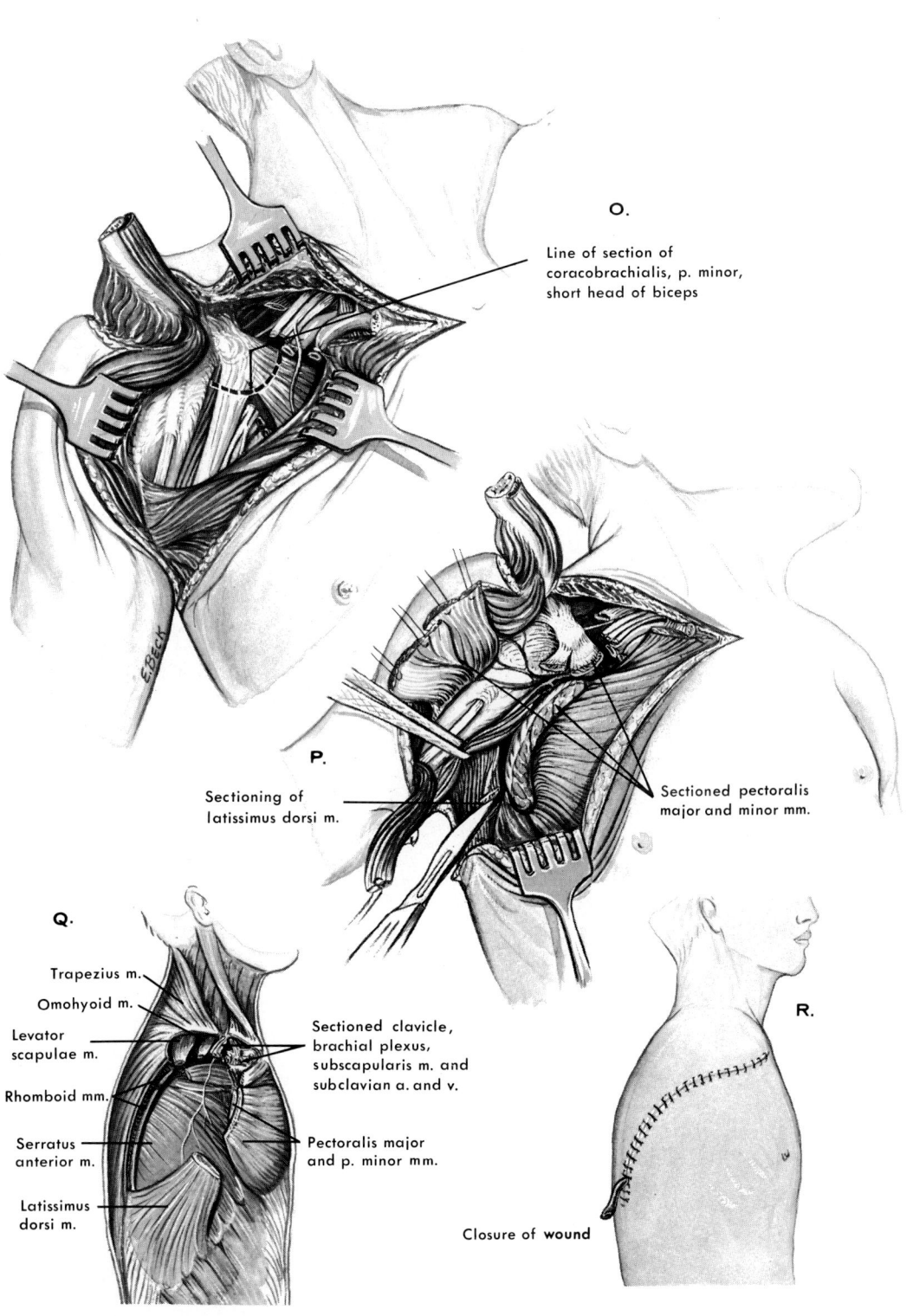

Disarticulation of the Shoulder

The patient is placed in semilateral position so that the posterior aspect of the affected shoulder, scapula, axilla, and the entire upper limb can be prepared and draped sterile.

A. The skin incision begins at the coracoid process and extends distally in the deltopectoral groove to the insertion of the deltoid muscle, and then is continued proximally along the posterior border of the deltoid muscle to terminate at the posterior axillary fold. A second incision in the axilla connects the anterior and posterior borders of the first incision.

B. In the deltopectoral groove, the cephalic vein is identified, ligated, and excised. The deltoid muscle is retracted laterally to expose the humeral attachment of the pectoralis major muscle, which is divided at its insertion and reflected medially. The coracobrachialis and short head of the biceps are divided at their origins from the coracoid process and are reflected distally.

Next, the deltoid muscle is detached from its insertion on the humerus and retracted proximally.

C. The axillary artery and vein and the thoracoacromial vessels are identified, isolated, doubly ligated with 0-silk suture, and divided. The thoracoacromial artery is a short trunk branching from the anterior surface of the axillary artery. Its origin is usually covered by the pectoralis minor muscle. The median, ulnar, musculocutaneous, and radial nerves are identified, isolated, pulled distally, and divided with a sharp knife, then allowed to retract beneath the pectoralis minor muscle.

Plate 48. Disarticulation of the Shoulder

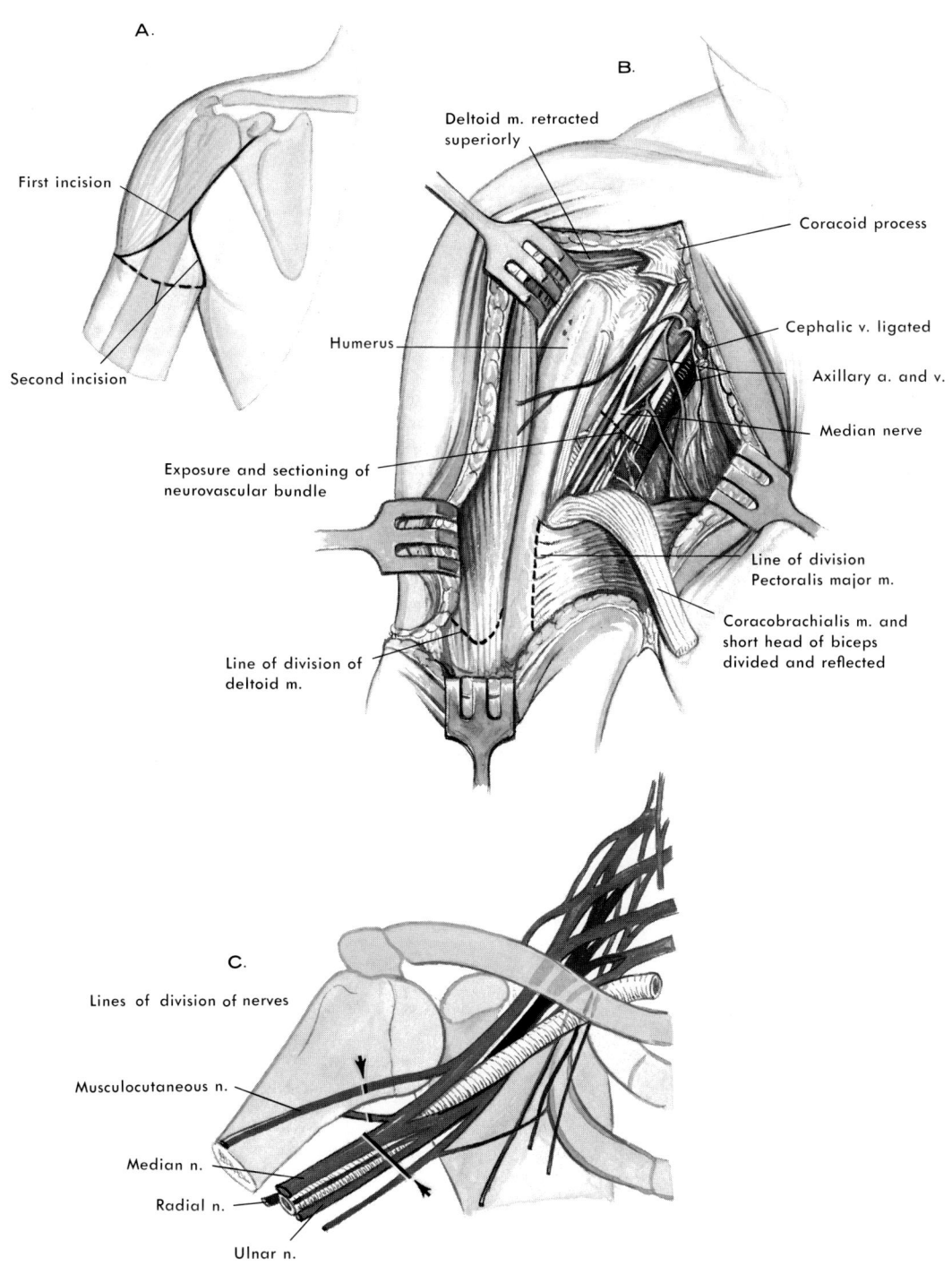

Amputation Through the Arm

The patient is placed in supine position with a sandbag under the shoulder that is to be operated on. A sterile Esmarch tourniquet is applied on the axillary region for hemostasis.

A. Anterior and posterior skin flaps are fashioned so that they are equal in length and 1 cm. longer than half the diameter of the arm at the intended level of amputation. The subcutaneous tissue and deep fascia are divided in line with the skin incision and the wound flaps are retracted.

B and **C.** The brachial artery and vein are identified, doubly ligated, and divided. The median and ulnar nerves are isolated, pulled distally, sectioned with a sharp knife, and allowed to retract proximally. The muscles in the anterior compartment of the arm are divided 1.5 cm. distal to the site of bone division, and the muscle mass beveled distally.

Plate 49. Amputation Through the Arm

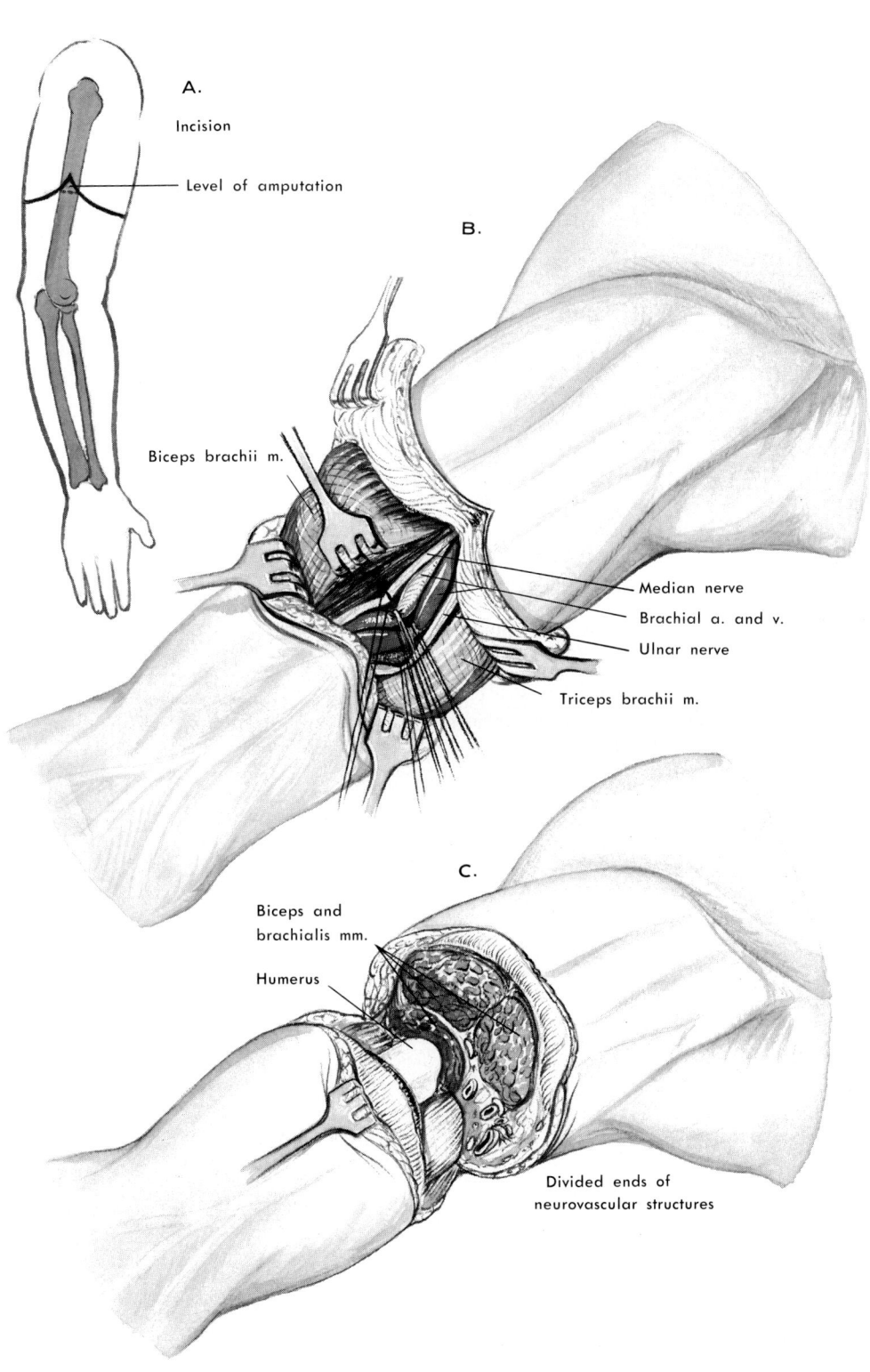

Amputation Through the Arm (Continued)

D. The radial nerve is isolated, pulled distally, and sectioned with a sharp knife. The deep brachial vessels are doubly ligated and divided. The triceps brachii muscle is sectioned 3 to 4 cm. distal to the level of the bone section, and beveled to form a skin flap.

E. The humerus is divided and the bone end is made smooth with a rasp.

F. The distal end of the triceps muscle is brought anteriorly and sutured to the deep fascia of the anterior compartment muscles. Catheters are inserted for closed suction and the wound is closed with interrupted sutures.

Plate 49. Amputation Through the Arm

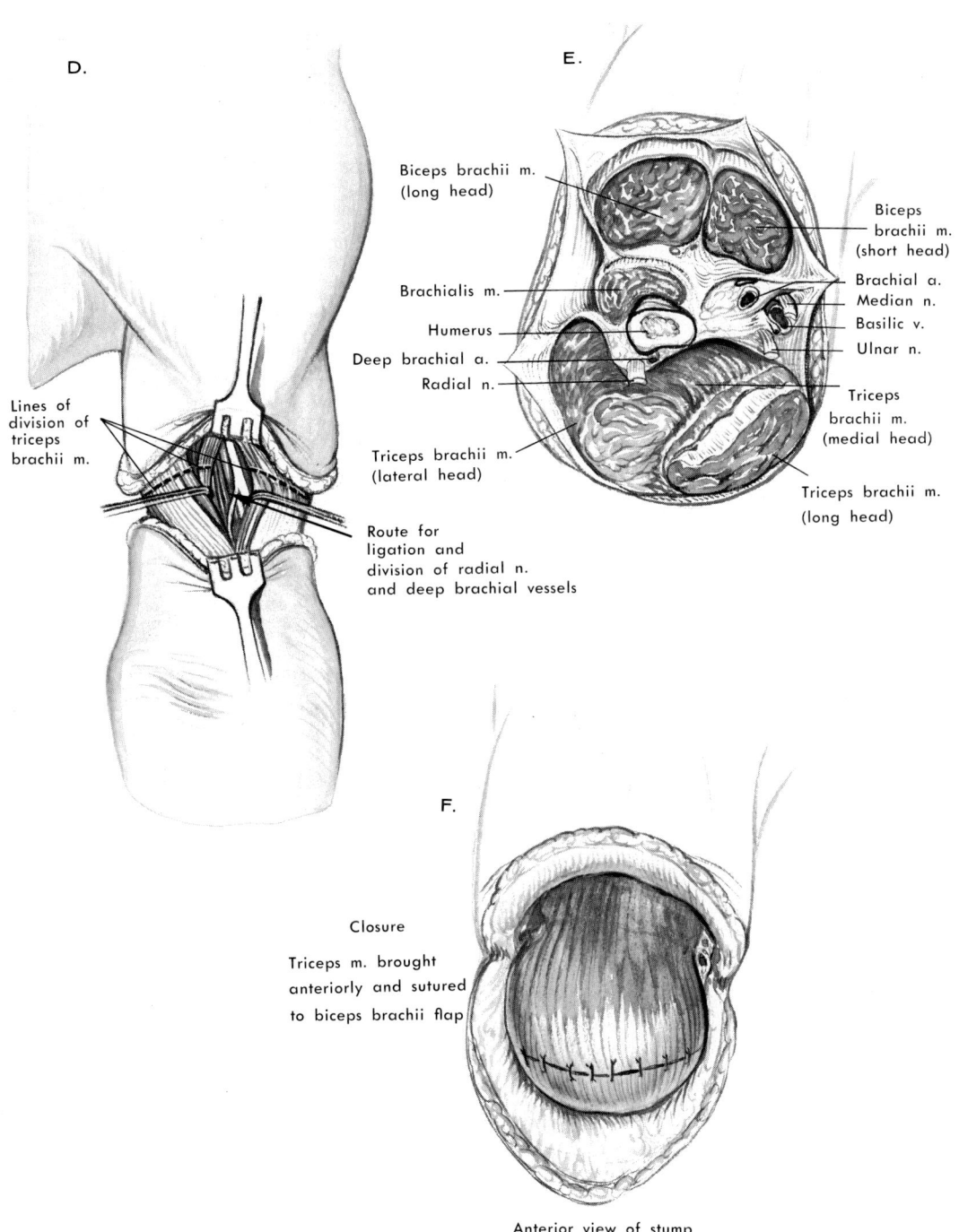

Disarticulation of the Elbow

The operation is performed with a pneumatic tourniquet on the proximal arm.

A. The anterior and posterior skin flaps are fashioned equal in length to the medial and lateral epicondyles of the humerus, which serve as the medial and lateral proximal points. The lower margin of the posterior flap is 2.5 cm. distal to the tip of the olecranon; the distal margin of the anterior flap is immediately inferior to the insertion of the biceps tendon on the tuberosity of the radius.

B. The wound flaps are undermined and reflected 3 cm. proximal to the level of the epicondyles of the humerus. The lacertus fibrosus is sectioned. The common flexor muscles of the forearm are divided at their origin from the medial epicondyle of the humerus, elevated extraperiosteally, and reflected distally.

C and D. The brachial vessels and the median nerve on the medial aspect of the biceps tendon are exposed. The brachial vessels are doubly ligated and divided proximal to the joint level. The median nerve is pulled distally, divided with a sharp knife, and allowed to retract proximally. The ulnar nerve is dissected free in its groove behind the medial epicondyle, drawn distally, and sharply sectioned. The biceps tendon is detached from its insertion on the radial tuberosity.

The radial nerve is isolated in the interval between the brachioradialis and brachialis muscles; the nerve is pulled distally and divided with a sharp knife; the brachialis muscle is divided at its insertion to the coronoid process.

Plate 50. Disarticulation of the Elbow

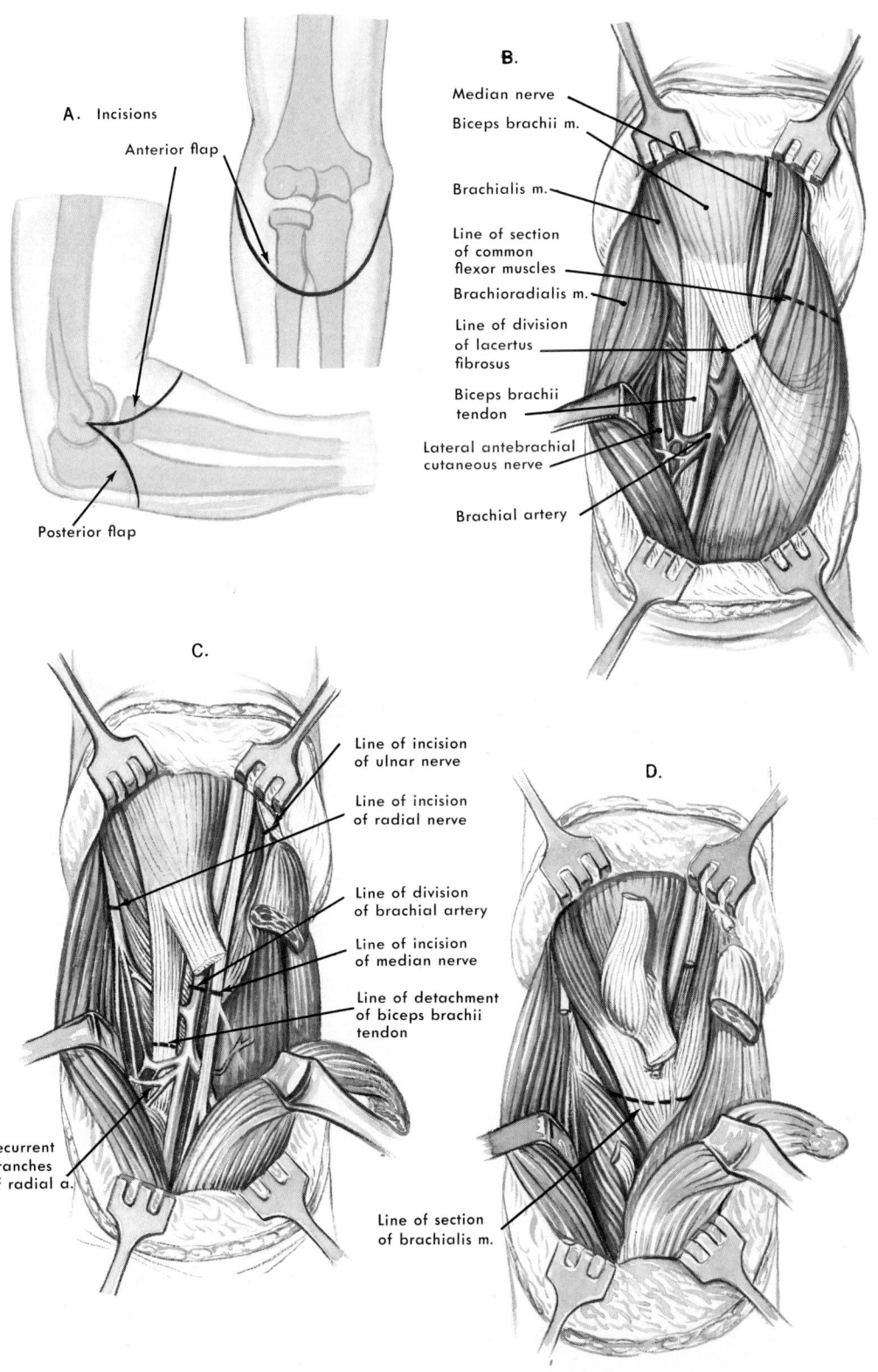

Disarticulation of the Elbow (Continued)

E and **F.** The brachioradialis and common extensor muscles are sectioned transversely about 4 to 5 cm. distal to the joint line. Following detachment of the triceps tendon at its insertion near the tip of the olecranon process, division of the common extensor muscles of the forearm is completed.

G and **H.** The capsule and ligaments of the elbow joint are divided and the forearm is removed. The tourniquet is released and complete hemostasis is obtained.

I. The triceps tendon is sutured to the brachialis and biceps tendons. The proximal segment of the extensor muscles of the forearm is brought laterally and sutured to the triceps tendon. The wound flaps are approximated with interrupted sutures. Catheters are placed in the wound for closed suction.

Plate 50. Disarticulation of the Elbow

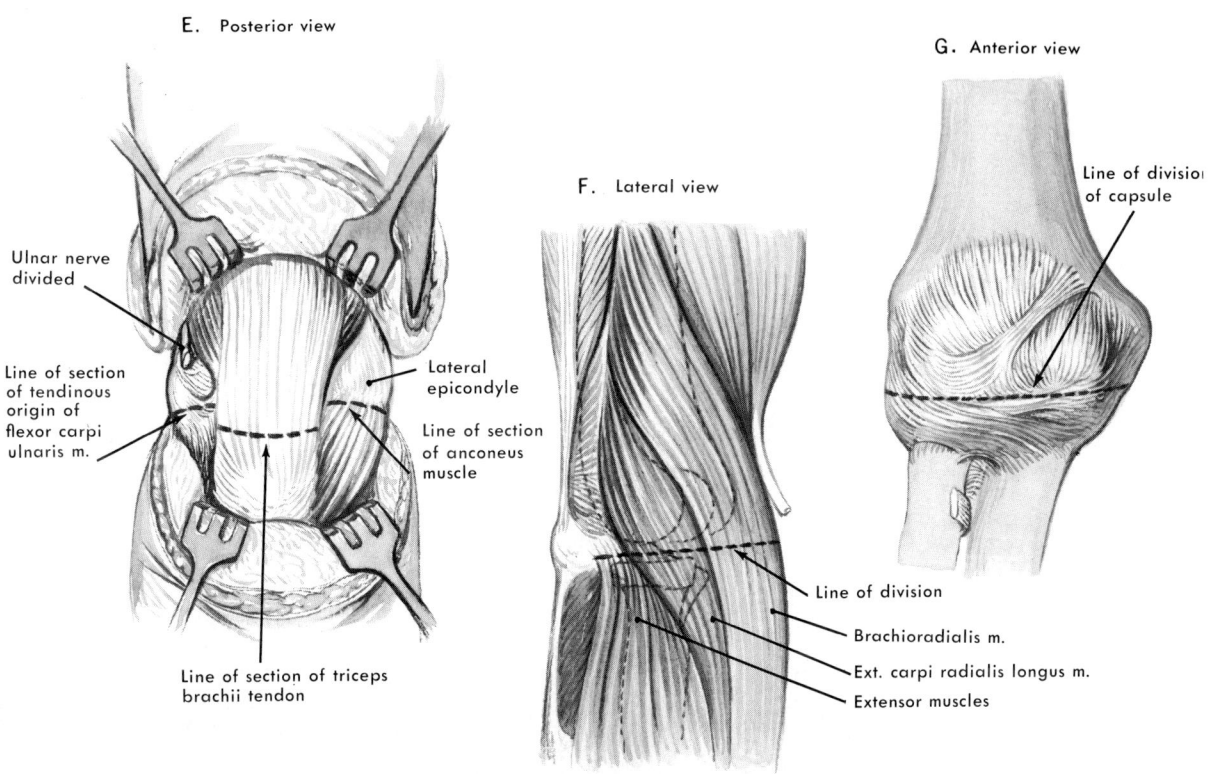

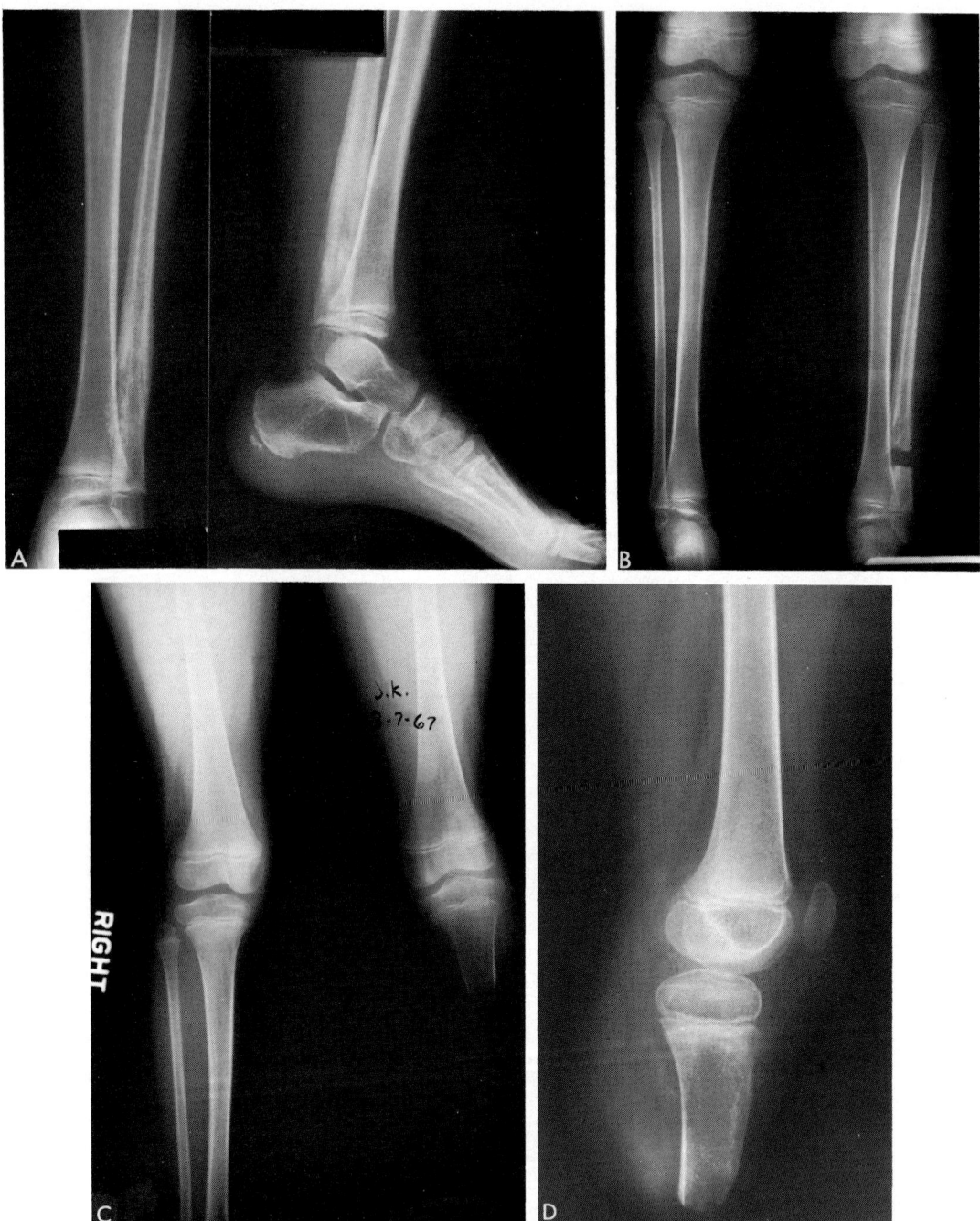

FIGURE 3–332. *Osteogenic sarcoma of distal left fibula in a five-and-one-half-year-old Caucasian girl.*

The child complained of local pain of about one month's duration. **A.** Initial radiograms of left leg show a destructive lesion of the distal metaphysis of the fibula with periosteal new bone formation and soft-tissue swelling. Skeletal survey, chest radiograms, intravenous pyelogram, and bone marrow examination were normal. Histologic examination of biopsy tissue disclosed the tumor to be osteogenic sarcoma. **B.** Radiograms of both legs. Note the segmental defect in distal left fibula showing the area of biopsy. A total of 5,000 r irradiation to the area was administered during a period of four weeks; 1,000 r was given before biopsy. The fibula was resected in toto, and a below-knee amputation was performed 3½ inches distal to the joint line. **C** and **D.** Postamputation radiograms. She had immediate prosthetic fitting and was walking the day following the operation. Monthly follow-up radiograms of chest and skeletal survey were normal until August, 1967 (ten months following amputation) when metastatic lesions developed in left lower and right lower lobes.

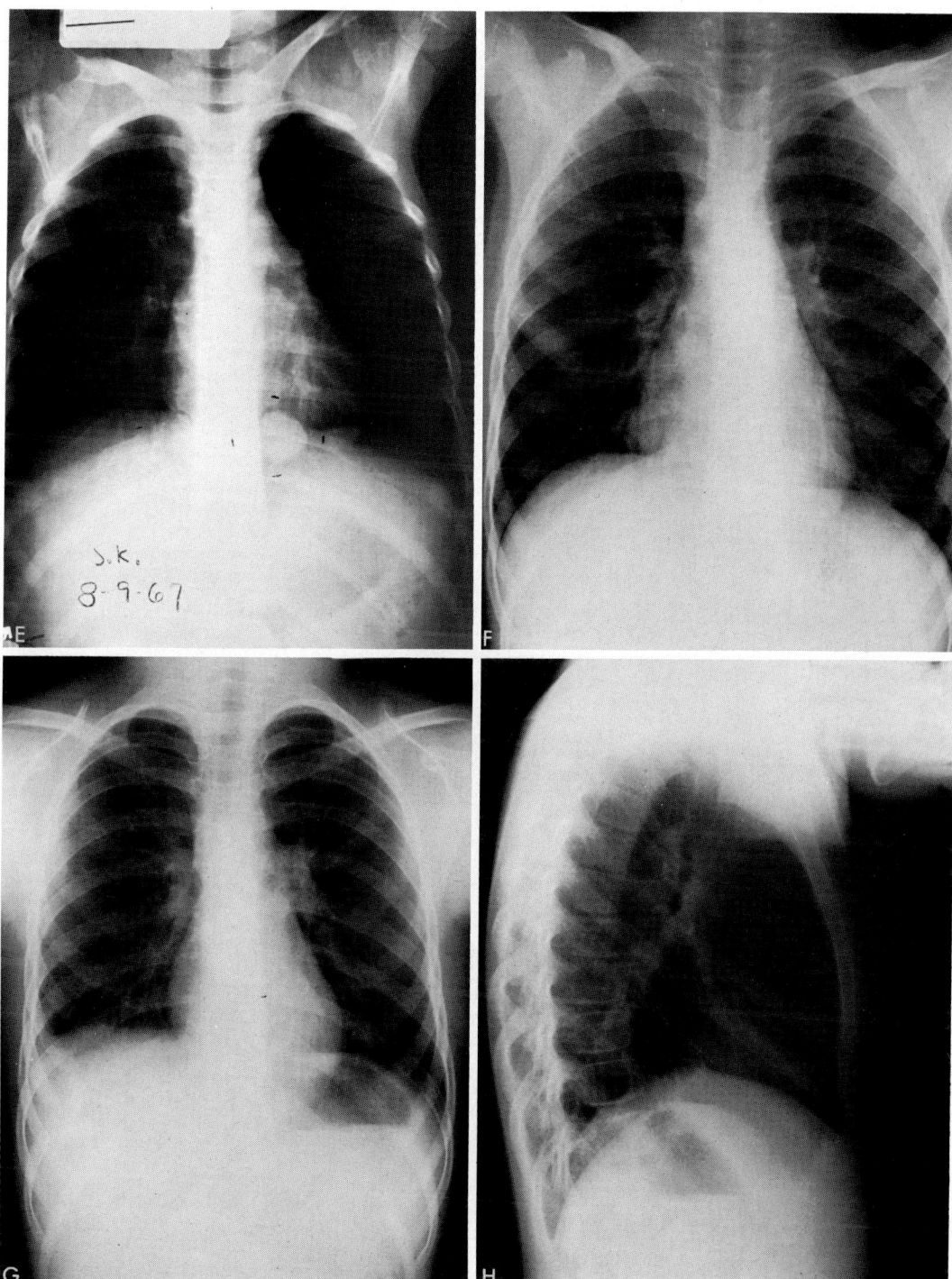

FIGURE 3–332 Continued. *Osteogenic sarcoma of distal left fibula in a five-and-one-half-year-old Caucasian girl.*

E and F. Chest radiograms showing the metastases. Radiograms of the chest were repeated in one and two months. New foci of metastases did not develop and the three lesions remained stationary. Wide segmental resection of the lung lesions was performed in two stages, in October and November, 1967. She had a smooth postoperative course. G and H. Radiograms of chest three years following excision of metastases. There is no evidence of any recurrence of tumor. The child performs normally with no physical limitations.

amputation. Other factors in making the decision are the general condition of the patient and his immediate prognosis as shown by failure of response to chemotherapy and rapidity of progression of the lung lesions.

If pulmonary metastases develop after amputation while adjuvant chemotherapy is in progress, the drugs may have to be changed. When a metatastic lesion is solitary, and sometimes when a maximum of only two or three foci of metastasis are present and remain stationary, a thoracotomy and wide excision are performed (Fig. 3–332).[9, 118, 120, 129, 150, 155] Attempts to control pulmonary metastases by radiotherapy have been disappointing, as an effective dose will destroy the normal lung tissue and cause pulmonary fibrosis.

References

1. Ackerman, A. J.: Multiple osteogenic sarcoma. Report of two cases. A.J.R., 60:623, 1948.
2. Aegerter, E., and Kirkpatrick, J. A.: Orthopaedic Diseases. 4th Ed. Philadelphia, Saunders, 1975, p. 519.
3. Allen, C. V., and Stevens, K. R.: Preoperative irradiation for osteogenic sarcoma. Cancer, 31:1364, 1973.
4. Amstutz, H. C.: Multiple osteogenic sarcoma. Metastatic or multicentric? Cancer, 24:923, 1969.
5. Ayala, A. G., and Zaronosa, J.: Primary bone tumors; percutaneous needle biopsy. Radiologic-pathologic study of 222 biopsies. Radiology, 149:675, 1983.
6. Azouz, E. M., Esseltine, D. W., Chevalier, L., and Gledhill, R. B.: Radiological evaluation of osteosarcoma. J. Can. Assoc. Radiol., 33:167, 1982.
7. Bacci, G., Picci, P., Calderoni, P., Figus, E., and Borghi, A.: Full-lung tomograms and bone scanning in the initial work-up of patients with ostogenic sarcoma. A review of 126 cases. Eur. J. Cancer, Clin. Oncol., 18:967, 1982.
8. Barwick, K. W., Huvos, A. F., and Smith, H.: Primary osteogenic sarcoma of the vertebral column. Cancer, 46:595, 1980.
9. Beattie, E. J.: The management of pulmonary metastasis in children with osteogenic sarcoma with resection combined with chemotherapy. Cancer, 35:618, 1975.
10. Beck, D.: Tumoral biology of osteosarcoma. Chir. Pediatr., 26:203, 1985.
11. Bertoni, F., Present, D., and Enneking, W. F.: Osteosarcoma of the jaw arising in fibrous dysplasia—case report (meeting abstract). Second General Meeting of the International Association of Oral Pathologists. Amsterdam, June, 1984, p. 31.
12. Blumberg, J. M., and Hofner, R.: Primary osteogenic sarcoma following irradiation (abstract). Am. J. Pathol., 28:563, 1952.
13. Bleyer, W. A., Haas, J. E., Feigl, P., Greenlee, T. K., Schaller, R. T., Jr., Morgan, A., Pendergrass, T. W., Johnson, F. L., Bernstein, I. D., Chard, R. L., Jr., and Hartmann, J. R.: Improved 3-year survival in osteosarcoma: Efficacy of adjunctive chemotherapy. J. Bone Joint Surg., 64-B:233, 1982.
14. Brady, T. J., Rosen, B. R., Pykett, I. L., McGuire, M. H., Mankin, H. J., and Rosenthal, D. I.: NMR imaging of leg tumors. Radiology, 149:181, 1983.
15. Brostom, L. A., Harris, M. A., Simon, M. A., Cooperman, D. R., and Nilsonne, U.: The effect of biopsy on survival of patients with osteosarcoma. J. Bone Joint Surg., 61-B:209, 1979.
16. Cabitza, P., and Mapelli, S.: Osteosarcoma multicentrico: Presentazio ne di un caso e revisione della letteratura. Ital. J. Orthop. Traumatol., 7:263, 1981.
17. Cade, S.: Osteogenic sarcoma, a study based on 133 patients. J. R. Coll. Surg., 1:79, 1955.
18. Campanacci, M., and Cervellati, G.: Osteosarcoma. A review of 345 cases. Ital. J. Orthop. Traumatol., 1:5, 1975.
19. Campanacci, M., and Costa, P.: Total resection of the distal femur or proximal tibia for bone tumors. J. Bone Joint Surg., 61-B:455, 1979.
20. Campanacci, M., and Laus, M.: Local recurrence after amputation for osteosarcoma. J. Bone Joint Surg., 62-B:201, 1980.
21. Campanacci, M., and Pizzoferrato, A.: Osteosarcoma emorragico. Chir. Organi Mov., 60:409, 1971.
22. Campanacci, M., Bacci, G., Pagano, P., and Giunti, A.: Multiple drug chemotherapy for the primary treatment of osteosarcoma of the extremities. J. Bone Joint Surg., 62-B:93, 1980.
23. Campanacci, M., Bertoni, F., Campanna, R., and Cervellati, C.: Central osteosarcoma of low-grade malignancy. Ital. J. Orthop. Traumatol., 7:71, 1981.
24. Campbell, C. J., Cohen, J., and Enneking, W. F.: New therapies for osteogenic sarcoma. J. Bone Joint Surg., 57-A:143, 1975.
25. Chang, P.: Progress in the treatment of osteosarcoma. Med. Clin. North Am., 61:1027, 1977.
26. Chuang, V. P., Benjamin, R., Jaffe, N., Wallace, S., Ayala, A. G., Murray, J., Charnsangavej, C., and Soo, C. S.: Radiographic and angiographic changes in osteosarcoma after intraarterial chemotherapy. A.J.R., 139:1065, 1982.
27. Coffre, C., Vanel, D., Contesso, G., Kalifa, C., Dubousset, J., Genin, J., and Masselot, J.: Problems and pitfalls in the use of computed tomography for the local evaluation of long bone osteosarcoma. Report on 30 cases. Skeletal Radiol., 13:147, 1985.
28. Coley, B.: Osteosarcoma. In Neoplasms of Bone and Related Conditions. 2nd Ed. New York, Hoeber, 1960, p. 270.
29. Cortes, E. P., Holland, J. F., Wang, J. J., Sinks, L. F., Blom, J., Senn, H., Bank, A., and Glidewell, O.: Amputation and Adriamycin in primary osteosarcoma. N. Engl. J. Med., 291:998, 1974.
30. Coventry, M. B., and Dahlin, D. C.: Osteogenic sarcoma. J. Bone Joint Surg., 39-A:741, 1957.
31. Cremin, B. J., Heselson, N. G., and Webber, B. L.: The multiple sclerotic osteogenic sarcoma of early childhood. Br. J. Radiol., 49:416, 1976.
32. Cruz, M., Coley, B. L., and Stewart, F. W.: Postradiation bone sarcoma. Cancer, 10:72, 1957.
33. Dahlin, D. C.: Pathology of osteosarcoma. Clin. Orthop., 111:23, 1975.
34. Dahlin, D. C.: Bone Tumors. 3rd Ed. Springfield, Ill., Thomas, 1978, pp. 226–273, 376–377.
35. Dahlin, D. C., and Coventry, M. B.: Osteogenic sarcoma: A study of 600 cases. J. Bone Joint Surg., 49-A:101, 1967.
36. Dahlin, D. C., and Unni, K. K.: Osteosarcoma of bone and its important recognizable varieties. Am. J. Surg. Pathol., 1:61, 1977.
37. Dal Monte, A.: Osteosarcoma of the proximal femur and humerus in children treated by resection, endoprosthesis and complementary chemotherapy. Ital. J. Orthop. Traumatol., 9:151, 1983.
38. Denton, J. W., Manes, E., Dunham, W. K., and Salter, M.: Preoperative regional chemotherapy and rapid-fraction irradiation for sarcomas of the soft tissues and bone. Surg. Gynecol. Obstet., 158:545, 1984.
39. De Santos, L. A., and Edeiken, B.: Purely lytic osteosarcoma. Skeletal Radiol. 9:1, 1982.

40. De Santos, L. A., Bernardino, M. E., and Murray, J. A.: Computed tomography in the evaluation of osteosarcoma: Experience with 25 cases. A.J.R., 132:535, 1979.
41. De Santos, L. A., Goldstein, H. M., and Wallace, S.: Computed tomography in musculoskeletal neoplasms. Radiology, 128:89, 1978.
42. De Santos, L. A., Murray, J. A., and Ayala, A. G.: The value of percutaneous needle biopsy in the management of primary bone tumors. Cancer, 43:735, 1979.
43. De Santos, L. A., Murray, J. A., and Finkelstein, J. B.: The radiographic spectrum of periosteal osteosarcoma. Radiology, 127:123, 1978.
44. Destouet, J. M., Gilula, L. A., and Murphy, W. A.: Computed tomography of long bone osteosarcoma. Radiology, 131:439, 1979.
45. Dowdle, J. A., Winter, R. B., and Dehner, L. P.: Postradiation osteosarcoma of the cervical spine in childhood. A case report. J. Bone Joint Surg., 59-A:969, 1977.
46. Drompp, B. W.: Bilateral osteosarcoma in the phalanges of the hand. A solitary case report. J. Bone Joint Surg., 43-A:199, 1961.
47. Edeiken, J., and Hodes, P. J.: In Roentgen Diagnosis of Diseases of Bone. 3rd Ed. Baltimore, Williams & Wilkins, 1981.
48. Eilber, F. R., Townsend, C., and Morton, D. L.: Osteosarcoma. Results of treatment employing adjuvant immunotherapy. Clin. Orthop., 111:94, 1975.
49. Ellman, H., Gold, R. H., and Mirra, J. B.: Roentgenographically benign but rapidly lethal diaphyseal osteosarcoma. J. Bone Joint Surg., 56-A:1265, 1974.
50. Enneking, W. F., and Kagan, A.: "Skip" metastases in osteosarcoma. Cancer, 36:2192, 1975.
51. Enneking, W. F., and Kagan, A.: The implications of "skip" metastases in osteosarcoma. Clin. Orthop., 111:33, 1975.
52. Enneking, W. F., and Kagan, A.: Transepiphyseal extension of osteosarcoma: Incidence, mechanism and implications. Cancer, 41:1526, 1978.
53. Enneking, W. F., and Shirley, P. D.: Resection arthrodesis for malignant lesions about the knee. J. Bone Joint Surg., 59-A:223, 1977.
54. Enneking, W. F., and Springfield, D. S.: Osteosarcoma. Orthop. Clin. North Am., 8:785, 1977.
55. Enneking, W. F., Spanier, S. S., Goodman, M. A.: Surgical staging of musculoskeletal sarcoma. J. Bone Joint Surg., 62-A:1039, 1980.
56. Epstein, B. S.: The vertebral column. In Hodes, P. J. (ed.): Atlas of Tumor Radiology. Chicago, Year Book, 1974, p. 3.
57. Espinosa, G. A., and Platt, H.: Two cases of osteosarcoma of the spine arising from pagetic bone. Applied Radiol., 12:59, 1983.
58. Farr, G. H., Huvos, A. G., Marcove, B. C., Higinbotham, N. L., and Foote, F. W., Jr.: Telangiectatic osteogenic sarcoma. Cancer, 34:1150, 1974.
59. Fechner, R. E., Huvos, A. G., Mirra, J. M., Spjut, H. J., and Unni, K. K.: A symposium on the pathology of bone tumours. In Sommers, S. A., and Rosen, P. P., (eds.): Pathology Annual, Part One. Norwalk, Conn., Appleton-Century-Crofts, 1984.
60. Fielding, J. W., Fietti, V. G., Hughes, J. E. O., and Gabriellian, J. -C. Z.: Primary osteogenic sarcoma of the cervical spine. J. Bone Joint Surg., 58-A:892, 1976.
61. Fitzgerald, R. H., Jr., Dahlin, D. C., and Sim, F. H.: Multiple metachronous osteogenic sarcoma. Report of twelve cases with two long-term survivors. J. Bone Joint Surg., 55-A:595, 1973.
62. Foci, A., and Barile, L.: Il sarcoma osteogenico sclerosante a localizazione multipla. Arch. Putti Chir. Organi Mov., 26:409, 1971.
63. Friedman, M. A., and Carter, S. K.: Therapy of osteogenic sarcoma: Current status and thoughts for future. J. Surg. Oncol., 4:482, 1972.
64. Gehan, E. A., Sutow, W. W., and Uribe-Botero: Osteosarcoma. The M. D. Anderson Hospital Experience 1950–1974. Prog. Cancer Res. Ther., 1:271, 1976.
65. Genieser, N. B., and Firooznia, H.: Bone scanning—osteogenic sarcoma. Correlation with surgical pathology. A.J.R., 124:83, 1975.
66. Geschickter, C. F.: Osteogenic sarcoma. Arch. Surg., 24:602, 1932.
67. Ghadially, F. N., and Mehta, P. N.: Ultrastructure of osteogenic sarcoma. Cancer, 25:1457, 1970.
68. Gherlinzoni, F., Antoci, B., and Canale, V.: Case report 250: Multicentric osteosarcomata (osteosarcomatosis). Skeletal Radiol., 10:281, 1983.
69. Giunti, A., and Laus, M.: Sarcomi in Morbo de Paget. Ital. J. Orthop. Traumatol., 5:325, 1979.
70. Greditzer, H. G., McLeod, R. A., Krishnan, K. U., and Beabout, J. W.: Bone sarcomas in Paget's disease. Radiology, 156:327, 1983.
71. Green, W. T.: Recent experience with treatment of osteogenic sarcoma. J. Bone Joint Surg., 40-A:1437, 1958.
72. Greenfield, G. B.: Radiology of Bone Diseases. 3rd Ed. Philadelphia, Lippincott, 1986.
73. Greenfield, G. B.: General concepts and pathology of tumors of osseous origin. In Ranninger, R., (ed.): Encyclopedia of Medical Radiology. Vol. V(6): Bone Tumors. Berlin, Heidelberg, New York, Springer-Verlag, 1977, p. 23.
74. Harmon, T. P., and Morton, K. S.: Osteogenic sarcoma in four siblings. J. Bone Joint Surg., 48-B:493, 1966.
75. Heaston, D. K., and Gelman, M. L.: Case report 41. Telangiectatic osteogenic sarcoma. Skeletal Radiol., 2:117, 1977.
76. Heelan, R. T.: Computed tomography of lower extremity tumors. A.J.R., 132:933, 1979.
77. Hill, P.: Local recurrence in primary osteosarcoma of the femur. Br. J. Surg., 60:40, 1973.
78. Hingorani, C. B., and Sharma, O. P.: Osteosarcoma. A roentgenographic study. Indian J. Cancer, 10:285, 1973.
79. Hudson, T. M., Schiebler, M., Springfield, D. S., Hawkins, I. F., Jr., Enneking, W. F., and Spanier, S. S.: Radiologic imaging of osteosarcoma: Role in planning surgical treatment. Skeletal Radiol., 10:137, 1983.
80. Huvos, A. G., Higinbotham, N. L., and Miller, T. J.: Bone sarcoma arising in fibrous dysplasia. J. Bone Joint Surg., 54-A:1047, 1972.
81. Huvos, A. G., Rosen, G., and Marcove, R. C.: Primary osteogenic sarcoma. Arch. Pathol. Lab. Med., 101:14, 1977.
82. Huvos, A. G., Butler, A., and Bretsky, S.: Osteogenic sarcoma in the American black. Cancer, 52:1959, 1983.
83. Jacobs, P. A.: Limb salvage and rotationplasty for osteosarcoma in children. Clin. Orthop., 188:217, 1984.
84. Jaffe, H. L.: Osteogenic sarcoma of bone. Clin. Orthop., 7:27, 1956.
85. Jaffe, H. L.: Tumors and Tumorous Conditions of the Bones and Joints. Philadelphia, Lea & Febiger, 1958, p. 256.
86. Jaffe, N.: The potential for an improved prognosis with chemotherapy in osteogenic sarcoma. Clin. Orthop., 113:111, 1975.
87. Jaffe, N., and Watts, H. G.: Multidrug chemotherapy in primary treatment of osteosarcoma. J. Bone Joint Surg., 58-A:634, 1976.
88. Jaffe, N., Frei, E., III, Traggis, D., and Bishop, Y.:

Adjuvant methotrexate and citrovorum-factor treatment of osteogenic sarcoma. N. Engl. J. Med., *291*:994, 1974.
89. Jaffe, N., Link, M. P., Cohen, D., Traggis, D., Frei, E., III, Watts, H., Beardsley, G. P., and Abelson, H. T.: High-dose methotrexate in osteogenic sarcoma. Natl. Cancer Inst. Monogr., *56*:201, 1981.
90. Jeffree, G. M., Price, C. H. G., and Sissons, H. A.: The metastatic patterns of osteosarcoma. Br. J. Cancer, *32*:87, 1975.
91. Johnston, J. O., Harries, T. J., and Alexander, C. E.: Limb salvage procedure for neoplasms about the knee by spherocentric total knee arthroplasty and autogenous autoclaved bone grafting. Clin. Orthop., *181*:137, 1983.
92. Jones, E. T., Kuhns, L. R., and Arbor, A.: Pitfalls in the use of computed tomography for musculoskeletal tumors in children. J. Bone Joint Surg., *63-A*:1297, 1981.
93. Kaufman, S. L., and Stout, A. P.: Extraskeletal osteogenic sarcomas and chondrosarcomas in children. Cancer, *16*:432, 1963.
94. Kesselring, F. O. H. W.: Radiological aspects of classic primary osteosarcoma. Value of some radiological investigations. Diagn. Imaging, *51*:78, 1982.
95. Kotz, R., and Salzer, M.: Rotation-plasty for childhood osteosarcoma of the distal part of the femur. J. Bone Joint Surg., *64-A*:959, 1982.
96. Kumpan, W., Lechner, G., Wittich, G. R., Salzer-Kuntschik, M., Delling, G., Kotz, R., Hajek, P., and Sekera, J.: The angiographic response of osteosarcoma following pre-operative chemotherapy. Skeletal Radiol., *15*:96, 1986.
97. Kuo, K. N., Gitelis, S., Sim, F. H., Pritchard, D., Chao, E., Rostoker, W., Galante, J. O., and McDonald, P.: Segmental replacement of long bones using titanium fiber metal composite following tumor resection. Clin. Orthop., *176*:108, 1983.
98. Kyriakos, M., and Murphy, W. A.: Concurrence of metaphyseal fibrous defect and osteosarcoma. Report of a case and review of the literature. Skeletal Radiol., *6*:179, 1981.
99. Larsson, S., and Lorentzon, R.: The geographic variation of the incidence of malignant primary bone tumors in Sweden. J. Bone Joint Surg., *56-A*:592, 1974.
100. Larsson, S., and Lorentzon, R.: The incidence of malignant primary bone tumors in relation to age, sex, and site. J. Bone Joint Surg., *56-B*:534, 1976.
101. Laus, M.: Osteosarcoma multicentrico. Ital. J. Orthop. Traumatol., *6*:245, 1980.
102. Levine, A. M., and Chretien, P.: Deep venous occlusion as the initial presentation of osteogenic sarcoma of the sacrum. A case report. J. Bone Joint Surg., *61-A*:775, 1979.
103. Lichtenstein, L.: Bone Tumors. 5th Ed. St. Louis, Mosby, 1977, pp. 220–252.
104. Lindbom, A., Soderberg, G., and Spjut, H. J.: Osteosarcoma. A review of 96 cases. Acta Radiol., *56*:1, 1961.
105. Lodwick, G. S.: Case report 169: Low-grade osteosarcoma of the tibia. Skeletal Radiol., *7*:139, 1981.
106. Lowbeer, L.: Multifocal osteosarcomatosis. A rare entity. Bull. Pathol., *9*:52, 1968.
107. McDougall, R., and Kriss, J. P.: Screening for bone metastases. J.A.M.A., *231*:46, 1975.
108. McKenna, R. J., Schwinn, C. P., and Higinbotham, N. L.: Osteogenic sarcoma in children. Calif. Med., *103*:165, 1965.
109. McKenna, R. J., Schwinn, C. P., Soong, K. Y., and Higinbotham, N. L.: Osteogenic sarcoma arising in Paget's disease. Cancer, *17*:42, 1964.
110. McKenna, R. J., Schwinn, C. P., Soong, K. Y., and Higinbotham, N. L.: Sarcomata of the osteogenic series (osteosarcoma, fibrosarcoma, parosteal osteogenic sarcoma and sarcoma arising in abnormal bone). J. Bone Joint Surg., *48-A*:1, 1966.
111. McKillop, J. H., Etcubanas, E., and Goris, M. L.: The indications for and limitations of bone scintigraphy in osteogenic sarcoma: A review of 55 patients. Cancer, *48*:1133, 1981.
112. McLaughlin, R. E., and Miller, C. W.: Osteosarcoma in siblings. J. Bone Joint Surg., *59-A*:261, 1977.
113. McMaster, J. H., Ferguson, R. J., and Weinert, C. R., Jr.: The host immune response in human osteosarcoma. Clin. Orthop., *111*:76, 1975.
114. Madsen, E. H.: Lymph node metastases from osteoblastic osteogenic sarcoma visible on plain films. Skeletal Radiol., *4*:216, 1979.
115. Mail, J. T., Cohen, M. D., Mirkin, L. D., and Provisor, A. J.: Response of osteosarcoma to preoperative intravenous high dose methotrexate chemotherapy: CT evaluation. A.J.R., *144*:89, 1985.
116. Malawer, M. M., and Dunham, W. K.: Skip metastases in osteosarcoma: Recent experience. J. Surg. Oncol., *22*:236, 1983.
117. Malpas, J. S.: Advances in the treatment of osteogenic sarcoma. J. Bone Joint Surg., *57-B*:267, 1975.
118. Marcove, R. C., and Lewis, M. M.: Prolonged survival in osteogenic sarcoma with multiple pulmonary metastases. J. Bone Joint Surg., *55-A*:1516, 1973.
119. Marcove, R. C., and Rosen, G.: "En block" resections for osteogenic sarcoma. Cancer, *45*:3040, 1980.
120. Marcove, R. C., Martini, N., and Rosen, G.: The treatment of pulmonary metastasis in osteogenic sarcoma. Clin. Orthop., *111*:65, 1975.
121. Marcove, R. C., Mike, V., Hajek, J. V., Levin, A. G., and Hutter, R. V. P.: Osteogenic sarcoma under the age of twenty-one. A review of one hundred forty-five operative cases. J. Bone Joint Surg., *52-A*:411, 1970.
122. Marion, J., Burgers, V., Breur, K., van Dobbenburgh, O. A., Hazebroek, F., Vos, A., and Voute, P. A.: Role of metastatectomy without chemotherapy in the management of osteosarcoma in children. Cancer, *45*:1664, 1980.
123. Marsh, H. O., and Choi, C. -B.: Primary osteogenic sarcoma of the cervical spine originally mistaken for benign osteoblastoma. A case report. J. Bone Joint Surg., *52-A*:1467, 1970.
124. Marsh, B., Flynn, L., and Enneking, W. F.: Immunologic aspects of osteosarcoma and their applications to therapy. J. Bone Joint Surg., *54-A*:1367, 1972.
125. Martinez-Tello, F. J., and Navas-Palacios, J. J.: The ultrastructure of conventional, parosteal, and periosteal osteosarcomas. Cancer, *50*:949, 1982.
126. Matsuno, T., Krishman, K. O., McLeod, R. A., and Unni, K. K.: Telangiectatic osteogenic sarcoma. Cancer, *38*:2538, 1978.
127. Merryweather, R., Middlemiss, J. H., and Sanerkin, N. G.: Malignant transformation of osteoblastoma. J. Bone Joint Surg., *62-B*:381, 1980.
128. Mignami, G.: Un caso di sarcoma osteogenico sclerosante a localizazione multipla. Arch. Putti Chir. Organi Mov., *4*:454, 1954.
129. Miller, C. W.: Growth characteristics of pulmonary metastases from osteosarcoma. Clin. Orthop., *116*:70, 1976.
130. Miller, C. W., and McLaughlin, R. E.: Osteosarcoma in siblings. Report of two cases. J. Bone Joint Surg., *59-A*:261, 1977.
131. Mock, D., and Rosen, I. B.: Osteosarcoma in irradiated fibrous dysplasia (clinical conference). J. Oral Pathol., *15*:1, 1986.
132. Moore, G. E., Gerner, R. E., and Brugarolas, A.: Osteogenic sarcoma. Surg. Gynecol. Obstet., *136*:359, 1973.
133. Naiken, V. S., Tellem, M., and Meranze, D. R.:

Osteogenic sarcoma of the ilium occurring in the region of the sacroiliac joint. Report of a case occurring in an elderly man in the absence of Paget's disease. J. Bone Joint Surg., 45-A:778, 1963.
134. Nilsonne, U.: Limb-preserving radical surgery for malignant bone tumors. Clin. Orthop., 191:21, 1984.
135. Ohno, T., Abe, M., Tateishi, A., Kato, K., Miki, H., Sekine, K., Veyama, H., Hasegawa, O., and Obara, K.: Osteogenic sarcoma. A study of 130 cases. J. Bone Joint Surg., 57-A:397, 1975.
136. Patel, D. V., Hammer, R. A., Levin, B., and Fisher, M. A.: Primary osteogenic sarcoma of the spine. Skeletal Radiol., 12:276, 1984.
137. Paushter, D. M., Borkowski, G. P., Buonocore, E., Belhobek, G. H., and Marks, K. E.: Digital subtraction angiography for preoperative evaluation of extremity tumors. A.J.R., 141:129, 1983.
138. Pendergrass, E. P., Lafferty, J. O., and Horn, R. C.: Osteogenic sarcoma and chondrosarcoma with special reference to the roentgen diagnosis. A.J.R., 54:234, 1945.
139. Picci, P., Gherlinzoni, F., and Guerra, A.: Intracortical osteosarcoma. Rare entity or early manifestation of classic osteosarcoma? Skeletal Radiol., 9:255, 1983.
140. Pho, R. W. H., Lim, S. M. L., and Satku, K.: Late metastases from osteogenic sarcoma. A case report. J. Bone Joint Surg., 67-A:147, 1985.
141. Porretta, C. A., Dahlin, D. C., and Janes, J. M.: Sarcoma in Paget's disease of bone. J. Bone Joint Surg., 39-A:1314, 1957.
142. Pratt, C., Shanks, E., Histo, O., Rivera, G., Smith, J., and Kumar, A. P. M.: Adjuvant multiple drug chemotherapy for osteosarcoma of the extremity. Cancer, 39:51, 1977.
143. Present, D., Bertoni, F., and Enneking, W. F.: Osteosarcoma of the mandible arising in fibrous dysplasia. A case report. Clin. Orthop., 204:238, 1986.
144. Price, C. H. G.: The grading of osteogenic sarcoma. Br. J. Cancer, 6:46, 1952.
145. Price, C. H. G.: Osteogenic sarcoma: Analysis of survival and its relationship to histologic grading and structure. J. Bone Joint Surg., 43-B:300, 1961.
146. Price, C. H. G., and Truscott, D. E.: Multifocal osteogenic sarcoma. J. Bone Joint Surg., 39-B:524, 1957.
147. Price, C. H. G., Zhuber, K., Salzer-Kunschik, M., Salzer, M., Willert, H. G., Immencamp, M., Groh, P., Matejorsky, Z., and Keyl, W.: Osteosarcoma in children. J. Bone Joint Surg., 57-B:341, 1975.
148. Pritchard, D. J., Finkel, M. P., and Reilly, C. A., Jr.: The etiology of osteosarcoma. A review of current considerations. Clin. Orthop., 111:14, 1975.
149. Roberts, C. W., and Roberts, C. P.: Concurrent osteogenic sarcoma in brother and sisters. J.A.M.A., 105:181, 1935.
150. Rosen, G., Tefft, M., Martinez, A., Cham, W., and Murphy, M. L.: Combination chemotherapy and radiation therapy in the treatment of metastatic osteogenic sarcoma. Cancer, 35:622, 1975.
151. Rosen, G., Marcove, R. C., Huvos, A. G., Caparros, B. J., Lane, J. M., Nirenberg, A., Cacavio, A., and Groshen, S.: Primary osteogenic sarcoma: Eight year experience with adjuvant chemotherapy. J. Cancer Res. Clin. Oncol., 106(Suppl.):55, 1983.
152. Rosen, G., Caparros, B., Huvos, A. G., Kosloff, C., Nirenberg, A., Cacavio, A., Marcove, R. C., Lane, J. M., Mehta, B., and Urban, C.: Pre-operative chemotherapy for osteogenic sarcoma: Selection of postoperative adjuvant chemotherapy based on the response of the primary tumor to preoperative chemotherapy. Cancer, 49:1221, 1982.
153. Salzar, M., Knahr, K., and Kotz, R.: Treatment of osteosarcomata of the distal femur by rotation plasty. Arch. Orthop. Trauma Surg., 99:131, 1981.
154. Salzer-Kuntschik, M., Delling, G., Beron, G., and Sigmund, R.: Morphological grades of regression in osteosarcoma after polychemotherapy—Study COSS 80. J. Cancer Res. Clin. Oncol., 106(Suppl.):21, 1983.
155. Sandler, M. S., Heyman, S., and Watts, R. L.: Localization of 99mTc methylene diphosphonate within synovial fluid in osteosarcoma. A.J.R., 143:349, 1984.
156. Schajowicz, F.: Current trends in the diagnosis and treatment of malignant bone tumors. Clin. Orthop., 180:220, 1983.
157. Schaller, R. T., Jr., Haas, J., Schaller, J., Morgan, A., and Bleyer, A.: Improved survival in children with osteosarcoma following resection of pulmonary metastases. J. Pediatr. Surg., 17:546, 1982.
158. Schimke, R. N., Lowman, J. T., and Cowan, G. A. B.: Retinoblastoma and osteogenic sarcoma in siblings. Cancer, 34:2077, 1974.
159. Scranton, P. E., Jr., DeCicco, F. A., Totten, R. S., and Yunis, E. J.: Prognostic factors in osteosarcoma: A review of 20 years' experience at the University of Pittsburgh Health Center Hospitals. Cancer, 36:2179, 1975.
160. Shah, I. C., Arlen, M., and Miller, T.: Osteogenic sarcoma developing after radiotherapy for retinoblastoma. Am. Surg., 40:485, 1974.
161. Sherman, M., and Irani, R. N.: Osteogenic sarcoma. Two cases of unexpectedly long survival. J. Bone Joint Surg., 44-A:561, 1962.
162. Shirkhoda, A., Jaffe, N., Wallace, S., Aayala, A., Lindell, M., and Zornoza, J.: Computed tomography of osteosarcoma after intra-arterial chemotherapy. A.J.R., 144:95, 1985.
163. Siddiqui, A. R., and Ellis, J. H.: "Cold spot" on bone scan at the site of primary osteosarcoma. Eur. J. Nucl. Med., 7:480, 1982.
164. Silverman, G.: Multiple osteogenic sarcoma. Arch. Pathol., 21:88, 1936.
165. Sim, F. H., Ivins, J. C., and Pritchard, D.: Osteosarcoma: New developments in diagnosis and treatment. J. Bone Joint Surg., 61-B:513, 1979.
166. Sim, F. H., Cupps, R. E., Dahlin, D. C., and Ivins, J. C.: Postradiation sarcoma of bone. J. Bone Joint Surg., 54-A:1479, 1972.
167. Simon, M. A.: Rotation-plasty for childhood osteosarcoma of the distal part of the femur (letter). J. Bone Joint Surg., 65-A:566, 1983.
168. Simon, M. A.: Causes of increased survival of patients with osteosarcoma: Current controversies. J. Bone Joint Surg., 66-A:306, 1984.
169. Simon, M. A., and Bos, G. D.: Epiphyseal extension of metaphyseal osteosarcoma in skeletally immature individuals. J. Bone Joint Surg., 62-A:195, 1980.
170. Sinks, L. F., and Mindell, E. R.: Chemotherapy of osteosarcoma. Clin. Orthop., 111:101, 1975.
171. Smith, J., Heelan, R. T., Huvos, A. G., Caparros, B., Rosen, G., Irmacher, G., and Caravelli, J. F.: Radiographic changes in primary osteogenic sarcoma following intensive chemotherapy: Radiological-pathological correlation in 63 cases. Radiology, 143:355, 1982.
172. Sonneland, P. R., and Unni, K. K.: Case report 258. High-grade "surface" osteosarcoma arising from femoral shaft. Skeletal Radiol., 11:77, 1984.
173. Spjut, H. J., Dorfman, H. D., Fechner, R. E., and Ackerman, L. V.: tumors of bone and cartilage. In Atlas of Tumor Pathology. Fascicle 5. Washington, D.C., Armed Forces Institute of Pathology, 1971, p. 174.
174. Sundaram, M., Herbold, D. R., and McGuire, M. H.: Case report 370: Low-grade (well-differentiated) intramedullary osteosarcoma. Skeletal Radiol., 15:338, 1986.
175. Swaney, J. J.: Familial osteogenic sarcoma. Clin. Orthop., 97:64, 1973.

176. Sweetnam, R.: Amputation in osteogenic sarcoma. J. Bone Joint Surg., 55-B:189, 1973.
177. Sweetnam, R.: The surgical management of primary osteosarcoma. Clin. Orthop., 111:57, 1975.
178. Sweetnam, R., Knowelden, J., and Seddon, H.: Bone sarcoma: Treatment by irradiation, amputation or a combination of the two. Br. Med. J., 2:363, 1971.
179. Taylor, W. F., Ivins, J. C., Dahlin, D. C., Edmonson, J. H., and Pritchard, D. J.: Trends and variability in survival from osteosarcoma. Mayo Clin. Proc., 53:695, 1978.
180. Tobias, J. D., Pratt, B., Parham, D. M., Green, A. A., and Rao, B.: The significance of calcified regional lymph nodes at the time of diagnosis of osteosarcoma. Orthopedics, 8:49, 1985.
181. Towbin, R. B., Ballard, E. T., and Crawford, A. H.: Muscle necrosis simulating recurrent osteosarcoma. A case report. J. Bone Joint Surg., 62-A:1024, 1980.
182. Unni, K. K.: Case report 136. Central low-grade osteosarcoma of the tibia. Skeletal Radiol., 6:65, 1981.
183. Unni, K. K., Dahlin, D. C., McLeod, R. A., and Pritchard, D. J.: Intraosseous well-differentiated osteosarcoma. Cancer, 40:1337, 1977.
184. Van der Heul, R. O., and Von Ronnen, J. R.: Juxtacortical osteosarcoma. Diagnosis, differential diagnosis, treatment and an analysis of eighty cases. J. Bone Joint Surg., 49-A:415, 1967.
185. Varela-Duran, J., and Dehner, L. P.: Postirradiation osteosarcoma in childhood. A clinicopathologic study of three cases and review of the literature. Am. J. Pediatr. Hematol. Oncol., 2:263, 1980.
186. Voegeli, E., and Uehlinger, E.: Arteriography in bone tumors. Skeletal Radiol., 1:3, 1976.
187. Weinfeld, M. S., and Dudley, H. R., Jr.: Osteogenic sarcoma. A follow-up study of the 94 cases observed at the Massachusetts General Hospital from 1920 to 1960. J. Bone Joint Surg., 44-A:269, 1962.
188. Wilimas, J., Barrett, G., and Pratt, C.: Osteosarcoma in very young children. Clin. Pediatr., 16:548, 1977.
189. Winkler, K., Beron, G., Kotz, R., Salzer-Kuntschik, M., Beck, J., Beck, W., Brandies, W., Ebell, W., Erttmann, R., Guebel, O., Havers, W., Henze, G., Hinderfeld, L., Hoecker, P., Jobke, A., Jurgens, H., Kabisch, H., Landbeck, G., Preusser, P., Prindull, G., Ramach, W., Ritter, J., Sekera, J., Treuner, J., and Wust, G.: Adjuvant chemotherapy in osteosarcoma—effects of cisplatinum, BCD, and fibroblast interferon in sequential combination with HD-MTX and Adriamycin. Preliminary results of the COSS-80 study. J. Cancer Res. Clin. Oncol., 106(Suppl.):1, 1983.
190. Witkin, G. B., Guilford, W. B., and Siegal, G. P.: Osteogenic sarcoma and soft tissue myxoma in a patient with fibrous dysplasia. Clin. Orthop., 204:245, 1986.
191. Wold, L. E., Unni, K. K., Raymond, A. K., and Dahlin, D. C.: High grade surface osteosarcoma (abstract). Lab. Invest., 48:94A, 1983.
192. Xipell, J. M., and Rush, J.: Case report 340: Well differentiated intraosseous osteosarcoma of the left femur. Skeletal Radiol., 14:312, 1985.

Parosteal Osteogenic Sarcoma

This low-grade osteosarcoma develops in the paraosseous space between the periosteum and overlying muscle of the diaphysis of a major long bone, extending along its longitudinal axis. It has a definite predilection for the distal femur and proximal tibia, and occurs in young adults and adolescents. It is more common in the male. Parosteal osteogenic sarcoma is a slow-growing but malignant tumor.

The clinical finding is a hard, fixed mass on the external surface of the affected bone. Local tenderness and pain are minimal. Radiographs will disclose a long, dense, homogeneous bony mass that is fusiform in shape and separated from the subjacent cortex by a thin radiolucent line. Computed tomography will delineate the structural details of the lesion and the fissure between the tumor and underlying bone. Scintigraphy with technetium-99m will show increased uptake.

In the differential diagnosis of parosteal osteogenic sarcoma one should consider sessile osteochondroma and myositis ossificans. In the bone scan with technetium-99m there is minimal increase in uptake in exostoses. In parosteal osteogenic sarcoma there is no cleft, the bony tumor is connected to and is part of the underlying bone. Myositis ossificans is characterized by the mature bone peripherally and immature, poorly mineralized tissue centrally.

Parosteal osteogenic sarcoma is a Stage IA low-grade malignant lesion, and it remains so for a long time. It does not invade the overlying muscle, rather it pushes the muscle away. As it enlarges it extends into the cortex of underlying bone.

Treatment consists of wide excision or amputation.

References

1. Aakhus, T., and Stokke, T.: Parosteal sarcoma. A.J.R., 111:579, 1971.
2. Aegerter, E., and Kirkpatrick, J. A., Jr.: Orthopedic Diseases: Physiology, Pathology, Radiology. 4th Ed. Philadelphia, Saunders, 1975, p. 530.
3. Ahuja, S. C., Villacin, A. B., Smith, J., Bullough, P. G., Huvos, A. G., and Marcove, R. C.: Juxtacortical (parosteal) osteogenic sarcoma. J. Bone Joint Surg., 59-A:632, 1977.
4. Amendola, M. A., Glazer, G. M., Agha, F. P., Francis, I. R., Weatherbee, L., and Martel, W.: Myositis ossificans circumscripta: Computed tomographic diagnosis. Radiology, 149:775, 1983.
5. Bertoni, F., Boriani, S., Laus, M., and Campanacci, M.: Periosteal chondrosarcoma and periosteal osteosarcoma. Two distinct entities. J. Bone Joint Surg., 64-B:370, 1982.
6. Campanacci, M., Picci, P., Gherlinzoni, F., Guerra, A., Bertoni, F., and Neff, J. R.: Parosteal osteosarcoma. J. Bone Joint Surg., 66-B:313, 1984.
7. Copeland, M. M.: Parosteal osteoma: Differential diagnosis and treatment. In Tumors of Bone and Soft Tissue. A Collection of Papers. Presented at the Eighth Annual Clinical Conference in Cancer, 1963, at The University of Texas M. D. Anderson Hospital and Tumor Institute, Houston, Texas. Chicago, Year Book, 1965, pp. 201–218.
8. Copeland, M. M., and Geschickter, C. F.: The treatment of parosteal osteoma of bone. Surg. Gynecol. Obstet., 108:537, 1959.

9. Dahlin, D. C.: Bone Tumors. 3rd Ed. Springfield, Ill., Thomas, 1978, Chap. 20, p. 261.
10. deSantos, L. A., Bernardino, M. E., and Murray, J. A.: Computed tomography in the valuation of osteosarcoma: Experience with 25 cases. A.J.R., 132:535, 1979.
11. deSantos, L. A., Murray, J. A., Finkelstein, J. B., Spjut, H. J., and Ayala, A. G.: The radiographic spectrum of periosteal osteosarcoma. Radiology, 127:123, 1978.
12. Destouet, J. M., Gilula, L. A., and Murphy, W. A.: Computed tomography of long-bone osteosarcoma. Radiology, 131:439, 1979.
13. Dwinnell, L. A., Dahlin, D. C., and Ghormley, R. K.: Parosteal (juxtacortical) osteogenic sarcoma. J. Bone Joint Surg., 36-A:732, 1954.
14. Edeiken, J.: Roentgen Diagnosis of Disease of Bone. 3rd Ed. Baltimore, Williams & Wilkins, 1981, p. 209.
15. Edeiken, J., Farrell, C., Ackerman, L. V., and Spjut, H. J.: Parosteal sarcoma. A.J.R., 111:579, 1971.
16. Enneking, W. F.: Musculoskeletal Tumor Surgery. New York, Churchill-Livingstone, 1983, p. 1075.
17. Farmlett, E., and Fishman, E. K.: Case Report 300: Parosteal osteosarcoma arising from the proximal end of the left radius. Skeletal Radiol., 13:89, 1985.
18. Farr, G. H., and Huvos, A. G.: Juxtacortical osteogenic sarcoma. An analysis of fourteen cases. J. Bone Joint Surg., 54-A:1205, 1972.
19. Geschickter, C. F., and Copeland, M. M.: Parosteal osteoma of bone: A new entity. Ann. Surg., 133:790, 1951.
20. Green, P. W. B., Ilardi, C. F., Bitter, J. J., and Dee, R. D.: Case Report 260: Parosteal osteosarcoma of the pubis. Skeletal Radiol., 11:141, 1984.
21. Harkess, J. W.: Parosteal osteosarcoma. Am. Surg., 30:730, 1964.
22. Johnson, R. J.: Parosteal osteosarcoma. Clin. Orthop., 68:78, 1970.
23. Kricun, M. E., and Stead, J.: Case Report 289: "Cystic" parosteal osteosarcoma. Skeletal Radiol., 12:227, 1984.
24. Lawson, J. P., and Barwick, K. W.: Case Report 162: Periosteal osteosarcoma of rib. Skeletal Radiol., 7:63, 1981.
25. Lepine, E., Jean, J. P., Proulx, C., and Lamarche, J.: Parosteal osteogenic sarcoma: A study of four cases. Can. J. Surg., 25:229, 1982.
26. Levine, E., DeSmet, A. A., and Huntrakoon, M.: Juxtacortical osteosarcoma: A radiologic and histologic spectrum. Skeletal Radiol., 14:38, 1985.
27. Levine, E., Lee, K. R., Neff, J. R., Makled, N. F., Robinson, R. G., and Preston, D. F.: Comparison of computed tomography and other imaging modalities in the evaluation of musculoskeletal tumors. Radiology, 131:431, 1979.
28. Lorentzon, R., Larsson, S. E., and Boquist, L.: Parosteal (juxtacortical) osteosarcoma. J. Bone Joint Surg., 62-B:86, 1980.
29. Luck, J. V., Jr., Luck, J. V., and Schwinn, C. P.: Parosteal osteosarcoma: A treatment oriented study. Clin. Orthop., 153:92, 1980.
30. Mirra, J. M.: Bone Tumors. Diagnosis and Treatment. Philadelphia, Lippincott, 1980, p. 536.
31. Newland, J. R. and Ayala, A. G.: Parosteal osteosarcoma of the maxilla. Oral Surg., 43:727, 1977.
32. Orcutt, J., Ragsdale, B. D., Curtis, D. J., and Levine, M. I.: Misleading CT in parosteal osteosarcoma. A.J.R., 136:1233, 1981.
33. Probst, F. P.: Angiography in juxtacortical osteosarcomas. Case report with special reference to the differential diagnosis. Acta Radiol., 11:49, 1971.
34. Ranniger, K., and Altner, P. C.: Parosteal osteoid sarcoma. Radiology, 86:648, 1966.
35. Sammons, B. P., Sarkisian, S. S., and Krepela, M. C.: Juxtacortical osteogenic sarcoma. A.J.R., 79:592, 1958.
36. Scaglietti, O., and Calandriello, B.: Ossifying parosteal sarcoma. Parosteal osteoma or juxtacortical osteogenic sarcoma. J. Bone Joint Surg., 44-A:635, 1962.
37. Schajowicz, F.: Juxtacortical chondrosarcoma. J. Bone Joint Surg., 59-B:473, 1977.
38. Simon, M. A., and Kirchner, P. T.: Scintigraphic evaluation of primary bone tumors. J. Bone Joint Surg., 62-A:758, 1980.
39. Sirsat, M. V., and Doctor, V. M.: Parosteal (juxtacortical) osteogenic sarcoma: Emphasis on histopathology. Postgrad. Med., 11:191, 1965.
40. Smith, J., Ahuja, S. C., Huvos, A. G., and Bullough, P. G.: Parosteal (juxtacortical) osteogenic sarcoma. A roentgenological study of 30 patients. J. Can. Assoc. Radiol., 29:167, 1978.
41. Soloman, M. P., Biernacki, J., Slipper, M., and Rosen, Y.: Parosteal osteogenic sarcoma of the mandible. Arch. Otolaryngol., 101:754, 1975.
42. Spjut, H. J., Dorfman, H. D., Fechner, R. E., and Ackerman, L. V.: Tumors of bone and cartilage. In Atlas of Tumor Pathology, fascicle 5. Washington, D.C., U.S. Armed Forces Institute of Pathology, 1971, p. 166.
43. Stark, H. H., Jones, F. E., and Jernstrom, P.: Parosteal osteogenic sarcoma of a metacarpal bone. J. Bone Joint Surg., 53-A:147, 1971.
44. Stevens, G. M., Pugh, D. G., and Dahlin, D. C.: Roentgenographic recognition and differentiation of parosteal osteogenic sarcoma. A.J.R., 78:1, 1957.
45. Sundaram, M., Burdge, R. W., Martin, S. A., and Wolverson, M. K.: Case Report 142: Periosteal osteosarcoma of femur. Skeletal Radiol., 6:131, 1981.
46. Thrall, J. H., Geslien, G. E., Corcoron, R. J., and Johnson, M. C.: Abnormal radionuclide deposition patterns adjacent to focal skeletal lesions. Radiology, 115:659, 1975.
47. Unni, K. K., Dahlin, D. C., and Beabout, J. W.: Parosteal osteogenic sarcoma. Cancer, 37:2466, 1976.
48. van der Heul, R. O., and von Ronnen, J. R.: Juxtacortical osteosarcoma: Diagnosis, differential diagnosis, treatment, and an analysis of eighty cases. J. Bone Joint Surg., 49-A:415, 1967.
49. Wold, L. E., Unni, K. K., Beabout, J. W., and Pritchard, D. J.: High-grade surface osteosarcomas. Am. J. Surg. Pathol., 8:181, 1984.
50. Wold, L. E., Unni, K. K., Beabout, J. W., Sim, F. H., and Dahlin, D. C.: Dedifferentiated parosteal osteosarcoma. J. Bone Joint Surg., 66-A:53, 1984.
51. Wolfel, D. A., and Carter, P. R.: Parosteal osteosarcoma. A.J.R., 105:142, 1969.
52. Yaghmai, I.: Angiographic features of osteosarcoma. A.J.R., 129:1073, 1971.
53. Zeanan, W. R., and Hudson, T. M.: Myositis ossificans. Radiologic evaluation of two cases with diagnostic computed tomograms. Clin. Orthop., 168:187, 1982.

EWING'S SARCOMA

This uncommon primary malignant bone tumor was so named after Ewing, who first described it as a distinct entity in 1921.[31] He originally named it "diffuse endothelioma" or "endothelial myeloma," in accordance with his belief that it was derived from vasoformative tissue. There has been much ensuing debate, however, concerning its pathogenesis. The current view is that it arises either from the nonmesenchymal cells of bone marrow or primitive noncommitted mesenchymal cells.

Ewing's sarcoma is the second most common primary malignant tumor of bone found in children. Occasionally it is encountered in soft tissue as its primary site. It has a characteristic predilection for an age group between 10 and 15 years. If certain similar findings are encountered in a child under 5 years of age, neuroblastoma is the probable diagnosis; whereas, encountered in a patient over the typical age range, such findings may be considered to indicate metastatic carcinoma, and in one over 50 years, multiple myeloma. The tumor is more common in boys than in girls.

Localization of Ewing's sarcoma is often in the innominate bone, femur, humerus, fibula, clavicle, or tibia. In the long tubular limb bones, the lesion is situated in the diaphysis rather than in the metaphysis. Other infrequent sites in the trunk are a rib, scapula, or vertebra. Rarely it occurs in the bones of the hands or feet.[18, 26, 83, 124, 166, 167]

Pathologic Findings

On gross inspection the neoplasm appears as a whitish-gray soft mass that arises in the marrow spaces of the interior of the affected bone. Necrotic and hemorrhagic areas in the tumor are frequent. Anatomic findings show that involvement of the bone is much more extensive than is apparent in the radiograms, an observation that stresses the importance of irradiating the entire affected bone. The neoplastic tissue destroys and replaces the involved bone. The periosteum is elevated and often is perforated, a large soft-tissue mass extending well beyond the bony boundaries. The tumor is not encapsulated. When an innominate bone is involved, the soft-tissue mass will protrude into the pelvic and abdominal cavities.

Histologic examination discloses compact sheets of small polyhedral cells with pale cytoplasm and ill-defined boundaries. The nuclei are uniform, round or oval in shape, and contain scattered areas of chromatin (Fig. 3–333). There are a multitude of thin-walled vascular channels among a scanty stroma. The cytoplasmic material is PAS positive and diastase digestible. Occasional rosette or pseudo-rosette formations may be present. These cytologic findings simulate those of neuroblastoma or malignant lymphoma.

Extensive necrosis and degenerative changes may also confuse the picture. Hemorrhage may provoke a reparative inflammatory reaction to the tumor, a finding that may be misinterpreted as being a mere infection.

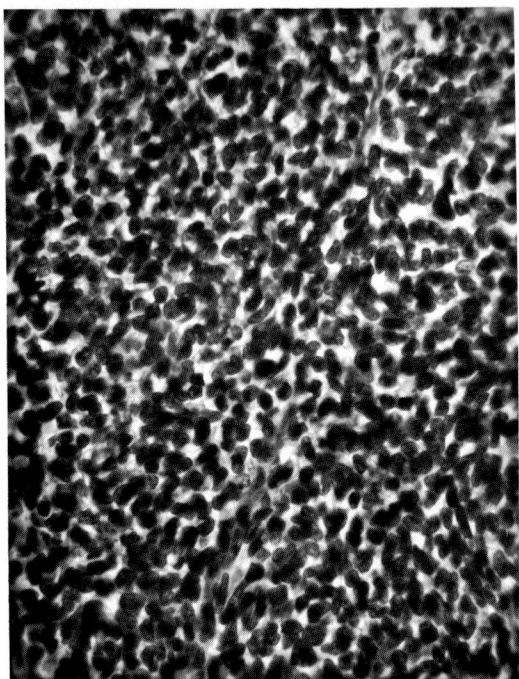

FIGURE 3–333. *Ewing's sarcoma—histologic findings.*

Photomicrograph shows the round cells, which are polyhedral with pale cytoplasm and small hyperchromatic nuclei ($\times$ 400).

Reticulin fibers are not a consistent feature of Ewing's sarcoma. Another distinguishing histochemical finding is the presence of glycogen in the cells of Ewing's sarcoma; in reticulosarcoma, the tumor cells do not contain glycogen.[132]

Ultrastructural studies have shown medium-sized cells, polygonal shape, oval nuclei, smooth nuclear envelope, abundant euchromatin, well-developed nucleolonema, scant membranous organelles, abundant hyaloplasmic glycogen, occasional lipid vacuoles, straight cell membranes, and primitive intercellular junctions.[6]

Clinical Picture

Local pain is the presenting complaint. Other symptoms depend on the site of the lesion. When a rib is involved, pleural effusion may be noted. Some degree of stiffness of the adjacent joint is common in cases of long bone affection. When the lumbar spine is the site of the lesion, the nerve trunks may be involved, producing sciatic pain, tingling sensations, or motor weakness. Rectal and urinary complaints may result when the neoplasm is located in an innominate bone and impinges on pelvic organs. On occasion the presenting feature is a pathologic fracture of a femur or tibia involved with Ewing's sarcoma.

On physical examination, one can usually palpate a tumor mass that is tender on pressure. It is larger than the bony lesion depicted in the radiogram, indicating that the neoplasm has violated the cortex and has spread extraosseously into the surrounding soft tissues. Characteristically the tumor rapidly increases in size. In about 50 per cent of cases, the presenting lesion is in some part of the innominate bone; if the pubis or ischium is involved, an elastic, irregular, globular mass may be palpated on rectal examination; or if the ilium is the site of the lesion, a tumor mass may be present in the lower quadrant of the abdomen or in the gluteal region.

Fever, secondary anemia, leukocytosis with a shift to the left, and an increase in the erythrocyte sedimentation rate are not infrequent, indicating a marked neovascular and inflammatory reaction to the tumor. These findings are hallmarks of a fulminating course. Malaise, lethargy, and progressive weight loss develop early in the course of the disease.

Radiographic Findings

The radiographic appearance is fairly characteristic, but not pathognomonic (Figs. 3–334 to 3–336). Mottled rarefaction of the spongiosa with permeation of the overlying cortex is the principal finding, reflecting bone destruction. The bone at the site of the lesion may show

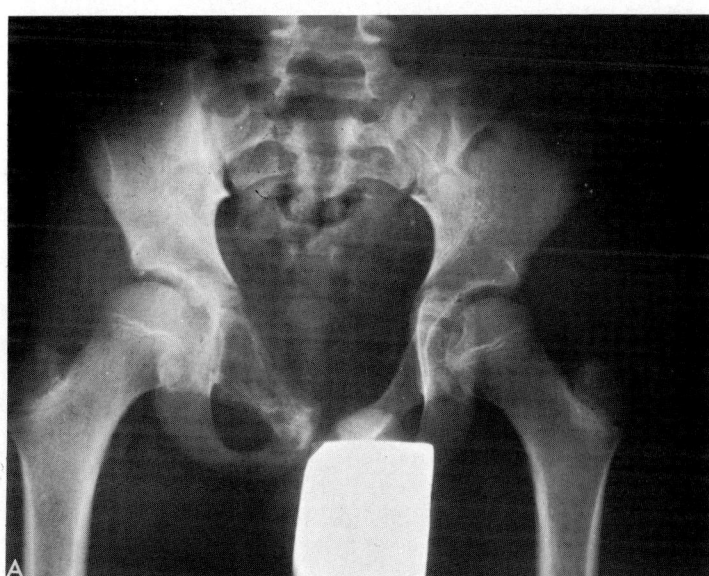

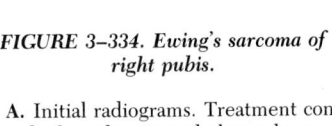

FIGURE 3–334. *Ewing's sarcoma of right pubis.*

A. Initial radiograms. Treatment consisted of irradiation and chemotherapy. B. Nine months later, some healing is apparent. The patient developed metastases, however, and died a year later.

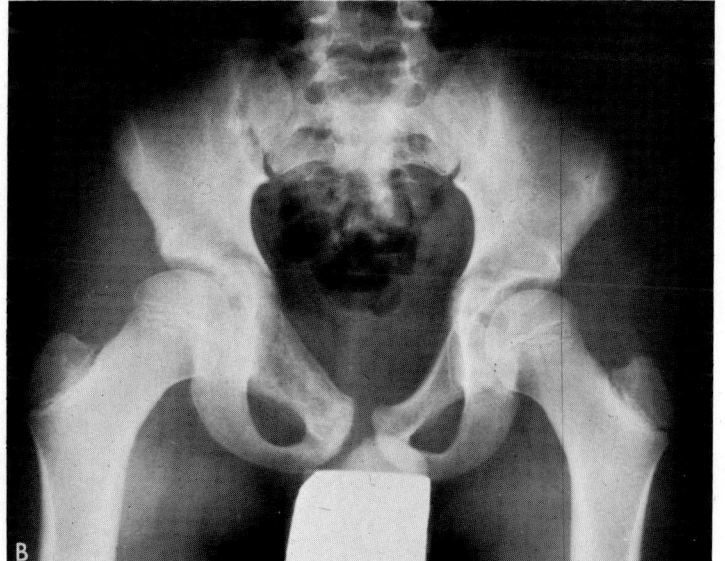

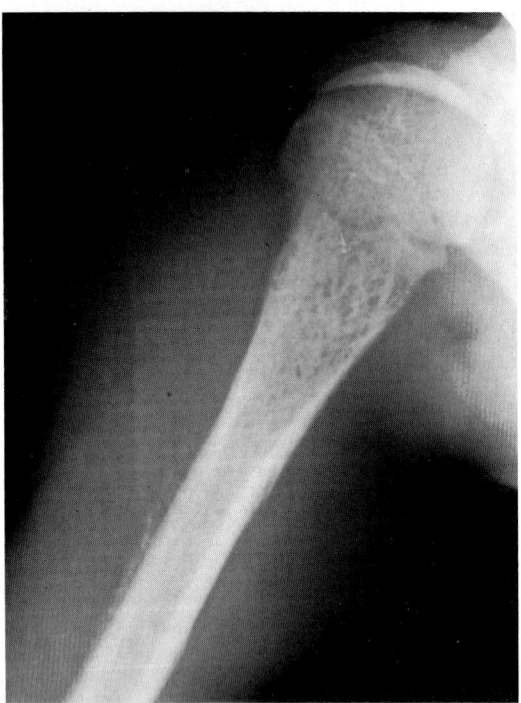

FIGURE 3–335. Ewing's sarcoma of humerus.

Note the mottled areas of rarefaction and subperiosteal reaction.

some expansion. Periosteal new bone formation, often of the laminated "onion-peel" form, is common, but is not specific for Ewing's sarcoma. A soft-tissue mass overlying the area of bone destruction is frequently seen in the radiogram, indicating that the neoplasm has perforated the cortex and has spread into the adjacent soft tissues. In the long bones, the lesion is diaphyseal in location and involvement is extensive. Pathologic fractures are rare.

In the differential diagnosis, one should consider conditions such as eosinophilic granuloma, reticulum-cell sarcoma, malignant lymphoma, "osteolytic" osteogenic sarcoma, metastatic neuroblastoma, leukemia, and osteomyelitis.

Staging

Prognostically the best method of staging Ewing's sarcoma is by the extent of involvement at the time of presentation. *Stage I* is solitary and intraosseous; *Stage II* is solitary and extraosseous; *Stage III* is multicentric but confined to the affected bones; *Stage IV* is Ewing's sarcoma with distant metastases at the time of presentation.

The stage is determined by the following studies. *Scintigraphy with technetium-99m* will show marked increased uptake at the site of involvement, which is more extensive than the lesion depicted in the conventional radiograph. The bone scan with technetium-99m is the best method of skeletal survey to detect metastases. Scintigraphy is the first step in staging after conventional radiography; it should be mandatory. *Linear tomography and computed tomography* will demonstrate the details of the radiolucent area (whether ossified or not, thereby differentiating Ewing's sarcoma from osteogenic sarcoma), the presence or absence of cortical destruction, the extent of the intraosseous involvement, and the degree of extraosseous soft-tissue spread. *Angiography* will, in the early arterial phase, show the extent of soft-tissue involvement, and in the late venous phase will depict the blush of neoplastic vasculature. *Nuclear magnetic resonance* has, in preliminary experience, shown itself to be very effective in delineating the extent of the tumor.

Diagnosis

Definitive diagnosis is made from histologic study of tissue sections obtained at open biopsy. Needle biopsy may be performed in surgically difficult accessible sites (such as vertebral bodies); this author, however, strongly recommends open biopsy. It is imperative that tissue obtained at biopsy be adequate. Radiographic control must be utilized to ensure that the biopsy is taken from the correct site. A frozen tissue section is also greatly helpful. Degenerative changes in the tumor may grossly resemble a purulent exudate; this, along with the radiographic findings, may easily lead one to confuse Ewing's sarcoma with osteomyelitis.

Prognosis

In the past the outlook for Ewing's sarcoma was poor, with an overall 10 per cent five-year survival rate. With the advent of combined chemotherapy and radiotherapy and skeletal adjuvant surgery, the prognosis is greatly improved with a five-year survival rate of 50 to 75 per cent.[67, 128]

Treatment

The tumor is radiosensitive, and irradiation markedly reduces the size of the lesion; it does not, however, completely eradicate the tumor as shown by the substantial rate of local recurrence in autopsy material.

Ewing's sarcoma responds to chemotherapy,

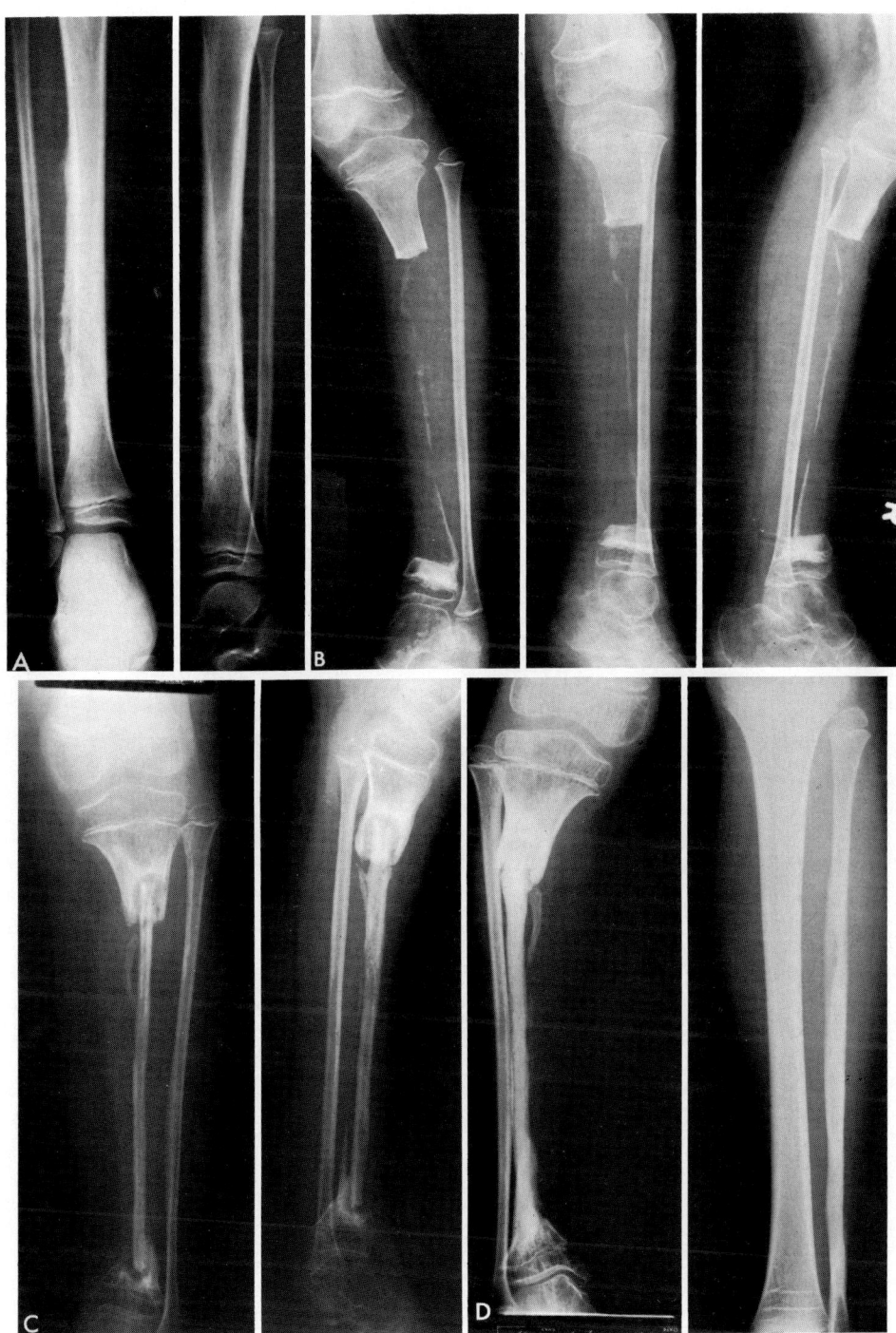

FIGURE 3–336. Ewing's sarcoma of right tibia in an eight-year-old girl.

A. Initial radiograms. The diagnosis was confirmed on biopsy; after 5,000 r irradiation, the tibial shaft was resected and the fibula from the opposite leg was used for bone graft. **B** and **C.** Immediate postoperative radiograms. The leg was supported in a cast for four months and then in a brace. **D.** Radiograms of legs two years later.

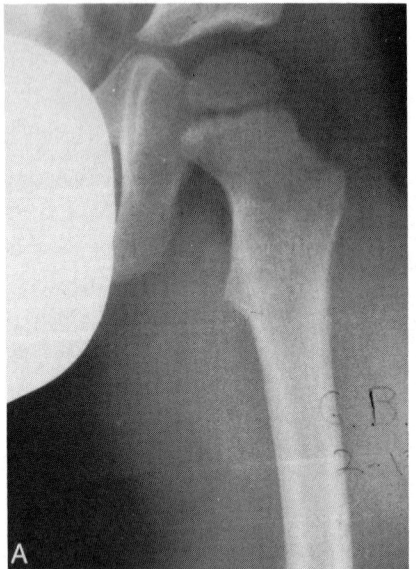 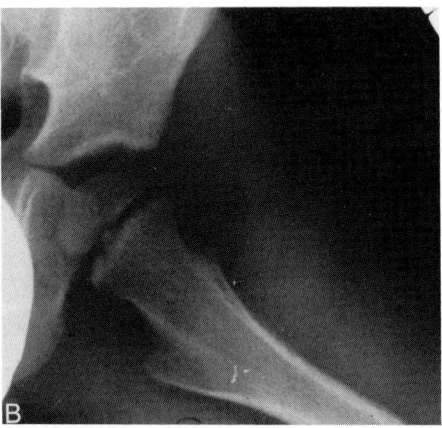

FIGURE 3–337. *Ewing's sarcoma of proximal femur in a five-year-old boy.*

A and **B.** Anteroposterior and lateral radiograph of the proximal femur showing subperiosteal reaction and mottling of the outer cortex.

which should be administered in all cases. At present, clinical experience has shown that the most effective methods of treatment, providing the best changes for complete supression of the tumor, are a combination of chemotherapy and irradiation; a combination of chemotherapy and surgical ablation; or in a few selected cases, a combination of the three—chemotherapy, irradiation, and surgical ablation.

Indications for surgical ablation of the involved part are: a bone that can be removed without great functional impairment and disability (such as fibula, clavicle, or scapula); a bone with a pathologic fracture through a large tumor, making it difficult or impossible to treat; a tumor that does not respond to irradiation; and a tumor in close proximity to the physis of a long bone (such as the distal femur or proximal tibia) in a young child in whom irradiation of the part will result in growth arrest and gross limb length disparity (Fig. 3–337).

In other instances chemotherapy combined with irradiation is the preferred method of treatment. There is a marked tendency for the neoplasm to extend longitudinally in the affected bone by direct infiltration; thus the field or irradiation should extend well beyond the limits of the radiographic extent of the tumor. A tumor dose of 5000 to 7000 r is delivered over a five- to seven-week period, using supravoltage equipment. Chemotherapy is administered by the oncologist.

Long bones, particularly the femur and humerus, are at high risk for pathologic fracture. When such a complication occurs, treatment consists of early internal fixation and, if necessary, bone grafting (Fig. 3–338).[147]

In the older child and adolescent with postirradiation growth retardation of the distal femur or proximal tibia, limb length equalization by epiphysiodesis of the contralateral distal femur or proximal tibia may be indicated.

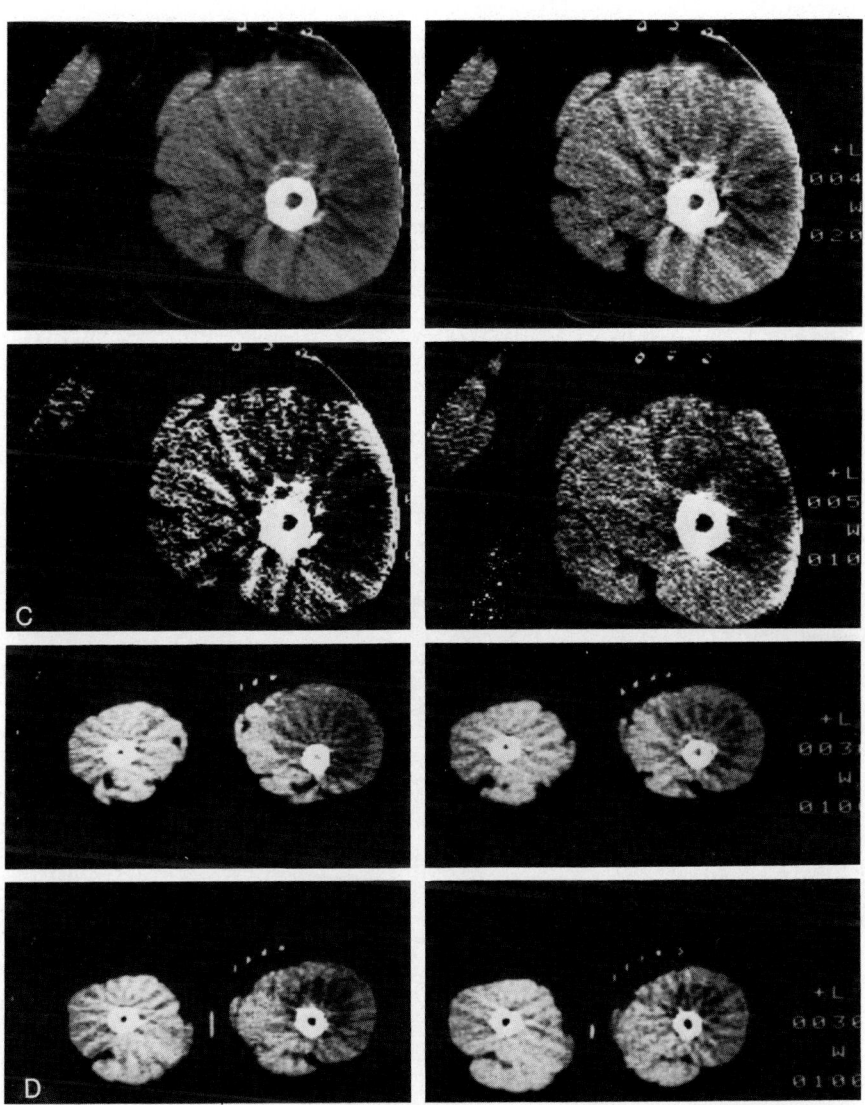

FIGURE 3–337 Continued. **C** and **D.** The CT scan showing cross sections of the bony and soft-tissue changes in the proximal femur. Treatment was by irradiation and chemotherapy.

Illustration continued on following page

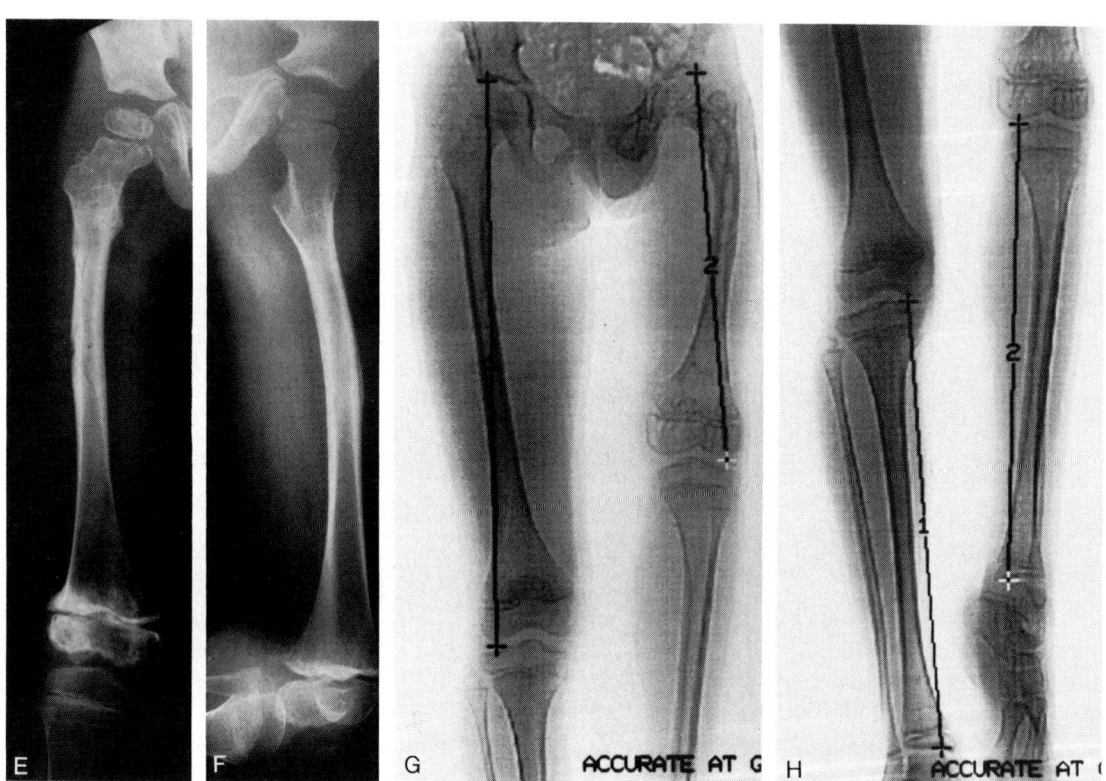

FIGURE 3–337 Continued. *Ewing's sarcoma of proximal femur in a five-year-old boy.*

FIGURE 3–337 Continued. **E** and **F.** Immediate postoperative radiograms. **G** and **H.** CT scan mensuration shows the marked lower limb length disparity due to postirradiation growth arrest of the proximal and distal femoral physes.

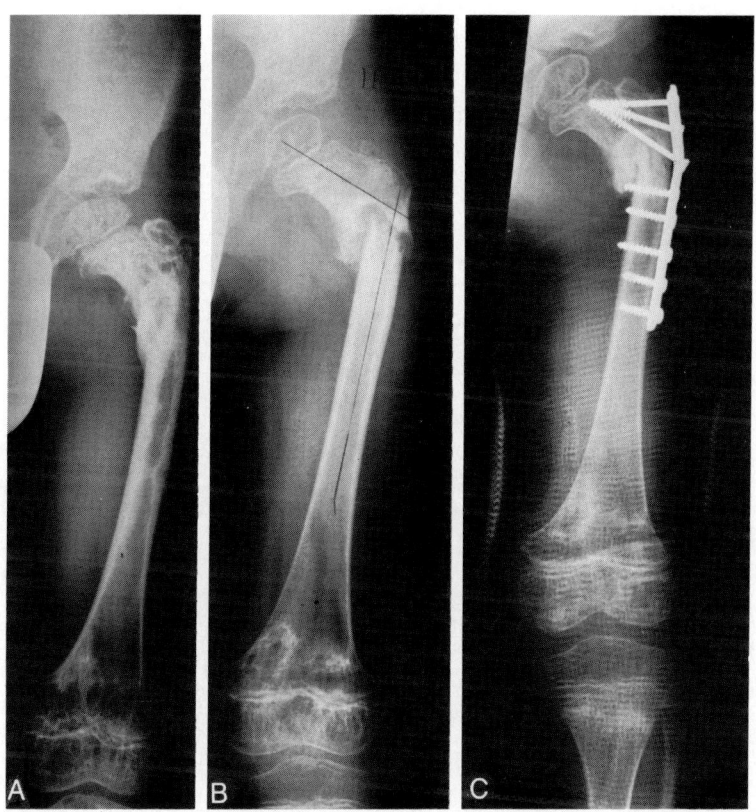

FIGURE 3–338. Subtrochanteric pathologic fracture in Ewing's sarcoma of the proximal femur treated by internal fixation with plate and screws.

A. Prefracture radiogram showing the sclerosis and radiolucent changes in bone. **B.** Anteroposterior radiogram of the femur with the subtrochanteric pathologic fracture. **C.** Postoperative anteroposterior radiogram. Internal fixation was with plate and screws.

When metastases develop they are irradiated when possible, and chemotherapy is continued. The outlook of Ewing's sarcoma with the regimen of therapy is markedly improved, and an increasing percentage of cases show apparent cure.

References

1. Bacci, G., Campanacci, M., and Pagani, P. A.: Adjuvant chemotherapy in the treatment of localized Ewing's sarcoma. J. Bone Joint Surg., 60-B:567, 1978.
2. Bacci, G., Picci, R., Gitelo, S., Borghi, A., and Campanacci, M.: The treatment of localized Ewing's sarcoma: The experience at the Istituto Ortopedico Rizzoli in 163 cases treated with and without adjuvant chemotherapy. Cancer, 49:1561, 1982.
3. Baird, R. J., and Krause, V. W.: Ewing's tumor: A review of 33 cases. Can. J. Surg., 6:136, 1963.
4. Barden, R. P.: The similarity of clinical and roentgen findings in children with Ewing's sarcoma (endothelial myeloma) and sympathetic neuroblastoma. A.J.R., 50:575, 1943.
5. Berger, P. E., and Kuhn, J. P.: Computed tomography of tumors of the musculoskeletal system in children. Radiology, 127:171, 1978.
6. Berthold, F., Kracht, J., Lampert, F., Millar, T. J., Muller, T. H., Reither, M., and Unsicker, K.: Ultrastructural, biochemical and cell-culture studies of a presumed extraskeletal Ewing's sarcoma with special reference to differential diagnosis from neuroblastoma. J. Cancer Res. Clin. Oncol., 103:293, 1982.
7. Bhansali, S. K., and Desai, P. B.: Ewing's sarcoma. Observations on 107 cases. J. Bone Joint Surg., 45-A:541, 1963.
8. Blakemore, J. R., and Stein, M.: Primary Ewing's sarcoma of the mandible: Report of a case. J. Oral Surg., 33:376, 1975.
9. Boyer, C. W., Jr., Brickner, T. J., Jr., and Perry, R. H.: Ewing's sarcoma. Case against surgery. Cancer, 20:1602, 1967.
10. Branson, J.: Ewing's tumor of a rib. Australas. Radiol., 20:341, 1976.
11. Brav, E. A., and Rechtman, A. M.: Primary endotheliomyeloma (Ewing's tumor) of the sacrum. J. Bone Joint Surg., 20:1034, 1938.
12. Buhnell, D., Shirazi, P., Khedkar, N., and Blank, J.: Ewing's sarcoma seen as a "cold" lesion on bone scans. Clin. Nucl. Med., 8:173, 1983.
13. Cabenela, M. E., Sim, F. H., Beabout, J. W., and Dahlin, D. C.: Osteomyelitis appearing as neoplasms. A diagnostic problem. Arch. Surg., 109:68, 1974.
14. Cade, S.: Bone sarcoma. J. R. Col. Surg. (Edinburgh), 12:85, 1967.
15. Caffey, J., and Silverman, F. N.: Pediatric X-ray Diagnosis. 7th Ed. Chicago, Year Book, 1979.
16. Campbell, W. C., and Hamilton, J. F.: Ewing's tumor (endothelial myeloma). J. Bone Joint Surg., 362:1018, 1938.
17. Carpenter, E. B., and Kirk, A. A.: Ewing's tumor occurring at the age of 7 months. Am. J. Surg., 83:584, 1952.
18. Cohen, J., Brown, K. A., and Grice, D. S.: Ewing's tumor of the talus (astragalus) simulating aseptic necrosis. J. Bone Joint Surg., 35-A:1008, 1953.
19. Coley, B. L.: Neoplasms of Bone and Related Conditions. Their Etiology, Pathogenesis, Diagnosis, and Treatment. 2nd Ed. New York, Hoeber, 1960, pp. 341–363.
20. Coley, B. L., Higinbotham, N. L., and Bowden, L.: Endothelioma of bone (Ewing's sarcoma). Ann. Surg., 128:533, 1948.
21. Colville, H. C., and Willis, R. A.: Neuroblastoma metastases in bones with a criticism of Ewing's endothelioma. Am. J. Pathol., 9:421, 1933.
22. Connor, C. L.: Endothelial myeloma. Ewing; report of 54 cases. Arch. Surg., 12:789, 1926.
23. Coombs, R. J., Zeiss, J., McCann, K., and Phillips, E.: Case report 360: Multifocal Ewing tumor of the skeletal system. Skeletal Radiol., 15:254, 1986.
24. Dahlin, D. C., Coventry, M. B., and Scanlon, P. W.: Ewing's sarcoma. A critical analysis of 165 cases. J. Bone Joint Surg., 43-A:185, 1961.
25. DeSantos, L. A., Goldstein, H. M., Murray, J. A., and Wallace, S.: Computed tomography in the evaluation of musculoskeletal neoplasms. Radiology, 128:89, 1978.
26. Dick, H. M., Francis, K. C., and Johnston, A. D.: Ewing's sarcoma of the hand. J. Bone Joint Surg., 53-A:345, 1971.
27. Dickman, P. S., Liotta, L. A., and Triche, T. J.: Ewing's sarcoma characterization in established cultures and evidence of its histogenesis. Lab. Invest., 47:375, 1982.
28. Dvorak, P. F., Vorlicky, L. N., and Nesbit, M. E.: Ewing's sarcoma of the rib, presenting as the superior mediastinal syndrome. Clin. Pediatr. (Phila.), 10:607, 1971.
29. Edeiken, J.: Roentgen Diagnosis of Diseases of Bone. 3rd Ed. Baltimore, Williams & Wilkins, 1981, p. 273.
30. Ellis, H. A.: Metabolic bone disease. In Anthony, P. P., and Macsween, R. N. M. (eds.): Recent Advances in Histopathology. Vol. II. Edinburgh, Churchill-Livingstone, 1981, p. 185.
31. Ewing, J.: Diffuse endothelioma of bone. Proc. N.Y. Pathol. Soc., 21:17, 1921.
32. Ewing, J.: A review and classification of bone sarcomas. Arch. Surg., 4:485, 1922.
33. Ewing, J.: Further report on endothelial myeloma of bone. Proc. N.Y. Pathol. Soc., 24:93, 1924
34. Ewing, J.; Neoplastic Diseases. A Treatise on Tumors. 4th Ed. Philadelphia, Saunders, 1940, pp. 360–370.
35. Falk, S., and Alpert, M.: The clinical and roentgen aspects of Ewing's sarcoma. Am. J. Med. Sci., 250:492, 1965.
36. Falk, S., and Alpert, M.: Five year survival of patients with Ewing's sarcoma. Surg. Gynecol. Obstet., 124:319, 1967.
37. Fernandez, C. H., Lindenberg, R. D., Sutown, W. W., and Samuels, M. L.: Localized Ewing's sarcoma. Treatment and results. Cancer, 34:143, 1974.
38. Foote, F. W., Jr., and Anderson, H. R.: Histogenesis of Ewing's tumor. Am. J. Pathol., 17:497, 1941.
39. Frankel, R. S., Jones, A. E., Cohen, J. A., et al.: Clinical correlation of 67-Ga and skeletal whole body radionuclide studies with radiography in Ewing's sarcoma. Radiology, 110:597, 1974.
40. Franken, E. A., Smith, J. A., and Smith, W. L.: Tumors of the chest wall in infants and children. Pediatr. Radiol., 6:13, 1977.
41. Fraumeni, J. F., Jr., and Glass, A. G.: Rarity of Ewing's sarcoma among U.S. Negro children. Lancet, 1:366, 1970.
42. Freeman, A. I., Sachatello, C., Gaeta, J., Shah, N. K., Wang, J. J., and Sinks, L. F.: An analysis of Ewing's tumor in children at Roswell Park Memorial Institute. Cancer, 29:1563, 1972.
43. Friedman, B., and Gold, H.: Ultrastructure of Ewing's sarcoma of bone. Cancer, 22:307, 1968.
44. Garand, R., Nomballais, F., Le Mevel, A., Mourand, E., and Le Mevel, B.: Acute myeloblastic leukemia following Ewing's sarcoma: Iatrogenic complication? (Author's translation.) Bull. Cancer (Paris), 68:25, 1981.
45. Garber, C. Z.: Reactive bone formation in Ewing's sarcoma. Cancer, 4:839, 1951.

46. Gehan, E. A., Nesbit, M. E., Jr., Burgert, E. O., Jr., Viettit, J., Tefft, M., Perez, C. A., Kissane, J., and Hempel, C.: Prognostic factors in children with Ewing's sarcoma. Natl. Cancer Inst. Monogr., 56:273, 1981.
47. Geschickter, C. F., and Maseritz, J. R.: Ewing's sarcoma. J. Bone Joint Surg., 21:26, 1939.
48. Gharpure, V. V.: Endothelial myeloma (Ewing's tumor of bone) Am. J. Pathol., 17:503, 1941.
49. Gilbert, E. F., Jones, B., and Majzoub, H. S.: Malignant hemangioendothelioma of bone in childhood. Am. J. Dis. Child., 121:410, 1971.
50. Gilula, L. A., Murphy, W. A., Tailor, C. C., and Pastel, R. B.: Computed tomography of the osseous pelvis. Radiology, 132:107, 1979.
51. Ginaldi, S., and De Santos, L. A.: Computed tomography in the evaluation of small round cell tumors of bone. Radiology, 134:441, 1980.
52. Goldstein, H., McNeil, B. J., Zufall, E., and Treves, S.: Is there still a place for bone scanning in Ewing's sarcoma? Concise communication. J. Nucl. Med., 21:10, 1980.
53. Gouliamos, A. D., Carter, B. L., and Emami, B.: Computed tomography of the chest wall. Radiology, 134:433, 1980.
54. Hamilton, J. F.: Ewing's sarcoma (endothelial myeloma). Arch. Surg., 41:29, 1940.
55. Harrison, H. N.: Ewing's sarcoma: Ten-year survivals. Report of a case with recurrent pulmonary metastases. Ann. Surg., 148:783, 1958.
56. Harrison, R. S.: Ewing's bone sarcoma. Br. J. Radiol., 7:580, 1934.
57. Hayes, F. A., Thompson, E. I., Hrizdala, E., O'Connor, D., and Green, A. A.: Chemotherapy as an alternative to laminectomy and radiation in the management of epidural tumor. J. Pediatr., 104:221, 1984.
58. Heald, J. H., Soto-Hall, R., and Hill, H. A.: Ewing's sarcoma. A.J.R., 91:1167, 1964.
59. Heaston, D. K., and Gelman, M. I.: Case report 74. Skeletal Radiol., 3:186, 1978.
60. Heelan, R. T., Watson, R. C., and Smith, J.: Computed tomography of lower extremity tumors. A.J.R., 132:933, 1979.
61. Herber, S. M., Kay, R., May, R., and Milner, R. D. G.: Growth of long term survivors of childhood malignancy. Acta Pediatr. Scand., 74:438, 1985.
62. Huntington, R. W., Henkelmann, C. R., and Franklin, R.: Atypical Ewing tumor in the sister of a patient with Ewing's tumor. Clinical and autopsy findings. J. Bone Joint Surg., 43-A:572, 1961.
63. Hurvitz, J. S., Harrison, M. R., and Weitzman, J. J.: Aneurysmal bone cyst mimicking Ewing's sarcoma of the rib. J. Pediatr. Surg., 12:1067, 1977.
64. Hustu, H. O., Pinkel, D., and Pratt, C. B.: Treatment of clinically localized Ewing's sarcoma with radiotherapy and combination chemotherapy. Cancer, 30:1522, 1972.
65. Hutter, R. V. P., Francis, K. C., and Foote, F. W., Jr.: Ewing's sarcoma in siblings. Report of the second known occurrence. Am. J. Surg., 107:598, 1964.
66. Jaffe, H. L.: The problem of Ewing's sarcoma of bone. Bull. Hosp. Joint Dis., 6:82, 1945.
67. Jaffe, H. L., Traggis, D., Sallan, S., and Cassady, J. R.: Improved outlook for Ewing's sarcoma with combination chemotherapy and radiation therapy. Cancer, 38:1925, 1976.
68. Jaffe, N.: Advances in the management of malignant bone tumors in children and adolescents. Pediatr. Clin. North Am., 32:801, 1985.
69. Jenkin, R. D. T.: Ewing's sarcoma—a study of treatment methods. Clin. Radiol., 17:97, 1966.
70. Jenkin, R. D. T.: Radiation treatment of Ewing's sarcoma and osteogenic sarcoma. Can. J. Surg., 20:530, 1977.
71. Jenkin, R. D. T., Rider, W. D., and Sonley, M. J.: Ewing's sarcoma. A trial of adjuvant total body irradiation. Radiology, 96:151, 1970.
72. Jentzsch, K., Binder, H., Cramer, H., Glaubiger, D. L., Kessler, R. M., Bull, C., Pomeroy, T. C., and Gerber, N. L.: Leg function after radiotherapy for Ewing's sarcoma. Cancer, 47:1267, 1981.
73. Johnson, R., and Humphreys, S. R.: Past failures and future possibilities in Ewing's sarcoma. Experimental and preliminary clinical results. Cancer, 23:161, 1969.
74. Johnson, R. E., and Pomeroy, T. C.: Evaluation of therapeutic results in Ewing's sarcoma. A.J.R., 123:583, 1975.
75. Joseph, W. L., and Fonkalsrud, E. W.: Primary rib tumors in children. Am. Surg., 38:338, 1972.
76. Joyce, M. J., Harmon, D. C., Mankin, H. J., Suit, H. D., Schiller, A. L., and Truman, J. T.: Ewing's sarcoma in female siblings. A clinical report and review of the literature. Cancer, 53:1959, 1984.
77. Kadin, M. E., and Bensch, K. G.: On the origin of Ewing's tumor. Cancer, 27:257, 1971.
78. Kahanovitz, N., Johanson, P. H., and Hirose, F. M.: Ewing's sarcoma presenting with a coexistent bacterial organism. A case report. J. Bone Joint Surg., 61-A:604, 1979.
79. Kissane, J. M., Askin, F. B., Nesbit, M. E., Vietti, T. J., Burgert, E. D., Jr., Cangir, A., Gehan, E. A., Perez, C. A., Pritchard, D. J., and Tefft, M.: Sarcomas of bone in childhood; pathologic aspects. Natl. Cancer Inst. Monogr., 56:29, 1981.
80. Klaassen, M.A., and Hoffman, G.: Ewing's sarcoma presenting as spondylolithesis. Report of a case. J. Bone Joint Surg., 69-A:1089, 1987.
81. Larsson, S. E., Boquist, L., and Bergdahl, L.: Ewing's sarcoma. A consecutive series of 64 cases diagnosed in Sweden 1958–1967. Clin. Orthop., 95:263, 1973.
82. Lattman, I.: A review of Ewing's tumor with case reports. Br. J. Radiol., 7:194, 1934.
83. Levin, N. B.: Ewing's sarcoma of the calcaneus. J. Foot Surg., 19:127, 1980.
84. Levine, E.: Computed tomography of musculoskeletal tumors. CRC Crit. Rev. Diagn. Imaging, 16:279, 1981.
85. Levine, E., and Levine, C.: Ewing tumor of rib: Radiologic findings and computed tomography contribution. Skeletal Radiol., 9:227, 1983.
86. Levine, E., Kyo Rak Lee, P. D., Neff, J. R., Maklad, N. F., Robinson, R. G., and Preston, D. F.: Comparison of computed tomography and other imaging modalities in the evaluation of musculoskeletal tumors. Radiology, 131:431, 1979.
87. Lewis, R. J., Marcove, R. C., and Rosen, G.: Ewing's sarcoma—functional effects of radiation therapy. J. Bone Joint Surg., 59-A:325, 1977.
88. Li, W. K., Lane, J. M., Rosen, G., Marcove, R. C., Capparos, R., Huvos, A., and Groshen, S.: Pelvic Ewing's sarcoma. Advances in treatment. J. Bone Joint Surg., 65-A:738, 1983.
89. Lichtenstein, L., and Jaffe, H. L.: Ewing's sarcoma of bone. Am. J. Pathol., 23:43, 1947.
90. Llombart-Bosch, A., Blache, R., and Peydro-Olaya, A.: Ultrastructural study of 28 cases of Ewing's sarcoma: Typical and atypical forms. Cancer, 41:1362, 1978.
91. Lombardi, F., Gasparini, M., Gianni, C., Petrillo, R., Tesoro-Tess, J. D., Volterrani, F., and Musumeci, R.: Ewing's sarcoma: An approach to radiologic diagnosis. Tumori, 65:389, 1979.
92. Neff, J. R.: Nonmetastatic Ewing sarcoma of bone: The role of surgical therapy. Clin. Orthop., 204:111, 1986.
93. McCormick, L. J., Dockerty, M. B., and Ghormley, R. K.: Ewing's sarcoma. Cancer, 5:85, 1952.
94. MacIntosh, D. J., Price, C. H. G., and Jeffree, G.

M.: Ewing's tumor. A study of behaviour and treatment in 47 cases. J. Bone Joint Surg., 57-B:331, 1975.
95. McKeen, E. A., Hanson, M. R., Mulvihill, J. J., et al.: Birth defects with Ewing's sarcoma (letter). N. Engl. J. Med., 309:1522, 1983.
96. McKenzie, A. H., and Day, F. G.: Eosinophilic granuloma of the femoral shaft simulating Ewing's sarcoma. J. Bone Joint Surg., 39-A:408, 1957.
97. MacLeod, R. A., Stephens, D. H., Beabout, J. W., Sheedy, P. F., II., and Hattery, R. R.: Computed tomography of the skeletal system. Semin. Roentgenol., 13:235, 1978.
98. McSwain, B., Byrd, B. F., Jr., and Inman, W. O., Jr.: Ewing's tumor. Surg. Gynecol. Obstet., 89:209, 1949.
99. Malangoni, M. A., Ofstein, L. C., Grosfeld, J. L., Weber, T. R., Eigen, H., and Baehner, R. L.: Survival and pulmonary function following chest wall resection and reconstruction in children. J. Pediatr. Surg., 15:906, 1980.
100. Marsden, H. B., and Steward, J. K.: Ewing's tumors and neuroblastomas. J. Clin. Pathol., 17:411, 1964.
101. Melnick, P. J.: Histogenesis of Ewing's sarcoma of bone; with postmortem report of a case. Am. J. Cancer, 19:353, 1933.
102. Mendenhall, C. M., Marcus, R. B., Jr., Enneking, W. F., Springfield, D. S., Thar, T. L., and Million, R. R.: The prognostic significance of soft tissue extension in Ewing's sarcoma. Cancer, 51:913, 1983.
103. Meyerding, H. W.: The diagnosis and treatment of Ewing's tumor (endothelial myeloma; solitary diffuse endothelioma; hemangio-endothelioma). Trans. West. Surg. Assoc., 48:183, 1938.
104. Morton, J. J.: Treatment of Ewing's sarcoma of bone. In Pack, G. T., and Livingston, E. M. (eds.): Treatment of Cancer and Allied Diseases. New York, Hoeber, 1940, pp. 2422–2436.
105. Naidich, D. P., Freedman, M. T., Bowerman, J. W., and Siegelman, S. S.: Computerized tomography in the evaluation of the soft tissue component of bony lesions of the pelvis. Skeletal Radiol., 3:144, 1978.
106. Navas-Palacio, J. J., Aparicio-Duque, R., and Valdes, M. D.: On the histogenesis of Ewing's sarcoma. An ultrastructural, immunohistochemical and cytochemical study. Cancer, 53:1882, 1984.
107. Neely, J. M., and Rogers, F. T.: Roentgenological and pathological considerations of Ewing's tumor of bone. A.J.R., 43:204, 1940.
108. Nesbit, M. E., Perez, C. A., Tefft, M., Burgert, E. O., Jr., Vietti, T. J., Kissane, J., Pritchard, D. J., and Gehan, E. A.: Multimodal therapy for the management of primary, non-metastatic Ewing's sarcoma of bone: An intergroup study. Natl. Cancer Inst. Monogr., 56:255, 1981.
109. Oberling, C.: Les reticulosarcomes et les reticuloendotheliosarcomes de la moelle osseuse (sarcomes d'Ewing). Bull. Assoc. Fr. Cancer, 17:259, 1928.
110. Oberling, C., and Railenau, C.: Nouvelles recherches sur les reticulosarcomes de la moelle osseuse (sarcomes d'Ewing). Bull. Assoc. Fr. Cancer, 21:333, 1932.
111. Olowu, A. O.: Ewing's sarcoma in a young Nigerian. Br. J. Radiol., 43:425, 1970.
112. Perez, C. A., Tefft, M., Nesbit, M., Burgert, E. O., Jr., Vietti, T., Kissane, J., Pritchard, D. J., and Gehan, E. A.: The role of radiation therapy in the management of non-metastatic Ewing's sarcoma of bone. Report of the intergroup Ewing's sarcoma study. Int. J. Padiatr. Oncol. Biol. Phys., 7:141, 1981.
113. Phelan, J. T., and Cabrera, A.: Ewing's sarcoma. Surg. Gynecol. Obstet., 118:795, 1964.
114. Phillips, R., and Higinbotham, N.: The curability of Ewing's endothelioma of bone in children. J. Pediatr., 70:391, 1967.
115. Pilepich, M. V., Vietti, T. J., Nesbit, M. E., Tefft, M., Kissane, J., Burgert, E. O., and Pritchard, D.: Radiotherapy and combination chemotherapy in advanced Ewing's sarcoma–Intergroup study. Cancer, 47:1930, 1981.
116. Pizzoli, G., Piana, G., and Rigamonti, D.: Ultrastructural diagnosis of Ewing's sarcoma. Arch. Sci. Med. (Torino), 137:477, 1980.
117. Pomeroy, T. C., and Johnson, R. E.: Combined modality therapy of Ewing's sarcoma. Cancer, 35:36, 1975.
118. Pomeroy, T. C., and Johnson, R. E.: Prognostic factors for survival in Ewing's sarcoma. A.J.R., 123:598, 1975.
119. Potdar, G. G.: Ewing's tumor. Clin. Radiol., 22:528, 1971.
120. Price, C. H. G.: A critique of Ewing's tumor of bone. In Price, C. H. G., and Ross, F. G. M. (eds.): Bone—Certain Aspects of Neoplasia (Colston Papers No. 24). London, Butterworth, 1973.
121. Prindull, G., Willert, H. G., and Notter, G.: Local therapy of rhabdomyosarcoma, osteosarcoma and Ewing's sarcoma of children and adolescents. Eur. J. Pediatr., 144:120, 1985.
122. Pritchard, D. J.: Surgical experience in the management of Ewing's sarcoma of bone. Natl. Cancer Inst. Monogr., 56:169, 1981.
123. Pritchard, D. J., Dahlin, D. C., Dauphine, R. T., Taylor, W. F., and Beabout, J. W.: Ewing's sarcoma. A clinicopathological and statistical analysis of patients surviving five years or longer. J. Bone Joint Surg., 57-A:10, 1975.
124. Reinus, W. R., Gilula, L. A., Shirley, S. K., et al.: Radiographic appearance of Ewing's sarcoma of the hands and feet. A.J.R., 144:331, 1985.
125. Reynolds, W. A., and Karo, J. J.: Radiologic diagnosis of metabolic bone disease. Orthop. Clin. North Am., 3:521, 1972.
126. Ridings, G. R.: Ewing's tumor. Radiol. Clin. North Am., 2:315, 1964.
127. Rose, J. S., Herman, G., Mendelson, D. S., and Ambinder, E. P.: Extraskeletal Ewing's sarcoma with computed tomography correlation. Skeletal Radiol., 9:234, 1983.
128. Rosen, G., Caparros, B., Mosende, C., McCormick, B., Huvos, A. G., and Marcove, R. C.: Curability of Ewing's sarcoma and considerations for future therapeutic trials. Cancer, 41:888, 1978.
129. Rosen, G., Wollner, N., Tan, C., Wu, S. J., Hajdu, S. I., Chan, W., D'Angio, G. J. D., and Murphy, M. L.: Disease-free survival in children with Ewing's sarcoma treated with radiation therapy and adjuvant four-drug sequential chemotherapy. Cancer, 33:384, 1974.
130. Rosenstock, J. G., Jones, P. M., Pearson, D., and Palmer, M. K.: Ewing's sarcoma, adjunct chemotherapy and pathologic fracture. Eur. J. Cancer, 14:799, 1978.
131. Roth, A., Touzet, P., and Rigault, P.: Association of Ewing's sarcoma with fibrous dysplasia of the tibia. Apropos of a case report. Rev. Chir. Orthop., 71:133, 1985.
132. Schajowicz, F.: Ewing's sarcoma and reticulum cell sarcoma of bone; with special reference to the histochemical demonstration of glycogen as an aid to differential diagnosis. J. Bone Joint Surg., 41-A:349, 1959.
133. Schajowicz, F.: Differential diagnosis of Ewing's sarcoma. In Price, C. H. G., and Ross, F. G. M. (eds.): Bone—Certain Aspects of Neoplasia, (Colston Papers No. 24). London, Butterworth, 1973.
134. Schifter, S., Vendelbo, L., Jensen, O. M., and Kaae, S.: Ewing's tumor following bilateral retinoblastoma. A case report. Cancer, 51:1746, 1983.

135. Schmidt, F. E., and Trummer, M. J.: Primary tumors of ribs. Ann. Thorac. Surg., 13:251, 1972.
136. Schmitt-Graff, A., Jurgens, H., Gobel, U., Ritter, J., Lubbesmeier, A., and Borchard, F.: Acute monocytic leukemia complicating combined-modality therapy for localized childhood Ewing's sarcoma. J. Cancer Res. Clin. Oncol., 102:93, 1981.
137. Schumacher, T. M., Genant, H. K., Korobkin, M., and Bovill, E. G., Jr.: Computed tomography. Its use in space-occupying lesions of the musculoskeletal system. J. Bone Joint Surg., 60-A:600, 1978.
138. Shahar, E., Frand, M., and Rotem, Y.: Ewing sarcoma simulating acute osteomyelitis. Harefuah, 98:167, 1980.
139. Sherman, R. S., and Soong, K. Y.: Ewing's sarcoma: Its roentgen classification and diagnosis. Radiology, 66:529, 1956.
140. Shirley, S. K., Gilula, L. A., Siegal, G. P., Foulkes, M. A., Kissane, J. M., and Askin, F. B.: Roentgenographic-pathologic correlation of diffuse sclerosis in Ewing's sarcoma of bone. Skeletal Radiol., 12:69, 1984.
141. Siegal, G. P., Dahlin, D. C., and Sim, F. H.: Osteoblastic osteogenic sarcoma in a 35-month-old girl. Am. J. Clin. Pathol., 63:886, 1975.
142. Siegal, G. P., Schoppe, J., Foulkes, M., Kissane, J. M., and Askin, F. B.: Ewing's sarcoma in the bones of the head and neck. Lab. Invest., 48:78, 1983.
143. Sim, F. H., Unni, K. K., Beabout, J. W., and Dahlin, D. C.: Osteosarcoma with small cells simulating Ewing's tumor. J. Bone Joint Surg., 61-A:207, 1979.
144. Simon, M. A., and Nachman, J.: The clinical utility of preoperative therapy for sarcomas. J. Bone Joint Surg., 68-A:1458, 1986.
145. Simonati, A., Vio, M., Iannucci, A. M., Bricolo, A., and Rizzuto, N.: Lumbar epidural Ewing sarcoma. Light and electron microscopic investigation. J. Neurol., 225:67, 1981.
146. Sirsat, M. V.: Some uncommon tumours in childhood. Indian J. Child Health, 10:7, 1961.
147. Springfield, D. S., and Pagliarulo, C.: Fractures of long bones previously treated for Ewing's sarcoma. J. Bone Joint Surg., 67-A:477, 1985.
148. Steinberg, G. G.: Ewing's sarcoma arising in a unicameral bone cyst. Case report. J. pediatr. Orthop., 5:97, 1985.
149. Stout, A. P.: A discussion of the pathology and histogenesis of Ewing's tumor of bone marrow. A.J.R., 50:334, 1943.
150. Swenson, P. C.: The roentgenologic aspects of Ewing's tumor of bone marrow. A.J.R., 50:343, 1943.
151. Swenson, P. C., and Teplick, J. G.: An unusual case of Ewing's sarcoma. Radiology, 45:594, 1945.
152. Taber, D. S., Libshitz, H. I., and Cohen, M. A.: Treated Ewing sarcoma: Radiographic appearance in response, recurrence, and new primaries. A.J.R., 140:753, 1983.
153. Tefft, M.: Treatment of Ewing's sarcoma with radiation therapy. Int. J. Radiol. Oncol. Biol. Phys., 7:277, 1981.
154. Tefft, M., Lattin, P. B., Jereb, B., Cham, W., Ghavimi, F., Rosen, G., Ehelby, P., Marcove, R., Murphy, M. L., and D'Angio, G. J.: Acute and late effects on normal tissues following combined chemo- and radiotherapy for childhood rhabdomyosarcoma and Ewing's sarcoma. Cancer, 37:1201, 1976.
155. Teitelbaum, S. L.: Tumors of the chest wall. Surg. Gynecol. Obstet., 129:1059, 1969.
156. Thomas, P. R., Foulkes, M. A., Gilula, L. A., Bergert, E. O., Evans, R. G., Kissane, J., Nesbit, M. E., Pritchard, D. J., Tefft, M., and Vietti, T. J.: Primary Ewing's sarcoma of the ribs: A report from the intergroup Ewing's sarcoma. Cancer, 51:1021, 1983.
157. Uehlinger, E., Botsztejn, C., and Schinz, H. R.: Ewings-sarkom und Knochenretikulosarkom: Klinik, Diagnose und Differential-Diagnose. Oncologia, 1:193, 1948.
158. Valls, J.: Ewing's sarcoma (abstract). J. Bone Joint Surg., 30-B:728, 1948.
159. Vanel, D., Contesso, G., Couanet, D., Piekarski, J. D., Sarrazin, D., and Masselot, J.: Computed tomography in the evaluation of 41 cases of Ewing's sarcoma. Skeletal Radiol., 9:8, 1982.
160. Vogt-Moykopf, I., and Krumhaar, D.: Management of primary rib tumors. Surg. Gynecol. Obstet., 125:1239, 1967.
161. Vohra, V. G.: Roentgen manifestations in Ewing's sarcoma. A study of 156 cases. Cancer, 20:727, 1967.
162. Wang, C. C., and Schulz, M. D.: Ewing's sarcoma—a study of 50 cases treated at the Massachusetts General Hospital. N. Engl. J. Med., 248:571, 1953.
163. Watt, I.: Radiology in the diagnosis and management of bone tumours. J. Bone Joint Surg., 67-B:520, 1985.
164. Weinstein, J. B., Siegel, M. J., and Griffith, R. C.: Spinal Ewing's sarcoma: Misleading appearances. Skeletal Radiol., 11:262, 1984.
165. Weis, L., Heelan, R. T., and Watson, R. C.: Computed tomography of orthopedic tumors of the pelvis and lower extremities. Clin. Orthop., 130:254, 1978.
166. Weissman, S. L., Salama, R., Papo, Y., and Loewenthal, M.: Ewing's tumor of the talus misdiagnosed as avascular necrosis. A case report. J. Bone Joint Surg., 48-A:333, 1966.
167. Wientroub, S., Michels, H., Baratz, M., Shile, R., and Salama, R.: Ewing's tumor of the cuboid bone simulating avascular necrosis. J. Bone Joint Surg., 61-A:951, 1979.
168. Willis, R. A.: Metastatic neuroblastoma in bone presenting the Ewing syndrome, with a discussion of "Ewing's sarcoma." Am. J. Pathol., 16:317, 1940.
169. Wilner, D.: Radiology of Bone Tumors and Allied Disorders. Philadelphia, Saunders, 1982.
170. Wilson, J. S., Korobkin, M., Genant, H. K., and Bovill, E. G.: Computed tomography of musculoskeletal disorders. A.J.R., 131:55, 1978.
171. Zucker, J. M., Henry-Amar, M., Sarrazin, D., Blache, R., Patte, C., and Schweisguth, O.: Intensive systemic chemotherapy in localized Ewing's sarcoma in childhood. A historical trial. Cancer, 52:415, 1983.

CHONDROSARCOMA

Chondrosarcoma occurs primarily in the adult; it is rarely encountered in the adolescent and almost never in a child. There are four different types of chondrosarcoma: primary, secondary, mesenchymal, and dedifferentiated. The great majority of cases are primary or secondary chondrosarcoma. The mesenchymal and dedifferentiated types are extremely rare. The concern of the pediatric orthopedic surgeon is the secondary chondrosarcoma that arises from either osteochondroma or enchondroma—benign cartilaginous lesions of childhood. The sarcomatous change takes place in adult life. About one fourth to one third of all chondrosarcomas are of the secondary type. Malignant transformation is more common in multiple hereditary exostosis and multiple enchondromatosis (Ollier's or Maffucci's syndrome) than in solitary exostosis or enchondroma. In exostosis, malignant transformation takes place more commonly in the regions of the pelvic or shoulder girdle, whereas the enchondromas that become malignant are usually located in the metaphyses of long bones. The chondrosarcoma is peripheral in the case of exostosis and central in that of enchondroma. The presenting complaint is a dull aching pain in the centrally located chondrosarcoma; the clinical picture of a peripheral chondrosarcoma is a mass or deformity of the limb.

Radiographic and Imaging Findings

Radiographic features of secondary chondrosarcoma show evidence of the pre-existing benign cartilaginous lesion—i.e., exostosis or enchondroma. These have been described earlier in this chapter. In brief, in osteochondroma, sarcomatous proliferation of the cartilage cells occurs from the cartilaginous cap that extends and protrudes into the surrounding soft parts. The process is indolent, and the sarcoma low-grade in nature. For a long time the radiographic picture of chondrosarcoma shows an irregular mass of calcification of varying density around the periphery of the exostosis with minimal or no permeative reaction of the underlying cortex. Eventually there will be increased radiolucency of the underlying bone, indicating destruction. Radiographically it may be difficult to differentiate chondrosarcomatous change of a sessile osteochondroma from parosteal osteogenic sarcoma; features indicating chondrosarcoma are speckled calcification, a lobulated appearance, and radiolucent destruction of underlying bone.

When an enchondroma undergoes malignant transformation into chondrosarcoma radiographic features manifest themselves early in the form of vaguely marginated areas of radiolucency that extend into the surrounding cancellous bone. With progressive increase in the tumor's size, the endosteum develops scalloped areas of destruction. Gradually the surrounding cortex is eroded. The calcified areas of central enchondroma are intermixed with areas of radiolucency indicating permeative destruction. Endosteal reactive bone may form as an internal Codman's triangle—which appears in the radiograph as reactive bone with its base along the endosteal surface of the cortex and its apex pointing toward the medullary canal.

Linear tomography will depict small areas of radiolucency with poor permeative borders, it will assist in distinguishing calcification from ossification; it will also estimate the extent of intraosseous involvement. *Computed tomography* and *nuclear magnetic resonance imaging* are of great value in delineating the thickness, irregularity and calcification of the cartilaginous cap of secondary chondrosarcoma of an exostosis and also the internal details of malignant transformation of an enchondroma. They will distinguish the painful adventitious bursa overlying an exostosis from an indolent chondrosarcoma. Computed tomography will clearly depict the intraosseous and soft-tissue extent of the lesion and will reflect the relationship of the lesion to bone. The CT scan is vital in surgical staging, as it will show the extent of excision of the tissue needed in order to achieve the desired margin.

Bone scanning with technetium-99m will show increased uptake at sites of mineralization. The increase in uptake is greater in high-grade lesions. Serial scanning may show progressive increase in uptake of the radionuclide.

Angiography is performed to detect proximity to neurovascular structures as a step in operative planning.

Pathology

On gross inspection chondrosarcoma has a lobulated appearance and seems to consist of gray unmineralized cartilage intermixed with chalky-calcified cartilage. It feels firm on palpation. There may be areas of necrosis and degeneration.

Histologic appearance varies with the grade and stage of the lesion. The malignant chondrocytes with double nuclei can be readily recognized. In low-grade lesions the cell-matrix ratio is low (i.e., relatively more matrix than cells) with the malignant chondrocytes grouped in small clusters among wide areas of chondroid matrix. In high-grade lesions the cell-matrix ratio is high with no clustering pattern; the hyperchromatic chondrocytes are multinuclear and show numerous mitoses.

Treatment

Surgical ablation of the involved part with the surgical margin depending on the stage of the disease is the treatment. Limb preservation is possible in most cases. The prognosis for survival is good.

Primary, mesenchymal, and dedifferentiated chondrosarcomas do not occur in children and adolescents. These are comprehensively discussed in the references.

References

1. Anderson, R. L., Popowitz, L., and Li, J. K. H.: An unusual sarcoma arising in a solitary osteochondroma. J. Bone Joint Surg., *51-A*:1199, 1969.
2. Arnold, P. G., and Pairolero, P. C.: Chondrosarcoma of the manubrium. Resection and reconstruction with pectoralis major muscle. Mayo Clin. Proc., *53*:54, 1978.
3. Bahr, A. L., and Gayler, B. W.: Cranial chondrosarcomas. Radiology, *124*:151, 1977.
4. Barnes, R., and Catto, M.: Chondrosarcoma of bone. J. Bone Joint Surg., *48-B*:729, 1966.
5. Bennett, G. E., and Berkheimer, G. A.: Malignant degeneration in a case of multiple benign exostoses. With a brief review of the literature. Surgery, *10*:781, 1941.
6. Bertoni, F., Present, D., Picci, P., and Bacchini, P.: Case report 301: Dedifferentiated chondrosarcoma of the upper end of the humerus. Skeletal Radiol., *13*:228, 1985.
7. Bessler, W.: Malignant potentialities of skeletal chondromas. Schweiz. Med. Wochenschr., *96*:461, 1966.
8. Blaylock, R. L., and Kempe, L. G.: Chondrosarcoma of the cervical spine. Case report. J. Neurosurg., *44*:500, 1976.
9. Block, R. S., and Burton, R. I.: Multiple chondrosarcomas in a hand: A case report. J. Hand Surg., *2*:310, 1977.
10. Buckwater, J. A.: The structure of human chondrosarcoma proteoglycans. J. Bone Joint Surg., *65-A*:958, 1983.
11. Burnett, K., and Staple, T. W.: Case report 134: Mesenchymal chondrosarcoma of the right side of the pelvis and thigh. Skeletal Radiol., *6*:58, 1981.
12. Burrows, H. J., Wilson, J. N., and Scales, J. T.: Excision of tumors of the humerus and femur with restoration by internal prosthesis. J. Bone Joint Surg., *57*:148, 1975.
13. Campanacci, M.: Giant-cell tumor and chondrosarcoma: Grading, treatment and results (studies of 209 and 131 cases). Recent Results Cancer Res., *54*:257, 1976.
14. Campanacci, M., Bertoni, F., and Capanna, R.: Dedifferentiated chondrosarcoma. Ital. J. Orthop. Traumatol., *5*:331, 1979.
15. Carpenter, E. B.: Resection of the proximal third of the femur for chondrosarcoma in a child: Replacement with a metallic prosthesis: A case report. J. Bone Joint Surg., *61-A*:628, 1979.
16. Coley, B. L.: Neoplasms of Bone. 2nd Ed. New York, Hoeber, 1960, p. 322.
17. Coley, B. L., and Higinbotham, N. L.: Secondary chondrosarcoma. Ann. Surg., *139*:547, 1954.
18. Copeland, M. M., and Geschicter, C. F.: Chondroid tumors of bone: Benign and malignant. Ann. Surg., *129*:724, 1949.
19. Cruickshank, A. H.: Chondrosarcoma of a phalanx with cutaneous metastases. J. Pathol. Bacteriol., *57*:144, 1945.
20. Culver, J. E., Jr., Sweet, D. E., and McCue, F. C.: Chondrosarcoma of the hand arising from a preexistent benign solitary enchondroma. Case report and pathologic description. Clin. Orthop., *113*:128, 1975.
21. Dahlin, D. C.: Bone Tumors. 3rd Ed. Springfield, Ill., Thomas, 1978.
22. Dahlin, D. C., and Beabout, J. W.: Dedifferentiation of low grade chondrosarcomas. Cancer, *28*:461, 1971.
23. Dahlin, D. C., and Henderson, E. D.: Chondrosarcoma. A surgical and pathological problem. Review of 212 cases. J. Bone Joint Surg., *38-A*:1025, 1956.
24. Dahlin, D. C., and Henderson, E. D.: Mesenchymal chondrosarcoma: Further observations on a new entity. Cancer, *15*:410, 1962.
25. Dahlin, D. C., and Salvador, A. H.: Chondrosarcomas of bones of the hands and feet—a study of 30 cases. Cancer, *34*:755, 1974.
26. Dowling, E. A.: Mesenchymal chondrosarcoma. J. Bone Joint Surg., *46-A*:747, 1964.
27. Eriksson, A. I., Schiller, A., and Mankin, H. J.: The management of chondrosarcoma of bone. Clin. Orthop., *153*:44, 1980.
28. Evans, H. L., Ayala, A. G., and Romsdahl, M. M.: Prognostic factors in chondrosarcoma of bone. Cancer, *40*:818, 1977.
29. Ford, L. T., and Ramsey, R. H.: Chondrosarcoma of the pelvis and shoulder girdle. South. Med. J., *55*:901, 1962.
30. Frassica, F. J., Unni, K. K., and Sim, F. H.: Case report 347: Dedifferentiated chondrosarcoma: Grade 4 fibrosarcoma arising in Grade 1 chondrosarcoma (femur). Skeletal Radiol., *15*:77, 1986.
31. Gallegher, P., Sanerkin, N. G., and Ratliff, A. H.: Chondrosarcoma: A study of 47 cases in the Bristol Bone Tumor Registry (abstract). J. Bone Joint Surg., *60-B*:442, 1978.
32. Geschickter, C. F., and Copeland, M. M.: Tumors of Bone. 3rd Ed. Philadelphia, Lippincott, 1949, pp. 111–122.
33. Ghormley, R. K.: Chondromas and chondrosarcomas of the scapula and the innominate bone. Arch. Surg., *63*:48, 1951.
34. Gitelis, S., Bertoni, F., Picci, P., and Campanacci, M.: Chondrosarcoma of bone. The experience at the Instituto Orthopedico Rizzoli. J. Bone Joint Surg., *63-A*:1248, 1981.
35. Goldenberg, R. R.: Chondrosarcoma. Bull. Hosp. Joint Dis., *15*:30, 1964.
36. Goldman, R. L.: Mesenchymal chondrosarcoma, a rare malignant chondroid tumor usually primary in bone. Report of a case arising in extraskeletal soft tissue. Cancer, *20*:1494, 1967.
37. Grabias, S., and Mankin, H. J.: Chondrosarcoma arising in histologically proved unicameral bone cyst. J. Bone Joint Surg., *56-A*:1501, 1974.
38. Habal, M. B., Snyder, H. H., Jr., and Murray, J. E.: Chondrosarcoma of the hand. Am. J. Surg., *125*:775, 1973.
39. Haber, M. H., Alter, A. H., and Wheelock, M. C.: Tumors of the hand. Surg. Gynecol. Obstet., *121*:1073, 1965.
40. Halawa, M., and Aziz, A. A.: Chondrosarcoma in fibrous dysplasia of the pelvis. A case report and review of the literature. J. Bone Joint Surg., *66-B*:760, 1984.
41. Hermann, G., Sacher, M., Lanzieri, C. F., Anderson, P. J., and Rabinowitz, J. G.: Chondrosarcoma of the spine: An unusual radiographic presentation. Skeletal Radiol., *14*:178, 1985.
42. Hertz, I., Hermann, G., Shafir, M., and Keller, R. J.: Case report 239: Chondrosarcoma of the left humerus with metastases (suggestive of the differentiated chondrosarcoma) to scapular lymph nodes and jejunum at multiple sites. Skeletal Radiol., *10*:126, 1983.
43. Higinbotham, N. L., Marcove, R. C., and Casson, P.: Hemipelvectomy: Clinical study of 100 cases with five-year follow-up on sixty patients. Surgery, *39*:706, 1966.
44. Hiki, Y., and Mankin, H. J.: Radical resection and allograft replacement in the treatment of bone tumors. J. Jpn. Orthop. Assoc., *54*:475, 1980.
45. Hudson, T. M., Manaster, B. J., Springfield, D. S., Spanier, S. S., Enneking, W. F., and Hawkins, I. F., Jr.: Radiology of medullary chondrosarcoma: Preoperative treatment planning. Skeletal Radiol., *10*:69, 1983.

46. Huvos, A. G.: Bone Tumors. Philadelphia, Saunders, 1979, pp. 206–237.
47. Huvos, A. G., Rosen, G., Dabska, M., and Marcove, R. C.: Mesenchymal chondrosarcoma. A clinicopathologic analysis of 35 patients with emphasis on treatment. Cancer, 51:1230, 1983.
48. Jacobs, P.: Case report 7: Highly malignant chondrosarcoma of unknown origin, with tumor emboli of the inferior vena cava and main pulmonary artery. Skeletal Radiol., 1:109, 1976.
49. Jaffe, H. J.: Tumors and Tumorous Conditions of the Bones and Joints. Philadelphia, Lea & Febiger, 1958, p. 314.
50. Jakobson, E., and Spjut, H. J.: Chondrosarcoma of the bones of the hand. Report of 3 cases. Acta Radiol., 54:426, 1960.
51. Jaworsski, R. C.: Dedifferentiated chondrosarcoma. An ultrastructural study. Cancer, 53:2674, 1984.
52. Johnson, J. T.: Reconstruction of the pelvic ring following tumor resection. J. Bone Joint Surg., 60-A:747, 1978.
53. Kahn, L. B.: Chondrosarcoma with dedifferentiated foci. Cancer 37:1365, 1976.
54. Knight, J. D. S.: Sarcomatous change in three brothers with diaphyseal aclasia. Br. Med. J., 1:1013, 1960.
55. Krantz, S., and Gay, B. B., Jr.: Primary chondrosarcoma of the occipital bone. A.J.R., 69:598, 1953.
56. Lansche, W. E., and Spjut, H. J.: Chondrosarcoma of the small bones of the hand. J. Bone Joint Surg., 40-A:1139, 1958.
57. Levy, W. M., Aegerter, E. E., and Kirkpatrick, J. A., Jr.: The nature of cartilaginous tumors. Radiol. Clin. North Am., 2:327, 1964.
58. Lewis, M. M., Marcove, R. C., and Bullough, P. G.: Chondrosarcoma of the foot. Cancer, 36:568, 1975.
59. Lichtenstein, L.: Bone Tumors. 5th Ed. St. Louis, Mosby, 1977, pp. 186–219.
60. Lichtenstein, L., and Bernstein, D.: Unusual benign and malignant chondroid tumors of bone. Survey of some mesenchymal cartilage tumors and malignant chondroblastic tumors, including few multicentric ones, as well as many atypical benign chondroblastomas and chondromyxoid fibromas. Cancer, 12:1142, 1959.
61. Lichtenstein, L., and Goldman, R. L.: Cartilage tumors in soft tissues, particularly in the hand and foot. Cancer, 17:1203, 1964.
62. Lichtenstein, L., and Jaffe, H. L.: Chondrosarcoma of bone. Am. J. Pathol., 19:553, 1943.
63. Lindbom, A., Soderberg, G., and Spjut, H. J.: Primary chondrosarcoma of bone. Acta Radiol., 55:81, 1961.
64. Lobe, J.: On 35-S therapy of chondrosarcoma. Radiobiol. Radiother., 16:207, 1975.
65. Longstreth, H. P., Blanco, P., and Sanes, S.: Myxochondrosarcoma of the talus. J. Bone Joint Surg., 30-A:774, 1948.
66. McCarthy, E. F., and Dorfman, H. D.: Chondrosarcoma of bone with dedifferentiation: A study of eighteen cases. Hum. Pathol., 13:36, 1982.
67. McFarland, G. B., Jr., McKinley, L. M., and Reed, R. J.: Dedifferentiation of low grade chondrosarcomas. Clin. Orthop., 122:157, 1977.
68. McLaughlin, R. E., Wang, G. J., Ritchie, W. P., and Sweet, D. E.: Protracted survival in chondrosarcoma despite an unusual metastasis that regressed spontaneously. J. Bone Joint Surg., 61-A:137, 1979.
69. Mankin, H. J., Brendze, S., and Trahan, C.: Cell population and kinetics in human chondrosarcomas. Trans. Orthop. Res. Soc., 5:153, 1980.
70. Mankin, H. J., Cantley, K. P., Lippiello, L., Schiller, A. L., and Campbell, C. J.: The biology of human chondrosarcoma. I. Description of the series, grading, and biochemical analyses. J. Bone Joint Surg., 62-A:160, 1980.
71. Mankin, H. J., Cantley, K. P., Schiller, A. L., and Lipiello, L.: The biology of human chondrosarcoma. II. Variation in chemical composition among types and subtypes of benign and malignant cartilage tumors. J. Bone Joint Surg., 62-A:176, 1980.
72. Marcove, R. C.: Chondrosarcoma: Diagnosis and treatment. Orthop. Clin. North Am., 8:811, 1977.
73. Marcove, R. C., and Francis, K. C.: Chondrosarcoma and altered carbohydrate metabolism. N. Engl. J. Med., 268:1399, 1963.
74. Marcove, R. C., and Huvos, A. G.: Cartilaginous tumors of the ribs. Cancer, 27:794, 1971.
75. Marcove, R. C., and Khafagy, M. M.: Total femur and knee replacement using a metallic prosthesis. Mem. Hosp. Clin. Bull., 4:69, 1974.
76. Marcove, R. C., Lewis, M. M., and Huvos, A. G.: En bloc upper humeral interscapulothoracic resection: The Tikhoff-Linberg procedure. Clin. Orthop., 124:219, 1977.
77. Marcove, R. C., Shoji, H., and Arlen, M.: Altered carbohydrate metabolism in cartilaginous tumors. Contemp. Surg., 5:53, 1974.
78. Marcove, R. C., Stovell, P. B., Huvos, A. G., and Bullough, P. G.: The use of cryosurgery in the treatment of low and medium grade chondrosarcoma—a preliminary report. Clin. Orthop., 122:147, 1977.
79. Marcove, R. C., Mike, V., Hutter, R. V. P., Huvos, A. G., Shoji, H., Miller, T. R., and Kosloff, R.: Chondrosarcoma of the pelvis and upper end of the femur. An analysis of factors influencing survival time in 113 cases. J. Bone Joint Surg., 56-A:561, 1972.
80. Menanteau, B. P., and Dilenge, D.: Angiographic findings in chondrosarcoma. J. Can. Assoc. Radiol., 28:193, 1977.
81. Mirra, J. M., and Marcove, R. C.: Fibrosarcomatous dedifferentiation of primary and secondary chondrosarcoma. J. Bone Joint Surg., 56-A:285, 1974.
82. Monro, R. S., and Golding, J. S. R.: Chondrosarcoma of the ilium complicating hereditary multiple exostoses. Br. J. Surg., 39:73, 1951.
83. Morton, J. J., and Mider, C. B.: Chondrosarcoma. Ann. Surg., 126:895, 1947.
84. Netherlands Committee on Bone Tumours: Radiological Atlas of Bone Tumours. Vol. 1. Baltimore, Williams & Wilkins, 1966, pp. 75–110.
85. Nielsen, H. K. L., Veth, R. P. H., Oldhoff, J., Schraffordt Koops, H., and Scales, J. T.: Resection of a peri-acetabular chondrosarcoma and reconstruction of the pelvis. A case report. J. Bone Joint Surg., 67-B:413, 1985.
86. Norman, A., and Sissons, H. A.: Radiographic hallmarks of peripheral chondrosarcoma. Radiology, 15:589, 1984.
87. O'Neal, L. W., and Ackerman, L. V.: Chondrosarcoma of bone. Cancer, 5:551, 1952.
88. Ottolenghi, C. E., and Petracchi, L. J.: Chondromyxosarcoma of the calcaneus. Report of a case of total replacement of involved bone with a homogenous refrigerated calcaneus. J. Bone Joint Surg., 35-A:211, 1953.
89. Pachter, M. R., and Albert, M.: Chondrosarcoma of the foot skeleton. J. Bone Joint Surg., 46-A:601, 1964.
90. Palmier, T. J.: Chondrosarcoma of the hand. J. Hand Surg., 9-A:332, 1984.
91. Parrish, F. F.: Allograft replacement of all or part of the end of a long bone following excision of a tumor: Report of twenty-one cases. J. Bone Joint Surg., 55-A:1, 1973.
92. Patel, M. R., Pearlman, H. S., Engler, J., and Wollowick, B. S.: Chondrosarcoma of the proximal phalanx of the finger. J. Bone Joint Surg., 59-A:401, 1977.
93. Pavon, S. J., Bullough, P. G., and Marcove, R. C.: Mesenchymal chondrosarcoma. N.Y. State J. Med., 71:1662, 1971.
94. Pepe, A. J., Kuhlmann, R. F., and Miller, D. B.:

Mesenchymal chondrosarcoma. A case report. J. Bone Joint Surg., 59-A:256, 1977.
95. Peltier, L. L.: The treatment of chondrosarcoma. Prog. Clin. Cancer, 2:289, 1966.
96. Phelan, J. T., and Cabrera, A.: Chondrosarcoma of bone. Surg. Gynecol. Obstet., 119:42, 1964.
97. Phemister, D. B.: Chondrosarcoma of bone. Surg. Gynecol. Obstet., 50:216, 1930.
98. Phemister, D. B.: Chondrosarcoma of bone. Surg. Gynecol. Obstet., 70:355, 1940.
99. Pinstein, M. L., Sebes, J. I., and Scott, R. L.: Transarticular extension of chondrosarcoma. A.J.R., 142:779, 1984.
100. Pope, T. L., Jr., McLaughlin, R., Wanebo, H. J., Williamson, B. R. J., and Fechner, R. E.: Case report 281: Low grade cartilaginous tumor with "skip" lesion. Skeletal Radiol., 12:134, 1984.
101. Reiter, F. B., Ackerman, L. V., and Staple, T. W.: Central chondrosarcoma of the appendicular skeleton. Radiology, 105:525, 1972.
102. Robb, J. A.: Chondrosarcoma of bone with "dedifferentiation." Hum. Pathol., 13:964, 1982.
103. Roberg, O. T., Jr.: Chondrosarcoma. The relation of structure and location to the clinical course. Surg. Gynecol. Obstet., 61:68, 1935.
104. Romsdahl, M. M., Evans, H. L., and Ayala, A. G.: Surgical treatment of chondrosarcoma. In MD Anderson Hospital and Tumor Institute. Management of Primary Bone and Soft Tissue Tumors. Chicago, Year Book, 1977.
105. Rywlin, A. M.: Chondrosarcoma of bone with "dedifferentiation." Hum. Pathol., 13:963, 1982.
106. Salvador, A. H., Beabout, J. W., and Dahlin, D. C.: Mesenchymal chondrosarcoma. Cancer, 28:605, 1971.
107. Sanerkin, N. G., and Gallagher, P.: A review of the behavior of chondrosarcoma of bone. J. Bone Joint Surg., 61-B:395, 1979.
108. Sbarbaro, J. L., Jr., and Straub, L. R.: Chondrosarcoma in a phalanx. Report of a case. Am. J. Surg., 100:751, 1960.
109. Schajowicz, F.: Juxtacortical chondrosarcoma. J. Bone Joint Surg., 59-B:473, 1977.
110. Schajowicz, F., and Bessone, J. E.: Chondrosarcoma in three brothers. J. Bone Joint Surg., 49-A:129, 1967.
111. Schajowicz, F., and Cambiaggi, J. E.: Chondrosarcoma de mano. Bol. Trab. Soc. Argent. Ortop. Traumatol., 25:191, 1961.
112. Scott, W. W., Fishman, E. K., and Lubbe, W. J.: Case report 259: Chondrosarcoma of the right trapezoid bone. Skeletal Radiol., 11:137, 1984.
113. Shellito, J. G., and Dockerty, M. B.: Cartilaginous tumors of the hand. Surg. Gynecol. Obstet., 86:465, 1948.
114. Smith, W. S., and Simon, M. A.: Segmental resection for chondrosarcoma. J. Bone Joint Surg., 57-A:1097, 1975.
115. Solomon, L.: Chondrosarcoma in hereditary multiple exostosis. S. Afr. Med. J., 48:671, 1974.
116. Spjut, H. J., Dorfman, H. D., Fechner, R. E., and Ackerman, L. V.: Atlas of Tumor Pathology, Second Series, Fascicle 5. Tumors of Bone and Cartilage. Washington, D.C., Armed Forces Institute of Pathology, 1971, pp. 84–116.
117. Steel, H. H.: Partial or complete resection of the hemipelvis: An alternative to hind quarter amputation for periacetabular chondrosarcoma of the pelvis. J. Bone Joint Surg., 60-A:719, 1978.
118. Steiner, B.: Total spondylectomy in chondrosarcoma arising from the 7th thoracic vertebra. J. Bone Joint Surg., 52-B:288, 1971.
119. Steiner, G., Greenspan, A., and Jahss, M.: Myxoid chondrosarcoma of the os calcis: A case report. Foot Ankle, 5:84, 1984.
120. Steiner, O. C., Mirra, J. M., and Bullough, P. G.: Mesenchymal chondrosarcoma. A study of the ultrastructure. Cancer, 32:926, 1973.
121. Sun, T. C., Swee, R. G., Shives, T. C., and Unni, K. K.: Chondrosarcoma in Maffucci's syndrome. J. Bone Joint Surg., 67-A:1214, 1985.
122. Thompson, V. P., and Steggall, C. T.: Chondrosarcoma of proximal portion of femur treated by resection and bone replacement; six year result. J. Bone Joint Surg., 38-A:357, 1957.
123. Tiwisina, T.: Dyschondroplasie (Ollier) mit multiplen Haemangiomen und ortlicher maligner Entartung (Chondrosarkom). Beitr. Klin. Chir., 188:8, 1954.
124. Unni, K. K., Dahlin, D. C., Beabout, J. W., and Sim, F. H.: Chondrosarcoma: Clear-cell variant. A report of sixteen cases. J. Bone Joint Surg., 58-A:676, 1976.
125. Vanel, D., Coffre, C., Zemoura, L., and Oberlin, O.: Chondrosarcoma in children subsequent ot other malignant tumours in different locations. Skeletal Radiol., 11:96, 1984.
126. Weiland, A. J., Daniel, R. K., and Riley, L. H., Jr.: Application of free vascularized bone graft in the treatment of malignant or aggressive bone tumors. Johns Hopkins Med. J., 140:85, 1977.
127. Wilkinson, R. H., and Kirkpatrick, J. A.: Case report 14. Low grade chondrosarcoma of femur in a child. Skeletal Radiol., 1:127, 1976.
128. Williamson, A. W.: A case of chondrosarcoma of the fifth metatarsal. Br. J. Surg., 48:337, 1960.
129. Wilson, P. D., Jr., and Lance, E. M.: Surgical reconstruction of the skeleton following segmental resection for bone tumors. J. Bone Joint Surg., 47-A:1629, 1965.
130. Wood, W., and Mankin, H. J.: Pelvic resection as an alternative to hemipelvectomy in the treatment of malignant tumors. In press.
131. Wu, K. K., and Kelly, A. P.: Periosteal (juxtacortical) chondrosarcoma: Report of a case occurring in the hand. J. Hand Surg., 2:314, 1977.
132. Wu, K. K., Frost, H. M., and Guise, E. E.: A chondrosarcoma of the hand arising from an asymptomatic benign solitary enchondroma of 40 years' duration. J. Hand Surg., 8:317, 1983.

FIBROSARCOMA AND MALIGNANT FIBROUS HISTIOCYTOMA

These are rare lesions that do not occur in children.

METASTATIC TUMORS OF BONE

Neuroblastoma

Neuroblastoma is a malignant round-cell tumor that is common in infants and children under five years of age. It arises from any part of the sympathetic nervous system, usually from the medulla of the adrenal gland. Metastatic spread is via the lymphatic and hematogenous routes, with the liver, lymph nodes, and skeleton being predilected sites. The bony metastases are usually multiple, though on occasion, there may be a single focus.

In the radiogram the metastatic bone lesions are characterized by "punched-out" osteolytic

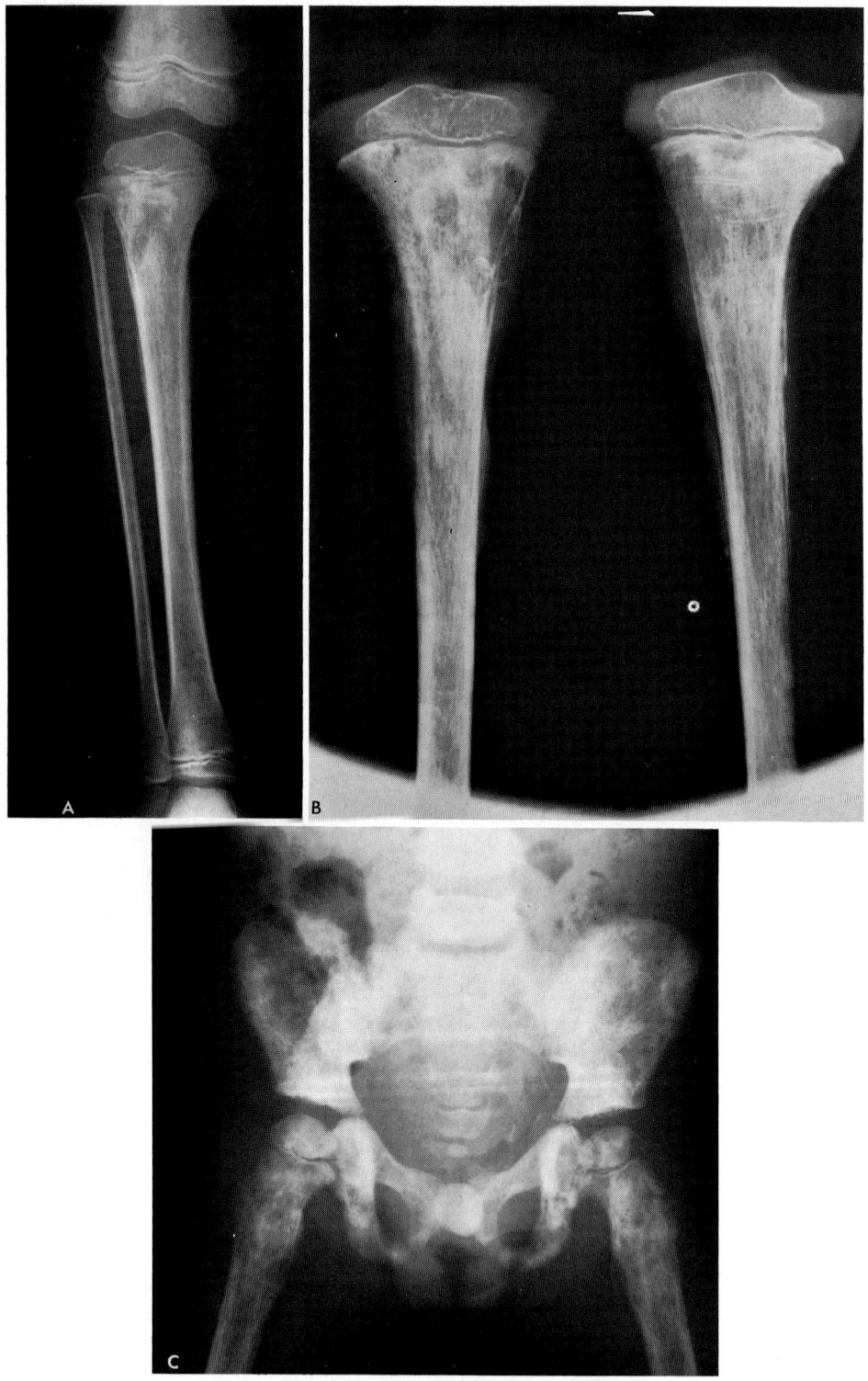

FIGURE 3–339. Bone metastasis from neuroblastoma.

A to **C.** Radiograms of right leg, of disarticulated tibiae (obtained at autopsy), and of pelvis show multiple rarefying destructive lesions.

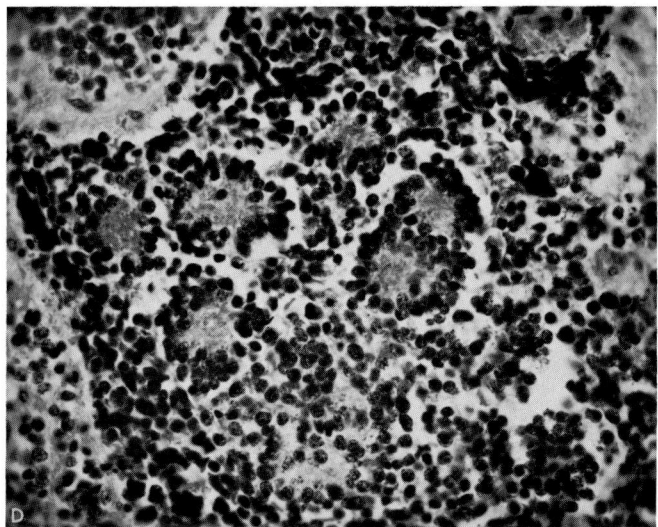

FIGURE 3–339 Continued. Bone metastasis from neuroblastoma.

D. Photomicrograph showing the histologic appearance of the tissue removed from a metastatic area (× 400). Note the roundish tumor cells and the rosette formations.

areas with some reactive new bone formation (Figs. 3–339 and 3–340). Cranial bones show extensive mottling and separation of the sutures. Pathologic fractures may occur.

A solitary lesion may be mistaken for a primary neoplasm of bone, such as Ewing's sarcoma. Bone marrow smears will disclose neoplastic cells in the presence of skeletal metastases. Another diagnostic aid in neuroblastoma is the finding of elevated levels of catecholamines and their metabolites (3-methoxy-4-hydroxymandelic acid (VMA) and homovanillic acid (HVA) in the urine.

Treatment of neuroblastoma consists of surgical excision of the tumor and postoperative irradiation, combined with chemotherapeutic agents such as vincristine sulfate and cyclophosphamide (Cytoxan). The rate of cure is about 30 per cent. When neuroblastoma has metastasized to bone the prognosis is very grave, the condition being almost uniformly fatal.

Wilms' Tumor (Nephroblastoma)

This presents as an abdominal mass usually in infants and children under three years of age. Treatment consists of prompt, radical nephrectomy. The tumor may occur bilaterally, and the presence and function of the opposite kidney should be established by intravenous pyelography. Actinomycin D and irradiation are given following surgery. Metastases to the skeleton may occur (Fig. 3–341). The overall survival rate is 30 to 50 per cent; in patients under one year of age, however, the survival rate is approximately 80 per cent.

References

NEUROBLASTOMA

1. Altman, A. J., and Baehner, R. L.: Favorable prognosis for survival in children with coincident opso-myoclonus and neuroblastoma. Cancer, 37:846, 1976.
2. Anders, D., Kindermann, G., and Pfeifer, U.: Metastasizing fetal neuroblastoma with involvement of the placenta simulating fetal erythroblastosis. J. Pediatr., 82:50, 1973.
3. Anderson, O. W.: Neuroblastoma with skeletal metastases and apparent recovery. Am. J. Dis. Child., 83:782, 1953.
4. Arenson, E. B., Jr., Hutter, J. J., Restuccia, R. D., and Holton, C. P.: Neuroblastoma in father and son. J.A.M.A., 235:727, 1976.
5. Aterman, K., and Schueller, E. F.: Maturation of neuroblastoma to ganglioneuroma. Am. J. Dis. Child., 120:217, 1970.
6. Beck, S. M., Jr., and Howard, P. J.: Neuroblastoma. Am. J. Dis. Child., 82:325, 1951.
7. Berger, P. E., Kuhn, J. P., and Munschauer, R. W.: Computed tomography and ultrasound in the diagnosis and management of neuroblastoma. Radiology, 128:663, 1978.
8. Bond, J. V.: Abdominal pain caused by metastatic neuroblastoma. Clin. Oncol., 1:97, 1975.
9. Boyd, W.: Three tumors arising from neuroblasts. Arch. Surg., 12:1031, 1926.
10. Breslow, N., and McCann, B.: Statistical estimation of prognosis for children with neuroblastoma. Cancer Res., 31:2098, 1971.
11. Carter, T., Gabrielson, T., and Abell, M.: Mechanism of split cranial sutures in metastatic neuroblastoma. Radiology, 91:467, 1968.
12. Chatten, J., and Voorhess, M. L.: Familial neuroblastoma. N. Engl. J. Med., 277:1230, 1967.

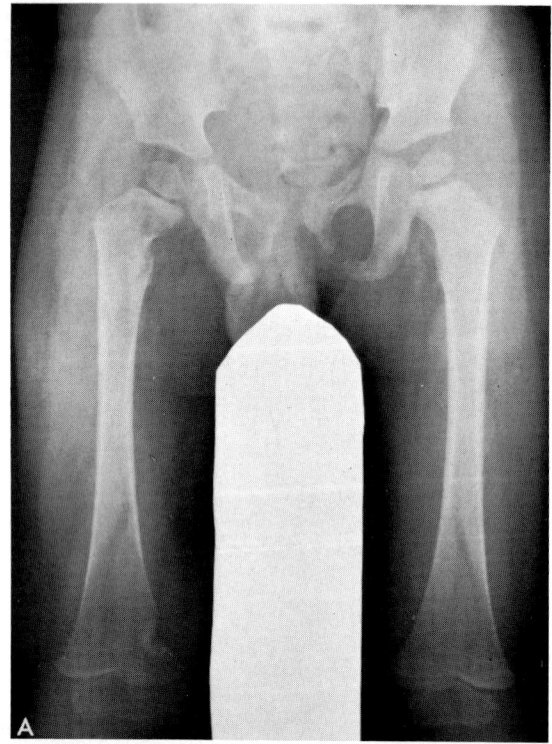
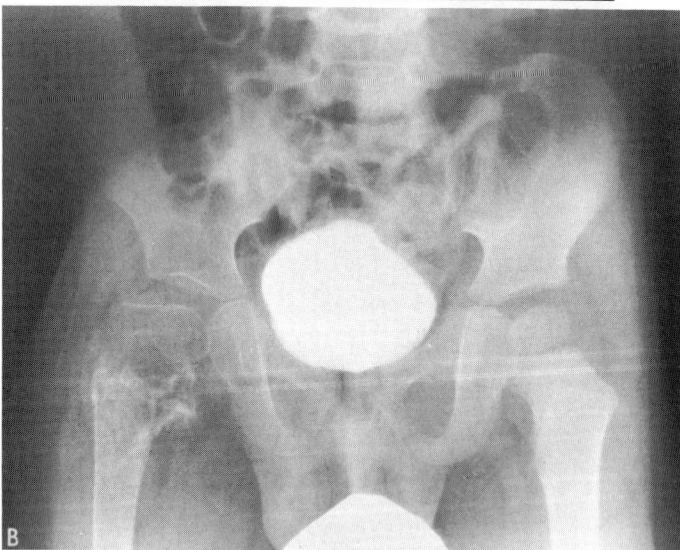

FIGURE 3–340. Neuroblastoma in a three-year-old boy who complained of pain in the right thigh of six weeks' duration.

A. Radiograms of femora showing the rarefying destructive lesions on the medial aspect of right femoral neck and distal metaphysis. **B.** Radiogram of hips a month later. Despite chemotherapy and irradiation, the area of bone destruction has rapidly increased in size.

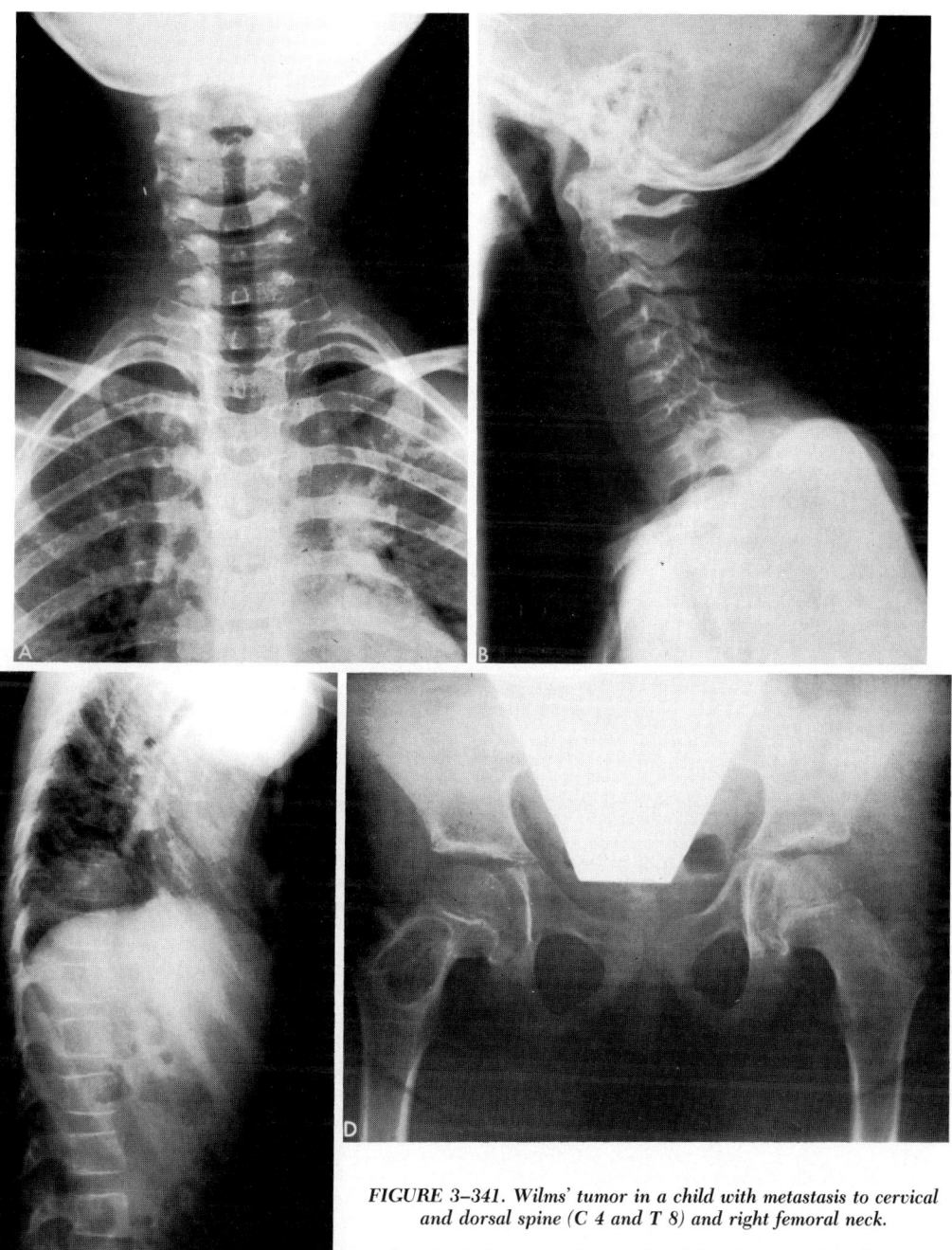

FIGURE 3–341. Wilms' tumor in a child with metastasis to cervical and dorsal spine (C 4 and T 8) and right femoral neck.

A to **D**. Radiograms of cervical and dorsal spine and both hips.

13. Chont, L. K.: Neuroblastoma and its roentgen diagnosis: Report of 8 cases. A.J.R., 46:809, 1941.
14. Colville, H. C., and Willis, R. A.: Neuroblastoma metastases in bones, with criticism of Ewing's endothelioma. Am. J. Pathol., 9:421, 1933.
15. D'Angio, G. J., Evans, A. E., and Koop, C. E.: Special pattern of widespread neuroblastoma with a favorable prognosis. Lancet, 1:1046, 1971.
16. D'Angio, G. J., Loken, M., and Nesbit, M.: Radionuclear (75Se) identification of tumor in children with neuroblastoma. Radiology, 93:615, 1969.
17. Dargeon, H. W.: Problems in the prognosis of neuroblastoma. A.J.R., 83:551, 1960.
18. Dargeon, H. W.: Neuroblastoma. J. Pediatr., 61:456, 1962.
19. Evans, A. E.: Neuroblastoma. Some children are best left on their own. Medical World News, p. 23, May 7, 1971.
20. Evans, A. E., D'Angio, G. J., and Randolph, J.: A proposed staging for children with neuroblastoma. Cancer, 27:374, 1971.
21. Evans, A. E., Blore, J., Hadley, R., and Tanindi, S.: The LaBrosse spot test: A practical aid in the diagnosis and management of children with neuroblastoma. Pediatrics, 47:913, 1971.
22. Excelby, P.: Solid tumors in children. Wilms' tumor, neuroblastoma and soft tissue sarcomas. CA, 28:146, 1978.
23. Farber, S.: Neuroblastoma (abstract). Am. J. Dis. Child., 60:749, 1940.
24. Farber, S.: Chemotherapy of disseminated neuroblastoma in children. Am. J. Dis. Child., 82:239, 1951.
25. Farber, S., Gross, R., and Martin, L.: Neuroblastoma sympatheticum. Pediatrics, 23:1179, 1959.
26. Feldman, J. A., and Morales, J. O.: Gallium scanning for neuroblastoma. J. Pediatr. Surg., 10:553, 1975.
27. Friedland, G. W., and Crowe, J. E.: Neuroblastoma and other adrenal neoplasms. In Parker, B. R., and Castellino, R. A. (eds.): Pediatric Oncologic Radiology. St. Louis, Mosby, 1977, p. 267.
28. Goldring, D.: Neuroblastoma sympatheticum with metastases. J. Pediatr., 38:231, 1951.
29. Griff, L. C., and Griff, R. E.: Neuroblastoma: Emphasis on the mediastinal neuroblastoma. A.J.R., 103:19, 1968.
30. Gross, R. E., Farber, S., and Martin, L. W.: Neuroblastoma sympatheticum: A study and report of 217 cases. Pediatrics, 23:1179, 1959.
31. Guin, G. H., Gilbert, E. F., and Jones, B.: Incidental neuroblastoma in infants. Am. J. Clin. Pathol., 51:126, 1969.
32. Hamilton, P. K.: Neuroblastoma of spinal cord. Am. J. Clin. Pathol., 21:846, 1951.
33. Hansman, C. F., and Girdany, B. R.: The roentgenographic findings associated with neuroblastoma. J. Pediatr., 51:621, 1957.
34. Harrison, J., Myers, M. Rowen, M., and Vermund, H.: Results of combination chemotherapy, surgery and radiotherapy in children with neuroblastoma. Cancer, 34:485, 1974.
35. Hauser, H.: Radiosensitive neuroblastoma. A.J.R., 31:234, 1934.
36. Helson, L., and Namerow, D. M.: Clinical observation on neuroblastoma diagnosis. Clin. Bull. MSKCC, 1972.
37. Helson, L., Watson, R. C., Benua, R. S., et al.: F-18 radioisotope scanning of metastatic bone lesions in children with neuroblastoma. A.J.R., 115:191, 1972.
38. Henle, C. -B.: Roentgen findings in neuroblastoma. A.J.R., 20:414, 1928.
39. Hinton, P., and Buschke, R.: Neuroblastoma in children: 42 cases. Radiol. Clin. Biol., 37:19, 1968.
40. Holmes, G. W., and Dresser, R.: Roentgenologic observations in neuroblastoma. J.A.M.A., 91:1246, 1928.
41. Hope-Stone, H. F.: Extra-adrenal neuroblastoma. Br. J. Surg., 48:424, 1961.
42. Howmam-Giles, R. B., Gilday, D. L., and Ash, J. M.: Radionuclide skeletal survey in neuroblastoma. Radiology, 131:497, 1979.
43. James, D. H., Hustu, O., Wrenn, E. L., and Pinkel, D.: Combination chemotherapy of childhood neuroblastoma. J.A.M.A., 194:103, 1965.
44. Judisch, J. M., and McIntyre, P. A.: Recognition of metastatic neuroblastoma by scanning the reticuloendothelial system. Johns Hopkins Med. J., 130:83, 1972.
45. Kadish, S., Goodman, M., and Wang, C. C.: Olfactory neuroblastoma. Cancer, 37:1571, 1976.
46. Karsner, H. T.: Distribution of metastases of neuroblastoma of adrenal. Trans. Assoc. Am. Phys., 57:209, 1942.
47. Kaufman, R. A., Thrall, J. H., Keyes, J. W., Brown, M. L., and Zakem, J. F.: False negative bone scans in neuroblastoma metastatic to the ends of the long bones. A.J.R., 130:131, 1978.
48. Keating, J. W., and Cromwell, L. D.: Remote effects of neuroblastoma. A.J.R., 131:299, 1978.
49. Kelly, F.: Prognosis in extra-abdominal neuroblastoma. Acta Radiol., 6:100, 1967.
50. Kincaid, O. W., Hodgson, J. R., and Dockerty, M. B.: Neuroblastoma: Roentgenologic and pathologic study. A.J.R., 78:420, 1957.
51. King, R. L., Storaasli, J. P., and Bolande, R. P.: Neuroblastoma: Review of 28 cases and presentation of 2 cases with metastases and long survival. A.J.R., 85:733, 1961.
52. Klein, J.: Neuroblastoma of the adrenal, with multiple metastases. Am. J. Med. Sci., 184:491, 1932.
53. Koop, C. E.: Role of surgery in resectable, non-resectable and metastatic neuroblastoma. J.A.M.A., 205:157, 1968.
54. Koop, C. E.: Neuroblastoma: Two-year survival and treatment correlations. J. Pediatr. Surg., 3:178, 1968.
55. Koop, C. E., and Schnauffer, L.: The management of abdominal neuroblastoma. Cancer, 35:905, 1975.
56. Koop, C. E., Kiesewetter, W. B., and Horn, R. C., Jr.: Neuroblastoma in childhood—an evaluation of surgical management. Pediatrics, 16:652, 1955.
57. Koop, C. E., Kiesewetter, W. B., and Horn, R. C., Jr.: Neuroblastoma in childhood. Surgery, 38:272, 1955.
58. Kouyoumdjian, A. O., and McDonald, J. J.: Association of congenital adrenal neuroblastoma with multiple anomalies. Cancer, 4:784, 1951.
59. Kwartin, B., and Twis, J. R.: Malignant neuroblastoma. Am. J. Dis. Child., 34:61, 1927.
60. Larimer, R. C.: Neuroblastoma (sympathogonioma) of the adrenal in the newborn infant. J. Pediatr., 34:365, 1949.
61. Lederer, M.: Neuroblastoma of the adrenal gland. J. Cancer Res., 10:377, 1926.
62. Lehman, E. P.: Adrenal neuroblastoma in infancy—fifteen year survival. Ann. Surg., 95:473, 1932.
63. Oberman, H. A., and Rice, D. H.: Olfactory neuroblastomas. Cancer, 38:2494, 1976.
64. Parsons, P. B., and Platt, L.: Calcification in abdominal neuroblastoma. Report of two cases. A.J.R., 44:175, 1940.
65. Pascual-Castroviejo, I., Lopez-Martin, V., Rodriguez-Costa, T., and Pascual-Pascual, J. I.: Radiological and anatomical aspects of the cranial metastasis of neuroblastomas. Neuroradiology, 9:33, 1975.
66. Phillips, R.: Neuroblastoma. Ann. R. Coll. Surg. Engl., 12:29, 1953.
67. Pochedly, C.: Neuroblastoma. Littleton, Mass., Publishing Science Group, 1976.
68. Priebec, C. J., and Clatworthy, H. W.: Neuroblastoma. Arch. Surg., 95:538, 1967.
69. Redman, J. L., Agerty, H. J. A., Barthmaier, O. F., and Fisher, H. R.: Adrenal neuroblastoma. Am. J. Dis. Child., 56:1097, 1938.
70. Reilly, D., Nesbit, M. E., and Krivit, W.: Cure of

three patients who had skeletal metastases in disseminated neuroblastoma. Pediatrics, 41:47, 1968.
71. Ritter, S. A.: Neuroblastoma of the intestine. Am. J. Pathol., 1:519, 1925.
72. Roberts, F. F., and Lee, K. R.: Familial neuroblastoma presenting as multiple tumors. Radiology, 118:133, 1975.
73. Rosenfield, N., and Treves, S.: Osseous and extraosseous uptake of fluorine-18 and technetium 99m polyphosphate in children with neuroblastoma. Radiology, 111:127, 1974.
74. Rosengren, J. -E., Jing, B. -S., Wallace, S., and Danzigler, J.: Radiographic features of olfactory neuroblastoma. A.J.R., 132:945, 1979.
75. Ross, P.: Calcification in liver metastases from neuroblastoma. Radiology, 85:1074, 1965.
76. Rypins, E. L.: Roentgen diagnosis of neuroblastoma in children. A.J.R., 37:325, 1937.
77. Schneider, K. M., Becker, J. M., and Krasna, I. H.: Neonatal neuroblastoma. Pediatrics, 36:359, 1965.
78. Seaman, W. B., and Eagleton, M. D.: Radiation therapy of neuroblastoma. Radiology, 68:1, 1957.
79. Sinks, L. F., and Woodruff, M. W.: Chemotherapy of neuroblastoma. J.A.M.A., 205:161, 1968.
80. Startz, I. S., and Abrams, J.: Neuroblastoma: A childhood type of malignant tumor of the sympathetic nervous system. Radiology, 30:232, 1938.
81. Sturtevant, C. N., and Kelly, T. C.: Neurocytoma of the left suprarenal gland; with metastases to liver, skull and bones. Am. J. Dis. Child., 33:590, 1927.
82. Sutow, W. W.: Prognosis of neuroblastoma in childhood. Am. J. Dis. Child., 96:299, 1958.
83. Tefft, M., and Wittenborg, M. H.: Radiotherapeutic management of neuroblastoma in childhood. J.A.M.A., 205:159, 1968.
84. Wahl, H. R.: Neuroblastomata; with study of a case illustrating the three types that arise from sympathetic system. J. Med. Res., 30:205, 1914.
85. Williams, C. M., and Greer, M.: Homovanillic acid and vanilmandelic acid in diagnosis of neuroblastoma. J.A.M.A., 183:134, 1963.
86. Wilner, D: Radiology of Bone Tumors and Allied Disorders. Philadelphia, W. B. Saunders, 1982.
87. Wittenborg, M. H.: Roentgen therapy in neuroblastoma: Review of 73 cases. Radiology, 54:679, 1950.
88. Wong, K. Y., Hanenson, I. B., and Lampkin, B. C.: Familial neuroblastoma. Am. J. Dis. Child., 121:415, 1971.
89. Wright, J. H.: Neurocytoma or neuroblastoma: A kind of tumor not generally recognized. J. Exp. Med., 12:556, 1910.
90. Wyatt, G. M., and Farber, S.: Neuroblastoma sympatheticum; roentgenological appearances and radiation treatment. A.J.R., 46:485, 1941.
91. Young, L. W., Rubin, P., and Hanson, R. E.: The extra-adrenal neuroblastoma: High radiocurability and diagnostic accuracy. A.J.R., 108:75, 1970.

WILMS' TUMOR

1. Aron, B. S.: Wilms' tumor: A clinical study of eighty-one patients. Cancer, 33:637, 1974.
2. Beckwith, J. B., and Palmer, N. F.: Histopathology and prognosis of Wilms' tumor. Cancer, 41:1937, 1978.
3. Berdon, W. E., Wigger, H. J., and Baker, D. H.: Benign tumors to be distinguished from Wilms' tumor: Report of three cases. A.J.R., 118:18, 1973.
4. Boxer, L. A., and Smith, D. L.: Wilms' tumor prior to onset of hemihypertrophy. Am. J. Dis. Child., 120:564, 1970.
5. Breslow, N. E., Palmer, N. F., Hill, L. R., Buring, J., and D'Angio, G. J.: Wilms' tumor: Prognostic factors for patients without metastases at diagnosis. Cancer, 41:1577, 1978.
6. Cassady, J. R., Jaffe, N., Paed, D., and Filler, R. M.: The increasing importance of radiation therapy in the improved prognosis of children with Wilms' tumor. Cancer, 39:825, 1977.
7. Cope, J. R., Roylance, J., and Gordon, I. R.: The radiological features of Wilms' tumour. Clin. Radiol., 23:331, 1972.
8. D'Angio, G. J.: Management of children with Wilms' tumor. Cancer, 30:1528, 1972.
9. Dickey, J. B., and Chandler, L. R.: Embryoma of the kidney in children. Pediatrics, 4:197, 1949.
10. Edelstein, G., Webb, R. S., Romsdahl, M. M., and Arboit, J. M.: Extrarenal Wilms' tumor. Am. J. Surg., 109:509, 1965.
11. Exelby, P.: Solid tumors in children. Wilms' tumor, neuroblastoma and soft tissue sarcomas. CA, 28:146, 1978.
12. Fleming, I. D., and Johnson, W. W.: Clinical and pathologic staging as a guide in the management of Wilms' tumor. Cancer, 26:660, 1970.
13. Griffel, M.: Wilms' tumor in New York State. Cancer, 40:3140, 1977.
14. Grossman, H.: Observing the growth of Wilms' tumor. Radiology, 121:697, 1976.
15. Heaston, D. K., Libshitz, H. I., and Chan, R. C.: Skeletal effects of megavoltage irradiation in survivors of Wilms' tumor. A.J.R., 133:389, 1979.
16. Hunig, R., and Kinser, J.: Ultrasonic diagnosis of Wilms' tumors. A.J.R., 117:119, 1973.
17. Kaufman, R. A., Holt, J. F., and Heidelberger, K. P.: Calcification in primary and metastatic Wilms' tumor. A.J.R., 130:783, 1978.
18. Meadows, A. T., Litchtenfeld, J. L., and Koop, C. E.: Wilms' tumor in three children of a woman with congenital hemihypertrophy. N. Engl. J. Med., 291:23, 1974.
19. Meng, C., and Elkin, M.: Angiographic manifestations of Wilms' tumor. A.J.R., 105:95, 1969.
20. Merten, D. F., Yang, S. S., and Bernstein, J.: Wilms' tumor in adolescence. Cancer, 37:1532, 1976.
21. Mixter, C. G.: Malignant tumors of the kidney in infancy and childhood. Ann. Surg., 96:1017, 1932.
22. Pearson, D., Duncan, W. B., and Pointon, R. C. S.: Wilms' tumours: A review of 96 consecutive cases. Br. J. Radiol., 37:154, 1964.
23. Perlman, M., Levin, M., and Wittels, B.: Syndrome of fetal gigantism, renal hamartomas, and nephroblastomatosis with Wilms' tumor. Cancer, 35:1212, 1975.
24. Peterman, M. G.: Suprarenal tumor with metastases. Am. J. Dis. Child., 43:655, 1932.
25. Schneider, B., Sagerman, R. H., Wolff, J. A., and Santulli, T. V.: Wilms' tumor: The evolution of a treatment program. A.J.R., 108:92, 1970.
26. Swenson, O.: Wilms' tumor and neuroblastoma. In Pediatric Surgery. New York, Appleton-Century-Crofts, 1969, p. 874.
27. Wara, W. M., Margolis, L. W., Smith, W. B., Kushner, J., and deLorimier, A.: Treatment of metastatic Wilms' tumor. Radiology, 112:695, 1974.
28. Westra, P., Kieffer, S. A., and Mosser, D. G.: Wilms' tumor. A.J.R., 100:214, 1967.
29. Wolff, J. A.: Advances in the treatment of Wilms' tumor. Cancer, 35:901, 1975.
30. Wolff, J. A., Krivit, W., Newton, W. A., Jr., and D'Angio, G. J.: Single versus multiple dose actinomycin D therapy of Wilms' tumor. Pediatr. Radiol., 3:81, 1975.
31. Wolff, J. A., D'Angio, G., Hartman, J., Krivit, W., and Newton, W. A., Jr.: Long-term evaluation of single versus multiple courses of actinomycin-D therapy of Wilms' tumor. N. Engl. J. Med., 290:84, 1974.
32. Woodard, J. R., Gay, B. B., and Rutherford, C. R., Jr.: The incipient Wilms' tumor. Pediatr. Radiol., 3:81, 1975.

4. Joints

A *joint* is defined as the connection between any of the rigid components of the skeleton. It is classified by the type of tissue that unites the parts as *synostosis* (bone), *syndesmosis* (fibrous tissue), *synchondrosis* (cartilage), or *diarthrosis* (synovium).

Orthopedic surgery is primarily concerned with the diarthrodial, or synovial, joints. A diarthrodial joint has hyaline cartilage covering its articular ends and synovial membrane lining its interior. Synovial membrane is a specially adapted connective tissue that forms the synovial fluid, which serves to lubricate the joint and provide nourishment to the articular cartilage. Synovium normally does not cover articular cartilage. The bones are held together by a fibrous capsule and by ligaments, which, along with the motor strength of activating muscles and the shape of the articular surfaces, give the joint stability.

Synovial fluid is a dialysate of plasma that contains a sulfate-free mucopolysaccharide called hyaluronic acid, a substance most probably secreted by the synovial cells. The exact mechanism of production of hyaluronic acid is not fully understood. Absorption from the joint cavity takes place through the semipermeable synovial membrane, and the route of removal is primarily vascular, though it may be lymphatic.[1, 8] Particles over 100 mµ in diameter have difficulty in crossing the synovial barrier. The combination of the highly viscous fluid and the shape of the articular body ends protects the hyaline cartilaginous surfaces from extreme physical stress from body weight and muscular forces.[11, 12]

The articular surfaces of synovial joints are incongruous, and they do not fit perfectly throughout the whole range of motion, only parts of their opposing ends being in contact in any one position. Therefore, the size of the intra-articular spaces through which the synovial fluid circulates during motion changes. This also permits the development of intra-articular hydrostatic pressure, which keeps the joint surfaces apart, with an intervening thin film of synovial fluid rather than the hyaline cartilage absorbing the forces of friction.

Intra-articular pressure in normal and abnormal joints has been studied by several authors.[4, 9, 10, 20]

The positions of minimum intra-articular pressure were determined by the simple manometric method by Eyring and Murray.[9] In the hip joint this was found to be 30 to 65 degrees of flexion, 15 degrees of abduction, and 15 degrees of lateral rotation. Intra-articular pressure was increased by extension, wide abduction, and medial rotation of the hip. In the knee, the pressure was minimal in a broad range of midflexion (25 to 60 degrees); hyperextension elevated the intra-articular pressure. In the ankle the position of minimal pressure was 15 degrees of plantar flexion, with the subtalar joint in midposition. In the shoulder joint the position of minimal pressure was one of neutral flexion, neutral rotation, and 30 to 65 degrees of abduction. In the elbow joint the pressure was minimal between 30 and 70 degrees of flexion—this was independent of pronation and supination of the forearm. In the wrist, the pressure was minimal in the neutral position.[21]

That articular cartilage derives the greater part of its nutrition from synovial fluid was suggested by the observation of Strangeways, who noted that loose bodies in joints increase in size as a result of growth of their cartilaginous portion.[21] In the immature skeleton, the articular cartilage receives its nutrition by diffusion of nutrients from the synovial fluid in the joint cavity as well as from the underlying cancellous bone. In the mature skeleton, however, synovial fluid is the only source of nutrition, the "tidemark" at the osteochondral junction serving as a permanent barrier between the articular cartilage and subchondral bone.[3, 16]

More detailed review of the structure, mechanics, and pathophysiology of diarthrodial joints is to be found in the essays of Barnett and Hamerman and their associates.[2, 13, 14]

DIAGNOSTIC CONSIDERATIONS

Symptoms arising from a joint are ordinarily associated with motion and with the stresses of standing and walking. Pain is an outstanding feature, as joints have numerous nerve endings in the synovial membrane and capsule. Oversecretion of synovial fluid produces distention of the joint capsule. Excess of synovial fluid can be easily seen and palpated in superficial joints. In later stages of inflammation, proliferation and general thickening of the synovium take place, which can be detected by careful palpation. Frequently, active and passive motion of the joint will be limited.

Muscle spasm, a visceromotor reflex response to painful stimuli, is common. Usually it is more predominant in the flexor muscle groups, producing flexion deformity. Muscle atrophy of antagonists to those in spasm occurs early, lasting for the duration of the joint disease and often persisting after it is over. If a weight-bearing joint is affected, the child will walk with an antalgic limp.

Ultrasonography will depict fluid in the joint and distention of the joint capsule.[22] Radiograms in the acute inflammatory stage will disclose distention of the capsule with excessive effusion, and later xeroradiography will detect synovial thickening. Narrowing of the articular space occurs with softening and erosion of the cartilage. The subjacent bone will become atrophic and decalcified as a result of a destructive process in the joint, as in villonodular synovitis. With extreme destruction of the joint, raw cancellous bone may be exposed, and fibrous or bony ankylosis may result. In some cases with chronic irritation the adjacent bone may respond with sclerosis and osteophytic new bone formation. Osteocartilaginous loose bodies may form when a piece of cartilage or bone breaks loose into the joint.

Joint Fluid Analysis

Examination of synovial fluid is an important tool in the differential diagnosis of joint disease. Aspiration of a joint should be performed under rigid aseptic conditions. The area should be washed with Betadine or some other surgical soap for ten minutes, painted with tincture of Betadine, and then draped adequately to ensure sterility. Mask and gloves are worn, and assistants should be available to control the apprehensive child.

The anatomic approach for aspiration of various joints is illustrated in Figure 4–1. It is best to utilize an 18-gauge lumbar puncture needle with a stylet inside. A local anesthetic, such as 1 per cent lidocaine (Xylocaine) or procaine, is used.

Gross Appearance. The gross appearance of the joint fluid often gives important information. Normal synovial fluid is clear and colorless or straw-colored. In the course of aspiration, blood vessels may be punctured and sanguineous streaks may be found in the joint fluid. This uneven distribution of blood in the syringe is distinguishable from that of acute traumatic hemarthrosis, in which the fluid is entirely sanguineous. In chronic hemarthrosis the fluid may be xanthochromatic. With inflammation the joint fluid becomes turbid. The greater the degree of inflammation, the more turbid is the synovial effusion. The fluid from a pyogenic joint has the creamy or grayish appearance of frank pus. In rheumatoid arthritis the fluid may be clear in the early stages, but as inflammation increases, it becomes turbid in appearance. The fluid in acute gout is milky white because of its urate content. In degenerative arthritis, the joint fluid is almost normal in appearance.

Viscosity and Mucin Clot. The concentration and quality of hyaluronate give viscosity to the synovial fluid. The Ostwald viscosimeter measures the viscosity of synovial fluid relative to water. A simple, but gross, method of measurement is to drip the synovial fluid slowly, drop by drop, from the aspirating syringe to observe how it will "string," i.e., the length of the string

Table 4-1. Synovial Findings in Joint Affections

	Group I Noninflammatory			Group II Noninfectious Inflammatory	
	Normal	Traumatic Arthritis	Degenerative Joint Disease	Systemic Lupus Erythematosus	Pigmented Villonodular Synovitis
Appearance	Straw or clear yellow	Clear yellow, bloody, or xanthochromatic	Clear yellow	Straw	Xanthochromatic
Clarity	Transparent	Transparent or turbid	Transparent	Slightly cloudy	Turbid
Viscosity	Normal	Normal	Normal	Normal or decreased	Normal
Mucin clot	Good	Good	Good	Good or fair	Good
Total WBC	200 or less	2,000 or less (few to many RBC)	1,000 or less	5,000 (10% DNA particles)	3,000 or less (some RBC)
Polys (%)		less than 20	less than 20		less than 20
Crystals	Negative	Negative	Negative	Negative	Negative
"R.A." or "L.E." cells	Negative	Negative	Negative	"L.E." cells	Negative
Bacteria	Negative	Negative	Negative	Negative	Negative
Glucose—difference between levels in joint fluid and blood	20 mg./100 ml.	20 mg./100 ml.	20 mg./100 ml.	20 to 30 mg./100 ml	20 mg./100 ml.
Total proteins	1.8 gm./100 ml.	3.3 gm./100 ml.	3.0 gm./100 ml.	3.2 gm./100 ml.	3.0 gm./100 ml.
Albumin (%)	60–70	60	60	60	57
Gamma globulin (%)	14	16	16	15	17
Immunoglobulin		Normal	Normal	Elevated	Normal
Complement—total and B_1-C		Normal	Normal	Decreased	Negative
Latex fixation and sensitized sheep cell agglutination	Negative	Negative	Negative	Occasionally positive	Negative

made by a drop before it separates. Another way is to place a drop of synovial fluid between the thumb and forefinger and open and close them. If the fluid feels sticky and the fingers can be separated at least an inch before the string breaks, the viscosity is *normal*. The viscosity is *decreased* when the fluid strings less than 1 inch. It is classified as *poor* when the fluid feels watery and does not string out.

The quality of mucin is assayed by the mucin precipitation test or the "Ropes test." The mucin precipitation test is performed by adding 0.1 ml. of synovial fluid to 4 ml. of distilled water and allowing the clot to form. In the Ropes test, a few drops of synovial fluid are added to 5 to 10 ml. of 5 per cent solution of acetic acid. Four grades are recognizable, namely, *normal*, in which the mucin precipitate obtained is a tight, ropy clump and remains together suspended on top in a clear solution; *fair*, a soft mass that strings out, sticks, but remains loosely intact in a very slightly cloudy solution; *poor*, small friable masses in a cloudy solution; and *very poor*, a few flecks in a cloudy solution.

Microscopic Examination. The total leukocyte count of normal synovial fluid is usually less than 300 per cubic millimeter. Normally it does not contain erythrocytes. Physiologic saline solution is used to dilute the joint fluid, as the acid in the ordinary white cell counting solution will clot the mucin. The anticoagulated specimen is drawn in a leukocyte count pipette to the 0.5 mark and diluted to the 11 mark. A regular hemacytometer is used, and cells are counted as for a standard leukocyte count.

A differential leukocyte count is made as follows: A drop of the centrifuged cellular sediment is smeared and stained with Wright's or modified Giemsa stain. Two hundred cells are counted. Mononuclear cells (monocytes, lymphocytes) constitute the greater proportion of leukocytes; the polymorphonuclear leukocytes are normally less than 25 per cent.

Cytoplasmic inclusions are composed of immunoglobulins, rheumatoid factors, and components of the complement system. Ordinary light microscopy or a phase-optical system is utilized to visualize the cellular inclusions in a wet preparation of joint fluid. The wet preparation is supravitally stained with a drop of Sternheimer-Malbin stain, or direct immunofluorescent staining techniques may be used. The joint fluid cells containing cellular inclusions were once thought to be diagnostic for rheumatoid arthritis and were called "rheumatoid arthritis cells"; they have since, however, been described in joint fluids from other conditions.

Polarized light microscopy is used to demonstrate crystals in joint fluid. These are of two

		Group III		
		Severe Noninfectious Inflammatory	Infectious Inflammatory	
Rheumatic Fever	Gout	Rheumatoid Arthritis	Pyogenic Arthritis	Tuberculous Arthritis
Yellow	Yellow to turbid milky	Yellow to greenish	Grayish or bloody	Yellow
Slightly cloudy	Cloudy	Cloudy	Turbid purulent	Cloudy
Decreased	Decreased	Decreased to poor	Decreased to poor	Decreased to poor
Good	Poor	Poor	Poor	Poor
10,000	10,000–14,000	15,000 (1,000–60,000)	60,000	20,000
50	60–70	55	90	60
Negative	Urate + (in pseudogout, calcium pyrophosphate)	Negative	Negative	Negative
Negative	Negative	"R.A." cells	Negative	Negative
Negative	Negative	Negative	Positive	Positive
20 mg./100 ml.	20 mg./100 ml.	30 mg./100 ml. or more	30–50 mg./100 ml.	30–50 mg./100 ml.
3.0 gm./100 ml.	5 gm./100 ml.	4.1 gm./100 ml.	4.2 gm./100 ml.	4.2 gm./100 ml.
60	70	42	45	45
14	9	25	25	25
Normal or slightly elevated	Normal	Elevated	Normal	Normal
Normal	Normal or elevated	Decreased	Normal	Normal
Negative	Negative	Positive	Negative	Negative

types: uric acid crystals (seen in gout) and calcium pyrophosphate crystals (seen in pseudogout or articular chondrocalcinosis).

Glucose. The difference between the levels in the joint fluid and the blood is the important determination. The upper limit of the normal difference is about 20 mg./100 ml. It is best to perform the aspiration while the patient is fasting, as there is normally a physiologic lag of glucose transport across the synovial membrane. In severe inflammatory joint disease, such as tuberculosis, pyogenic arthritis, or acute rheumatoid arthritis, the synovial fluid sugar level is characteristically lowered. This results from both the glucolytic properties of the leukocyte and the presence of bacterial organisms that utilize sugar.

Proteins. The concentration of proteins in normal synovial fluid is low (about 30 per cent of that of serum) because of the physiologic barrier of the synovial membrane. It seems the size of molecules is an important factor in the passage of proteins across the synovial membrane. The level of total proteins is usually 1.8 gm./100 ml., of which 70 per cent is albumin and about 7 per cent is alpha-2 globulin. In normal synovial fluid, fibrinogen is absent, and the fluid will not clot. In acute inflammatory and infectious effusions, the permeability of the synovial membrane increases and the protein content and pattern of synovial fluid will be similar to that of the serum. Inflammatory synovial fluid will clot because it contains fibrinogen as well as other clotting factors.

In synovial fluid analysis 5 to 10 ml. of joint fluid is placed in a plain test tube, which is centrifuged. The clear supernatant portion is saved for determination of gamma globulin, immunoglobulin, complement (total and B1–C), and latex fixation. The same determinations are performed on a matched serum specimen obtained from the patient.

The details of the synovial fluid examination are individualized, depending on the reason for joint aspiration. Ropes and Bauer have classified joint affections into three groups on the basis of the synovial fluid findings and have set up levels for normal and various abnormal conditions. This work is summarized in Table 4–1.

Group I includes degenerative arthritis, traumatic arthritis, and neuropathic arthropathy. It is characterized by an increased amount of fluid with no significant change in the leukocyte count, sugar concentration, or the quality of mucin.

Group III is characterized by severe inflammation of the synovial membrane and includes pyogenic arthritis, tuberculous infections, and acute rheumatoid arthritis. In these the mucin is of poor quality, and the synovial fluid glucose

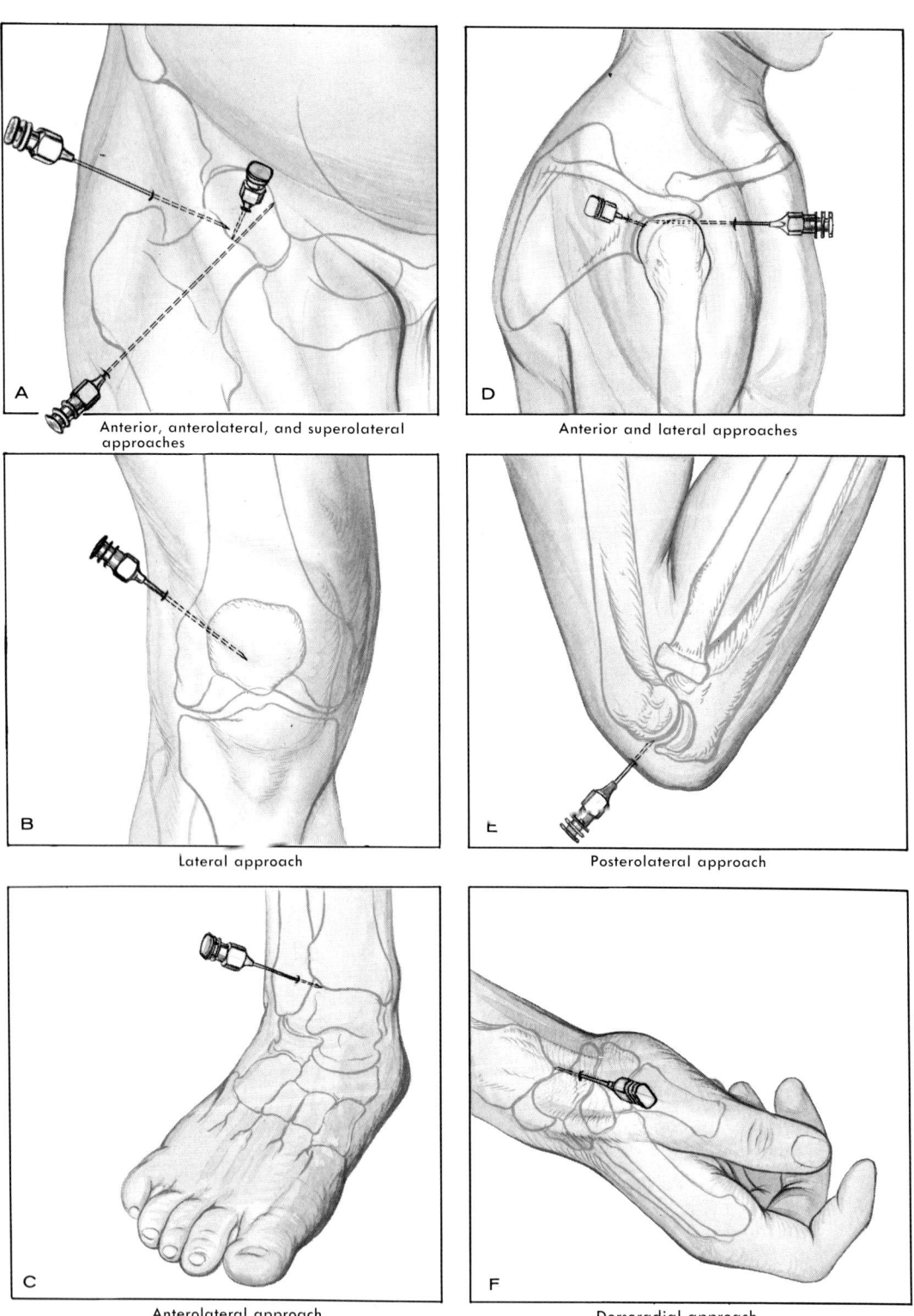

FIGURE 4–1. *Routes of aspiration of joints.*

level is markedly lowered. The leukocyte count is elevated. In pyogenic arthritis the average leukocyte count is 60,000 with 90 per cent polymorphonuclear neutrophils; in tuberculous arthritis, the average leukocyte count is 15,000 with 55 per cent polymorphonuclear neutrophils, though it may vary between 1,000 and 60,000, depending on the degree of acute inflammation.

Group II includes systemic lupus erythematosus, gout, pigmented villonodular synovitis, and acute rheumatic fever. In these the synovial fluid findings are mixed, constituting an intermediate category between Groups I and III.

References

1. Adkins, E. W. O., and Davies, D. V.: Absorption from the joint cavity. Q. J. Exp. Physiol., 30:147, 1940.
2. Barnett, C. H., Davies, D. V., and MacConaill, M. A.: Synovial Joints. Their Structure and Mechanics. Springfield, Ill., Thomas; London, Clowes & Sons, 1961.
3. Brower, T. D., Akakoshi, Y., and Orlie, P.: The diffusion of dyes through articular cartilage in vivo. J. Bone Joint Surg., 44-A:456, 1962.
4. Caughney, D. E., and Bywaters, E. G. L.: Joint fluid pressure in chronic knee effusions. Ann. Rheum. Dis., 22:106, 1963.
5. Cohen, A. S. (ed.): Laboratory Diagnostic Procedures in Rheumatic Diseases. Boston, Little, Brown, 1968.
6. Cracchiolo, A., III, Barnett, E., and Pearson, C.: Joint Fluid Analysis, Synovial Research Laboratories, Division of Orthopedic Surgery and Division of Rheumatology, U.C.L.A. Medical Center, 1970.
7. Curtiss, P. H.: Changes produced in the synovial membrane and synovial fluid by disease. J. Bone Joint Surg., 46-A:873, 1961.
8. Edlund, T.: Studies on absorption of colloids and fluid from rabbit knee joint. Acta Physiol. Scand., 18:Suppl. 62:1–108, 1949.
9. Eyring, E. J., and Murray, W. R.: Effect of joint position on the pressure of intra-articular effusion. J. Bone Joint Surg., 46-A:1235, 1964.
10. Favreau, J. C., and Laurin, C. A.: Joint effusion and flexion deformities. Can. Med. Assoc. J., 88:575, 1963.
11. Gardner, E.: Physiology of movable joints. Physiol. Rev., 30:127, 1950.
12. Gardner, E.: Physiological mechanism of movable joints. A.A.O.S. Instruct. Course Lect., 10:251, 1953.
13. Hamerman, D., and Schubert, M.: Diarthrodial joints—an essay. Am. J. Med., 33:555, 1962.
14. Hamerman, D., Rosenberg, L. C., and Schubert, M.: Diarthrodial joints revisited. J. Bone Joint Surg., 52-A:725, 1970.
15. Jessar, R.: The synovial fluid. In Hollander, J. H. L. (ed.): Arthritis and Allied Conditions. 7th Ed. Philadelphia, Lea & Febiger, 1966, p. 76.
16. Maroudas, A., Bullough, P., Swanson, S. A. V., and Freeman, M. A. R.: The permeability of articular cartilage. J. Bone Joint Surg., 50-B:166, 1968.
17. Miller, J. A., Jr.: Joint paracentesis from an anatomic point of view. I. Shoulder, elbow, wrist and hand. Surgery, 40:993, 1956.
18. Miller, J. A., Jr.: Joint paracentesis from an anatomic point of view. II. Hip, knee, ankle and foot. Surgery, 41:999, 1957.
19. Ropes, M. W., and Bauer, W.: Synovial Fluid Changes in Joint Disease. Cambridge, Mass., Harvard University Press, 1953.
20. Soto-Hall, R., Johnson, L. H., and Johnson, R. A.: Variations in the intraarticular pressure of the hip joint in injury and disease. J. Bone Joint Surg., 46-A:509, 1964.
21. Strangeways, T. S. P.: Observation on the nutrition of articular cartilage. Br. Med. J., 1:661, 1920.
22. Wingstraad, H.: Ultrasonography in hip joint effusion. Report of a child with transient synovitis. Acta Orthop. Scand., 55:469, 1984.

ACUTE SUPPURATIVE ARTHRITIS (Septic Joint)

Acute suppurative or septic arthritis is an inflammation of the joint caused by pus-forming organisms. Historically the crippling effects of pyarthrosis were recognized by Smith in 1874.[207] In the literature, septic arthritis is sometimes referred to as "Tom Smith's arthritis." Previously, in 1743, Hunter had described the destruction of articular cartilage in septic arthritis.[92]

Septic arthritis occurs in all age groups, but is primarily seen in neonates, infants, and children between two and three years of age. It is two to three times more frequent in the male. The hip joint is most commonly involved, with the knee and elbow affected next in order of frequency; however, any joint may be the site of sepsis. Occasionally more than one joint may be infected.

Pathogenesis*

The bacteria gain entrance to the joint by one of three routes: *hematogenous*, in which the organisms become seeded in the synovia via the blood stream from a distant focus of infection, such as a furuncle, infected abrasion, or upper respiratory or middle ear infection; *direct extension* of infection from an adjacent focus, such as osteomyelitis (in infants osteomyelitis of the proximal femoral metaphysis is intracapsular, and often it is the source of contamination of the hip joint and septic arthritis; the upper metaphysis of the humerus is also intracapsular, and metaphyseal abscess may spread into the shoulder joint); and *direct inoculation* of pathogenic organisms during joint aspiration or arthrotomy or by an accidental

---

*Written with Ellen G. Chadwick, M.D., Assistant Professor of Pediatrics, Northwestern University Medical School, and Attending Physician, The Children's Memorial Hospital, Chicago, Illinois; and by Stanford L. Shulman, M.D., Professor of Pediatrics and Head, Division of Infectious Disease, The Children's Memorial Hospital, Chicago, Illinois.

wound. Femoral venipuncture and accidental penetration of the joint may be the route of bacterial infection of the hip.

Etiologic Organism. The pathogenic organism may be *Staphylococcus aureus*, *Streptococcus hemolyticus* (Group B), *Hemophilus influenzae*, pneumococcus, gonococcus, meningococcus, colon bacillus, salmonella, brucella, and a variety of other rare organisms. In the past 15 years, due to long-term hyperalimentation, prolonged intravenous catheterization, and the use of potent antibiotics for critically ill infants, *Candida albicans* has emerged as a pathogen. The predominance of the type of organism depends on the age of the patient and epidemiologic factors, i.e., "hospital-acquired" infection while in the hospital or "community-acquired" in which the child becomes symptomatic at home.

In the neonate the leading pathogen is *S. aureus*. Jackson and Nelson reported the pathogenic organism in 15 neonates less than one month of age to be: *S. aureus* (36 per cent), group B streptococcus (21 per cent), and a variety of gram-negative organisms (28 per cent).[94] Dan, in a retrospective study of 92 cases of septic arthritis in infants less than three months of age (average age 21 days) reviewed the English literature between 1960 and 1979 and found the predominant organism to be *S. aureus* (46.3 per cent), followed by streptococci (25.3 per cent), gram-negative bacilli (9.5 per cent), candida species (9.5 per cent), *Neisseria gonorrhoeae* (7.3 per cent), and *H. influenzae* (2 per cent). Epidemiologically, 52 of the 92 cases were hospital-acquired infections and the other 40 cases were community-acquired.[38]

In the "hospital-acquired" infection group, staphylococci were the most frequent pathogens (62 per cent), followed by candida species (17 per cent), gram-negative bacilli (13 per cent), and streptococci and *H. influenzae* (4 per cent each). The candidal and *H. influenzae* arthritides tended to display polyarticular involvement. The majority of these patients had predisposing factors including prematurity, premature rupture of membranes, cesarean section, Rh incompatibility requiring exchange transfusion, or respiratory distress syndrome. Many underwent invasive procedures such as catheterization of the umbilical vessels (25 cases) and femoral venipuncture (16 cases). Contiguous osteomyelitis was diagnosed in 34 of 52 "hospital-acquired" cases. Twenty-seven per cent of the infants died from their infections, and the majority of the survivors developed deformities of the musculoskeletal system.[38]

The infants with "community-acquired" infection were in general good health, and the average age of onset of infection was 21.9 days. The predominant organisms affecting this group were streptococci, particularly group B (52 per cent), staphylococci (25 per cent), *N. gonorrhoeae* (17 per cent), and gram-negative bacilli (5 per cent). Contiguous osteomyelitis was present in 66 per cent of cases. The mortality rate was very low in this group.

In infants and children *one month to three years old*, *H. influenzae* is the predominant pathogen causing septic arthritis. A review of 337 patients between the ages of one month and five years with acute suppurative arthritis revealed the following bacterial etiologies: *H. influenzae* (31 per cent), streptococci (12 per cent), *S. aureus* (11 per cent), gram-negative organisms (10 per cent), and unknown (35 per cent).[94]

In children *over three years* septic arthritis is largely caused by the same organisms as those found in adults. In one series of 120 cases of suppurative arthritis in children over five years, 33 per cent were due to *S. aureus*, followed by hemolytic streptococci in 18 per cent, *N. gonorrhoeae* in 7 per cent, and unknown in 34 per cent. A literature review of 73 patients between the ages of 2 and 14 years with nongonococcal septic arthritis reported similar results: *S. aureus* in 42 per cent, hemolytic streptococci in 26 per cent, gram-negative bacilli in 14 per cent, *S. pneumoniae* in 7 per cent, and *H. influenzae* in 5 per cent. All of the *H. influenzae* disease occurred in children less than three years of age.[64] The etiology of septic arthritis by age group is given in Table 4–2.

Rare and unusual organisms are the etiologic agent when there is immunodeficiency or alteration of the patient's immunologic status by systemic disease or treatment with corticosteroids or when there has been penetration of the joint by a foreign body.[212]

In about one fourth to one third of the reported cases of septic arthritis no causative organism can be identified.

Pathology

The synovial membrane becomes edematous, swollen, and hyperemic and produces an increased amount of synovial fluid, which distends the joint. The synovial fluid may be thin and cloudy, and contains leukocytes of the polymorphonuclear type, the count in the early stages usually being higher than 50,000 per cubic millimeter. The pathogenic bacteria may be

Table 4–2. Bacterial Pathogens of Septic Arthritis

	Common (Per cent)	Uncommon	Rare
Neonates	S. aureus (36) Group B streptococcus (21)	Enteric bacilli Candida N. gonorrhoeae	H. influenzae
One month to three years	H. influenzae (31) Streptococcus (12) S. aureus (11)	Gram-negative bacilli	(Unknown in one third of cases)
Over three years	S. aureus (42) Hemolytic streptococci (26)	Gram-negative bacilli N. gonorrhoeae	S. pneumoniae H. influenzae (Unknown in one fourth of cases)

demonstrated on smear and Gram stain. The sugar content of the synovial fluid is decreased, but its protein content is elevated.

Within a few days, with persistence of infection, frank pus accumulates in the joint cavity. Destructive and degenerative changes soon take place in the hyaline articular cartilage. This destruction of cartilage occurs first and is most extensive at points of contact between opposing articular surfaces, such as the central portions of weight-bearing joints. The synovial membrane is eventually replaced by granulation tissue that fills the denuded areas. Infection may extend to underlying bone. Fibrin within the joint clots and produces pockets of pus and formation of adhesions that restrict joint motion.[26]

Pathologic subluxation or dislocation, especially of the hip joint, may occur when there is marked distention of the lax joint capsule (Fig. 4–2). Pus contained within the thick anatomic barriers of a joint will lead to increased intraarticular pressure. In the hip joint this may cause avascular necrosis of the femoral head due to tamponade of the retinacular blood vessels. If the infection remains uncontrolled, it may progress to fibrous or bony ankylosis of the joint (Fig. 4–3).

Pathophysiology of Cartilage Destruction. Phemister incubated articular cartilage with pus from a tuberculous infection, a suspension of staphylococcal organisms, and normal saline for 40 hours at 55° C. The hyaline cartilage incubated in pus obtained from pyogenic infection was completely digested in from 3 to 24 hours, whereas, in the control preparations, changes did not occur. Phemister believed the chondrolysis to be caused by enzymes in the pus, possibly derived from the polymorphonuclear leukocytes.[168] On incubating cartilage with polymorphonuclear leukocyte autolysate at 37° C. and 56° C., Keefer and associates found that only at a temperature of 56° C. are cartilage changes produced. At normal body temperature (37° C.) no appreciable changes occurred.[104] Lack proposed that staphylokinase produced by bacteria converted plasminogen to plasmin, which then exerted its proteolytic effect.[106] In vitro studies by Curtiss and Klein showed that collagen loss was a prerequisite for visible cartilage destruction.[34, 36] In vivo experiments in dogs with septic arthritis demonstrated a loss of chondroitin sulfate. The possible role of lysosomes was postulated.[34, 221]

The chemical sequence of events in degradation and destruction of cartilage is as follows: *first* there is significant loss of cartilage matrix. Experimentally in infected rabbit joints this takes place in five days following instillation of infection. The *second* event is loss of collagen, which experimentally takes place after nine days.[39] The cartilage matrix may break down by the action of several enzymes: by lysosomal enzymes that may be released from cartilage, neutrophils, or synovium; plasmin-plasmogen activated by staphylokinase; and extracellular proteolytic enzymes produced by *Staphylococcus aureus*.*

Mechanical wear and tear also causes cartilage destruction experimentally and clinically in the human. This is supported by the finding of greater wear of cartilage on the central contact areas of septic joints.[35]

Following loss of ground substance the external gross appearance of the articular cartilage may be unaltered, but on mechanical testing it is less stiff and more flexible.[35]

The effect of antibiotics on the destruction of cartilage in experimental infectious arthritis was studied by Smith and associates. After inoculating *Staphylococcus aureus* into the knee joints of rabbits, inducing septic arthritis, they measured the extent to which antibiotic therapy with

---

*See references: lysosomal enzymes, 43, 51, 96, 160; proteolytic enzymes from S. aureus, 3, 107.

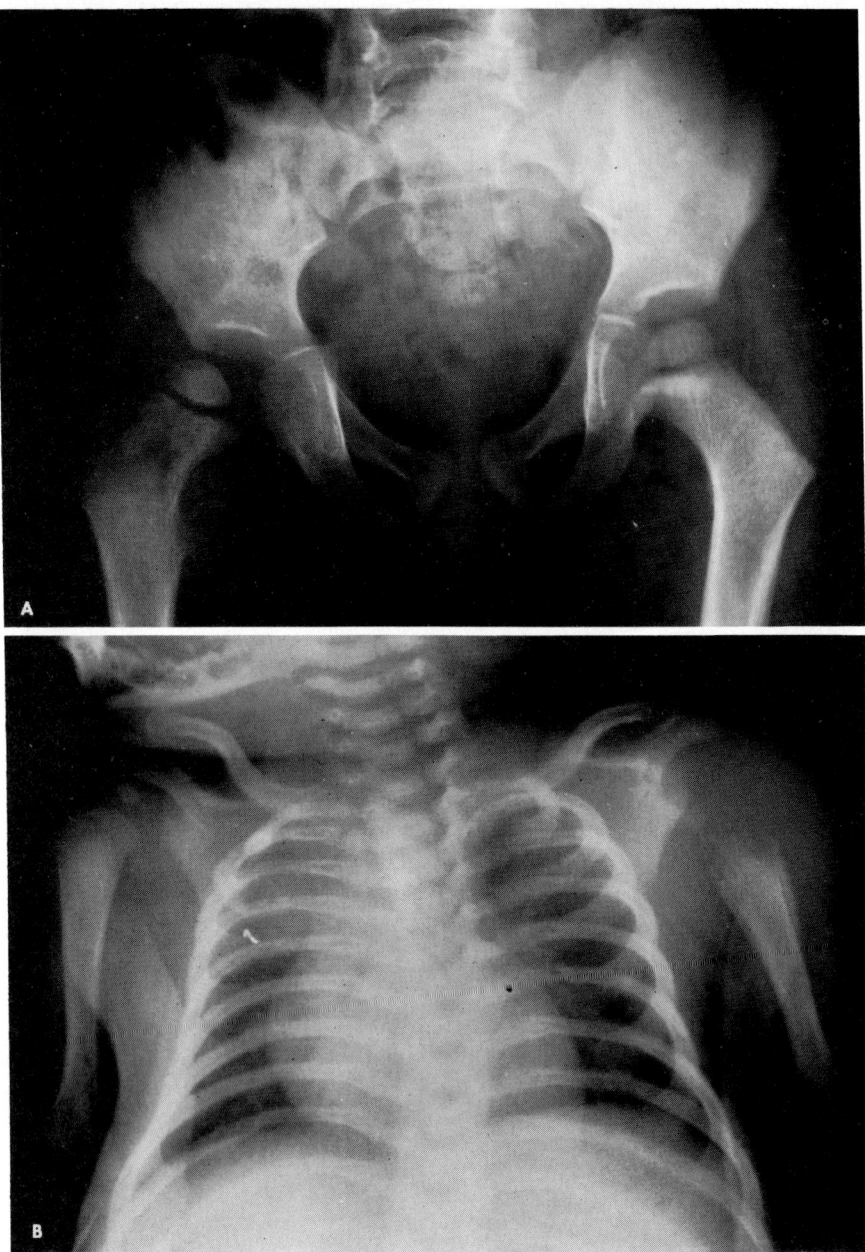

FIGURE 4–2. *Pathologic subluxation secondary to pyogenic arthritis.*

A. Septic arthritis of the right hip with subluxation. Note the osteomyelitis of the femoral neck. **B.** Subluxation of the left shoulder with osteomyelitis of the proximal humerus.

cefaronide altered the degradation of cartilage; this was quantified by analysis for glycosaminoglycan and collagen. In spite of prompt antibiotic therapy, prolonged destruction of articular cartilage occurred. Three weeks after the infection was produced, the cartilage had lost more than half its glycosaminoglycan, whether the antibiotic therapy had been started at one, two, or seven days after infection. Beginning the antibiotic treatment one day after infection reduced overall loss of collagen by 37 per cent and decreased the area of erosion of the infected articular sufaces. When antibiotic treatment was begun at 4, 8, or 12 hours after infection, the loss of glycosaminoglycan averaged 18 per cent. Prophylaxis with antibiotics completely prevented any degradation of the cartilage.[205]

The effect of lavage of septic joints in rabbits

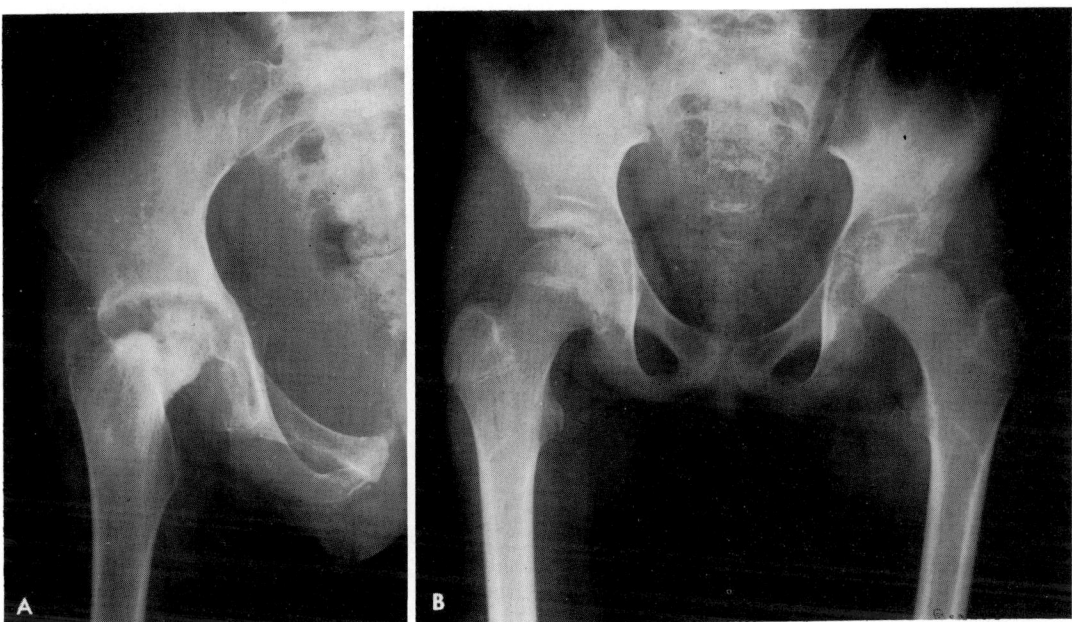

FIGURE 4–3. *Ankylosis of the hip secondary to pyogenic arthritis.*

A. Fibrous ankylosis. **B.** Bony ankylosis.

was studied by Daniel and associates. All the animals were treated with systemic procaine penicillin. One group of the animals had surgical lavage at four and seven days after bacterial inoculation. There was no significant loss of collagen (two weeks after inoculation) in this group of animals in contrast to those with unlavaged septic joints, in which there was definite loss of collagen. Lavage, however, delayed but did not prevent loss of collagen. Eleven weeks after the joint was rendered sterile there was evidence of the inflammatory process. The pathogenic factors of continued cartilage destruction may be an immunologic disease of the articular cartilage initiated by the septic process, a perpetuation of the inflammatory process due to tissue-fixed bacterial products, or the inability of degraded chondrocytes to replace the depleted matrix.[13, 17, 39, 40]

Clinical Picture

A history of recent injury or antecedent infection such as otitis media or skin infection may be obtained in most cases.

The onset of symptoms is usually acute. Pain in the affected joint is the most prominent complaint. If the lower limb is involved, the child walks with an antalgic limp, and soon weight-bearing becomes so painful that he may not be able to walk at all. The child is apprehensive, irritable, anorexic, and feverish. Temperature may be as high as 104° or 105° F. In the newborn infant systemic manifestations may be minimal or absent.

Examination discloses the infected joint to be warm and swollen, a result of excessive effusion and distention of the joint capsule. The joint (in response to increased hydrostatic pressure due to effusion) is held in a position of minimum intra-articular pressure; protective muscle spasm will force it into varying degrees of flexion. The hip will be in 30 to 65 degrees of flexion, 15 degrees of abduction, and 10 to 15 degrees of lateral rotation. The ankle will be in 10 to 20 degrees of plantar flexion; the knee and elbow in 30 to 60 degrees of flexion. The wrist will be in neutral position; the shoulder in 30 to 65 degrees of abduction, neutral flexion, and neutral rotation.

Imaging Findings

Radiography. Distention of the joint capsule with fluid and increased opacity within the joint is the initial finding in the radiograms. The periarticular fat and muscle shadows will be displaced by the capsular distention. There may be loss of soft-tissue planes. In the hip joint the femoral head may be displaced laterally or even subluxated (Fig. 4–4). In the knee, ankle, and elbow there may be increased distance between the subchondral bony ends. It is always best to assess these radiographic findings by compari-

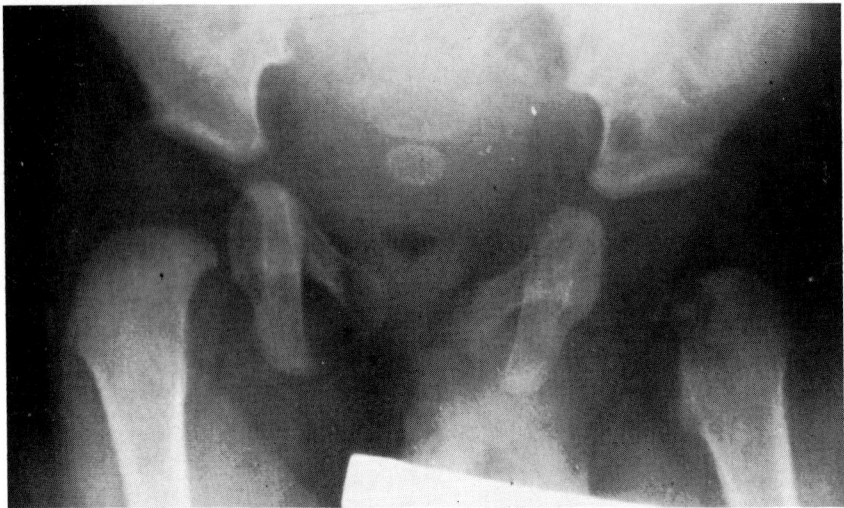

FIGURE 4–4. Septic arthritis of left hip.
Lateral subluxation and area of rarefaction in the femoral neck are evident.

son with the contralateral normal limb. *Always look for evidence of osteomyelitis of adjacent bone.* In the hip joint is there evidence of rarefaction of the metaphysis of the femoral neck? With delayed diagnosis there may be erosion or even disappearance of the ossific nucleus of the epiphysis.

In the hip traction views, the presence of a radiolucent gas shadow will rule out effusion in the joint; absence of a vacuum phenomenon does not, however, confirm the presence of effusion.[128]

Ultrasonography. This is the best way to detect fluid in the joint. Ultrasound can also assist in locating a site for accurate aspiration. Ultrasound control is of definite value when decompressing loculated fluid collections in pyarthrosis by aspiration. Sequential examinations of a joint by ultrasonography will record the diminishing or increasing volume of pus in the joint.[68]

Radionuclide Imaging. Technetium-99m diphosphonate imaging will show increased periarticular uptake due to synovial inflammation and consequent local hyperemia and increased blood flow. If there is associated osteomyelitis, e.g., in the proximal femoral metaphysis in septic arthritis of the hip, there will be intense focal accumulation of the radionuclide. Pinhole and SPECT imaging are of great value in detecting associated osteomyelitis.

Imaging with gallium-67 citrate is performed in doubtful cases when further assessment is required. Gallium-67 citrate tends to localize primarily in the inflammatory tissue as it is bound to serum proteins and labels the white blood leukocytes.[112, 113]

Borman and associates used gallium-67 citrate scintigraphy to study 34 children with presumptive acute osteomyelitis or septic arthritis. The accuracy of the technique was 91 per cent, but, because of the large radiation dose, they did not recommend its routine use.[15]

A white blood cell scan in which the patient's own leukocytes are labeled with a radioactive tagging agent (Inoxine 111) can distinguish an active infectious process from other conditions; it is not ordinarily used except in complex cases.[170]

Diagnosis

Infection should be suspected in any acute joint disease. A painful, swollen joint that is markedly limited in motion and that also displays clinical and laboratory signs of sepsis should be suspected of being infected and should be aspirated to confirm the diagnosis.

Aspiration of joints should be performed under strict aseptic conditions. The child should be properly sedated and restrained to make the procedure as painless as possible. An 18- or 20-gauge lumbar puncture needle with a stylet is used. The routes of aspiration of various joints are illustrated in Figure 4–1.[133, 134] Insert the needle into the joint through the easiest access route through the site of maximal fluctuation. Avoid areas of cellulitis in order to prevent the danger of infecting a joint containing sterile sympathetic effusion. The hip joint is difficult to aspirate. The procedure is best performed under image intensifier control in the radiology department or in the operating room. In the hip, the *adductor* approach is preferred by this author. With the hips in flexion–abduction–lateral rotation the needle is inserted immediately posterior to the adductor longus tendon pointing to the sternum. The use of image intensifier x-ray makes the technique relatively simple. When the anterior approach is used, the needle is inserted at right angles to the skin, ½ inch lateral to the femoral artery and ½ inch distal to Poupart's ligament. The femoral artery is used as a guide, as it usually lies beneath the middle of the ligament. In the lateral approach, the needle is inserted perpendicular to the lateral surface of the thigh at a point immediately superior and lateral to the tip of the greater trochanter. It is directed horizontally and medially toward the lateral surface of the ilium. When the needle touches bone, it is withdrawn ½ inch, the hip is adducted, and the needle is advanced distally and medially at an angle of from 45 to 60 degrees. One has to feel his way, so to speak, into the distended capsule, being careful not to penetrate the articular surfaces, in order to avoid spread of infection into bone. The tip of the needle should always be double-checked to ensure that it is not broken. A stylet inside prevents such an accident and also serves to avoid plugging of the needle with thickened synovium and fibrin. At the end of aspiration and after adequate material has been obtained for culture, a radiopaque dye is introduced into the joint, particularly in the hip, for permanent verification and recording that the needle was in the hip joint. The dye is bacteriocidal—do not instill prior to obtaining material for culture. When attempted hip joint aspiration is dry, use air for verification of the site of the tip of the needle.

When the joint contains little fluid or the fluid is very thick, one may introduce 1 ml. of sterile normal saline into the joint and reaspirate it. The joint fluid is then cultured, and smears are made with Gram stain to identify the causative organism under the microscope.

Gram stain of purulent joint effusions is positive in approximately 30 per cent of cases.[14] Counterimmunoelectrophoresis or latex agglutination may rapidly detect the presence of the bacterial antigens of *H. influenzae*, meningococcus, pneumococcus, and group B streptococcus.[41, 130] To improve the yield of positive cultures from joint fluid, 0.5 to 1.0 ml. of joint fluid may be injected into a blood culture bottle to dilute the antibacterial effect of white blood cells and other factors that may prevent bacterial growth on routine cultures.

Do not be misled by the gross appearance of the joint fluid. A clear fluid may be infected and full of bacteria, whereas a turbid fluid may be found in a noninfectious inflammation such as rheumatoid arthritis. Demonstration of the presence of bacteria on Gram stain not only strengthens the diagnosis but also aids in the selection of the antibiotic to be used. Sensitivity studies should always be performed.

In the early stages the joint fluid may be serosanguineous. Within a few days it becomes cloudy with an elevated cell count (usually between 15,000 and 200,000 per millimeter) and a high polymorphonuclear leukocyte differential count. The joint fluid sugar is reduced, averaging 50 mg./100 ml. less than the blood sugar. The mucin, measured on the acid precipitation test, is poor to very poor.

Definitive diagnosis of septic arthritis is made by positive synovial fluid or tissue culture; however, in a certain percentage of the cases pathogenic organisms do not grow. In the absence of a positive culture the criteria utilized for diagnosis are aspiration of gross or microscopic pus from the joint or histologic findings in the synovial biopsy specimen consistent with an acute inflammatory process. Other findings that favor the diagnosis of septic arthritis are joint irritability and effusion with increased local heat, radiographic and radionuclide imaging changes consistent with septic arthritis, systemic response of fever and elevation of erythrocyte sedimentation rate, subsidence of symptoms and signs on empiric antibiotic therapy and surgical drainage, and absence of other possible pathologic diagnosis.

Differential Diagnosis

In the differential diagnosis one should consider osteomyelitis, acute rheumatoid arthritis, transient synovitis, tuberculous arthritis, acute rheumatic fever, cellulitis, and hemarthrosis. *Osteomyelitis*, particularly if associated with sympathetic effusion in the adjacent joint, presents a difficult problem in differential diagnosis, as most of its signs and symptoms resemble those of suppurative arthritis. In osteomyelitis the maximal point of tenderness is over the metaphysis, whereas in septic arthritis it is directly over the joint line. On gentle examination of the joint, motion is much less restricted and less painful in osteomyelitis than it is in septic arthritis. The limb as a whole is more swollen in osteomyelitis; in septic arthritis, it is the joint that is swollen. It is often necessary to aspirate the joint in order to make the diagnosis. One should exercise considerable caution not to contaminate a clean joint from an infected focus in the metaphysis. The joint fluid of sympathetic effusion of osteomyelitis will be straw-colored, with only a few thousand leukocytes.

In *acute transient* and *traumatic synovitis* systemic manifestations are absent, and the motion of the affected joint is relatively less limited and is less painful. If there is severe limitation of joint motion and the radiograph and ultrasonograms disclose marked distention of the joint capsule or lateral displacement of the femoral head, the joint should be aspirated despite the absence of fever and leukocytosis.

Rheumatoid arthritis may involve only one joint. Its onset, as a rule, however, is gradual, and usually the child is not acutely ill. The affected joint has a better range of motion, is not as tender, and is less swollen than in septic arthritis. The total leukocyte count in rheumatoid arthritis may be as high as that in septic arthritis, but the differential count will disclose many fewer polymorphonuclear cells. Mucin is poor in both conditions. Gram stain and culture, however, are negative in rheumatoid arthritis, and the glucose content is not diminished as much as in septic joint.

The hot, red, swollen and painful joints and high temperature of *rheumatic fever* may be mistaken for suppurative arthritis. Fleeting migratory joint involvement and cardiac manifestations are the hallmarks of rheumatic fever. Its response to an adequate dose of salicylates is dramatic, with relief of swelling and pain in the joints and return of temperature and pulse rate to normal. Salicylates should not, however, be given as a diagnostic test until sepsis has been ruled out, as their administration will only cloud the picture and cause delay in treatment of a pyogenic joint.

In *cellulitis* there are local skin redness and edema with a greater area of local tenderness. The adjacent or subjacent joint has relatively more range of motion and is less painful than in septic arthritis. Often in cellulitis there is associated lymphadenopathy.

Hemarthrosis may be the first presentation of a bleeding disorder such as hemophilia. This is rare, but occasionally it poses a problem in differential diagnosis. In *Henoch-Schönlein purpura* one or more joints may be swollen and painful prior to the appearance of skin manifestations. In the hip joint one always has to consider *Legg-Calvé-Perthes disease* in the differential diagnosis.

Treatment

Suppurative arthritis is a serious disease; it degrades articular cartilage and destroys the joint, causing crippling deformity. It should be treated immediately as an emergency. The importance of the urgency of *adequate* treatment cannot be overemphasized; delay causes loss of proteoglycans and collagen.

The goals of treatment are: *first*, control of sepsis and sterilization of the joint by administration of appropriate antibiotics; *second*, evacuation of the fibrin, debris, and bacterial products associated with infection by adequate drainage of the joint; *third*, provision of support to the joint to relieve pain and to prevent deformity due to muscle spasm; and *fourth*, restoration of normal function and anatomic configuration to the joint.

ANTIBIOTIC THERAPY*

The purpose of antibiotic therapy is to kill the pathogenic bacteria and control the infection. The antibiotics chosen should be effective in type, dose, and duration of administration. They should be administered early without waiting for determination of the pathogenic organism; antibiotics should not, however, be given before blood is obtained and the joint aspirated for culture and Gram stain. These preliminary studies to isolate the organism may be negative. Ordinarily it takes two days for sensitivity of organisms to antibiotics to be determined. In some cases the bacterial cause may be unknown. In a series of 45 patients with clinical diagnoses of acute septic arthritis, Nade could not identify the pathogenic organism in 19 of the cases. In the joint aspirates the causative organism was determined in 62 per cent (16 of 26 joints), whereas when pus was found on arthrotomy, organisms were grown in 83 per cent (15 of 18 joints).[143] Therefore, there is a period when initial antibiotic therapy is given empirically. The "best guess" as to appropriate choice of antibiotic is based on knowledge of the predominant pathogens responsible for septic arthritis in the three major age groups in children and the type of organism (when seen)

---

*Contributed by Ellen G. Chadwick, M.D., Assistant Professor of Pediatrics, Northwestern University Medical School, and Attending Physician, The Children's Memorial Hospital, Chicago, Illinois; and by Stanford L. Shulman, M.D., Professor of Pediatrics Northwestern University Medical School, and Head, Division of Infectious Disease, The Children's Memorial Hospital, Chicago, Illinois.

on Gram stain of the fluid aspirated from the joint. It should be noted, however, that microbiologic and epidemiologic data should be monitored constantly and that the most appropriate antibiotic for initial use will vary from time to time and place to place. Strains of bacteria resistant to various antibiotics are constantly developing, differing from one geographic area to another. Newer and more effective antibiotics are being developed.

Antibiotic therapy should consist of a penicillinase-stable penicillin such as nafcillin (75 to 100 mg. per kilogram per day divided every 6 to 8 hours, in neonates less than seven days of age) to provide coverage for staphylococci, streptococci, and gonococci, in conjunction with an aminoglycoside such as amikacin or gentamicin to treat gram-negative organisms. It should be noted that this regimen will not treat the rare case of *H. influenzae* arthritis. If single antibiotic therapy is desirable, a second- or third-generation cephalosporin such as ceftriaxone or cefuroxime may be considered. These newer antibiotics can achieve high levels in the joint fluid that greatly exceed the minimum inhibitory concentrations for the likely pathogens. They tend to be well tolerated and do not carry the risk of nephro- or ototoxicity common to the aminoglycosides. Candidal infections should be considered carefully in the hospitalized neonate who has been subjected to invasive procedures, particularly indwelling vascular catheters, and appropriate fungal cultures should be performed. In most instances Candida grows on routine agar media so that special media are not routinely required. Fungal arthritis requires treatment for six weeks with amphotericin B; the toxicity of this drug demands that a firm diagnosis be made prior to institution of therapy.

When an organism is isolated from an infected joint and its antibiotic sensitivities are determined, the single most effective parenteral antibiotic with the narrowest spectrum and fewest side effects should be used. In infants and children one month to three years of age, initial antibiotic therapy should include coverage for *H. influenzae* as well as staphylococci and streptococci. Appropriate choices would be a second- or third-generation cephalosporin such as cefuroxime, cefotaxime, or ceftriaxone.

For children older than three years, a penicillinase-resistant pencillin such as nafcillin or a first- or second-generation cephalosporin such as cephalothin or cefuroxime is chosen.

When an etiologic agent has been isolated, the single most effective antibiotic with the fewest side effects should be administered. The general principles of antibiotic therapy in septic arthritis are given in Table 4–3. The antibiotic options for initial therapy are given in Table 4–4. Antibiotic dosage is given in Table 4–5.

Route and Duration of Administration. Initially antibiotics should be administered through the parenteral (intravenous) route. Depending on the clinical response and whether the joint is drained or not, the intravenous antibiotics are given parenterally for two to three weeks. Then they are administered orally for another two to three weeks. The duration of treatment is shorter when a joint is surgically drained, i.e., intravenous for 10 to 14 days followed by oral for two to three weeks. It is longer if there is associated osteomyelitis—a total of 6 to 12 weeks, 3 weeks of intravenous, followed by 3 to 9 weeks of oral. In the literature, recommendation for duration of antibiotic therapy is empirical; it is not based on scientific studies. Contraindications to oral antibiotic therapy are given in Table 4–6.

The most important determinant of penetration of antibiotics through the synovial barrier is the concentration of the antibiotic in the serum. When oral antibiotics are given it is vital to monitor their serum levels and determine the serum bacteriocidal titer by tube dilution methods.

Systemic administration of antibiotics can achieve adequate therapeutic levels of antibiotics in the joint. Drutz and associates reviewed the literature and showed that penicillin, methicillin, streptomycin, vancomycin, kanamycin,

Table 4–3. *Antibiotic Therapy of Septic Arthritis: General Principles*

Bactericidal antibiotics preferred
Large doses needed (usually parenteral administration)*
Broad initial coverage for organisms suspected on basis of patient's age
Change to single best agent when pathogen identified
Adequate length of therapy

*See text for exceptions.

Table 4–4. *Options for Initial Antibiotic Therapy of Acute Bone and Joint Infections in Children*

Age	Antibiotics
<2 mo.	Nafcillin + aminoglycoside
	Nafcillin + moxalactam
	Ceftriaxone
	Cefuroxime
>2 mo., <3 yr.	Ceftriaxone
	Cefuroxime
	Cefotaxime
	Nafcillin + ampicillin
>3 yr.	Nafcillin

Table 4–5. Antibiotic Dosages for Pediatric Bone and Joint Infections

	Dose/Day	Interval	Route of Administration
Ampicillin	200 mg./kg.	q. 6 hr.	I.V., I.M.
Penicillin	100,000 U./kg.	q. 4–6 hr.	I.V., I.M.
Nafcillin	200 mg./kg.	q. 6 hr.	I.V.
Gentamicin	7.5 mg./kg.	q. 8 hr.	I.V., I.M.
Amikacin	15 mg./kg.	q. 12 hr.	I.V., I.M.
Moxalactam	225 mg./kg.	q. 8 hr.	I.V.
Ceftriaxone	75 mg./kg.	q. 12 hr.	I.V., I.M.
Cefotaxime	150 mg./kg.	q. 8 hr.	I.V.
Cefuroxime	75 mg./kg.	q. 8 hr.	I.V.
Cephalothin	150 mg./kg.	q. 4–6 hr.	I.V.
Carbenicillin	400–600 mg./kg.	q. 4–6 hr.	I.V.
Piperacillin	200–300 mg./kg.	q. 4 hr.	I.V.
Ethambutol	25 mg./kg.	q.d.	P.O.
Streptomycin	15 mg./kg.	q.d.	I.M.
INH	10–20 mg./kg.	q.d.	P.O.
Rifampin	15–20 mg./kg.	b.i.d.	P.O.
Amphotericin B	1 mg./kg.*	over 6 hr.	I.V.

*Consult pharmacy for initial dosing regimen.

chloramphenicol, and tetracycline, when given in sufficient dosage, readily cross the synovial barrier, and can achieve adequate concentration in the joint fluid. Only erythromycin did not reach adequate therapeutic levels.[46]

Nelson compared joint fluid levels of antibiotics following intravenous and intramuscular administration with those obtained by intra-articular administration. With penicillin, methicillin, ampicillin, and cephalothin the levels were the same as or even higher than those obtained by injecting the antibiotic directly into the joint.[147]

This author does not recommend intra-articular administration of antibiotics, except during initial diagnostic aspiration of a joint suspected to be septic. At the end of the procedure the joint is thoroughly irrigated—first with normal saline solution, and then with a local antibiotic solution such as 1 per cent neomycin or penicillin (10,000 units per milliliter). At the end of irrigation, several milliliters of the antibiotic solution are left in the joint. Systemic antibiotics are immediately administered intravenously.

*Table 4–6. Contraindications to Oral Antibiotic Therapy**

Inability to swallow and/or retain medication
Etiologic agent not established
Inability of laboratory to perform analysis of serum bactericidal activity
Infection with agent for which no effective oral therapy exists (e.g., *Pseudomonas aeruginosa*)
Failure of patient to demonstrate clinical response to parenteral antibiotics

*From Jackson, M. A., and Nelson, J. D.: Etiology and medical management of acute suppurative bone and joint infections in pediatric patients. J. Pediatr. Orthop., 2:313, 1982. Reprinted by permission.

DRAINAGE OF JOINT

In order to evacuate bacterial products and infectious debris, surgical drainage of the affected joint is indicated in most patients. On occasion, however, the infection is diagnosed early, the disease is of short duration, and the organism is very sensitive to the antibiotic (as are meningococci and streptococci). In these cases response to conservative treatment may be dramatic, with immediate relief of local pain and tenderness, rapid increase in motion, fall of elevated temperature to normal, and subsidence of local symptoms such as effusion and synovial thickening. These patients will not require surgical drainage. In borderline cases, the joint should be reaspirated and irrigated, and cultures should be taken to check sterility. Do not administer antibiotics intra-articularly, as a high concentration may itself provoke an inflammatory reaction and be very painful. The joints that respond to conservative management are protected in plastic splints or bivalved casts, and active and passive exercises are performed until full function is restored.

Surgical drainage of the infected joint is indicated when pus is obtained on initial diagnostic aspiration or when there is no dramatic response to antibiotic therapy. One has to make a decision as to the method of drainage: repeated aspiration and irrigation, endoscopic lavage through the arthroscope, drainage through open arthrotomy, or a closed-drainage or closed-suction-drainage irrigation system.

In the older cooperative patient and for the superficial joints such as the knee, aspiration and irrigation may be an adequate form of treatment when serosanguineous fluid (not pus) is obtained on aspiration and the septic joint does not respond to simple antibiotic therapy. The drawbacks of repeated aspiration and irrigation are the pain induced by the procedure, the uncertainty of results, the recurrence of effusion and tension within the joint, the necessity for multiple punctures to evacuate loculated pockets of pus, and the difficulty of removing pus that is often thick and cannot be aspirated adequately.[164]

Drainage Through the Arthroscope. This is an effective way to lavage superficial large joints such as the knee, ankle, elbow, and shoulder. Through the arthroscope the joint can be thoroughly inspected and lavaged, and loculation can be disrupted and debris completely evacuated. Also, one can perform synovial biopsy and, if necessary, synovectomy. Tubes can be inserted for continuous drainage or continuous tube irrigation.[58] It is best to insert four tubes into the joint so that, in case some of the drains become obstructed, the drainage irrigation system is preserved for the planned duration. Arthroscopic drainage of the septic joint is best performed under general anesthesia. The operative incisional scars are small and cosmetically very acceptable. This author finds drainage lavage of pyoarthrosis of the knee, shoulder, ankle, and elbow very effective; it is highly recommended. Associated osteomyelitis, however, requires open arthrotomy and exploration and drainage of the osteomyelitic focus.

Drainage Through Open Arthrotomy. All infected hips should be drained by open arthrotomy as soon as the diagnosis is established. The hip is a deeply located joint and is difficult to aspirate without producing mechanical injury to the femoral head. After a few days of sepsis, a thick, fibrinous exudate will form that cannot be evacuated by aspiration. If the hip is not decompressed the increased intra-articular pressure will cause tamponade of retinacular vessels and avascular necrosis of the femoral head. Adequate drainage of the hip through the arthroscope is difficult; the distention of the joint required for arthroscopy may cause tamponade of blood vessels and increase the risk of avascular necrosis. Distention of the joint capsule and the associated muscle spasm will dislocate the hip. The operative technique of surgical drainage of the hip through Ober's posterior approach is illustrated in Plate 51. Some surgeons may prefer to drain the hip through the anterolateral surgical approach.

Following arthrotomy, open drainage should not be performed; it is obsolete. Closed suction drainage is carried out with or without irrigation. This author recommends simple closed drainage with adequate diameter catheters to prevent plugging. Simple closure of the wound without drainage is not recommended. Intra-articular antibiotics should not be administered.

LOCAL CARE OF JOINT

As soon as suppurative arthritis is definitely suspected, the joint should be supported by splints or skin traction. Counterpoised traction is used when possible. When the hip or knee is involved, split Russell traction is employed; for the shoulder, modified Dunlap traction; and for the elbow, traction on the forearm. Traction, whose use in septic arthritis cannot be overemphasized, has the following advantages over a cast: it relieves muscle spasm, diminishes pain, separates the joint surfaces, prevents compression of hyaline articular cartilage, allows early mobilization and restoration of function of the joint, and corrects and prevents deformity. When the wrist or ankle is involved, a plaster splint is utilized for immobilization. Providing the joint with rest and stability relieves pain and muscle spasm and prevents contractural deformity.

Active and passive exercises are performed to increase motor strength of the muscles controlling the joint and the range of joint motion. The weight-bearing joints are protected by crutches until they attain anatomic and functional normality.

Prognosis

The prognosis of septic arthritis is determined by several factors.[49, 70, 121, 139]

First is the length of *time between onset* of symptoms and *initiation of treatment*. The importance of early diagnosis cannot be overemphasized. Pus, especially under pressure in a closed space, has a necrotizing effect on hyaline cartilage, causing irreparable destruction of the joint.

Second is the *joint involved*; the prognosis is poor if the hip is the affected site. Third is the presence of *associated osteomyelitis*, which makes the prognosis poorer.

Finally, there is the *age of the patient*. Infants have a worse prognosis than do older children. This is because the hip joint is more often involved in infants, and there is a longer delay in diagnosis because systemic response to the infection is lacking.

With early recognition, adequate therapy, and meticulous postoperative care, the prognosis for joint function is good.

Surgical Drainage of the Hip Through Ober's Posterior Approach

OPERATIVE TECHNIQUE

A. The skin incision is made in line with the middle of the femoral neck, starting 1 inch distal to the tip of the greater trochanter and extending proximally toward the posterior superior iliac spine.

B. With scissors the fibers of the gluteus maximus muscle are bluntly separated in line with the skin incision. If branches of the gluteal vessels are encountered, they are ligated and divided. The sciatic nerve, lying in a layer of fatty tissue in the medial angle of the incision, is identified and protected from injury. The distended capsule is exposed by retracting the short rotator muscles. If wider exposure is necessary, the short rotator muscles can be detached from the trochanter.

C. and **D.** The capsule and synovial membrane are incised throughout their posterosuperior length, and, if necessary, also transversely in the superomedial portion. The joint is thoroughly irrigated with normal saline and then with appropriate antibiotic solution to remove all fibrinous debris. The synovial membrane and capsule are sutured with 00 Vicryl to the surrounding soft tissues and gluteal fascia. One or two plastic tubes of small diameter are sutured with 00 Vicryl to the "marsupialized" capsule. The tubes are placed into the joint, but not between the femoral head and the acetabulum.

E. The soft tissues and skin are closed primarily. The egress tube is connected to a low Gomko wall suction unit or to a Hemovac evacuator. Closed suction irrigation of the joint with antibiotics is not recommended; therefore, this author does not insert an ingress tube as shown in the illustration.

Upon leaving the operating room the infant is immediately replaced in counterpoised bilateral split Russell traction with the hips in wide abduction.

POSTOPERATIVE CARE

Active and passive exercises should be performed by the patient several times a day while in traction to gradually develop motion of the hip joint. Periodic roentgenograms of the hip are taken in traction to determine the relationship of the femoral head to the acetabulum and also the subsidence of effusion and synovial thickening. Traction is continued for at least three weeks postoperatively until the affected hip has full range of motion and synovial thickening has subsided.

The patient is discharged home in a bivalved one-and-one-half hip spica cast, maintaining the affected hip in 30 to 40 degrees of abduction and neutral rotation. Active and passive range-of-motion exercises are performed out of the cast several times a day, and the periods out of the cast are gradually increased. Weight-bearing, such as crawling or standing, is not permitted for six weeks; then walking is resumed gradually, the hip being protected with a three-point crutch gait. Early weight-bearing causes compression of the softened hyaline cartilage and consequent degenerative arthritis in later life.

Plate 51. Surgical Drainage of the Hip Through Ober's Posterior Approach

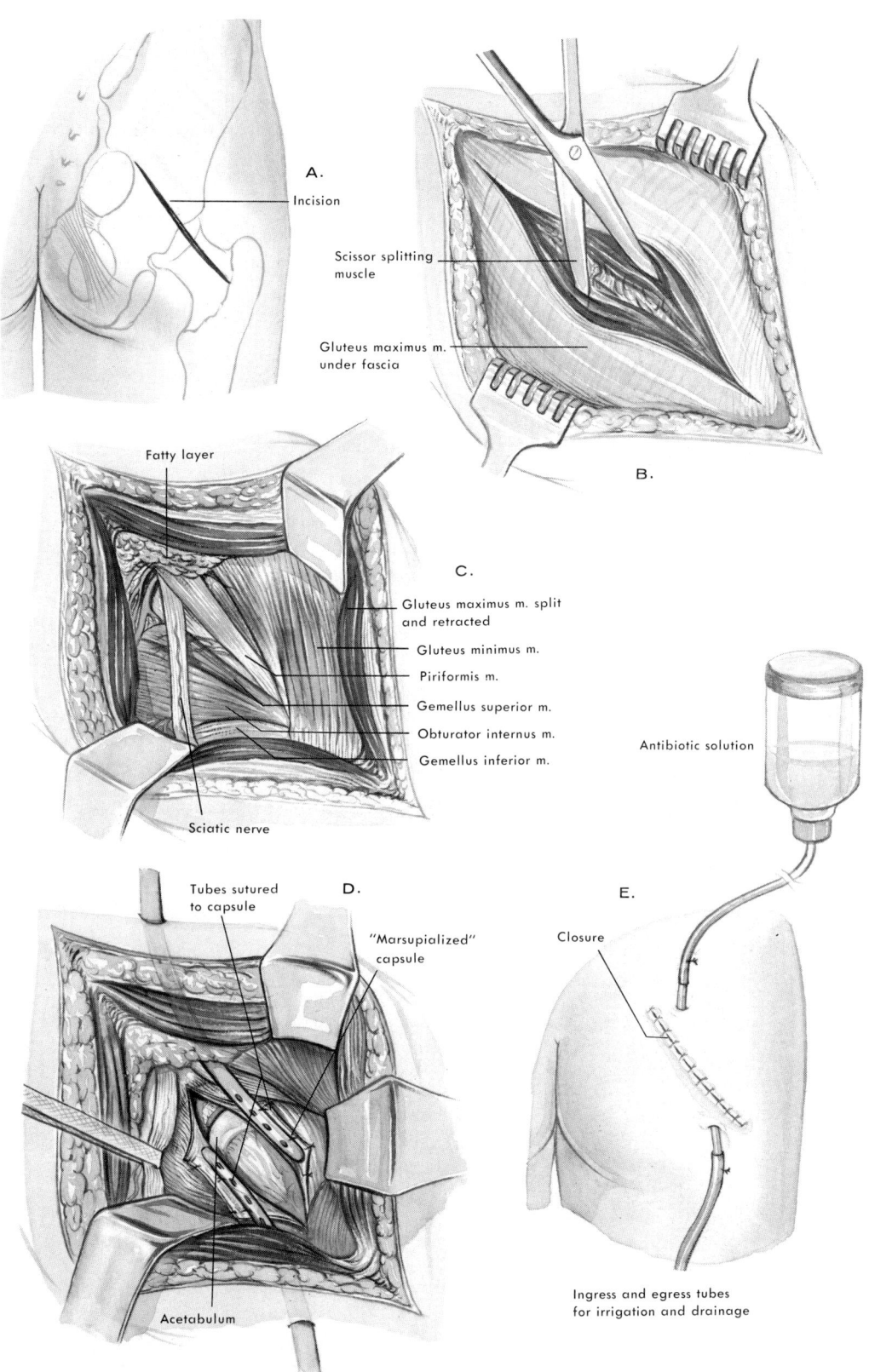

Septic Arthritis of the Hip in the Newborn and Infant

Septic arthritis of the hip is a serious problem and is discussed separately in order to stress several factors: the often-delayed diagnosis, the urgency of immediate surgical drainage, the importance of diligent postoperative care, and the consequent irreparable damage to the hip joint if inadequately treated.*

Sepsis of the hip joint is hematogenous. From the metaphysis of the neck of the femur, an osteomyelitic focus can break through the cortex and liberate pus into the hip joint (Fig. 4–5). This is the common route of infection. In some cases, however, the organisms may reach the joint by lodging primarily in the synovial membrane.

Clinical Features. Fever is not the usual finding of septicemia in infancy, especially during the neonatal period. One cannot overemphasize this lack of systemic reaction in the newborn with sepsis. Septicemia should be suspected in an infant who has an open wound or focus of infection, one who is irritable, refuses to feed, or fails to gain or maintain weight. When septicemia is present, the limbs should be carefully and frequently examined for localization of infection in bones or joints.

The septic hip joint is held in the position of minimum hydrostatic pressure, i.e., moderate flexion (45 to 60 degrees), slight abduction (10 to 20 degrees), and some lateral rotation (10 to 15 degrees). Passive motions of the affected hip are painful and limited in range. On palpation of the hip anteriorly and posteriorly there is local tenderness, as shown by increase in the intensity of the cry. The proximal thigh, the inguinal region, and the buttocks are edematous and swollen. With subluxation and dislocation, asymmetry of the gluteal, thigh, and popliteal creases will develop (Fig. 4–6).

Imaging Findings. Ultrasonography will show fluid in the hip joint. Radiograms of the hips show soft-tissue swelling, capsular distention, and varying degrees of lateral displacement of the proximal femur (indicating subluxation) (Fig. 4–7 A). Pathologic dislocation of the hip may occur. Later in the course of the disease, areas of rarefaction in the metaphysis of the femoral neck may develop, and subperiosteal new bone may form along the proximal femoral shaft as a result of associated osteomyelitis.

---

*See references 19, 48, 49, 70, 75, 90, 114, 121, 139, 152, 155, 180, 222.

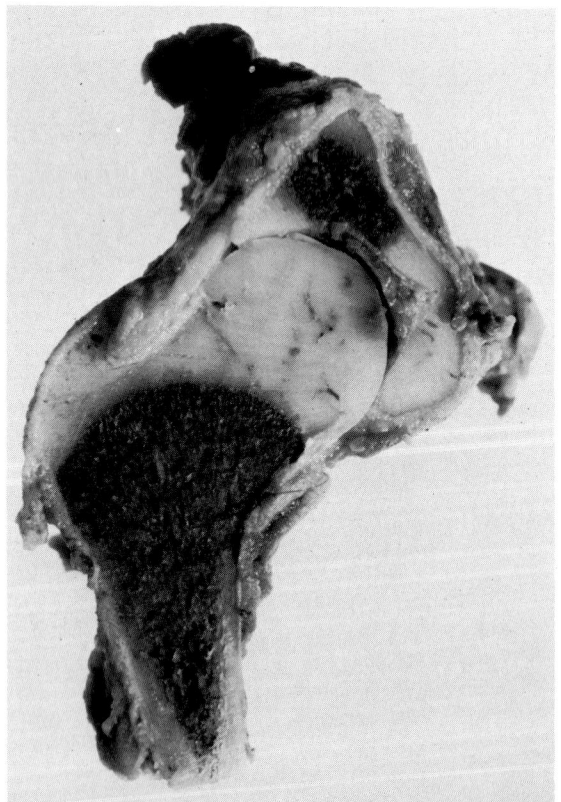

FIGURE 4–5. Gross specimen of the hip joint of an infant.

Note that the metaphysis of the femoral neck is intracapsular.

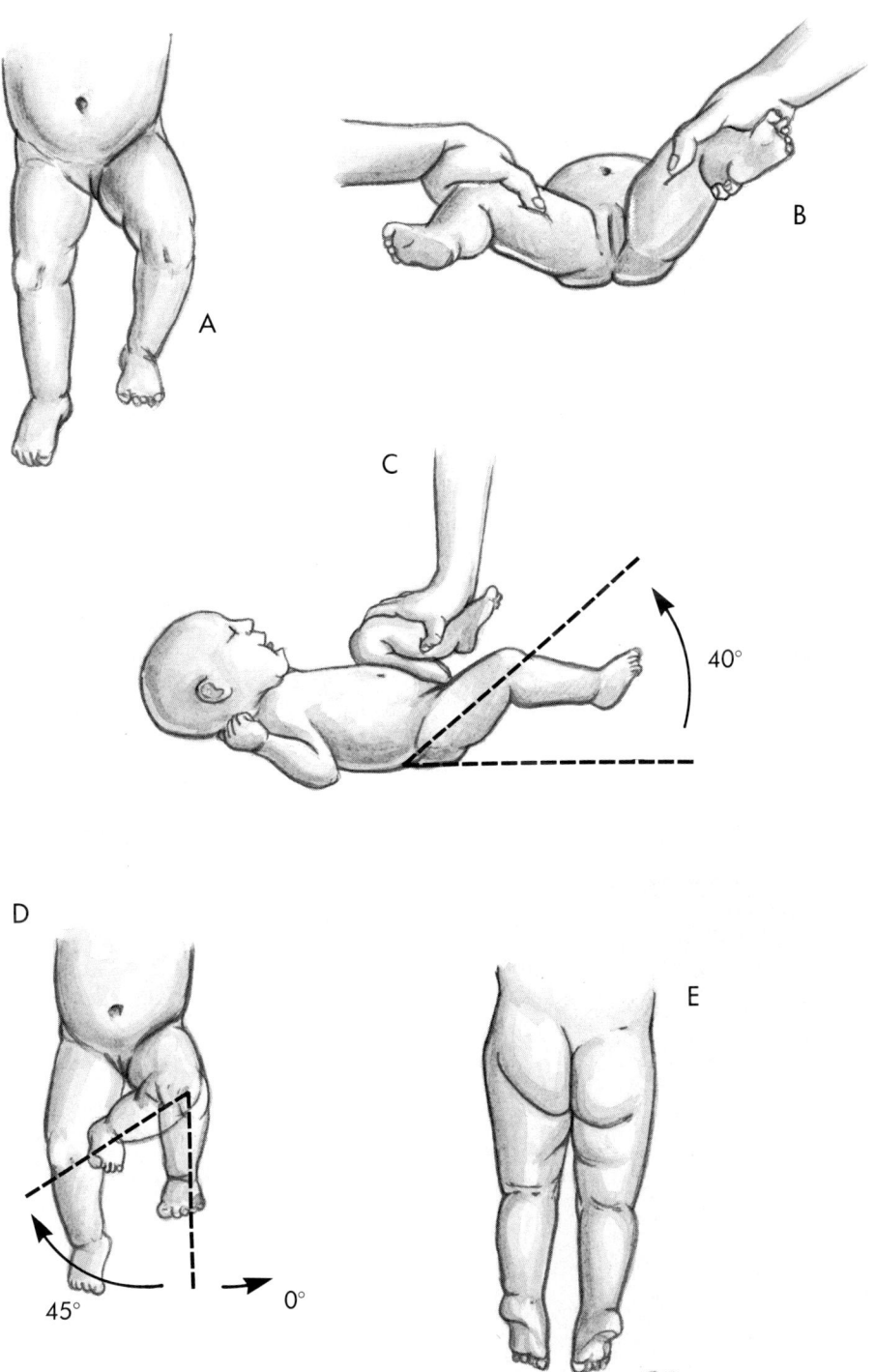

FIGURE 4-6. Physical findings in suppurative arthritis of the hip.

A. The acutely inflamed hip is held in the position of comfort—that of minimum hydrostatic pressure. Note the edematous and swollen proximal thigh, and inguinal and gluteal regions. **B.** Limitation of and resistance to passive hip abduction. **C.** Passive hip extension is limited. **D.** Limited medial rotation in flexion. **E.** Asymmetry of gluteal, thigh, and popliteal creases has developed with subluxation of the hip.

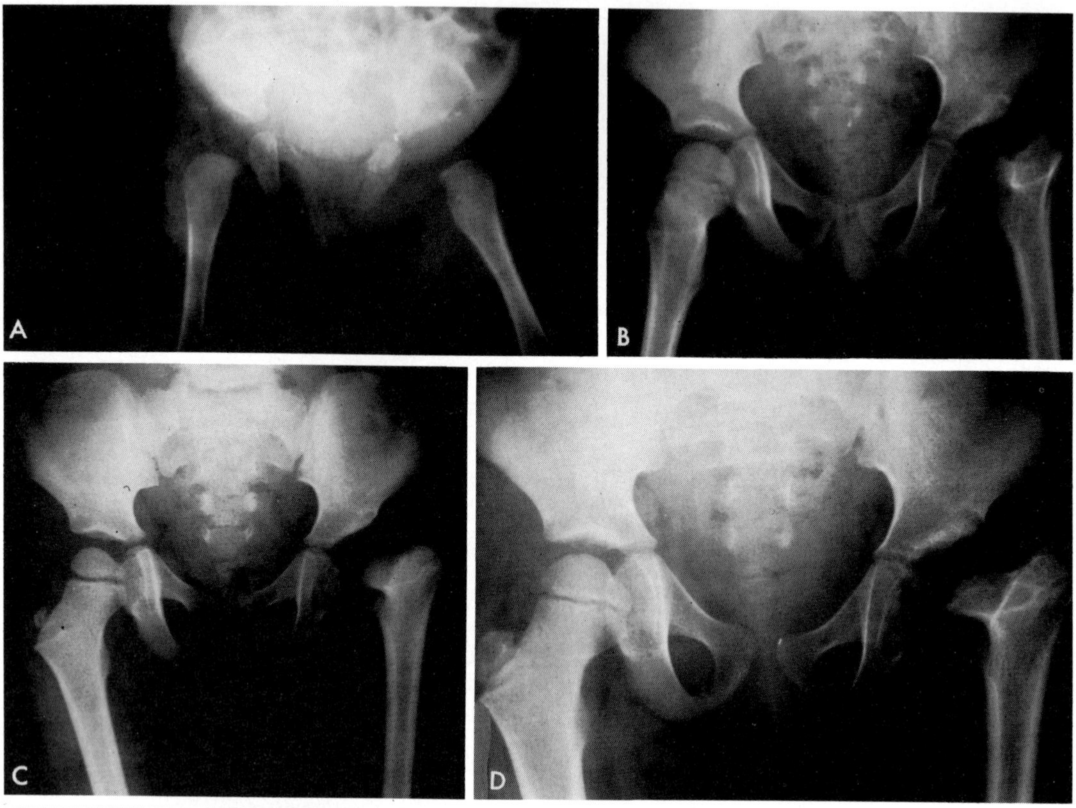

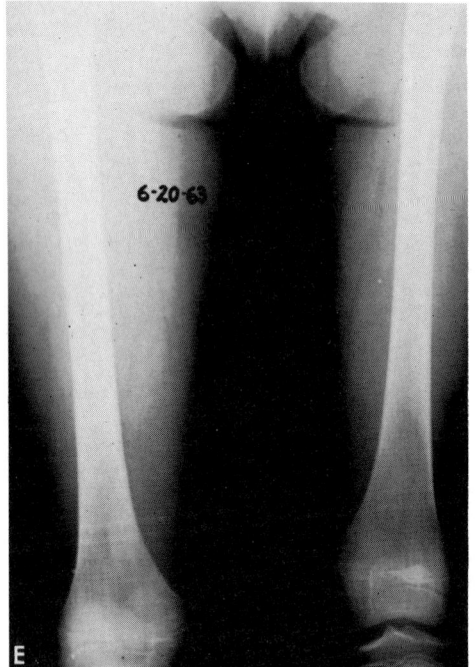

FIGURE 4–7. *Suppurative arthritis of the left hip in a three-month-old infant.*

Onset was at four weeks of age. Erroneous diagnosis of fibrocystic disease and thrombophlebitis resulted in a two-month delay in diagnosis. **A.** Radiograms of hips show marked effusion of left hip with lateral subluxation. **B** to **D.** Serial radiograms of hips show failure of ossification of the femoral head (due to avascular necrosis) and the development of coxa vara. **E.** Teleoradiograms taken nine and one half years after onset of sepsis in left hip. There is a 3.9-cm. shortening of left femur. A subtrochanteric abduction osteotomy was performed four years earlier. The left hip has functional range of motion. Skeletal growth of lower limbs is being followed, and the plan is to perform distal femoral epiphyseodesis on the right at the appropriate age.

A bone scan with technetium-99m will disclose intense increased focal uptake in the metaphysis of the femoral neck if there is associated osteomyelitis. A gallium-67 citrate scan will show generalized increased periarticular uptake. Occasionally computed tomography is performed to rule out both osteomyelitis of the acetabulum or femoral neck and posterior or anterior dislocation of the hip.

Laboratory Findings. The total white blood

count and differential count may often be normal; one should not be deceived by this lack of systemic response.

Treatment. As soon as the possibility of septic hip is suspected, the joint is aspirated to confirm the diagnosis and the hip joint is drained. The operative technique of drainage of the hip through the posterior approach is illustrated in Plate 51. The anterolateral approach is utilized if there is associated osteomyelitis of the femoral neck or if the hip is subluxated or dislocated. When the approach is anterolateral, particularly if the femoral head is displaced, it is important to immobilize it in abduction, medial rotation, and some flexion in order to prevent anterior dislocation.

Complications. *Avascular necrosis of the femoral head* is caused by tamponade of retinacular vessels with increased hydrostatic pressure in the hip joint. Initially it can be detected in the bone scan with technetium-99m by lack of uptake of the radionuclide. Later, necrosis of the femoral head is recognized in the radiogram by the absence or loss of its ossification center (see Fig. 4–7). Avascular necrosis of the femoral head is treated by protecting the affected hip from forces of weight-bearing—first, in a bivalved hip spica cast or hip abduction splint, and later, as the child gets older, in an ambulatory hip containment splint such as the Scottish-Rite orthosis.

Coxa magna is a frequent sequela of septic avascular necrosis. With arrest of growth of the capital femoral epiphyseal plate and continued growth from the greater trochanteric apophysis, a varying degree of *relative overgrowth of the greater trochanter* and shortening of the femoral neck occur (Fig. 4–8). The result is gluteus medius–short leg limp. The greater trochanter may abut the lateral wall of the ilium, limiting hip abduction. Arrest of the greater trochanteric apophysis or distal lateral transfer of the greater trochanter is indicated in such cases.

Coxa vara may result. If it is severe, an abduction osteotomy of the proximal femur is performed to correct it.

Lower limb length discrepancy is a common complication that is treated by epiphysiodesis of the longer leg at the appropriate age, if it is of clinical significance. In inadequately treated cases, *fibrous ankylosis* of the hip joint may result (Fig. 4–9).

Pathologic dislocation results from marked effusion and increased intra-articular pressure (Fig. 4–10). All these hips are drained, and at operation an open reduction of the hip is performed. The reduction is maintained in a solid hip spica cast for two to three weeks. The cast is later bivalved, and gentle passive and active exercises are performed to develop motion in the joint.

With delayed diagnosis, the cartilaginous femoral head may be destroyed and the femoral neck may have disintegrated into a "nubbin." The result is an unstable hip with lateral and proximal migration of the femur and flexion-adduction contracture of the hip. Failure of growth from the capital femoral physis causes progressive shortening of the femur. The child walks with a short leg and gluteus medius or Trendelenburg lurch. The hip joint becomes progressively stiff and painful. In such an instance, the greater trochanter is placed in the acetabulum and the hip abductors are transferred distally. In four to six weeks, a varization osteotomy is performed to establish a physiologic femoral neck-shaft angle.

Colonna developed a greater trochanteric arthroplasty in which the greater trochanteric apophysis is placed in the acetabulum, and the gluteus medius and minimus muscles are transferred distally on the femoral shaft to improve their motor function.[28] Initially Colonna used the greater trochanteric hip arthroplasty for treatment of ununited fractures of the femoral neck. The use of Colonna's hip arthroplasty to treat pathologic dislocation of the septic hip with destroyed femoral head was described by Lloyd Roberts, who also recommended varus osteotomy of the upper femoral shaft to improve hip abductor leverage.[115, 117] The Colonna procedure with varus subtrochanteric osteotomy was performed in a three and one half–year–old child by Weissman and in a three-year-old child by Stetson and associates with follow-up of 6½ years and 11 years, respectively.[208, 222] In both cases the hip joints were located but ankylosed. Rigault and associates reported their experience with ten greater trochanteric arthroplasties, six of which were for femoral heads destroyed by septic arthritis. The results of these six operations were: no motion in two hips, fair range of motion in two, and in the remaining two cases, follow-up too short to assess.[177] Westin, in 1970, reported 17 greater trochanteric arthroplasties, six of which were performed for sequelae of septic arthritis; he termed the procedure the "stick femur reconstruction." In 1980 the results of Westin's cases from the Shriner's Hospital for Crippled Children, Los Angeles, were published by Freeland, Sullivan and Westin. The average follow-up of these patients was 11 years, and 14 patients were followed to skeletal maturity or

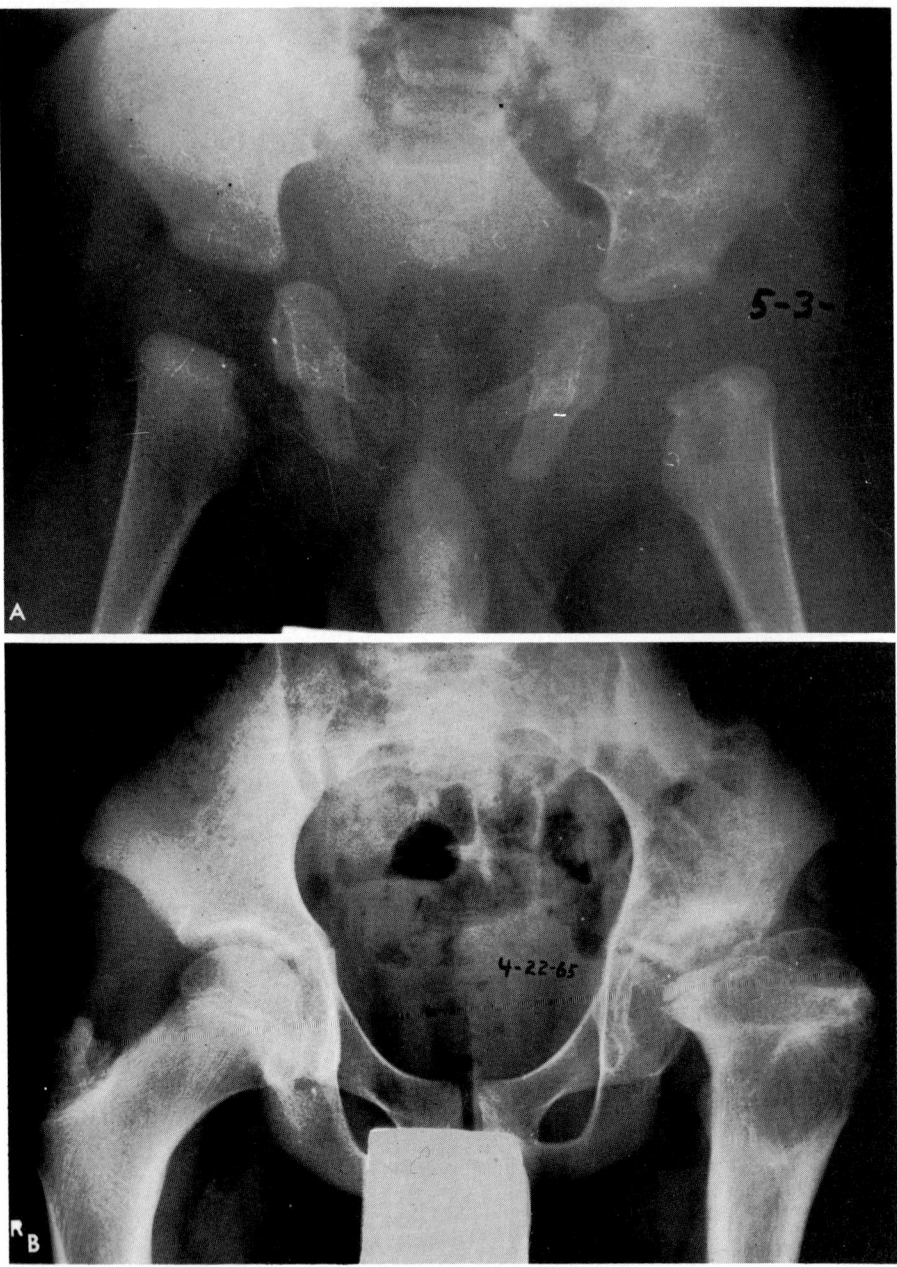

FIGURE 4–8. *A two-month-old infant with septic arthritis of left hip and osteomyelitis of femoral neck.*

The child was treated with antibiotics only for four weeks. **A.** Initial radiograms of the hips show the marked effusion with lateral subluxation and an area of radiolucency in the metaphysis of the femoral neck. **B.** Radiograms of the hips taken at 11 years of age. Note the short and markedly broadened left femoral neck with loss of most of the capital epiphysis and persistence of subluxation of the hip. There is limitation of motion of the left hip and 2.1 cm. shortening of left femur.

longer. In Group I, consisting of four patients with greater trochanteric arthroplasty alone, good initial stability gradually deteriorated as subluxation occurred, accompanied by a proportionate return of abductor limp, loss of hip motion, and an increased rate of degenerative changes in the joint. Group II, consisting of eight patients who had either acetabuloplasty or innominate osteotomy in addition to greater trochanteric arthroplasty, had only slightly improved hip containment and results similar to those in Group I. Spontaneous ankylosis of the hip occurred in six of the patients in those two groups; this may have been due to loss of articular cartilage and exposed cancellous bone due to previous sepsis, reaming of the cartilage

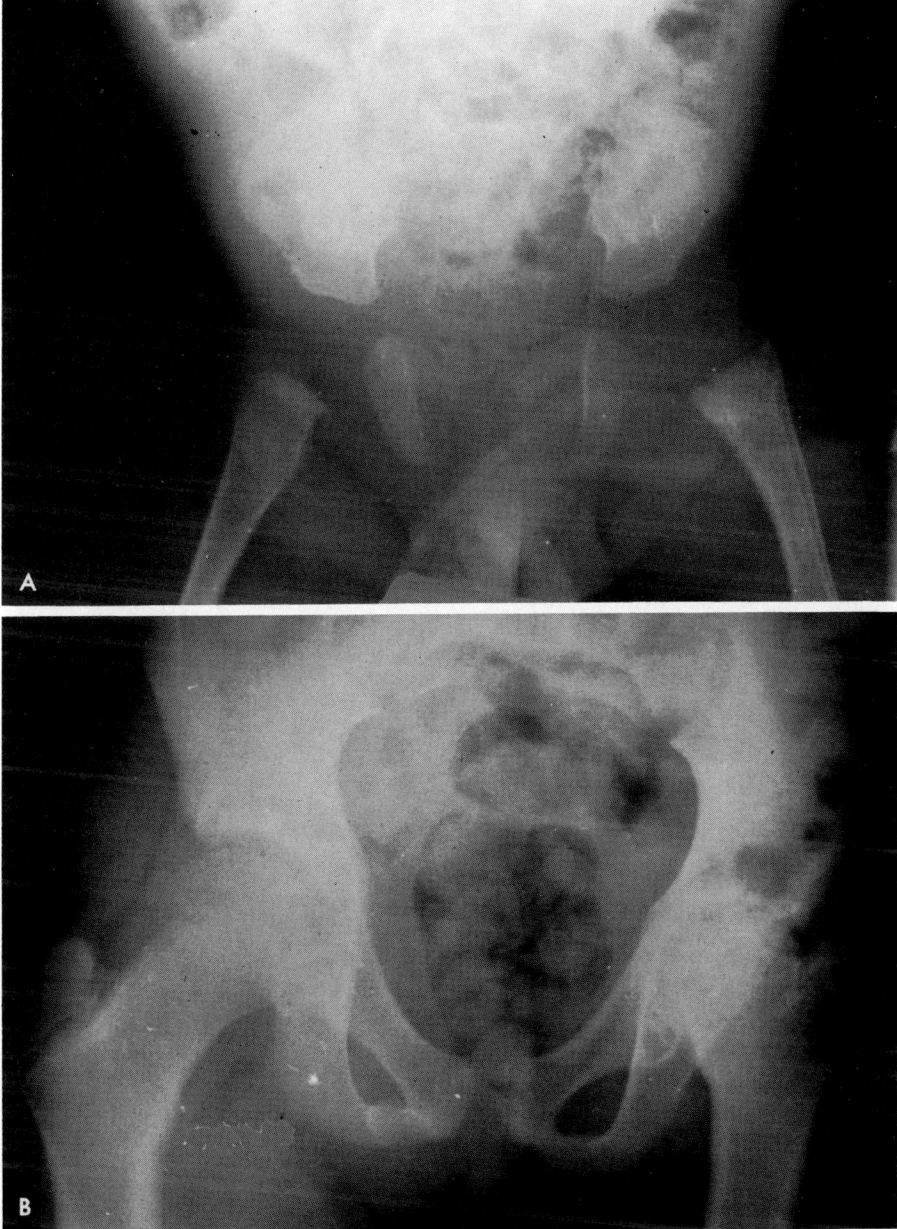

FIGURE 4-9. *Septic arthritis of left hip with osteomyelitis of proximal femur in a newborn infant.*

Six-week delay in diagnosis was due to lack of systemic reaction. The child was treated with antibiotics for one month and immobilization in a hip spica cast for three months. **A.** Radiograms of hips show effusion in left hip with lateral subluxation and osteomyelitis of left proximal femur. **B.** Radiograms of hips taken 11 years later show the hip joint ankylosed in 40 degrees flexion and 20 degrees adduction. Growth from the capital femoral epiphysis has stopped. The greater trochanteric apophysis has continued to grow and is abutting the lateral surface of the ilium. There is 3-cm. shortening of the left femur.

of the acetabulum at the time of arthroplasty, and increased articular pressure. In Group III (four patients) greater trochanteric arthroplasty and proximal femoral osteotomy were performed; and in Group IV greater trochanteric arthroplasty, proximal femoral osteotomy, and innominate osteotomy were performed. Best results were obtained in the 5 patients in Groups III and IV, who had supplemental proximal femoral varus osteotomy to decompress the hip and decrease the need for acetabular reconstruction and deepening.[56]

Combined Acute Osteomyelitis and Septic Arthritis. Failure to detect the pressure of acute

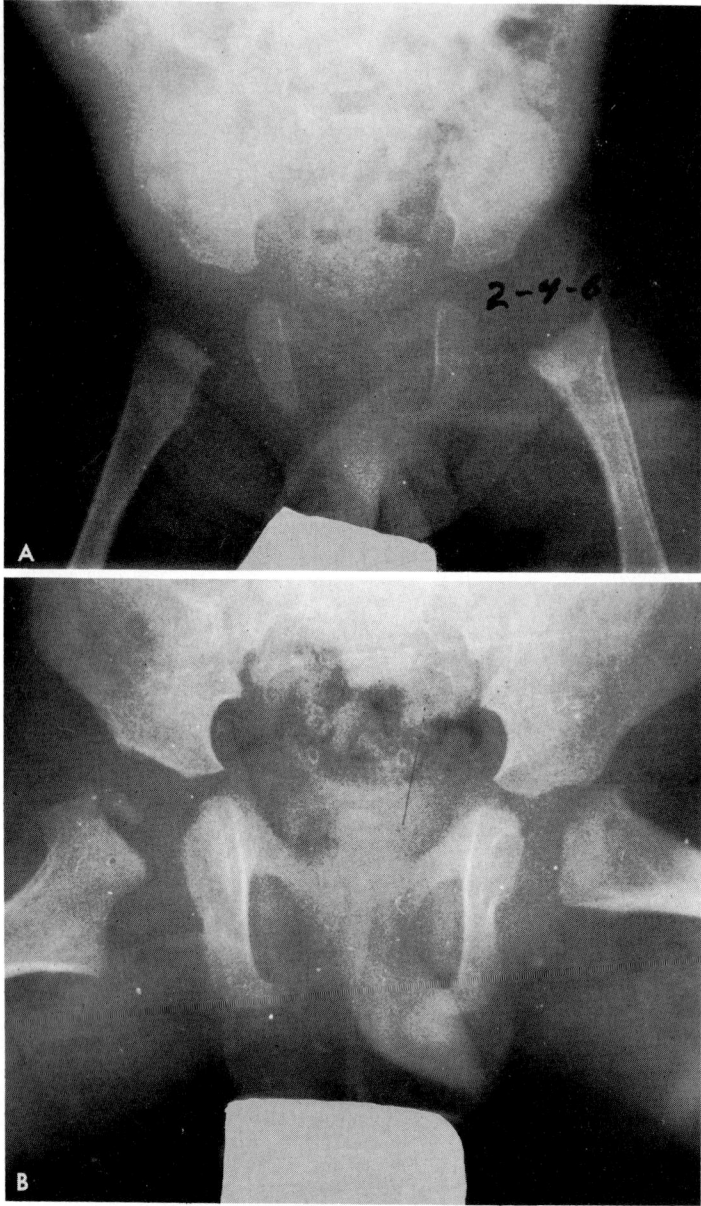

FIGURE 4–10. Septic arthritis of left hip with osteomyelitis of proximal femur in a two-month-old infant.

Onset of suppurative arthritis was at birth, but recognition was delayed because of misdiagnosis of thrombophlebitis due to exchange transfusion. **A.** Initial radiogram. Treatment was with antibiotics and abduction splint. **B.** Radiogram of hips at one and one half years of age. Note the posterior dislocation of the left hip. At arthrotomy the femoral head was found to be disintegrated to a small nubbin and dislocated posteriorly. The greater trochanter was placed into the acetabulum and maintained in a hip spica cast.

osteomyelitis when draining a septic joint, particularly the hip, can result in failure of positive response to treatment. Scintigraphy with technetium-99m and gallium citrate has made it relatively simple to rule out association of osteomyelitis with septic arthritis. Always ask the question—is the infection mixed—bone and joint or joint only? When draining a septic hip when associated osteomyelitis of the femoral neck is suspected, it is best to use the anterolateral approach; it permits better visualization and palpation of the femoral neck and bone drilling for decompression of the abscess. In such a case antibiotic therapy should be continued for a minimum of six weeks, at least three weeks of which should be parenteral.

Septic Arthritis Superimposed on Pre-Existing Joint Disease

A joint damaged by a disease process may become the site for a septic process. Rheumatoid arthritis, avascular necrosis, Charcot (neuropathic) joints, gout, and hypercortisonism are conditions that predispose joints to a septic process.[71, 85, 100, 105, 123, 129, 141] It is vital to have a high degree of clinical suspicion in these conditions; in order to make the diagnosis the painful inflamed joint should be aspirated. Early diagnosis and immediate adequate treatment are crucial in order to prevent irreparable damage to the affected joint.

References

1. Alderson, M., Speers, D., Emslie, K., and Nade, S.: Acute haematogenous osteomyelitis and septic arthritis—a single disease. A hypothesis based upon the presence of transepiphyseal blood vessels. J. Bone Joint Surg., 68-B:268, 1986.
2. Ang-Fonte, G. Z., Rozboril, M. B., and Thompson, G. R.: Changes in nongonococcal septic arthritis. Drug abuse and methicillin-resistant Staphylococcus aureus. Arthritis Rheum., 28:210, 1985.
3. Arvidson, S., Holme, T., and Lindholm, B.: The formation of extracellular proteolytic enzymes by Staphylococcus aureus. Acta Pathol. Microbiol. Scand. [B.], 80:835, 1972.
4. Asnes, R. S., and Arendar, G. M.: Septic arthritis of the hip: A complication of femoral venipuncture. Pediatrics, 38:837, 1966.
5. Atkinson, L. S., Halford, J. G., Jr., Burton, O. M., and Moorhead, S. R., Jr.: Septic and aseptic arthritis complicating varicella. J. Fam. Pract., 12:917, 1981.
6. Badgely, C. E.: Study of the end-results in 113 cases of septic hips. J. Bone Joint Surg., 18:1047, 1936.
7. Baitch, A.: Recent observations of acute suppurative arthritis. Clin. Orthop., 22:157, 1962.
8. Balboni, V. G., Shapiro, I. M., and Kydd, P. M.: The penetration of penicillin into joint fluid following intramuscular administration. Am. J. Med. Sci., 210:588, 1945.
9. Bardenheier, J. A., III, Morgan, H. C., and Stamp, W. G.: Treatment and sequelae of experimentally-produced septic arthritis. Surg. Gynecol. Obstet., 120:249, 1966.
10. Bird, H. A., and Ring, E. F.: Thermography and radiology in the localization of infections. Rheumatol. Rehabil., 17:103, 1978.
11. Bliznak, J., and Ramsey, J.: Emphysematous septic arthritis due to Escherichia coli. J. Bone Joint Surg., 58-A:138, 1976.
12. Bobechko, W. P.: Autoimmune reactions of articular cartilage. Orthop. Surg. Traumatol. Int. Cong. Series 291, SICOT, 1972.
13. Bobechko, W. P., and Mandel, L.: Immunology of cartilage in septic arthritis. Clin. Orthop., 108:84, 1975.
14. Borella, L., Goobar, J. E., Summit, R. I., and Clark, G. M.: Septic arthritis in childhood. J. Pediatr., 62:742, 1963.
15. Borman, T. R., Johnson, R. A., and Sherman, F. C.: Gallium scintigraphy for diagnosis of septic arthritis and osteomyelitis in children. J. Pediatr. Orthop., 6:317, 1986.
16. Bowler, J., Drvaric, D. M., Roberts, J. M., and Burke, S. W.: Kawasaki syndrome presenting as pyarthrosis of the hip. A case report. J. Bone Joint Surg., 68-A:467, 1986.
17. Braude, A. I., Jones, J. L., and Douglas, H.: The behavior of Escherichia coli endotoxin (somatic antigen) during infectious arthritis. J. Immunol., 90:297, 1963.
18. Broughton, R. A., Wilson, H. D., Goodman, N. L., and Hedrick, J. A.: Septic arthritis and osteomyelitis caused by an organism of the genus rhodococcus. J. Clin. Microbiol., 13:209, 1981.
19. Bryson, A. F.: Treatment of pathologic dislocation of the hip after suppurative arthritis in infants. J. Bone Joint Surg., 30-B:449, 1943.
20. Bynum, D. K., Nunley, J. A., Goldner, J. L., and Martinez, S.: Pyogenic arthritis. Emphasis on the need for surgical drainage of the infected joint. South. Med. J., 75:1232, 1982.
21. Cauchoix, J., and Duprae, J.: La synovectomie dans le traitement des arthrites suppurées du genou. Mem. Acad. Chir., 88:569, 1962.
22. Chacha, P. B.: Suppurative arthritis of the hip joints in infancy. J. Bone Joint Surg., 53-A:538, 1971.
23. Chang, M. J., Controni, G., and Rodriquez, W. J.: Ampicillin-resistant Hemophilus influenzae type B septic arthritis in children. Clin. Pediatr., (Phila.), 20:139, 1981.
24. Chusid, M. J., and Sty, J. R.: Pneumococcal arthritis and osteomyelitis in children. Clin. Pediatr., (Phila.), 20:105, 1981.
25. Chusid, M. J., Jacobs, W. M., and Sty, J. R.: Pseudomonas arthritis following puncture wounds of the foot. J. Pediatr., 94:429, 1979.
26. Clawson, D. K., and Dunn, A. W.: Management of common bacterial infections of bones and joints. J. Bone Joint Surg., 49-A:164, 1967.
27. Colchero, F. R., Orst, G., and Vidal, J.: Scarification: Its role in the treatment of chronic fistulated pyogenic osteoarticular infection. Int. Orthop., 6:263, 1982.
28. Colonna, P. C.: A new type of reconstruction operation for old ununited fracture of the neck of the femur. J. Bone Joint Surg., 17:110, 1935.
29. Compere, E. L., Metzger, W. I., and Rathindra, N. M.: The treatment of pyogenic bone and joint infections by closed irrigation (circulation) with a non-toxic detergent and one or more antibiotics. J. Bone Joint Surg., 49-A:614, 1967.
30. Conway, J. J.: Radionuclide bone imaging in pediatrics. Pediatr. Clin. North Am., 24:701, 1977.
31. Cooke, C. P., III, Levinsohn, E. M., and Baker, B. E.: Septic hip in pelvic fractures with urologic injury: A case report, review of the literature and discussion of the pathophysiology. Clin. Orthop., 147:253, 1980.
32. Coy, J. T., III, Wolf, C. R., Brower, T. D., and Winter, W. G.: Pyogenic arthritis of the sacroiliac joint. Long-term follow-up. J. Bone Joint Surg., 58-A:845, 1976.
33. Curtiss, P. H., Jr.: Destruction of articular cartilage in septic arthritis. I. In vitro studies. J. Bone Joint Surg., 45-A:797, 1963.
34. Curtiss, P. H., Jr.: Cartilage damage in septic arthritis. Clin. Orthop., 64:87, 1969.
35. Curtiss, P. H., Jr.: The pathophysiology of joint infections. Clin. Orthop., 96:129, 1973.
36. Curtiss, P. H., Jr., and Klein, L.: Destruction of articular cartilage in septic arthritis. I. In vivo studies. J. Bone Joint Surg., 49-A:797, 1963.
37. Dal Monte, A., Capelli, A., and Donzelli, O., et al.: Trochanteroplasty in the treatment of infantile septic

arthritis of the hip. Ital. J. Orthop. Traumatol., 10:145, 1984.
38. Dan, M.: Septic arthritis in young infants: Clinical and microbiologic correlations and therapeutic implications. Rev. Infect. Dis., 6:147, 1984.
39. Daniel, D., Akeson, W., Amiel, D., Ryder, M., and Boyer, J.: Lavage of septic joints in rabbits: Effects of chondrolysis. J. Bone Joint Surg., 58-A:393, 1976.
40. Daniel, D., Boyer, J., Green, S., Amiel, D., and Akeson, W.: Cartilage destruction in experimentally produced Staphylococcus aureus joint infections. Surg. Forum, 24:479, 1973.
41. DeLucas, P. A., Gutman, L. T., and Ruderman, R. J.: Counterimmunoelectrophoresis of synovial fluid in the diagnosis of septic arthritis. J. Pediatr. Orthop., 5:167, 1985.
42. Dick, H. M., and Tietjen, R.: Humeral lengthening for septic neonatal growth arrest. Case report. J. Bone Joint Surg., 60-A:1138, 1978.
43. Dingle, J. T.: The role of lysosomal enzymes in skeletal tissue. J. Bone Joint Surg., 55-B:87, 1973.
44. Dorff, G., Ziolkowski, J. S., and Rytel, M. W.: Detection by counterimmunoelectrophoresis of pneumococcal antigen from synovial fluid in septic arthritis. Arthritis Rheum., 18:613, 1975.
45. Dorff, G. J., Frerichs, L., Zabransky, R. J., Jacobs, P., and Spankus, J. D.: Musculoskeletal infections due to Mycobacterium kansasii. Clin. Orthop., 136:244, 1978.
46. Drutz, D. J., Schaffner, W., Hillman, J. W., and Koenig, M. G.: The penetration of penicillin and other antimicrobials into joint fluid. Three case reports with a reappraisal of the literature. J. Bone Joint Surg., 49-A:1415, 1967.
47. Egund, N., Wingstrand, H., Forsberg, L., Pettersson, H., and Sunden, G.: Computed tomography and ultrasonography for diagnosis of hip joint effusion in children. Acta Orthop. Scand., 57:212, 1986.
48. Eyre-Brook, A. L.: Septic arthritis of the hip and osteomyelitis of the upper end of the femur in infants. J. Bone Joint Surg., 42-B:11, 1960.
49. Fabry, G., and Meire, E.: Septic arthritis of the hip in children: Poor results after late and inadequate treatment. J. Pediatr. Orthop., 3:461, 1983.
50. Feigin, R. D., Pickering, L. K., Anderson, D., Keeney, R. E., and Shackleford, P. C.: Clindamycin treatment of osteomyelitis and septic arthritis in children. Pediatrics, 55:213, 1975.
51. Fessel, J. M., and Chrisman, O. D.: Enzymatic degradation of chondromucoprotein by cell-free extracts of human cartilage. Arthritis Rheum., 7:398, 1964.
52. Finsterbusch, A., Argaman, M., and Backs, T.: Bone and joint perfusions with antibiotics in the treatment of experimental staphylococcal infections in rabbits. J. Bone Joint Surg., 52-A:1424, 1970.
53. Fitzgerald, R. H., Jr.: Antimicrobial therapy for the musculoskeletal system. Instr. Course Lect., 31:1, 1982.
54. Fitzgerald, R. H., Jr., Rosenblatt, J. E., Tenney, J. H., et al.: Anaerobic septic arthritis. Clin. Orthop., 164:141, 1982.
55. Fraser, G. L.: Treatment of nongonococcal bacterial septic arthritis. Drug Intell. Clin. Pharm., 151:531, 1981.
56. Freeland, A. E., Sullivan, D. J., and Westin, G. W.: Greater trochanteric hip arthroplasty in children with loss of the femoral head. J. Bone Joint Surg., 62-A:1351, 1980.
57. Freiberg, J. A., and Perlman, R.: Pelvic abscesses associated with acute purulent infection of the hip joint. J. Bone Joint Surg., 18:417, 1936.
58. Gainor, B. J.: Instillation of continuous tube irrigation in the septic knee at arthroscopy: A technique. Clin. Orthop., 183:96, 1984.

59. Gamble, J. G., Rinsky, L. A., and Bleck, E. E.: Acetabular osteomyelitis in children. Clin. Orthop., 186:71, 1984.
60. Gelman, M. I., and Ward, J. R.: Septic arthritis: A complication of rheumatoid arthritis. Radiology, 122:17, 1977.
61. Gerard, Y., Lamarque, B., Segal, P., Bedoucha, J. S., and Schernberg, F.: La place de la synovectomie dans le traitement des arthrites aiguës a pyogènes. Rev. Rhum., 44:741, 1977.
62. Gillespie, R.: Septic arthritis of childhood. Clin. Orthop., 96:152, 1973.
63. Girdlestone, G. R.: Acute pyogenic arthritis of the hip; operation giving free access and effective drainage. 1943. Clin. Orthop., 170:3, 1982.
64. Goldenberg, D. L., and Cohen, A. S.: Acute infectious arthritis. A review of patients with nongonococcal joint infections (with emphasis on therapy and prognosis). Am. J. Med., 60:369, 1976.
65. Goldenberg, D. L., and Reed, J. I.: Bacterial arthritis. N. Engl. J. Med., 312:764, 1985.
66. Goldenberg, D. L., Reed, J. I., and Rice, P. A.: Arthritis in rabbits induced by killed Neisseria gonorrhoeae and gonococcal lipopolysacharide. J. Rheumatol., 11:3, 1984.
67. Goldenberg, D. L., Brandt, K. D., Cohen, A. S., and Cathcart, E. S.: Treatment of septic arthritis. Comparison of needle aspiration and surgery as initial modes of joint drainage. Arthritis Rheum., 18:83, 1975.
68. Gompels, B. M., and Darlington, L. G.: Septic arthritis in rheumatoid disease causing bilateral shoulder dislocation: Diagnosis and treatment assisted by grey scale ultrasonography. Ann. Rheum. Dis., 40:609, 1981.
69. Griffin, P. P.: Bone and joint infections in children. Pediatr. Clin. North Am., 14:533, 1967.
70. Griffin, P. P., and Green, W. T.: Hip joint infections in infants and children. Orthop. Clin. North Am., 9:123, 1978.
71. Gristina, A. G., Rovere, G. D., and Shoji, H.: Spontaneous septic arthritis complicating rheumatoid arthritis. J. Bone Joint Surg., 56-A:1180, 1974.
72. Gutowicz, I. F., and Doenning, D. A.: Septic hip in a child. J. Fam. Pract., 12:841, 1981.
73. Habermann, E. T., and Friedenthal, R. B.: Septic arthritis associated with avascular necrosis of the femoral head. Clin. Orthop., 134:325, 1978.
74. Hall, B. B., Rosenblatt, J. E., and Fitzgerald, R. H., Jr.: Anaerobic septic arthritis and osteomyelitis. Orthop. Clin. North Am., 15:505, 1984.
75. Hallel, T., and Salvati, E. A.: Septic arthritis of the hip in infancy, end result study. Clin. Orthop., 132:115, 1978.
76. Hampton, O. P., Jr.: Observations on the management of suppurative arthritis of the knee joint. Am. J. Surg., 74:631, 1947.
77. Hampton, O. P., Jr.: Wounds of joints. Surg. Clin. North Am., 38:1517, 1958.
78. Harcke, H. T.: Bone imaging in infants and children: A review. J. Nucl. Med., 19:324, 1978.
79. Hardinge, K., Cleary, J., and Charnley, J.: Low-friction arthroplasty for healed septic and tuberculous arthritis. J. Bone Joint Surg., 61-B:144, 1979.
80. Harmon, P. H.: Surgical treatment of the residual deformity from suppurative arthritis of the hip occurring in young children. J. Bone Joint Surg., 24:576, 1942.
81. Harmon, P. H., and Adams, C. O.: Pyogenic coxitis; end-results and consideration of diagnosis and treatment. Surg. Gynecol. Obstet., 78:371, 1944.
82. Heberling, J. A.: A review of two hundred and one cases of suppurative arthritis. J. Bone Joint Surg., 23:917, 1941.

83. Herndon, W. A., Knauer, S., Sullivan, A., and Gross, R. H.: Management of septic arthritis in children. J. Pediatr. Orthop., 6:576, 1986.
84. Herrell, W. E., Nichols, D. R., and Heilman, D. H.: Penicillin. Its usefulness, limitations, diffusion and detection, with analysis of 150 cases in which it was employed. J.A.M.A., 125:1003, 1944.
85. Hess, R. J., and Martin, J. H.: Pyarthrosis complicating gout. J.A.M.A., 218:592, 1971.
86. Hirsh, H. L., Feffer, H. L., and Neil, C. B.: A study of the diffusion of penicillin across the serous membranes of joint cavities. J. Lab. Clin. Med., 31:535, 1946.
87. Hofmann, A., Wyatt, R., and Bybee, B.: Septic arthritis of the knee in a 12-year-old hemophiliac. J. Pediatr. Orthop., 4:498, 1984.
88. Houghton, G. R.: Septic arthritis of the hip in a hemophiliac. Report of a case. Clin. Orthop., 129:223, 1977.
89. Howard, J. B., Highgenboten, C. L., and Nelson, J. D.: Residual effects of septic arthritis in infancy and childhood. J.A.M.A., 235:932, 1976.
90. Howard, P. J.: Sepsis in normal and premature infants with localization in the hip joint. Pediatrics, 20:279, 1957.
91. Hunka, L., Said, S. E., MacKenzie, D. A., Rogala, E. J., and Cruess, R. L.: Classification and surgical management of the severe sequelae of septic hips in children. Clin. Orthop., 171:30, 1982.
92. Hunter, W.: Of the structure and diseases of articulating cartilage. Phil. Trans. R. Soc. London, 42:514, 1743.
93. Inge, G., and Liebdt, F. L.: The treatment of acute suppurative arthritis. Report of 36 cases treated by operation. Surg. Gynecol. Obstet., 60:86, 1935.
94. Jackson, M. A., and Nelson, J. D.: Etiology and medical management of acute suppurative bone and joint infections in pediatric patients. J. Pediatr. Orthop., 2:313, 1982.
95. James, A. E., Wagner, H. N., and Cooke, R. E. (eds.): Pediatric Nuclear Medicine. Philadelphia, Saunders, 1974, pp. 102, 513–519.
96. Janoff, A., and Blondin, J.: Depletion of cartilage matrix by a neutral protease fraction of human leukocyte lysosomes (35040). Proc. Soc. Exp. Biol. Med., 135:302, 1970.
97. Jarrett, M. P., Grossman, L., Sadler, A. H., and Grayzel, A. I.: The role of arthroscopy in the treatment of septic arthritis. Arthritis Rheum., 24:737, 1981.
98. Jocson, C. T.: The diffusion of antibiotics through the synovial membrane. J. Bone Joint Surg., 37-A:107, 1955.
99. Jones, R., Jr., and Roberts, L.: Acute osteomyelitis of the upper end of the femur. Surg. Gynecol. Obstet., 65:753, 1937.
100. Karten, I.: Septic arthritis complicating rheumatoid arthritis. Ann. Intern. Med., 70:1147, 1969.
101. Kawashima, M., Torisu, T., Kamo, Y., et al.: The treatment of bone and joint infections by closed irrigation-suction. Clin. Orthop., 148:240, 1980.
102. Kaye, J. J.: Bacterial infections of the hips in infancy and childhood. Curr. Probl. Radiol., 3:17, 1973.
103. Kaye, J. J., Winchester, P. H., and Freiberg, R. H.: Neonatal septic "dislocation" of the hip: True dislocation or pathological epiphyseal separation? Radiology, 114:671, 1975.
104. Keefer, C. S., Holmes, W. F., Jr., and Myers, W. K.: The inhibition of tryptic digestion of cartilage by synovial fluid in patients with various types of arthritis. J. Clin. Invest., 14:131, 1935.
105. Kellgren, J. H., Ball, J., Fairbrother, R. W., and Barnes, K. L.: Suppurative arthritis complicating rheumatoid arthritis. Br. Med. J., 1:1193, 1958.
106. Lack, C. H.: Chondrolysis in arthritis. J. Bone Joint Surg., 41-B:384, 1959.
107. Lack, C. H., and Rogers, H. J.: Action of plasmin on cartilage. Nature, 182:948, 1958.
108. Lafuente Martinez, D., Bonilla Velasco, F. A., Sampedro Alvarez, J., and Mendez Lozano, A.: Septic arthritis caused by Serratia marcescens (Letter). Arthritis Rheum., 24:567, 1981.
109. Lancaster, S. J., and Cummings, R. J.: Hip aspiration: Verification of needle position by air arthrography. J. Pediatr. Orthop., 7:91, 1987.
110. Langenskiöld, A., and Salenius, P.: Epiphysiodesis of the greater trochanter. Acta Orthop. Scand., 38:199, 1967.
111. L'Episcopo, J. B.: Stabilization of pathological dislocation of the hip in children. J. Bone Joint Surg., 18:737, 1936.
112. Lisbona, R., and Rosenthal, L.: Observations on the sequential use of 99m Tc-phosphate complex and 67-Ga imaging in osteomyelitis, cellulitis and septic arthritis. Radiology, 123:123, 1977.
113. Lisbona, R., and Rosenthal, L.: Radionuclide imaging of septic joints and their differentiation from periarticular osteomyelitis and cellulitis in pediatrics. Clin. Nucl. Med., 2:337, 1977.
114. Lloyd Roberts, G. C.: Suppurative arthritis of infancy. Some observations upon prognosis and management. J. Bone Joint Surg., 42-B:706, 1960.
115. Lloyd Roberts, G. C.: Some aspects of orthopaedic surgery in childhood. Ann. R. Coll. Surg., 57:25, 1975.
116. Lloyd Roberts, G. C.: Some aspects of orthopaedic surgery in childhood. Bull. Hosp. Joint Dis., 76:37, 1976.
117. Lloyd Roberts, G. C.: Septic arthritis in infancy. Int. Orthop., 2:97, 1978.
118. Lloyd Roberts, G. C.: Septic arthritis in infancy. Aust. Paediatr. J., 15 (special issue):41, 1979.
119. Lovell, W. W.: Infection of the knee joint by Clostridium welchii. J. Bone Joint Surg., 28:398, 1946.
120. Lowery, C. E., and Stern, P. J.: Septic dislocation of the hip with extension of emphysema. Clin. Orthop., 178:241, 1983.
121. Lunseth, P. A., and Heiple, K. G.: Prognosis in septic arthritis of the hip in children. Clin. Orthop., 139:81, 1979.
122. McCarroll, J. R.: Isolated staphylococcal infection of the sternoclavicular joint. Clin. Orthop., 156:149, 1981.
123. McConville, J. H., Pototsky, R. S., Calia, F. M., and Pachas, W. N.: Septic and crystalline joint disease, a simultaneous occurrence. J.A.M.A., 231:841, 1975.
124. McElvenny, R. T.: The use of closed circulation of suction in the treatment of chronically infected, acutely infected, and potentially infected wounds. Am. J. Orthop., 3:86, 1961.
125. McElvenny, R. T.: The use of closed circulation of suction in the treatment of chronically infected, acutely infected, and potentially infected wounds. Part II. Am. J. Orthop., 3:154, 1961.
126. McGinty, J. B.: Editorial. J. Bone Joint Surg., 65-A:287, 1983.
127. McNee, J.: An unusual case of Clostridium welchii infection. J. Bone Joint Surg., 48-B:512, 1966.
128. Martel, W., and Poznanski, A. K.: The value of traction during roentgenography of the hip. Radiology, 94:497, 1970.
129. Martin, J. R., Root, H. S., Kim, S. O., and Johnson, L. G.: Staphylococcus suppurative arthritis occurring in neuropathic knee joints. Arthritis Rheum., 8:389, 1965.
130. Merritt, K., Boyle, W. E., Jr., Dye, S. K., and Porter, R. E.: Counter immunoelectrophoresis in the diagnosis of septic arthritis caused by Hemophilus

influenzae. Report of two cases. J. Bone Joint Surg., 58-A:414, 1976.
131. Middleton, W. D., and McAlister, W. H.: Hip joint fluid in the presence of the vacuum phenomenon. Pediatr. Radiol., 16:171, 1986.
132. Mielants, H., Dhondt, E., Goethals, L., Verbruggen, G., and Veys, E.: Long-term functional results of the non-surgical treatment of common bacterial infections of joints. Scand. J. Rheumatol., 11:101, 1982.
133. Miller, J. A., Jr.: Joint paracentesis from an anatomic point of view. I. Shoulder, elbow, wrist, and hand. Surgery, 40:993, 1956.
134. Miller, J. A., Jr.: Joint paracentesis from an anatomic point of view. II. Hip, knee, ankle, and foot. Surgery, 41:999, 1957.
135. Mitchell, G. P.: Management of acquired dislocation of the hip in septic arthritis. Orthop. Clin. North Am., 11:51, 1980.
136. Morgan, H. C., Hertel, R. C., and Stamp, W. G.: Quantitative barrier of synovium to penicillin. Arch. Surg., 87:450, 1963.
137. Morgan, H. C., Stamp, W. G., and Nickel, J. S.: Quantitative barriers of infected synovium to penicillin. South. Med. J., 58:710, 1965.
138. Morrey, B. F., Bianco, A. J., and Rhodes, K. H.: Suppurative arthritis of the hip in children. J. Bone Joint Surg., 78-A:388, 1976.
139. Morrissy, R. T.: Bone and joint sepsis in children. Instr. Course Lect., 31:49, 1982.
140. Murray, I. P. C.: Photopenia in skeletal scintigraphy of suspected bone and joint infection. Clin. Nucl. Med., 7:13, 1982.
141. Myers, A. R., Miller, L. M., and Pinals, R. S.: Pyarthrosis complicating rheumatoid arthritis. Lancet, 2:714, 1969.
142. Myles, A. B.: Pyogenic arthritis presenting as a ruptured popliteal cyst. Ann. Rheum. Dis., 38:578, 1979.
143. Nade, S.: Acute septic arthritis in infancy and childhood. Aust. Paediatr. J., 11:145, 1975.
144. Nade, S.: Acute septic arthritis in infancy and childhood. J. Bone Joint Surg., 65-B:234, 1983.
145. Nade, S., Robertson, F. W., and Taylor, T. K. F.: Antibiotics in the treatment of acute osteomyelitis and acute septic arthritis in children. Med. J. Aust., 2:703, 1974.
146. Nagel, D. A., Albright, J. A., and Hollingsworth, J. R.: Studies on the pathophysiology of some host defense factors in staphylococcal arthritis in the rabbit and on the relationship of septic inflammation to infection rate. Yale J. Biol. Med., 39:119, 1966.
147. Nelson, J. D.: Antibiotic concentrations in septic joint effusions. N. Engl. J. Med., 284:349, 1971.
148. Nelson, J. D.: The bacterial etiology and antibiotic management of septic arthritis in infants and children. Pediatrics, 50:437, 1972.
149. Nelson, J. D., and Koontz, W. C.: Septic arthritis in infants and children: A review of 117 cases. Pediatrics, 38:966, 1966.
150. Nelson, J. D., Bucholz, R. W., Kusmiesz, H., and Shelton, S.: Benefits and risks of sequential parenteral-oral cephalosporin therapy for suppurative bone and joint infections. J. Pediatr. Orthop., 2:255, 1982.
151. Newman, J. H.: Review of septic arthritis throughout the antibiotic era. Ann. Rheum. Dis., 35:198, 1976.
152. Nicholson, J. T.: Pyogenic arthritis with pathological dislocation of the hip in infants. J.A.M.A., 141:827, 1947.
153. Nitsche, J. F., Vaughan, J. H., Williams, G., and Curd, J. G.: Septic sternoclavicular arthritis with Pasteurella multocida and Streptococcus sanguis. Arthritis Rheum., 25:467, 1982.
154. Ober, R.: Posterior arthrotomy of the hip joint. Report of five cases. J.A.M.A., 83:1500, 1924.
155. Obletz, B. E.: Acute suppurative arthritis of the hip in the neonatal period. J. Bone Joint Surg., 42-A:23, 1960.
156. Obletz, B. E.: Suppurative arthritis of the hip joint in infants. Clin. Orthop., 22:27, 1962.
157. O'Connor, R. L.: Arthroscopy. Philadelphia, Lippincott, 1977, pp. 93–96.
158. Ogden, J. A.: Pediatric osteomyelitis and septic arthritis: The pathology of neonatal disease. Yale J. Biol. Med., 52:423, 1979.
159. Orchard, R. A., and Stamp, W. G.: Early treatment of induced suppurative arthritis. Clin. Orthop., 59:287, 1968.
160. Oronsky, A., Ignarro, L., and Perper, R.: Release of cartilage mucopolysaccharide-degrading neutral protease from human leukocytes. J. Exp. Med., 138:461, 1973.
161. Ory, E. M., Meads, M., Brown, B., Wilcox, C., and Finland, M.: Penicillin levels in serum and in some body fluids during systemic and local therapy. J. Lab. Clin. Med., 30:809, 1945.
162. Oyemade, G. A.: Presenting features of septic arthritis of the hip in Nigerian children. Trop. Geogr. Med., 32:145, 1980.
163. Parker, R. H., and Schmid, F. R.: Antibacterial activity of synovial fluid during therapy of septic arthritis. Arthritis Rheum., 14:96, 1971.
164. Paterson, D. C.: Acute suppurative arthritis in infancy and childhood. J. Bone Joint Surg., 52-B:474, 1970.
165. Paterson, D.: Septic arthritis of the hip joint. Etiology, pathology, clinical features and diagnosis. Orthop. Clin. North Am., 9:135, 1978.
166. Peltola, H., Vahvanen, V., and Aalto, K.: Fever, C-reactive protein and erythrocyte sedimentation rate in monitoring recovery from septic arthritis: A preliminary study. J. Pediatr. Orthop., 4:170, 1984.
167. Petersen, S., Knudsen, F. U., Andersen, E. A., and Egeblad, M.: Acute haematogenous osteomyelitis and septic arthritis in childhood. A 10-yr review and follow-up. Acta Orthop. Scand., 51:45, 1980.
168. Phemister, D. B.: Changes in the articular surfaces in tuberculosis and in pyogenic infections of joints. A.J.R., 12:1, 1924.
169. Phemister, D. B.: The effect of pressure on articular surfaces in pyogenic and tuberculous arthritis and its bearing on treatment. Ann. Surg., 80:481, 1924.
170. Propst-Proctor, S. L., Dillingham, M. F., McDougall, I. R., and Goodwin, D.: The white blood cell scan in orthopedics. Clin. Orthop., 168:157, 1982.
171. Pulaski, E. J., and Tubbs, R. S.: Inhibitory effects of kanamycin and diffusion into various body fluids. Antibiot. Med. Clin. Therap., 6:589, 1959.
172. Rapp, G. F., Griffith, R. S., and Hebble, W. M.: The permeability of traumatically inflamed synovial membrane to commonly used antibiotics. J. Bone Joint Surg., 48-A:1534, 1966.
173. Rashkoff, E. S., Burkhalter, W. E., and Mann, R. J.: Septic arthritis of the wrist. J. Bone Joint Surg., 65-A:824, 1983.
174. Reich, R. S.: Purulent arthritis. J. Bone Joint Surg., 10:554, 1928.
175. Rhodes, K. H.: Antibiotic management of acute osteomyelitis and septic arthritis in children. Orthop. Clin. North Am., 6:915, 1975.
176. Riegels-Nielsen, P., and Jensen, J. S.: Septic arthritis of the knee. Five cases treated with synovectomy. Acta Orthop. Scand., 55:657, 1984.
177. Rigault, P., Lagrange, J., Pouliquen, J. C., Guyonvarch, G., Lewalle, J., and Mullier, J.: La trochantéroplastie: Opération de sauvetage dans les mutilations de la tête et du col du fémur chez l'enfant. Indications, technique et résultats à propos de 10 cas. Rev. Chir. Orthop., 59:565, 1973.
178. Robinson, S. C.: Bacillus cereus septic arthritis following arthrography. Clin. Orthop., 145:237, 1979.

179. Rosenberg, D., Baskies, A. M., Deckers, P. J., Leiter, B. E., Ordia, J. I., and Yablon, I. G.: Pyogenic sacroiliitis. An absolute indication for computerized tomographic scanning. Clin. Orthop., 184:128, 1984.
180. Ross, D. W.: Acute suppurative arthritis of the hip in premature infants. J.A.M.A., 156:303, 1954.
181. Roy, S., and Bhawan, J.: Ultrastructure of articular cartilage in pyogenic arthritis. Arch. Pathol., 99:44, 1975.
182. Rubinow, A., Spark, E. C., and Canoso, J. J.: Septic arthritis in a Charcot joint. Clin. Orthop., 147:203, 1980.
183. Russell, A. S., and Ansell, B. M.: Septic arthritis. Ann. Rheum. Dis., 31:40, 1972.
184. Ryeen, A. C., Schean, A., and Agell, B. O.: A case of septic arthritis in multiple joints due to Bacteroides fragilis in a patient with rheumatoid arthritis. Acta Orthop. Scand., 49:98, 1978.
185. Saklatvala, J., and Sarsfield, S. J.: Lymphocytes induce resorption of cartilage by producing catabolin. Biochem. J., 202:275, 1982.
186. Salter, R. B., Bell, R. S., and Keeley, F. W.: The protective effect of continuous passive motion on living articular cartilage in acute septic arthritis: An experimental investigation in the rabbit. Clin. Orthop., 159:223, 1981.
187. Salter, R. B., Hamilton, H. W., Wedge, J. H., Tile, M., Torode, I. P., O'Driscoll, S. W., Murnaghan, J. J., and Saringer, J. H.: Clinical application of basic research on continuous passive motion for disorders and injuries of synovial joints: A preliminary report of a feasibility study. J. Orthop. Res., 1:325, 1984.
188. Samilson, R. L., Bersani, F. A., and Watkins, M. B.: Acute suppurative arthritis in infants and children. The importance of early diagnosis and surgical drainage. Pediatrics, 21:798, 1958.
189. Schaad, U. B., McCracken, G. H., Jr., and Nelson, J. D.: Pyogenic arthritis of the sacroiliac joint in pediatric patients. Pediatrics, 66:375, 1980.
190. Schiller, M., Donnelly, P. J., Melo, J. C., and Raff, M. J.: Clostridium perfringens septic arthritis. Report of a case and review of the literature. Clin. Orthop., 139:92, 1979.
191. Schmidt, D., Mubarak, S., and Gelberman, R.: Septic shoulders in children. J. Pediatr. Orthop., 1:67, 1981.
192. Schurman, D. J., and Wheeler, R.: Gram negative bone and joint infection: Sixty patients treated with amikacin. Clin. Orthop., 134:268, 1978.
193. Schurman, D. J., Johnson, B. L., Jr., and Amstutz, H. C.: Knee joint infections with Staphylococcus aureus and micrococcus species. Influence of antibiotics, metal debris, bacteremia, blood, and steroids in a rabbit model. J. Bone Joint Surg., 57-A:40, 1975.
194. Schurman, D. J., Kajiyama, G., and Nagel, D. A.: Escherichia coli infections in rabbit knee joints. The pharmacological and antibacterial effects of intramuscular antibiotics. J. Bone Joint Surg., 62-A:620, 1980.
195. Schurman, D. J., Mirra, J., Ding, A., and Nagel, D. A.: Experimental E. coli arthritis in the rabbit. A model of infectious and post-infectious inflammatory synovitis. J. Rheumatol., 4:118, 1977.
196. Scoles, P. V., and Aronoff, S. C.: Antimicrobial therapy of childhood skeletal infections. J. Bone Joint Surg., 66-A:1487, 1984.
197. Scott, J. E., and Harrison, D. H.: Septic arthritis in association with primary lymphoedema. Acta Orthop. Scand., 47:676, 1976.
198. Severin, E.: Arthrography in sequelae to acute infectious arthritis of the hips of young children. Acta Chir. Scand., 93:389, 1946.
199. Siffert, R. S.: The effect of the juxta-epiphyseal pyogenic infection on epiphyseal growth. Clin. Orthop., 10:131, 1957.
200. Singson, R. D., Berdon, W. E., Feldman, F., Denton, J. R., Abramson, S., and Baker, D. H.: "Missing" femoral condyle: An unusual sequela to neonatal osteomyelitis and septic arthritis. Radiology, 161:359, 1986.
201. Smith, A. DeF.: Treatment of suppurative arthritis of the hip by antibiotics. Bull. Hosp. Joint Dis., 12:459, 1951.
202. Smith, R. L., and Schurman, D. J.: Comparison of cartilage destruction between infectious and adjuvant arthritis. J. Orthop. Res., 1:136, 1983.
203. Smith, R. L., and Schurman, D. J.: Bacterial arthritis. A staphylococcal proteoglycan-releasing factor. Arthritis Rheum., 29:1378, 1986.
204. Smith, R. L., Merchant, T. C., and Schurman, D. J.: In vitro cartilage degradation by Escherichia coli and Staphylococcus aureus. Arthritis Rheum., 25:441, 1982.
205. Smith, R. L., Schurman, D. J., Kajiyama, G., Mell, M., and Gilkerson, E.: The effect of antibiotics on the destruction of cartilage in experimental infectious arthritis. J. Bone Joint Surg., 69-A:1063, 1987.
206. Smith, R. T., Platou, E. S., and Good, R. A.: Septicemia of the newborn. Current status of the problem. Pediatrics, 17:549, 1956.
207. Smith, T.: On the acute arthritis of infants. St. Bart. Hosp. Rep., 10:189, 1874.
208. Stetson, J. W., DePonte, R. J., and Southwick, W. O.: Acute septic arthritis of the hip in children. Clin. Orthop., 56:105, 1968.
209. Stewart, I. M., Swinson, D. R., and Hardinge, K.: Pyogenic arthritis presenting as a ruptured popliteal cyst. Ann. Rheum. Dis., 38:181, 1979.
210. Sullivan, J. A., Vasileff, T., and Leonard, J. C.: An evaluation of nuclear scanning in orthopedic infections. J. Pediatr. Orthop., 1:73, 1981.
211. Thompson, G. R., Ferreyra, A., and Brackett, R. G.: Acute arthritis complicating rubella vaccination. Arthritis Rheum. 14:19, 1971.
212. Torg, J. S., and Lammot, T. R.: Septic arthritis of the knee due to Clostridium welchii. J. Bone Joint Surg., 50-A:1233, 1968.
213. Torholm, C., Hedstrom, A.-A., Sunden, G., and Lidgren, L.: Synovectomy in bacterial arthritis. Acta Orthop. Scand., 54:748, 1983.
214. Tuazon, C. U.: Teichoic acid antibodies in osteomyelitis and septic arthritis caused by Staphylococcus aureus. J. Bone Joint Surg., 64-A:762, 1982.
215. Tucker, J. L., and Tepper, W. R.: Intra-articular penicillin treatment of suppurative arthritis in infants and children. J. Pediatr., 29:711, 1946.
216. Tuli, S. M., and Mukherjee, S. K.: Excision arthroplasty for tuberculous and pyogenic arthritis of the hip. J. Bone Joint Surg., 63-B:29, 1981.
217. Viek, P.: Concentration of sodium nafcillin in pathological synovial fluid. Antimicrob. Agents Chemother., p. 379, 1962.
218. Viek, P., and Santangelo, S. C.: Pyarthrosis: A surgical emergency. J. Int. Coll. Surg., 37:88, 1962.
219. Viggiano, D. A., Garrett, J. C., and Clayton, M. L.: Septic arthritis presenting as olecranon bursitis in patients with rheumatoid arthritis. J. Bone Joint Surg., 62-A:1011, 1980.
220. Watkins, M. B., Samilson, R. L., and Winters, D. M.: Acute suppurative arthritis. J. Bone Joint Surg., 38-A:1313, 1956.
221. Weissman, G., and Spilberg, I.: Breakdown of cartilage protein polysaccharide by lysosomes. Arthritis Rheum., 11:162, 1968.
222. Weissman, S. L.: Transplantation of the trochanteric epiphysis into the acetabulum after septic arthritis of the hip. J. Bone Joint Surg., 49-A:1647, 1967.
223. Wellman, H. N., Siddiqui, A., Mail, J. T., and Georgi, P.: Choice of radiotracer in the study of bone or joint infection in children. Ann. Radiol., 26:411, 1983.

223a. Westin, G. W.: The stick femur. Paper presented in Chicago, Illinois, 1970.
224. White, H.: Roentgen findings of acute infectious disease of the hip in infants and children. Clin. Orthop., 22:34, 1962.
225. Whitesides, T. E., and Shufflebarger, H.: Septic dislocation of the hip in infants. J. Bone Joint Surg., 53-A:1245, 1971.
226. Wientroub, S., Lloyd Roberts, G. C., and Fraser, M.: The prognostic significance of the triradiate cartilage in suppurative arthritis of the hip in infancy and early childhood. J. Bone Joint Surg., 63-B:190, 1981.
227. Wiley, J. J., and Fraser, G. A.: Septic arthritis in childhood. Can. J. Surg., 22:326, 1979.
228. Wilkens, R. M., and Wiedel, J. D.: Septic arthritis of the knee in a hemophiliac. A case report. J. Bone Joint Surg., 65-A:267, 1983.
229. Wilson, N. I. L., and DiPaola, M.: Acute septic arthritis in infancy and childhood. 10 years' experience. J. Bone Joint Surg., 68-B:584, 1986.
230. Wingstrand, H., Egund, N., Lidgren, L., and Sahlstrand, T.: Sonography in septic arthritis of the hip in the child: Report of four cases. J. Pediatr. Orthop., 7:206, 1987.
231. Wittels, N. P., Donley, J. M., and Burkhalter, W. E.: A functional treatment method for interphalangeal pyogenic arthritis. J. Hand Surg., 9:894, 1984.
232. Wolff, J. A., Jr., Tuomanen, E. I., and Greenberg, I. D.: Radionuclide joint imaging: Acute rheumatic fever simulating septic arthritis. Pediatrics, 65:339, 1980.
233. Wood, B. P.: The vanishing epiphyseal ossification center: A sequel to septic arthritis of childhood. Radiology, 134:387, 1980.

LYME ARTHRITIS

Lyme disease is caused by the spirochete *Borrelia burgdorferi* and is transmitted by the tick *Ixodes dammini* (deer tick) or a related ixodid tick. Arthritis is the presenting manifestation in the majority of cases. The infection is endemic in certain areas of North America, primarily in southern New England, the middle-Atlantic states, Wisconsin, and California. It has been described in 19 countries. Lyme disease characteristically develops in the summer and autumn—periods when the ticks are very active.

Clinical Features

The arthritis is preceded in about half the cases by a characteristic rash—erythema chronicum migrans. The appearance of the rash is striking; it may escape notice by the patient, however. Half the affected children will definitely recollect being bitten by a tick. Prodromal systemic illness in the form of low-grade fever, stiff neck, or headache is present in about 40 per cent of cases.

The arthritis is pauciarticular, usually affecting one or a few large joints. The knee is the most common site, being involved in over 95 per cent of cases. Other joints that can be affected are the elbow, hip, ankle, shoulder, sternoclavicular, and interphalangeal. The arthritis follows the skin rash or prodromal systemic symptoms, usually within a few months (with a range from one week to 12 months). The synovitis manifests itself as joint swelling, increased local heat, joint tenderness, and pain on extremes of motion. When the knee, hip, or ankle is involved, the patient is able to bear weight and walk on the affected lower limb with an antalgic limp. The typical pattern of synovitis is brief and intermittent. If untreated, however, it becomes chronic.

Other clinical features of Lyme disease are meningitis or neurologic disease in the form of nerve palsy such as Bell's, and cardiac involvement, particularly conduction defect.

Diagnosis

Elevated titers of IgM and IgG antibodies against *Ixodes dammini* will establish the diagnosis of Lyme disease. A nonspecific finding is elevation of the erythrocyte sedimentation rate. In its initial stages Lyme disease should be differentiated from the monarticular or pauciarticular form of juvenile rheumatoid arthritis. This may be difficult. The attacks of Lyme arthritis are usually brief and self-limited, but that of juvenile rheumatoid arthritis is unremitting for at least six weeks. Chronic iridocyclitis does not occur in Lyme arthritis. This author has made the erroneous diagnosis of juvenile rheumatoid arthritis in several cases of Lyme arthropathy. It is strongly recommended that in the diagnostic work-up of the pauciarticular form of juvenile rheumatoid arthritis, serologic tests be performed to rule out Lyme disease.

Pyogenic septic arthritis is another entity to be differentiated from Lyme disease. In bacterial arthritis, the affected joint is acutely painful, red, and hot, and the patient is unable to bear weight on the lower limbs if the knee or hip is involved. In septic arthritis, joint fluid cultures are positive in 70 per cent of cases. Synovial fluid analysis is ordinarily not of great assistance in differentiating the two because in both conditions the leukocyte count is elevated with neutrophilia. The erythrocyte sedimentation rate is elevated in both. In case of doubt the arthritis should be treated as if septic, pending the results of serologic tests for Lyme disease, which should be available within one to two weeks.

Treatment

Therapy consists of administration of antibiotics—penicillin or tetracycline alone. Initially, when the arthritic symptoms are mild, penicillin may be given orally (phenoxymethyl penicillin) 50 mg/kg/day for four weeks. If tetracycline is administered, the dosage is 30 mg/kg/day. If the arthritis fails to respond to oral antibiotics, or if it is acute, the parenteral route is employed. Intravenous penicillin G or benzathine penicillin is given for ten days. Antibiotics do prevent or attenuate subsequent attacks. They should be administered for at least one month in order to minimize the risk of recurrence with exacerbation of the arthritis.

References

1. Benach, J. L., Bosler, E. M., Hanrahan, J. P., Coleman, J. L., Habicht, G. S., Bast, T. F., Cameron, D. J., Ziegler, J. L., Barbour, A. G., Burgdorfer, W., Edelman, R., and Kaslow, R. A.: Spirochetes isolated from the blood of two patients with Lyme disease. N. Engl. J. Med., 308:740, 1983.
2. Bowen, G. S., Griffin, M., Hayne, C., Slade, J., Schulze, T. L., and Parkin, W.: Clinical manifestations and descriptive epidemiology of Lyme disease in New Jersey, 1978 to 1982. J.A.M.A., 251:2236, 1984.
3. Burgdorfer, W., Barbour, A. G., Hayes, S. F., Benach, J. L., Grunwalt, E., and Davis, J. P.: Lyme disease: A tick-borne spirochetosis? Science, 216:1317, 1982.
4. Centers for Disease Control: Update: Lyme disease—United States. M.M.W.R., 33:268, 1984.
5. Craft, J. E., Grodzicki, R. L., and Steere, A. C.: Antibody response in Lyme disease, evaluation of diagnostic tests. J. Infect. Dis., 149:789, 1984.
6. Cristofaro, R. L., Appel, R. H., Gelb, R. I., and Williams, C. L.: Musculoskeletal manifestations of Lyme disease. J. Pediatr. Orthop., 7:527, 1987.
7. Culp, R. W., Eichenfield, A. H., Davidson, R. S., Drummond, D. S., Christofersen, M. R., and Goldsmith, D. P.: Lyme arthritis in children. J. Bone Joint Surg., 69-A:96, 1987.
8. Doughty, R. A.: Lyme disease. Musculoskeletal disease. Pediatr. Rev. 6:20, 1984.
9. Lawson, J. P., and Steere, A. C.: Roentgenologic findings in Lyme arthritis: Roentgenologic findings. Radiology, 154:37, 1985.
10. Pachner, A. R., and Steere, A. C.: The triad of neurologic manifestations of Lyme disease: Meningitis, cranial neuritis and radiculoneuritis. Neurology, 35:47, 1985.
11. Reik, L., Steere, A. C., Barthenhagen, N. H., Shope, R. E., and Malawista, S. E.: Neurologic abnormalities of Lyme disease. Medicine (Baltimore), 58:281, 1979.
12. Ross, A. H., and Benach, J. L.: Lyme arthritis in children. Arthritis Rheum. (Suppl.), 26:S35, 1983.
13. Russell, H., Sampson, J. S., Schmid, G. P., Wilkinson, H. W., and Plikaytis, B.: Enzyme-linked immunosorbent assay and indirect immunofluorescence for Lyme disease. J. Infect. Dis., 149:465, 1984.
14. Schmid, G. P., Horsley, R., Steere, A. C., Hanrahan, J. P., Davis, J. P., Bowen, G. S., Osterholm, M. T., Weisfeld, J. S., Hightower, A. W., and Broome, C. V.: Surveillance of Lyme disease in the United States. 1982. J. Infect. Dis., 151:1144, 1985.
15. Steere, A. C., and Malawista, S. E.: Cases of Lyme disease in the United States: Locations correlated with the distribution of Ixodes dammini. Ann. Intern. Med., 91:730, 1979.
16. Steere, A. C., Broderick, T. F., and Malawista, S. E.: Erythema chronicum migrans and Lyme arthritis. Epidemiologic evidence for a tick vector. Am. J. Epidemiol., 108:312, 1978.
17. Steere, A. C., Malawista, S. E., Newman, J. H., Spieler, P. N., and Bartenhagen, N. H.: Antibiotic therapy in Lyme disease. Ann. Intern. Med., 93:1, 1980.
18. Steere, A. C., Brinckerhoff, C. E., Miller, D. J., Drinker, J., Harris, E. D., Jr., and Malawista, S. E.: Elevated levels of collagenase and prostaglandin E2 from synovium associated with erosion of cartilage and bone in a patient with chronic Lyme arthritis. Arthritis Rheum., 23:591, 1980.
19. Steere, A. C., Gibofsky, A., Patarroyo, M. E., Winchester, R. J., Hardin, J. A., and Malawista, S. E.: Chronic Lyme arthritis: Clinical and immunogenetic differentiation from rheumatoid arthritis. Ann. Intern. Med., 90:896, 1979.
20. Steere, A. C., Malawista, S. E., Hardin, J. A., Ruddy, S., Askenase, P. W., and Andiman, W. A.: Erythema chronicum migrans and Lyme disease: The enlarging clinical spectrum. Ann. Intern. Med., 86:685, 1977.
21. Steere, A. C., Batsford, W. P., Weinberg, M., Alexander, J., Berger, H. J., Wolfson, S., and Malawista, S. E.: Lyme carditis: Cardiac abnormalities of Lyme disease. Ann. Intern. Med., 93:8, 1980.
22. Steere, A. C., Green, J., Schoen, R. T., Taylor, E., Hutchinson, G. J., Rahn, D. W., and Malawista, S. E.: Successful parenteral penicillin therapy of established Lyme arthritis. N. Engl. J. Med., 312:868, 1985.
23. Steere, A. C., Hutchinson, G. J., Rahn, D. W., Sigal, L. H., Craft, J. E., DeSanna, E. T., and Malawista, S. E.: Treatment of the early manifestations of Lyme disease. Ann. Intern. Med., 99:22, 1983.
24. Steere, A. C., Malawista, S. E., Snydman, D. R., Shope, R. E., Andiman, W. A., Ross, M. R., and Steele, F. M.: Lyme arthritis: An epidemic of oligoarticular arthritis in children and adults in three Connecticut communities. Arthritis Rheum., 20:7, 1977.
25. Steere, A. C., Grodzicki, R. L., Kornblatt, A. N., Craft, J. E., Barbour, A. G., Burgdorfer, W., Schmid, G. P., Johnson, E., and Malawista, S. E.: The spirochetal etiology of Lyme disease. N. Engl. J. Med., 308:733, 1983.
26. Steere, A. C., Bartenhagen, N. H., Craft, J. E., Hutchinson, G. J., Newman, J. H., Rahn, D. W., Sigal, L. H., Spieler, P. N., Stenn, K. S., and Malawista, S. E.: The early clinical manifestations of Lyme disease. Ann. Intern. Med., 99:76, 1983.

GONOCOCCAL ARTHRITIS

Gonococcal arthritis is caused by metastatic invasion of the joint by the gonococcus, usually from a recent or inadequately treated gonorrheal urethritis. The arthritis, which usually develops two to four weeks following the initial infection, may be polyarticular or monarticular. The knees, ankles, wrists, and sternoclavicular joints are the most frequently affected sites.

The disease usually begins as fleeting pains in multiple joints accompanied by fever and malaise quite similar to those at the onset of rheumatic fever. In a few days, the obvious infection settles in a single joint, which becomes hot, red, extremely tender, swollen, tense, and very painful on motion. The acute inflammation may spread to the adjacent tendons and bursae. Often there is a history of gonorrheal infection or a concomitant urethritis. In the more chronic cases, systemic reaction is usually minimal and multiple joints are involved. Gonorrheal arthritis may be associated with dermatitis.[18, 20]

A mother may have primary gonococcal infection of her genitourinary tract that may be asymptomatic or in which symptoms may be so slight as to go unnoticed. Such maternal infection may be transmitted from mother to infant. Gonococcal arthritis-dermatitis may manifest itself in the form of erythematous papules surrounded by a hemorrhagic or vesiculopustulous lesion that may precede the joint involvement. When both skin and joint are involved, the condition is referred to as gonococcal arthritis-dermatitis (GADS).[22]

Diagnosis is made by bacteriologic study of the aspirated joint fluid and of the urethral or vaginal discharge. The gonococcal organism can often be identified in the joint fluid within the first week of infection; in the course of the disease, however, joint cultures are negative. In such subacute or chronic cases, immunofluorescent methods for the detection of gonococcal antibodies and gonococcal complement fixation tests are of some aid in diagnosis. Gonorrheal arthritis should be distinguished from Reiter's syndrome, which consists of the triad of polyarthritis, urethritis, and conjunctivitis. Reiter's syndrome is rare in childhood; it is a form of nongonococcal urethritis, probably caused by a virus.

In gonococcal arthritis, destruction of articular cartilage is rapid, as shown by the disappearance of articular cartilage space in the radiogram.

Treatment should be immediate to prevent destruction and permanent damage to the joint. Penicillin is specific and very effective in the treatment of gonococcal arthritis. It is administered through the intramuscular route in doses of 2,000,000 to 3,000,000 units per day. The joint is aspirated and thoroughly lavaged with normal saline, following which 10,000 to 50,000 units of aqueous penicillin is instilled into it. On occasion, the gonococci may be penicillin-resistant; in such an instance, sulfonamide is administered orally along with intramuscular streptomycin. Surgical drainage of the joint (except the hip) is ordinarily not necessary. Local care of the affected joint is similar to that in septic arthritis.

References

1. Angevine, C. D., Hall, C. B., and Jacox, R. F.: A case of gonococcal osteomyelitis. A complication of gonococcal arthritis. Am. J. Dis. Child., 130:1013, 1976.
2. Baddeley, P., and Shardlow, J. P.: Antenatal gonococcal arthritis. J. Obstet. Gynaecol. Br. Commw., 80:186, 1973.
3. Barr, J., and Danielsson, D.: Disseminated gonococcal infections (gonococcal septicemia). In Danielsson, D. (ed.): Genital Infections and Their Complications. Stockholm, Almqvist & Wiksell, 1975, pp. 77–84.
4. Barrett-Connor, E.: Gonorrhea and the pediatrician. Am. J. Dis. Child., 125:233, 1973.
5. Cooperman, M. B.: Gonococcus arthritis in infancy. A clinical study of forty-four cases. Am. J. Dis. Child., 33:932, 1927.
6. Cooperman, M. B.: End results of gonorrheal arthritis. A review of seventy cases. Am. J. Surg., 5:241, 1928.
7. Cramolini, G. M., and Litt, I. F.: The pharynx as the only positive culture site in an adolescent with disseminated gonorrhea. J. Pediatr., 100:644, 1982.
8. Fink, C. W.: Gonococcal arthritis in children. J.A.M.A., 194:237, 1965.
9. Fitzhugh, A. S., and Nasca, R. J.: Gonococcal arthritis in a two-week-old infant treated by arthrotomy. J. Arkansas Med. Soc., 71:302, 1975.
10. Gerster, J. C., and Perroud, H.: Joint manifestations of gonorrhea, secondary syphilis and Reiter's syndrome. Rev. Med. Suisse Romande, 98:103, 1978.
11. Gregory, J. E., Chisom, J. L., and Meadows, A. T.: Gonococcal arthritis in an infant. Br. J. Vener. Dis., 48:306, 1972.
12. Henderson, R.: Recommended treatment schedules for gonorrhea—1974. Arch. Dermatol., 11:317, 1975.
13. Holmes, K. K., Count, G. W., and Beaty, H. N.: Disseminated gonococcal infection. Ann. Intern. Med., 74:979, 1971.
14. Israel, K. S., Rissing, K. B., and Brooks, G. F.: Neonatal and childhood gonococcal infections. Clin. Obstet. Gynecol., 18:143, 1975.
15. Keiser, H., Ruben, F. L., Wolinsky, E., and Kushner, I.: Clinical forms of gonococcal arthritis. N. Engl. J. Med., 279:234, 1968.
16. Kleiman, M. B., and Lamb, G. A.: Gonococcal arthritis in a newborn infant. Pediatrics, 52:285, 1973.
17. Kutscher, E., Southern, P. M., Jr., and Sanford, J. P.: Clinical significance of lincomycin-resistant Neisseria gonorrhoeae. Antimicrob. Agents Chemother., 8:331, 1968.
18. Lightfoot, R. W., Jr., and Gotschlich, E. C.: Gonococcal disease. Am. J. Med., 56:327, 1974.
19. Ludivico, C. L., and Myers, A. R.: Survey for immune complexes in disseminated gonococcal arthritis-dermatitis syndrome. Arthritis Rheum., 22:19, 1979.
20. Moen, F.: Gonorrheic arthritis and Reiter's syndrome. Tidsskr. Nor. Laegeforen., 97:1638, 1977.
21. Nazarian, L. F.: The current prevalence of gonococcal infections in children. Pediatrics, 39:372, 1967.
22. Nussbaum, M., Scalettar, H., and Shenker, I. R.: Gonococcal arthritis-dermatitis (GADS) as a complication of gonococcemia in adolescents. Clin. Pediatr., 14:1037, 1975.
23. Ogiela, D. M., and Peimer, C. A.: Acute gonococcal flexor tenosynovitis—case report and literature review. J. Hand Surg., 6:470, 1981.
24. Rubinow, A.: Septic arthritis of the hip caused by Neisseria gonococcae. Clin. Orthop., 181:115, 1983.
25. Rytter, M., and Gast, W.: Diagnosis and therapy of the extragenital manifestations of gonorrhea. Z. Gesamte Inn. Med., 35:304, 1980.
26. Sharp, J. T.: Editorial: Gonococcal infection and arthritis. Arthritis Rheum., 17:511, 1974.
27. Siefert, M. H., Miller, A. C., and Warin, A. P.: Benign gonococcal arthritis with cutaneous lesions. Ann. Rheum. Dis., 32:392, 1973.
28. Starck, V.: Complications of gonorrhea. Nord. Med., 76:811, 1966.
29. Svanbom, M., Bengtsson, E., Strandell, T., and Tanveall, G.: Benign gonococcemia with skin lesions and arthritis. Scand. J. Infect. Dis., 2:191, 1970.

30. Tindall, E. A., Adams, J., Yulich, J., and Bergin, J.: Gonococcal osteomyelitis complicating septic arthritis. J.A.M.A., 250:2671, 1983.
31. Wolff, C. B., Goodman, H. V., and Vahrman, J.: Gonorrhea with skin and joint manifestations. Br. Med. J., 2:271, 1970.

TUBERCULOUS ARTHRITIS

Tuberculosis of bones and joints is a granulomatous inflammation caused by *Mycobacterium tuberculosis*. It is a localized and destructive disease that is usually blood-borne from a primary focus such as infected peribronchial or mesenteric lymph nodes. The infection may be either of the human or the bovine type. In countries where raw milk is used extensively, bovine transmission is common, whereas in areas where milk is pasteurized and there is rigid control of dairy herds, the bovine type is extremely rare and the human type is more common.

The incidence of tuberculosis has greatly declined in the past three decades owing to the discovery of antituberculous drugs and the enforcement of strict public health measures such as pasteurization and the reporting and isolation of patients with active tuberculosis. Not too long ago, tuberculosis used to be the most common disease affecting the skeleton; this is still true in certain areas of the world. Even in economically well-developed countries it is still prevalent. Tuberculosis of bones and joints is more common in children, though it may occur at any age.

Pathology

The invasion of a joint by the tubercle bacillus may occur by direct hematogenous infection of the synovial membrane (synovial tuberculosis) or by indirect spread from a focus in an adjacent bone, e.g., in the metaphysis or epiphysis. Tuberculous osteomyelitis is characterized by destruction of bone with little or no tendency for new bone formation. The tuberculous bone focus spreads with increasing centrifugal destruction of surrounding bone, finally breaking into the joint. The synovial membrane reacts first by excessive secretion of fluid and later by proliferation, thickening, studding of its inner surface with tubercles, and fibrosis of its outer surface (Fig. 4–11).

The tuberculous granulation tissue soon covers the hyaline articular cartilage as a pannus that eventually destroys the underlying articular cartilage and subchondral bone. The destruction of articular surfaces is most extensive around the periphery in areas where tuberculous granulations involve the synovial membrane.

With progression of the disease, increasing amounts of caseous necrotic material and tuberculous exudate are produced. Soon, with increasing intraosseous or intra-articular pressure, the bony cortex or joint capsule will perforate and the so-called "cold abscess" will form. These tuberculous abscesses are so named because of the absence of acute inflammation. They spread by dissecting along tissue planes between muscles or between muscle sheaths, being limited by the deep fascia. With increasing tension the deep fascia perforates and the abscess becomes subcutaneous. A thick fibrous wall lines the tuberculous abscess, which contains serum along with caseous necrotic tissue, tubercle bacilli, and degenerating leukocytes. If the original focus remains active and these abscesses remain untreated, they will rupture externally through the skin to form sinuses, the results being the inevitable secondary infection by pyogenic bacteria, and complete destruction of the affected joint.

Clinical Features

Tuberculous arthritis is insidious in its onset; it is often monarticular (90 per cent of cases) in its involvement.

Typically, the child appers generally ill, is easily fatigued, and has evident weight loss. A family history of tuberculosis or a personal history of cervical adenitis or pleurisy may be obtained.

If the lesion is in the lower limb, for instance, in the hip, the initial symptom may be a slight limp due to discomfort. The affected joint will be stiff, and soon the "night-cries" develop; because irritation from the process is low-grade, muscle spasm protects the part quite satisfactorily during the day, but when the child is asleep the protective action of the muscles is lost, and on motion, pain is produced; hence, the cry.

Local physical signs vary according to the joint involved. The vertebral column is the most common site, the next in order of frequency being the hip, knee, ankle, sacroiliac, shoulder, and wrist joints. In tuberculous spondylitis, the child is presented with the complaint of a painful and stiff back. He walks with a protective gait in which he keeps his back hyperextended and he steps lightly. The typical kyphosis develops as bone destruction progresses and the vertebral bodies collapse. If the disease remains unchecked over a long period of time, the so-called "cold abscess" may be clinically

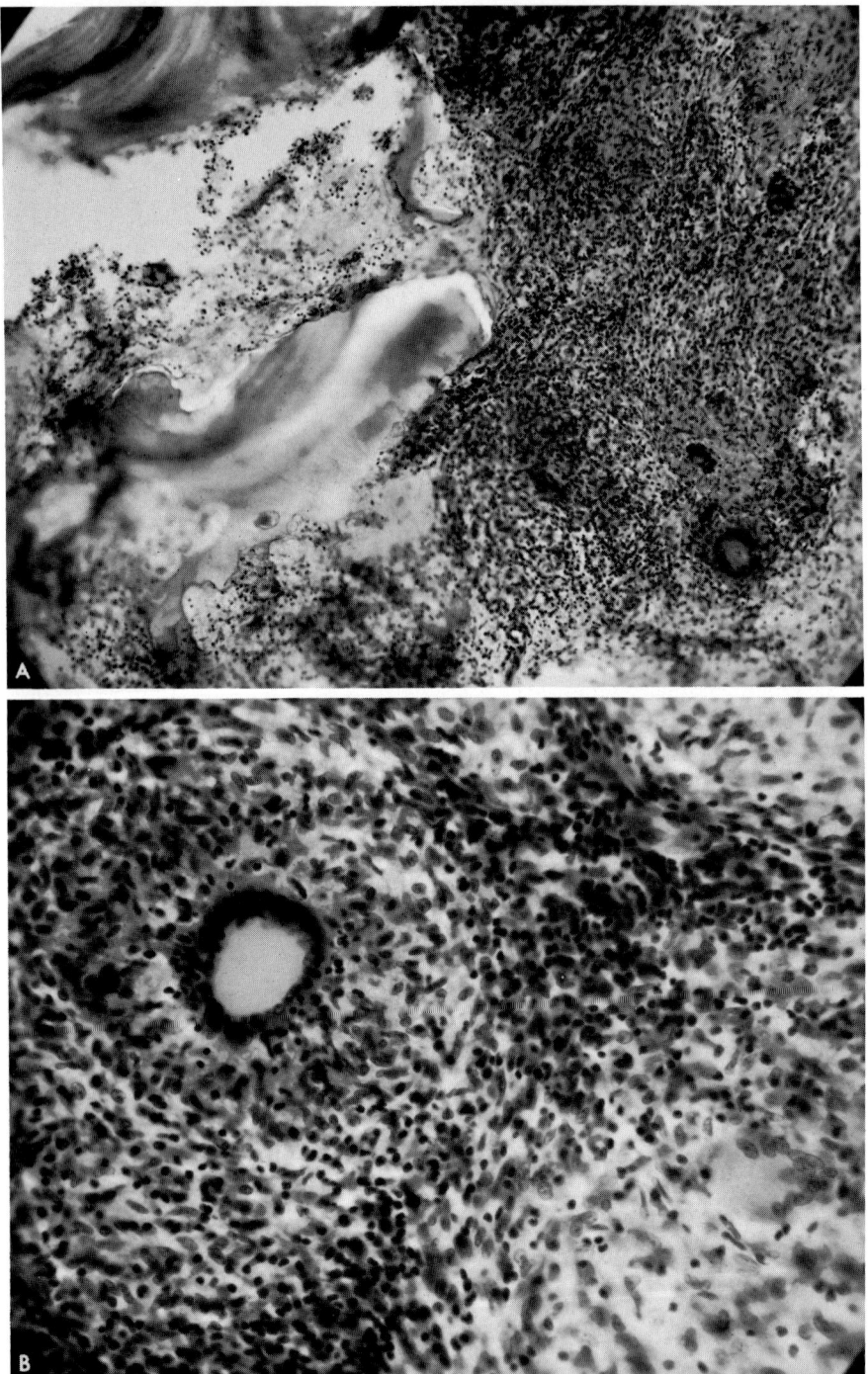

FIGURE 4–11. Microscopic picture of tuberculous arthritis.

A. × 100. B. × 250. Hematoxylin and eosin stain. Note the granulomatous inflammation and the Langhans giant cells.

recognizable in the form of a psoas abscess from a lesion of the lumbar spine.

In superficial joints, such as the knee or elbow, synovial thickening and effusion present as a fullness or bogginess. This may be difficult to detect in the deep joints such as the hip. Local heat and redness are usually absent, and tenderness is minimal. Muscle atrophy is usually marked and is often present in the early stages. Joint motion is usually limited. Temperature elevation is ordinarily not marked.

Radiographic Features

The earliest findings in the radiograms are regional bone atrophy, soft-tissue swelling, and capsular distention (Fig. 4–12). These changes are due to synovitis and are nonspecific. As a rule, the bone decalcification in tuberculous arthritis is widespread, extending 3 to 5 cm. from the joint.

The joint space is widened and is preserved until late in the course of the disease. Destruction of the hyaline cartilage by the tuberculous granulation tissue is a slow process. Eventually, with progression of the disease, the articular cartilage space will gradually narrow. This is in contrast to suppurative arthritis, in which the destruction of articular cartilage and narrowing of the joint space take place early in the course of the disease.

In joints such as the hip, in which there is a congruous and accurate fit of the opposing articular surfaces, the hyaline cartilage is eroded by the tuberculous granulation tissue in its

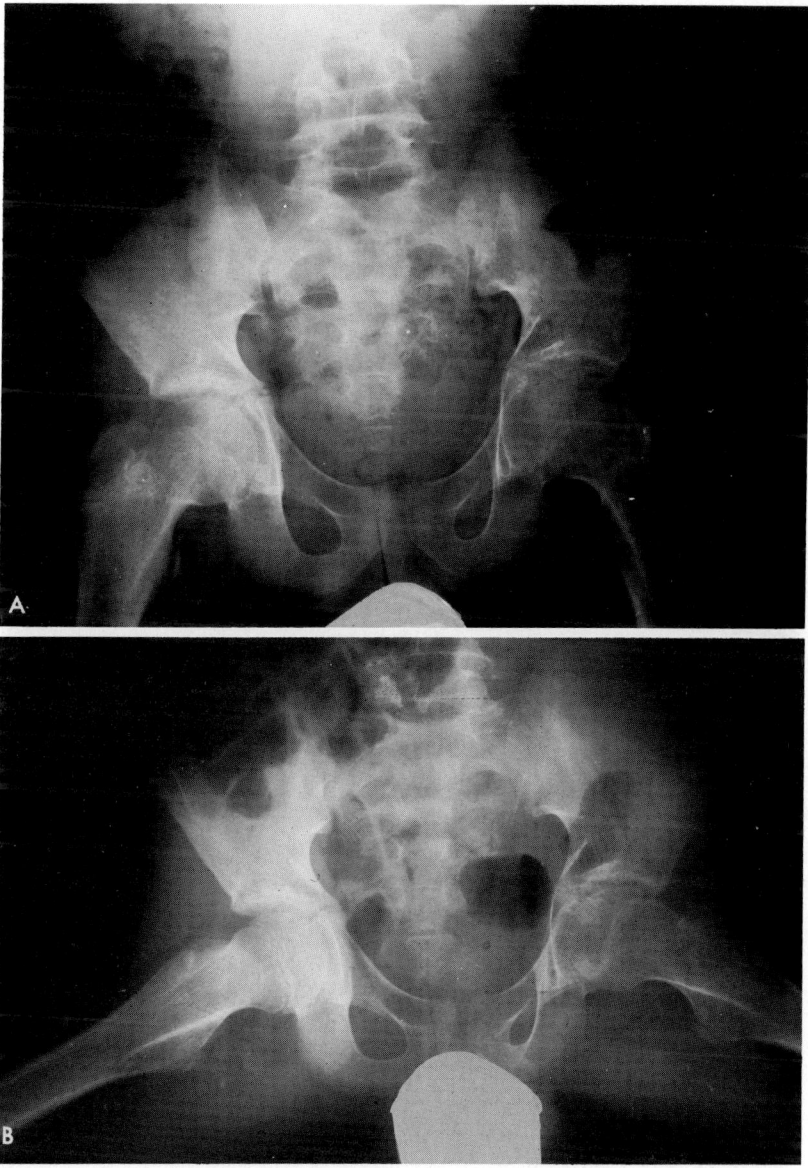

FIGURE 4–12. Tuberculous arthritis of left hip.

Radiograms showing regional bone atrophy.

periphery where there is little or no contact or pressure (Fig. 4–13). In articulations with incongruous articular surfaces, such as the knee, noncontact areas are diffusely distributed and the tuberculous granulation tissue destroys articular cartilage wherever the noncontact areas are, centrally or peripherally.

Bone destruction may be seen in the epiphysis or metaphysis as areas of radiolucency in which the normal trabecular structure of bone has disappeared. In primary synovial tuberculosis the infection spreads from the joint to the subchondral bone of the contiguous epiphysis; hence, the pattern of bone destruction is usually peripheral and is present in noncontact areas. When affection of the joint is secondary to a tuberculous focus in the epiphysis or metaphysis the areas of bone destruction may be anywhere and are not distributed peripherally in the noncontact portions. In tuberculous arthritis, if there is involvement of the ends of both bones of a joint, the destructive foci are usually directly opposite each other.

Reactive new bone formation is characteristically absent in the early stages of tuberculous arthritis; it is only in the late healing stages that it develops. Sequestra may occasionally be present.

If tuberculous arthritis remains untreated, the entire articular cartilage will eventually be eroded and extensive destruction of subjacent bone will take place, resulting in gross deformity of the joint (Fig. 4–14). Abscesses are usually seen early in tuberculous spondylitis in the form of paravertebral or psoas abscesses.

Laboratory Findings

The general findings are those of a chronic illness. Hypochromic anemia is common. The leukocyte count may be normal, or there may be slight leukocytosis. An elevated erythrocyte sedimentation rate and positive tubercular skin test are almost always present. Evidence of associated visceral tuberculosis (lungs, kidneys, lymph nodes) is the rule, as demonstrated by findings in the chest radiogram, in the intravenous pyelogram, or in the flat plate of the abdomen.

The synovial fluid shows an elevated leukocyte count, a lowered sugar level, and poor mucin. The leukocyte count usually averages 20,000 per cubic millimeter, though it may vary between 3,000 and 100,000 cells. The differential leukocyte count will disclose a predominance of polymorphonuclears (60 per cent) with 20 per cent lymphocytes and 20 per cent monocytes. Tubercle bacilli may be seen on microscopic examination of sediment of the joint fluid. A finding of great help in differential diagnosis is the marked reduction or absence of glucose in the synovial fluid. Cultural studies

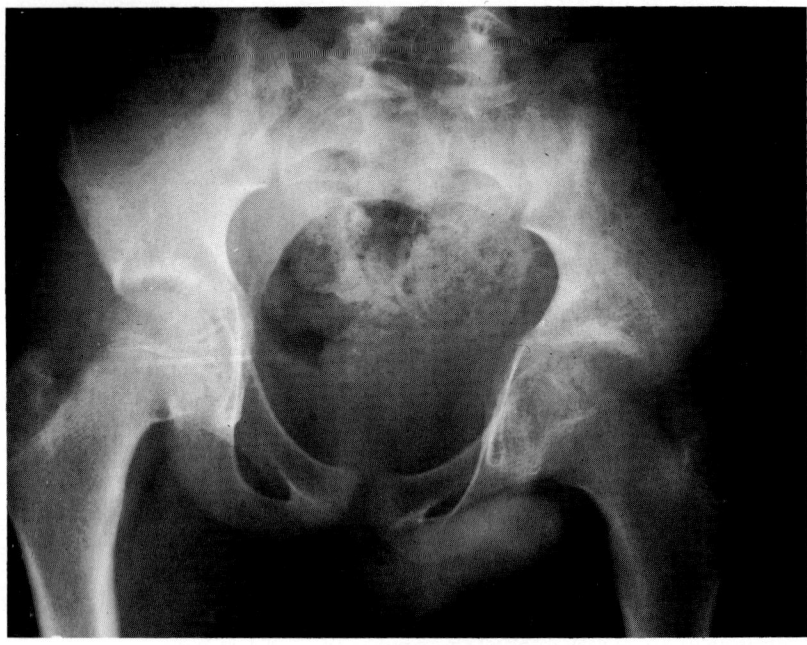

FIGURE 4–13. Tuberculous arthritis of left hip.

Note the erosion of hyaline articular cartilage.

and guinea pig inoculations will be positive for tuberculosis.

The diagnosis is also confirmed by histologic examination of synovial tissue obtained by exploratory arthrotomy or by biopsy of enlarged regional lymph nodes.

Treatment

In the past, treatment consisted of bed rest, possibly of several years' duration, with immobilization of the diseased part in a cast, in traction, or on a frame. Then, when the lesion started healing as a result of the patient's immunologic defenses, the involved segment of the spine or the affected joint was fused in functional position, a method that was considered to be the only certain means of arresting the disease.

At present, early diagnosis and the use of antituberculous drugs have radically improved the prognosis of tuberculous arthritis. Joint function is salvaged by means of excision of the focus of infection; this is followed by prolonged administration of antituberculous drugs, which have greatly diminished the chances of recurrence.

Treatment consists of general medical measures, chemotherapy, local conservative orthopedic care, and surgery.

General Medical Measures. These consist of bed rest and a well-balanced nutritious diet containing adequate amounts of protein, minerals, and vitamins. A cheerful and optimistic attitude is essential for providing positive psychologic support to the child. School work and, to a limited degree, ordinary activities of daily living are permitted.

Antituberculous Drugs. The objective of chemotherapy of tuberculosis is to achieve sterilization of the tuberculous lesion. Of the various chemotherapeutic agents, isoniazid (isonicotinic acid hydrazide, INH) and rifampin are the standard, commonly used drugs. In bone and joint tuberculosis and whenever resistance to INH is anticipated, a third drug is added for the first two months. In children, possible third drugs are pyrazinamide, streptomycin, and ethambutol. (When children have acquired the tuberculous organism from foreign-born adults, the incidence of resistance to INH can be as high as 15 per cent.) Other drugs that have shown antituberculous efficacy are kanamycin, capreomycin, ethionamide, and cycloserine—these chemotherapeutic agents are used only in

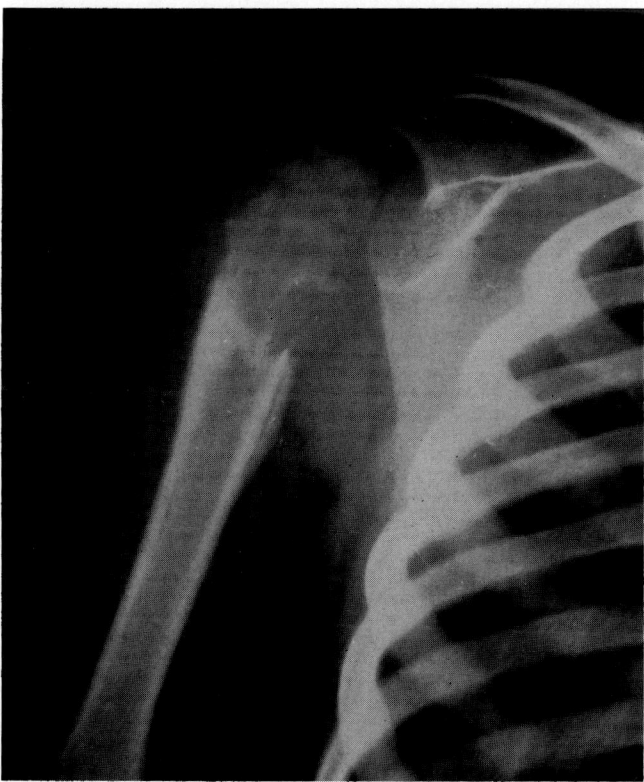

FIGURE 4–14. Tuberculosis of right shoulder, showing extensive bone destruction.

patients infected with resistant strains of tubercle bacilli.

Duration of drug therapy should be 9 to 12 months. For the first four to eight weeks of this regimen, INH and rifampin are administered daily. The total daily dosage of INH is 10 to 20 mg. per kg. of body weight, depending upon the severity of infection. The total daily dosage should not exceed 300 mg. The daily dosage of rifampin is 10 to 15 mg. per kg. of body weight, with a maximum daily dosage of 600 mg. The third drug given daily may be pyrazinamide (daily dosage of 15 to 30 mg. per kg. of body weight, with a maximum of 2 gm.), or ethambutol (total daily dosage of 15 to 25 mg. per kg. of body weight, with a maximum of 2.5 gm.). The use of streptomycin should be reserved for special cases, as emergence of resistance to streptomycin by the tubercle bacillus is usually rapid, and labyrinthine disorders and deafness are toxic complications. Streptomycin is administered by intramuscular injection in a total daily dosage of 20 to 40 mg. per kg. of body weight. The total daily dose should not exceed 1 gm.

After this initial four- to eight-week period of daily triple-drug therapy, a combination of INH and rifampin is given twice weekly. The total dosage, twice weekly, of INH is 20 to 40 mg. per kg. (maximum 900 mg.), and that of rifampin is 10 to 20 mg. per kg., with a maximum of 600 mg. For the third drug, the twice-weekly dosage of pyrazinamide is 50 to 70 mg. per kg. of body weight, and that of ethambutol is 50 mg. per kg. of body weight.

Rifampin and INH are given orally; however, they may be administered parenterally when the patient is vomiting. INH is available in tablets (50 mg., 100 mg., and 300 mg.) and in syrup (50 mg. per 50 ml.). Rifampin is available in capsules (150 mg. and 300 mg.) and in syrup (formulated from capsules in 10 mg. per ml.). Pyrazinamide is available in tablets of 500 mg., and ethambutol in tablets (100 mg. and 400 mg.).

The adverse and toxic reactions of INH are mild hepatic enzyme elevation, hepatitis, peripheral neuritis, and allergic reactions; those of rifampin are orange discoloration of secretions and urine, nausea, vomiting, hepatitis, febrile reaction, and thrombocytopenia. Pyrazinamide may cause hypouricemia and is hepatotoxic. Ethambutol can cause optic neuritis (reversible), decreased visual acuity, decreased red-green color discrimination, gastrointestinal disturbance, and allergic reaction.

During the course of chemotherapy of tuberculosis, spontaneous emergence of drug-resistant mutants can occur. The response to therapy should be carefully monitored both clinically and by appropriate radiographic and laboratory studies.

Local Conservative Care. The affected joint is put to rest in a functional position as soon as the diagnosis is suspected. The type of protection used depends upon the joint involved; when the hip or knee is affected, split Russell traction is applied; modified Dunlap traction is used with the shoulder; and a bivalved cast when the elbow, wrist, or ankle is involved. Gentle active and passive exercises are performed several times a day to preserve and increase range of motion of the affected joint.

Surgical Measures—Synovectomy and Curettage. Often when the diagnosis of tuberculous arthritis is made, the disease process is well advanced with extensive synovial involvement. After a preliminary period of chemotherapy of four to six weeks, synovectomy with excision of tuberculous granulomatous tissue is performed. If there is osseous involvement, the tuberculous foci in the epiphysis and metaphysis are curetted under radiographic control, exercising great caution not to damage the growth plate. The pannus covering the soft articular cartilage is gently wiped off with a moist sponge. The tourniquet is released before closure so that hemostasis may be effected. The wound is closed primarily and the limb is replaced in traction or a bivalved cast. As soon as the patient is comfortable, exercises are reinstated to increase range of motion of the affected joint.

Postoperatively there is usually dramatic improvement in the general condition of the patient. Temperature and erythrocyte sedimentation rate revert to normal, the patient's appetite improves, and he begins to gain weight. The inflamed joint, in turn, shows striking improvement; the synovial thickening and effusion rapidly diminish, muscle spasm disappears, range of joint motion increases, and the radiolucent aras of bone destruction begin to reossify.

The protection of the affected joint is continued for at least three months and antituberculous drugs are administered for 12 to 18 months following the operation.

Arthrodesis of a joint may still be indicated if it is greatly distorted with destruction of articular cartilage and bone. For technical details the reader is referred to the voluminous literature on the subject.* In the past, extra-

---

*See references 4–7, 9, 14, 16, 19, 20, 36, 41, 57, 72, 81, 82, 95–97, 114, 124, 171, 194, 219.

articular methods of fusion were used in order not to open an infected area; however, with effective chemotherapeutic agents, such techniques have become unnecessary.

Tuberculosis of the Spine

Tuberculosis of the vertebral column was first described by Percivall Pott as a painful kyphotic deformity of the spine associated with paraplegia.[162] The condition is since often referred to as Pott's disease. The spine is the most common site of skeletal tuberculosis, accounting for 50 per cent of the cases. Any level of the spine may be involved, the lower thoracic region being the most common segment; next in decreasing order of frequency are the lumbar, upper dorsal, cervical, and sacral regions.

In the past, tuberculous spondylitis used to be a disease of early childhood, usually between three and five years of age. Recently, however, with improved public health measures, this age incidence has changed, and adults are more frequently affected.

Tuberculous spondylitis warrants individual consideration because of certain significant differences between it and tuberculous arthritis of the limbs.*

Pathology. The initial focus of infection usually begins in the cancellous bone of the vertebral body and only occasionally in the posterior neural arch, transverse process, or subperiosteally deep to the anterior longitudinal ligament in front of the vertebral body (Fig. 4–15). The area of infection gradually enlarges and spreads to involve two or more adjacent vertebrae by extension beneath the anterior longitudinal ligament or directly across the intervertebral disc. Occasionally there may be multiple foci of involvement separated by normal vertebrae, or the infection may be disseminated to distant vertebrae via the paravertebral abscess.

The vertebral bodies lose their mechanical strength as a result of progressive destruction under the force of body weight and eventually collapse with the intervertebral joints and the posterior neural arch intact; thus, an angular kyphotic deformity is produced, the severity of which depends upon the extent of destruction, the level of the lesion, and the number of vertebrae involved. In the thoracic region the kyphosis is most marked because of the normal dorsal curvature; in the lumbar area it is slight because of the normal lumbar lordosis in which most of the body weight is transmitted posteriorly and collapse is partial; and in the cervical spine, collapse is minimal, if present at all, because most of the body weight is borne through the articular processes.

Healing takes place by gradual fibrosis and calcification of the granulomatous tuberculous tissue. Eventually the fibrous tissue is ossified, with resulting bony ankylosis of the collapsed vertebrae.

Paravertebral *abscess formation* occurs in almost every case. With collapse of the vertebral body, tuberculous granulation tissue, caseous matter, and necrotic bone and bone marrow are extruded through the bony cortex and accumulate beneath the anterior longitudinal ligament. These cold abscesses gravitate along the fascial planes and present externally at some distance from the site of the original lesion (Fig. 4–16). In the lumbar region the abscess gravitates along the psoas fascial sheath and usually points into the groin just below the inguinal ligament. In the thoracic region, the longitudinal ligaments limit the abscess, which is seen in the radiogram as a fusiform radiopaque shadow at or just below the level of the involved vertebra; if under great tension, it may rupture into the mediastinum, where it may be walled off to form the "bird's nest" type of paravertebral abscess. Occasionally, a thoracic abscess may reach the anterior chest wall in the parasternal area by tracking via the intercostal vessels. The prevertebral fascia limits the cervical abscess, which may burst into the retropharyngeal area or gravitate laterally on each side of the neck.

Paraplegia results from compression of the cord by the abscess, by the caseating or granulating mass, or by the posteriorly protruding border of the intervetebral disc or edge of bone. Other contributory factors may be thrombosis of the local vessels and edema of the cord. It occurs most often in the mid- or upper-thoracic region, where the kyphosis is most acute, the spinal canal is narrow, and the spinal cord is relatively large. In the literature it is described as occurring in 6 to 25 per cent of the reported cases, but recently, with early diagnosis and effective treatment, the incidence has become greatly diminished.

Clinical Features. The onset of Pott's disease is usually insidious and of slow evolution. Initial symptoms are vague, consisting of generalized malaise, easy fatiguability, loss of appetite and weight, and loss of desire to play outdoors. There may be an afternoon or evening fever.

---

*See references 2, 8, 11, 16, 23, 26, 30, 31, 33, 37, 39, 40, 45–49, 52, 59, 61, 62, 70, 72, 74, 76, 78, 88, 94, 97, 103, 106, 107, 109, 141, 144, 153, 166, 170, 172, 175, 177, 178, 181, 187–198, 200, 208, 209, 212, 214.

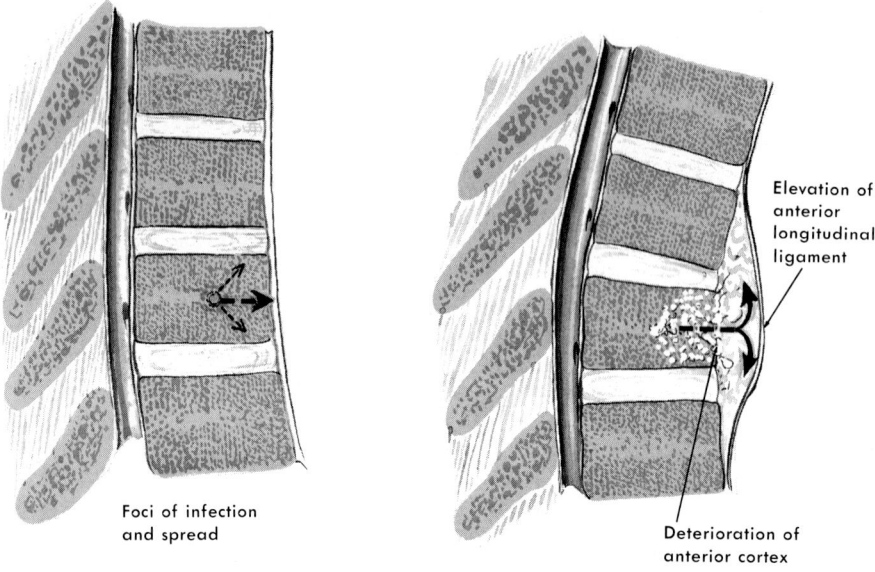
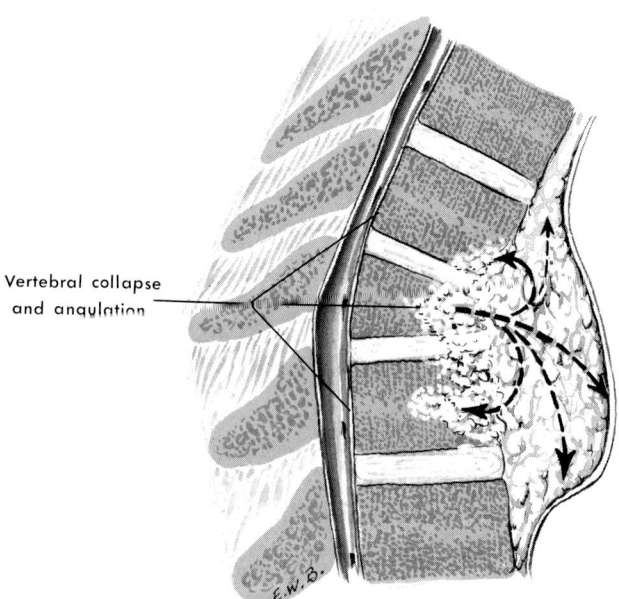

FIGURE 4–15. *Pathogenesis of tuberculous spondylitis.*

Backache is usually minimal; it may be referred segmentally.

Muscle spasm in the affected region of the spine is a constant finding. The spine is held rigid. When picking an object up from the floor, the patient flexes his hips and knees, keeping the spine in extension (Fig. 4–17). Motion of the spine is limited in all directions. Spasm of the paravetebral muscles in the lumbar region is also elicited by passive hyperextension of the hips with the patient in prone position—this also puts stretch on the iliopsoas muscle, which is in spasm and contracture owing to psoas abscess.

A kyphos in the thoracic region may be the first noticeable sign. As the kyphos increases, the ribs will crowd together and a barrel chest deformity will develop. When the lesion is

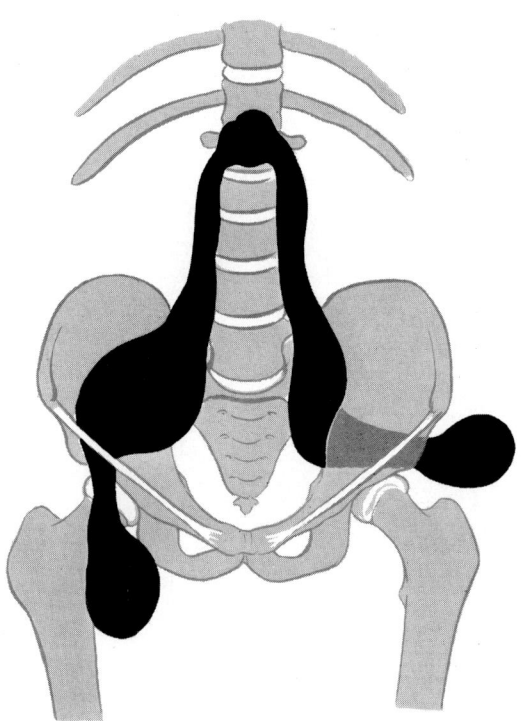

FIGURE 4–16. Abscess formation in Pott's disease.

Diagrammatic representation of the various courses that a tuberculous abscess arising from the thoracolumbar spine may take. (After Calott.)

situated in the cervical or lumbar spine, a flattening of the normal lordosis is the initial finding.

On gentle percussion or pressure over the spinous process of the affected vertebrae, tenderness is often present. The abscesses may be palpated as fluctuant swellings in the groin, iliac fossa, retropharynx, or on the side of the neck, depending upon the level of the lesion.

The gait of the child with Pott's disease is peculiar, reflecting the protective rigidity of the spine. His steps are short, as he is trying to avoid any jarring of his back. In tuberculosis of the cervical spine, he holds his neck in extension and supports his head with one hand under the chin and the other over the occiput. If the level is in the lumbodorsal area and a psoas abscess is present, the patient walks with his knees and hips in flexion and supports the spine by placing his hands over the thighs. If paraplegia develops, there will be spasticity of the lower limbs with hyperactive deep tendon reflexes, a spastic gait, a varying degree of motor weakness, and disturbances of bladder and anorectal function.

Radiographic Features. In tuberculous spondylitis the radiographic findings are suggestive, but not pathognomonic. In addition to the routine anteroposterior and lateral views of the spine, linear tomograms, CAT scan, and nuclear magnetic resonance imaging are used to delineate bone and spinal cord pathology in detail. Also, in the radiographic study of the patient who is suspected of having tuberculosis, chest radiograms and an intravenous pyelogram are taken to rule out other foci of systemic disease.

The vertebral body depicts the initial changes; it becomes rarefied with loss and haziness of its bone trabecular pattern. Soon the vertebral body expands and its borders are indistinct. With progressive destruction of bone the vertebral body collapses (Figs. 4–18 and 4–19). The intervertebral disc space first narrows and later is obliterated. Paraspinal abscesses may be seen quite early, presenting as fusiform or rounded shadows of water density.

In the differential diagnosis one should consider suppurative spondylitis, leukemia, Hodgkin's disease, eosinophilic granuloma, aneurysmal bone cyst, and Ewing's sarcoma. All these conditions may cause destruction and collapse of the vertebral body, narrowing and obliteration of intervertebral disc spaces, and paraspinal soft-tissue swelling.

Scheuermann's disease is easy to differentiate because there is no rarefaction of the vertebral bodies except in the superior and inferior angles

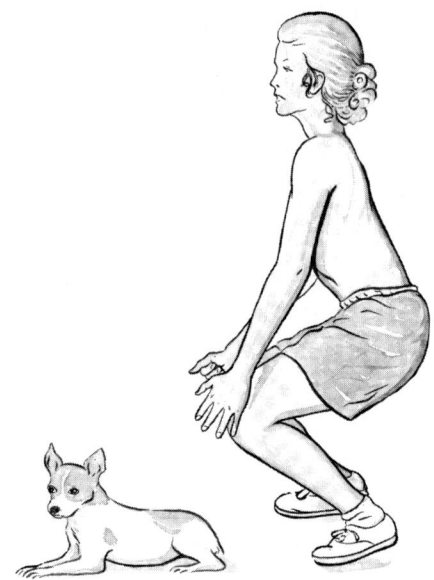

FIGURE 4–17. A child with tuberculous spondylitis.

When picking an object from the floor, because of rigidity of the spine she flexes her hips and knees, keeping the spine in extension.

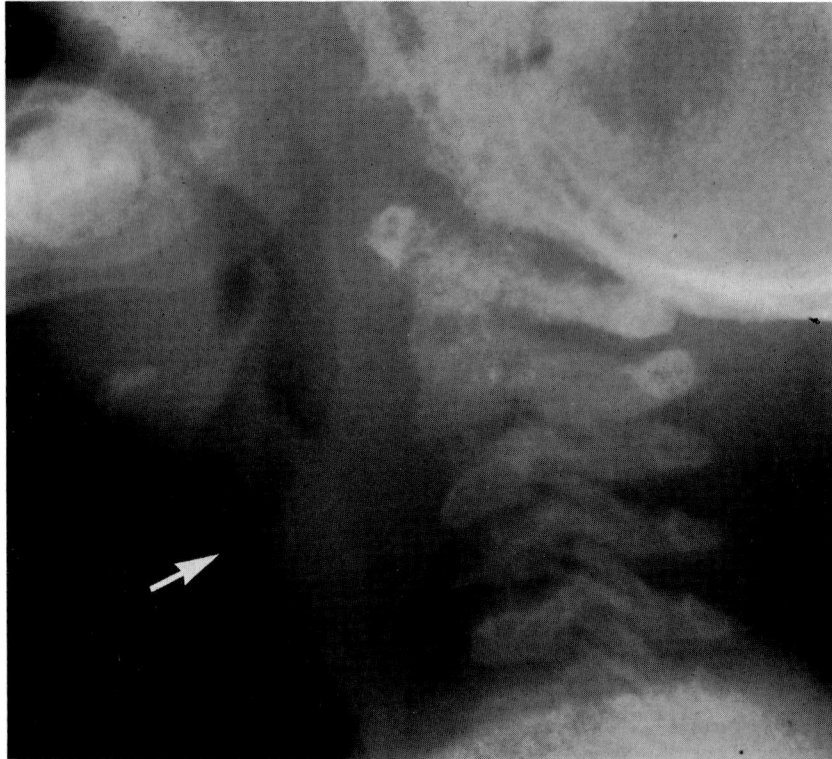

FIGURE 4–18. *Tuberculosis of cervical spine.*

Note the destruction of the fourth cervical vertebra and the retropharyngeal abscess.

of their anterior portion and paraspinal abscesses are not formed.

Treatment. As soon as the diagnosis of tuberculous spondylitis is suspected, the patient is placed in recumbency and his spine is protected in extension in a bivalved body cast. The hips are included in the cast if the lumbar spine is affected. Immobilization of the spine in a plaster of Paris cast or a plastic splint is imperative, as it serves to prevent motion and diminishes the likelihood of further compression and deformity.

Chemotherapy is initiated immediately. After four to six weeks of chemotherapy the tuberculous focus is eradicated directly through an anterior approach. The necrotic, caseating area containing fragments of dead bone and granulation tissue is evacuated, and the resulting cavity is packed with autogenous bone graft. The technical details have been described by Hodgson and Stock.[99, 101] This direct radical approach eradicates the disease focus, provides raw bleeding surface (facilitating local access of chemotherapeutic agents), promotes rapid healing, and achieves early stabilization of the spine by fusing together the affected vertebrae. Posterior spinal fusion is performed only when bone consolidation is delayed or does not take place through the anterior approach.

Paraplegia in Tuberculous Spondylitis. Paraplegia is a serious complication of tuberculosis of the spine. Its incidence is reported to be 10.6 per cent by Hodgson et al., though in the series of Cleveland, 29 per cent of the patients developed paraplegia.[126, 171] With early diagnosis and effective treatment the incidence is markedly decreasing. It is more common under ten years of age (about two thirds of the cases). There is no sex predilection.

Sorrel-Dejerine classified paraplegia of Pott's disease into *early onset paraplegia*, occurring in less than two years from the onset of the disease, and *late onset paraplegia*, arising after this time.[188] Seddon and Butler modified the classification of Sorrel into three types.[35, 175, 177, 178] In *Type I*, the onset is typically early, occurring within the first two years of disease, and is associated with active disease. The paralysis is usually complete but diminishes with complete recovery. *Type II* also begins early and is associated with active disease; however, it persists permanently, even if the tuberculous infection becomes completely quiescent. *Type III* is of late onset and may or may not improve.

Hodgson and associates gave the following

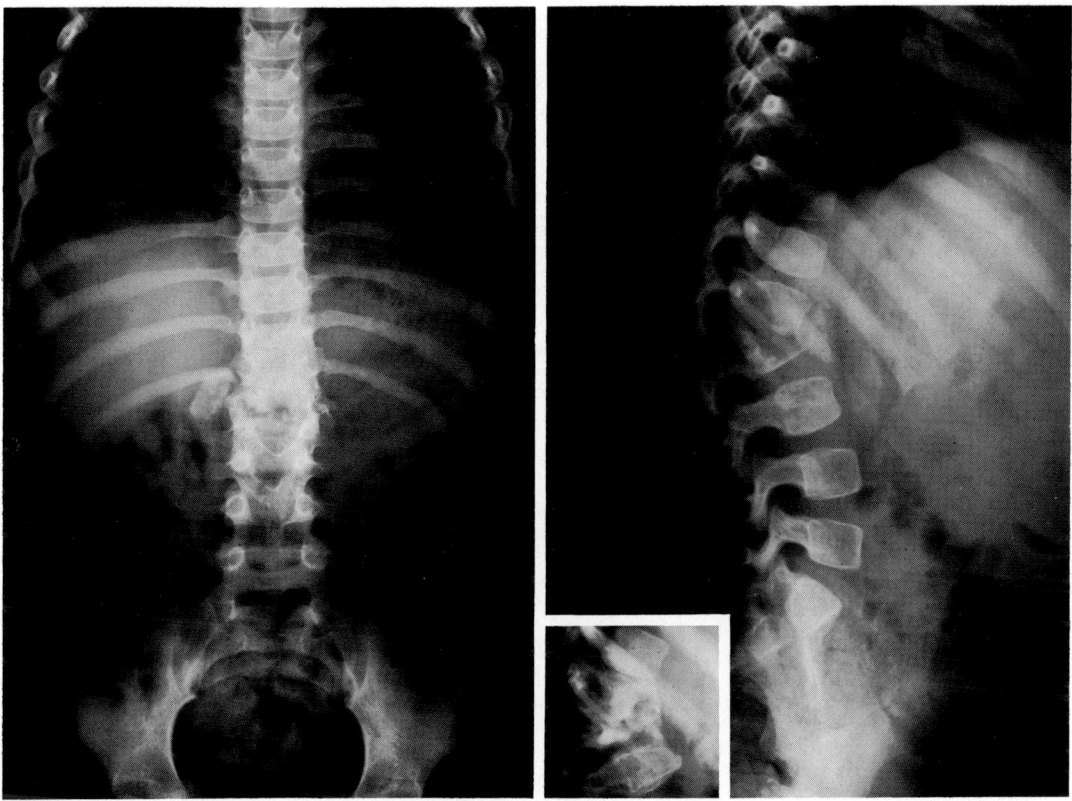

FIGURE 4–19. Tuberculous spondylitis.

First and second lumbar vertebrae are involved. Note collapse of the vertebral bodies, obliteration of intervertebral disc interspace, and localized kyphosis.

practical classification based on its pathogenesis.[102]

Paraplegia of active disease resulting from external compression of the cord and the dura by caseating pus, bony sequestra, sequestered disc, subluxation and dislocation of the vertebrae, or tuberculous granulation tissue in the spinal canal. Clinically, these patients have a varying degree of spasticity of their lower limbs, but do not have involuntary muscle spasms and withdrawal reflex. The prognosis is good in this type, with good recovery to be expected following surgery.

Paraplegia of active disease due to tuberculous disease within the cord. The dura has been penetrated by the tuberculosis, producing tuberculous meningomyelitis or tuberculous arachnoiditis. Clinically, these patients have severe spasticity with involuntary muscle spasm and withdrawal reflex. The prognosis in this type is poor and varies with the extent of damage to the cord. In general, urinary and fecal incontinence, the presence of sensory disturbances, and paraplegia are ominous hallmarks.

Paraplegia of healing due to fibrosis of the meninges and the granulation tissue or the meninges and pressure on the cord.

Paraplegia from other rare causes, such as thrombosis of vessels supplying the cord.

When signs of paraplegia are found, a lumbar puncture is performed with a Queckenstedt test, cell count, and determination of total protein level to assess the severity of block. Myelography is used in selected cases to determine whether the block is partial or complete. At present, magnetic resonance imaging is performed first; it is noninvasive and depicts in detail the spinal cord and bone pathology. Hodgson and associates recommend immediate evacuation of the tuberculous focus and decompression of the cord through an anterior approach, followed by local bone grafting to stabilize the spine. They caution that a policy of mere observation may cause permanent paraplegia.

Hodgson and associates condemn laminectomy as a primary procedure in the treatment of Pott's paraplegia on the basis that excision of the lamina and posterior neural elements removes the only supporting structure remaining in the presence of the anterior disease.[102] The only indication for laminectomy is when paraplegia is due to laminar disease or involvement of the cord, or when paraplegia persists after anterior decompression and successful fusion, and myelography shows a block.

References

1. Aabye, R.: Tuberculous osteomyelitis of the patella. Acta Chir. Scand., *111*:409, 1956.
2. Adams, Z. B.: Tuberculosis of the spine in children. A review of sixty-three cases from the Lakeville State Sanatorium. J. Bone Joint Surg., *22*:860, 1940.
3. Ahern, R. T.: Tuberculosis of the femoral neck and greater trochanter. J. Bone Joint Surg., *40-B*:406, 1958.
4. Ahlberg, A.: Radical operative treatment of the tuberculous hip. A report of 112 cases. J. Bone Joint Surg., *30-A*:550, 1948.
5. Albee, F. H.: Transplantation of a portion of the tibia into the spine for Pott's disease. J.A.M.A., *57*:885, 1911.
6. Albee, F. H.: Bone Graft Surgery. Philadelphia, Saunders, 1915.
7. Albee, F. H.: The bone-graft operation for tuberculosis of the spine. Twenty years of experience. J.A.M.A., *94*:1417, 1930.
8. Alexander, G. L.: Neurological complications of spinal tuberculosis. Proc. R. Soc. Med., *39*:730, 1945–46.
9. Allen, A. R., and Stevenson, A. W.: The results of combined drug therapy and early fusion in bone tuberculosis. J. Bone Joint Surg., *39-A*:32, 1957.
10. Allred, S. W., and Minear, W. L.: Statistical study of tuberculosis of the bones and joints in children. Am. Surg., *18*:58, 1952.
11. Alpero, B. J., and Palmer, H. D.: Compression of the spinal cord due to tuberculosis abscess. Report of case of Pott's disease with direct extension from lung to spinal canal. Am. J. Surg., *24*:163, 1934.
12. Arafiles, R. P.: A new technique of fusion for tuberculous arthritis of the elbow. J. Bone Joint Surg., *63-A*:1396, 1981.
13. Babhulkar, S. S., Tayade, W. B., and Babhulkar, S. K.: Atypical spinal tuberculosis. J. Bone Joint Surg., *66-B*:239, 1984.
14. Badgley, C. E., and Hammond, G.: Tuberculosis of the hip. J. Bone Joint Surg., *24*:135, 1942.
15. Bailey, H., Sister Mary Gabriel, Hodgson, A. R., and Shin, J. S.: Tuberculosis of the spine in children. J. Bone Joint Surg., *54-A*:1633, 1972.
16. Bakalim, G.: Tuberculous spondylitis. A clinical study with special reference to the significance of spinal fusion and chemotherapy. Acta Orthop. Scand., Suppl. 47, 1960.
17. Benkeddache, Y., and Gottesman, H.: Skeletal tuberculosis of the wrist and hand: A study of 27 cases. J. Hand Surg., *7*:593, 1982.
18. Bickel, W. H.: Tuberculosis of bones and joints. Proc. Staff Meet. Mayo Clin., *28*:370, 1953.
19. Bosworth, D. M. L.: Femoro-ischial transplantation. J. Bone Joint Surg., *24*:38, 1942.
20. Bosworth, D. M.: Treatment of bone and joint tuberculosis in children. J. Bone Joint Surg., *41-A*:1255, 1959.
21. Bosworth, D. M.: Treatment of tuberculosis of bone and joint. Bull. N.Y. Acad. Med., *35*:167, 1959.
22. Bosworth, D. M., and Graul, W. R.: Amputation for tuberculosis of joints. A study of the therapeutic and prognostic value. J. Bone Joint Surg., *31-A*:194, 1949.
23. Bosworth, D. M., and Levine, J.: Tuberculosis of the spine. An analysis of cases treated surgically. J. Bone Joint Surg., *31-A*:267, 1949.
24. Bosworth, D. M., and Wright, H. A.: Streptomycin in bone and joint tuberculosis. J. Bone Joint Surg., *34-A*:255, 1952.
25. Bosworth, D. M., Della Pietra, A., and Farrell, R. F.: The classic streptomycin in tuberculosis bone and joint lesions with mixed infection and sinuses. Clin. Orthop., *116*:2, 1976.
26. Bosworth, D. M., Della Pietra, A., and Rahilly, G.: Paraplegia resulting from tuberculosis of the spine. J. Bone Joint Surg., *35-A*:735, 1953.
27. Bosworth, D. M., Wright, H. A., and Fielding, J. W.: The treatment of bone and joint tuberculosis: Effect of Isonicotinyl-2-isopropyl hydrazine. A preliminary report. J. Bone Joint Surg., *34-A*:761, 1952.
28. Bosworth, D. M., Wright, H. A., Fielding, J. W., and Wilson, H.: The use of isoniazid in the treatment of bone and joint tuberculosis. J. Bone Joint Surg., *35-A*:577, 1953.
29. Brant-Zawadski, M., Burke, V. D., and Jeffrey, R. B.: CT in the evaluation of spine infection. Spine, *8*:358, 1983.
30. Brodin, H.: Myelography with water-soluble contrast medium in lumbar and sacrolumbar tuberculous spondylitis. Acta Orthop. Scand., *21*:259, 1951.
31. Brooks, W. D. W.: Paravertebral abscess with rupture into the pleura. Br. J. Tuberc., *36*:49, 1942.
32. Bryan, W. J., Doherty, J. H., Jr., and Sculco, T. P.: Tuberculosis in a rheumatoid patient. A case report. Clin. Orthop., *171*:206, 1982.
33. Burke, H. E.: The pathogenesis of Pott's disease. Trans. Am. Clin. Climatol. Assoc., *59*:122, 1948.
34. Bush, D. C., and Schneider, L. H.: Tuberculosis of the hand and wrist. J. Hand Surg., *9-A*:391, 1984.
35. Butler, R. W.: Paraplegia in Pott's disease, with special reference to the pathology and etiology. Br. J. Surg., *22*:738, 1935.
36. Campos, O. P.: Bone and joint tuberculosis and its treatment. J. Bone Joint Surg., *37-A*:937, 1955.
37. Cauchoix, J., Cotrel, Y., and Morel, G.: Traitement moderne du mal Pott. Rev. Prat., *6*:1049, 1956.
38. Chandler, F. A., and Fox, T. A.: Amputation for the discrepancy of limb length in tuberculosis of the hip. J. Bone Joint Surg., *31-A*:420, 1949.
39. Chandler, F. A., and Page, M. A.: Tuberculosis of the spine. J. Bone Joint Surg., *22*:851, 1940.
40. Charcot, J. M.: Paraplegie par mal de Pott. Gaz. Hôp. (Paris), *56*:483, 1883.
41. Charnley, J., and Baker, S. L.: Compression arthrodesis of the knee. J. Bone Joint Surg., *34-B*:187, 1952.
42. Chow, S. P., and Yau, A.: Tuberculosis of the knee—a long term follow-up. Int. Orthop., *4*:87, 1980.
43. Chung, S. M., Kim, N. H., Kim, Y. A., Kang, E. S., and Park, B. M.: Clinical studies of tuberculosis of the spine. Yonsei Med. J., *19*:96, 1978.
44. Cleveland, M.: Surgical treatment of joint tuberculosis. Surg. Gynecol. Obstet., *61*:503, 1935.
45. Cleveland, M.: Tuberculosis of the spine. A clinical study of 203 patients from Sea View and St. Luke's Hospital. Am. Rev. Tuber., *41*:215, 1940.
46. Cleveland, M.: Treatment of tuberculosis of the spine. J. Bone Joint Surg., *22*:824, 1940.
47. Cleveland, M., and Bosworth, D. M.: The pathology of tuberculosis of the spine. J. Bone Joint Surg., *24*:527, 1942.
48. Cleveland, M., Bosworth, D. M., Fielding, J. W., and Smyruis, P.: Fusion of the spine for tuberculosis in children. J. Bone Joint Surg., *40-A*:91, 1958.
49. Compere, E. L., and Garrison, M.: Correlation of

pathologic and roentgenographic findings in tuberculosis and pyogenic infection of the vertebrae. The fate of the intervertebral disk. Ann. Surg., *104*:1038, 1936.
50. Cortese, M., Cavliere, G., De Toni, T., Bagnara, V., Naselli, A., and Duillo, M. T.: Tuberculosis of the hand in childhood. Minerva Pediatr., *34*:761, 1982.
51. Crofton, J.: The chemotherapy of tuberculosis. Br. Med. Bull., *16*:55, 1960.
52. Dalechamps, J.: Chirurgie Française. 3rd. Ed. Paris, 1610.
53. Davidson, A. J., and Horwitz, M. T.: Resection of the elbow joint. Surgery, *3*:226, 1938.
54. Davies, P. D. O., Humphries, M. J., Byfield, S. P., Nunn, A. J., Darbyshire, J. H., Citron, K. M., and Fox, W.: Bone and joint tuberculosis. A survey of notifications in England and Wales. J. Bone Joint Surg., *66-B*:326, 1984.
55. DeMarchi, E.: Resection of the os pubis and os ischii for tuberculosis. Arch. Orthop., *60*:1, 1948.
56. DeRoy, M. S., and Fisher, H.: The treatment of tuberculosis bone disease by surgical drainage combined with streptomycin. J. Bone Joint Surg., *34-A*:299, 1952.
57. Dobson, J.: Arthrodesis in tuberculosis of the hip joint. An analysis of fifty cases. J. Bone Joint Surg., *30-B*:95, 1948.
58. Dobson, J.: Prognosis in tuberculosis of the hip. Analysis of the results of the treatment and of the factors which influence the end-results. J. Bone Joint Surg., *33-B*:149, 1951.
59. Dobson, J.: Tuberculosis of the spine. An analysis of the results of conservative treatment and of the factors influencing the prognosis. J. Bone Joint Surg., *33-B*:517, 1951.
60. Donovan, M. S., and Sosman, M. C.: Tuberculosis of the greater trochanter and its bursa. A.J.R., *48*:719, 1942.
61. Dott, N. M.: Skeletal traction and anterior decompression in the management of Pott's paraplegia. Edinburgh Med. J., *54*:620, 1947.
62. Doub, H. P., and Badgley, C. E.: Roentgen signs of tuberculosis of the vertebral body. A.J.R., *27*:827, 1932.
63. Dowd, C. F., Sartoris, D. J., Haghighi, P., and Resnick, D.: Case report 344. Tuberculous spondylitis resulting in atlantoaxial dislocation. Skeletal Radiol., *15*:65, 1986.
64. Duncan, G. A.: Skeletal and extra-skeletal tuberculous lesions associated with joint tuberculosis. J. Bone Joint Surg., *19*:64, 1937.
65. Enarson, D. A., Fujii, M., Nakielna, E. M., and Grzbowski, S.: Bone and joint tuberculosis: A continuing problem. Can. Med. Assoc. J., *120*:139, 1979.
66. Erlacher, P. J.: The radical operative treatment of bone and joint tuberculosis. J. Bone Joint Surg., *17*:536, 1935.
67. Evans, D.: The diagnosis and treatment of skeletal tuberculosis. Br. J. Clin. Pract., *12*:811, 1958.
68. Evans, E. T.: Tuberculosis of the bones and joints. J. Bone Joint Surg., *34-A*:267, 1952.
69. Fang, D., Leong, J. C. Y., and Fang, H. S. Y.: Tuberculosis of the upper cervical spine. J. Bone Joint Surg., *65-B*:47, 1983.
70. Fellander, M.: Radical operation for tuberculosis of the spine. Acta Orthop. Scand., Suppl. 19, 1955.
71. Ferguson, A. B.: Roentgenography of tuberculosis of the joints. J. Bone Joint Surg., *19*:653, 1937.
72. Fraser, J.: Tuberculosis of the spinal column. Edinburgh Med. J., *36*:133, 1929.
73. Fraser, J.: Tuberculosis of the Bones and Joints. Edinburgh Medical Series. London, A. & C. Black, 1937.
74. Friedman, B.: Chemotherapy of tuberculosis of the spine. J. Bone Joint Surg., *48-A*:451, 1956.
75. Garber, E. K., and Bluestone, R.: Case report 138. Tuberculous arthritis of the knee with "cold abscess" communicating with the knee joint. Skeletal Radiol., *6*:75, 1981.
76. Garceau, G. J., and Brash, T. A.: Pott's paraplegia. J. Bone Joint Surg., *33-A*:87, 1950.
77. Ghormley, R. K.: Chemotherapy in bone and joint tuberculosis. J. Bone Joint Surg., *34-A*:254, 1952.
78. Ghormley, R. K., and Bradley, J. I.: Prognostic signs in the x-rays of tuberculous spines in children. J. Bone Joint Surg., *10*:796, 1928.
79. Gibney, V. P.: Compression paraplegia in Pott's disease of the spine, based on the analysis of seventy-four cases. J. Nerv. Ment. Dis., *24*:195, 1897.
80. Gill, G. G.: The cause of discrepancy in length of the limb following tuberculosis of the hip in children. J. Bone Joint Surg., *26*:272, 1944.
81. Girdlestone, G. R.: Tuberculosis of Bone and Joint. London, Oxford University Press, 1940.
82. Girdlestone, G. R., and Somerville, E. W.: Tuberculosis of Bone and Joint. London, Oxford University Press, 1952.
83. Griffiths, D. I.: Pott's paraplegia and its operative treatment. J. Bone Joint Surg., *35-B*:487, 1953.
84. Griffiths, D. I., Seddon, H. J., and Roaf, R.: Pott's paraplegia. New York and London, Oxford University Press, 1956.
85. Griffiths, D. L. L.: The treatment of spinal tuberculosis. *In* McKibbin, B. (ed.), Recent Advances in Orthopedics, No. 3. Edinburgh, London, and New York, Churchill-Livingstone, 1979, pp. 1–17.
86. Griffiths, D. L.: Tuberculosis of the spine: A review. Adv. Tuberc. Res., *20*:92, 1980.
87. Gruca, A.: The treatment of quiescent tuberculosis of the hip joint by excision and "dynamic" osteotomy. J. Bone Joint Surg., *32-B*:174, 1950.
88. Hallock, H., and Jones, J. B.: Tuberculosis of the spine. An end-result study of the effects of the spine-fusion operation in a large number of patients. J. Bone Joint Surg., *36-A*:219, 1954.
89. Halsey, J. P., Reeback, J. S., and Barnes, O. G.: A decade of skeletal tuberculosis. Ann. Rheum. Dis., *41*:7, 1982.
90. Hardinge, K., Cleary, J., and Charnley, J.: Low-friction arthroplasty for healed septic and tuberculous arthritis. J. Bone Joint Surg., *61-B*:144, 1979.
91. Harris, R. I., and Couthard, H. S.: Prognosis in bone and joint tuberculosis. J. Bone Joint Surg., *24*:382, 1942.
92. Harris, R. I., Couthard, H. S., and Dewar, F. P.: Streptomycin in the treatment of bone and joint tuberculosis. Clinical analysis of 118 lesions. J. Bone Joint Surg., *34-A*:279, 1952.
93. Hartung, E. F.: Tuberculous arthritis. J.A.M.A., *158*:818, 1955.
94. Henderson, M. D.: Tuberculosis of the spine. End results of operative treatment. Surg. Gynecol. Obstet., *24*:600, 1917.
95. Hibbs, R. A.: An operation for stiffening the knee joint. Ann. Surg., *53*:404, 1911.
96. Hibbs, R. A.: Treatment of tuberculosis of joints of the lower extremities by operative fusion. J. Bone Joint Surg., *12*:749, 1930.
97. Hibbs, R. A., and Risser, J. C.: Treatment of vertebral tuberculosis by spine fusion operation. A report of 286 cases. J. Bone Joint Surg., *10*:805, 1928.
98. Hodgson, A. R., and Smith, T. K.: Tuberculosis of the wrist. Clin. Orthop., *183*:73, 1982.
99. Hodgson, A. R., and Stock, F. E.: Anterior spine fusion. Br. J. Surg., *44*:266, 1956.
100. Hodgson, A. R., and Stock, F. E.: Anterior spine fusion for the treatment of tuberculosis of the spine. J. Bone Joint Surg., *42-A*:295, 1960.
101. Hodgson, A. R., Stock, F. E., Fang, H. S. Y., and Ong, G. B.: Anterior spinal fusion. The operative

approach and pathologic findings in 412 patients with Pott's disease of the spine. Br. J. Surg., 48:172, 1960.
102. Hodgson, A. R., Yau, A., Kwon, J. S., and Kim, D.: A clinical study of 100 consecutive cases of Pott's paraplegia. Clin. Orthop., 36:128, 1964.
103. Hoover, M. J., Jr.: The treatment of tuberculous psoas abscess. South. Surg., 16:729, 1950.
104. Hsu, L. C. S., and Leong, J. C. Y.: Tuberculosis of the lower cervical spine (C2 to C7). A report of 40 cases. J. Bone Joint Surg., 66-B:1, 1984.
105. Isaacson, A. S., and Whitehouse, W. M.: Spontaneous sacroiliac obliteration in patients with tuberculosis. J. Bone Joint Surg., 31-A:306, 1949.
106. Ito, H., Tsuchiya, J., and Asami, G.: A new radical operation for Pott's disease. J. Bone Joint Surg., 16:499, 1934.
107. Johnson, R. W., Jr., Hillman, J. W., and Southwick, W. O.: The importance of direct surgical attack upon lesions of the vertebral bodies, particularly in Pott's disease. J. Bone Joint Surg., 35-A:17, 1953.
108. Jones, W. C., III, and Miller, W. E.: Skeletal tuberculosis 1963. South. Med. J., 57:964, 1964.
109. Karlen, A.: Early drainage of paraspinal tuberculosis abscesses in children. J. Bone Joint Surg., 41-B:491, 1959.
110. Katayama, R., Itami, Y., and Marumo, E.: Treatment of hip and knee joint tuberculosis, an attempt to retain motion. J. Bone Joint Surg., 44-A:897, 1962.
111. Kemp, H. B. S., Jackson, J. W., Jeremiah, J. D., and Cook, J.: Anterior fusion of the spine for infective lesions in adults. J. Bone Joint Surg., 55-B:715, 1973.
112. Kerri, O., and Martini, M.: Tuberculosis of the knee. Int. Orthop., 9:153, 1985.
113. Kim, Y., Han, D., and Park, B.: Total hip arthroplasty for tuberculous coxarthrosis. J. Bone Joint Surg., 69-A:718, 1987.
114. Kirkaldy-Willis, W. H.: Ischio-femoral arthrodesis of the hip joint. An analysis of fifty cases. J. Bone Joint Surg., 32-B:187, 1950.
115. Kondo, E., and Yamada, K.: End results of focal debridement in bone and joint tuberculosis and its indications. A study of 830 patients including comparison of results with and without streptomycin. J. Bone Joint Surg., 39-A:27, 1957.
116. Konstam, P. G., and Blesovsky, A.: The ambulant treatment of spinal tuberculosis. Br J Surg., 50.20, 1062.
117. Kovalenko, D. G., Milovanova, E. M., and Kovalenko, K. N.: Current aspects of the treatment of osteoarticular tuberculosis in children. Probl. Tuberk., 1:50, 1982.
118. Kovalenko, D. G., Milovanova, E. M., and Kovalenko, K. N.: New state of surgery of osteoarticular tuberculosis in children. Probl. Tuberk., 6:47, 1982.
119. Kumar, K.: A clinical study and classification of posterior spinal tuberculosis. Int. Orthop., 9:147, 1985.
120. Lau, J. H. K., Leong, J. C. Y., and Stroebel, A. B.: A longitudinal study of antibody titres to Antigen 6 in patients with bone and joint tuberculosis. Int. Orthop., 7:205, 1983.
121. Leff, A., Lester, T. W., and Addington, W.: Tuberculosis—a chemotherapeutic triumph but a persistent socioeconomic problem. Arch. Intern. Med., 139:1375, 1979.
122. Lorin, M. I., Hsu, K. H., and Jacob, S. C.: Treatment of tuberculosis in children. Pediatr. Clin. North Am., 30:333, 1983.
123. Lynch, A. F.: Tuberculosis of the greater trochanter. A report of eight cases. J. Bone Joint Surg., 64-A:185, 1982.
124. McCarroll, H. R., and Heath, R. D.: Tuberculosis of the hip in children. J. Bone Joint Surg., 29:889, 1947.
125. McKee, D. F., Barr, W. M., Bryan, C. S., and Lunceford, E. M., Jr.: Primary aspergillosis of the spine mimicking Pott's paraplegia. J. Bone Joint Surg., 66-A:1481, 1984.
126. McNeur, J. C., and Pritchard, A. E.: Tuberculosis of the greater trochanter. J. Bone Joint Surg., 37-B:246, 1955.
127. Manzella, J. P., Vanvoris, L. P., and Hruska, J. F.: Isolated calcaneal tuberculosis osteomyelitis. A case report. J. Bone Joint Surg., 61-A:946, 1979.
128. Martin, N. S.: Tuberculosis of the spine: A study of the results of treatment during the last twenty-five years. J. Bone Joint Surg., 53-B:613, 1970.
129. Martini, M., and Gottesman, H.: Results of conservative treatment in tuberculosis of the elbow. Int. Orthop., 4:83, 1980.
130. Martini, M., Adjrad, A., and Daoud, A.: Tuberculous osteoarthritis of the foot and ankle joint. Int. Orthop., 8:203, 1984.
131. Martini, M., Benkeddache, Y., and Gottesman, H.: Tuberculosis of the upper limb joints. Int. Orthop., 10:17, 1986.
132. Medical Research Council Working Party on Tuberculosis of the Spine: A controlled trial of plaster-of-Paris jackets in the management of ambulant outpatient treatment of tuberculosis of the spine in children on standard chemotherapy. Tubercle, 54:261, 1973.
133. Medical Research Council, 1st Report: Seddon, H., Sir (Chairman), Fox, W., Konstam, P. G., Scadding, J. G., Stott, H., Sutherland, I., Tall, R., and Griffiths, D. L.: A controlled trial of ambulant out-patient treatment and in-patient rest in bed in the management of tuberculosis of the spine in young Korean patients on standard chemotherapy. J. Bone Joint Surg., 55-B:678, 1973.
134. Medical Research Council Working Party on Tuberculosis of the Spine: A controlled trial of debridement and ambulatory treatment in the management of tuberculosis of the spine in patients on standard chemotherapy. A study in Bulawayo, Rhodesia. J. Trop. Med. Hyg., 77:72, 1974.
135. Medical Research Council, 4th Report: A controlled trial of anterior spinal fusion and debridement in the surgical management of the spine in patients on standard chemotherapy. A study in Hong Kong. Br. J. Surg., 61:853, 1974.
136. Medical Research Council Working Party on Tuberculosis of the Spine: A five year assessment of controlled trials of inpatient and out-patient treatment and of plaster-of-Paris jackets for tuberculosis of the spine in children on standard chemotherapy. J. Bone Joint Surg., 58-B:399, 1976.
137. Medical Research Council Working Party on Tuberculosis of the Spine: Five-year assessments of controlled trials of ambulatory treatment, debridement and anterior spinal fusion in the management of tuberculosis of the spine. J. Bone Joint Surg., 60-B:163, 1978.
138. Medical Research Council Working Party on Tuberculosis of the Spine: 7th Report. A controlled trial of anterior spinal fusion and debridement in the surgical management of tuberculosis of the spine in patients on standard chemotherapy: A study in two centres in South Africa. Tubercle, 59:79, 1978.
139. Medical Research Council: National survey of tuberculosis notifications in England and Wales, 1978/79: Report from the Medical Research Council Tuberculosis and Chest Diseases Unit. Br. Med. J., 281:895, 1980.
140. Medical Research Council Working Party on Tuberculosis of the Spine: A 10-year assessment of a controlled trial comparing debridement and anterior spinal fusion in the management of tuberculosis of the spine in patients on standard chemotherapy in Hong Kong. J. Bone Joint Surg., 64-B:393, 1982.
141. Menard, V.: Etude Pratique sur le Mal de Pott. Paris, Masson et Cie, 1900.

142. Mennonna, P., Sottini, M., and Briani, S.: One case report of quadriparesis from tuberculous infection of the cervical spine. J. Neurosurg. Sci., 18:278, 1974.
143. Mercer, W.: The management of the tuberculous hip joint. J. Bone Joint Surg., 36-A:1123, 1954.
144. Meyerding, H. W.: Tuberculosis of the spine. Treatment and results. J. Bone Joint Surg., 22:840, 1940.
145. Misgar, M. S., Nazir, A. M., and Tsering, N.: Partial synovectomy in the treatment of tuberculosis of the knee. Int. Surg., 67:53, 1982.
146. Moon, M. S., Rhee, S. K., Lee, K. S., and Kim, S. S.: A natural course of a dislocated healed tuberculous hip in a child. A case report. Clin. Orthop., 190:154, 1984.
147. Mora, F. B., and Llamedo, L. P.: Experimental studies on the treatment of bone and joint tuberculosis with dihydrosteptomycin and isonicotinic acid hydrazide. J. Bone Joint Surg., 37-A:156, 1955.
148. Moula, T., Fowles, J. V., Kassab, M. J., and Sliman, N.: Pott's paraplegia: A clinical review of operative and conservative treatment in 63 adults and children. Int. Orthop., 5:23, 1981.
149. Mukopadhaya, B., and Mishra, N. K.: Treatment of tuberculous sinuses and abscesses of osteoarticular origin. J. Bone Joint Surg., 39-B:326, 1957.
150. Naim-ur-Rahmann: Atypical forms of spinal tuberculosis. J. Bone Joint Surg., 62-B:162, 1980.
151. Newton, P., Sharp, J., and Barnes, K. L.: Bone and joint tuberculosis in Greater Manchester 1969–79. Ann. Rheum. Dis., 41:1, 1982.
152. Nicholson, R. A.: Twenty years of bone and joint tuberculosis in Bradford: A comparison of the disease in the indigenous and Asian populations. J. Bone Joint Surg., 56-B:760, 1974.
153. Norcross, J. R.: Compression of the spinal cord due to direct extension from a tuberculous pulmonary abscess. J. Bone Joint Surg., 30-A:492, 1948.
154. Orell, S.: The radical treatment of bone and joint tuberculosis. Acta Orthop. Scand., 21:187, 1951.
155. Papvasiliou, V. A., and Petropoulous, A. V.: Bone and joint tuberculosis in childhood. Acta Orthop. Scand., 52:1, 1981.
156. Parke, W., Colvin, G. S., and Almond, A. H. G.: Premature epiphyseal fusion at the knee joint in tuberculous disease of the hip. J. Bone Joint Surg., 31-B:63, 1949.
157. Paus, B.: The changed pattern of bone and joint tuberculosis in Norway. Acta Orthop. Scand., 48:277, 1977.
158. Peacock, J. E., Jr.: Colonic perforation with thigh abscess: An unusual presentation of tuberculous spondylitis. South. Med. J., 75:623, 1982.
159. Phemister, D. B.: Changes in the articular surfaces in tuberculosis and pyogenic infection of joints. A.J.R., 12:1, 1924.
160. Phemister, D. B.: Effect of pressure on articular surfaces in pyogenic and tuberculous arthritides and its bearing on treatment. Ann. Surg., 80:481, 1924.
161. Phemister, D. B., and Hatcher, H. C.: Correlation of pathologic and roentgenologic findings in the diagnosis of tuberculous arthritis. A.J.R., 29:736, 1933.
162. Pott, P.: Remarks on that Kind of Palsy of the Lower Limbs which is Frequently Found to Accompany Curvature of the Spine and is Supposed to be Caused by it, Together with its Method of Cure. The Chirurgical Works. London, Lowndes, 1779.
163. Ratliff, A. H. C.: Tuberculosis of the femoral neck in childhood. J. Bone Joint Surg., 39-A:1365, 1957.
164. Research Committee of the British Thoracic and Tuberculosis Association: A tuberculosis survey in England and Wales 1971: The influence of immigration and country of birth upon notifications. Tubercle, 54:249, 1973.
165. Research Committee of the British Tuberculosis Association: Tuberculosis among immigrants to England and Wales: A national survey in 1965. Tubercle, 47:145, 1966.
166. Rich, E. A.: The paralysis of Pott's disease. J. Bone Joint Surg., 12:112, 1930.
167. Rich, E. A.: The Pathogenesis of Tuberculosis. 2nd Ed. Springfield, Ill., Thomas, 1951.
168. Roaf, R.: Tuberculosis of the hip joint. J. Bone Joint Surg., 33-B:147, 1951.
169. Robins, R. H. C.: Tuberculosis of the wrist and hand. Br. J. Surg., 54:211, 1967.
170. Rosenheim, S.: On the pathological changes in the spinal cord in a case of Pott's disease. Johns Hopkins Hosp. Bull., 9:240, 1898.
171. Sanchis-Olmos, V.: Skeletal Tuberculosis. Baltimore, Williams & Wilkins, 1948.
172. Scott, J. C.: Treatment of tuberculosis of the spine. J. Bone Joint Surg., 37-B:367, 1955.
173. Scott, J. E., and Taor, W. S.: The changing pattern of bone and joint tuberculosis. J. Bone Joint Surg., 64-B:250, 1982.
174. Seddon, H. J.: Pott's paraplegia: Prognosis and treatment. Br. J. Surg., 22:769, 1935.
175. Seddon, H. J.: Fatal case of empyema secondary to a tuberculous spinal abscess. Proc. R. Soc. Med., 29:1662, 1936.
176. Seddon, H. J.: Treatment of tuberculous disease of the spine. Proc. R. Soc. Med., 31:951, 1938.
177. Seddon, H. J.: The pathology of Pott's paraplegia. Proc. R. Soc. Med., 39:723, 1946.
178. Seddon, H. J.: Pott's paraplegia. In Platt, H. (ed.): Modern Trends in Orthopedics (Second Series). New York, Hoeber, 1956, p. 220.
179. Shea, J. M.: Bilateral tuberculous osteomyelitis of medial humeral condyles. Infection secondary to cutaneous inoculation. J.A.M.A., 247:821, 1982.
180. Silva, J. F.: A review of patients with skeletal tuberculosis treated at the University Hospital, Kuala Lumpur. Int. Orthop., 4:71, 1980.
181. Simpson, T. W., and Grobbelaar, B. G.: Rupture of the aorta complicating tuberculosis of the spine. J. Bone Joint Surg., 37-B:614, 1955.
182. Smith, A. DeF.: The early diagnosis of joint tuberculosis. J.A.M.A., 83:1569, 1924.
183. Smith, A. DeF.: The pathology of joint tuberculosis in its early stages. Arch. Surg., 12:740, 1926.
184. Smith, A. DeF.: The treatment of bone and joint tuberculosis. J. Bone Joint Surg., 37-A:1214, 1955.
185. Soholt, S. T.: Tuberculosis of the sacroiliac joint. A review of seventy-five cases. J. Bone Joint Surg., 31-A:119, 1951.
186. Somerville, E. W., and Wilkinson, M. C. (eds.): Girdlestone's Tuberculosis of Bone and Joint. New York, Oxford University Press, 1965.
187. Somerville, E. W., and Wishart, J.: Pott's disease of the spine with rupture of the aorta. J. Bone Joint Surg., 30-B:327, 1948.
188. Sorrel-Dejerine, Y.: Contribution à l'Etude des Paraplegies Pottiques. Paris, 1925.
189. Spiller, W. G.: A microscopic study of the spinal cord in two cases of Pott's disease. Johns Hopkins Hosp. Bull., 9:125, 1898.
190. Stevenson, F. H.: The chemotherapy of orthopaedic tuberculosis. J. Bone Joint Surg., 22:878, 1940.
191. Stevenson, F. H.: Chemotherapy and tuberculosis of bone and joint. Tubercle, 38:355, 1957.
192. Stevenson, F. H., Cholmeley, J. A., and Jory, H. I.: Tuberculosis of the hip in children, seven years use of chemotherapy. Tubercle, 38:164, 1957.
193. Stevenson, F. H., Cholmeley, J. A., and Jory, H. I.: Tuberculosis of the knee: Results of chemotherapy between 1948 and 1956. Tubercle, 39:1, 1958.
194. Stratford, B.: The Trumble graft. A review of thirty-six cases. J. Bone Joint Surg., 35-B:247, 1953.

195. Strange, F. C.: The prognosis in sacroiliac tuberculosis. Br. J. Surg., 50:561, 1963.
196. Sundararaj, G. D., and Selvapandian, A. J.: Tuberculosis of the hip with urinary fistulas—a case report. Br. J. Surg., 70:241, 1983.
197. Svivastava, T. P.: Tuberculosis of the Elbow Joint. Proceedings of the Combined Congress of the International Bone and Joint Tuberculosis Club and Indian Orthopaedic Association, Madras, India. Indian Orthop. J., 12:26, 1983.
198. Sweet, P. P., Bennett, G. E., and Street, D. M.: Pott's disease. J. Bone Joint Surg., 22:878, 1940.
199. Swift, W. E.: Frozen section diagnosis of tuberculous joints. J. Bone Joint Surg., 18:641, 1936.
200. Swift, W. E.: End results of the spine-fusion operation for tuberculosis of the spine. J. Bone Joint Surg., 22:815, 1940.
201. Tuli, S. M., and Mukherjee, S. K.: Excision arthroplasty for tuberculosis and pyogenic arthritis of the hip. J. Bone Joint Surg., 63-B:29, 1981.
202. Tupman, G. S.: A case of tuberculosis of the ischium. J. Bone Joint Surg., 35-B:590, 1953.
203. United States Department of Health Education and Welfare: Extrapulmonary tuberculosis in the United States. HEW Publication No. (CDC)78–8360. Atlanta, DHEW, 1978.
204. Versfeld, G. A., and Solomon, A.: A diagnostic approach to tuberculosis of bones and joints. J. Bone Joint Surg., 64-A:446, 1982.
205. Wang, L. X.: Peroral focal debridement for treatment of tuberculosis of the atlas and axis. Chin. J. Orthop., 1:207, 1981.
206. Weaver, P., and Lifeso, R. M.: The radiological diagnosis of tuberculosis of the adult spine. Skeletal Radiol., 12:178, 1984.
207. Weber, R.: Tuberculose du Genou. Etude des possibilités de guérison avec conservation de la mobilité. Rev. Chir. Orthop., 58:587, 1977.
208. Weinberg, J. A.: The surgical excision of psoas abscesses resulting from spinal tuberculosis. J. Bone Joint Surg., 39-A:17, 1957.
209. White, J. F.: Case of caries of dorsal vertebrae, with an abscess communicating with the lungs, and expectoration of bone. Philadelphia, Med. Exam., 4:213, 1841.
210. Wilkinson, M. C.: Synovectomy and curettage in the treatment of tuberculosis of joints. J. Bone Joint Surg., 35-B:209, 1953.
211. Wilkinson, M. C.: Chemotherapy of tuberculosis of bones and joints. J. Bone Joint Surg., 36-B:23, 1954.
212. Wilkinson, M. C.: The treatment of tuberculosis of the spine by evacuation of the paravertebral abscess and curettage of the vertebral bodies. J. Bone Joint Surg., 37-B:382, 1955.
213. Wilkinson, M. C.: Partial synovectomy and curettage in treatment of tuberculosis of the hip. J. Bone Joint Surg., 39-B:66, 1957.
214. Wilkinson, M. C.: Treatment of tuberculosis of the spine. Br. Med. J., 2:280, 1959.
215. Wilkinson, M. C.: Partial synovectomy in the treatment of tuberculosis of the knee. J. Bone Joint Surg., 44-B:34, 1962.
216. Wilkinson, M. C.: Tuberculosis of the hip and knee treated by chemotherapy, synovectomy and debridement. J. Bone Joint Surg., 51-A:1343, 1969.
217. Wilson, J. N.: Tuberculosis of the elbow. A study of thirty-one cases. J. Bone Joint Surg., 35-B:551, 1953.
218. Wolfgang, G. L.: Tuberculosis joint infection. Clin. Orthop., 136:257, 1978.
219. Yu, H. I.: Tuberculosis of the hip. A follow-up study of fifty-eight cases with special reference to fusion results in young children. J. Bone Joint Surg., 33-A:131, 1951.

SYPHILITIC JOINT DISEASE

In children with congenital syphilis, two types of joint disease may be encountered: namely, Parrot's syphilitic osteochondritis and Clutton's joints.

Parrot's syphilitic osteochondritis occurs in the first three months of life in infants with congenital syphilis. It is a form of epiphysitis that affects the upper limbs more often than the lower. The shoulders, wrists, and knees are frequent sites. The cartilage and bone undergo a gelatinous change and disintegrate, forming a greenish-yellow fluid. The juxtaepiphyseal regions are swollen and tender. Complete epiphyseal separation may occur (Parrot's pseudoparalysis). Radiograms will disclose widening of the articular cartilage space, irregularity of the physis, periosteal thickening, cupping of the metaphysis, and decalcification of adjacent bones. Wassermann reaction of the aspirated fluid is strongly positive. Treatment consists of adequate doses of penicillin for the syphilis and appropriate splinting of the affected limbs. With early diagnosis and treatment, recovery of the joint is complete. In late and inadequately treated cases, epiphyseal growth is disturbed, with resultant shortening or asymmetrical deformities of the limb.

Clutton's joints are a late manifestation of congenital syphilis, occurring in children between 6 and 16 years of age. The condition develops insidiously as a painless symmetrical hydrarthrosis of the knees. Occasionally, the elbows may be affected. There is no fever, and the children ambulate quite well.[2, 5] Radiograms will disclose the synovial effusion. The joint fluid will show leukocytosis of 10,000 to 45,000 (primarily lymphocytes). Following paracentesis, the joint fluid accumulates rapidly. The arthritis runs its natural course to spontaneous recovery within a few years with no permanent damage to the joint. It does not respond to antibiotic therapy.

References

1. Bandirali, G. R., and Pratesi, A. C.: Su alcuni casi di sifilde ossea congenita precoce di recente osservazione. Ann. Radiol. Diagn., 36:349, 1963.
2. Borella, L., Goobar, J. E., and Clark, G. M.: Synovitis of the knee joints in late congenital syphilis, Clutton's joints. J.A.M.A., 180:190, 1962.
3. Caffey, J.: Syphilis of the skeleton in early infancy. A.J.R., 42:637, 1937.
4. Canalla, P.: A case of bilateral and symmetrical bone syphilis of the humerus. Ital. J. Orthop. Traumatol., 3:257, 1977.

5. Clutton, H. H.: Symmetrical synovitis of the knee in hereditary syphilis (reprint). Clin. Orthop., 57:5, 1968.
6. Coblentz, D. R., Cimini, R., Mikity, V. G., and Rosen, R.: Roentgenographic diagnosis of congenital syphilis in the newborn. J.A.M.A., 212:1063, 1970.
7. Cremin, B. J., and Fisher, R. M.: The lesions of congenital syphilis. Br. J. Radiol., 43:333, 1970.
8. Drucker, M. G., and Mankin, H. J.: Congenital syphilis in 1970: A case report. Bull. Hosp. Joint Dis., 31:132, 1970.
9. Dzebolo, N. N.: Congenital syphilis: An unusual presentation. Radiology, 136:372, 1980.
10. Fiumara, N. J.: Syphilis in newborn children. Clin. Obstet. Gynecol., 18:183, 1975.
11. Fleming, T. C., and Bardenstein, M. B.: Congenital syphilis. J. Bone Joint Surg., 53-A:1648, 1971.
12. Horodniceanu, C., Grunebaum, M., Volovitz, B., and Nitzan, M.: Unusual bone involvement in congenital syphilis mimicking the battered child syndrome. Pediatr. Radiol., 7:232, 1978.
13. Jones, D.: Syphilitic disorders of the spine. Report of two cases. J. Bone Joint Surg., 52-B:724, 1970.
14. Krugman, S., and Katz, S. L.: Infectious Diseases of Children. St. Louis, Mosby, 1981.
15. McCracken, G. H., and Kaplan, J. M.: Penicillin treatment for congenital syphilis. J.A.M.A., 228:855, 1974.
16. McDonald, R.: Congenital syphilis has many faces. Clin. Pediatr., 9:110, 1970.
17. Oppenheimer, E. H., and Hardy, J. B.: Congenital syphilis in the newborn infant: Clinical and pathological observations in recent cases. Johns Hopkins Med. J., 129:63, 1971.
18. Robinson, R. C. V.: Congenital syphilis. Arch. Dermatol., 99:559, 1969.
19. Rosenfeld, S. R., Weinert, C. R., Jr., and Kahn, B.: Congenital syphilis. A case report. J. Bone Joint Surg., 65-A:115, 1983.
20. Solomon, A., and Rosen, E.: The aspect of trauma in the bone changes of congenital lues. Pediatr. Radiol., 3:175, 1975.
21. Solomon, A., and Rosen, E.: Focal osseous lesions in congenital lues. Ped. Radiol., 7:36, 1978.
22. Tan, K. L.: The re-emergence of early congenital syphilis. Acta Paediatr. Scand., 62:601, 1973.
23. Tight, R. R., and Warner, J. F.: Skeletal involvement in secondary syphilis detected by bone scanning. J.A.M.A., 235:2326, 1976.
24. Toohey, J. S.: Skeletal presentation of congenital syphilis: Case report and review of the literature. J. Pediatr. Orthop., 5:104, 1985.
25. Wechselberg, K., and Schneider, J. D.: Morbiditat und klinische Symptomatik der konnatalen Lues im Sauglingsalter. Deutsche Med. Wochenschr., 95:1976, 1970.
26. Wilkinson, R. H., and Heller, R. M.: Congenital syphilis: Resurgence of an old problem. Pediatrics, 47:27, 1971.

ARTHRITIS ASSOCIATED WITH VIRAL DISEASE

Joint pain and effusion may occur in a number of viral diseases such as rubella, mumps, chickenpox, glandular fever (Epstein-Barr virus), cytomegalic virus, hepatitis B, adenovirus—especially 7, influenza, arbovirus, herpes zoster, and simple herpes.* The viral arthropathies tend to be mild, polyarticular, and relatively benign, resolving spontaneously within a few weeks and leaving no residual deformity. The synovitis appears to be caused by deposition of immune complexes, which have been detected in both synovial fluid and serum.[37] Treatment is symptomatic; no special orthopedic treatment is required.

Arthritis associated with rubella is the most common. It may develop in children receiving rubella virus vaccine. It usually is encountered in teenage girls, who complain of fleeting joint pains and swelling. The joints of the hand and knee are the common sites. Carpal tunnel syndrome can develop in children. The arthritis may precede, accompany, or follow the rash. The finding of occipital lymphadenopathy prior to the appearance of the rash helps in clinical diagnosis of rubella. The laboratory demonstration of a rising titer against rubella in the serum will make the definitive diagnosis. Treatment is symptomatic. Arthritis may persist for some time after recovery from rubella.

In viral arthritis associated with mumps the large joints are involved. The presence of parotitis will assist in making the diagnosis.[20] In varicella the arthritis is pauciarticular.[4, 10, 11, 13, 24, 25, 30, 39, 40]

In acute viral hepatitis, particularly Type B, arthralgia is present in about 50 per cent of cases as a feature of an associated serum sickness–like syndrome.[2, 28]

References

1. Adebonojo, F. O.: Monoarticular arthritis: Unusual manifestation of infectious mononucleosis. Clin. Pediatr., 11:549, 1972.
2. Alarcon, G. S., and Townes, A. S.: Arthritis in viral hepatitis: Report of two cases and review of the literature. Johns Hopkins Med. J., 132:1, 1973.
3. Balfour, H. H., Jr., Groth, K. E., and Edelman, C. K.: RA27/3 rubella vaccine. A four-year follow-up. Am. J. Dis. Child., 134:350, 1980.
4. Borgenicht, L.: Varicella arthritis (letter). Pediatrics, 66:649, 1980.
5. Brna, J. A., and Hall, R. F., Jr.: Acute monarticular herpetic arthritis. A case report. J. Bone Joint Surg., 66-A:623, 1984.
6. Chambers, R. J., and Bywaters, E. G. L.: Rubella synovitis. Ann. Rheum. Dis., 22:263, 1963.
7. Chatterjee, R. N.: Incidence of arthritis in smallpox. Indian Med. Gaz., 85:49, 1950.
8. Cooper, L. Z., Ziring, P. R., and Weiss, H. J.: Transient arthritis after rubella vaccination. Am. J. Dis. Child., 118:218, 1969.
9. Devereaux, M. D., and Hazelton, R. A.: Acute monarticular arthritis in association with herpes zoster (letter). Arthritis Rheum., 26:236, 1983.
10. DiLiberti, J. H., Bartel, S. J., Humphrey, T. R., and Pang, A. W.: Acute monarticular arthritis in association with varicella. Clin. Pediatr., 16:663, 1977.
11. Evers, K. G., Zippel, C., and Kruger, J.: Varicella

---

*See references: rubella, 3, 6, 8, 14, 16–19, 21–23, 26, 31, 33, 34, 36; mumps, 20; chickenpox, 4, 10, 11, 13, 24, 25, 30, 39, 40; hepatitis B, 2, 28, 29; herpes zoster, 9, 27; simple herpes, 5, 12, 29.

arthritis—a rare complication of varicella (author's transl.). Monatsschr. Kinderheilkd., 128:147, 1980.
12. Friedman, H. M., Pincus, T., Gibilisco, P., Baker, D., Glazer, J. P., Plotkin, S. A., and Schumacher, H. R.: Acute monoarticular arthritis caused by herpes simplex virus and cytomegalovirus. Am. J. Med., 69:241, 1980.
13. Gupta, S. K., and Srivastava, T. P.: Roentgen features of skeletal involvement in smallpox. Australas. Radiol., 17:205, 1973.
14. Hildebrandt, H. M., and Massab, H. F.: Rubella synovitis in a one-year-old patient. N. Engl. J. Med., 274:1428, 1966.
15. Hyer, F. Y., and Gottlieb, N. L.: Rheumatic disorders associated with viral infections. Semin. Arthritis Rheum., 8:17, 1978.
16. Johnson, R. E., and Hall, A. P.: Rubella arthritis. N. Engl. J. Med., 258:743, 1958.
17. Kantor, T. G., and Tanner, M.: Rubella, arthritis and rheumatoid arthritis. Arthritis Rheum., 5:378, 1962.
18. Kilroy, A. W., Schaffner, W., Fleet, W. F., Jr., Lefkowitz, L. B., Jr., and Karzon, D. T.: Two syndromes following rubella immunization. Clinical observations and epidemiological studies. J.A.M.A., 214:2287, 1970.
19. Kuhn, L. R., Slovis, T., Hernandez, R., and Poznanski, A. K.: Knee maturation as a differentiating sign between congenital rubella and cytomegalovirus infections. Pediatr. Radiol., 6:36, 1977.
20. Lass, R., and Shepard, E.: Mumps arthritis. Br. Med. J., 2:1613, 1961.
21. Lee, P. R., Barnett, A. F., Scholer, J. F., Bryner, S., and Clark, W. H.: Rubella arthritis: Study of 20 cases. Calif. Med., 93:125, 1960.
22. Lerman, S. J., Nankervis, G. A., Heggie, A. D., and Gold, E.: Immunologic response, virus excretion and joint reactions with rubella vaccine. Ann. Intern. Med., 74:67, 1971.
23. Lewis, G. W.: Polyarthritis in rubella. Rheumatism, 10:66, 1954.
24. Margolis, H. S., Subbarao, K., Pitt, M. J., and Boyer, J.: Case report 58. Residual osteoarticular lesions due to smallpox, with secondary degenerative joint disease. Skeletal Radiol., 2:261, 1978.
25. Mulhern, L. M., Friday, G. A., and Perri, J. A.: Arthritis complicating varicella infection. Pediatrics, 48:827, 1971.
26. Ogra, P. L., and Herd, J. K.: Arthritis associated with induced rubella infection. J. Immunol., 107:810, 1971.
27. Remafedi, G., and Muldoon, R. L.: Acute monarticular arthritis caused by herpes simplex virus type I. Pediatrics, 72:882, 1983.
28. Schumacher, H. R., and Gall, E. P.: Arthritis in acute hepatitis and chronic active hepatitis. Pathology of the synovial membrane with evidence for the presence of Australia antigen in synovial membranes. Am. J. Med., 57:655, 1974.
29. Shelly, W. B.: Herpetic arthritis associated with disseminate herpes simplex in a wrestler. Br. J. Dermatol., 103:209, 1980.
30. Shuper, A., Mimouni, M., Mukamel, M., and Varsano, I.: Varicella arthritis in a child. Arch. Dis. Child., 55:568, 1980.
31. Singleton, E. B., Rudolph, A. J., Rosenberg, H. S., and Singer, D. B.: The roentgenographic manifestations of the rubella syndrome in newborn infants. A.J.R., 97:82, 1966.
32. Smith, J. W., and Sanford, J. P.: Viral arthritis. Ann. Intern. Med., 67:651, 1967.
33. Spruance, S. L.: Recurrent joint symptoms in children vaccinated with HPV-77DK12 rubella vaccine. J. Pediatr., 80:413, 1972.
34. Spruance, S. L., and Smith, C. B.: Joint complications associated with derivatives of HPV-77 rubella vaccine. Am. J. Dis. Child., 122:1051, 1971.
35. Srivastava, A. N.: Orthopaedic complications of smallpox. J. Bone Joint Surg., 48-B:183, 1966.
36. Thompson, G. R., Ferreyra, A., and Brackett, R. G.: Acute arthritis complicating rubella vaccination. Arthritis Rheum., 14:19, 1971.
37. Utsinger, F.: Immunologic study of arthritis associated with adenovirus infection. Arthritis Rheum., 20:138, 1977.
38. Van, H., Souter, S., and Utsinger, P. D.: Viral arthritis. Clin. Rheum. Dis., 4:225, 1978.
39. Ward, J. R., and Bishop, B.: Varicella arthritis. J.A.M.A., 212:1954, 1970.
40. Younes, R. P., and Freeman, D.: Chicken pox with associated arthritis. Clin. Pediatr. (Phila.), 22:649, 1983.

FUNGUS INFECTIONS OF JOINTS

Mycotic diseases are rare in childhood. Actinomycosis, blastomycosis, and coccidioidomycosis are occasionally complicated by involvement of one or more large joints. Such a possibility should be considered when there is a resistant chronic synovitis with progressive destruction of adjacent bone. Diagnosis is made by bacteriologic studies and often by histologic examination of biopsy tissue. Treatment consists of synovectomy and curettage of bone lesions with administration of amphotericin B—a potent antifungus antibiotic. On occasion, the disease is eradicated by amputation. *Histoplasma capsulatum* may infect joints, giving findings similar to tuberculosis.

References

1. Adler, S., Randall, J., and Plotkin, S.: Candida osteomyelitis and arthritis in a neonate. Am. J. Dis. Child., 123:595, 1972.
2. Aidem, H. P.: Intra-articular amphotericin B in the treatment of coccidioidal synovitis of the knee. J. Bone Joint Surg., 50-A:1663, 1968.
3. Altner, P. C., and Turner, R. R.: Sporotrichosis of bones and joints. Review of the literature and report of six cases. Clin. Orthop., 68:138, 1970.
4. Bayer, A. S., Scott, V. J., and Guez, L. B.: Fungal arthritis. III. Sporotrichal arthritis. Semin. Arthritis Rheum., 9:66, 1979.
5. Chang, A. C., Destouet, J. M., and Murphy, W. A.: Musculoskeletal sporotrichosis. Skeletal Radiol., 12:23, 1984.
6. Chmel, H., Grieco, M. H., and Zickel, R.: Candida osteomyelitis. Report of a case. Am. J. Med. Sci., 266:299, 1973.
7. Crevasse, I., and Ellner, P. D.: An outbreak of sporotrichosis in Florida. J.A.M.A., 173:29, 1960.
8. Crout, J. E., Brewer, N. S., and Tompkins, R. B.: Sporotrichosis arthritis. Clinical features in seven patients. Ann. Intern. Med., 86:294, 1977.
9. de Beurmann, L.: On sporotrichosis. Br. Med. J., 2:289, 1912.
10. DeHaven, K. E., Wilde, A. H., and O'Duffy, J. D.: Sporotrichosis arthritis and tenosynovitis. J. Bone Joint Surg., 54-A:874, 1972.
11. Duran, J. R., Coventry, M. B., and Weed, L. A.:

Sporotrichosis. Twenty-three cases in the upper extremity. J. Bone Joint Surg., 39-A:1330, 1977.
12. Emmons, C. W., Binford, C. H., Utz, J. P., and Kwon-Chung, K. J.: Sporotrichosis. In Medical Mycology, 3rd Ed. Philadelphia, Lea & Febiger, 1977, p. 407.
13. Farha, S. J., and Fort, C. R.: An unusual sporotrichosis infection. Am. Surg., 30:335, 1964.
14. Gladstone, J. L., and Littman, M. L.: Osseous sporotrichosis. Failure of treatment with potassium iodide and sulfadimethoxine and success with amphotericin B. Am. J. Med., 51:121, 1971.
15. Groff, D. B.: Complications of intravenous hyperalimentation in newborns and infants. J. Pediatr. Surg., 4:460, 1969.
16. Haapasaar, J., Essen, R. V., Kahanpaa, A., Kostiala, A. A., Holmberg, K., and Ahlqvist, J.: Fungal arthritis simulating juvenile rheumatoid arthritis. Br. Med. J. (Clin. Res.), 285:6346, 1982.
17. Hart, P. D., Russell, E., Jr., and Remington, J. S.: The compromised host and infection. II. Deep fungus infections. J. Infect. Dis., 120:169, 1969.
18. Hernandez, A. D.: Sporothrix schenckii Part III. Infectious diseases and their etiologic agents. In Mandell, G. L., Douglas, R. G., and Bennett, J. E. (eds.): Principles and Practice of Infectious Diseases. New York, Wiley, 1979, p. 2015.
19. Herve, F., Drouhet, E., Dupont, B., Barois, A., and Beneux, J.: Fungal osteoarthritis of the knee joint with destruction treated with ketoconazole. Arch. Fr. Pediatr., 40:309, 1983.
20. Hurley, D. L., Balow, J. E., and Fauci, A. S.: Experimental disseminated candidiasis. II. Administration of glucocorticosteroids, susceptibility to infection, and immunity. J. Infect. Dis., 132:393, 1975.
21. Isacson, M., Noah, Z., Faber, J., Herishano, Y., and Gottfried, L.: Use of 5-fluorocytosine in systemic candidiasis in infancy. Arch. Dis. Child., 47:954, 1972.
22. Kahn, M. I., Goss, G., Gotsman, A., et al.: Sporotrichosis arthritis. South Afr. Med. J., 64:1099, 1983.
23. Klein, J. D., Yamauchi, T., and Horlick, S. P.: Neonatal candidiasis, meningitis and arthritis. Observations and a review of the literature. J. Pediatr., 81:31, 1972.
24. Kumar, R., Smissen, E., and Jorizzo, J.: Systemic sporotrichosis with osteomyelitis. J. Can. Assoc. Radiol., 35:84, 1984.
25. Levinsky, W. J.: Sporotrichal arthritis. Report of a case mimicking gout. Arch. Intern. Med., 129:118, 1972.
26. Lurie, H. I.: Five unusual cases of sporotrichosis from South Africa showing lesions in muscles, bones and viscera. Br. J. Surg., 50:585, 1963.
27. Lynch, P. J., Voorhees, J. J., and Harrell, E. R.: Systemic sporotrichosis. Ann. Intern. Med., 73:23, 1970.
28. Marmor, L., and Peter, J. B.: Candida arthritis of the knee joint. Clin. Orthop., 118:133, 1976.
29. Marrocco, G. R., Tihen, W. S., Goodnough, C. P., et al.: Granulomatous synovitis and osteitis caused by Sporothrix schenkii. Am. J. Clin. Pathol., 64:345, 1975.
30. Molstad, B., and Strom, R.: Multiarticular sporotrichosis. J.A.M.A., 240:556, 1978.
31. Noble, H. B., and Lyne, E. D.: Candida osteomyelitis and arthritis from hyperalimentation therapy. J. Bone Joint Surg., 56-A:825, 1974.
32. Noyes, F. R., McCabe, J. D., and Fekety, F. R.: Acute candida arthritis. Report of a case and use of amphotericin B. J. Bone Joint Surg., 55-A:169, 1973.
33. Poplack, D. G., and Jacobs, S. A.: Candida arthritis treated with amphotericin B. J. Pediatr., 87:989, 1975.
34. Pruitt, A. W., Achord, J. L., Fales, F. W., and Patterson, J. H.: Glucose-galactose malabsorption complicated by monilial arthritis. Pediatrics, 43:106, 1969.
35. Schwarz, J.: What's new in mycotic bone and joint diseases. Pathol. Res. Pract., 178:617, 1984.
36. Seelig, M. S.: The role of antibiotics in the pathogenesis of candida infections. Am. J. Med., 40:887, 1966.
37. Serstock, D. S., and Zinneman, H. H.: Pulmonary and articular sporotrichosis. J.A.M.A., 223:1291, 1975.
38. Sotelo-Ortiz, F.: Chronic coccidioidal synovitis of the knee joint. J. Bone Joint Surg., 37-A:49, 1955.
39. Svirsky-Fein, S., Langer, L., Milbauer, B., Khermosh, O., and Rubinstein, E.: Neonatal osteomyelitis caused by Candida tropicalis. Report of two cases and review of the literature. J. Bone Joint Surg., 61-A:455, 1979.
40. Toone, E. C., Jr., and Kelly, J.: Joint and bone disease due to mycotic infection. Am. J. Med. Sci., 231:263, 1956.
41. Utz, J. P.: Sporotrichosis. Rev. Infect. Dis., 2:625, 1980.
42. Wall, B. A., Weinblatt, M. E., Darnall, J. T., and Muss, H.: Candida tropicalis arthritis and bursitis. J.A.M.A., 248:1098, 1982.
43. Webster, F. S., and Wilander, D.: Chronic sporotrichal synovitis of the knee. J. Bone Joint Surg., 39-A:207, 1957.
44. Weitzner, R., Mak, E., and Lertratanakul, Y.: Articular sporotrichosis. Ann. Intern. Med., 87:382, 1977.
45. Winter, T. Q., and Pearson, K. D.: Systemic sporotrichosis. Radiology, 104:579, 1972.
46. Yacobucci, G. N., and Santilli, M. D.: Sporotrichosis of the knee: A case report. Orthopedics, 9:387, 1986.
47. Yousefzadeh, D. K., and Jackson, J. H.: Neonatal and infantile candidal arthritis with or without osteomyelitis: A clinical and radiographical review of 21 cases. Skeletal Radiol., 5:77, 1980.

ACUTE TRANSIENT SYNOVITIS OF THE HIP

Acute transient synovitis of the hip is a nonspecific inflammatory and self-limited condition. It is the most common cause of a painful hip in children under ten years of age. Other synonyms used include acute toxic synovitis of the hip, "observation hip," irritable hip, coxitis fugax, coxitis serosa seu simplex, and acute transient epiphysitis.

In 1892, Lovett and Morse first described this clinical entity as an ephemeral hip disease in which the symptoms disappeared within a few weeks or months.[37]

Since then numerous reports have been given in the literature on this benign category of inflammatory hip disease in children, stressing its benign clinical course, differential diagnosis, and sequelae.[1–64]

Boys are more frequently affected than girls, the ratio varying from 3:2 to 5:1 in the literature. The age group most commonly affected is that between three and six years, but the disorder can occur in infancy and early adolescence. The right hip is slightly more commonly affected than the left; in about 4.5 per cent of cases, involvement is bilateral.[27]

Etiology

The cause of the condition is unknown. Trauma, infection, and allergy have been con-

Table 4–7. Differential Diagnosis of Acute Transient Synovitis of the Hip

Septic Arthritis
  Suspect if (1) Fever (2) Elevated white blood count and erythrocyte sedimentation rate (3) Acute pain and spasm about hip (4) Lateral displacement of femoral head with widening of medial joint space in radiograph (5) Marked effusion in hip as shown by ultrasonography
  Perform diagnostic aspiration of hip joint with child appropriately sedated and restrained under image intensifier radiographic control for verification that needle was in hip joint
  Avoid pitfall of waiting two or three days pending clinical course and results of investigations

Legg-Calvé-Perthes Disease
  Suspect if (1) "Irritability" of hip does not subside within a week (2) Recurrent episode of synovitis (3) Short stature with delay of skeletal maturation (4) Ossific nucleus of femoral head of affected hip is smaller than contralateral normal hip; is there a subchondral fissure in the femoral head?
  Perform bone scintigraphy with technetium-99m—if Perthes' disease it will show partial or total absence of uptake of radionuclide in femoral head
  Avoid pitfall of not following synovitis of the hip. Examine clinically and make radiographs two months and six months after initial episode

Juvenile Rheumatoid Arthritis (monarticular or pauciarticular disease)
  Suspect if (1) Symptoms and signs persist for more than 10–14 days (2) In presence of macular rash, fever, lymphadenopathy, and tumefaction of digits (3) Eye findings such as iridocyclitis
  Perform laboratory investigations such as ESR, rheumatoid factor (IgM and IgG), nuclear antibodies (ANA) and immune complexes. Note—negative serum findings do not rule out juvenile rheumatoid arthritis.
  Obtain consultation with pediatric immunologist

Rheumatic Fever (Very rare in North America, but does occur)
  Suspect (1) Sustained fever (2) Erythema marginatum (3) Migratory arthralgia. Rule out endocarditis and pericarditis.
  Obtain pediatric consultation

Slipped Capital Femoral Epiphysis (in adolescent with pre-slip or minimal chronic slip)
  Suspect if (1) Limitation of hip flexion (extension deformity) (2) Lateral hip rotation on flexion
  Obtain (1) True lateral of upper end of femur "blanch" sign (Steel) (2) *Look for* AP projection (3) Scintigraphy with technetium-99m will show increased uptake at capital femoral physis (4) CT scan will clearly demonstrate posterior slip

Idiopathic Chondrolysis of Hip (in early stages)
  Suspect if (1) Flexion deformity of the hip (2) Limitation of hip motion in all planes (3) Narrowing of articular cartilage space in conventional radiograph
  Obtain bone scan with technetium-99m. It will show increased uptake in both femoral head and acetabulum

Miscellaneous Rare Conditions
  Gaucher's disease
  Osteoid osteoma of femoral head
  Leukemia

The hip joint is decompressed only when there is definite widening of the joint space with lateral displacement of the femoral head and marked limitation of hip motion. These cases require diagnostic aspiration of the joint to rule out sepsis.

To prevent recurrence of synovitis it is best to continue the non-weight-bearing regimen (either bed rest or crutches) at home for seven to ten days after normal hip motion is restored. As a routine measure, it is recommended that the child be re-examined in two weeks to determine whether there is any recurrence prior to resuming full weight-bearing and normal activity. Radiograms of the hips in both anteroposterior and lateral views should be repeated in two and four to six months to rule out aseptic necrosis of the femoral head.

Recurrent episodes of acute transient synovitis of the hip do occur sometimes, particularly in "allergic" children and following streptococcal infection or upper respiratory viral infection.

Sequelae

Legg-Perthes disease may develop several months following an episode of transient synovitis of the hip. The recorded incidence in the literature varies from 2.5 per cent (Haueisen) to 10 per cent (Jacobs).[27, 34]

It has been proposed that increased hydrostatic pressure in the hip joint secondary to synovitis will cause tamponade of retinacular vessels and avascular necrosis of the femoral head. The diagnosis of Legg-Perthes disease is usually made two to six months following the initial episode of acute transient synovitis.

Kallio and associates, in a prospective study of 119 children with transient synovitis of the hip with a follow-up of one year, did not find a single case of Legg-Calvé-Perthes disease. They believed that the reported cases in the literature represented misdiagnosis of early Legg-Calvé-Perthes disease as transient synovitis of the hip.[35]

Sharwood, in a long-term follow-up (average of 8.2 years with a minimum of 5 years and a maximum of 15 years) of 101 children with irritable hip syndrome found one case of Legg-Calvé-Perthes disease and one case of coxa magna; these two patients had prolonged symptoms and radiologic abnormalities on admission.[49]

This author recommends clinical and radiographic examination of the hips in children with transient synovitis of the hip at two and six months after the initial episode. Routine scintigraphy with technetium-99m is not recommended; bone scanning is performed when there are recurrent episodes of synovitis of the hip, when irritability of the hip does not subside following a period of bed rest and traction, when there is marked delay in skeletal maturation, and when suspicion of Legg-Calvé-Perthes disease is suggested by the smaller size of the ossific nucleus of the femoral head of the symptomatic hip.

With the inflammatory hypervascularity and the consequent increased blood supply to the epiphysis, growth of the epiphysis may be stimulated, causing enlargement of the capital femoral epiphyses. Valderrama, in a study of the late sequelae of the "observation hip" syndrome, found a varying degree of coxa magna, simple broadening of the femoral head, and osteoarthritis in the radiograms of 12 of 23 patients.[55]

References

1. Adams, J. A.: Transient synovitis of the hip joint in children. J. Bone Joint Surg., 45-B:471, 1963.
2. Anderson, J., and Stewart, A. M.: The significance of the magnitude of the medial hip joint space. Br. J. Radiol., 43:238, 1970.
3. Anonymous: Transient synovitis and Perthes disease (Editorial). Br. Med. J., 62:2, 1973.
4. Belmonte, A. C.: Over voorbijgaande, goedaardige "Coxitis" (Coxitis fugax). Nederl. T. Geneesk., 75:5, 1931.
5. Berger, H.: Intermittent hydrarthrosis with an allergic basis. J.A.M.A., 112:240, 1939.
6. Blockey, N. J., and Porter, B. B.: Transient synovitis of hip. A virological investigation. Br. Med. J., 4:557, 1968.
7. Bradford, E. H.: Treatment of hip disease. Am. J. Orthop. Surg., 9:354, 1912.
8. Brown, I.: A study of the "capsular" shadow in disorders of the hip in children. J. Bone Joint Surg., 57-B:175, 1975.
9. Butler, R. W.: Transitory arthritis of the hip-joint in childhood. Br. Med. J., 1:951, 1933.
10. Caravias, D. E.: The significance of the so-called "irritable hips" in children. Arch. Dis. Child., 31:415, 1956.
11. Carty, H., Maxted, M., Fielding, J. A., Gulliford, P., and Owen, R.: Isotope scanning in the "irritable hip syndrome". Skeletal Radiol., 11:32, 1984.
12. Donaldson, W. F.: Transient synovitis of the hip joint. Pediatr. Clin. North Am., 2:1073, 1955.
13. Drey, L.: A roentgenographic study of transitory synovitis of the hip joint. Radiology, 60:588, 1953.
14. Dzioba, R. B., and Barrington, T. W.: Transient monoarticular synovitis of the hip joint in adults. Clin. Orthop., 126:190, 1977.
15. Edwards, E. G.: Transient synovitis of the hip joint in children. Report of thirteen cases. J.A.M.A., 148:30, 1952.
16. Fairbank, H. A. T.: Discussion on non-tuberculous coxitis in the young. Br. Med. J., 2:828, 1926.
17. Ferguson, A. B., Jr.: Synovitis of the hip and Legg-Perthes disease. Clin. Orthop., 4:180, 1954.
18. Finder, J. G.: Transitory synovitis of the hip joint in childhood. J.A.M.A., 107:3, 1936.
19. Fox, K. W., and Griffin, L. L.: Transient synovitis of the hip joint in children. Tex. State J. Med., 52:15, 1956.
20. Gershuni, D. H., and Axer, A.: Synovitis of the hip joint—an experimental model in rabbits. J. Bone Joint Surg., 56-B:69, 1974.
21. Gershuni, D. H., and Kuei, S. C.: Articular cartilage deformation following experimental synovitis in the rabbit hip. J. Orthop. Res., 1:313, 1984.
22. Gershuni, D. H., Axer, A., and Siegel, B.: Localized regressive articular cartilage changes in the hip of the rabbit following an induced synovitis. Acta Orthop. Scand., 50:179, 1979.
23. Gershuni, D. H., Axer, A., and Hendel, D.: Arthrographic findings in Legg-Calvé-Perthes disease and transient synovitis of the hip. J. Bone Joint Surg., 60-A:457, 1978.
24. Gershuni, D. H., Amiel, D., Gonsalves, M., and Akeson, W. H.: The biochemical response of rabbit articular cartilage matrix to induced talcum synovitis. Acta Orthop. Scand., 52:599, 1981.
25. Gledhill, R. B. and McIntyre, J. M.: Transient synovitis and Legg-Calvé-Perthes disease; a comparative study. Can. Med. Assoc. J., 100:311, 1969.
26. Hardinge, K.: The etiology of transient synovitis of the hip in childhood. J. Bone Joint Surg., 52-B:101, 1970.
27. Haueisen, D. C., Weiner, D. S., and Weiner, S. D.: The characterization of "transient synovitis of the hip" in children. J. Pediatr. Orthop., 6:11, 1986.
28. Hermel, M. B., and Albert, S. M.: Transient synovitis of the hip. Clin. Orthop., 22:21, 1962.
29. Hermel, M. B., and Sklaroff, D. M.: Roentgen changes in transient synovitis of the hip joint. Arch. Surg., 68:364, 1954.
30. Heyman, S., Goldstein, H. A., Crowley, W., and Treves, S.: The scintigraphic evaluation of hip pain in children. Clin. Nucl. Med., 5:109, 1980.
31. Illingworth, C. M.: One hundred twenty-eight limping children with no fracture, sprain, or obvious cause. Clin. Pediatr., 17:139, 1978.
32. Illingworth, C. M.: Recurrences of transient synovitis of the hip. Arch. Dis. Child., 58:620, 1983.
33. Jacobs, B. W.: Early recognition of osteochondrosis of the capital epiphysis of femur. J.A.M.A., 172:527, 1960.
34. Jacobs, B. W.: Synovitis of the hip in children and its significance. Pediatrics, 47:558, 1974.
35. Kallio, P., Ryoppy, S., and Kunnamo, I.: Transient synovitis and Perthes' disease. J. Bone Joint Surg., 68-B:898, 1986.
36. Kloiber, R., Pavlosky, W., Portner, O., and Gartke, K.: Bone scintigraphy of hip joint effusions in children. A.J.R., 140:995, 1983.

37. Lovett, R. W., and Morse, J. L.: A transient or ephemeral form of hip-disease, with a report of cases. Boston Med. Surg. J., 127:161, 1892.
38. Lucas, L. S.: Painful hips in children. A.A.O.S. Instruct. Course Lect., 5:144, 1948.
39. McMurray, B.: A report of six cases of coxa magna following synovitis of the hip joint. Br. J. Radiol., 20:477, 1947.
40. Miller, O. L.: Acute transient epiphysitis of the hip joint. J.A.M.A., 96:575, 1931.
41. Mukherjee, K.: Transient non-specific synovitis of the hip joint. Br. J. Clin. Pract., 24:137, 1970.
42. Nachemson, A., and Scheller, S.: A clinical and radiological follow-up study of transient synovitis of the hip. Acta Orthop. Scand., 40:479, 1969.
43. Neuhauser, E. B. D., and Wittenborg, M. H.: Synovitis of the hips in infancy and childhood. Radiol. Clin. North Am., 1:13, 1963.
44. Palm, E. T.: Transient synovitis of the hip in children. Am. J. Orthop., 4:50, 1962.
45. Rauch, S.: Transient synovitis of the hip joint in children. Am. J. Dis. Child., 59:1245, 1940.
46. Reichman, S.: Roentgenologic soft tissue appearances in hip joint disease. Acta Radiol. (Diagn.) (Stockh.)., 6:167, 1967.
47. Rosenberg, N. J., and Smith, E. E.: Transient synovitis of the hip. J. Pediatr., 48:776, 1956.
48. Rothschild, H. B., Russ, J. D., and Wasserman, C. F.: Corticotropins in the treatment of transient synovitis of the hip in children. J. Pediatr., 49:33, 1956.
49. Sharwood, P. F.: The irritable hip syndrome in children. A long-term follow-up. Acta Orthop. Scand., 52:633, 1981.
50. Spock, A.: Transient synovitis of the hip joint in children. Pediatrics, 24:1042, 1959.
51. Tachdjian, M. O., and Grana, L.: Response of the hip joint to increased intra-articular hydrostatic pressure. Clin. Orthop., 61:199, 1968.
52. Thulin, W. J.: Transient synovitis of the hip joint in children. Rocky Mt. Med. J., 54:238, 1957.
53. Todd, A. H.: Discussion on the differential diagnosis of nontuberculous coxitis in children and adolescents. Proc. R. Soc. Med., 18:31, 1925.
54. Tudor, R. B.: Hip synovitis in children. Lancet, 80:51, 1960.
55. Valderrama, J. A. F. de: The observation hip" syndrome and its late sequelae. J. Bone Joint Surg., 45-B:462, 1963.
56. Vandeputte, L., Mulier, J. C., and Mulier, F.: Transient synovitis of the hip in children. Acta Orthop. Belg., 37:186, 1971.
57. Vera Cruz, P. G.: Transient synovitis of the hip joint. Proc. Child. Hosp. Washington, D.C., 13:28, 1957.
58. Vidigal, E. C., and daSilva, O. L.: Observation hip. Acta Orthop. Scand., 52:191, 1981.
59. Vidigal, E. C.: Transient arthritis of the hip in children (a study of 74 cases). Ital. J. Orthop. Traumatol., 10:237, 1984.
60. Wilson, D. J., Green, D. J., and McLarnon, J. C.: Arthrosonography of the painful hip. Clin. Radiol., 35:17, 1984.
61. Wingstrand, H.: Ultrasonography in hip joint effusion. Report of a child with transient synovitis. Acta Orthop. Scand., 55:469, 1984.
62. Wingstrand, H., Bauer, G. C. H., Brismar, J., Carlin, N. O., Pettersson, H., and Sunden, G.: Transient ischemia of the proximal femoral epiphysis in the child. Acta Orthop. Scand., 56:197, 1985.
63. Wingstrand, H., Egund, N., Carlin, N. O., Forsberg, L., Gustafson, T., and Sunden, G.: Intracapsular pressure in transient synovitis of the hip. Acta Orthop. Scand., 56:204, 1985.

RHEUMATOID ARTHRITIS

Rheumatoid arthritis in children is a generalized systemic disease of which arthritis is but one manifestation. Still, in his classic description of 22 cases in children, emphasized the florid form of the disease with fever, lymphadenopathy, and splenomegaly.[337] Rheumatoid arthritis of childhood is often referred to as "Still's disease"; it was, however, originally described by Cornil in 1864.[103] The term *rheumatoid disease* is perhaps more appropriate.[119]

Incidence

The incidence of juvenile rheumatoid arthritis is about three new cases annually in a general population of 100,000 under 15 years of age.[141] There is some geographic variation; for example, in Finland, Laaksonen estimated an annual incidence of six to eight children per 100,000 of the population under 15 years of age.[209] It is more common in the female (70 per cent of cases).

Rheumatoid disease may begin at any age, the average time of onset being six years of age. It starts most frequently in the one- to four-year age group, with another rise of incidence of onset toward the age of puberty (9- to 14-year age group).

Etiology

The exact pathogenesis of rheumatoid arthritis is unknown. The following plausible causative factors have been proposed:

Autoimmune Disease. This theory is supported by the presence of a large number of nonspecific immunologic changes. It is believed that the inflammatory process of rheumatoid arthritis results from depression of a macroglobulin, an antibody-like rheumatoid factor within the joint, which causes release of lysosomal enzymes, the accelerated release of which initiates and perpetuates damage to the joint.

Heredity. Familial incidence of rheumatoid arthritis is reported to be 23 per cent by Edstrom, 30 per cent by Sairanen, and 40.78 per cent by Laaksonen.[115, 209, 291] Brewer and Fahlberg, however, in reviewing the literature, concluded that a genetic relationship with the increased familial incidence is lacking, and that, rather, the possibility of exogenous environmental factors as an etiologic agent should be seriously considered.[62]

The occurrence of juvenile rheumatoid arthritis in both members of monozygotic twins was reported by Baum and Fink, who reviewed ten monozygotic twin sets and found the incidence of concordance to be 30 per cent.[39]

Climatic Factors. It is well known that a rapid increase of humidity and rapid decrease of barometric pressure will cause a flare-up of arthritis. It is also common experience that arthritis is ameliorated in a warm, dry climate.

Infection. That rheumatoid arthritis represents a direct infection with an organism such as Mycoplasma, Bedsonia, or a virus has been proposed. *Mycoplasma fermentans* was isolated in 31 of 79 specimens of synovial fluid from patients with active rheumatoid arthritis. Further work by Williams, using leukocyte migration inhibition tests, disclosed that leukocytes from 29 of 43 patients with established rheumatoid arthritis were inhibited by a preparation of *M. fermentans* membrane. This was not observed in the control normal subjects. Gold salts and antimalarial drugs are effective in the treatment of rheumatoid arthritis and also strongly inhibit the growth of *M. fermentans*. These observations support the possible role of this organism in the pathogenesis of rheumatoid disease.[362]

A previous infection, usually one that is of the upper respiratory system, has been reported in about one fifth to three fifths of the patients.[36, 104, 114, 263] Rahal and associates suggested that rheumatoid arthritis is caused by adenoviral infection; there have, however, been no other reports of early viral infection.[271] The streptococcal agglutination reaction is increased in a significant number of these children; this may reflect an increased immune responsiveness.

Stress Reaction. A history of physical or psychic injury within four to six weeks of onset of illness is not uncommon.

Pathology

The pathologic changes of rheumatoid arthritis are not limited to the musculoskeletal system alone. The condition is a systemic disease of mesenchymal tissues, and may affect the collagen and connective tissue of any organ system.

The reactions of synovial tissue are nonspecific. The histologic picture of rheumatoid arthritis is not pathognomonic for the disease. Identical responses may occur from an adjacent tumor, from mechanical irritation of a torn semilunar cartilage, or in simple degenerative joint disease.[312] Thus, a positive diagnosis of rheumatoid arthritis cannot be made from microscopic sections alone. The total clinical and pathologic picture should be considered.

Joint Changes. These are characterized by a nonsuppurative inflammation that is acute initially, following which it passes through subacute and chronic stages and results in a mass of scar tissue.

Synovitis. The disease, as a rule, first manifests itself in the synovium, which becomes edematous and hypervascular, allowing migration of the leukocytes into the synovial tissues and joint fluid. The predominant infiltrating cells are small lymphocytes, which tend to aggregate in follicles; in the very early acute stage of the disease, however, numerous polymorphonuclear leukocytes may be found (Fig. 4–21). This exudative inflammatory reaction results in the formation of excessive synovial fluid. As mucin production is inadequate, the fluid is thin and watery. With progression of the inflammation, the synovial cells proliferate, and the synovium becomes thickened, forming nodules and villi that project into the joint spaces. Formation of synovial cysts may also occur during this acute stage of synovitis.

As the synovitis persists, fibrinoid degeneration and granulomatous changes begin in the hypertrophied synovium. In time a membrane of granulation tissue is formed, which grows over the hyaline articular cartilage as a pannus. Rice bodies form when the precipitated deposits of fibrin break loose into the joint. The capsule thickens and undergoes fibrotic changes, becoming inelastic and causing limitation of joint motion.

Bone and Cartilage Changes. The inflammatory reaction begins initially in the subchondral osseous tissue and at the attachments of the capsule, where the bone in the metaphyseal regions is eroded by the granulation tissue. As the pannus spreads over the articular surfaces, it destroys the hyaline cartilage. The subchondral bone undergoes destruction from both sides. The hypervascularity of inflammation and disuse causes osteoporosis. Accelerated epiphyseal growth and new periosteal formation adjacent to the inflamed joint may occur.

With progression of the disease, the proliferated synovium and the pannus fill the articular cavity. Fibrous ankylosis results when the opposing joint surfaces join by the proliferated collagenous tissue; bony ankylosis may take place when the dense collagen tissue of the pannus ossifies.

Acute tenosynovitis may be the initial manifestation of rheumatoid disease.[183, 193] Arthritis and tenosynovitis not infrequently begin con-

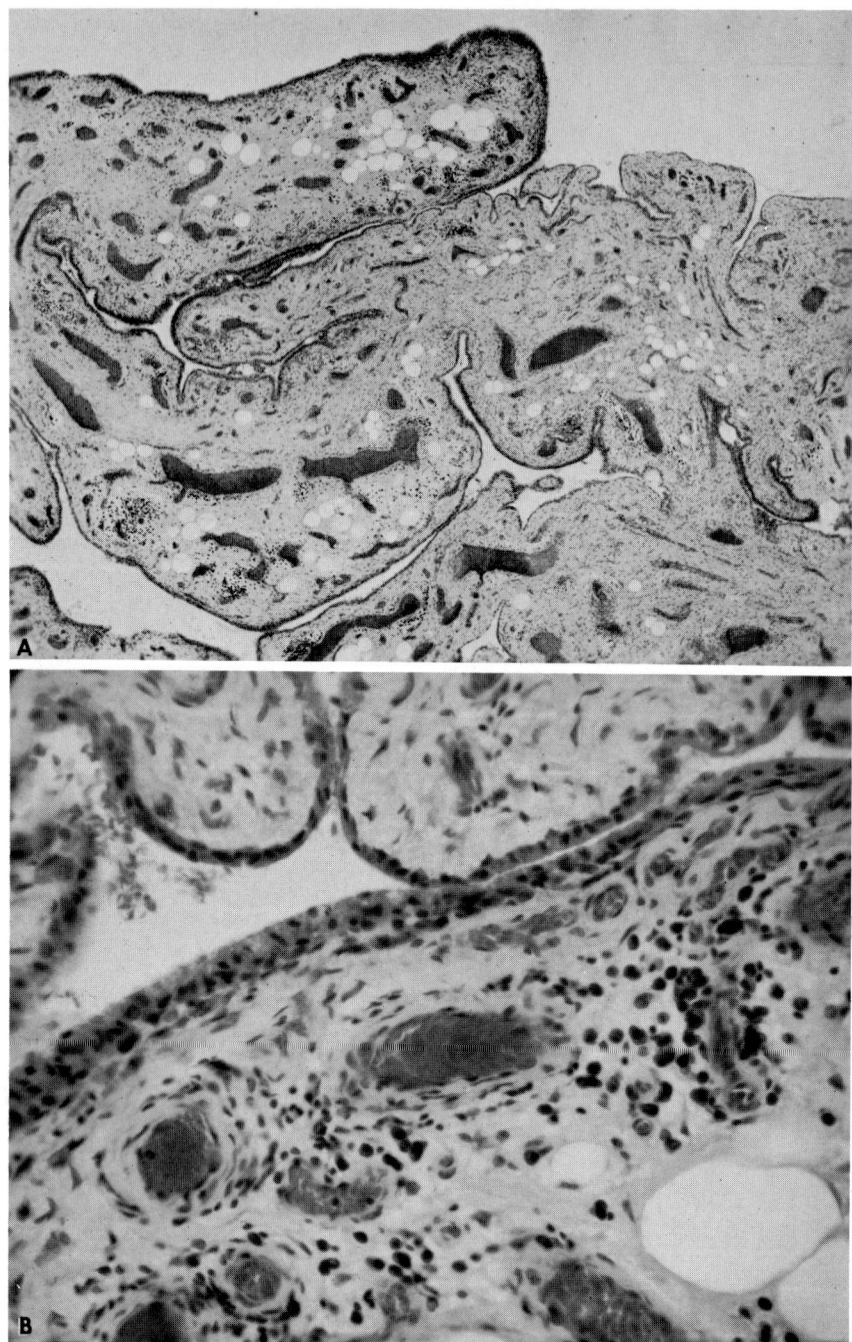

FIGURE 4–21. *Histologic appearance of synovium in rheumatoid arthritis.*

A. × 100. B. × 250.

currently; on occasion, however, tenosynovitis may precede joint symptoms by several weeks or months. The histopathologic changes of rheumatoid inflammation of tendon sheaths are similar to those of synovial tissue of joints. The granulation tissue of tenosynovitis presents as a gray jelly that fills the synovial sheath and infiltrates the enclosed tendon. The lubricating mechanism of the sheath is lost. Soon attritional and inflammatory changes develop in the tendon, which thickens, becomes yellow in color, and undergoes mucoid degeneration. Nodular masses may form in the tendon. Spontaneous rupture of the affected tendon occurs as a result of attrition and direct involvement.

Rheumatoid nodule is rare in children, but when present is pathognomonic of the disease.[75] The extensor surfaces of the elbows and knees are common sites. The nodules are usually firm masses in the subcutaneous tissues, varying in diameter from 4 mm. to several centimeters. Occasionally they may become fluctuant and drain. The histologic picture of rheumatoid nodule is characteristic. The central nodule with fibrinoid degeneration is surrounded by fibroblasts arranged in palisade formation (Fig. 4–22).

Inflammation of skeletal muscles may occur with diffuse scattering of follicles of lymphocytes. The pleura, pericardium, and peritoneum may be affected by an exudative inflammatory reaction. Iridocyclitis may develop. Significant kidney involvement is not a feature of rheumatoid disease. Renal biopsies have shown minimal nonspecific involvement, but kidney function is not impaired unless amyloidosis is present as a complication. The histologic picture of rheumatoid rash is that of a few inflammatory cells surrounding dilated vessels of subepithelial tissues without extravasation of erythrocytes.

Clinical Features

Rheumatoid arthritis in children varies greatly in its clinical manifestations, type of onset, course, and prognosis. The many variants of the disease may be arbitrarily grouped into pauciarticular arthritis, polyarthritis with minimal systemic manifestations, and severe systemic rheumatoid disease with polyarthritis.

Pauciarticular Arthritis. This type is characterized by involvement of few large joints with minimal or no systemic manifestations and is occasionally associated with tumefaction of a digit. The prefix *pauci* is derived from the Latin paucus, meaning "few," and the term *pauciarticular arthritis* was first used by Green to distinguish it from the severe generalized form.[150]

The joints of the lower limbs are involved more often than those of the upper limbs, with

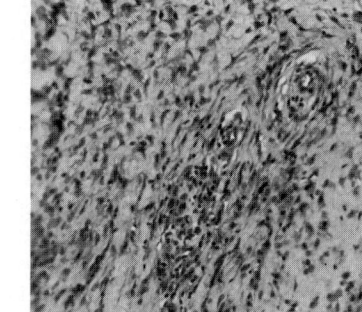

FIGURE 4–22. Microscopic appearance of rheumatoid nodule.

Note the focus of fibrinoid degeneration surrounded by fibroblasts arranged in palisade formation.

the knee and ankle being the two most common. The hip, elbow, wrist, and subtalar joints are other sites of affection. Fingers and toes are involved in some children, with tumefaction of an entire digit (Fig. 4–23). In about 50 per cent of patients, involvement is monarticular; in 25 per cent two joints are affected, and in 18 per cent three joints may be affected. When at onset involvement is monarticular the pauciarticular pattern frequently will develop within weeks to months and at most within one year. The cases in which more than two or three joints are involved tend to have initially higher erythrocyte sedimentation rates and raised immunoglobulin levels.

The condition is more common in girls, the female to male ratio being 7:3. The age incidence is greatest between two and four years, with onset of over 50 per cent of cases coming before the fourth year. The disease, however, may begin at any time between 4 months and 15 years of age.

The joint inflammation has an insidious onset with swelling, stiffness, and some local pain. An antalgic limp may be the presenting complaint if the lower limb is involved. When the subtalar joint is affected, inversion of the heel and toeing-in may be the initial manifestations. Pain on motion and local tenderness are usually minimal. On palpation the synovium will be found to be thickened and boggy. In the acute stage, palpable effusion is present. The synovium remains thickened as long as the disease is active. Limitation of motion and varying degrees of flexion deformity are present in all affected joints. The degree of muscle atrophy depends on the severity and duration of involvement. Overgrowth of a limb results from the chronic synovitis and increased circulation to the physis.

Systemically, these children are not ill; they do not have fever, hepatosplenomegaly, rash, or subcutaneous nodules.

The peripheral leukocyte count is normal. The erythrocyte sedimentation rate may be normal or slightly or moderately elevated. A child with pauciarticular arthritis with onset at a young age with antinuclear antibodies is at great risk of developing chronic iridocyclitis.

The clinical course of the disease is benign. It is characterized by exacerbations and remissions but with minimal functional improvement. The inflammation of the joints can be controlled easily. Amyloidosis does not develop. Eye involvement with iridocyclitis is the serious problem. The active period of the disease lasts approximately 2 years and 9 months (the minimum being 3 months and the maximum 11 years). In about 50 per cent of patients, the duration is less than two years.[150]

Juvenile ankylosing spondylitis may have a pauciarticular onset. In this form the age of onset is usually nine years or later, and there is definite sex predilection for the male. There is often a positive family history. The joints of the lower limb—hips, knees, and ankles—are the ones commonly affected; joints of the upper limb (with the exception of the elbow) are relatively spared. After a few years backache develops. Initially the sacroiliac joints appear normal in the radiograph, but bone scan with technetium-99m may show increased local uptake. Occasionally atlantoaxial subluxation may be the presenting feature. In about 25 per cent of cases acute iridocyclitis may affect one or both eyes. In this form of pauciarticular arthritis with juvenile ankylosing spondylitis there is an apparent excess of HLA–B27.

Polyarthritis With Minimal Systemic Manifestation. In this form, multiple joints are diffusely involved; symptoms of systemic disease are minimal. There are two peaks in the age distribution of polyarthritis: the *first* from one to three years, in which the polyarthritis often follows a systemic illness and there is no sex predilection; and a *second* from eight to ten years, in which females are more commonly affected. Any joint in the body may be affected. Frequent sites are the wrists, subtalar and midtarsal joints of the feet, hips, elbows, shoulders, proximal interphalangeal joints of fingers and toes, cervical spine, and temporomandibular joints. The affected joints are warm, tender, painful on motion, and swollen, with synovial thickening and effusion. Limitation of range of joint motion is almost always present; this is initially caused by protective muscle spasm and later by destruction of articular cartilage and fibrosis. The affected children have a typical apprehensive appearance, and they guard their painful limbs against movement. Symptoms arising in the temporomandibular joint are often referred to as "earache," and those from the sternoclavicular and costochondral joints as "chest pain." On occasion, hoarseness and laryngeal stridor may result from inflammation of the cricoarytenoid joints. Subcutaneous nodules may develop occasionally at the elbows or heels, over vertebrae or occiput, and in the flexor tendons of the hands and feet. Cervical spine involvement with fusion of the apophyseal joints will result in limitation of neck motion. Affection of the temporomandibular joint will cause failure of development of the lower jaw and result in a receding chin.

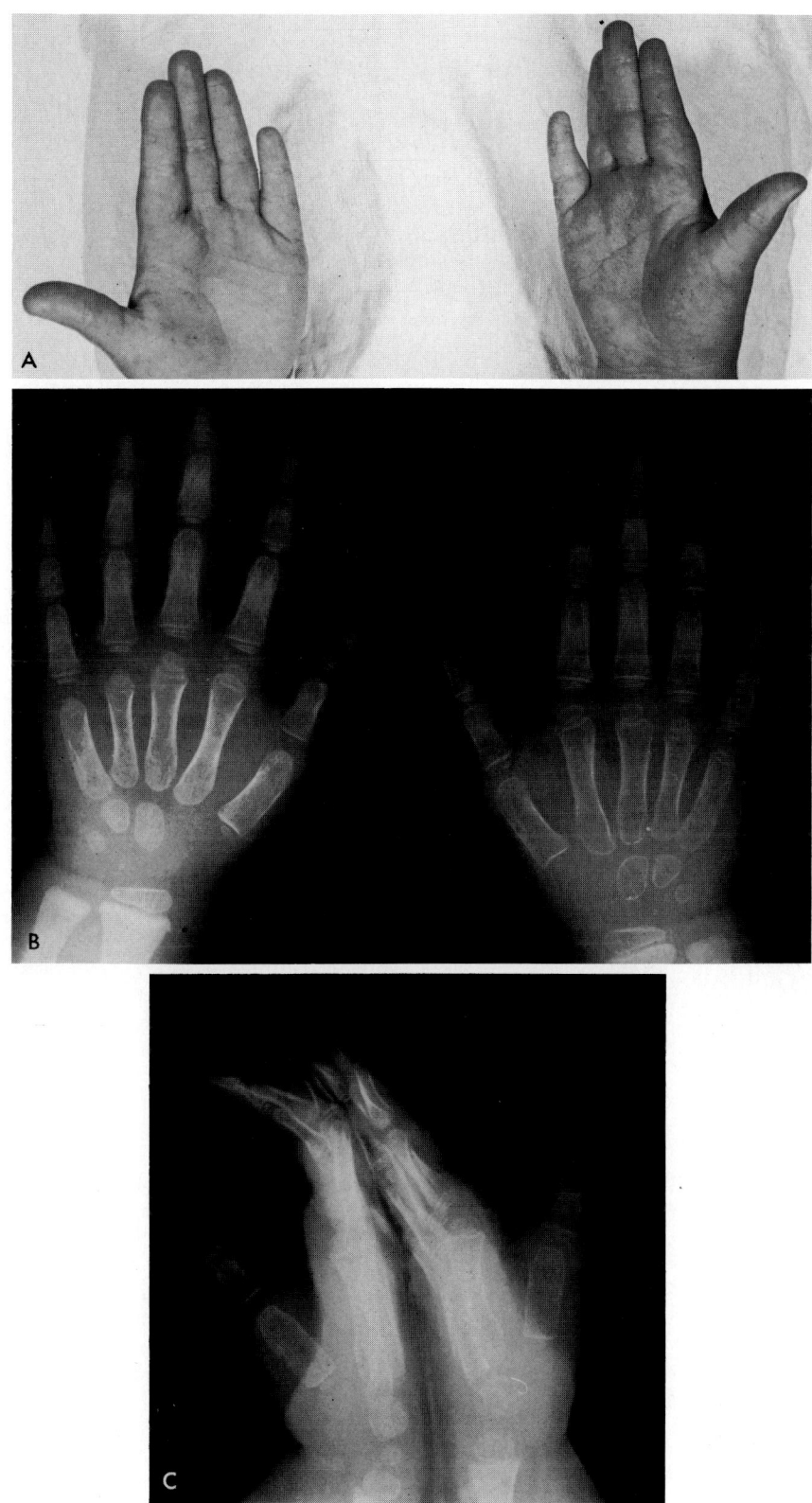

FIGURE 4–23. Pauciarticular arthritis in a two-year-old child.
Note tumefaction of right thumb. **A.** Clinical appearance. **B** and **C.** Radiograms.

The onset of polyarthritis is usually insidious, though it may be sudden in some. The clinical course of the disease is chronic and may last many years with periods of partial remission of minimal joint involvement interspersed with acute exacerbations.

Systemic Rheumatoid Disease With Polyarthritis. This type often begins acutely with severe systemic manifestations and polyarthritis. It usually runs an explosive clinical course with acute exacerbations lasting from several weeks to several months, followed by partial remissions of several months' to several years' duration. Occasionally, this form may run a relentless course with continuous activity and no remission, resulting in severe debility.

Fever usually has an abrupt onset; the fever pattern is quotidian with one or two daily rises from normal to 104° or 105° F. Less frequently, the fever may be remittent or low-grade and sustained. These bouts of fever may not respond to salicylates or antibiotics and may persist for days, weeks, or months. The affected child, especially if under five years of age, shows signs of severe inflammation and is listless and irritable.

Hepatosplenomegaly and *generalized lymphadenopathy* are frequently present. These enlargements are usually not tender and last from a few days to several months. Enlarged inflamed mesenteric nodes may cause abdominal pain and distention, suggesting an acute surgical abdominal disorder. Splenomegaly is less frequent than lymphadenopathy. Persistent hepatomegaly or lymphadenopathy is rare. Liver function tests do not disclose any abnormality. Portal hypertension may be a rare complication.

Pericarditis with enlargement of the heart and abnormalities of the S-T segment and T waves in the electrocardiogram may be detected in 10 per cent of patients. Myocarditis is rare, and endocarditis does not develop.[108, 220] The course of rheumatoid carditis is benign and ordinarily is not complicated by heart failure or constrictive pericarditis. Nonspecific chest or abdominal pain may occur as a result of inflammation of the pleura or peritoneum. Encephalitic manifestations occasionally develop.

Rheumatoid rash occurs in half to three fourths of children with systemic rheumatoid disease. It ordinarily appears during febrile episodes and is an important diagnostic clue to the nature of the disease. The individual lesions are salmon pink, discrete, maculopapular, circular or circinate, and nonurticarial and usually develop over the thighs, arms, axilla, trunk, and occasionally over the face. Typically the

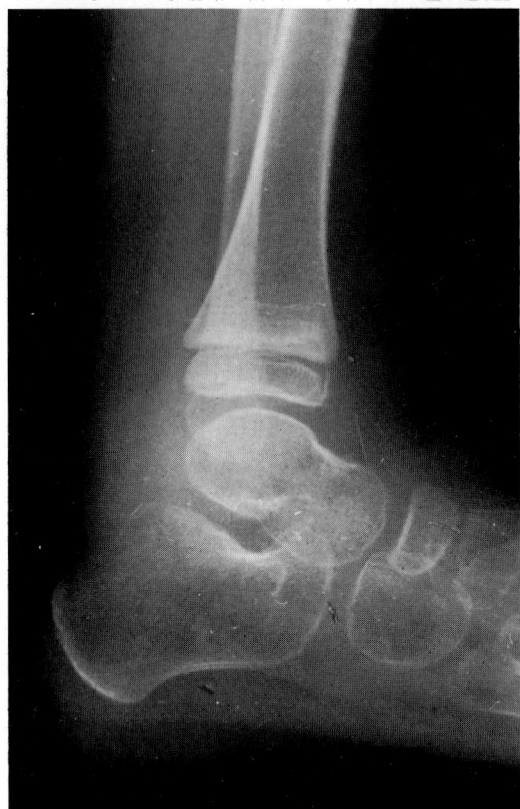

FIGURE 4–24. Rheumatoid arthritis of left ankle.

Radiogram shows soft-tissue swelling and capsular distention.

rash is recurrent and fleeting; it may appear during examination of the patient and disappear within a few hours. The rash is most florid at sites of rubbing or pressure or where skin has been subjected to slight pressure from underclothing. Light scratching along susceptible sites will bring out the rash (the Koebner phenomenon). Occasionally papular rashes and erythema multiforme may be encountered in rheumatoid arthritis.

Subcutaneous nodules may be palpated near the olecranon process of the elbows, along the anterior border of the tibia, or near the flexor or extensor tendons of the wrist or fingers. On palpation they are not tender and should be differentiated from enlarged lymph nodes.[75]

Chronic iridocyclitis and *amyloidosis* are serious problems in rheumatoid arthritis.

Ocular inflammation occurs in 2 to 2.5 per cent of children with rheumatoid disease. Ordinarily it affects the iris and ciliary body (iridocyclitis), but may extend posteriorly to involve the uveal tract (uveitis). The mean age of onset is about four years. In 65 per cent of these cases both eyes are affected, the contralateral eye becoming inflamed either within a

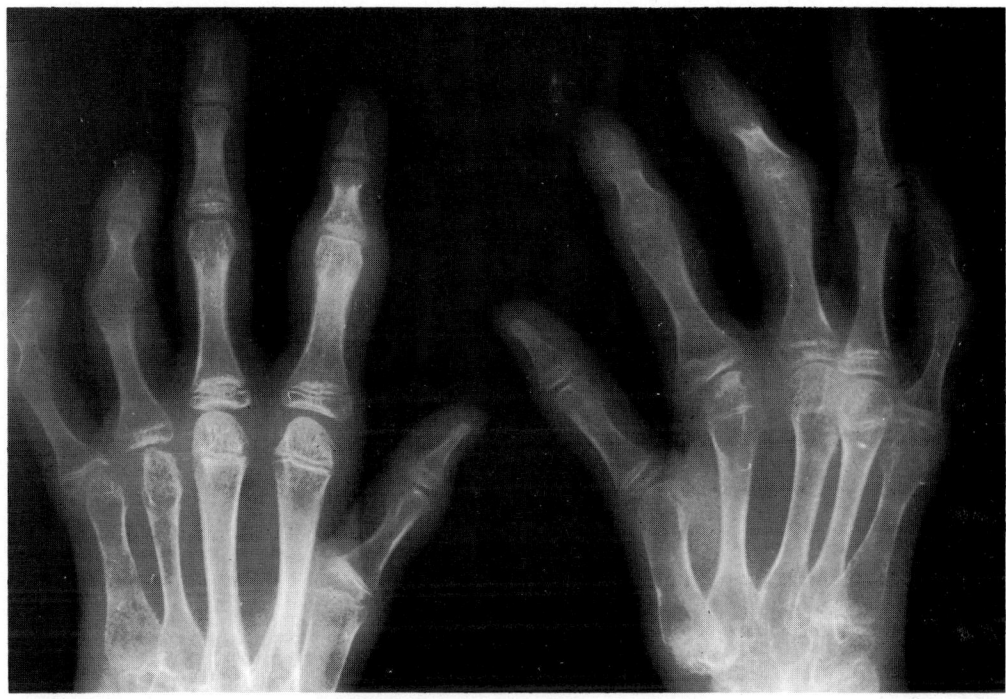

FIGURE 4–25. Rheumatoid arthritis of hands.
Radiogram shows soft-tissue thickening around proximal interphalangeal joints.

few months or not at all. In 90 per cent of cases of rheumatoid arthritis that are complicated by chronic iridocyclitis the serologic tests are positive for antinuclear antibodies.[294] In fact, children with pauciarticular arthritis and a strongly positive antinuclear antibody titer are at great risk of developing iridocyclitis. The onset of iridocyclitis is insidious and not related to the severity of systemic or local joint manifestations. Pain and conjunctivitis are minimal or absent. Asymmetry of the pupils and diminution of vision are the findings that draw attention to the condition. Slit lamp examination will disclose nongranulomatous fibrinous inflammation of the iris.[53, 324, 355] Periodic ophthalmologic examinations are imperative for early detection. Treatment of iridocyclitis consists of local potent corticosteroid drops and mydriatics. Untreated cases develop scarring and adhesions about the iris, band keratopathy, and cataracts, which are serious complications that interfere with vision. Uveitis may result in glaucoma.

Amyloidosis is a grave complication that is rare in North America, but in Great Britain occurs in about 7.5 per cent of cases.[10] It manifests itself by the development of proteinuria and hypertension. Ordinarily IgG and C-reactive protein levels are high in patients who develop amyloidosis. Treatment consists of measures to control the activity of the rheumatoid disease.[11] Death in rheumatoid disease is due to amyloidosis or to lethal complications of therapy.

Radiographic Findings

The earliest radiographic manifestations reflect the acute synovitis and the response to the inflammatory hyperemia. Thus, soft-tissue swelling, capsular distention, and periarticular osteoporosis are the initial findings in the radiograms (Figs. 4–24 and 4–25). These changes are nonspecific. Juxta-articular periosteal new bone formation, particularly in the phalanges and metatarsals, is not uncommon (Fig. 4–26).

With progression of the disease, the articular cartilage space narrows owing to destruction of the hyaline articular cartilage by the pannus. The shadow of the subchondral bony plate disappears. Soon erosive changes produce notchlike defects in bone, especially in the carpal bones. Epiphyseal growth may be accelerated or retarded (Fig. 4–27). The diameter of long bones is often decreased. With disuse, the muscle mass shadow becomes smaller or thinner.

In the late stages, the articular spaces completely disappear, obliterated by fibrous or bony ankylosis (Fig. 4–28).

In the cervical spine, erosion of the odontoid

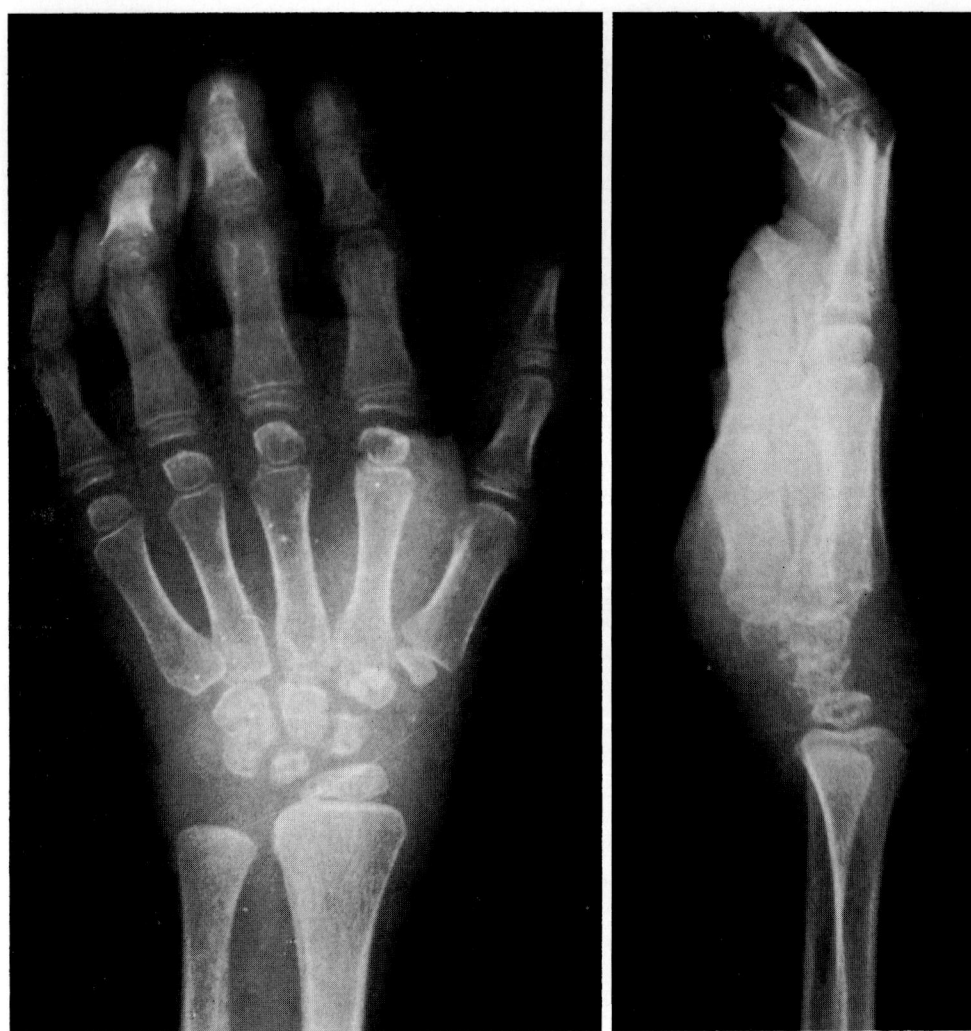

FIGURE 4–26. Radiograms of hand with rheumatoid arthritis. Note the juxta-articular new bone formation in the phalanges.

process and atlantoaxial subluxation may occur.[124, 240] Other changes in the spine are narrowing and eventual fusion of the apophyseal joints and calcification or ossification of the longitudinal ligaments.

Bone scan with technetium-99m will disclose minimal increased uptake in both sides of the joint. *Computed tomography* will clearly show the soft-tissue changes and the degree of osseous involvement. *Ultrasonography* will depict the fluid and soft-tissue changes in the joint.

Laboratory Findings*

In laboratory investigation of arthritis in children the indicated studies are:

---

*See references 57, 74, 199, 314, 345, 353, 354, 360, 367, 370.

Hemoglobin, white blood cell, differential, and platelet counts and erythrocyte sedimentation rate.

Bleeding and clotting times (when a bleeding disorder such as hemophilia is suspected).

Blood cultures (if suppurative arthritis is considered in differential diagnosis).

Agglutination test for IgM.

Rheumatoid factor test (latex or other).

Antinuclear antibody tests.

Identification of antibodies to Brucella, Salmonella, and the like.

Synovial fluid analysis and culture.

Synovial membrane histologic examination and culture.

Tuberculosis test.

It is best to plan ahead for all necessary studies and avoid multiple venous punctures.

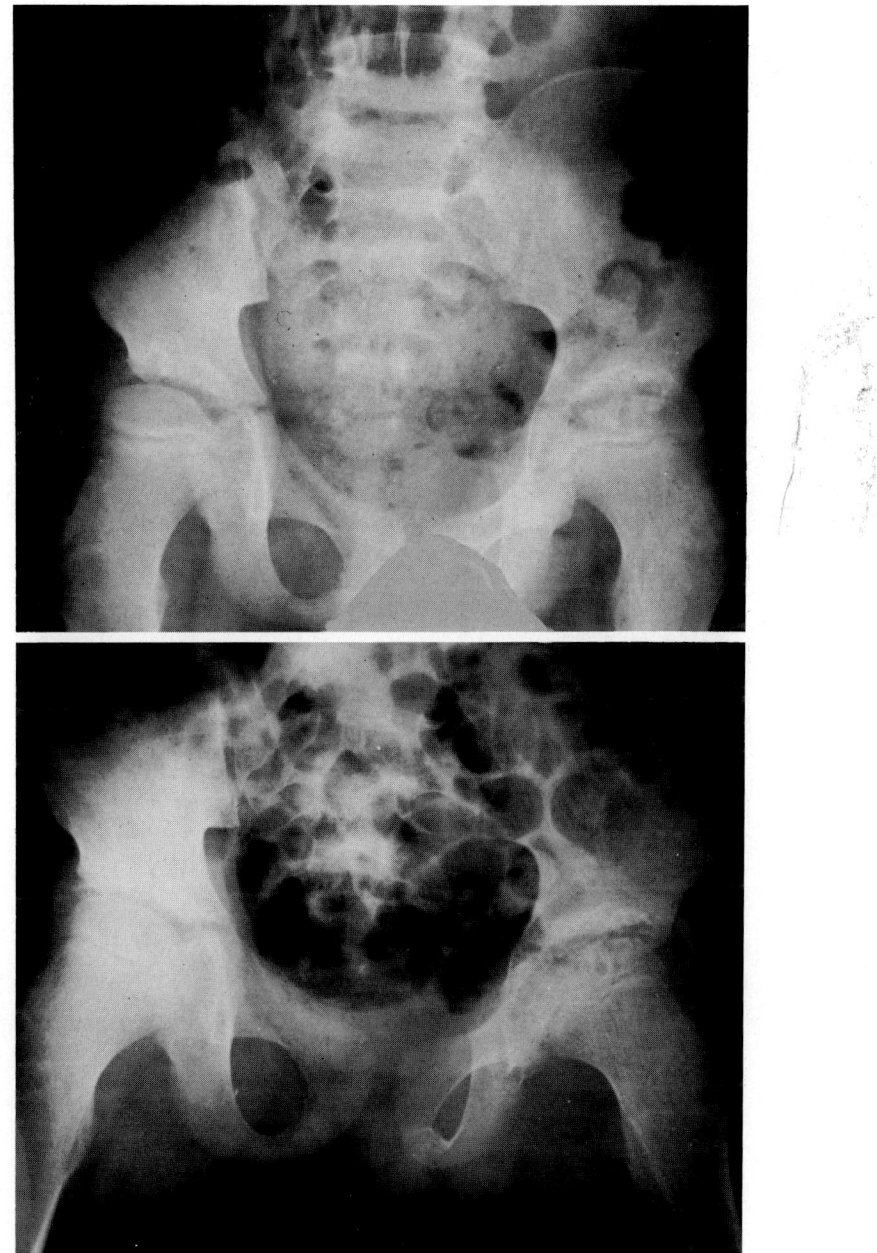

FIGURE 4–27. *Rheumatoid arthritis of both hips.*

Note the coxa magna on the right. In the left femoral head the subchondral bony plate has disappeared and there are erosive changes in the ossific nucleus. There is marked limitation of motion of both hips.

Store a small amount of serum for further studies (such as identification of viral antibodies) if necessary.

A swollen inflamed joint requires aspiration for synovial fluid analysis and culture; the procedure should be performed under strict aseptic conditions and under local anesthesia with the child adequately sedated. Make it as atraumatic as possible for the frightened, restless young child. If a hip joint is aspirated, image intensifier radiographic control will facilitate the procedure and ensure that the hip joint is penetrated properly; do not inject radiopaque dye before cultures are taken. Initially verify the position of the needle in the joint by air arthrography.

Synovial biopsy for histologic study and culture is best carried out through the arthroscope.

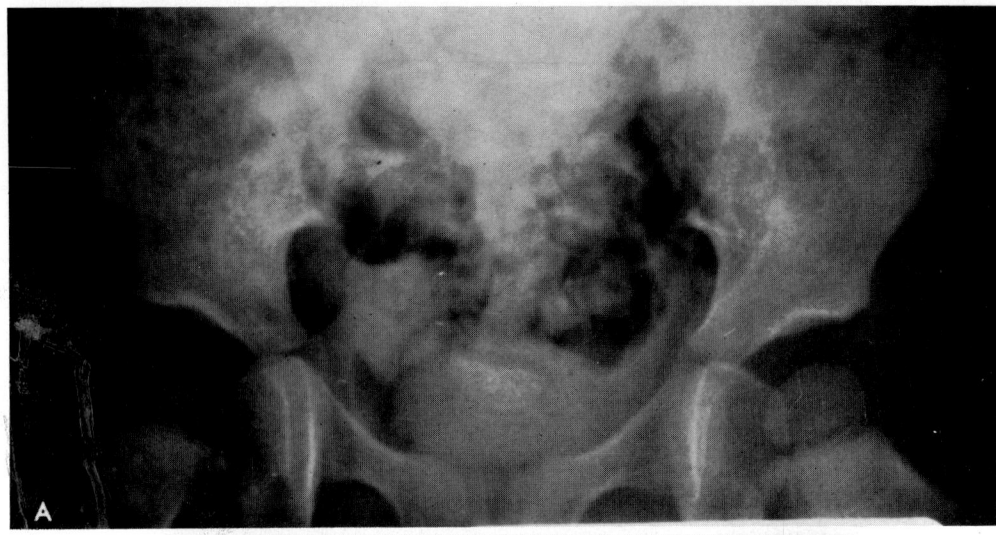
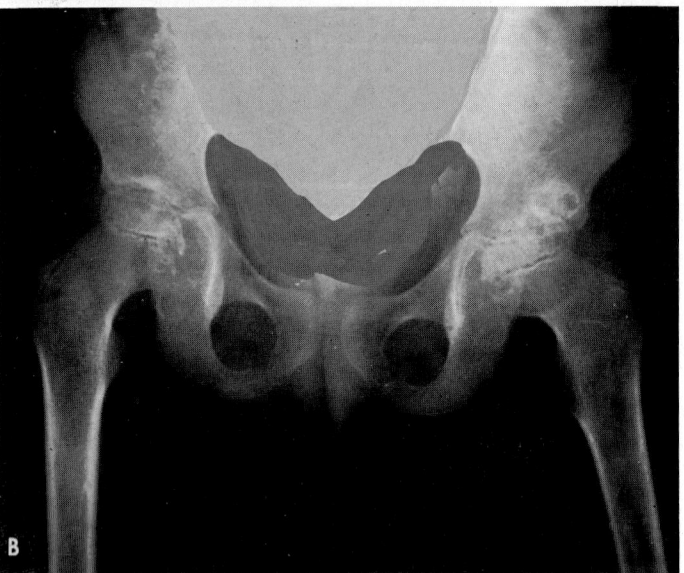

FIGURE 4–28. Rheumatoid arthritis of both hips.

A. Initial radiogram. **B.** Radiogram of hips taken three years later. The child was allowed to be ambulatory without protection of the hips. Note the destructive changes with fibrous ankylosis on the right and bony ankylosis on the left.

This method is ideal for visualizing the affected joint and obtaining the tissue from the proper site. General anesthesia is required for arthroscopy, which is performed in the operating room.

There are no pathognomonic laboratory findings for rheumatoid disease. During the active phase, the erythrocyte sedimentation rate generally is elevated and the C-reactive protein test is often positive. Depending upon the acuteness of inflammation, a slight leukocytosis with an increase of predominantly polymorphonuclear leukocytes is not uncommon. Occasionally, leukemoid reaction with white blood counts as high as 80,000 per cubic millimeter may occur. A moderate hypochromic normocytic anemia is common and is unresponsive to iron.[112, 134, 218, 278] A nonspecific finding is the alteration of serum proteins with a decrease in albumin and an increase in alpha and gamma globulin fractions. Antinuclear factors may be found in some affected children.

Rheumatoid factor is a 19 S macrogammaglobulin, which is demonstrated by the latex, sensitized sheep cell agglutination, or bentonite particle test. The tests are positive in only about 10 per cent of children with rheumatoid arthritis, but in adults, 60 to 80 per cent are positive.

The reason for this low incidence of positive rheumatoid factor in children is unknown. Children with systemic lupus erythematosus, scleroderma, or polyarteritis nodosa may also have a positive rheumatoid factor. The synovial fluid findings are shown in Table 4–1.

The laboratory findings vary depending on whether the illness is severe systemic rheumatoid disease with polyarthritis, polyarthritis with minimal systemic manifestation, or simple pauciarticular arthritis.

In systemic rheumatoid arthritis (Still's disease) there is polymorphonucleocytosis, elevation of the platelet count, high erythrocyte sedimentation rate (usually 100 mm. or more), and low hemoglobulin level (10 gm. or less). All the immunoglobulin levels are elevated, and immune complexes can frequently be detected; however, these are nonspecific changes and not diagnostic for rheumatoid arthritis. The detection of IgM rheumatoid factor by a poorly positive latex test is uncommon. The finding of antinuclear antibodies in systemic rheumatoid disease is rare.

In polyarthritis (i.e., five or more joints involved) with minimal systemic disease the test for IgM rheumatoid factor is positive in 10 per cent of cases and negative in the remaining 90 per cent. Other laboratory findings are intermediate; the sedimentation rate is elevated to 60 to 70 mm. The white blood count is raised to 15,000 with primarily polymorphonuclear leukocytosis, and the hemoglobin level is 10 to 12 gm. The immunoglobulins are slightly or moderately increased, and antinuclear antibodies are present in a small percentage of cases.

In pauciarticular arthritis the laboratory changes are minimal except in cases in which antinuclear antibodies are present in the serum, which is often associated with chronic iridocyclitis.

Treatment

In the management of the child with rheumatoid arthritis, it is imperative to employ a multidisciplinary approach in which the pediatrician, orthopedic surgeon, hematologist, physical and occupational therapists, psychologist, and social worker collaborate closely.

The activity of rheumatoid arthritis may persist for many years. During this period of active disease, vigilant and detailed care of the whole child should be provided. The objectives of orthopedic treatment are to prevent and correct contractural deformation of joints and growth deformities of bones. One should not forget, however, the proper development of the mind, intellectual and emotional stimulation, and educational pursuits. The child should attend school. Medical and orthopedic care should be provided in the natural home environment with periods of hospitalization as brief as possible.

Rest. During the acute inflammatory stage, local and general rest are necessary. The inflamed joints should be protected from weight-bearing; continuous and prolonged immobilization, however, leads to disuse atrophy of muscles and bone. Rest and motion are both essential to the health of joints, and a physiologic compromise between the two should be chosen, tailored to the individual needs of the patient.

Diet. A well-balanced, nutritious diet with an ample supply of proteins, minerals, and vitamins is prescribed. The intake of meat, milk, cream, eggs, cheese, butter, and fresh fruits is encouraged, as rheumatoid arthritis is a chronic wasting disease and anorexia is a further cause of weight loss.

Obesity is a problem in some patients, as it may put additional stress on the involved weight-bearing joints. Excess body weight should be controlled by a strict diet.

The parents should understand that dietary deficiencies or excesses do not have any etiologic bearing in rheumatoid arthritis. The use of "folk medicine" such as cranberry juice, garlic, radishes, or various molasses mixtures should be discouraged.

Drug Therapy

In selecting the appropriate drug to control activity of the disease one should consider the possible side effects, the presence or absence of systemic involvement, and the pattern of the course of the disease process. If one or two joints are affected a simple analgesic anti-inflammatory agent is administered; whereas when multiple joints are affected with systemic disease, initially high-dosage salicylates or other potent anti-inflammatory drugs are given; if these fail to suppress the acute inflammatory disease, early use of steroids is considered. One should constantly weigh the beneficial value of a drug against its potential serious toxic effect. Refrain from use of steroids and gold unless it is absolutely necessary.

Analgesic Anti-Inflammatory Agents. *Salicylates*, of which aspirin (acetylsalicylic acid) is the most useful and generally effective anti-inflammatory agent in the treatment of rheumatoid arthritis, will alleviate pain, give a feeling of well-being, lower fever, diminish effusion and synovial thickening of joints, and increase the range of joint motion.[110, 143, 171, 255, 269, 340, 349, 363]

Ordinarily prednisone is the steroid prescribed at a dosage of 10 to 20 mg. per single dose every 48 hours. In the acutely ill child a 40 mg. dose may be given initially, and the dosage then gradually tapered.

Intra-articular steroid therapy may be administered judiciously on occasion into a large joint, particularly the knee, hip, ankle, shoulder, wrist, or elbow. It will temporarily alleviate the acute inflammation and help to obtain functional range of motion. Following intrasynovial injection of corticosteroid, the joint should be protected in a splint, and active and passive exercises performed. Often with relief of pain, physical activity is increased, and the affected osteoporotic joints are further damaged by stress fractures. The injudicious and frequent use of corticosteroids in weight-bearing joints should be condemned.

Slow-Acting Drugs. *Gold salts* are effective in the treatment of rheumatoid arthritis in the adult.[41, 66, 292] Experience with their use in children is limited; however, gold does not appear to be more toxic in children than in adults. Sodium aurothiomalate is the gold preparation preferred by Brewer and Ansell. At present, two gold salts are available for injection: Sodium aurothiomalate (Myochrysine) and aurothioglucose (Solganal).

Myochrysine should be administered only by intramuscular injection, preferably intragluteally. The pediatric dose of Myochrysine is proportional to the adult dose on a weight basis. After the initial dose of 10 mg., the recommended dose for children is 1 mg. per kg. of body weight, not to exceed 50 mg. for a single injection. Myochrysine is continued until the cumulative dose reaches 1 gm. unless toxicity or major clinical improvement occurs. It causes more pain on injection, and patients experience a higher incidence of nitritoid reactions (flushing and dizziness) after injection than with doses of Solganal.

Solganal is administered to children 6 to 12 years of age in doses equivalent to one fourth the adult dose, governed chiefly by body weight but not to exceed 25 mg. per dose. It is not approved by the FDA for children under six years of age. Solganal suspension should be injected intramuscularly, preferably intragluteally, never intravenously! In adults, the first dose is 10 mg., the second and third doses are 25 mg., and the fourth and subsequent doses 50 mg. The interval between doses is one week.

It is important that a patient who receives gold lie down for ten minutes following injection.

There is an oral form of gold now available (Auranofin). It is not yet approved by the FDA for use in children under 12 years of age. The dosage is 0.1 to 0.2 mg. per kg. per day. The oral gold therapy is not as effective as intramuscular administration.

Gold salts are toxic drugs, causing bone marrow depression, nephritis, dermatitis, irritation of the gastrointestinal tract, and disturbance of the central nervous system. Occasionally they may exacerbate the arthritis. Brewer and associates state that the toxicity of gold is less than that of steroids and certainly does not preclude its use when indicated.[63] A hemogram and urinalysis are performed at weekly intervals when gold is being administered.

Chloroquine is effective in suppressing systemic rheumatoid disease; however, its use is not recommended because of the possible occurrence of irreversible retinal damage.[294] Methotrexate is now tried in selected children with rheumatoid arthritis who are recalcitrant to other therapy and do not respond to nonsteroidal anti-inflammatory medications. However, long-term results are still not available, and a multicenter pediatric study is currently in progress.

Immunosuppressant Therapy. These agents may be tried in the severely systemically ill child who fails to respond or has serious side effects from corticosteroids or gold therapy.

Azathioprine in a daily dosage of 2.5 mg. per kilogram of body weight is useful. Chlorambucil is effective in controlling disease activity in those cases complicated by amyloidosis.

ORTHOPEDIC MANAGEMENT

Conservative Therapy.* Local care of a joint is very essential, as it determines the end result when the disease becomes quiescent. Basic principles of care include rest of the joint, relief of muscle spasm, prevention of deformity, and maintenance of motion (as effected by traction, plastic splints or bivalved casts, local heat, and active and passive exercises).

The modality of treatment depends on the stage of the disease, the degree of inflammation, and the type and severity of deformity. In the beginning, during the acute phase, it is best to admit the child to the hospital for thorough evaluation and initiation of treatment. When the hip or knee is involved, split Russell traction is applied with the horizontal force directed along the longitudinal axis of the leg and the vertical force placed behind the proximal tibia

---

*See References 151, 201, 248, 274, 286, and 358.

(not the distal femur). Buck's traction should not be used, as it produces posterior subluxation of the tibia (Fig. 4–29). While the child is in traction, active assisted exercises should be performed several times a day. Following correction of the deformity, the joint should be supported in a bivalved cast, which holds it in corrected position and prevents recurrence of deformity. The limb is removed from the cast for exercises several times a day.

When the wrist, ankle, or elbow is involved, a plastic splint is used initially, providing support, relieving muscle spasm, and preventing deformity. Again, the limb should be taken out

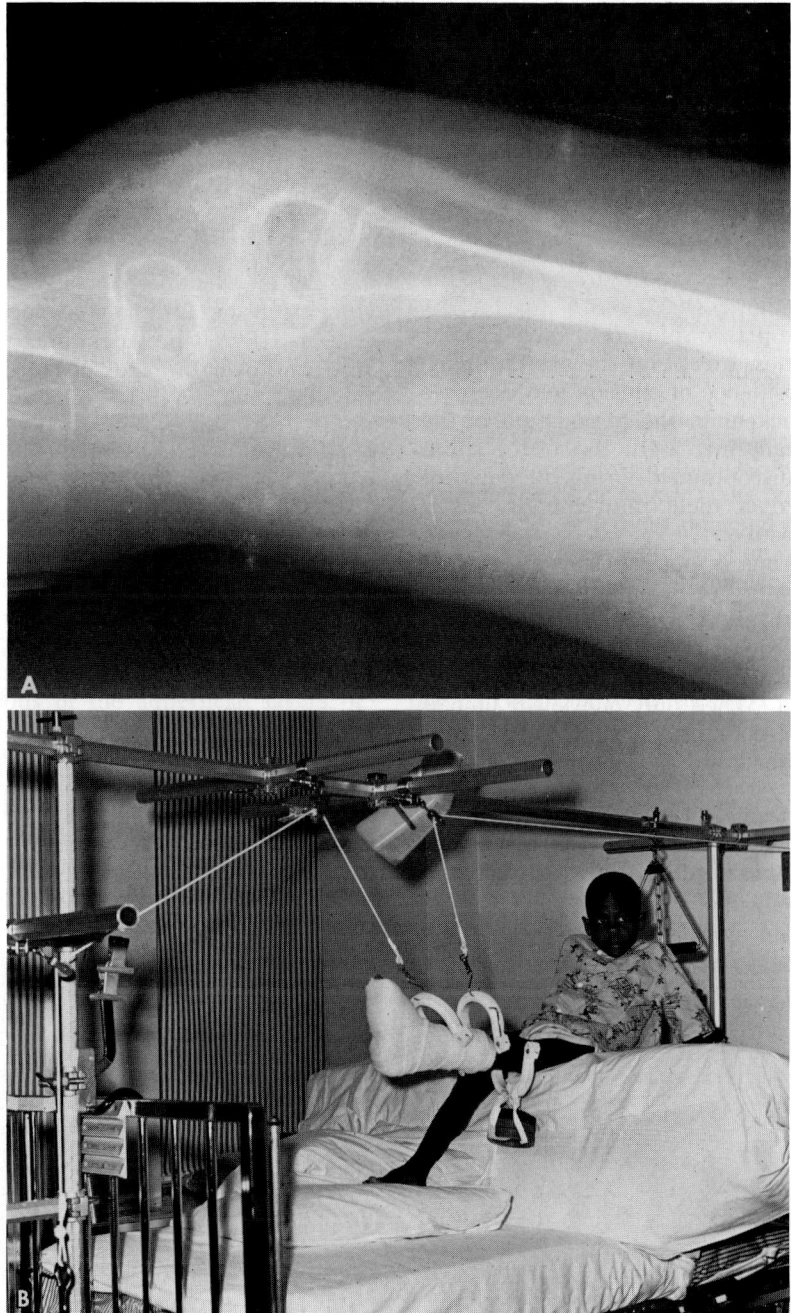

FIGURE 4–29. Posterior subluxation of the knee in rheumatoid arthritis.

A. Radiogram. **B.** Conservative method of reduction of posterior subluxation of the tibia by skeletal traction.

destruction.[368, 372] Following removal of the diseased synovial tissue, a new, relatively normal one regenerates in its place. Histologic studies after synovectomy have demonstrated excellent preservation of articular cartilage.[136, 178] Synovial fluid is the source of articular cartilage nutrition and joint lubrication. Restoration of normal synovial tissue is paramount to normal joint function.

As reported in the literature, the results of synovectomy have been favorable; it prevents progressive destruction of the joint, improves function, and ameliorates the patient's general condition. The synovectomized joints will usually remain unaffected by subsequent flare-ups of the disease at other sites. Recurrence of synovitis occurs in children in whom synovectomy was performed during a phase of great disease activity, particularly those with polyarticular and systemic disease.[289]

Operative Technique. Synovectomy is best performed through the arthroscope. In the hands of an experienced surgeon and with proper instrumentation, a subtotal synovectomy can be carried out with relative ease. The scars of the portals of entry of the arthroscope and instrumentation are small and cosmetically pleasing. As complete a synovectomy as possible is carried out. Care should be taken not to damage the growth plates and hyaline articular cartilage. All visible synovial tissue is excised, including that covering the anterior and posterior cruciate and collateral ligaments and the posterior fossa, and the synovial pannus covering the tibial plateau. The menisci are not excised unless they are torn and irreparable. The hyaline articular cartilage is inspected and graded as to stage of deterioration—visual grading by inspection through the arthroscope is much more reliable than radiologic grading. After thorough irrigation of the wound, closed suction tubes are inserted to minimize hemarthrosis and swelling of the joint. A Robert Jones compression dressing is applied. Isometric exercises for the quadriceps and hamstring muscles are started the first postoperative day. As soon as the patient is comfortable (usually the third or fourth postoperative day) active assisted and gentle passive range of motion exercises are performed.

When lack of cooperation and poor motivation are problems, a continuous passive motion machine is applied seven to ten days postoperatively. If, within three to four weeks after operation, range of joint motion has not been obtained the joint is gently manipulated and mobilized under general anesthesia. Do not cause stress fracture! Document it by appropriate pre- and postmanipulation radiograms. Then the joint motion is maintained in a continuous passive motion machine, and an intensive program of active and passive exercises is begun. It will take several months and sometimes almost a year to obtain maximum results of synovectomy. It is surprising how much joint function improves with persistent physical therapy.

Synovectomy of the ankle or elbow through an arthroscope is difficult and technically demanding, but possible; however, synovectomy of the hip is often performed through an open arthrotomy.

Soft-Tissue Release. Muscle tendon lengthening, tenotomy, capsulotomy, or capsulectomy is indicated to correct fixed contractural deformity of joints that fail to respond to conservative measures. The objectives of soft-tissue release are to relieve muscle spasm, correct deformity, and decompress the joint to relieve pain and provide greater range of joint motion. It is preferable to perform simple musculotendinous fractional or Z-plasty tendon lengthening or tenotomy and not to perform the more extensive capsulotomy or capsulectomy unless necessary. It is difficult to predict the course of the disease and eventual prognosis in an individual patient. If the activity of the disease subsides after soft-tissue release, the improved function may be permanent, and even if the rheumatoid disease activity persists or becomes exacerbated a more functional position of the joint is achieved for activities of daily living. Swann and Ansell reviewed the results of soft-tissue release of the hips in juvenile rheumatoid arthritis. Eighty-nine psoas and adductor tenotomies were performed; pain was relieved and range of motion and function improved in all; in addition, in half the patients there was radiologic evidence of improvement. In their experience psoas and adductor tenotomy was simple, safe, and effective in treatment of contractural deformity of the hips in juvenile rheumatoid arthritis. They recommended that it be done first, before resorting to a more extensive open capsulectomy or synovectomy.[344]

Bone and Joint Procedures. These are indicated to correct deformities and to restore mobility in stiff, totally damaged joints. Malalignment of long bones is corrected by rotational or angular osteotomies. Severe genu valgum may be corrected by medial physeal stapling of the distal femur or the proximal tibia or both at the appropriate skeletal age.

Lower Limb Length Disparity. It may be significant in monarticular and pauciarticular arthritis. When the rheumatoid disease develops after the age of nine years, rapid premature closure of the physis adjacent to the involved joint may occur; in such an instance there will be marked shortening of the involved limb. Overgrowth of the involved limb occurs when the disease develops before the age of nine. In the lower limb, Simon and associates found that the overgrowth never exceeded 3 cm. The greater disparity developed within the first three to four years and either increased very slowly thereafter, remained level, or decreased. This pattern of lower limb length disparity in monarticular arthritis emphasizes the importance of close follow-up of the growth pattern.[317] Physeal arrest of the longer limb is performed after thorough calculations when lower limb length disparity is significant (see Chapter 7).

Total Joint Replacement. This is indicated in the polyarthritic form with or without severe systemic disease. Prosthetic implants in the young growing patient have their definite drawbacks: problems of component wear and fatigue, aseptic loosening, implant rejection, long-term toxic effects of the cement, and possible growth after the insertion of the implant. The rheumatoid adolescent who requires total joint replacement, however, is underweight and his physical activity is restricted; therefore he exerts less stress on the components, and wear is minimal. Most of these patients have been receiving corticosteroid therapy to control the severe systemic manifestations of the disease; the corticosteroids cause skeletal growth retardation with premature physeal closure; therefore, continued growth after insertion of the prosthesis usually is not a problem.

Ruddlesdin and associates reported the results of 75 total hip replacements in 42 children with juvenile chronic arthritis. The age range was 11 to 17 years at the time of operation. Many of the hip joints had active disease with severe pain and marked stiffness, limiting the child's physical capacity and ability to walk. Half the children were still growing and continued to grow after operation. There were marked improvement of range of movement that was maintained during later follow-up, dramatic relief of pain, and increased walking ability. The strides made in social development for independence of living were very rewarding. The complications included one hip dislocation, which was successfully reduced; one hematoma, which was absorbed spontaneously; one lateral popliteal nerve palsy; which recovered spontaneously in one year; and one femoral component loosening, which was revised with excellent result. There were no cases of infection.[287]

Singsen and associates reported similar good results in 26 total hip replacements for juvenile chronic arthritis in 14 children between 12 and 18 years of age.[319]

Colville and Raunio reported the results of 59 Charnley low-friction arthroplasties of the hip in 41 patients with a mean follow-up of 30 months and mean age of 30.5 years. The result with regard to pain relief was excellent in 90 per cent and good in 10 per cent. Mobility was significantly improved in all but two patients who developed ectopic bone formation. Total hip replacement in a child with juvenile rheumatoid arthritis is technically demanding and very difficult. With carefully selected patients and detailed preoperative planning in the hands of the experienced surgeon, the results are worthwhile.[98]

Total Knee Arthroplasty. The knee joints may be destroyed by rheumatoid disease with severe functional impairment despite adequate physical therapy, traction, soft-tissue release, and synovectomy. Total knee arthroplasty should be considered when the foregoing therapeutic measures have been employed but failed to prevent joint destruction. Almost all the patients requiring total joint replacement have polyarticular rheumatoid arthritis, and often the hips are painful and deformed in flexion-adduction contracture. The hip should be operated on first when total hip replacement is also indicated, because it is very difficult to rehabilitate the knee in the presence of a deformed and painful hip, whereas it is feasible to rehabilitate the hip joint in the presence of a stiff and deformed knee. Also at the time of hip surgery, the contracted biarticular muscles that cross the hip and knee are released. Severe flexion deformity of the knee is treated preoperatively by serial stretching extension casts. This will reduce the extent of soft-tissue release needed at operation.[293]

Often in the young patient, custom-made small prosthetic components are required. Preoperative planning is crucial. When total knee replacement is performed, often patellar resurfacing is indicated; this obviates the problem of postoperative patellofemoral pain. In order to achieve optimum results it is crucial to have cooperation from and motivation on the part of the patient. This author recommends preoperative psychologic or psychiatric assessment. Some chronically disabled adolescents intensely fear losing parental support and becoming independent; despite the fact that they are able to walk, they choose wheelchair mobility.

Temporomandibular joint and cervical spine

involvement make intubation of these patients difficult during anesthesia. Obtain flexion-extension radiographs of the cervical spine to rule out atlantoaxial instability. The anesthesiologist and sometimes an endoscopist should be consulted preoperatively. Often the fiberoptic laryngoscope has to be utilized.

It is beyond the scope of this book to discuss operative technique in detail. A straight anterior incision that crosses the medial third of the patella should be used. Angular and flexion deformities are corrected by appropriate soft-tissue release. Posterior cruciate ligaments are preserved whenever possible. Knee instability due to insufficiency of capsule and ligaments is managed by using a more constraining prosthesis.

Sarokhan and associates reported the results of 29 total knee arthroplasties in 17 patients with juvenile rheumatoid arthritis. The average age at operation was 23 years (range 13 to 39 years). The average follow-up was 5 years (range 2 to 11 years). Postoperative follow-up revealed dramatic relief of discomfort, the arc of knee motion increased by an average of 34 degrees, and in all but one knee the angular deformity corrected to 0 to 10 degrees of valgus angulation. All but one patient became a limited- to full-community ambulator. Postoperative complications consisted of one late deep infection and posterior tibial subluxation. Postoperative manipulation was required in 21 of the 29 knees. The study of Sarokhan and associates shows that total knee arthroplasty in juvenile rheumatoid arthritis provides marked improvement in knee function and in the quality of life.[293]

Cervical Fusion. This is indicated when there is instability with neurologic deficit. Ordinarily, surgery is not indicated because simple support of the cervical spine will stabilize it and prevent progressive subluxation. An exception to this is the occurrence of rheumatoid arthritis in Down syndrome and other conditions with excessive ligamentous hyperlaxity such as Ehlers-Danlos syndrome. The combination of the two makes the cervical spine very unstable, and it is strongly recommended that surgical intervention be carried out to prevent neurologic deficit.

References

1. Aiden, M. P., and Baker, L. D.: Synovectomy of the knee joint in rheumatoid arthritis. J.A.M.A. 187:4, 1964.
2. Alarcon-Segovia, O., and Ward, L. E.: Charcot-like arthropathy in rheumatoid arthritis. J.A.M.A., 193:136, 1965.
3. Albright, J. A., Albright, J. P., and Odgen, J. A.: Synovectomy of the knee in juvenile rheumatoid arthritis. Clin. Orthop., 106:48, 1975.
4. Allin, R. E., and Lawton, D. S.: The management of juvenile chronic polyarthritis. The Association of Paediatric Chartered Physiotherapists, 1968.
5. American Rheumatism Association Committee: Diagnostic criteria for rheumatoid arthritis. 1958 Revision. Ann. Rheum. Dis., 18:49, 1959.
6. Andrews, L. G.: Myelopathy due to atlanto-axial dislocation in a patient with Down's syndrome and rheumatoid arthritis. Dev. Med. Child Neurol., 23:356, 1981.
7. Ansell, B. M.: Treatment of juvenile chronic polyarthritis. Clin. Rheum. Dis., 1:443, 1975.
8. Ansell, B. M.: Joint manifestations in children with juvenile chronic polyarthritis. Arthritis Rheum., 20:Suppl. 2:204, 1977.
9. Ansell, B. M.: Heberden Oration 1977. Chronic arthritis in childhood. Ann. Rheum. Dis., 37:107, 1978.
10. Ansell, B. M.: Juvenile spondylitis and related disorders. In Moll, J. M. H. (ed.): Ankylosing Spondylitis. Edinburgh, Churchill Livingstone, 1980, pp. 120–136.
11. Ansell, B. M.: Rheumatic Disorders in Childhood. Postgraduate Pediatric Series. London, Boston, Butterworths, 1980.
12. Ansell, B. M.: Rehabilitation in juvenile chronic arthritis. Clin. Rheum. Dis., 7:469, 1981.
13. Ansell, B. M.: Juvenile chronic arthritis. In Hart, F. D. (ed.): Drug Treatment of Rheumatic Diseases. 2nd Ed. London, M.T.P. Press, 1982, pp. 185–195.
14. Ansell, B. M., and Bywaters, E. G.: Growth in Still's disease. Ann. Rheum. Dis., 15:295, 1956.
15. Ansell, B. M., and Bywaters, E. G.: Prognosis in Still's disease. Bull. Rheum. Dis., 9:189, 1959.
16. Ansell, B. M., and Bywaters, E. G. L.: Alternate-day corticosteroid therapy in juvenile chronic polyarthritis. J. Rheumatol., 1:176, 1974.
17. Ansell, B. M., and Hall, M. A.: Penicillamine in chronic arthritis in childhood. J. Rheumatol., 7:112, 1981.
18. Ansell, B. W., and Kent, P. A.: Radiological changes in juvenile chronic polyarthritis. Skeletal Radiol., 1:129, 1977.
19. Ansell, B. M., and Simpson, C.: The effect of penicillamine on growth as height in juvenile chronic polyarthritis. Proc. R. Soc. Med., 70:123, 1977.
20. Ansell, B. M., and Swann, M.: The management of chronic arthritis of children. J. Bone Joint Surg., 65-B:536, 1983.
21. Ansell, B. M., and Wood, P. H. N.: Prognosis in juvenile chronic polyarthritis. Clin. Rheum. Dis., 2:397, 1976.
22. Ansell, B. M., Bywaters, E. G., and Lawrence, J. S.: A family study in Still's disease. Ann. Rheum. Dis., 21:243, 1962.
23. Ansell, B. M., Hanna, B., Moran, H., Hall, M. A., and Engler, C.: Naproxen in juvenile chronic polyarthritis. Eur. J. Rheumatol. Inflamm., 2:79, 1979.
24. Anttila, R., and Laaksonen, A. L.: Renal disease in juvenile rheumatoid arthritis. Acta Rheumatol. Scand., 15:99, 1969.
25. Arden, G. P., and Ansell, B. M.: Surgical Management of Juvenile Chronic Polyarthritis. London, Academic Press; New York, Grune & Stratton, 1978.
26. Arden, G. P., Ansell, B. M., and Hunter, M. J.: Total hip replacement in juvenile chronic polyarthritis and ankylosing spondylitis. Clin. Orthop., 84:130, 1972.
27. Arnett, F. C., Bias, W. B., and Stevens, M. B.: Juvenile-onset chronic arthritis. Clinical and roentgenographic features of a unique HLA-B27 subset. Am. J. Med., 69:369, 1980.
28. Arthritis Foundation Committee on Evaluation of

Synovectomy: Multicenter evaluation of synovectomy in the treatment of rheumatoid arthritis. Report of results at the end of three years. Arthritis Rheum., 20:765, 1977.
29. Arthritis and Rheumatism Council and British Orthopaedic Association: Controlled trial of synovectomy of knee and metacarpophalangeal joints in rheumatoid arthritis. Ann. Rheum. Dis., 35:437, 1976.
30. Athreya, B. H., Moser, G., Cecil, H. S., and Myers, A. R.: Aspirin-induced hepatoxicity in juvenile rheumatoid arthritis—a prospective study. Arthritis Rheum., 18:347, 1975.
31. Aufranc, W. E.: Constructive Surgery of the Hip. St. Louis, Mosby, 1962.
32. Bache, C.: Mandibular growth and dental occlusion in juvenile rheumatoid arthritis. Acta Rheumatol. Scand., 10:142, 1964.
33. Badley, B. W. D., and Ansell, B. M.: Fractures in Still's disease. Ann. Rheum. Dis., 19:135, 1960.
34. Baker, F.: Rheumatoid arthritis. Present day physical therapy. Calif. Med., 92:330, 1960.
35. Baldurrsson, H., and Gustafson, M.: Total radiation dosage from x-ray examinations in rheumatoid arthritis and other chronic skeletal diseases. A study of two cases. Acta Orthop. Scand., 48:138, 1977.
36. Barkin, R. E.: The clinical course of juvenile rheumatoid arthritis. Bull. Rheum. Dis., 3:19, 1952.
37. Barkin, R., Stillman, S., and Potter, T.: The spondylitis of juvenile rheumatoid arthritis. N. Engl. J. Med., 253:1107, 1955.
38. Barry, P. E., and Stillman, J. S.: Characteristics of juvenile rheumatoid arthritis: Its medical and orthopedic management. Orthop. Clin. North Am., 6:641, 1975.
39. Baum, J., and Fink, C. W.: Juvenile rheumatoid arthritis in monozygotic twins: A case report and review of the literature. Arthritis Rheum., 11:33, 1968.
40. Baum, J., and Gutowska, G.: Death in juvenile rheumatoid arthritis. Arthritis Rheum., 20:Suppl. 2:253, 1977.
41. Bayles, T. B.: Gold salt therapy in rheumatoid arthritis. Med. Clin. North Am., 45:1230, 1961.
42. Beales, J. G., Keen, J. H., and Holt, P. J. L.: The child's perception of the disease and the experience of pain in juvenile chronic arthritis. J. Rheumatol., 10:61, 1983.
43. Bennet, G., Zeller, J., and Bauer, W.: Subcutaneous nodules of rheumatoid arthritis with rheumatic fever. Arch. Pathol., 30:70, 1940.
44. Bernstein, B. H., Takahashi, M., and Hanson, V.: Cardiac involvement in juvenile rheumatoid arthritis. J. Pediatr., 85:313, 1974.
45. Bernstein, B. H., Singsen, B. H., Koster-King, K., and Hanson, V.: Aspirin induced hepatoxicity and its effect on juvenile rheumatoid arthritis. Am. J, Dis. Child., 33:659, 1977.
46. Bernstein, B. H., Forrester, D., Singsen, B., Koster-King, K., Kornreich, H., and Hanson, V.: Hip joint restoration in juvenile rheumatoid arthritis. Arthritis Rheum., 20:1099, 1977.
47. Bernstein, B. H., Stobie, D., Singsen, B. H., Koster-King, K., Korneich, H. K., and Hanson, V.: Growth retardation in juvenile rheumatoid arthritis (JRA). Arthritis Rheum., 20:212, 1977.
48. Bhettay, E., and Thomson, A. J.: Double-blind study of ketoprofen and indomethacin in juvenile chronic arthritis. South Afr. Med. J., 54:276, 1978.
49. Bianco, A. J., Jr., and Peterson, H. A.: Juvenile rheumatoid arthritis. Orthop. Clin. North Am., 2:745, 1971.
50. Bille, B. S. V.: Kronisk Polyatrit hos barn och dess guldbehendling. Nord. Med., 37:307, 1948.
51. Bisla, R. S., Inglis, A. E., and Ranawat, C. S.: Joint replacement surgery in patients under thirty. J. Bone Joint Surg., 58-A:1098, 1976.
52. Black, R. I., Oglesby, R. B., Sallman, I., and Bunim, J. J.: Posterior subcapsular cataracts induced by corticosteroids in patients with rheumatoid arthritis. J.A.M.A., 174:166, 1960.
53. Blegvad, O.: Iridocyclitis and disease of the joints in children. Acta Ophthalmol., 19:219, 1941.
54. Blockey, N. J., Gibson, A. A., and Goel, K. M.: Monoarticular juvenile rheumatoid arthritis. J. Bone Joint Surg., 62-B:368, 1980.
55. Blodgett, F. M., Burgin, L., Iezzoni, D., Gribetz, D., and Talbot, N. B.: Effects of prolonged cortisone therapy on statural growth, skeletal maturation and metabolic status of children. N. Engl. J. Med., 254:636, 1956.
56. Bloom, J., and Rubin, J. H.: Transient pulmonary manifestations in rheumatoid arthritis. Can. Med. Assoc. J., 63:355, 1950.
57. Boziecevish, J., Bunim, J. J., Freund, J., and Ward, S. B.: Bentonite flocculation test for rheumatoid arthritis. Proc. Soc. Exp. Biol. Med. (N.Y.), 97:180, 1958.
58. Brattstrom, M.: Asymmetry of ossification and rate of growth of long bones in children with unilateral juvenile gonarthritis. Acta Rheumatol. Scand., 9:102, 1963.
59. Brattstrom, H., and Holgersson, S.: Synovectomy of the hip joint. In Munthe, E. (ed.): EULAR bulletin, Monography series No. 3. Basel, EULAR Publishers, 1978, p. 177.
60. Brattstrom, M., and Sundberg, J.: Juvenile rheumatoid gonarthritis. I. Clinical and roentgenological study. Acta Rheumatol Scand., 11:266, 1965.
61. Brewer, E. J., Jr.: Juvenile Rheumatoid Arthritis. Philadelphia, Saunders, 1970.
62. Brewer, E. J., and Fahlberg, W. J.: In Lamont-Havers, R. W., and Wagner, B. M. (eds.): Proceedings of the Conference on Effects of Chronic Salicylate Administration. New York, National Institutes of Health, 1966, pp. 26–39.
63. Brewer, E. J., Giannini, E. H., and Person, D. A.: Juvenile Rheumatoid Arthritis. 2nd Ed. Philadelphia, Saunders, 1981.
64. Brewer, E. J., Jr., Bass, J., Baum, J., Cassidy, J. T., Fink, C., Jacobs, J., Hanson, V., Levinson, J. E., Schaller, J., and Stillman, J. S.: Current proposed revision of JRA criteria. Arthritis Rheum., 20:195, 1977.
65. Brewerton, E. J., Jr.: HLA-B27 and the inheritance of susceptibility to rheumatic disease. Arthritis Rheum., 19:656, 1976.
66. Brown, R. A. P., and Currie, J. P.: Observations on gold therapy. Br. Med. J., 1:916, 1953.
67. Bryan, W. J., Doherty, J. H., Jr., and Sculo, T. P.: Tuberculosis in a rheumatoid patient. A case report. Clin. Orthop., 171:206, 1982.
68. Bunim, J., Burch, T. A., and O'Brien, W.: Influence of genetic and environmental factors on the occurrence of rheumatoid arthritis and rheumatoid factor in American Indians. Bull. Rheum. Dis., 14:349, 1964.
69. Burch, T. A., O'Brien, W., and Bunim, J.: Family and genetic studies of rheumatoid arthritis and rheumatoid factor in Blackfeet Indians. Am. J. Public Health, 54:1184, 1964.
70. Bywaters, E. G. L.: The early radiologic signs of rheumatoid arthritis. Bull. Rheum. Dis., 11:231, 1960.
71. Bywaters, E. G. L.: The present status of steroid treatment in rheumatoid arthritis. Proc. R. Soc. Med., 58:649, 1965.
72. Bywaters, E. G. L.: The management of juvenile chronic polyarthritis. Bull. Rheum. Dis., 27:882, 1976.
73. Bywaters, E. G. L., and Ansell, B. M.: Monarticular arthritis in children. Ann. Rheum. Dis., 24:116, 1965.

74. Bywaters, E. G. L., Carter, M. E., and Scott, F. E.: Differential agglutination titre (D.A.T.) in juvenile rheumatoid arthritis. Ann. Rheum. Dis., 18:225, 1959.
75. Bywaters, E. G. L., Glynn, L. E., and Zeldis, A.: Subcutaneous nodules of Still's disease. Ann. Rheum. Dis., 17:278, 1958.
76. Cabot, A., and Becker, A.: The cervical spine in rheumatoid arthritis. Clin. Orthop., 131:130, 1978.
77. Calabro, J. J.: Other extra-articular manifestations of juvenile rheumatoid arthritis. Arthritis Rheum., 20:Suppl. 2:237, 1977.
78. Calabro, J. J., and Garg, S. L.: Psoriatic arthritis in children. Arthritis Rheum., 16:117, 1973.
79. Calabro, J. J., and Marchesano, J. M.: Prognosis in juvenile rheumatoid arthritis. Arthritis Rheum., 8:434, 1965.
80. Calabro, J. J., and Marchesano, J. M.: Juvenile rheumatoid arthritis. Current concepts. N. Engl. J. Med., 277:696, 1967.
81. Calabro, J. J., Holgerson, W. B., Sonpal, G. M., and Khoury, M. I.: Juvenile rheumatoid arthritis: A general review and report of 100 patients observed for 15 years. Semin. Arthritis Rheum., 5:257, 1976.
82. Campbell, R. D., and Straub, L. R.: Surgical considerations for rheumatoid disease in the forearm and wrist. Am. J. Surg., 109:361, 1965.
83. Cassidy, J. T.: Juvenile rheumatoid arthritis. In Kelly, W. N., Harris, E. D., Ruddy, S., and Sledge, C. B. (eds.): Textbook of Rheumatology. Philadelphia, Saunders, 1980, pp. 1279–1305.
84. Cassidy, J. T.: Textbook of Pediatric Rheumatology. New York, Wiley, 1982.
85. Cassidy, J. T., and Martel, W.: Juvenile rheumatoid arthritis: Clinicoradiologic correlations. Arthritis Rheum., 20:Suppl. 2:207, 1977.
86. Cassidy, J. T., and Valkenberg, H. A.: A five year prospective study of rheumatoid factor tests in juvenile rheumatoid arthritis. Arthritis Rheum., 10:83, 1976.
87. Cassidy, J. T., Brody, G. L., and Martel, W.: Monoarticular juvenile rheumatoid arthritis. J. Pediatr., 70:867, 1967.
88. Cervical-spine involvement in rheumatoid arthritis (Editorial). Lancet, 1:586, 1973.
89. Chandler, G. N., and Wright, V.: Deleterious effects of intra-articular hydrocortisone. Lancet, 2:661, 1958.
90. Chandler, H. P., and Dickson, D. B.: Total hip replacement in the young patient. A.A.O.S. Instruct Course Lect., 23:184, 1974.
91. Chandler, H. P., Reinick, F. T., Wixson, R. L., and McCarthy, J. C.: Total hip replacement in patients younger than thirty years old. A five-year follow-up study. J. Bone Joint Surg., 63-A:1426, 1981.
92. Chaplin, D., Pulkki, T., Saarimaa, A., and Vainio, K.: Wrist and finger deformities in juvenile rheumatoid arthritis. Acta Rheumatol. Scand., 15:206, 1969.
93. Charnley, J.: The long-term results of low-friction arthroplasty of the hip performed as a primary intervention. J. Bone Joint Surg., 54-B:61, 1972.
94. Clayton, M. L.: Surgery of the forefoot in rheumatoid arthritis. Clin. Orthop., 16:136, 1960.
95. Clemens, L. E., Albert, L. E., and Ansell, B. M.: HLA studies in IgM rheumatoid factor positive childhood arthritis. Ann. Rheum. Dis., 42:431, 1983.
96. Cleveland, S. E., Reitman, E. E., and Brewer, E. J.: Psychological factors in juvenile rheumatoid arthritis. Arthritis Rheum., 8:1152, 1965.
97. Colver, T.: The prognosis in rheumatoid arthritis in childhood. Arch. Dis. Child., 12:253, 1937.
98. Colville, J., and Raunio, P.: Total hip replacement in juvenile rheumatoid arthritis. Analysis of 59 hips. Acta Orthop. Scand., 50:197, 1979.
99. Conaty, J. P., and Mongan, E. S.: Cervical fusion in rheumatoid arthritis. J. Bone Joint Surg., 63-A:1218, 1981.
100. Copeland, S. A., and Taylor, J. G.: Synovectomy of the elbow in rheumatoid arthritis. The place of excision of the head of the radius. J. Bone Joint Surg., 61-B:69, 1979.
101. Copeman, W. S. C.: Textbook of Rheumatic Diseases. 4th Ed. London, Livingstone, 1969.
102. Corner, B. D.: Reiter's syndrome in childhood. Arch. Dis. Child., 25:398, 1950.
103. Cornil, V.: Memoire sur des coincidences pathologiques du rhumatisme articulaire chronique. C. R. Mem. Soc. Biol. (Paris), 3:3, 1864.
104. Coss, J. A., Jr., and Boots, R. H.: Juvenile rheumatoid arthritis. A study of fifty-six cases with a note on skeletal changes. J. Pediatr., 29:143, 1946.
105. Crowe, W., Hauselman, C., Shear, E., Miller, E. H., Balz, G. P., and Levinson, J. E.: Total hip arthroplasty in children with juvenile rheumatoid arthritis (abstract). Arthritis Rheum., 22:602, 1979.
106. Dale, I.: The treatment of juvenile rheumatoid arthritis with azathioprine. Scand. J. Rheumatol., 1:125, 1972.
107. DeBlecourt, J. J., and Veenstra, S. M.: Transverse lesion in a patient with juvenile rheumatoid arthritis caused by subluxation of some cervical vertebrae. Acta Rheumatol. Scand., 6:251, 1960.
108. Debre, R., Broca, R., and Lamy, M.: Forme endocarditique de la maladie de Still. Arch. Med. Enf., 33:212, 1930.
109. Diamantberger, S.: Du rhumatisme nouveau (polyarthrite déformante) chez l'enfant. Thèse, Paris, 1890.
110. Dixon, A. St. J., et al. (eds.): Salicylates: An International Symposium. Boston, Little, Brown, 1962.
111. Donovan, W. H.: Physical measures in the treatment of juvenile rheumatoid arthritis. Arthritis Rheum., 20:553, 1977.
112. Ebaugh, F. G., Peterson, R. E., Rodman, G. P., and Bunim, J. J.: The anemia of rheumatoid arthritis. Med. Clin. North Am., 39:489, 1955.
113. Edmonds, J., Metzger, A., Teraswaki, P., Bluestone, R., Ansell, B., and Bywaters, E. G. L.: HL-A antigen W27 in juvenile chronic polyarthritis. Ann. Rheum. Dis., 33:576, 1974.
114. Edstrom, G.: Rheumatoid arthritis in children. A clinical study. Acta Paediatr. (Uppsala), 34:334, 1947.
115. Edstrom, G.: Rheumatoid arthritis and Still's disease in children. A survey of 161 cases. Arthritis Rheum., 1:497, 1958.
116. Edstrom, G., and Gedda, P. O.: Clinic and prognosis of rheumatoid arthritis in children. Acta Rheumatol. Scand., 3:129, 1957.
117. Eichenblat, M., Hass, A., and Kessler, I.: Synovectomy of the elbow in rheumatoid arthritis. J. Bone Joint Surg., 64-A:1074, 1982.
118. Ellefsen, F.: Prognosen ved den juvenile reumatiske polyartritt. Tidsskr. Nor. Laegeforen., 83:530, 1963.
119. Ellman, P., and Ball, R. E.: "Rheumatoid disease" with joint and pulmonary manifestations. Br. Med. J., 2:816, 1948.
120. Endresen, G. K. H., Hoyeraal, H. M., and Kass, E.: Platelet count and disease activity in juvenile rheumatoid arthritis. Scand. J. Rheumatol., 6:237, 1977.
121. Engen, T. J.: Adjustable knee or elbow extension orthosis: A new orthotic development. Orthot. Prosthet. Appl. J., March, 1961.
122. Eyring, E. J.: The therapeutic potential of synovectomy in juvenile rheumatoid arthritis. Arthritis Rheum., 11:688, 1968.
123. Eyring, E. J., Longert, A. L., and Bass, J. C.: Synovectomy in juvenile rheumatoid arthritis. J. Bone Joint Surg., 52-A:831, 1970.
124. Ferguson, A. B.: Roentgenographic features of rheumatoid arthritis. J. Bone Joint Surg., 18:297, 1936.
125. Ferlic, D. C., Clayton, M. L., Leidholt, J. D., and Gamble, W. E.: Surgical treatment of the symptom-

atic unstable cervical spine in rheumatoid arthritis. J. Bone Joint Surg., 57-A:349, 1975.
126. Fink, C. W., Baum, J., Paradies, L. H., and Carrell, B. C.: Synovectomy in juvenile rheumatoid arthritis. Ann. Rheum. Dis., 28:612, 1969.
127. Fisher, D. A., Panos, T. C., and Melby, J. C.: Intermittent corticosteroid therapy of juvenile rheumatoid arthritis. Arthritis Rheum. Dis., 19:95, 1960.
128. Fiszman, P., Ansell, B. M., and Renton, P.: Radiological assessment of knees in juvenile chronic arthritis (juvenile rheumatoid arthritis). Scand. J. Rheumatol., 10:145, 1981.
129. Flatt, A. E.: The Care of the Rheumatoid Hand. 2nd Ed. St. Louis, Mosby, 1970.
130. Forestier, J., Jacqueline, F., and Canet, L.: Le rhumatisme inflammatoire chronique de l'enfant. (Etude clinique et radiologique.) Rhumatologie, 11:51, 1959.
131. Forsyth, C. C.: Calcification of digital vessels in a child with rheumatoid arthritis. Arch. Dis. Child., 35:296, 1960.
132. Fowler, R. L., and Berg, E.: Synovectomies in moderately to severely involved rheumatoid knees: An alternative to implant arthroplasty. South. Med. J., 70:181, 1977.
133. Francon, F., Forestier, J., and Robert, P.: Radiographies d'un cas de syndrome de Chauffard-Still. J. Radiol., 21:5, 1937.
134. Freireich, E. J., Ross, J. F., Bayles, T., Emerson, C. P., and Finch, S. C.: Radioactive iron metabolism and erythrocyte survival studies of the mechanism of the anemia associated with rheumatoid arthritis. J. Clin. Invest., 36:1043, 1957.
135. Fried, J. A., Athreya, B., and Gregg, J. R.: The cervical spine in juvenile rheumatoid arthritis. Clin. Orthop., 179:102, 1983.
136. Fujita, H.: A study of synovectomy of the knee joint in rheumatoid arthritis: follow-up study of 127 synovectomized joints and histopathological observation on the regenerated rheumatoid synovium. Cent. Jpn. J. Orthop. Traumatol., 18:1117, 1975.
137. Furst, C., Smiley, W. K., and Ansell, B. M.: Steroid cataract. Ann. Rheum. Dis., 25:364, 1966.
138. Fyfe, W. M.: Rheumatoid arthritis in childhood. Glasgow Med. J., 36:102, 1955.
139. Gariepy, R., Demers, R., and Laurin, C. A.: The prophylactic effect of synovectomy of the knee in rheumatoid arthritis. Can. Med. Assoc. J., 94:1349, 1966.
140. Garrett, A. L., and Campbell, C.: Synovectomy in children. In Cruess, R. L., and Nelson, M. (eds.): Surgery of Rheumatoid Arthritis. Philadelphia, Lippincott, 1971, pp. 111–116.
141. Gauchat, R. D., and May, C. D.: Early recognition of rheumatoid disease with comments on treatment. Pediatrics, 19:672, 1957.
142. Geens, S.: Synovectomy and debridement of the knee in rheumatoid arthritis. Part I. Historical review. J. Bone Joint Surg., 51-A:617, 1969.
143. Ginsberg, J. M.: Protective effect of salicylate on cartilage degeneration. J. Bone Joint Surg., 57-A:831, 1970.
144. Goel, K. M., Rawson, S. P., and Shanks, R. A.: Radiological assessment of fifty patients with juvenile rheumatoid arthritis: Correlation with clinical and laboratory abnormalities. Pediatr. Radiol., 2:51, 1974.
145. Good, R. A., Rotstein, J., and Mazzitello, W. F.: The simultaneous occurrence of rheumatoid arthritis and agammaglobulinemia. J. Lab. Clin. Med., 49:343, 1957.
146. Granberry, W. M.: Synovectomy in juvenile rheumatoid arthritis. Arthritis Rheum., 20:561, 1977.
147. Granberry, G. M.: Soft tissue release in children with juvenile rheumatoid arthritis. Arthritis Rheum., 20:565, 1977.
148. Granberry, W. M., and Brewer, E. J.: Early surgery in juvenile rheumatoid arthritis. A.A.O.S. Instruct. Course Lect., 23:32, 1974.
149. Granberry, W. M., and Brewer, E. J.: Results of synovectomy in children with rheumatoid arthritis. Clin. Orthop., 101:120, 1981.
150. Griffin, P. P., Tachdjian, M. O., and Green, W. T.: Pauciarticular arthritis in children. J.A.M.A., 184:145, 1963.
151. Grokoest, A. W.: Juvenile rheumatoid arthritis. Am. J. Occup. Ther., 19:152, 1965.
152. Grokoest, A. W., Snyder, A. I., and Ragan, C.: Some aspects of juvenile rheumatoid arthritis. Bull. Rheum. Dis., 8:147, 1957.
153. Grokoest, A. W., Snyder, A. I., and Schlaeger, R.: Juvenile Rheumatoid Arthritis. Boston, Little, Brown, 1961.
154. Grossman, B. J., Ozoa, N. F., and Arya, S. C.: Problems in juvenile rheumatoid arthritis. Med. Clin. North Am., 49:33, 1965.
155. Halla, J. T., Fallahi, S., and Hardin, J. G.: Nonreducible rotational head tilt and atlantoaxial lateral mass collapse. Clinical and roentgenographic features in patients with juvenile rheumatoid arthritis and ankylosing spondylitis. Arch. Intern. Med., 143:471, 1983.
156. Halley, D. K., and Charnley, J.: Results of low friction arthroplasty in patients thirty years of age or younger. Clin. Orthop., 112:180, 1975.
157. Hanson, V., Drexler, E., and Kornreich, H.: The relationship factor to age of onset in juvenile rheumatoid arthritis. Arthritis Rheum., 12:82, 1969.
158. Hanson, V., Kornreich, H., and Drexler, E.: Rheumatoid factor in children with lupus erythematosus. Am. J. Dis. Child., 112:28, 1966.
159. Hanson, V., Kornreich, H., Bernstein, B., King, K. K., and Singsen, B.: Prognosis of juvenile rheumatoid arthritis. Arthritis Rheum., 20:279, 1977.
160. Harnagel, E. E.: Long-term use of prednisone and prednisolone in juvenile rheumatoid arthritis. Am. J. Dis. Child., 97:426, 1959.
161. Harris, H. A.: Growth of long bone in childhood, with special refferrence to certain bony striations of metaphysis and to role of vitamins. Arch. Intern. Med., 38:785, 1926.
162. Hatherley, E.: Uveitis and band-shaped keratitis in a case of Still's disease. Proc. R. Soc. Med., 44:978, 1951.
163. Heinmann, W. G., and Freiberger, R. H.: Avascular necrosis of the femoral and humeral heads with high-dose corticosteroid therapy. N. Engl. J. Med., 263:672, 1960.
164. Heller, H., Gafni, J., Michaeli, D., Shahin, N., Sohar, E., Ehrlich, G., Karten, I., and Sokoloff, L.: The arthritis of familial Mediterranean fever (FMF). Arthritis Rheum., 9:1, 1966.
165. Hellstrom, B.: The diagnosis and course of rheumatoid arthritis and benign aseptic arthritis in children. Acta Paediatr. (Uppsala), 50:329, 1961.
166. Hensinger, R. N., DeVito, P. D., and Ragsdale, C. G.: Changes in the cervical spine in juvenile rheumatoid arthritis. J. Bone Joint Surg., 68-A:189, 1986.
167. Herness, D., and Makin, M.: Articular damage in familial Mediterranean fever. J. Bone Joint Surg., 57-A:265, 1975.
168. Hewitt, D., Westropp, C. K., and Acheson, R. M.: Oxford Child Health Survey. Effect of childish ailments on skeletal development. Br. J. Prev. Soc. Med., 9:179, 1955.
169. Heywood, A. W.: Supramalleolar osteotomy in the management of the rheumatoid hindfoot. Clin. Orthop., 177:76, 1983.
170. Holgersson, S., Brattstrom, H., Mogensen, B., and Lidgren, L.: Arthroscopy of the hip in juvenile chronic arthritis. J. Pediatr. Orthop., 1:273, 1981.

171. Holt, P. R.: Measurements of gastrointestinal blood loss in subjects taking aspirin. J. Lab. Clin. Med., 56:717, 1960.
172. Hopkins, J. S.: Lower cervical rheumatoid subluxation with tetraplegia. J. Bone Joint Surg., 49-B:46, 1967.
173. Ibrahim, J.: Die chronische Arthritis im Kindesalter. Z. Orthop. Chir., 34:213, 1914.
174. Isaacson, A. S.: Operative procedures on patients with juvenile rheumatoid arthritis. A.A.O.S. Instruct. Course Lect., 23:37, 1974.
175. Isdale, I. C.: Hip disease in juvenile rheumatoid arthritis. Ann. Rheum. Dis., 29:603, 1970.
176. Isdale, I. C., and Bywaters, E. G. L.: The rash of rheumatoid arthritis and Still's disease. Q. J. Med., 25:377, 1956.
177. Isdale, I. C., and Conlon, P. W.: Atlanto-axial subluxation. A six-year follow-up report. Ann. Rheum. Dis., 30:387, 1971.
178. Ishikawa, H., and Ziff, M.: Electron microscopic observations of immunoreactive cells in the rheumatoid synovial membrane. Arthritis Rheum., 19:1, 1976.
179. Ishikawa, H., Ohno, O., and Hirohata, K.: The purpose and significance of the synovectomy in rheumatoid arthritis: An immunohistological study of regenerated synovial membrane. Clin. Orthop., 14:17, 1979.
180. Ishikawa, H., Ohno, O., and Hirohata, K.: Long-term results of synovectomy in rheumatoid patients. J. Bone Joint Surg., 68-A:198, 1986.
181. Iveson, M., Nanda, B. S., Hancock, J. A. H., Pownall, P. J., and Wright, V.: Reiter's disease in three boys. Ann. Rheum. Dis., 34:364, 1975.
182. Jacobs, J. C.: Sudden death in arthritic children receiving large doses of indomethacin. J.A.M.A., 199:932, 1967.
183. Jacobs, J. H., Hess, E. W., and Beswick, I. P.: Rheumatoid arthritis presenting as tenosynovitis. J. Bone Joint Surg., 39-B:288, 1957.
184. Jacqueline, F., Buojot, A., and Canet, L.: Involvement of the hips in juvenile rheumatoid arthritis. Arthritis Rheum., 4:500, 1961.
185. Jakubowski, S.: Present status of prophylactic synovectomy. In Munthe, E. (ed.): EULAR Bulletin, Monograph series No. 3. Basel, EULAR Publishers, 1978, pp. 175–177.
186. Jakubowski, S., and Rusczcynska, J.: The possibility of surgical treatment in cases of juvenile rheumatoid arthritis. Acta Rheumatol. Scand., 13:113, 1967.
187. Jani, L., and Waigand, D.: Synovectomy of the knee joint in juvenile rheumatoid arthritis. Reconstr. Surg. Traumatol., 12:35, 1971.
188. Jensen, C. M.: Synovectomy with resection of the distal ulna in rheumatoid arthritis of the wrist. Acta Orthop. Scand., 54:754, 1983.
189. Johnson, N. J., and Dodd, K.: Juvenile rheumatoid arthritis. Med. Clin. North Am., 39:459, 1955.
190. Jones, M. C.: Arthritis and arthralgia in infection with Mycoplasma pneumoniae. Thorax, 25:748, 1970.
191. Kampner, S., and Ferguson, A. B.: Efficacy of synovectomy in juvenile rheumatoid arthritis. Clin. Orthop., 88:94, 1972.
192. Kanski, J. J.: Anterior uveitis in juvenile rheumatoid arthritis. Arch. Ophthalmol., 95:1794, 1977.
193. Kellgren, J. H., and Ball, J.: Tendon lesions in rheumatoid arthritis. Ann. Rheum. Dis., 9:48, 1950.
194. Kelly, M.: The correction and prevention of deformity in rheumatoid arthritis. Can. Med. Assoc. J., 81:827, 1959.
195. Kelsey, W. M., and Sharyj, M.: Fatal hepatitis probably due to indomethacin. J.A.M.A., 199:586, 1967.
196. Kennedy, A. C., Smith, D. A., Buchanan, W. W., Anderson, J. B., and Jasani, M. K.: Bone loss in patients with rheumatoid arthritis. Scand. J. Rheumatol., 4:73, 1975.
197. Kienbock, R.: Über infantile chronische Polyarthritis. Fortschr. Geb. Röntgenstr., 23:343, 1915.
198. Kienbock, R.: Über schwere infantile Polyarthritis chronica und ihre Folgezustande. Allgemeiner Wachstumsstillstand und Mikromelie. "Pseudo-Achondroplasie". Fortschr. Geb. Röntgenstr., 30:258, 1922.
199. Kievits, J. H., Goslings, J., Schuit, R. E., and Humans, W.: Rheumatoid arthritis and the positive LE cell phenomenon. Ann. Rheum. Dis., 15:211, 1956.
200. Klassen, R. A., Parlasca, R. J., and Bianco, A. J., Jr.: Total joint arthroplasty in children and adolescents. Mayo Clin. Proc., 54:579, 1979.
201. Knott, M.: Neuromuscular facilitation in the treatment of rheumatoid arthritis. J. Am. Phys. Ther. Assoc., 44:737, 1964.
202. Knutsson, F.: Roentgenological early symptoms and healing phenomena in chronic rheumatoid arthritis. Acta Radiol. (Stockh.), 24:121, 1943.
203. Kobayashi, I., and Ziff, M.: Electron microscopic studies of lymphoid cells in the rheumatoid synovial membrane. Arthritis Rheum., 16:471, 1973.
204. Kornblum, D., Clayton, M. L., and Nash, H. H.: Nontraumatic cervical dislocations in rheumatoid spondylitis. J.A.M.A., 149:431, 1952.
205. Koster, M. S., and Jansen, M., discussed by Corner, B. D.: Reiter's syndrome in childhood. Arch. Dis. Child., 25:398, 1950.
206. Kuhns, J. G.: The foot in chronic arthritis. Clin. Orthop., 16:141, 1960.
207. Kuhns, J. G., and Swaim, L. T.: Disturbances of growth in chronic arthritis in children. Am. J. Dis. Child., 43:1118, 1932.
208. Kulka, J. P., Bocking, D., Ropes, M. W., and Bauer, W.: Early joint lesion of rheumatoid arthritis. Arch. Pathol., 59:129, 1955.
209. Laaksonen, A. I.: A prognostic study of juvenile rheumatoid arthritis. Acta Paediatr. Scand. Suppl. 166, 1966.
210. Laaksonen, A. L., and Laine, V.: A comparative study of joint pain in adult and juvenile rheumatoid arthritis. Ann. Rheum. Dis., 20:386, 1961.
211. Laaksonen, A. L., Koskiahde, V., and Juva, K.: Dosage of antimalarial drugs for children with juvenile rheumatoid arthritis and systemic lupus erythematosus. A clinical study with determination of serum concentration of chloroquine and hydroxychloroquine. Scand. J. Rheumatol., 3:103, 1974.
212. Lachiewicz, P. F., McCaskill, B., Inglis, A., Ranawat, C. S., and Rosenstein, B. D.: Total hip arthroplasty in juvenile rheumatoid arthritis. Two to eleven year results. J. Bone Joint Surg., 68-A:502, 1986.
213. Laine, H., and Mikkelsen, O. A.: Epiphyseal stapling in juvenile rheumatoid gonarthritis. Acta Rheumatol. Scand., 14:317, 1968.
214. Lang, A. G., and Klassen, R. A.: Cup arthroplasties in teenagers and children. J. Bone Joint Surg., 59-A:444, 1977.
215. Laurin, C. A., DeMarchias, J., Daziano, L., Gariepy, R., and Derome, A.: Long-term results of synovectomy of the knee in rheumatoid patients. J. Bone Joint Surg., 56-A:521, 1974.
216. Laurin, C. A., and Favreau, J. C.: Rheumatoid disease in children. Can. Med. Assoc. J., 89:288, 1963.
217. Levinson, J. E., Baum, J., Brewer, E. J., Fink, C., Hanson, V., and Schaller, J.: Comparison of tolmetin sodium and aspirin in the treatment of juvenile rheumatoid arthritis. J. Paediatr., 91:799, 1977.
218. Lewis, S. M., and Porter, I. H.: Erythrocyte survival in rheumatoid arthritis. Ann. Rheum. Dis., 19:54, 1960.
219. Lewis-Fanning, E.: Report on an inquiry into the aetiological factors associated with rheumatoid arthritis. Ann. Rheum. Dis., 9:Suppl., 1956.
220. Lietman, P. S., and Bywaters, E. G. L.: Pericarditis

in juvenile rheumatoid arthritis. Pediatrics, 32:856, 1963.
221. Linclau, L. A., Winia, W. P., and Korst, J. K.: Synovectomy of the elbow in rheumatoid arthritis. Acta Orthop. Scand., 54:935, 1983.
222. Lindberg, I. F.: Juvenile rheumatoid arthritis. A followup of 75 cases. Arch. Dis. Child., 39:576, 1964.
223. Lindsley, C. B., and Schaller, J. G.: Arthritis associated with inflammatory bowel disease in children. J. Pediatr., 84:16, 1974.
224. Lockie, L. M.: Steroid therapy in rheumatoid arthritis. J.A.M.A., 170:1063, 1959.
225. Lockie, L. M., and Norcross, B. M.: Juvenile rheumatoid arthritis. Pediatrics, 2:694, 1948.
226. London, P. S.: Synovectomy of knee in rheumatoid arthritis. J. Bone Joint Surg., 37-B:392, 1955.
227. Lourie, H., and Stewart, W. A.: Spontaneous atlantoaxial dislocation. A complication of rheumatoid disease. N. Engl. J. Med., 265:677, 1961.
228. Ludwig, A. O.: Psychogenic factors in rheumatoid arthritis. Bull. Rheum. Dis., 2:15, 1952.
229. McEwin, C., Ziff, M., Carmel, P., Ditata, D., and Tanner, M.: The relationship to rheumatoid arthritis of its so-called variants. Arthritis Rheum., 1:481, 1958.
230. McGovern, J. P., and Merritt, D. H.: Sarcoidosis in childhood. Adv. Pediatr., 8:97, 1956.
231. McGraw, R. W., and Rusch, R. M.: Atlanto-axial arthrodesis. J. Bone Joint Surg., 55-B:482, 1973.
232. McMaster, M.: Synovectomy of the knee in juvenile rheumatoid arthritis. J. Bone Joint Surg., 54-B:263, 1972.
233. Maddison, P. J., and Bacon, P. A.: Vitamin D deficiency, spontaneous fractures, and osteopenia in rheumatoid arthritis. Br. Med. J., 4:433, 1974.
234. Makela, A. L.: Naproxen in the treatment of juvenile rheumatoid arthritis; metabolism, safety and efficacy. Scand. J. Rheumatol., 6:193, 1977.
235. Makela, A. L.: Dosage of salicylates for children with juvenile rheumatoid arthritis: A prospective clinical trial with three different preparations of acetylsalicylic acid. Acta Paediatr. Scand., 68:423, 1979.
236. Manheimer, R. H., Greene, K. R., and Kroll, F.: Juvenile rheumatoid arthritis in New York City. Arch. Pediatr., 76:173, 1959.
237. Margulies, M. E., Katz, I., and Rosenberg, M.: Spontaneous dislocation of the atlanto-axial joint in rheumatoid spondylitis. Recovery from quadriplegia following surgical decompression. Neurology, 5:290, 1955.
238. Marmor, L.: Synovectomy of the knee. Clin. Orthop., 44:151, 1966.
239. Marmor, L.: Surgery in Rheumatoid Arthritis. Philadelphia, Lea & Febiger, 1967.
240. Martel, W., Holt, J. F., and Cassidy, J. T.: Roentgenologic manifestations of juvenile rheumatoid arthritis. A.J.R., 88:400, 1962.
241. Martin, G. M., Lowman, E. W., and Kammerer, W. H.: Physical medicine in rheumatoid arthritis. Arthritis Rheum., 6:177, 1963.
242. Meyerowitz, S., Jacox, R. F., and Hess, D. W.: Monozygotic twins discordant for rheumatoid arthritis: A genetic, clinical and psychological study of eight sets. Arthritis Rheum., 11:1, 1968.
243. Middlemiss, J. H.: Juvenile rheumatoid arthritis (Still's disease). Proc. R. Soc. Med., 44:805, 1951.
244. Miele, J. F., Piasio, M. A., and Goldberg, M. J.: Orthopedic deformity occurring in Down syndrome patients with juvenile rheumatoid arthritis. J. Bone Joint Surg., 10:130, 1986.
245. Milch, R. A. (ed.): Surgery of Arthritis. Baltimore, Williams & Wilkins, 1964.
246. Miller, D. S.: Monarticular arthritis of children. Med. Clin. North Am., 49:49, 1965.
247. Miller, J. J., and French, J. W.: Myocarditis in juvenile rheumatoid arthritis. Am. J. Dis. Child., 131:205, 1977.
248. Moesmann, G.: Factors precipitating and predisposing to rheumatoid arthritis as illustrated by studies on monozygotic twins. Acta Rheumatol. Scand., 5:291, 1959.
249. Mogensen, B., Svantesson, H., and Lidgren, L.: Surface replacement of the hip in juvenile chronic arthritis. Scand. J. Rheumatol., 10:269, 1981.
250. Mogensen, B., Brattstrom, H., Svantesson, H., and Lidgren, L.: Soft tissue release of the hip in juvenile chronic arthritis. Scand. J. Rheumatol., 12:17, 1983.
251. Mogensen, B., Brattstrom, H., Ekelund, L., Svantesson, H., and Lidgren, L.: Synovectomy of the hip in juvenile chronic arthritis. J. Bone Joint Surg., 64-B:295, 1982.
252. Moore, T. L., and Weiss, T. D.: Treatment of juvenile rheumatoid arthritis. Bull. Rheum. Dis., 32:21, 1982.
253. Moos, R. H.: Personality factors associated with rheumatoid arthritis. A review. J. Chronic Dis., 17:41, 1964.
254. Moran, H. M., Ansell, B. M., Mowbray, J. F., Levinsky, R. J., and Soothill, J. R.: Antigen antibody complexes in the serum of patients with juvenile chronic arthritis. Arch. Dis. Child., 54:120, 1979.
255. Muir, A., and Cossar, I. A.: Aspirin and gastric hemorrhage. Lancet, 1:539, 1959.
256. Munthe, E. (ed.): Care of rheumatic children. EULAR Bulletin Monograph Series No. 3. Basel, EULAR Publishers, 1978.
257. Murray, W. R.: Juvenile rheumatoid arthritis. Curr. Pract. Orthop. Surg., 6:171, 1975.
258. Nathan, F. F., and Bickel, W. H.: Spontaneous axial subluxation in a child as the first sign of juvenile rheumatoid arthritis. J. Bone Joint Surg., 50-A:1675, 1968.
259. Neumann, H. W., and Weber, C.: Synovektomien bei der juvenilen Rheumatoid Arthritis. Beitr. Orthop. Traumatol., 25:468, 1978.
260. Newman, R. J., and Fitton, J. M.: Conservation of metatarsal heads in surgery of rheumatoid arthritis of the forefoot. Acta Orthop. Scand., 54:417, 1983.
261. Nomenclature and classification of arthritis in children. European League against Rheumatism. EULAR Bull. 4 (Basel), 1977.
262. Norcross, B. M.: Treatment of connective tissue diseases with a new non-steroid compound (indomethacin). Arthritis Rheum., 6:290, 1963.
263. O'Driscoll, S., and O'Driscoll, M.: Osteomalacia in rheumatoid arthritis. Ann. Rheum. Dis., 39:1, 1980.
264. Pahle, J. A., Kass, E., and Munthe, E.: Orthopaedic surgery for childhood arthritis. Clin. Rheum. Dis., 4:425, 1978.
265. Pellicci, P. M., Ranawat, C. S., Tsairis, P., and Bryan, W. J.: A prospective study of the progression of rheumatoid arthritis of the cervical spine. J. Bone Joint Surg., 63-A:342, 1981.
266. Peltier, L. F.: The classic: Concerning arthritis deformans juvenilis. Professor Georg C. Perthes. Clin. Orthop., 158:5, 1981.
267. Pettersson, H., and Rydholm, U.: Radiologic classification of knee joint destruction in juvenile chronic arthritis. Pediatr. Radiol., 14:419, 1984.
268. Petty, B. G., Zahka, K. G., and Berstein, M. T.: Aspirin hepatitis associated with encephalopathy. J. Pediatr., 93:881, 1978.
269. Pierson, R. N., Jr., Holt, P. R., Watson, R. M., and Keating, R. P.: Aspirin and gastrointestinal bleeding. Am. J. Med., 31:259, 1961.
270. Porter, B. B., Richardson, C., and Vainio, K.: Rheumatoid arthritis of the elbow. The results of synovectomy. J. Bone Joint Surg., 56-B:427, 1974.
271. Rahal, J. J., Millian, S. J., and Noviega, E. R.: Coxsackie virus and adenovirus infection; association

with acute febrile and juvenile rheumatoid arthritis. J.A.M.A., 235:2496, 1976.
272. Rawson, A. J., Abelson, N. M., and Hollander, J. L.: Studies on the pathogenesis of rheumatoid joint inflammation. II. Intracytoplasmic particulate complexes in rheumatoid synovial fluids. Ann. Intern. Med., 62:281, 1965.
273. Reimann, H. R.: Periodic disease; a probable syndrome including periodic fever, benign paroxysmal peritonitis, cyclic neutropenia and intermittent arthralgia. J.A.M.A., 136:239, 1948.
274. Rhinelander, F. W.: The effectiveness of splinting and bracing on rheumatoid arthritis. Arthritis Rheum., 2:270, 1959.
275. Rhinelander, F. W., and Ropes, M. W.: Adjustable casts in the treatment of joint deformities. J. Bone Joint Surg., 27:311, 1945.
276. Richardson, B., and Stobo, J. D.: The major histocompatibility complex antigens in rheumatoid arthritis and juvenile arthritis. Bull. Rheum. Dis., 31:21, 1981.
277. Riley, M. J., Ansell, B. M., and Bywaters, E. G. L.: Radiological manifestations of ankylosing spondylitis according to age at onset. Ann. Rheum. Dis., 30:138, 1971.
278. Roberts, F. D., Hagedorn, A. B., Slocumb, C. H., and Owen, C. A.: Evaluation of the anemia of rheumatoid arthritis. Blood, 21:470, 1963.
279. Roles, N. C.: Synovectomy of the knee. In Arden, G. P., and Ansell, B. M. (eds.): Surgical Management of Juvenile Chronic Polyarthritis. London, Academic Press; New York, Grune & Stratton, 1978, pp. 75–91.
280. Roles, N. C., Arden, G. P., and Ansell, B. M.: Synovectomy of the knee in juvenile chronic arthritis. (Abstract). J. Bone Joint Surg., 60-B:138, 1978.
281. Rombouts, J. J., and Rombouts-Lindemans, C.: Involvement of the hip in juvenile rheumatoid arthritis. Acta Rheumatol. Scand., 17:248, 1971.
282. Ropes, M. W., Bennett, G. A., Cobb, S., Jacox, R., and Jessar, R. A.: 1958 Revision of diagnostic criteria for rheumatoid arthritis. Bull. Rheum. Dis., 9:175, 1958.
283. Rosberg, G., and Laine, V.: Natural history of radiological changes of knee joint in juvenile rheumatoid arthritis. Acta Paediatr. Scand., 56:671, 1967.
284. Rosenberg, E. F., Baggenstoss, A. H., and Hench, P. S.: The causes of death in thirty cases of rheumatoid arthritis. Ann. Intern. Med., 20:903, 1944.
285. Rothschild, B. M., and Hanissian, A. S.: Severe generalized (Charcot-like) joint destruction in juvenile rheumatoid arthritis. Clin. Orthop., 155:75, 1981.
286. Rotstein, J.: Simple Splinting. Philadelphia, Saunders, 1965.
287. Ruddlesdin, C., Ansell, B. M., Arden, G. P., and Swann, M.: Total hip replacement in children with juvenile chronic arthritis. J. Bone Joint Surg., 68-B:218, 1986.
288. Rydholm, U., Boegard, T., and Lidgren, L.: Total knee replacement in juvenile chronic arthritis. Scand. J. Rheumatol., 14:329, 1985.
289. Rydholm, U., Elborgh, R., Ranstam, J., Schroder, A., Svantesson, H., and Lidgren, L.: Synovectomy of the knee in juvenile chronic arthritis. A retrospective, consecutive followup study. J. Bone Joint Surg., 68-B:223, 1986.
290. Sack, K. E., and Miller, C.: Examining adults and children for rheumatic disease. J. Musculoskelet. Med., 3:19, 1986.
291. Sairanen, E.: On micrognathia in juvenile rheumatoid arthritis. Acta Rheumatol. Scand., 10:133, 1964.
292. Sairanen, E., and Laaksonen, A. L.: The toxicity of gold therapy in children suffering from rheumatoid arthritis. Ann. Pediatr. Fenn., 8:105, 1962.
293. Sarokhan, A. J., Scott, R. D., Thomas, W. H., Sledge, C. B., Ewald, F. C., and Cloos, D. W.: Total knee arthroplasty in juvenile rheumatoid arthritis. J. Bone Joint Surg., 65-A:1071, 1983.
294. Sataline, L. R., and Farmer, H.: Impaired vision after prolonged chloroquine therapy. N. Engl. J. Med., 266:346, 1962.
295. Schaller, J. G.: Histo-compatibility antigens in childhood onset arthritis. J. Pediatr., 88:926, 1976.
296. Schaller, J. G.: Ankylosing spondylitis of childhood. Arthrit. Rheum., 20:398, 1977.
297. Schaller, J. G.: Arthritis and immunodeficiency. Arthrit. Rheum., 20:443, 1977.
298. Schaller, J. G.: The seronegative spondyloarthropalsies of childhood. Clin. Orthop., 143:76, 1979.
299. Schaller, J. G., and Wedgwood, R. J.: Classification of juvenile rheumatoid arthritis. New Engl. J. Med., 277:1374, 1967.
300. Schaller, J. G., and Wedgwood, R. J.: Juvenile rheumatoid arthritis: a review. Pediatrics, 50:940, 1972.
301. Schaller, J. G., Bitnum, S., and Wedgwood, R. J.: Ankylosing spondylitis with childhood onset. J. Pediat., 74:505, 1969.
302. Scharf, J., Levy, J., Benderly, A., and Nahir, M.: Pericardial tamponade in juvenile rheumatoid arthritis. Arthrit. Rheum., 19:760, 1976.
303. Schlesinger, B. E.: Rheumatoid arthritis in the young. Br. Med. J., 2:197, 1949.
304. Schlesinger, B. E., Forsyth, C. C., White, R. H., Smellie, J. M., and Stroud, C. E.: Observations on the clinical course and treatment of one hundred cases of Still's disease. Arch. Dis. Child., 36:65, 1961.
305. Schnitzer, T. J., and Ansell, B. M.: Amyloidosis in juvenile chronic polyarthritis. Arthritis Rheum., 20:245, 1977.
306. Schutt, A. H., and Martin, G. M.: Rehabilitation medicine for the patient with arthritis. Orthop. Clin. North Am., 2:623, 1971.
307. Scott, P. J., Ansell, B. M., and Huskisson, E. C.: Measurement of pain in juvenile chronic polyarthritis. Ann. Rheum. Dis., 36:186, 1977.
308. Scott, R. D., and Sledge, C. B.: The surgery of juvenile rheumatoid arthritis. In Kelly, W. N., Harris, E. D., Ruddy, S., and Sledge, C. B. (eds.): Textbook of Rheumatology, Philadelphia, Saunders, 1980, pp. 2014–2019.
309. Scott, R. D., Sarokhan, A. J., and Dalziel, R.: Total hip and total knee arthroplasty in juvenile rheumatoid arthritis. Clin. Orthop., 182:90, 1984.
310. Sharp, J., and Purser, D. W.: Spontaneous atlanto-axial dislocation in ankylosing spondylitis and rheumatoid arthritis. Ann. Rheum. Dis., 20:47, 1961.
311. Sherk, H. H., Pasquariello, P. S., and Watters, W. C.: Multiple dislocations of the cervical spine in a patient with juvenile rheumatoid arthritis and Down's syndrome. Clin. Orthop., 162:37, 1982.
312. Sherman, M. S.: The nonspecificity of synovial reactions. Bull. Hosp. Joint Dis., 12:110, 1951.
313. Shore, A., and Ansell, B. M.: Juvenile psoriatic arthritis—an analysis of 60 cases. J. Pediatr., 100:529, 1982.
314. Short, C. L., Bauer, W., and Reynolds, W. E.: Rheumatoid Arthritis. Cambridge, Harvard University Press, 1957.
315. Sievers, K., Ahvonen, P., Aho, K., and Wager, O.: Serological patterns in juvenile rheumatoid arthritis. Rheumatism, 19:88, 1963.
316. Sills, E. M.: Errors in diagnosis of juvenile rheumatoid arthritis. Johns Hopkins Med. J., 133:88, 1973.
317. Simon, S., Whiffen, J., and Shapiro, F.: Leg-length discrepancies in monoarticular and pauciarticular juvenile rheumatoid arthritis. J. Bone Joint Surg., 63-A:209, 1981.
318. Singsen, B. H., Bernstein, B. H., Koster-King, K. G., Glovsky, M. M., and Hanson, V.: Reiter's syn-

319. Singsen, B. H., Isaacson, A. S., Bernstein, B. H., Patzakis, M. J., Kornreich, H. K., King, K. K., and Hanson, V.: Total hip replacement in children with arthritis. Arthritis Rheum., 21:401, 1978.
320. Skoglund, R. R., Schanberger, J. E., and Kaplan, J. M.: Cyclophosphamide therapy for severe juvenile rheumatoid arthritis. Am. J. Dis. Child., 121:531, 1971.
321. Sledge, C. B.: Joint replacement surgery in juvenile rheumatoid arthritis. Arthritis Rheum., 20:567, 1977.
322. Sliwinsky, A. J., and Zvaifler, N. J.: In vivo synthesis of IgG by rheumatoid synovium. J. Lab. Clin. Med., 76:304, 1970.
323. Smiley, J. D., Sachs, C., and Ziff, M.: In vitro synthesis of immunoglobulin by rheumatoid synovial membrane. J. Clin. Invest., 47:624, 1968.
324. Smiley, W. K.: The eye changes of Still's disease. Proc. R. Soc. Med., 51:597, 1958.
325. Smiley, W. K., and Kanski, J. J.: In Arden, G. P., and Ansell, B. M. (eds.): Surgical Management of Juvenile Chronic Polyarthritis. London, Academic Press; New York, Grune & Stratton, 1978, p. 235.
326. Smiley, W. K., May, E., and Bywaters, E. G. L.: Ocular presentations of Still's disease and their treatment. Ann. Rheum. Dis., 16:371, 1957.
327. Smith, P. H., Benn, R. T., and Sharp, J.: Natural history of rheumatoid cervical luxations. Ann. Rheum. Dis., 31:431, 1972.
328. Smith-Peterson, M. N.: Arthroplasty of the hip. J. Bone Joint Surg., 21:269, 1939.
329. Sneh, E., Pras, M., Michaeli, D., Shahin, H., and Gafni, J.: Protracted arthritis in familial Mediterranean fever. Rheum. Rehabil., 16:102, 1977.
330. Sokoloff, L.: The pathology of rheumatoid arthritis and allied disorders. In Hollander, J. L. (ed.): Arthritis and Allied Conditions. 7th Ed. Philadelphia, Lea & Febiger, 1966.
331. Somerville, E. W.: Flexion contractures of the knee. J. Bone Joint Surg., 42-B:730, 1960.
332. Stastny, P., and Fink, C. W.: Different HLA-D associations in adult and juvenile rheumatoid arthritis. J. Clin. Invest., 63:124, 1979.
333. Stecher, R. M.: Hereditary factors in arthritis. Med. Clin. North Am., 39:499, 1955.
334. Stecher, R. M., Hersh, A. H., Solomon, W. M., and Wolpaw, R.: The genetics of rheumatoid arthritis: Analyses of 224 families. Am. J. Hum. Genet., 5:118, 1953.
335. Steinbrocker, O., and Argyros, T. G.: Phenylbutazone as a therapeutic agent in rheumatic disease. Arthritis Rheum., 3:368, 1960.
336. Steinbrocker, O., Traeger, C. H., and Batterman, R. C.: Therapeutic criteria in rheumatoid arthritis. J.A.M.A., 140:659, 1949.
337. Still, G. F.: On a form of chronic joint disease in children. Med. Chir. Trans., 80:47, 1897.
338. Stillman, J. S., and Barry, P. E.: Juvenile rheumatoid arthritis: Series 2. Arthritis Rheum., 20:Suppl. 2:171, 1977.
339. Stovell, P. B., Ahuja, S. C., and Inglis, A. E.: Pseudarthrosis of the proximal femoral epiphysis in juvenile rheumatoid arthritis. J. Bone Joint Surg., 57-A:860, 1975.
340. Stubbe, L.: Occult blood in feces after administration of aspirin. Br. Med. J., 5104:1062, 1958.
341. Sury, B.: Rheumatoid Arthritis in Children. A Clinical Study. Thesis. Copenhagen, Munksgaard, 1952.
342. Sury, B.: Late prognosis in juvenile rheumatoid arthritis (Still's disease). Atti del X Congresso della lega internazionale contro il Reumatismo, Torino, 1961.
343. Swann, M.: Management of lower limb deformities. In Arden, G. P., and Ansell, B. M. (eds.): Surgical Management of Juvenile Chronic Polyarthritis. London, Academic Press, 1978, pp. 97–115.
344. Swann, M., and Ansell, B. M.: Soft-tissue release of the hips in children with juvenile chronic arthritis. J. Bone Joint Surg., 68-B:404, 1986.
345. Sydnes, O. A.: On the electrophoretic estimated serum proteins in relation to the latex test and Waaler's test in rheumatoid arthritis. Acta Rheumatol. Scand., 9:237, 1963.
346. Taylor, A. R., Mukerjea, S. K., and Rana, N. A.: Excision of the head of the radius in rheumatoid arthritis. J. Bone Joint Surg., 58-B:485, 1976.
347. Towner, S. R., Michet, C. J., O'Fallon, W. M., and Nelson, A. M.: The epidemiology of juvenile rheumatoid arthritis in Rochester, Minnesota, 1960–1979. Arthritis Rheum., 26:1208, 1983.
348. Troncy, R.: La maladie de Still chez l'enfant; étude critique. Thèse. Faculte de Medecine et de Pharmacie de Lyon, 1950.
349. Ungar, G., Damgaard, E., and Hummel, F. P.: Action of salicylates and related drugs on inflammation. Am. J. Physiol., 171:545, 1952.
350. Valeyos, E., Leidholt, J., and Smyth, C.: Arthropathy associated with steroid therapy. Ann. Intern. Med., 64:759, 1966.
351. Van, H., Souter, S., and Utsinger, P. D.: Viral arthritis. Clin. Rheum. Dis., 4:225, 1978.
352. Van Metre, T. E., Niermann, W. A., and Rosen, L. J.: A comparison of cortisone, prednisone, and other adrenal cortical hormones. J. Allergy, 31:531, 1960.
353. Vanace, P.: Results of the latex agglutination and inhibition tests in children with rheumatoid arthritis. Am. J. Dis. Child., 102:777, 1961.
354. Vaughn, J. H.: The rheumatoid factors. In Hollander, J. L. (ed.): Arthritis and Allied Conditions, 7th Ed. Philadelphia, Lea & Febiger, 1966, p. 88.
355. Vesterdal, E., and Sury, B.: Iridocyclitis and band-shaped corneal opacity in juvenile rheumatoid arthritis. Acta Ophthalmol., 28:322, 1950.
356. Walsh, H.: Some clinical features of juvenile rheumatoid arthritis. Med. J. Aust., 49:507, 1962.
357. Ward, L. E., Polley, H. F., Slocumb, C. H., and Heuch, P. S.: Cortisone in treatment of rheumatoid arthritis. J.A.M.A., 152:119, 1953.
358. Watkings, A. L.: Therapeutic exercise in rheumatoid arthritis. Arthritis Rheum., 2:21, 1959.
359. Werne, S.: Spontaneous dislocation of the atlas (as a complication of rheumatoid arthritis). Acta Rheumatol. Scand., 3:101, 1957.
360. Wilkinson, M., and Jones, B. S.: Serum and synovial fluid proteins in arthritis. Ann. Rheum. Dis., 21:51, 1962.
361. Wilkinson, V. A.: Juvenile chronic arthritis in adolescence: Facing the reality. Int. Rehabil. Med., 3:11, 1980.
362. Williams, M. H.: Recovery of Mycoplasma from rheumatoid synovial fluid. In Duthie, J. J. R., and Alexander, W. R. M. (eds.): Rheumatic Diseases. Baltimore, Williams & Wilkins, 1968, p. 172.
363. Wood, P. H. N.: Salicylates. Bull. Rheum. Dis., 13:297, 1963.
364. Wood, P.: Special meeting on nomenclature and classification of arthritis in children. In Munthe, E. (ed.): EULAR Bulletin, Monograph series No. 3. Basel, EULAR Publishers, 1978, p. 47.
365. Wood, P. H. N.: Criteria for chronic arthritis of childhood immunogenetics in rheumatology. Int. Congr. Ser., 602:159, 1982.
366. Young, A., Kinsella, P., and Boland, P.: Stress fractures of the lower limb in patients with rheumatoid arthritis. J. Bone Joint Surg., 63-B:239, 1981.
367. Ziff, M.: The agglutination reaction as a diagnostic aid in rheumatoid arthritis. Bull. Rheum. Dis., 7:13, 1956.

368. Ziff, M.: Pathophysiology of rheumatoid arthritis. Fed. Proc., 32:131, 1973.
369. Ziff, M.: Immunological aspects of rheumatoid synovitis—25 years. Arthritis Rheum., 20:Suppl.:s31–s33, 1977.
370. Ziff, M., and Baum, J.: Laboratory findings in rheumatoid arthritis. In Hollander, J. L. (ed.): Arthritis and Allied Conditions. 7th Ed. Philadelphia, Lea & Febiger, 1966, p. 236.
371. Ziff, M., Contreras, V., and McEwen, C.: Spondylitis in postpubertal patients with rheumatoid arthritis of juvenile onset. Ann. Rheum. Dis., 15:40, 1956.
372. Zvaifler, N. J.: The immunopathology of joint inflammation in rheumatoid arthritis. Adv. Immunol., 16:265, 1973.

GOUT

Gout is a congenital disturbance of uric acid metabolism that is inherited as an autosomal dominant trait. It is primarily a disease of adults, only occasionally occurring in children. Hyperuricemia is 20 times as frequent in men as in women. Deposition of uric acid in various mesenchymal tissues results in an inflammatory response.

Hyperuricemia is present in Lesch-Nyhan syndrome, which is characterized by mental retardation, choreoathetoid movements, scissoring of lower limbs, and self-mutilation. The condition is caused by an enzyme defect in hypoxanthine guanine phosphoribosyltransferase activity.

The clinical picture of gout in children is similar to that of adults. It is characterized by acute and recurring attacks of severely painful arthritis; deposition of sodium urate (tophi) in the articular, periarticular, and subcutaneous tissues; and in the late advanced stages of the disease by cardiovascular lesions, nephritis with urinary calculi, and frequently severe crippling. Radiograms of the joints in the early stages are usually normal, but later will show areas of bone erosion. The uric acid level of the blood will be elevated.

Treatment of gout in children is the same as that of adults. Most cases of gout can be controlled with medicinal treatment. In the late stages of the disease, tophaceous destruction of tendons, ligaments, and bone may be avoided by carefully selected surgical procedures. Excision and curettage of tophi are indicated when they interfere with the function of tendons and joints, when they encroach upon nerves, or when they threaten to cause skin necrosis and ulceration. In the latter case, the tophi may become so large and unsightly as to interfere with wearing of shoes and gloves.

On occasion, amputation of the toes may be necessary. Other procedures that may be employed include partial resection of tendons, resection of joints, arthroplasty, or arthrodesis of painful joints.

References

1. Akizuki, S.: A population study of hyperuricaemia and gout in Japan. Analysis of sex, age, and occupational differences in thirty-four thousand people living in Nagano Prefecture. Ryumachi, 22:201, 1982.
2. Friedman, M., and Byers, S.: Increased renal excretion of urate in young patients with gout. Am. J. Med., 9:31, 1950.
3. Hoyningen-Huene, C.: Gout and glycogen storage disease in preadolescent brothers. Arch. Intern. Med., 118:471, 1966.
4. Larmon, W. A., and Kurtz, J. F.: The surgical management of chronic tophaceous gout. J. Bone Joint Surg., 40:743, 1958.
5. Laroche, C., Cremer, G. A., Sereni, D., and Auscher, C.: Familial juvenile gout caused by partial HGPRT deficiency with neurologic manifestations; a variant of the Lesch-Nyhan syndrome? Bull. Mem. Acad. R. Med. Belg., 135:219, 1980.
6. Riley, I.: Gout and cerebral palsy in a three-year-old boy. Arch. Dis. Child., 35:293, 1960.
7. Rosenthal, I., Gaballah, S., and Rafelson, M.: Gout in infancy manifested by renal failure. Pediatrics, 33:251, 1964.
8. Simmonds, H. A., Cameron, J. S., Potter, C. F., Warren, D., Gibson, T., and Farebrother, D.: Renal failure in young subjects with familial gout. Adv. Exp. Med. Biol., 122-A:15, 1980.
9. Talbott, J.: Selected aspects of acute and gouty arthritis. An internist's interpretation of an orthopedist's experiences with gout and gouty arthritis. J. Bone Joint Surg., 40-A:994, 1958.

HEMOPHILIA

Hemophilia, a genetically determined disorder, is characterized by abnormality of the coagulation mechanism due to functional deficiency of a specific factor, namely VIII or IX.

Since Biblical times the crippling deformities of the musculoskeletal system and death resulting from uncontrolled hemorrhage are well depicted in the pages of history. Talmudic writings of 200 A.D. state that a child whose siblings had bled excessively after circumcision was excused from the ritual.[104] Queen Victoria of England transmitted the gene through her daughters to the ruling families of Russia, Spain, and Austria.

The name *hemophilia*, coined by Hopff in 1828, means blood loving. Wright is credited with being the first to demonstrate the prolonged clotting time in the disorder.[220] The deficient substance was isolated by Patek and Taylor in 1937—they named it antihemophilic globulin.[156]

Definite advances have been made in the management of hemophilia in the past four decades. The treatment of the coagulation defect became relatively simple with the advent of preservation of plasma from which fractions were obtained. The rise in incidence of acquired immunodeficiency syndrome (AIDS) in 1981, however, created horrendous problems in the management of hemophiliac patients.

Incidence

It is estimated to be 1 per 10,000 male births in the United States of America, and 0.8 per 10,000 male births in England.[11, 52]

Classification and Inheritance

The hemophilias may be subclassified as follows:

Hemophilia A. "Classic hemophilia" results from a congenital deficiency of factor VIII—antihemophilic factor (AHF) or antihemophilic globulin (AHG). This type comprises about 80 per cent of cases and is caused by a gene carried on the X chromosome. It occurs in the male and is transmitted by asymptomatic female carriers. A female could be affected if her mother were a carrier and her father a hemophiliac; this, however, is very rare.

Hemophilia B. "Christmas disease" is due to a deficiency of factor IX (plasma thromboplastin component [PTC] or Christmas factor). Its clinical manifestations are quite similar to those of classic hemophilia. The hereditary transmission is also by an X-linked recessive gene. This type is the cause of about 15 per cent of cases.

Von Willebrand's Disease. In this bleeding disorder both factor VIII deficiency and platelet functional abnormality are present. It is inherited as an autosomal dominant trait, occurring in both males and females. The bleeding disorder is relatively mild.

Factor VIII, a glycoprotein with a molecular weight of two million, is composed of subunits of about 200,000 molecular weight. All these subunits contain carbohydrate and are held together by disulfide bonds.[103, 167] The precoagulant sex-linked hemophiliac defect is located on the lighter protein portion of the glycoprotein, whereas the autosomal dominant von Willebrand defect is related to the larger molecular weight carbohydrate moiety of the molecule.[133]

Clinical Picture

Uncontrolled hemorrhage and repeated episodes of bleeding are the hallmarks of hemophilia. The severity of the disease varies from patient to patient, but it is constant in any one patient. Clinical manifestations of hemophilia A and B are similar; they depend on the blood levels of factor VIII or IX. The level of hemostasis is normal when the blood level of either factor is 50 to 100 per cent of normal. When the functional plasma level of the factor is *25 to 50 per cent* of normal the hemophilia is *mild*; excessive bleeding occurs only after major trauma or during surgery; when the plasma level of the factor is *5 to 25 per cent* of normal, the hemophilia is *moderate*; severe uncontrolled bleeding occurs after minor injury or during an operative procedure; when it is *1 to 5 per cent* of normal the hemophilia is *moderately severe* with major hemorrhage taking place after minor injury or unrecognized mild trauma. When the plasma levels of factor VIII or IX are below *1 per cent*, the hemophilia is considered *very severe*; clinically there are repeated spontaneous hemorrhages into joints and bleeding into deep soft tissues.

Abnormal bleeding may occur in any area of the body. Joints are the most frequent sites of repeated hemorrhage; the sites next in frequency are muscles and soft tissues. In the severe hemophiliac the abnormal bleeding tendency may manifest itself in the neonatal period or early infancy. Ordinarily the ecchymosis and soft-tissue bleeding are minor, resorb relatively readily, and are not detected by the parents. When the infant begins to crawl and begins to bump into objects, or when he attempts to stand and falls, abnormal bleeding into joints and soft tissues is noted by the parents. At this stage the infant is usually seen by the pediatrician. It is crucial to have a high index of suspicion for hemophilia in order to prevent serious consequences of invasive treatment such as aspiration of joints. About three fourths of bleeding sustained by hemophiliacs is into either the joints, the deep soft tissues, or both.

Hemophilic Arthropathy

Site of Involvement. The weight-bearing joints are most commonly affected, with frequency of involvement being, in descending order: knee, elbow, shoulder, ankle, wrist, and hip. The vertebral column is rarely involved. Any joint, however, may be the site of pathologic change.

Pathophysiology. This was initially described by Konig.[112] There are an initial stage of synovial reaction to the bleeding into the joint and a later stage of cartilage degeneration and joint destruction. Following injury, the synovial vessels rupture, and blood accumulates in the joint. Bleeding continues until the intra-articular hy-

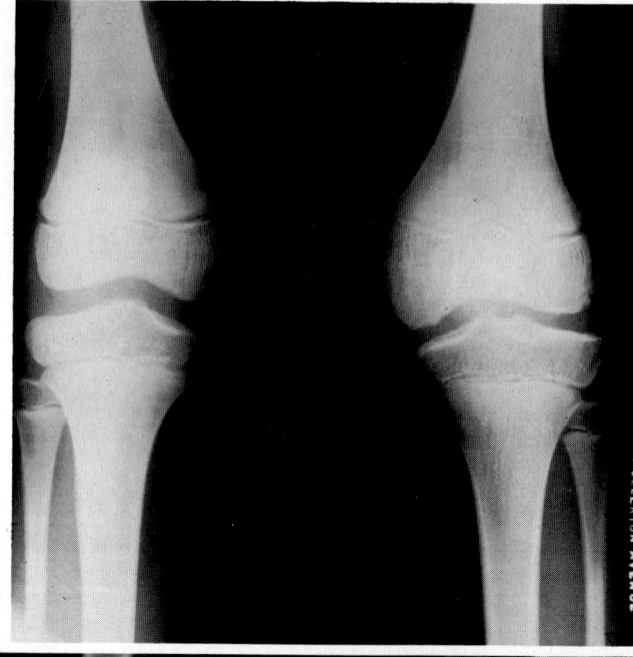

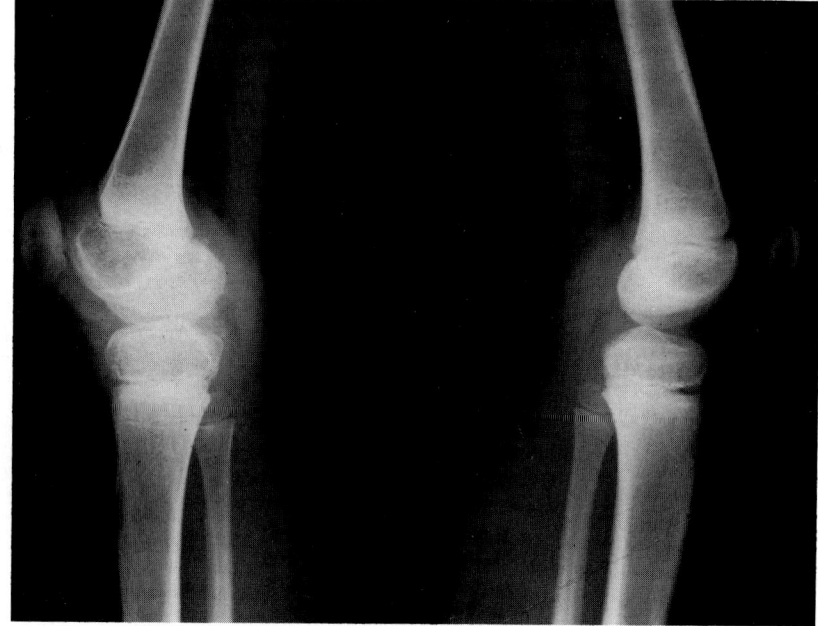

FIGURE 4–32. Hemophilic arthropathy of left knee.

Radiograms show the chronic synovitis and enlargement of distal femoral epiphysis.

drostatic pressure exceeds that of the arterial and capillary pressure in the synovium. The resultant tamponade of the synovial vessels causes ischemia of the synovium and subchondral bone.

With repeated hemorrhage, hyperplasia and fibrosis of the synovium will occur. Pannus formation by the proliferating synovial tissue will erode the hyaline cartilage peripherally, and compression of its opposing cartilaginous surfaces will result in degeneration of articular cartilage centrally. Articular cartilage is also degraded by the action of proteolytic enzymes—lysosomal proteases, acid phosphatase, and cathepsin D. Prostaglandin levels are also elevated in hemophilic arthropathy. There is an inflammatory process that invades and destroys cartilage. Loss of joint motion and contractural

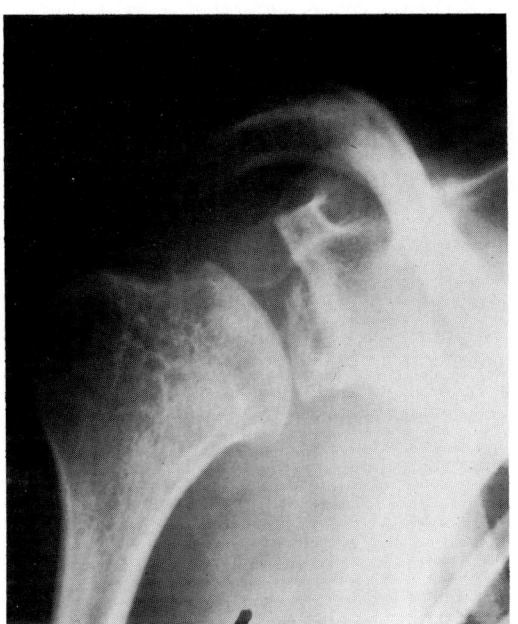

FIGURE 4–33. *Hemophilic arthropathy of shoulder.*

deformity due to capsular-synovial fibrosis follows. Local ischemia will cause formation of subchondral bone cysts.

Repeated hemarthrosis causes marked dilatation of the capsular and epiphyseal vessels. The resultant hyperemia and increased circulation to the part will result in enlargement of the epiphysis and increased longitudinal length of the limb. Stimulation of growth may be asymmetrical, resulting in valgus or varus deformity. Shortening of a limb may be produced by early closure of the physis. Osteoporosis and muscle atrophy are common.

Clinical Findings. These depend on the severity of hemorrhage and whether the hemarthrosis is acute, subacute, or chronic. In *acute hemarthrosis* pain and swelling with distention of the joint capsule are the principal findings. A history of injury may not be elicited. With cessation of bleeding the intensity of pain decreases. The joint will assume the position of minimal discomfort, which will also be the position of minimal intra-articular pressure. The hip joint, for example, is held in 30 to 65 degrees of flexion, 15 degrees of abduction, and 15 degrees of lateral rotation. Extension, wide abduction, and medial rotation of the hip are limited and painful, as they increase intra-articular hydrostatic pressure. The knee joint is held in flexion with marked restriction of range of motion, caused by protective spasm, pain, and the hemarthrosis. Local tenderness and increased heat are present. The overlying skin will be tense and shiny. The intense pain of acute hemarthrosis subsides rapidly after the administration of factor VIII or IX.

Subacute hemarthrosis develops after several episodes of bleeding into the joint. Pain is minimal. The synovium is thickened and boggy. Restriction of joint motion is moderate. Subacute hemarthrosis does not respond rapidly to administration of clotting factor. *Chronic hemarthrosis* develops after six months of involvement. Progressive destruction of the joint takes place, with the end stage being a fibrotic, stiff, totally destroyed joint.[11]

Radiographic Findings. Radiograms will disclose soft-tissue swelling due to distention of the joint capsule. With repeated hemorrhage and resultant chronic synovitis there may be osteoporosis, enlargement of the epiphysis, subchondral cysts, narrowing of the articular cartilage space, and formation of peripheral osteophytes (Figs. 4–32 to 4–34). The final phase of hemophilic arthropathy is fibrous ankylosis (Fig. 4–35).

On the basis of radiographic findings and the degree of cartilage destruction, Arnold and Hilgartner classified hemophilic arthropathy into five stages (Table 4–9).

In *Stage I* there is only soft-tissue swelling, but no skeletal abnormalities.

Stage II is characterized by overgrowth and osteoporosis of the epiphysis, but joint integrity is maintained—there are no bone cysts and no

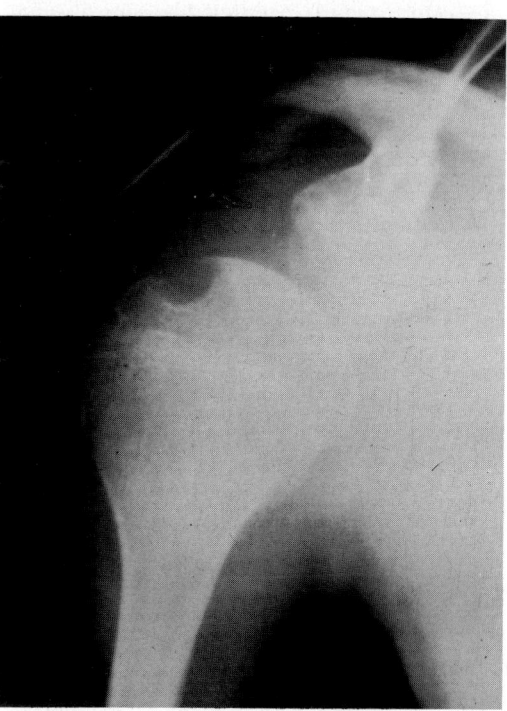

FIGURE 4–34. *Hemophilic arthropathy of shoulder.*

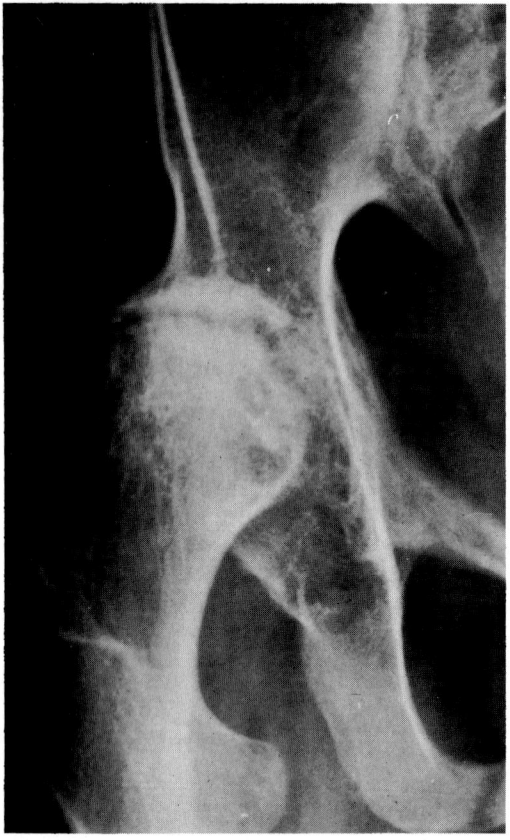

FIGURE 4–35. *Fibrous ankylosis of hip as a result of hemophilic arthropathy.*

narrowing of the articular cartilage space. The radiologic Stage II parallels the clinical stage of subacute hemophilic arthropathy.

In *Stage III* there is minimal to moderate joint space narrowing with subchondral cysts, which occasionally communicate with the joint space. There is widening of the intercondylar

Table 4–9. *Radiographic Staging of Hemophilic Arthropathy**

Stage I	Soft tissue swelling No skeletal abnormality
Stage II	Overgrowth and osteoporosis of epiphysis Integrity of joint maintained
Stage III	Mild to moderate joint narrowing Subchondral cysts Patellar squaring Widening of intercondylar notch of knee and trochlear notch of elbow
Stage IV	Severe narrowing of joint space with cartilage destruction Other osseous changes very pronounced
Stage V	Total loss of joint space with fibrous ankylosis Severe incongruity of articular structures with marked irregular epiphyseal overgrowth

*Modified from Arnold, W. D., and Hilgartner, M. W.: Hemophilic arthropathy. Current concepts of pathogenesis and management. J. Bone Joint Surg., 59-A:287, 1977.

notch of the knee and the trochlear notch of the ulna. In the knee there may be squaring of the patella. In Stage III the articular cartilage is still preserved, indicating that with treatment hemophilic arthropathy is still reversible.

In *Stage IV* there is destruction of articular cartilage with severe narrowing of the joint space. The other osseous changes found in Stage III—i.e., subchondral cysts, patellar squaring, and widening of intercondylar or trochlear notch—are more pronounced.

Stage V is characterized by total loss of joint space with fibrous ankylosis of the joint. There is marked incongruity of the articular structures with severe irregular hypertrophy of the epiphysis.

Soft-Tissue Bleeding

Following a direct injury, a large hematoma may accumulate in the subcutaneous tissues. The blood usually is absorbed spontaneously; occasionally ulceration occurs, commonly on the forehead, the olecranon process, or the prepatellar area. This type of superficial hematoma usually remains fluid and fluctuant for a long time. Superficial soft-tissue hemorrhage in the form of ecchymosis is common, especially in the severe hemophiliac; it is of no clinical significance.

Intramuscular and Intermuscular Hemorrhage. In the lower limb the most common site of bleeding is the quadriceps (44 per cent), followed by the triceps surae (35 per cent), anterior compartment (7 per cent), adductors of the thigh (7 per cent), hamstrings (6 per cent), and sartorius (1 per cent).[13] In the upper limb the most common site of bleeding is the deltoid (24 per cent), followed by wrist and finger flexors in the forearm (23.5 per cent), brachioradialis (19.5 per cent), biceps (14 per cent), wrist and finger extensors in the forearm (11 per cent), and triceps (8 per cent).[165] The presenting complaint is pain on movement or at rest.

Hemorrhage in the quadriceps muscle on occasion may be painless and present only as "stiffness" or "weakness" of the knee. Physical findings consist of local tenderness and swelling with limitation of motion of the adjacent joints. Bleeding in the detoid muscle will restrict shoulder motion—especially abduction and to some extent a varying degree of rotation, flexion, and extension of the shoulder. Bleeding in the forearm flexors will restrict motion of the fingers, wrist, or elbow either alone or in combination.

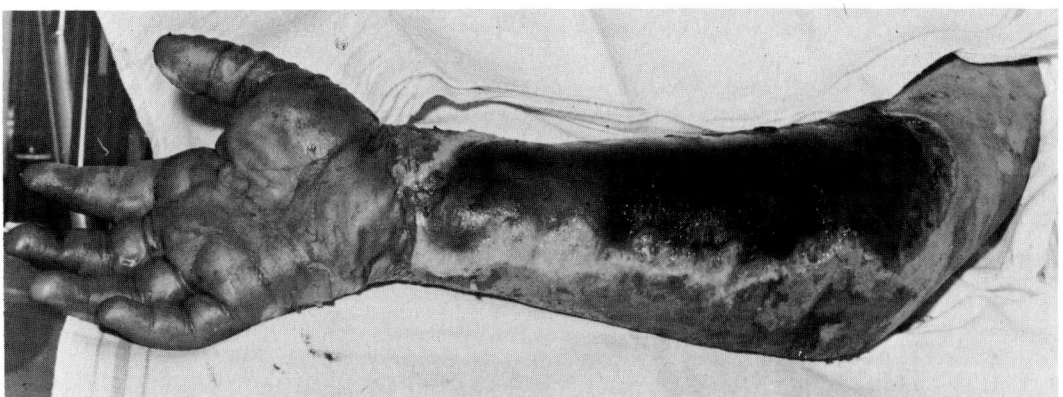

FIGURE 4–36. Volkmann's ischemic contracture of the forearm following fracture of both bones in a hemophilic boy.

Hemorrhage into the iliopsoas muscle or retroperitoneum may mimic a variety of surgical or medical emergencies such as appendicitis or renal colic.

Ischemia and fibrosis of muscles with subsequent myostatic contracture result from bleeding within muscles or among muscles contained in a firm fascial compartment.[119, 137, 138, 145] Hemorrhage within the calf muscles will produce fixed equinus deformity. Bleeding in the volar surface of the forearm may produce Volkmann's ischemic contracture with flexion deformity of the digits and wrists (Fig. 4–36).

Ultrasound.[26, 109, 114, 136, 154, 179, 211, 216, 217] Diagnostic ultrasound is carried out routinely in hemophiliac patients in whom hemorrhage into joints or soft tissues is suspected. It is noninvasive and can be performed at the bedside with minimal disturbance of the patient. The use of a jelly block reduces the amount of skin contact; skin pressure by the probes is minimal, and the procedure does not cause further bleeding from injudicious handling of the patient.

Hemorrhage into superficial joints—such as the knee, elbow, ankle, or wrist—is readily determined by physical examination. The diagnostic value of ultrasound is in identification of bleeding into the hip, shoulder, and deep soft tissues such as the iliopsoas or retroperitoneum (Fig. 4–37). Effusions into these deep anatomic sites are readily detected by ultrasound.

The echo pattern varies with the duration and anatomic site of the hemorrhage. In the soft tissues a hematoma initially displays increased echogenicity as compared with surrounding soft tissues; within three to four days relatively echo-free areas develop in the bleeding site; ordinarily in ten days the established hematoma is relatively echo-free. A soft-tissue hematoma may be of uniform texture, separating muscle planes; or it may interdigitate with muscle fibers, giving a mottled texture with poorly defined margins. On follow-up ultrasound examination the intramuscular hematoma may have resolved spontaneously, or progressively liquified, with decreased internal echoes and development of well-defined borders. A sudden increase in echogenicity indicates a fresh hemorrhage.

The echo pattern of bleeding into joints depicts a mixture of echo-free fluid within the

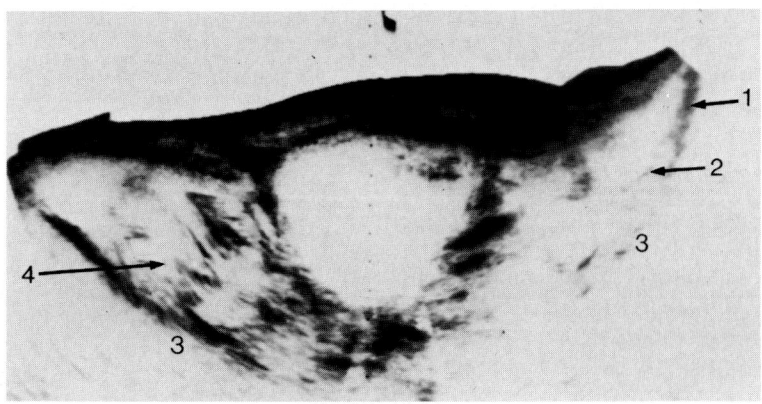

FIGURE 4–37. Ultrasonographic findings in soft-tissue bleeding in the iliopsoas muscle on the right.

1. Normal iliopsoas. 2. Fascial plane. 3. Iliac bone. 4. Bleed in the iliopsoas.

joint and a variable amount of echogenic material floating free. In its very initial stage, hemarthrosis is sometimes uniformly echogenic; this is dissimilar to the echo-free appearance of joint effusions from other causes such as toxic synovitis or septic arthritis.

Nerve Palsy

Neurapraxia in hemophilia is primarily due to compression from the hematoma. The femoral nerve is most frequently involved, as it is in a closed, rigid compartment limited by the iliacus fascia. The psoas sheath is easily distensible. Brower and Wilde reported six cases of femoral nerve palsy, and Goodfellow and associates described 20 cases of femoral nerve compression.[29, 69] The nerve next most frequently affected is the median nerve. The ulnar, radial, sciatic, peroneal, and lateral femoral cutaneous nerves may also be involved.[43, 120]

A history of injury, such as twisting of the limb or strenuous use, may be obtained in some cases. Pain is the presenting complaint and is soon followed by weakness of the affected muscle groups.

In femoral nerve palsy, the hip is held in moderate flexion and some lateral rotation. Extension and medial rotation of the hip are limited and painful. On palpation a tender mass in the iliac fossa extending to the iliac crest and groin may be present. There will be anesthesia or hypoesthesia in the areas of the cutaneous distribution of the femoral nerve. Quadriceps paralysis in varying degrees is often present. Ultrasound and computed tomography will demonstrate the iliacus hematoma. With adequate factor replacement the natural course is one of gradual and steady recovery, usually within 12 months.*

Hemophilic Pseudotumor

The term *hemophilic pseudotumor* refers to a progressive cystic swelling involving the musculoskeletal system. It is caused by uncontrolled hemorrhage within a confined space. The hematoma increases in size and causes pressure necrosis and erosion of surrounding tissues. The subjacent bone is frequently involved.[11]

The entity was first described by Starker in 1918, and in the subsequent 70 years fewer than 100 cases have been reported.[192] It occurs only in severely affected hemophiliacs who have a functional clotting factor level of below 1 per cent. In these severe hemophiliacs the estimated incidence is 1 to 2 per cent.

Valderrama and Matthews have described the three ways in which such hemophilic cysts may develop.

The *simple cyst* occurs within the fascial envelope of a muscle or muscles and is confined by the tendinous attachments. No bone changes are seen on the radiograms. It usually remains localized under the muscle fascia, though it may extend between muscle and fascia to point internally or through the skin.

The second type of cyst occurs in a muscle with wide and firm fibrous periosteal attachment and may eventually cause cortical thinning because of compressive interference with the periosteal and outer cortical blood supply.

In the third type, the pseudotumor originates as a subperiosteal hemorrhage, and progressively strips the periosteum from the cortex until it is limited by the aponeurotic or tendinous attachments. The overlying muscle is raised or destroyed.[207] Most hemophilic pseudotumors are caused by subperiosteal hemorrhage. Occasionally one may arise from intraosseous hemorrhage.[97]

In the past, intramedullary bleeding was thought to be a common cause of hemophilic pseudotumor.[1, 85, 97] It was proposed that uncontrolled intraosseous hemorrhage increases the intramarrow pressure and causes necrosis of the marrow and inner cortex of the bone. With progressive bleeding and increasing pressure the cortex perforates, causing elevation of the periosteum and bone necrosis. Pathologic examination of large hemophilic pseudotumors has, however, failed to demonstrate bone necrosis or resorption of the inner part of the cortex. Trueta cites MacMahon and Blackburn's case of cystic expansion of the metacarpal bone as a pseudotumor that probably had an intramedullary origin.[134, 205]

The most common location of pseudotumors is in the thigh, which is the site in 50 per cent of cases. Next in frequency are the abdomen, pelvis, and tibia (Fig. 4–38 A).[85] It may also occur in the hand (Fig. 4–38 B).[18] Pseudotumor involving the calcaneus may cause marked erosion of the calcaneal tuberosity.[36, 113]

A bone involved by pseudotumor may undergo pathologic fracture. In the days prior to adequate factor replacement pseudotumors caused death in the majority of patients. Involved limbs have been amputated in the past. Valderrama and Matthews observed that localization of these tumors is related to the powerful

---
*See references 1, 8, 18, 28, 44, 54, 61, 74, 85, 91, 117, 134, 173, 176, 193.

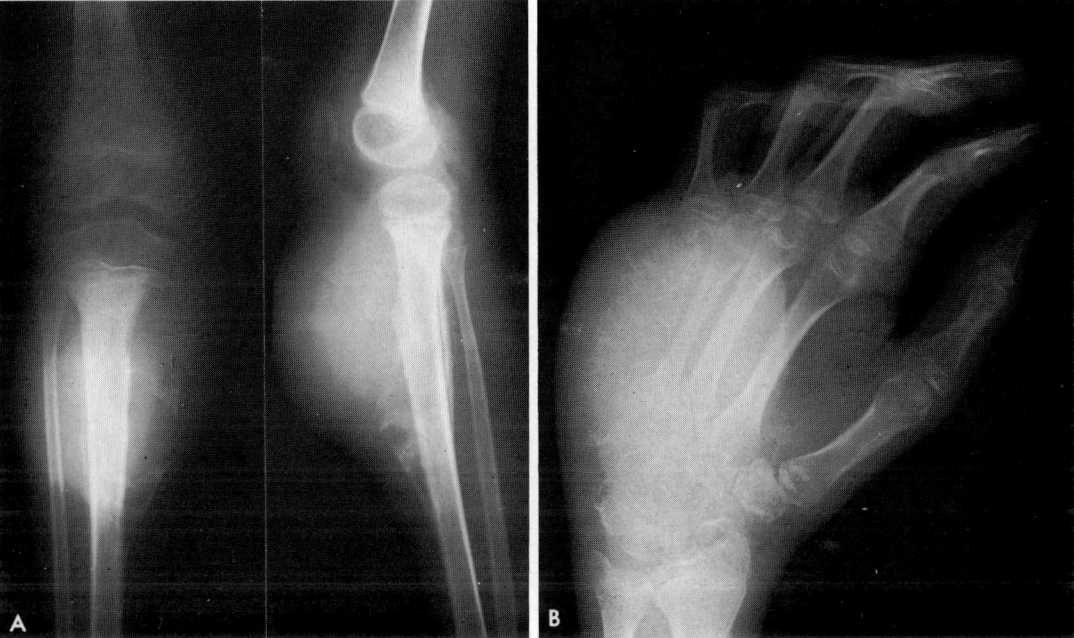

FIGURE 4–38. Hemophilic pseudotumor.

A. Of the tibia. B. Of the hand.

muscle groups of the quadriceps femoris, triceps surae, gluteus maximus, and iliopsoas muscles, which have firm attachments between their fibers and the periosteum but not to any great extent with the bone itself. These muscles also have profuse vascular connections with the underlying periosteum and bone. Hemorrhage from these injured vessels will easily detach and elevate the periosteum.

Hemophilic pseudotumor is essentially an expanding hematoma. Computed tomography will demonstrate that the lesion is of fluid consistency and will depict its true extent, bone destruction, and extraosseous abnormality.[158] Nuclear magnetic resonance imaging is also of great value in delineating the nature and extent of the pseudotumor. It is imperative that a hemophilic tumor not be mistaken for a malignant or expanding benign bone tumor. It should not be aspirated nor should a biopsy be taken for diagnosis, particularly without appropriate preoperative correction of functional factor deficiency.

Fractures

Fractures in hemophilia do occur; they may result from trauma or be pathologic after trivial injury. They are most common in the lower limb, especially in patients with stiff knees, who sustain supracondylar fracture of the femur. Hematomas may be large, especially following femoral fractures. In cases of fracture of either the bones of the forearm or the tibia, uncontrolled bleeding into a closed fascial compartment may lead to Volkmann's ischemic contracture (see Fig. 4–36).

Dislocations

Intra-articular bleeding in the hip will stretch the joint capsule and cause subluxation and eventual dislocation of the hip. Floman and Niska reported a six-year-old boy with hemophilia A who developed a spontaneous posterior dislocation of the hip due to repeated intra-articular bleeding. The prognosis of such dislocation is poor. In this patient, despite immediate reduction, the hip became ankylosed.[59] In the literature other cases of hip dislocation in hemophilia are reported by Teitelbaum, Driessen, and Boardman and English.[25, 51, 201]

Bleeding in the hip joint is rare in hemophilia, but a serious problem. Increased intra-articular pressure in addition to stretching the joint capsule will cause avascular necrosis of the femoral head with eventual joint space narrowing, subchondral irregularity and cyst formation, collapse of the femoral head, osteoarthrosis and arthrokatadysis.[178, 201]

Myositis Ossificans

Ectopic ossification in hemophilia, first described by Hutcheson, develops as a result of inter- or intramuscular bleeding.[92] Heterotopic bone formation around the hip joint will cause restriction of hip motion.[121] In the past it was thought to be a rare complication in hemophilia, but in a radiographic survey by Vas and associates it was found in 15 per cent of patients; in most of their cases the disability was minimal.[209]

Treatment

The care of the hemophiliac with musculoskeletal disorders requires a multidisciplinary approach consisting of a team of a hematologist, orthopedic surgeon, physical therapist, nurse clinician, medical psychologist, social worker, and geneticist. There should be immediate access to a laboratory capable of performing accurate factor VIII or IX assays and detecting factor antibodies. Factor material should be readily available for replacement therapy. The creation of multidisciplinary hemophilia clinics in children's hospitals has relatively simplified the care of hemophiliac children. In this section the management of bleeding into the locomotor system is discussed.

MEDICAL MANAGEMENT

The objective of medical management is control of bleeding by hemostasis, achieved by replacement of the deficient factor with concentrate of the clotting factors obtained from fresh frozen plasma. The use of concentrates allows administration of adequate amounts of factor in a small volume, thereby avoiding the dangers of circulatory overload. For factor VIII deficiency (hemophilia A and von Willebrand's disease) the concentrate used contains factor VIII and fibrinogen. Cryoprecipitate is protein that precipitates in fresh frozen plasma when it is thawed at 4° C.; it is rich in factor VIII and is readily prepared and stored in ordinary blood banks. Lyophilized cryoprecipitates are commercially prepared with a greater degree of purification and removal of fibrinogen; these commercial products are better standardized, are safer, and are easily administered.

For factor IX deficiency (hemophilia B) the concentrate used contains a high level of factor IX and low levels of factors II, VII, and X; it is manufactured as the prothrombin complex from human plasma. The commercially available products Konyne (Cutter) and Proplex (Hyland) are standardized, lyophilized, and readily soluble for use.

Both types of concentrates have the potential for causing acquired immunodeficiency syndrome (AIDS) by transmission of the infectious virus via the infused blood products. Other troublesome side effects of these transfusion products are hepatitis, fever, allergic reactions, headache, abdominal pain, and occasional development of disseminated intravascular coagulation.

Factor Replacement. The dosage required to replace a factor deficiency depends on the patient's weight and plasma volume. The hematologist makes the calculations and is in charge of administration of the factor. The orthopedic surgeon, however, should be aware that 20 to 30 minutes after administration of the antihemophilic factor the plasma level will rise. The biologic half-life of factor VIII is 6 to 12 hours, whereas that of factor IX is 8 to 18 hours.

In the management of bleeding into joints, muscles, and soft tissue, the dose of factor VIII or IX is calculated to raise the plasma level to 30 per cent of normal. In severe hemarthrosis it may be desirable to raise the plasma level to 40 per cent of normal.

Inhibitors of factor VIII and IX develop as a result of the immunologic response of the human body.[214] A low titer of inhibitors may be circumvented by high dosage of factor VIII infusion. Other methods to overcome this life-threatening problem are the administration of prednisone and cyclophosphamide or the use of concentrations of prothrombin-activated material or of plasmaphoresis.

Early Bleeding into Muscles and Soft Tissues. Early treatment of bleeding into muscles and soft tissues by self-administration of factor VIII or IX by the hemophiliacs or their parents at home has become effective. The dose of factor is calculated to raise the level to 30 to 40 per cent of normal. The part is splinted in comfortable neutral position in foam pillows or soft appliances. If the hemorrhage is in the lower limb, weight-bearing is restricted by crutches or eliminated by confinement to bed or wheelchair. As soon as the acute symptoms of pain and muscle spasm have subsided the affected limb is gradually mobilized under cover of factor replacement. With early treatment (within two to three hours) the hemorrhage in the muscles will usually resolve within three to five days. Hemorrhages in the quadriceps femoris and biceps brachii take the longest time to resolve.[13, 65]

Hemarthrosis. Acute bleeding into joints

should be considered an emergency requiring immediate attention. With proper education, instructions as to dosage schedules, and communication between the physician, nurse clinician, and parents, many patients can be treated at home by themselves or by a family member. Immediate treatment of bleeding into joints results in less arthropathy and minimizes the extent of joint destruction. Home care therapy permits factor replacment as soon as a bleeding episode takes place. This type of patient self-help has, however, the disadvantage of inadequate follow-up, possibility of transmission of hepatitis to a family member, and increased risk of infection due to lack of appropriate sterile technique in handling of materials.[123, 124] The parents should be instructed, if the bleeding is severe with marked distention of the joint, to bring the child to the hospital within four hours of the onset of hemorrhage. It cannot be overemphasized that delay in adequate treatment is the primary cause of crippling joint deformity in hemophilia. A minimal or moderate intra-articular hemorrhage may not be so painful at the onset, and the child will continue to use and bear weight on the affected limb, causing continuous or intermittent progressive bleeding into the joint. Within a few days the joint will become markedly swollen, very painful, and inflamed by reaction to the blood and will develop fixed flexion contracture. Initially, in the event of associated bleeding into the periarticular tissues and muscles, pain and muscle spasm will be marked from the onset; the patient will be apprehensive of moving the limb and will be forced to rest and to seek medical attention.

The affected joint is temporarily immobilized in a molded, well-padded splint in a position of rest and minimum hydrostatic pressure. This position varies with each joint—for example, for the knee, it is 35 to 45 degrees of flexion; and for the elbow, 50 to 60 degrees of flexion. There are commercially available semiflexible splints (such as the Jordan splint) that provide partial immobilization and moderate compression.

Compression is effectively achieved with a rubber sponge over the site of hemorrhage and an elastic bandage. A second bandage may be applied intermittently over the first one to increase tension. Distal circulation should be carefully watched. Under no circumstances should a circular plaster cast be used; the swelling underneath will obstruct the blood flow and cause gangrene. The limb should be elevated to reduce hydrostatic venous pressure. Cold compresses in the form of ice bags are applied over the affected joint. The clotting defect is corrected by intravenous administration of antihemophilic factor.

Analgesics. It is best not to give analgesics or sedatives to allay pain and apprehension, as with such a chronic disease, addiction can easily become a problem. Also, the course of the bleeding is best assessed by the patient, and under heavy analgesia he will be unable to give proper warning of continued bleeding. Diminution of severity of pain is the first indication of cessation of hemorrhage. The circumference of the joint is measured at intervals to determine whether there is any progressive distention of the joint capsule. Also, analgesic drugs that contain aspirin, guaiacolate, and antihistamines inhibit platelet aggregation and prolong the bleeding time. Do not give such medications and produce a secondary bleeding disorder! If the pain is intolerable and does not respond to factor replacement and splinting, pain medications to be given are propoxyphene (Darvon), acetaminophen (Tylenol), codeine, or methadone.

Aspiration. The joint should be aspirated and decompressed if there is severe hemarthrosis with marked distention of the joint capsule. Hemarthrosis is harmful to joint physiology. It would be desirable to evacuate all the blood, but this is not possible. Loculation and clot formation impede aspiration and are relative contraindications. The acute bleeding episode should be of less than 24 hours' duration. During the past decade, aspiration of joints has been performed less and less owing to the efficacy of early diagnosis and immediate effective treatment by factor replacement. Aspiration of the joint should be performed under strict aseptic conditions in the operating room and under local anesthesia. Factor VIII or IX is administered intravenously and will reach an effective blood level 20 to 30 minutes later. This is the time to aspirate the joint, not after two or three infusions have already been given, because aspiration will be unsuccessful owing to thickening and clotting of the blood. Aspiration is performed with an 18-gauge lumbar puncture needle with a stylet. Do not make more than one or at most two puncture wounds with the needle. The joint is irrigated with normal saline solution until the return is clear. Intra-articular administration of corticosteroids is not indicated. The compression dressing and posterior splint are reapplied.

Administration of the factor is continued for three to seven days following cessation of bleeding. At this time, physical therapy to mobilize the joint is initiated. First isometric muscle exercises are begun. These are followed by gentle active assisted exercises, first with gravity eliminated and then against gravity. Between exercises the limb is protected in an appropriate splint. The range of motion of the affected joint is progressively increased. Weight-bearing joints are protected with crutches with a three-point gait. Full weight-bearing is not permitted for a minimum of two weeks, and longer if necessitated by limitation of joint motion and muscle weakness. It is imperative that transition to activity be gradual.

Subacute Hemophilic Arthropathy. Repeated episodes of bleeding into a joint in a relatively short time will result in synovial hypertrophy and persistent effusion. This is best managed nonoperatively by immobilization of the joint in a well-padded splint and with factor replacement. Ordinarily the majority of subacute hemarthroses will resolve over a period of three to four weeks with this regimen of therapy. Do not attempt to evacuate clots. Isometric exercises are performed to maintain muscle tone and strength. Initially, passive range of motion is not allowed. Partial weight-bearing with crutches is permitted. With resolution of synovitis and effusion the patient is gradually allowed to return to normal function.

If the subacute hemarthrosis fails to respond to three weeks of partial immobilization, physical therapy, and factor replacement, prednisone or a similar steroid is given for one week in the appropriate dosage. Prolonged immobilization of the affected joint should be avoided, as it will result in marked muscle atrophy and restriction of joint motion. If the knee is involved, quadriceps atrophy will cause joint instability leading to repeated trauma and bleeding.

Support of the lower limb in orthotic devices is indicated when motor power of the quadriceps or triceps surae muscle is less than fair or when flexion deformity of the knee or equinus deformity of the ankle is present to such a degree that mechanical insufficiency of the lower limb predisposes the child to fall and sustain repeated injury. Rubbing and recurrent trauma to the opposite thigh or leg by the medial caliper is a real problem; it will cause soft-tissue bleeding. Only a lateral upright is used. A well-padded plastic orthosis should be used whenever possible. When flexion deformity of the knee or equinus deformity of the ankle develops, appropriate splinting is utilized at night to keep the part out of the position of deformity.

During the stage of subacute hemarthrosis prophylactic factor replacement is administered in conjunction with an intensive physical therapy program. Graduated progressive resistive active and gentle passive range of motion exercises are performed immediately after infusion of the factor in the evening and the following morning. The patient is allowed to swim and perform ordinary physical activities of daily living. Contact sports should be avoided.

Chronic Hemophilic Arthropathy. This can be prevented in most cases by effective and immediate treatment of acute hemarthrosis. The importance of prevention of chronic arthropathy with intra-articular fibrosis, cartilage destruction, and joint stiffness cannot be overemphasized.

In the management of chronic hemophilic arthropathy, four modalities of treatment are available: physical therapy, orthoses, traction and other corrective appliances, and surgery. The objective is to correct joint deformity and to restore function.

Nonsurgical Management. Nonoperative measures should always be employed prior to surgery. In flexion deformities of the knee and hip, a period of continuous traction is effective in relieving muscle spasm and increasing range of motion. Initially traction forces are in the line of deformity and are gradually altered to achieve correction. Split Russell traction is utilized by the author; the vertical force is exerted by a sling placed under the proximal tibia when the knee is involved; with the hip, the sling support is under the distal thigh. In the case of lateral rotation contracture of the hip, a medial rotation strap is added to the thigh. Houghton and Duthie recommend the use of reverse dynamic slings to correct flexion deformity of the knee and elbow.[89]

Prophylactic protection with antihemophilic factor is usually not required while the child is in traction. Once a neutral or a nearly neutral position is obtained, well-padded plastic splints are used to maintain the part in the corrected position. Active exercises are begun to increase muscle power and range of motion of the joints. It is best to refrain from forceful passive stretching exercises.

If functional range of motion is not achieved after two or three weeks of traction, a wedging cast is applied. Posterior subluxation of the knee may be prevented by applying an extension-desubluxation hinge; it will lift the proximal tibia anteriorly as the knee is extended.[130, 151, 153, 194] For safety, the antihemophilic factor is administered when the cast is wedged. When full knee extension is achieved the knee is immobilized for a period of seven to ten days, a plastic splint is utilized to maintain the correction, and physical therapy in the form of active exercises is begun. Gradually partial weight-bearing and three-point crutch gait are permitted. If bleeding occurs during this period of training, it is controlled by intravenous administration of antihemophilic factor. Crutch support is discontinued and full weight-bearing is allowed when there is functional range of joint motion and at least fair strength of the quadriceps muscle.

Management of flexion contracture of the elbow follows the same principles as that of the knee. Equinus deformity of the ankle is treated by a dorsiflexion wedging cast. Forceful manipulation of a joint under general anesthesia is not recommended.

SURGICAL TREATMENT

If deformities caused by hemarthrosis cannot be corrected by conservative closed methods, one should not hesitate to perform open operations. If equinus deformity is very severe and rigid, tendo Achillis lengthening is indicated. Fractional lengthening of the hamstrings combined with posterior capsulotomy is performed for flexion contracture of the knee. On occasion, one may have to resort to osteotomy of the distal femur, tilting it anteriorly to correct flexion deformity of the knee.

Open surgery has become relatively safe, provided the clotting mechanism is restored to near normal by the administration of antihemophilic factor, which should be continued for three weeks, with sutures removed on the fourteenth to sixteenth day postoperatively. Wounds and bone heal normally in hemophilic patients.

Hematologic Management. Prior to surgery the hematologist determines the factor level and performs tests to rule out the presence of factor inhibitors. During surgery and the first postoperative day, the factor level should be raised to 100 per cent by infusion of factor concentrate. During the first postoperative week, the factor level is maintained at 50 per cent, and subsequently for the first postoperative month at 30 to 40 per cent by daily infusions of factor concentrate.

Synovectomy. The objective of synovectomy is to prevent progression of hemophilic arthropathy. The *rationale* for synovectomy in hemophilic arthropathy is based on the following considerations: mechanically the vulnerability to trauma of the highly vascular synovial tissue is diminished by its excision, and biochemically hemophilic synovial tissue has a high level of fibrinolytic activity that tends to prolong the bleeding episodes.[196, 197] Also, the hypertrophic synovial tissue in hemophilia contains increased levels of acid phosphatase and cathepsin D, which are further elevated during bleeding episodes; these proteolytic enzymes destroy hyaline articular cartilage.[79, 80, 213] The chronic synovial inflammation is perpetuated by the elevated levels of prostaglandin E and polymorphonuclear leukocytes (due to chemotactic properties of the enzymes). Also, hemosiderin deposition in the synovium interferes with the production of collagenases, which may cause death of chondrocytes.

Indications. Synovectomy of peripheral joints, particularly of the knee, is indicated in patients with a history of severe recurrent hemarthrosis (two or three major bleeding episodes per month), and those who fail to respond to aggressive medical management for a period of at least six months. Specifically, the latter is a prophylactic factor-replacement program raising factor level to 30 to 40 per cent of normal (factor replacement administered every other day in hemophilia A and every third day in hemophilia B) and administration of systemic steroids (prednisone given in doses of 1 mg. per kilogram of body weight for one to two months). The use of intra-articular steroids is not recommended. Other indications are failure of response to orthopedic nonsurgical treatment consisting of physical therapy and protection with crutches and orthoses, and radiographic Stage II or Stage III hemophilic arthropathy—in stages IV and V synovectomy is ineffective and contraindicated.

Operative Technique.[146] Synovectomy of the knee is performed as follows: The procedure is carried out under tourniquet ischemia. The surgical approach to the *knee* is through a long medial parapatellar incision; it begins 5 cm. above the superior border of the patella and extends to the medial border of the patella and then to the medial border of the proximal tibial tubercle. Throughout the operation electrocautery is utilized to maintain strict hemostasis. The subcutaneous tissue, fascia, and capsule are divided, and the knee joint is thoroughly inspected. The proliferative synovial tissue is excised—first, from the suprapatellar pouch, then from the medial and lateral recesses of the knee and intercondylar notch, including that around the cruciate ligaments, and lastly the menisci. Caution! Preserve the coronary ligaments. The synovial tissue on the articular cartilage is removed gently with a moist sponge. Do not disturb the growth of the distal femoral physis. Next, irrigate the joint copiously with antibiotic solution, and apply Gelfoam mixed with a solution of injectable saline and thrombin over the denuded tissues. Pack the wound with moist lap pads, and after application of several layers of Ace bandages for compression, release the tourniquet. Five to ten minutes later, the wound is inspected and thorough hemostasis is obtained. The previously applied Gelfoam is removed, and the wound is closed in layers. Suction drainage is always inserted. A bulky compression dressing is applied, and the limb is immobilized in an above-knee plaster of Paris posterior splint. The suction drainage is removed in two or three days.

This author has no personal experience with synovectomy of peripheral joints through the arthroscope in chronic hemophilic arthropathy. Technically, it is demanding and difficult to secure hemostasis, and operating time may be unduly prolonged.

Postoperative Care. Isometric quadriceps and hamstring strengthening exercises are begun immediately. Active range of motion exercises should not be commenced early because they may result in massive hemarthrosis. Seven to ten days postoperatively gentle active assisted and passive range of motion exercises are started. Toe-touch weight-bearing with crutch protection is allowed as tolerated. Passive range of knee motion is carried out with a continuous passive motion (CPM) machine 14 days following surgery—in the beginning for several hours of the day during waking hours to ensure there is no bleeding into the joint, then for gradually increasing periods. The third week postoperatively the limb should be in the continuous passive motion machine all night and part of the day. Active exercises are performed intensively to develop quadriceps function. Gradually full weight-bearing is allowed.

Problems and Complications. Postoperative loss of range of joint motion due to adhesions of the patellofemoral and tibiofemoral joints is a common and challenging problem following synovectomy for hemophilic arthropathy. In the series of 13 patients reported by Montane and associates knee motion was reduced in 11 patients (85 per cent); the average loss of range was 41 degrees. In the younger patients (less than 11 years) the postoperative loss of joint motion was greater owing to lack of motivation and poor cooperation with the postoperative physical therapy program. One of their young patients subsequently required knee arthrodesis.[146] Manucci and associates reported marked decrease in joint motion, particularly flexion, in 8 of their 15 patients.[141] Kay and associates found decreased knee motion following surgery in nine patients, three of whom required postoperative manipulation under anesthesia; one of these patients sustained a supracondylar fracture of the femur during manipulation, but in the other two patients there was significant improvement of motion.[105] Arnold and Hilgartner recommended manipulation of the knee two to three weeks after synovectomy if joint motion was lost, and they stressed the importance of increasing factor levels to nearly 100 per cent of normal.[11] The stage of arthropathy, the adequacy of control of intra-articular bleeding at surgery and postoperatively, the degree of quadriceps and hamstring atrophy, and the motivation of and cooperation by the patient are important factors in determining final range of motion. Intensive and prolonged physical therapy and the use of continuous passive motion are vital following synovectomy.

Massive bleeding may occur in the joint during the immediate postoperative period following synovectomy or during the habilitation phase of treatment. This may require aspiration or surgical arthroscopic evacuation of the hematoma.

Despite these complications the results reported in the literature indicate that chronic recurrent hemarthrosis and the pain in chronic hemophilic arthropathy can be effectively eliminated after open synovectomy, which also appears to slow the pace of progression of the disease.*

Synoviorthesis. Chemical and radioisotope synovectomy has been tried in the treatment of chronic hemophilic arthropathy.[9, 63, 196] The results have been dubious; at present surgical synovectomy is the procedure of choice.

Total Joint Replacement and Arthrodesis. Deciding between total joint replacement and arthrodesis is difficult; it should be individualized. Disabling pain is the prime indication for surgery. If involvement is unilateral and the opposite lower limb is relatively normal, this author prefers arthrodesis. In bilateral knee involvement total joint replacement is indicated with Stage IV or Stage V arthropathy when persistent knee pain is definitely due to joint derangement; there should be at least 45 degrees of knee motion. Arnold and Hilgartner

---

*See references 32, 37, 53, 105, 126, 129, 141, 146, 150, 160, 187, 196, 197.

reported the results of five total knee joint replacements in hemophiliac patients; relief of pain was impressive, and functional range of motion was preserved without serious complications.[11] Other encouraging results were reported by Lachiewicz and associates, by London and associates, by McCollough and associates, by Marmor, and by Small and associates.[115, 126, 129, 139, 142, 181] Goldberg and associates reported the results of 13 total knee arthroplasties of the semicontainment type in ten patients with hemophilia A with a follow-up of two to six and a half years. All patients had had severe pain, requiring crutches or wheelchairs for ambulation. The results were graded as excellent or good in four, fair in eight, and poor in one (who required arthrodesis). They recommended total knee arthroplasty when arthrodesis was the only other alternative.[68]

Total hip replacement is indicated in Stage IV or Stage V hemophilic arthropathy when pain is persistent with severe disability not relieved by conservative measures.[45, 161] Arthroplasty of the elbow has been reported.[182]

Arthrodesis of the ankle, subtalar and midtarsal joints in the foot, shoulder, or knee may be indicated when these joints are destroyed. The surgical technique is the same as in normal patients with the exception that percutaneous pins should not be utilized in hemophiliacs, as they require factor replacement at moderate levels until the pins are removed.[88, 156]

Neurapraxia is treated by factor replacement therapy in doses to attain factor levels of 80 to 100 per cent of normal for 48 hours after onset of hemorrhage; the dose is tapered to maintain a level of 40 per cent for one to two weeks. The limb is splinted. Gentle physical therapy is performed seven days after the bleeding episode. Occasionally decompression of the entrapped nerve may have to be performed.[120]

Fractures[25, 26, 39, 57, 107]

These usually heal in the normal time. Factor replacement should be to the level of 40 to 60 per cent of normal on the day of fracture and the following day; subsequently it should be 20 to 30 per cent for seven or more days depending on the degree of associated soft-tissue injury.[57] Whenever possible fractures are treated by closed reduction and immobilization in a cast. Do not use pins for skeletal traction, as they require prolonged replacement therapy. External fixators should be avoided. Open reduction and internal fixation are carried out when closed methods are not appropriate.

Pseudotumors

If surgical intervention is planned, it is recommended that angiography, CAT scan, and nuclear magnetic resonance imaging be performed in order to provide accurate anatomic detail of adjacent vessels.[117] The pseudotumor per se is avascular.[199] The surgical extirpation of a hemophilic pseudotumor requires careful preoperative planning and extensive dissection.[74, 162, 173]

Radiotherapy has been utilized to control expanding hematoma of hemophilic pseudotumors; irradiation will cause new bone formation and sclerosis of the cystic cavity. Its use may be considered in surgically inaccessible sites; it is important to shield the physis in order not to cause growth disturbance.[82] Amputation of a limb may be indicated when the patient is seen quite late and in a case in which deformity is so severe that the limb is of no use.[24, 40, 175]

In conclusion, with early treatment and proper collaboration between the hematologist and orthopedic surgeon, deformities and crippling in hemophilia can be prevented and corrected.

References

1. Abell, J. M., Jr., and Bailey, R. W.: Hemophilic pseudo-tumor. Arch. Surg., *81*:569, 1960.
2. Abildgaard, C. F.: Current concepts in the management of hemophilia. Semin. Hematol., *12*:223, 1975.
3. Abildgaard, C. F., Britton, M., and Harris, J.: Use of prothrombin complex concentrate (Konyne) in the treatment of hemophilic patients with factor VIII inhibitors. J. Pediatr., *88*:200, 1976.
4. Abildgaard, C. F., Penner, J. A., and Watson-Williams, E. J.: Anti-inhibitor coagulant complex (Autoplex) for treatment of factor VIII inhibitors in hemophilia. Blood, *56*:978, 1980.
5. Ackroyd, C. E., and Dinley, R. J.: The locked patella. An unusual complication of haemophilia. J. Bone Joint Surg., *58-B*:511, 1976.
6. Ahlberg, A.: Haemophilia in Sweden. VII. Incidence, treatment, and prophylaxis of arthropathy and other musculoskeletal manifestations of haemophilia A and B. Acta Orthop. Scand., Suppl. 77, 1965.
7. Ahlberg, A.: Treatment and prophylaxis of arthropathy in severe hemophilia. Clin. Orthop., *53*:135, 1967.
8. Ahlberg, A.: On natural history of hemophilic pseudotumor. J. Bone Joint Surg., *57-A*:1133, 1975.
9. Ahlberg, A., and Petterson, H.: Synoviorthesis with radioactive gold in hemophiliacs. Clinical and radiological follow-up. Acta Orthop. Scand., *50*:513, 1979.
10. Arnold, W. D.: Synovectomy. Ann. N.Y. Acad. Sci., *240*:338, 1975.
11. Arnold, W. D., and Hilgartner, M. W.: Hemophilic arthropathy. Current concepts of pathogenesis and management. J. Bone Joint Surg., *59-A*:287, 1977.
12. Aronstram, A., Rainsford, S. G., and Painter, M. J.: Patterns of bleeding in adolescents with severe haemophilia A. Br. Med. J., *1*:469, 1979.
13. Aronstram, A., Browne, R. S., Wassef, M., and Hamad, Z.: The clinical features of early bleeding into

the muscles of the lower limb in severe hemophiliacs. J. Bone Joint Surg., 65-B:19, 1983.

14. Aronstram, A., McLellan, D. S., Mbatha, P. S., and Wassef, M.: The use of an activated factor IX complex (Autoplex) in the management of haemarthroses in haemophiliacs with antibodies to factor VIII. Clin. Lab. Haemot., 4:231, 1982.

15. Aronstram, A., Wassef, M., Hamad, Z., and Aston, D. L.: The identification of high-risk elbow hemorrhages in adolescents with severe hemophilia A. J. Pediatr., 98:776, 1981.

16. Aronstram, A., Wassef, M., Hamad, Z., and Aston, D. L.: The identification of high risk knee bleeds in adolescents with severe hemophilia A. Clin. Lab. Haemotol., 4:17, 1982.

17. Aronstram, A., Wassef, M., Choudhury, D. P., Turk, P. M., and McLellan, D. S.: Double-blind controlled trial of three dosage regimens in treatment of haemarthroses in haemophilia A. Lancet, 1:169, 1980.

18. Bayer, W. L., Shea, J. D., Curiel, D. C., Szeto, I. L. F., and Lewis, J. H.: Excision of pseudocyst of the hand in a hemophiliac (PTC deficiency). J. Bone Joint Surg., 51-A:1423, 1969.

19. Becker, F.: Sarkom vortauschende sog. Reoptionsgeschwulst bei Haemophilie. Zentralbl. Chir., 69:1133, 1942.

20. Belloir, A., Didier, D., and Weill, F.: Etude ultrasonographique des hématomes retropéritoneaux et abdomino-pelviens. J. Radiol., 64:621, 1983.

21. Biggs, R.: The Treatment of Haemophilia A and B and Von Willebrand's Disease. Oxford, Blackwell, 1978, pp. 127–152.

22. Biggs, R., and MacFarlane, R. G.: The Treatment of Haemophilia and Other Coagulation Disorders. Oxford, Blackwell, 1966.

23. Biggs, R., and Rizza, C. R.: The control of haemostasis in haemophilic patients. In The Treatment of Haemophilia A and B and Von Willebrand's Disease. Oxford, Blackwell, 1978.

24. Blalock, A.: Amputation of arm of patient with hemophilia. J.A.M.A., 99:1777, 1932.

25. Boardman, K. P., and English, P.: Fractures and dislocations in hemophilia. Clin. Orthop., 148:221, 1980.

26. Boni, M., and Ceciliani, L.: Fractures in haemophilia. Ital. J. Orthop. Traumatol., 2:301, 1976.

27. Boone, D. C.: Long term management of the hemophilic patient with emphasis on musculoskeletal complications. Prog. Phys. Ther., 1:138, 1974.

28. Brant, E. E., and Jordan, H. H.: Radiological aspects of hemophilic pseudotumors in bone. A.J.R., 115:525, 1972.

29. Brower, T. D., and Wilde, A. H.: Femoral neuropathy in hemophilia. J. Bone Joint Surg., 48-A:487, 1966.

30. Buchanan, G. R.: Hemophilia. Pediatr. Clin. North Am., 27:309, 1980.

31. Bullock, W., and Fildes, P.: Haemophilia. In Francis Galton Laboratory for National Eugenics: Treasury of Human Inheritance. London, University of London, 1911.

32. Bussi, L., Silvello, L., Baudd, F., and DeCataldo, F.: Results of synovectomy of the knee in haemophilia. Haemotologica (Pavia), 59:81, 1974.

33. Caffey, J., and Schlesinger, E. R.: Certain effects of hemophilia on the growing skeleton. Some roentgenographic observations on overgrowth and dysgenesis of the epiphysis associated with chronic hemarthrosis. J. Pediatr., 16:549, 1940.

34. Cambouroglou, G., Papathanassiou, B., Koutoulidis, C., Bossinakou, I., and Mandalaki, T.: Hemophilic arthropathy surveyed with whole-body gamma-camera scintigraphy. Acta Orthop. Scand., 47:607, 1979.

35. Chantseva, E. A., and Kashulin, A. M.: Use of the Volkov-Oganesian apparatus in treating hemophilic osteoarthritis of the knee joint. Ortop. Travmatol. Protez., 2:39, 1982.

36. Chen, Y. F.: Bilateral hemophilic pseudotumors of the calcaneus and cuboid treated by irradiation. J. Bone Joint Surg., 47:517, 1965.

37. Clark, M. W.: Knee synovectomy in hemophilia. Orthopaedics, 1:285, 1978.

38. Collins, D. H.: Haemosiderosis and haemochromatosis of synovial tissues. J. Bone Joint Surg., 33-B:436, 1951.

39. Coventry, M. B., Owen, C. A., Jr., Murphy, T. R., and Mills, S. D.: Survival of patient with hemophilia and fracture of the femur. J. Bone Joint Surg., 41-A:1392, 1959.

40. Crandon, J. H., Staudinger, L., Jr., and Friedman, E.: Midthigh amputation in a patient with hemophilia. N. Engl. J. Med., 249:657, 1953.

41. Creveld, S., von Hoedemaeker, P. J., Kingma, M. J., and Wagenvoort, C. A.: Degeneration of joints in haemophiliacs under treatment by modern methods. J. Bone Joint Surg., 53-B:296, 1971.

42. Crock, H. V., and Boni, V.: The management of orthopedic problems in haemophiliacs. A review of twenty-one cases. Br. J. Surg., 48:8, 1960.

43. Culver, J. E., Jr.: Combined posterior interosseous and ulnar nerve compression in a hemophiliac. Bull. Hosp. Joint Dis., 39:103, 1978.

44. Cunning, H. J.: The surgery of haemophilia cysts. In Biggs, R., and MacFarlane, R. G., (eds.): Treatment of Haemophilia and Other Coagulation Disorders. Oxford, Blackwell, 1966.

45. D'Ambrosia, R. D., Neimann, K. M. W., O'Grady, L., and Scott, C. W.: Total hip replacement for patients with hemophilia and hemorrhagic diathesis. Surg., Gynecol., Obstet., 139:381, 1974.

46. Dallman, P. R., and Pool, J. G.: Treatment of hemophilia with factor VIII concentrates. N. Engl. J. Med., 278:199, 1968.

47. DePalma, A. F.: Guiding principles in the surgery of haemophilic patients. In Tocantins, L. M. (ed.): Progress in Haemotology, Vol. I. New York, Grune & Stratton, 1956, p. 103.

48. DePalma, A. F.: Hemophilic arthropathy. Clin. Orthop., 52:145, 1974.

49. DeVore, G. R., Mahoney, M. J., and Hobbins, J. C.: Antenatal diagnosis of haemoglobinopathies, haemophilia, von Willebrand's disease, Duchenne's muscular dystrophy and chronic granulomatous disease by fetal blood analysis. Clin. Obstet. Gynaecol., 7:41, 1980.

50. Diamond, L. K., Green, W. T., and Chandler, H. P.: Hemophilia: Medical and orthopedic management. Postgrad. Med., 34:271, 1963.

51. Driessen, A. P. P. M.: Arthropathies in Haemophiliacs. Groningen, Van-Grocum Company B. V.-Assen, 1973.

52. Duthie, R. B., Matthews, J. M., Rizza, C. R., and Steel, W. M.: The Management of Musculoskeletal Problems in the Haemophilias. Oxford, Blackwell, 1972.

53. Dyszy-Laube, B., Kaminski, W., Gizycka, I., Kaminska, D., Sekowska, J., and Ludert, E.: Synovectomy in the treatment of haemophilic arthropathy. J. Pediatr. Surg., 9:123, 1984.

54. Echternacht, A. P.: Pseudotumor of bone in hemophilia. Radiology, 41:565, 1943.

55. Edwards, J. H.: Carrier detection. Prog. Clin. Biol. Res., 103:15, 1982.

56. Eyring, E. J., Bjornson, D. R., and Close, J. R.: Management of hemophilia in children. Clin. Orthop., 40:95, 1965.

57. Feil, E., Bentley, G., and Rizza, C. R.: Fracture management in patients with haemophilia. J. Bone Joint Surg., 56-B:643, 1974.

58. Firor, W. M., and Woodhall, B.: Hemophiliac pseudotumor: Diagnosis, pathology and surgical treatment of hemophilic lesions of the smaller bones and joints. Bull. Johns Hopkins Hosp., 59:237, 1936.
59. Floman, Y., and Niska, M.: Dislocation of the hip joint complicating repeated hemarthrosis in hemophilia. J. Pediatr. Orthop., 3:99, 1983.
60. Fraenkel, G. J.: Surgery in haemophilia. J. R. Coll. Surg. Edinb., 3:54, 1957.
61. Fraenkel, G. J., Taylor, K. B., and Richards, W. C. D.: Haemophilic blood cysts. Br. J. Surg., 46:383, 1959.
62. France, W. G., and Wolf, P.: Treatment and prevention of chronic hemorrhagic arthropathy and contractures in haemophilia. J. Bone Joint Surg., 47-B:247, 1965.
63. Gamba, G., Grignani, G., and Ascari, E.: Synoviorthesis versus synovectomy in the treatment of recurrent haemophilic haemarthrosis: Long-term evaluation. Thromb. Haemost., 45:127, 1981.
64. Gershuni, D. H., Axer, A., and Siegel, B.: Localized regressive articular cartilage changes in the hip of the rabbit following an induced synovitis. Acta Orthop. Scand., 50:179, 1979.
65. Ghormley, R. K., and Clegg, R. S.: Bone and joint changes in hemophilia. J. Bone Joint Surg., 30-A:589, 1948.
66. Gilbert, M. S.: Musculoskeletal manifestations of haemophilia. Mt. Sinai J. Med., 44:339, 1977.
67. Gilchrist, G. S., Hagedorn, A. B., and Stauffer, R. N.: Severe degenerative joint disease in mild and moderately severe haemophilia. J.A.M.A., 238:2383, 1977.
68. Goldberg, V. M., Heiple, K. G., Ratnoff, O. D., Kurczynski, E., and Arvan, G.: Total knee arthroplasty in classic hemophilia. J. Bone Joint Surg., 63-A:695, 1981.
69. Goodfellow, J. W., Fearn, C. B. d'A., and Matthews, J. M.: Iliacus hematoma: A common complication in hemophilia. J. Bone Joint Surg., 49-B:748, 1967.
70. Gordon, E. M., Berkowitz, R. J., Strandjord, S. E., Kurczynski, E. M., Goldberg, J. S., and Coccia, P. F.: Burkitt lymphoma in a patient with classic hemophilia receiving factor VIII concentrates. J. Pediatr., 103:75, 1983.
71. Greene, W. B.: Use of continuous passive slow motion in the postoperative rehabilitation of difficult pediatric knee and elbow problems. J. Pediatr. Orthop., 3:419, 1983.
72. Greer, R. B., III: Operative management of hemophilic arthropathy. Orthopedics, 3:135, 1980.
73. Greer, R. B., III, and Ballard, J. O., 3rd.: Musculoskeletal bleeding in hemophilia. Pediatr. Ann., 11:521, 1982.
74. Hall, M. R. P., Handley, D. A., and Webster, C. U.: The surgical treatment of haemophilic blood cysts. J. Bone Joint Surg., 44-B:781, 1962.
75. Handelsman, J. E.: The knee joint in hemophilia. Orthop. Clin. North Am., 10:139, 1979.
76. Hasiba, U., Scranton, P. E., Lewis, J. H., and Spero, J. A.: Efficacy and safety of ibuprofen for hemophilic arthropathy. Arch. Intern. Med., 140:1583, 1980.
77. Heim, M., Horoszowski, H., and Martinowitz, U.: Leg length inequality in hemophilia. Clin. Pediatr., 24:600, 1985.
78. Heim, M., Horoszowski, H., Martinowitz, U., Seligsohn, U., and Engel, J.: Haemophiliac hands–a three year followup study. Hand, 14:333, 1982.
79. Hilgartner, M. W.: Pathogenesis of joint changes in hemophilia. In Committee on Prosthetic Research and Development: Comprehensive Management of Musculoskeletal Disorders in Hemophilia. Washington, D.C., Natl. Acad. Sci., 1973, pp. 33–36.
80. Hilgartner, M. W.: Hemophilic arthropathy. Adv. Pediatr., 21:139, 1974.
81. Hilgartner, M. W.: Home care for hemophilia: Current state of the art. Scand. J. Haematol., 30:58, 1977.
82. Hilgartner, M. W., and Arnold, W. D.: Hemophilic pseudotumor treated with replacement therapy and radiation. Report of a case. J. Bone Joint Surg., 57-A:1145, 1975.
83. Hoaglund, F. T.: Experimental hemarthrosis: The response of canine knees to injections of autologous blood. J. Bone Joint Surg., 49:285, 1967.
84. Hofmann, A., Wyatt, R., and Bybee, B.: Septic arthritis of the knee in a 12-year-old hemophiliac. J. Pediatr. Orthop., 4:498, 1984.
85. Horwitz, H., Simon, N., and Bassen, F. A.: Haemophilic pseudotumor of the pelvis. Br. J. Radiol., N.S., 32:51, 1959.
86. Hoskinson, J., and Duthie, R. B.: Management of musculoskeletal problems in the hemophilias. Orthop. Clin. North Am., 9:455, 1978.
87. Houghton, G. R.: Septic arthritis of the hip in a hemophiliac. Report of a case. Clin. Orthop., 129:223, 1977.
88. Houghton, G. R., and Dickson, R. A.: Lower limb arthrodesis in haemophilia. J. Bone Joint Surg., 60-B:387, 1978.
89. Houghton, G. R., and Duthie, R. B.: Orthopedic problems in hemophilia. Clin. Orthop., 138:197, 1979.
90. Hurri, L., Silvers, K., and Oka, M.: Intra-articular osmic acid in rheumatoid arthritis. Acta Rheumatol. Scand., 9:20, 1963.
91. Hussey, H. H.: Editorial. Hemophilic pseudotumor of bone. J.A.M.A., 232:1040, 1975.
92. Hutcheson, J.: Peripelvic new bone formation in hemophilia. Radiology, 109:529, 1973.
93. Hutchinson, R. J., Penner, J. A., and Hensinger, R. N.: Antiinhibitor coagulant complex (Autoplex) in hemophilia inhibitor patients undergoing synovectomy. Pediatrics, 71:631, 1983.
94. Ingram, G. I. C., Matthews, J. A., and Bennett, A. E.: A controlled trial of joint aspiration in acute haemophilic haemarthrosis. Br. J. Haematol., 23:649, 1972.
95. Ingram, G. I. C., Brozovic, M., and Slater, N. G. P.: Bleeding Disorders: Investigation and Management. 2nd Ed. Oxford, Blackwell, 1982.
96. Inwood, M. J., Killackey, B., and Startup, S. J.: The use and safety of ibuprofen in the hemophiliac. Blood, 61:709, 1983.
97. Ivins, J. C.: Bone and joint complications of hemophilia. In Brinkhous, K. M. (ed.): Hemophilia and Hemophilioid Diseases. International Symposium. Chapel Hill, N.C.: University of North Carolina Press, 1957, p. 225.
98. Johnson, J. B., Davis, T. W., and Bullock, W. H.: Bone and joint changes in hemophilia, a long-term study in 12 Negro subjects. Radiology, 63:64, 1954.
99. Jordan, H. H.: Haemophilic Arthropathies. Springfield, Ill., Thomas, 1959.
100. Kahn, M.: Hip joint changes in hemophilia. Radiology, 22:286, 1934.
101. Kasper, C. K.: Postoperative thrombosis in hemophilia (letter). N. Engl. J. Med., 289:160, 1973.
102. Kasper, C. K., and Rapaport, S. I.: Bleeding times and platelet aggregation after analgesics in hemophilia. Ann. Intern. Med., 77:189, 1972.
103. Kass, L., Ratnoff, O. D., and Leon, M. A.: Studies on the purification of antihemophilic factor (factor 8) 1. Precipitation of antihemophilic factor by concanavalin. Am. J. Clin. Invest., 48:351, 1969.
104. Katznelson, J. L.: Hemophilia with special reference to the Talmud. Hebrew Med. J., 1:163, 1958.
105. Kay, L., Stainsby, D., Buzzard, B., Fearns, M., Hamilton, P. J., Owen, P., and Jones, P.: The role of synovectomy in the management of recurrent hemarthroses in haemophilia. Br. J. Haematol., 49:53, 1981.

106. Keefer, C. S., and Myers, W. K.: Hemophilic arthritis. N. Engl. J. Med., 208:1183, 1933.
107. Kemp, H. S., and Matthews, J. M.: The management of fractures in haemophilia and Christmas disease. J. Bone Joint Surg., 50-B:351, 1968.
108. Key, J. A.: Hemophilic arthritis (bleeder's joints). Ann. Surg., 95:198, 1932.
109. Kinnas, P. A., Woodham, C. H., and MacLarnon, J. C.: Ultrasonic measurements of haematomata of joints and soft tissues in the haemophiliac. Scand. J. Haematol., Suppl. 40:225, 1984.
110. Kisker, C. T., and Burke, C.: Double-blind studies on the use of steroids in the treatment of acute hemarthrosis in patients with hemophilia. N. Engl. J. Med., 282:639, 1970.
111. Koch, B., Cohen, S., Luban, N. C., and Eng, G.: Hemophiliac knees: Rehabilitation techniques. Arch. Phys. Med. Rehabil., 63:379, 1982.
112. Konig, F.: Die Gelenkerkrankungen bie Bluten mit besonderer Berucksichtigung der Diagnose. Samml. Klin. Bort. Chir. Nos. 1–25, Leipzig, 1890–1894.
113. Krill, C. E., Jr., and Mauer, A. M.: Pseudotumors of calcaneus in Christmas disease. J. Pediatr., 77:848, 1970.
114. Kumari, S., Fulco, J. D., Karayalcin, G., and Lipton, R.: Gray scale ultrasound: Evaluation of iliopsoas hematomas in hemophiliacs. A.J.R., 133:103, 1979.
115. Lachiewicz, P. F., Inglis, J. N., Insall, J. N., Sculco, T. P., Hilgartner, M. W., and Bussell, J. B.: Total knee arthroplasty in hemophilia. J. Bone Joint Surg., 67-A:1361, 1985.
116. Lack, C. H.: Chondrolysis in arthritis. J. Bone Joint Surg., 41-B:384, 1959.
117. Lae Thomas, M., and Walter, H. L.: The angiographic findings in a haemophilic pseudotumor of bone. Australas. Radiol., 21:346, 1977.
118. Lamy, M.: L'aspect radiologique des ostéo-arthropathies hémophiliques. Bull. Mem. Soc. Med. Hôp. Paris, 58:45, 1942.
119. Lancourt, J. E., Gilbert, M. S., and Posner, M. A.: Management of bleeding and associated complications of hemophilia in the hand and forearm. J. Bone Joint Surg., 59-A:451, 1977.
120. Large, D. F., Ludlam, C. A., and Manicol, M. F.: Common peroneal nerve entrapment in a hemophiliac. Clin. Orthop., 181:165, 1983.
121. Lazerson, J., Nagel, D. H., and Becker, J.: Myositis ossificans as a complication of severe hemophilia A. In Comprehensive Management of Musculoskeletal Disorders in Hemophilia. Washington, D.C.: Natl. Acad. Sci., 1973.
122. Le Balc'h, T., Ebelin, M., Laurian, Y., Lambert, T., Verroust, F., and Larrieu, M.-J.: Synovectomy of the elbow in young hemophilic patients. J. Bone Joint Surg., 69-A:264, 1987.
123. Levine, P. H.: Efficacy of self-therapy in hemophilia. A study of 72 patients with hemophilia A and B. N. Engl. J. Med., 291:1381, 1974.
124. Levine, P. H., and Britten, A. F. H.: Supervised patient-management of hemophilia. A study of 45 patients with hemophilia A and B. Ann. Intern. Med., 78:195, 1973.
125. Lieberg, O. U., Penner, J. A., and Bailey, R. W.: Fibrosarcoma presenting as a pseudotumor of hemophilia. Report of an unusual case. J. Bone Joint Surg., 57-A:422, 1975.
126. London, J. T., Kattlove, H., Louie, J. S., Forster, G. L.: Synovectomy and total joint arthroplasty for recurrent hemarthroses in the arthropathic joint in hemophilia. Arthritis Rheum., 20:1543, 1977.
127. Lyons, J. B.: Femoral nerve lesions in haemophilia. J. Irish Med. Assoc., 32:110, 1953.
128. McCollough, N. C., III, Lovitt, J., Enis, J. E., Niemann, K. M. W., and Loughlin, E. C.: Major surgery of the knee joint in hemophilia. Paper presented at A.A.O.S. meeting, Las Vegas, Nevada, Feb. 1977.
129. McCollough, N. C., III, Enis, J. E., Lovitt, J., Lian, E. C. Y., Niemann, K. M. W., and Loughlin, E. C., Jr.: Synovectomy or total replacement of the knee in hemophilia. J. Bone Joint Surg., 61-A:69, 1979.
130. McDaniel, W. J.: A modified subluxation hinge for use in hemophilic knee flexion contractures. Clin. Orthop., 103:50, 1974.
131. McDonald, E. J., and Lozner, E. L.: Hemophilic arthritis. Roentgenographic studies in fifteen adult patients with hemophilia. A.J.R., 49:405, 1943.
132. MacKay, S. R.: Early management of joint and soft tissue bleeding. In Committee on Prosthetics Research and Development, National Academy of Science (eds.): Comprehensive Management of Musculoskeletal Disorders in Hemophilia. Washington, D.C., Natl. Acad. Sci., 1973, p. 72.
133. McKee, P. A., Anderson, J. C., and Switzer, M. E.: Recent advances in hemophilia. Ann. N. Y. Acad. Sci., 240:8, 1975.
134. MacMahon, J. S., and Blackburn, C. R. B.: Haemophilic pseudotumor. A report of a case treated conservatively. Aust. N.Z. J. Surg., 29:129, 1960.
135. McMillan, C. W., Diamond, L. K., and Surgenor, P. M.: Treatment of classic hemophilia. The use of fibrogen rich in factor VIII for hemorrhage and for surgery. N. Engl. J. Med., 265:224, 1961.
136. McVerry, B. A., Voke, J., Vicary, F. R., and Dormandy, K. M.: Ultrasonography in the management of haemophilia. Lancet, 1:872, 1977.
137. Madigan, R. R.: Acute compartment syndrome in hemophiliac. A case report (letter). J. Bone Joint Surg., 64-A:313, 1982.
138. Madigan, R. R., Hanna, W. T., and Wallace, S. L.: Acute compartment syndrome in hemophilia. A case report. J. Bone Joint Surg., 63-A:1327, 1981.
139. Magone, J. B., Dennis, D. A., and Weiss, L. D.: Total knee arthroplasty in chronic hemophilic arthropathy. Orthopedics, 9:653, 1986.
140. Mainardi, C. L., Levine, P. H., Werb, Z., and Harris, E. D., Jr.: Proliferative synovitis in hemophilia: Biochemical and morphologic observations. Arthritis Rheum., 21:137, 1978.
141. Mannucci, P. M., De Franchis, R., Torri, G., and Pietrogrande, V.: Role of synovectomy in haemophilic arthropathy. Isr. J. Med. Sci., 13:983, 1977.
142. Marmor, L.: Total knee replacement in hemophilia. Clin. Orthop., 125:192, 1977.
143. Medrea, O., Antonescu, D., Andronescu, S., Filipescu, G., Ionescu, T., and Lupescu, A.: The surgical treatment of haemophilic arthropathy. Rev. Chir. Orthop., 67:107, 1981.
144. Miller, E. H., Flessa, H. C., and Glueck, H. I.: The management of deep soft tissue bleeding and hemarthrosis in hemophilia. Clin. Orthop., 82:92, 1972.
145. Moneim, M. S., and Gribble, T. J.: Carpal tunnel syndrome in hemophilia. J. Hand Surg., 9:580, 1984.
146. Montane, I., McCollough, N. C., and Lian, E. C. Y.: Synovectomy of the knee for hemophilic arthropathy. J. Bone Joint Surg., 68-A:210, 1986.
147. Montgomery, R. R., and Hathaway, W. E.: Acute bleeding emergencies. Pediatr. Clin. North Am., 27:327, 1980.
148. Morrissette, L.: Hémophilie et manifestations articulaires. Un. Med. Can., 73:662, 1944.
149. Newcomber, N. B.: The joint changes in hemophilia. Radiology, 32:573, 1939.
150. Nichol, R. O., and Menelaus, M. B.: Synovectomy of the knee in hemophilia. J. Pediatr. Orthop., 6:330, 1986.
151. Niemann, K. M. W.: Surgical correction of flexion deformities in hemophilia. Am. Surg., 37:685, 1971.

152. Niemann, K. M. W.: Pathogenesis of hemophilic arthropathy. In Comprehensive Management of Musculoskeletal Disorders in Hemophilia. Washington, D.C.: Natl. Acad. Sci., 1972.
153. Niemann, K. M. W.: Lower extremity contractures resulting from hemophilia. South. Med. J., 67:437, 1974.
154. Nowotny, C., Niessner, H., Thaler, E., and Lechner, K.: Sonography: A method for localizing of hematomas in hemophiliacs. Haemostasis, 5(3):129, 1976.
155. Otto, J. C.: An account of an haemorrhagic disposition existing in certain families. Repository N.Y., 6:1, 1803.
156. Patek, A. J., and Taylor, F. H. L.: Some properties of a substance obtained from normal human plasma effective in accelerating the coagulation of hemophilic blood. J. Clin. Invest., 16:113, 1937.
157. Patel, M. R., Pearlman, H. S., and Lavine, L. S.: Arthrodesis in hemophilia. Clin. Orthop., 86:168, 1972.
158. Pettersson, H., and Ahlberg, A.: Computed tomography in hemophilic pseudotumor. Acta Radiol. (Diagn.), (Stockh.), 23:453, 1982.
159. Pettersson, H., Ahlberg, A., and Nilsson, I. M.: A radiologic classification of hemophilic arthropathy. Clin. Orthop., 149:153, 1980.
160. Pietrogrande, V., Dioguard, N., and Mannucci, P. M.: Short-term evaluation of synovectomy in haemophilia. Br. Med. J., 2:378, 1972.
161. Post, M.: Hemophilic arthropathy of the hip. Orthop. Clin. North Am., 11:65, 1980.
162. Post, M., and Telfer, M. C.: Surgery in hemophilic patients. J. Bone Joint Surg., 57-A:1135, 1975.
163. Post, M., Watts, G., and Telfer, M.: Synovectomy in hemophilic arthropathy. Clin. Orthop., 202:139, 1986.
164. Prip Buus, C. E.: Articular changes in hemophilia. Acta Radiol., 16:503, 1935.
165. Railton, G. T., and Aronstam, A.: Early bleeding into upper muscles in severe haemophilia. J. Bone Joint Surg., 69-B:100, 1987.
166. Ratnoff, O. D.: Bleeding Syndromes: A Clinical Manual. Springfield, Ill., Thomas, 1960.
167. Ratnoff, O. D., Kass, L., and Lang, P. D.: Studies on the purification of antihemophilic factor (factor 8) 2. Separation of partially purified antihemophilic factor by gel filtration of plasma. Am. J. Clin. Invest., 48:957, 1969.
168. Reinecke, and Wohlwill, F.: Über hämophile Gelenkerkrankung. Arch. Klin. Chir., 154:425, 1929.
169. Richardson, M. L., Helms, C. A., Vogler, J. B., III, and Genant, H. K.: Skeletal changes in neuromuscular disorders mimicking juvenile rheumatoid arthritis and hemophilia. A.J.R., 143:893, 1984.
170. Rizza, C. R.: Haemophilia A and B. Prescribers J., 24:71, 1984.
171. Robins, R. C., and Murrell, J. S.: Traumatic ischaemia in a haemophiliac. Report of a case of prolonged haemostasis with cryoprecipitate during decompression and skin grafting. J. Bone Joint Surg., 53-B:112, 1971.
172. Robinson, H. J., Jr., and Granda, J. L.: Prostaglandins in synovial inflammatory disease. Surg. Forum, 25:467, 1974.
173. Rosenthal, R. L., Graham, J. J., and Selirio, E.: Excision of pseudotumor with repair by bone graft of pathological fracture of the femur in hemophilia. J. Bone Joint Surg., 55-A:827, 1973.
174. Sancho, F. G.: Experimental model of haemophilic arthropathy with high pressure haemarthrosis. Int. Orthop., 4:57, 1980.
175. Schuster, J. L.: Mid-thigh amputation in a hemophiliac. J. Bone Joint Surg., 36-A:144, 1954.
176. Schwartz, E.: Hemophilic pseudotumor of bone. Radiology, 75:795, 1960.
177. Scoles, P. V., and King, D.: Traumatic aneurysm of the descending geniculate artery: A complication of suction drainage in synovectomy for hemophilic arthropathy. Clin. Orthop., 150:245, 1980.
178. Serre, H., Izran, P., Simon, L., and Rogues, J. M.: Les attients de la hanche au cours de l'hémophilie. Marseille Med., 106:483, 1969.
179. Shirkhoda, A., Mauro, M. A., Staab, E. V., and Blatt, P. M.: Soft-tissue hemorrhage in hemophilia patients: Computed tomography and ultrasound study. Radiology, 147:811, 1983.
180. Sinclair, W. F., and McCollough, N. C., III: Orthopedic management in hemophilia. In Committee on Prosthetics Research and Development, National Academy of Science (eds.): Comprehensive Management of Musculoskeletal Disorders in Hemophilia. Washington, D.C., Natl. Acad. Sci., 1973, p. 88.
181. Small, M., Steven, M. M., Freeman, P. A., Lowe, G. D. O., Belch, J. J. F., Forbes, C. A., and Prentice, C. R. M.: Total knee arthroplasty in hemophiliac arthritis. J. Bone Joint Surg., 65-B:163, 1983.
182. Smith, M. A., Savidge, G. F., and Fountain, E. J.: Interposition arthroplasty in the management of advanced haemophilic arthropathy of the elbow. J. Bone Joint Surg., 65-B:436, 1983.
183. Smith, M. A., Urquhart, D. R., and Savidge, G. F.: The surgical management of varus deformity in haemophilic arthropathy of the knee. J. Bone Joint Surg., 63-B:261, 1981.
184. Sneppen, O., Beck, H., and Holsteen, V.: Synovectomy as a prophylactic measure in recurrent haemophilic haemarthrosis. Acta Paediatr. Scand., 67:491, 1978.
185. Soeur, R.: The synovial membrane of the knee in pathological conditions. J. Bone Joint Surg., 31:317, 1949.
186. Solis-Cohen, L., and Levine, S.: Bone and joint changes in hemophilia. A.J.R., 31:487, 1937.
187. Soreff, J.: Joint debridement in the treatment of advanced hemophilic knee arthropathy. Clin. Orthop., 191:179, 1984.
188. Soreff, J., and Blomback, M.: Arthropathy in children with severe hemophilia A. Acta Paediatr. Scand., 69:667, 1980.
189. Spear, C. V., Mason, J. A., Williamson, S. R., Neff, R. S., Comeaux, L. J., and Gwathmey, F. W.: Undiagnosed bleeding states and medical treatment. Clin. Orthop., 134:249, 1978.
190. Speer, D. P.: Early pathogenesis of hemophilic arthropathy. Evolution of the subchondral cyst. Clin. Orthop., 185:250, 1984.
191. Staas, W. E., Jr., Ditunno, J. F., Jr., Gartland, J. J., and Shapiro, S. S.: Lower extremity amputation in hemophilia. Case report and review of surgical principles. J. Bone Joint Surg., 54-A:1514, 1972.
192. Starker, L.: Knochenusur durch ein hamophiles, subperiosteles Hamatom. Mitt. Grenzgeb. Med. Chir., 31:381, 1918–1919.
193. Steel, W. M., Duthie, R. B., and O'Connor, B. T.: Haemophilic cysts. J. Bone Joint Surg., 51-B:614, 1969.
194. Stein, H., and Dickson, R. A.: Reversed dynamic slings for knee flexion contractures in the hemophiliac. J. Bone Joint Surg., 57-A:282, 1975.
195. Stein, H., and Duthie, R. B.: The pathogenesis of chronic haemophilic arthropathy. J. Bone Joint Surg., 63-B:601, 1981.
196. Storti, E., and Ascari, E.: Surgical and chemical synovectomy. Ann. N.Y. Acad. Sci., 240:316, 1975.
197. Storti, E., Traldi, A., Tosatti, E., and Davoli, P. G.: Synovectomy, a new approach to haemophilic arthropathy. Acta Haematol. (Basel), 41:193, 1969.
198. Strauss, H. S.: Acquired circulating anticoagulants in haemophilia A. N. Engl. J. Med., 281:866, 1969.
199. Sundaram, M., Wolverson, M. K., Joist, J. H., Raiz,

M. A., and Rao, B. J.: Case report 133. Hemophilic pseudo-tumor of iliac and soft tissue. Skeletal Radiol., 6:54, 1981.
200. Tarnay, T. J.: Surgery in the Hemophiliac. Springfield, Ill., Thomas, 1968.
201. Teitelbaum, S.: Radiologic evaluation of the hemophilic hip. Mt. Sinai J. Med., 44:400, 1977.
202. Thomas, H. B.: Some orthopedic findings in 98 cases of hemophilia. J. Bone Joint Surg., 18:140, 1936.
203. Thomas, P., Hepburn, B., Kim, H. C., and Saidi, P.: Nonsteroidal anti-inflammatory drugs in the treatment of hemophilic arthropathy. Am. J. Hematol., 12:131, 1982.
204. Torri, G., Motta, F., and Lozej, E.: Arthropathy and deformity of the hemophiliac knee in children, with particular reference to femoral-rotular articulation. Evaluation and results. Pediatr. Med. Chir., 5:21, 1983.
205. Trueta, J.: The orthopedic management of patients with hemophilia and Christmas disease. In Biggs, R., and McFarlane, R. G. (eds.): Treatment of Hemophilia and Other Coagulation Disorders. Oxford, Blackwell, 1966.
206. Trueta, J.: Studies in the Development and Decay of the Human Frame. Philadelphia, Saunders, 1968, p. 238.
207. Valderrama, J. A. F. de, and Matthews, J. M.: The hemophilic pseudotumor or hemophilic subperiosteal hematoma. J. Bone Joint Surg., 47-B:256, 1965.
208. Van Creveld, S., Hoedemaeker, P. J., Kingma, M. J., and Wagenvoort, C. A.: Degeneration of joints in haemophiliacs under treatment by modern methods. J. Bone Joint Surg., 53-B:296, 1971.
209. Vas, W., Cockshott, W. P., Martin, R. F., Pai, M. K., and Walker, I.: Myositis ossificans in hemophilia. Skeletal Radiol., 7:27, 1981.
210. Voke, J., Madgwick, C., and Dormandy, K.: Haemophilia Centre Handbook. Sevenoaks, Immuno, 1978.
211. Wallis, J., van Kaick, G., Schimpf, K., and Zeltsch, P.: Ultraschalldiagnostik von Muskelhämartomen bei Hämophiliepatienten. R.O.F.O., 134:153, 1981.
212. Warrier, A. I., and Lusher, J. M.: DDAVP: A useful alternative to blood components in moderate hemophilia A and von Willebrand disease. Lancet, 1:213, 1983.
213. Weissman, G., and Spilberg, I.: Breakdown of cartilage proteinpolysaccharide by lysosomes. Arthritis Rheum., 11:162, 1968.
214. White, G. C., II, McMillan, C. W., Blatt, P. M., and Roberts, H. R.: Factor VIII inhibitors: A clinical overview. Am. J. Hematol., 13:335, 1982.
215. Wilkins, R. M., and Wiedel, J. D.: Septic arthritis of the knee in a hemophiliac. A case report. J. Bone Joint Surg., 65-A:267, 1983.
216. Wilson, D. J., Green, D. J., and MacLarnon, J. C.: Arthrosonography of the painful hip. Clin. Radiol., 35:17, 1984.
217. Wilson, D. J., McLardy-Smith, P. D., Woodham, C. H., and MacLarnon, J. C.: Diagnostic ultrasound in haemophilia. J. Bone Joint Surg., 69-B:103, 1987.
218. Winston, M. E.: Haemophiliac arthropathy of the hip. J. Bone Joint Surg., 34-B:412, 1952.
219. Wood, K., Omer, A., and Shaw, M. T.: Hemophilic arthropathy. A combined radiological and clinical study. Br. J. Radiol., 42:498, 1969.
220. Wright, A. E.: On a method of determining the condition of blood coagulability for clinical and experimental uses. Br. Med. J., 2:223, 1893.
221. Zimbler, S., McVerry, B., and Levine, P.: Hemophilic arthropathy of the foot and ankle. Orthop. Clin. North Am., 76:985, 1976.

NEUROPATHIC JOINT DISEASE (Charcot Joint)

Charcot, in 1868, described a bizarre destruction of the knee joints with indolent swelling and instability in patients with tabes dorsalis, proposing that the disease resulted from traumatization of a joint deprived of sensation.[4] Steindler subdivided the condition into the destructive, atrophic, and hypertrophic proliferative forms.[50]

Charcot-like changes in joints are seen in patients who have absence or depression of pain and proprioceptive sensation and who take part in extended continuous physical activity. Consequently their joints sustain repeated trauma. In children, neurologic conditions causing neuropathic arthropathy are congenital insensitivity to pain, peripheral nerve injuries, and diabetic neuropathy, as well as a variety of chronic diseases of the spinal cord that lead to sensory disturbances of the limbs. In myelomeningocele, absence of pain sensation is associated with flaccid paralysis and marked limitation of physical activity; thus, owing to associated severe osteoporosis, the bone and joint changes present a different picture.

The joints involved vary with the different etiologic conditions. In congenital insensitivity to pain and diabetic neuropathy, the destructive changes occur primarily in the tarsal and metatarsal joints, less commonly in the ankle, and rarely in the knee. In syringomyelia, the joints involved are those of the shoulder and elbow, whereas in tabes dorsalis, the knee, hip, ankle, and thoracolumbar spine are frequent sites of the disease.

Clinicopathologic Features

When a limb with normal sensation is injured the joint affected with severe sprain or hemarthrosis is protected from further trauma by pain. In the absence of pain and proprioceptive sensation, however, the joint continues to be active and is repeatedly injured. Synovial effusion and hemarthrosis are aggravated and, together with the abnormal stresses on the joint, cause extreme stretching and weakening of the capsule and supportive ligaments. Local hyperemia causes bone atrophy and resorption. Cartilage destruction, bone erosion, and minute fractures soon follow. Reparative response results in the formation of callus and metaplastic changes in surrounding traumatized soft tissues. With repeated injury, the joint becomes totally disorganized, subluxation ensues, and severe degenerative changes take place.

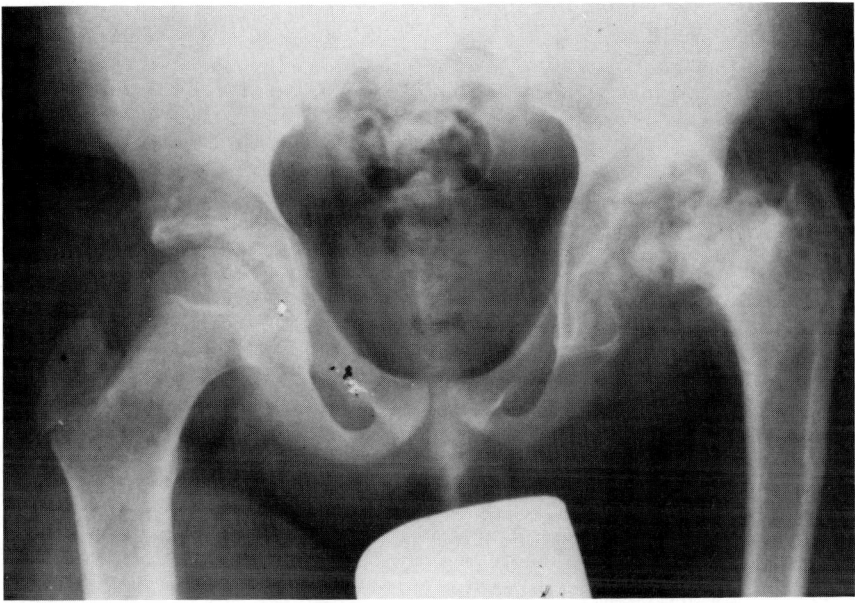

FIGURE 4–39. *Pathologic fracture of the neck of the left femur with subluxation of hip in a ten-year-old boy with congenital insensitivity to pain.*

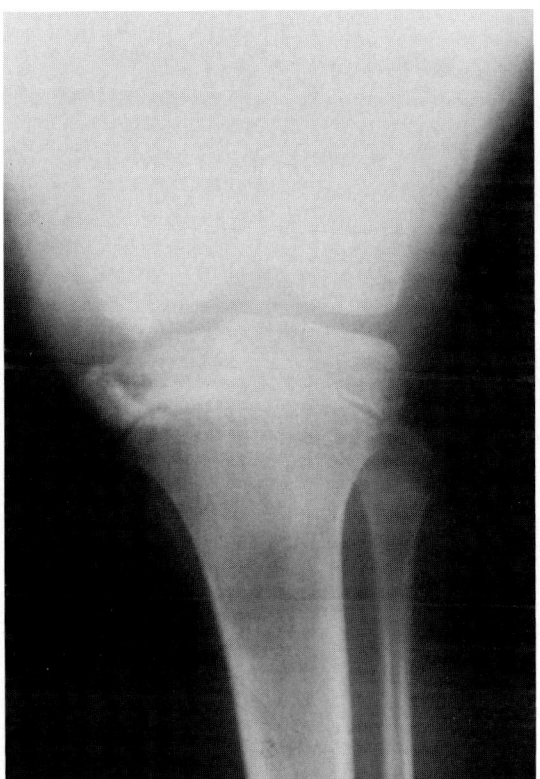

FIGURE 4–40. *Neuropathic disease of the right knee.*

Note the multiple loose bodies and the destruction and subluxation of the joint.

Clinically, the affected joints are boggy, tense, swollen, nontender, and have an excessively abnormal range of motion. The local triad of swelling, instability, and absence of pain is nearly always suggestive of Charcot joint.

Radiographic Findings

The neurotrophic joint will show varying degrees of destructive and hypertrophic changes. There is loss of articular cartilage, fragmentation and absorption of subchondral bone, and osseous proliferation of the articular margins. The bone overgrowth may be enormous, bizarre in configuration, and so great as to surround the joint as a spongy mass. The periarticular soft tissues are thickened and contain scattered calcifications. Pathologic fractures involving the articular surface are common, as are irregular loose bodies within the joint (Figs. 4–39 and 4–40).

Treatment

The affected joints are protected from repeated injury and the stresses of weight-bearing. For the ankle and foot, a patellar weight-bearing ankle-foot orthosis is worn. Progression of the disease is usually delayed with conservative management. Surgical measures are directed toward stabilization of the joint by arthrodesis. Often internal fixation and synovectomy are indicated to achieve union. However, fusion is difficult to achieve in neuropathic joints; adjacent joints develop wear and tear owing to abnormal stresses. In the feet, bony prominences may be excised to facilitate shoe wear.

References

1. Abell, J. M., Jr., and Hayes, J. T.: Charcot knee due to congenital insensitivity to pain. J. Bone Joint Surg., 46-A:1287, 1964.
2. Blanford, A. T., Keane, S. P., McCarthy, A. J., and Abers, J. W.: Idiopathic Charcot joint of the elbow. Arthritis Rheum., 21:723, 1978.
3. Boynton, E. L., Paley, D., Gross, A. E., Silverstein, E., and Goldberg, M. R.: False aneurysm in a Charcot hip. J. Bone Joint Surg., 68-A:462, 1986.
4. Charcot, J. M.: Sur quelques arthropathies qui paraissent dépendre d'une lésion du cerveau ou de la moelle épinière. Arch. Physiol. Norm. Pathol., 1:161, 1868.
5. Charcot, J. M., and Marie, P.: Sur une forme particulière d'atrophie musculaire progressive, souvent familiale, débutant par les pieds et les jambes et atteignant plus tard les mains. Rev. Méd. (Paris), 6:97, 1886.
6. Chillag, K. J., and Stevens, D. B.: Idiopathic neurogenic arthropathy. A case report. J. Pediatr. Orthop., 5:597, 1985.
7. Das, P. C., Banerji, A., Roy, A., and Basu, S.: Neurogenic arthropathies (Charcot joints). J. Indian Med. Assoc., 54:368, 1970.
8. Degenhardt, D. P., and Goodwin, M. A.: Neuropathic joints in diabetes. J. Bone Joint Surg., 42-B:769, 1960.
9. Delano, P. J.: The pathogenesis of Charcot joints. A.J.R., 56:189, 1946.
10. Dimon, J. H., Funk, F. J., Jr., and Wells, R. E.: Congenital indifference to pain with associated orthopedic abnormalities. South. Med. J., 58:524, 1965.
11. Drennan, J. C.: Hereditary and motor sensory neuropathies. In Lovell, W. W., and Winter, R. B. (eds.): Pediatric Orthopedics. 2nd Ed. Philadelphia, Lippincott, 1986, pp. 329–331.
12. Dyck, P. J., and Lambert, E. H.: Lower motor and primary sensory neuron diseases with peroneal muscular atrophy. Part I. Neurologic, genetic, and electrophysiologic findings in hereditary polyneuropathies. Part II. Neurologic, genetic, and electrophysiologic findings in various neuronal degenerations. Arch. Neurol., 18:603, 1968.
13. Dyck, P. J., and Stevens, J. C.: Charcot joints associated with normal cutaneous sensation. Trans. Am. Neurol. Assoc., 101:240, 1976.
14. Dyck, P. J., Stevens, J. C., O'Brien, P. C., Oviatt, K. F., Lais, A. C., Coventry, M. B., and Beabout, J. W.: Neurogenic arthropathy and recurring fractures with subclinical inherited neuropathy. Neurology, 33:357, 1983.
15. Eichenholtz, S. N.: Charcot Joints. Springfield, Ill., Thomas, 1966.
16. Eloesser, L.: On the nature of neuropathic affections of the joints. Ann. Surg., 66:201, 1917.
17. Fath, M. A., Hassanein, M. R., and James, J. I.: Congenital absence of pain. A family study. J. Bone Joint Surg., 65-B:186, 1983.
18. Feindel, W.: Note on the nerve endings in a subject with arthropathy and congenital absence of pain. J. Bone Joint Surg., 35-B:402, 1953.
19. Fitzgerald, J. A. W.: Neuropathic arthropathy secondary to atypical congenital indifference to pain. Proc. R. Soc. Med., 61:663, 1968.
20. Ford, F. R., and Wilkins, L.: Congenital universal insensitivity to pain. A clinical report of three children with discussion of the literature. Bull. Johns Hopkins Hosp., 62:448, 1938.
21. Gherlinzoni, F., and Gherlinzoni, G.: Neurogenic joint disease secondary to congenital insensitivity to pain. Ital. J. Orthop. Traumatol., 8:487, 1982.
22. Goodman, M. A., and Swartz, W.: Infection in a Charcot joint. Case report. J. Bone Joint Surg., 67-A:642, 1985.
23. Gore, R. J.: Multiple Charcot joints. J. Am. Geriatr. Soc., 17:525, 1969.
24. Greider, T. D.: Orthopedic aspects of congenital insensitivity to pain. Clin. Orthop., 172:177, 1983.
25. Harding, A. E., and Thomas, P. K.: The clinical features of hereditary motor and sensory neuropathy types I and II. Brain, 103:259, 1980.
26. Heiple, K. G., and Cammarn, M. R.: Diabetic neuropathy with spontaneous peritalar fracture-dislocation. A report of two cases. J. Bone Joint Surg., 48-A:1176, 1966.
27. Helms, C. A., Chapman, G. S., and Wild, J. H.: Charcot-like joints in calcium pyrophosphate dihydrate deposition disease. Skeletal Radiol., 7:55, 1981.
28. Horwitz, T.: Bone and cartilage debris in the synovial membrane. Its significance in the early diagnosis of neuroarthropathy. J. Bone Joint Surg., 30-A:579, 1948.
29. Hovwen, H.: A case of neuropathic arthritis caused by indifference to pain. J. Bone Joint Surg., 43-B:314, 1961.
30. Johnson, J. T. H.: Neuropathic fractures and joint injuries. J. Bone Joint Surg., 49-A:1, 1967.
31. Katz, I., Rabinowitz, J. G., and Dziadiw, R.: Early changes in Charcot's joints. A.J.R., 86:965, 1961.
32. King, E. J. S.: On some aspects of the pathology of hypertrophic Charcot's joints. Br. J. Surg., 18:113, 1930.
33. MacEwen, G. D., and Floyd, G. C.: Congenital insensitivity to pain and its orthopedic implications. Clin. Orthop., 68:100, 1970.
34. Mazar, A., Herold, H. Z., and Vardy, P. A.: Congenital sensory neuropathy with anhidrosis. Orthopedic complications and management. Clin. Orthop., 118:184, 1976.
35. Meyn, M., Jr., and Yablon, I. G.: Idiopathic arthropathy of the elbow. Clin. Orthop., 97:90, 1973.
36. Mooney, V., and Mankin, A. J.: A case of congenital insensitivity to pain with neuropathic arthropathy. Arthritis Rheum., 9:820, 1966.
37. Murray, R. O.: Congenital indifference to pain with special reference to skeletal changes. Br. J. Radiol., 30:2, 1957.
38. Murray, T. J.: Congenital sensory neuropathy. Brain, 96:387, 1973.
39. Newman, J. H.: Spontaneous dislocation in diabetic neuropathy. J. Bone Joint Surg., 61-B:484, 1979.
40. Norman, A., Robbins, H., and Milgram, J. E.: The acute neuropathic arthropathy—a rapid, severely disorganizing form of arthritis. Radiology, 90:1159, 1968.
41. Ogden, T. E., Robert, F., and Carmichael, E. A.: Some sensory syndromes in children: Indifference to pain and sensory neuropathy. J. Neurol. Neurosurg. Psychiatry, 22:267, 1959.
42. Petrie, J. G.: A case of progressive joint disorders caused by insensitivity to pain. J. Bone Joint Surg., 35-B:399, 1953.
43. Riley, C. M., Day, R. L., Greely, D. McL., and Langford, W. S.: Central autonomic dysfunction with defective lacrimation. Pediatrics, 3:468, 1949.
44. Robinson, S. C., and Sweeney, J. P.: Cauda equina lipoma presenting as acute neuropathic arthropathy of the knee. Clin. Orthop., 178:210, 1983.
45. Rose, G. K.: Arthropathy of the ankle in congenital indifference to pain. J. Bone Joint Surg., 35-B:408, 1953.

46. Rubinow, A., Spark, E. C., and Canoso, J. J.: Septic arthritis in a Charcot joint. Clin. Orthop., *147*:203, 1980.
47. Ryckewaert, A., and Naveau, B.: Osteoarticular diseases from J. M. Charcot to present time. Rev. Neurol. (Paris), *138*:997, 1982.
48. Shands, A. R., Jr.: Neuropathies of the bones and joints: Report of a case of an arthropathy of the ankle due to a peripheral nerve lesion. Arch. Surg., *20*:614, 1930.
49. Silverman, F. N., and Gilden, J. J.: Congenital insensitivity to pain: A neurologic syndrome with bizarre skeletal lesions. Radiology, *72*:176, 1959.
50. Steindler, A.: The tabetic arthropathies. J.A.M.A., *96*:250, 1931.
51. van der Houwen, H.: A case of neuropathic arthritis caused by indifference to pain. J. Bone Joint Surg., *43-B*:314, 1961.
52. Weinberg, E. D.: The treatment of Charcot joints. South. Med. J., *23*:527, 1930.
53. Yoslow, W., Becker, M. H., Bartels, J., and Thompson, W. A. L.: Orthopaedic defects in familial dysautonomia. J. Bone Joint Surg., *53-A*:1541, 1971.

OSTEOCHONDRITIS DISSECANS

Osteochondritis dissecans is a condition in which a segment of articular cartilage with its underlying subchondral bone gradually separates from the surrounding osteocartilaginous tissue. The separation of the fragment may be partial or complete. The osteochondral segment may remain in situ, it may become partially detached, or it may become completely detached and lodge in the contiguous joint as a loose body. The term *dissecans* is derived from the prefix *dis*, meaning "from," and *secare*, "to cut out." It is important to differentiate the word *dissecans* from *desiccans*, the latter being derived from *desiccare*, "to dry up."

Historical Background

Ambrose Paré removed loose bodies from joints in 1558.[175] The disease was first described in 1870 by Sir James Paget, who called it "quiet necrosis."[170] The name *osteochondritis dissecans* was given in 1887 by König, who believed that necrosis of part of the articular bone surface was caused by trauma and that this was followed by "dissecting inflammation," which eventually caused the fragment to separate.[117] During the early part of this century various modalities of treatment of osteochondritis dissecans were recommended: simple observation, restriction of physical activity, non-weight-bearing by crutch protection, immobilization, and surgery in the form of simple drilling, transfixing with pins, bone grafting, and removal of the partially or completely detached osteochondral fragment.

Osteochondritis dissecans has been described as a disease of the young adult. Green and Banks, in 1953, pointed out that it is not uncommon in children.[81] They stressed not only the importance of distinguishing the childhood form from the adult type of osteochondritis but also that in the young patient with open physes treatment should be conservative, as the outlook for healing is excellent.

The advent of arthroscopic surgery in the 1970's opened new vistas in management of osteochondritis dissecans. It allowed direct visualization of the lesion, drilling of the base of the osteochondral fragment, stabilization of partially separated fragments with Kirschner wires or bone graft, and atraumatic removal of loose bodies without open arthrotomy. Scintigraphy in the 1980's assisted in the follow-up of cases treated conservatively and determination of which cases required surgical treatment.

Etiology

The exact cause of osteochondritis dissecans remains a matter of conjecture; no pathogenetic theory is fully accepted. Heredity, constitutional predisposition, ischemia, and trauma are etiologic factors to be considered. The etiology is most probably multifactorial.

Heredity and Constitutional Predisposition. There are many examples of familial incidence mentioned in the literature. Wagoner and Cohn described osteochondritis dissecans of the knee in a boy, his father, a paternal uncle, and his two brothers.[220] Stougaard, in 1964, reported a family in which ten members of the second and third generations were involved.[207] Neilson, in a survey of osteochondritis dissecans of the humeral capitellum, found the incidence to be 4.1 per cent of 1,000 men who were otherwise normal; the incidence in male relatives of affected men, however, was 14.6 per cent.[161] Petrie reported a family study in which 34 patients with osteochondritis dissecans and 86 of their first-degree relatives were examined clinically and radiologically. Only one relative was found to have osteochondritis dissecans. Association with other forms of osteochondritis, endocrine abnormalities, and dwarfism could not be demonstrated. Petrie concluded that the common form of osteochondritis dissecans is not familial; this is in contradiction to previous reports that osteochondritis dissecans can appear in a familial form.[177]

Multiple joint involvement in the same patient is not uncommon, indicating a constitutional factor in its etiology.[220] White reported multiple osteochondritis dissecans in association hip, shoulder (humeral head or glenoid fossa), and patella may also be involved. Involvement of the lateral tibial plateau in a 12-year-old boy is reported by Towbin and associates.[214] Characteristically, there is a particular site on the articular surface of each joint that is affected, examples being the lateral surface of the medial femoral condyle in the knee, the capitellum in the elbow, the superior surface of the talus in the ankle, and the superior area of the capital femoral epiphysis in the hip.

Clinical Picture

The usual presenting complaints are intermittent pain in the joint on strenuous physical activity, stiffness, swelling, clicking, and occasional locking. In weight-bearing joints, an antalgic limp is frequent. At times, the condition is asymptomatic until the osteochondritis dissecans fragment becomes completely detached, falls into the joint, and causes locking. When the knee joint is involved, "giving way" of the knee is a frequent complaint.

Physical findings depend on the joint involved, the duration of the disease, and whether or not the fragment has become detached. On examination, an important finding is localized tenderness over the lesional area. This is usually over the lateral surface of the medial femoral condyle and is best elicited by deep pressure over the lesion with the knee acutely flexed. When the medial femoral condyle is the site of the lesion, the patient will toe out; lateral rotation of the tibia prevents the tibial spine from impinging on the lateral surface of the medial femoral condyle.

Wilson described a sign that is probably diagnostic of osteochondritis dissecans of the knee; in the literature it is often referred to as Wilson's sign. With the patient in supine position, the affected knee is flexed to a right angle, the leg is medially rotated fully, and then the knee is gradually extended. At 30 degrees of flexion, the patient will complain of pain over the anterior aspect of the medial femoral condyle. The pain is relieved on lateral rotation of the leg.[225]

Atrophy of the controlling muscles is common. There may be synovial thickening, hydrarthrosis, and limited joint motion. On rare occasions a detached loose body may be palpated in the knee joint.

In the ankle, the usual complaint is pain on weight-bearing; the pain is usually intermittent and aggravated by strenuous physical activity such as running and sports. Antalgic limp is frequent. There may be episodes of "locking" in the ankle joint or a sensation of "missing" a step. At times, the condition is asymptomatic.

Physical findings depend on the stage in the course of the disease and whether or not the fragment has become detached. The important finding is localized tenderness over the lesional area, detected by markedly plantar-flexing the ankle joint and palpating the medial and lateral corners of the dome of the talus. Pressure can be exerted on the dome of the talus by rotating the leg inward and outward while the foot remains on the floor in plantar flexion and inversion, then in dorsiflexion and eversion. When the fragment is displaced in the joint there will be effusion and synovial thickening of the ankle, clicking, and restriction of range of motion. Atrophy of the calf is common.

Imaging Findings

Radiography. The radiographic picture is diagnostic. A well-circumscribed fragment of subchondral bone is demarcated from the sur-

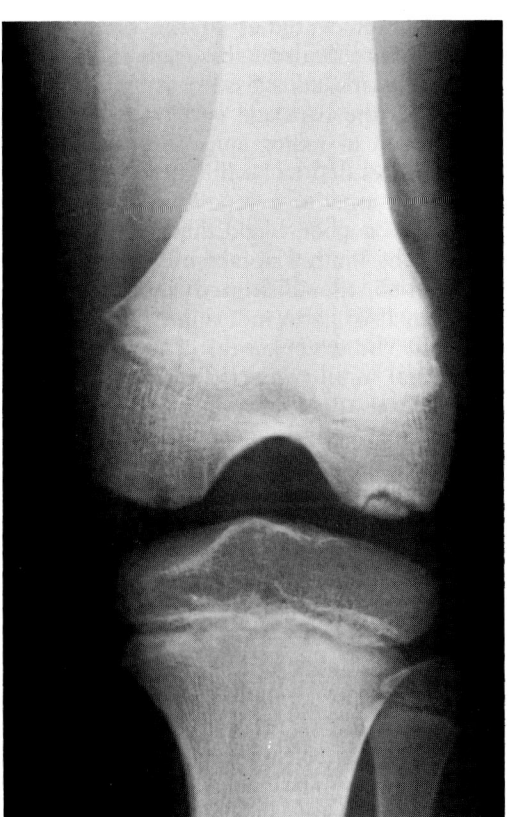

FIGURE 4–41. Osteochondritis dissecans of the knee.

Typical radiographic appearance. A fragment of subchondral bone is demarcated by a radiolucent saucer-shaped line.

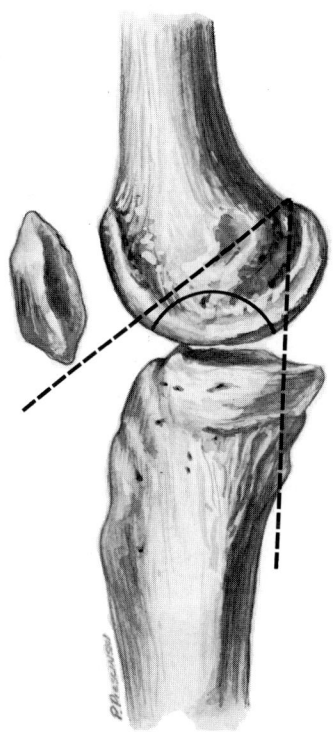

FIGURE 4–42. *Drawing of true lateral projection of knee; method of topographic location of osteochondritis dissecans of medial femoral condyle.*

Table 4–10. *Radiographic Classification of Osteochondritis Dissecans Involving Femoral Condyles**

Topographic location
Medial femoral condyle
Central
Centrolateral
Inferocentral
Lateral femoral condyle
Inferocentral
Posterior
Size—in millimeters
Involvement of weight-bearing area
Weight-bearing
Non-weight-bearing

*From Guhl, J.: Osteochondritis dissecans. *In* Shahriaree, H. (ed.): O'Connor's Textbook of Arthroscopic Surgery. Philadelphia, J. B. Lippincott Co., 1984, p. 211. Reprinted by permission.

The weight-bearing area of the medial femoral condyle is within the boundaries of two intersecting lines, one projected from the posterior femoral shaft and the second projected across the femoral groove.

rounding femoral condyle or affected bone by a radiolucent saucer- or crescent-shaped line (Fig. 4–41). The affected bone may appear denser than the surrounding parent bone. As the fragment separates, the continuity of subchondral bone is distorted, and a "crater" or depression is seen at the site of separation. The detached loose body in the joint, which receives nutrition from the synovial fluid, will continue to grow. Radiopacity of the osteochondritic fragment is due to subchondral bone with articular cartilage, secondary calcification in degenerating articular cartilage, new bone formation following revascularization, and calcification in new surface layers of cartilage and bone.[150]

Special views may be necessary to visualize the lesion. In the knee, for example, the common site of osteochondritis dissecans is the posterolateral aspect of the medial femoral condyle. A routine anteroposterior radiographic view will not show it, so a posteroanterior tunnel or notch view should be made to bring the posterior portion of the femoral condyles and the intercondylar notch into relief. A true lateral view of the knee is made; it is vital that the tibial spine does not overlap the osteochondritic lesion. The purpose of the lateral projection is to determine the topographic location of the lesion—whether it is in the weight-bearing or non-weight-bearing area. The weight-bearing area of the *medial* femoral condyle in the lateral view is outlined—bounded by two intersecting lines—one projected from the posterior femoral shaft, and the second a line projected across the femoral groove (Fig. 4–42).

When describing osteochondritis dissecans of the femoral condyle, one should describe its

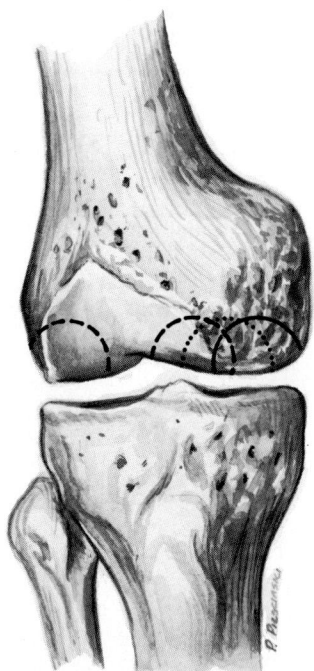

FIGURE 4–43. *Drawing illustrating possible topographic locations of osteochondritis dissecans in femoral condyles.*

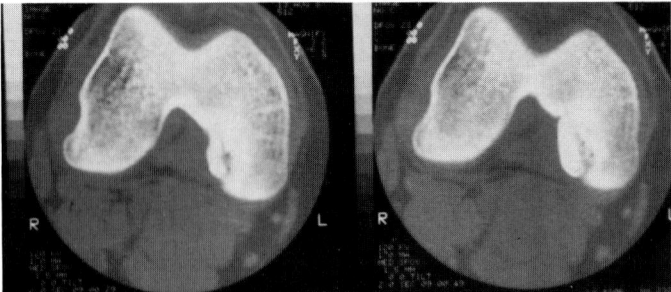

FIGURE 4–44. *Osteochondritis dissecans.*

CT scan of the knee showing osteochondritis dissecans of the medial femoral condyle. Note the clear delineation of the extent of the lesion; the fragment is partially detached.

topographic location, give its size in millimeters, and state whether it is a weight-bearing or a non-weight-bearing area (Fig. 4–43) (Table 4–10).

Irregularity of ossification of the distal femoral epiphyses is normal and should not be mistaken for osteochondritis dissecans. Between the ages of two and six years, the epiphyses have an irregular and ragged outline. Separate small foci of ossification may appear beyond the margin of the main ossific nucleus, simulating loose bodies.[37, 183, 204] Radiologically, the irregular ossification of the femoral condyles has been divided into three groups by Caffey. Group I shows varying degrees of roughening of the margins and, occasionally, small separate foci of calcification; Group II has larger marginal irregularities with specific indentations; and Group

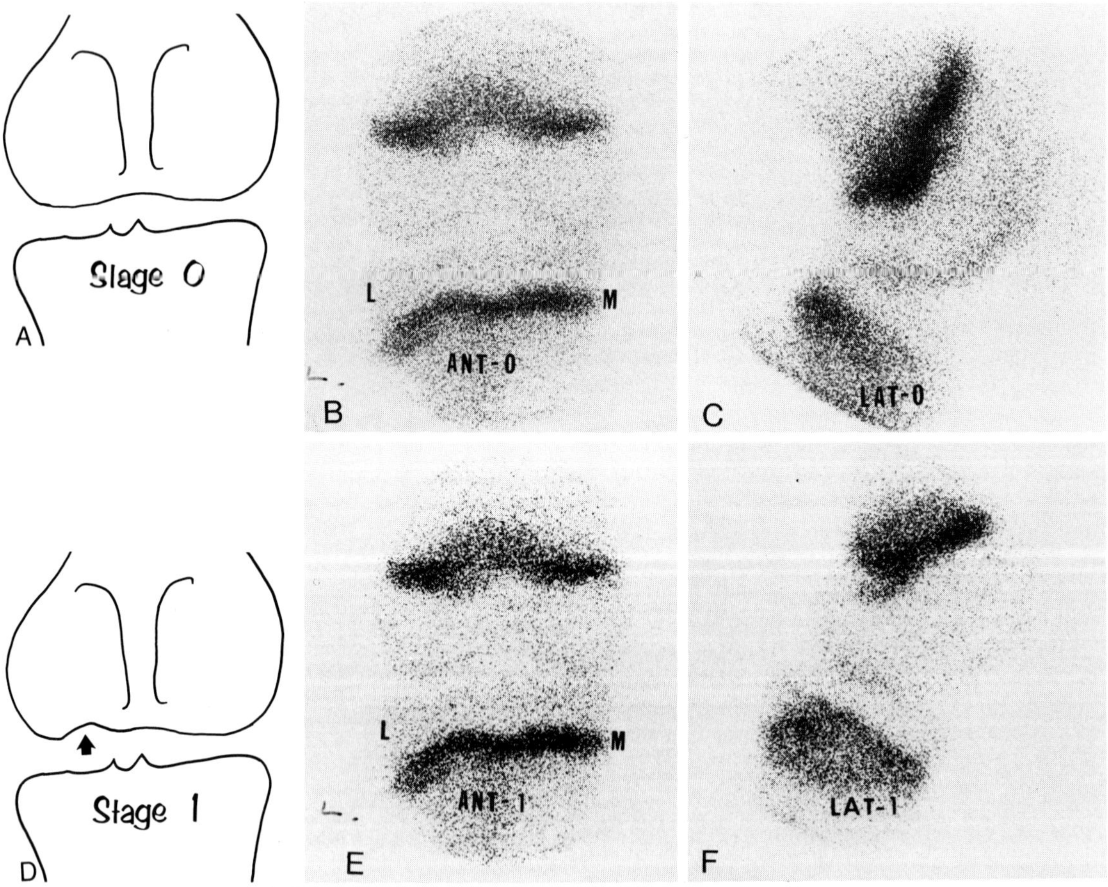

FIGURE 4–45. *Scintigraphic classification of osteochondritis dissecans.*

A to **C**. Stage 0. Line drawing of scintigraphic findings and bone imaging with technetium-99m (anteroposterior and lateral projections) of a normal knee. **D** to **F**. Stage 1. Line drawing and scintigraphic findings of osteochondritis dissecans are normal; the x-rays, however, will show a characteristic defect.

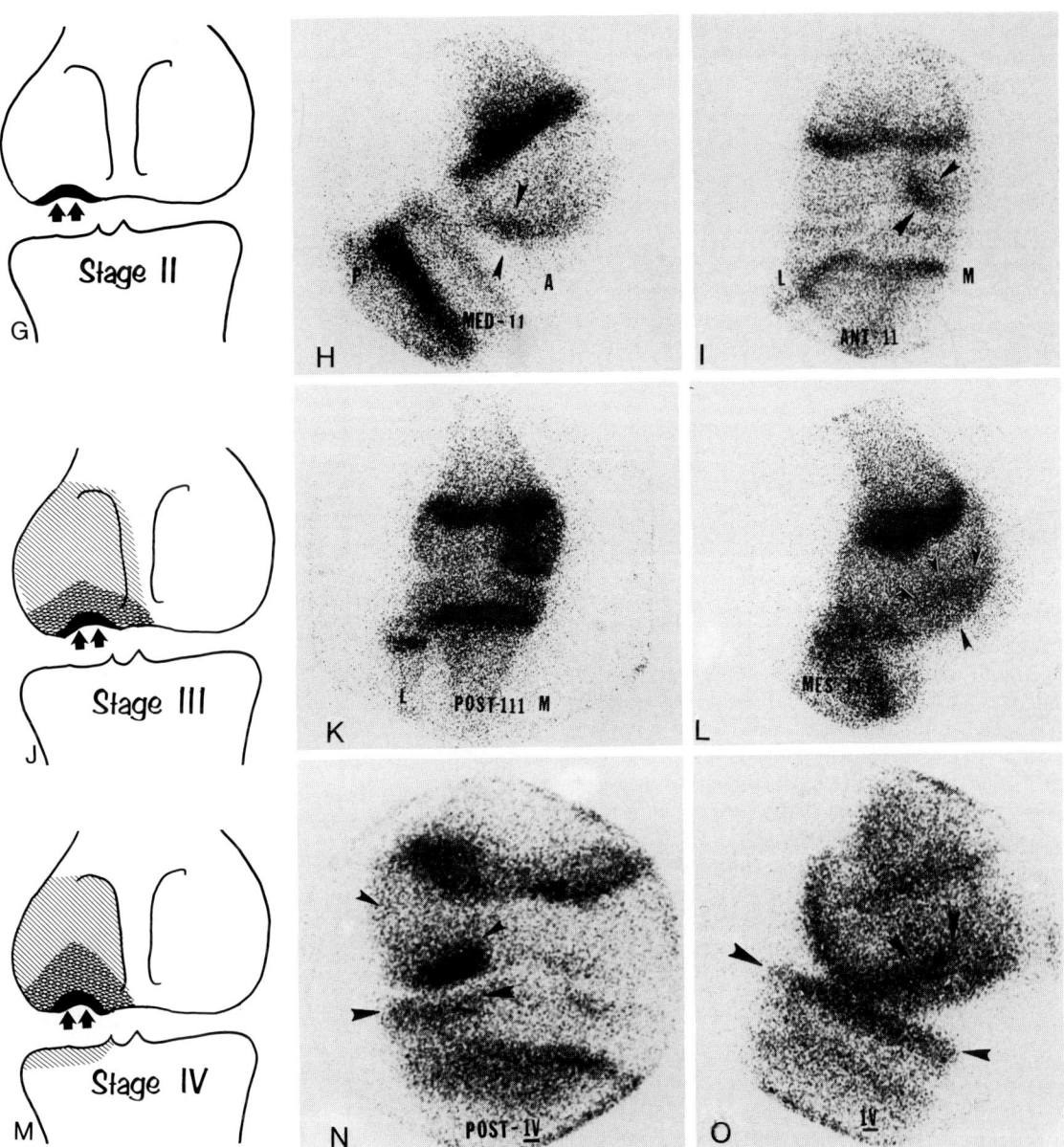

FIGURE 4–45 *Continued. Scintigraphic classification of osteochondritis dissecans.*

G to I. Stage 2. Note the increased focal uptake at the site of the osteochondritic defect. J to L. Stage 3. Note the increased local uptake at the site of the osteochondritis dissecans plus increased activity in the femoral condyle immediately around the lesion. M to O. Stage 4. Same as Stage 3 plus increased activity of the juxtaarticular tibial plateau. (From Cahill, D. K., and Berg, B. C.: 99m-Technetium phosphate compound joint scintigraphy in the management of juvenile osteochondritis dissecans of the femoral condyles. Am. J. Sports Med. 11:329, 1983. Reprinted by permission.)

III has marginal irregularities with an independent island of bone in the marginal crater similar to osteochondritis dissecans in older children.[37]

In the ankle, special views may be necessary. Oblique-lateral views of the ankle are essential. In some cases additional information can be obtained by lateral and anteroposterior linear tomography.

Computed Tomography. The CT scan is of great value in diagnosis and assessment of osteochondritis dissecans (Fig. 4–44). It makes possible a definitive diagnosis when plain radiographs and linear tomography are inconclusive, and it also determines the precise location and true extent of the lesion and sometimes reveals whether the fragment is detached completely or partially, thereby assisting in planning rational operative management.[233]

Arthrography. Routine use of arthrography

*Table 4–11. Scintigraphic Activity Profile with Technetium-99m in Osteochondritis Dissecans of the Femoral Condyles as Correlated with Radiographic and Clinical Findings**

Stage	Increased Uptake in Femoral Condyle	Increased Uptake in Tibia (Juxtaarticular)	Radiographic Defect	Clinical Pain– Local Tenderness
0	−	−	−	−
I	−	−	+	−
II	+	−	+	±
III	+	−	+	+
IV	+	+	+	+

*From Cahill, B. R., and Berg, B. C.: 99m-Technetium phosphate compound joint scintigraphy in the management of juvenile osteochondritis dissecans of the femoral condyles. Am. J. Sports Med., 11:329, 1983. Reprinted by permission.

is not indicated in the knee. In the hip and ankle joints it is of value in determining the looseness of the fragment; i.e., the dye will pass from the intra-articular cartilaginous area beneath an osseous loose body.

Bone Scanning With Technetium-99m. This shows localized increased activity at the site of the lesion. It is vital to use a pinhole collimator to image the involved area. In the knee, anterior, posterior, lateral, and medial projections are made. The image can be enhanced by computer assistance.

Cahill and Berg studied osteochondritis dissecans of the femoral condyles in 18 patients, in seven of whom both knees were involved. The average age of the patients was 12.9 years. The scintigrams were repeated at six-week intervals until the lesion healed. According to the level of scintigraphic activity (in 95 scans) they proposed the following scintigraphic classification of osteochondritis dissecans (Fig. 4–45).[38]

In *Stage 0* the scintigraphic and radiographic findings are those of a *normal* knee.

Stage I shows scintigraphic findings that are normal, but the radiograph depicts a characteristic osteochondritic defect.

The *Stage II* bone scan shows increased focal uptake at the site of the osteochondritic defect.

In *Stage III* the bone scan shows increased local uptake at the site of the osteochondritis dissecans plus increased activity in the femoral condyle immediately around the lesion. The radiograph shows the typical osteochondritis dissecans lesion.

Stage IV has the same scintigraphic activity as Stage III in the femoral condyle plus increased activity of the juxta-articular tibial plateau. The radiograph shows the typical findings of osteochondritis dissecans.

Clinically Stages 0 and I are asymptomatic; Stage II may or may not be associated with pain; Stage III and Stage IV are symptomatic with pain and local tenderness at the site of the lesion.[38] The scintigraphic activity profile and its correlation with radiographic and clinical findings are summarized in Table 4–11.

With healing of the osteochondritis dissecans the increased uptake progressively decreases.

The routine use of bone imaging for osteochondritis dissecans is not recommended by this author. It is performed when the diagnosis is uncertain and anomalies of ossification of the femoral condyles are to be ruled out; in the latter, the scintigraphic appearance will be normal. The second indication is when there is failure of response to conservative management and the decision must be made as to whether surgical intervention is required to enhance the process of healing.

Nuclear magnetic resonance imaging will depict the lesion very clearly and is of great value in delineating the cartilage surface. This author recommends its use in osteochondritis dissecans of the hip and in problem cases if decision-making as to surgical management is needed.

Osteochondritis Dissecans of the Talus

Berndt and Harty reviewed the literature pertaining to this uncommon lesion in 1959 and found two cases of loose bodies in the ankle joint, 30 cases of flake fractures, and 151 cases of osteochondritis dissecans (8 with bilateral involvement), giving a total of 191 lesions.[22] Of the publications they examined, only three reported more than four cases; namely Ray and Coughlin, 13 cases; DiGinder, 19 cases; and Roden and associates, 55 cases.[55, 181, 187] Since then Bourrel and co-workers have reported nine cases in 1972; Kerr, nine cases in 1973; and Scharling, 19 cases in 1978.[29, 112, 192] Males are affected twice as frequently as females.

The site of the lesion is in either the upper medial or the upper lateral angle of the dome of the talus; occasionally it may appear in both medial and lateral angles of the same talus. It is not seen in the middle third of the trochlea. In the 19 cases reported by Scharling the lesions were medial in 13, lateral in 5, and both medial and lateral in 1.[192]

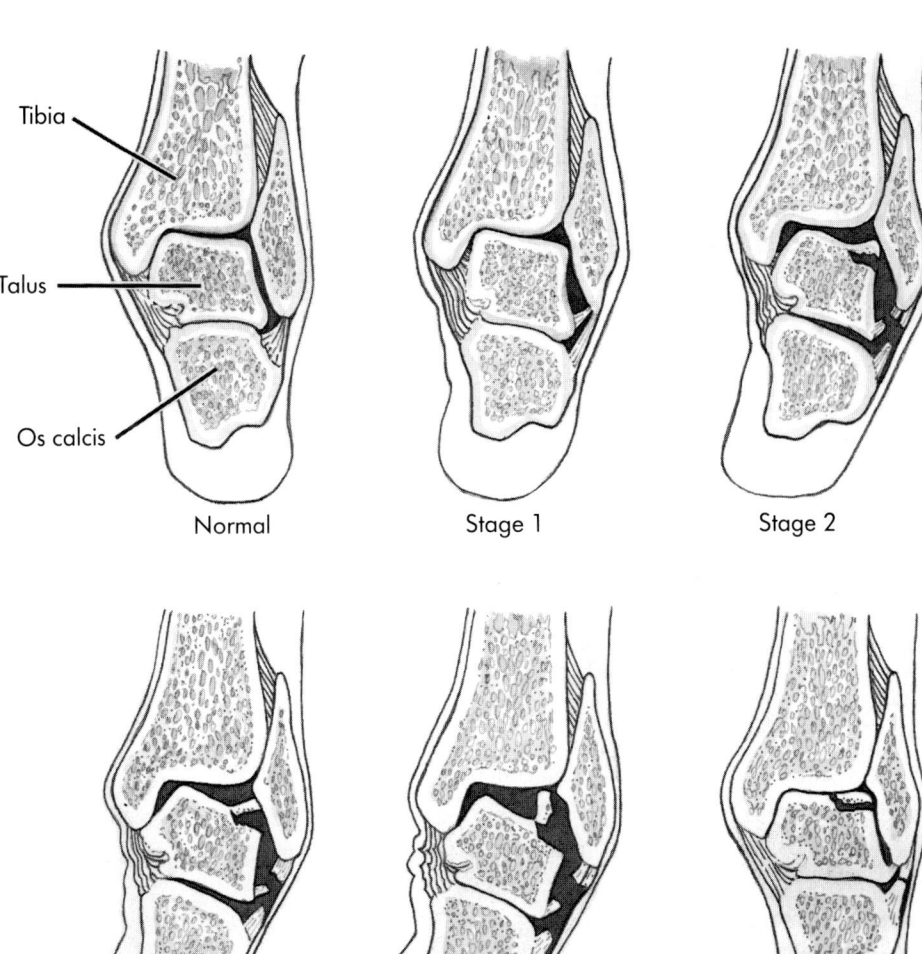

FIGURE 4–46. *Diagram showing mechanism of fracture of lateral border of the dome of the talus (see text).*

(From Berndt, A. L., and Harty, M.: Transchondral fractures (osteochondritis dissecans) of the talus. J. Bone Joint Surg., 41-A:988, 1959. Reprinted by permission.)

In the literature, a definite distinction is made between the lateral and medial lesions. It is generally accepted that osteochondritis dissecans of the lateral angle of the talus are of traumatic origin, whereas injury is not a causative factor in the medially localized lesions. Eskesen proposed that osteochondritis dissecans located in the lateral angle of the dome of the talus is a transchondral fracture.[64] Rasmussen published a report of one case of osteochondritis dissecans localized laterally in the talus that definitely followed an injury.[180] Roden and associates, Berndt and Harty, and O'Donoghue support the theory of the traumatic genesis of lateral angle lesions of the talus.[22, 165, 187] The role of injury in the etiology of medial lesions is not clear; Myhre does not feel that trauma is a causative factor.[159]

In the series of Scharling, in five of the six cases with changes in the upper lateral angle of the talus, symptoms had started following trauma; the sixth patient had a history of severe injury seven and a half years earlier, but the symptoms had not developed until five years later. Of the medially localized lesions, only 5 of 14 had a history of trauma.[192]

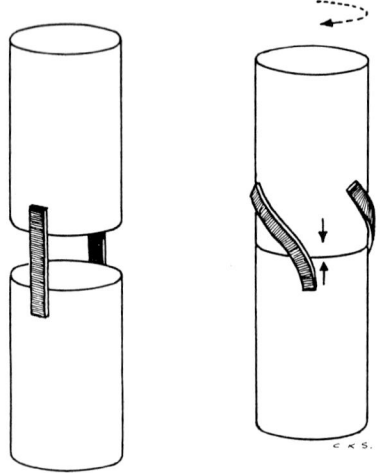

FIGURE 4–47. *Diagram showing mechanism of transchondral fracture of the medial border of the dome of the talus. With the foot in plantar flexion and inversion, lateral rotation of the tibia exerts compression on the medial upper border of the dome of the talus.*

(From Berndt, A. L., and Harty, M.: Transchondral fractures (osteochondritis dissecans) of the talus. J. Bone Joint Surg., 41-A:988, 1959. Reprinted by permission.)

Berndt and Harty have studied the mechanism of transchondral fractures of the dome of the talus. In the lateral lesions, as the foot is inverted, the lateral border of the dome of the talus is compressed against the fibula (Fig. 4–46). At first, *Stage I*, the fibular collateral ligament is intact. In *Stage II* further inversion of the foot ruptures the lateral ligament and causes avulsion with a chip of transchondral bone. In *Stages III and IV* the fragment is completely detached and may remain in place or may be displaced by inversion.

Transchondral fracture of the medial border of the talar dome occurs when, with the foot in plantar flexion and inversion, lateral rotation of the tibia exerts compression on a small area of the medial upper border of the dome of the talus (Fig. 4–47). In *Stage I* the collateral ligaments remain intact. Greater force pushes the posteroinferior lip of the tibia so that it rides medially across the superiorly turned margin of the talus, gouging out an osteochondral chip. In *Stage II* the fragment is partially detached, in *Stage III* it is completely detached, and in *Stage IV* it is displaced within the joint (Fig. 4–48).[22]

Radiographic findings of osteochondritis dissecans of the dome of the talus are shown, those of the lateral corner in Figure 4–49, and those of the medial corner in Figure 4–50.

Treatment

The objectives of treatment are to improve blood supply to the fragment, to promote and expedite healing of the lesion, and to prevent detachment of the fragment.

The type of treatment depends on the age of the patient and the anatomic status of the osteochondritic lesion—whether it is intact, early separated, or partially detached—and whether the crater and detached osteochondritic loose body are salvageable or unsalvageable. The size and topographic location of the lesion and the joint involved are additional factors in decision-making.

NONSURGICAL MANAGEMENT

Treatment in children under 12 years of age is nonoperative and without arthroscopy unless the fragment has become detached. It is vital to distinguish anomalous ossification centers from osteochondritis dissecans—if in doubt, bone imaging with technetium-99m is performed. True undetached osteochondritis dissecans in children usually will heal without surgical intervention, provided the joint is protected from the stresses of weight-bearing.[81] When the lesion is in a non-weight-bearing area or it involves only a portion of the weight-bearing area of a joint it is observed with serial radiograms made every six to eight weeks to determine its natural course. Protection from weight-bearing is not required in such cases, unless the lesion begins to separate and symptoms persist.

The type of appliance utilized to relieve weight-bearing forces varies according to the joint affected. In the knee, an above-knee cylinder plaster cast is applied to eliminate pressure on the lesion caused by walking. The angle of flexion at the knee is predetermined by taking lateral views of the knee in varying degrees of flexion to demonstrate the angle at which weight-bearing forces are not transmitted or are minimally transmitted to the affected area. For a lesion of the talus, a below-knee cast is applied, whereas when the femoral head is involved, crutches are given, or a hip orthosis is utilized to maintain the hip joint in a position in which weight-bearing forces across the lesion are minimal. For an involved knee or ankle, after a six-week period of immobilization, a plastic removable splint may be used. Exercises are performed several times a day to increase muscle strength and range of joint motion.

Weight-bearing is gradually resumed, with crutches providing partial support. Often a pe-

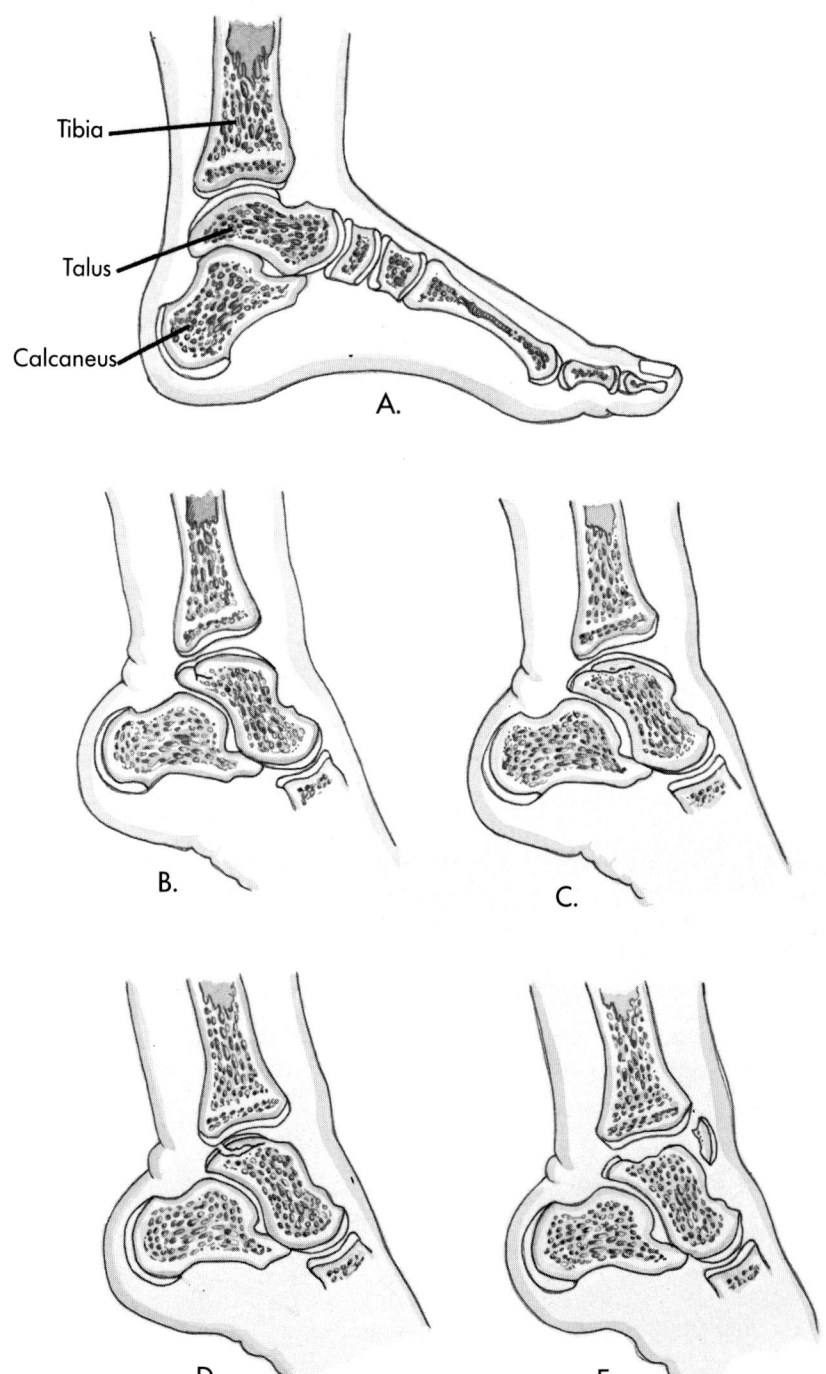

FIGURE 4–48. *Diagram showing mechanism of injury of medial border of the dome of the talus.*

A. Normal. **B.** Stage 1. When the ankle is in plantar flexion and the foot inverts lateral rotation of the tibia produces a small area of compression. Note that the collateral ligaments are intact. **C.** Stage 2. Greater exertion of forces causes the posteroinferior lip of the tibia to ride medially across the superomedial margin of the talus; the result is an osteochondral chip that is partially detached. **D.** Stage 3. The osteochondral fragment is completely detached. **E.** Stage 4. The detached fragment is displaced within the joint. (Redrawn from Berndt, A. L., and Harty, M.: Transchondral fractures [osteochondritis dissecans] of the talus. J. Bone Joint Surg., *41-A*:988, 1959.)

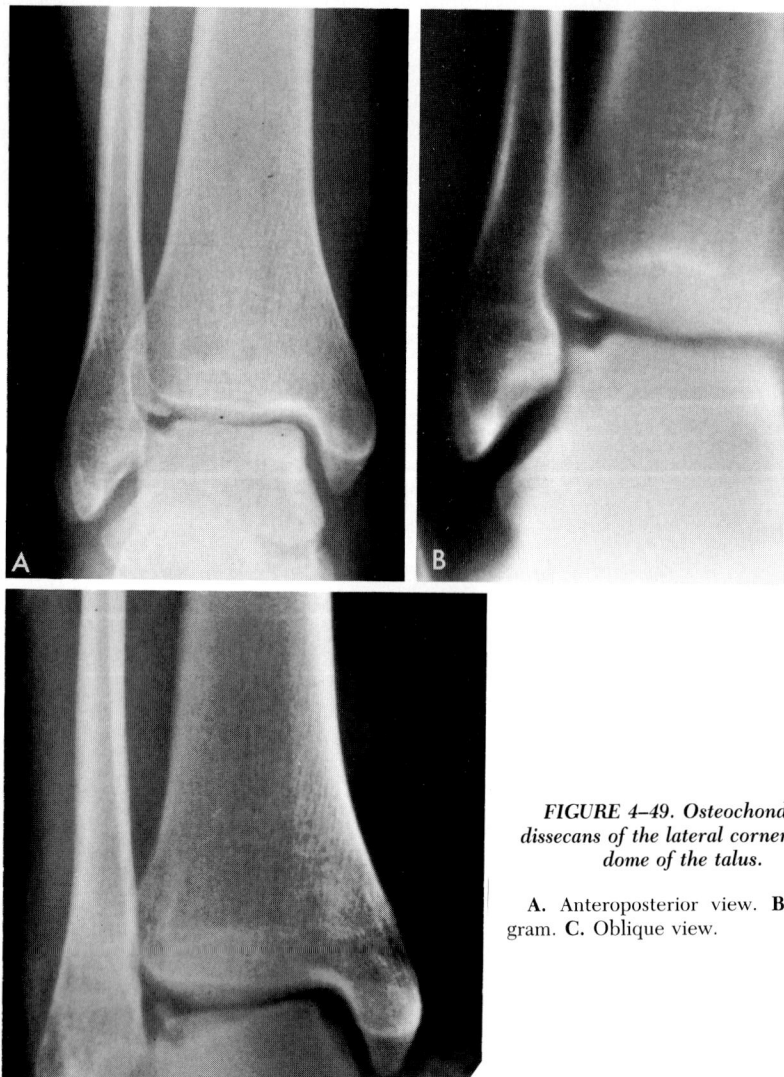

FIGURE 4–49. Osteochondritis dissecans of the lateral corner of the dome of the talus.

A. Anteroposterior view. **B.** Tomogram. **C.** Oblique view.

riod of three months is required for healing of the lesion; in seven to ten months, it may be hardly visible in the radiogram. In about one year, no abnormalities can be visualized.

Unfortunately, not every osteochondritis dissecans lesion in a child under 12 years of age heals; sometimes the fragments separate and become partially or completely detached. When separation begins and the lesion fails to respond to nonsurgical measures this author recommends bone imaging with technetium-99m and computed tomographic studies. Conventional radiographs give a crude depiction of the pathologic state of the lesion, whereas the CT scan will determine whether the lesion is healing or becoming detached. When the lesion is healing, scintigraphy with technetium-99m will show increased uptake. When osteochondritis dissecans in a child fails to respond to nonsurgical management, arthroscopic examination and drilling of the osteochondritic lesion are recommended.

ARTHROSCOPY

Arthroscopy is vital in assessment of osteochondritis dissecans. It directly visualizes the involved area and determines its exact location and size, and probing determines the degree of articular cartilage separation.

Indications. Initially arthroscopy is indicated in osteochondritis dissecans in patients 12 years of age and older in whom the weight-bearing

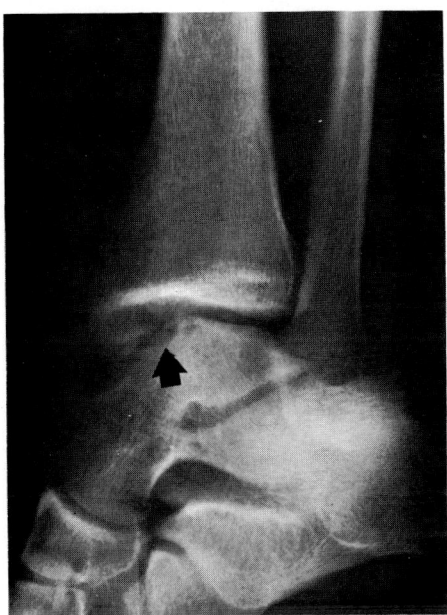

FIGURE 4–50. *Osteochondritis dissecans of medial corner of the dome of the talus.*

Oblique radiograph of the ankle.

area is involved with a lesion over 1 cm. in diameter. Arthroscopic examination is also indicated when the diagnosis is made late, and the lesion has partially separated and produces symptoms. In children under 12 years of age arthroscopic examination is performed when, after an adequate period of nonsurgical treatment, there is no radiographic or clinical evidence of improvement, or if the lesion becomes partially or completely detached.

Technique. Arthroscopy should be performed under general anesthesia in a hospital operating room under strict aseptic conditions. First, the entire joint is thoroughly examined; it is vital to rule out the presence of other associated pathologic conditions, such as meniscal tears or chondromalacia of the patella. Next, the osteochondritic lesion is carefully assessed. Osteochondritis dissecans may be classified as intact, early separated, partially detached, salvageable

Table 4–12. *Arthroscopic Classification of Osteochondritis Dissecans**

1. Intact lesion
2. Early-separated lesion
3. Partially detached lesion
4. Salvageable craters and loose bodies
5. Unsalvageable craters and loose bodies

*From Guhl, J.: Osteochondritis dissecans. *In* Shahriaree, H. (ed.): O'Connor's Textbook of Arthroscopic Surgery. Philadelphia, J. B. Lippincott Co., 1984. Reprinted by permission.

craters and loose bodies, and unsalvageable craters and loose bodies (Table 4–12). Treatment varies according to the progressive stage of the osteochondritic lesion.

In the *intact lesion* the articular cartilage surface is irregular, but there is no break in its continuity as demonstrated visually and by careful probing.

In the *early separated lesion* in addition to softness, fibrillation, and irregularity of the articular cartilage surface there is a partial break of the periphery of the lesion and mobility of the fragment. The *partially detached lesion* is hinged on one edge to adjacent articular cartilage and, in probing, a trapdoor effect can be demonstrated. With the *salvageable loose body* the crater is not more than several weeks old, and the ulcer is fresh with smooth edges. With the *unsalvageable loose body* the crater is filled with fibrous tissue with irregular edges; the detached osteochondral fragment has inadequate bone for reattachment or healing. There may be several loose bodies.

The *intact lesion* is treated by multiple drilling of the transarticular cartilage with an 0.062 smooth Kirschner wire, which is introduced through a small arthroscopic sleeve (a needle-scope cannula). Do not drill through the weight-bearing area of the lesion. It is desirable, if possible, to drill from a non-weight-bearing area. The drill is kept perpendicular to the articular surface; therefore inferocentral lesions of the femoral condyles are drilled from the same side, whereas centrolateral lesions are drilled from the opposite side of the lesion. Caution is exercised to avoid injury to the distal femoral physis and neurovascular structures.

The *early separated lesion* is treated by in situ pinning through the arthroscope. Two or more divergent 0.062 Kirschner wires (preferably smooth) are used for internal fixation. The pins are driven through the lesion into the femoral condyle, aiming at its posterosuperior flare. The protruded proximal part of the pin is attached to a power drill and withdrawn retrograde. The last few millimeters of the pin are withdrawn under direct visualization through the arthroscope until the intra-articular ends of the pins are flush with the surface of the articular cartilage. Multiple drill holes are made in the osteochondritic fragment down to bleeding bone to promote healing. The periphery of the osteochondritic lesion is carefully examined through the arthroscope to ensure that all fibrous tissue is excised. The pins are cut so they protrude only a few millimeters from the posterosuperior flare of the femoral condyles to expedite their later removal.

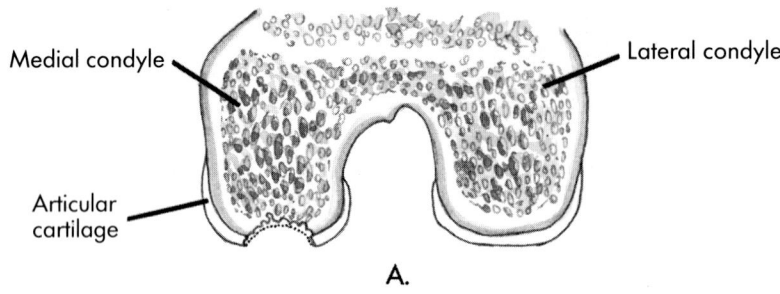

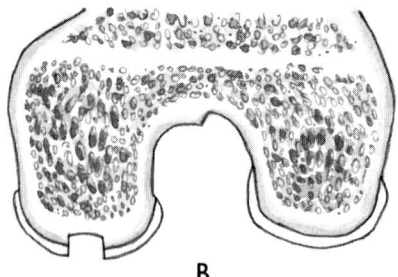
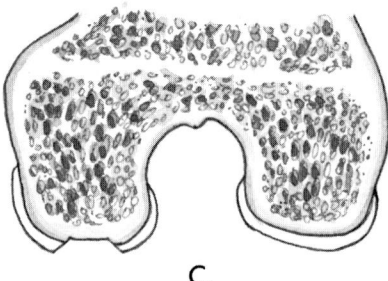

FIGURE 4–51. *Diagram showing methods of treatment of the crater when the osteochondritic loose body is unsalvageable and is removed.*

A. Spongialization—the fibrous tissue and underlying subchondral bone are excised down to bleeding cancellous bone. **B.** Trephination—the edges of the defect are cut perpendicular to the articular surface. **C.** Saucerization—in which the edges of the defect are tapered. Do not perform!

The *partially detached lesion* is treated by flipping the fragment out of the way and debriding the base of the lesion of all fibrous tissue down to bleeding bone. One may use a combination of curets, dental burs, or motorized shavers for debriding fibrous tissue. The base of the crater is then drilled, and the fragment is replaced and pinned with two or more divergent Kirschner wires. Be sure that the periphery of the osteochondritic fragment is congruous with adjacent articular cartilage.

The *salvageable loose body* is treated by curetting the base of the crater down to bleeding bone. The loose fragment is grasped, its undersurface is debrided of fibrous tissue, and then the fragment is reduced into its crater and pinned with two or more divergent Kirschner wires.

The *unsalvageable loose body* is removed through the arthroscope. The crater can be managed with one of the following methods. The best method is spongialization, as proposed by Ficat and associates, in which the fibrous tissue and underlying subchondral bone are removed down to bleeding cancellous bone (Fig. 4–51 A).[66] Another technique is trephining, in which the edges of the defect are cut at right angles to the articular surface. This enhances more uniform ingrowth of fibrocartilage into the defect without interfering with the normal articular surface (Fig. 4–51 B). Saucerization, in which the edges of the defect are tapered, is not recommended (Fig. 4–51 C).

Postoperative Care. After drilling, the knee is immobilized in an above-knee cylinder cast with the foot and ankle free and the knee in the appropriate degree of flexion to relieve pressure on the femoral condyles. Crutches are utilized to prevent weight-bearing. The period of immobilization depends on the age of the patient and the size of the osteochondritic lesion. In the young adolescent and in those with small lesions (less than 1 cm. in diameter), four weeks of immobilization is adequate. Older patients who are skeletally mature require eight weeks of immobilization and protection from weight-bearing. When there is radiographic evidence of early healing the cast is removed, and exercises are performed to develop normal range of joint motion and motor strength of

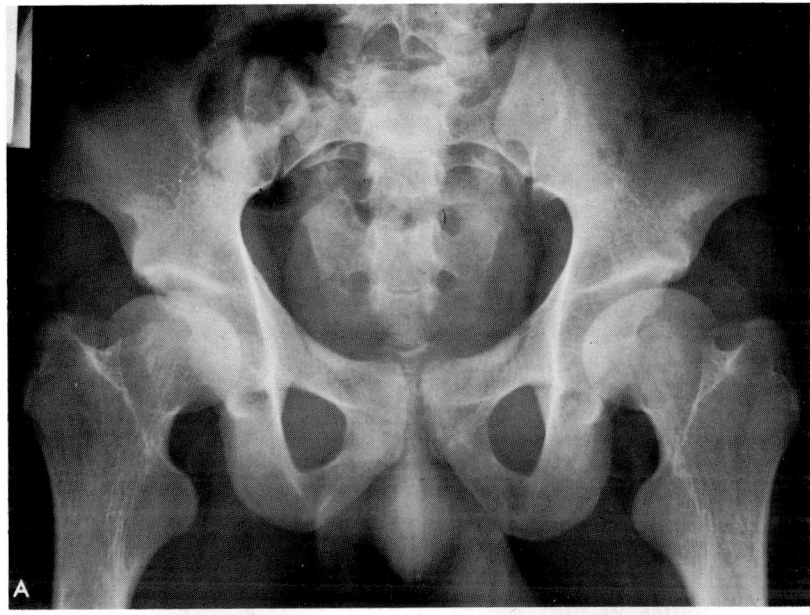

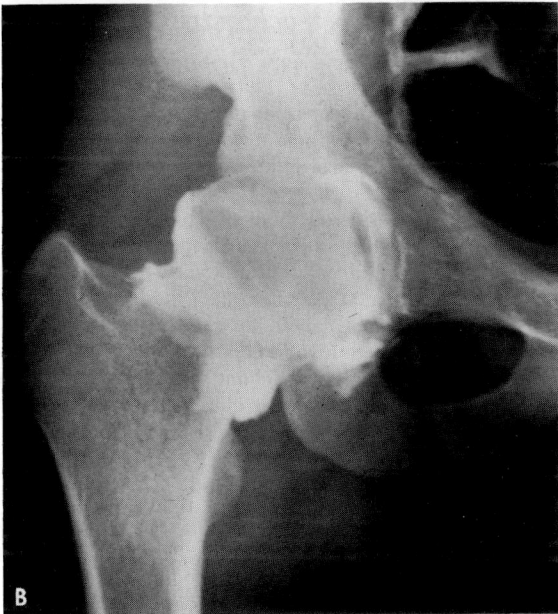

FIGURE 4–52. Osteochondritis dissecans of the hip.

A. Anteroposterior radiograms of both hips. Note the lesion on the superior surface of the right femoral head. **B.** Arthrogram of same hip showing that the fragment is not detached.

muscles. Physical activity and sports are restricted until there is adequate healing, with mature bone trabeculae traversing the defect. Occasionally, in recalcitrant lesions that fail to heal, a follow-up arthroscopic examination and repeat drilling of the lesion may be necessary.

When the fragment is internally fixed with Kirschner wires, the limb is immobilized in a cast, and weight-bearing is prevented by protecting with crutches for eight weeks until there is radiographic evidence of healing. The pins are then removed, and active assisted and passive exercises are performed to develop range of motion of the joint and muscle strength. Full weight-bearing is not allowed until there is radiographic evidence of adequate healing as evidenced by mature bone trabeculae traversing the defect (at about four months). Resumption of normal physical and sports activities is individualized.

Text continued on page 1534

Exposure of the Angles of the Dome of the Talus for Excision of Osteochondritis Dissecans (Continued)

MEDIAL CORNER OF THE DOME OF THE TALUS

To expose the medial corner of the dome of the talus an osteotomy of the medial malleolus is required.

E. A medial incision about 7 to 9 cm. long is made centered over the medial malleolus. The subcutaneous tissue and deep fascia are divided in line with the skin incision.

F. The level of the ankle joint and the tip of the medial malleolus are identified. If the *distal tibial physis* is still open it should *not* be *injured*. The capsule of the ankle joint is opened by a transverse incision. The line of osteotomy of the medial malleolus is in line with the ankle joint.

G. The distal part of the medial malleolus is exposed subperiosteally. If the distal physis of the tibia is open, a transverse incision is made; if closed, a longitudinal incision.

H. Then a transverse osteotomy of the medial malleolus is performed at the level of the ankle joint. By rotating the medial malleolus downward 90 degrees and forcefully abducting the foot, the ankle joint and superior surface of the talus are visualized.

I. After excision of the osteochondritic fragment the medial malleolus is anatomically reduced and internally fixed with two or three *smooth* pins when the distal tibial physis is open, or with a single metal screw in the skeletally mature ankle. The capsule of the ankle joint and the wound are closed. A below-knee cast is applied for six weeks. The healing of the osteotomized malleolus is not a problem.

Plate 52. Exposure of the Angles of the Dome of the Talus for Excision of Osteochondritis Dissecans

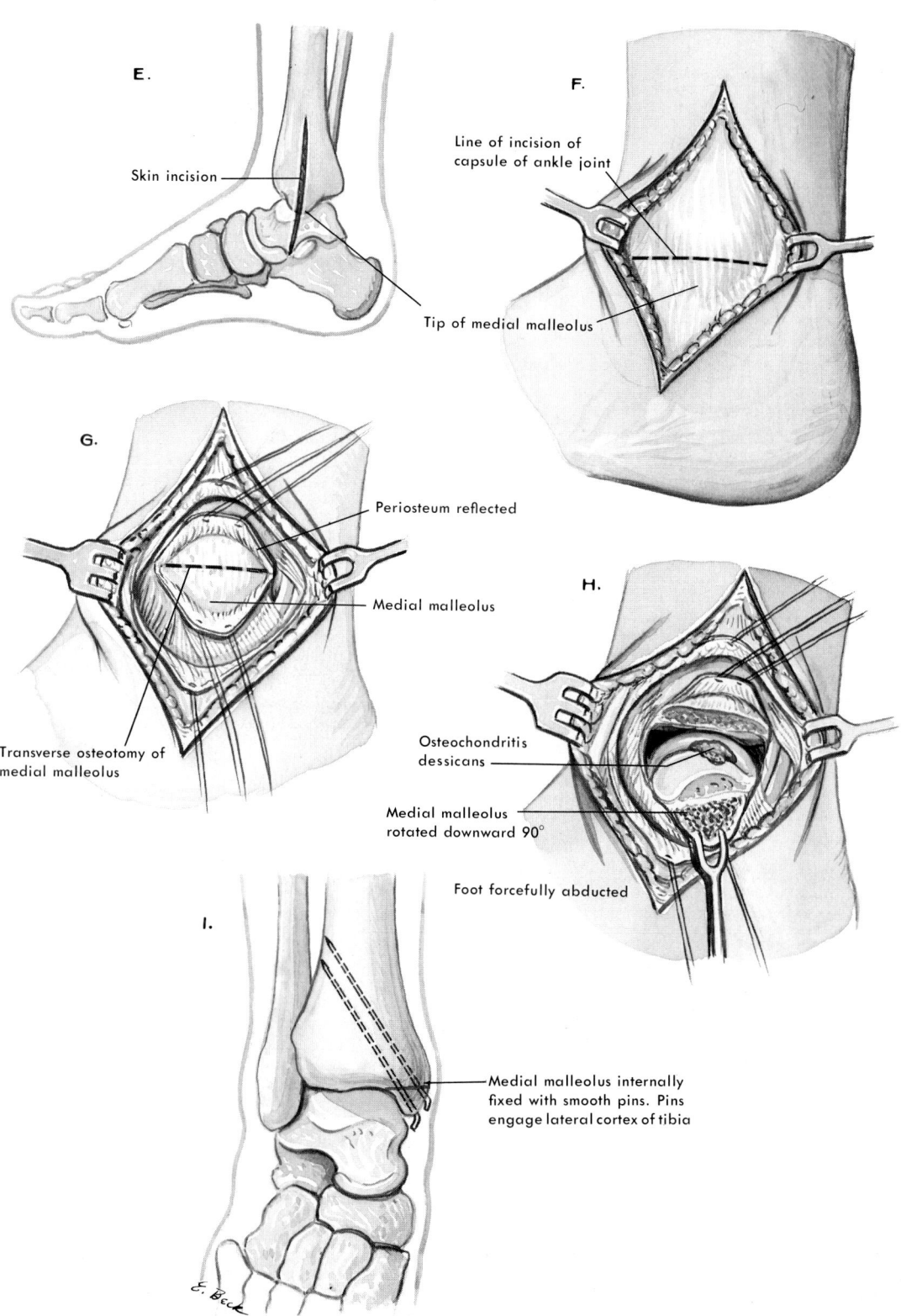

When the unsalvageable loose body is removed and the crater is debrided, immediate motion of the knee is crucial. Protected weight-bearing is permitted early, and full weight-bearing is allowed as soon as the joint is asymptomatic.

OPEN SURGICAL TREATMENT

Arthrotomy is recommended when grafting of the base of the crater and reshaping of the osteochondritic fragment for a congruous fit are required. Also, open arthrotomy is indicated when there are multiple loose fragments or the anatomic site of the lesion makes access with arthroscopic instrumentation difficult.

Operative Technique. In the knee, an anteromedial incision is used for lesions of the medial femoral condyle and an anterolateral incision for those of the lateral condyle. The loose osteochondritic fragment is removed, and its under surface carefully debrided of all fibrous tissue. The crater is curetted and drilled until bleeding cancellous bone is exposed. The tourniquet should be released at this stage to be sure that the prepared bed at the crater is bleeding. After hemostasis, the tourniquet is reinflated, and the loose bone fragment is grafted into the bed of the crater and fixed internally with divergent Kirschner wires. This author recommends the use of threaded wires. The intra-articular ends of the wires should be flush with the articular cartilage surface, and their proximal ends should protrude only a few millimeters out of the femoral condyles and deep into subcutaneous tissue for ease of later removal. The limb is immobilized. The pins are removed four to six weeks after surgery. Weight-bearing is not allowed until there is radiographic evidence of union of the fragment to underlying bone.[140]

When the ankle is involved, inaccessible lesions may require osteotomy of the medial malleolus for surgical exposure. The technique of surgical exposure of the lateral and medial angles of the dome of the talus is described and illustrated in Plate 52. The rest of the preparation of the bed and grafting is the same as for knee lesions.

Perfect repositioning of the displaced fragment so that it is flush with the rest of the articular surface is technically difficult. If the fragment is placed too deeply, a defect in the articular surface will still persist, whereas if the fragment projects, it creates an irregularity and incongruity of the joint, damaging a normal articular area of the corresponding opposing bone. This technique also requires a second operation for removal of the pins.

Osteochondritis Dissecans of the Hip

This presents a difficult problem. The lesion is usually located in the superolateral portion of the femoral head (Fig. 4–52). It may be a sequela of Legg-Perthes disease. If the fragment is not loose, conservative management is recommended. The hip is protected with crutches with a three-point toe-touch gait for six months. If healing does not take place, operative intervention may be required. The early separated lesion is treated by multiple drilling, but the partially detached fragment should be fixed internally. Often, one must dislocate the hip for proper visualization and exposure of the lesion. The type of internal fixation utilized varies according to the experience of the surgeon. It may be with screws, which are countersunk, or by multiple Kirschner wires. If it is in the weight-bearing portion, this author recommends an intertrochanteric osteotomy to tilt and rotate the site of involvement to a non-weight-bearing area. This will definitely expedite healing and prevent collapse.

References

1. Aichroth, P.: Osteochondritis dissecans of the knee. A clinical survey. J. Bone Joint Surg., 53-B:440, 1971.
2. Aichroth, P.: Osteochondral fractures and their relationship to osteochondritis dissecans of the knee. An experimental study in animals. J. Bone Joint Surg., 53 B:448, 1071.
3. Alexander, A. H., and Lichtman, D. M.: Surgical treatment of transchondral talar-dome fractures (osteochondritis dissecans). Long-term follow-up. J. Bone Joint Surg., 62-A:646, 1980.
4. Almgard, L. E., and Wikstad, I.: Late results of surgery for osteochondritis dissecans of the knee joint. Acta Chir. Scand., 127:588, 1964.
5. Altenstrasser, F.: Zur operativen Behandlung der Osteochondrosis dissecans des Huftgelenkes. Arch. Orthop. Unfallchir., 60:148, 1966.
6. Anderson, D. V., and Lyne, E. D.: Osteochondritis dissecans of the talus: Case report on two family members. J. Pediatr. Orthop., 4:356, 1984.
7. Anderson, W. J., and Guilford, W. B.: Osteochondritis dissecans of the humeral head. An unusual cause of shoulder pain. Clin. Orthop., 173:166, 1983.
8. Andren, L., Carstam, N., and Linden, B.: Osteochondritis dissecans and brachymesophalangia: A hereditary syndrome. J. Hand Surg., 3:117, 1978.
9. Andrews, T. A., Spivey, J., and Lindebaum, R. H.: Familial osteochondritis dissecans and dwarfism. Acta Orthop. Scand., 52:519, 1981.
10. Archer, V. W., and Peterson, C. H.: Osteochondritis dissecans. South. Med. J., 23:611, 1930.
11. Arcomand, J. P., Kamhi, E., Karas, S., and Moriarty, V. J.: Transchondral fractures and osteochondritis dissecans of talus. N.Y. State J. Med., 78:2183, 1978.
12. Aronsson, H.: Über Osteochondritis dissecans im Fussgelenk. Zentralbl. Chir., 69:312, 1942.
13. Auffray, Y., and Kraft, F.: Ostéochondrite primitive de la hanche. Evolution et prognostic des spontanément centrées. Rev. Chir. Orthop., 58:303, 1972.

14. Auld, C. D., and Chesney, R. B.: Familial osteochondritis dissecans and carpal tunnel syndrome. Acta Orthop. Scand., 50:727, 1979.
15. Axhausen, G.: Die Aetiologie der Kohler'schen Erkrankung der Metatarsalkopfchen. Beitr. Klin. Chir., 126:451, 1922.
16. Bandi, W.: Über die Ätiologie der Osteochondritis dissecans. Helv. Chir. Acta, 18:221, 1951.
17. Bandi, W., and Allgower, M.: Zur Therapie der Osteochondritis dissecans. Helv. Chir. Acta, 26:552, 1959.
18. Barbieri, L., and Bononi, E.: Considerazioni etiopathogenetiche sulle osteocondrosi giovanili. Minerva Orthop., 20:119, 1969.
19. Bauer, R.: Mechanical factors relating to osteochondritis dissecans of the hip. Verh. Dtsch. Ges. Orthop., 55:374, 1968.
20. Beck, W., and Saffar, H.: Osteochondroses dissecans des Kniegelenks bei Scheibenmeniskus. Beitr. Klin. Chir., 218:270, 1970.
21. Bennett, G. A., and Bauer, W.: A study of the repair of articular cartilage and the reaction of normal joints of adult dogs to surgically created defects of articular cartilage, "joint mice," and patellar displacement. Am. J. Pathol., 8:499, 1932.
22. Berndt, A. L., and Harty, M.: Transchondral fractures (osteochondritis dissecans) of the talus. J. Bone Joint Surg., 41-A:988, 1959.
23. Bernstein, M. A.: Osteochondritis dissecans. J. Bone Joint Surg., 7:319, 1925.
24. Bigelow, D. R.: Juvenile osteochondritis dissecans. J. Bone Joint Surg., 57-B:530, 1975.
25. Boldero, J. L., and Mitchell, G. P.: Osteochondritis of the superior tibial epiphysis. J. Bone Joint Surg., 36-B:114, 1954.
26. Boni, V.: Osteocondrite dissecante dell'anca. Arch. Putti Chir. Organi Mov., 6:151, 1955.
27. Bonnin, J. G.: Osteochondritis dissecans and torn lateral meniscus. Br. J. Surg., 33:380, 1946.
28. Bots, R. A., and Slooff, T. J.: Arthroscopy in the evaluation of operative treatment of osteochondrosis dissecans. Orthop. Clin. North Am., 10:685, 1979.
29. Bourrel, P., Maistre, B., Palinacci, J. C., Gourul, J. C., and Jardin, M.: Ostéochondrite de l'astragale. A propos de 9 observations. Rev. Chir. Orthop., 58:609, 1972.
30. Brickey, P. A., and Grow, J. B.: Osteochondritis dissecans. Report of cases involving elbow, ankle and metatarsophalangeal joint. Am. J. Surg., 48:463, 1940.
31. Brown, R. T.: Costochondritis in adolescents. J. Adolesc. Health Care, 1:198, 1981.
32. Bruckl, R., Rosemeyer, B., and Thiermann, G.: Osteochondrosis dissecans of the knee. Results of operative treatment in juveniles. Arch. Orthop. Trauma. Surg., 102:221, 1984.
33. Buchner, L., and Rieger, H.: Konnen freie Gelenkkorper durch Trauma entstehen. Arch. Klin. Chir., 116:460, 1921.
34. Burge, M., Dolanc, B., Jenny, H., and Morscher, E.: Therapy and results in osteochondritis dissecans of the knee joint. Orthopaede, 9:320, 1980.
35. Burr, R. C.: Osteochondritis dissecans. Can. Med. Assoc. J., 41:232, 1939.
36. Buxton, R. A., and McCullough, C. J.: Healing of osteochondritis dissecans following congenital dislocation of the hip: Report of a case. Clin. Orthop., 147:157, 1980.
37. Caffey, J., Madell, S. H., Royer, C., and Morales, P.: Ossification of the distal femoral epiphysis. J. Bone Joint Surg., 40-A:647, 1958.
38. Cahill, B. R., and Berg, B. C.: 99m-Technetium phosphate compound joint scintigraphy in the management of juvenile osteochondritis dissecans of the femoral condyles. Am. J. Sports Med., 11:329, 1983.
39. Camera, R.: Osteocondrite giovanile del capitello radiale. Minerva Ortop., 5:376, 1954.
40. Cameron, H. U., Piliar, R. M., and MacNab, I.: Fixation of loose bodies in joints. Clin. Orthop., 100:309, 1974.
41. Campbell, C., and Ranawat, C.: Osteochondritis dissecans: The question of etiology. J. Trauma, 6:201, 1966.
42. Canale, S. T., and Belding, R. H.: Osteochondral lesions of the talus. J. Bone Joint Surg., 62-A:97, 1980.
43. Carroll, N. C., and Mubarak, S. J.: Juvenile osteochondritis dissecans of the knee. J. Bone Joint Surg., 59-B:506, 1977.
44. Casscells, S. W.: The place of arthroscopy in the diagnosis and treatment of internal derangement of the knee: An analysis of 1000 cases. Clin. Orthop., 151:135, 1980.
45. Chiroff, R. T., and Cooke, C. P., III: Osteochondritis dissecans: A histologic and microradiographic analysis of surgically excised lesions. J. Trauma, 15:689, 1975.
46. Chironi, P.: In tema di osteochondrite della rotula. Minerva Ortop., 5:140, 1954.
47. Clanton, T. O., and DeLee, J. C.: Osteochondritis dissecans. History, pathophysiology and current treatment concepts. Clin. Orthop., 167:50, 1982.
48. Cobey, M. C.: Osteochondritis dissecans of the astragalus. Milit. Surg., 93:184, 1943.
49. Cobey, M. C.: Traumatic avascular necrosis of the astragalus. Clin. Orthop., 81:180, 1971.
50. Convery, F. R., Akeson, W. Y., and Keown, G. H.: The repair of large osteochondral defects. Clin. Orthop., 82:253, 1972.
51. Conway, F. M.: Osteochondritis dissecans: Description of stages of the condition and its probable traumatic etiology. Am. J. Surg., N.S., 38:691, 1937.
52. Crysler, W. E., and Morton, H. S.: Osteochondritis dissecans of the supratrochlear septum of the humerus. A.J.R., 54:41, 1945.
53. Dawson, C. W.: Osteochondritis dissecans: A discussion of two similar lesions. Arch. Surg., 46:635, 1943.
54. Debeyre, J., Goutallier, D., and Ghopin, D.: L'ostéochondrite disséquante du femur. Rev. Chir. Orthop., 59:381, 1973.
55. DeGinder, W. L.: Osteochondritis dissecans of the talus. Radiology, 65:590, 1955.
56. De Santis, E., and Fabbriciani, C.: Osteochondrosis dissecans of the knee in juveniles. Arch. Putti Chir. Organi Mov., 31:35, 1981.
57. Devas, M.: Stress avulsions and osteochondritis. In Stress Fractures. London, Churchill Livingstone, 1975, pp. 190–211.
58. Dexel, M., and Jehle, U.: Results in the operative treatment of osteochondrosis dissecans of the knee joint (author's transl.). Orthopaede, 10:87, 1981.
59. Dini, P.: Localizzazioni rare dell'osteocondrite dei metatarsi. Arch. Putti, 15:280, 1961.
60. Dinkel, L.: Der seltene Befund einer Osteochondritis Dissecans am Fibularenrand der Talusrolle. Fortschr. Geb. Röntgenstr., 115:265, 1971.
61. Edelstein, G. M.: Osteochondritis dissecans with spontaneous resolution. J. Bone Joint Surg., 36-B:343, 1954.
62. Editorial: Osteochondritis dissecans. Lancet, 2:243, 1976.
63. Edwards, D. H., and Bentley, G.: Osteochondritis dissecans of the patella. J. Bone Joint Surg., 59-B:58, 1977.
64. Eskesen, B.: En sjaelden intraartikulaer talus-fractur. Nord. Med., 16:436, 1942.
65. Fairbanks, H. A. T.: Osteo-chondritis dissecans. Br. J. Surg., 21:67, 1933.
66. Ficat, P., Arlet, J., and Mazieres, B.: Osteochondritis and osteonecrosis of the lower end of the femur:

Interest of functional investigation of the marrow. Sem. Hôp. Paris, 51:1907, 1975.
67. Ficat, R. P., Ficat, C., Gedeon, P., and Toussaint, J. B.: Spongialization: A new treatment for diseased patellae. Clin. Orthop., 144:74, 1979.
68. Fontaine, R.: Ostéochondrite disséquante bilaterale de tête fémorale. Rev. Chir. Orthop., 39:342, 1953.
69. Francon, E.: L'ostéochondrite disséquante de la hance (maladie de Koenig de la tête fémorale). Rev. Rhum., 2:770, 1935.
70. Fraser, W. N. C.: Familial osteochondritis dissecans. J. Bone Joint Surg., 48-B:598, 1966.
71. Freehafer, A. A.: Osteochondritis dissecans following Legg-Calvé-Perthes disease. J. Bone Joint Surg., 42-A:777, 1960.
72. Freiberg, A. H.: Osteochondritis dissecans. J. Bone Joint Surg., 5:13, 1923.
73. Freiberg, A. H., and Woolley, P. G.: Osteochondritis dissecans: Concerning its nature and relation to formation of joint mice. Am. J. Orthop. Surg., 8:477, 1910.
74. Freund, E.: Osteochondritis dissecans of the head of the femur. Arch. Surg., 39:323, 1939.
75. Gade, E. A.: Zur operativen Frühbehandlung der Osteochondrosis dissecans des Kniegelenkes. Z. Orthop., 114:233, 1976.
76. Gardiner, T. B.: Osteochondritis dissecans in three members of one family. J. Bone Joint Surg., 37-B:139, 1955.
77. Genovesi, A.: L'osteocondrosi dissecante del capitello del radio. Minerva Ortop., 7:463, 1955.
78. Gillespie, N. F., and Day, B.: Bone peg fixation in the treatment of osteochondritis dissecans. Clin. Orthop., 125:130, 1979.
79. Goldman, A. B., Hallel, T., Salvati, E. M., and Freiberg, R. H.: Osteochondritis dissecans complicating Legg-Perthes disease. A report of four cases. Radiology, 121:561, 1976.
80. Green, J. P.: Osteochondritis dissecans of the knee. J. Bone Joint Surg., 48-B:82, 1966.
81. Green, W. T., and Banks, H. H.: Osteochondritis dissecans in children. J. Bone Joint Surg., 35-A:26, 1953.
82. Grepl, J., and Eckert, V.: Dissecant osteochondrosis of the ankle joint (author's transl.). Acta Chir. Orthop. Traumatol. Cech., 49:66, 1982.
83. Greville, N. R.: Osteochondritis dissecans: Treatment by bone grafting. South. Med. J., 57:886, 1964.
84. Gschwend, N., Munzinger, U., and Lohr, J.: Our method of extra-articular dissected fixation in osteochondrosis dissecans of the knee (author's transl.). Orthopaede, 10:83, 1981.
85. Guelpa, G., Chamay, A., and Lagier, R.: Bilateral osteochondritis dissecans of the carpal scaphoid. A radiological and anatomical study of one case. Int. Orthop., 4:25, 1980.
86. Guhl, J.: Arthroscopic treatment of osteochondritis dissecans. Preliminary report. Orthop. Clin. North Am., 10:671, 1979.
87. Guhl, J.: Arthroscopic treatment of osteochondritis dissecans. Clin Orthop., 167:65, 1982.
88. Guhl, J.: Osteochondritis dissecans. In Casscells, S. W. (ed.): Arthroscopy Diagnostic and Surgical Practice. Philadelphia, Lea & Febiger, 1984, pp. 113–120.
89. Guhl, J.: Osteochondritis dissecans. In Shahriaree, H. (ed.): O'Connor's Textbook of Arthroscopic Surgery. Philadelphia, Lippincott, 1984, pp. 211–226.
90. Guhl, J. F.: Update in the treatment of osteochondritis dissecans. Orthopedics, 7:1744, 1984.
91. Guicciardi, E., Rusconi, U., and Valli, F.: Considerazioni sulla ossificazione dell'acetabolo nell'anca lussata sede di osteocondrite post-riduttiva. Minerva Ortop., 20:93, 1969.
92. Guilleminet, M., and Barbier, J. M.: Osteochondritis dissecans of the hip. J. Bone Joint Surg., 39-B:268, 1957.
93. Hallel, T., and Salvati, E. A.: Osteochondritis dissecans following Legg-Calvé-Perthes disease. Report of three cases. J. Bone Joint Surg., 58-A:708, 1976.
94. Hanley, W. B., McKusick, V. A., and Barranco, F. T.: Osteochondritis dissecans with associated malformations in two brothers. A review of familial aspects. J. Bone Joint Surg., 49-A:925, 1967.
95. Harbin, M., and Zollinger, R.: Osteochondritis of the growth centres. Surg. Gynecol. Obstet., 51:145, 1930.
96. Harding, W. G., 3rd: Diagnosis of osteochondritis dissecans of the femoral condyles: The value of the lateral x-ray view. Clin. Orthop., 123:25, 1977.
97. Harms, H.: Osteochondritis Dissecans an der Talusrolle. Zentralbl. Chir., 54:1017, 1927.
98. Hay, B. M.: Two cases of osteochondritis dissecans affecting several joints. J. Bone Joint Surg., 32-B:361, 1950.
99. Hermadsson, I.: Über die Osteochondritis dissecans des Femurkopfes. Acta Radiol., 25:269, 1944.
100. Hermans, G. P.: Osteochondritis dissecans of the elbow joint (author's transl.). Orthopaede, 10:335, 1981.
101. Hermanson, R. H.: Bilateral osteochondritis dissecans of the knee. Radiology, 47:349, 1946.
102. Herzberger, M., Schuler, P., and Rossak, K.: Osteochondrosis dissecans of the patella (author's transl.). Z. Orthop., 120:268, 1982.
103. Hicks, G. B. T.: Osteochondritis of the tarsal second cuneiform bone. Br. J. Radiol., 26:214, 1953.
104. Hughston, J. C., Hergenroeder, P. T., and Courtenay, B. G.: Osteochondritis dissecans of the femoral condyles. J. Bone Joint Surg., 66-A:1340, 1984.
105. Hutchinson, R. G.: Osteochondritis dissecans. Records of some unusual cases. Br. J. Radiol., 16:147, 1943.
106. Ilfeld, F. W., and Rosen, V.: Osteochondritis of the first metatarsal sesamoid. Clin. Orthop., 85:38, 1972.
107. Irani, R. N., Karasick, D., and Karasick, S.: A possible explanation of the pathogenesis of osteochondritis dissecans. J. Pediatr. Orthop., 4:358, 1984.
108. Jenkins, S. A.: Osteochondritis dissecans of the hip. J. Bone Joint. Surg., 40-B:827, 1958.
109. Johnson, E. W., Jr., and McLeod, T. L.: Osteochondral fragments of the distal end of the femur fixed with bone pegs. Report of two cases. J. Bone Joint Surg., 59-A:677, 1977.
110. Katz, J. F., and Siffert, R. S.: Osteochondritis dissecans in association with Legg-Calvé-Perthes disease. Int. Orthop., 3:189, 1979.
111. Kennedy, J. C., Grainger, R. W., and McGraw, R. W.: Osteochondral fractures of the femoral condyles. J. Bone Joint Surg., 48-B:436, 1966.
112. Kerr, T. S.: Osteochondritis dissecans of the talus. Proc. R. Soc. Med., 66:517, 1973.
113. King, D.: Osteochondritis dissecans. J. Bone Joint Surg., 14:535, 1932.
114. King, D., and Richards, V.: Osteochondritis dissecans of the hip. J. Bone Joint Surg., 22:327, 1940.
115. Kleinberg, S.: Bilateral osteochondritis dissecans of the patella. J. Bone Joint Surg., 31-A:185, 1949.
116. Kolp, W., and Jaster, D.: Operative treatment of osteochondritis dissecans of the knee joint. Beitr. Orthop. Traumatol., 27:212, 1980.
117. König, F.: Ueber freie Korper in den Gelenken. Dtsch. Z. Chir., 27:90, 1887–1888.
118. König, F.: Zur Frage der Osteochondritis Dissecans. Zentralbl. Chir., 32:809, 1905.
119. König, F.: Osteochondritis dissecans (Teilnekrose an den Gelenkenden). Arch. Klin. Chir., 142:600, 1926.
120. Lacroix, P.: L'ostéochondrite disséquante. Rev. Belge Sci. Med., 13:78, 1941.
121. Langenskiöld, A.: Can osteochondritis dissecans arise

as a sequel of cartilage fracture in early childhood? Acta Chir. Scand., *109*:206, 1955.
122. Langer, F., and Percy, E. C.: Osteochondritis dissecans and anomalous centres of ossification: A review of 80 lesions in 61 patients. Can. J. Surg., *14*:208, 1971.
123. Langer, M., and Langer, R.: Diagnosis and follow-up study of osteochondrosis dissecans tali (author's transl.). Unfallheilkunde, *84*:37, 1981.
124. Langton, C. D.: Some points in the diagnosis of osteochondritis of the knee. Proc. R. Soc. Med., *35*:206, 1942.
125. Lee, C. K., and Mercurio, C.: Operative treatment of osteochondritis dissecans in situ by retrograde drilling and cancellous bone graft: A preliminary report. Clin. Orthop., *158*:129, 1981.
126. Lewin, P.: Epiphyses. Their growth development. Injuries and disease. Am. J. Dis. Child., *37*:141, 1929.
127. Linden, B.: The incidence of osteochondritis dissecans in condyles of the femur. Acta Orthop Scand., *47*:664, 1976.
128. Linden, B.: Osteochondritis dissecans of the femoral condyles. J. Bone Joint Surg., 59-A:769, 1977.
129. Linden, B., and Nilsson, B. E.: Strontium-85 uptake in knee joints with osteochondritis dissecans. Acta Orthop. Scand., *47*:668, 1976.
130. Linden, B., and Nilsson, B. E.: Chondrocalcinosis following osteochondritis dissecans in the femur condyles. Clin. Orthop., *130*:223, 1978.
131. Linden, B., and Telhag, H.: Morphology and crystal composition of chondrocalcinosis after osteochondritis dissecans. Clin. Orthop., *123*:243, 1977.
132. Linden, B., and Telhag, H.: Osteochondritis dissecans: A histologic and autoradiographic study in man. Acta Orthop. Scand., *18*:682, 1977.
133. Lindholm, S., and Pylkkanen, P.: Internal fixation of the fragments of osteochondritis dissecans of the knee by means of a bone pin. Acta Chir. Scand., *140*:626, 1974.
134. Lindholm, S., Pylkkanen, P., and Oesterman, K.: Fixation of osteochondral fragments in the knee joint. Clin. Orthop., *126*:256, 1977.
135. Lindholm, T.: Osteochondritis dissecans of the knee. Ann. Chir., *63*:69, 1974.
136. Lindholm, T. S., and Osterman, K.: Internal fixation of the fragment of osteochondritis dissecans in the hip using bone transplants. A report of two cases. J. Bone Joint Surg., 62-B:43, 1980.
137. Lindholm, T. S., and Osterman, K.: Long-term results after transfixation of an osteochondritis dissecans fragment to the femoral condyle using autologous bone transplants in adolescent and adult patients. Arch. Orthop. Trauma Surg., *97*:225, 1980.
138. Lindholm, T. S., Osterman, K., and Vankka, E.: Osteochondritis dissecans of the elbow, ankle and hip: A comparison survey. Clin. Orthop., *148*:245, 1980.
139. Lindholm, T. S., Vankka, E., and Osterman, K.: Radiographically observed growth of fragment in juvenile osteochondritis dissecans. Acta Orthop. Belg., *48*:504, 1982.
140. Lipscomb, P. R., Jr., Lipscomb, P. R., Sr., and Bryan, R. S.: Osteochondritis dissecans of the knee with loose fragments. Treatment by replacement and fixation with readily removed pins. J. Bone Joint Surg., 60-A:235, 1978.
141. Litt, R., and Moyersoen, J.: Ostéochondrite disséquante du genou. Traitement par forage. Acta Orthop. Belg., *39*:507, 1973.
142. Lofgren, L.: Spontaneous healing of osteochondritis dissecans in children and adolescents. Acta Chir. Scand., *106*:460, 1953.
143. Lorenz, E.: Die Reimplantation freier Gelenkkorper bei der Osteochondrosis dissecans an Kniegelenk. 63. Kongress der Deutschen Gesellschaft fur Orthopädie und Traumatologie. Sept., 1976. Z. Orthop., *115*:469, 1977.
144. McCullough, C. J., and Venugopal, V.: Osteochondritis dissecans of the talus: The natural history. Clin. Orthop., *144*:264, 1979.
145. Magiera, J.: Case report of osteochondritis dissecans of the patella of both knee joints. Beitr. Orthop. Traumatol., *17*:314, 1970.
146. Mann, M.: Arthroscopy of the knee joint in the diagnosis and follow-up observation of osteochondritis dissecans. Endoscopy, *12*:275, 1980.
147. Marks, K. L.: Flake fracture of the talus progressing to osteochondritis dissecans. J. Bone Joint Surg., 34-B:90, 1952.
148. Mensor, M. C., and Melody, G. F.: Osteochondritis dissecans of ankle joint. J. Bone Joint Surg., *23*:903, 1941.
149. Milgram, J. W.: The development of loose bodies in human joints. Clin. Orthop., *124*:292, 1977.
150. Milgram, J. W.: Radiological and pathological manifestations of osteochondritis dissecans of the distal femur. Radiology, *126*:305, 1978.
151. Miller, L. F., and Hilkevitch, A.: Osteochondritis dissecans of the shoulder. A.J.R., *63*:223, 1950.
152. Mitsunaga, M. M., Adishian, D. A., and Bianco, A. J., Jr.: Osteochondritis dissecans of the capitellum. J. Trauma, *22*:53, 1982.
153. Mollan, R. A. B.: Osteochondritis dissecans of the knee. Acta Orthop. Scand., *48*:517, 1977.
154. Morris, M. L., and McGibbon, K. C.: Osteochondritis dissecans following Legg-Calvé-Perthes disease. J. Bone Joint Surg., 44-B:562, 1962.
155. Moulonguet, P.: Ostéochondrite disséquante de la hanche (maladie de Koenig de la tête fémorale). Bull. Mem. Soc. Nat. Chir., *58*:471, 1932.
156. Mubarak, S. J., and Carroll, N. C.: Familial osteochondritis dissecans of the knee. Clin. Orthop., *140*:131, 1979.
157. Mubarak, S. J., and Carroll, N. C.: Juvenile osteochondritis dissecans of the knee: Etiology. Clin. Orthop., *157*:200, 1981.
158. Muller, W.: Osteochondritis dissecans. *In* Hastings, D. E. (ed.): The Knee: Ligament and Articular Cartilage Injuries. Berlin, Springer-Verlag, 1978, pp. 135–142.
159. Myhre, H.: On osteochondritis dissecans trochleae tali. Acta Radiol., *20*:272, 1939.
160. Nagura, S.: The so-called osteochondritis dissecans of Koenig. Clin. Orthop., *18*:100, 1960.
161. Neilson, N. A.: Osteochondritis dissecans capituli humeri. Acta Orthop. Scand., *4*:307, 1933.
162. Novotny, H.: Preventive and conservative treatment of osteochondritis dissecans. Acta Orthop. Scand., *21*:40, 1951.
163. Novotny, H.: Osteochondritis in two brothers. The pre- and developed state. Acta Radiol., *37*:493, 1952.
164. Nuvemann, M., and Contzen, H.: Unusual extension and localization of osteochondrosis dissecans on the patella. R.O.E.F.O., *133*:335, 1980.
165. O'Donoghue, D. H.: Chondral and osteochondral fractures. J. Trauma, *6*:469, 1966.
166. O'Farrell, T. A., and Costello, B. G.: Osteochondritis dissecans of the talus. The late results of surgical treatment. J. Bone Joint Surg., 64-B:494, 1982.
167. Osterman, K., and Lindholm, T. S.: Osteochondritis dissecans following Perthes' disease. Clin. Orthop., *152*:247, 1980.
168. Outerbridge, R. E.: Osteochondritis dissecans of the posterior femoral condyle. Clin. Orthop., *175*:121, 1983.
169. Paatsama, S., Rokkanen, P., and Tussila, J.: Etiological factors in osteochondritis dissecans. Acta Orthop. Scand., *46*:906, 1975.
170. Paget, J.: On production of some of the loose bodies in joints. St. Bart. Hosp. Rep., *6*:1, 1870.

171. Painter, C. F.: Infraction of the second metatarsal head. Boston Med. Surg. J., *184*:533, 1921.
172. Pantazopoulos, T., and Exarchou, E.: Osteochondritis dissecans of the patella. J. Bone Joint Surg., 53-A:1205, 1971.
173. Pantazopoulos, T., Matsoukas, J., Gavras, M., Nikiforidis, P., and Hartofilakidis-garofalidis, G.: Osteochondritis dissecans following coxa plana. Acta Orthop. Scand., *43*:532, 1972.
174. Pappas, A. M.: Osteochondrosis dissecans. Clin. Orthop., *158*:59, 1981.
175. Paré, A.: Oeuvres Complètes. Tome III. Paris, Balliere, 1840–1841, p. 32.
176. Pavlansky, R.: Traitment de l'ostéochondrite dissécente a l'aide d'une greffe osseuse corticale. Rev. Chir. Orthop., *59*:681, 1973.
177. Petrie, P. W. R.: Aetiology of osteochondritis dissecans. J. Bone Joint Surg., *59-B*:366, 1977.
178. Phillips, H. O., and Grubb, S. A.: Familial multiple osteochondritis dissecans. Report of a kindred. J. Bone Joint Surg., *67-A*:155, 1985.
179. Phillips, M. N., and Start, R. F.: Osteochondritis dissecans of the carpal scaphoid. Br. J. Radiol., *38*:633, 1965.
180. Rasmussen, K. B.: Osteochondritis dissecans—et bidrag til sporgsmalet om aetiologien. Nord. Med., *28*:2088, 1945.
181. Ray, R. B., and Coughlin, E. J., Jr.: Osteochondritis dissecans of the talus. J. Bone Joint Surg., *29*:697, 1947.
182. Rehbein, F.: Die Enstehung der Osteochondritis dissecans. Arch. Klin. Chir., *265*:69, 1950.
183. Ribbing, S.: The hereditary multiple epiphyseal disturbance and its consequences for the aetiogenesis of local malacias—particularly the osteochondrosis dissecans. Acta Orthop. Scand., *24*:286, 1955.
184. Rideout, D. F., Davis, S., and Navani, S. V.: Osteochondritis dissecans patellae. Br. J. Radiol., *39*:673, 1966.
185. Rinaldi, E.: Treatment of osteochondritis dissecans and cartilaginous fractures of the knee by osteocartilaginous autografts. Ital. J. Orthop. Traumatol., *8*:17, 1982.
186. Roberts, M., and Hughes, R.: Osteochondritis dissecans of the elbow joint. J. Bone Joint Surg., *32-B*:348, 1950.
187. Roden, S., Tillegard, P., and Unander-Scharin, L.: Osteochondritis dissecans and similar lesions of the talus. Acta Orthop. Scand., *23*:51, 1953.
188. Rogers, W. M., and Gladstone, H.: Vascular foramina and arterial supply of the distal end of the femur. J. Bone Joint Surg., *32-A*:867, 1950.
189. Rombold, C.: Osteochondritis dissecans of the patella. J. Bone Joint Surg., *18*:230, 1936.
190. Rosenberg, N. J.: Osteochondral fractures of the lateral femoral condyle. J. Bone Joint Surg., *46-A*:1013, 1964.
191. Sawtell, R. O.: Irregular ossification of the extremities of boys and girls. A.J.R., *25*:330, 1931.
192. Scharling, M.: Osteochondritis dissecans of the talus. Acta Orthop. Scand., *49*:89, 1978.
193. Seidenstein, H.: Osteochondritis dissecans of the knee. Spontaneous healing in children. Bull. Hosp. Joint Dis., *18*:123, 1957.
194. Shands, A. R., Jr.: Regeneration of hyaline cartilage in joints. An experimental study. Arch. Surg., *22*:137, 1931.
195. Shipp, F. L.: Osteochondritis dissecans. Surg. Clin. North Am., *32*:713, 1952.
196. Smillie, I. S.: Treatment of osteochondritis dissecans. J. Bone Joint Surg., *37-B*:723, 1955.
197. Smillie, I. S.: Treatment of osteochondritis dissecans. J. Bone Joint Surg., *39-B*:248, 1957.
198. Smillie, I. S.: Osteochondritis Dissecans. Edinburgh, Livingstone; Baltimore, Williams & Wilkins, 1960.
199. Smillie, I. S.: Injuries of the Knee Joint. Edinburgh, Livingstone, 1970.
200. Smith, A. D.: Osteochondritis of the knee joint. J. Bone Joint Surg., *42-A*:289, 1960.
201. Smith, G. R., Winquist, R. A., Allan, T. N. K., and Northrop, C. H.: Subtle transchondral fractures of the talar dome: A radiological perspective. Radiology, *124*:667, 1977.
202. Smith, R. B., and Nevelos, A. B.: Osteochondritis occurring at multiple sites. Acta Orthop. Scand., *51*:445, 1980.
203. Soeur, R.: L'ostéochondrite disséquante reactions de la membrane synoviale. Rev. Chir. Orthop., *37*:5, 1951.
204. Sontag, L. W., and Pyle, S. I.: Variations in the calcification pattern in epiphyses. Their nature and significance. A.J.R., *45*:50, 1941.
205. Stein, G. H., Ikins, R. G., and Lowry, F. C.: Osteochondritis dissecans. Am. J. Surg., *64*:328, 1944.
206. Stougaard, J.: The hereditary factor in osteochondritis dissecans. J. Bone Joint Surg., *43-B*:256, 1961.
207. Stougaard, J.: Familial occurrence of osteochondritis dissecans. J. Bone Joint Surg., *46-B*:542, 1964.
208. Strange, T. B.: Osteochondritis dissecans. Am. J. Surg., *63*:144, 1944.
209. Sutro, C. J.: Perthes' disease complicated by so-called osteochondritis dissecans. Bull. Hosp. Joint Dis., *39*:42, 1978.
210. Szepesi, K.: Ein Fall einer Zweiseitigen Osteochondritis Juvenilis der Trochlea Humeri. Arch. Orthop. Unfallchir., *70*:340, 1971.
211. Tallqvist, G.: The reaction to mechanical trauma in growing articular cartilage. Acta Orthop. Scand., Suppl. 53, 1962.
212. Tivnon, M. C., Anzel, S. H., and Waugh, T. R.: Surgical management of osteochondritis dissecans of the capitellum. Am. J. Sports Med., *4*:121, 1976.
213. Tobin, W. C.: Familial osteochondritis dissecans with associated tibia vara. J. Bone Joint Surg., *39-A*:1091, 1957.
214. Towbin, J., Towbin, R., and Crawford, A.: Osteochondritis dissecans of the tibial plateau. A case report. J. Bone Joint Surg., *64-A*:783, 1982.
215. Trias, A., and Ray, R. D.: Juvenile osteochondritis of the radial head. J. Bone Joint Surg., *45-A*:576, 1963.
216. Trillat, A.: Considerations sur les ostéochondrites disséquantes du genou. Acta Orthop Belg., *39*:505, 1973.
217. Van DeMark, R. E.: Osteochondritis dissecans with spontaneous healing. J. Bone Joint Surg., *34-A*:143, 1952.
218. Van Der Weyer, F. A. A.: Osteochondritis dissecans. J. Bone Joint Surg., *46-B*:574, 1964.
219. Vaughan, C. E., and Stapleton, J. G.: Osteochondritis dissecans of the ankle. Radiology, *49*:72, 1947.
220. Wagoner, G., and Cohn, B. N. E.: Osteochondritis dissecans. A resume of the theories of etiology and the consideration of heredity as an etiologic factor. Arch. Surg., *23*:1, 1931.
221. Walsh, T. D.: Costochondritis (letter). N. Engl. J. Med., *297*:1071, 1977.
222. White, J.: Osteochondritis dissecans in association with dwarfism. J. Bone Joint Surg., *39-B*:261, 1957.
223. Wiberg, G.: Spontanheilung von Osteochondritis dissecans im Kniegelenk. Acta Chir. Scand., *85*:421, 1941.
224. Wiberg, G.: Spontaneous healing of osteochondritis dissecans in the knee joint. Acta Orthop. Scand., *14*:270, 1943.
225. Wilson, J. N.: A diagnostic sign in osteochondritis dissecans of the knee. J. Bone Joint Surg., *49-A*:477, 1967.
226. Wolbach, S. B., and Allison, N.: Osteochondritis dissecans. Arch. Surg., *16*:1176, 1928.

227. Woodward, A. H., and Bianco, A. J.: Osteochondritis dissecans of the elbow. Clin. Orthop., 110:35, 1975.
228. Woodward, A. H., and Decker, J. S.: Osteochondritis dissecans following Legg-Perthes' disease. South. Med. J., 69:943, 1976.
229. Yeung, D. W.: Radionuclide imaging in osteochondritis dissecans. Clin. Nucl. Med., 6:122, 1981.
230. Yuan, H. A., Cady, R. B., and DeRosa, C.: Osteochondritis dissecans of the talus associated with subchondral cysts. Report of three cases. J. Bone Joint Surg., 61-A:1249, 1979.
231. Zellweger, H., and Ebnother, M.: A familial skeletal disorder with multilocular aseptic bone necrosis, and with osteochondritis dissecans in particular. Helv. Paediatr. Acta., 6:95, 1951.
232. Zeman, S. C., and Nielson, M. W.: Osteochondritis dissecans of the knee. Orthop. Rev., 7:101, 1978.
233. Zinman, C., and Reis, N. D.: Osteochondritis dissecans of the talus: Use of high resolution computed tomography scanner. Acta Orthop. Scand., 53:697, 1982.
234. Ziv, I., and Carroll, N. C.: The role of arthroscopy in children. J. Pediatr. Orthop., 2:243, 1982.
235. Zsernaviczky, J.: Hyperproteinamie als mögliche Ursache der Osteochondritis dissecans. Z. Orthop., 115:35, 1977.

DISCOID MENISCUS

Discoid meniscus is an abnormality in which the cartilaginous meniscus of the knee is discoid rather than semilunar in shape. The condition was first reported by Young in 1889.[82] Kroiss is credited as having first associated "snapping knee" with discoid meniscus.[46]

The lateral meniscus is most frequently affected, though on occasion, the condition may occur in the medial meniscus.* Involvement is often bilateral. There is no sex predilection.

The condition is diagnosed comparatively rarely, and it may often go unrecognized. The incidence of discoid cartilage in patients operated on for suspected cartilage tears was reported by Smillie to be 29 in 1,300. Only one of these was the medial meniscus.[72] Nathan and Cole found 30 discoid menisci among 1,219 menisci (2.4 per cent) that were surgically removed in the Hospital for Joint Diseases in New York; 27 were on the lateral side and 3 on the medial; in one knee both medial and lateral menisci were discoid.[61] Dickason and associates, in a retrospective study, examined 14,731 menisci; of the 8,040 medial menisci 10 (0.12 per cent) were discoid; and of the 6,691 lateral menisci 102 (1.5 per cent) were discoid.[16]

Familial incidence of discoid lateral meniscus has been reported by Dashefsky.[15] Bilateral lateral discoid meniscus in identical twins has been described by Gebhardt.[32]

---

*See references 5, 7, 11, 16, 18, 60, 61, 65, 66, 68, 72, and 81.

Pathogenesis

In the past, discoid cartilage was thought to be caused by an arrest in development and persistence of the fetal state. Smillie, in 1948, originally proposed that there are three types of discoid lateral meniscus—primitive, intermediate, and infantile.[72]

The *primitive type* is a complete disc. Opposing movement between the superior and inferior surfaces of the meniscus causes stress and damage within its substance. The inferior surface of the meniscus tears away, and the superior surface sinks into the depressions and holes, developing ridges. It is the movement of the femoral condyle over these ridges that produces the snapping sensation and sound. The hypermobility of the posterior part of the lateral meniscus with medial displacement and catching between the femoral condyle and tibial plateau causes the loud click. The *intermediate type* is less thick in the center and smaller in size, but complete. It tears in the same way as the primitive type. The *infantile type* is discoid in shape but of normal size, exhibiting tears that take place in a normally shaped meniscus.[72]

Smillie originally believed discoid meniscus was caused by failure of gradual absorption of the central portion of the complete plate during later fetal life. Embryologic studies of the knee, however, have shown that in the early phase of development there is an undifferentiated mass of mesenchyme between the cartilaginous precursors of the femur and tibia. Toward the end of the second month, the intermediate mesenchymal plate or blastemic matrix breaks down to form a space between the two bones. Some parts of the mesenchyme persist to form the fibrocartilages and other intra-articular structures such as the cruciate ligaments. When the joint space is developing, the central part of the mesenchymal plate is absorbed, and the menisci from the very beginning of their formation have the basic adult semilunar shape. At no phase of fetal development does the fibrocartilage have a disclike appearance.[31, 42, 43, 48, 68] In view of this evidence, Smillie later retracted the theory of persistence of the fetal state in the etiology of discoid meniscus.[73]

Ross, Tough, and English believed that discoid cartilage is a congenital lesion due to abnormal development, fibrocartilage being laid down in mesenchyme that normally disappears in the formation of a joint.[68]

Kaplan proposed the following etiology of discoid meniscus. At operation, he found that in individuals with discoid meniscus there is no attachment of the posterior horn of the lateral meniscus to the tibial plateau, but instead the meniscofemoral ligament (ligament of Wrisberg) joins the posterior horn of the meniscus to the lateral surface of the medial femoral condyle. This is a normal finding in all animals in which the usual functional position of the knee is one of flexion. In the human knee, however, which is predominantly used in the extended position, this occurs rarely as an anatomic anomaly. In such individuals, because of the short meniscofemoral ligament, the lateral meniscus is not permitted to glide forward when the knee is extended, but instead it is pulled into the intercondylar area. On flexion of the knee, it returns to its usual position. The constant mediolateral motion and irritation of the lateral meniscus transforms the initially normal semilunar cartilage into a thick fibrocartilaginous mass, which assumes a solid irregular form.[42, 43] Nathan and Cole reported a discoid lateral meniscus in a four-month-old infant, but they believed the presence of a discoid meniscus in a very young patient is not inconsistent with this theory of abnormal stresses on a hypermobile meniscus because there is knee motion in utero.[61]

Watanabe and associates classified three types of discoid meniscus as visualized through the arthroscope.[78, 79] First is the *Wrisberg-ligament type* in which the lateral meniscus has no attachment to the tibial plateau posteriorly; its only posterior attachment is through the lateral meniscofemoral ligament (or the ligament of Wrisberg), which is taut and does not accommodate the normal flexion and extension of the knee. The hypermobility of the posterior part of the lateral meniscus results in its secondary hypertrophic thickening. This type corresponds to Kaplan's description of discoid meniscus. It is clinically symptomatic. In the second, or *complete type*, the attachments of the lateral meniscus are intact; there is no meniscal hyperlaxity or abnormal motion associated with flexion and extension of the knee. The menisci are disc-shaped, covering the entire tibial plateau. This type corresponds to the abnormal embryologic developmental type. The *incomplete type* differs from the complete type only in size.

Dickhaut and DeLee reported the arthroscopic findings in 347 knees with symptoms attributed to meniscal lesions. Six patients had the Wrisberg-ligament type of discoid lateral meniscus; all six had abnormal meniscal mobility symptoms typical of the "snapping-knee" syndrome. They were treated by arthroscopic lateral meniscectomy. Twelve patients had the complete type of discoid lateral meniscus with normal intact tibial attachments. All 12 knees had no symptoms attributable to the discoid lateral meniscus. There was no meniscal laxity and no tears. The complete type of discoid lateral meniscus was an incidental finding at arthroscopy. They stressed the importance of distinguishing the asymptomatic complete type from the symptomatic hypermobile Wrisberg-ligament type.[17]

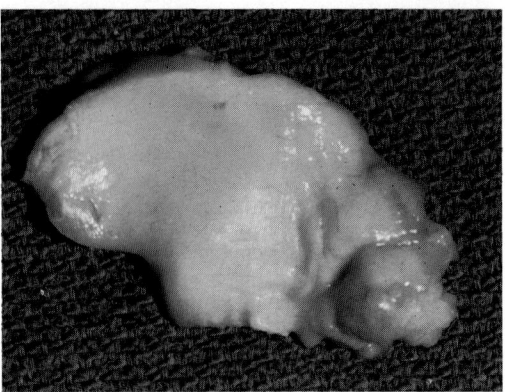

FIGURE 4–53. *Discoid lateral meniscus.*

Pathology

The affected meniscus is a solid mass of fibrocartilage, oval or roughly circular in shape, and varying in thickness from 0.5 to 1.3 cm. (Fig. 4–53).[40] The corresponding surface of the tibial plateau will be almost entirely covered by the discoid meniscus, which at its inner margin is attached throughout its length along the intercondylar space and cruciate ligaments. Occasionally its anterior horn and body will be a solid mass, whereas the posterior horn will be normal.

Cystic degeneration with centrally located cavities is not uncommon. Histologic examination has shown some degree of mucoid degeneration in all specimens, indicating that the menisci were subjected to increased wear. Horizontal or longitudinal tears of the meniscus may occur as a result of injury.

Clinical Features

The mere presence of a disc-shaped cartilage does not cause disability. The condition is often asymptomatic in infancy and early childhood. By the sixth or eighth year of life the child may complain of "snapping" or a "click" in the knee and vague symptoms such as "giving way" or "catching." Symptoms may be precipitated by a recent injury, especially in the adolescent.

On examination the abnormality is palpable, and a loud "clunk" is audible during the last 15 to 20 degrees of extension of the flexed knee; it is produced by the lateromedial movement of the semilunar cartilage. On extension of the knee joint, the lateral meniscus, which is not fixed posteriorly to the tibia, does not remain in place under the lateral femoral condyle but is dislocated medially onto the intercondylar space by the pull of the short meniscofemoral ligament. During flexion the ligament relaxes, and the lateral meniscus is replaced in its usual position by the contracting popliteus and coronary ligaments.[42, 43]

On palpation of the fully flexed knee a fullness may be detected in the lateral parapatellar area at the joint line. Atrophy of the thigh, joint effusion, and synovial thickening are significantly absent. Unless connected with an injury, there is no functional disability. On occasion, forced hyperextension of the knee may elicit pain on the lateral aspect of the joint.

In the differential diagnosis of discoid meniscus one should consider the following conditions that cause snapping knee in infancy and childhood: meniscal cyst, congenital subluxation of the tibiofemoral joint, abnormal movement of the popliteus tendon, snapping of the tendons about the knee, and subluxation or dislocation of the proximal tibiofibular joint or of the patellofemoral joint.[6, 51]

Imaging Findings

In the plain radiographic films widening of the lateral joint space may be found when the discoid lateral meniscus is unusually thick. It is best noted when comparable views of both knees are taken on the same plate (Fig. 4–54). Other radiographic findings suggestive of discoid lateral meniscus are flattening of the lateral femoral condyle (giving a squared-off appearance) and cupping of the lateral aspect of the tibial plateau.[20]

Contrast arthrography (especially double-contrast) is of definite value in the diagnosis of discoid meniscus. A water soluble contrast agent (10 to 12 ml.) is injected into the infrapatellar synovial space through a lateral approach. Anteroposterior, lateral oblique, medial oblique, posteroanterior, and lateral projections are taken. The midportion of the lateral meniscus is best visualized in the posteroanterior projection, as this view depicts the femorotibial articulation best, and the lateral meniscal wedge is not obscured by the posteriorly situated popliteal bursa. The diagnosis of discoid meniscus is made when the meniscus can be demonstrated extending to the intercondylar notch separating the cartilages of the lateral femoral condyle and lateral tibial plateau. The normal lateral and medial menisci are half-moon-shaped with a sharp triangular outline and extend centrally toward the intercondylar notch 1.5 cm.

Magnetic resonance imaging will clearly depict the configuration of the menisci; its only drawback is the cost. It is highly recommended by this author, as it is noninvasive, painless, and without radiation risk. This author prefers MRI to CT scan.

Treatment

Biomechanically the menisci in the knee joint are vital in compensating for the incongruity between the femur and tibia, in load bearing, in the distribution of joint pressure, as a shock absorber, for stabilization of the knee, in provision of rotation, in spreading of synovial fluid, and in nutrition of articular cartilage. An intact meniscus transmits 70 to 90 per cent of the total load across the knee joint.[70, 71] Therefore, it is desirable to preserve the meniscus (even a part of it) whenever possible.

Maquet and associates experimentally determined femorotibial weight-bearing contact areas; in the normal knee they ranged from 20 sq. cm. at full extension to 11 sq. cm. at 90 degrees of flexion, whereas after tibial meniscectomy these areas were reduced to 12 sq. cm. in full extension and 6 sq. cm. in 90 degrees of flexion. It is obvious that the menisci form a substantial part of the weight-bearing surface of the knee even in 90 degrees of flexion.[56]

Experimental and clinical studies have shown that degenerative changes following partial resection of the meniscus are minimal, whereas following total meniscectomy they are marked.[1, 29, 53, 55]

In the treatment of discoid meniscus in children a conservative nonoperative method of management is recommended, especially if pain and functional disability are minimal. Conservative measures consist of a short period of immobilization of the knee followed by restriction of physical activity and progressive exercises for the quadriceps. Some discoid menisci in children are clinically silent. They require no treatment, just periodic observation.

If the knee locks frequently or persistently and the degree of pain and the functional dis-

Text continued on page 1549

Excision of Discoid Lateral Meniscus by Direct Lateral Approach

OPERATIVE TECHNIQUE

A. Diagrammatic representation of gross anatomy of discoid lateral meniscus.

B. The surgical approach is described by Bruser.*

With the tourniquet on the proximal thigh, the patient is placed in the supine position and his lower limb is prepared and draped so that full motion of the knee is permitted without contamination of the operative area.

The affected knee is acutely (fully) flexed so that the heel almost touches the buttocks. This position also flexes the hip 80 degrees, relaxing the taut fibers of the iliotibial band. The skin incision is made over the lateral joint line, beginning at the patellar ligament anteriorly and ending at a point midway between the fibular head and the lateral femoral condyle. The subcutaneous tissue is divided and the wound edges are retracted with sharp rakes.

C. The shiny fibers of the iliotibial band are exposed; they lie almost parallel to the skin incision and the joint line. The fascial fibers are split or, if necessary, divided. The lateral (or fibular) collateral ligament traverses longitudinally in the posterior end of the fascial incision. Caution should be exercised so that the ligament is not divided inadvertently.

D. With a blunt right-angled knee retractor the lateral ligament and popliteus tendon are retracted posteriorly. The capsule and synovium are divided at the joint line along the superior margin of the discoid lateral meniscus.

---

*Bruser, D. M.: A direct lateral approach to the lateral compartment of the knee joint. J. Bone Joint Surg., *42–B*:348, 1960.

Plate 53. Excision of Discoid Lateral Meniscus by Direct Lateral Approach

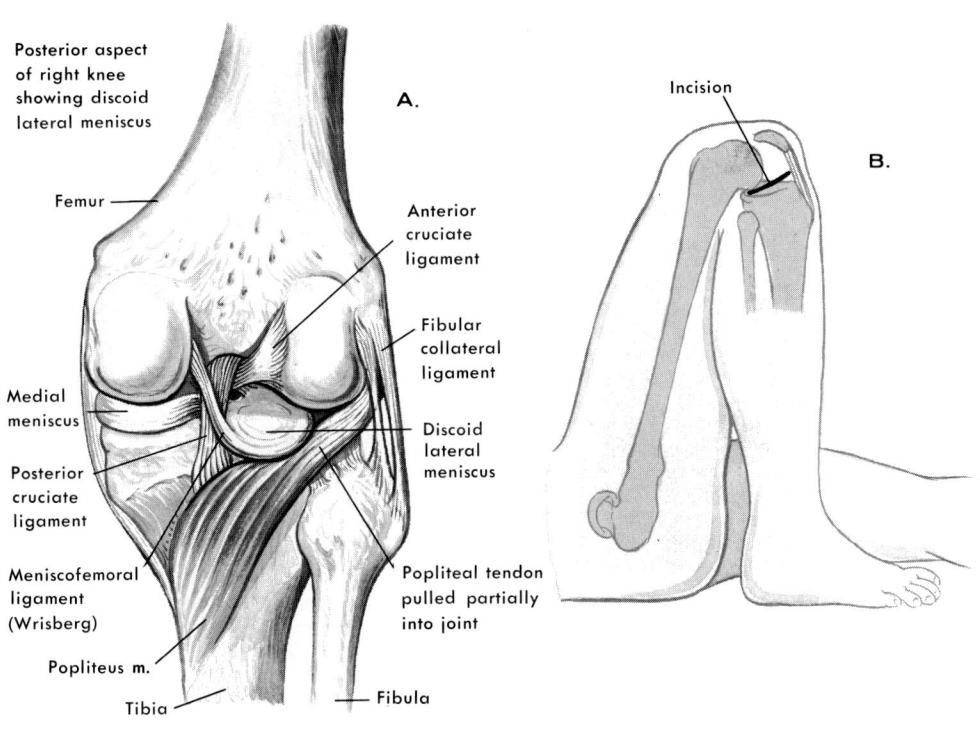

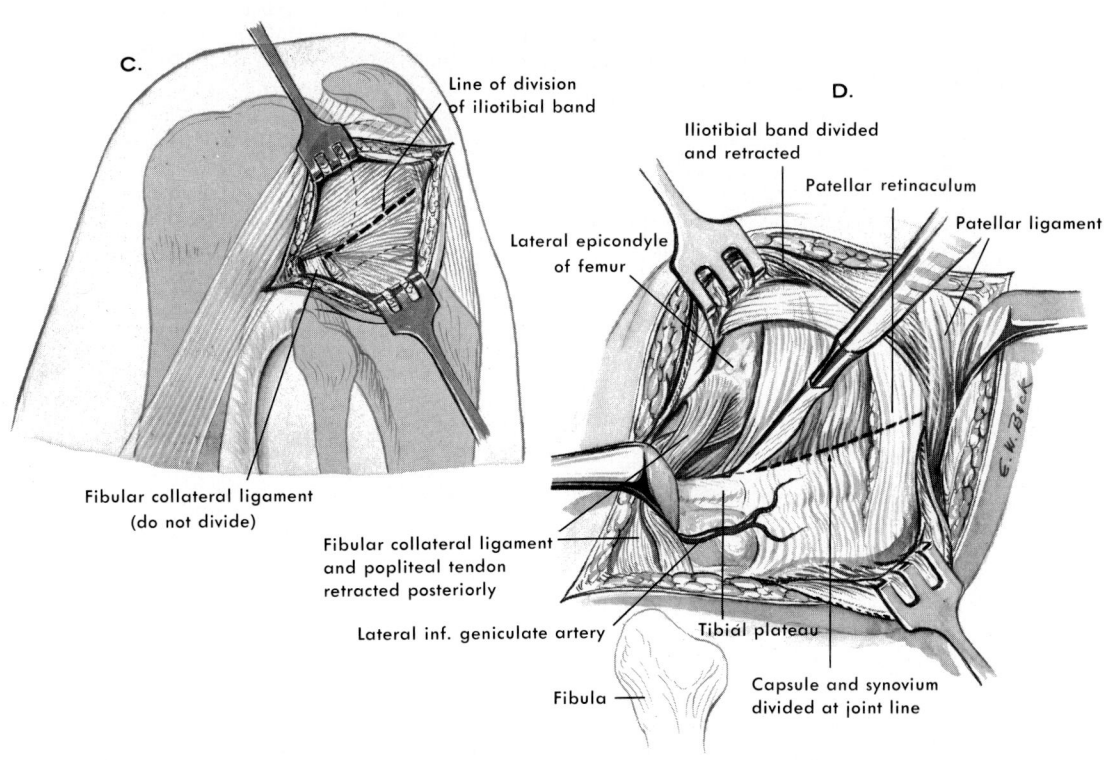

1543

Excision of Discoid Lateral Meniscus by Direct Lateral Approach (Continued)

E to H. Certain anatomical details should be considered next. The normal lateral meniscus is attached on the superior articular surface of the tibia at two sites, on the anterior and posterior aspects of the lateral intercondylar tubercle. Also, the ligament of Wrisberg or the meniscofemoral ligament connects the posterior horn of the lateral meniscus to the lateral surface of the medial femoral condyle, traversing obliquely behind the posterior cruciate ligament. (Humphry's ligament is the anterior branch of Wrisberg's ligament, and it runs in front of the anterior surface of the posterior cruciate ligament.)

When the knee is flexed Wrisberg's ligament is relaxed, whereas the posterior cruciate ligament is relaxed during flexion and extension and runs almost vertically along the posterior midline. The discoid lateral meniscus, according to Kaplan, does not have a posterior tibial attachment and is connected to the medial femoral condyle by the meniscofemoral ligament. When the knee is in extension the discoid lateral meniscus is displaced posteromedially in the intercondylar area; in flexion it returns to its usual position. The popliteus tendon is attached anterior to the origin of the lateral ligament.

It is also important to remember that the popliteal artery is located 1 cm. posterior to the ligament of Wrisberg and that the lateral inferior genicular artery passes outside the synovium between the fibular collateral ligament and the posterolateral aspect of the meniscus. Injury to these vessels must be avoided. If inadvertently the genicular vessels are divided, they must be ligated to prevent hemarthrosis.

Plate 53. Excision of Discoid Lateral Meniscus by Direct Lateral Approach

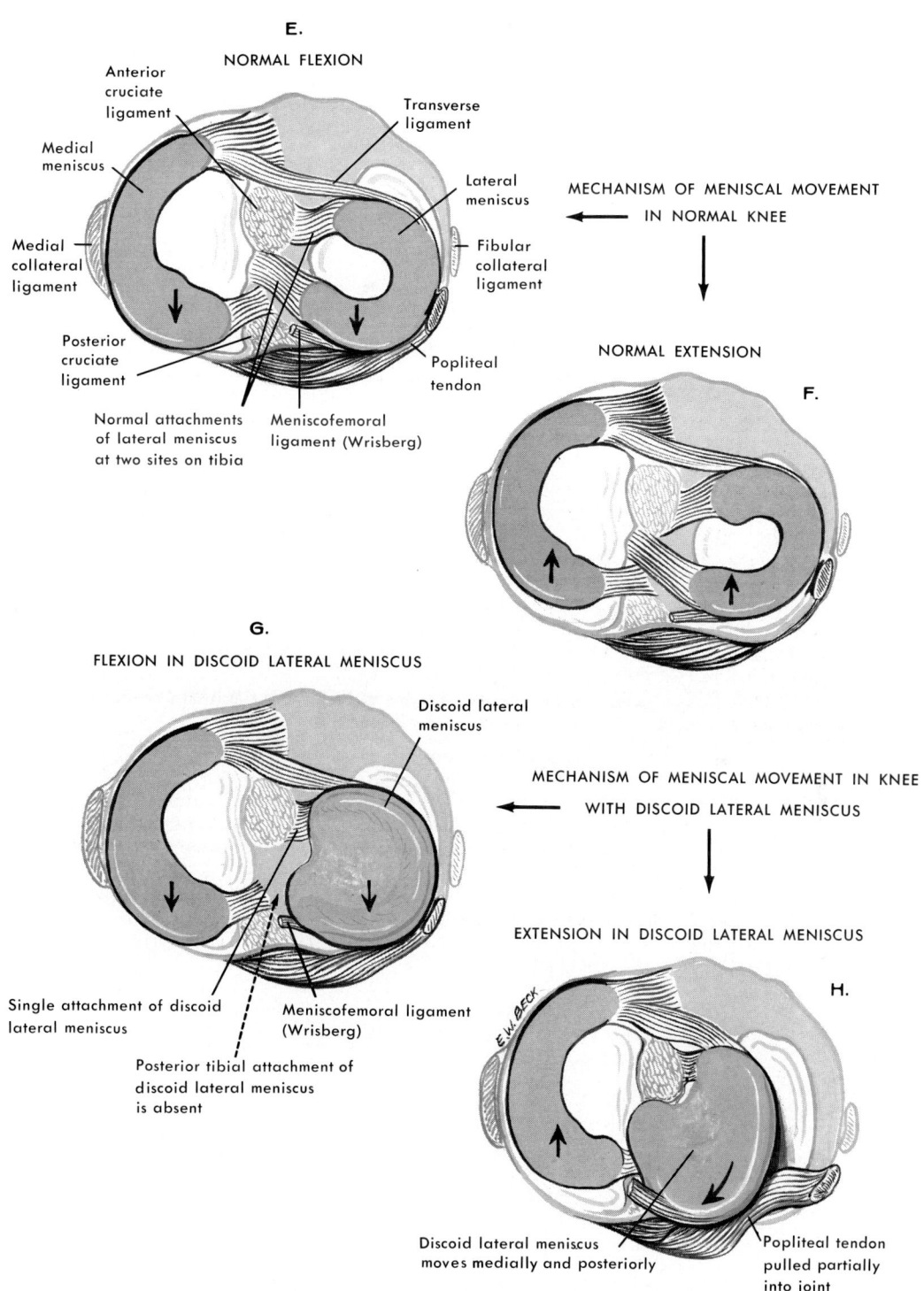

1545

Excision of Discoid Lateral Meniscus by Direct Lateral Approach (Continued)

I and **J.** By sharp dissection the lateral meniscus is freed from its anterior, medial, and peripheral attachments. Forcibly bending the knee inward will aid in visualization of the central portion of the joint. Posteriorly, the meniscus is freed by division of Wrisberg's ligament. After removal of the cartilage the lateral compartment of the joint is thoroughly inspected with the knee in flexion and extension; namely, the anterior and posterior cruciate ligaments, the popliteus tendon, the lateral femoral and tibial condyles, the lateral collateral ligament, and the lateral half of the articular surface of the patella. The tourniquet is released and complete hemostasis is obtained.

With the knee in 90 degrees of flexion the synovial membrane is closed with continuous plain catgut suture.

K. The knee is then extended, and the fascia is closed with interrupted sutures. The subcutaneous tissue and skin are closed in the usual manner. A compression dressing is applied. Protection of the joint with a posterior plaster of Paris cast or a light cylinder cast is not necessary, as the lateral collateral ligament is not divided.

POSTOPERATIVE CARE

Exercises are begun on the day surgery is performed; they consist of quadriceps setting, hamstring setting, and straight leg raising. Several days postoperatively the patient is allowed partial weight-bearing with crutches, and activities are gradually increased as they are tolerated.

Within seven to ten days (as soon as the soft tissues have healed) the knee is gently mobilized by side-lying flexion and extension exercises to redevelop muscle strength in the quadriceps, hamstrings, and triceps surae. These are continued until normal motor power and full range of knee motion are obtained.

Plate 53. Excision of Discoid Lateral Meniscus by Direct Lateral Approach

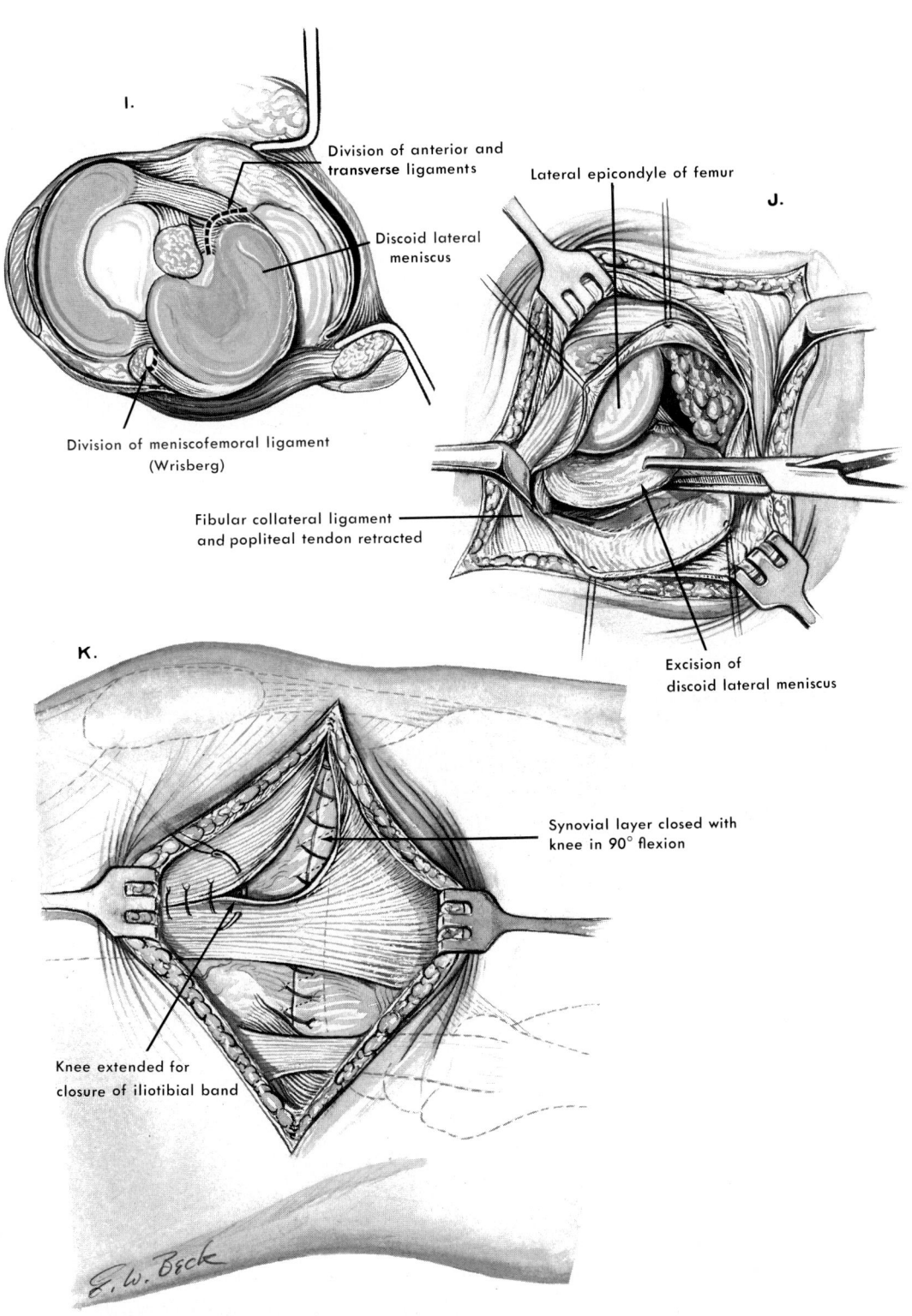

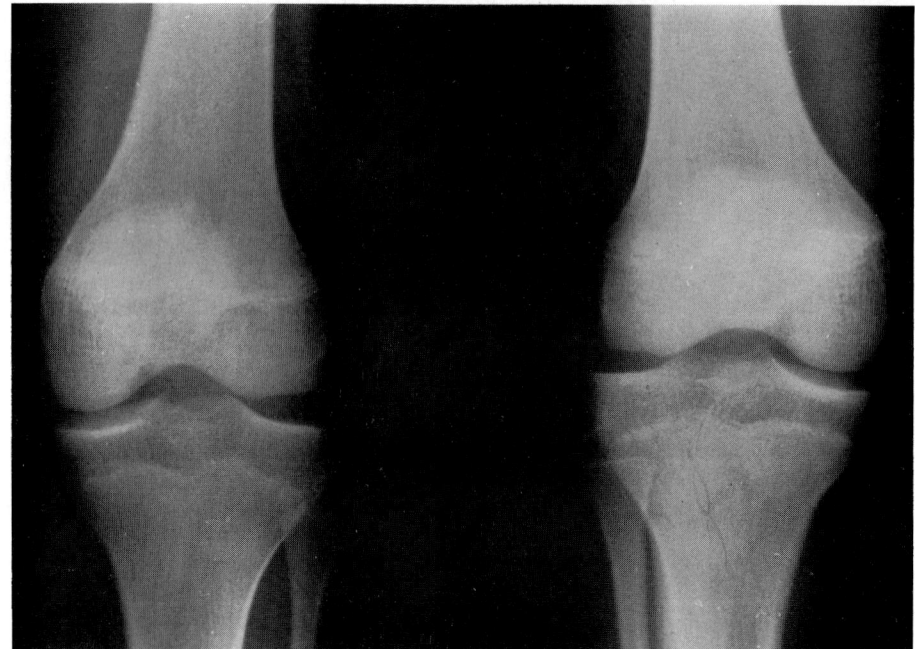

FIGURE 4–54. Widening of lateral joint space of the right knee as a result of thick discoid lateral meniscus.

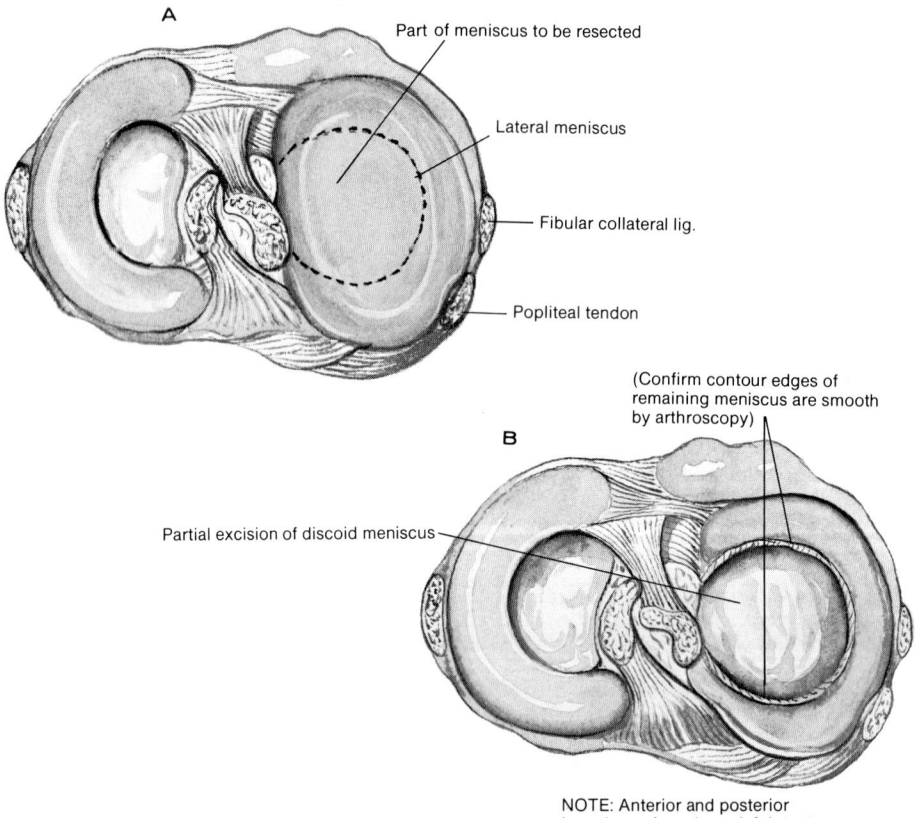

FIGURE 4–55. Diagram of partial resection of discoid meniscus.

A. The line of incision. Note that the posterior and anterior attachments of the meniscus are left intact. **B.** After partial resection, the residual part of the meniscus left in the knee should be free of tears and degeneration. Its anterior, posterior, and capsular attachments should be intact, and there should be no hypermobility. (Redrawn after Fujikawa, K., Iseki, F., and Mikuri, Y.: Partial resection of the discoid meniscus in the child's knee. J. Bone Joint Surg., *63-B*:391, 1981.)

ability are severe, partial or complete excision of the discoid meniscus is indicated. Prior to surgical intervention diagnostic arthroscopy is carried out to delineate the pathologic changes and the type of discoid meniscus. Some surgeons may prefer to perform double-contrast arthrography first and then diagnostic arthroscopy, as general anesthesia is required for arthroscopy in children, whereas arthrography can be performed under local anesthesia. This author recommends magnetic resonance imaging instead of double-contrast arthrography.

Partial resection of the discoid meniscus is preferred when it is of the complete or incomplete type with minimal tearing and slight degeneration; its capsular attachments should be intact, and the meniscus should not be hypermobile (the Wrisberg type). These requisites are determined prior to surgery by diagnostic arthroscopy and double-contrast arthrography. Recently, MRI has been utilized for delineating this pathology. For partial resection of the discoid meniscus often an open arthrotomy is required. With the knee flexed 90 degrees a 4 cm. long anterolateral incision is made. The femoral surface of the discoid meniscus usually appears normal; degenerative changes and minimal tears are often within its structure or on the tibial surface. By fingertip palpation moving from the periphery toward the center, the sagittal line of irregularity is determined. With a sharp knife the meniscus is excised along this irregular border. Its anterior and posterior attachments are left intact. The anterior incised part is pulled toward the intercondylar fossa, and partial resection of the central and posterior parts is completed with scissors and knife. The excised part of the meniscus is circular in outline, converting the discoid meniscus to a semicircular half-moon shape (Fig. 4–55). Next, using an arthroscope through the wound, the meniscus left behind is carefully inspected for possible tears and degeneration; its posterior, anterior, and capsular attachments should be intact. If it is torn, degenerated, or loose it should be completely excised.

Excision of the entire meniscus is performed when it is of the Wrisberg type (hypermobile) or when it is torn and there is marked degeneration. The details of the operative technique are described and illustrated in Plate 53.

Arthroscopic excision of the discoid lateral meniscus is difficult, but can be performed by the experienced surgeon. Initially the anterior portion of the meniscus is removed; this provides clearer visualization and more space for manipulation of surgical instruments.[37]

References

1. Aarstrand, T.: Treatment of meniscal rupture of the knee joint. A follow-up examination of material where only the ruptured part of the meniscus has been removed. Acta Chir. Scand., 107:146, 1954.
2. Abrams, R. C.: Meniscus lesions of the knee in young children. J. Bone Joint Surg., 39-A:194, 1957.
3. Anderson, H.: Histochemical studies on the histogenesis of the knee joint and superior tibio-fibular joint in human foetuses. Acta Anat., 46:279, 1961.
4. Aufranc, O. E.: Approach of the knee joint by release of the lateral ligaments. Clin. Orthop., 55:97, 1967.
5. Basmajian, J. V.: A ring-shaped medial semilunar cartilage. J. Bone Joint Surg., 34-B:638, 1952.
6. Beals, R. K.: The "snapping knee" of infancy. J. Bone Joint Surg., 60-A:679, 1978.
7. Berson, B. L., and Herman, G.: Torn discoid meniscus of the knee in adults. Four case reports. J. Bone Joint Surg., 61-A:303, 1979.
8. Bhaduri, T., and Glass, A.: Meniscectomy in children. Injury, 3:176, 1972.
9. Bruser, D. M.: A direct lateral approach to the lateral compartment of the knee joint. J. Bone Joint Surg., 42-B:348, 1960.
10. Casscells, S. W.: The place of arthroscopy in the diagnosis and treatment of internal derangement of the knee: An analysis of 1000 cases. Clin. Orthop., 151:135, 1980.
11. Cave, E. F., and Staples, O. S.: Congenital discoid meniscus: A cause of internal derangement of knee. Am. J. Surg., 54:371, 1941.
12. Clark, C. R., and Ogden, J. A.: Development of the menisci of the human knee joint. Morphological changes and their potential role in childhood meniscal injury. J. Bone Joint Surg., 65-A:538, 1983.
13. Cotto, H.: Kindlicher Meniscusschaden. Hefte Unfallheilkd., 128:59, 1976.
14. Cox, J. S., Nye, C. E., Schaefer, W. W., and Woodstein, I. J.: The degenerative effects of partial and total resection of the medial meniscus in dog's knees. Clin. Orthop., 109:178, 1975.
15. Dashefsky, J. H.: Discoid lateral meniscus in three members of a family. Case reports. J. Bone Joint Surg., 53-A:1208, 1971.
16. Dickason, J. M., Del Pizzo, W., Blazina, M. F., Fox, J. M., Friedman, M. J., and Snyder, S. J.: A series of ten discoid medial menisci. Clin. Orthop., 168:75, 1982.
17. Dickhaut, S. C., and DeLee, J. C.: The discoid lateral meniscus syndrome. J. Bone Joint Surg., 64-A:1068, 1982.
18. Dwyer, F. C., and Taylor, C.: Congenital discoid internal cartilage. Br. Med. J., 2:287, 1945.
19. Ellis, V. H.: Congenital abnormality of the external semilunar cartilage. Lancet, 1:1359, 1932.
20. Engber, W. D., and Mickelson, M. R.: Cupping of the lateral tibial plateau associated with a discoid meniscus. Orthopaedics, 4:904, 1981.
21. Fahmy, N. R., Williams, E. A., and Noble, J.: Meniscal pathology and osteoarthritis of the knee. J. Bone Joint Surg., 65-B:24, 1983.
22. Fairbank, H. A. T.: Internal derangement of the knee in children and adolescents. Proc. R. Soc. Med., 30:427, 1937.
23. Fairbank, T. J.: Knee joint changes after meniscectomy. J. Bone Joint Surg., 30-B:664, 1948.
24. Fairbank, T. J., and Jamieson, E. S.: A complication of lateral meniscectomy. A false aneurysm on the inferior lateral genicular artery. Two cases. J. Bone Joint Surg., 33-B:567, 1951.
25. Ferrone, J. D., Jr.: Congenital deformities about the knee. Orthop. Clin. North Am., 7:323, 1976.

26. Finder, J. G.: Discoid external semilunar cartilage. A cause of internal derangement of the knee joint. J. Bone Joint Surg., 16:804, 1934.
27. Fisher, A. G. T.: The disk-shaped external semilunar cartilage. Br. Med. J., 1:688, 1936.
28. Freiberger, R. H., Killoran, P. J., and Cardena, G.: Arthrography of the knee by double contrast method. A.J.R., 97:736, 1966.
29. Fujikawa, K., Iseki, F., and Mikura, Y.: Partial resection of the discoid meniscus in the child's knee. J. Bone Joint Surg., 63-B:391, 1981.
30. Fujikawa, K., Tomatsu, T., Matsu, K., Koiae, A., Tanaka, Y., and Iseki, F.: Morphologicial analysis of meniscus and articular cartilage in the knee joint by means of arthrogram. J. Jpn. Orthop. Assoc., 52:203, 1978.
31. Gardner, E., and O'Rahilly, R.: The early development of the knee joint in staged human embryos. J. Anat., 102:289, 1968.
32. Gebhardt, M. C., and Rosenthal, R. K.: Bilateral lateral discoid meniscus in identical twins. J. Bone Joint Surg., 61-A:1110, 1979.
33. Goodfellow, J. W.: Closed meniscectomy (editorial). J. Bone Joint Surg., 65-B:373, 1983.
34. Gray, D. J., and Gardner, E.: Prenatal development of the human knee and superior tibiofibular joints. Am. J. Anat., 86:235, 1952.
35. Hall, F. M.: Arthrography of the discoid lateral meniscus. A.J.R., 128:993, 1977.
36. Haveson, S. B., and Rein, B. I.: Lateral discoid meniscus of the knee: Arthrographic diagnosis. A.J.R., 109:581, 1970.
37. Ikeuchi, H.: Arthroscopic treatment of the discoid lateral meniscus. Technique and long-term results. Clin. Orthop., 167:19, 1982.
38. Jackson, J. P.: Degenerative changes in the knee after meniscectomy. Br. Med. J., 2:525, 1968.
39. Jaroschy, W.: Der Scheibenförmig Meniscus Lateralis Genu als Ursache des Schnellen den Knies. Beitr. Klin. Chir., 161:139, 1935.
40. Jeannopoulos, C. L.: Observations on discoid menisci. J. Bone Joint Surg., 32-A:649, 1950.
41. Jones, F. B.: The discoid or congenital abnormality of the interarticular fibrocartilage of the knee joint. Part 2. Liverpool Med. Chir. J., 213:78, 1935.
42. Kaplan, E. B.: The embryology of the menisci of the knee joint. Bull. Hosp. Joint Dis., 16:111, 1955.
43. Kaplan, E. B.: Discoid lateral meniscus of the knee joint: Nature, mechanism, and operative treatment. J. Bone Joint Surg., 39-A:77, 1957.
44. Kettelkamp, D. B., and Jacobs, A. W.: Tibiofemoral contact area—determination and implications. J. Bone Joint Surg., 54-A:349, 1972.
45. Kobayashi, A.: Discoid meniscus of the knee joint. Clin. Orthop. Surg. Jpn., 10:10, 1975.
46. Kroiss, F.: Die Verletzungen der Kniegelenkozwischenknorfel und ihrer Verbindungen. Beitr. Klin. Chir., 66:598, 1910.
47. Kulowski, J., and Rickett, H. W.: The relation of discoid meniscus to cyst formation and joint mechanics. J. Bone Joint Surg., 29:990, 1947.
48. Levine, E. F., and Blazina, M. E.: Investigations of the lateral meniscus. Surg. Forum, 17:443, 1966.
49. Lidge, R. T.: Meniscal derangement: Unusual cases. Orthop. Clin. North Am., 10:659, 1979.
50. Lindblum, K.: Arthrography of knee: Roentgenographic and anatomic study. Acta Radiol., Suppl. 74, 1948.
51. Lloyd, E. I.: Clicking knee in childhood. Lancet, 1:525, 1933.
52. Lugli, T.: Conventional radiographic findings in discoid meniscus. Ann. Radiol. Diagn., 39:18, 1966.
53. McGinty, J. B., Geuss, L. F., and Marvin, R. A.: Partial or total meniscectomy. J. Bone Joint Surg., 59-A:763, 1977.
54. Maknoon, A. S.: Congenital discoid meniscus (snapping knee). West Va. Med. J., 68:123, 1972.
55. Manzione, M., Pizzutilo, P. D., Peoples, A. B., and Scheneizer, P. A.: Meniscectomy in children: A long-term follow-up study. Am. J. Sports Med., 11:111, 1983.
56. Maquet, P. G., Van de Berg, A. J., and Simonet, J. C.: Femorotibial weight-bearing areas: Experimental determinations. J. Bone Joint Surg., 57-A:766, 1975.
57. Meekison, D. M.: Discoid lateral meniscus of the knee joint with rupture and cyst formation. Br. J. Surg., 28:135, 1940.
58. Middleton, D. S.: Congenital disc-shaped lateral meniscus with snapping knee. Br. J. Surg., 24:246, 1936.
59. Moon, N. F.: Discoid lateral meniscus. Rocky Mt. Med. J., 65:61, 1968.
60. Murdoch, G.: Congenital discoid medial semilunar cartilage. J. Bone Joint Surg., 38-B:564, 1956.
61. Nathan, P. A., and Cole, S. C.: Discoid meniscus. A clinical and pathologic study. Clin. Orthop., 64:107, 1969.
62. Nemoto, H. N.: Study on discoid meniscus of the knee. Nigata Med. J., 64:404, 1950.
63. Ober, F. R.: Discoid cartilage, trigger knee. Surgery, 6:24, 1939.
64. Resnick, D., Goergen, T. G., Kay, J. J., Ghelman, B., and Woody, P. R.: Discoid medial meniscus. Radiology, 12:3 Pt. 1:575, 1976.
65. Riachi, E., and Phares, A.: An unusual deformity of the medial semilunar cartilage. J. Bone Joint Surg., 45-B:146, 1963.
66. Richmond, D. A.: Two cases of discoid medial cartilage. J. Bone Joint Surg., 40-B:268, 1958.
67. Ritchie, D.: Meniscectomy in children. J. Bone Joint Surg., 47-B:596, 1965.
68. Ross, J. A., Tough, I. C. K., and English, T. A.: Congenital discoid cartilage. Report of a case of discoid medial cartilage, with an embryological note. J. Bone Joint Surg., 40-B:262, 1958.
69. Ross, W. T.: Injury to the popliteal artery during meniscectomy. Report of a case. J. Bone Joint Surg., 33-B:571, 1951.
70. Seedhom, B. B.: Transmission of the load in the knee joint with special reference to the role of the menisci. Part 1. Anatomy, analysis and apparatus. Eng. Med., 8:207, 1979.
71. Seedhom, B. B., and Hargreaves, D. J.: Transmission of the load in the knee joint with special reference to the role of the menisci. Part II. Experimental results, discussion and conclusion. Eng. Med., 8:220, 1979.
72. Smillie, I. S.: The congenital discoid meniscus. J. Bone Joint Surg., 30-B:671, 1948.
73. Smillie, I. S.: Injuries of the Knee Joint. 4th Ed. Baltimore, Williams & Wilkins, 1970, pp. 39–97.
74. Snellman, O., and Stentrom, R. H.: Congenital discoid meniscus of the knee joint. Ann. Paediatr. Fenn., 6:124, 1960.
75. Takao, T.: An experimental study on the development of osteoarthritis of the knee joint with special reference to the degree of resection of the meniscus. J. Jpn. Orthop. Assoc., 45:731, 1971.
76. Vahvanen, V., and Aalto, K.: Meniscectomy in children. Acta Orthop. Scand., 50:6 Pt. 2:791, 1979.
77. Walker, P. S., and Erkman, J.: The role of the menisci in force transmission across the knee. Clin. Orthop., 109:184, 1975.
78. Watanabe, M.: Arthroscopy of the knee joint. In Helfet, A. J. (ed.): Disorders of the Knee. Philadelphia, Lippincott, 1974.
79. Watanabe, M., Takeda, S., and Ikeuchi, H.: Atlas of Arthroscopy. 2nd Ed. Tokyo, Igaku Shoin, 1969.
80. Watson-Jones, R.: Specimen of internal semilunar cartilage as a complete disc. Proc. R. Acad. Med., 23:68, 1930.

81. Weiner, B., and Rosenberg, N.: Discoid medial meniscus: Association with bone changes in the tibia. J. Bone Joint Surg., 56-A:171, 1974.
82. Young, R. B.: The external semilunar cartilage as a complete disc. In Cleland, J., MacKay, J. Y., and Young, R. B. (eds.): Memoirs and Memoranda in Anatomy. London, Edinburgh, Williams & Norgate, 1889, p. 179.
83. Zaman, M., and Leonard, M. A.: Meniscectomy in children: Results in 59 knees. Injury, 12:425, 1981.

SNAPPING OF POPLITEUS TENDON

Snapping of the knee may be caused by abnormal movement of the popliteus tendon over the lateral femoral condyle during flexion and extension of the joint. If it is demonstrated that the popliteus tendon is the cause of the snapping of the knee, and if the snapping is functionally disabling, it is sectioned or segmentally resected.

RECURRENT MOMENTARY LATERAL SUBLUXATION OF THE TIBIOFEMORAL JOINT

Painful, spontaneous, audible popping (or "jumping") of one or both knees may occur in infants and children because of lateral displacement of the tibiofemoral joint. This entity was first reported by Beals in 1978 in three cases, all girls.[1] This author has observed this in two patients, one girl and one boy. Both joint laxity and knee flexion are required for the subluxation; it appears to be caused by an isolated contraction of the biceps femoris muscle in association with capsular laxity. In the lateral radiograph there is no appreciable alteration in the position of the proximal fibula in relation to the tibia. There is an audible and palpable intraarticular double click, which corresponds to the subluxation and relocation of the tibiofemoral joint. It may occur when the infant or child is awake or asleep (waking up the baby, crying). Radiograms in the anteroposterior projection will show lateral subluxation of the tibiofemoral joint. The proximal tibiofibular articulation is normal.

Treatment

Part-time splinting of the knee in extension will provide symptomatic relief of the painful, irritable knee. A conservative, nonsurgical approach to management is recommended. As the child gets older and the joint capsular hyperlaxity diminishes, the episodes of involuntary subluxation cease; the child may, however, subluxate the joint voluntarily for attention. Sectioning or fractional elongation of the biceps tendon is not necessary.

Reference

1. Beals, R. K.: The snapping knee of infancy. J. Bone Joint Surg., 60-A:679, 1978.

RECURRENT SUBLUXATION OR DISLOCATION OF THE PATELLA

Recurrent dislocation of the patella is relatively uncommon. When it does occur, displacement is almost always lateral. It may be congenital, developmental, or post-traumatic.

Recurrent subluxation of the patella is quite common, involvement being predominantly in females; in the experience of Goldthwait, it occurred almost entirely in girls or women.[55, 56] In Macnab's series, 40 of 46 patients were females.[120] Bowker and Thompson reported the female-to-male ratio to be 3:1.[14] Hughston reported that 58 per cent of his patients were female.[81]

A definite familial tendency is present in recurrent subluxation of the patella. Bowker and Thompson found that 12 of their 48 patients had similarly afflicted relatives, with multiple generation involvement in ten of the families.[14]

Etiology

Various causes should be considered:
Ligamentous Laxity. Laxity of the medial capsule of the knee is a definite factor. A high incidence of ligamentous laxity in patients with recurrent subluxation of the patella was shown by DePalma and by Carter and Sweetnam.[17, 35] Heywood, in his series of 54 patients, found generalized ligamentous laxity in 19 patients, laxity of knee ligaments in only 5 patients, and lateral mobility of the patella (all other joints being stable) in 30 patients.[75] A higher incidence of recurrent dislocation of the patella is present in children with generalized affections with ligamentous laxity, such as osteogenesis imperfecta, arachnodactyly, or the Ehlers-Danlos syndrome.

Contracture of Lateral Patellar Soft Tissues and Abnormal Attachments of Iliotibial Tract.

Lateral patellar soft-tissue contracture is a definite pathogenic factor in most cases. The lateral patellar retinaculum and patellofemoral ligament are taut. The vastus lateralis may be contracted, hypertrophied, and inserted low. The iliotibial tract, a thickened strip of fascia lata, normally inserts to the lateral condyle of the tibia. On the lateral side of the thigh, it gives origin to the lateral intermuscular septum and is reinforced in its distal portion by fibers that blend with the aponeurosis of the vastus lateralis. Occasionally, taut strands from the iliotibial band are attached to the upper pole or lateral border of the patella or both. On the Ober test, these fascial bands may be seen on the lateral aspect of the thigh. The iliotibial tract lies anterior to the axis of motion of the fully extended knee, but when the knee is flexed, it passes behind that axis. Thus, during flexion of the knee, the patella will be displaced laterally if it is attached to the iliotibial tract. If the patella is firmly held in the intercondylar groove, the knee could not flex beyond that angle at which the iliotibial tract passes posterior to the axis of knee motion.[92] Malattachments of the iliotibial tract in recurrent dislocation of the patella have been reported by Ober, Smillie, and Jeffreys.[92, 142, 159] This abnormality of attachment and contracture of the iliotibial band are important pathologic causes of recurrent subluxation of the patella.

In excessive lateral patellar pressure syndrome the patella is tilted laterally without actual lateral subluxation (displacement). The abnormal pull of the contracted lateral soft tissues tilts the patella but is not strong enough to subluxate or dislocate it.[42, 43]

Muscle Imbalance. Atrophy, weakness, or a high oblique insertion of the vastus medialis is a factor in most patients. The vastus medialis is a dynamic medial stabilizer of the patella.[110, 126] It is important that it be strengthened and that a dynamic balance between vastus medialis and vastus lateralis be provided.[176]

The orientation of the vastus lateralis and the vastus lateralis obliquus and its tendinous insertions into the lateral retinaculum and patella may create a dynamic lateral force-vector on the patella and contribute to patellofemoral malalignment. In the study of Hallisey and associates, three distinct patterns were noted: First, the vastus lateralis obliquus muscle originated beneath the main muscle belly of the vastus lateralis and then circled distally and anteriorly to insert obliquely on the vastus lateralis portion of the quadriceps tendon; second, its fibers did not always completely join the quadriceps tendon. Rather, they crossed inferiorly to interdigitate with the superficial oblique fibers of the lateral retinaculum; and third, the vastus lateralis portion of the quadriceps tendon did not always travel completely over the patella to join the patellar ligament. Instead, some fibers interdigitated with the superficial oblique fibers of the lateral retinaculum and received the vastus lateralis obliquus muscle without contributing to the patellar ligament.[65]

Rotatory and Angular Malalignment of the Lower Limb. Femoral antetorsion, lateral tibiofibular torsion, and genu valgum will displace the insertion of the patellar ligament laterally and cause valgus position of the quadriceps mechanism. Determination of the Q angle (i.e., the angle formed between the patellar tendon with a vertical line extended distally from the center of the inferior pole of the patella) provides information as to the rotatory-angular forces that act to produce lateral subluxation of the patella.

A High-Riding Patella. This is the so-called patella alta. In Osgood-Schlatter's disease with elongation of the patellar tendon, the normal buttressing effect of the lateral femoral condyle, which serves to check the tendency to lateral patellar displacement, will be lost. A *congenital hypoplasia* and *flattening of the lateral femoral condyle* will have similar effects.

Injury. Injury undoubtedly plays a role in a certain number of patients. A traumatic lateral dislocation inadequately treated will result in stretching and weakening of the medial capsule of the knee and insufficiency of the vastus medialis, predisposing to recurrent lateral subluxation.

Classification

Subluxation and dislocation of the patella may be classified as follows: (1) *congenital dislocation*, which may be fixed or recurrent; as (2) *chronic or habitual developmental subluxation or dislocation*; as (3) *post-traumatic recurrent lateral subluxation or dislocation*; as (4) *recurrent subluxation or dislocation due to* (a) *high-riding patella* (patella alta), characterized by lateral displacement of the knee in extension (the patellar tendon position and femoral sulcus are often normal in this type), (b) an increased Q angle with rotatory-angular malalignment, or (c) a shallow femoral sulcus; or as (5) *recurrent lateral subluxation or dislocation*, which may comprise an excessive lateral compression syndrome with a contracted lateral

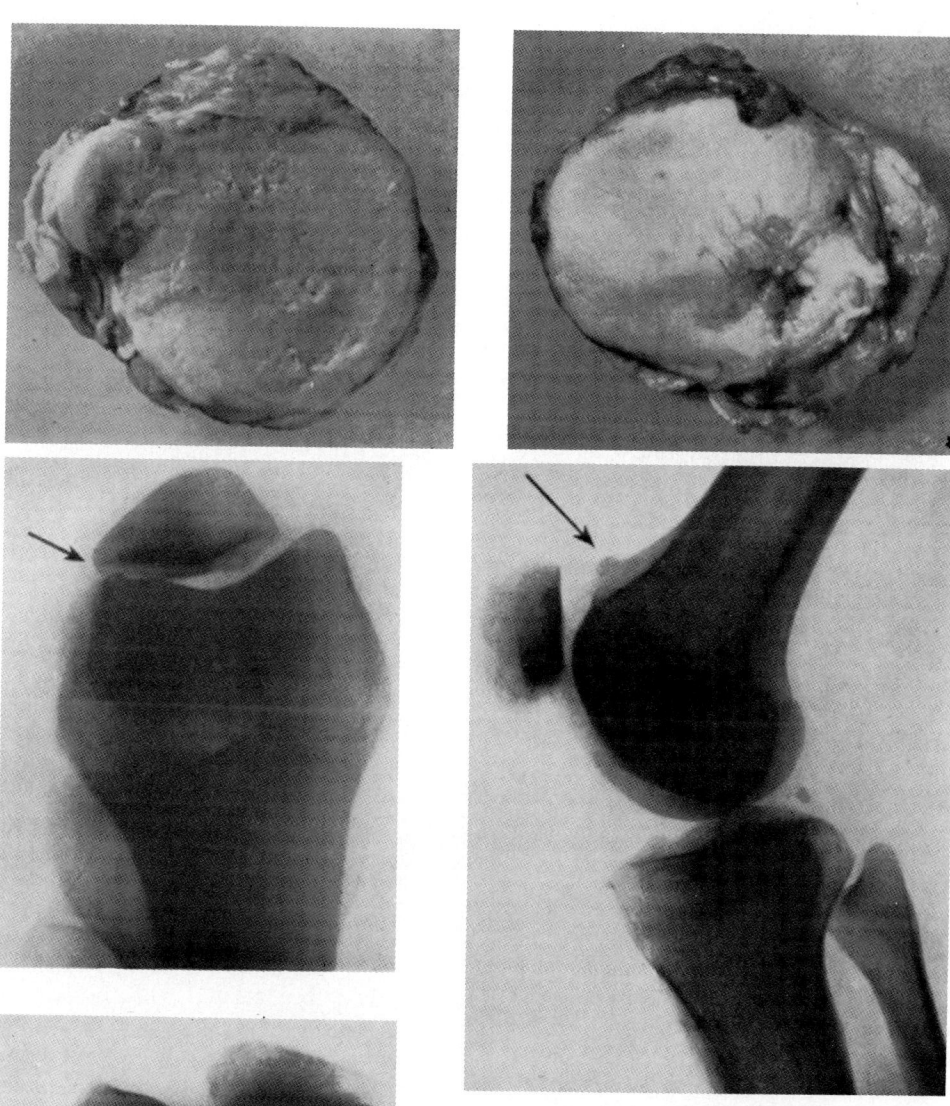

FIGURE 4–56. Stages of degenerative changes in recurrent dislocation of the patella.

A. *Stage I.* Note the fibrillation of the articular cartilage of the patella. **B.** *Stage II.* There is greater wear and tear of the articular cartilage of the patella. Note the crater on its medial facet and exposure of the underlying eburnated bone. **C** and **D.** *Stage III.* Tangential and lateral radiogram of the knee joint showing the onset of patellofemoral arthritis. Erosion of the lateral femoral condyle is evident in the tangential view. Note in the lateral radiogram the spur of bone heaped up in relation to the superior border of the patellar facet of the femur. **E.** *Stage IV.* The marked patellofemoral arthritis and loss of the medial ridge of the patella is evident in this tangential radiogram of the knee. (From Macnab, I.: Recurrent dislocation of the patella. J. Bone Joint Surg., *34-A*:960, 1952. Reprinted by permission.)

Illustration continued on following page

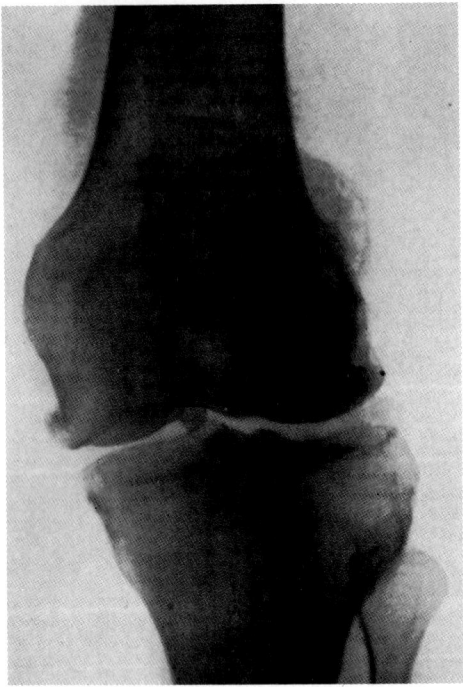

FIGURE 4–56 Continued. Stages of degenerative changes in recurrent dislocation of the patella.

F. *Stage V.* Anteroposterior radiogram of the knee showing generalized degenerative arthritis of the knee joint. (From Macnab, I.: Recurrent dislocation of the patella. J. Bone Joint Surg., 34-A:960, 1952. Reprinted by permission.)

patellar and knee soft tissues but a normal femoral sulcus and patellar tendon position, or an increased Q angle with malalignment of the entire quadriceps mechanism.

Pathology

The recurrent abnormal excursions of the patella that occur with flexion and extension of the knee cause progressive degeneration of the patellofemoral joint. The medial side of the patella undergoes the greatest degree of trauma and increasing degeneration with lateral dislocation of the patella. Macnab has subdivided the pathologic changes into five stages.[120]

Stage I. In this initial stage, the changes are confined to the patella, which shows fibrillation and heaping up of the articular cartilage in its medial facet (Fig. 4–56 A). The radiographic findings are within normal limits.

Stage II. A greater amount of degeneration of the articular surface of the patella occurs in this stage. With attrition, the underlying eburnated bone is exposed, and loose bodies may form on the medial edge of the patella (Fig. 4–56 B). Radiograms will depict these degenerative changes.

Stage III. Patellofemoral arthritis begins to develop with progressive attrition of the articular cartilage of the patella and opposing femur. The subchondral bone becomes exposed and eburnated, with spurs of bone forming at the superior border of the patellar surface of the femur (Fig. 4–56 C and D).

Stage IV. Patellofemoral arthritis is marked, with loss of the median ridge of the patella and planing off and flattening of the femoral surface (Fig. 4–56 E).

Stage V. When recurrent dislocation of the patella remains untreated over a period of years, osteoarthritic changes progress to involve the femorotibial joint, resulting in generalized arthritis of the knee (Fig. 4–56 F).

Clinical Picture

Recurrent Lateral Subluxation. The typical patient is a teenage girl who becomes physically active in junior high school physical education or gymnastics. The presenting complaint is peripatellar or retropatellar pain precipitated by physical activities that require knee flexion and extension. The cause of pain is eccentric impingement of the patella against the lateral femoral condyle during knee flexion, as such motion exerts both compressive and shearing forces.[87, 144] Sometimes the pain is diffuse and nondescript—"The knee just hurts all over."

The knee may "give way"; this may be followed by effusion. Locking and popping of the

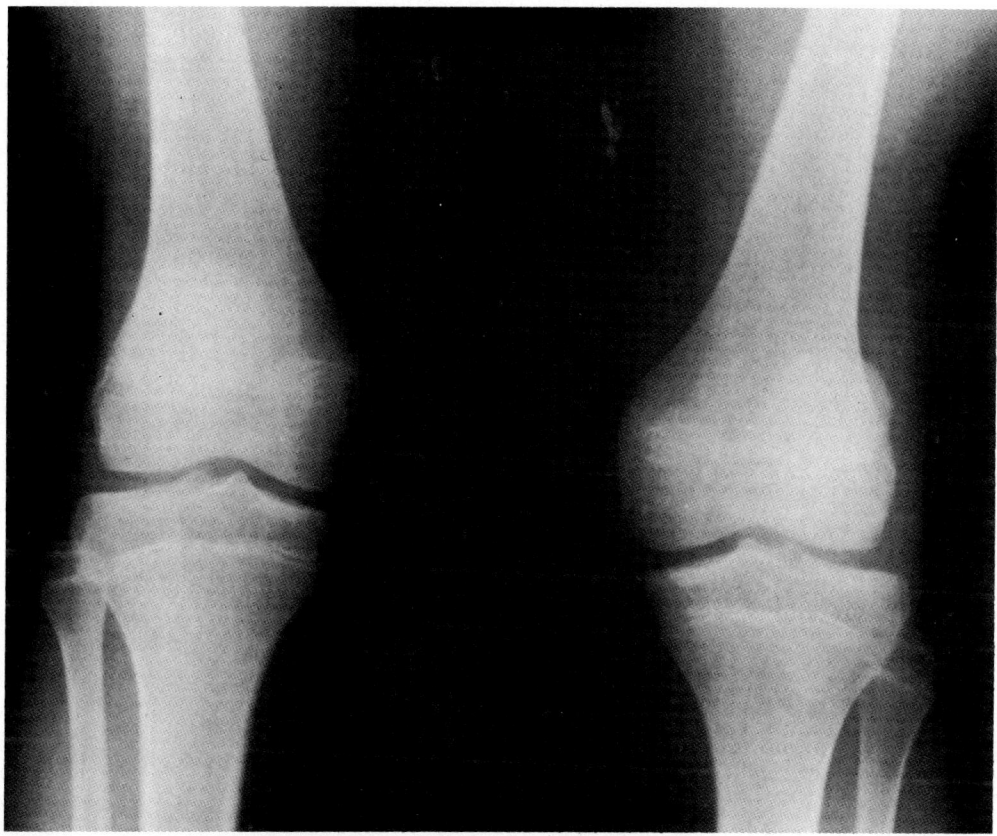

FIGURE 4–57. *Anteroposterior radiograms of both knees in a child with recurrent dislocation of the left patella, which is located in an abnormally lateral position.*

knee are other complaints. The locking usually is apparent and not true with sustained restriction of knee extension; the knee motion toward full extension is momentarily checked when the patella is displaced laterally in semi-flexion, and as the subluxated patella slips back into the intercondylar groove of the femur, the knee extends fully. When there is chondromalacia, the patient complains of a sensation of grating.

Recurrent Dislocation of the Patella. Often this patient is seen between acute episodes. The actual dislocation is precipitated by sudden contraction of the quadriceps muscle with the tibia in lateral rotation and the knee in extension or slight flexion. At the time of the dislocation, the patient may fall down. With frequent dislocations, the intensity of pain and disability diminish.

On examination, first inspect the *position of the patella* with the patient sitting relaxed on the examining table with her knees flexed 90 degrees. In the involved case the posture of the patella will be lateral. In complete extension of the knee the patella slips medially and relocates in the femoral intercondylar groove. On flexion it is displaced laterally. The malalignment of the patellofemoral joint is a *dynamic process*—observed with knee motion. It should be noted, however, that when recurrent subluxation of the patella is due to a high-riding patella with elongation of the patellar tendon, the patella will be displaced laterally with the knee in extension owing to loss of the buttress of the lateral femoral condyle.

Second, the *stability of the patellofemoral joint* is tested by attempting to displace the patella laterally. With the knee flexed 30 degrees and the quadriceps relaxed, exert laterally directed pressure with both thumbs pressing on the medial side of the patella. Frequently the patient becomes fearful and uncomfortable when the patella reaches the point of maximum displacement and will resist and seize the examiner's hand to prevent manipulative dislocation.[38] She attempts to straighten her knee to replace the patella in its relatively normal position. This is referred to as *Fairbank's apprehension test.* When the patella is displaced laterally with the knee in complete extension, the sense of apprehension is not elicited, as the

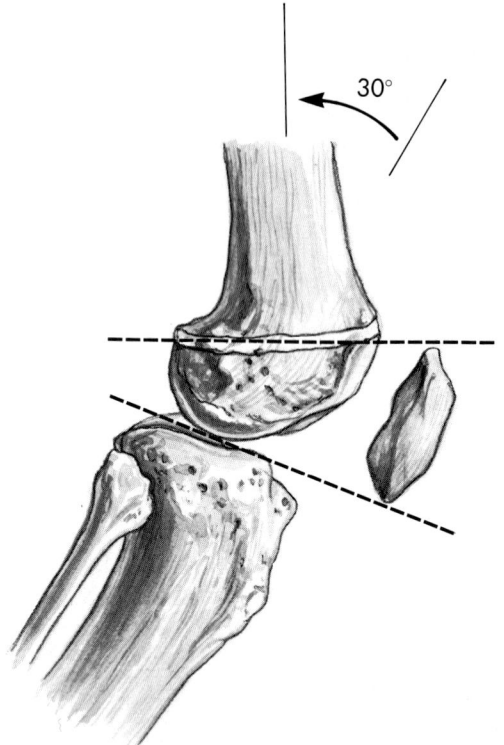

FIGURE 4–58. *Normal resting position of the patella as seen in the lateral radiographic view of the knee, made with the knee in 30 degrees of flexion.*

Note that the patella is between the anterior projections of the intercondylar notch line and the metaphyseal plate line (central part of the physis).

patella moves readily on the flat condylar and supracondylar surface of the femur and not across the highest point of the lateral condyle.[81]

Third, there may be limitation of medial excursion of the patella with the knee in extension with a palpable sensation of tautness of the lateral soft tissues.

Fourth, there will be tenderness on palpation over the medial retinaculum and on compression of the patella. Pain elicited by manual pressure on the patella is most probably due to compression of the synovial membrane, not the articular cartilage.

Genu valgum and lateral torsional deformity of the tibia are usually present. The patellar tendon may insert laterally with abnormal increase of the Q angle. The tendon may be elongated with a high-riding patella (patella alta). In chronic recurrent subluxation of the patella there may be effusion and synovial thickening. On occasion the knee may not fully extend passively because of hamstring spasm.

Radiographic Findings

Dislocation of the patella is readily visualized in the radiograph; patellar subluxation, however, is difficult to demonstrate.

Radiographic study of the knee with the clinical diagnosis of patellofemoral subluxation should include anteroposterior and lateral views with the knee in complete extension, a tunnel or a notch view, and special axial or tangential projections for visualization of the patellofemoral joint. The purpose of taking anteroposterior and lateral views is to show the abnormally high position of the patella and the presence of genu valgum as well as other possible structural abnormalities such as hypoplasia of the femoral condyles and other concomitant lesions (Fig. 4–57). The notch view will assist in detecting possible cartilaginous loose bodies.

Blumensaat recommends that the lateral projection of the knee be made with the knee in 30 degrees of flexion.[12] In this view, normally the patella should rest between the anterior projections of the intercondylar notch line (roof of the intercondylar notch) and the metaphyseal plate line (central part of the physis), and the upper end of the patella should reach almost to the projection of the intercondylar notch line (Fig. 4–58).[81]

An infrapatellar axial or tangential view is vital for visualization of the patellofemoral joint. It should be pointed out that recurrent subluxation of the patella is a dynamic process; the diagnosis is made clinically. Inappropriately made radiographs may appear completely normal. All the films should be diligently scrutinized for the presence of osteocartilaginous loose bodies. In the literature a number of radiographic techniques have been described.[43, 120, 133]

Macnab has pointed out that a routine "skyline view," taken with the knee in full flexion, shows the tibial surfaces of the femoral condyles and an oblique view of the patella. He recommends taking the tangential view with the knee flexed 40 degrees for clear depiction of the patellofemoral joint (Fig. 4–59).[120] In this view one can clearly visualize the relationship of the patella to the distal end of the femur, early degenerative changes of the medial facet of the patella, and narrowing of the joint space.

Hughston recommended the following technique for the infrapatellar view: with the patient prone the cassette is placed underneath both knees and the lower part of the thighs; the patient's feet rest on the x-ray tube, with her

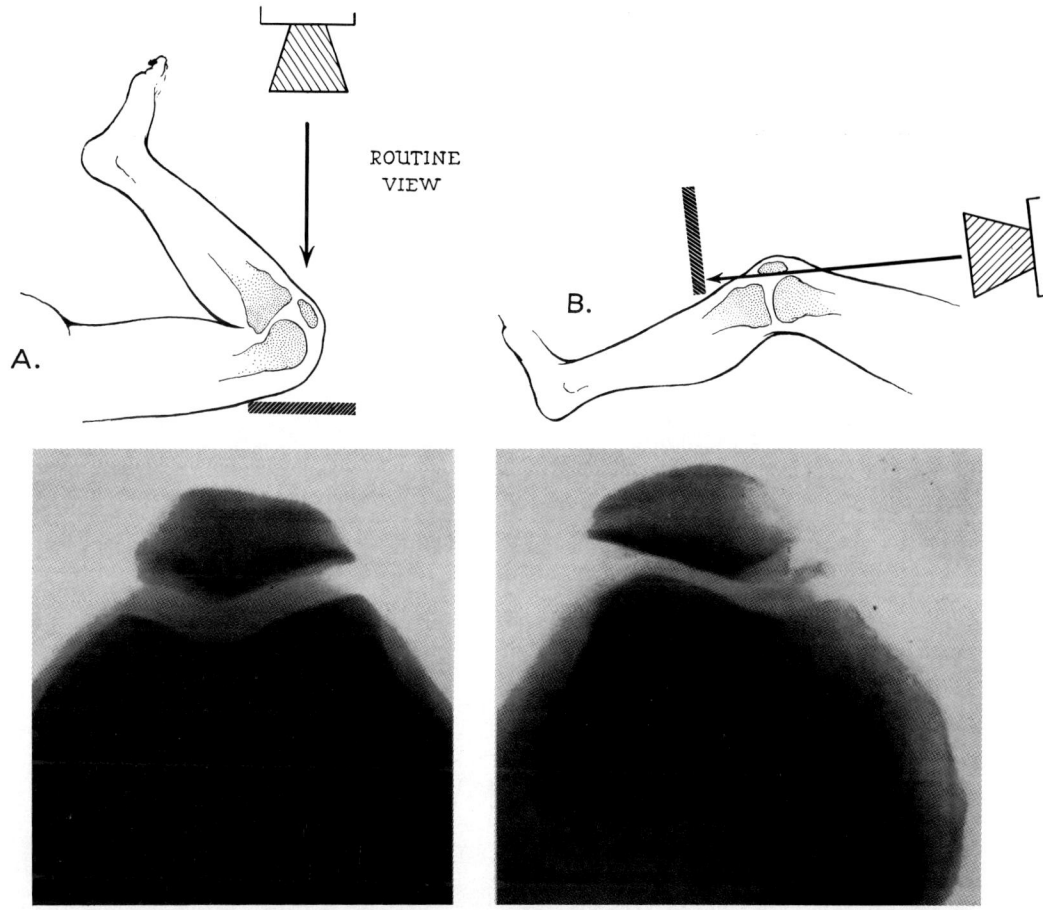

FIGURE 4–59. *Radiographic view recommended by Macnab for recurrent dislocation of the patella.*

A. The routine "skyline view," which shows the tibial surface of the femoral condyles and an oblique projection of the patella. **B.** The tangential view of the patellofemoral joint taken with the knee flexed 40 degrees. **C.** Radiogram of the normal patellofemoral joint made with the knee in 40 degrees of flexion. **D.** Radiogram of the patellofemoral joint in a case with recurrent dislocation of the patella. Note the loose bodies in relation to the medial edge of the laterally subluxated patella. (From Macnab, I.: Recurrent dislocation of the patella. J. Bone Joint Surg., 34-A:958, 1952. Reprinted by permission.)

legs in neutral rotation and the knees flexed 50 to 60 degrees. The x-ray tube is angled 45 degrees from the vertical and directed along the anterior border of the tibia toward the infrapatellar region (Fig. 4–60).[81]

Laurin and associates recommended that the patient be placed supine, the knees flexed 20 to 30 degrees, the x-ray tube between the ankles, and the cassette held proximal to the knees and perpendicular to the x-ray beam. The x-ray beam is directed cephalad so that it is almost parallel to the anterior border of the tibia and parallel to the plane of the proximal part of the patellofemoral joint space (Fig. 4–61). Special apparatus is not required to stabilize the cassette, which is in close proximity to the patella.[109]

Merchant and associates described a radiographic technique for analysis of patellofemoral congruence. The patient is placed supine on the x-ray table with the knees flexed 45 degrees. By slight elevation of the knees the femora are kept horizontal and parallel with the table surface. The x-ray tube and collimator are raised over the patient and angled distally 30 degrees from the horizontal; thereby a beam-to-femur angle of 30 degrees is provided. The cassette is placed 12 inches below the knees, resting on the tibiae and at a right angle to the x-ray beam. Rotation of the legs into neutral position is maintained by appropriate strapping. Both knees are exposed simultaneously. The quadriceps muscle should be relaxed during exposure (Fig. 4–62).[133]

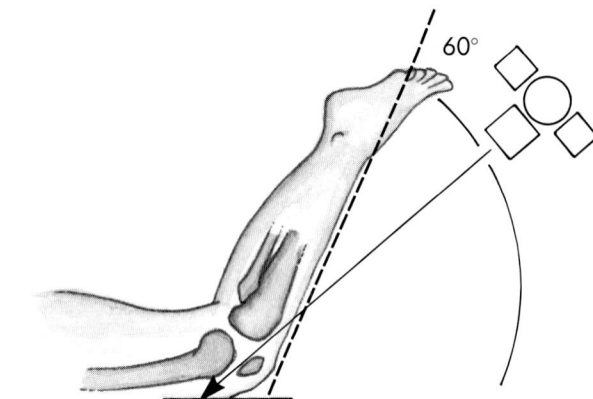

FIGURE 4–60. *Hughston technique for infrapatellar axial or tangential projection.*

FIGURE 4–61. *Laurin technique for infrapatellar axial or tangential projection.*

(Redrawn after Laurin, C. A., Levesque, H. P., Dussault, R., Labelle, H., and Peides, J. P.: The abnormal lateral patellofemoral angle: A diagnostic roentgenographic sign of recurrent patellar subluxation. J. Bone Joint Surg., 60-A:55, 1978.)

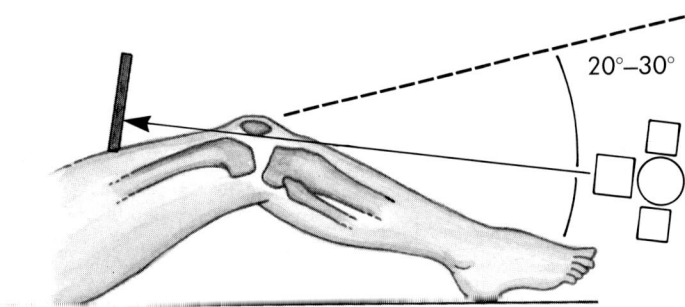

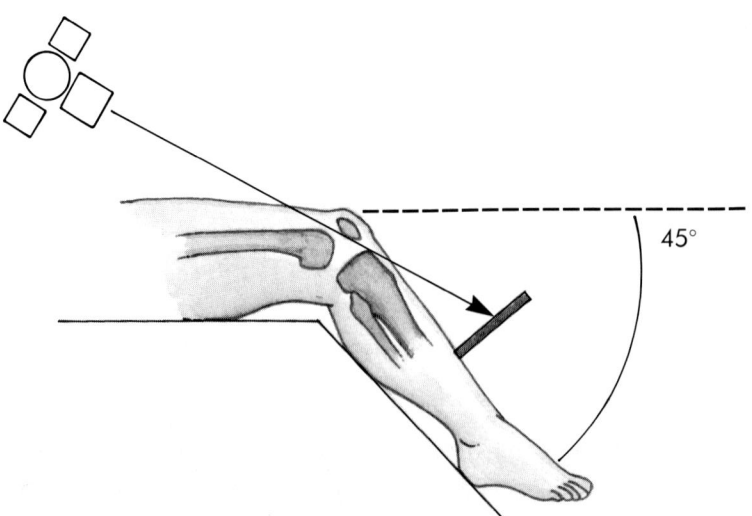

FIGURE 4–62. *Diagram of Merchant technique for radiography of patellofemoral joints in axial projection.*

(Redrawn after Merchant, A. C., Mercer, R. L., Jacobsen, R. H., and Cool, C. R.: Roentgenographic analysis of patellofemoral congruence. J. Bone Joint Surg., 56-A:1391, 1974.)

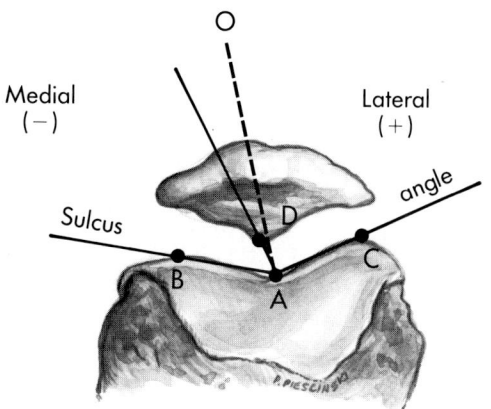

FIGURE 4–63. *The congruence angle.*

To measure the congruence angle: Find the highest point of the medial (B) and lateral (C) condyles and the lowest point of the intercondylar sulcus (A). (A clear plastic straight edge is helpful.) The angle, BAC, is the sulcus angle. Bisect the sulcus angle to establish the zero reference line, AO. Find the lowest point on the articular ridge of the patella (D). (A straight edge held parallel to the horizontal axis of the patella helps.) Project line AD. The angle DAO is the congruence angle. (Redrawn after Merchant, A. C., Mercer, R. L., Jacobsen, R. H., and Cool, C. R.: Roentgenographic analysis of patellofemoral congruence. J. Bone Joint Surg., 56-A:1391, 1974.)

The relationship of the patella to the intercondylar sulcus is determined by the *congruence angle*, which is measured as follows: First, draw the *sulcus angle* by bisecting the highest points of the medial (B) and lateral (C) condyles of the femur and the lowest point of the intercondylar sulcus (A). Second, locate and mark the lowest point on the articular ridge of the patella (D). Third, establish a zero reference line by bisecting the sulcus angle (line AO). Fourth, project a line from the apex of the sulcus angle through the lowest point of the articular ridge of the patella (line AD). The angle measured between these two lines (lines AO and AD) is the congruence angle (Fig. 4–63). If the apex of the patellar articular ridge is lateral to the zero line, the congruence angle is designated positive; if it is medial, the congruence angle is negative. In the normal patellofemoral joint the average congruence angle is minus 6 degrees with a standard deviation of 11 degrees. Any congruence angle greater than +16 degrees is abnormal, indicating lateral patellofemoral subluxation in 95 per cent of cases.

The *lateral patellofemoral angle* of Laurin is measured as follows: First, draw a line between the anterior summits of the lateral and medial femoral condyles (A–A1), and second, draw a straight line between the limits of the lateral patellar facet (B–B1). The angle formed by these two lines (A–A1 and B–B1) is the lateral patellofemoral angle, which is always anterior to the line A–A1 (Fig. 4–64). In the *normal* patellofemoral joint the lateral patellofemoral angle is *open laterally* (in the series of 100 normal knees it was open laterally in 97 and parallel in the other 3). In lateral subluxation of the patella the lateral patellofemoral angle was zero (the two lines were parallel) in 80 per cent or open medially (in 20 per cent). According to Laurin and associates, when the two lines are parallel or open medially the lateral patellofemoral angle is an accurate radiographic indicator of lateral subluxation of the patella.[109]

Computed tomography will depict accurately the anatomic congruence of the patellofemoral joint; it is performed with the knee in full extension and at 10 and 30 degrees of flexion with the quadriceps first relaxed and then contracted.[97] Its routine use is not recommended because of the cost and the exposure to irradiation.

In a *laterally tilted patella* there are increased

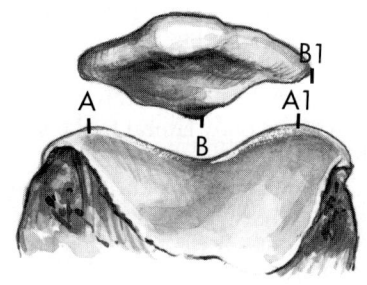

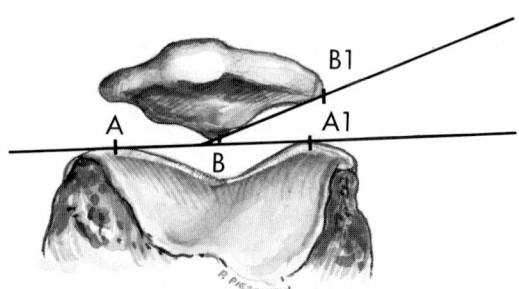

FIGURE 4–64. *The lateral patellofemoral angle.*

Line A–A1 passes through the limits of the femoral sulcus and line B–B1, through the limits of the lateral patellar facet. The lateral patellofemoral angle is formed by the lines A–A1 and B–B1. Note that the lateral patellofemoral angle is always situated anterior to (above) line A–A1. (Redrawn after Laurin, C. A., Levesque, H. P., Dussault, R., Labelle, H., and Peides, J. P.: The abnormal lateral patellofemoral angle: A diagnostic roentgenographic sign of recurrent patellar subluxation. J. Bone Joint Surg., 60-A:55, 1978.)

Quadriceps-plasty for Recurrent Dislocation of the Patella (Green)

OPERATIVE TECHNIQUE

A. The surgical approach is by two longitudinal skin incisions. The first incision is medial, beginning 3 cm. medial and 4 cm. proximal to the superior pole of the patella and extending distally to terminate at a point 2 cm. distal and 1 cm. medial to the proximal tibial tubercle. The lateral longitudinal skin incision begins at the joint line 2 cm. lateral to the lateral margin of the patellar tendon and extends proximally for a distance of 1 to 10 cm. In this drawing a J shaped incision is illustrated; its use is not recommended by this author because the operative scar is ugly. The subcutaneous tissue and superficial fascia are divided and the skin flaps are developed medially and laterally to expose the quadriceps muscle, patella, patellar tendon, patellar retinaculum, joint capsule, and iliotibial band.

B and C. Starting at a level 1½ inches proximal to the lateral femoral condyle, a 3-inch segment of the fascia lata and the lateral intermuscular septum are excised. Next, abnormal attachments of the iliotibial band are divided, and the vastus lateralis muscle is widely mobilized from the deep surface of the fascia lata and its origin from the femur to allow free medial displacement of the patella. During this procedure, several muscular branches of the perforating arteries may be encountered, requiring coagulation or ligation.

Plate 54. Quadriceps-plasty for Recurrent Dislocation of the Patella (Green)

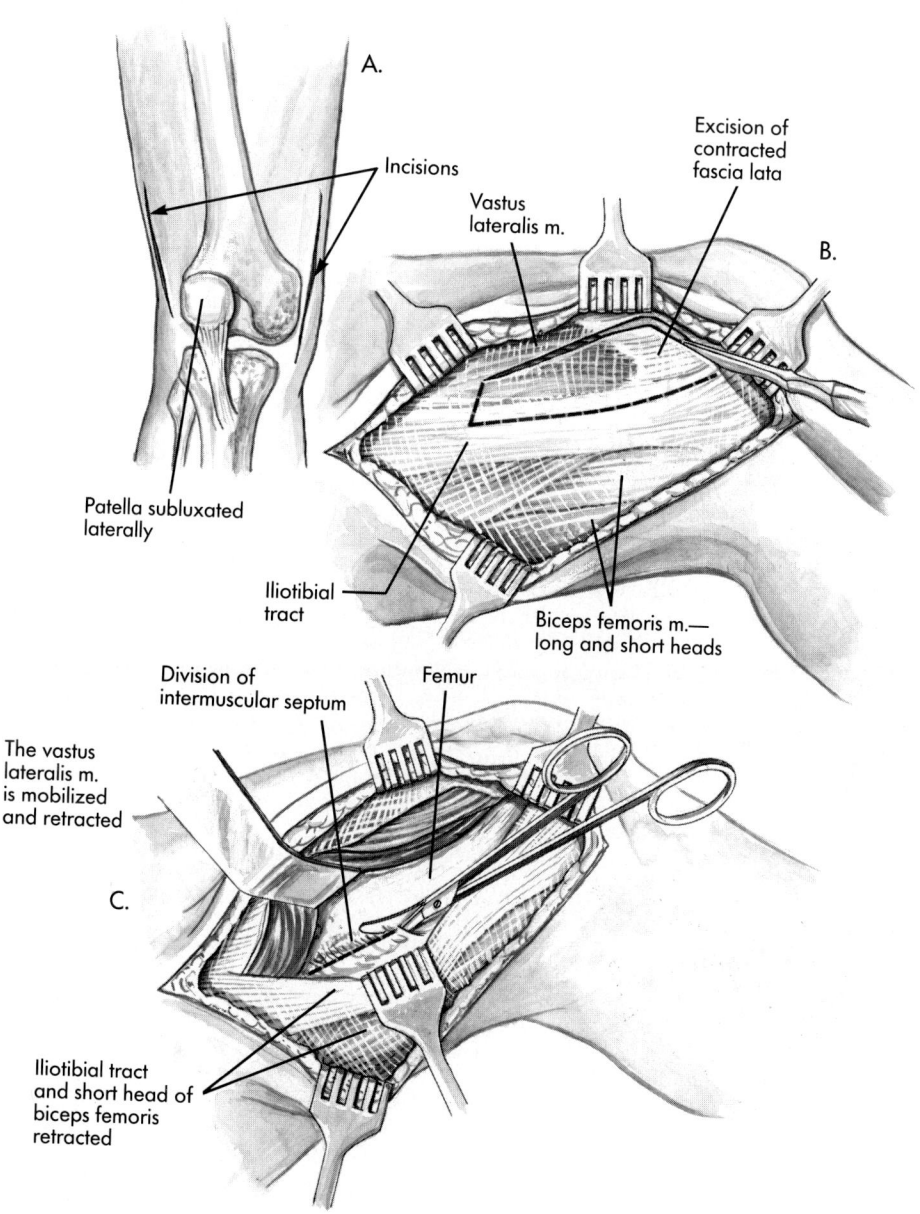

Quadriceps-plasty for Recurrent Dislocation of the Patella (Green) (Continued)

D and **E.** The contracted iliotibial tract, patellar retinaculum, and lateral joint capsule are then longitudinally divided in their posterolateral portion to allow medial displacement of the patella. The lax medial joint capsule and patellar retinaculum are longitudinally incised, to be reefed later. The insertion of the vastus medialis, with its tendinous fibers and the periosteum of the patella, is detached from the medial and superior border of the patella by U-shaped incisions in the superoranterior and posteroinferior margins of the muscle. The synovial membrane is not incised unless visualization of the interior of the joint for loose bodies or chondromalacia of the patella is indicated. Next, the patella is displaced medially and the medial joint capsule is imbricated and tightly closed by reefing sutures. With the knee in complete extension, the medial patellar retinaculum is also imbricated by reefing sutures.

F. The superficial surface of the anterolateral third of the inferior half of the patella is then roughened with curved osteotomes and curet. The vastus medialis tendon is transferred laterally and distally deep to the patellar bursa and sutured to the lateral border of the patellar tendon. The wounds are closed in layers and a well-molded long leg cylinder cast is applied with the knee in neutral or 5 degrees flexed position.

POSTOPERATIVE CARE

Immobilization in the solid cast is continued for a period of three to four weeks. During this time the patient is permitted to walk with crutches with a three-point partial weight-bearing gait. Quadriceps muscle strength is maintained by isometric exercises in the solid cast. Then the cast is removed, and knee motion and muscle strength are gradually developed by flexion-extension exercises. A knee orthosis holding the patella in reduced anatomic position and the knee in neutral extension is worn during the day for four weeks. Protection with crutches is continued until there is fair strength of the quadriceps muscle and 90 degrees of knee flexion.

Plate 54. Quadriceps-plasty for Recurrent Dislocation of the Patella (Green)

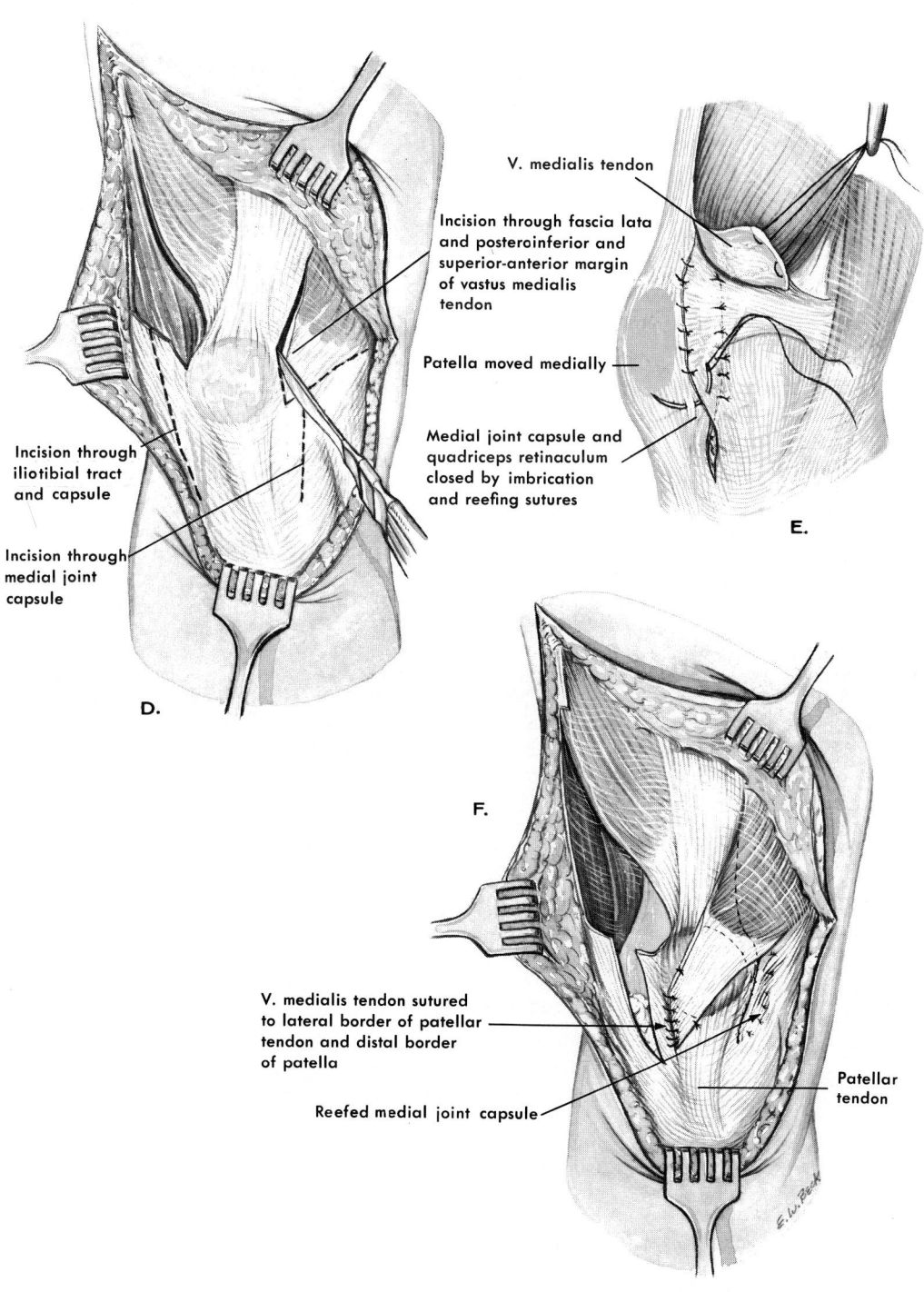

Goldthwait-Hauser Procedure for Recurrent Lateral Dislocation of the Patella

OPERATIVE TECHNIQUE

A. An anteromedial incision is made, starting 2 cm. medial to the superior pole of the patella and extending distally to 3 cm. distal and 1 cm. medial to the proximal tibial tubercle. In this drawing, a U-shaped incision is illustrated over the anterior aspect of the knee; cosmetically the scar is ugly; therefore, this author does not recommend its use. The subcutaneous tissue and fascia are divided in line with the skin incision and the wound edges are retracted. Avoid injury to the infrapatellar branch of the saphenous nerve.

B. A longitudinal incision is made on each side of the patellar tendon, which is dissected free from its underlying fat pad. The patellar tendon should be left intact and attached at its insertion to the proximal tibial tubercle.

C. A rectangular block of bone (1 by 2 cm.) is resected from the tibial tuberosity at the site of insertion of the patellar tendon. The distal part is undercut as a wedge, following the method of McKeever.* The joint capsule is incised on the medial and lateral side of the patella. The synovial membrane is left intact. The joint is not opened unless there are indications for inspection of the deep surfaces of the patella, menisci, and cruciate ligaments (such as patellar crepitation and locking of the knee). Next, a site for transplantation of the bone block is selected; it is 2 cm. medial and 1.5 to 2 cm. distal from its original location. The patella should lie between the femoral condyles in its normal position. A solid strut of bone should be present between the two blocks, in order to prevent fracture. It is best to use sharp drill points to control the extent of osteotomy. Too distal a position should be avoided, unless the patella was riding high. The periosteum is incised longitudinally and a similar-sized rectangular block of bone is removed.

D. The first block of bone with the patellar tendon attached to it is firmly inserted and countersunk into the space created by removal of the second block. The bone block is transfixed internally with a screw, which should engage the posterior cortex of the tibia. The periosteum is closed with interrupted sutures, which should pass through the patellar tendon. The medial capsule is imbricated and reefed with interrupted sutures. The lateral capsule is left open. The second block of bone is inserted into the space created at the original site of patellar tendon insertion. The subcutaneous tissues and skin are closed in the routine manner, and the limb is immobilized in an above-knee cylinder cast with the foot and ankle free.

POSTOPERATIVE CARE

The patient is allowed to be ambulatory with crutches with a three-point partial weight-bearing gait as soon as he is comfortable. Quadriceps setting exercises are begun the day of operation. At four weeks, the cast is removed and radiograms are taken to determine the healing of the transplanted bone block. At this time, bony union is usually solid enough to allow side-lying knee flexion and extension exercises. A knee immobilizer holding the knee in extension is used for two to three weeks during walking. Then full weight-bearing is allowed. Quadriceps exercises are continued until full motor strength is regained. Full knee flexion may be difficult for some patients; hence, it is imperative to emphasize knee flexion as well extension in the rehabilitation program.

---

*McKeever, D. C.: Recurrent dislocation of the patella. Clin. Orthop., 3:55, 1954.

Plate 55. Goldthwait-Hauser Procedure for Recurrent Lateral Dislocation of the Patella

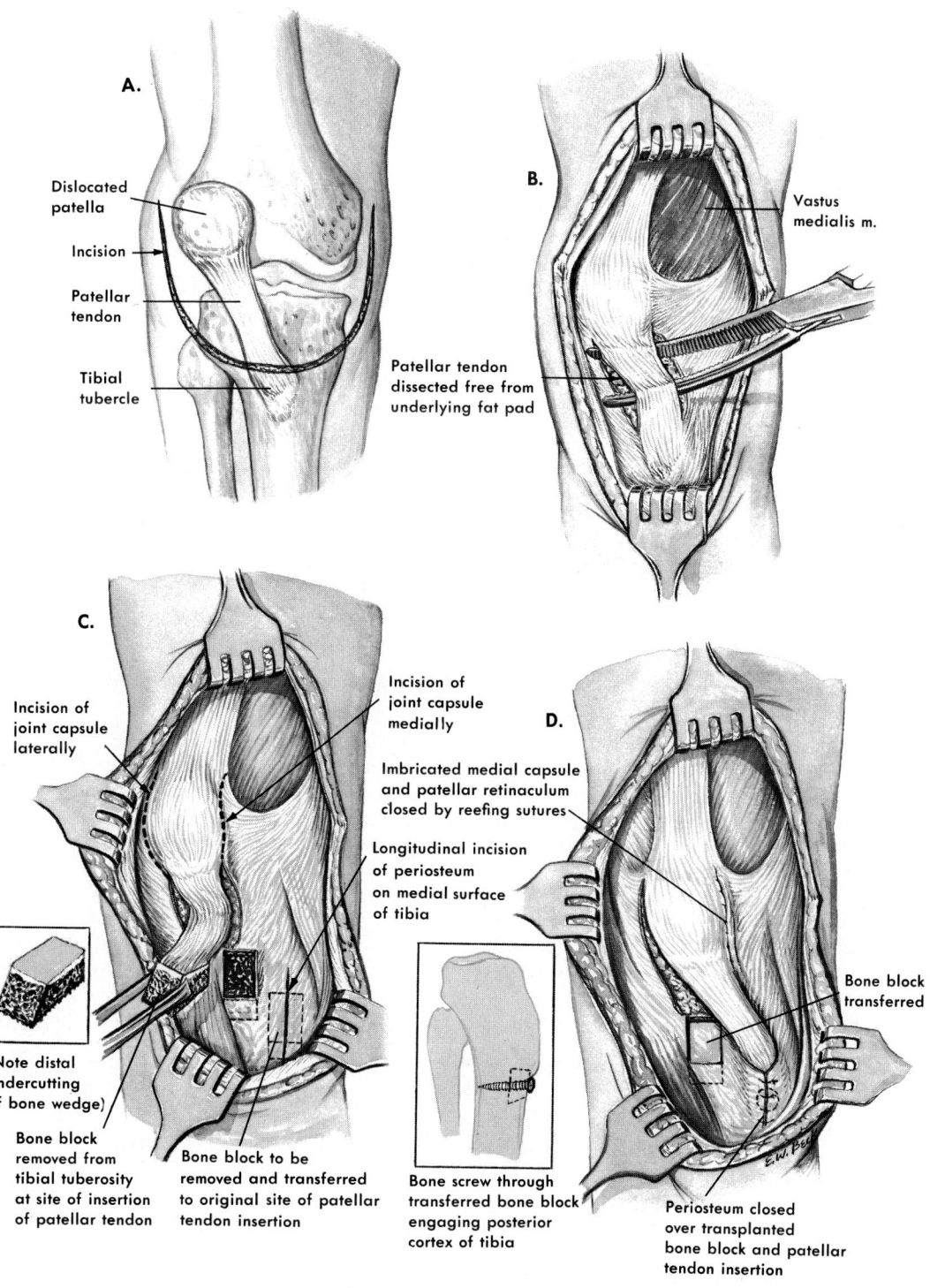

Table 4–13. Physical Signs in Recurrent Lateral Subluxation-Dislocation of the Patella

Tenderness over patellar facets and femoral condyles
Positive apprehension test
Positive patellar compression test
Quadriceps atrophy
Actual lateral displacement of patella with extension of knee
Patellofemoral crepitus
Limitation of medial passive mobility of patella with knee in extension and quadriceps femoris relaxed
Limited range of knee motion

tive and preferably isometric, not isotonic. If there is associated contracture of the iliotibial band and lateral patellar retinaculum, it is passively stretched. Descending and climbing stairs, bicycle riding, contact sports, and other strenuous physical activities are curtailed. Flexed, loaded positions of the knee should be avoided. If associated synovitis and chondromalacia are causing pain, anti-inflammatory medication is given. This author prefers simple salicylates (enteric coated in patients with sensitive gastric mucosa). Other anti-inflammatory drugs such as Naprosyn (250 mg. or 375 mg. tablets—one tablet twice a day with meals) or Tolectin (100 or 200 mg. tablets—one tablet twice a day with meals) may be given; dosage is individualized according to the response and toxic reactions to the medications. Do not combine salicylates with other anti-inflammatory medications. Finally, weight reduction of an obese patient is recommended.

When recurrent subluxation is severe and associated chondromalacia moderate, again this author recommends a trial period of the foregoing conservative measures. It is true that early surgical intervention can prevent degenerative arthritis of the patellofemoral joint; it is also surprising how well teenage girls do with simple conservative management. In this author's experience about 75 per cent of patients will gain symptomatic relief with nonoperative management.

Operative measures are carried out when an adequate trial of conservative management fails to relieve symptoms. Prior to surgery, diligently re-evaluate the knee to rule out other causes of continued symptoms of malalignment. Is there a symptomatic plica? Beware of the psychologically unstable teenager who complains of pain in the knee with minimal or moderate lateral subluxation of the patellofemoral joint; treat this one nonoperatively! Pain is subjective. Look for concrete physical signs (Table 4–13). Thoroughly examine the knee by appropriate radiographs for patellar tilting, subluxation, and patellofemoral joint incongruity.

SURGICAL PROCEDURES

Lateral Patellar Retinacular Release. This procedure is indicated when thickened and contracted lateral soft tissues are the cause of lateral tilting and displacement of the patella and excessive lateral pressure syndrome. It should be pointed out, however, Mr. Peter Williams noted in his patients with habitual lateral subluxation of the patella, that they primarily had contracture of the vastus lateralis and rarely of the iliotibial band. Examine the knee thoroughly! Is the Ober test positive? Is there contracture of the lateral patellar retinaculum as shown by restriction of passive medial mobility of the patella? Are there weakness of the vastus medialis and stretching and weakness of the medial aspect of the knee joint? Study the radiographs carefully—is there lateral patellar tilt and subluxation?

Indications for lateral patellar retinacular release are: first, a history of chronic, intermittent anterior knee pain aggravated by physical activities that involve flexion and extension of the knee; second, typical physical findings of lateral subluxation of the patella due to contracture of lateral parapatellar soft tissues (see Table 4–13); third, radiographic confirmation of lateral patellar subluxation or tilting; fourth, failure to respond to a trial period of adequate conservative management; and fifth, arthroscopic determination of lateral patellar subluxation and compression.[134]

This author strongly stresses that simple clinical demonstration of lateral subluxation of the patella is *not* an indication for diagnostic arthroscopy and lateral release.

In the past lateral retinacular release was an open or limited open surgical procedure with excellent or good results in 75 to 85 per cent of cases. Willner excised a strip of fascia in seven knees with 100 per cent success in all.[177] Merchant and Mercer performed an open release of the lateral retinaculum in 20 knees with 85 per cent good results.[132] Ficat and Hungerford reported 76 per cent good or excellent results by open lateral retinacular release in 174 knees.[43] Larson and associates, and later Ceder and Larson, found 82 and 81 per cent excellent or good results following Z-plasty lengthening of the lateral retinaculum.[20, 108] Chen and associates designed a closed technique of lateral release by the use of a specially designed flanged knife, which blindly sectioned the taut soft tissues percutaneously.[21, 22]

Arthroscopic Lateral Patellar Retinacular Release. At present, lateral release is performed through the arthroscope; it is a simple, effective

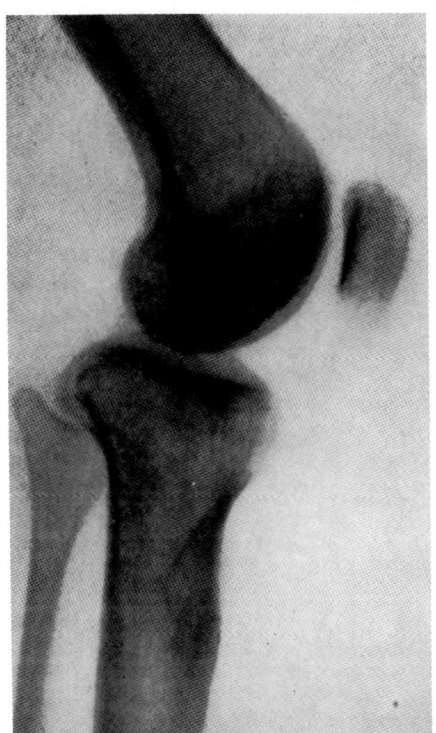

FIGURE 4-67. *Lateral roentgenogram of the knee of a patient who in childhood had tibial tubercle transfer for recurrent dislocation of the patella.*

Note the forward tilting of the tibial plateau secondary to premature arrest of growth of anterior portion of proximal tibial epiphysis. (From Macnab, I.: Recurrent dislocation of the patella. J. Bone Joint Surg., 34-A:966, 1952. Reprinted by permission.)

method of sectioning the contracted thickened lateral soft tissues.[134] It has the following advantages: It visualizes patellar tracking without the distortion that can ensue from arthrotomy. It will detect any other associated pathologic conditions in the knee, such as a torn meniscus. Complete release of the lateral deforming forces allows dynamic realignment of the patella in the femoral trochlea. The surgical scars are minimal and cosmetically very pleasing. Finally, the postoperative morbidity is relatively minimal as compared with open arthrotomy. In order to prevent bleeding, salicylates should be withheld three weeks preoperatively and for three weeks after surgery.

Arthroscopic lateral patellar release is contraindicated when there is marked ligamentous hyperlaxity with recurrent dislocation of a high-riding patella and when there is advanced degenerative arthritis of the patellofemoral joint. A Q angle greater than 20 degrees is an ominous sign, as it indicates severe malalignment of the quadriceps mechanism. In such an instance, simple lateral release is inadequate; a thorough open realignment of the quadriceps mechanism should be performed.

Operative Technique. The operative procedure is performed as outpatient surgery but under general anesthesia and tourniquet ischemia. The entire lower limb is prepared and draped as for major open surgical procedures. The importance of asepsis during the entire operation cannot be overemphasized. The portal of entry of the arthroscope usually is inferolateral; it could be superolateral if so desired, as there is no difference in the observed tracking of the patella. When inserting the arthroscope inferolaterally do not do so too close to the patellar tendon, as the pressure of the arthroscope may decrease the tendency for lateral tracking. Keep to the middle of the anterolateral sulcus, away from the tendon!

First, a complete methodical diagnostic arthroscopic examination is performed to evaluate the entire knee. Rule out associated injuries to the menisci and the presence of loose bodies. Inspect the femoral condyles and deep surface of the patella for chondromalacia.

The degree of chondromalacia is classified by Metcalf as follows: Grade 0—normal, a smooth, firm articular surface; Grade I—a central softening but no surface breakdown; Grade II—minimal fissuring and fragmentation of the articular surface; Grade III—significant (moderate) fibrillation, fragmentation, or fissuring involving less than half of the articular surface of the patella; and Grade IV—severe fissuring and fibrillation involving more than 50 per cent of the surface area and ulceration exposing subchondral bone.[134]

Next, tracking of the patella in the intercondylar sulcus is observed. The knee is flexed 90 degrees and extended, and the patellofemoral articular relationship is noted. Normally the central ridge of the patella seats in the trochlear groove of the femur during the first 45 degrees of flexion. Patellar tracking malalignment is present when the patella rides laterally during the initial 45 degrees of knee flexion, i.e., the central ridge of the patella tracks along the lateral femoral condyle, concomitantly tilting the patella laterally. The patellofemoral joint space is widened medially, and laterally the lateral facet and central ridge of the patella press against the lateral femoral condyle (this is referred to as Casscell's sign).[19]

In severe lateral tracking of the patella, its lateral facet overhangs the lateral condylar ridge; this is best seen with the arthroscope through the inferolateral port.

Prior to lateral release a long-acting local anesthetic agent (20 ml. of 0.5 per cent bupivacaine [Marcaine] with epinephrine) is injected into contracted lateral soft tissues; this measure provides additional hemostasis after release of the tourniquet and relieves immediate postoperative pain.

Then contracted lateral soft tissues are released by either of two methods: either subcutaneously with heavy Mayo-type scissors or with special arthroscopy scissors. It is important to divide the patellar retinaculum, synovium, and lower part of the insertion of the vastus lateralis muscle. At the superolateral margin of the patella the scissors curve medially to section the insertion of the vastus lateralis.

Next, the arthroscope is reinserted through the inferolateral portal and the adequacy of release is checked by inspection of patellofemoral motion. Further release may have to be done proximally and distally in order to provide congruity of both the medial and lateral patellar facets with the respective condyles of the femur. Patellar shaving is performed when there is Grade II or III chondromalacia. Recently, laser-assisted abrasion chondroplasty has been explored in the management of chondromalacia of the patella. Hemovac suction tubes are inserted. A Jones compression dressing is applied, and the tourniquet is released.

Postoperative Care. It is the custom of this author to admit the patient to the hospital overnight. The next morning the Hemovac suction tubes are removed. A less clumsy compression dressing is applied, and the patient is allowed to be up and around with three-point crutch gait with partial weight-bearing on the limb that was operated. Isometric quadriceps exercises are performed several times a day.

Seven to ten days postoperatively, side-lying knee flexion-extension exercises are commenced. Crutch protection is discontinued in 7 to 10 days, once the patient has developed adequate muscle strength and is comfortable. The dressing is removed, and a patellar immobilizer is used for two to preferably three weeks after surgery. This slower protective rehabilitation program has prevented effusion of the knee, and the postoperative course has become smoother. Three weeks after surgery an aggressive physical therapy program consisting of progressive resistive exercises is instituted. The patient is allowed gradual resumption of normal activity six to eight weeks after surgery when the symptoms have subsided and the motor strength of the knee muscles is normal.

Realignment of Quadriceps Mechanism. In the literature numerous surgical procedures have been described. These include both proximal and distal realignments.[31] The objective of surgery is to achieve and maintain congruous reduction of the patellofemoral joint by correcting the pathogenic factors by: (1) releasing contracted lateral soft-tissue structures; (2) tautening lax medial soft tissues (i.e., capsule and patellar retinaculum) by plication; (3) establishing dynamic mediolateral balance of muscle forces acting on the patella (i.e., mobilizing contracture of the distal insertion of the vastus lateralis and advancing the insertion of the vastus medialis distally and laterally); (4) correcting the increased Q angle (which is caused by excessive femoral antetorsion, excessive lateral tibiofibular torsion and genu valgum) by medial advancement of the patellar tendon; (5) lowering the high-riding patella (patella alta) by distal transfer of the patellar tendon; and (6) strengthening excessively lax, poor quality medial soft tissues by tenodesis of the semitendinosus to the patella and the patellar tendon. A variety of modifications of surgical techniques have been developed to achieve these goals.

Proximal Realignment of Entire Quadriceps. This is indicated in the treatment of recurrent lateral subluxation or dislocation of the patella when conservative nonoperative treatment or partial proximal realignment by lateral release alone has failed. The technique recommended by this author is the same as that described by Green and is illustrated in Plate 54.

When there is patella alta with increased Q angle, the proximal tibial tubercle is transferred medially and distally to realign the quadriceps pull. The surgical procedure described by Goldthwait and popularized by Hauser is illustrated in Plate 55. The proximal tibial tubercle should not be transferred in children and adolescents with open physes and apophyses because such a procedure will arrest growth from the anterior portion of the proximal tibial epiphysis, resulting in anterior tilting of the tibial plateau and genu recurvatum (Fig. 4–67). Another hazard is distal migration of the patella with the tibial tubercle, causing patellofemoral incongruity and early degenerative arthritis (Fig. 4–68). Furthermore, the transplanted tubercle may be pulled out like a traction apophysis and present as a large mass of bone at its new site (Fig. 4–69). Medial transfer of the tibial tubercle will often produce excessive lateral rotation of the tibia. Another serious complication of the Goldthwait-Hauser procedure is the anterior compartment syndrome. Wall reported 11 such cases; in two of the patients,

Text continued on page 1578

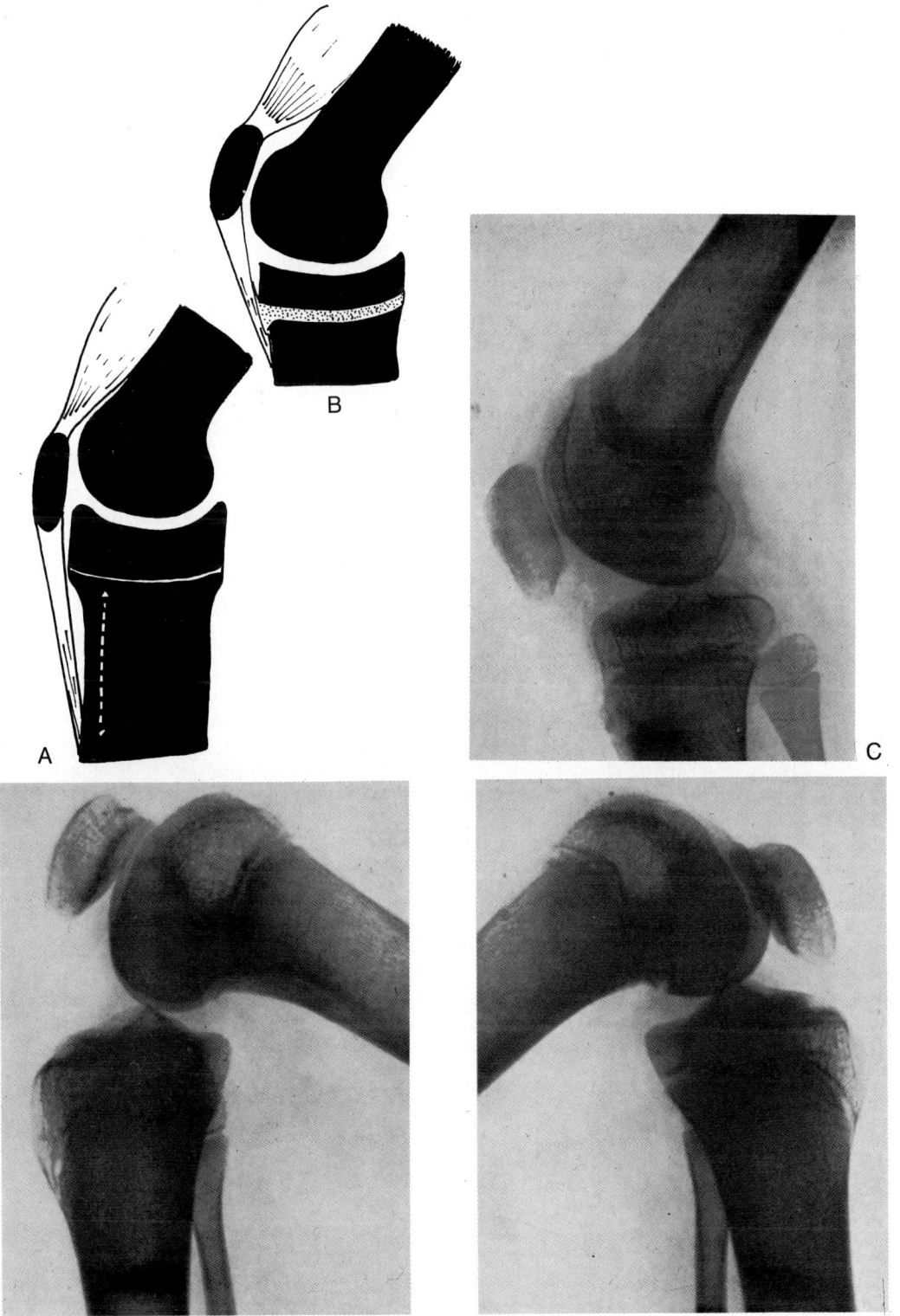

FIGURE 4–68. Migration of tibial tubercle when transferred during childhood.

A and **B**. Diagrammatic illustration. **C** to **E**. Radiograms depicting the distal migration of the right patella with the transferred tibial tubercle. **C** is immediately postoperative at age of nine years. **D** (right knee) and **E** (left knee) are radiograms taken three years later showing the distal migration of the transferred tubercle (its site is translucent) on the right, pulling the patella down with it. (From Macnab, I.: Recurrent dislocation of the patella. J. Bone Joint Surg., 34-A:964–965, 1952. Reprinted by permission.)

Semitendinosus Tenodesis for Recurrent Lateral Subluxation of Patellofemoral Joint

OPERATIVE TECHNIQUE

A. First, make a 4 to 5 cm. long longitudinal incision over the proximal aspect of the lower third of the thigh, centered over the course of the semitendinosus tendon. The fusiform muscle of the semitendinosus ends a little below in the middle of the thigh in a long, rounded tendon that lies on the external surface of the semimembranosus. Identify the semitendinosus tendon by palpation and flexion-extension of the knee. Subcutaneous tissue and fascia are divided in line with the skin incision. Caution! Do not injure the posterior femoral cutaneous nerve—in the back of the thigh it descends usually more laterally, medial to the biceps tendon.

B and **C.** The semitendinosus tendon is sectioned at its musculotendinous junction; its muscle belly is sutured to the semimembranosus.

D. Next identify and follow the distal stump of the semitendinosus tendon to its insertion. It curves around the medial condyle of the tibia superficial to the medial collateral ligament of the knee, from which it is separated by a bursa. Pull on the semitendinosus tendon and palpate its tendon at its insertion. Make a 3 to 4 cm. oblique skin incision along the course of the tendon below the knee joint over the anteromedial aspect of the upper leg. Caution! Do not injure the infrapatellar branch of the saphenous nerve.

E. The semitendinosus tendon is attached to the upper part of the medial surface of the tibia, posterior to the attachment of the sartorius and inferior to that of the gracilis. It is suprising how often the novice orthopedic resident has trouble identifying the semitendinosus tendon at its insertion. The semitendinosus tendon is delivered into the distal wound and left attached distally. If indicated, the synovium is incised and the interior of the knee joint is inspected. Determine the degree of chondromalacia—if marked or severe, shave the degenerated retropatellar articular cartilage. Inspect for possible loose bodies in the knee joint; if any is present, remove it.

Plate 56. Semitendinosus Tenodesis for Recurrent Lateral Subluxation of Patellofemoral Joint

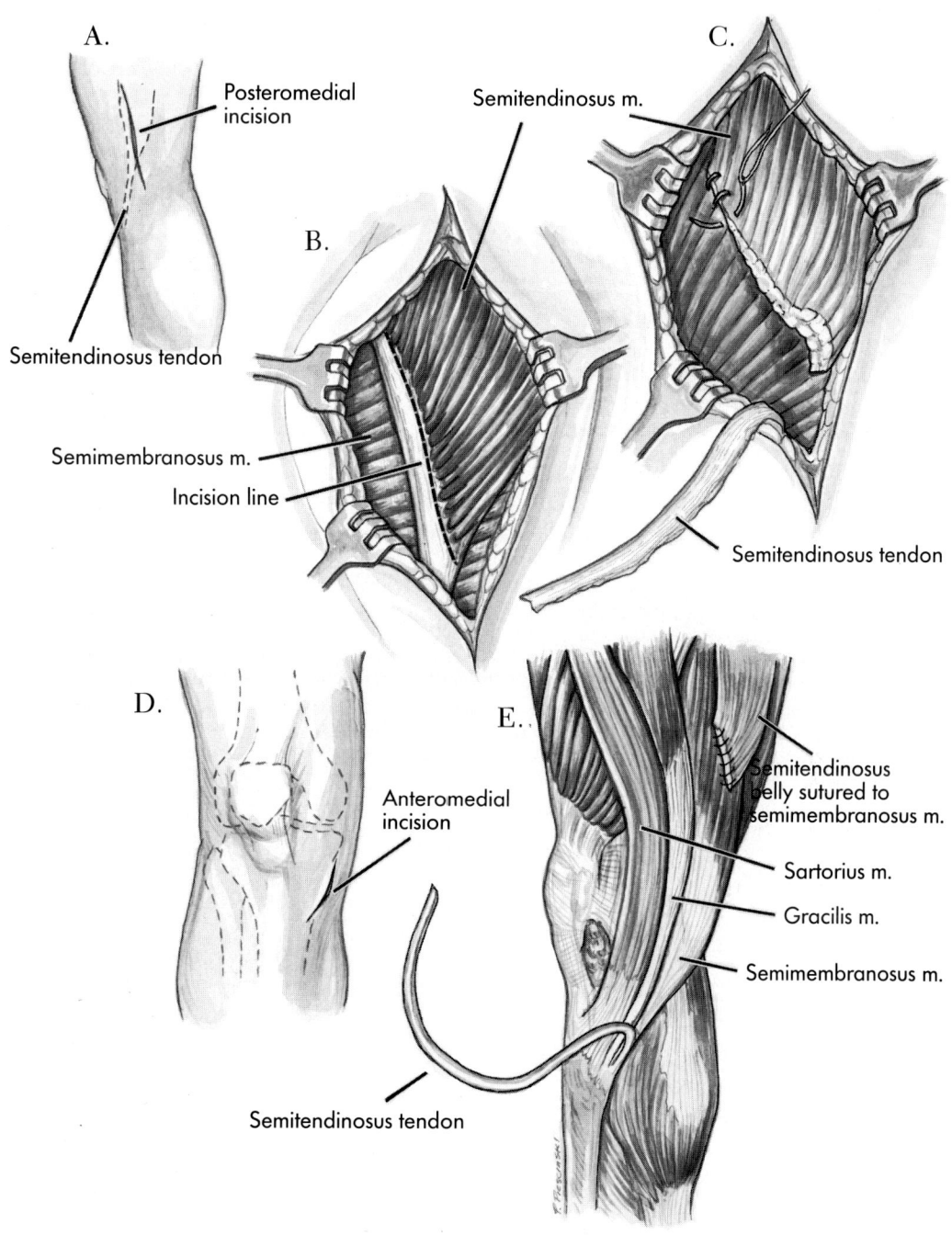

Semitendinosus Tenodesis for Recurrent Lateral Subluxation of Patellofemoral Joint *(Continued)*

F. Next, make a medial parapatellar incision beginning 4 to 5 cm. proximal and 3 cm. medial to the superior pole of the patella. Extend it distally to terminate 2 cm. distal to the knee joint line and 2 cm. medial to the patellar tendon. The subcutaneous tissue and superficial fascia are divided in line with the skin incision. Avoid injury to the infrapatellar branch of the saphenous nerve.

G. The lateral and medial skin flaps are dissected and mobilized, exposing the anterior surface of the patella, patellar tendon, medial and lateral patellar retinaculi, vastus medialis, rectus femoris, vastus lateralis, and joint capsule. The lateral patellar retinaculum is divided to mobilize the patella medially; if the lateral joint capsule is contracted, it is also sectioned.

H. Next, an oblique hole is drilled across the patella in the line of tenodesis. Do not damage the articular cartilage on the deep surface of the patella!

I. The semitendinosus tendon is passed through the hole in the patella from its medial to its lateral side.

Plate 56. Semitendinosus Tenodesis for Recurrent Lateral Subluxation of Patellofemoral Joint

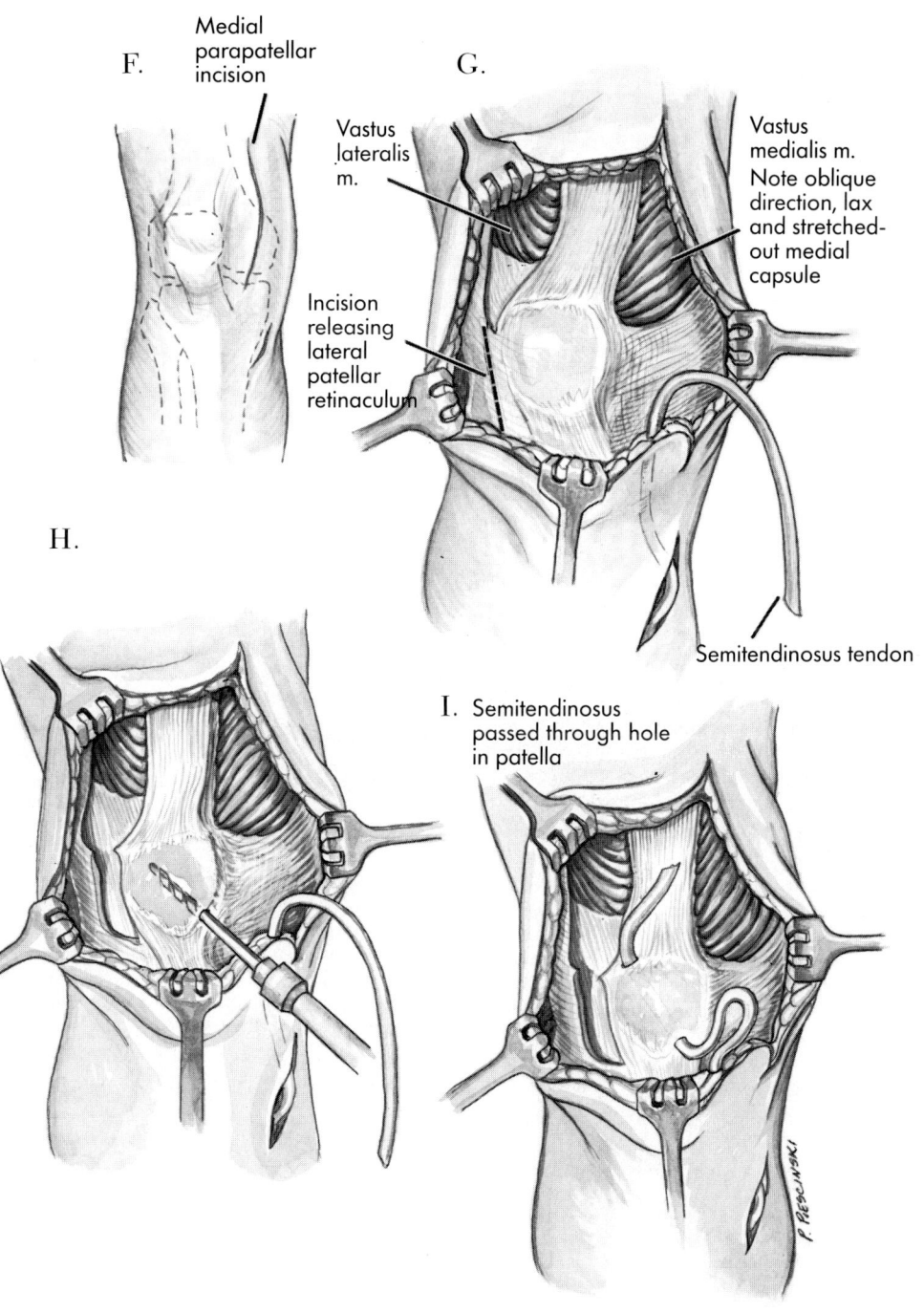

Semitendinosus Tenodesis for Recurrent Lateral Subluxation of Patellofemoral Joint (Continued)

J. The patella is pulled down medially and distally and, while held there, the semitendinosus tendon is sewn back to itself; thereby the pull of the quadriceps is directed in line with the intercondylar notch of the femur. The patellar insertion is a yoke of inverted U.

K. The semitendinosus patellar tenodesis is combined with plication of the medial capsule and medial patellar retinaculum and realignment of the quadriceps mechanism. The vastus lateralis is released, and the vastus medialis is advanced distally and laterally. The oblique course of vastus medialis is corrected to a transverse course. If the patellar tendon is slack, it is tautened by distal-medial transfer of its lateral half; the medial half of the patellar tendon is shortened by plication.

POSTOPERATIVE CARE

The knee is immobilized in an above-knee cylinder cast for four to six weeks. The patient is allowed to be ambulatory with crutches with a three-point partial weight-bearing gait. Isometric exercises of the quadriceps femoris and hamstrings are begun the day of surgery. At four to six weeks postoperatively, the cast is removed. This author admits the patient to the hospital for intensive physical therapy; active exercises (gravity eliminated and then against gravity) are performed to increase motor strength of the quadriceps femoris, hamstrings, and triceps surae. Side-lying active assisted knee flexion-extension exercises are performed to increase range of knee flexion. An above-knee orthosis is applied, holding the knee in extension and the patella in its relocated anatomic position. Initially the orthosis is worn day and night, except for exercise periods, and then its use is gradually decreased. When quadriceps femoris motor strength is normal and the knee has full range of motion, the use of the orthosis is discontinued. Running, jumping, and contact sports are not allowed for 6 to 12 months. The two failures that this author had were due to falls and injury in the immediate postoperative period. The importance of a meticulous physical therapy program to restoration of normal knee function cannot be overemphasized. Trauma to the knee should be avoided.

Plate 56. Semitendinosus Tenodesis for Recurrent Lateral Subluxation of Patellofemoral Joint

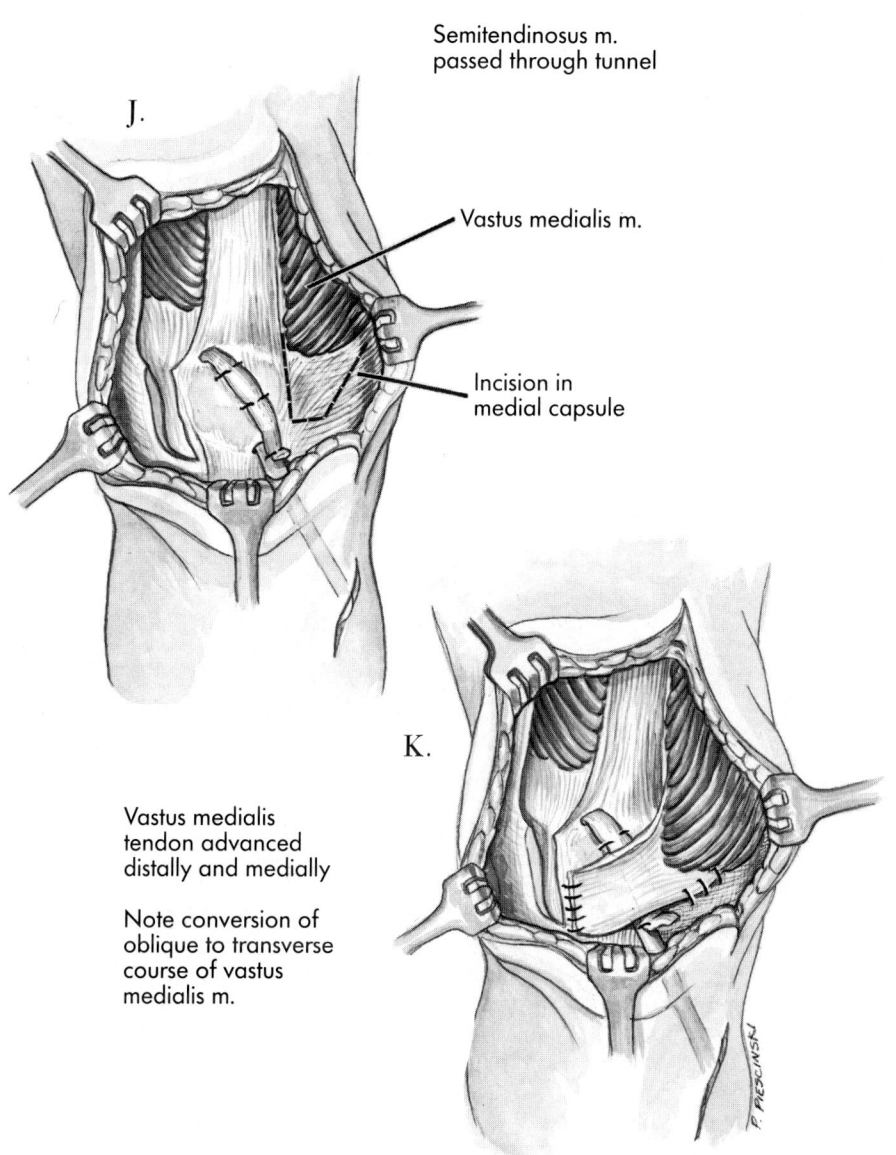

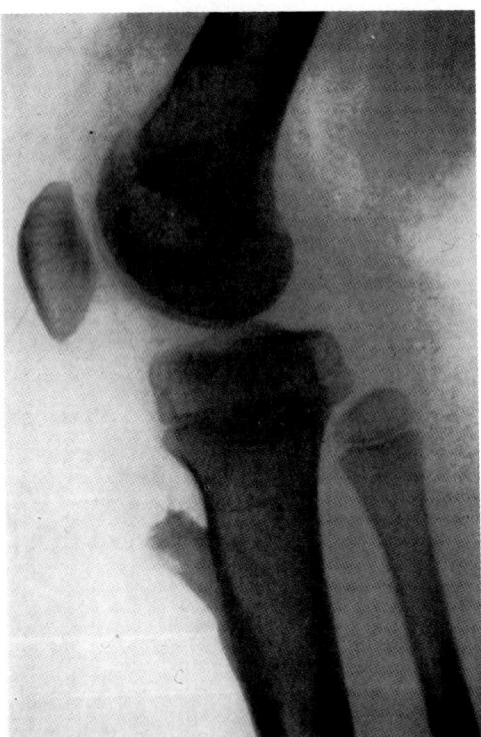

FIGURE 4–69. *Traction effect of the transplanted tubercle.*

It has been pulled out like a traction apophysis, forming a large mass of bone. (From Macnab, I.: Recurrent dislocation of the patella. J. Bone Joint Surg., 34-A:966, 1952. Reprinted by permission.)

above-knee amputation was subsequently required because of complete muscle necrosis. The anterior tibial recurrent vessels have numerous leash-like branches that terminate along the lateral border of the tibial tubercle. When these vessels are inadvertently divided they retract laterally and distally under the fascia and within the muscles of the anterior compartment. Continued postoperative hemorrhage from them results in an ischemic compartment syndrome in the leg.

Distal transfer of the patellar tendon may increase patellar compression. Crosby and Insall compared the long-term results of distal realignment by proximal tibial tubercle transfer with those of soft-tissue quadriceps realignment. The incidence of degenerative arthritis was disturbingly high after 69 tibial tubercle transfers, whereas in 12 soft-tissue proximal realignments there was not a single case of late degenerative arthritis.[31] It is evident that distal advancement of the patellar tendon may actually increase the incidence of osteoarthritis. This author strongly recommends caution in distal transfers of the proximal tibial tubercle; he has not performed the procedure during the past 20 years. It is best to lower the patella in its anatomic position and keep it there by tenodesis of the semitendinosus to the patella and to shorten the lax patellar tendon by imbrication.

Semitendinosus Tenodesis for Recurrent Lateral Subluxation of Patellofemoral Joint. *Indications* are when recurrent subluxation or dislocation of the patellofemoral joint is associated with a high-riding patella and when there is marked generalized ligamentous hyperlaxity, familial or as in Down's syndrome, Marfan's syndrome, or Ehler-Danlos syndrome. The operative technique is described and illustrated in Plate 56.

The results of the Galeazzi-Dewar procedure as reported in the literature are good.[4, 36, 64, 130] For success, however, it is vital *first* to realign the malaligned quadriceps femoris by adequate mobilization of the vastus lateralis, complete lateral release of the patellar retinaculum and capsule (if necessary), distal and lateral advancement of the vastus medialis, and plication of the medial capsule. *Second*, the semitendinosus tendon should be sutured under tension and anchored firmly to bone; and *third*, because the patellar tendon will become slack when the patella is lowered, it is important to tauten the lax tendon. Cosmesis of the operative scars is an important consideration; do not employ transverse or midline incisions, as they stretch and become wide and unsightly.

Postoperative peripatellar pain is due to persistence of chondromalacia. It is hoped that reestablishment of the correct anatomic relationship of the patella to the femoral condyles will arrest or sometimes reverse the degenerative process in the patellofemoral joint. When, at surgery, the degree of chondromalacia is marked or severe, it is wise to shave the patella.

Numbness in the distribution of the saphenous nerve is due to traction injury or inadvertent division of the nerve. Identify the saphenous nerve, particularly its infrapatellar branch, and protect it from iatrogenic injury. It is surprising how often a relatively minor, but so important, detail is ignored when making parapatellar incisions. If a resultant neuroma causes pain, further surgery is required; the neuroma is excised, and the saphenous nerve is repaired.

Treatment of Associated Chondromalacia. When chondromalacia of the patella is *mild*, simple realignment of the quadriceps is adequate to improve the symptoms. The chondromalacia will improve or show no progression.

When the chondromalacia is *moderate* or *severe* preliminary arthroscopy may be performed in order to determine whether arthroscopic surgery or arthrotomy during the realignment procedure is required for appropriate treatment of the chondromalacia. *Moderate chondromalacia* can be managed by arthroscopic shaving. *Severe* or incompletely shaved cases of moderate chondromalacia are best treated by a modified Maquet procedure—elevation of the proximal tibial tubercle will decompress the patellofemoral joint and relieve the symptoms.[47, 124, 125] The Maquet procedure should not be performed when the proximal tibial physis and apophysis are still open. In *severe degeneration of the patella* with osteoarthritis of the knee, excision of the patella may be required; this is considered with realignment of the quadriceps to prevent recurrent subluxation of the patellar tendon.

References

1. Albee, F. H.: The bone graft wedge in the treatment of habitual dislocation of the patella. Med. Rec., 88:257, 1915.
2. Albee, F. H.: Orthopedic and Reconstructive Surgery, Industrial and Civilian. Philadelphia, Saunders, 1919, p. 624.
3. Andersen, P. T.: Treatment of recurrent dislocation of the patella by the method of McCaroll and Schwartzmann. Acta Chir. Scand., 117:252, 1959.
4. Baker, R. H., Carroll, N., Dewar, F. P., and Hall, J. E.: The semitendinosus tenodesis for recurrent dislocation of the patella. J. Bone Joint Surg., 54-B:103, 1972.
5. Baksi, D. P.: Restoration of dynamic stability of the patella by pes anserinus transposition. A new approach. J. Bone Joint Surg., 63-B:399, 1981.
6. Bauer, F. C. H., Wredmark, T., and Isberg, B.: Krogius tenoplasty for recurrent dislocation of the patella. Failure associated with joint laxity. Acta Orthop. Scand., 55:267, 1984.
7. Bauer, W., and Bennett, G. A.: Joint changes resulting from patellar displacement and their relation to degenerative joint disease. J. Bone Joint Surg., 19:667, 1937.
8. Bentley, G.: Chondromalacia patella. J. Bone Joint Surg., 52-A:221, 1970.
9. Bevan, A. D.: Dislocation of patellae. Surg. Clin. North Am., 4:929, 1920.
10. Bigos, S. J., and McBride, G. G.: The isolated lateral retinacular release in the treatment of patellofemoral disorders. Clin. Orthop., 186:75, 1984.
11. Blazina, M. E., Fox, J. M., Carlson, G. J., and Jurgutis, J. J.: Patella baja. A technical consideration in evaluating results of tibial tubercle transplantation. J. Bone Joint Surg., 57-A:1027, 1975.
12. Blumensaat, C.: Die Lageabweichungen und Verrenkungen der Kniescheibe. Ergebn. Chir. Orthop., 31:147, 1938.
13. Bose, K.: Personal communication.
14. Bowker, H. H., and Thompson, E. B.: Surgical treatment of recurrent dislocation of the patella. A study of 48 cases. J. Bone Joint Surg., 46-A:1451, 1964.
15. Brattstrom, H.: Shape of the intercondylar groove normally and in recurrent dislocation of patella. A clinical and x-ray anatomical investigation. Acta Orthop. Scand., Suppl. 68, 1964.
16. Brown, D. E., Alexander, A. H., and Lichtman, D. M.: The Elmslie-Trillat procedure: Evaluation in patellar dislocation and subluxation. Am. J. Sports Med., 12:104, 1984.
17. Carter, G., and Sweetnam, R.: Familial joint laxity and recurrent dislocation of the patella. J. Bone Joint Surg., 40-B:664, 1958.
18. Carter, G., and Sweetnam, R.: Recurrent dislocation of the patella and of the shoulder. J. Bone Joint Surg., 42-B:721, 1960.
19. Casscells, S. W.: The arthroscope in the diagnosis of disorders of the patello-femoral joint. Clin. Orthop., 144:45, 1979.
20. Ceder, L. C., and Larson, R. L.: Z-plasty lateral retinacular release for the treatment of patellar compression syndrome. Clin. Orthop., 144:110, 1979.
21. Chen, C., Helal, B., King, J., and Roper, B. A.: Lateral retinacular release in chondromalacia patellae. Int. Rev. Rheumatol., 33:35, 1976.
22. Chen, S. C., and Ramanathan, E. B.: The treatment of patellar instability by lateral release. J. Bone Joint Surg., 66-B:344, 1984.
23. Chrisman, O. D., Snook, G. A., and Wilson, T. C.: A long-term prospective study of the Hauser and Roux-Goldwaite procedures for recurrent patellar dislocation. Clin. Orthop., 144:27, 1979.
24. Cofield, R. H., and Bryan, R. S.: Acute dislocations of the patella. Results of conservative treatment. J. Trauma, 17:526, 1977.
25. Cole, W. H., and Williamson, G. A.: Chronic recurrent dislocation of the patella. J.A.M.A., 102:357, 1934.
26. Coleman, H. M.: Recurrent osteochondral fracture of the patella. J. Bone Joint Surg., 30-B:153, 1948.
27. Conn, H. R.: A new method of operative reduction for congenital luxation of the patella. J. Bone Joint Surg., 7:370, 1925.
28. Cotta, H.: On therapy of habitual patellar luxation. Arch. Orthop. Unfallchir., 51:265, 1959.
29. Cox, J. S.: An evaluation of the Elmslie-Trillat procedure for management of patellar dislocations and subluxations: Preliminary report. Am. J. Sports Med., 4:72, 1976.
30. Cox, J. S.: Evaluation of the Roux-Elmslie-Trillat procedure for knee extensor realignment. Am. J. Sports Med., 10:303, 1982.
31. Crosby, E. B., and Insall, J.: Recurrent dislocation of the patella. Relation of treatment to osteoarthritis. J. Bone Joint Surg., 58-A:9, 1976.
32. Davis, C. B.: Recurrent dislocation of the patella. Surg. Clin. North Am., 3:291, 1919.
33. DeCesare, W. F.: Late results of Hauser procedure for recurrent dislocation of the patella. Clin. Orthop., 140:137, 1979.
34. Delgado-Martins, H.: A study of the position of the patella using computerized tomography. J. Bone Joint Surg., 61-B:443, 1976.
35. DePalma, A. F.: Diseases of the Knee. Philadelphia, Lippincott, 1954.
36. Dewar, F. P., and Hall, J. E.: Recurrent dislocation of the patella. J. Bone Joint Surg., 39-B:798, 1957.
37. Dickson, J. A.: Recurrent dislocation of the patella. Surg. Clin. N. Amer., 16:997, 1936.
38. Dimon, J. H., III: Apprehension test for subluxation of the patella. Clin. Orthop., 103:39, 1974.
39. Dougherty, J., Wirth, C. R., and Akbarnia, B. A.: Management of patellar subluxation. A modification of Hauser's technique. Clin. Orthop., 115:204, 1976.
40. Dowd, G. S. E., and Bentley, G.: Radiographic assessment in patellar instability and chondromalacia patellae. J. Bone Joint Surg., 68-B:297, 1986.

41. Dugdale, T. W., and Renshaw, T. S.: Instability of the patellofemoral joint in Down's syndrome. J. Bone Joint Surg., 68-A:405, 1986.
42. Ficat, P., Ficat, C., and Bailleux, A.: Syndrome d'hyperpression extrême de la rotula (SHPE). Son intérêt pour la connaissance de l'arthrose. Rev. Chir. Orthop., 61:39, 1975.
43. Ficat, R. P., and Hungerford, D. S.: Disorders of the Patellofemoral Joint. Baltimore, Williams & Wilkins, 1977.
44. Fielding, J. W., Liebler, W. A., Urs, D., Wilson, S. A., and Publisi, A.: Tibial tubercle transfer. A long range follow-up study. Clin. Orthop., 144:43, 1979.
45. Finsterbush, A.: Rotation knee strain resulting in patellar dislocation. An experimental study in rabbits. Clin. Orthop., 169:259, 1982.
46. Fiume, M.: La rotulopessi secondo Galeazzi nella lussazione recidivante di rotula. Minerva Ortop., 5:171, 1954.
47. Fondren, F. B., Goldner, J. L., and Bassett, F. H., III: Recurrent dislocation of the patella treated by the modified Roux-Goldthwait procedure. A prospective study of forty-seven knees. J. Bone Joint surg., 67-A:993, 1985.
48. Fox, T. A.: Dysplasia of the quadriceps mechanism: Hypoplasia of the vastus medialis muscle as related to the hypermobile patella syndrome. Surg. Clin. North Am., 55:199, 1975.
49. Fulkerson, J. P.: The etiology of patellofemoral pain in young, active patients. A prospective study. Clin. Orthop., 179:129, 1983.
50. Fulkerson, J. P., and Gossling, H. R.: Anatomy of the knee joint lateral retinacular. Clin. Orthop., 153:183, 1980.
51. Galeazzi, R.: Nouve applicazioni del trapianto muscolare e tendineo. Arch. Ortop., 38:1922, 1921.
52. Gallie, W. E., and LeMesurier, A. B.: Habitual dislocation of the patella. J. Bone Joint Surg., 6:575, 1924.
53. Garnier, C.: Les luxations de la rotule en dehors des luxations traumatiques récentes. Rev. Orthop., 36:444, 1950.
54. Goldthwait, J. E.: Dislocation of the patella. Trans. Am. Orthop. Assoc., 8:237, 1895.
55. Goldthwait, J. E.: Permanent dislocation of the patella. The report of a case of twenty year's duration, successfully treated by transplantation of the patellar tendon, with the tubercle of the tibia. Ann. Surg., 29:62, 1899.
56. Goldthwait, J. E.: Slipping or recurrent dislocation of the patella: With the report of eleven cases. Boston Med. Surg. J., 150:169, 1904.
57. Goodfellow, J. W., Hungerford, D. S., and Zindel, M.: Patello-femoral mechanics and pathology. I. Functional anatomy of the patello-femoral joint. J. Bone Joint Surg., 58-B:287, 1976.
58. Goutallier, D., Bernageau, J., and Lecodunnec, B.: The measurement of the tibial tuberosity. Patella groove distanced technique and results. Rev. Chir. Orthop., 64:423, 1978.
59. Goymann, V., and Buck, F.: Operative treatment of recurrent dislocation of the patella by Bruckner. Z. Orthop., 114:64, 1975.
60. Grana, W. A., and O'Donoghue, D. H.: Patellar-tendon transfer by the slot-block method for recurrent subluxation and dislocation of the patella. J. Bone Joint Surg., 59:736, 1977.
61. Grana, W. A., Hinkley, B., and Hollingsworth, S.: Arthroscopic evaluation and treatment of patellar malalignment. Clin. Orthop., 186:122, 1984.
62. Green, W. T.: Recurrent dislocation of the patella. Its surgical correction in the growing child. J. Bone Joint Surg., 47-A:1670, 1965.
63. Grimes, H. A.: Subluxating and luxating patellae. J. Arkansas Med. Soc., 72:173, 1975.
64. Hall, J. E., Micheli, L. J., and McNamara, G. B., Jr.: Semitendinosus tenodesis for recurrent subluxation or dislocation of the patella. Clin. Orthop., 144:31, 1979.
65. Hallisey, M. J., Doherty, N., Bennett, W. F., and Fulkerson, J. P.: Anatomy of the junction of the vastus lateralis tendon and the patella. J. Bone Joint Surg., 69-A:545, 1987.
66. Hampson, W. G. J., and Hill, P.: Late results of transfer of the tibial tubercle for recurrent dislocation of the patella. J. Bone Joint Surg., 57-B:209, 1975.
67. Harrison, M. H. M.: The results of realignment operation for recurrent dislocation of the patella. J. Bone Joint Surg., 37-B:559, 1955.
68. Harrison, M. H. M.: The results of a realignment operation for recurrent dislocation of the patella. Clin. Orthop., 18:96, 1960.
69. Harwin, S. F., and Stern, R. E.: Subcutaneous lateral retinacular release for chondromalacia patellae. A preliminary report. Clin. Orthop., 156:207, 1981.
70. Hauser, E. D. W.: Total tendon transplant for slipping patella, a new operation for recurrent dislocation of the patella. Surg. Gynecol. Obstet., 66:199, 1938.
71. Hejgaard, N., Skive, L., and Perrild, C.: Recurrent dislocation of the patella. Treatment by a modification of the method of McCarroll and Schwartzmann. Acta Orthop. Scand., 511:673, 1980.
72. Henche, H. R.: Recurrent dislocation of the patella and prearthrosis of the patello-femoral joint. Z. Orthop., 111:523, 1973.
73. Henry, J. H., and Craven, P. R.: Surgical treatment of patellar instability: Indications and results. Am. J. Sports Med., 9:82, 1981.
74. Henry, J. H., and Crosland, J. W.: Conservative treatment of patellofemoral subluxation. Am. J. Sports Med., 7:12, 1979.
75. Heywood, A. W. B.: Recurrent dislocation of the patella. A study of its pathology and treatment in 106 knees. J. Bone Joint Surg., 43-B:508, 1961.
76. Hinze, M.: Surgery of the recurrent and habitual patella luxation using Bruckner's method. Beitr. Orthop. Traumatol., 18:51, 1971.
77. Hochheim, B.: Clinical results following surgically managed habitual and recurrent patella luxations. Beitr. Orthop. Traumatol., 25:299, 1978.
78. Hoffa, A.: Zur Behandlung der habituellen patellar Luxation. Arch. Klin. Chir., 59:543, 1899.
79. Horwitz, M. T.: Recurrent or habitual dislocation of the patella. A critical analysis of twenty cases. J. Bone Joint Surg., 19:1027, 1937.
80. Huebscher, C.: Ueber Operationen bei habituellen Luxation der Kniescheibe. Z. Orthop. Chir., 24:1, 1909.
81. Hughston, J. C.: Subluxation of the patella. J. Bone Joint Surg., 50-A:1003, 1968.
82. Hughston, J. C.: Reconstruction of the extensor mechanism for subluxating patella. J. Sports Med., 1:6, 1972.
83. Hughston, J. C., and Stone, M. M.: Recurring dislocations of the patella in athletes. South. Med. J., 57:623, 1964.
84. Hungerford, D. S., and Barry, M.: Biomechanics of the patellofemoral joint. Clin. Orthop., 144:9, 1979.
85. Hvid, I., and Andersen, L. I.: The quadriceps angle and its relation to femoral torsion. Acta Orthop. Scand., 53:577, 1982.
86. Insall, J., and Salvati, E.: Patella position in the normal knee joint. Radiology, 101:101, 1971.
87. Insall, J., Bullough, P. G., and Burstein, A. H.: Proximal "tube" realignment of the patella for chondromalacia patellae. Clin. Orthop., 144:63, 1979.
88. Insall, J., Falvo, K. A., and Wise, D. W.: Chondromalacia patellae. A prospective study. J. Bone Joint Surg., 58-A:1, 1976.

89. Insall, J., Goldberg, V., and Salvati, E.: Recurrent dislocation and the high-riding patella. Clin. Orthop., 88:67, 1972.
90. Jackson, R. W.: Etiology of chondromalacia patella. A.A.O.A. Instr. Course Lect., 25:39, 1976.
91. Jacobsen, K., and Bertheussen, K.: The vertical location of patella. Fundamental views on the concept patella alta, using a normal sample. Acta Orthop. Scand., 45:436, 1974.
92. Jeffreys, T. E.: Recurrent dislocation of the patella due to abnormal attachment of the ilio-tibial tract. J. Bone Joint Surg., 45-B:7401, 1963.
93. Jones, J. B., Francis, K. C., and Mahoney, J. R.: Recurrent dislocating patella—a long-term follow-up study. Clin. Orthop., 20:230, 1961.
94. Juliusson, R., and Markhede, G.: A modified Hauser procedure for recurrent dislocation of the patella. A long-term follow-up story with special reference to osteoarthritis. Arch. Orthop. Trauma Surg., 103:42, 1984.
95. Kapel, O.: The operative treatment of recurrent and chronic dislocation of the patella with special reference to the operations of Krogius and Goldthwait. Acta Chir. Scand., 77:201, 1935.
96. Katauka, O.: Surgery of habitual dislocation of the patella. Shujutsu, 25:473, 1971.
97. Kettlekamp, D. B.: Management of patellar malalignment. J. Bone Joint Surg., 63-A:1344, 1981.
98. Kettlekamp, D. B., and DeRosa, G. P.: Surgery of the patellofemoral joint. A.A.O.S. Instr. Course Lect., 25:27, 1976.
99. Khastigian, H. A., Evanski, P. M., and Waugh, T. R.: Body type and rotational laxity of the knee. Clin. Orthop., 130:228, 1978.
100. Kimberlin, G. E.: Radiological assessment of the patellofemoral articulation and subluxation of the patella. Radiol. Technol., 45:129, 1973.
101. Krogius, A.: Zur Operative Behandlung der habituellen Luxation der Kniescheibe. Zentralbl. Chir., 31:254, 1904.
102. Krompinger, W. J., and Fulkerson, J. P.: Lateral retinacular release for intractable lateral retinacular pain. Clin. Orthop., 179:191, 1983.
103. Kummel, B.: Tibiofemoral incongruity in association with patellar instability. Clin. Orthop., 155:97, 1981.
104. Kummel, B., and Crutchlow, W. P.: Stabilization of the subluxating patella by semitendinous transfer to the lateral third of the infrapatellar tendon. Am. J. Sports Med., 5:194, 1977.
105. Labelle, H., Peides, J. P., Levesque, H. P., Fauteux, P., and Laurin, C. A.: Evaluation of patellar position by tangential x-ray visualization. Union Med. Can., 105:870, 1976.
106. Lancourt, J. E., and Christini, J. A.: Patella alta and patella infera—their etiological role in patellar dislocation, chondromalacia and apophysitis of the tibial tubercle. J. Bone Joint Surg., 57-A:1112, 1975.
107. Larsen, E., and Lauridsen, F.: Conservative treatment of patellar dislocations. Influence of evident factors on the tendency to redislocation and the therapeutic results. Clin. Orthop., 171:131, 1982.
108. Larson, R. L., Cabaud, H. E., Slocum, D. B., James, S. L., Keenan, T., and Hutchinson, T.: The patellar compression syndrome: Surgical treatment by lateral release. Clin. Orthop., 134:158, 1978.
109. Laurin, C. A., Levesque, H. P., Dussault, R., Labelle, H., and Peides, J. P.: The abnormal lateral patellofemoral angle: A diagnostic roentgenographic sign of recurrent patellar subluxation. J. Bone Joint Surg., 60-A:55, 1978.
110. Leach, R. E.: Malalignment syndromes of the patella. A.A.O.S. Instr. Course Lect., 25:49, 1976.
111. Lieb, F. J., and Perry, J.: Quadriceps function: An electromyographic study under isometric conditions. J. Bone Joint Surg., 53-A:749, 1971.
112. MacAusland, W. R., and Sargent, A. F.: Recurrent dislocation of the patella. With reports of sixteen cases. Surg. Gynecol. Obstet., 35:35, 1922.
113. McCall, R. E., and Gavioli, R. L.: Patellar malalignment syndrome. South. Med. J., 74:1056, 1981.
114. McCarroll, H. R., and Schwartzmann, J. R.: Lateral dislocation of the patella, correction by simultaneous transplantation of the tibial tubercle and semitendinosus tendon. J. Bone Joint Surg., 27:446, 1945.
115. McFarland, B.: Excision of patella for recurrent dislocation. J. Bone Joint Surg., 30-B:158, 1948.
116. McGinty, J. B., and McCarthy, J. C.: Endoscopic lateral retinacular release. A preliminary report. Clin. Orthop., 158:120, 1981.
117. McKeever, D. C.: Transplantation of the tibial tubercle. J. Bone Joint Surg., 33-A:478, 1951.
118. McKeever, D. C.: Recurrent dislocation of the patella. Clin. Orthop., 3:55, 1954.
119. McManus, F., Rang, M., and Heslin, D. J.: Acute dislocation of the patella in children. The natural history. Clin. Orthop., 139:88, 1976.
120. Macnab, I.: Recurrent dislocation of the patella. J. Bone Joint Surg., 34-A:957, 1952.
121. Madigan, R., Wissinger, H. A., and Donaldson, W. F.: Preliminary experience with a method of quadricepsplasty in recurrent subluxation of the patella. J. Bone Joint Surg., 57-A:600, 1975.
122. Makin, M.: Osteochondral fracture of the lateral femoral condyle. J. Bone Joint Surg., 33-A:262, 1951.
123. Malgaigne, J. F.: Mémoire des déterminations des diverses espèces de luxations de la rotule, leurs signes, et leur traitement. Gaz. Méd. Paris, 1836.
124. Maquet, P. G. J.: Biomechanics of the Knee. New York, Springer, 1976, p. 137.
125. Maquet, P.: Mechanics and osteoarthritis of the patellofemoral joint. Clin. Orthop., 144:70, 1979.
126. Mariani, P. P., and Caruso, I.: An electromyographic investigation of subluxation of the patella. J. Bone Joint Surg., 61-B:169, 1979.
127. Marion, J., and Barcat, J.: Les luxations de la rotule en dehors des luxations traumatiques récentes. Rev. Chir. Orthop., 36:181, 1950.
128. Martinez, S., Korobkin, M., Fondren, F. B., and Goldner, J. L.: A device for computed tomography of the patellofemoral joint. A.J.R., 140:400, 1983.
129. Martinez, S., Korobkin, M., Fondren, F. B., Hedlund, L. W., and Goldner, J. L.: Diagnosis of patellofemoral malalignment by computed tomography. J. Comput. Assist. Tomogr., 7:1050, 1983.
130. Marziani, R.: Sulla lussazione della rotula e sul suo trattamento operativo. Arch. Ortop., 46:797, 1930.
131. Merle d'Aubigne, R.: Les luxations de la rotule en dehors des luxations traumatiques récentes. Rev. Orthop., 36:437, 1950.
132. Merchant, A. C., and Mercer, R. L.: Lateral release of the patella. A preliminary report. Clin. Orthop., 103:40, 1974.
133. Merchant, A. C., Mercer, R. L., Jacobsen, R. H., and Cool, C. R.: Roentgenographic analysis of patellofemoral congruence. J. Bone Joint Surg., 56-A:1391, 1974.
134. Metcalf, R. W.: An arthroscopic method for lateral release of subluxating or dislocating patella. Clin. Orthop., 167:9, 1982.
135. Micheli, L. J., and Stanitski, C. L.: Lateral patellar retinacular release. Am. J. Sports Med., 9:330, 1981.
136. Milgram, J. E.: Tangential osteochondral fracture of the patella. J. Bone Joint Surg., 25:271, 1943.
137. Miller, G. F.: Familial recurrent dislocation of the patella. J. Bone Joint Surg., 60-B:203, 1978.
138. Moore, B. H.: A case of hereditary recurrent dislocation of the patella. J. Bone Joint Surg., 12:654, 1930.
139. Nagayama, Y., and Hasegawa, O.: Therapeutic expe-

rience in habitual dislocation of the patella with special reference to postoperative x-ray findings. Orthop. Surg., (Tokyo), 21:533, 1970.
140. Norman, O., Egund, N., Ekelund, L., and Runow, A.: The vertical position of the patella. Acta Orthop. Scand., 54:908, 1983.
141. Ober, F. R.: Slipping patella or recurrent dislocation of the patella. J. Bone Joint Surg., 17:774, 1935.
142. Ober, F. R.: Recurrent dislocation of the patella. Am. J. Surg., 43:497, 1939.
143. Outerbridge, R. E.: The etiology of chondromalacia patellae. J. Bone Joint Surg., 43-B:752, 1961.
144. Outerbridge, R. E., and Dunlop, J. A.: The problem of chondromalacia patellae. Clin. Orthop., 110:177, 1975.
145. Provenzano, K. W.: Congenital dislocation of the knee. N. Engl. J. Med., 236:360, 1947.
146. Rauschning, W., and Amici, F., Jr.: Surgical treatment of recurrent subluxation of the patella in athletes. Ital. J. Orthop. Traumatol., 8:167, 1982.
147. Reider, B., Marshall, J. L., and Ring, B.: Patellar tracking. Clin. Orthop., 157:143, 1981.
148. Reider, B., Marshall, J. L., and Warren, R. F.: Clinical characteristics of patellar disorders in athletes. Am. J. Sports Med., 9:270, 1981.
149. Roux: Luxation habituelle de la rotule. Rev. Chir., 8:682, 1888.
150. Roux, C.: The classic. Recurrent dislocation of the patella: Operative treatment. Clin. Orthop., 144:4, 1979.
151. Runow, A.: The dislocating patella. Etiology and prognosis in relation to generalized joint laxity and anatomy of the patellar articulation. Acta Orthop. Scand. (Suppl.), 202:1, 1983.
152. Rutt, A.: Various forms of patella dislocation and their pathological mechanisms. Z. Orthop., 110:235, 1972.
153. Sarkar, S. D.: Central dislocations of the patella. J. Trauma, 21:409, 1981.
154. Savastano, A. A., and Cronin, R. J.: Recurrent subluxation of the patella. Int. Surg., 60:25, 1975.
155. Scheller, S., and Martenson, L.: Traumatic dislocation of the patella. A radiographic investigation. Acta Radiol., (Suppl.) 306, 1974.
156. Schneider, D.: Arthroscopy and arthroscopic surgery in patellar problems. Orthop. Clin. North Am., 13:407, 1982.
157. Seedorff, K.: Habitual dislocation of the patella treated operatively ad modum Goldthwait. Acta Orthop. Scand., 16:203, 1946.
158. Slocum, B., Slocum, D. B., Devine, T., and Boone, E.: Wedge resection for treatment of recurrent luxation of the patella: A preliminary report. Clin. Orthop., 164:48, 1982.
159. Smillie, I. S.: Ligamentous injury and subluxation of the patella. J. Bone Joint Surg., 41-B:214, 1959.
160. Southwick, W. O., Becker, G. E., and Albright, J. A.: Dovetail patellar tendon transfer for recurrent dislocating patella. J.A.M.A., 203:665, 1968.
161. Soutter, R.: A new operation for slipping patella. J.A.M.A., 82:1261, 1924.
162. Soutter, R.: A new operation for slipping patella. N. Engl. J. Med., 209:59, 1933.
163. Teal, F.: Treatment of dislocation of the patella. Clin. Orthop., 3:61, 1954.
164. Thompson, F. R., and Bosworth, D. M.: Recurrent dislocations of the patella. Am. J. Surg., 73:335, 1947.
165. Trillat, A., DeJour, J., and Louette, A.: Diagnostic et traitement des subluxations récidiventes de la rotula. Rev. Chir. Orthop., 50:813, 1964.
166. Turba, J. E., Walsh, W. M., and McLeod, W. D.: Long term results of extensor mechanism reconstruction. A standard for evaluation. Am. J. Sports Med., 7:91, 1979.
167. Venker VanHaagen, A. J.: Transplantation of the tibial crest in the surgical correction of dislocation of the patella in dogs. Tijdschr. Diergeneeskd., 100:251, 1975.
168. Villiger, K. J.: Modified bridle-plasty in recurrent luxation of the patella. Chirurg, 49:223, 1978.
169. Wagner, L. C.: A plastic operation for relief of recurrent slippings and dislocation of the patella. J. Bone Joint Surg., 14:332, 1932.
170. Wall, J. J.: Compartment syndrome as a complication of the Hauser procedure. J. Bone Joint Surg., 61-A:185, 1979.
171. Walmsley, R.: Development of patella. J. Anat., 74:360, 1940.
172. West, F. E., and Soto-Hall, R.: Recurrent dislocation of the patella in the adult. End results of patellectomy with quadricepsplasty. J. Bone Joint Surg., 40-A:386, 1958.
173. Wiberg, G.: Roentgenographic and anatomic studies on the femoropatellar joint. Acta Orthop. Scand., 12:319, 1941.
174. Wiles, P., and Bremer, R. A.: Chondromalacia of the patella. J. Bone Joint Surg., 42-B:65, 1960.
175. Wiles, P., and Devas, M. B.: Chondromalacia of the patella. J. Bone Joint Surg., 38-B:95, 1956.
176. Williams, P. F.: Quadriceps contracture. J. Bone Joint Surg., 50-B:278, 1968.
177. Willner, P.: Recurrent dislocation of the patella. Clin. Orthop., 69:213, 1970.
178. Wilson, J. C.: Silk ligament in habitual dislocation or slipping of the patella. Am. J. Surg., 39:144, 1925.
179. Zimbler, S., Smith, J., Scheller, A., and Banks, H. H.: Recurrent subluxation and dislocation of the patella in association with athletic injuries. Orthop. Clin. North Am., 11:755, 1980.

POPLITEAL CYST

Popliteal cyst is a soft-tissue swelling in the posterior aspect of the knee that has become distended with gelatinous fluid and transilluminates. It is commonly located on the medial side just distal to the popliteal crease under the medial head of the gastrocnemius. Tumorous lesions in the popliteal region of the knee in association with chronic rheumatic arthritis were reported by Adams in 1840.[2] Fouchet, in 1856, when he described the pathology of popliteal cysts, believed them to be bursae distended with fluid as a result of chronic irritation.[18] Baker, in 1887, however, proposed that these swellings represented herniations of the knee joint space.[3] The condition is referred to in the literature as gastrocnemio-semimembranosus bursae, semimembranosus bursae, synovial cysts, posterior herniae of the knee joint, and commonly by the eponym *Baker's cyst*. Burleson, Bickel, and Dahlin prefer the term *popliteal cyst*, since regardless of where they originate, these lesions behave alike clinically and pathologically, and have the same indications for treatment.[8]

The condition is not infrequent in children, being twice as common in boys as in girls. It is most often unilateral.

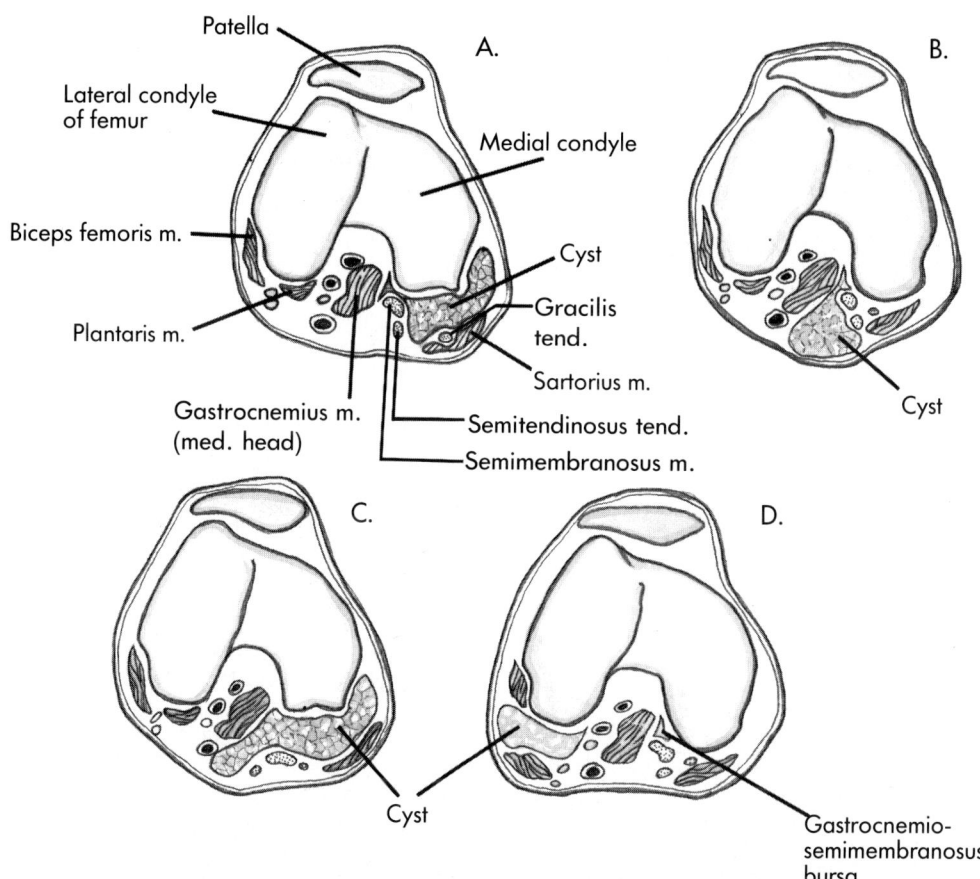

FIGURE 4–70. Cross sections of the knee illustrating gastrocnemius-semimembranosus bursa and popliteal cyst.

A. Semimembranosus bursa cyst. **B.** Gastrocnemius bursa cyst. **C.** Gastrocnemio-semimembranosus bursa cyst. **D.** Atypical popliteal cyst and normal gastrocnemius-semimembranosus bursa. (Redrawn after Lee, K. R., Tines, S. C., Price, H. I., Batnitzky, S., and Dwyer, S. J. 3rd.: The computed tomographic findings of popliteal cysts. Skeletal Radiol. 10:26, 1983.)

Pathologic Findings

The cysts may be either bursal or hernial in origin.[8, 39] The gastrocnemius-semimembranosus bursa is the most common site of their formation (Fig. 4–70). Proximally the gastrocnemius-semimembranosus bursa extends around the inner border of the origin of the medial head of the gastrocnemius, partially covering the muscle superficially; it extends transversely over the deep surfaces of the gastrocnemius and semimembranosus muscles and then reflects onto the articular capsule over the upper part of the medial condyle of the femur.[59] Sometimes popliteal cysts arise in the semimembranosus bursa or in the bursa deep to the medial head of the gastrocnemius. Rarely they are laterally located. Occasionally a cyst may extend into the calf of the leg.

Burleson, Bickel, and Dahlin described the operative findings in 83 popliteal cysts that were totally excised in 82 patients.[8] About 55 per cent of these cysts seemed to arise from bursae, 31 per cent from herniae, and 13 per cent from indeterminate sites. The hernial cysts protruded abnormally through the posterior capsule of the knee, and frequently they were medial in location, sometimes midline, and very occasionally laterally situated. In about two thirds of the cases, the cyst communicated with the knee joint.

Histopathologically, the cysts may be described as *fibrous, synovial, inflammatory*, or *transitional*. Such classifications are arbitrary, since the evidence indicates that these are basically variations of the same type. The *fibrous cysts* have a well-outlined limiting wall, which has a smooth-to-glistening inner surface and consists of fibrous tissue that is largely hyalinized. Rice bodies may be found near the surface lining (Fig. 4–71 A). The synovial cysts have a thicker wall (2 to 5 mm.), which is less

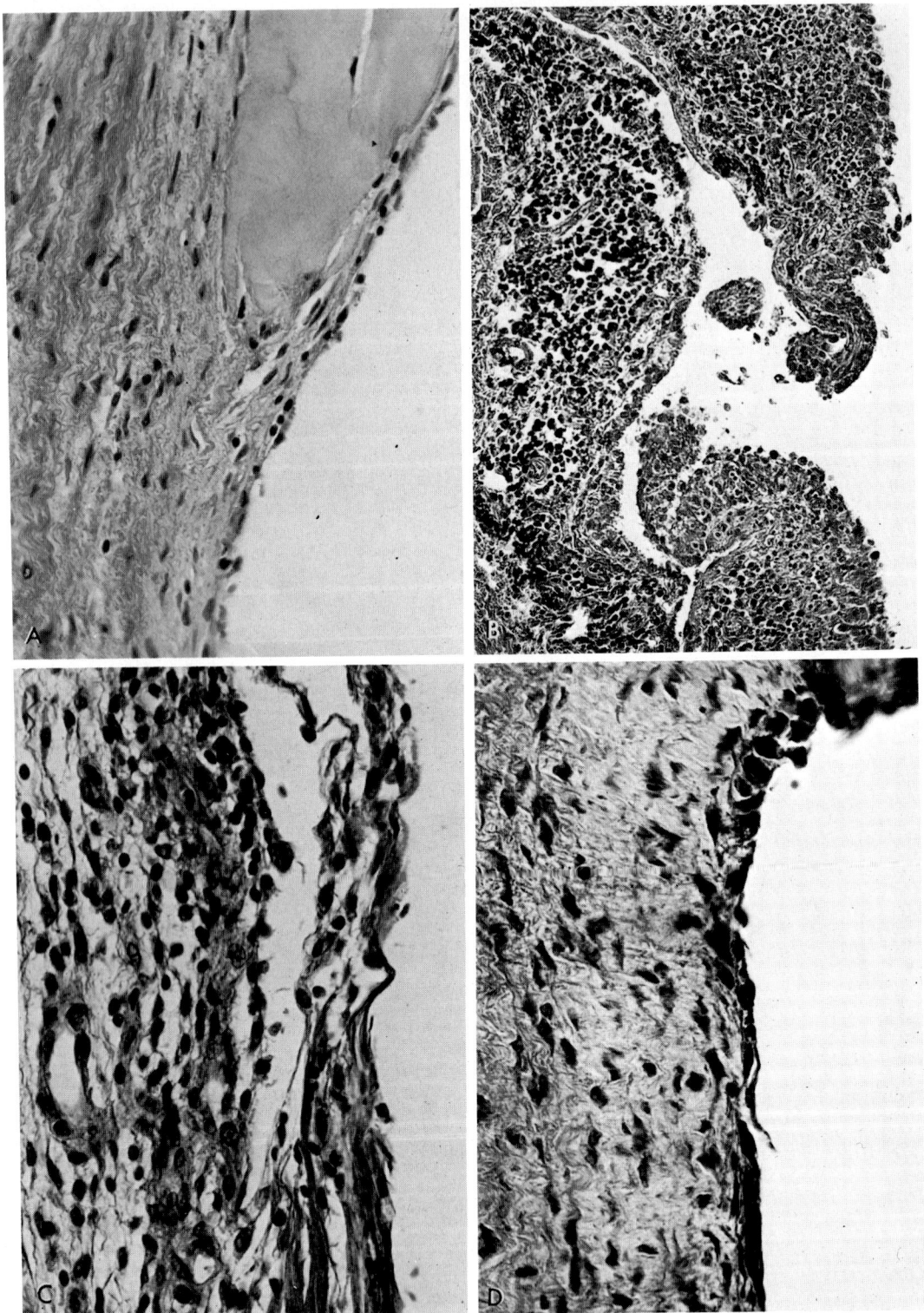

FIGURE 4–71. The four histopathologic types of popliteal cyst.

A. *Fibrous cyst.* The lining wall (1 to 2 mm. thick) consists of fibrous tissue that is largely hyalinized with flattened cells on its innermost surface. Note that hyalinized rice body is present (hematoxylin and eosin, × 300). **B.** *Synovial cyst.* The lining is thicker, with synovium-like cells and villous formation. Note the round-cell infiltration (hematoxylin and eosin, × 140). **C.** *Inflammatory cyst.* Note the fibrinous surface and infiltration with histiocytes, plasma cells, and lymphocytes (hematoxylin and eosin, × 400). **D.** *Transitional cyst.* The lining cells are synovium-like near the top and fibroblastic below. (From Burleson, R. J., Bickel, W. H., and Dahlin, D. C.: Popliteal cyst. A clinicopathological survey. J. Bone Joint Surg., 38-A:1265, 1956. Reprinted by permission.)

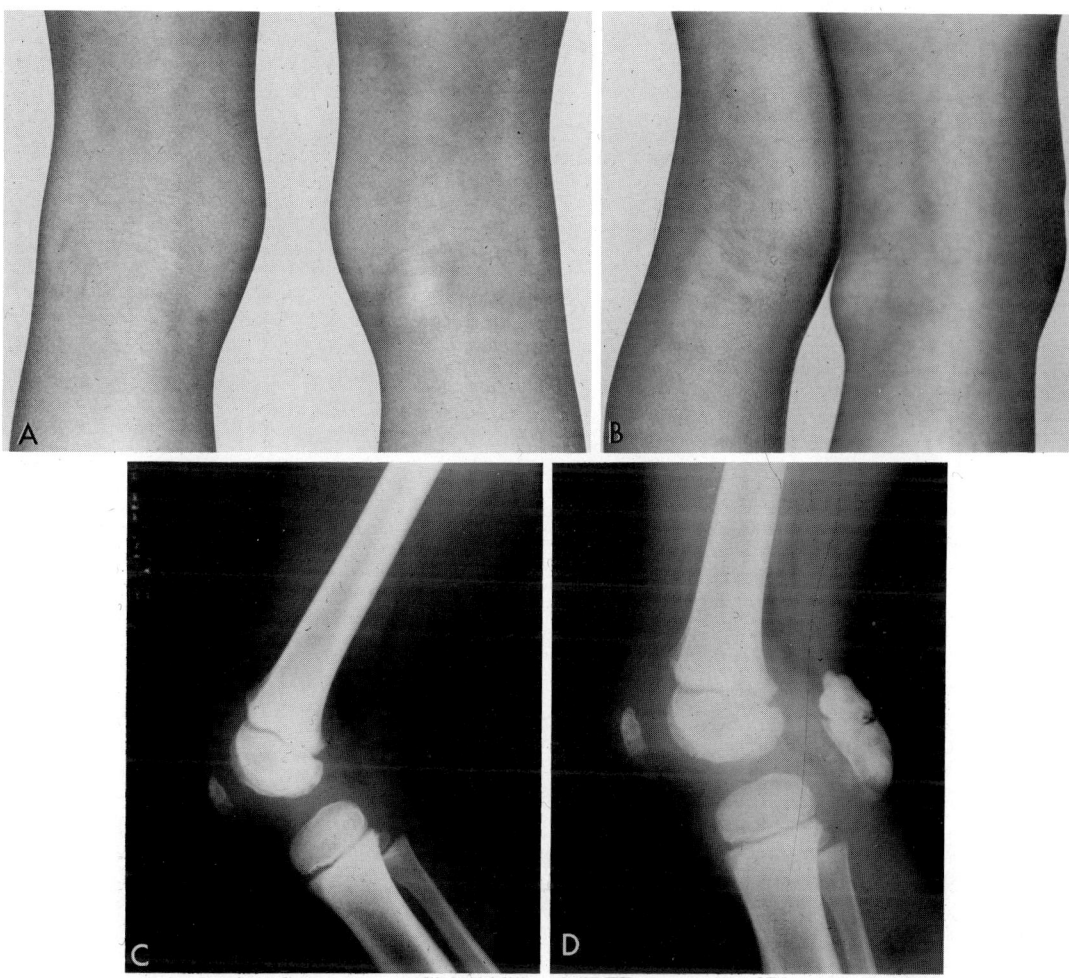

FIGURE 4–72. *Popliteal cyst.*

A and **B.** Clinical appearance. **C** and **D.** Plain and contrast lateral radiograms.

shiny, with villous formation. The fibrous connective tissue in the wall is less dense, and its surface is lined with synovium-like cells. There is round-cell infiltration (Fig. 4–71 B). The *inflammatory cysts* have a very thick wall and appear shaggy from adherent fibrinous exudate. Infiltration by lymphocytes, plasma cells, histiocytes, and even polymorphonuclear cells is seen in varying degrees. Areas of metaplasia into cartilaginous and osteoid elements may also be encountered (Fig. 4–71 C). The *transitional cyst* represents a form that is partially fibrinous and partially synovial in type, indicating a basic similarity in all the cyst types (Fig. 4–71 D).

Rauschning and associates classified 30 surgically excised popliteal cysts on the basis of 12 idiopathic and 18 symptomatic lesions; mean age of patients was 44.4 years with a range of 16 to 73 years. On light and scanning electron microscopic examination they found considerable histopathologic variation. Although there was no valid distinction between the two types of cyst, they advised thorough pathologic examination of all excised popliteal cysts in order to rule out malignancy and other inflammatory disorders.[47]

Clinical Picture

In children, the presence of a mass in the posterior aspect of the knee is the presenting complaint. Associated symptoms of derangement of the knee are usually absent, in contrast to findings in the adult. On occasion there may be stiffness and local pain. The swelling is located distal to the popliteal crease, becoming prominent when the knee is hyperextended and disappearing when it is flexed. The mass is hard, firm, and can be transilluminated (Fig. 4–72). The knee joint should be carefully ex-

Excision of Popliteal Cyst

The patient preferably should be in prone position with a pneumatic tourniquet placed on the proximal thigh.

A. The skin incision is oblique and centered directly over the swelling; it should *not* cross the popliteal crease.

The anatomical relationship of vessels and nerves in the popliteal areas in shown in this cross-section of the knee.

B. Subcutaneous tissue and deep fascia are divided and the protruding mass is exposed. Every effort should be made not to rupture the cyst, as this will make it difficult to determine its outline and to dissect it to its pedicle or its point of contact with the joint. Excision of the sac should be complete to prevent recurrence. The knee is flexed, relaxing the hamstrings and both heads of the gastrocnemius.

The proper plane of dissection depends upon the site of the cyst. If it is located between the semimembranosus and the medial head of the gastrocnemius, the interval between the muscles is exposed by appropriate retraction. In this plane, neuromuscular structures should be avoided.

C and D. With scissors and sharp knife dissection, the cyst is separated and traced to its base, which may be attached to the capsule synovium. The entire cyst is removed by division of the pedicle at its base.

E. Tight closure of any opening in the capsule is unnecessary, although, if possible, it is carried out. The wound is closed in layers. A compression dressing is applied and the child is allowed to be ambulatory as soon as possible.

Plate 57. Excision of Popliteal Cyst

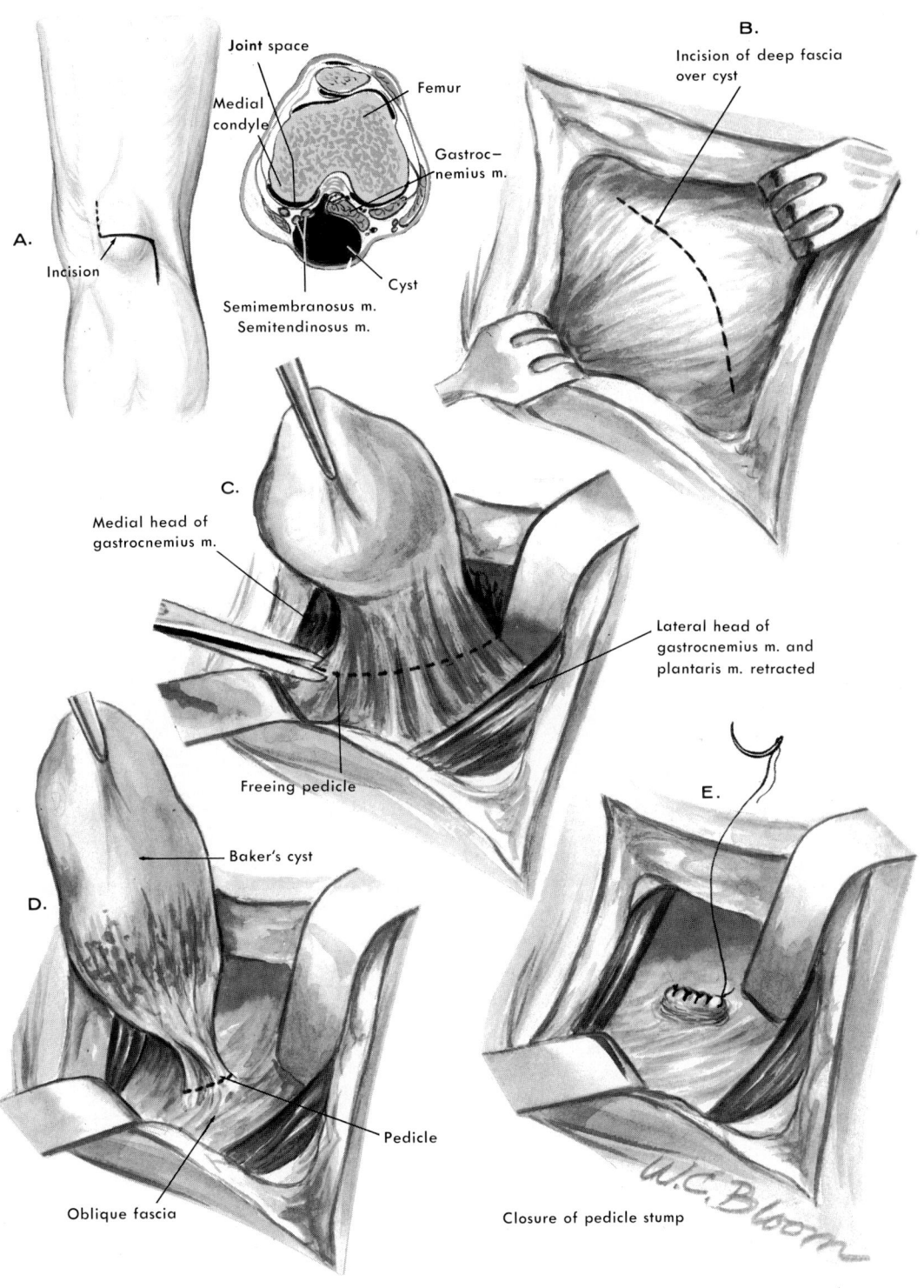

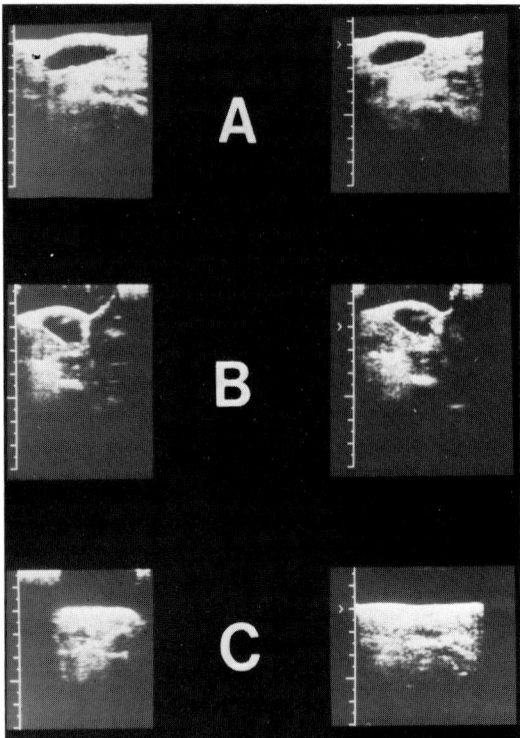

FIGURE 4–73. *Ultrasonography of both knees with popliteal cyst on the right.*

A and **B.** Sagittal images showing large echo-free mass in the popliteal fossa of the right knee. **C.** The normal left knee.

amined for signs of internal derangement and arthritis.

Diagnosis

Swelling in the popliteal region is initially evaluated by *conventional radiography* in the anteroposterior, lateral, and oblique projections; it will disclose soft-tissue swelling of fluid density and, also, rule out pathologic osseous changes such as osteochondroma.

Ultrasonography is a reliable and effective tool in assessing a popliteal mass. Ultrasound can distinguish between fluid and solid mass. Different images are created by transmission of high-frequency sound waves; the fluid-filled popliteal cyst is depicted as an echo-free space, as shown in Figure 4–73, whereas solid tissue is echogenic. Transverse and longitudinal images are formulated as "slices." Popliteal cysts are best shown by sagittal ultrasound image projections. Spatial relations of the mass to popliteal structures can be determined. "Realtime" images can show arterial pulsation. Ultrasonography is performed as an outpatient procedure; it is quick and noninvasive. Following conventional radiography this author strongly recommends ultrasonography in diagnostic assessment of a popliteal soft-tissue mass. Its only limitation is that it cannot depict a popliteal cyst that is completely ruptured.[5, 10, 51]

Computed tomography and nuclear magnetic resonance imaging will clearly show that the cyst is of fluid density with a well-defined thin wall with or without central septum or septa. In special cases computed tomography may be combined with arthrography of the knee (with the CT scan performed immediately after arthrography). Nuclear magnetic resonance imaging will show the popliteal cyst and its relationship to adjacent structures and the knee joint. It is safe, accurate, noninvasive, and without radiation hazard. Its drawback is the cost and complexity.[27]

Arthrography is rarely indicated in children with popliteal cysts. It is performed occasionally when the cyst is abnormal in its location and there is suspicion of associated intra-articular disease such as cystic degeneration of the lateral meniscus. Double contrast agents (20 ml. of room air and 10 ml. of 75 per cent Hypaque) are injected. After repeated flexion and extension of the knee under the image intensifier the condition of the meniscus and other intra-articular structures is determined. Popliteal cysts are best visualized in the lateral projection. Radiographs are made for permanent recording. An anatomic communication between the gastrocnemius-semimembranosus bursa and the knee joint is present in many patients, but arthrography demonstrates this communication

Table 4–14. Diagnostic Steps in Assessing Popliteal Swelling

Clinical history and physical examination
  Does it transilluminate?
  Does it pulsate?
  Where is it located? (most popliteal cysts of childhood are medial; if lateral or unusual location, be cautious!)
  Does it have any solid feel on palpation? (beware of tumor!)
Conventional radiography
Ultrasonography (typical popliteal cyst shows as echo-free space)
Computed tomography; nuclear magnetic resonance imaging (do not perform routinely, only in suspicious cases)
Arthrography (if communication with knee joint is suspected)
Arteriography or venography (if diagnostic clues indicate aneurysm or popliteal varices)
Aspiration biopsy (when in doubt as to nature of mass)

only when a joint effusion has been present for a significant length of time. Acute internal derangements of the knee in children and adolescents rarely are associated with cysts identifiable in the arthrogram, but when a popliteal cyst is not present it is most unusual to be able to demonstrate a communication between the joint space and the gastrocnemius-semimembranosus bursa.[60] Steps in the diagnosis of popliteal cyst are summarized in Table 4–14.

In the *differential diagnosis* various entities should be considered. A lipoma in the popliteal region is distinguished by the radiolucent shadow it gives in the radiogram. Aneurysm is characterized by the pulsations it transmits; if these pulsations are present, arteriography is indicated. Popliteal varices may present a diagnostic problem, which will be settled by venography. Thrombophlebitis, neuroma, nerve ganglia, semimembranosus hypertrophy, and enlarged lymph nodes are other conditions to consider in the differential diagnosis. A popliteal cyst may contain an osteochondral mass.[15, 55, 61] Pigmented villonodular synovitis and inflammatory conditions in the knee joint such as rheumatoid arthritis, tuberculosis, brucellosis, or a pyogenic abscess may cause a cystic swelling in the popliteal area. Pigmented villonodular synovitis or tears or cystic degeneration of the posterior portion of the meniscus are not usually seen in children, though in adults they may be the original site of disease. Occasionally malignant tumors may clinically simulate popliteal cysts. Bogumill and associates report fibrosarcoma, synovial sarcoma, and fibrous histiocytoma masquerading as popliteal cysts. All three of these malignant tumors, however, occurred in adults and they were located in the lateral portion of the popliteal fossa. *Popliteal cyst usually arises in the medial part of the fossa; when it is located laterally one should be suspicious.* Also, the presence of solid components in a mostly cystic mass should serve as a warning of the possibility of a malignant growth. If there is doubt as to the nature of the mass, aspiration will settle the diagnosis. Popliteal cysts contain gelatinous fluid.

Treatment

Operative removal of popliteal cysts in children is seldom required. MacMahon, in a review of 42 popliteal cysts that were not operated on in children followed for six months to six years, reported spontaneous disappearance of the cysts in 25 and decrease in size in 8. The average time for disappearance of the cyst was ten months. Only two cysts increased in size. He recommended a nonsurgical conservative approach of simple observation.[38] Dinham reviewed the natural history of 120 popliteal cysts in children; of the 71 untreated cysts, 51 (73 per cent) disappeared spontaneously during a mean period of 20 months; of the 50 cysts that were operated on, 21 recurred in a mean period of 7 months; three of the children with recurrences had more than one further operation. One patient had five operations, and the popliteal cyst was still present. Dinham also recommended a conservative nonoperative management of asymptomatic popliteal cyst.[16] Disadvantages of surgery are the cost of unnecessary admission to hospital and surgery, risk of anesthesia, a disfiguring operative scar, and definite high rate of postoperative recurrence. In the literature, recurrence after operation was reported by Jefferson, Haggert, and Burleson et al.[8, 24, 28]

Surgical excision of the cyst is indicated if, after a period of two to three years of observation, it does not regress, but instead remains large or increases in size and continues to cause symptoms. The operation technique of excision of popliteal cyst is described and illustrated in Plate 57. After the cyst is excised it is important to transect the specimen in the operating room before closure of the wound. When solid or unusual masses are found they should be examined by frozen section before the wound is closed. Aspiration of the cyst and instillation of hydrocortisone is not recommended, as the cyst will almost always recur.

References

1. Adams, J., Yulich, J., and Bergin, J.: Ruptured Baker's cyst simulating thrombophlebitis (letter). J.A.M.A., 241:358, 1979.
2. Adams, R.: Chronic rheumatic arthritis of the knee joint. Dublin J. Med. Sci., 17:520, 1840.
3. Baker, W. M.: On the formation of synovial cysts in the leg in connection with disease of the knee joint. St. Bart. Hosp. Rep., 13:245, 1877.
4. Baker, W. M.: The formation of abnormal synovial cysts in connection with the joints. St. Bart. Hosp. Rep., 21:177, 1885.
5. Beals, R. K., Lee, T. G., Knochel, J. Q., and Henderson, S.: Ultrasound as a diagnostic aid in the evaluation of popliteal swelling. Clin. Orthop., 149:220, 1980.
6. Bogumill, G. P., Bruno, P. D., and Barrick, E. F.: Malignant lesions masquerading as popliteal cysts. A report of three cases. J. Bone Joint Surg., 63-A:474, 1981.
7. Bryan, R. S., DiMichelle, J. D., and Ford, G. L., Jr.: Popliteal cysts. Arthrography as an aid to diagnosis and treatment. Clin. Orthop., 50:203, 1967.
8. Burleson, R. J., Bickel, W. H., and Dahlin, D. C.:

Popliteal cyst. A clinicopathological survey. J. Bone Joint Surg., 38-A:1265, 1956.
9. Burman, M.: Semimembranosus bursitis. J.A.M.A., 124:29, 1944.
10. Carpenter, J. R., Hattery, R. R., Hunder, G. G., Byran, R. S., and McLeod, R. A.: Ultrasound evaluation of the popliteal space—comparison with arthrography and physical examination. Mayo Clin. Proc., 51:498, 1976.
11. Childress, H. M.: Popliteal cysts associated with undiagnosed posterior lesions of the medial meniscus. J. Bone Joint Surg., 36-A:1233, 1954.
12. Childress, H. M.: Popliteal cysts and posterior lesions of the medial meniscus. Clin. Orthop., 18:136, 1960.
13. Cooper, R. A.: Computerized tomography (body scan) of Baker's cysts. J. Rheumatol., 5:184, 1978.
14. Cravener, E. K.: Hernia of the knee joint (Baker's cyst). J. Bone Joint Surg., 14:186, 1932.
15. de Benedetti, M., Waugh, T. R., and Evanski, P. M.: A popliteal cyst with a large osteochondral mass. J. Bone Joint Surg., 61-A:147, 1979.
16. Dinham, J. M.: Popliteal cysts in children. J. Bone Joint Surg., 57-B:69, 1975.
17. Eyanson, S., McFarlane, J. D., and Brandt, K. D.: Popliteal cyst mimicking thrombophlebitis as the first indication of knee disease. Clin. Orthop., 144:215, 1979.
18. Fouchet, E.: Mémoire sur les kystes de la région poplitée. Arch. Gén. Méd., 2:313, 1856.
19. Fullerton, A.: The surgical anatomy of the synovial membrane of the knee-joint. Br. J. Surg., 4:191, 1916.
20. Gompels, B. M., and Darkington, L. G.: Evaluation of popliteal cysts and painful calves with ultrasonography; comparison with arthrography. Ann. Rheum. Dis., 4:355, 1982.
21. Griffiths, H. T., Elston, C. W., Colton, C. L., and Swannel, A. J.: Popliteal masses masquerading as popliteal cysts. Ann. Rheum. Dis., 43:60, 1984.
22. Gristina, A. G., and Wilson, P. D.: Popliteal cysts in adults and children. A review of 90 operative cases. J. Bone Joint Surg., 45-A:1552, 1963.
23. Guerra, J., Jr., Newell, J. D., Resnick, D., and Danzig, L. A.: Gastrocnemius-semimembranosus bursal region of the knee. A.J.R., 136:593, 1981.
24. Haggart, G. E.: Synovial cyst of the popliteal space. Clinical significance and treatment. Ann. Surg., 188:438, 1943.
25. Hermann, G., Yeh, H., Lehr-Janus, C., and Berson, B. L.: Diagnosis of popliteal cyst: Double contrast arthrography and sonography. A.J.R., 137:369, 1981.
26. Hoffman, B. K.: Cystic lesions of the popliteal space. Surg., Gynecol. Obstet., 116:551, 1963.
27. Hull, R. G., Rennie, J. A. N., Eastmond, C. J., Hutchison, J. M. S., and Smith, F. S.: Nuclear magnetic resonance (NMR) tomographic imaging for popliteal cysts in rheumatoid arthritis. Ann. Rheum. Dis., 43:56, 1984.
28. Jefferson, G.: Bilateral Baker's cysts: Recurrence after operation. Proc. R. Soc. Med., 13:162, 1920.
29. Kattapuram, S. V.: Case report 181. Calcified popliteal cyst (Baker's cyst). Skeletal Radiol., 7:279, 1982.
30. Kessler, I., and Sillberman, Z.: The development of popliteal cysts: An arthrographic study. Clin. Orthop., 18:149, 1960.
31. Khan, M. A., and Ganuza, C.: Ruptured popliteal cysts and thrombophlebitis (letter). Arthritis Rheum., 20:1560, 1977.
32. Kilcoyne, R. F., Imray, T. J., and Stewart, E. T.: Ruptured Baker's cyst simulating acute thrombophlebitis. J.A.M.A., 240:1517, 1978.
33. Krag, D. N., and Stansel, H. C.: Popliteal cyst producing complete arterial occlusion. A case report. J. Bone Joint Surg., 64-A:1369, 1982.
34. Kuhn, H. M., and Hemphill, J. E.: Baker's cyst.

Posterior herniation of the knee joint. Radiology, 42:237, 1942.
35. Lee, K. R., Tines, S. C., Price, H. I., DeSmet, A. A., and Neff, J. R.: The computed tomographic findings of popliteal cysts. Skeletal Radiol., 10:26, 1983.
36. Levitin, P. M.: Diagnosis of Baker's cyst (letter). J.A.M.A., 236:253, 1976.
37. Levitin, P. M.: Dissecting popliteal cyst: An unusual complication of Reiter's syndrome. South. Med. J., 69:1522, 1976.
38. MacMahon, E. B.: Baker's cysts in children—is surgery necessary? J. Bone Joint Surg., 55-A:1311, 1973.
39. Meyerding, W. H., and Van Demark, R. E.: Posterior horns of the knee (Baker's cyst, popliteal cyst, semimembranosus bursitis, medial gastrocnemius bursitis and popliteal bursitis). J.A.M.A., 122:858, 1943.
40. Miller, A.: Ruptured Baker's cyst and thrombophlebitis (letter). J.A.M.A., 241:564, 1979.
41. Moore, M., Jr.: Popliteal varices simulating Baker's cyst. South. Surg., 14:1, 1948.
42. Nakano, K. K.: Entrapment neuropathy from Baker's cyst. J.A.M.A., 239:135, 1978.
43. O'Dell, J. R., Andersen, P. A., Hollister, J. R., and West, S. G.: Anterior tibial mass; an unusual complication of popliteal cysts. Arthritis Rheum., 27:113, 1984.
44. Patrone, N. A., and Ramsdell, C. M.: Baker's cyst and venous thrombosis. South. Med. J., 74:768, 1981.
45. Prescott, S. M., Pearl, J. E., and Tikoff, G.: Pseudopseudothrombophlebitis: Ruptured popliteal cyst with deep vein thrombosis (letter). N. Engl. J. Med., 299:1192, 1978.
46. Rauschning, W.: Popliteal cysts and their relationship to the gastrocnemio-semimembranosus bursa. Studies on the surgical and functional anatomy. Acta Orthop. Scand. (Suppl.), 179:1, 1979.
47. Rauschning, W., Fredriksson, B. A., and Wilander, E.: Histomorphology of idiopathic and symptomatic popliteal cysts. Clin. Orthop., 164:306, 1982.
48. Rennebohm, R. M., Towbin, R. B., Crowe, W. E., and Levinson, J. E.: Popliteal cysts in juvenile rheumatoid arthritis. A.J.R., 140:123, 1983.
49. Resnick, D., and Niwayama, G.: Diagnosis of Bone and Joint Disorders with Emphasis on Articular Abnormalities. Philadelphia, Saunders, 1981, p. 594.
50. Rosenthal, D. I., Schwartz, A. N., and Schiller, A. L.: Case report 170: Subperiosteal synovial cyst of the knee. Skeletal Radiol., 7:142, 1981.
51. Rudikoff, J. C., Lynch, J. J., Phillips, E., and Clapp, P. R.: Ultrasound diagnosis of Baker's cyst. J.A.M.A., 235:1054, 1976.
52. Schlenker, J. D., Johnston, K., and Wolkoff, J. S.: Occlusion of popliteal artery caused by popliteal cysts. Surgery, 76:833, 1974.
53. Scott, W. N., Jacobs, B., and Lockshin, M. D.: Posterior compartment syndrome resulting from a dissecting popliteal cyst. Case report. Clin. Orthop., 122:189, 1977.
54. Shepard, J. R., and Helms, C. A.: Atypical popliteal cyst due to lateral synovial herniation. Radiology, 140:66, 1981.
55. Smillie, I. S.: Injuries of the Knee Joint. 4th Ed. Baltimore, Williams & Wilkins, 1970.
56. Symeonides, P. P., and Paschaloglou, C.: Localised hypertrophy of the semimembranosus muscle simulating popliteal cyst. J. Bone Joint Surg., 52-B:337, 1970.
57. Trecco, F., de Paulis, F., Masciocchi, C., Bonanni, G., Beomonte Zobol, B., Caloisi, V., Romanini, L., and Passariello, R.: Clinical interpretation of cysts in the popliteal space using computerized tomography. Ital. J. Orthop. Traumatol., 10:511, 1984.
58. Wheeler, P. H.: Popliteal hernia. Trans. N. Engl. Surg. Soc., 30:172, 1949.
59. Wilson, P. D., Eyre-Brook, A. L., and Francis, J. D.:

A clinical and anatomical study of the semimembranosus bursa in relation to popliteal cyst. J. Bone Joint Surg., *20-A*:963, 1938.
60. Wolfe, R. D., and Colloff, B.: Popliteal cysts. An arthrographic study and review of the literature. J. Bone Joint Surg., *54-A*:1057, 1972.
61. Zadek, I.: Osteochondromatosis of a popliteal bursa. Bull. Hosp. Joint Dis., *5*:12, 1944.

SYNOVIAL CHONDROMATOSIS

Synovial chondromatosis is a condition characterized by the formation of metaplastic and multiple foci of cartilage in the intimal layer of the synovial membrane of a joint. It also occurs in bursae and tendon sheaths.[48, 53] The term *synovial osteochondromatosis* is used when the lesional cartilage is ossified.

This benign neoplasm is very rare and usually occurs in persons over 40 years of age and only occasionally in adolescents. It is twice as common in the male as in the female. The etiology of the condition is unknown. Trauma has been postulated as a possible stimulus of metaplasia of the synovial cells into chondrocytes.

Ordinarily only one joint is involved, usually a large synovial joint. The knee is the commonest site; next in order of frequency of involvement are the hip, ankle, elbow, and wrist.

Arthrotomy reveals the synovium to be thickened and studded by innumerable small, firm, flat or slightly raised, grayish white nodules (Fig. 4–74 A). These cartilaginous or osteocartilaginous foci may become pedunculated and detached from the affected membrane, entering the joint cavity as loose bodies. Histologic studies disclose numerous foci of cartilaginous metaplasia of the synovium, which may be calcified or ossified (Fig. 4–74 B).

Clinical complaints consist of pain, swelling, and stiffness of the affected joint—locking may be a symptom when there are loose bodies. Months or years may elapse before a patient seeks treatment. On examination, the synovial membrane is observed to be thickened and the joint limited in its range of motion. Other physical signs that can be elicited are crepitus and palpable loose bodies.

Radiograms disclose multiple areas of stippled calcification in and around the affected joint when the lesion is cartilaginous, in which case the findings are those of capsular distention and synovial thickening (Fig. 4–75).

Treatment consists of simple removal of the loose bodies and partial synovectomy. Extensive and complete synovectomy is impractical and usually not necessary. The condition has a definite tendency to eventual resolution.

References

1. Aumont: Corps étrangers ostéo-cartilagenous d'une bourse séreuse axillaire. Mém. Acad. Chir., *64*:1423, 1938.
2. Ballet, F. L., Watson, H. K., and Ryer, J.: Synovial chondromatosis of the distal radioulnar joint. J. Hand Surg., *9-A*:590, 1984.
3. Bennett, G. A.: Reactive and neoplastic changes in synovial tissue. Proc. Inst. Med. Chicago, *18*:26, 1950.
4. Bloom, R., and Pattinson, J. N.: Osteochondromatosis of the hip joint. J. Bone Joint Surg., *33-B*:80, 1951.
5. Cahuzac, J. B., Lebarbier, P., Germaneau, J., and Pasquie, M.: La chondratose synoviale de l'enfant (à propos de 4 observations). Chir. Pediatr., *20*:89, 1979.
6. Calandriello, B., and Nigrisoli, P.: Articular synovial microchondromatosis. Ital. J. Orthop. Traumatol., *8*:67, 1982.
7. Carey, R. P.: Synovial chondromatosis of the knees in childhood. A report of two cases. J. Bone Joint Surg., *65-B*:444, 1983.
8. Chevrier: Fibro-chondromatose du prolongement synovial bicipital. Bull. Mem. Soc. Nat. Chir., *58*:565, 1932.
9. Coventry, M. B., Harrison, E. G., and Martin, J. F.: Benign synovial tumors of the knee: A diagnostic problem. J. Bone Joint Surg., *48-A*:1350, 1966.
10. Drennan, J. C.: Juvenile osteochondromatosis. Orthop. Trans., *3*:115, 1979.
11. Dunn, A. W., and Whisler, J. H.: Synovial chondromatosis of the knee with associated extracapsular chondromas. J. Bone Joint Surg., *55-A*:1747, 1973.
12. Dunn, E. J., McGavran, M. H., Nelson, P., and Greer, R. B., III: Synovial chondromasarcoma. Report of a case. J. Bone Joint Surg., *56-A*:811, 1974.
13. Eisenberg, K. S., and Johnston, J. O.: Synovial chondromatosis of the hip joint presenting as an intrapelvic mass. J. Bone Joint Surg., *54-A*:176, 1972.
14. Freund, E.: Chondromatosis of joints. Arch. Surg., *34*:670, 1937.
15. Goldman, R. L., and Lichtenstein, L.: Synovial chondrosarcoma. Cancer, *17*:1233, 1964.
16. Henderson, M. S., and Jones, H. T.: Loose bodies in joints and bursae due to synovial osteochondromatosis. J. Bone Joint Surg., *5*:400, 1923.
17. Holm, C. L.: Primary synovial chondromatosis of the ankle. J. Bone Joint Surg., *58-A*:878, 1976.
18. Jaffe, H. L.: Tumors and Tumorous Conditions of the Bones and Joints. Philadelphia, Lea & Febiger, 1958, pp. 558–576.
19. Jeffreys, T. E.: Synovial chondromatosis. J. Bone Joint Surg., *49-B*:530, 1967.
20. Jones, H. T.: Loose body formation in synovial osteochondromatosis with special reference to etiology and pathology. J. Bone Joint Surg., *6*:407, 1924.
21. Khermosh, O., and Weissman, S. L.: Synovial osteochondromatosis of the ankle. Harefuah, *84*:219, 1973.
22. King, J. W., Spjut, H. G., Fechner, R. E., and Vanderpool, D. W.: Synovial chondrosarcoma of the knee joint. J. Bone Joint Surg., *49-B*:1389, 1967.
23. Levinson, E. D., Pillsbury, S. L., and Ozonoff, M. B.: Case report: Synovial chondromatosis of the ankle with extracapsular extension. Skeletal Radiol., *7*:219, 1981.
24. Leydig, S. M., and Odell, R. T.: Synovial osteochondromatosis. Surg. Gynecol. Obstet., *89*:457, 1949.
25. Lichtenstein, L.: Tumors of synovial joints, bursae and tendon sheaths. *In* Lichtenstein, L. (ed.): Bone Tumors. 5th Ed. St. Louis, Mosby, 1977, pp. 428–452.
26. Lichtenstein, L., and Goldman, R. L.: Cartilage tumors in soft tissues, particularly in the hand and foot. Cancer, *17*:1203, 1964.
27. Lyritis, G.: Synovial chondromatosis of the inferior radioulnar joint. Acta Orthop. Scand., *47*:373, 1976.

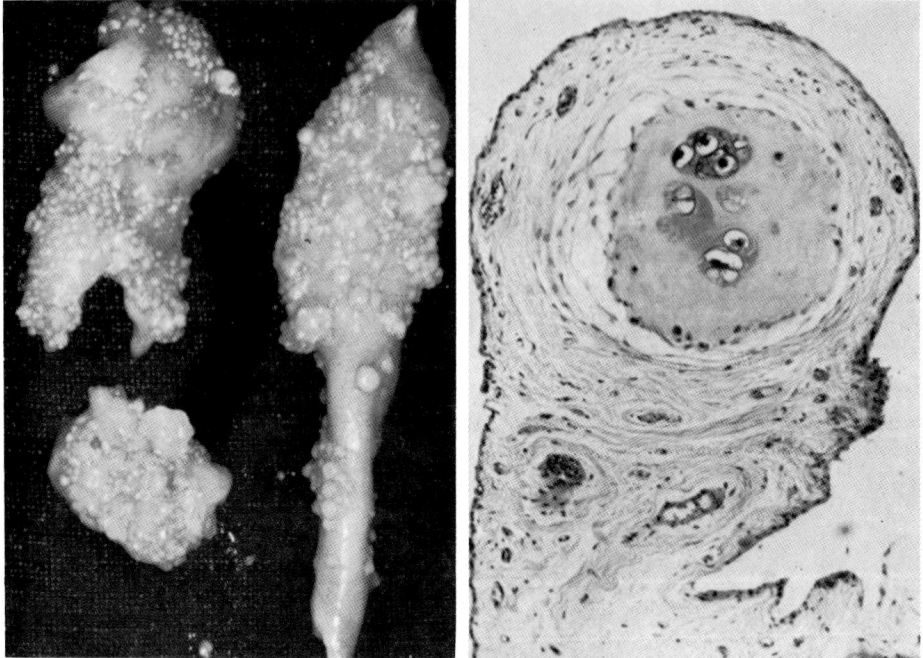

FIGURE 4–74. Synovial chondromatosis.

A. Gross appearance of an excised synovium of the knee joint. Note the innumerable small and slightly raised grayish-white nodules in the thickened synovium. **B.** Histologic picture showing cartilaginous metaplasia of the synovium, which is calcified. (From Jeffreys, T.: Synovial chondromatosis. J. Bone Joint Surg., *49-A*:534, 1967. Reprinted by permission.)

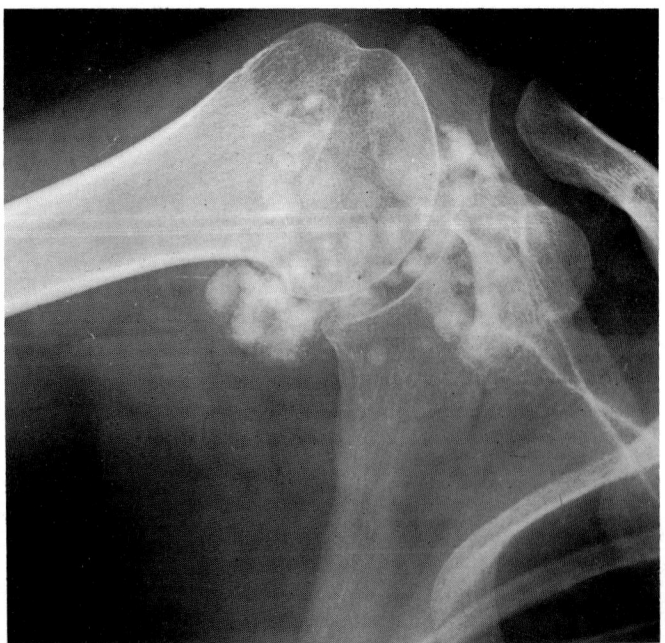

FIGURE 4–75. Synovial chondromatosis of the shoulder.

Radiogram shows the multiple stippled calcifications in and around the joint.

28. McCarthy, E. F., and Dorfman, H. D.: Primary synovial chondromatosis. An ultrastructural study. Clin. Orthop., *168*:178, 1982.
29. McIvor, P. R., and King, D. E.: Osteochondromatosis of the hip joint. J. Bone Joint Surg., *44-A*:87, 1962.
30. Milgram, J. W.: Synovial osteochondromatosis: A histopathological study of 30 cases. J. Bone Joint Surg., *59-A*:792, 1977.
31. Milgram, J. W.: Synovial osteochondromatosis in association with Legg-Calvé-Perthes disease. Clin. Orthop., *145*:179, 1979.
32. Milgram, J. W., and Addison, R. G.: Synovial osteochondromatosis of the knee. Chondromatous recurrence with possible chondromasarcomatous degeneration. J. Bone Joint Surg., *58-A*:264, 1976.
33. Milgram, J. W., and Pease, C. W.: Synovial osteochondromatosis in a young child. A case report. J. Bone Joint Surg., *62-A*:1021, 1980.
34. Mullins, F., Berard, C. W., and Eisenberg, S. H.: Chondrosarcoma following synovial chondromatosis. A case study. Cancer, *18*:1180, 1965.
35. Murphy, A. F., and Wilson, J. N.: Tenosynovial osteochondroma of the hand. J. Bone Joint Surg., *40-A*:1236, 1958.
36. Murphy, F. P., Dahlin, D. C., and Sullivan, C. R.: Articular synovial chondromatosis. J. Bone Joint Surg., *44-A*:77, 1962.
37. Mussey, R. D., Jr., and Henderson, M. S.: Osteochondromatosis. J. Bone Joint Surg., *31-A*:619, 1949.
38. Nixon, J. E., Frank, G. R., and Chambers, G.: Synovial osteochondromatosis with report of four cases, one showing malignant change. U.S. Armed Forces Med. J., *11*:1434, 1960.
39. Pelker, R., Drennan, J. C., and Ozonoff, M. B.: Juvenile synovial chondromatosis of the hip. J. Bone Joint Surg., *65-A*:552, 1983.
40. Prager, R. J., and Mall, J. C.: Arthrographic diagnosis of synovial chondromatosis. A.J.R., *127*:344, 1976.
41. Rao, J. P., Spingola, C., Mastromonaco, E., and Villacin, A.: Synovial osteochondromatosis. Computerized axial tomography, frozen section and arthrography in diagnosis and management. Orthop. Rev., *15*:245, 1986.
42. Rixford, E.: Osteochondromatosis. Ann. Surg., *92*:673, 1930.
43. Rockey, H. C.: Trigger-finger due to a tenosynovial osteochondroma. J. Bone Joint Surg., *45-A*:387, 1963.
44. Roques, C. F., Amigues, H., Puget, J., et al.: Métastase synoviale du genou, premier symptôme d'un cancer de l'estomac. Rev. Méd. Toulouse, *10*(3):235, 1974.
45. Sabanas, A. E., and Ghormley, R. K.: Hemangioma of the knee complicated by synovial chondromatosis. Report of a case. Proc. Staff Meet. Mayo Clin., *30*:171, 1955.
46. Savino, A. W., and Kuo, K. N.: Synovial chondromatosis in association with Turner's syndrome: A case report. Clin. Orthop., *144*:183, 1979.
47. Sim, F. H., Dahlin, D. C., and Ivins, J. C.: Extraarticular synovial chondromatosis. J. Bone Joint Surg., *59-A*:492, 1977.
48. Symeonides, P.: Bursal chondromatosis. J. Bone Joint Surg., *48-B*:371, 1966.
49. Varma, D. P., and Ramakrishna, Y. J.: Synovial chondromatosis of the shoulder. Aust. N.Z. J. Surg., *46*:44, 1976.
50. Villacin, A.: Primary and secondary synovial chondrometaplasia. Hum. Pathol., *10*:439, 1979.
51. Wee, G. C., Torres, A., Jack, L. D., and Russell, H. E.: Synovial chondromatosis of the ankle. Case report. Mo. Med., *68*:781, 1971.
52. Wilmoth, C. L.: Osteochondromatosis. J. Bone Joint Surg., *23*:367, 1941.
53. Zadek, I.: Osteochondromatosis of a popliteal bursa. Bull. Hosp. Joint Dis., *5*:12, 1944.

PIGMENTED VILLONODULAR SYNOVITIS

In this relatively rare condition, the synovial membrane undergoes a proliferative reaction, with its surface becoming nodular, villous, and brownish in color.[1-78] The term *pigmented villonodular synovitis* was introduced by Jaffe, Lichtenstein, and Sutro in 1941.[33] The etiology of the condition is unknown; an inflammatory process is favored by most authors. Young adults are most often affected, though it may be seen in adolescents and occasionally in children.

Involvement is usually monarticular. The knee joint is the most usual site, and the fingers, feet, ankles, hips, wrists, and shoulders are affected in decreasing order of frequency. Involvement of the lumbar vertebral facet joint has been reported by Campbell and Wells.[9] Multifocal involvement is rare; a case in a child is described by Walls and Nogi.[73]

Clinical complaints consist of pain and swelling of the affected joint. The proliferated synovial membrane may get caught between the articular bone ends and cause locking. Limitation of joint motion is common. Incidental trauma may aggravate the symptoms.

The radiograms will commonly disclose irregular synovial thickening. There will be erosions of the articular ends of the bones, especially in the hip or ankle joints, which are tautly compartmentalized. Both sides of the joint are affected by single or confluent clusters of cystlike areas. In the knee the site of bone involvement is usually in the intercondylar regions of the femur and tibia.[24, 51] On occasion the lytic bone lesions may occur at a distance from the subchondral bone. Bone involvement in the knee may be confined to only one side of the joint, such as the proximal end of the tibia and fibula, or to isolated lesions in the femoral condyles. Long-standing pigmented villonodular synovitis may extensively involve the distal end of the femur with lytic lesions without apparently involving the tibia in the plain radiograph.[57]

The diseased tissue penetrates bone by infiltrating and extending through the vascular foramina. The lytic areas in bone are most common where the vascular foramina are largest and most numerous.[62]

In the hip the lytic bone lesion may appear aggressive, involving the femoral head and superomedial and inferior areas of the acetabulum. Computed tomography will depict the lesions, which are usually bordered by thin margins of sclerosis.

Contrast arthrography will disclose multiple filling defects of the synovium, which are quite typical of pigmented villonodular synovitis.[30, 59] Arteriography has been utilized to detect the synovial changes.[36]

Angiography will show richly vascularized tumorlike lesions with early filling of the veins and irregularity of the vessels.

On aspiration of the affected joint, a dark brown or frankly serosanguinous fluid is obtained, which is of diagnostic significance provided there is no history of recent severe trauma and hemorrhage into the joint.

Gross appearance on arthroscopy and arthrotomy is quite typical. The synovial membrane will be diffusely thickened and brownish red in color, with sessile or pedunculated nodules covering its surface. On biopsy (best performed through the arthroscope) and histologic examination the tissue consists of a stroma of reticulin and collagen fibers, in which are found foam cells, multinucleated giant cells, and hemosiderin deposits.

In the differential diagnosis chronic monarticular rheumatoid arthritis, synovial hemangiomatosis, low-grade infectious arthritis, and other inflammatory joint conditions, such as tuberculosis, should be considered.

The lytic destruction of bone in pigmented villonodular synovitis may simulate giant cell tumor. Histologic diagnosis may be difficult as there are many lesions in bone that contain giant cells. Hemosiderin granules within macrophages and stromal cells may be present in both giant cell tumors and pigmented villonodular synovitis. In giant cell tumor the classic stroma is composed of plump ovoid or spindle cells that lack clear cytoplasmic borders; these stromal cells are dispersed throughout the specimen. In pigmented villonodular synovitis the giant cells usually aggregate in areas of hemorrhage and fibrosis. The confluent diffuse lytic bone lesions in pigmented villonodular synovitis may also be suggestive of aneurysmal bone cyst.

Treatment

This consists of synovectomy, total if possible. It is best performed through the arthroscope by a surgeon well experienced in operative arthroscopy. Recurrence after surgery is common in pigmented villonodular synovitis. It is best to inform the parents and patient preoperatively of the recalcitrant nature of the disease.

In recurrent cases with extensive bone involvement and joint destruction, radiation therapy in relatively small doses over a period of two to three weeks may be indicated. It has been used in the past with relief of symptoms. Radiation therapy is not utilized today except in extreme cases because of the reported complications.[2, 4, 38, 44]

A long course of the disease and numerous recurrences with marked bone and soft-tissue involvement and severe functional disability may necessitate amputation.[37]

References

1. Arthaud, J. B.: Pigmented nodular synovitis: Report of 11 lesions in nonarticular locations. Am. J. Clin. Pathol., 511:517, 1972.
2. Atmore, W. G., Dahlin, D. C., and Ghormley, R. K.: Pigmented villonodular synovitis. A clinical and pathologic study. Minn. Med., 39:196, 1956.
3. Bhawan, J., Joris, I., Cohen, N., and Majno, G.: Microcirculatory changes in posttraumatic pigmented villonodular synovitis. Arch. Pathol. Lab. Med., 104:328, 1980.
4. Bobechko, W. P., and Kostuik, J. P.: Childhood villonodular synovitis. Can. J. Surg., 11:480, 1968.
5. Bonacina, P., Pessina, R., Percudani, W., Villa, L., and Bonfanti, R.: Pigmented villonodular synovitis: Research methods and differential diagnostic problems. Chir. Ital., 33:170, 1981.
6. Breimer, C. W., and Freiberger, R. H.: Bone lesions associated with villonodular synovitis. A.J.R., 79:618, 1958.
7. Burnett, R. A.: A cause of erroneous diagnosis of pigmented villonodular synovitis. J. Clin. Pathol., 29:17, 1976.
8. Byers, P. D., Cotton, R. E., Deacon, O. W., Lowy, M., Newman, P. H., Sissons, H. A., and Thomson, A. D.: The diagnosis and treatment of pigmented villonodular synovitis. J. Bone Joint Surg., 50-B:290, 1968.
9. Campbell, A. J., and Wells, I. P.: Pigmented villonodular synovitis of a lumbar vertebral facet joint. J. Bone Joint Surg., 64-A:145, 1982.
10. Carr, C. R., Berley, F. V., and Davis, W. C.: Pigmented villonodular synovitis of the hip joint. A case report. J. Bone Joint Surg., 36-A:1007, 1954.
11. Cavina, C., Cossi, C. G., Pagliazzi, A., Giorgi, B., Grasso, A., and Cosenza, M.: Evaluation of double contrast arthrography in pigmented villonodular synovitis of the knee. Ital. J. Orthop. Traumatol., 10:121, 1984.
12. Chung, S. M. K., and James, J. M.: Diffuse pigmented villonodular synovitis of the hip joint. J. Bone Joint Surg., 47-A:293, 1965.
13. Cockshott, W. P., and Evans, K. T.: The place of soft tissue arteriography. Br. J. Radiol., 37:367, 1964.
14. Crawford, G. P., and Offerman, R. J.: Pigmented villonodular synovitis in the hand. Hand, 12:282, 1980.
15. Danzig, L. A., Gershuni, D. H., and Resnick, D.: Diagnosis and treatment of diffuse pigmented villonodular synovitis of the hip. Clin. Orthop., 168:42, 1982.
16. De Santis, E., Di Giovanni, C., and De Vecchis, L.: Pigmented villonodular synovitis in its articular manifestations. A review of 19 cases. Arch. Putti Chir. Organi Mov., 32:351, 1982.
17. DeSanto, D. A., and Wilson, P. D.: Xanthomatous tumors of joints. J. Bone Joint Surg., 21:531, 1939.
18. Donde, R., and Funding, J.: Pigmented villonodular synovitis. A follow-up study. Scand. J. Rheumatol., 9:172, 1980.

19. Dorwart, R. H., Genant, H. K., Johnston, W. H., and Morris, J. M.: Pigmented villonodular synovitis of the shoulder: Radiologic-pathologic assessment. A.J.R., 143:886, 1984.
20. Dorwart, R. H., Genant, H. K., Johnston, W. H., and Morris, J. M.: Pigmented villonodular synovitis of synovial joints: Clinical, pathologic and radiographic features. A.J.R., 143:877, 1984.
21. Fisk, G. R.: Hyperplasia and metaplasia in synovial membrane. Ann. R. Coll. Surg. Eng., 11:157, 1952.
22. Friedman, M., and Schwartz, E. E.: Irradiation therapy of pigmented villonodular synovitis. Bull. Hosp. Joint Dis., 18:19, 1957.
23. Fyfe, I. S., and MacFarlane, A. U.: Pigmented villonodular synovitis of the hand. Hand, 12:179, 1980.
24. Gaubert, J., Mazabraud, A., Verdie, J. C., and Cheneau, J.: Les synovites villo-nodulaires hémo-pigmentées des grosses articulations. Rev. Chir. Orthop., 60:265, 1974.
25. Gehweiler, J. A., and Wilson, J. W.: Diffuse biarticular pigmented villonodular synovitis. Radiology, 93:845, 1969.
26. Ghormley, R. K., and Romness, J. O.: Pigmented villonodular synovitis (xanthomatosis) of the hip joint. Proc. Staff Meet. Mayo Clin., 29:171, 1954.
27. Granowitz, S. P., and Mankin, H. J.: Localized pigmented villonodular synovitis. Report of five cases. J. Bone Joint Surg., 49-A:122, 1967.
28. Granowitz, S. P., D'Antonio, J., and Mankin, H. L.: The pathogenesis and long term end results of pigmented villonodular synovitis. Clin. Orthop., 114:335, 1976.
29. Greenfield, M. M., and Wallace, K. M.: Pigmented villonodular synovitis. Radiology, 54:350, 1950.
30. Halpern, A. A., Donovan, T. L., Horowitz, B., and Nagel, D.: Arthrographic demonstration of pigmented villonodular synovitis of the knee. Clin. Orthop., 132:193, 1978.
31. Hoaglund, F. T.: Experimental hemarthrosis. J. Bone Joint Surg., 49-A:285, 1967.
32. Jaffe, H. L.: Tumors and Tumorous Conditions of the Bones and Joints. Philadelphia, Lea & Febiger, 1958, pp. 534–545.
33. Jaffe, H. L., Lichtenstein, L., and Sutro, C. J.: Pigmented villonodular synovitis, bursitis and tenosynovitis. Arch. Pathol., 31:731, 1941.
34. Jergenson, H. E., Mankin, H. J., and Schiller, A. J.: Diffuse pigmented villonodular synovitis of the knee mimicking primary bone neoplasms. A report of two cases. J. Bone Joint Surg., 60-A:825, 1978.
35. Johansson, J. E., Ajjoub, S., Coughlin, L. P., Wener, J. A., and Cruess, R. L.: Pigmented villonodular synovitis of joints. Clin. Orthop., 163:159, 1982.
36. Kaufman, R. A., Towbin, R. B., Babcock, D. S., and Crawford, A. H.: Arthrosonography in the diagnosis of pigmented villonodular synovitis. A.J.R., 139:396, 1982.
37. Kindblom, L. G., and Guterberg, B.: Pigmented villonodular synovitis involving bone. J. Bone Joint Surg., 60-A:830, 1978.
38. Larmon, W. A.: Pigmented villonodular synovitis. Med. Clin. North Am., 49:141, 1965.
39. Lequesne, M., Nicholas, J. L., Kerboull, M., and Postel, M.: Pigmented villonodular synovitis of the hip joint. A report of six cases with review of the literature (author's transl.). Int. Orthop., 4:133, 1980.
40. Leszlzynki, J.: Pigmented villonodular synovitis in multiple joints. Ann. Rheum. Dis., 34:269, 1975.
41. Lewis, R. W.: Roentgen diagnosis of pigmented villonodular synovitis and synovial sarcoma of the knee joint. A preliminary report. Radiology, 49:26, 1947.
42. Lindenbaum, B. L., and Hunt, T.: An unusual presentation of pigmented villonodular synovitis. Clin. Orthop., 122:263, 1977.
43. Lowenstein, M. B., Smith, J. R., and Cole, S.: Infrapatellar pigmented villonodular synovitis: Arthrographic detection. A.J.R., 135:279, 1980.
44. McMaster, P. E.: Pigmented villonodular synovitis with invasion of bone. J. Bone Joint Surg., 42-A:1170, 1960.
45. Mikhailova, L. N., Rodionova, S. S., and Berman, A. M.: Electron microscope study of pigmented villonodular synovitis. Arkh. Patol., 45:33, 1983.
46. Miller, W. E.: Villonodular synovitis: Pigmented and nonpigmented variations. South. Med. J., 75:1084, 1982.
47. Minear, W. L.: Xanthomatous joint tumors. J. Bone Joint Surg., 33-A:451, 1951.
48. Mirra, J. M., Finerman, G., and Lindholm, S.: Diffuse pigmented villonodular synovitis in association with Paget's disease of bone. Report of a case. Clin. Orthop., 149:305, 1980.
49. Moroni, A., Innao, V., and Picci, P.: Pigmented villonodular synovitis of the hip. A study of 9 cases. Ital. J. Orthop. Traumatol., 9:331, 1983.
50. Myers, B. W., and Masi, A. T.: Pigmented villonodular synovitis and tenosynovitis: A clinical epidemiologic study of 166 cases and literature review. Medicine (Baltimore), 59:223, 1980.
51. Nilsonne, U., and Moberger, G.: Pigmented villonodular synovitis of joints. Histological and clinical problems in diagnosis. Acta Orthop. Scand., 40:448, 1969.
52. Pandey, S., and Pandey, A. K.: Pigmented villonodular synovitis with bone involvement. Arch. Orthop. Trauma. Surg., 98:217, 1981.
53. Pantazopoulos, T., Stavrou, Z., Stamos, C., Kehayas, G., and Hartofilakidis-Garofalidis, G.: Bone lesions in pigmented villonodular synovitis. Acta Orthop. Scand., 46:579, 1975.
54. Patel, M. R., and Zinberg, E. M.: Pigmented villonodular synovitis of the wrist invading bone—report of a case. J. Hand Surg., 9-A:854, 1984.
55. Peterson, L. F. A., Johnson, E. W., Jr., and Woolner, L. B.: Extra-articular pigmented villonodular synovitis of the knee. Report of a case. Am. J. Clin. Pathol., 30:158, 1958.
56. Present, D. A., Bertoni, F., and Enneking, W. F.: Case report 348. Pigmented villonodular synovitis arising from bursa of the pes anserinus muscle, with secondary involvement of the tibia. Skeletal Radiol., 15:236, 1986.
57. Probst, F. P.: Extra-articular pigmented villonodular synovitis affecting bone. The role of angiography as an aid in its differentiation from similar bone destroying conditions. Radiologe, 13:436, 1973.
58. Rao, A. S., and Vigorita, V. J.: Pigmented villonodular synovitis (giant-cell tumor of the tendon sheath and synovial membrane). A review of eighty-one cases. J. Bone Joint Surg., 66-A:76, 1984.
59. Rein, B. I., Bilodeau, L. P., and Johanson, P.: Arthrography and arteriography in pigmented villonodular synovitis of the knee. A.J.R., 92:1322, 1964.
60. Schajowicz, F., and Blumenfield, I.: Pigmented villonodular synovitis of the wrist with penetration into bone. J. Bone Joint Surg., 50-B:312, 1968.
61. Schumacher, H. R., Lotke, P., Athreya, B., and Rothfuss, S.: Pigmented villonodular synovitis: Light and electron microscopic studies. Semin. Arthritis Rheum., 12:32, 1982.
62. Scott, P. M.: Bone lesions in pigmented villonodular synovitis. J. Bone Joint Surg., 50-B:306, 1968.
63. Shafer, S. J., and Larmon, W. A.: Pigmented villonodular synovitis. A report of seven cases. Surg. Gynecol. Obstet., 92:574, 1951.
64. Shives, T. C., and Ivins, J. C.: Case report 140. Pigmented villonodular synovitis (PVC) right hip. Skeletal Radiol., 6:123, 1981.
65. Smith, J. H., and Pugh, D. C.: Roentgenographic

aspects of articular pigmented villonodular synovitis. A.J.R., 87:1146, 1962.
66. Snook, G. A.: Pigmented villonodular synovitis with bony invasions: A report of two cases. J.A.M.A., 230:410, 1963.
67. Soeur, R.: The synovial membrane of the knee in pathologic conditions. J. Bone Joint Surg., 31-A:317, 1949.
68. Steckel, R. J.: Usefulness of extremity arteriography in special situations. Radiology, 86:293, 1966.
69. Sutton, D.: Arteriography. Edinburgh, Livingstone, 1962.
70. Tartaglia, L., and Chiroff, R. T.: Diffuse pigmented villonodular synovitis. An indication for total hip replacement in the young patient. Clin. Orthop., 115:172, 1976.
71. Torisu, T., Iwabuchi, R., and Kamo, Y.: Pigmented villonodular synovitis of the elbow with bony invasion. Case report. Clin. Orthop., 94:275, 1973.
72. Vigorita, V. J.: Pigmented villonodular synovitis-like lesions in association with rare cases of rheumatoid arthritis, osteonecrosis and advanced degenerative joint disease. Report of five cases. Clin. Orthop., 183:115, 1984.
73. Walls, J. P., and Nogi, J.: Multifocal pigmented villonodular synovitis in a child. J. Pediatr. Orthop., 5:229, 1985.
74. Wiss, D. A.: Recurrent villonodular synovitis of the knee. Successful treatment with yttrium-90. Clin. Orthop., 169:139, 1982.
75. Woods, C., Jr., Alade, C. O., Anderson, V., and Ashby, M. E.: Pigmented villonodular synovitis of the knee presenting as a loose body. A case report. Clin. Orthop., 129:230, 1977.
76. Wright, C. J. E.: Benign giant cell synovioma. An investigation of 85 cases. Br. J. Surg., 38:257, 1951.
77. Young, J. M., and Hudacek, A. G.: Experimental production of pigmented villonodular synovitis in dogs. Am. J. Pathol., 30:799, 1954.
78. Zwierzchowski, H.: Development of bone changes in pigmented villo-nodular synovitis of joints. Chir. Narzadow Ruchu Ortop. Pol., 36:535, 1971.

HEMANGIOMA OF SYNOVIAL MEMBRANE

Synovial hemangioma is a rare lesion that is most probably a hamartoma or a congenital vascular malformation rather than a true neoplasm. It is seen in adolescents and young adults, though often the joint symptoms date back to early childhood. The commonest site is the knee; other joints that are occasionally affected include the ankle, elbow, and shoulder.

Symptoms consist of intermittent pain and periodic swelling of the joint, usually without obvious cause. There may be a history of locking if the knee joint is involved. On examination, often an exquisitely tender mass can be palpated; the tumor is soft and doughy, increasing in size on elevation. Muscle atrophy about the joint is marked. In atrophy of the synovial hemangioma of the knee, atrophy of the quadriceps muscle is extreme and is an important diagnostic clue. Limitation of joint motion may be present. Other associated findings may be the presence of cutaneous hemangiomas and leg length discrepancy.

Radiograms are usually normal and do not usually show calcification. There may be varying degrees of osteoporosis.

Arthrotomy may reveal hemangiomas that are diffuse or localized. The typical gross appearance is that of a grapelike mass underneath a shiny synovial covering (Fig. 4–76 A). Histologically, most synovial hemangiomas are of the mixed capillary and cavernous types, though purely venous and capillary types can occur (Fig. 4–76 B).

Treatment consists of thorough excision of the lesion. This is easily accomplished in the localized form; in the diffuse type, however, it is difficult but should be attempted. The lesions can recur, and in such cases, radiation therapy is given.

References

1. Bennett, G. E., and Cobey, M. C.: Hemangioma of joints. Report of five cases. Arch. Surg., 38:487, 1939.
2. Bouchut, E.: Tumeur érectile de l'articulation du genou. Gaz. Hôp., 29:379, 1856.
3. Cobey, M. C.: Hemangioma of joints. Arch. Surg., 46:465, 1943.
4. DePalma, A. F., and Mauler, G. G.: Hemangioma of synovial membrane. Clin. Orthop., 32:93, 1964.
5. Galimberti, A.: Angioma sinoviale. Arch. Ortop., 79:95, 1961.
6. Halborg, A., Hansen, H., and Sneppen, H. O.: Haemangioma of the knee joint. Acta Orthop. Scand., 39:1223, 1968.
7. Harmon, P. H.: Hemangioma of synovial membrane of the knee joint cured by synovectomy. Arch. Surg., 47:359, 1943.
8. Hunt, A. H., and Todd, I. P.: Cavernous haemangioma of the knee joint. J. Bone Joint Surg., 33-B:106, 1951.
9. Jacobs, J. E., and Lee, F. W.: Hemangioma of the knee joint. J. Bone Joint Surg., 31-A:831, 1949.
10. Karlholm, S., and Stjernsward, J.: Hemangioma of the knee joint. Acta Orthop. Scand., 33:306, 1963.
11. Koch, R. A., and Jackson, D. W.: Juxtaarticular hemangioma of the knee associated with medial synovial plica. A case report. Am. J. Sports Med., 9:265, 1981.
12. Larsen, I. J., and Landry, R. M.: Hemangioma of the synovial membrane. J. Bone Joint Surg., 51-A:1210, 1969.
13. Lewis, R. C., Jr., Coventry, M. B., and Soule, E. H.: Hemangioma of the synovial membrane. J. Bone Joint Surg., 41-A:264, 1959.
14. Linson, M. A., and Posner, I. P.: Synovial hemangioma as a cause of recurrent knee effusions. J.A.M.A., 242:2214, 1979.
15. Randelli, M.: Sull'angioma della sinoviale. Arch. Ortop., 74:353, 1961.
16. Reeves, B.: Hemangioma of the knee joint. Proc. R. Soc. Med., 59:705, 1966.
17. Seimon, L. P., and Hekmat, F.: Synovial hemangioma of the knee. Case report. J. Pediatr. Orthop., 6:356, 1986.
18. Wallace, G. T., and Ghormley, R. K.: Cavernous hemangioma of the knee. Proc. Staff. Meet. Mayo Clin., 18:177, 1943.

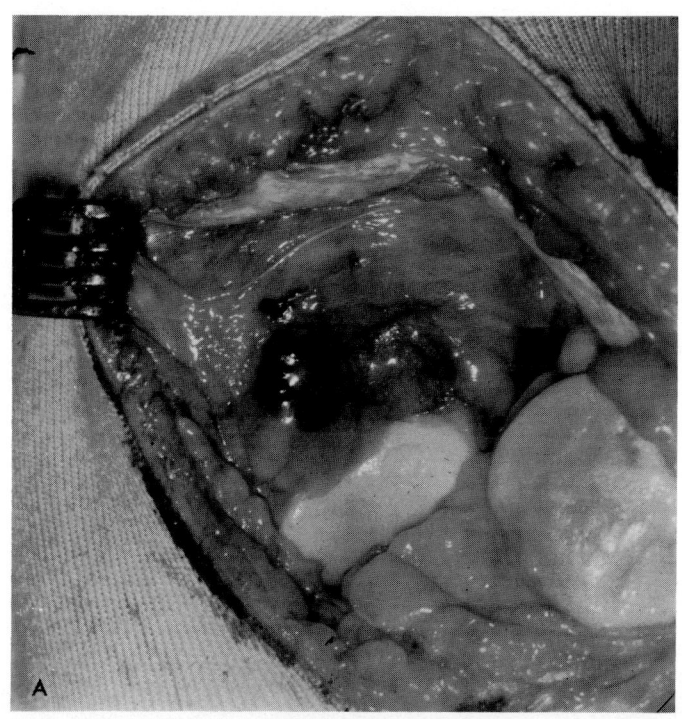
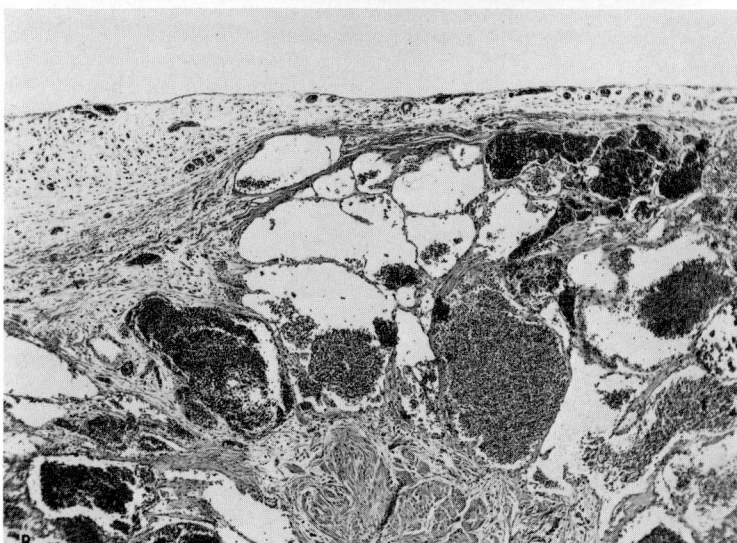

FIGURE 4–76. Hemangioma of synovial membrane.

A. Gross appearance. Note the dark grape-like mass in the subsynovial tissue. **B.** Histologic section showing the abundant cavernous spaces filled with erythrocytes (hematoxylin and eosin, ×50). (From Coventry, M. B., Harrison, E. G., and Martin, J. F.: Benign synovial tumors of the knee: A diagnostic problem. J. Bone Joint Surg., 48-A:1350, 1966. Reprinted by permission.)

19. Zadek, I.: Painful knee due to hemangioma (cured by operation). Bull. Hosp. Joint Dis., 6:29, 1945.

INTRA-ARTICULAR LIPOMA

Lipoma of synovial tissues is a rare tumor originating in the mesenchymal fat cells. Lipomas are often arborescent, with multiple limbs and segments. Their size varies and they are usually slightly encapsulated. Local abnormal swelling is the only clinical finding. They do not cause pain or dysfunction of the joint. The knee is the commonest site of affection. Treatment by surgical excision is usually not indicated.

SYNOVIAL SARCOMA
(Synovioma)

Synovial sarcoma, a highly malignant soft-tissue tumor, originates from synovial tissues but is usually found beyond the confines of the capsule in the para-articular soft tissues of the limbs. The majority of patients are young adults, though the tumor may occur in adolescents and children. The majority of the tumors (85 per cent) are located around the thigh, knee, or hip, or in the shoulder, arm, or elbow. At these sites the synoviomas are large, bulky, and fast-growing; they may be painful. Their sarcomatous nature is suspected at the outset. In about 15 per cent of cases synovioma is located in the hands and feet; in these distal sites the tumors present as small, superficial, soft, fixed masses that grow slowly (or may increase or decrease in size); their sarcomatous nature is not suspected initially. In the hands and feet the tumor may be present for months or a year before diagnosis is made.

Regional lymph node metastasis is not uncommon. The involved nodes are hard, fixed, and nontender, and they enlarge rapidly.

Diagnosis and Staging

Radiograms will disclose the soft-tissue mass, which may show spotty radiopacity representing focal calcification taking place in the tumor tissue.

Scintigraphy with technetium-99m shows increased uptake in the tumor due to microcalcification and revascularization of synovial sarcoma. The zone about the synovium depicts a very active increased reactive uptake. The involved bone and lymph nodes show increased activity.

Computed tomography will depict the soft-tissue tumor and delineate its extent of spread—whether intracompartmental or extracompartmental.

Angiography is of great value in staging. In the early arterial phase there is an active vascular reaction in the soft-tissue tumor and the metastasized regional lymph nodes; in the late venous phase a tumor blush will be visualized.

In gross appearance, the tumor is a semifirm, somewhat encapsulated lesion that measures from 1 to 4 cm. in diameter. The histologic findings consist of closely intermingled fibrosarcomatous and synovial components. The cytologic hallmark of synovioma is the primitive or mesenchymal spindle connective tissue cells lining spaces and clefts, which may contain mucin (Fig. 4–77). Occasionally, the cells are more cylindrical and arranged around spaces resembling cells of epithelial origin.

Treatment

It depends upon the anatomic site and stage of the neoplasm. Small Stage I tumors in the hands or feet are treated by wide excision; if they recur a wide amputation is performed. The large proximally located synovial sarcomas are usually Stage II—they are treated by radical excision.

Postoperative radiation is definitely palliative. The value of chemotherapy is as yet undetermined.

References

1. Archer, I. A., Brown, R. B., and Fitton, J. M.: Epithelioid sarcoma in the hand. J. Hand Surg., 9-B:207, 1984.
2. Ariel, I. M., and Hartley, J.: Level of amputation for patients with soft tissue sarcomas of the extremities as determined by isotopic lymphangiography. Bull. Hosp. Joint Dis., 37:34, 1976.
3. Baretta, G., Bonadonna, G., Bajetta, E., et al.: Combination chemotherapy with DTIC (NSC 45388) in advanced malignant melanoma, soft tissue sarcomas, and Hodgkin's disease. Cancer Treat. Rep., 60:205, 1976.
4. Benjamin, R. S., Gottlieb, J. A., Baker, L. H., et al.: Cyvadic vs. Cyvadact—a randomized trial of cyclophosphamide (Cy), vincristine (V), and adriamycin (A), plus dacarbazine (DIC) or actinomycin-D (DACT), in metastatic sarcomas. Proc. Am. Assoc. Cancer Res. ASCO, 17:256, 1976.
5. Bogumil, G. P., Bruno, P. D., and Barrick, E. F.: Malignant lesions masquerading as popliteal cysts. A report of three cases. J. Bone Joint Surg., 63-A:474, 1981.
6. Buck, P., Mickelson, M. R., and Bonfiglio, M.: Synovial sarcoma: A review of 33 cases. Clin. Orthop., 156:211, 1981.
7. Cadman, N. L., Soule, E. H., and Kelly, P. J.: Synovial

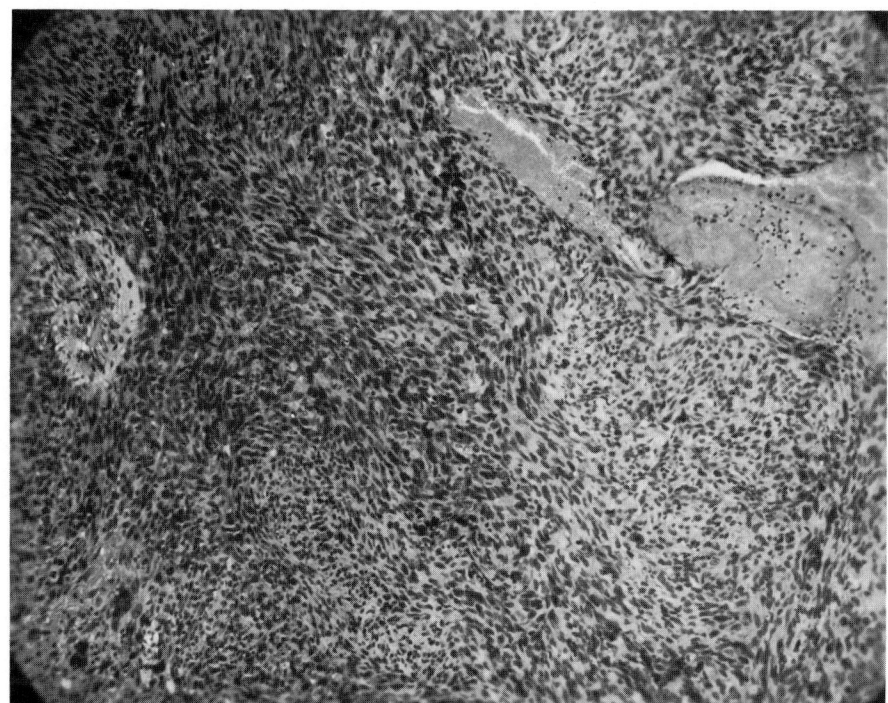

FIGURE 4-77. *Histologic picture of synovioma (× 100).*

sarcoma: An analysis of 134 tumors. Cancer, 18:613, 1965.
8. Campanacci, M., Bertoni, F., and Laus, M.: Soft tissue sarcoma of the hand. Ital. J. Orthop. Traumatol., 7:313, 1981.
9. De Santis, E., Rosa, M. A., Oransky, M., and Sanguinetti, C.: Experimentally induced synovial sarcoma. Int. Orthop., 5:37, 1981.
10. Enneking, W. F., and Shirley, P. D.: Resection-arthrodesis for malignant and potentially malignant lesions about the knee using an intramedullary rod and local bone grafts. J. Bone Joint Surg., 59-A:223, 1977.
11. Greene, T. L., and Strickland, J. W.: Fibroma of tendon sheath. J. Hand Surg., 9-A:758, 1984.
12. Haagensen, C. D., and Stout, A. P.: Synovial sarcoma. Ann. Surg., 120:826, 1944.
13. Hadju, S. I., Shiu, M. H., and Fortner, J. C.: Tendosynovial sarcoma. A clinicopathological study of 136 cases. Cancer, 39:1201, 1977.
14. Hoeffel, J. C., Rolain, G., Preaut, J., et al.: Pseudotumoral aspect of posttraumatic digital synovitis. Am. J. Surg., 134:416, 1977.
15. Ichinose, H., Hoerner, H. E., and Derbes, V. J.: Minute synovial sarcoma in the occult non-palpable phase. A case report. J. Bone Joint Surg., 60-A:836, 1978.
16. Ichinose, H., Wickstrom, J. K., Hoerner, H. E., and Derbes, V. L.: The early clinical presentation of synovial sarcoma. Clin. Orthop., 142:185, 1979.
17. Ishii, S., Yamawaki, S., Saki, T., Usui, M., Ubayama, Y., Minami, A., Yagi, T., Isu, K., and Kobayashi, M.: Characteristics of human soft tissue sarcomas in xenografts and in vitro. Clin. Orthop., 173:251, 1983.
18. Israels, S. J., Chan, H. S., Daneman, A., and Weitzman, S. S.: Synovial sarcoma in childhood. A.J.R., 142:803, 1984.
19. Johnson, R. J., and Garvie, N.: Case report 121: Synovioma (synovial sarcoma) of left knee. Skeletal Radiol., 5:185, 1980.
20. Johnston, A. D., and Parisien, M. V.: Soft tissue tumors about the knee. Orthop. Clin. North Am., 10:263, 1979.
21. Kaufman, J., and Tsukada, Y.: Synovial sarcoma with brain metastasis. Report of a case responding to supervoltage irradiation and review of the literature. Cancer, 38:96, 1976.
22. Lindberg, R. D., Martin, R. M., and Rohmsdahl, M. M.: Surgery and postoperative radiotherapy in the treatment of soft-tissue sarcomas in adults. A.J.R., 123:123, 1975.
23. Lucas, G. L., and Sponsellar, P. D.: Synovial chondrometaplasia of the hand: Case report and review of the literature. J. Hand Surg., 9-A:269, 1984.
24. McClain, E. J., and Wissinger, H. A.: The acute carpal tunnel syndrome: Nine case reports. J. Trauma, 16:75, 1976.
25. MacKenzie, D. H.: Synovial sarcoma. A review of 58 cases. Cancer, 19:169, 1966.
26. McNeer, G. P., Cantin, J., Chu, F., et al.: The effectiveness of radiation therapy in the management of sarcoma of the soft somatic tissues. Cancer, 22:391, 1968.
27. Mayer, D. P., Clancy, M., Bonakdarpour, A., Peterson, R. O., and Steel, H. H.: Case report 152: Synovial sarcoma of the knee. Skeletal Radiol., 6:221, 1981.
28. Morton, D. L., Eilber, F. R., Townsend, C. M., et al.: Limb salvage from a multi-disciplinary treatment approach for skeletal and soft-tissue sarcomas of the extremity. Ann. Surg., 184:268, 1976.
29. Murray, J. A.: Synovial sarcoma. Orthop. Clin. North Am., 8:963, 1977.
30. Pack, G. T., and Ariel, I. M.: Synovial sarcoma (malignant synovioma): A report of 60 cases. Surgery, 28:1047, 1950.
31. Patchefsky, A. S., Goriano, R., and Kostianovsky, M.: Epithelioid sarcoma: Ultrastructural similarity to nodular synovitis. Cancer, 39:143, 1977.
32. Pinedo, H. M., and Kenis, Y.: Chemotherapy of ad-

vanced soft tissue sarcomas in adults. Cancer Treat. Rev., 4:67, 1977.
33. Robertson, D. I., and Hogg, G. R.: Chordoid sarcoma: Ultrastructure evidence supporting a synovial origin. Cancer, 45:520, 1980.
34. Rosenberg, S. A., Kent, H., Costa, J., et al.: Prospective randomized evaluation of the role of limb-sparing surgery, radiation therapy, and adjuvant chemoimmunotherapy in the treatment of adult soft-tissue sarcomas. Surgery, 84:62, 1978.
35. Russell, W. O., Cohen, J., Enzinger, F., et al.: A clinical and pathologic staging system for soft-tissue sarcomas. Cancer, 40:1562, 1977.
36. Ryan, J. R., Baker, L. H., and Benjamin, R. S.: The natural history of metastatic synovial sarcoma: Experience of the Southwest Oncology group. Clin. Orthop., 164:257, 1982.
37. Schiffman, R.: Epithelioid sarcoma and synovial sarcoma in the same knee. Cancer, 45:158, 1980.
38. Shiraishi, S., Ohkubo, Y., and Saito, T.: Regression of multiple osseous metastatic renal cell carcinoma. Clin. Orthop., 138:246, 1979.
39. Shiu, M. H., Castro, E. B., Hadju, S. I., et al.: Surgical treatment of 297 soft-tissue sarcomas of the lower extremity. Ann. Surg., 123:577, 1975.
40. Shiu, M. H., McCormack, P. M., Hadju, S. I., et al.: Surgical treatment of tendosynovial sarcoma. Cancer, 43:889, 1979.
41. Simon, M. A., and Enneking, W. F.: Management of soft-tissue sarcomas of the extremities. J. Bone Joint Surg., 58-A:317, 1976.
42. Simon, M. A., Spanier, S. S., and Enneking, W. F.: Management of adult soft-tissue sarcomas of the extremities. Surg. Annu., 11:363, 1979.
43. Sugarbaker, P. H., Weiss, C. M., Davidson, D. D., and Roth, Y. F.: Increasing phantom limb pain as a symptom of cancer recurrence. Cancer, 54:373, 1984.
44. Suit, H. D., and Russell, W. O.: Soft part tumors. Cancer, 39:830, 1977.
45. Suit, H. D., Russell, W. O., and Martin, R. G.: Management of patients with sarcoma of soft-tissue in an extremity. Cancer, 31:1247, 1973.
46. Suit, H. D., Russell, W. O., and Martin, R. G.: Sarcoma of soft-tissue; Clinical and histopathologic parameters and response to treatment. Cancer, 35:1478, 1975.
47. Suit, H. D., Proppe, K. H., Mankin, H. J., et al.: Preoperative radiation therapy for sarcoma of soft tissue. Cancer, 47:2269, 1981.
48. Sutro, C. J.: Synovial sarcoma of the soft parts of the 1st toe: Recurrence after a 35 year interval. Bull. Hosp. Joint Dis., 37:105, 1976.
49. Thunold, J., and Baug, G.: Synovial sarcoma: A case report. Acta Orthop. Scand., 47:231, 1976.
50. Urist, M. R., Grant, T. T., Lindholm, T. S., Mirra, J. M., Hirano, H., and Finerman, G. A. M.: Induction of new bone formation in the host bed by human bone-tumor transplants in athymic nude mice. J. Bone Joint Surg., 61-A:1207, 1979.
51. Varela-Duran, J., and Enzinger, F. M.: Calcifying synovial sarcoma. Cancer, 50:345, 1982.
52. Waag, K. L., et al.: Synovial sarcoma in childhood. Z. Kinderchir., 39:Suppl. 1:48, 1984.
53. Wittels, M., Ghandur-Mnaymneh, L., and Mnaymneh, W.: Giant cell tumor of tendon sheath developing at the site of tendon laceration. Clin. Orthop., 169:207, 1982.
54. Wright, P. H., Sim, F. H., Soule, E. H., and Taylor, W. F.: Synovial sarcoma. J. Bone Joint Surg., 64-A:112, 1982.

Index

Note: Page numbers in *italics* refer to illustrations; page numbers in boldface refer to surgical plates. Page numbers followed by the letter t refer to tables.

A

Abdominal circumference, in relation to age, in females, 78t
　in males, 77t
Abduction, definition of, 33
Abductor digiti quinti manus transfer of Littler, 2057, **2070–2071**
Abductor pollicis brevis, congenital absence of, 288–289, *288–290*
Abscess, in tuberculosis of spine, 1449, *1451*
Acetabular augmentation, Staheli's, in congenital dysplasia of hip in adolescent, 522–526, *524–525*
Acetabular index, in congenital dysplasia of hip, 322
　preoperative, in Salter's innominate osteotomy, 414–415
Acetabular torsion, computed tomography of, in congenital dysplasia of hip, 364, *366–367*
Acetabuloplasty, in congenital dysplasia of hip, 422–423
Acetabulum, in congenital dysplasia of hip in adolescent, 468, *469*
　labrum of, rose thorn in arthrography of, 351–352, *352*
　torn, in Legg-Calvé-Perthes disease, 988
　primary dysplasia of, in congenital dysplasia of hip, 302
　secondary dysplasia of, in congenital dysplasia of hip, 311–312
Achard's syndrome, Marfan's syndrome vs., 839
Achilles tendon, anterior advancement of, 1675, *1675*, **1678–1679**, *1680*
　sliding lengthening of, 1666, *1667*, **1668–1669**, *1670*
　subcutaneous lengthening of, 1666, *1671*
　transfer of, in talipes equinovarus, 2512
　Z-lengthening of, 1666, *1671*
Achondrogenesis, 730
Achondroplasia, 720–727
　clinical picture in, 721, *722–725*, *726*
　diagnosis in, 726–727
　etiology of, 721
　pathology in, 721
　prognosis and treatment in, 727

Achondroplasia (*Continued*)
　pseudoachondroplasia vs., 751t
　radiographic findings in, 722–727, *726*
Acidosis, in vitamin D refractory rickets, 908, 910
Acrocephalosyndactylism, 236–240, *237–239*
Acrocephalosyndactyly, 855–856
Acromioclavicular dislocation, 3041
Acromion process, fracture of, 3044
Actinomycosis, of bone, 1129
Adamantinoma, 1301–1304
　clinical features of, 1301
　differential diagnosis of, 1301
　pathologic findings in, 1301, *1303*
　radiography in, 1301, *1302–1303*
　treatment of, 1303–1304
Adams' forward bending test, in scoliosis, 2275–2277, *2276*
Adduction, definition of, 33
Adductor longus, in gait, 14
Adductor magnus, in gait, 14
Adductor myotomy, and obturator neurectomy, of Banks and Green, **1638–1641**
Adductor pollicis, release of, **1726–1729**, *1730*
Adiadochokinesia, in cerebral palsy, 1613
A-frame, in myelomeningocele, 1855, *1856*
Africoid talus, 2416, *2619*
Age, normal measurements in relation to, female, 78t
　male, 77t
Airway, in anesthesia, in juvenile rheumatoid arthritis, 69
Alpha-fetoprotein, in antenatal testing for myelomeningocele, 1776
Ambulation. See *Gait*.
Amikacin, in septic arthritis, 1424t
Aminoaciduria, in vitamin D refractory rickets, 908, 910
Amniocentesis, in myelomeningocele, 1776
Amphotericin B, in septic arthritis, 1424t
Ampicillin, in septic arthritis, 1424t
Amputation, below-knee, **1350–1353**
　elbow disarticulation, **1376–1379**
　forequarter (Littlewood), **1354–1367**
　hemipelvectomy (Banks and Coleman), **1318–1325**

Amputation *(Continued)*
  hip disarticulation, **1326–1335**
  in bone tumor, 1159, *1160*
  ischial-bearing above-knee (mid-thigh), **1336–1345**
  knee disarticulation, **1346–1349**
  shoulder disarticulation, **1368–1371**
  through arm, **1372–1375**
Amstutz and Wilson's osteotomy, in coxa vara, *594*, 595
Amyloidosis, in rheumatoid arthritis, 1473
Analgia, congenital or hereditary, 1992–1999
Anemia, 1135–1139
  Cooley's, 1136–1139, *1137–1138*
  Fanconi's, 1135
  Mediterranean, 1136–1139, *1137–1138*
  preoperative, 67
Anesthesia, in arthrogryposis, 69
  in cerebral palsy, 70
  in Duchenne's muscular dystrophy, 68
  in hemophilia, 71
  in juvenile rheumatoid arthritis, 69
  in kyphoscoliosis, 70–71
  in muscular dystrophy, 68
  in myelomeningocele, 69
  in myotonia, 68
  in osteogenesis imperfecta, 68–69
  in sickle cell disease, 71
  malignant hyperthermia syndrome in, 71–73
  preoperative assessment for, 67–68
  preoperative consultation in, 74
  risks of, 75
Angular deformity, terminology in, 31–32
Ankle. See also under individual disorders.
  ball-and-socket, congenital, 2631–2632, *2632*
  flail, in myelomeningocele, 1817
  fracture of, 3302–3336
    anatomic classification of, 3303
    classification and mechanism of injury in, 3303–3323
    complications of, 3331–3336
      lateral rotation deformity as, 3335
      premature closure of physis as, 3331–3335, *3332–3334*
      valgus deformity as, 3335–3336, *3335–3336*
    mechanistic classification of, 3303, 3306, 3316
      in pronation-eversion-lateral rotation injury, 3316, *3319–3320*
      in supination-inversion injury, 3306, *3307–3314*
      in supination-lateral rotation fracture, 3306, 3316, *3316–3318*
      in supination-plantar flexion injury, 3306, *3314–3315*
    of Carothers and Crenshaw, *3305*, 3306
    of Dias and Tachdjian, 3306, 3309t
    of Tillaux in adolescent, 3316, 3321, *3321–3322*
    treatment of, 3323, 3327–3331
      in adolescent fracture of Tillaux, 3330, *3331*
      in epiphyseal separation, 3327
      in pronation-eversion-lateral rotation injury, 3330, *3330*
      in supination-inversion injury, 3328, *3328*
      in supination-lateral rotation injury, *3329*, 3330
      in supination-plantar flexion injury, 3328–3330, *3329*
    triplane of distal tibia, 3321, 3323, *3323–3327*
  in arthrogryposis multiplex congenita, 2099
  in cerebral palsy, 1660–1705. See also *Cerebral palsy, foot and ankle in.*
  in multiple exostosis, 1173, *1178–1179*
  in myelomeningocele, 1795–1817
  in poliomyelitis, 1937–1957

Ankle *(Continued)*
  motion in gait of, 11, *11*
  paralytic deformities of, tendon transfers for, 1940t–1941t
  position of minimal intra-articular pressure for, 1410
  valgus, in myelomeningocele, 1804–1805, *1805*, **1806–1807**, *1808–1809*
Ankle-foot orthosis–posterior splint, in myelomeningocele, 1855
Ankylosing spondylitis, juvenile, pauciarticular, 1470
Ankylosis, fibrous, in hemophilic arthropathy, 1497, *1498*
  in septic arthritis in neonate hip, 1431, *1433*
  of lower limb joints, gait in, 24
Antalgic limp, 24
Antenatal diagnosis, in myelomeningocele, 1776
Anterior horn cell degeneration, electromyography in, 65
Apert's syndrome, 236–240, *237–239*, 855–856
  tarsal coalition in, 2581, *2584*
Apophyseodesis, Langenskiöld's, of greater trochanter, 441–442, **444–449**
Apophysis, vertebral, slipped, 2404
Apophysitis, of os calcis, 1016
Arachnodactyly. See also *Marfan's syndrome*.
  congenital contractural, 837–839
    clinical features of, 837–839, *838–839*
    differential diagnosis of, 839
    treatment of, 839
Arm. See also *Forearm; Limb*.
  epiphyseal closure in, *61*
  epiphyseal ossification in, *60*
  in cerebral palsy, 1717, 1722–1747. See also *Cerebral palsy, arm in*.
  length of, measurement of, 31
  longitudinal deficiencies of, 105, *110–111*
  terminal transverse deficiencies of, 105, *108*
  wringer injury to, 3210–3211
Arnold-Chiari malformation, 1980t
Around the world hip motion machine, in Legg-Calvé-Perthes disease, 977, *978*
Arthritis, gonococcal, 1441–1442
  in viral disease, 1459
  Lyme, 1440–1441
  pyogenic, joint fluid analysis in, 1414t
    Legg-Calvé-Perthes disease vs., 957
  rheumatoid, 1466–1486. See also *Rheumatoid arthritis*.
  septic, 1415–1435
    acute transient synovitis vs., 1464t
    antibiotic therapy in, 1422–1424, 1423t–1424t
    cartilage destruction in, 1417–1419
    clinical picture in, 1419
    community-acquired, 1416
    diagnosis of, 1420–1421
    differential diagnosis of, 1421–1422
    etiologic organisms in, 1416, 1417t
    hospital-acquired, 1416
    in neonatal hip, 1428–1435
      clinical features of, 1428, *1429*
      complications of, 1431
      gross pathology in, 1428, *1428*
      imaging in, 1428–1430, *1430*
      laboratory findings in, 1430–1431
      osteomyelitis and, 1433–1434
      surgical therapy in, 1431–1434
      treatment of, 1431
    in pre-existing joint disease, 1435
    in pyogenic osteomyelitis, 1103
    joint drainage in, 1424, **1425–1426**, 1427
      arthroscope in, 1427
      arthrotomy in, 1427

Volume 1, pgs. 1–687; Volume 2, pgs. 688–1600; Volume 3, pgs. 1601–2404; Volume 4, pgs. 2405–3373

Arthritis (Continued)
        technique for hip in, **1425–1426**
    joint fluid analysis in, 1421
    local joint care in, 1427
    Lyme disease vs., 1440
    pathogenesis of, 1415–1416
    pathology of, 1416–1419, *1418–1419*
    prognosis in, 1427
    radiography in, 1419–1420, *1420*
    radionuclide imaging in, 1420
    treatment of, 1422–1427
    ultrasonography in, 1420
  traumatic, joint fluid analysis in, 1413t
  tuberculous, 1443–1454
    clinical features of, 1443–1445
    joint fluid analysis in, 1414t
    laboratory findings in, 1446–1447
    of spine, 1449–1454. See also *Tuberculosis, of spine.*
    pathology in, 1443, *1444*
    radiography in, 1445–1446, *1445–1446*
    treatment of, 1447–1449
      conservative, 1448
      drug therapy in, 1447–1448
      general medical, 1447
      surgical, 1448–1449
Arthrogryposis multiplex congenita, 2086–2114
  anesthesia in, 69
  classification of, 2087, 2097
    amyoplasia in, 2087, *2089–2096*
    areas of involvement in, 2088t
    distal involvement in, 2087, 2097
    joint contractures with body involvement in, 2097
    joint contractures with central nervous system dysfunction in, 2097
    limb involvement in, 2087, *2089–2096*, 2097
  etiology of, 2086–2087
  historical, 2086
  neurogenic subtypes in, 2098
  pathology in, 2097–2098
  talipes equinovarus in, 2452, *2452*
  treatment of, 2098–2114
    elbow in, 2101–2103, *2102*, **2104–2111**
      anterior transfer of triceps brachii in, 2103, **2104–2107**
      pectoralis major transfer for flexor paralysis in, 2103, **2108–2111**
    fingers in, 2113
    foot-ankle in, 2099
    hip in, 2100–2101
    knee in, 2099–2100
    spine in, 2113–2114
    thumb in, 2112–2113
    wrist in, 2112
Arthro-ophthalmopathy, hereditary progressive, 716
Arthroscopy, 59
Aseptic necrosis, in congenital dysplasia of hip in adolescent, 469
  of bone, 689
  of proximal femur, due to Pavlik harness treatment, 339
ASNIS guided screw system, in slipped femoral capital epiphysis, 1032–1033, **1034–1043**
Asphyxiating thoracic dysplasia, 737, *738*
Asthma, preoperative precautions in, 67
Asynergy, in cerebral palsy, 1613
Ataxia, cerebellar, gait in, 26
  Friedreich's, gait in, 26
  in cerebral palsy, 1612–1613
  spinal, gait in, 26
Ataxia telangiectasia, 1980t

Ataxic gait, 26
Athetosis, in cerebral palsy, 1612
Atlantoaxial joint, instability of, in Down's syndrome, 891–892
  rotatory subluxation of, 3345
Atlas, anterior dislocation of, with fracture of odontoid process, 3345
Atrophy, muscle, 1411
Avascular necrosis, due to Salter's innominate osteotomy, 418
  in sickle cell disease, 1144
  in slipped femoral capital epiphysis, 1068–1073
  of femoral head, in septic arthritis in neonate hip, 1431

B

Baker horizontal calcaneal osteotomy, 1703, *1704*
Baker technique, of gastrocnemius lengthening, 1667, *1673*
Balance, in cerebral palsy, 1613
Banks and Coleman hemipelvectomy, in osteogenic sarcoma, **1318–1325**
Banks and Green obturator neurectomy and adductor myotomy, **1638–1641**
Barlow's test, 314, *315*
Barr erector spinae transfer, in gluteus maximus paralysis, *1926*, 1926–1927
Basilar impression, 2232
Basilar invagination, 2232
Bassen-Kornzweig syndrome, 1980t
Batchelor subtalar extra-articular arthrodesis, 1700–1702, *1701*
Battered child, 3366–3370, *3368–3370*
Below-knee amputation, in osteogenic sarcoma, **1350–1353**
Biceps brachii tendon rerouting of Zancolli, 2057, **2058–2061**
Biceps femoris, in gait, 14
Bilhaut-Cloquet procedure, in preaxial polydactyly, *254*, 255
Biopsy, in bone tumor, 1161
  in eosinophilic granuloma of bone, 1284
  in osteogenic sarcoma, 1315
Birth history, 3–4
Birth injury, 3352–3357. See also *Obstetrical injury.*
Birth order, in congenital dysplasia of hip, 303
Blastomycosis, of bone, 1129
Bleb theory, in Sprengel's deformity, 136–137
Blood chemistry, normal, 93t–94t
Blood loss, in kyphoscoliosis surgery, 70
Blood values, normal, 92t
Blount's disease, 2835–2848. See also *Tibia vara.*
  genu varum vs., 2824, 2826t
Body righting reflex, 51
Bone, 688–1409
  aneurysmal cyst of, 1251–1255. See also *Bone cyst, aneurysmal.*
  aseptic necrosis of, 689
  dysplasia of. See also individual types.
    biochemical studies in, 700–701
    bone biopsy in, 701
    history and physical examination in, 695, *696–699*, 700
    roentgenography in, 700
    terminology and classification of, 690, 690t, *691–692*, 693t–694t, 694–695

Bone *(Continued)*
    fibrous defect of, 1246–1249, *1247*
    fungal infection of, 1129–1130
    growth of, 2852–2867. See also *Growth*.
    infection of. See *Osteomyelitis*.
    long, fracture of shaft of, obstetrical, 3353
        longitudinal growth of, 2852
        radiography for measurement of, 2867–2870, *2868–2870*
    modeling of, terminology in, *691*
    physiologic responses of, 688–690, *689*
        circulatory disturbances and, 689
        function and, 688, *689*
        injury (repair) and, 689–690
        muscular action and, 688
        radiation and, 690
        use and disuse and, 688–689
    radionuclide imaging of, 59
    syphilis of, 1124–1125, *1124–1126*
    tuberculosis of, 1127–1128, *1127–1128*
Bone aspiration, in pyogenic osteomyelitis, 1093
Bone cyst, aneurysmal, 1251–1255
    age and sex distribution in, 1252
    bone imaging in, 1255
    clinical features in, 1252
    complications of, 1255
    diagnosis of, 1255
    etiology of, 1251–1252
    of metatarsal, 2780, *2785*
    pathology in, 1252, *1253*
    radiography in, 1252, *1254*, 1254–1255
    sites of involvement in, 1252
    treatment of, 1255
    unicameral bone cyst vs., 1261
unicameral, 1258–1272
    aneurysmal bone cyst vs., 1261
    clinical findings in, 1259
    complications of, 1270–1272, *1271*
    differential diagnosis in, 1261, 1264
    enchondroma vs., 1264
    eosinophilic granuloma vs., 1261, 1264
    epiphyseal involvement in, 1271–1272
    etiology of, 1258–1259
    giant cell tumor vs., 1264
    growth retardation in, 1271
    malignant change in, 1271
    of hindfoot, 2780, *2786–2787*
    pathologic fracture in, 1270–1271, *1271*
    pathology in, 1259, *1260*
    radiography in, 1259–1261, *1261–1263*
    sites of involvement in, 1258
    solitary fibrous dysplasia vs., 1264
    treatment of, 1264–1270
        corticosteroids in, 1264–1265
        curettage and bone grafting in, **1266–1269**, 1270
        decompression by multiple drilling in, 1265, 1270
        subtotal resection and bone grafting in, 1270
Bone infarction, in sickle cell disease, 1140, *1141*
Bone tumor, 1150–1161
    amputation in, 1159, *1160*
    anatomic site of, 1151–1152, 1152t–1153t
    angiography in, 1155
    biopsy in, 1161
    classification of, 1150, 1150t
    clinical picture in, 1150–1151
    computed tomography in, 1155
    host tissue response in diagnosis of, 1154t
    intravenous pyelography in, 1155
    isotope scans in, 1153–1155

Bone tumor *(Continued)*
    gallium-67 citrate in, 1154–1155
    technetium polyphosphonate in, 1154
    laboratory tests in, 1155–1156
    liver-spleen scan in, 1155
    local surgical procedures in, 1159, *1160*
    lymphangiography in, 1155
    magnetic resonance imaging in, 1155
    principles of surgical management of, 1158–1159, 1159t, *1160*
    radiographic features in, 1151–1153
    staging of, *1156–1157*, 1156–1158, 1157t–1158t
    surgical margins and excision type in, 1159, 1159t
    surgical margins and pathology of, 1159, 1159t
    treatment of, 1159–1161
Borden, Spencer, and Herndon's osteotomy, in coxa vara, 595
Boston brace, in scoliosis, 2300–2301, *2301*
Bowing, angulation of, 31–32
Boyes technique, 2057, **2072–2073**
Brachial plexus palsy, obstetrical, 2009–2079
    classification of, 2009–2010
    clinical features of, 2010–2011, *2012–2013*
    differential diagnosis of, 2013–2014
    elbow in, 2022–2023, *2024–2025*, 2046, 2053
    Erb-Duchenne type, 2011
    etiology of, 2009, *2010–2011*
    forearm in, 2023, *2026*, 2026–2027, 2053, **2054–2055**, 2057, **2058–2079**
        abductor digiti quinti manus transfer of Littler for, 2057, **2070–2071**
        biceps brachii tendon rerouting of Zancolli for, 2057, **2058–2061**
        Boyes technique for, 2057, **2072–2073**
        extensor pollicis brevis tendon transfer to extensor tendon of ulna for, 2057, **2074–2075**
        index finger abduction restoration of Phalen for, 2057, **2076–2077**
        intermetacarpal bone block for thenar paralysis in, 2057, **2078–2079**
        soft tissue release for supination deformity of, 2053, **2054–2055**, 2057
        thumb opposition restoration of Brand for, 2057, **2068–2069**
        thumb opposition restoration of Riordan for, 2057, **2062–2067**
    Klumpke type, 2011
    prognosis and natural history of, 2013
    shoulder in, asynergy or dyskinesia of, 2014
        classification of sequelae of, 2014, 2015t
        Green's modified Sever-L'Episcopo procedure for, 2028, **2030–2039**
        lateral rotation-abduction contracture of, 2021, *2022*, 2046, *2047*, 2052
        lateral rotation osteotomy of humerus in, 2046, **2048–2051**
        latissimus dorsi and teres major transfer to rotator cuff for, 2029, **2042–2045**
        medial rotation-adduction contracture of, 2014, *2016–2021*, 2027–2029, **2030–2041**
        pure abduction contracture of, 2021–2022, *2023*, 2046
        Putti's scapular elevation sign in, 2014, *2016–2018*
        residual deformities of, 2014, 2021–2022
        subscapularis muscle recession at origin for, 2028–2029, **2040–2041**
        total flaccid paralysis of, 2022
Brachioradialis transfer, for thumb abduction and extension, **1734–1737**

Brachymesophalangy, 283
Brachymetacarpalia, 283
Brachymetatarsia, 2633, *2634–2636*, 2637
Brachytelephalangy, 283
Brain, in myelomeningocele, 1778
Brand thumb opposition restoration, 2057, **2068–2069**
Braumann's angle, 3066, *3066*
Breech posture, development of, 2422, *2423*
Breech presentation, in congenital dysplasia of hip, 302–303, *303*
Brevicollis, 128–136. See also *Klippel-Feil syndrome*.
Brown's fibulofemoral arthroplasty, in congenital longitudinal deficiency of tibia, 643, *645*, **646–649**
Brucellar osteomyelitis, 1123–1124
Bryant's traction, in congenital dysplasia of hip, 343, *344*
  in femoral shaft fracture, *3256–3259*, 3256–3261
  modified, in femoral shaft fracture, *3261*, 3261–3262
Buck-Gramcko technique, **262–267**
Buckminister Brown brace, in congenital torticollis, *119*
Bunion, *2626–2628*, 2626–2629
  dorsal, in poliomyelitis, 1945, *1946–1948*, *1950–1951*
Bursitis, 2181–2182
  infectious or suppurative, 2182
  traumatic, 2181–2182

C

Cadence, 6
Café-au-lait spots, in fibrous dysplasia, 1229
  in neurofibromatosis, 1290, *1290*
Caffey's disease, 817–824. See also *Cortical hyperostosis, infantile*.
Caffey's sign, in Legg-Calvé-Perthes disease, 949
Caisson disease, 689
Calcaneal lateral wedge resection, of Dwyer, in pes cavus, 2700–2701, **2702–2703**
Calcaneal osteotomy, Baker's horizontal, 1703, *1704*
  Dwyer's, 1702–1703
  in talipes equinovarus, 2517, **2518–2519**, 2520–2521
Calcaneocuboid synostosis, 2579
Calcaneofibular tenodesis, in myelomeningocele, 1805, **1806–1807**
Calcaneonavicular coalition, 2601, **2602–2607**, 2608
Calcaneus, fracture of, 3341
  in talipes equinovarus, 2435
  unicameral bone cyst of, 2780, *2786*
Calcification, of intervertebral disc, 2391–2393, *2392*
Calcinosis, of foot, 2780, *2780*
Calcium, vitamin D metabolism and, 897–898
Callotasis, for lengthening of femur, 2896
  for lengthening of tibia, 2896, **2960–2971**
Campanacci syndrome, 1242–1246, *1243–1245*
Campylodactyly, 284–285
  diagnosis of, 284–285, *285*
  disorders associated with, 284t
  etiology of, 284
  treatment of, 285, *286*
Camurati-Engelmann disease, 804–807, *805*
  clinical features of, 804
  differential diagnosis of, 806
  etiology and heredity in, 804
  infantile cortical hyperostosis vs., 806
  pathology in, 804, *805*
  radiography and scintigraphy in, 806
  treatment of, 806–807

Carbenicillin, in septic arthritis, 1424t
Cardiovascular system, in Klippel-Feil syndrome, 131
  in Marfan's syndrome, 832
Carpenter's syndrome, 856
Carpus, centralization over distal ulna of, 199–205, **200–203**
  stabilization of, in Madelung's deformity, 221
Cartilage, articular, nutrition of, 1411
  destruction of, in septic arthritis, 1417–1419
Cartilaginous exostosis, multiple, 1172–1190. See also *Exostosis, multiple*.
Caster cart, in myelomeningocele, 1855, *1855*
Cat-scratch fever, 1133
Cavovarus deformity, in arthrogryposis multiplex congenita, 2099
Cavovarus test, 2681, *2682–2683*
Cavus deformity, in myelomeningocele, *1816*, 1816–1817
Cefotaxime, in septic arthritis, 1424t
Ceftriaxone, in septic arthritis, 1424t
Cefuroxime, in septic arthritis, 1424t
Cellulitis, pyogenic osteomyelitis vs., 1092–1093
  septic arthritis vs., 1422
Cephalothin, in septic arthritis, 1424t
Cerebellar ataxia, dentate, 1980t
  gait in, 26, 1613
  hereditary, 1980t
Cerebellar disorders, differentiation of, 1602t-1603t, 1604
Cerebellar tumor, 1980t
Cerebral cortex, developmental changes in, 42
Cerebral palsy, 1605–1757
  anesthesia in, 70
  arm in, 1717, 1722–1747
    abduction contracture of shoulder in, 1747, *1747*, *1754*
    cosmetic appearance of, 1717, 1722, *1722*
    finger deformities in, 1738–1744
      flexion, 1738–1739, *1740–1743*
      swan-neck, 1739, *1744*
      Swanson sublimis tenodesis of proximal interphalangeal joints in, 1739, *1744*
    flexion deformity of elbow in, 1746–1747
    flexion deformity of wrist in, *1744–1745*, 1744–1746, **1748–1753**
    function of, 1717
    Green's flexor carpi ulnaris transfer in, 1746, **1748–1753**
    preoperative assessment of, 1717
    pronation contracture of forearm in, 1746
    thumb-in-palm deformity of, 1722–1738
      adductor myotomy of thumb in, 1730, **1732–1733**
      adductor pollicis release in, **1726–1729**, 1730
      bivalved long arm cast in, 1730, *1730*
      brachioradialis transfer in, **1734–1737**
      extensor pollicis longus rerouting in, 1731
      metacarpophalangeal capsulorrhaphy in, 1731, 1738
      opponens splint in, 1724, *1725*
      tendon transfers for thumb motor function in, 1730–1731
      treatment of, 1724–1738
      types of, 1722–1724, *1724*
  classification of, 1605t-1608t, 1605–1608
    American, 1605, 1605t
    Crothers and Paine's, 1606, 1608t
    Ingram and Balf's, 1606, 1608t
    Minear's, 1606, 1607t
    Perlstein's, 1606, 1606t
  clinical features of, 1614–1620
    epilepsy in, 1616

Cerebral palsy (Continued)
  extrapyramidal, 1617–1620, 1619
  intelligence and speech in, 1616
  sensory deficits in, 1615–1616
  spastic diplegia in, 1616–1617
  spastic hemiplegia in, 1614–1615, 1614–1616
  spastic quadriplegia in, 1617, 1618
 definition of, 1605
 distribution of paralysis in, 1606, 1608
 drooling in, 1756–1757
 etiology of, 1608–1610
  birth injury in, 1608–1609
   hypoxic, 1609
   toxic, 1609
   traumatic, 1609
  developmental malformations in, 1609–1610
  neurologic sequelae of, 1610t
  postnatal causes of, 1610
 foot and ankle in, 1660–1705
  conservative management of, 1663, 1665
  equinovalgus in, 1661, 1663, 1663
   treatment of, 1692–1703
  equinovarus in, 1663, 1664
   treatment of, 1680–1692
  equinus deformity in, 1660–1661, 1661–1662
   treatment of, 1665–1680
  hip and knee flexion contracture and, 1663, 1666
  surgical treatment of, 1665–1705
   anterior heel cord advancement in, 1675, 1675, **1678–1679**, 1680
   anterior transfer of posterior tibial tendon in, 1680–1681, 1686, 1686–1687
   Baker's horizontal calcaneal osteotomy in, 1703, 1704
   Dwyer's calcaneal osteotomy in, 1702–1703
   extensor hallucis longus rerouting in, 1680, **1682–1685**
   gastrocnemius lengthening of Baker technique in, 1667, 1673
   gastrocnemius lengthening of Vulpius technique in, 1666–1667, 1672
   gastrocnemius recession of Silverskiöld in, 1667, 1673
   gastrocnemius recession of Strayer in, 1667, 1674
   in calcaneus deformity, 1703, 1705
   in equinovalgus, 1692–1703
   in equinovarus, 1680–1692
   in equinus deformity, 1665–1680
   in forefoot and toe involvement, 1703, 1705
   peroneus brevis fractional lengthening in, 1693
   proximal gastrocnemius recession in, 1674, 1675
   sliding heel cord lengthening in, 1666, 1667, **1668–1669**, 1670
   sliding lengthening of posterior tibial tendon in, 1680, 1681
   split transfer of anterior tibial tendon in, 1687, 1692, 1692
   split transfer of posterior tibial tendon in, 1686–1687, 1688–1691
   subcutaneous lengthening of Achilles tendon in, 1666, 1671
   subtalar extra-articular arthrodesis of Batchelor in, 1700–1702, 1701
   subtalar extra-articular arthrodesis of Grice in, 1693, **1694–1697**, 1698–1699, 1698–1700
   tibial neurectomy in, 1674–1675, **1676–1677**
   Z-lengthening of Achilles tendon in, 1666, 1671
  testing triceps surae in, 1660–1661, 1661
  tibial muscle voluntary contraction in, 1663, 1665

Cerebral palsy (Continued)
  toe-toe-gait in, 1661, 1662
 hip in, 1627–1660
  adduction-flexion deformity of, 1628–1630, 1629–1632
  flexion-adduction deformity of, treatment of, 1637, **1638–1641**, 1642–1643, 1644–1645
  medial rotation deformity of, 1630, 1633, 1634
  subluxation and dislocation of, 1633–1637
   clinical features of, 1635–1637
   pathogenesis of, 1634–1635, 1635–1636
   prevalence of, 1633, 1633t
  surgical management of, 1627–1628
  treatment of, 1637–1660
   adductor myotomy and obturator neurectomy of Banks and Green in, **1638–1641**
   arthrodesis or arthroplasty in, 1648
   conservative, 1637
   derotation osteotomy of femur in, 1651, 1660
   Girdlestone procedure in, 1647–1648
   in anterior dislocation, 1648, 1650
   in dislocation, 1646–1647, 1647–1649
   in flexion-adduction deformity, 1637, **1638–1641**, 1642–1643, 1644–1645
   in medial rotation deformity, 1650–1651, **1652–1659**, 1660
   in subluxation, 1645–1646
   intrapelvic obturator neurectomy in, 1645
   pelvic obliquity due to, 1660
   posterior transfer of hip adductors to ischium in, 1637, 1643, 1644–1645
   posterior transfer of tensor fasciae latae and sartorius in, 1650–1651, **1652–1657**
   posterolateral transfer of semitendinosus tendon in, 1651
   problems and complications of, 1660
   rectus femoris release in, 1637, 1642
   Steel's anterior advancement of gluteus medius and minimus insertion in, 1651, **1658–1659**
 knee in, 1705–1717
  Chandler patellar advancement technique in, 1717, 1718–1721
  extension contracture of, 1714–1716
   positive Ely test in, 1714, 1715
   rectus femoris release in, 1714–1715
   rectus femoris tendon transfer in, 1715–1716
   subtalar extra-articular stabilization in, 1716
  flexion deformity of, 1706–1714
   assessment in, 1706–1707, 1706–1707
   Egger's hamstring transfer in, 1712, 1712–1713
   fractional lengthening of hamstring in, **1708–1711**, 1712
   Holt method for hamstring contracture in, 1706, 1706
   proximal hamstring release in, 1713–1714
   straight leg raising in, 1706, 1706
   treatment of, 1707–1714
  patellar tendon elongation and quadriceps femoris insufficiency in, 1717
 management principles in, 1620–1627
  adequacy of postoperative care in, 1621–1622
  casting and splinting in, 1626–1627
  drug therapy for muscle relaxation in, 1627
  general, 1620
  interdependence of lower extremity and trunk in, 1622–1623, 1622–1626
  kinetic electromyography and gait analysis in, 1623
  nonoperative, 1623–1627
  orthosis in, 1627
  physical therapy in, 1623–1626

Cerebral palsy *(Continued)*
  reflex maturation and motor level development in, 1621
  surgical, 1620
  type and timing of surgical procedures in, 1622
  type of involvement in, 1620–1621
  walking prognosis in, 1621
 neurophysiologic considerations in, 1610–1613
  ataxia in, 1612–1613
  athetosis in, 1612
  hyperkinesia in, 1611–1612
  motor strength combinations in, 1611t
  rigidity in, 1613
  spasticity in, 1610–1611, 1611t
  tremor in, 1612
 neurosurgical therapy in, 1755–1757
 prevalence of, 1613–1614
 scoliosis in, 1747, 1755, *1755–1756*
Cerebrospinal fluid values, normal, 94t
Cervical fusion, in rheumatoid arthritis, 1486
Cervical ribs, in pseudarthrosis of clavicle, 168
Cervical spine, congenital anomalies of, 2230–2236
 pedicles and facets of, congenital absence of, 2236
 spondylolisthesis of, 2236
Cervical vertebrae, congenital synostosis of, 128–136. See also *Klippel-Feil syndrome.*
 fusion with occiput of, 2232–2233
Chandler patellar advancement technique, 1717, *1718–1721*
Charcot joint, 1512–1514, *1513*
 in congenital indifference to pain, 1999, *1999*
Charcot-Marie-Tooth disease, 1983–1986, *1984–1985*
Cheilectomy, in Legg-Calvé-Perthes disease, 984
Chest circumference, in relation to age, in females, 78t
 in males, 77t
Chiari type II and III deformity, in myelomeningocele, 1778
Chiari's innominate osteotomy, in congenital hip dysplasia in adolescent, 503–506
 advantages of, 504, *504*
 complications of, 506
 contraindications in, 506
 disadvantages of, 504
 illustrative cases of, *507*
 indications of, *505*, 505–506
 technique in, **508–517**
Chiari's medial displacement osteotomy, in focal deficiency of proximal femur, 566–569, *567*
Chloroquine, in rheumatoid arthritis, 1480
Chondral fracture, mechanism of, 1516
Chondroblastoma, benign, *1200*, 1200–1201
Chondrodysplasia, in Ellis–van Creveld syndrome, 730, 736
 metaphyseal, 737, *739, 740*
Chondrodysplasia calcificans punctata, 708–715
 Conradi-Hünermann disease in, *712–714*, 715
 rhizomelic form of, 708–709, *709–711*, 715
Chondroectodermal dysplasia, 730, *731–753*, 736
Chondrolysis, in slipped femoral capital epiphysis, 1062–1068. See also *Femoral capital epiphysis, slipped, chondrolysis in.*
 of hip, acute transient synovitis vs., 1464t
Chondroma, periosteal, 1199
Chondromalacia, in recurrent subluxation or dislocation of patella, 1578–1579
Chondromatosis, synovial, 1591, *1592*
Chondromyxoid fibroma, 1203–1205, *1204*
Chondrosarcoma, 1399–1400
 osteochondroma vs., 1170t

Chorionic gonadotropin therapy, slipped femoral capital epiphysis due to, 1022
Chronic granulomatous disease of childhood, 1133, *1134*
Cincinnati incision, in talipes equinovarus, 2483
Circumflex artery, medial, in congenital dysplasia of hip, 311
Clavicle, anatomy of, 3030
 fracture of, 3030–3037
  complications of, 3036–3037
  diagnosis of, 3032–3033
   at birth, 3032
   in infancy and childhood, 3032–3033, *3033–3034*
  mechanism of injury in, 3030–3032
  pathologic anatomy in, *3031*, 3032
  treatment of, 3033–3036
   in birth fracture, 3033–3034
   in older children and adolescents, 3034–3036, *3035–3036*
   in young children, 3034
   recumbent, 3036
 in cleidocranial dysostosis, 840, *841*
 morcellation of, in Sprengel's deformity, 145
 ossification of, 3030
 physeal separation of medial end of, 3038–3040, *3039*
 pseudarthrosis of, 168–174
  clinical findings in, 168–169, *169–170*
  etiology of, 168
  radiographic findings in, 169
  surgical repair of, **172, 173**
  treatment of, 169–174
 pyogenic osteomyelitis of, 1106
Clavus durus, 2789
Clavus mollis, 2789, *2790*
Claw toes, 2715–2717, *2716*
 in myelomeningocele, *1816*, 1816–1817
Cleft hand, 279–282
Cleidocranial dysostosis, 840–843
 clinical and roentgenographic features of, 840–843, *841–842*
 etiology of, 840
 inheritance in, 840
 treatment of, 843
Cleidocranial dysplasia, pycnodysostosis vs., 800t
Clinodactyly, 285–286, *286*, 287t
Clubfoot. See *Talipes equinovarus.*
Clutton's joints, 1458
Coccidioidomycosis, of bone, 1129–1130
Cogwheel rigidity, in cerebral palsy, 1613
Collagen, in osteogenesis imperfecta, 759
Colonna greater trochanteric arthroplasty, in septic arthritis of neonatal hip, 1431–1434
Compartment syndrome, 3099–3103
 diagnosis of, 3100–3101, *3101–3102*
 incidence and mechanism of, 3099
 pathophysiology in, 3099–3100
 treatment of, 3101–3103
Complaint, presenting, 3
Computed tomography, 59
Concentric contraction, of muscle, 14
Congenital deformities, 104–687. See also individual types.
 classification of, 104–112
 glossary of terminology in, 109t
 postural deformities vs., 2421, 2422t
Congruence angle, in recurrent subluxation or dislocation of patella, 1559, *1559*
Conradi-Hünermann disease, *712–714*, 715
Constriction band syndrome, congenital, 111

Constriction ring syndrome, 291–297
    classification of, 294, 296
    clinical picture in, 291–294, *291–296*
    etiology of, 291
    treatment of, 294, 296
Contraction, concentric, of muscle, 14
    eccentric, of muscle, 14
Cooley's anemia, 1136–1139, *1137–1138*
Coracoid process, fracture of, 3044
Cornelia de Lange syndrome, 861
Corns, of foot, 2789, *2790*
Cortical hyperostosis, infantile, 817–824
    clinical features of, 819
    complications of, 824
    diagnosis of, 819
    differential diagnosis of, 819t
    etiology of, 817
    pathology in, 817–819, *818*
    roentgenography in, 819, *820–823*
    treatment of, 824
Corticosteroids, in unicameral bone cyst, 1264–1265
Cotrel-Dubousset instrumentation, in scoliosis, 2319, *2319–2320*
Coventry lag screw, 395
Coxa breva, 588, *591*
    in Legg-Calvé-Perthes disease, 983, *984*
Coxa magna, in septic arthritis in neonate hip, 1431, *1432*
Coxa valga, 31–32
    in hip dislocation in cerebral palsy, 1634–1635
    in multiple exostosis, 1173, *1179–1180*
Coxa vara, 32
    developmental, 583–605
        age for operative intervention in, 592
        Amstutz and Wilson's osteotomy in, *594*, 595
        biomechanics of, 584–588, *585–586*
        Borden, Spencer, and Herndon's osteotomy in, 595
        clinical features of, *587–589*, 588
        congenital vs., 583
        coxa breva vs., 588, *591*
        differential diagnosis of, 588
        Haas osteotomy in, 592–593
        heredity in, 584, *584*
        Hilgenreiner epiphyseal (HE) angle in, 592, *593*
        incidence of, 584
        Langenskiöld's osteotomy in, 593–595, *594*
        MacEwen and Shands' osteotomy in, 595–597, *596–597*
        pathogenesis of, 584
        Pauwels' intertrochanteric Y osteotomy in, *599–601*, 600–601, **602–605**
        radiographic findings in, 588, *590*
        terminology in, 583
        treatment of, 588–605
        valgus intertrochanteric osteotomy of proximal femur in, 597–600, *598*
    in multiple epiphyseal dysplasia, 703, 706
    in septic arthritis in neonate hip, 1431
Craig splint, in congenital dysplasia of hip, 340–341, *341*
Craniocarpotarsal dysplasia, *851*, 852
Craniodiaphyseal dysplasia, 826
Craniofacial dysplasia, 855
Craniometaphyseal dysplasia, 826
Cretinism, 927–929, *928*
Cri-du-chat syndrome, 896–897
Crossed extension reflex, 47–49, *49*
Crouzon's syndrome, 856
Cryptococcus neoformans, of bone, 1130
Cubitus valgus, 31

Cubitus valgus *(Continued)*
    in fracture of lateral condyle of humerus, 3117–3118, 3118
    in supracondylar fracture of humerus, 3079–3081, *3081–3082*
Cubitus varus, 31
    in fracture of lateral condyle of humerus, 3119
    in supracondylar fracture of humerus, 3079–3081, *3081–3082*, **3084–3091**
Cuboid, accessory bone at, 2416
    fracture of, 3342
    unicameral bone cyst of, 2780, *2787*
Cubonavicular synostosis, 2579
Cuneiform, accessory bone at, 2416
    fracture of, 3342
Cyst, bone, aneurysmal, 1251–1255. See also *Bone cyst, aneurysmal.*
    unicameral, 1258–1272. See also *Bone cyst, unicameral.*
    popliteal, 1582–1589. See also *Popliteal cyst.*
Cystine storage disease, in vitamin D refractory rickets, 910
Cytoplasmic inclusions, in joint fluid analysis, 1413

D

Dactylitis, tuberculous, 1127, *1128*
Deafness, in Klippel-Feil syndrome, 131
    in osteogenesis imperfecta, 769
Deficiency, congenital, classification of, 106t–107t
    longitudinal, of limbs, 105, *110–111*
    terminal transverse, of limbs, 105, *108*
Deformity, angular, terminology in, 31–32
    congenital. See *Congenital deformities;* individual types.
    examination of, 27–32
Déjérine-Sottas disease, 1988–1989
Degenerative joint disease. See *Arthritis.*
Deltoid muscle, fibrosis of, 2122
    paralysis of, Saha trapezius transfer for, 1958, *1958*
    release of, at insertion, 1747, *1754*
Denis Browne hip abduction splint, in congenital dysplasia of hip, 341, *342*, 357
Dentate cerebellar ataxia, 1980t
Dermatomyositis, 2159–2164. See also *Polymyositis.*
Desmoplastic fibroma, 1250
Development. See also *Growth.*
    arrest of, 105, *108–111*
    motor, evaluation of, 90t–91t
Diabetes mellitus, peripheral neuropathy in, 2085
    preoperative precautions in, 67
Diapers, triple, in congenital dysplasia of hip, 341, *342*
Diaphyseal dysplasia, progressive, 804–807, *805*
    clinical features of, 804
    differential diagnosis in, 806
    etiology and heredity in, 804
    infantile cortical hyperostosis vs., 806
    osteopetrosis vs., 797
    pathology in, 804, *805*
    radiography and scintigraphy in, 806
    treatment of, 806–807
Diarthrosis, 1410
Diastrophic dysplasia, 752–756
    clinical picture in, 752–756, *753–754*
    differential diagnosis of, 756
    pathogenesis and pathology of, 752

Diastrophic dysplasia *(Continued)*
  radiography in, 756
  treatment in, 756
Digital gigantism, 277, *278*
Digitus minimus varus, congenital, 2653, 2655, *2658–2660*, 2661, **2662–2663**
Diplegia, 1606
  spastic, 1606, 1616–1617. See also *Cerebral palsy.*
Discitis, 2394–2401
  clinical findings in, 2394–2395, *2395*
  diagnosis of, 2397–2399, 2399t, *2400*
  imaging findings in, *2393–2398*, 2395–2396
  laboratory findings in, 2396
  pathogenesis of, 2394
  treatment of, 2399–2401
Discoid meniscus, 1539–1549. See also *Meniscus, discoid.*
Dislocation. See individual joint.
Down's syndrome, 890–895
  atlantoaxial instability in, 891–892
  dislocation of hip in, 892, *894*, 895
  maternal age and, 891t
  patellofemoral joint dislocation in, 895
  radiography in, 891, *891–893*
  treatment of, 891–895
Drooling, in cerebral palsy, 1756–1757
Drop-foot gait, 24
Drummond system, in scoliosis, 2318–2319
Duchenne muscular dystrophy. See *Muscular dystrophy, Duchenne.*
Dunn femoral head reduction by femoral neck shortening, in slipped femoral capital epiphysis, 1047, **1048–1055**, 1062
DuPont jacket, in scoliosis, *2301*, 2301–2302
Dwarfism, diastrophic, 752–756. See also *Diastrophic dysplasia.*
  dystrophic, talipes equinovarus in, *2452*, *2454*, 2455
  pituitary, *926*, 926–927
  terminology in, 694
  thanatophoric, 730, *731*
Dwyer calcaneal lateral wedge resection, in pes cavus, 2700–2701, **2702–2703**
Dwyer calcaneal osteotomy, 1702–1703
  in talipes equinovarus, 2517, **2518–2519**, 2520–2521
Dwyer instrumentation, in scoliosis, 2320, **2332–2353**
Dyggve-Melchior-Clausen disease, 757–758
Dynamic stress method, in congenital dysplasia of hip, 324, *324*
Dysautonomia, familial, 1995, 1996t–1997t, 1998–1999
Dyschondroplasia, 1195, *1196–1198*
Dysdiadochokinesia, in cerebral palsy, 1613
Dysmetria, in cerebral palsy, 1613
Dysostosis multiplex, in mucopolysaccharidosis, 865–867, *866*
Dysplasia, congenital, of hip, 297–526. See also *Hip, congenital dysplasia of.*
  ectodermal, in Ellis–van Creveld syndrome, 736
  epiphyseal, multiple, 701–707. See also *Epiphyseal dysplasia, multiple.*
  fibrous, 1228–1239. See also *Fibrous dysplasia.*
  metaphyseal, 825–826, *826–828*
  osteopetrosis vs., 797
Dysplasia epiphysealis hemimelica, *712–714*, 716, *717–718*, 719
Dyssynergy, in cerebral palsy, 1613
Dystelephalangy, 287, *287*
Dystrophia myotonica, *2138–2140*, 2138–2141
Dystrophia ophthalmoplegia, progressive, 2138
Dystrophic gait, 26

E

Eccentric contraction, of muscle, 14
Ectodermal dysplasia, in Ellis–van Creveld syndrome, 736
Ectopia lentis, in Marfan's syndrome, 832
Ectromelia, 105
Egger's hamstring transfer, *1712*, 1712–1713
Ehlers-Danlos syndrome, 861–864, *862–863*
Elbow. See also individual disorders of.
  disarticulation of, in osteogenic sarcoma, **1376–1379**
  dislocation of, 3124–3134
    classification of, 3125t
    complications of, 3131–3134
      heterotopic bone formation and myositis ossificans as, 3133
      median nerve, *3132*, 3132–3133
      recurrence as, 3133–3134, *3134*
      ulnar nerve, 3131–3132
      vascular, 3131
    diagnosis of, 3125
    mechanism of injury and pathologic anatomy of, 3125, *3126–3130*
    treatment of, 3128–3131
  flexion deformity of, in cerebral palsy, 1746–1747
  in arthrogryposis multiplex congenita, 2101–2103, *2102*, **2104–2111**
  in hereditary onycho-osteodystrophy, 845, *846*
  in obstetrical brachial plexus palsy, 2022–2023, *2024–2025*
  in poliomyelitis, 1959, 1962–1971
  position of minimal intra-articular pressure for, 1410–1411
  pulled, 3148–3151
    diagnosis of, 3149–3150
    mechanism of injury and pathologic anatomy in, 3148–3149, *3149–3150*
    treatment of, 3150–3151
  range of motion of, 33, *34*
  Steindler flexorplasty of, 1959, *1962*, 1962–1963
  synostosis of, congenital, *177–179*, 179
Electrical current, faradic, 64
  galvanic, 64
Electrical stimulation, in congenital pseudarthrosis of tibia, 666–667, 678–681
Electrodiagnosis, 59, 64–65
Electromyography, 64–65
Elephantiasis, in neurofibromatosis, 1290, *1292*
Ellis test, 31
Ellis–van Creveld syndrome, 730, *731*–753, 736
Ely test, in spastic cerebral palsy, 1628, *1631*, 1714, *1715*
Enchondroma, solitary, 1191–1194
  clinical picture in, 1191, *1191*
  differential diagnosis of, 1193
  radiography in, *1192*, 1192–1193
  surgical pathology in, *1193*, 1193–1194
  treatment of, 1194
  unicameral bone cyst vs., 1264
Enchondromatosis, multiple, 1195, *1196–1198*
Endobone, in osteopetrosis, *796*, 796
Endocrinopathy, slipped femoral capital epiphysis due to, 1022
Engen's adjustable extension orthosis, in rheumatoid arthritis, 1482, *1483*
Englemann's disease, osteopetrosis vs., 797
Eosinophilic granuloma, of bone, 1278, 1281–1286
  age and sex in, 1278

Volume 1, pgs. 1–687; Volume 2, pgs. 688–1600; Volume 3, pgs. 1601–2404; Volume 4, pgs. 2405–3373

Eosinophilic granuloma (Continued)
  biopsy in, 1284
  bone scan in, 1284
  clinical picture in, 1278, 1281
  diagnosis of, 1284
  differential diagnosis of, 1284
  radiography in, 1281–1284, *1282–1283*
  site of involvement in, 1278
  treatment of, 1285–1286
    percutaneous injection of methylprednisone sodium in, 1285
    radiation in, 1286
    surgical curettage in, 1285
  vertebra plana in, 1281–1282, *1283*
  unicameral bone cyst vs., 1261, 1264
Epilepsy, in cerebral palsy, 1616
Epiphyseal dysgenesis, in hypothyroidism, 928
Epiphyseal dysplasia, multiple, 701–707
  clinical features of, 701, 703
  coxa vara in, 703, *706*
  hands in, 703, *707*
  inheritance in, 701
  Legg-Calvé-Perthes disease vs., 703, *705*, 958, *959–960*
  pathology in, 701, *702–703*
  radiography and differential diagnosis in, 703, *704–707*
  treatment of, 703, 707
Epiphyseal extrusion index, of Green, in Legg-Calvé-Perthes disease, 963, *963*
Epiphyseal growth plate, definition of, 932
  injury to, 3026
Epiphysis. See also individual bone.
  in unicameral bone cyst, 1271–1272
  lower limb, appearance of centers of ossification of, 62
    closure of, 63
  pressure, 2852
  traction, 2852
  upper limb, appearance of centers of ossification of, 60
    closure of, 61
Eppright's periacetabular osteotomy, in congenital dysplasia of hip in adolescent, 503, *503*
Equilibrium, tests for maturation of, 55, *56*
Equinus deformity. See under *Talipes*.
Erector spinae, in gait, 14, 15
Erector spinae transfer, of Barr, in gluteus maximus paralysis, *1926*, 1926–1927
Estrogen, metabolism of, in congenital dysplasia of hip, 302
Ethambutol, in septic arthritis, 1424t
Eversion, definition of, 33
Ewing's sarcoma, 1387–1396
  clinical picture in, 1388–1389
  diagnosis in, 1390
  pathologic findings in, 1388, *1388*
  prognosis in, 1390
  radiography in, 1389–1390, *1389–1391*
  staging in, 1390
  treatment in, 1390–1396, *1392–1395*
Examination, 4–57. See also individual parts.
  neurologic, 42–55
  of deformities, 27–32
  of gait, 5–27
  of motor power–muscle testing, 40–42
  of motor system, 55–57
  of range of joint motion, 32–40
  of stance and posture, 4–5
Exostosis, multiple, 1172–1190
  clinical features of, 1173, *1174–1180*, 1180

Exostosis (Continued)
  inheritance of, 1172
  lengthening of humerus in, 1184, *1185*
  localization of, 1172
  pathology in, 1172–1173
  proximal fibular excision in, 1184, *1186–1189*
  radiography in, 1180, *1181–1182*
  sarcomatous transformation in, 1184, 1190
  treatment of, 1180–1184, *1183–1185*, **1186–1189**
  ulnar drift of wrist in, 1180, 1183, *1184*
  Z-step cut lengthening of ulna in, 1183–1184, *1185*
  subungual, of toe, 2780, *2788*
Exostosis bursata, 1165
Extension, definition of, 33
Extensor digitorum longus, in gait, 14
Extensor hallucis longus, in gait, 14
  rerouting through anterior tibial tendon of, 1680, **1682–1685**
Extensor pollicis brevis tendon transfer, to extensor tendon of ulna, 2057, **2074–2075**
Extensor pollicis longus, rerouting of, in cerebral palsy, 1731
Extensor thrust reflex, 49
External oblique abdominal muscle, transfer to greater trochanter, in myelomeningocele, 1836
Extrapyramidal disorders, 1602t–1603t, 1604

F

Face, asymmetry of, in congenital torticollis, 113, *114*
Fairbank's apprehension test, in recurrent subluxation or dislocation of patella, 1555
Familial dysautonomia, 1995, 1996t–1997t, 1998–1999
Familial periodic paralysis, electrical testing in, 64
Fanconi's anemia, 1135
Faradic current, 64
Fascia lata transfer to lumbodorsal fascia, of Hogshead, in gluteus maximus paralysis, 1927, *1928*
Fasciculations, 65
Femoral artery, pseudoaneurysm of, in osteochondroma, 1167, 1170
Femoral capital epiphysis, slipped, 1016–1073
  acute transient synovitis vs., 1464t
  anatomic factors preventing, 1017–1018, *1018*
  avascular necrosis in, 1068–1073
    bone grafting in, 1072–1073
    diagnosis of, 1068, 1070
    hip arthrodesis in, 1070, *1071*, 1072
    hip joint resurfacing in, 1072
    prevention of, 1068
    Sugioka's transtrochanteric derotation osteotomy in, 1070, *1070*
  chondrolysis in, 1062–1068
    bone scan in, 1066, *1067*
    clinical picture in, 1066
    etiology of, 1062–1063
    hip arthrodesis in, 1068, *1068*
    incidence of, 1063, 1063t
    natural history of, 1066
    pathology in, 1063
    radiography in, 1066, *1067*
    risk factors in, 1063, 1063t
    treatment of, 1067–1068, *1068*
  classification of, 1017
  clinical picture in, 1026–1028, *1027*
  complications of, 1062–1073

Femoral capital epiphysis (Continued)
  etiology of, 1017–1022, *1018–1023*
    chorionic gonadotropin therapy in, 1022
    endocrinopathies in, 1022
    growth hormone and, 1019, *1020–1021*
    growth spurt in, 1018–1019
    hypothyroidism in, 1019, 1022
    mammillary processes in, 1018
    perichondrial ring in, 1017
    physeal contour in, 1018
    physeal inclination angle in, 1018
    physeal thickness in, 1018
    renal failure in, 1022, *1023*
    transepiphyseal collagen fibers in, 1017–1018
  incidence and epidemiology of, 1016–1017
  inheritance in, 1022
  measurement of slipping in, 1028, *1030–1031*, 1031
  pathology in, 1022–1026, *1024–1026*
  radiography in, 1028, *1029–1030*
  Southwick method for femoral head-shaft angle in, 1028, 1031, *1031*
  stress fracture after treatment of, *1072*, 1073
  treatment of, 1031–1062
    cast immobilization in, 1031–1032
    Dunn femoral head reduction by femoral neck shortening in, 1047, **1048–1055**, 1062
    epiphysiodesis with autogenous bone graft in, 1033, 1044
    femoral neck and head remodeling in, 1044, *1045*
    in acute or chronic slip, 1047, **1048–1055**
    in acute slip, 1044, 1046, *1046*
    in anterior slip, 1047, 1062
    in situ pin fixation with ASNIS system in, 1032–1033, **1034–1043**
    in valgus slip, 1047
    Kramer femoral neck osteotomy in, 1062, **1064–1065**
    osteotomy in, 1062
    sex hormone therapy in, 1032
    Southwick trochanteric triplane osteotomy in, **1056–1061**, 1062
    subtrochanteric osteotomy after growth plate closure in, 1062
Femoral distal epiphysis, fracture of, 3274–3281
  diagnosis of, 3275
  mechanism of injury and pathologic anatomy in, 3274–3275
  problems and complications in, 3281
  radiography in, 3275, *3276–3278*
  treatment of, 3275–3281
    in abduction type, 3275, 3279
    in hyperextension type, 3279
    in hyperflexion type, 3279–3281, *3280*
  separation of, obstetrical, 3353–3354
Femoral head, avascular necrosis of, in septic arthritis in neonate hip, 1431
  cartilaginous, CT appearance of, 357–358, *358*
  in arthrography of congenital dysplasia of hip, 352
  lateral displacement of, measurement of, 320, *320*
  reduction by Dunn's femoral neck shortening, in slipped femoral capital epiphysis, 1047, **1048–1055**, 1062
  superior and posterior dislocation of, mechanism of, 1635, *1636*
Femoral head–shaft angle, Southwick method for, in slipped femoral capital epiphysis, 1028, 1031, *1031*
Femoral neck, fracture of, 3231–3245
  classification of, 3231, 3232, 3232t
  complications of, 3237, 3242–3245
    aseptic necrosis as, 3237, 3242–3244, *3243*

Femoral neck (Continued)
    coxa vara as, 3244
    delayed union and nonunion as, 3244–3245
    premature epiphyseal fusion as, 3244
  diagnosis of, 3233
  displaced transcervical or cervicotrochanteric, 3237, *3240*
  intertrochanteric, 3237, *3241–3242*
  mechanism of injury in, 3231–3233
  transepiphyseal, 3236–3237
  treatment of, 3233–3237, 3236t
    manipulative reduction and cast immobilization in, 3235–3236
    Whitman's reduction in, 3233, *3234*
  undisplaced transcervical or cervicotrochanteric, 3237, *3238–3239*
  osteomyelitis of, Legg-Calvé-Perthes disease vs., 957
Femoral neck and head remodeling, in slipped femoral capital epiphysis, 1044, *1045*
Femoral neck osteotomy, Kramer's, in slipped femoral capital epiphysis, 1062, **1064–1065**
Femoral neck–shaft angle, in developmental coxa vara, 586, *586*
  in different age groups, *584*
Femoral nerve injury, due to Pavlik harness treatment, 340
  due to Salter's innominate osteotomy, 418
Femoral osteotomy, distal supracondylar extension, in myelomeningocele, 1819, *1820*
  in congenital hip dysplasia, 392–422
    biomechanics of, 394, 395
    Coventry lag screw in, 395
    indications for, 392
    intertrochanteric, 395
    Lloyd Roberts technique for, 395, **402–403**
    preoperative assessment in, 392–393, *393*
    prerequisites for, 392
    Salter's technique for, 395–422. See also *Salter's innominate osteotomy.*
    subtrochanteric, 393, 395
    Wagner technique for, 394, 395, **396–401**
  in coxa vara, Amstutz and Wilson's technique for, *594*, 595
    Borden, Spencer, and Herndon's technique for, 595
    Haas technique in, 592–593
    Langenskiöld's technique in, 593–595, *594*
    MacEwen and Shands' technique in, 595–597, *596–597*
    Pauwels' intertrochanteric Y technique in, *599–601*, 600–601, **602–605**
    valgus intertrochanteric, 597–600, *598*
  in Legg-Calvé-Perthes disease, 981–982, *982–983*
  in medial rotation deformity of hip, 1651, 1660
  proximal extension, in myelomeningocele, *1838*, 1838–1839
Femoral retroversion, in congenital dysplasia of hip, computed tomography in, 364, *365*
Femoral shaft, fracture of, 3248–3268
  complications of, 3266–3268
    angular deformity as, 3268
    limb length discrepancy as, 3266–3268
  diagnosis in, 3255
  pathologic anatomy in, 3248, *3249–3254*, 3255
  treatment of, 3255–3266
    90–90 degree skeletal traction in, 3262–3263, *3263–3264*
    Bryant's traction in, 3256–3259, *3256–3261*
    closed reduction and cast immobilization in, 3262, 3266
    in older children, 3262–3266
    in preadolescent and adolescent age group, 3266

Femoral shaft *(Continued)*
    modified Bryant's traction in, *3261*, 3261–3262
    Russell skin traction in, 3264–3266, *3267*
    suspension traction in, 3264, *3265*
    up to two years of age, 3255–3262
Femoral torsion, 2800–2810
  clinical features of, 2801–2803, *2802–2805*
  in congenital dysplasia of hip, computed tomography in, 361, *363–365*, 364
  in resubluxation of reduced hip, 391
  measurement of, 2803–2805
    clinical method for, 2803
    imaging methods for, 2803–2805
    radiographic methods for, 2805, *2806–2809*
  natural course of, 2799, 2800–2801, *2801*
  treatment of, 2805–2810
    conservative, 2805–2806
    operative, 2806, 2809–2810
Femur, axial rotation of, in gait, 12
  congenital abnormalities of, 552t–553t, 554
  congenital aplasia of, 583
  congenital hypoplasia of, *582*, 582–583
  congenital longitudinal deficiency of, 553–554
  distal, epiphysiodesis of, **2878–2881**
  fetal development of, 555t
  in congenital dysplasia of hip in adolescent, 468–469, *470*
  lengthening of, by callotasis, 2896, **2942–2859**
    in leg length inequality, 2892–2893
    Wagner method for, 2896, *2897*, **2898–2921**
  proximal, aseptic necrosis of, due to Pavlik harness treatment, 339
  focal deficiency of, 554–576
    Aitken classification of, 554–561, *556–562*
    associated anomalies in, 561, *563–564*, 564
    bilateral, 565–566
    Chiari's medial displacement osteotomy in, 566–569, *567*
    clinical presentation in, *563 564*, 564 565
    Gillespie and Torode classification of, 554
    King's knee fusion in, 571, 576, *577*, **578–579**
    malrotation of lower limb in, 566
    pelvifemoral instability in, 566–569, *567*
    prosthesis in, *568–570*, 569–570
    serial radiography in, 559, 561, *562*
    Torode and Gillespie rotation-plasty in, 571, **572–575**, *576*
    treatment of, 565–579
    unilateral, 566–576
    Van Nes rotation-plasty in, 570–571
  in congenital dysplasia of hip, 311–312
  superior displacement of, measurement of, 320, *320–321*
  shortening of, in leg length inequality, 2889–2892, *2890–2891*
  Wasserstein lengthening of, 2896, *2994*
Fetus, hypoxia of, in cerebral palsy, 1609
Fever, cat-scratch, 1133
  in rheumatoid arthritis, 1472
  rheumatic, acute transient synovitis vs., 1464t
  joint fluid analysis in, 1414t
  Legg-Calvé-Perthes disease vs., 957
Fibrillation potentials, 65
Fibrinogen, in joint fluid analysis, 1414
Fibrodysplasia ossificans progressiva, 857–860, *858–860*
  clinical features of, 857–858, *858*
  pathology in, 857
  prognosis and treatment in, 860
  radiographic findings in, 858, *859–860*

Fibroma, chondromyxoid, 1203–1205, *1204*
  desmoplastic, 1250
  recurrent, digital, 2770–2773
Fibroma molluscum, in neurofibromatosis, 1290, *1291*
Fibrosarcoma, 1403
  of foot, 2780, *2783*
Fibrosis, of deltoid muscle, 2122
  of quadriceps muscle, 2122, *2123–2124*
  of sternocleidomastoid muscle, in congenital torticollis, 112–113
Fibrous ankylosis, in hemophilic arthropathy, 1497, *1498*
  in septic arthritis in neonate hip, 1431, *1433*
Fibrous defect, of bone, 1246–1249, *1247*
Fibrous dysplasia, 1228–1239
  bone scan in, 1234, *1235*
  café-au-lait spots in, 1229
  clinical findings in, 1228–1229, *1229*
  computed tomography in, 1234, *1236*
  etiology of, 1228
  incidence of, 1228
  localization of, 1228
  malignant transformation in, 1239
  natural course of, 1234
  nonskeletal manifestations of, 1229–1230
  pathologic fracture in, 1237, *1238–1239*
  pathology in, 1230–1231, *1230–1231*
  radiography in, 1231, *1232–1233*
  sexual precocity in, 1229–1230
  solitary, unicameral bone cyst vs., 1264
  treatment of, 1234–1239
Fibrous histiocytoma, malignant, 1403
Fibrous metaphyseal defect, 1247–1249, *1248*
Fibula, congenital longitudinal deficiency of, 620–636
  associated anomalies in, 624, *625*
  calculation of shortening at maturity in, 624
  classification of, *621–622*, 621–623
  diagnosis in, 623–624, *623–626*
  differential diagnosis in, 624
  foot in, 623, *623*
  foot preservation technique in, 634
  Gurca's bifurcation technique in, 634–636, *635*
  in proximal focal femoral deficiency, 561
  pathogenesis of, 620–621
  Syme amputation in, 626–629, **630–633**
  treatment of, 624–636
  type II, treatment options in, 626–628, *627–628*
  congenital posteromedial angulation of, 651–656
    clinical presentation in, 652, *652*
    progressive length discrepancy in, 652, *653*
    radiography in, 652, *654–655*
    treatment of, 653, 656
  congenital pseudarthrosis of, 685, *686*
  distal, accessory ossification center of, 2416
  distal epiphysis of, ossification of, 3302, *3303*
  fracture of, in older children and adolescents, 3298, *3300*
  in multiple exostosis, 1173, *1178–1179*
  osteofibrous dysplasia of, 1242–1246, *1243–1245*
  osteogenic sarcoma of, 2780, *2788*
  paraxial hemimelia of, 620–636. See also Fibula, *congenital longitudinal deficiency of.*
  proximal, epiphysiodesis of, **2882–2885**
    excision of, in multiple exostosis, 1184, *1186–1189*
  stress fracture of, 3362
Fibular transplant, free vascularized, in congenital pseudarthrosis of tibia, 677–678, *678–680*
Fick method, in radiography of hip flexion deformity, 1630

Volume 1, pgs. 1–687; Volume 2, pgs. 688–1600; Volume 3, pgs. 1601–2404; Volume 4, pgs. 2405–3373

Filum terminale, lipoma of, clinical features of, 1873–1874, *1874*
  embryology and pathology of, 1873, *1873*
Fingernails, in hereditary onycho-osteodystrophy, 845, *846*
Fingers, deformities of, 284–290
  in cerebral palsy, 1738–1744
  fracture of, 3205, *3206–3208*, 3209
  hypoplastic, 283
  in arthrogryposis multiplex congenita, 2113
  index, pollicization of, **262–267**
  little, duplication of, ablation of, **246–249**
  polydactyly of. See *Polydactyly*.
  recurrent fibroma of, 2770–2773
  ring and long, technique for separation of, **228–233**
  swan-neck deformity of, in cerebral palsy, 1739, 1744
  syndactyly of. See *Syndactyly*.
Flaccid paralysis, chart for muscle examination in, 81t–82t
Flexion, definition of, 33
Flexor carpi ulnaris transfer, Green's, 1746, **1748–1753**
Flexor digitorum longus, in gait, 14, *15*
Flexor digitorum sublimis, transfer to thumb of, 289
Flexor pollicis brevis, congenital absence of, 288–289, *288–290*
Flexor pollicis longus, congenital absence of, 288–289, *288–290*
  stenosing tendovaginitis of, 272–273
Foot. See also under individual disorders.
  accessory bones of, 2412–2420, *2413*
  cleft, congenital (lobster claw), 2637, *2638–2642*
  congenital deformities of. See under *Talipes*.
  development and ossification of, 2406–2408, *2407–2410*
  dorsiflexion of, muscles in, 1938
  eversion of, muscles in, 1938
  flat. See *Pes planovalgus*.
  fracture of, 3339–3343
    calcaneus in, 3341
    lateral process of talus in, 3341
    Lisfranc's tarsometatarsal fracture-dislocation in, 3341–3342, *3341–3342*
    metatarsal in, 3342–3343, *3343*
    navicular, cuboid, cuneiform in, 3342
    os peroneum in, 3343
    talar body in, 3339–3341, *3340*
    talar neck in, 3339
    tuberosity of fifth metatarsal in, 3343
  functional considerations in, 2405
  in arthrogryposis multiplex congenita, 2099
  in cerebral palsy, 1660–1705. See also *Cerebral palsy, foot and ankle in*.
  in congenital longitudinal deficiency of fibula, 623, *623*
  in myelomeningocele, 1795–1817
  in poliomyelitis, 1937–1957
  inversion of, muscles in, 1938
  normal, growth of, *2411*, 2411–2412, 2412t
  paralytic deformities of, tendon transfers for, 1940t–1941t
  plantar flexion of, muscles in, 1938
  postural deformities of, 2421–2427. See also under *Talipes*.
  range of motion of, 36
  rocker-bottom, 2461–2462, *2464*
  skin and nail lesions of, 2789–2791
  tumors of, 2766–2780
    bone, 2780
    calcinosis as, 2780, *2780*
    fibrosarcoma as, 2780, *2783*
    foreign body granuloma as, 2780, *2781*

Foot *(Continued)*
  ganglion as, 2766–2768, *2768–2770*
  hemangioma as, 2768, *2771–2776*
  lipoma as, 2766, *2767*
  lymphangiectasis as, 2768, *2770, 2777*
  nerve sheath, 2773, *2778*
  pigmented villonodular synovitis as, 2780, *2781*
  synovioma as, 2780, *2783*
  xanthomatosis, *2779, 2780*
Foot motion, in gait, 11, *11*
Force plate, in gait, *8*, 8–9
Forearm. See also *Arm*.
  Monteggia equivalent lesions of, 3178–3179
  pronation contracture of, in cerebral palsy, 1746
  supination contracture of, in poliomyelitis, 1971
Foreign body granuloma, of foot, 2780, *2781*
Forequarter amputation (Littlewood), in osteogenic sarcoma, **1354–1367**
Fracture. See also specific bone.
  butterfly, 3014
  greenstick, 3014
  in children, 3013
  oblique, 3014
  pathologic, 3366
    in fibrous dysplasia, 1237, *1238–1239*
    in osteopetrosis, 797, *797–798*
    in pyogenic osteomyelitis, 1103
    in sickle cell disease, 1144
    in unicameral bone cyst, 1270–1271, *1271*
  spiral, 3014
  stress, 3359–3363
    clinical findings in, 3360
    differential diagnosis of, 3363
    in slipped femoral capital epiphysis, *1072*, 1073
    pathogenesis of, 3360
    radiography in, 3360–3363, *3361–3362*
    sites of involvement of, 3360
    treatment of, 3363
  torus, 3014
  transverse, 3014
Freeman-Sheldon syndrome, *851*, 852
  talipes equinovarus in, 2455, *2456*
Freiberg's infraction, 1006–1008, *1006–1009*
Frejka pillow, in congenital dysplasia of hip, 341, *342*
Friedreich's ataxia, 1978–1981, 1980t
  gait in, 26
Fungal infection, of bone, 1129–1130
  of joints, 1460

G

Gage and Winter's traction stations, in congenital dysplasia of hip, 345, *346–347*
Gait, analysis of, 26–27
  antalgic, 24
  ataxic, 26
  axial rotation in, 12–13
  calcaneus, 22–24, *25*
  cerebellar ataxic, 1613
  clinical appraisal of, 18
  cycle of, *6, 7*
  determinants of, 9–12
    foot and ankle motion as, 11, *11*
    knee flexion as, 10–11, *11*
    knee motion as, 12, *12*
    lateral displacement of pelvis as, 12, *13*

Gait *(Continued)*
  pelvic rotation as, 9, 9–10
  pelvic tilt as, 10, *10*
 drop-foot, 24
 dystrophic, 26
 force plate in, 8, *8–9*
 gluteus medius lurch, 22, *23*
 gravity effects on, 8, *8–9*
 in bilateral congenital dysplasia of hip, 328, *328–329*
 in equinus deformity, 9
 in hamstring contracture, 1706, *1707*
 in myelomeningocele, 1792–1795
 in spastic hemiplegia, 1615
 in spastic paraplegia, 25
 in talipes equinus, 1661, *1662*
 in tuberculosis of spine, 1451
 maturational development of, 14–18, *16–22*
  in one-year-old, 16, *16–17*
  in three-year-old, 16–18, *18–20*
  in six-year-old, 18, *20–22*
 muscle action in, 13–14, *15*
 muscle weakness and, 18, 22–24, *23–25*
 neurologic deformities and, 24–26
 pathologic, 18–26
 penguin, 26
 sensory ataxic, 1613
 spastic, 25–26
 stance phase of, 6, *7–8*
 steppage, 24
 structural deformities of bones and joints and, 24
 swing phase of, 6, *7–8*
Galant's reflex, 49, *50*
Galleazzi sign, in congenital dysplasia of hip, *326*, 327
Galleazzi test, 31
Galvanic current, 64
Ganglion, of foot, 2766–2768, *2768–2770*
Gastrocnemius, in gait, 14, *15*
Gastrocnemius lengthening, of Baker technique, 1667, *1673*
 of Vulpius technique, 1666–1667, *1672*
Gastrocnemius recession, of Silverskiöld, 1667, *1673*
 of Strayer, 1667, *1674*
 proximal, 1674, *1675*
Gastrocnemius-soleus, paralysis of, gait in, 22–24, 25
Gaucher's disease, 882–886
 bone manifestations of, 883–885, *884–885*
 cells in, 882, *883*
 clinical features of, 882–883
 etiology of, 882
 heredity in, 882
 treatment of, 885–886
Genetic factors, in congenital dysplasia of hip, 304–306
Gentamicin, in septic arthritis, 1424t
Genu recurvatum, 617–618
 congenital dislocation and subluxation of knee vs., 612
 in arthrogryposis multiplex congenita, 2100
 in cerebral palsy, 1716–1717
 in poliomyelitis, 1934–1937, *1935–1936*
Genu valgum, developmental, 2827–2834
  clinical findings in, 2827, *2827*
  differential diagnosis of, 2827–2828
  treatment of, 2828–2834
   angular deformity vs. growth remaining in, 2830, *2831*, 2831t
   female vs. male in, 2829, *2829*
   in adolescent, 2828–2829
   orthosis in, 2828
   osteotomy of distal femur in, 2832–2834

Genu valgum *(Continued)*
   stapling and epiphysiodesis of distal femur or proximal tibia in, 2829–2832
  in arthrogryposis multiplex congenita, 2100
  in myelomeningocele, 1821
  measurement of, 32, *32*
 Genu varum, in myelomeningocele, 1821
  measurement of, 32
  pathologic conditions causing, 2824t
  physiologic, 2822–2827
   differential diagnosis of, 2824t, 2824–2826, 2826t
   familial, 2822, *2823*
   radiography in, 2824, *2825*
   rickets vs., 2824, 2826
   tibia vara (Blount's disease) vs., 2824, 2826t
   treatment of, 2826–2827
Giant cell tumor, unicameral bone cyst vs., 1264
Gibbus, 2185
Gigantism, 927
 digital, 277, *278*
 of limb, 110–111
Glenohumeral joint. See *Shoulder*.
Glenoid cavity, hypoplasia of, congenital, 175–176, *176*
 retrotorsion or antetorsion of, congenital, 176
Glucose, joint fluid levels vs. blood levels, 1414
Gluteus maximus, in gait, 14, *15*
 paralysis of, gait in, 22
 in poliomyelitis, 1925–1927, *1926*, *1928*
Gluteus medius, in congenital dysplasia of hip, 310–311, *311*
 in gait, 14, *15*
 paralysis of, gait in, 22, *23*
 in poliomyelitis, 1925
Gluteus medius and minimus insertion, Steel's anterior advancement of, 1651, **1658–1659**
Gluteus medius lurch, 22, *23*
Gluteus minimus, in congenital dysplasia of hip, 310–311, *311*
 in gait, 14, *15*
Gold salts, in rheumatoid arthritis, 1400
Goldthwait-Hauser procedure, in recurrent patellar dislocation, **1566–1567**
Gonococcal arthritis, 1441–1442
Gorham's massive osteolysis, 791
Gout, 1494
 joint fluid analysis in, 1414t
Gowers' sign, in Duchenne muscular dystrophy, 2132, *2133*
Gracilis muscle, contracture of, test for, 1628
 in gait, 14
Granuloma, eosinophilic. See *Eosinophilic granuloma*.
 foreign body, of foot, 2780, *2781*
Granulomatous disease of childhood, chronic, 1133, *1134*
Gravity, gait and, 8, *8–9*
Green-Anderson growth remaining method, in epiphysiodesis, 2871–2872
Greene's quadriceps-plasty, in recurrent patellar dislocation, **1563–1566**
Green's epiphyseal extrusion index, in Legg-Calvé-Perthes disease, 963, *963*
Green's flexor carpi ulnaris transfer, 1746, **1748–1753**
Green's modified Sever-L'Episcopo procedure, 2028, **2030–2039**
Green's scapuloplasty, modified, in Sprengel's deformity, *147*, 148–160, **149–161**
Grice subtalar extra-articular arthrodesis, 1693, **1694–1697**, *1698–1699*, 1698–1700
Growth, 2852–2867
 of long bones, 2852

Volume 1, pgs. 1–687; Volume 2, pgs. 688–1600; Volume 3, pgs. 1601–2404; Volume 4, pgs. 2405–3373

Growth (Continued)
  prediction charts for, 2864, 2864–2867, 2865t
  rate of, 2852–2854, 2853, 2854t
  relative height, length of femur and tibia vs. skeletal age and, 2854, 2855t–2857t, 2858–2863
  relative maturity and, 2854, 2864
Growth hormone, slipped femoral capital epiphysis due to, 1019, 1020–1021
Growth plate, epiphyseal, definition of, 932
  injury to, 3026
  physeal, definition of, 932
Guillain-Barré syndrome, 2003–2004
Gurca's bifurcation technique, in congenital longitudinal deficiency of fibula, 634–636, 635

H

Haas osteotomy in, in coxa vara, 592–593
Hallux rigidus, 2758–2765
  clinical features of, 2759–2760, 2761–2762
  etiology of, 2758–2759, 2759
  radiography in, 2760, 2763
  treatment of, 2760, 2764–2765, 2764–2765
Hallux valgus, congenital, 2626–2628, 2626–2629
  in cerebral palsy, 1705
Hallux valgus interphalangeus, 2661, 2661, 2664–2665
Hallux varus, congenital, 2649–2650, 2649–2651
Hammer toe, 2667, **2668–2669**, 2670
  in cerebral palsy, 1705
Hamstring, Egger's transfer of, 1712, 1712–1713
  fractional lengthening of, **1708–1711**, 1712
  proximal release of, 1713–1714
Hamstring contracture, gait in, 1706, 1707
  Holt method for, 1706, 1706
Hand, cleft, 279–282
  centripetal suppression theory of, 280, 281
  classifications of, 280
  clinical presentation in, 280, 282
  syndromes associated with, 279, 280t
  treatment of, 282
  V-shaped defect in, 279, 280
  hypoplastic, 283
  in multiple epiphyseal dysplasia, 703, 707
  thumb-clutched, 270
Hand grasp reflex, 42–45, 44
Hand-Schüller-Christian disease, 1278, 1280–1281
Harrington instrumentation, in scoliosis, 2317, 2317, **2322–2331**
Harrison's groove, 899
Head circumference, in relation to age, in females, 78t
  in males, 77t
Hearing loss, in Klippel-Feil syndrome, 131
Heart disease, congenital, in Ellis–van Creveld syndrome, 736
Heel cord. See Achilles tendon.
Height, in relation to age, in females, 78t
  in males, 77t
  total and sitting, 696–699
Hemangioma, of foot, 2768, 2771–2776
  of synovial membrane, 1596, 1597
Hemarthrosis, in hemophilia, 1502–1503
  septic arthritis vs., 1422
Hematology values, normal, 92t
Hemimelia, 105
Hemipelvectomy (Banks and Coleman), in osteogenic sarcoma, **1318–1325**

Hemiplegia, 40, 1606
  double, 1606
  spastic, 1614–1615, 1614–1616. See also Cerebral palsy.
Hemivertebra, segmented, 2197–2198, 2198
  semisegmented and nonsegmented, 2198, 2198
Hemoglobinopathy, 1136
Hemophilia, 1494–1507
  anesthesia in, 71
  arthropathy in, 1495–1498
    clinical findings in, 1497
    fibrous ankylosis in, 1497, 1498
    pathophysiology in, 1495–1497
    radiography in, 1496–1498, 1497–1498, 1498t
    site of involvement in, 1495
  classification and inheritance of, 1495
  clinical picture in, 1495
  dislocation in, 1501
  fracture in, 1501
  historical, 1494–1495
  incidence of, 1495
  myositis ossificans in, 1502
  nerve palsy in, 1500
  pseudotumor in, 1500–1501, 1501
  soft tissue bleeding in, 1498–1499, 1499
  treatment of, 1502–1507
    medical, 1502–1505
      analgesia in, 1503
      aspiration in, 1503–1504
      casting in, 1504–1505
      factor replacement in, 1502
      in chronic arthropathy, 1504
      in early bleeding into soft tissue, 1502
      in hemarthrosis, 1502–1503
      in subacute arthropathy, 1504
      traction in, 1504–1505
    surgical, 1505–1507
      hematologic, 1505
      of fracture, 1507
      of neuropraxia, 1507
      of pseudotumor, 1507
      synovectomy in, 1505–1506
      synoviorthesis in, 1506
      total joint replacement and arthrodesis in, 1506–1507
  ultrasound in, 1499, 1499–1500
  Volkmann's ischemic contracture in, 1499, 1499
Hemophilus influenzae, in septic arthritis, 1416
Henoch-Schönlein purpura, septic arthritis vs., 1422
Hepatosplenomegaly, in rheumatoid arthritis, 1472
Hereditary disorders. See individual types.
Heredopathia atactica polyneuritiformis, 1990–1991
Herniated intervertebral disc, 2402
Herpes zoster, 2006–2007
Hilgenreiner epiphyseal (HE) angle, 592, 593
Hilgenreiner's line, in congenital dysplasia of hip, 319, 319
  in quantitation of traction effectiveness, 345, 346
Hindbrain dysfunction, in myelomeningocele, 1791
Hip, abduction and lateral rotation deformity of, in myelomeningocele, 1839–1840
  abduction contracture of, congenital, 549–551, 549–552
    cast immobilization in, 551–552
    passive stretching exercises in, 551, 551
    test for, 27, 30
  abduction of, 33, 35, 36
  acute transient synovitis of, 1461–1465. See also Synovitis, acute transient, in hip.

Hip (Continued)
  adduction contracture, due to Pavlik harness treatment, 339
  adduction deformity of, in myelomeningocele, 1840–1841
  adduction-flexion deformity of, in cerebral palsy, 1628–1630, *1629–1632*
  adductor paralysis in, iliopsoas transfer in, 1825–1826, *1827*, **1828–1835**, 1836
  adductor transfer in, in cerebral palsy, 1637, *1643*, 1644–1645
  ankylosis of, in septic arthritis, 1417, *1419*
  arthrodesis of, in slipped femoral capital epiphysis, 1068, *1068*, 1070, *1071*, 1072
  aspiration of, technique in, 1420–1421
  chondrolysis of, acute transient synovitis vs., 1464t
  congenital dysplasia of, 297–526
    after walking, 327–330, *328–330*
      gait in, 24, *328*, 328–329
      Trendelenburg test in, 329, *329*
    at birth to two months, 312–326, 330–341
      abduction contracture of contralateral hip in, 314, 316
      acetabular index in, 322
      associated deformities in, 316
      Barlow's test in, 314, *315*
      clinical findings in, 312–316
      closed reduction in, 331, **332–333**
      Craig or Ilfeld splint in, 340–341, *341*
      Denis Browne hip abduction splint in, 341, *342*
      diagnosis of, 312–326
      dynamic stress method in, 324, *324*
      Frejka pillow in, 341, *342*
      H distance in, *321*, 321
      high-risk infants in, 316–317
      Hilgenreiner's line or Y line in, 319, *319*
      measurement of lateral displacement of femoral head in, 320, *320*
      negative radiogram in, *317*, 317–318
      Ombredanne's line in, 319, *319*
      Ortolani test in, 312–314, *313*
      Pavlik harness in, 331–340. See also *Pavlik harness.*
      Perkin's line in, 319, *319*
      positioning for radiography in, *318*, 318–319
      postnatal dislocation in, 317
      radiographic findings in, 317–322
      Shenton's or Menard's line in, 320, *320–321*
      spica cast evaluation in, 326
      static (nonstress) technique of Graf in, 322–324, *323–324*
      Thomas test in, 314, *316*
      treatment of, 330–341
      triple diapers in, 341, *342*
      U figure or teardrop shadow of Koehler in, *321*, 321
      ultrasonographic classification of, 324–325, *325*
      ultrasonographic findings in, 322–326
      ultrasonographic screening in, 325–326
      Von Rosen (Malmö) splint in, 340, *341*
    at three to twelve months, 326–327, *326–328*, 341–468
      acetabuloplasty in, 422–423
      antenatal (teratologic), 379, *390–391*
      anteroposterior arthrogram in, *348*, 349
      arthrography indications in, 346–347
      arthrography of capsule in, 350–351, *350–351*
      arthrography of labrum and limbus in, 351–352, *352*
      arthrography technique in, 347–350, *348–349*
      Bryant's traction in, 343, *344*
      closed reduction in, 346
      computed tomography of acetabular configuration in, 364, *366–367*
      computed tomography of capsule constriction in, 359, *360–361*
      computed tomography of femoral torsion in, 361, *363–365*, 364
      computed tomography of lateral displacement in, 358, *358*
      computed tomography of pin protrusion in, 361, *363*
      computed tomography of posterior displacement in, 358–359, *359*
      computed tomography of pulvinar in, 361, *362*
      femoral osteotomy in, 392–422. See also *Femoral osteotomy; Salter's innominate osteotomy.*
      femoral shortening and derotation osteotomy in, 379, *379*, **388–389**
      Gage and Winter's traction stations in, 345, *346–347*
      Galleazzi sign in, *326*, 327
      hip spica cast application technique in, 353–357, *354–355*
      hip spica cast positioning in, 352–353
      Hughes arthrography technique in, 350
      Mitchell arthrography technique in, 350
      Nélaton's line in, 327, *327*
      open reduction via anterolateral approach in, *378*, 378–379, **380–387**
      open reduction via medial approach in, 364–367, **368–377**, 378
      Pauwel's modified osteotomy with greater trochanter transfer in, 442, **462–465**, 466, *468*
      Pemberton's pericapsular innominate osteotomy in, 423–424, **425–432**, 433–442
      plain radiography in, 357, *357*
      preliminary traction in, 342–346
      removable orthosis in, 357
      resubluxation or redislocation in, 379, 391–392
      shallow acetabulum correction in, 422–442
      skeletal traction in, 343–345, *344*
      skin traction technique in, 345–346
      split Russell's traction in, 342–343, *343*, 345–346
      treatment of, 341–468
      Wagner's distal and lateral transfer of greater trochanter in, 442–443, **450–457**, *466*
      Wagner's intertrochanteric double osteotomy in, 442, **460–461**, 466, *467*
      Wagner's lateral advancement of greater trochanter in, 442, 443, **458–459**
  classification of, 298, 300
    dislocatability in, 298
    dislocation in, 298
    subluxatability in, 298, 300
    teratologic, 298
    typical, 298, 300
  definition of, 298
  etiology of, 301–306
    birth order in, 303
    breech presentation in, 302–303, *303*
    critical periods in, 301–302
    familial incidence in, 304–305
    genetic factors in, 304–306
    in utero malposition in, 302–304, *303–305*
    ligamentous laxity in, 302
    oligohydramnios in, 303, *304*

Hip *(Continued)*
    postnatal environmental factors in, 306, *306*
    primary acetabular dysplasia in, 302
    seasonal influence in, 306
    sex incidence in, 305–306
    side involved in, 303–304, *305*
  in adolescent, 468–526
    acetabulum in, 468, *469*
    biomechanics of joint pressure in, 470, *472*
    Chiari's innominate osteotomy in, 503–517. See also *Chiari's innominate osteotomy.*
    classification of, 474
    Eppright's periacetabular osteotomy in, 503, *503*
    femur in, 468–469, *470*
    Hopf's double innominate osteotomy in, 474–475
    Kawamura's medial displacement dome pelvic osteotomy in, 506, 518–519, *518–519*
    osteoarthritis in, 469–470, *471*
    pain in, 473
    periacetabular triple innominate osteotomy in, 493, **494–501**, *502*
    preoperative assessment in, 473, *474*
    Salter's innominate osteotomy in, 474
    shelf operation in, 519–525, *521–525*
    Staheli's acetabular augmentation in, 522–526, *524–525*
    Steele's triple innominate osteotomy in, 475, **482–491**, 493
    subchondral bone in acetabulum in, 473, *473*
    surgical indications in, 470, 473, *473*
    surgical procedures for, 474–526
    Sutherland's double innominate osteotomy in, 474–475, **476–481**, *492*
    Tönnis's triple innominate osteotomy in, 493
    Wagner type I periacetabular osteotomy in, 493, *502*, 503
    Wagner type II periacetabular osteotomy in, 503, *503*
    Wagner type III periacetabular osteotomy in, 503, *503*
    Wilson's shelf procedure in, 520–522, *521–523*
  incidence of, 300–301, 301t
  pathology of, 306–312
    acetabulum in, 311–312
    barriers to reduction in, 307–310, *309–310*
    capsular adhesions in, 308–309, *309*
    iliopsoas tendon in, 308, *309*
    in dislocatability, 306, *307*
    in irreducible dislocation, 306–307, *308*
    in subluxatability, 306, *307*
    ligamentum teres in, 309
    limbus in, 309–310, *310*
    medial circumflex artery in, 311
    pelvifemoral muscles in, 310–311, *311*
    proximal femur in, 311
    pulvinar in, 309
  disarticulation of, in osteogenic sarcoma, **1326–1335**
  dislocation of, due to Pavlik harness treatment, 339–340
    in cerebral palsy, 1633–1637. See also *Cerebral palsy, hip in.*
    treatment of, 1646–1647, *1647–1649*
    in Down's syndrome, 892, *894*, 895
    in myelomeningocele, 1821–1836
    traumatic, 3212–3227
      central, 3224
      circumduction method of Bigelow in, 3222–3224, *3223*
      complications and problems in, 3226–3227
      diagnostic features in, 3216–3219, *3219–3220*

Hip *(Continued)*
      direct method of Allis in, 3221–3222, *3222*, 3224, *3225*
      fracture and, 3224
      gravity method of Stimson in, 3220–3221, *3221*
      mechanism of injury in, 3214–3216, *3215–3217*
      pathologic anatomy in, 3216, *3218*
      postoperative care in, 3224
      recurrent, 3226–3227
      treatment of, 3219–3224
      types of, 3212–3214, *3212–3214*
  embryology of, 297–298, *299–300*
  extension of, 33–36, *36*
  flexion-adduction deformity of, in cerebral palsy, treatment of, 1637, **1638–1641**, *1642–1643*, 1644–1645
  flexion deformity of, in myelomeningocele, 1836–1839
    posture in, 1623, *1624*
    tests for, 27, *28–29*
  hinged abduction of, in Legg-Calvé-Perthes disease, 983–984, *985*
  in arthrogryposis multiplex congenita, 2100–2101
  in cerebral palsy, 1627–1660. See also *Cerebral palsy, hip in.*
  in myelomeningocele, 1821–1841. See also *Myelomeningocele, hip in.*
  in poliomyelitis, 1921–1931. See also under *Poliomyelitis.*
  medial rotation deformity of, in cerebral palsy, 1630, 1633, *1634*
    treatment of, 1650–1651, **1652–1659**, 1660
  osteochondritis dissecans of, *1533*, 1534
  pathologic dislocation of, in septic arthritis, 1431, *1434*
  pathologic subluxation of, in septic arthritis, 1417, *1418*
  position of minimal intra-articular pressure for, 1410
  range of motion of, 33–36, *35–36*
  rotation in extension of, 33, *35*
  rotation in flexion of, 33, *35*
  septic arthritis of, in neonate, 1428–1435. See also *Arthritis, septic, in neonatal hip.*
  subluxation of, due to Pavlik harness treatment, 339–340
    in cerebral palsy, 1633–1637. See also *Cerebral palsy, hip in.*
    treatment of, 1645–1646
    in myelomeningocele, 1821–1836
  surgical drainage of, through Ober's posterior approach, **1425–1426**
  total replacement of, in rheumatoid arthritis, 1485
  tuberculosis of, Legg-Calvé-Perthes disease vs., 957–958, *958*
Histiocytoma, malignant fibrous, 1403
Histiocytosis X, 1274–1286
  classification of, 1274
  eosinophilic granuloma of bone in, 1278, 1281–1286. See also *Eosinophilic granuloma, of bone.*
  etiology of, 1275
  Hand-Schüller-Christian disease in, 1278, *1280–1281*
  Letterer-Siwe disease in, 1276–1278, *1277–1279*
  pathologic features of, 1275–1276, *1275–1276*
  pathology in, 1275–1276, *1275–1276*
History, birth, 3–4
  orthopedic, 2–4
  form for, 95t–103t
  prenatal, 3
Hitchhiker's thumb, 752, *753*
Hodgkin's disease, 1147, *1148*
Hogshead fascia lata transfer to lumbodorsal fascia, in gluteus maximus paralysis in, 1927, *1928*
Holt method for hamstring contracture, 1706, *1706*

Homocystinuria, 888–889
  Marfan's syndrome vs., 839, 889t
Hopf's double innominate osteotomy, in congenital dysplasia of hip in adolescent, 474–475
Horn cell, anterior, degeneration of, electromyography in, 65
Hughes arthrography technique, in congenital dysplasia of hip, 350
Humeral capitellum, osteochondritis of, 1013–1014, *1015*
Humerus, distal epiphysis of, displacement of, obstetrical, 3354, *3355–3356*
  distal physis of, fracture-separation of, 3105–3107, *3106–3107*
  lateral condyle of, fracture of, 3108–3119
    avascular necrosis in, 3119
    complications of, 3116–3119
    cubitus valgus due to, *3117–3118*, 3118
    cubitus varus due to, 3119
    delayed union of, 3116
    diagnosis of, 3109–3110
    mechanism of injury and pathology of, 3109, *3109–3111*
    nerve palsy in, 3119
    nonunion of, 3116
    premature physeal closure due to, 3116–3118
    treatment of, 3110–3116, **3112–3115**
  lateral rotation osteotomy of, 2046, **2048–2051**
  medial epicondyle of, fracture of, 3121–3123, *3122*
  neck of, excessive retroversion or anteversion of, 179
  proximal, congenital varus deformity of, 176
  proximal physis of, fracture of, 3046–3050
    diagnosis of, 3047, *3048*
    mechanism of injury in, 3046
    pathologic anatomy of, 3047
    treatment of, 3047–3050, *3050*
  shaft of, fracture of, 3052–3057
    diagnosis of, 3054
    mechanism of injury in, 3052–3054, *3053*
    pathologic anatomy in, 3054, *3055*
    treatment of, 3054–3057, *3055–3057*
  supracondylar fracture of, 3058–3092
    complications of, 3079–3092
      carrying angle change as, 3079–3081, *3080*
      joint stiffness as, 3092
      malunion (cubitus varus or valgus) as, 3079–3081, *3081–3082*, **3084–3091**
      myositis ossificans as, 3092
      neural, 3081–3083
      vascular, 3083, 3092
    diagnosis of, 3064–3066
    mechanism of injury and classification of, 3058–3062, *3059–3061*
    pathologic anatomy of, 3062
      extension type, *3059–3060*, 3062
      flexion type, *3061*, 3062
    radiography in, *3063–3067*, 3066–3067
    treatment of, 3067–3079
      emergency splinting in, 3067–3068
      in moderately displaced fractures, 3068–3070, *3069*
      in severely displaced fractures, 3070–3075, *3071–3074*
      in undisplaced or minimally displaced fractures, *3064–3065*, 3068
      open reduction in, 3075–3079
      skeletal traction in, 3075, *3076–3078*
  Wagner diaphyseal lengthening of, 1184, *1185*
Hunter syndrome, 875
Hurler syndrome, 867–875

Hurler syndrome (*Continued*)
  characteristic features of, 876
  clinical features of, 867–868, *870–872*
  pathologic and laboratory findings in, 867
  radiography in, 868–869, *873–874*
  treatment of, 875
Hyaluronic acid, in synovial fluid, 1410
Hydrocephalus, in myelomeningocele, 1790
Hypercalcemia, idiopathic, infantile, 925
Hyperextension, definition of, 33
Hyperglycinuria, in vitamin D refractory rickets, 910
Hyperkalemic periodic paralysis, 2172–2173
Hyperkinesia, in cerebral palsy, 1611–1612
Hyperostosis, infantile cortical, Camurati-Engelmann disease vs., 806
  progressive diaphyseal dysplasia vs., 806
Hyperparathyroidism, primary, 931
Hyperphosphatasia, idiopathic, 816–817
Hyperthermia, malignant, 71–73, 103t
Hypertrichosis, in spinal dysraphism, 1873–1874, *1874*
Hypertrophic interstitial neuritis, 1988–1989
Hypervitaminosis A, 920–922, *921*
Hypervitaminosis D, 923–925, *924*
Hypochondroplasia, 729
Hypokalemic periodic paralysis, 2172
Hypoparathyroidism, idiopathic, 929
Hypophosphatasia, 741–745
  clinical and roentgenographic findings in, 742–743, *742–745*
  differential diagnosis of, 743
  inheritance in, 741–742
  laboratory findings in, 743
  mild adult, 745
  pathology in, 742
  treatment of, 743
Hyporeflexia, in cerebral palsy, 1613
Hypothyroidism, 927–929, *928*
  Legg-Calvé-Perthes disease vs., 958, *961–962*
  slipped femoral capital epiphysis due to, 1019, 1022
Hypotonic child syndrome, 1906t
Hypoxia, fetal, in cerebral palsy, 1609

I

Ibuprofen, in rheumatoid arthritis, 1479
Ilfeld splint, in congenital dysplasia of hip, 340–341, *341*
Iliopsoas, in gait, 14
Iliopsoas tendon, hip capsule constriction due to, 359, *360–361*
  in irreducible congenital dysplasia of hip, 308, *309*
Iliopsoas transfer, in paralysis of hip adductors, 1825–1826, *1827*, **1828–1835**, 1836
Iliotibial band, attachment to iliac crest of, 1921, *1922*
Iliotibial tract, in recurrent subluxation or dislocation of patella, 1552
Ilium, pyogenic osteomyelitis of, 1106–1107
Ilizarov two-level tibial lengthening, 2896, **2972–2989**, 2992–2993
Immobilization, in double hip spica cast, 3262
Index finger abduction restoration of Phalen, 2057, **2076–2077**
Indomethacin, in rheumatoid arthritis, 1479
Infant, acute pyogenic osteomyelitis in, 1094, 1095t
  development of locomotion in, 14
  septic arthritis of hip in, 1428–1435. See also *Arthritis, septic, in neonatal hip.*
Infantile cortical hyperostosis, 817–824. See also *Cortical hyperostosis, infantile.*

Volume 1, pgs. 1–687; Volume 2, pgs. 688–1600; Volume 3, pgs. 1601–2404; Volume 4, pgs. 2405–3373

Infarction, bone, in sickle cell disease, 1140, *1141*
Infection, of bone. See *Osteomyelitis*.
Infraction, Freiberg's, 1006–1008, *1006–1009*
INH, in septic arthritis, 1424t
  in tuberculous arthritis, 1448
Intelligence, in cerebral palsy, 1616
  in myelomeningocele, 1790–1791
Intermetacarpal bone block for thenar paralysis, 2057, **2078–2079**
Interphalangeal joint, flexion deformity of, 1738–1739, **1740–1743**
  proximal, Swanson sublimis tenodesis of, 1739, 1744
Interstitial neuritis, hypertrophic, 1988–1989
Intertrochanteric double osteotomy, Wagner's, 442, **460–461**, 466, *467*
Intertrochanteric osteotomy, abduction-extension, in Legg-Calvé-Perthes disease, 984, *985*
Intervertebral disc, calcification of, 2391–2393, *2392*
  discitis of, 2394–2401. See also *Discitis*.
  herniated, 2402
Intra-articular lipoma, 1598
Intracranial tumor, 1771–1773, *1772*
  clinical features in, 1771
  diagnostic considerations in, 1771–1772
  pathologic considerations in, 1771, *1772*
  treatment of, 1772–1773
Intramedullary rod fixation, in osteogenesis imperfecta, 778–782, *780–781*
Intraspinal tumor, 1887–1902
  cerebrospinal fluid findings in, 1892
  clinical picture in, 1887–1888, *1888–1891*
  differential diagnosis of, 1892–1893, *1894–1895*
  radiographic findings in, 1888–1889, 1892, *1892*
  treatment of, 1893, *1896–1901*, 1902
Intrauterine fracture, 3354, 3357
Intrauterine posture, development of, 2421–2422, *2423*
Inversion, definition of, 33
Involucrum, in osteomyelitis, 1084
Iridocyclitis, in rheumatoid arthritis, 1472–1473
Ischial-bearing above-knee amputation, in osteogenic sarcoma, **1336–1345**
Ischiopubic osteochondritis, 1016

J

Jack toe-raising test, 2724, *2728*
Japas V-osteotomy of tarsus, 2691, **2694–2698**
Jarcho-Levin syndrome, 2199
Jeune's disease, 737, *738*
Joint fluid analysis, 1411–1415
  glucose in, 1414
  gross appearance in, 1411
  in individual joint disorders, 1413t–1414t
  microscopic examination in, 1413–1414
  protein in, 1414
  routes of joint aspiration in, 1411, *1412*
  viscosity and mucin clot in, 1411, 1413
Joints, 1410–1600. See also individual types.
  Clutton's, 1458
  diagnostic considerations for, 1411–1415
  fungal infection of, 1460
  of lower limb, ankylosis of, gait in, 24
  positions of minimal intra-articular pressure for, 1410–1411
  range of motion of, 32–40, *34–41*

Joints (*Continued*)
  routes of aspiration of, 1411, *1412*
Juvenile ankylosing spondylitis, pauciarticular, 1470
Juvenile rheumatoid arthritis. See *Rheumatoid arthritis*.

K

Kalamchi and MacEwen classification, of ischemic necrosis, 438–441, *441*
Kalamchi's modification of Salter innominate osteotomy, 419–422, *421–423*
Kawamura's medial displacement dome pelvic osteotomy, 506, 518–519, *518–519*
Kinetic power, 40
King's knee fusion, in focal deficiency of proximal femur, 571, 576, 577, **578–579**
Kirner deformity, 286–287, *287*
Kirschner wire, in congenital longitudinal deficiency of radius, 204
  migration of, due to Salter's innominate osteotomy, 418
Klinefelter's syndrome, 897
Klippel-Feil syndrome, 128–136
  clinical features and anomalies of, 128–132, 129t, *129–130*
  etiology of, 128
  in Sprengel's deformity, 138, *142–143*
  roentgenographic features of, *129–132*, 132–133
  treatment of, 133
Knee. See also under *Genu*.
  congenital dislocation and subluxation of, 609–615
    associated deformities in, 610
    diagnosis of, 611–612, *612–614*
    etiology of, 609–610, *610*
    genu recurvatum vs., 612
    grades of severity in, 611, *611–612*
    heredity in, 610
    incidence of, 609
    pathologic findings and clinical features in, 610–611
    treatment of, 612–615, *616–617*
  disarticulation of, in osteogenic sarcoma, **1346–1349**
  extension contracture of, in cerebral palsy, 1714–1716
  extension or hyperextension of, in myelomeningocele, 1820–1821
  flail, in poliomyelitis, 1937, *1938*
  flexion deformity of, in cerebral palsy, 1706–1714
    in myelomeningocele, 1818–1820
    in poliomyelitis, 1922, 1934, *1934*
  flexion of, in gait, 10–11, *11*
  in arthrogryposis multiplex congenita, 2099–2100
  in cerebral palsy, 1705–1717. See also *Cerebral palsy, knee in*.
  in hereditary onycho-osteodystrophy, 845, *846*
  in myelomeningocele, 1818–1821
  in poliomyelitis, 1930–1937
  medial instability of, due to Pavlik harness treatment, 340, *340*
  motion of, in gait, 12, *12*
  osteochondral fracture of, 3282–3283
  position of minimal intra-articular pressure for, 1410
  subluxation of, in poliomyelitis, 1922
  synovectomy of, 1505–1506
  talipes equinus effects on, 1930, *1931*
  total arthroplasty of, in rheumatoid arthritis, 1485–1486
  valgus deformity of, in poliomyelitis, 1922
Knee fusion, King's, in focal deficiency of proximal femur, 571, 576, 577, **578–579**

Knee-lock, double, 11
Kniest disease, 757
Knock-knee. See *Genu valgum.*
Köhler's disease, of tarsal navicular, 1003–1005, *1004*
Kramer femoral neck osteotomy, in slipped femoral capital epiphysis, 1062, **1064–1065**
Kugelberg-Welander disease, 1904
Kyphoscoliosis, 2185
　anesthesia in, 70–71
　in osteogenesis imperfecta, 769, *770*
Kyphosis, congenital, 2207–2211
　　classification of, 2207–2208, *2208*
　　clinical picture in, 2208–2209, *2210*
　　differential diagnosis of, 2209
　　natural history of, 2209
　　treatment of, 2209–2211
　in intraspinal tumor, 1893, *1898–1899*
　in myelomeningocele, 1848–1852
　in neurofibromatosis, *1296*
　in scoliosis, 2288, *2289*
　Scheuermann's juvenile, 2380–2388. See also *Scheuermann's juvenile kyphosis.*
　terminology in, 2185

L

Labyrinthine righting reflex, 53
Lag screw, Coventry, 395
Landau reflex, 50–51
Langenskiöld fibular-tibial synostosis, in congenital pseudarthrosis of fibula, 685, *686*
Langenskiöld greater trochanteric apophyseodesis, 441–442, **444–449**
Langenskiöld osteotomy, in coxa vara, 593–595, *594*
Larsen's syndrome, 852–854, *853–854*
　talipes equinovarus in, 2455, *2457*
Latissimus dorsi and teres major transfer to rotator cuff, 2029, **2042–2045**
Latissimus dorsi transfer, for elbow in poliomyelitis, 1967, *1967–1970*
Leg. See also *Limb.*
　alignment of, physiologic evolution of, 2820–2822, *2821–2022*
　ankylosis of joints of, gait in, 24
　cutaneous sensation in, segmental innervation of, 1779, *1780*
　development and ossification of, 2406–2408, *2407–2410*
　duplication of long bones of, 686, *687*
　epiphyseal closure in, *63*
　epiphyseal ossification in, *62*
　length inequality of, 2850–3001
　　causes of, 2850, 2851t
　　epiphysiodesis in, 2871–2887
　　　complications of, 2876, 2887
　　　Green-Anderson growth remaining method in, 2871–2872
　　　Moseley's straight-line graph in, 2872–2876, *2873–2874*
　　　of distal femur, **2878–2881**
　　　of proximal tibia and fibula, **2882–2885**
　　　percutaneous, 2876
　　　results of, *2877,* 2886–2887
　　　White-Menelaus rule of thumb method in, 2872
　　examination in, 27, 31, *31*
　　femoral lengthening in, 2892–2893

Leg *(Continued)*
　　femoral shortening in, 2889–2892, *2890–2891*
　　gait in, 24
　　growth prediction charts in treatment planning for, *2864,* 2864–2867, 2865t
　　in femoral shaft fracture, 3266–3268
　　in Legg-Calvé-Perthes disease, 982–983
　　in rheumatoid arthritis, 1484–1485
　　in septic arthritis, 1431
　　intra- and postoperative problems in, 2991, 2995t, 2996–3001
　　　axial deviation as, 2999–3000
　　　compartment syndrome as, 2996
　　　delayed consolidation and nonunion as, 3001
　　　during corticotomy, 2996
　　　joint stiffness as, 2999
　　　joint subluxation and dislocation as, 2998–2999
　　　mental disturbance as, 3001
　　　muscle contracture as, 2997, *2997–2998*
　　　muscle weakness as, 2998
　　　neurologic compromise as, 2998
　　　premature consolidation as, 3000–3001
　　　screw or pin tract infection as, 2996–2997
　　　stress fracture and plastic bowing as, 3001
　　　vascular disorders as, 2998
　　limb lengthening in, 2893–2991
　　　biologic principles of, 2893–2894
　　　contraindications in, 2894–2895
　　　femoral lengthening by callotasis in, 2896, **2942–2859**
　　　Ilizarov two-level tibial lengthening in, 2896, **2972–2989,** *2992–2993*
　　　indications for, 2894
　　　methods for, 2895–2896
　　　requisites in, 2894
　　　soft-tissue release in femur in, 2895
　　　soft-tissue release in tibia in, 2895
　　　tibial lengthening by callotasis in, 2896, **2960–2971**
　　　Wagner femoral lengthening in, 2896, 2897, **2898–2921**
　　　Wagner tibial diaphyseal lengthening in, 2896, **2922–2941**
　　　Wasserstein femoral and tibial lengthening in, 2896, *2994*
　　physeal stapling in, 2887–2888, 2888t
　　radiography for measurement of, 2867–2870
　　　CT scan in, 2870, *2870*
　　　orthoroentgenography in, 2867–2870, *2868–2869*
　　　slit scanography in, 2867
　　　teleoroentgenography in, 2867, *2868*
　　scoliosis due to, 2191, *2194,* 2196
　　tibial lengthening in, 2893
　　tibial shortening in, 2888–2889
　　treatment principles in, 2871–2893
　length of, actual, measurement of, 27, *31*
　　apparent, measurement of, 27, *31*
　longitudinal deficiencies of, 105, *110–111*
　malalignment of, in recurrent subluxation or dislocation of patella, 1552
　muscles of, in gait, 13–14, *15*
　　innervation of, 85t
　neurosegmental innervation of, 1780, *1781*
　reflexes and joint movements of, neurosegmental innervation of, 1780, *1781*
　terminal transverse deficiencies of, 105, *108*
　torsional deformities of, 2791–2800. See also *Femoral torsion; Tibial torsion.*
　　etiology of, 2792–2794
　　heredity in, 2793

Volume 1, pgs. 1–687; Volume 2, pgs. 688–1600; Volume 3, pgs. 1601–2404; Volume 4, pgs. 2405–3373

Leg *(Continued)*
    persistent postnatal malposture in, 2793–2794
    persistent fetal alignment in, 2792–2793
    sitting habits in, 2794, *2795*
    sleeping habits in, 2793–2794
  pathophysiology in, 2791–2792
  rotation of limb bud in, 2792
  torsional profile in, 2794–2800
    foot deformities in, 2800, 2800t–2801t
    foot-progression angle in, 2794–2795, *2796*
    medial and lateral hip rotation in, 2795, *2796–2797*, *2798*
    thigh-foot angle in, 2798, *2798*
    transmalleolar axis angle in, 2798–2800, *2799*
Leg straightening reflex, 49
Legg-Calvé-Perthes disease, 933–988
  acute transient synovitis vs., 1464t
  associated anomalies in, 935
  bilateral, 958
  bone dysplasia vs., 958, *959–960*
  Caffey's sign in, 949
  classification of, 965–970
    Catterall's, 966, 966t, 969–970, *969–970*
    partial head type in, 966, *967*
    Salter's, 970
    total head type in, 966, *968*
  clinical manifestations of, 943
  constitutional factors in, 934–935
  deformity in, 943, *944–945*
  differential diagnosis of, 956–958, *958–962*
  etiology of, 935–936
  head at risk signs in, 965t
  hereditary factors in, 934
  histochemistry in, 939
  history of, 933
  hypothyroidism vs., 958, *961–962*
  incidence of, 934, 934t
  infection vs., 957
  juvenile rheumatoid arthritis vs., 957
  magnetic resonance imaging in, 956, *957*
  morphology in, 939
  natural history of, 958, 960
  pathogenesis of, 939, 943, *943–945*
  pathology of, 936–943, *937–945*
    in initial stage, 936, *937–938*
    in reparative stage, 939, *942*
    in resorption stage, 936, 939, *940–941*
  prognosis in, 960–965
    Dickens and Menelaus's method for, 963, *964*
    disease stage and, 965
    extent of involvement and, 960, 963
    femoral head protrusion in, 963, *963–964*
    Green's epiphyseal extrusion index in, 963, *963*
    hip motion loss and, 965
    metaphyseal changes and, 964–965, *965*
    obesity and, 965
    patient age and, 960
    physeal growth disturbance and, 963–964, *964*
  radiography in, 943, *946–953*, 949
  rheumatic fever vs., 957
  technetium-99m bone scan in, 949, 952, 953t, *954–956*, 956, 956t
  toxic synovitis vs., 956–957
  treatment of, 970–988
    containment by orthosis in, 972–977
      ambulatory devices in, 972, 972t
      around the world hip motion machine in, 977, *978*
      discontinuation of, 977
      Newington abduction orthosis in, 972–973, *974*

Legg-Calvé-Perthes disease *(Continued)*
      nonambulatory devices in, 972, 972t
      Petrie abduction cast in, 975
      prerequisites for, 975–977
      problems during, 977, *978*
      Roberts orthosis in, 973–974
      Scottish-Rite orthosis in, 972, *973*
      trilateral socket hip containment orthosis in, 974–975, *975–976*
    containment by surgery in, 977–982
      femoral osteotomy in, 981–982, *982–983*
      indications for, 979, *979–980*
      Salter's innominate osteotomy in, 979–981, *980–981*
    guidelines for selection of, 970–971
    initial phase of, 971
    objectives of, 970
    reconstructive, 982–988
      abduction-extension intertrochanteric osteotomy in, 984, *985*
      cheilectomy in, 984
      in greater trochanter overgrowth and coxa breva, 983, *984*
      in hinged abduction of hip, 983–984, *985*
      in lower limb length inequality, 982–983
      incongruous hip in, 984–986, *986*
      osteochondritis dissecans in, 986–988, *987–988*
      torn acetabular labrum in, 988
    second phase of, 971–982
    tuberculosis of hip vs., 957–958, *958*
    tumors vs., 958
Legg-Perthes disease, multiple epiphyseal dysplasia vs., 703, *705*
Léri-Weill syndrome, 213
Lesch-Nyhan syndrome, congenital indifference to pain vs., 1998–1999
Letterer-Siwe disease, 1276–1278, *1277–1279*
Leukemia, 1146, *1146–1147*
Leukocyte count, in joint fluid analysis, 1413
Levator scapulae, transfer of, in supraspinatus paralysis, 1959, *1960*
Ligamentous hyperflexibility, tests for, 2277, 2280
Ligamentum teres, in arthrography of congenital dysplasia of hip, 352
  in congenital dysplasia of hip, 309
Limb. See also *Arm; Leg.*
  congenital deficiency of, classification of, 106t–107t
  constriction bands of, 111
  duplication of, 110
  failure of differentiation of parts of, 105
  failure of formation of parts of, 105, *108–111*
  longitudinal deficiencies of, 105, *110–111*
  lower. See *Leg.*
  overgrowth of, 110–111
  terminal transverse deficiencies of, 105, *108*
  undergrowth of, 111
  upper. See *Arm.*
Limbus, in congenital dysplasia of hip, 309–310, *310*
Limp. See also *Gait.*
  antalgic, 24
  in short leg, 24
Lipoma, intra-articular, 1598
  intraosseous, of os calcis, 2780, *2787*
  of filum terminale, clinical features of, 1873–1874, *1874*
    embryology and pathology of, 1873, *1873*
  of foot, 2766, *2767*
  subcutaneous, with interdural stalk, 1873
Lipomyelomeningocele, 1871–1897
  clinical features of, 1873–1874, *1874*

Lipomyelomeningocele (Continued)
    diagnosis of, 1874–1875, *1875*
    embryology and pathology in, 1871–1873, *1872*
    neurosurgical management of, 1875–1878, *1876–1877*
        concurrent skin appendage in, 1877–1878
        deterioration after, 1878
        orthopedic management of, 1878–1879
        postoperative results of, 1878
        removing mass in, *1876*, 1877
        tilted placode in, 1877
Lisfranc's tarsometatarsal fracture-dislocation, 3341–3342, *3341–3342*
Littler abductor digiti quinti manus transfer, 2057, **2070–2071**
Littlewood forequarter amputation, **1354–1367**
Lloyd Roberts intertrochanteric oblique osteotomy, 395, **402–403**
Lobster claw deformity, 280, *281*. See also *Hand, cleft.*
Lobster claw foot, 2637, *2638–2642*
Locomotion. See also *Gait.*
    in infant, 14
Lordoscoliosis, 2185
Lordosis, in myelomeningocele, 1836, *1837*, 1841–1843, *1842*
    in poliomyelitis, 1922–1923
    in scoliosis, 2288, *2289*
    terminology in, 2185
Lower limb. See *Leg.*
Lower motor neuron disease, electrical testing in, 64
Lumbar disc syndrome, pyogenic osteomyelitis of, 1106–1107
Lumbar pedicle aplasia, congenital, 2229–2230
Lumbar vertebrae, compression fracture of, 3345, *3346*
Lumbosacral agenesis, 2212–2228
    classification of, 2213, *2214–2217*
    clinical picture in, 2213–2217, *2218–2226*
    etiology of, 2212
    pathologic findings in, 2212–2213
    radiography in, 2217–2218
    treatment of, 2218–2221, 2227–2228
Lupus erythematosus, systemic, joint fluid analysis in, 1413t
Luque double L-rod instrumentation, in scoliosis, 2319–2320, *2321*
Lurch, gluteus medius, 22, 23
Lyme arthritis, 1440–1441
Lymphadenopathy, in rheumatoid arthritis, 1472
Lymphangiectasis, of foot, 2768, 2770, 2777
Lymphoma, 1147, *1148*
Lymphosarcoma, 1147, *1148*

M

Macrodactylism, of toes, 2651, *2652–2654*
Macrodactyly, 277, *278*
Madelung's deformity, 210–222
    clinical features of, 211, *212*
    diagnosis of, 213
    differential diagnosis of, 213, *213*
    etiology of, 211
    pathologic anatomy in, 211
    treatment of, 213–221
        carpal stabilization in, 221
        control of distal radial asymmetrical growth in, 214–215, 215
        operative, clinical results of, *220*

Madelung's deformity (Continued)
    shortening of ulna in, 214–215
    ulnar head resection and distal radial open-wedge osteotomy in, **216–219**
Maffucci's syndrome, 1195, *1196–1198*
Malabsorption syndrome, vitamin D deficiency rickets and, 903–904
Malignant hyperthermia syndrome, 71–73
    counseling in, 73
    diagnosis of, 72
    incidence of, 71
    pathophysiology of, 71–72
    signs of, 103t
    susceptibility to, surgery in, 73
    treatment of, 72–73, 103t
Malleolus, medial, accessory ossification center of, 2416, *2418*
Mallet toe, 2670–2671, *2671*
    in cerebral palsy, 1705
Malmö splint, in congenital dysplasia of hip, 340, *341*
Marfan's syndrome, 829–836
    Achard's syndrome vs., 839
    clinical features of, 829–833, *830–833*, 832t
    differential diagnosis of, 833–834, 834t
    etiology of, 829
    forme fruste, 833
    heredity in, 829
    homocystinuria vs., 839, 889t
    treatment in, 834–836, *835*
Maroteaux-Lamy syndrome, 875
Marrow, hyperplasia of, in sickle cell disease, 1140, *1141*
Maturation, neurophysiologic, reflexes of, 86t–89t
McArdle's syndrome, 2174–2175
McFarland bypass procedure, in congenital longitudinal deficiency of tibia, 644, *650*
McFarland's posterior bypass autogenous bone graft procedure, in congenital pseudarthrosis of tibia, 662–666, *665–666*
McKay technique for dorsal bunion, in poliomyelitis, 1945, *1946–1948*, *1950–1951*
Measurements, normal, in relation to age, in females, 78t
    in males, 77t
Mediterranean anemia, 1136–1139, *1137–1138*
Megalodactyly, 277, *278*
Mehta's rib-vertebral angle, 2285, 2288, *2288–2289*
Melnick-Needles syndrome, 826, 829
Melorheostosis, 808–812
    clinical features of, 809, *810*
    differential diagnosis in, 809
    etiology of, 808
    pathology of, 808–809
    radiography in, 809, *810–811*
    treatment of, 809, 812
Menard's line, in congenital dysplasia of hip, *320*, 320–321
Meninges, in myelomeningocele, 1777–1778
Meningocele, 1773–1774. See also *Myelomeningocele.*
    neurosurgical treatment of, 1786–1790
Meniscus, discoid, 1539–1549
    clinical features in, 1540–1542
    complete type, 1540
    imaging in, *1541*, 1542
    infantile, 1539
    intermediate, 1539
    pathogenesis of, 1539–1540
    pathology in, 1540, *1540*
    primitive, 1539
    treatment of, 1542, **1543–1548**, 1549
    Wrisberg-ligament type, 1540

Menkes syndrome, 864
Metacarpal, fracture of, 3205, *3206–3208*, 3209
  hypoplastic, 283
Metacarpophalangeal capsulorrhaphy, in cerebral palsy, 1731, 1738
Metacarpophalangeal joint, flexion deformity of, 1738–1739, **1740–1743**
Metaphyseal blanch sign of Steel, in slipped femoral capital epiphysis, 1028, *1030*
Metaphyseal chondrodysplasia, 737, *739*, 740
  cartilage-hair hypoplasia (McKusick type), 740
  Jansen type, 737
  Schmid type, 737, *739*
  Spahr-Hartmann type, 737, 740
  treatment of, 740
  variations of, 740
Metaphyseal defect, fibrous, 1247–1249, *1248*
Metaphyseal dysplasia, 825–826, *826–828*
  osteopetrosis vs., 797
Metaphysitis, syphilitic, *1124*, 1125
Metastasis, pulmonary, in osteogenic sarcoma, 1316–1317, *1380–1381*, 1382
Metatarsal, accessory bone at, 2416, *2419*
  aneurysmal bone cyst of, 2780, *2785*
  fracture of, 3342–3343, *3343*
  Freiberg's infraction of, 1006–1008, *1006–1009*
  osteochondritis dissecans of, 2759, *2759*
  short, congenital, 2633, *2634–2636*, 2637
Metatarsal osteotomy, in talipes equinovarus, 2524
Metatarsus adductus, congenital, 2612
  postural, 2426, *2427*, 2614
Metatarsus primus varus, congenital, *2626–2628*, 2626–2629
Metatarsus varus, congenital, 2612–2619
  clinical features of, 2612, *2614*
  diagnosis of, 2614
  experimental production of, 2612, *2613*
  functional, 2614
  in congenital dysplasia of hip, 316
  in talipes equinovarus, 2531, *2531*, 2538
  treatment of, 2614–2619
   nonoperative, 2615, *2616–2618*
   surgical, 2615, 2619, **2620–2625**
Metatropic dysplasia, 757
Methylprednisone sodium, percutaneous injection of, 1285
Microdactylism, of toes, 2651, 2653
Mid-thigh amputation, in osteogenic sarcoma, **1336–1345**
Milch cuff resection, in Madelung's deformity, **216–219**
Milch method, in radiography of hip flexion deformity, 1630
Milwaukee brace, in Scheuermann's juvenile kyphosis, 2386, *2387*
  in scoliosis, *2296*, 2296–2300
Mitchell arthrography technique, in congenital dysplasia of hip, 350
Möbius syndrome, talipes equinovarus in, 2455, *2458*
Monoplegia, 40, 1606
Monteggia equivalent lesions of forearm, 3178–3179
Monteggia fracture-dislocation, 3151–3179
  classification of, *3152–3156*, 3158
  complications of, 3168, 3178
   malunion as, 3178
   nerve palsy as, 3168
   radiohumeral fibrous ankylosis as, 3178
   radioulnar synostosis as, 3178
   recurrence as, 3168, 3178
   Volkmann's ischemic contracture as, 3178

Monteggia fracture-dislocation *(Continued)*
  diagnosis of, *3161*, 3161–3163
  mechanism of injury in, *3157*, 3158, *3159–3160*, 3161
  treatment of, 3163–3168
   operative, 3163, **3164–3167**, 3168, **3170–3177**
   reduction in, *3162*, 3163
Moro reflex, 45, *46*
Morquio syndrome, 875–878
  clinical features of, 875–877
  prognosis in, 877–878
  radiography in, 877
  treatment of, 878
Moseley's straight-line graph, in epiphysiodesis, 2872–2876, *2873–2874*
Motor and sensory neuropathy, hereditary, 1982–1986
  classification of, 1982–1983
  types I and II, 1983–1986, *1984–1985*
Motor development, evaluation of, 90t–91t
Motor evaluation, 55–57
Motor neuron disease, lower, electrical testing in, 64
Motor power, testing of, 40–42
Moxalactam, in septic arthritis, 1424t
Mubarak's wick catheter tissue pressure method, 3100
Mucin precipitation test, 1413
Mucopolysaccharidosis, 865–878
  clinical and radiographic features of, 865–867, *866*
  differential diagnosis of, 867, 868t–869t
  dysostosis multiplex in, 865–867, *866*
  type I (Hurler syndrome), 867–875. See also *Hurler syndrome*.
  type II (Hunter syndrome), 875
  type III (Sanfilippo syndrome), 875
  type IV (Morquio syndrome), 875–878
  type V (Sheie syndrome), 875
  type VI (Maroteaux-Lamy syndrome), 875
Multiple enchondromatosis, 1195, *1196–1198*
Multiple epiphyseal dysplasia, 701–707. See also *Epiphyseal dysplasia, multiple*.
Multiple exostosis, 1172–1190. See also *Exostosis, multiple*.
Multiple sclerosis, differential diagnosis of, 1980t
Muscle, accessory, 2120, *2121–2122*
  atrophy of, 1411
  chart for examination of, in flaccid paralysis, 81t–82t
   in spastic paralysis, 79t–80t
  concentric contraction of, 14
  congenital absence of, 2119
  disorders of, differentiation of, 1601–1604, 1602t–1603t
  eccentric contraction of, 14
  in gait, 13–14, *15*
  of leg, innervation of, 85t
  of shoulder girdle, innervation of, 84t
  response to injury or disease of, 1604
  spasm of, 1411
   involuntary, 1
  spasticity of, 1610–1611, 1611t
  strength of, grading of, 83t
  testing of, 40–42
Muscular dystrophy, 2126–2151
  Becker, 2135
  biochemistry in, 2130–2132
   aldolase in, 2131
   body fluid changes in, 2130–2131
   creatine and creatinine in, 2130–2131
   creatine kinase in, 2131
   muscle changes in, 2131–2132
   serum enzyme changes in, 2131
  classification of, 2127–2128
  congenital, 2136

Muscular dystrophy *(Continued)*
  definition of, 2126–2127
  diagnosis of, 2141, *2145*
  differential diagnosis of, 2142t–2144t
  distal, 2136–2138
  Duchenne, 2132–2135
    anesthesia in, 68
    clinical course in, 2134
    clinical features in, 2132–2134, *2133*
    electromyographic findings in, 2134
    Gowers' sign in, 2132, *2133*
    heredity in, 2132
    laboratory findings in, 2134
    muscle biopsy in, 2134–2135
  electromyography in, 65
  Emery-Dreifuss, 2135
  etiology of, 2128
  facioscapulohumeral (Landouzy and Déjérine), 2136, *2137*
  histologic changes in, 2128–2130, *2129*
  historical, 2127
  limb girdle, 2135–2136
  pathology in, 2128–2130, *2129*
  polymyositis vs., 2144t
  scapuloperoneal, 2136
  screening and genetic counseling in, 2151
  treatment of, 2141–2151
    functional classification in, 2144
    loss of ambulation and, 2144
    orthoses in, 2150
    scapulocostal stabilization in, **2146–2149**, 2151
    surgical, 2150–2151
Myasthenia gravis, 2177–2179
  clinical features of, 2178
  diagnosis of, 2178–2179
  electrical testing in, 64
  etiology of, 2177
  incidence of, 2177
  juvenile, 2178
  neonatal persistent, 2178
  neonatal transient, 2178
  prognosis in, 2179
  treatment of, 2179
Myelocystocele, 1879
Myelodysplasia, 1773
  in myelomeningocele, 1778
Myelomeningocele, 1773–1858
  ambulation in, 1792–1795, *1793–1794*
    factors in potential for, 1792–1793
    subdivisions of, 1792
  anesthesia in, 69
  antenatal diagnosis of, 1776
    amniocentesis in, 1776
    ultrasonography in, 1776
  clinical features of, 1778–1780, *1779–1781*
  congenital anomalies with, 1780–1781, 1782t
  embryology in, 1774
  etiology of, 1774
  foot and ankle in, 1795–1817
    calcaneofibular tenodesis in, 1805, **1806–1807**
    flaccid vs. spastic paralysis in, 1795
    flail ankle in, 1817
    neurosegmental level of lesion in, 1796–1797, *1796–1798*
    paralytic congenital convex talipes valgus in, 1811–1816, *1814–1815*
    posterior tibial tendon transfer to os calcis in, 1799, **1800–1803**, 1804
    talipes calcaneus in, 1798–1799, **1800–1803**, 1804

Myelomeningocele *(Continued)*
    talipes cavus in, *1816*, 1816–1817
    talipes equinovarus in, 1805, 1809–1811, *1809–1812*
    talipes equinus in, 1811, *1813*
    treatment objectives in, 1797–1798
    types of, 1795, 1795t
    valgus ankle in, 1804–1805, *1805*, **1806–1807**, *1808–1809*
    Wiltse triangular osteotomy of distal tibial diaphysis in, 1805, *1809*
  fractures in, 1852–1854
    clinical features of, 1853
    etiology of, 1852–1853
    radiographic features of, 1853
    treatment of, 1853
  heredity in, 1775–1776
  hip in, 1821–1841
    abduction and lateral rotation deformity of, 1839–1840, *1840*
    adduction deformity of, 1840–1841
    flexion deformity of, 1836–1839
      extension osteotomy of proximal femur in, *1838*, 1838–1839
      lordosis in, 1836, *1837*
      orthosis in, 1837
      soft-tissue release of contracture in, 1837–1838
      treatment in, 1836–1839
    sublocation-dislocation of, 1821–1841
      diagnosis of, 1822
      external oblique abdominal muscle transfer to greater trochanter in, 1836
      iliopsoas transfer in, 1825–1826, *1827*, **1828–1835**, 1836
      in older child, 1825
      muscle paralysis patterns in, 1821–1822, *1822–1824*
      treatment principles in, 1822–1825
  incidence of, 1774
  knee in, extension or hyperextension contracture of, 1820–1821
    flexion deformity of, 1818–1820
      clinical and biochemical implications of, 1818–1819
      etiology of, 1818
      supracondylar distal femoral extension osteotomy in, 1819–1820, *1820*
      treatment of, 1819–1820
    genu valgum in, 1821
    genu varum in, 1821
  neurosurgical treatment of, 1786–1792
    hindbrain dysfunction in, 1791
    hydrocephalus in, 1790
    intelligence and, 1790–1791
    meningocele in, 1786–1790
      care of exposed tissue in, 1788
      early closure of, 1786–1788
      follow-up and late deterioriation in, 1789–1790
      postoperative care in, 1789
      preservation of neural tissue in, 1788
      reconstruction of neural tissue in, 1788–1789, *1789*
    mortality in, 1791–1792
    perceptual motor deficiency and, 1790–1791
    urinary incontinence in, 1791
  orthopedic management in, 1792–1795
  orthotics and habilation in, 1854–1858
    for standing, 1855–1856, *1856*
    in infant, 1855, *1855*
    in lower lumbar level lesion, 1857–1858
    in sacral level lesion, 1858
    in thoracic level lesion, 1856–1857
    in upper lumbar level lesion, 1857, *1857*

Myelomeningocele (*Continued*)
  wheelchairs in, 1858
  pathogenesis of, 1775
  pathology in, 1776–1778
    basic deformity in, 1776–1777, *1777*
    brain in, 1778
    meninges in, 1777–1778
    peripheral roots in, 1778
    skin in, 1777
    spinal cord in, 1778
    vertebrae in, 1778
  spine in, 1841–1852
    kyphosis in, 1848–1852
      balanced vs. unbalanced, 1848, 1848–1849, *1849*, *1849–1850*
      congenital, 1848–1852
      radiography in, 1849, *1851*
      treatment of, 1849, *1851–1852*, 1852
    lordosis in, *1837*, 1841–1843, *1842*
      etiology of, 1841
      treatment in, 1841–1843
      types of, 1841, *1842*
    scoliosis in, 1843–1848
      etiology of, 1843, *1844–1846*
      orthosis in, 1843, 1847
      pseudarthrosis in, 1848
      surgical complications in, 1847–1848
      treatment of, 1843, 1847
  torsional deformities of tibia-fibula in, 1817–1818
  treatment principles in, 1781–1786
    outcome criteria and patient selection in, 1781–1785, *1783–1785*
    parents and, 1785–1786
    team approach in, 1786, *1787*
Myeloschisis, in myelomeningocele, 1778
Myochrysine, in rheumatoid arthritis, 1480
Myoglobinuria, idiopathic paroxysmal, 2175–2176
Myophosphorylase deficiency, 2174–2175
Myositis, 2159
  electromyography in, 65
  parasitic, 2168
  suppurative, 2167
  traumatic, 2168–2169
  viral, 2167
Myositis ossificans, in dislocation of elbow, 3133
  in hemophilia, 1502
  traumatic, 2169–2170, *2170*
Myositis ossificans progressiva, 857–860
  clinical features of, 857–858, *858*
  pathology in, 857
  prognosis and treatment of, 860
  radiographic findings in, 858, *859–860*
Myostatic contracture, 1, 42
Myotonia, electromyography in, 65
Myotonia congenita, 2141, 2157–2159, 2158t
  anesthesia in, 68
  electrical testing in, 64
Myotonia dystrophica, anesthesia in, 68
  electrical testing in, 64
Myotonic dystrophy, *2138–2140*, 2138–2141
  differential diagnosis of, 2158t

N

Nafcillin, in septic arthritis, 1424t
Nail-patella syndrome, 844–847, *846–847*

Naproxen, in rheumatoid arthritis, 1479
Navicular, fracture of, 3342
Neck righting reflex, 51
Necrosis, aseptic, in congenital dysplasia of hip in adolescent, 469
  of bone, 689
  of proximal femur, due to Pavlik harness treatment, 339
  avascular, due to Salter's innominate osteotomy, 418
    in sickle cell disease, 1144
    in slipped femoral capital epiphysis, 1068–1073
    of femoral head, in septic arthritis in neonate hip, 1431
Neimann-Pick disease, 887
Nélaton's line, in congenital dysplasia of hip, 327, *327*
Neonate, acute pyogenic osteomyelitis in, 1094, 1095t
  development of locomotion in, 14
  septic arthritis of hip in, 1428–1435. See also *Arthritis, septic, in neonatal hip.*
Nephroblastoma, 1405, *1407*
Nerve conduction velocity determinations, 65
Nerve palsy, in hemophilia, 1500
  obstetrical, 3354
Nerve sheath tumors, of foot, 2773, *2778*
Nerves, peripheral, of leg muscles, 85t
  of shoulder girdle muscles, 84t
Neural axis, congenital malformation of, 2199
Neural disorders, differentiation of, 1601, 1602t–1603t
Neurilemmoma, of foot, 2773, *2778*
Neuritis, peripheral, diffuse, nerve conduction velocity studies in, 65
Neuroblastoma, 1403–1405, *1404–1406*
Neurofibromatosis, 1289–1294
  clinical features of, 1290–1294
  congenital pseudarthrosis of tibia and, 657
  etiology of, 1289
  heredity in, 1289
  neoplasia in, 1293–1294
  pathology in, 1289, *1289*
  scoliosis in, 2362
  skeletal findings in, 1290–1293, *1293–1296*
  soft tissue findings in, 1290, *1290–1292*
  treatment of, 1294
Neurologic assessment, 42–55. See also under *Reflex.*
Neuromuscular excitability, tests of, 64–65
Neuromuscular system. See also individual parts and disorders.
  as functional unit, 1604
  levels of affection of, 1601–1604, 1602t-1603t
Neuropathic joint disease, 1512–1514, *1513*
Neurophysiologic maturation, reflexes of, 86t–89t
Nevus, in neurofibromatosis, 1290, *1291*
Newington abduction orthosis, in Legg-Calv*a*ce-Perthes disease, 972–973, *974*
Nievergelt-Pearlman syndrome, 2581, *2582–2583*
Nodule, rheumatoid, 1469, *1469*, 1472
Normokalemic periodic paralysis, 2172–2173

O

Ober's fasciotomy, in iliotibial band contracture, 1923–1925, *1924*
Ober's test, 27, *30*
Obstetrical brachial plexus palsy. See *Brachial plexus palsy, obstetrical.*

Obstetrical injury, 3352–3357
  depressed skull fracture as, 3354
  displacement of distal humeral epiphysis as, 3354, 3355–3356
  fracture of physis of long bones as, 3353
  fracture of shafts of long bones as, 3353
  in cerebral palsy, 1608–1609
  intrauterine fracture as, 3354, 3357
  nerve palsy as, 3354
  separation of distal femoral epiphysis as, 3353–3354
Obturator neurectomy, and adductor myotomy, of Banks and Green, **1638–1641**
  intrapelvic, in cerebral palsy, 1645
Occipital vertebrae, 2231
Occiput, congenital anomalies of, 2230–2236
Ocular dystrophy, 2138
Oculocerebral syndrome, in vitamin D refractory rickets, 910
Oculopharyngeal dystrophy, 2138
Odontoid process, absence of, 2234
  congenital anomalies of, 2233–2234
  fracture of, with anterior dislocation of atlas, 3345
  separate, 2233–2234, *2235*
Ogden and Bucholz classification, of ischemic necrosis, *433–440*, 434–438
Olecranon, fracture of, 3145, *3146–3147*
Oligohydramnios, in congenital dysplasia of hip, 303, *304*
Oligosyndactyly, 226, *226–227*
Ollier's disease, 1195, *1196–1198*
Ombredanne's line, in congenital dysplasia of hip, 319, *319*
Omohyoid muscle, contracture of, in congenital torticollis, 115
Onycho-osteodystrophy, hereditary, 844–847, *846–847*
  clinical features in, 845, *846–847*
  incidence of, 845
  inheritance in, 845
  treatment of, 847
Opponens pollicis, congenital absence of, 288–289, *288–290*
Opponens splint, in thumb-in-palm deformity, 1724, *1725*
Optical righting reflex, 53–55, *54*
Oral reflex, 55
Orofaciodigital syndrome, 864–865
Orthopedic examination, 4–57. See also *Examination.*
Orthopedic history, 2–4
  form for, 95t–103t
Orthopedics, definition and scope of, 1–2
Orthosis. See also individual type and disorder.
  in cerebral palsy, 1627
  in congenital scoliosis, 2202
  in congenital torticollis, *121*
  in genu valgum, 2828
  in idiopathic scoliosis, 2294–2302
  in infantile tibia vara, 2842–2843
  in Legg-Calvé-Perthes disease, 972–977
  in muscular dystrophy, 2150
  in myelomeningocele, 1854–1858
  in pes planovalgus, 2729–2731, *2731*
  in poliomyelitis, *1916*, 1916–1918
  in rheumatoid arthritis, 1482, *1483*
  in Scheuermann's juvenile kyphosis, 2386, *2387*
  in scoliosis, in myelomeningocele, 1843, 1847
Ortolani test, 312–314, *313*
  click vs. clunk in, 312–314
  technique in, 312, *313*
Os calcaneus secundarius, tarsal coalition vs., 2588, *2589*
Os calcis, accessory bone at, 2416

Os calcis *(Continued)*
  apophysitis of, 1016
  intraosseous lipoma of, 2780, 2787
Os peroneum, fracture of, 3343
Os trigonum, 2415, *2415–2417*
Os-in-os, in osteopetrosis, 796, *796*
Osgood-Schlatter disease, 1010–1013
  clinical picture in, 1010
  complications of, 1012–1013
  etiology of, 1010
  radiographic findings in, 1011, *1011*
  treatment of, 1011–1012
Ossiculum terminale, 2231
Ossification, epiphyseal, in lower limbs, *62*
  in upper limbs, *60*
Osteoarthritis, in congenital dysplasia of hip in adolescent, 469–470, *471*
Osteoblastoma, benign, 1220–1226
  age and sex predilection in, 1220
  clinical findings in, 1224
  complications of, 1225–1226
  differential diagnosis of, 1225
  location of, 1220
  pathology in, *1220*, 1224
  radiography in, *1221–1225*, 1225
  treatment of, 1225
Osteochondritis, ischiopubic, 1016
  of humeral capitellum, 1013–1014, *1015*
  Parrot's syphilitic, 1458
Osteochondritis dissecans, 1515–1534
  arthrography in, 1521–1522
  bone scan in, *1520–1521*, 1522, 1522t
  clinical picture in, 1518
  computed tomography in, *1520*, 1521
  etiology of, 1515–1517
    heredity and constitutional predisposition in, 1515–1516
    ischemia in, 1516
    tibial spine theory in, 1516 1517
    trauma in, 1516–1517
  historical, 1515
  in Legg-Calvé-Perthes disease, 986–988, *987–988*
  of hip, *1529*, 1534
  of metatarsal, 2759, *2759*
  of talus, 1522–1524, *1523–1527*, **1530–1533**
  pathology in, 1517
  radiography in, *1518–1519*, 1518–1521, 1519t
  sex and age predilection in, 1517
  site of involvement in, 1517–1518
  treatment of, 1524–1534
    arthroscopic, 1526–1527, 1527t
      in early separated lesion, 1527–1528
      in intact lesion, 1527
      in partially detached lesion, 1528
      in salvageable loose body, 1528
      in unsalvageable loose body, 1528, *1528*
      postoperative care in, 1528–1529, 1534
    nonsurgical, 1524–1526
    open surgical, **1530–1533**, 1534
Osteochondroma, 1163–1171
  chondrosarcoma vs., 1170t
  clinical picture in, 1165
  complications of, 1167, 1170–1171
  etiology of, 1164
  incidence and anatomic site of, 1164
  pathology in, 1164–1165, *1164–1165*
  pseudoaneurysm of femoral artery in, 1167, 1170
  radiography in, 1165, *1166–1167*
  secondary sarcomatous change in, 1170–1171

Osteochondroma *(Continued)*
  treatment of, 1165–1167, **1168–1169**
Osteochondromatosis, synovial, 1591
Osteochondrosis, 932. See also individual types.
  classification of, 932t
  sites of, 932t
Osteodysplasty, 826, 829
Osteofibrous dysplasia, of tibia and fibula, 1242–1246, *1243–1245*
  age and sex predilection in, 1242
  clinical features of, 1242
  differential diagnosis of, 1245–1246
  localization of, 1242
  pathology in, 1242, 1245, *1245*
  radiographic features of, 1242, *1243–1244*
  treatment of, 1246
Osteogenesis imperfecta, 758–782
  anesthesia in, 68–69
  classification and heredity in, 758–759, 760t
  clinical picture in, 761–763, 764–772, 769
  differential diagnosis in, 775–776
  gross anatomic findings in, 761, *761–763*
  hyperplastic callus formation in, 774–775, 776
  incidence of, 759
  laboratory findings in, 775
  medical treatment in, 776–777
  orthopedic treatment in, 777–782
    for kyphosis and scoliosis, 782
    intramedullary rod fixation in, 778–782, *780–781*
      complications of, 782
      extensible rod in, 778–779, 781–782
      Tiley-Albright technique in, 780, *781*
      Williams modification in, 780, *780*
    orthoses in, 777–778
    pneumatic trouser splints in, 778
  pathology in, 759–761, *760–763*
  prognosis in, 782, 782t
  radiography in, 769–774, *773–775*
Osteogenesis imperfecta tarda, idiopathic juvenile osteoporosis vs., 788
Osteogenic sarcoma, 1305–1382
  amputation through arm in, **1372–1375**
  anatomic location of, 1305–1306
  angiography in, 1313
  below-knee amputation in, **1350–1353**
  biopsy in, 1315
  bone scan in, 1313, *1315*
  chemotherapy in, 1316
  classification of, 1305
  clinical findings in, 1307
  computed tomography in, 1313, *1314*
  elbow disarticulation in, **1376–1379**
  forequarter amputation (Littlewood) in, **1354–1367**
  hemipelvectomy (Banks and Coleman) in, **1318–1325**
  hip disarticulation in, **1326–1335**
  histology in, 1306–1307, *1307*
  immediate amputation in, 1315–1316
  ischial-bearing above-knee (mid-thigh) amputation in, **1336–1345**
  knee disarticulation in, **1346–1349**
  laboratory findings in, 1313
  limb salvage in, 1317
  of fibula, 2780, 2788
  parosteal, 1386
  pathologic findings in, 1306–1307, *1306–1307*
  psychological support for amputation in, 1317
  pulmonary metastasis in, 1316–1317, *1380–1381*, 1382
  radiography in, 1307–1313, *1308–1312*
  shoulder disarticulation in, **1368–1371**

Osteogenic sarcoma *(Continued)*
  staging in, 1313–1315
  treatment plan in, 1316–1317
Osteoid osteoma, 1206–1216
  age and sex predilection in, 1206
  clinical findings in, 1207
  natural history of, 1215
  of talus, 2780, *2784*
  pathology of, 1207, *1208*
  radiography in, 1207, *1209–1214*, 1215
  sites of involvement in, 1206–1207
  treatment of, 1215–1216, *1216*
Osteolysis, Gorham's massive, 791
  idiopathic, 790–791, *791*
Osteomyelitis, brucellar, 1123–1124
  in septic arthritis of neonate hip, 1433–1434
  in sickle cell disease, 1140, 1144
  of femoral neck, Legg-Calvé-Perthes disease vs., 957
  pyogenic, 1081–1111
    acute, 1093–1097
      antibiotic therapy in, 1093t, 1093–1094, 1096t
      at over three years of age, 1094–1095
      at two months to three years of age, 1094–1095, 1095t
      contraindications to oral antibiotic therapy in, 1095t
      neonatal, 1094, 1095t
      organisms in, 1094, 1094t
      orthopedic management in, 1095–1096
      sequential parenteral-oral therapy in, 1095, 1095t
      subacute vs., 1099t
      surgical drainage in, 1096–1097, *1096–1098*
    bone aspiration in, 1093
    bone scan in, 1087, *1091*, 1091–1092
    cellulitis vs., 1092–1093
    chronic, 1099–1103, *1104*
    clinical picture in, 1084–1085
    complications of, 1103, *1105*, 1106
    diagnosis of, 1092–1093
    differential diagnosis of, 1092–1093
    etiology of, 1081–1082
    histology in, 1082, *1083*
    in calcaneus, 1107, *1108*, *1110*
    in clavicle, 1106
    in ilium, 1106–1107
    in lumbar disc syndrome, 1106–1107
    in pelvic bones, 1106–1107
    in sesamoid bones, 1109–1111, *1111*
    in spine, 1106
    in talus, 1107, *1109*
    in tarsal bones, 1107–1109, *1108–1110*
    in vertebrae, 1106
    laboratory findings in, 1092
    pathology in, 1082–1084, *1082–1084*
    radiography in, 1085–1087, *1086–1090*
    sites of involvement in, 1084, *1085*
    subacute, 1097–1099, 1099t, *1100–1103*
    treatment of, 1093–1103
  salmonella, 1120–1122, *1121–1122*
  septic arthritis vs., 1421–1422
  vaccinial, 1131–1133
  viral, 1131–1133
Osteomyelitis variolosa, 1131, *1132*
Osteopathia striata, 812–814, *813–814*
Osteopetrosis, 792–798
  complications of, 797, 797–798
  congenital (malignant), 792–793
  differential diagnosis of, 797
  Englemann's disease vs., 797
  etiology and pathology of, 793–794, *794*

Osteopetrosis (Continued)
    laboratory findings in, 796
    metaphyseal dysplasia vs., 797
    progressive diaphyseal dysplasia vs., 797
    pycnodysostosis vs., 797, 800t
    Pyle's disease vs., 797
    roentgenography in, 794–796, 795–797
    tarda (benign), 793
    treatment of, 798
Osteopoikilosis, 815, 815–816
Osteoporosis, idiopathic juvenile, 787–789
    clinical picture in, 787
    diagnosis in, 788–789
    etiopathology of, 787
    osteogenesis imperfecta tarda vs., 788
    roentgenographic findings in, 787, 788
    treatment of, 789
    in childhood, causes of, 789t
Otopalatodigital syndrome, 865
Outpatient surgery, 74–75
Overgrowth, of limb, 110–111
Oxyphenbutazone, in rheumatoid arthritis, 1479

P

Pain, congenital insensitivity to, 1992–1995, 1993–1995, 1996t–1997t
Panner's disease, 1013–1014, 1015
Pantalar arthrodesis, in poliomyelitis, 1955–1956
Parachute reflex, 51, 53
Paralysis, 40. See also Poliomyelitis.
    familial periodic, electrical testing in, 64
    flaccid, chart for muscle examination in, 81t–82t
    of gastrocnemius-soleus, gait in, 22–24, 25
    of gluteus maximus, gait in, 22
    of gluteus medius, gait in, 22, 23
    of quadriceps femoris, gait in, 22, 24
    of triceps surae, gait in, 22–24, 25
    periodic, 2172–2173
        familial or hypokalemic, 2172
        hyperkalemic, 2172–2173
        normokalemic, 2173
    spastic, chart for muscle examination in, 79t–80t
Paramyotonia congenita, 2141, 2158t
Paramyotonia of Eulenberg, 2158t
Paraplegia, 40, 1606
    in tuberculosis of spine, 1452–1454
Parapodium, in myelomeningocele, 1855, 1856
Parasitic myositis, 2168
Parastremmatic dysplasia, 757
Parents, in history taking, 2
Paresis, 40
Parosteal osteogenic sarcoma, 1386
Parrot's syphilitic osteochondritis, 1458
Patella, congenital absence of, 620, 621
    congenital bipartite or tripartite, 620
    congenital dislocation of, 618, 619, 1560–1561
    fracture of, 3284–3285, 3285
    recurrent subluxation or dislocation of, 1551–1579
        classification of, 1552–1554
        clinical picture in, 1554–1556
        etiology of, 1551–1552
            high-riding patella in, 1552
            iliotibial tract in, 1552
            injury in, 1552
            lateral patellar soft-tissue contracture in, 1551–1552

Patella (Continued)
    ligamentous laxity in, 1551
    lower limb malalignment in, 1552
    muscle imbalance in, 1552
    pathology in, 1553–1554, 1554
    radiography in, 1555–1561, 1556–1560
        Blumensaat's recommended view in, 1556, 1556
        congruence angle in, 1559, 1559
        Hughston's recommended view in, 1556–1557, 1558
        lateral patellofemoral angle in, 1559, 1559
        Laurin's recommended view in, 1557, 1558
        Macnab's recommended view in, 1556, 1557
        Merchant's recommended view in, 1557, 1558
    treatment of, 1560–1579
        arthroscopic lateral patellar retinacular release in, 1562, 1569–1570
        chondromalacia in, 1572, 1579
        in chronic developmental subluxation, 1561
        in congenital dislocation, 1560–1561
        in post-traumatic recurrent subluxation, 1561
        in subluxation with excessive lateral pressure, 1561–1562, 1562t
        lateral patellar retinacular release in, 1568
        quadriceps realignment in, **1562–1567**, 1569–1572, 1570, 1572
        semitendinosus tenodesis in, 1578, **1572–1577**
    traumatic dislocation of, 3282–3283
Patella alta, in Osgood-Schlatter disease, 1012–1013
    in recurrent subluxation or dislocation of patella, 1552
    measurements in, 1560, 1561
Patellar advancement technique, of Chandler, 1717, 1718–1721
Patellar retinacular release, lateral, arthroscopic, 1562, 1569–1570
Patellar tendon, elongation of, in cerebral palsy, 1717
    Osgood-Schlatter disease of, 1010–1013
Patellar tendon-bearing orthosis, in rheumatoid arthritis, 1482, 1483
Patellofemoral angle, lateral, in recurrent subluxation or dislocation of patella, 1559, 1559
Patellofemoral joint, dislocation of, in Down's syndrome, 895
Pathological dislocation, of hip, in septic arthritis, 1431, 1434
Pathologic fracture, 3359, 3366
    in fibrous dysplasia, 1237, 1238–1239
    in osteopetrosis, 797, 797–798
    in pyogenic osteomyelitis, 1103
    in sickle cell disease, 1144
    in unicameral bone cyst, 1270–1271, 1271
Pauwels' intertrochanteric Y osteotomy, in coxa vara, 599–601, 600–601, **602–605**
Pauwels' modified osteotomy, with distal and lateral greater trochanter transfer, 442, **462–465**, 466, 468
Pavlik harness, in congenital hip dysplasia, 331–340
    indications and contraindications for, 334, 334t
    mechanism of reduction in, 334
    method and technique of application in, 334, 336, 337–338
    treatment complications in, 339t, 339–340, 340
    treatment duration in, 338–339
    treatment problems in, 339, 339t
    treatment regimen in, 338–339
    zone of safety for, 334, 335
Pectoralis major transfer, for elbow flexor paralysis, 2103, **2108–2111**
Pectoralis minor transfer, in subscapularis muscle paralysis, 1959, 1961

Volume 1, pgs. 1–687; Volume 2, pgs. 688–1600; Volume 3, pgs. 1601–2404; Volume 4, pgs. 2405–3373

Pectoralis muscle transfer, for elbow in poliomyelitis, 1963–1964
Pelvic bones, pyogenic osteomyelitis of, 1106–1107
Pelvic obliquity, congenital, *549–551*, 549–552
Pelvic rotation, in gait, *9*, 9–10
Pelvic tilt, 2188, *2188*
  in gait, 10, *10*
Pelvifemoral muscles, in congenital dysplasia of hip, 310–311, *311*
Pelvis, fracture of, 3345–3350
  avulsion, 3347, *3349*
  isolated with stable pelvic ring, 3347
  unstable with disruption of pelvic ring, 3347, *3348*
  in hereditary onycho-osteodystrophy, 845, *846*
  in poliomyelitis, 1922–1923
  lateral displacement of, in gait, 12, *13*
Pember-Sal osteotomy, Westin's, 419, *419–420*
Pemberton's pericapsular innominate osteotomy, 423–442
  advantages of, 423–424
  age restrictions in, 424
  disadvantages of, 424
  extreme immobilization positions in, 424, *425*
  indications for, 424
  ischemic necrosis due to, 424, 433–442
    anatomic sites of compression in, *432*, 433
    Kalamchi and MacEwen classification of, 438–441, *441*
    management and prognosis in, 441–442, **444–465**
    Ogden and Bucholz classification of, *433–440*, 434–438
  prerequisites for, 424
  technique in, 424, **426–432**
Penguin gait, 26
Penicillin, in septic arthritis, 1424t
Perceptual motor deficiency, in myelomeningocele, 1790–1791
Periacetabular osteotomy, Eppright's, in congenital dysplasia of hip in adolescent, 503, *503*
  Wagner type I, in congenital dysplasia of hip in adolescent, 493, *502*, 503
  Wagner type II, in congenital dysplasia of hip in adolescent, 503, *503*
  Wagner type III, in congenital dysplasia of hip in adolescent, 503, *503*
Periacetabular triple innominate osteotomy, in congenital dysplasia of hip in adolescent, 493, **494–501**, *502*
Pericarditis, in rheumatoid arthritis, 1472
Perichondrial ring, injuries to, 3025–3026
Periodic paralysis, 2172–2173
Periosteal chondroma, 1199
Peripheral nerve roots, in myelomeningocele, 1778
Peripheral nerves, of leg muscles, 85t
  of shoulder girdle muscles, 84t
Peripheral neuropathy, 2085
Perkin's line, in congenital dysplasia of hip, 319, *319*
Peroneal muscle, paralysis of, 1938–1939, *1939*
Peroneal muscular atrophy, 1983–1986, *1984–1985*
  clinical picture in, 1983–1985, *1984–1985*
  diagnosis of, 1985–1986
  incidence of, 1983
  inheritance in, 1983
  pathology in, 1983
  treatment of, 1986
Peroneus brevis, fractional lengthening of, 1693
Peroneus longus, in gait, 14, *15*
Pes calcaneocavus, 2676
  treatment of, osteotomy of calcaneus in, 2701, *2704–2705*, 2705, **2706–2711**, *2712*

Pes cavovarus, 2674–2675
Pes cavus, 2671–2713
  clinical features of, *2672–2678*, 2674–2676
  congenital, 2676
  etiology and pathogenesis of, 2671–2674
    genetic factors in, 2674
    intrinsic muscle hyperactivity in, 2674
    intrinsic muscle paralysis in, 2673–2674
    isolated muscle weakness in, 2672
    muscle fibrosis and contracture in, 2674
    muscle imbalance in, 2671–2672
    triceps surae muscle in, 2674
  radiography in, 2676, *2679*
  simple, 2674
  treatment of, 2680–2713
    anterior tibial tendon transfer in, 2687, *2690*
    beak triple arthrodesis in, 2691, 2700, *2700–2701*
    cavovarus test in, 2681, *2682–2683*
    close-up lateral wedge osteotomy in, 2700–2701, **2702–2703**
    contracture release on plantar aspect in, **2684–2685**, 2686
    dorsal tarsal wedge osteotomy in, 2691, **2692–2693**
    dorsal wedge osteotomy of metatarsals in, 2691, *2698–2699*
    fusion of first metatarsocuneiform joint in, 2691
    hindfoot varus deformity in, 2701
    long toe extensor transfer in, 2686–2687, **2688–2689**
    opening-wedge osteotomy of medial cuneiform in, 2691
    sesamoidectomy in, 2705, 2713
    shoe insert in, 2680, *2680*
    subtotal talar excision in, 2713
    surgical indications in, 2680–2681, *2681–2683*, 2686
    V-osteotomy of tarsus in, 2691, **2694–2698**
    wedge resection and fusion of talonavicular and calcaneocuboid joints in, 2691
Pes deformities. See also under *Talipes.*
Pes equinocavus, 2676
Pes planovalgus, flexible, 2717–2755
  classification of, 2717, 2718t
  clinical features of, 2724, *2727–2728*, 2728
  radiographic analysis of, 2717–2724, *2718–2726*
  toe-raising test of Jack in, 2724, *2728*
  treatment of, 2728–2755
    Chambers procedure in, 2748, *2750*
    conservative, 2729–2731, *2730–2731*
    Evans operation in, 2754–2755
    in hindfoot valgus deformity, 2748–2755
    in naviculocuneiform sag, 2734–2736, *2736*, **2738–2747**
    in talonavicular sag, 2736–2737, *2737*, 2748, *2749*, **2752–2753**
    medial displacement osteotomy in, 2748, *2751*, *2751*, 2754
    orthotics in, 2729–2731, *2731*
    surgical indications in, 2731–2733, *2732*
    surgical procedures in, 2733t–2734t, *2733–2734*
Pes valgus, congenital convex, 2557–2577
  clinical features in, 2563–2566, *2565*
  differential diagnosis of, 2567
  etiology of, 2557–2561, *2558–2560*
  incidence of, 2557
  pathologic anatomy in, 2561–2563
    bone and joint changes in, *2561*, 2561–2562
    ligamentous changes in, 2562, *2562–2563*
    muscle and tendon abnormalities in, 2562–2563, *2564*

Pes valgus (Continued)
    radiography in, 2566–2567, 2566–2568
    terminology in, 2557
    treatment of, 2567–2577
        manipulative stretching in, 2568–2569
        open reduction in, 2569, **2570–2575**, 2576–2577
        options in, 2569t
Petrie abduction cast, in Legg-Calvé-Perthes disease, 975
Phalanges. See Fingers; Toes.
Phalen index finger abduction restoration, 2057, **2076–2077**
Phenylbutazone, in rheumatoid arthritis, 1479
Philippson's reflex, 49
Phocomelia, 105, *111*
Physeal growth plate, definition of, 932
Physeal stapling, in leg length inequality, 2887–2888, 2888t
Physical therapy, in cerebral palsy, 1623–1626
Physis, 3014–3027. See also individual bone.
    anatomy of, 3014–3015, *3015*
    blood supply to, 3016, *3016*, *3018–3020*, 3019
    compression injury to, 3021
    destruction of, in pyogenic osteomyelitis, 1103
    direct trauma effects on, 3015–3019, *3016*, 3017t
    fracture of, classification of, 3021–3026, *3022–3024*
        Aitken's, 3021–3022
        Foucher's, 3021
        Ogden's, *3024*, 3025
        Poland's, 3021, *3022*
        Salter and Harris', 3022–3025, *3023*
    healing after, 3016–3018
    incidence of, 3026, 3026t
    management of, 3026–3027
    ischemic effects on, 3019–3021
    of long bone, fracture of, obstetrical, 3353
Pigeon breast deformity, 899
Pigmented villonodular synovitis, 1593–1594
    joint fluid analysis in, 1413t
    of foot, 2780, *2781*
Pin protrusion, in congenital dysplasia of hip, 361, *363*
Piperacillin, in septic arthritis, 1424t
Pituitary dwarfism, *926*, 926–927
Placing reflex, 47, *47–48*
Plagiocephaly, in congenital dysplasia of hip, 316
    in idiopathic scoliosis, 2267, *2268*
Plantar grasp reflex, 45, *45*
Plantar wart, 2786–2790
Platybasia, 2231–2232
Pneumatic trouser splints, in osteogenesis imperfecta, 778
Poliomyelitis, 1910–1971
    anterior tibial, toe extensor, peroneal paralysis in, 1943, *1943*
    anterior tibial muscle paralysis in, 1941–1943, *1942*
    course of disease in, 1911
    dorsal bunion in, 1945, *1946–1948*, *1950–1951*
    elbow in, 1959, 1962–1971
        anterior triceps brachii transfer for, 1964, *1966*, 1967
        latissimus dorsi transfer in, 1967, *1967–1970*
        pectoralis minor muscle transfer for, 1964
        pectoralis muscle transfer for, 1963–1964
        Steindler flexorplasty in, 1959, *1962*, 1962–1963
        sternocleidomastoid transfer for, 1964, *1965*
        triceps brachii paralysis in, 1967, 1971
    foot and ankle in, 1937–1957
        ankle fusion and pantalar arthrodesis in, 1955–1956
        anterior or posterior bone block in, 1956–1957
        extra-articular subtalar arthrodesis in, 1955
        lateral transfer of anterior tibial tendon in, 1939, 1941
        muscle paralysis in, 1937–1946

Poliomyelitis (Continued)
        operative procedure for calcaneocavus deformity in, 1952, *1954*, 1955
        operative procedure for equinus deformity in, 1955
        operative procedure for valgus deformity in, 1952
        operative procedure for varus deformity in, 1952, *1953*
        stabilizing operations for, 1949t
        tendon transfers for, 1940t–1941t
        triple arthrodesis of, 1946, 1950, *1951*, 1952, *1953–1954*, 1955
    forearm in, 1971
    gluteus maximus paralysis in, 1925–1927, *1926*, *1928*
        Barr erector spinae transfer in, *1926*, 1926–1927
        Hogshead fascia lata transfer to lumbodorsal fascia in, 1927, *1928*
        motor evaluation in, 1925
        Sharrard iliopsoas transfer in, 1927
    gluteus medius paralysis in, 1925
    hip in, 1921–1931
        contralateral, subluxation of, 1922
        flexion, abduction, external rotation contracture of, 1921–1922
        lower limb deformity and, 1921–1922
        paralytic dislocation of, 1928–1930
            arthrodesis in, 1929–1930, *1930*
            treatment of, 1928–1929
        soft-tissue contracture in, 1921–1925
    iliotibial band contracture in, 1921–1925, *1922*
        external torsion of tibia and subluxation of knee in, 1922
        flexion, abduction, external rotation contracture of hip in, 1921–1922
        flexion and valgus deformity of knee and external torsion of tibia in, 1922
        pelvis and trunk in, 1922–1923
        positional pes varus in, 1922
        treatment of, 1923–1925
            conservative, 1923
            surgical, 1923–1925, *1924*
    knee in, 1930–1937
        flail, 1937, *1938*
        flexion deformity of, 1934, *1934*
        genu recurvatum of, 1934–1937, *1935–1936*
    pathology in, 1910–1911
    peroneal, extensor digitorum longus, extensor hallucis longus paralysis in, 1939, 1941
    peroneal muscle paralysis in, 1938–1939, *1939*
    quadriceps femoris paralysis in, 1930–1934, *1931–1932*
        gait in, 1930–1931, *1931*
        semitendinosus and biceps femoris tendon transfer in, 1931–1934, *1932*
    shoulder in, 1957–1959
        functional classification of muscles of, 1957–1958
        tendon transfer for, *1958*, 1958t, 1958–1959, *1960–1962*
    treatment principles in, 1911–1921
        in acute phase, 1911–1913
            in bulbar and respiratory involvement, 1912
            moist heat in, 1913
            muscle spasm in, 1912–1913
            patient positioning in, 1912
        in chronic phase, 1915–1921
            active hypertrophy exercises in, 1915–1916
            functional training in, 1916
            orthoses in, *1916*, 1916–1918
            passive stretching exercises in, 1916
            physical therapy in, 1915–1916
            postoperative care and training in, 1919–1921

Poliomyelitis (Continued)
    surgery in, 1918–1921
        tendon transfer in, 1918–1919
    in convalescent phase, 1913–1915
        contractural deformity and loss of function in, 1914–1915, *1915*
        exercise regimen in, 1913
        fatigue in, 1914
        motor activity patterns in, 1914
        muscle examination in, 1913–1914
        objectives of, 1913
    triceps surae muscle paralysis in, 1943–1946, *1944–1951*
    trunk in, 1957
Pollicization, of index finger, **262–267**
Polydactyly, 240–257
    central, 244, *245*
    in Ellis–van Creveld syndrome, 736
    incidence of, 240t, 240–241
    of toes, 2642, *2643–2648*
    postaxial, 241–242
        anomalies associated with, 241–242, 242t
        inheritance of, 241
        treatment of, 244, **246–249**
        types of, 241, *241*
    preaxial, 242–244
        Bilhaut-Cloquet procedure in, *254*, 255
        blood supply in, 242, *244*
        classification of, 242, *243*
        syndromes associated with, 244, 244t
        treatment of, 244, **250–253**
        with syndactyly, 242, *243*
Polymorphonuclear leukocytes, in joint fluid analysis, 1413
Polymyositis, 2159–2164
    age-sex in, 2160
    classification of, 2160
    clinical features of, 2161, *2162*, 2163t
    connective tissue disease and, 2160
    diagnosis of, 2163
    etiology of, 2160
    laboratory findings in, 2161–2162
    muscular dystrophy vs., 2144t
    neoplasia and, 2160
    pathology in, 2160–2161
    treatment of, 2163–2164
Polyradiculoneuritis, acute, 2003–2004
Polysyndactyly, 242
Popliteal cyst, 1582–1589
    clinical picture in, 1585, *1585*, 1588
    diagnosis of, 1588–1589, *1588*
    pathology of, 1583–1585, *1583–1584*
    treatment of, **1586–1587**, 1589
Popliteus tendon, snapping of, 1551
Porphyria, acute intermittent, 2085
Positive support response, 49
Postirradiation scoliosis, 2362
Postural deformities, clinical associations between types of, 2421, 2422t
    congenital malformations vs., 2421, 2422t
Posture. See also *Scoliosis*.
    development of, 2186–2187, *2186–2187*
    gradation of, 2189, *2189*
    in cerebral palsy, 1613
    in hip flexion deformity, 1623, *1624*
    in talipes calcaneus, 1623, *1626*
    in talipes equinus, 1623, *1625*
    normal, 2187–2189
    stable upright, requirements for, 1622, *1622*
    treatment for, 2189, *2190–2193*, 2191

Pott's disease. See *Tuberculosis, of spine.*
Prematurity, preoperative precautions in, 68
Prenatal history, 3
Presenting complaint, 3
Pronation, definition of, 33
Prone rectus test, in spastic cerebral palsy, 1628, *1631*
Prosthesis, in focal deficiency of proximal femur, *568–570*, 569–570
Protective extension of arms reflex, 51, *53*
Protein, in joint fluid analysis, 1414
Pseudarthrosis, of clavicle, 168–174
Pseudoachondroplasia, 749–752, *751*, 751t
    achondroplasia vs., 751t
Pseudoaneurysm, of femoral artery, in osteochondroma, 1167, 1170
Pseudoarthrosis, in scoliosis, 1848
Pseudoathetosis, in cerebral palsy, 1612
Pseudohypoparathyroidism, *930*, 930–931
Pseudometatropic dysplasia, 757
Pseudospondylolisthesis, 2238
Pseudotumor, in hemophilia, 1500–1501, *1501*
Psychomotor disorders, differentiation of, 1602t–1603t, 1604
Pterygium colli, in Klippel-Feil syndrome, 128
Pulmonary function, in kyphoscoliosis, 70
Pulmonary metastasis, in osteogenic sarcoma, 1316–1317, *1380–1381*, 1382
Pulvinar, in arthrography of congenital dysplasia of hip, 352, *353*
    in computed tomography of congenital dysplasia of hip, 361, *362*
    in congenital dysplasia of hip, 309
Purvis and Holder's dual onlay graft, in congenital pseudarthrosis of tibia, 661–662
Pycnodysostosis, 800, 800t, *801–803*
    cleidocranial dysplasia vs., 800t
    osteopetrosis vs., 797, 800t
Pyelography, intravenous, in Klippel-Feil syndrome, 131
Pyle's disease, 825–826, *826–828*
    osteopetrosis vs., 797
Pyogenic arthritis, joint fluid analysis in, 1414t
    Legg-Calvé-Perthes disease vs., 957
Pyramidal disorders, differentiation of, 1602t–1603t, 1604

Q

Quadriceps femoris, fibrosis of, 2122, *2123–2124*
    in gait, 14, *15*
    insufficiency of, in cerebral palsy, 1717
    paralysis of, gait in, 22, *24*
        in poliomyelitis, 1930–1934, *1931–1932*
    realignment of, in recurrent subluxation or dislocation of patella, **1562–1567**, *1569–1572*, 1570, 1572
Quadriplegia, 40, 1606
    spastic, 1617, *1618*. See also *Cerebral palsy.*

R

Rachischisis, 1774
Radial club hand, 188
Radial head, dislocation of, congenital, 184–187
    anterior, *184*, 185
    diagnosis of, 186–187

Radial head *(Continued)*
    posterior or lateral, 185, *185*
    treatment of, *186*, 187
  in obstetrical brachial palsy, 2022–2023, *2024–2025*, 2053, *2056*
  subluxation of, 3148–3151
    diagnosis of, 3149–3150
    mechanism of injury and pathologic anatomy in, 3148–3149, *3149–3150*
    treatment of, 3150–3151
Radiography, 59
Radionuclide bone imaging, 59
Radioulnar synostosis, congenital, 180–183, *181–183*
Radius, congenital longitudinal deficiency of, 188–206
  associated anomalies in, 188–189, 189t
  clinical findings in, 194–198, *196–197*
  etiology of, 188
  genetics of, 188
  incidence of, 188
  muscles in, 194
  nerves in, 194, *195*
  pathologic anatomy in, 189–194, *190–193*
  treatment of, 198–205
    alternative internal fixation techniques in, 204
    alternative surgical procedures in, 205
    centralization of carpus over distal ulna in, 199–205, **200–203**
    complications of, 205
    contraindication to surgery in, 204
    passive exercise and splinting in, 198, *199*
    radial lengthening in, 198
    results of, 204–205
  vessels in, 194
  distal, asymmetrical growth of, correction of, 215, 221
    bowing of, correction of, 215
    open-wedge osteotomy of, in Madelung's deformity, **216–219**
  distal physis of, fracture-separation of, 3202–3204, *3203*
  in multiple exostosis, 1173, *1176*, *1183*
  proximal physis and neck of, fracture of, 3137–3143
    classification of, 3139, 3139t, *3141*
    complications of, 3143
    diagnosis of, 3139–3140
    incidence of, 3137–3143
    mechanism of injury in, 3137–3139, *3138–3140*
    treatment of, 3140–3143
  ulna and, fracture of, 3181–3195
    diagnosis of, 3182
    displaced of middle third of forearm, 3185–3188
    greenstick of middle third of forearm, 3184–3185, *3185–3186*
    mechanism of injury and pathologic anatomy in, 3181–3182
    of distal third of forearm, 3187–3193, *3188*
    of proximal third of forearm, 3194, *3194*
    remodeling or malunion of, 3195, *3196–3199*
    treatment principles in, 3182–3183
    plastic deformation (traumatic bowing) of, 3194–3195
Range of motion, of elbow, 33, *34*
  of feet, 36
  of hip, 33–36, *35–36*
  of joints, 32–40, *34–41*
  of shoulder, 36–40, *37–41*
Rash, in rheumatoid arthritis, 1472
Reciprocating gait orthosis, in myelomeningocele, 1857, *1857*
Rectus femoris, Steel's technique for stretch reflex of, 1630, *1632*
Rectus femoris release, in cerebral palsy, 1714–1715

Rectus femoris tendon transfer, in cerebral palsy, 1715–1716
Reflex, 42–55
  body righting, 51
  crossed extension, 47–49, *49*
  extensor thrust, 49
  Galant's, 49, *50*
  hand grasp, 42–45, *44*
  labyrinthine righting, 53
  Landau, 50–51
  leg straightening, 49
  maturation of, *43*
  Moro, 45, *46*
  neck righting, 51
  of neurophysiologic maturation, 86t–89t
  optical righting, 53–55, *54*
  oral, 55
  parachute, 51, *53*
  Philippson's, 49
  placing, 47, *47–48*
  plantar grasp, 45, *45*
  protective extension of arms, 51, *53*
  righting, 51–55
  rooting, 55
  search, 55
  startle, 47
  sucking, 55
  tonic neck, 49–50, *51–52*
  walking or stepping, 47, *48*
  withdrawal, 49
Refsum's disease, 1990–1991
Renal failure, slipped femoral capital epiphysis due to, 1022, *1023*
Renal osteodystrophy, 910–916
  biochemical findings in, 912
  clinical features of, 911–912, *912*
  etiology of, 910–911
  medical treatment of, 916
  orthopedic treatment of, 916
  pathology in, 911, *911*
  radiography in, 912, *912–915*
Renal tubular acidosis, in vitamin D refractory rickets, 910
Reticuloendothelial neoplasia, 1146–1147
Rheumatic fever, acute transient synovitis vs., 1464t
  joint fluid analysis in, 1414t
  Legg-Calvé-Perthes disease vs., 957
Rheumatoid arthritis, 1466–1486
  anesthesia in, 69
  autoimmunity in, 1466
  bone and cartilage in, 1467–1469, *1469*
  clinical features of, 1469–1473
  drug therapy in, 1477–1480
    analgesic anti-inflammatory agents (salicylates) in, 1477–1479, 1478t
    immunosuppressants in, 1480
    nonsteroidal anti-inflammatory agents in, 1479
    slow-reacting drugs in, 1480
    steroids in, 1479–1480
  etiology of, 1466–1467
  heredity in, 1466–1467
  incidence of, 1466
  infection in, 1467
  joint fluid analysis in, 1414t
  laboratory findings in, 1474–1477
  Legg-Calvé-Perthes disease vs., 957
  orthopedic management of, 1480–1486
    bone and joint procedures in, 1484

Rheumatoid arthritis *(Continued)*
    cervical fusion in, 1486
    conservative, 1480–1482, *1481, 1483*
    lower limb length disparity in, 1484–1485
    soft-tissue release in, 1484
    surgical, 1482–1486
    synovectomy in, 1482–1484
    total joint replacement in, 1485
    total knee arthroplasty in, 1485–1486
  pathology in, 1467–1469, *1468–1469*
  pauciarticular, 1469–1470, *1471*
  polyarthritic, in minimal systemic manifestations, 1470–1472
    in systemic manifestations, 1472–1473
  radiography in, *1472–1476*, 1473–1474
  rheumatoid nodule in, 1469, *1469*
  synovitis in, 1467, *1468*
  treatment of, 1477–1486
Rheumatoid arthritis cells, in joint fluid analysis, 1413
Rheumatoid nodule, 1469, *1469*, 1472
Ribs, fusion of, 2199
Rib-vertebral angle of Mehta, 2285, 2288, *2288–2289*
Rickets, 897–916
  genu varum vs., 2824, 2826
  pathogenesis of, 897–898
  vitamin D deficiency, 898–904
    clinical findings in, 899, *900–902*
    malabsorption syndrome and, 903–904
    pathology of, 898–899, *899*
    radiography in, 899, *901*
    treatment of, 899, 903
  vitamin D refractory, 905–910
    acidosis in, 908, 910
    aminoaciduria in, 908, 910
    biochemical findings in, 906
    clinical features of, 905–906
    cystine storage disease and, 910
    heredity in, 905
    hyperglycinuria and, 910
    medical treatment of, 906–908
    oculocerebral syndrome and, 910
    orthopedic treatment of, 908
    radiography in, 906, *907*
    renal tubular acidosis and, 910
    surgical treatment of, 908, *909*
Rifampin, in septic arthritis, 1424t
  in tuberculous arthritis, 1448
Righting reflex, 51–55
Riley-Day syndrome, 1995, 1996t-1997t, 1998–1999
Riordan thumb opposition restoration, 2057, **2062–2067**
Risser sign, 2288, *2290*
Roberts orthosis, in Legg-Calvé-Perthes disease, 973–974
Rocker-bottom foot, in talipes equinovarus, 2461–2462, *2464*
Rooting reflex, 55
Ropes test, 1413
Rose thorn, in arthrography of acetabular labrum, 351–352, *352*
Rubinstein-Taybi syndrome, 865
Russell skin traction, in femoral shaft fracture, 3264–3266, *3267*
Russell split traction, in congenital dysplasia of hip, 342–343, *343*, 345–346

S

Saber shin, in congenital syphilis, 1125, *1126*
Sacrum, congenital absence of, 2212–2228. See also *Lumbosacral agenesis.*

Saha trapezius transfer, in deltoid paralysis, 1958, *1958*
Salicylates, in rheumatoid arthritis, 1477–1479, 1478t
Salmonella osteomyelitis, 1120–1122, *1121–1122*
Salter's innominate osteotomy, in congenital hip dysplasia, 395–422
  advantages of, 404
  age limits in, 404–405
  complications of, 418–419
  drawbacks of, 405
  for acetabular antetorsion, 415, *415–417*
  in adolescent, 474
  increased intra-articular pressure in, 417
  increased pelvifemoral muscle tension in, 417
  indications for, 404
  ipsilateral limb elongation in, 417
  Kalamchi's modification of, 419–422, *421–423*
  limitations on degree of correction in, 405, 412–417, *412–417*
  objective of, 395, 404, *404*
  open reduction with, 405
  operative technique in, 404, **406–411**
  preoperative acetabular index in, 414–415
  preoperative radiographic assessment in, 412–414, *412–414*
  prerequisites for, 417–418
  Westin's modification of, 419, *419–420*
  in Legg-Calvé-Perthes disease, 979–981, *980–981*
Sanfilippo syndrome, 875
Sarcoma, Ewing's, 1387–1396. See also *Ewing's sarcoma.*
  osteogenic, 1305–1382. See also *Osteogenic sarcoma.*
  of fibula, 2780, *2788*
  synovial, 1598, *1599*
Sartorius, and tensor fasciae latae, posterior transfer of, 1650–1651, **1652–1657**
  in gait, 14
Scapula, aplasia of, 176
  congenital high, 136–168. See also *Sprengel's deformity.*
  embryologic development of, 137
  fracture of, 3042–3044
    of acromion process, 3044
    of body, 3043
    of coracoid process, 3044
    of glenoid cavity, 3044
    of neck, 3043–3044
  nonunion of ossific centers of, 176, *177*
  ossification of, 3042–3043
  winging of, in Sprengel's deformity, 147
Scapulocostal stabilization, for scapular winging, **2146–2149**, 2151
Scapuloplasty, Green's, modified, in Sprengel's deformity, *147*, 148–160, **149–161**
Scheuermann's juvenile kyphosis, 2380–2388
  clinical features in, 2381–2383, *2382*
  definition of, 2380
  differential diagnosis of, 2383–2385
  etiology and pathogenesis of, 2380–2381
  incidence of, 2380
  natural history, course, prognosis of, 2385–2386
  pathology in, 2381
  radiography in, 2383, *2384–2385*
  treatment of, 2386–2388, *2387*
Sciatic nerve palsy, 2082–2084
  due to Chiari's innominate osteotomy, 506
  due to Salter's innominate osteotomy, 418
Sclera, in osteogenesis imperfecta, 763, 769
Sclerosis, multiple, differential diagnosis of, 1980t
Scoliosis, congenital, 2201–2205
  age of patient and prognosis in, 2202

Scoliosis (Continued)
  area involved in, 2202
  balanced vs. unbalanced, 2202, 2203–2204
  natural history of, 2201–2202
  severity of curve in, 2202, 2205
  specific anomaly in, 2200, 2201–2202
  treatment of, 2202–2205
    orthosis in, 2202
    surgical, 2202–2203, 2205
  definition of, 2265
  functional, in lower limb length disparity, 2191, 2194, 2196
  hysterical, 2196
  idiopathic, 2265–2362
    Adam's forward bending test in, 2275–2277, 2276
    age of onset and maturity in, 2272–2273
    backache in, 2273
    clinical features of, 2273–2282, 2274–2282
    curve pattern in, 2291–2293, 2292
    decompensation of spine in, 2273, 2275
    etiology of, 2268–2270
    flexibility of curve in, 2277, 2277
    genetic aspects of, 2267–2268, 2268
    infantile, 2356–2360
      diagnosis of, 2358
      natural progression-prognosis in, 2357–2358
      prevalence of, 2356–2357, 2357
      treatment of, 2358–2360, 2359
    juvenile, 2360, 2362
    mobility of sagittal curves in, 2277, 2278
    natural history and risk factors in, 2272t, 2272–2273
    pathology in, 2270–2271, 2270–2272
    photographic views in, 2281–2282, 2282
    plagiocephaly in, 2267, 2268
    posture and alignment of, 2273, 2274
    prevalence of, 2266
    radiography in, 2282–2291
      curve measurement in, 2284, 2295
      kyphosis and lordosis in, 2288, 2289
      Mehta's rib-vertebral angle in, 2285, 2288, 2288–2289
      radiation exposure in, 2282–2283
      skeletal maturity in, 2288, 2290–2291, 2291
      vertical wedging and rotation in, 2284–2285, 2286–2287
      views in, 2283–2284, 2284
    school screening for, 2266–2267
    sex predilection in, 2266
    sexual maturity in, 2279t, 2280–2281, 2280–2281
    shoulder level in, 1175, 2275
    standing and sitting height in, 2273, 2274
    treatment of, 2293–2356
      biofeedback in, 2293–2294
      Boston brace in, 2300–2301, 2301
      Cotrel-Dubousset instrumentation in, 2319, 2319–2320
      Drummond system in, 2318–2319
      Dwyer instrumentation in, 2320, **2332–2353**
      electrical stimulation in, 2294
      Harrington instrumentation in, 2317, 2317, **2322–2331**
      Harrington rods with sublaminar wires in, 2317–2318
      lower limb length equalization in, 2356
      Luque double L-rod instrumentation in, 2319–2320, 2321
      Milwaukee brace in, 2296, 2296–2300
      nonoperative, 2293–2294
      operative, 2302–2356

Scoliosis (Continued)
    orthotic, 2294–2302
    physical therapy in, 2293
    preoperative forcible correction in, 2304
    prominent rib hump resection in, 2320, 2354–2355, 2354–2356
    scapulectomy in, 2356
    spinal fusion in, 2304–2316, **2306–2315**
    spinal instrumentation in, 2316–2320, **2322–2353**, 2354–2356
    thoracolumbosacral orthoses in, 2300–2302, 3201
    Zielke instrumentation in, 2320, 2321
  in cerebral palsy, 1747, 1755, 1755–1756
  in intraspinal tumor, 1887, 1891, 1893, 1896–1897
  in Klippel-Feil syndrome, 128
  in Marfan's syndrome, 833, 833, 834
  in myelomeningocele, 1843–1848
  in neurofibromatosis, 1290, 1291, 1293, 1295, 2362
  lumbar, in poliomyelitis, 1922
  nonstructural, in pelvic obliquity, 2195, 2196
  paralytic, 2360–2361, 2362
  postirradiation, 2362
  postural, 2191
  terminology in, 2184–2185
Scottish-Rite orthosis, in Legg-Calvé-Perthes disease, 972, 973
Scurvy, 918–920
  clinical features in, 918
  diagnosis of, 919–920
  pathology in, 918
  radiography in, 918–919, 919
  treatment of, 920
Search reflex, 55
Semimembranosus tendon, in gait, 14
Semitendinosus and biceps femoris tendon transfer, in quadriceps femoris paralysis, 1931–1934, 1932
Semitendinosus tendon, in gait, 14
  posterolateral transfer of, to anterolateral aspect of femur, 1651
Semitendinosus tenodesis, in recurrent subluxation or dislocation of patella, 1578, **1572–1577**
Senior syndrome, 283
Sensory ataxic gait, 1613
Sensory neuropathy, acquired, 1996t–1997t
  congenital, 1996t–1997t, 1998
  familiar, with anhidrosis, 1996t–1997t, 1998
Sensory radicular neuropathy, hereditary, 1996t–1997t, 1998
Septic arthritis. See Arthritis, septic.
Sequestrum, in osteomyelitis, 1084
Serratus anterior, transfer of, in subscapularis muscle paralysis, 1959, 1960
Sesamoid bones, pyogenic osteomyelitis in, 1109–1111, 1111
Sever's disease, 1016
Sexual maturity, Tanner stages of, 2279t, 2280–2281, 2280–2281
Sheie syndrome, 875
Shelf operation, in congenital dysplasia of hip in adolescent, 519–525, 521–525
Shenton's line, in congenital dysplasia of hip, 320, 320–321
  in quantitation of traction effectiveness, 345, 346
Shin, saber, in congenital syphilis, 1125, 1126
Short-rib polydactyly syndrome, 730
Shoulder. See also under individual disorder.
  abduction and adduction of, 39, 39
  abduction contracture of, in cerebral palsy, 1747, 1747, 1754

Shoulder (Continued)
  disarticulation of, in osteogenic sarcoma, **1368–1371**
  dislocation of, congenital, 174–175, *175*
  elevation of, 36–39, *38*
  flexion and extension of, 39, *39*
  in obstetrical brachial plexus palsy, 2014, 2021–2022
  in poliomyelitis, 1957–1959, 1958t, *1958–1962*
  in Sprengel's deformity, 138, *139–140*
  position of minimal intra-articular pressure for, 1410
  range of motion of, 36–40, *37–41*
  rotation of, 39–40, *40*
Shoulder girdle, muscles in movement of, innervation of, 84t
Shrewsbury Swivel Walker, in myelomeningocele, 1856
Sickle cell disease, 1139–1144
  anesthesia in, 71
  bone infarction in, 1140, *1141*
  growth disturbance in, 1140
  hand-foot syndrome in, 1140, *1142–1143*
  marrow hyperplasia in, 1140, *1141*
  osteomyelitis in, 1140, 1144
  pathologic fractures in, 1144
  preoperative testing for, 67
  treatment of, 1144
Silverskiöld gastrocnemius recession, 1667, *1673*
Skeletal growth, 2852–2867. See also *Growth.*
Skull fracture, depressed, obstetrical, 3354
Slipped femoral capital epiphysis, 1016–1073. See also *Femoral capital epiphysis, slipped.*
Slipped vertebral apophysis, 2404
Sofield-Millar fragmentation and intramedullary fixation technique, in congenital pseudarthrosis of tibia, 662, 663
Soleus, in gait, 14, *15*
Solganal, in rheumatoid arthritis, 1480
Somatosensory evoked potentials, in kyphoscoliosis surgery, 70
Southwick method for femoral head-shaft angle, in slipped femoral capital epiphysis, 1028, 1031, *1031*
Southwick trochanteric triplane osteotomy, in slipped femoral capital epiphysis, **1056–1061**, 1062
Spasm, muscle, 1411
Spastic diplegia, 1606, 1616–1617. See also *Cerebral palsy.*
Spastic gait, 25–26
Spastic hemiplegia, *1614–1615*, 1614–1616. See also *Cerebral palsy.*
Spastic paralysis, chart for muscle examination in, 79t-80t
Spastic paraplegia, gait in, 25
Spastic quadriplegia, 1617, *1618*. See also *Cerebral palsy.*
Spasticity, in cerebral palsy, 1610–1611, 1611t
Spina bifida. See *Myelomeningocele.*
Spina bifida occulta, 1886–1887
Spina ventosa, 1127, *1128*
Spinal ataxia, gait in, 26
Spinal cord, in myelomeningocele, 1778
  tethered, 1879–1880
  tumor of, differential diagnosis of, 1980t
Spinal dysraphism, 1773, 1871–1880. See also individual types.
Spinal fusion, in scoliosis, 2304–2316, **2306–2315**
Spinal muscular atrophy, 1903–1908
  categories of, 1903
  clinical features of, 1903–1904
  differential diagnosis of, 1905, 1906t
  functional classification of, 1904
  genetic transmission of, 1903
  laboratory findings in, 1904–1905
  pathology of, 1903

Spinal muscular atrophy (Continued)
  treatment of, 1905, *1907*, 1908
Spine. See also *Lordosis; Scoliosis.*
  cervical, congenital anomalies of, 2230–2236
    pedicles and facets of, congenital absence of, 2236
    spondylolisthesis of, 2236
  congenital anomalies of, 2196–2200. See also individual types.
    associated anomalies in, 2199–2200
    classification of, 2197–2198, *2197–2199*
    defective formation as, 2197
    defective segmentation as, 2197, *2197*
    heredity in, 2198–2199
    segmented hemivertebra as, 2197–2198, *2198*
    semisegmented and nonsegmented hemivertebra as, 2198, *2198*
  curves of, terminology in, 2184–2185
  deformities of, classification of, 2183–2184
  disorders of, differentiation of, 1601, 1602t–1603t
  fracture of odontoid process with anterior dislocation of atlas in, 3345
  in arthrogryposis multiplex congenita, 2113–2114
  in myelomeningocele, 1841–1852. See also *Myelomeningocele, spine in.*
  lordosis in, *1837*, 1841–1843, *1842*
  osteoid osteoma of, 1216, *1216*
  pyogenic osteomyelitis of, 1106
  rotatory subluxation of atlantoaxial joint of, 3345
  thoracic and lumbar, compression fracture of vertebrae of, 3345, *3346*
  tuberculosis of, 1449–1454. See also *Tuberculosis, of spine.*
Spinocerebellar ataxia, hereditary, 1978–1981, 1980t
Spinomuscular disorders, differentiation of, 1601–1604, 1602t–1603t
Splint, Craig, in congenital dysplasia of hip, 340–341, *341*
  Denis Browne hip abduction, in congenital dysplasia of hip, 341, *342*, 357
  Ilfeld, in congenital dysplasia of hip, 340–341, *341*
  Malmö, in congenital dysplasia of hip, 340, *341*
  Von Rosen, in congenital dysplasia of hip, 340, *341*
Split Russell's traction, in congenital dysplasia of hip, 342–343, *343*, 345–346
Spondylitis, ankylosing, juvenile, pauciarticular, 1470
Spondyloepiphyseal dysplasia, 746–749
  congenital type, 746–749, *747–748*
  Legg-Calvé-Perthes disease vs., 958
  tarda type, 749
Spondylolisthesis, 2238–2256
  degenerative, 2239
  dysplastic, 2239–2241, *2240–2241*
  history and terminology in, 2238
  isthmic, 2239, 2241–2258
    age incidence of, 2242
    clinical features of, 2248, *2251*
    etiology of, 2242–2243, *2244*
    forward slipping in, 2245–2247, *2246–2250*
    genetic factors in, 2243–2245
    level of involvement in, 2245
    pathology in, 2245, *2245*
    radiography in, 2251–2252, *2253*
    risk factors for progression of, 2254t
    treatment of, 2252–2258
      anterior fusion in, 2257
      in situ fusion in, 2255, 2257
      indications for, 2255
      objectives in, 2255
      reduction in, 2256, 2257–2258, *2258*
  of cervical spine, 2236

Spondylolisthesis (Continued)
  pathologic, 2239
  traumatic, 2239
  types of, 2238–2239
Spondylolysis, 2238
  treatment of, 2254
Spondyloschisis, 2238
Spondylothoracic dysplasia, 2199
Sporotrichosis, of bone, 1130
Spotted bone, *815*, 815–816
Sprengel's deformity, 136–168
  bleb theory in, 136–137
  clinical features of, 138, *139–143*
  etiology of, 136–137
  grades of, 146
  Klippel-Feil syndrome and, 128, 138, *142–143*
  pathology of, *137*, 137–138
  radiographic findings in, 138, *141–142*
  treatment of, 138, 140, 144–165
    Cabanac's procedure in, 145
    clavicle morcellation in, 145
    conservative, 138, 140
    Green's procedure in, 144, *144*
    Koenig's procedure in, 140, 144
    McFarland's procedure in, 144
    modified Green's scapuloplasty in, *147*, 148–160, **149–161**
    Ober's procedure in, 140
    patient factors in surgical procedures for, 146
    Petrie's procedure in, 145
    Putti's procedure in, 140
    results of operative intervention in, 145–146
    Robinson's procedure in, 145
    Schrock's procedure in, 140
    Smith's procedure in, 140
    Woodward's operation in, 162–164, **163–165**
    Woodward's procedure in, 144–145
Staheli's acetabular augmentation, in congenital dysplasia of hip in adolescent, 522–520, *524–525*
Staphylococcus aureus, in septic arthritis, 1416
Startle reflex, 47
Static (nonstress) technique of Graf, in congenital dysplasia of hip, 322–324, *323–324*
Static power, 40
Steel's anterior advancement of gluteus medius and minimus insertion, 1651, **1658–1659**
Steel's metaphyseal blanch sign, in slipped femoral capital epiphysis, 1028, *1030*
Steel's technique for stretch reflex of rectus femoris, 1630, *1632*
Steel's triple innominate osteotomy, in congenital dysplasia of hip in adolescent, 475, **482–491**, *493*
Steinberg sign, in Marfan's syndrome, 832, *832*
Steindler flexorplasty, of elbow, 1959, *1962*, 1962–1963
Steinmann pin migration, due to Salter's innominate osteotomy, 418
Step length, 6
Steppage gait, 24
Stepping reflex, 47, *48*
Sternocleidomastoid muscle, division of distal attachment of, 122–124, **123–125**
  fibrosis of, in congenital torticollis, 112–113
  stretching exercises for, in congenital torticollis, 115–117, *116*
  transfer of, for elbow in poliomyelitis, 1964, *1965*
  in supraspinatus paralysis, 1959, *1961*
Stickler's syndrome, 716
Stiff-man syndrome, 2176
Strayer gastrocnemius recession, 1667, *1674*

Streeter's dysplasia, 291–297. See also *Constriction ring syndrome.*
  talipes equinovarus in, 2452, *2453*
Strength, muscle, grading of, 83t
Strength-duration curve, 64
Streptomycin, in septic arthritis, 1424t
Stress fracture, 3359–3363
  clinical findings in, 3360
  differential diagnosis of, 3363
  in slipped femoral capital epiphysis, *1072*, 1073
  pathogenesis of, 3360
  radiography in, 3360–3363, *3361–3362*
  sites of involvement of, 3360
  treatment of, 3363
Stride length, 6
Subchondral fracture, mechanism of, 1516
Subclavian artery, in pseudarthrosis of clavicle, 168
Sublimis tenodesis, of Swanson, of proximal interphalangeal joints, 1739, 1744
Subluxation. See individual joint.
Subscapularis muscle paralysis, transfer of pectoralis minor in, 1959, *1961*
  transfer of serratus anterior for, 1959, *1960*
Subscapularis muscle recession at origin, 2028–2029, **2040–2041**
Subtalar extra-articular arthrodesis, of Batchelor, 1700–1702, *1701*
  of Grice, 1693, **1694–1697**, *1698–1699*, 1698–1700
Subtalar extra-articular stabilization, in cerebral palsy, 1716
Subtalar joint, anatomy of, 2588, *2590–2592*
Subtrochanteric osteotomy, after growth plate closure, in slipped femoral capital epiphysis, 1062
Subungual exostosis, of toe, 2780, *2788*
Sucking reflex, 55
Sugioka's transtrochanteric derotation osteotomy, in slipped femoral capital epiphysis, 1070, *1070*
Supination, definition of, 33
Suppurative arthritis. See *Arthritis, septic.*
Suppurative myositis, 2167
Supraspinatus paralysis, levator scapulae transfer in, 1959, *1960*
  sternocleidomastoid transfer for, 1959, *1961*
Surgery, outpatient, 74–75
Sutherland's double innominate osteotomy, in congenital dysplasia of hip in adolescent, 474–475, **476–481**, *492*
Swan-neck deformity, of fingers, in cerebral palsy, 1739, 1744
Swanson sublimis tenodesis of proximal interphalangeal joints, 1739, 1744
Syme amputation, in congenital longitudinal deficiency of fibula, 626–629, **630–633**
Symphalangism, 273, 273t, 276, *276*
Synchondrosis, 1410
Syndactylism, of toes, 2653, *2655–2657*
Syndactyly, 222–236
  classification of, 222, *223*, 224t
  incidence of, 222
  inheritance of, 222
  polydactyly in, 242, *243*
  treatment of, 222–235
    arteriography in, 226, *234*
    four-flap Z-plasty in, 226, *234*
    separation between ring and long fingers in, **228–233**
    timing of surgery in, 222, *224–225*
    V-Y release with lateral Z's in, 226, *235*
Syndesmosis, 1410
Synkinesia, in Klippel-Feil syndrome, 131–132

Synostosis, 1410
  congenital, of cervical vertebrae, 128–136. See also *Klippel-Feil syndrome.*
  of elbow, congenital, 177–179, *179*
  radioulnar, congenital, 180–183, *181–183*
Synovectomy, in hemophilia, 1505–1506
  in rheumatoid arthritis, 1482–1484
  of knee, 1505–1506
Synovial chondromatosis, 1591, *1592*
Synovial fluid, 1410
  analysis of, 1411–1415. See also *Joint fluid analysis.*
  in septic arthritis, 1416–1417
  oversecretion of, 1411
Synovial membrane, 1410
  hemangioma of, 1596, *1597*
  in septic arthritis, 1416–1417
Synovial osteochondromatosis, 1591
Synovial sarcoma, 1598, *1599*
Synovioma, 1598, *1599*
  of foot, 2780, *2783*
Synovitis, acute transient, in hip, 1461–1465
    clinical picture in, 1462
    differential diagnosis in, 1462–1463, 1464t
    etiology of, 1461–1462
    imaging in, 1462, *1463*
    laboratory findings in, 1462
    septic arthritis vs., 1422
    sequelae of, 1464–1465
    treatment of, 1463–1464
  in rheumatoid arthritis, 1467, *1468*
  pigmented villonodular, 1593–1594
    joint fluid analysis in, 1413t
    of foot, 2780, *2781*
  toxic, Legg-Calvé-Perthes disease vs., 956–957
Syphilis, of bone, 1124–1125, *1124–1126*
  of joints, 1458
Syringomyelia, 1996t–1997t

T

Talipes calcaneocavus, operative correction of, 1952, *1954*, 1955
Talipes calcaneovalgus, in congenital dysplasia of hip, 316
  postural, 2423–2425, *2424*
Talipes calcaneus, as complication of talipes equinovarus, 2525, *2525*
  gait in, 22–24, *25*
  in cerebral palsy, 1703, *1705*
  in myelomeningocele, 1798–1799, **1800–1803**, 1804
  in poliomyelitis, 1944, *1944*
  posterior tibial tendon transfer to os calcis in, 1799, **1800–1803**, 1804
  posture in, 1623, *1626*
  pyogenic osteomyelitis in, 1107, *1108*, *1110*
Talipes deformities. See also under *Pes.*
Talipes equinovalgus, in anterior tibial muscle paralysis, 1941, *1942*
  in cerebral palsy, 1661, 1663, *1663*. See also *Cerebral palsy, foot and ankle in.*
  treatment of, 1692–1703
Talipes equinovarus, congenital, 2428–2541
    articular malalignments in, 2437–2439
      calcaneal-cuboidal relations in, 2439, *2439*
      navicular-talar relations in, 2438
      talar-calcaneal relations in, *2438*, 2438–2439

Talipes equinovarus (Continued)
    talar-tibular and fibular relations in, 2437–2438
  bony deformities in, 2434–2437
    calcaneus in, 2435
    forefoot and tibia in, 2435–2437
    talus in, 2434–2435, *2434–2437*
  clinical appearance in, 2447, *2449–2450*, 2450
  closed nonoperative management of, 2463–2475
    casting in, 2470–2471, *2472*
    closed reduction of dislocation in, *2468*, 2470
    complications of, 2474–2475, *2475*
    outflare shoes in, 2471, 2474, *2474*
    prewalker shoes in, 2471, *2473*
    Robert Jones adhesive strapping in, 2465, *2469*, 2470
    soft tissue manipulations in, 2465, *2466–2468*
  complications of, 2524–2541
    ankle equinus as, 2527
    ankle valgus as, 2526–2527
    anterior pes cavus as, 2538
    aseptic necrosis of navicular as, 2540
    aseptic necrosis of talus as, 2540
    calcaneus deformity in, 2525, *2525*
    distal fibular physis growth arrest as, 2527
    dorsal bunion as, 2539
    dorsal talonavicular subluxation as, 2529, 2529–2530
    first metatarsal physis growth arrest as, 2538–2539
    foot rigidity as, 2540
    forefoot abduction as, 2538
    hallux varus as, 2539
    hammer toe as, 2539
    lateral talonavicular subluxation as, 2530
    loss of reduction and recurrence as, 2541
    medial calcaneocuboid subluxation as, 2531
    medial talonavicular subluxation as, 2529
    metatarsus varus as, 2531, *2531*, 2538
    neurovascular, 2540
    of bone, 2539–2540
    pes planus as, 2530
    posterior pes cavus as, 2530
    posterior tibial physis growth arrest as, 2527
    restricted plantar flexion of ankle as, 2525–2526, *2526*
    restricted range of subtalar motion as, 2528
    supination at midfoot as, 2530–2531, **2532–3527**
    sustentaculum tali transection as, 2539
    talar head transection as, 2540
    valgus deformity of subtalar joint as, 2527–2528
    varus deformity of subtalar joint as, 2528
    wound dehiscence as, 2524–2525
    wound infection as, 2525
  diagnosis of, 2447–2455
  differential diagnosis of, 2450–2452, *2452*
  etiology of, 2430–2433
    arrested fetal development in, 2431t, 2431–2433, *2432*
    intrauterine mechanical factors in, 2430
    neuromuscular defect in, 2430–2431
    primary germ plasm defect in, 2433
  heredity in, 2428–2430, 2429t
  horizontal breach in, 2444–2445, *2445–2446*
  in arthrogryposis multiplex, 2452, *2452*
  in dystrophic dwarfism, 2452, *2454*, 2455
  in Freeman-Sheldon syndrome, 2455, *2456*
  in Larsen's syndrome, 2455, *2457*
  in Möbius syndrome, 2455, *2458*
  in Streeter's dysplasia, 2452, *2453*
  incidence of, 2428, 2429t

Talipes equinovarus *(Continued)*
  movements of calcaneus under talus in, 2442, *2443–2444*
  pathology in, 2433–2447
  postural clubfoot vs., 2450, 2451t
  radiography in, 2455–2462
    angle measurements in, 2455, 2455t, 2459–2462, *2460–2464*
    indications for, 2455
    positioning in, 2458–2459
    rocker-bottom foot in, 2461–2462, *2464*
    talocalcaneal index in, 2461
  soft-tissue changes in, 2440–2441, *2441*
  surgical division of soft tissue contracture in, 2445–2447, *2446–2447*
  surgical management of, 2475–2524
    Achilles tendon transfer in, 2512
    anterior tibial tendon transfer in, 2477
    bone procedures in, 2512–2524
    calcaneal osteotomy in, 2517, **2518–2519**, 2520–2521
    choice of procedures in, 2476, 2478t–2481t
    Cincinnati incision in, *2483*
    manipulation and cast retention in, 2522
    medial subtalar stabilization in, 2521
    metatarsal osteotomy in, 2524
    posterior tibial tendon transfer in, 2510–2512
    shortening of lateral column of foot in, 2512–2513, **2514–2515**, 2516–2617
    soft-tissue procedures in, 2476–2477, 2482t
    soft-tissue release in, 2522
    split anterior tibial tendon transfer in, 2510
    subtalar release by posteromedial and lateral approach in, **2484–2509**
    talectomy in, 2523–2524
    tarsal reconstruction in, 2522–2523
    tibial osteotomy in, 2524
    timing of, 2476
    triple arthrodesis in, 2521–2522
  synchronized movements of lower limb articulations in, 2442–2444, *2445*
  talocalcaneonavicular joint in, 2441–2442, *2442*
  treatment of, 2462–2524
  in arthrogryposis multiplex congenita, 2099
  in cerebral palsy, 1663, *1664.* See also *Cerebral palsy, foot and ankle in.*
    treatment of, 1680–1692
  in diastrophic dysplasia, 752, 754
  in muscular dystrophy, 2150
  in myelomeningocele, 1805, 1809–1811, *1809–1812*
  in poliomyelitis, 1943, *1943*
  postural, 2426–2427
    congenital vs., 2450, 2451t
Talipes equinus, effect on knee of, 1930, *1931*
  gait in, 9, 1661, *1662*
  in cerebral palsy, 1660–1661, *1661–1662.* See also *Cerebral palsy, foot and ankle in.*
    treatment of, 1665–1680
  in muscular dystrophy, 2150
  in myelomeningocele, 1811, *1813*
  inhibitory cast in, 1627
  operative correction of, 1955
  orthosis in, 1627
  posture in, 1623, *1625*
Talipes planovalgus, in congenital dysplasia of hip, 316
Talipes valgus, in arthrogryposis multiplex congenita, 2099
  operative correction of, 1952
  paralytic congenital convex, in myelomeningocele, 1811–1816, *1814–1815*

Talipes valgus *(Continued)*
  postural, 2425
Talipes varus, in poliomyelitis, 1922
  operative correction of, 1952, *1953*
  postural, 2425, *2426*
Talocalcaneal coalition, medial, 2579, *2580*, 2600–2601, *2601*
Talocalcaneonavicular joint, in talipes equinovarus, 2441–2442, *2442*
Talonavicular coalition, 2579
Talus, accessory bone at, 2416
  africoid, 2416, *2619*
  body of, fracture of, 3339–3341, *3340*
  in talipes equinovarus, 2434–2435, *2434–2437*
  lateral process of, fracture of, 3341
  neck of, fracture of, 3339
  osteochondritis dissecans of, 1522–1524, *1523–1527*, **1529–1532**
  osteoid osteoma of, 2780, *2784*
  pyogenic osteomyelitis in, 1107, *1109*
Tarsal bones, pyogenic osteomyelitis in, 1107–1109, *1108–1110*
Tarsal coalition, 2578–2608
  arthrography in, 2595–2596, *2599*
  classification of, 2579t, 2579–2581, *2580*
  clinical features in, 2585–2586, *2587*
  etiology of, 2581, 2585
  heredity in, 2581, 2585
  incidence of, 2578t, 2579
  os calcaneus secundarius vs., 2588, *2589*
  radiography in, 2586–2596
    cartilaginous bridge in, 2588, *2589*
    in apparent coalition, 2593, 2595, *2595–2598*
    lateral oblique axial view in, 2593, *2594*
    medial oblique axial view in, 2590, 2593, *2593–2594*
    oblique lateral dorsoplantar view in, 2590, *2593*
    oblique view in, 2586, 2588, *2588*
    secondary changes in, 2594, *2599*
    talocalcaneal joint in, 2588, *2590, 2591*
  subtalar joint anatomy and, 2588, *2590–2592*
  treatment of, 2596–2608, **2602–2607**
Tarsal navicular, accessory, 2412–2415, *2414–2415*
  accessory bone at, 2416
  Köhler's disease of, 1003–1005, *1004*
Tarsometatarsal fracture-dislocation, Lisfranc's, 3341–3342, *3341–3342*
Tarsus, Japas V-osteotomy of, 2691, **2694–2698**
Teardrop shadow of Koehler, in congenital dysplasia of hip, *321*, 321
Teeth, in osteogenesis imperfecta, 769, *769*
Tendovaginitis, stenosing, of flexor pollicis longus, 272–273
Tenosynovitis, in rheumatoid arthritis, 1467–1469
Tensor fascia latae, and sartorius, posterior transfer of, 1650–1651, **1652–1657**
  in gait, 14, *15*
Tensor fasciae latae, in gait, 14
Tetany, electrical testing in, 64
Tethered cord, 1879–1880
Tetraplegia, 40, 1606
Thalassemia, 1136–1139
  major, 1136–1139, *1137–1138*
  minor, 1136
Thanatophoric dwarfism, 730, *731*
Thenar paralysis, intermetacarpal bone block for, 2057, **2078–2079**
Thigh, measurement of length of, 27, 31
Thomas test, 27, *28*
  in congenital dysplasia of hip, 314, *316*

Thomas test *(Continued)*
    in spastic cerebral palsy, 1628, *1630*
Thomsen's disease, 64, 2157–2159, 2158t
Thoracic dysplasia, asphyxiating, 737, *738*
Thoracic vertebrae, compression fracture of, 3345
Thoracolumbosacral hip-knee-ankle-foot orthosis, in myelomeningocele, 1855, 1857
Thumb, adductor myotomy of, 1730, **1732–1733**
    congenital absence of, 261, 268, 269
    congenital clasped, 270–272
        anatomic and clinical findings in, 270, *270*
        classification of, 270
        incidence of, 270
        treatment of, 271
            splinting in, 271
            tendon transfer in, 271
    congenital longitudinal deficiency of, 260–269
        pollicization of index finger in, **262–267**
    duplicated, ablation of, **250–253**
    duplication of, 242–244. See also *Polydactyly.*
    floating, 268–269
    hitchhiker's, 752, *753*
    hypoplastic, 260, 268
    in arthrogryposis multiplex congenita, 2112–2113
    trigger, 272–273
        operative release of, **274–275**
    triphalangeal, 258–259, *265*
Thumb-in-palm deformity, in cerebral palsy, 1722–1738. See also *Cerebral palsy, arm in.*
Thumb opposition restoration of Brand, 2057, **2068–2069**
Thumb opposition restoration of Riordan, 2057, **2062–2067**
Thurston Holland's sign, 3025
Tibia, axial rotation of, in gait, 12–13
    congenital longitudinal deficiency of, 637–651
        Brown's fibulofemoral arthroplasty in, 643, *645*, **646–649**
        classification of, 637, *639–644*
        duplication of femur in, 637, *638*
        McFarland bypass procedure in, 644, *650*
        treatment of, 637–651
    congenital posteromedial angulation of, 651–656
        clinical presentation in, 652, *652*
        progressive length discrepancy in, 652, *653*
        radiography in, 652, *654–655*
        treatment of, 653, 656
    congenital pseudarthrosis of, 656–681
        amputation in, 676–677
        classification of, 658, *659–661*
        dual graft technique in, 667, **668–673**, *674*
        electrical stimulation in, 666–667, 678–681
        etiology of, 656–658
        free vascularized fibular transplant in, 677–678, *678–680*
        hereditary, 657
        incidence of, 656
        McFarland's posterior bypass autogenous bone graft procedure in, 662–666, *665–666*
        neurofibromatosis and, 657
        pathogenesis of, 657–658
        post-union complications in, 667, 675
        Purvis and Holder's dual onlay graft in, 661–662
        Sofield-Millar fragmentation and intramedullary fixation in, 662, *663*
        treatment of, 658–681
            in established pseudarthrosis, 667–681
            in pre-pseudarthrosis stage, 662–667
    diaphyseal lengthening in, Wagner method for, 2896, **2922–2941**

Tibia *(Continued)*
    fracture of, in older children and adolescents, 3298, *3300*
    Ilizarov two-level lengthening for, 2896, **2972–2989**, *2992–2993*
    in talipes equinovarus, 2435–2437
    intercondylar eminence of, fracture of, 3286–3290
        classification of, 3286–3287, *3287*
        clinical picture in, 3287–3288
        mechanism of injury in, 3286
        radiography in, 3288, *3288–3289*
        treatment of, 3288–3290
    lengthening of, by callotasis, 2896, **2960–2971**
        in leg length inequality, 2893
    osteofibrous dysplasia of, 1242–1246, *1243–1245*
    proximal, epiphysiodesis of, **2882–2885**
    shortening of, in leg length inequality, 2888–2889
    spiral fracture of, with intact fibula, 3295–3296, *3296–3297*
    stress fracture of, 3362, *3362*
    upper shaft of, greenstick fracture of, 3297–3298, *3299*
    Wasserstein lengthening of, 2896, *2994*
Tibia valga, in multiple exostosis, 1173, *1177*
Tibia vara, 2835–2848
    classification of, 2835–2836
    clinical picture in, 2837–2839, *2838*
    differential diagnosis of, 2841
    etiology of, 2836–2837
    genu varum vs., 2824, 2826t
    pathologic conditions causing, 2824t
    pathology in, 2837
    radiography in, *2839–2840*, 2839–2841
    treatment of, 2841–2848
        in adolescent disorder, 2846–2847, *2847–2848*
        in adult disorder, 2847–2848
        in infantile disorder, *2842–2844*, 2842–2846
Tibial diaphysis, distal, Wiltse triangular osteotomy of, 1805, *1809*
Tibial epiphysis, distal, in multiple exostosis, 1173, *1178*
    ossification of, 3302, *3303*
Tibial metaphysis, proximal, greenstick fracture of, 3297–3298, *3299*
Tibial muscle, anterior, in gait, 14
    paralysis of, 1941–1943, *1942*
    posterior, in gait, 14, *15*
Tibial neurectomy, in cerebral palsy, 1674–1675, **1676–1677**
Tibial osteotomy, in talipes equinovarus, 2524
Tibial physis, proximal, fracture of, 3290–3291, *3292*
Tibial tendon, anterior, lateral transfer of, in poliomyelitis, 1939, 1941
    posterior tibial transfer to os calcis of, 1799, **1800–1803**, 1804
    split transfer of, 1687, 1692, *1692*
    posterior, anterior transfer of, 1680–1681, 1686, *1686–1687*
        sliding lengthening of, 1680, *1681*
        split transfer of, 1686–1687, *1688–1691*
Tibial torsion, 2810–2817
    differential diagnosis of, 2816–2817
    external, in poliomyelitis, 1922
    measurement of, 2811–2816
        clinical methods of, 2812, *2813–2814*
        computed tomography in, 2815
        in anatomic specimen, 2811, *2811*
        in lateral torsion, 2816, *2816*
        in medial torsion, 2815–2816
        radiographic methods of, 2812, *2814*
        ultrasound in, 2815

Tibial torsion (Continued)
  medial, in myelomeningocele, 1817–1818
  treatment of, 2817
Tibial tubercle, apophysis of, avulsion fracture of, 3291–3294, *3293*
  proximal, Osgood-Schlatter disease of, 1010–1013
Tibiofemoral angle, development during growth of, 2820–2822, *2822*
Tibiofemoral joint, recurrent momentary lateral subluxation of, 1551
Tibiofibular torsion, lateral, in myelomeningocele, 1817
Tilting reactions, 55, *56*
Toeing-in, etiology of, 2817t
Toeing-out, etiology of, 2817t
Toenail, ingrowing, 2790–2791
Toe-raising test of Jack, 2724, *2728*
Toes, claw, 2715–2717, *2716*
  in myelomeningocele, *1816*, 1816–1817
  curly (varus), congenital, 2661, 2665, *2666*
  digitus minimus varus of, 2653, 2655, *2658–2660*, 2661, **2662–2663**
  divergent or convergent, 2653, *2657*
  hammer, 2667, **2668–2669**, *2670*
  hammer or mallet, in cerebral palsy, 1705
  macrodactylism of, 2651, *2652–2654*
  mallet, 2670–2671, *2671*
  microdactylism of, 2651, 2653
  phalanges of, 2416, 2420
  recurrent fibroma of, 2770–2773
  subungual exostosis of, 2780, *2788*
  supernumerary, 2642, *2643–2648*
  syndactylism of, 2653, *2655–2657*
Tolmetin, in rheumatoid arthritis, 1479
Tonic neck reflex, 49–50, *51–52*
Tönnis's triple innominate osteotomy, in congenital dysplasia of hip in adolescent, 493
Torode and Gillespie rotation-plasty, in focal deficiency of proximal femur, 571, **572–575**, *576*
Torticollis, congenital muscular, 112–128
  clinical findings in, *113–114*, 113–115
  diagnosis in, 115, 115t
  differential diagnosis of, 115t
  etiology of, 112
  in Klippel-Feil syndrome, 128
  operative technique in, 122–124, **123–125**
  pathology in, 112–113
  treatment in, 115–124, *116–121*, **123**, *125*
  in congenital dysplasia of hip, 316
  in intraspinal tumor, 1887, *1890*
Toxic neuropathy, 2085
Toxic synovitis, Legg-Calvé-Perthes disease vs., 956–957
Traction, 90–90 degree, in femoral shaft fracture, 3262–3264, *3263–3264*
  Bryant's, in congenital dysplasia of hip, 343, *344*
  in femoral shaft fracture, 3256–3259, *3256–3261*
  modified Bryant's, in femoral shaft fracture, 3261, *3261–3262*
  preliminary, in congenital dysplasia of hip, 342–346
  Russell skin, in femoral shaft fracture, 3264–3266, *3267*
  skeletal, of distal femur, in congenital dysplasia of hip, 343–345, *344*
  skin, in congenital dysplasia of hip, 345–346
  split Russell's, in congenital dysplasia of hip, 342–343, *343*, 345–346
  suspension, in femoral shaft fracture, 3264, *3265*
Traction stations, Gage and Winter's, in congenital dysplasia of hip, 345, *346–347*
Transtrochanteric derotation osteotomy, Sugioka's, in slipped femoral capital epiphysis, 1070, *1070*

Trapezius transfer, of Saha, in deltoid paralysis, 1958, *1958*
Traumatic arthritis, joint fluid analysis in, 1413t
Traumatic myositis, 2168–2169
Traumatic myositis ossificans, 2169–2170, *2170*
Trendelenburg test, delayed, in congenital dysplasia of hip in adolescent, 470
  in congenital dysplasia of hip, 329, *329*
Triceps brachii, anterior transfer of, Carroll's modification of Bunnell, 2103, **2104–2107**
  for elbow in poliomyelitis, 1964, *1966*, 1967
  paralysis of, in poliomyelitis, 1967, 1971
Triceps surae, in gait, 14, *15*
  paralysis of, gait in, 22–24, *25*
  in poliomyelitis, 1943–1946, *1944–1951*
  testing spasticity and contracture of, 1660–1661, *1661*
Trichorhinophalangeal dysplasia, 848, *849–850*
Trichorhinophalangeal syndrome, Legg-Calvé-Perthes disease vs., 958
Trigger thumb, 272–273
  operative release of, **274–275**
Trilateral socket hip containment orthosis, in Legg-Calvé-Perthes disease, 974–975, *975–976*
Triple diapers, in congenital dysplasia of hip, 341, *342*
Triplegia, 1606
Trisomy 8, 896
Trisomy 13–15, 896
Trisomy 18, 896, *896*
Trisomy 21, 890–895. See also *Down's syndrome.*
Trochanter, greater, avulsion fracture of, 3247–3248
  Colonna arthroplasty of, 1431–1434
  distal and lateral transfer of, modified Pauwel's osteotomy with, 442, **462–465**, *466*, *468*
  Langenskiöld's apophyseodesis of, 441–442, **444–449**
  overgrowth of, in Legg-Calvé-Perthes disease, 983, *984*
  Wagner's distal and lateral transfer of, 442–443, **450–457**, *466*
  Wagner's lateral advancement of, 442, 449, **450–459**
  lesser, avulsion fracture of, 3247, 3247–3248
  triplane osteotomy of, Southwick's, in slipped femoral capital epiphysis, **1056–1061**, 1062
Trunk incurvation, 49, *50*
Tuberculosis, of bone, 1127–1128, *1127–1128*
  of hip, Legg-Calvé-Perthes disease vs., 957–958, *958*
  of spine, 1449–1454
    abscess formation in, 1449, *1451*
    clinical features of, 1449–1451, *1451*
    paraplegia in, 1452–1454
    pathogenesis of, 1449, *1450*
    pathology in, 1449
    radiography in, 1451–1452, *1452–1453*
    treatment of, 1452
Tuberculous arthritis, 1443–1454. See also *Arthritis, tuberculous.*
  joint fluid analysis in, 1414t
Tumor, bone, 1150–1161. See also *Bone tumor*; individual types.
  intracranial, 1771–1773, *1772*
  intraspinal, 1887–1902. See also *Intraspinal tumor.*
  of foot, 2766–2780
Turner's syndrome, 897
  Madelung's deformity in, 213, *213*

U

U figure, in congenital dysplasia of hip, 321, *321*
Ulna, congenital longitudinal deficiency of, 206–209

Ulna (Continued)
  classification of, 207
  treatment of, 207–208, 208
  distal, centralization of carpus over, 199–205, **200–203**
  in multiple exostosis, 1173, 1176, 1183–1184, 1185
  radius and, fracture of, 3181–3195. See also *Radius, ulna and, fracture of.*
  shortening of, in treatment of Madelung's deformity, 214–215
  Z-step cut lengthening of, 1183–1184, 1185
Ulnar dimelia, 209–210, 210
Ulnar head, resection of, with distal radial osteotomy, in Madelung's deformity, **216–219**
Ultrasound, 59
Undergrowth, of limb, 111
Upper limb. See *Arm.*
Upper respiratory infection, preoperative precautions in, 68
Urinary incontinence, in myelomeningocele, 1791
Urinary tract, in Klippel-Feil syndrome, 128, 131
Uveitis, in rheumatoid arthritis, 1472–1473

V

Valgus, definition of, 31–32
Van Nes rotation-plasty, in focal deficiency of proximal femur, 570–571
Varus, definition of, 31–32
Verrucous hyperplasia, in neurofibromatosis, 1290, 1292
Vertebra plana, in eosinophilic granuloma of bone, 1281–1282, 1283
Vertebrae, cervical, congenital synostosis of, 128–136. See also *Klippel-Feil syndrome.*
  fusion with occiput of, 2232–2233
  in myelomeningocele, 1778
  lumbar, compression fracture of, 3345, 3346
  lumbosacral, congenital absence of, 2212–2228. See also *Lumbosacral agenesis.*
  occipital, 2231
  pyogenic osteomyelitis of, 1106
  thoracic, compression fracture of, 3345
Vertebral apophysis, slipped, 2404
Vitamin D, calcium metabolism and, 897–898
Volkmann's ischemic contracture, 3099–3103
  diagnosis of, 3100–3101, 3101–3102
  in hemophilia, 1499, 1499
  in Monteggia fracture-dislocation, 3178
  incidence and mechanism of, 3099
  pathophysiology of, 3099–3100
  treatment of, 3101–3103
von Recklinghausen's disease, 1289–1294. See also *Neurofibromatosis.*
Von Rosen splint, in congenital dysplasia of hip, 340, 341
Vulpius technique, of gastrocnemius lengthening, 1666–1667, 1672

W

Wagner diaphyseal lengthening of humerus, 1184, 1185
Wagner distal and lateral transfer of greater trochanter, 442–443, **450–457**, 466
Wagner femoral lengthening, 2896, 2897, **2898–2921**
Wagner intertrochanteric double osteotomy, 442, **460–461**, 466, 467

Wagner intertrochanteric oblique osteotomy, 394, 395, **396–401**
Wagner lateral advancement of greater trochanter, 442, 443, **458–459**
Wagner tibial diaphyseal lengthening, 2896, **2922–2941**
Wagner type I periacetabular osteotomy, in congenital dysplasia of hip in adolescent, 493, 502, 503
Wagner type II periacetabular osteotomy, in congenital dysplasia of hip in adolescent, 503, 503
Wagner type III periacetabular osteotomy, in congenital dysplasia of hip in adolescent, 503, 503
Wake up test, in kyphoscoliosis surgery, 70
Walking. See also *Gait.*
  reflex of, 47, 48
  velocity of, 6
Wart, plantar, 2786–2790
Wasserstein femoral and tibial lengthening, 2896, 2994
Weakness, 40
Weight, in relation to age, in females, 78t
  in males, 77t
Werdnig-Hoffmann disease. See *Spinal muscular atrophy.*
Westin's Pember-Sal osteotomy, 419, 419–420
Wheelchair, in myelomeningocele, 1858
Whistling face syndrome, 851, 852
White-Menelaus rule of thumb method, in epiphysiodesis, 2872
Whitesides tissue pressure measurement technique, 3100–3101
Wilmington TLSO, in scoliosis, 2301, 2301–2302
Wilms' tumor, 1405, 1407
Wilson's shelf procedure, in congenital dysplasia of hip in adolescent, 520–522, 521–523
Wiltse triangular osteotomy of distal tibial diaphysis, 1805, 1809
Winchester syndrome, 791
Withdrawal reflex, 49
Wolff's law, 688, 689
Woodward operation, in Sprengel's deformity, 162–164, **163–165**
Wormian bones, in osteogenesis imperfecta, 771, 774
Wrist, arthrodesis of, in congenital longitudinal deficiency of radius, 205
  flexion deformity of, in cerebral palsy, 1744–1745, 1744–1746
  in arthrogryposis multiplex congenita, 2112
  in multiple exostosis, 1173, 1176, 1180, 1183, 1183
  position of minimal intra-articular pressure for, 1411
Wryneck, 112. See also *Torticollis, congenital muscular.*

X

Xanthomatosis, of foot, 2779, 2780

Y

Y line, in congenital dysplasia of hip, 319, 319
Yount's fasciotomy, in iliotibial band contracture in, 1923–1925, 1924

Z

Zancolli biceps brachii tendon rerouting, 2057, **2058–2061**
Zielke instrumentation, in scoliosis, 2320, 2321